Principles and Practice of
PHYSICAL REHABILITATION

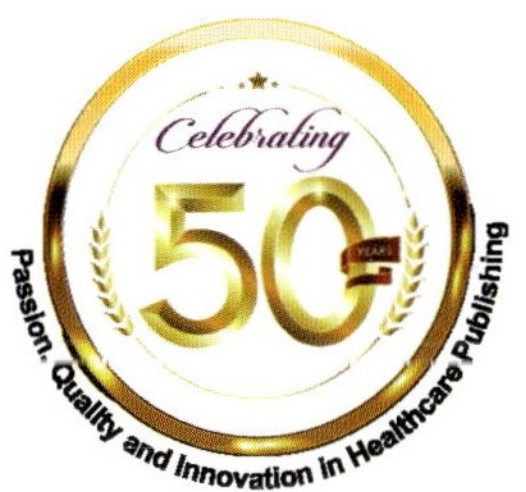

Principles and Practice of
PHYSICAL REHABILITATION

Neeta J Vyas PT PhD
Professor and Principal
IKDRC College of Physiotherapy
Gujarat University of Transplantation Sciences
Ahmedabad, Gujarat, India

Megha S Sheth PT MPT PhD Guide
Lecturer
SBB College of Physiotherapy
Ahmedabad, Gujarat, India

Srishti S Sharma PT PhD
Assistant Professor
CM Patel College of Physiotherapy
Kadi Sarva Vishwavidyalaya University
Gandhinagar, Gujarat, India

Priya S Rangey PT MPT PhD Scholar
Assistant Professor
LJ Institute of Physiotherapy
Ahmedabad, Gujarat, India

Foreword
Deepak Kumar PT PhD

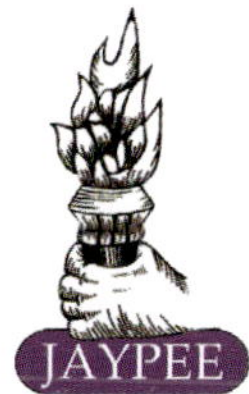

JAYPEE BROTHERS MEDICAL PUBLISHERS
The Health Sciences Publisher
New Delhi | London

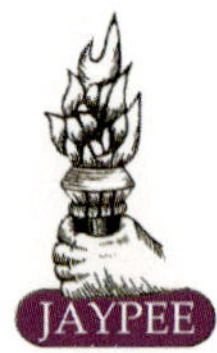 **Jaypee Brothers Medical Publishers (P) Ltd**

Headquarters

Jaypee Brothers Medical Publishers (P) Ltd
4838/24, Ansari Road, Daryaganj
New Delhi 110 002, India
Phone: +91-11-43574357
Fax: +91-11-43574314
Email: jaypee@jaypeebrothers.com

Overseas Office

J.P. Medical Ltd
83 Victoria Street, London
SW1H 0HW (UK)
Phone: +44 20 3170 8910
Fax: +44 (0)20 3008 6180
Email: info@jpmedpub.com

Website: www.jaypeebrothers.com
Website: www.jaypeedigital.com

© 2020, Jaypee Brothers Medical Publishers

The views and opinions expressed in this book are solely those of the original contributor(s)/author(s) and do not necessarily represent those of editor(s) of the book.

All rights reserved. No part of this publication may be reproduced, stored or transmitted in any form or by any means, electronic, mechanical, photocopying, recording or otherwise, without the prior permission in writing of the publishers.

All brand names and product names used in this book are trade names, service marks, trademarks or registered trademarks of their respective owners. The publisher is not associated with any product or vendor mentioned in this book.

Medical knowledge and practice change constantly. This book is designed to provide accurate, authoritative information about the subject matter in question. However, readers are advised to check the most current information available on procedures included and check information from the manufacturer of each product to be administered, to verify the recommended dose, formula, method and duration of administration, adverse effects and contraindications. It is the responsibility of the practitioner to take all appropriate safety precautions. Neither the publisher nor the author(s)/editor(s) assume any liability for any injury and/ or damage to persons or property arising from or related to use of material in this book.

This book is sold on the understanding that the publisher is not engaged in providing professional medical services. If such advice or services are required, the services of a competent medical professional should be sought.

Every effort has been made where necessary to contact holders of copyright to obtain permission to reproduce copyright material. If any have been inadvertently overlooked, the publisher will be pleased to make the necessary arrangements at the first opportunity. The **CD/DVD-ROM** (if any) provided in the sealed envelope with this book is complimentary and free of cost. **Not meant for sale.**

Inquiries for bulk sales may be solicited at: jaypee@jaypeebrothers.com

Principles and Practice of Physical Rehabilitation

First Edition: **2020**

ISBN 978-93-89776-79-9

Printed at: Samrat Offset Pvt. Ltd.

Dedicated to

"The Profession of Physical Therapy"

Foreword

The field of physical rehabilitation is ever growing and changing. Physical rehabilitation, in spite of being an essential component of health care, has been overlooked for the past several years. India has a huge population that suffers from some or the other form of disability, but there are a limited number of reliable resources available to give information about them.

The *Principles and Practice of Physical Rehabilitation* is a book that is the need of the physical therapy profession in current times. It is precise, concise and easily comprehensible. It gives complete clinical knowledge and information worthy for clinicians, academicians and students for the treatment of their valuable patients.

I have known the editors of the book *Principles and Practice of Physical Rehabilitation* for many years, and I feel proud to say that there can be no one better suited to write a book of this caliber. They have always prioritized the welfare of the students and the profession above anything else. Dr Neeta J Vyas, Dr Megha S Sheth, Dr Srishti S Sharma, and Dr Priya S Rangey are pillars in the field of physiotherapy, they are always looked upon for inspiration and have constantly contributed to the physiotherapy profession.

The contributors of the book are nationally recognized experts in their respective field, in which they have contributed not only with their constant perseverance and research work, but also by applying these methods into the most demanding case scenarios. The *Principles and Practice of Physical Rehabilitation* is positioned as a breakthrough book that will change the perspectives of the readers immensely. The book is aimed at easy learning for students to step into the world of physical therapy.

The book provides an insightful literature on physical rehabilitation in varied aspects. The book has sought to incorporate the common conditions keeping in mind the Indian subcontinent with literature majorly specific to India, and from other parts of the world. The book begins with a section on assessment and then describes strategies that can be incorporated in physiotherapy. The next section includes rehabilitation related to musculoskeletal, neurological, cardiac, pulmonary, women's health, endocrine and various other areas. Each chapter has been presented in detail to satisfy the eager mind to the fullest extent. The presentation of the chapters with learning objectives gives the reader an idea of what to expect from the chapter. Bullet format is aimed for easy learning. Case studies described at the end of the chapters of various conditions stimulate clinical thinking. The inclusion of review questions is helpful for the students for academic purposes. The presentation of the information in each chapter is simple and the chapters by themselves are all-inclusive.

This book is a testament of hard work, strong will and commitment. The book will prove to be a huge help to students, academicians and clinicians, in the field of physical therapy. It has been written with such clarity and flare that it will put the novice mind into a state of curiosity and eagerness to learn.

I sincerely believe that the book will achieve great success and respect. I am sure the students will find it as educating and enlightening as I found it to be. Best wishes galore!!

Deepak Kumar PT PhD
Director
Capri Institute of Manual Therapy
New Delhi, India

Contributors

Aashish Contractor MBBS MED FACSM
Director
Department of Rehabilitation and Sports Medicine
Sir HN Reliance Foundation Hospital and
Research Centre
Mumbai, Maharashtra, India

Ajit Dabholkar PT PhD
Professor
School of Physiotherapy
DY Patil University
Navi Mumbai, Maharashtra, India

Amit V Nagrale PT MPT PhD Scholar
Professor and Principal
Miraj Medical Center
College of Physiotherapy, Wanless Mission Hospital
Miraj, Maharashtra, India

Anjali Bhise PT PhD
Senior Lecturer
Principal In-Charge
Government Physiotherapy College
Ahmedabad, Gujarat, India

Anu Arora PT PhD
Associate Professor
School of Physiotherapy
DY Patil University
Navi Mumbai, Maharashtra, India

Asmita Karajgi PT PhD
Dean/Principal
The SIA College of Health Sciences
College of Physiotherapy
Dombivli, Maharashtra, India

Bijal Dodia PT MPT
Consultant Physiotherapist
Department of Rehabilitation and Sports Medicine
Sir HN Reliance Foundation Hospital and
Research Centre
Mumbai, Maharashtra, India

Chetali Paliwal PT MPT
Assistant Professor
Maharashtra University of Health Sciences
Nashik, Maharashtra, India

Deepak B Anap PT PhD
Professor and Head
DVVPF's College of Physiotherapy
Ahmednagar, Maharashtra, India

Dhara Sharma PT PhD
Senior Lecturer
Principal In-Charge
Khyati College of Physiotherapy
Ahmedabad, Gujarat, India

Dhruv Dave PT MPT PhD Scholar
Assistant Professor
Ashok and Rita Patel Institute of Physiotherapy
Anand, Gujarat, India

Dinesh Sorani PT PhD
Senior Lecturer
Principal In-Charge
Government Physiotherapy College
Jamnagar, Gujarat, India

Dipali Rana PT MPT
Lecturer
IKDRC College of Physiotherapy
Gujarat University of Transplantation Sciences
Ahmedabad, Gujarat, India

Harita Pultsya Vyas PT MPT
Lecturer
SBB College of Physiotherapy
Ahmedabad, Gujarat, India

Jaini Patel PT MPT
Deputy Consultant Physiotherapist
Department of Rehab and Sports Medicine
Sir HN Reliance Foundation Hospital and
Research Centre
Mumbai, Maharashtra, India

Mariya Jiandani PT MPT
Associate Professor
PT School and Centre
Seth GS Medical College and KEM Hospital
Mumbai, Maharashtra, India

Megha Jayswal PT MPT
Assistant Professor
College of Physiotherapy
Sumandeep Vidhyapeeth
Vadodara, Gujarat, India

Megha S Sheth PT MPT PhD Guide
Lecturer
SBB College of Physiotherapy
Ahmedabad, Gujarat, India

Neepa H Pandya PT MS
Professor
School of Physiotherapy
PP Savani University
Surat, Gujarat, India

Neeta J Vyas PT PhD
Professor and Principal
IKDRC College of Physiotherapy
Gujarat University of Transplantation Sciences
Ahmedabad, Gujarat, India

Nehal Shah PT PhD
Senior Lecturer
Principal-in-Charge
SBB College of Physiotherapy
Ahmedabad, Gujarat, India

Nipa Shah PT MPT
Lecturer
SBB College of Physiotherapy
Ahmedabad, Gujarat, India

Palak Mulji PT DPT
Moss Rehab
Einstein Health Network
Robert Wood Johnson University Hospital
New Brunswick, NJ, USA

Payal Gahlot PT MPT
Lecturer
SBB College of Physiotherapy
Ahmedabad, Gujarat, India

Prakash V PT PhD
Assistant Professor
Ashok and Rita Patel Institute of Physiotherapy
Charotar University of Science and Technology
Anand, Gujarat, India

Priyasingh Rangey PT MPT PhD Scholar
Assistant Professor
LJ Institute of Physiotherapy
Ahmedabad, Gujarat, India

R Harihara Prakash PT PhD
Professor and Principal
KM Patel Institute of Physiotherapy
Anand, Gujarat, India

Rutvik Purani PT MPT PhD Scholar
Lecturer
Khyati Institute of Physiotherapy
Ahmedabad, Gujarat, India

Saravanan M PT PhD
Associate Professor and Principal In-Charge
The Sarvajanik College of Physiotherapy
Surat, Gujarat, India

Sheshna Rathod PT PhD
Tutor-cum Physiotherapist
Government Physiotherapy College
Jamnagar, Gujarat, India

Shivani Verma PT MPT
Assistant Professor
Parul Institute of Physiotherapy
Vadodara, Gujarat, India

Shraddha Diwan PT PhD
Lecturer
SBB College of Physiotherapy
Ahmedabad, Gujarat, India

Shyam Ganvir PT PhD
Principal and Professor
DVVPF's College of Physiotherapy
Ahmednagar, Maharashtra, India

Srishti S Sharma PT PhD
Assistant Professor
CM Patel College of Physiotherapy
Kadi Sarva Vishwavidyalaya University
Gandhinagar, Gujarat, India

Sucheeta Golhar PT PhD
Principal and Professor
Maharashtra University of Health Sciences
Nashik, Maharashtra, India

Surendra Wani PT PhD
Associate Professor
Maharashtra University of Health Sciences
Nashik, Maharashtra, India

Suvarna Ganvir PT PhD
Professor and Head
Department of Neurophysiotherapy
DVVPF's College of Physiotherapy
Ahmednagar, Maharshtra, India

Tejashree Dabholkar PT PhD
Associate Professor
School of Physiotherapy
DY Patil University
Nerul, Maharshtra, India

Yagna Unmesh Shukla PT PhD
Senior Lecturer
Government Physiotherapy College
Ahmedabad, Gujarat, India

Zarna Ronak Shah PT PhD
Junior Lecturer
SBB College of Physiotherapy
Ahmedabad, Gujarat, India

Preface

Principles and practice of Physical Rehabilitation is a collaborative effort towards the development of knowledge and skills held by the young and tender minds of physical therapy students and the ever-learning clinicians and academicians. The book is designed to help the undergraduate as well as postgraduate students gain a wholesome experience of theoretical and practical world of physiotherapy. It aims to teach a comprehensive approach to the management of the young and adult patients. It incorporates an evidence-based practice approach towards rehabilitation, thus being a useful resource to students, academicians and clinicians.

India is a developing country and though we have overcome a ton of issues that we faced earlier, we are still on our path to development, making us susceptible to several other problems that are different from developed countries. Rehabilitation is the key to sustain the development we have achieved, to reduce the disabilities and handicaps faced by people and to limit the impairments and limitations faced by them. Not just India, but in several other countries too, physical rehabilitation forms one of the only possible elements to maintain health in the society.

The book consists of three sections: Section 1 dealing with the clinical decision making, ethics and assessment strategies, Section 2 incorporating intervention strategies and Section 3 including management strategies. Each chapter of the book is outlined based on the International Classification of Functioning, Disability and Health, thus aiding the students understand the concepts of each topic better. The book gives a comprehensive explanation of each pathology included in the book, encompassing the pathophysiology, clinical presentation and assessment and intervention strategies for the rehabilitation.

Evidence-based practice forms a vital component of the rehabilitation process in the present times and the focus of the book has been on the incorporation of such practice in the content of the book. Along with this, each chapter in the management section has case assignments included, to stimulate the students thinking to gain a clearer understanding of the assessment process and to test the clinical knowledge gained by them after the reading of the chapter. The case assignments are presented in a comprehensible format. Each chapter is entailed with review questions that have been formed after a thorough evaluation of the previously asked questions in the examinations of several universities of India.

A sound pedagogical format has been followed throughout the book. Vital information has been presented in boxes. Illustrations and clinical pictures have been provided to make the content uncomplicated for the reader. Information has been presented in the form of flowcharts and algorithms to make it more unambiguous. A display of an amalgamation of bulleted points and paragraphs has been used to present the information which makes it easier for the reader to understand. A plethora of particulars regarding various scales used for diagnostic and prognostic purposes has been provided along with the inclusion of several scales in the appendices.

The creation of something this comprehensive yet simple, requires hard work and dedication from a lot of people, which we have found amongst ourselves and the contributors we had the opportunity to work with. When first approached by the publication house for this project, it seemed to be an impossible task. But with great work, support and cooperation, this book has transitioned from just a thought to a reality. We are pleased to share this book with our readers and hope they enjoy and learn from it, as much as we did while making it. It is our hope that this small effort on our part can help in changing the outlook of young minds towards the profession of physical therapy.

Neeta J Vyas
Megha S Sheth
Srishti S Sharma
Priya S Rangey

Acknowledgments

We are thankful to The Almighty God to bless us all with such a great opportunity. It is only with God's grace that we got the opportunity to be a part of a substantial contribution in the field of physical therapy in India. We would like to extend our gratitude to all our teachers who have been the pathbreakers for us in this profession. As truly said "A teacher is like a candle that burns itself to light the world of others", our teachers have always been a constant source of inspiration and guidance for us to tread the path paved by them.

I would like to thank my parents who have been the reason of my existence and my achievements in life. No words can express the gratitude I feel towards my husband Dr Jayprakash Vyas, who has been a constant support throughout the drafting of this book. Heartfelt thanks to Khushboo and Jiya who have been the source of my smiles.

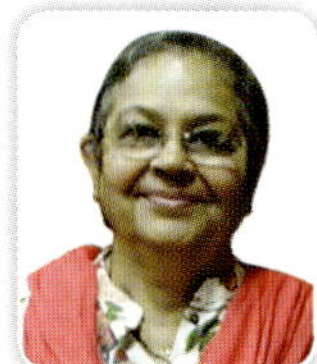

Neeta J Vyas

I am thankful to my parents, Mr Navnit Desai and Ms Aruna Desai, my in-laws Mr Bachubhai Sheth and Ms Veenaben Sheth for being a constant support. I would like to thank my husband Dr Sandeep Sheth who has always stood by me through thick and thin. I want to acknowledge my children, Siddharth and Shivani, who have always been a source of motivation and push I have required through the crucial phases of writing. I am thankful to my friends Dr Nehal Shah and Dr Neepa Pandya, who have always supported me and inspired me to never give up and keep moving through difficult times. My postgraduate student, Zishan Khan was always ready to do whatever I asked him with full enthusiasm. A special note of thanks to Ridham, Sonal, Sangita and Paresh for always being there. I am thankful to the entire team of SBB College of Physiotherapy, AMC MET Medical College, Ahmedabad, Gujarat, India.

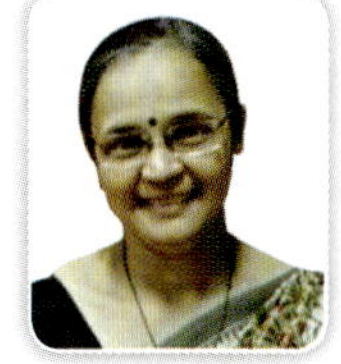

Megha S Sheth

Special thanks to my parents Mr Sanat Sharma and Ms Priti Sharma who always believed in my abilities and emphasized the importance of knowledge and education to me from the very beginning. If not for them, I would never have been what I am today. I also thank my brother Mr Udit Sharma for being there to help me in all the best possible ways. Huge thanks to my husband, Dr Rutvik Purani who has been my friend, my inspiration, my critic and the strongest pillar in my life. My sincere thanks to the Sharma and Purani family, for supporting me constantly. Also, a heartfelt thanks to CM Patel College of Physiotherapy, my undergraduate students and interns.

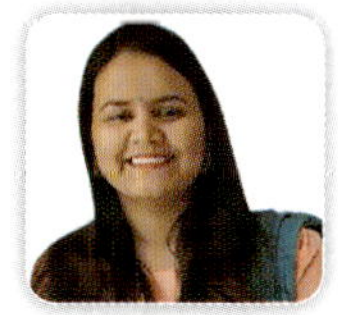

Srishti S Sharma

My first thanks goes to my parents Mr Bhagirath Singh Rangey and Ms Mina Rangey, who are the reason for my being and my life. It is because of their support and motivation that I have become capable of getting such a huge opportunity. I want to thank my brother, Mr Devrath Rangey who has been a constant source of nagging in my life, but all the while being a true driving force. My husband, Mr Pradeep Thakur, cannot be thanked enough for everything that he is for me. He is my best friend, my shoulder to cry on and my power source. Thank you for helping me meet my deadlines, for being so supportive when I ignored you, for letting me leave all work aside to focus just on my writing. I want to thank my in-laws Mr Chandan Singh Thakur and Ms Tara Thakur for making me feel so positive about myself. A heartfelt thanks to Priyanka Sharma, for being so proud of me and always being there for me whenever I needed you. A special thanks to my undergraduate students (Aarsh, Himani, Devanshi, Tithi, Dhiraj, Mohit, Riya, Saloni) and my staff members (Dr Mehul Panchal and Mr Jitendra Solanki). A note of thanks to the LJK Trust and LJ Institute of Physiotherapy for helping us.

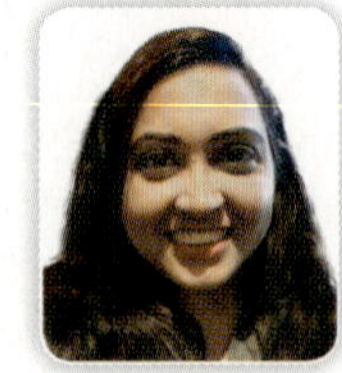

Priya S Rangey

This book has been a collaborative effort of several hard working and successful contributors. Each author has brought excellence to the book. Their academic as well as clinical expertise is reflected at every page turned. We thank Dr Aalap Shah, Dr Viral Shah and Dr Hardik Sharma for helping us with some of the pictures. We extend a kind word of gratitude to Dr Shivani Verma for providing help at every required step with utmost enthusiasm. We would like to thank the copyright holders who have provided permission to use scales. We also thank Dr Annamalai and the Indian Association of Physiotherapists for their support. We also want to express our gratitude towards Mr Sharad Patel for making this book a reality. We would like to acknowledge the support and understanding of our patients, who went out of their way to help us and give the readers a book that can be a wholesome experience.

We are very grateful to the whole team of M/s Jaypee Brothers Medical Publishers (P) Ltd, New Delhi, India, who helped and guided us, Shri Jitendar P Vij (Group Chairman), Mr Ankit Vij (Managing Director), Mr MS Mani (Group President), Dr Madhu Choudhary (Publishing Head–Education), Ms Pooja Bhandari (Production Head), Ms Sunita Katla (Executive Assistant to Group Chairman and Publishing Manager), Dr Sneha Kashyap (Development Editor), Mr Rajesh Sharma (Production Coordinator), Ms Seema Dogra (Cover Visualizer), Mr Laxmidhar Padhiary and Ms Geeta Rani (Proofreader), Mr Kapil Dev Sharma and Mr Jagvir Tomar (Typesetter), Mr Armaan Ali (Graphic Designer), and their team members, for all their support to work in this project and make it a success.

Contents

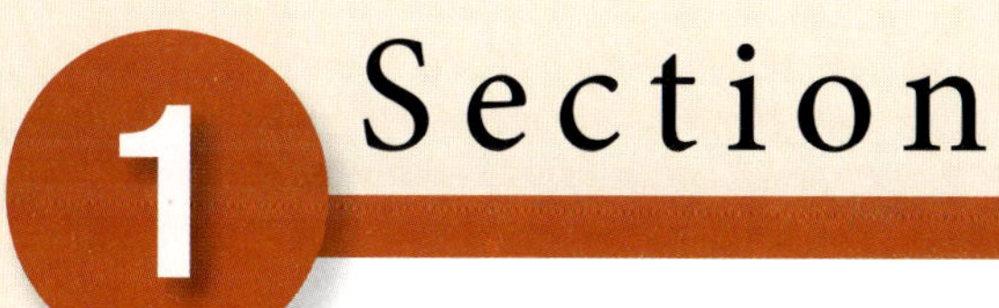

Evaluation Strategies

1 CHAPTER

Clinical Decision-making in Physiotherapy

Nehal Shah, Megha S Sheth

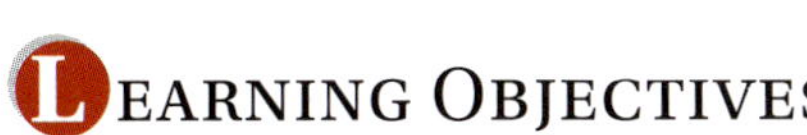

LEARNING OBJECTIVES

After reading this chapter, the readers should be able to:

- Understand clinical reasoning and clinical decision-making and its need in physiotherapy
- Learn the definition of clinical reasoning and the core dimensions of clinical reasoning
- Understand the key steps in the process of clinical decision-making
- Identify the important and unimportant elements in the assessment that should be documented
- Identify the factors affecting clinical decision-making
- Know the potential errors that can happen in the process of clinical decision-making
- Understand the importance of evidence-based medicine in physiotherapy management
- Understand the components of ICF in clinical decision-making and its framework
- Link the assessment with goals and formulate goals of physiotherapy management based on the interpretation of the assessment
- Understand the role of a physical therapist in planning effective treatment and developing a plan of care (POC) involving patient participation
- Understand documentation in physiotherapy

CHAPTER OUTLINE

- Clinical decision-making/clinical reasoning
  - What is clinical decision-making?
  - WCPT definition of clinical reasoning
  - What is clinical reasoning?
  - Process of clinical decision-making
  - Nature of clinical reasoning
  - Core dimensions
  - Other dimensions
  - Factors affecting clinical decision-making
- Errors in clinical reasoning
- Process of clinical reasoning
- Expert versus novice in clinical decision-making
- Developing the plan of care involving patient participation
- International Classification of Functioning, Disability and Health
- Evidence-based practice
  - Why evidence-based practice?
  - What is evidence-based practice?
- Assessment
  - Hypothesis-oriented algorithm for clinicians (HOAC) model
  - Writing a diagnosis for physiotherapy management
- Goals and management
- Documentation

INTRODUCTION

Principles and Practices of Physical Rehabilitation describes assessment and management of various conditions for physiotherapists, in clinical setup, hospitals, and community over the entire course of a person's rehabilitation. Physiotherapy is a health-care profession wherein assessment and management of a patient is involved. However, apart from this, what is more important for a therapist in the course of rehabilitation is the clinical reasoning (CR) and ability to establish an appropriate diagnosis. Physiotherapists are involved in more complex scenarios of conditions and diseases across the community and are hence imposed with circumstances that may involve difficult decision-making situations. It therefore makes it necessary for them to develop good clinical decision-making (CDM) skills. Clinical evaluation and standardized outcome measures are used by therapists for coming to a clinical diagnosis, and competency in this aspect can be maximized with use of effective CDM.

> **BOX 1.1:** Vision statement developed by American Physical Therapy Association.
>
> "By 2020, Physical therapy will be provided by physical therapists who are DOCTORS of physical therapy, recognized by consumers and other health-care professionals as the practitioners of choice to whom consumers have direct access for the diagnosis of, intervention for and prevention of impairments, functional limitations and disabilities related to **movement, function and health**."

With appropriate assessment, a physiotherapist can follow clinical practice guidelines for evaluation and diagnosis.

Physiotherapy practices have undergone revolutionary shift in past two decades from a referral and prescribed practice to a thoughtful practice with independence in making decisions regarding treatment. Majority of the countries across the globe have started recognizing physiotherapy as an independent practice **(Box 1.1)**.

CLINICAL DECISION-MAKING/CLINICAL REASONING

What is Clinical Decision-making?

In routine physiotherapy practice, we come across many patients whom we assess and decide the treatment. After few days of treatment, we tend to reassess the patient and make appropriate changes in the treatment. This is CDM in simple words. Physiotherapy tool box contains a plethora of treatment techniques ranging from electrophysical agents, basic exercises to most advanced manual therapy. CDM involves decision of apt tool of treatment from the tool box.

WCPT Definition of Clinical Reasoning

CR/CDM is a process in which the physical therapist, interacting with the patient and others (such as family members or others providing care), helps patients/clients structure meaning, goals, and health management strategies based on clinical data, patient/client choices, and professional judgment and knowledge. Thus CR is not only what the therapist knows or decides, but it also involves the patient and maybe relatives.

What is Clinical Reasoning?

CR can be described as follows:
- CR is the process of drawing conclusions based upon known or presumed facts and assists in the development of an accurate diagnosis and prognosis.
- It is the process of thinking that the practice of physiotherapy is guided by "Clinical reasoning is the foundation of professional clinical practice. In the absence of sound clinical reasoning, clinical practice becomes a technical operation requiring direction from a decision-maker."

—Higgs, Jones.

In clinical encounters, rarely is all the information available. Not all patients fit into the classical textbook conditions. Many responsible factors rule patient's presenting conditions. This is the situation where thorough knowledge and CR skills come into play. Assessment skills should be sound in order to come to a conclusion in such cases. More data must be gathered, and the clinician must deal with contradictory, confusing, imperfect, and even inaccurate information.

- The hallmark of processional competence is the capacity to reason in the presence of uncertainty and to find solutions to ill-defined problems.
  CR is the way clinicians think about the problems they deal with in clinical practice.
- It involves **clinical judgments** (deciding what is wrong with a patient) and **CDM** (deciding what to do).
- **Tanner** in 2006 conceptualizes CR as the process by which clinical judgments are made by **selecting** from alternatives, weighing evidence, using intuition, and by pattern recognition.

Process of Clinical Decision-making

It is a logical process by which clinicians decide the treatment of patients, which includes the following steps:
1. *Collect cues:* This is the part where one assesses the patients, subjectively and objectively.
2. *Process the information:* From the collected information, a judgment is made from the outcomes of the assessment such as range of motion assessment or manual muscle testing and analysis of the findings.
3. *Come to an understanding of a patient problem or situation:* This is a final outcome and physiotherapy diagnosis that is at the end of the assessment, which enables one to understand the patient as a whole.
4. *Plan and implement interventions:* Physiotherapy diagnosis enables one to understand the culprit structures and functions that have caused the problem. This can enable better planning of treatment strategies and executing them.
5. *Evaluate outcomes:* It is important to know whether the treatment strategy applied is apt or not, which comes from re-evaluating the patient periodically and regularly. This also helps one to decide a change in the treatment protocol as a means of progression.
6. *Reflect on and learn from the process:* **Every patient is a learning encyclopedia for a clinician.** The entire process of patient assessment and management is a new experience encountered, which can enable him/her to polish himself for the next patient, learning from good steps taken and also the mistakes made.

CR is not a linear process but can be conceptualized as a cycle of linked clinical encounters (Higgs and Jones). It is a **context-dependent** way of thinking and decision-making in professional practice to guide practice actions. So there are no fixed steps to diagnosis or management in physiotherapy but an individualized decision needs to be made for each patient. It involves the construction of narratives **to make sense of the multiple factors** and interests pertaining to the current reasoning task. CR utilizes core dimensions of:

- Practice knowledge
- Reasoning
- Metacognition/Cognition

CR is the mental activity involved in arriving at a diagnosis and management plan. It includes activity such as history taking or physical examination. CR is also called a practice decision-making. It encompasses professionalism (autonomy, responsibility, and accountability). Decision-making in conditions of uncertainty needs to be made by reasoning out. Experts and novices need to:

- Process multiple variables
- Contemplate priorities
- Negotiate interests of various participants
- Also think about ethics

Through experience CR becomes a chosen model of practicing rather than a process. CR is at the heart of practice thinking. Ability to reason clinically demonstrates how practitioner/learner has assimilated, integrated, and included all various sets of knowledge they have developed cognitively and experientially.

Applying this definition and explaining it in simple terms, let us see one example. A 25-year-old female computer operator suffers from neck pain of insidious onset. Can with this much information the physiotherapy treatment be started? The answer will be "NO." Majority of us would say patient needs to be assessed thoroughly before beginning treatment. The assessment that is done are the cues we collect and the differential diagnosis we make and rule out certain diagnosis and consider some diagnosis are the CR process we adopt to come to a final diagnosis. The final diagnosis and the treatment strategies adopted make a complete CDM process. This entire process depends on many factors that range from knowledge and experience of the therapist, his/her understanding of recent evidence regarding the condition under treatment, and also on the patient's level of understanding and patient as a whole. The CR model is shown in **Figure 1.1**.

Nature of Clinical Reasoning

Nature of CR can be described as follows:

- Some patients come to us with typical complaints described in textbooks, but some of the patients come to physiotherapy with vague complaints.
- Problems are ill structured; there is incomplete information or the information is dynamic in nature (complaints keep changing).
- The decision-making environment is changing, goals may be shifting, ill-defined, or competing goals (movement and rest indicated at the same time).
- Elements of time pressure and personal stress influence decisions.

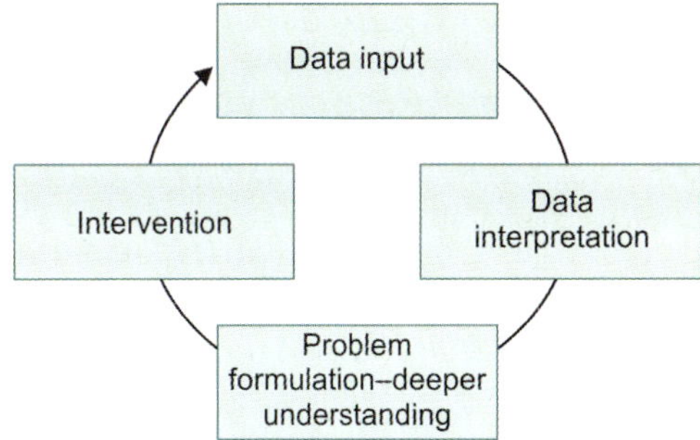

Fig. 1.1: Clinical reasoning model.

There are multiple interacting goals where one intervention can target many problems or multiple interventions are needed to achieve one goal. Multiple players act together, as members of the rehabilitation team, and a coordinated work among all is necessary to achieve best results. Organizational goals and norms cannot be overlooked during decision-making.

Core Dimensions

One needs the following dimensions for the process of CR.

Knowledge

A strong base from theory and experience is the basis of CR. Without knowledge of the condition and management strategies, a therapist will not be able to reason out a possible diagnosis and an appropriate management. Knowledge here does not imply only textbook knowledge. It involves knowledge about the recent advances and practices of the disease under consideration. Past experiences with the patients also help enhance knowledge, which will be practical in such cases.

Cognition

This involves thinking skills, to analyze, synthesize, and evaluate data. These skills are utilized to process clinical data against discipline-specific knowledge in consideration of patients' needs and problems. This implies that there is a need for a holistic approach toward the patient and disease under consideration. Concluding neck pain as Trapezitis or a discogenic problem and calling the patient daily for physiotherapy treatment reflects knowledge. But understanding the cause of trapezitis and treating the cause with ergonomic advice and modifications, understanding psychological and social aspects of the patient, and incorporating appropriate measures to take care of those factors reflects the cognition level of the treating physiotherapist.

Metacognition

Metacognition skills allow a bridge to be made between knowledge and cognition. Skills include:

- Self-awareness
- Identifying limitations
- Preparedness for unexpected findings

Taking the above example of trapezitis, if the patient is not getting better or worsening after the treatment, there is a need to refer the patient back to the consultant or the patient needs to undergo some investigations, and physiotherapy treatment till then may be stopped. This understanding reflects metacognition level of the therapist. To keep giving different treatments to the patient without any improvement is professionally and ethically incorrect. Hence, one needs to develop strong metacognition skills.

Other Dimensions

The following dimensions were added because of growing expectations of consumers. Compliant-dependent patients are now replaced by informed health-care consumers in today's health-care sector.

Mutual Decision-making

This includes the role of both therapist and patient to make common goals. Considering the above case of trapezitis, considering the spasm in the upper trapezius muscle, majority of the physiotherapists would prefer giving ice pack or cryotherapy. Theoretically, both ice and heat applications work well on muscle spasm and there have been many debates regarding the choice of application of these agents. But it has been seen that every patient is different in terms of tolerating cold therapy and heat therapy; hence, they may have different preferences. At such instances, if the therapist and the patient reach a mutual decision (keeping contraindications of each in mind) regarding what to apply, the results would be better and would also have more patient satisfaction, which is a key to cure any patient.

Contextual Interaction

The role of environment in causing the problem and modifying the environment for the solution needs to be analyzed. For occupation-related trapezitis, apart from giving physical agents, it is necessary to take care of the workplace environment and make modifications there. Modifying the work pattern and workplace furniture plays a vital role in prevention and cure of such conditions.

Task Impact

One needs to understand the influence of the problem in the patient's daily activities and participation in society. Due to excessive use of technology and gadgets, trapezitis is one of the commonest and alarming conditions seen. Treating that muscle spasm symptomatically will give excellent results for short term. But recurrence cannot be controlled. The cause of such myofascial pain syndromes is a lot related to faulty ergonomics at workplace and home. Working postures, stress, and anxiety play a vital role in aggravating such syndromes. If this is not addressed properly, the pain can hamper and affect the lifestyle of the patient.

> **BOX 1.2:** Factors influencing clinical decision-making.
> - Practitioner factors such as frames of reference, individual capabilities, experience
> - Four key capabilities: Cognitive, emotional, social, and reflexive
> - Task attributes such as difficulty, complexity, stability, and uncertainty
> - Should be within a broader contextual ethos, with dimensions particular to the practice in the specific workplace

Factors Affecting Clinical Decision-making

CDM is a complex process and is usually contextually dependent. It consists of a core process, which depends upon many factors **(Box 1.2)**.

- **Attributes of the decision-makers,** such as their capabilities, confidence, self-efficacy, emotions, frames of reference, and degree of expertise influence decision-making.
    - *Cognitive capabilities* are needed to identify and collect relevant information (task and contextual) and process this data in order to make decisions in focal areas of problems, intervention, interaction, and evaluation.
    - *Metacognitive capabilities* refer to the awareness of the process of decision-making and factors that influence one's decision-making.
    - *Emotional capabilities* mean the awareness of emotions and when they are impacting decision-making, particularly awareness of self-efficacy.
    - *Social capabilities* are needed to interact effectively with others in the decision-making context and critically learn from others.

  The decision-maker's level of expertise is extremely important factor influencing the process of CDM, with experts being considered as superior decision-makers making decisions that are faster and more accurate.

- **Attributes of external context** that influence the process of CDM are the contextual factors such as environment and human behavior, which are dynamic and variable. According to the changing environment, CDM may need to be modified and include social, professional, organizational, and physical and environmental dimensions.

Errors in Clinical Reasoning

It is easy to make errors in the process of CR. Errors in CR are frequently linked to errors in cognition. They are associated with habits of thinking and practice of the therapist. The same information can be analyzed differently by two therapists and the difference is more apparent if one is an expert in the field and the other a novice. The following are common errors that can occur in decision-making **(Box 1.3).**

BOX 1.3: Possible causes for errors.

- Insufficient knowledge base
- Poor cognitive skills
- Lack of metacognition
- Validity and reliability of the information collected not high

---

1. **Ascertainment bias:**
   - It is easy to make assumptions early in the evaluation process, based on a single symptom or based on the doctor's notes.
   - It is important to keep an open mind to assimilate all the information and get a clear picture only at the end.
   - Being biased towards a certain diagnosis makes us ascertain the same with our findings. It can also happen that the present complaint of the patient may not be because of the known condition. The problem occurs with overemphasis on the findings. Being biased to a diagnosis from the beginning of the evaluation makes the therapist overemphasize on certain weak positive findings and ignore other findings, which do not clearly fit into the picture.
   - This leads to incorrect interpretation related to logic. It is very easy to misinterpret a statement by the patient to mean something that fits your logic and ignore comments or findings that do not fit according to logic.
   - The best example to this bias, which we commonly encounter in practice, is the patient suffering from low back pain who comes with MRI done. The MRI report may say that there is a prolapsed intervertebral disk (PIVD) encroaching upon exiting nerve roots. This gives a bias in the therapist's mind that the patient has got PIVD. Hence, the treating therapist does not look beyond PIVD even if movement bias or other findings do not favor PIVD. The therapist does not completely evaluate the patient to rule out a muscular cause or any other cause, which was a possible cause for pain.

2. **Anchoring:**
   - Not considering enough hypotheses before locking a particular conclusion is also commonly seen. From the beginning, one thinks that this is the cause of the problem and not exploring other possibilities may lead to an incorrect diagnosis.
   - It becomes difficult to see anything outside the most familiar patterns.
   - When knowledge is limited one cannot see beyond the common conclusions, which can lead to an error in diagnosis. This happens because of lack of awareness of other conditions.
   - Patterns become rigid and it is difficult to recognize variations.
   - This is again an error in assuming the diagnosis too early in the evaluation process so that small variations in the pattern are not noticed. A focus on favorite patterns leads to them being identified with insufficient information.
   - Considering the same example of PIVD mentioned above and reasoning out ahead, even if the MRI was done 3 months back, therapist's mind gets fixed with the diagnosis of PIVD and fails to remember the natural course of healing of a bulged disk. Hence, he/she fails to diagnose other causes of low back pain. Second, there may exist the fixed idea of looking at the patient with a textbook mindset trying to find textbook manifestations and fixed patterns of affection. So with the biased mind with MRI suggesting PIVD and the textbook documented clinical features, one does not think or identify that the present symptoms of the patient could be because of sacroiliac joint (SIJ) problem or even quadratus lumborum syndrome, which has the characteristics of the same pain and referral pain. This leads to an error in making a diagnosis.

3. **Confirmation bias:** Common errors regarding confirmation bias are:
   - Failing to sample enough information leads to an error in diagnosis.
   - Each finding during the evaluation confirms the biased diagnosis.
   - While assessing the patient, one needs to be very careful to gather and analyze every possible information.
   - Again considering the same PIVD example, the moment one gets biased with the MRI report, he/she fails to assess movement bias or observe movement patterns. This gives a confirmation bias and one misses the diagnosis of conditions such as myofascial syndrome of low back or SIJ problem.

4. **Biasing information collected:**
   - This is again similar to the above points where there is rejection of findings that the therapist thinks are not related to the condition.
   - Most patients have a lot to say regarding their problems. Misinterpretation of noncontributory information can also lead to making this error.
   - During subjective assessment of patient such as taking history, the approach of the therapist at times becomes subjective. He/she usually processes the information given by the patient depending on his/her biases and past experiences. In this, one either misses out an important and specific information such as pain in low back while bending or getting up from a bent position, which is an important cue. Or he/she floods oneself with unwanted information such as family issues, which makes him/her believe that the patient's problem is a psychosomatic one.

5. **Error in detecting relationships:**
   - There could be coexistence of two conditions.
   - A patient can have two coexisting conditions such as cervical radiculopathy and carpal tunnel

syndrome. Failing to identify this double crush syndrome can lead to ineffective treatment.

- Knowing a relationship occurs, deducing they are causally related, can lead to errors in diagnosis.
- An example is the presence of yellow discoloration of nails seen with cigarette smoking. And cigarette smoking is known to cause cancer. Assuming yellow nails to be a sign of cancer is an error.

6. **Overconfidence bias:**
   - Having qualified to become a therapist increases our confidence.
   - We start to believe we know more than we do and act with incomplete information. The medical field is so vast; there would be plenty of information and knowledge that we lack. Also the medical field is dynamic, with ideas and beliefs changing frequently.
   - With increasing experience, our biases also increase in experience. There is a very thin line between confidence and overconfidence; hence, it is important to keep an open mind while looking at a patient.
   - Experienced clinicians are more prone to get overconfidence bias especially if they fail to go through recent advances. At the same time, a novice is equally likely to get this bias when he is not competently experienced to look at certain complicated cases and yet does not want to take suggestions and may at times make mistakes with basic concepts.

7. **Premature closure:**
   - Accepting a diagnosis before it is fully verified leads to missed diagnosis.
   - Listening to the patient partially and concluding a diagnosis with incomplete examination, because a diagnosis is assumed, leads to premature closure of the assessment.
   - Few possible differential diagnoses are then considered.
   - Looking at the MRI and concluding as PIVD leads to premature closure without even exploring other probable causes of the same symptoms such as piriformis syndrome, SIJ problem, or even a peripheral neuropathy.

8. **Diagnostic momentum:**
   - Once labels are attached, they get stickier, and other possibilities are excluded.
   - Formation of one idea for a possible diagnosis again leads to a bias for that possibility, and other possible differential diagnoses are eliminated quickly.
   - MRI report concluding PIVD, the orthopedician commenting as PIVD gives a diagnostic momentum. Patient's Google doctor approach strengthens this momentum and by the time patient visits a therapist, diagnosis is fixed and that makes

everyone devoid of exploring further to reach to another differential diagnosis and proving it.

Process of Clinical Reasoning

To practice CR, a therapist needs three interrelated skills:
1. Scanning
2. Gathering
3. Critical appraisal.

These three thinking skills stress on analysis by a therapist and emphasize the role of a physiotherapist in CDM, rather than instrumental competence by a computer or machine.

Scanning

The following need to be taken care of in scanning phase:
- During the scanning phase, a therapist should act with apprehension.
- An initial sweep through the information should be conducted to draw a bigger picture.
- One must decide boundaries, such that all possible diagnoses are thought of.
- Then scan the familiar patterns that are grounded in past experiences.
- New or unusual configurations should be looked for to avoid errors in diagnosis. Decide cues to be attended to, whether they are familiar or unfamiliar ones.

Gathering

A therapist should proceed with adequate information considering the following points:
- One should gather all available information, knowledge, and ideas related to the case, by exploring interpretative resources and analytic protocols available.
- Management for the patient can be based on the clinical practice guidelines of various associations that are systematically developed statements that include recommendations intended to optimize patient care.
- Information can also be from teachings in the class or from your own intuition. One should analyze the gathered information and correlate with relevant responses in the case.

Appraisal

Appraisal is the next process to follow:
- Scanning and gathering is followed by appraisal. Sort through the interpretations and see which fits in the situation.
- Depending on the reasoning take informed action. Appropriate reasoning is important in this phase.
- Judge the accuracy and validity of assumptions made. Judging is based on past experiences and following clinical protocols. One has to judge closeness to fit in the current situation and then take action.

Process of Appraisal

Ideas are what we have heard from authorities such as teachers, institution, and notes. We accept this information unquestioningly. There is a need to find evidence and to recheck textbooks, and this is called clinical appraisal. If our assumptions are justified we will feel confident. If the assumptions are flawed we need to reframe the assumptions.

Clinical appraisal should be done through:
1. Our experiences and teachers' views—most important sources of information to interpret against.
2. Patients' eyes—patients may or may not interpret our actions in the way we mean them to.
3. Our colleagues' experiences—open up versions of events we have experienced.

The above three are critical mirrors. Gain their perspective. Appraisal may suggest dynamics and causes that make more sense. It also provides emotional sustenance. Same problems may be faced by others. Clinical appraisal allows us to stand outside situations and see what we do from a wider perspective. It helps us develop a well-grounded rationale for our actions.

Expert versus Novice in Clinical Decision-making

It is a human tendency to visit a subject expert as far as medical science is concerned. But there will always be a debate on whom to consider an expert—the one who is into practice since years with less clinical exposure, or the one who has acquired greater clinical skills because of higher patient exposure maybe in fewer years. But in general, one needs to have a superior knowledge base and adequate clinical exposure to be an expert because the expert is expected to generate a high-quality hypothesis. On the other hand, a novice in the practice is thorough with the textbooks, may not be able to encompass greater clinical skills or the high-quality hypothesis, and application will be missing.

Clinical expert is known to have superiority in the following:
- Content knowledge
- Practical knowledge
- Technical skills
- Application of general principles or theory
- Critical analysis

Listening to the patients and trying to understand their nonverbal gestures play a vital role in understanding his sufferings and giving the best possible outcome. An expert develops intense focused connection with patient, verbal and nonverbal, and uses *clinical patterns* and *inductive reasoning* to develop a diagnosis. He is comfortable with the uncertainty of not knowing the immediate diagnosis and will not jump into assumptions, which is not the case with a novice. A novice may have a perspective that not giving an immediate diagnosis will prove him inefficient.

Management becomes more efficient and effective when imparted by an expert because treatment is given depending on "seeing" the clinical pattern. Treatment strategies usually focus on treating one or two primary issues depending on the priority of attention, which contradicts treatment strategies adopted by a novice who is usually enthusiastic.

There has been a paradigm shift in the way an expert is looked upon. Former paradigm accepted unsystematic observations based on basics and experience alone. Now an expert needs to follow a systematic approach according to clinical practice guidelines.

The Danger of Relying on Experience Alone

"Making the same mistakes with increasing confidence over an impressive number of years." Is that 25 years of experience or 1 year of experience repeated 25 times?

Hence, the new paradigm does not believe only in intuition but is also based on understanding rules to interpret the literature and actually believing in more objective tools, which are evidence based.

Developing the Plan of Care Involving Patient Participation

Whether physiotherapy should be patient-centered health care or it should be evidence-based practice is debatable. There needs to be a collaboration between patient and therapist during the management process. Collaboration and communication are as important as delivering care. Patient may seem to agree with the therapist but this may not be genuine, when the decisions are made only by the therapist (**Box 1.4**).

Collaboration leads to:
- Patient being well informed of what is going to happen during physiotherapy.
- Patient feeling involved.
- Patient feeling more satisfied.
- Patient feeling valued.

Collaboration also supports:
- Ethical issues—autonomy, nonmaleficence
- Legal issues regarding informed consent
- Cultural safety

Decision-making roles are dynamic and change according to condition of patient. Patients are better informed and want to know their options and be involved in decision-making and self-management. **Table 1.1** shows the difference in the patient of older times and the characteristics of the present patients.

Patients coming to physiotherapy have clear expectations and know what they want. These goals may clash with physical therapy (PT) expectations. The collaborative physiotherapist endorses values of inclusion

---

BOX 1.4: Essential elements of shared decision-making.

- Defining the problem
- Presenting the options
- Identifying patient values and preferences
- Identifying therapist knowledge
- Clarifying understanding

Table 1.1: Difference in the patient of older times and that of the present times.

Old patient	New patient
• Patient • Passive role • Receiver of health care • Physiotherapy had a clinical context—the difference is in relationship patterns	• Client • Active role • Informed customer—seeking to buy best available health-care options • Physiotherapy now has a professional approach—market-based, service provision

and power sharing and is an advocate of critical social science approach. Thus physiotherapy is both an art and science where one integrates biomedical facts with patient's perceptions of health-care needs and condition. Thus it is important to first consider scientific knowledge—nothing can replace this, and then understand the social beliefs and patient knowledge.

INTERNATIONAL CLASSIFICATION OF FUNCTIONING, DISABILITY AND HEALTH

The International Classification of Functioning, Disability and Health, known more commonly as ICF, provides a standard language and framework for the description of health and health-related states. In more recent times, ICF frameworks are being used in CDM. **Box 1.5** summarizes common ICF terminologies.

The ICF conceptualizes the level of functioning of an individual as a dynamic interaction between her or his health conditions, environmental factors, and personal factors. It is considered as a biopsychosocial model of disability, based on an integration of the social and medical models of disability. Each component contains hierarchically arranged domains. These are sets of related physiological functions, anatomical structures, actions, tasks, areas of life, and external influences **(Box 1.5)**.

Activity limitations and participation restrictions are graded as capacity and performance qualifier, respectively. *Capacity qualifier* focuses on limitations that are inherent or intrinsic features of the person themselves. These limitations should be direct manifestations of an individual's health state, without any assistance. *Performance qualifier* measures the difficulty the respondent experiences in doing things, assuming that they want to do them. Toward the end of each assessment, list of such activity limitations and participation restrictions should be made, which enables the therapist to put assessment in context and provides the focus for selecting relevant aspects of functioning and disability for assessment **(Table 1.2)**. (More about ICF is described in Chapter 8).

EVIDENCE-BASED PRACTICE

Consequences of not keeping up to date make a clinician lag in optimal practice behaviors. Ultimately clinical

BOX 1.5: Terminologies in International Classification of Functioning, Disability and Health.

- Body functions are physiological functions of body systems (including psychological functions)
- Body structures are anatomical parts of the body such as organs, limbs and their components
- Impairments are problems in body function or structure such as a significant deviation or loss
- Activity is the execution of a task or action by an individual
- Activity limitations are difficulties an individual may have in executing activities
- Participation is involvement in a life situation
- Participation restrictions are problems an individual may experience in involvement in life situations
- Contextual factors represent the entire background of an individual's life and living situation
- Environmental factors comprise of the physical, social, and attitudinal environment in which people live and conduct their lives such as social attitudes, architectural characteristics, legal and social structures, as well as climate and terrain
- Personal factors include gender, age, coping styles, social background, education, profession, past and current experience, overall behavior pattern, character, and other factors that influence how disability is experienced by the individual
- Performance qualifier describes what an individual does in his or her current environment
- Capacity qualifier describes an individual's ability to execute a task or an action

practice may become opinion driven and patients may be denied best care. In the modern era of technology-driven people, this make patients selectively know more than clinicians and this calls for a grave need to update and follow evidence-based practice.

Why Evidence-based Practice?

There are 30,000 biomedical journal articles published per year with a 7% increase each year. There are over 3,200 physiotherapy articles published per year. To keep up to date, a clinician would need to read approximately 10 articles per day. If two articles are read per day, after 1 year a clinician would be approximately 4 years behind. This points towards the fact that the world is moving too fast and so there is a need to keep pace with the best possible clinical practices using most recent evidence-based strategies. **Table 1.3** shows the levels of evidence of published literature.

What is Evidence-based Practice?

Evidence-based practice is "the integration of best research evidence with clinical expertise and patient values". In the clinical scenario, evidence-based practice does not mean only reading these evidences and following them blindly. One needs to amalgamate clinical expertise with recent advances and involve patients in decision-making to enable better patient outcomes.

Table 1.2: List of impairments, activity, and participation domains according to ICF.

Impairments (body function)

Mental functions	Functions of the digestive, metabolic, and endocrine systems
Sensory functions and pain	Genitourinary and reproductive functions
Voice and speech functions	Neuromusculoskeletal and movement-related functions
Functions of the cardiovascular, hematological, immunological, and respiratory systems	Functions of the skin and related structures

Impairments (body structure)

Structure of the nervous system	Structures related to the digestive, metabolic, and endocrine systems
The eye, ear, and related structures	Structure related to genitourinary and reproductive systems
Structures involved in voice and speech	Structures related to movement
Structure of the cardio-vascular, immunological, and respiratory systems	Skin and related structures

Activities and participation

Learning and applying knowledge	Domestic life
General tasks and demands	Interpersonal interactions and relationships
Communication	Major life areas
Mobility	Community, social and civic life
Self-care	Any other activity and participation

Table 1.3: Levels of evidence.

Level 1	Systematic review or a number of RCTs (meta-analysis) that substantially agree (do not have significant statistical variation)
Level 2	• Individual RCT with narrow confidence window (size of treatment effect precisely defined) • Observational study with dramatic effect
Level 3	Nonrandomized controlled cohort study
Level 4	Case–control, case-series, or historically controlled studies
Level 5	Mechanism-based reasoning (expert opinion)

(RCTs: randomized controlled trials)

ASSESSMENT

The first step in determining health status is assessing the patient. By talking to the patient a therapist gathers

BOX 1.6: Activities needed to perform a systematic assessment.

- **Collect data**—subjective and objective assessment
- **Verify data**—confirming the findings with the laboratory findings or findings of the consultant
- **Organize data**—to get information on structural and functional affections
- **Identify patterns**—to come to a physiotherapy diagnosis
- **Report and record data**—to compare it with successive assessment for progression.

information. Then with the objective assessment, observation and thorough examination, the therapist gathers all the "puzzle pieces." This helps to make a clear picture of patient's health problems and make a final physiotherapy diagnosis. Patient management largely depends on how accurately assessment is done taking care of smallest possible problems. Assessment needs to be complete, accurate, making sense of patterns that can lead to confirmatory conclusions and identifying the source of the problem, the culprit structure, and the functional affection due to it **(Box 1.6)**.

Hypothesis-oriented Algorithm for Clinicians (HOAC) Model

It is the process of generating hypothesis during the entire process of assessment and management. One can say HOAC is a structured thought process for developing patient care. This process helps in formulating a diagnosis stepwise and enables most effective patient care. It enables us to modify the diagnosis based on the on-going assessment and helps to narrow the differential diagnosis. This algorithm is problem based and question driven, which are usually close-ended questions, mainly replied by "Yes" or "No." One may need to use alternative questions as well. It is a sequential event that keeps on asking questions and receiving answers until the final outcome is achieved.

Case Example

A patient complains of tingling and numbness in the hand. This can be because of entrapment of some upper limb nerves or radiculopathy. If we confirm entrapment syndrome, we may need to find out the site of entrapment as well. If we apply HOAC, questions come as:

- Is the tingling numbness over the course of the median nerve?—the answer will be either a "Yes" or "No."
- If the answer is "Yes," the second question will be "is it involving the palm?"
- If the answer is "Yes," the affection of median nerve is at elbow and if the answer is "No," the affection of median nerve is at wrist.
- If the answer to the first question is "No," then we need to apply alternative hypothesis considering ulnar nerve as culprit structure.
- So the second question in such a scenario will be "is it along the course of ulnar nerve?"

12

- If the answer is "Yes," then the second question will be "is it involving dorsum of hand?"
- If the answer to that is "Yes," the compression of the ulnar nerve is across elbow and if the answer is "No," the compression of the ulnar nerve is around wrist.

Hence by such simple logical questions asked, one can narrow the differential diagnosis. At all stages, one needs to keep asking the question and after getting the final hypothesis, one last question one can ask will be "can there be anything else?"

At the end of HOAC, one comes to a final diagnosis of the patient which we need to modify and formulate a physiotherapy diagnosis according to ICF guidelines.

Writing a Diagnosis for Physiotherapy Management

Diagnosis in physiotherapy is different than a medical diagnosis. Physiotherapy diagnosis encompasses even the functional aspect of the disease and which we as physiotherapists can address. Physiotherapy diagnosis can be in a paragraph form because it includes all structural and functional alterations or inabilities developed due to a disease process. Back pain and shoulder pain are not diagnoses—they are symptoms of a structural affection. Cervical or lumbar spondylosis is a radiological finding and not a physiotherapy diagnosis. We as physiotherapists cannot alter the radiological findings like osteophytes. But we can treat pain, postural alteration, and affected length–tension relationship of muscles caused due to that and we can improve functional ability of the patient, which is affected because of the pain.

Case example: A middle-aged female complaining of acute low back pain with pain radiating to (rt) lower limb.

- *Medical diagnosis:* Herniated disk
- *Physical therapy diagnosis*: Low back pain due to spasm over (rt) lumbar paraspinal region with active myofascial triggers point over quadratus lumborum Right-sided radiculopathy prevents the patient from walking for more than 50 meters.
- *Physical and functional diagnosis:* A 30-year-old housewife suffering from acute herniated disk at L-5-S-1 level with paraspinal spasm and active myofascial trigger point over (rt) quadratus lumborum and (rt) L.L. radiculopathy with pain in the back and along the course of the sciatic nerve (rt) as a primary impairment. She is unable to walk for more than 50 meters. She is not able to do her household work and not able to move out to buy household things.

It is ultimately patient care that is important and it is for effective management that one undergoes the above-mentioned process of assessment, hypothesis generation, and formulating a diagnosis. Formulating physiotherapy diagnosis will enable a physiotherapist to decide the culprit structure and function we need to address for treating the patient. For most efficient treatment, we need to set goals for patient care.

GOALS AND MANAGEMENT

Setting up appropriate goals and their management is a very important step to be taken:

1. Goals give us a roadmap to treatment strategy. Goals need to be specific. Setting goals is a way to focus attention on what we want in our patient.
2. Depending upon the assessment and diagnosis, one needs to prioritize certain treatments and delay certain other treatments and hence make an entire package of treatment that encompasses physical, mental, social, and environmental aspects.
3. Goals must be realistic and achievable. We cannot set a goal of losing 20 kg in a month.
4. Priority in a treatment depends on primary and structural impairment. We also need to check with the feasibility of treatment that we wish to give.
5. One needs to set short- and long-term goals. Short-term goals are aimed at working on primary and structural impairment. They can be achieved quickly, e.g., pain relief, improving range of motion. Short-term goals aid in achieving long-term goals. Long-term goals may take months and years to be achieved depending on the condition. They are more directed toward functional gain in a patient, e.g., making a patient of fracture walk full weight-bearing without support or getting him back to work after a stroke.

Once we set goals we decide treatment strategies to fulfill these goals. A wide range of treatment options available enable a physiotherapist to provide better patient care. With increasing research and advances each day, it is mandatory for a clinician to be updated with all hands on skills as well. Collaborating evidence-based practice with clinical experience and expertise will enable the best patient care.

DOCUMENTATION

The following points describe the necessity of proper documentation:

- Documentation is an important part of evaluation and management.
- It provides evidence for reimbursement and quality assurance.
- It is a form of legal record, which can be used later.

Documentation can be in various forms as shown in **Box 1.7**.

BOX 1.7: Forms of documentation.

- Progress notes
- Report of patient's PT treatment sessions
- Proof of treatment plan that is being carried out and its effectiveness in the form of outcome measures
- Documentation of treatment progression focused on goals of management

---

BOX 1.8: Points to be included in documentation.

- Treatment provided
- Equipment used and/or provided
- Patient status
- Progress or regression
- Functional outcome
- Progress note may utilize any format, i.e., SOAP format

BOX 1.9: Documentation for description of function.

- Equipment needed
- Distance, height, length, times, weights, and repetitions
- Environment: Level, linoleum, carpet, ramp, and chair with and without armrests
- Cognitive status: Understand, able to follow directions, one step instruction, two step instruction, and memory

---

BOX 1.10: Documentation for description of treatment.

- Modality, exercise, and activity
- Dosage, repetitions, distance, intensity, and time
- Equipment needed
- Settings for the equipment TENS and US
- Tissue or area to be treated
- Purpose of treatment
- Patient position
- Duration, frequency, and breaks

Guidelines provided by American Physical Therapy Association suggest inclusion of points shown in **Box 1.8** when doing documentation.

Documentation can be for description of function or for treatment as shown in **Boxes 1.9 and 1.10**.

SUMMARY

To summarize, one can say that CR is a thought process adopted by clinicians throughout the assessment process for CDM, which is the final outcome of the process. This enables a clinician to identify the culprit structure, functions affected due to that culprit structure and deliver the apt treatment targeting the culprit structure. First one needs to consider scientific knowledge—nothing can replace this. Social beliefs, patient knowledge, and contributing factors then are considered in the formation of goals that are negotiated between therapist and patient for successful management.

Review Questions

1. What is clinical reasoning?
2. What is the need to understand clinical decision-making?
3. Describe the process of clinical decision-making.
4. What are the errors that can be made during clinical reasoning?
5. What should be included in documentation in physiotherapy?

BIBLIOGRAPHY

1. Cohn E. Fieldwork education: shaping a foundation for clinical reasoning. Am J Occup Ther. 1989;43(4):240-4.
2. Collins LF, Affeldt J. Bridging the clinical reasoning gap. OT Pract. 1996;1(8):33-5.
3. Edwards I, Jones M, Carr J, et al. Clinical reasoning strategies in physical therapy. Phys Ther. 2004;84:312-35.
4. Elstein AS, Shulman LS, Sprafka SA. Medical problem solving, a ten-year retrospective. Eval Health Prof. 1990;13:5-36.
5. Hadorn DC, Baker D, Hodges JS, et al. Rating the quality of evidence for clinical practice guidelines. J Clin Epidemiol. 1996;49:749-54.
6. Higgs J. Developing clinical reasoning competencies. Physiotherapy. 1992;78(8):575-81.
7. Hoffman K. A comparison of decision-making by "expert" and "novice" nurses in the clinical setting, monitoring patient hemodynamic status post abdominal aortic aneurysm surgery. Sydney, NSW: University of Technology; 2007.
8. ICF checklist. Available from http://www.who.int/classifications/icf/training/icfchecklist.pdf.
9. Jensen GM, Shepard KF, Hack LM. The novice versus the experienced clinician: insights into the work of the physical therapist. Phys Ther. 1990;70:314-23.
10. Johnson EJ. Expertise and decision under uncertainty: performance and process. In: Chi MTH, Glaser R, Farr MJ (Eds). The nature of expertise. Hillsdale, NJ: Lawrence Erlbaum; 1988. pp. 209-28.
11. Jones M, Rivett D. Clinical reasoning for manual therapists. Edinburgh: Butterworth Heinemann; 2004.
12. Jones MA. Clinical reasoning in manual therapy. Phys Ther. 1992;72:875-84.
13. Kempainen RR, Migeon MB, Wolf FM. Understanding our mistakes: a primer on errors in clinical reasoning. Med Teach. 2003;25(2):177-81.
14. Martinuzzi A, Salghetti A, Betto S, et al. The international classification of functioning disability and health, version for children and youth as a road-map for projecting and programming rehabilitation in a neuropediatric hospital unit. J Rehabil Med. 2010;42:49-55.
15. Mattingly C. What is clinical reasoning? Am J Occup Ther. 1991;45(11):979-86.
16. Milidonis KM, Godges JJ, Jensen GM. Nature of clinical practice for specialists in orthopedic physical therapy. J Orthop Sports Phys Ther. l999;29 (4):240-7.
17. O'Donnell M. A skeptic's medical dictionary. 1997.
18. Scott I. Teaching clinical reasoning: a case-based approach. In: Higgs J, Jones M (Eds). Clinical reasoning in the health professions, 2nd edition. Oxford: Butterworth-Heinemann; 2000. (2) (PDF) The clinical reasoning characteristics of diagnostic experts. Available from https://www.researchgate.net/publication/10644625_The_clinical_reasoning_characteristics_of_diagnostic_experts. [Accessed January 8, 2020].
19. Tanner CA. Thinking like a nurse: a research-based model of clinical judgment in nursing. J Nurs Educ. 2006;6(45):204-11.
20. World Health Organization (WHO). ICF Checklist, Version 2.1a, clinician form for International Classification of Functioning, Disability and Health. Geneva, Switzerland; 2003. Available from www.who.int/classifications/icf/training/icfchecklist.pdf. [Accessed March 4, 2011].

Ethics in Physiotherapy

Megha S Sheth, Neeta J Vyas

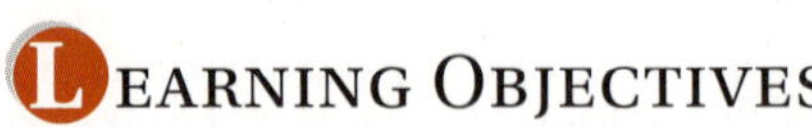

LEARNING OBJECTIVES

After reading this chapter, the readers should be able to:
- ◆ Understand what is ethics and its role in physiotherapy
- ◆ Identify the principles and rules influencing ethical practice of physiotherapy
- ◆ Describe situations where ethical conflicts arise and apply guidelines to resolve them
- ◆ Get an idea of Code of Ethics put forward by the Indian Association of Physiotherapists

CHAPTER OUTLINE

- Principles of ethics
  - Autonomy
  - Beneficence
  - Nonmaleficence
  - Justice
- Rules of ethics
- Application of values in rehabilitation
- Ethical rules and guidelines by the Indian Association of Physiotherapists
- Rights of patients
- Therapists rights
- Ethics in research
  - Information to the volunteer
  - Guide to ethical research

INTRODUCTION

Medicine is a humane art. In comparison to other professions such as engineering which deals with machines and computers, physiotherapy as physiotherapists as a profession deals with lives of human beings. We are into clinical reasoning to understand the problems the management of problems and into decision making about the diagnosis and intervention. We aim to decrease suffering of a person. As a profession, we are all into physiotherapy to earn a living. But we need to understand the importance of values to take our profession further. In physiotherapy, we have an oath similar to Hippocrates oath in Western medicine which states that we should practice ethically.

Ethics is the inner force that provides standards of practice. It is the difference in knowing the right thing and doing the right thing.

Each profession has its Code of Ethics and so does physiotherapy. Code of Ethics is a set of moral norms developed by a professional group. The World Confederation of Physical Therapy (WCPT) and the Indian Association of Physiotherapy (IAP) provide Code of Ethics for practicing physiotherapy. Ethics includes:

1. Providing honest quality care to a patient
2. Respecting rights, knowledge, and skills of colleagues and other health professionals.

Ethics needs to be applied to or followed in all fields of practice of physiotherapy.
1. Clinical practice
2. Research
3. Teaching

PRINCIPLES OF ETHICS

There are four moral principles which form the foundation of health care ethics:
1. Autonomy
2. Beneficence
3. Nonmaleficence
4. Justice

Three ethical rules follow these principles and complete the code:
1. Veracity
2. Confidentiality
3. Fidelity

Autonomy

"Auto" means self and "nomy" means rules. It is the right to choose for one's life. The patient has the right to choose the treatment which he thinks or finds suitable. A prerequisite for this principle is that the patient be provided accurate and relevant information. Information should be regarding the condition and the management options with the benefits and harm of the options. Once the patient has been provided the information, he/she should be in a position to make a choice of the treatment. Evidence-based practice now considers the patient to have an important role in decision making.

Beneficence

This means doing what is best for the patient. A physiotherapist should work in a manner benefitting to patient. This is especially important when the patient is at risk of harm. One should exercise sound judgment in deciding the cause of the problem and then making a decision regarding the management. The therapist should show professional competence in all decisions taken in benefit of the patient. It is the duty of a physiotherapist to promote high standards of practice. WCPT recognizes physical therapists as autonomous professionals who should have the freedom to exercise their professional judgment and decision making within the scope of physiotherapy practice. India is still working on laws regarding autonomous practice by physiotherapists. We need to work to take the profession a step further. The World Health Organization (WHO) now advocates first-hand practice by physiotherapists. This needs us to follow all principles of ethics.

Nonmaleficence

The word means "Do no harm." We should work in such a way that we prevent harm and not injure a patient. In physiotherapy, an error of "not doing good" to a patient is acceptable in comparison to "doing harm". Respect privacy of the patient with regards to exposure of body parts and always take prior permission. Harm should not be physical only, but psychological trauma should also be avoided too.

Justice

Justice needs to be followed in the following areas:

- **Fairness**: Be fair in behavior toward all patients. Do not be biased toward any patient.
- **Distributive**: Therapist resources such as time and skills should be equally distributed.
- **Compensatory**: If some injustice has been done to the patient, knowingly or unknowingly, compensation should be provided, e.g. causing a burn with short-wave diathermy (SWD), increasing the pain with an inappropriate exercise, more than what is usual should be taken care of. Compensatory management should be provided without extra costs.
- **Procedural**: The same procedure should be followed for all patients. There should be no discrimination based on paying capacity or social acquaintances.

RULES OF ETHICS

The below rules follow the principles explained earlier:

Veracity: The meaning of veracity is truthfulness. The therapist should be truthful about the condition, about how much the therapist knows of the condition. This rule follows autonomy and beneficence. One needs to inform the patient about the problem, the treatment options, and the prognosis so that the patient can make a decision regarding the treatment. One also needs to be truthful about one's knowledge so that we can benefit the patient and prevent harm. The question is always about how much truth to tell, should someone else tell truth about the condition or whether the patient should be informed that the condition may not get better.

Confidentiality and privacy: Be trustworthy. The patient should be able to place trust in the therapist regarding his/her complaints. One cannot disclose confidential or private information of patients or colleagues. Always comply with laws when advocating treatment or especially when doing research. Respect the rights and dignity of the person. Provide compassionate care.

Fidelity: Means faithfulness to patient and colleagues even when they disagree. This follows from the principle of beneficence.

APPLICATION OF VALUES IN REHABILITATION

Therapists, patients, and relatives may differ in goals of rehabilitation. Conflicts in daily practice include:

1. Reimbursement and allocation of scarce resources
2. Determination of rehabilitation goals
3. Compromised decision-making capacity in patients
4. Concerns about confidentiality, patient–practitioner relationship
5. Conflicts among treatment team
6. Duties, rights, and concerns of family members
7. Selection of patients and termination of treatment

Callahan describes five factors that are responsible for ethical tensions in practice:

1. Newer technology—new, expensive but effective technology makes it difficult to restrict the use, e.g. renal dialysis
2. Expensive medical resources—improved emergency care, ICUs increase the cost of healthcare
3. Expanded role of public—people coming up with problems rather than denying the existence of medical conditions
4. Language of rights—equal opportunities to be provided to people with disabilities who have a right to make their own decision
5. Increasing concern of quality of life—of the survivors because of extended medical interventions.

Table 2.1: Solving problems—in any ethical situations.

Problem	Possible solutions
Gather all the facts of the situation	SWD, metal implant
Decide principles involved	Beneficence, fidelity, nonmaleficence
Clarify professional duties	Do no harm, truthfulness, obey all laws
Describe consequences of all actions	SWD may harm the patient and implant
Be practical	What is a greater risk?
Decide the action	Avoid SWD and give another modality such as hot packs

(SWD: short-wave diathermy)

Ethical situations: They can occur daily. How much to ask as treatment charges? Is it right to charge more from someone who can afford higher charges? On the other hand, do we charge less from someone who needs physiotherapy but may not be able to financially afford it? Till now, we do not have standard charges, this problem may stay. It is important to provide standard care to all patients irrespective of treatment charges.

Ethical problem: The therapist can clearly differentiate right from wrong. We come across patients who over and above charges made, give gifts at regular intervals. Not to treat a patient in such a situation with special regard is a problem. It is natural to give more time to such patient's which is against ethical principles. Treating a large number of patients who come to the clinic or hospital is also an ethical problem and not doing justice to them when understaffed or overburdened is also a problem that can be faced.

Ethical dilemma: This happens when two or more principles conflict with each other and choice of best action is not clear. A situation where you know what's right for the patient but it is not advised—beneficence V/S fidelity. A lot of times, because we still follow referral practice, a contraindicated modality may be advised to the patient, e.g. SWD advised in a condition with metal implant where it is not be given **(Table 2.1)**.

ETHICAL RULES AND GUIDELINES BY THE INDIAN ASSOCIATION OF PHYSIOTHERAPISTS

- Provide honest quality care.
- Competent—know the skills that are needed to provide appropriate treatment.
- Accountable—you should be responsible for whatever happens to the patients.
- Treatment in interest of patient—patient should be the first priority. Exercise sound judgment.
- Refer patient to appropriate specialist when needed.
- Maintain secrecy of disease except during professional meets and case discussions.
- Provide accurate information to patient and concerned relatives. Appropriate information—the patient should be made aware of all correct and relevant information regarding the condition and treatment options. In case the therapist is unaware about certain updates or techniques, it should be made known to the patient.
- Prior consent should be taken, if treatment has side effects or if it is risky.
- No fee splitting/cut practice—especially if it means getting patients who do not need physiotherapy.
- Keep updated—science is ever changing. One should be aware of recent updates in the field.
- Contribute to development of profession—social responsibility.
- No activity against profession.
- Maintain high standards of professional conduct—dressing, talking in clinics.
- Follow physiotherapy practice according to the Code of Ethics. IAP code of Ethics given in **Appendix A** and is WCPT Code of Ethics described in **Appendices B and C**.

RIGHTS OF PATIENTS

The medical field has been transformed into a health industry where patients have become clients who seek services. The following are the rights of these clients during their treatment based on the principles of ethics:

- **Cultural morals/values should be respected:** A female patient may refuse exposure of a body part to a male therapist on grounds of religious or cultural beliefs.
- **Privacy:** Privacy needs to be respected. A patient needs to be informed about the procedure of treatment and permission needs to be taken.
- **Confidentiality:** All information about the patient should be kept confidential and not disclosed or discussed without prior permission.

THERAPISTS RIGHTS

There is a need for the physiotherapist to protect himself/herself. So, for safe practice, a therapist must:

- Fully understand laws (consumer protection)
- Refuse to give treatment if not in best interest of patient
- Practice professional independence and autonomy
- Refer to other qualified persons as and when need arises
- Consult other practitioner to develop suitable plan of care.

Proper documentation is needed to protect ourselves from legal issues that may arise in certain situations.

ETHICS IN RESEARCH

Research has become compulsory in the field of physiotherapy in India, more for jobs and promotions. Research should not be done at the cost of patient's time and resources without consent. It should fulfill the following:

- **Essentiality:** The research being conducted should be essential, for the betterment of patient or for society. Not only in interest of therapist.

- **Methodically correct:** The therapist should be proficient in the therapy being provided and the research method being used. The research should be meaningful with a sound research design and based on rational theoretical principles. Professionally fair treatment should be given to all participants in experimental and control groups.
- **Contributing to field:** The research should add new information to whatever is existing in the field. The researcher is obliged to prioritize questions important to society (not funding agents).
- **Risk minimization:** There should be no to minimum physical, psychological, or social risk for the participant taking part in the study.
- **Responsibility/accountability/honesty:** The researcher should be accountable for any positive or negative outcome of the study and should provide a compensation of a better treatment at the end of the study intervention especially in case of negative results.
- **Professional competence:** He/she should be competent to manage whatever happens during the study period in the manner best suited to the participant.

The researcher is obliged to publish the findings of the research.

Information to the Volunteer

The participation is voluntary in the study. Privacy, confidentiality should be maintained. The participant is invited and well informed. Explanation of what will be done, how long it will take, side effects if any, why are they being selected, if information has been withheld, benefits of study should be provided. A written informed consent should be given by participant, with no inducements, monetary or otherwise, for participation. Community consent if needed should be obtained in certain situations. Exploitation of any economic class of people should not be there and monetary incentive to participate should be avoided. Compensation for the time and travel may be given. Placebo group should not be deprived of any form of treatment. They can be placed in a waiting group and given the treatment at the end of the study.

Guide to Ethical Research

The following provide guidance for conducting ethical research:

- International Code of Ethics for Biomedical Research—Declaration of Helsinki, 1975
- Indian Council of Medical Research—ICMR
- Ethical Guidelines for Biomedical Research on Human Subjects in 2000
- Institutional Ethics Committee.

SUMMARY

Science, assessment, intervention, and other theories can be taught in classes or read in books. Values are inborn or learnt through life a part coming from the family and in the developing school years. Moral challenges will come during practice and compliance of ethical principles should be the aim of a practitioner. The extent to which they can be followed in the present intimidating health environment with financial restrains and technological advancements needs to be seen. Serial evaluation of self may help in achieving a balance in all goals.

BIBLIOGRAPHY

1. Callahan D. Personal communication (Telephone conversation, January 21, 1998).
2. Frontera WR, DeLisa JA. Physical medicine & rehabilitation: principles and practice, 5th edition. Philadelphia, PA: Wolters Kluwer/Lippincott Williams and Wilkins Health; 2010.
3. Kirschner K, Stocking C, Wagner L, et al. Ethical issues identified by rehabilitation clinicians. Arch Phys Med Rehabil. 2001;82:S2-8.
4. O'Sullivan SB, Schmitz TJ. Physical Rehabilitation. 4th edition. FA Davis Company, Jaypee Publisher; 2006.
5. Sackett DL, Strauss SE, Richardson WS, et al. Evidence-based medicine: how to practice and teach EBM, 2nd edition. Edinburgh: Churchill Livingstone; 2000.
6. Wcpt.org. (2017). Policy statement: autonomy. World Confederation for Physical Therapy. [online] Available from https://www.wcpt.org/policy/ps-autonomy. [Accessed August 31, 2019].
7. Zhang D, Cheng Z. Medicine is a humane art—the basic principles of professional ethics in Chinese medicine. Hastings Cent Rep. 2000;30(4):S8-12.

APPENDIX A: ETHICAL RULES AND GUIDELINES BY THE INDIAN ASSOCIATION OF PHYSIOTHERAPISTS*

GENERAL RESPONSIBILITIES

- Physiotherapists shall provide honest quality care, competent and accountable professional consultancy, therapeutic and otherwise, as 1st contact practitioner to any person who may seek or may be in need of the same.
- The physiotherapists shall administer only such treatment that is in the interest of the patient with the responsibility for the exercise of sound judgment with diligence.
- The physiotherapists shall respect the dignity and basic rights of the patients and professional colleagues.
- The physiotherapists shall refer the patient to the appropriate specialists whenever the problems/symptoms of the diseases of the patient so demand.
- The physiotherapists shall maintain secrecy of the patient's disease and shall not divulge the same to any other individual except to professional colleagues during scientific case discussions/meetings.
- The physiotherapists shall provide accurate information to the patient or to the next relative if required about the problem and specific physiotherapy management of that individual's problems if required.
- The physiotherapy management shall have the prior consent of the patient/relative if the procedure adopted involves risk of any damage to the tissue, organ system or any side effects/complications after explaining the same accurately.
- The physiotherapists shall comply with the laws governing the patient's rights and cause.
- The physiotherapists shall not solicit patients through fee splitting. It shall be based upon their individual competence and ability in accordance with the accepted scientific standards.
- The physiotherapists shall constantly strive to keep himself/herself abreast of the recent and latest scientific developments related to physiotherapy and add to the knowledge fund.
- The physiotherapists shall not indulge in or associate with any activity that goes against the dignity, honor and development of the profession.
- The physiotherapists shall contribute to the planning and development of professional services which address the health needs of the community.
- Maintain high standards of professional conduct.
- Follow ethical practices outlined in the Code of Ethics. Strive to follow the ethical practices outlined in the Principles for Physiotherapy Education and practice norms.
- Balance the wants, needs, and requirements of program patients, institutional policies, laws, and sponsors.

Members' ultimate concern must be the long-term well-being of physiotherapy education and practice norms.

- Resist pressures (personal, social, organizational, financial, and political) to use their influence inappropriately and refuse to allow self- aggrandizement or personal gain to influence their professional judgments.
- Seek appropriate guidance and direction when faced with ethical dilemmas.
- Make every effort to ensure that their services are offered only to individuals and organizations with a legitimate claim on these services.

In Their Professional Preparation and Development, Members Shall

- Accurately represent their areas of competence, education, training, and experience.
- Recognize the limits of their expertise and confine themselves to performing duties for which they are properly educated, trained, and qualified, making referrals when situations are outside their area of competence.
- Be informed of current developments in their fields, and ensure their continuing development and competence.
- Stay abreast of laws and regulations that affect their clients.
- Stay knowledgeable about world events that impact Physiotherapy education and practice program patients.
- Stay knowledgeable about differences in cultural and value orientations.
- Actively uphold IAP's Ethical Rules and Guidelines when practices that contravene it become evident.

In Relationship with Students, Scholars, and Other Members Shall

- Understand and protect the civil and human rights of all individuals.
- Not discriminate with regard to race, color, national origin, ethnicity, sex, religion, sexual orientation, marital status, age, political opinion, immigration status, or disability.
- Recognize their own cultural and value orientations and be aware of how those orientations affect their interactions with people from other cultures.
- Demonstrate awareness of, sensitivity to, and respect for other education and practice systems, values, beliefs, and cultures.

---

*(*Courtesy:* The Indian Association of Physiotherapists)

- Not exploit, threaten, coerce or sexually harass others.
- Not use one's position to proselytize.
- Refrain from invoking governmental or institutional regulations in order to intimidate patients in matters not related to their status.
- Maintain the confidentiality, integrity, and security of patients' records and of all communications with treatment program: Members shall secure permission of the individuals before sharing information with others inside or outside the organization, unless disclosure is authorized by law or institutional policy or is mandated by previous arrangement.
- Inform patients of their rights and responsibilities in the context of the institution and the community.
- Respond to inquiries fairly, equitably, and professionally.
- Provide accurate, complete, current and unbiased information.
- Refrain from becoming involved in personal relationships with patients when such relationships might result in either the appearance or the fact of undue influence being exercised on the making of professional judgments.
- Accept only gifts that are of nominal value and that do not seem intended to influence professional decisions, while remaining sensitive to the varying significance and implications of gifts in different cultures.
- Identify and provide appropriate referrals for patients who experience unusual levels of emotional difficulty.
- Provide information, orientation, and support services needed to facilitate patient's adaptation to a new education and practice and cultural environment.

In Professional Relationships, Members Shall

- Show respect for the diversity of viewpoints among colleagues, just as they show respect for the diversity of viewpoints among their clients.
- Refrain from unjustified or unseemly criticism of fellow members, other programs and other organizations.
- Use their office, title, and professional associations only for the conduct of official business.

- Uphold agreements when participating in joint activities and give due credit to collaborators for their contributions.
- Carry out, in a timely and professional manner, any IAP responsibilities they agree to accept.

In Administering Programs, Members Shall

- Clearly and accurately represent the identity of the organization and the goals, capabilities, and costs of programs.
- Recruit individuals, paid and unpaid, who are qualified to offer the instruction or services promised, train and supervise them responsibly, and ensure by means of regular evaluation that they are performing acceptably and that the overall program is meeting its professed goals.
- Encourage and support participation in professional development activities.
- Strive to establish standards, activities, instruction, and fee structures that are appropriate and responsive to patient's needs.
- Provide appropriate orientation, materials, and on-going guidance for patients.
- Provide appropriate opportunities for students to observe and to join in mutual inquiry into cultural differences.
- Take appropriate steps to enhance the safety and security of patients.
- Strive to ensure that the practices of those with whom one contracts do conform to IAP's Code of Ethics and the Principles for Physiotherapy Education and practice.

In Making Public Statements, Members Shall

- Clearly distinguish, in both written and oral public statements, between their personal opinions and those opinions representing IAP, their own institutions or other organizations.
- Provide accurate, complete, current, and unbiased information.

APPENDIX B: DECLARATION OF PRINCIPLES OF ETHICS BY WCPT

ETHICAL PRINCIPLES*

The World Confederation for Physical Therapy (WCPT) expects physical therapists to:

1. Respect the rights and dignity of all individuals
2. Comply with the laws and regulations governing the practice of physical therapy in the country in which they practice
3. Accept responsibility for the exercise of sound judgement
4. Provide honest, competent and accountable professional services
5. Provide quality services
6. Be entitled to a just and fair level of remuneration for their services
7. Provide accurate information to patients/clients[1], to other agencies and the community about physical therapy and the services physical therapists provide
8. Contribute to the planning and development of services which address the health needs of the community

Date adopted:	Originally adopted at the 13th General Meeting of WCPT June 1995. Revised and re-approved at the 16th General Meeting of WCPT June 2007
Date for review:	2011
Related WCPT Policies:	Declaration of Principle: Patients'/clients' rights in physical therapy Endorsement: Rights of the child Endorsement: The United Nations Standard Rules on the equalisation of opportunities for persons with disabilities

---

*World Confederation for Physical Therapy, 2007

[1] The term patient/client is used in this document as a generic term to refer to individuals and groups of individuals who can benefit from physical therapy interventions/treatments

APPENDIX C: WCPT DECLARATION ON ETHICAL PRINCIPLES

RESPONSIBILITIES OF WCPT AND ITS MEMBER ORGANIZATIONS

Member organizations have a duty to publish, promote and circulate their Code of Ethics or Code of Conduct for the benefit of their members, the general public, employers, governments and government agencies.

Member organizations have appropriate procedures for monitoring the practice of their members, disciplinary procedures and sanctions for members whose practice falls outside their Code of Ethics or Code of Conduct.

The WCPT will assist National Physical Therapy Organizations with the development of their own Code of Ethics or Code of Conduct.

INTERPRETING WCPT'S ETHICAL PRINCIPLES*

The following is intended to assist WCPT member organizations and individual physical therapists in interpreting WCPT's Ethical Principles. The information may be useful background for organisations developing their own codes of ethics or guides to ethical conduct which are consistent with WCPT's Ethical Principles and reflect national circumstances.

Ethical Principle 1

- Physical therapists respect the rights and dignity of all individuals.
- All persons who seek the services of physical therapists have the right to service regardless of age, gender, race, nationality, religion, ethnic origin, creed, color, sexual orientation, disability, health status or politics.
- Patients/clients have the right to:
  - Services of good quality
  - Information
  - Informed consent
  - Confidentiality
  - Access to data
  - Health education
  - Choose who, if anyone, should be informed on his/her behalf.
- Physical therapists have the absolute responsibility to ensure that their behavior is at all times professional, ensuring that the potential for misconduct cannot arise.
- Physical therapists have the right to expect co-operation from their colleagues.
- Physical therapists shall apply sound business principles when dealing with suppliers, manufacturers and other agents.

Ethical Principle 2

- Physical therapists comply with the laws and regulations governing the practice of physical therapy in the country in which they work.
- Physical therapists will have a full understanding of the laws and regulations governing the practice of physical therapy.
- Physical therapists have the right to refuse to treat or otherwise intervene when in their opinion the service is not in the best interests of the patient/client.

Ethical Principle 3

- Physical therapists accept responsibility for the exercise of sound judgment
- Physical therapists are professionally independent and autonomous practitioners.
- Physical therapists make independent judgments in the provision of services for which they have knowledge and skills and for which they can be held accountable.
- For each individual accepted for service, physical therapists undertake appropriate examination/evaluation to allow the development of a diagnosis.
- In light of the diagnosis and other relevant information about the patient/client, especially the patient's/client's goals, physical therapists plan and implement the intervention.
- When the goals have been achieved or further benefits can no longer be obtained, the physical therapist shall inform and discharge the patient/client.
- When the diagnosis is not clear or the required intervention/treatment is beyond the capacity of the physical therapist, the physical therapist shall inform the patient/client and provide assistance to facilitate a referral to other qualified persons.
- Physical therapists shall not delegate any activity which requires the unique skill, knowledge and judgment of the physical therapist.
- The physical therapist will consult with the referring medical practitioner if the treatment program or a continuation of the program is not in accord with the judgement of the physical therapist.

Ethical Principle 4

- Physical therapists provide an honest, competent and accountable professional service.
- Physical therapists ensure patients/clients understand the nature of the service being provided, especially the anticipated costs, both time and financial.

*Reproduced with permission from the World Confederation for Physical Therapy

- Physical therapists undertake a continuous, planned, personal development program designed to maintain and enhance professional knowledge and skills.
- Physical therapists maintain adequate patient/client records to allow for the effective evaluation of the patient's/client's care, as well as the evaluation of the physical therapist's practice.
- Physical therapists do not disclose any information about a patient/client to a third party without the patient's/client's permission or prior knowledge, unless such disclosure is required by law.
- Physical therapists participate in peer review and other forms of practice evaluation, the results of which shall not be disclosed to another party without the permission of the physical therapist.
- Physical therapists shall maintain adequate data to facilitate service performance measurement and shall make that data available to other agents as required by mutual agreement.
- The ethical principles governing the practice of physical therapy shall take precedence over any business or employment practice, where such conflict arises the physical therapist shall attempt to rectify the matter, seeking the assistance of the national physical therapy association if required.
- Physical therapists shall not allow their services to be misused.

Ethical Principle 5

- Physical therapists are committed to providing quality services
- Physical therapists shall be aware of the currently accepted standards of practice and undertake activities which measure their conformity.
- Physical therapists shall participate in ongoing education to enhance their basic knowledge and to provide new knowledge.
- Physical therapists shall support research that contributes to improved patient/client services.
- Physical therapists shall support quality education in academic and clinical settings.
- Physical therapists engaged in research shall abide by the current rules and policies applying to the conduct of research on human subjects shall ensure:
  - The consent of subjects
  - Subject confidentiality
  - Safety and well-being of subjects
  - Absence of fraud and plagiarism
  - Full disclosure of support
  - Appropriate acknowledgement of assistance
  - That any breaches of the rules are reported to appropriate authorities.
- Physical therapists shall share the results of their research freely, especially in journals and conference presentations.

- Physical therapists in the role of employer shall:
  - Ensure all employees are properly and duly qualified, ensuring compliance with statutory requirements
  - Apply current management principles and practices to the conduct of the service, with particular attention to appropriate standards of personnel management
  - Ensure implementation and monitoring of appropriate policies and procedures
  - Ensures appropriate evaluation and audit of clinical practice
  - Provide adequate opportunities for staff education and personal development based on effective performance appraisal.

Ethical Principle 6

- Physical therapists are entitled to a just and fair level of remuneration for their services.
- Physical therapists should ensure that their own fee schedules are based on reasonable considerations.
- Physical therapists should attempt to ensure that third-party fee schedules are based on reasonable considerations.
- Physical therapists shall not use undue influence for personal gain.

Ethical Principle 7

- Physical therapists provide accurate information to patients/clients, other agencies and the community about physical therapy and about the services physical therapists provide.
- Physical therapists shall participate in public education program, providing information about the profession.
- Physical therapists have a duty to inform the public and referring professionals truthfully about the nature of their service so individuals are more able to make a decision about the use of the service.
- Physical therapists may advertise their services.
- Physical therapists shall not use false, fraudulent, misleading, deceptive, unfair or sensational statements or claims.
- Physical therapists shall claim only those titles which correctly describe their professional status.

Ethical Principle 8

- Physical therapists contribute to the planning and development of services which address the health needs of the community.
- Physical therapists have a duty and an obligation to participate in planning services designed to provide optimum community health services.
- Physical therapists are obliged to work toward achieving justice in the provision of health services for all people.

Musculoskeletal Assessment

Saravanan M

LEARNING OBJECTIVES

After reading this chapter, the readers should be able to:
- Understand how anatomy and biomechanics influence the assessment process.
- Understand the purpose of performing musculoskeletal examination.
- Know the components of musculoskeletal examination.
- Understand the nuances of history taking and keen observation.
- Develop a thorough knowledge of the influence of pathomechanics on the assessment process.
- Understand an easy approach to detailed and comprehensive physical examination.
- Understand the procedures used to test specific tissue types in musculoskeletal examination.
- Understand the interpretation of various diagnostic imaging techniques used for musculoskeletal assessment.
- Describe the process of differential diagnoses.

CHAPTER OUTLINE

- Subjective examination
  - History taking
  - Detailed pain assessment
- Objective examination
  - Observation
  - Posture assessment
  - Gait assessment
  - Physical assessment
  - Palpation
  - Sensory examination and reflexes
  - Motor examination
  - Functional assessment
  - Musculoskeletal imaging
  - Electrodiagnosis
- Brief note on differential diagnosis

INTRODUCTION

The aim of musculoskeletal assessment is to provide an accurate, systematic, up-to-date, easily accessible approach to detailed and comprehensive physical examination of the musculoskeletal system, in approaching the problems of the patient.

Accuracy of a diagnosis depends on:
- Knowledge of anatomy and biomechanics
- Ability to listen to history
- Keen observation
- Appropriately systemized examination
- Thorough knowledge of pathomechanics and possible mechanism of injury
- Understanding of interpretation of diagnostic imaging techniques
- Basics of differential diagnosis

An understanding of the difference between assessment and evaluation becomes imperative as most students or therapists are trained well in assessing the patients but fail to evaluate.

- Assessment is defined as a process of appraising or the act of gauging a quality. It is a process of collecting, reviewing, and using data for the purpose of improvement in current performance. It is formative in nature and provides feedback and areas of improvement. For example, when range of motion (ROM) is measured, assessment refers to the ROM in degrees and based on that provides the basic idea of whether the joint is normal, hypo- or hypermobile.

- Evaluation focuses on making a judgment about values or numbers obtained from the process of assessment and is performed to determine the degree to which goals are attained. It is described as an act of concluding on the basis of the set of standards and determines the extent to which the set objectives are achieved. Based on the above example on ROM assessment, the evaluation focuses on the possible reason for restriction and the inabilities of the patient due to reduced joint ROM such as difficulties in activities of daily living (ADL) or occupation-related difficulties.

While assessment is process-oriented, evaluation is product-oriented. In musculoskeletal examination, assessment leads to a physical diagnosis and evaluation completes the functional diagnosis.

Documentation of patient care is an integral component of any examination procedure and appropriate methods to improve documentation skills of therapists become significant in clinical practice and in healthcare education.

The Goodman screening model can be used as a reference to conduct a screening evaluation for patients with musculoskeletal conditions **(Box 3.1).**

This model facilitates therapists to:

- Identify chief and secondary associated problems.
- Identify and rule out information that is inconsistent with the present complaints of the patient.
- Generate a logical hypothesis regarding the complaints of the patients.
- Formulate a working manageable diagnosis.
- Determine whether the patient requires referral or consultation from an expert other than a physiotherapist.

The screening procedure is initiated through the patient interview process, and based on the complaints, they are verified during the physical examination. The subjective information provided by the patient is compared and correlated with the objective findings so that any movement impairments related to the musculoskeletal system and/or neuromuscular system are identified. This also rules out the probable systemic involvement which might require expert referral.

Risk factor assessment forms an integral part of disease prevention. Since physiotherapists are involved in primary prevention, they play a major role in general health promotion by identifying and preventing a target condition in a population that is prone to get affected. Therapists should be trained and educated on identifying risk factors that will help them to establish interventions targeting dysfunction and disability leading to functional rehabilitation of patients.

SOAP Format

One of the most common methods used for documenting musculoskeletal problems of patients is the SOAP notes, which stand for subjective, objective, assessment, and plan.

The following are essential for a proper diagnosis:

- Accuracy of examination
- Concise representation of information
- Clarity in documenting

Above all, it is mandatory to understand that a therapist should assess and reassess patients on demand. It begins from the first patient contact, where the therapist performs an initial assessment, followed by reassessments after administration of a treatment technique, to evaluate the effectiveness of the treatment technique. Both subjective and objective methods of reassessment after treatment and before the beginning of a new or modified treatment, improve the ability of the therapist to judge the efficacy of the treatment method.

Based on this, musculoskeletal assessment can be summarized by following a systematic, organized and step by step approach as mentioned below:

1. Subjective examination
   a. Patient history
   b. Pain assessment
2. Objective examination
   a. Observation and palpation
   b. Physical assessment
3. Evaluation
   a. Functional assessment
   d. Diagnostic imaging and special tests

SUBJECTIVE EXAMINATION

Subjective examination can be described as follows:

- This is perhaps the most important part and one of the most undervalued components in musculoskeletal examination among therapists. While most of the students and therapists focus on objective clinical testing in musculoskeletal conditions, subjective examination including history taking is clearly one of the key aspects of evaluation that will lead to clinical reasoning.
- Detailed history taking and subjective examination would be of help to therapists to formulate provisional hypothesis on the condition prior to clinical testing of objective measures, provide an insight on the potential causes of the patient's symptoms and would form the basis for a strong objective examination.
- It is also a primary means of establishing a direct therapeutic relationship with patients, which is the key to success in clinical consultation as it improves adherence of patients to treatment.
- Accuracy of information is the main objective behind a subjective examination, and it depends on the quality

---

BOX 3.1: Goodman screening model.

- Subjective examination
  - Past medical history
  - Personal and family history
- Risk factor assessment
- Objective findings
  - Clinical presentation
- Evaluation
  - Associated signs and symptoms of systemic disease
  - Review of systems

<table>
<tr><td>BOX 3.2: Signs and symptoms in subjective examination.</td></tr>
</table>

Symptoms: Subjective evidence of disease or disorder, a phenomenon experienced by the patient affected by the disease or disorder

Signs: Objective evidence of a disease or disorder, a phenomenon detected, tested, elicited or measured by therapist or clinician

of communication between the therapist and the patient. It also depends on the ability of the therapist to ask pertinent questions based on clinical reasoning. **Box 3.2** represents the basic difference between signs and symptoms that indicate a potential medical condition.

History Taking

Prior to taking history of the present condition of the patient, it is essential to include the age, occupation, and details related to living environment, health status, functional status, and activity levels as there is a linear relationship of these factors to musculoskeletal symptoms. It also includes careful listening to chief complaints provided by the patient, and underlying mechanism or cause if known as explained by the patient. A preferable method of documenting the history part should be reporting it in the words of the patient avoiding medical jargon.

The components of subjective examination include but are not limited to the following as provided in **Table 3.1.**

Musculoskeletal conditions are mostly mechanical in nature. Questions related to:

- Onset and duration of symptoms
- Presence of trauma, pattern
- Characteristics or changes in the presentation of symptoms as experienced by the patient
- Any preoccurrence or reoccurrence of the symptoms
- Presence or absence of any acute or chronic systemic illness.
- Family history of prediagnosed conditions
- ADL and functional activities that are probably affected by the symptoms
- History of medications or drugs
- Socioeconomic background of the patient
- Any history of surgery
- Occupational and ergonomic factors, prolonged positions, repetitive use, training errors such as excess loading, techniques specific to sports or other occupation-related, footwear and intrinsic biomechanical factors (including weight gain) are all highly relevant.

It is always advisable to use a standard format to fill the personal and family history of the patient. **Table 3.2** provides the possible explanation of factors that are associated with specific disease conditions or disorders.

Table 3.1: Components of subjective examination.

Category	Description
General demographics	• Age • Gender • Race/ethnicity • Education
Social history	• Cultural beliefs and behaviors • Family resources • Social interactions, activities • Support system
Occupational history	• Current and prior occupation • Level of functioning in occupation • Social and recreational activities
Developmental history	• Past issues in growth and development • Dominance of limbs (upper and lower)
Living environment	• Living environment and support systems • Community activities in living environment • Devices, equipment used in living environment
General health status	• Self-perception of health status • Levels of physical functions • Psychological functions (mental capability and cognitive stability) • Self-perception of one's role in social and community function
Social and health habits	• Health risk habits (smoking, alcohol, or drug abuse) • Level of physical fitness
Family history	Familial risk factors to health
Past medical/ surgical history	• Musculoskeletal • Neuromuscular • Cardiovascular • Endocrine/metabolic • Obstetric/gynecological (in women) • Psychological
Core interview	
HOPI	Chief complaints
Subjective assessment	• Pain and symptom assessment • Medical treatment undertaking/taken • Medications • Sleep history

(HOPI: history of present illness)

This part of history taking is also important because it helps the therapist to take a decision by distinguishing between the health issues of the patient that they as a therapist can treat and health issues that need to be referred to other appropriate healthcare professional, which are beyond the scope of the therapist. Any presence of yellow and/or red flags either during the subjective examination or elicited during physical examination also should be an indication for further testing and referral.

Table 3.2: Factors and its possible association with disease conditions.

Factor	Possible explanation
Old age	• Degenerative conditions common with aging • ROM restrictions as a result of aging
Gender	
Female	• Osteoporosis • Gynecological conditions • Rheumatoid arthritis (women > men)
Male	Ankylosing spondylitis (men > women)
Gender and age	• A 30-year-old man less likely to have prostate cancer as compared to 60 years old • Middle-aged or elderly female more likely to have osteoporosis than young women due to hormonal deficiency of menopause
Living environment	• Does the patient need any assistive device or manual assistance as per their living environment due to the disease or disorder?
Health status	• Presence of any preexisting systemic disease, which has been diagnosed earlier
Occupational and leisure activities	• Effect of occupational load and/or leisure activity load on the condition • Possible need to reduce the intensity of the activity or delay in resumption of the activity
Family status	Is there enough support to perform the activities required in daily living? Can there be support to perform the exercises at home?

(ROM: range of motion)

Since pain is one of the most common symptoms that makes the patient visit physiotherapist most of the time and can be considered a subjective phenomenon, a detailed pain assessment is inevitable in most musculoskeletal conditions under subjective examination. It is however mandatory to objectively record the intensity of pain using any of the available outcome measures.

Detailed Pain Assessment

(Also see the Chapter 10: Pain Assessment and Management).

Since pain is often the primary symptom complained by most of the patients with musculoskeletal disorders, pain assessment is an integral part of physiotherapy screening. Pain is not only a sensory or a perceptual experience, but it also has behavioral, physiological, and psychological dimensions to it. Hence, pain assessment should address the complexity and multidimensionality of pain experience and should include the measurement of both sensory and emotional dimensions. Along with the aforementioned

Table 3.3: Various dimensions of pain and possible assessment parameters.

Dimension	Assessment parameter
Physiological	Location, onset, associated factors, duration, type of pain
Sensory	Intensity, quality, pattern
Affective	Distress, anxiety, depression, mental state, perception of suffering, irritability
Cognitive	Meaning of pain, thought processes, coping strategies, knowledge, attitudes, beliefs, previous treatments, and positive or negative influencing factors
Behavioral	Communication with others, interpersonal relationships, activities of daily living, behaviors (pain-related, preventive, or controlling), use of medications, sleep and rest patterns, and fatigue
Sociocultural	Ethnocultural background; family and social life; work and home responsibilities; environment; familial attitudes, beliefs, and behaviors; and personal attitudes and beliefs

factors, most importantly therapists need to identify and recognize pain patterns that are characteristic of systemic disease. Pain assessment should be ongoing (occurring at regular intervals), individualized, and documented so that all involved in the patient's care understand the pain problem. The multidimensions of pain that are useful in assessing a patient's pain are listed in **Table 3.3.**

A detailed pain assessment includes identification of the following dimensions related to pain experience:
- Onset and duration
- Quality
- Location and distribution
- Intensity
- Aggravating and relieving factors
- Functional impairment due to pain

Onset and Duration of Pain

Onset and duration of pain involve the following:
- This refers to the mechanism of injury or etiology of pain if identifiable by the patient.
- It can be abrupt/sudden or insidious/gradual, acute or chronic and with the presence of trauma can lead the therapists in a proper direction.
- Acute pain is mostly of sudden onset and is limited in duration and is usually a response to tissue damage, which includes bones or muscles. It has a short duration of mostly less than 1 month and has an intensity that is generally variable.
- Whereas chronic pain lasts longer (generally 3 months or longer) is associated with long-term illness and can be considered as a defining characteristic of a condition like fibromyalgia. Chronic pain is generally resistant to some forms of treatment and mostly described as constant.

Quality of Pain

Quality of pain is explained below:
- The quality of pain is described in a purely subjective manner.
- Describing the character of pain is often difficult, especially if it is a new or unique sensation that has never been experienced by the patient.
- Shooting, electrical, or burning sensations are characteristic of neuropathic pains, while nociceptive pains are more likely to be described as aching, dull, cramping, or throbbing.
- This part of pain assessment also includes the pattern of pain—constant, intermittent, sudden, gradual and diurnal variations of pain.

Location and Distribution of Pain

Description of the location and distribution of pain is as follows:
- Location of patient's pain is an important dimension in pain assessment as it helps to identify the region affected.
- Pain can be specifically localized to injured anatomic structure similar to most nociceptive pain that occurs due to musculoskeletal injuries.
- Pain of neural origin is typically confined to the sensory distribution of the affected nerve.
- Localization of pain can be misleading in patients with referred pain where the pain is perceived in anatomic locations remote from the site of pathology.
- Most patients have more than one site of pain. Thus it is important to ask patients, "Where is your pain?" or "Do you have pain in more than one area?" The pain that the patient may be referring to may be different than the one conceived by the therapist. Having the patient point to the painful area can be more specific and help to determine interventions. The most common method used to identify the location of pain is pain drawing or the body diagram (map) for pain location.

Table 3.4 describes the most common sites of pain source and the related region(s) of pain referral.

Table 3.4: Common sites of referred pain and its source.	
Pain source	**Region of referred pain**
Upper cervical facets	Occiput, vertex, and frontal head
Lower cervical facets	Shoulder, neck
Pancreas	Mid back
Kidney	Low thoracic and/or upper lumbar
Prostate/uterus	Low back
Lumbar facets	Buttock, groin, thigh, calf
Sacroiliac joints	Buttock, groin, thigh, calf

Intensity of Pain

As mentioned earlier, since pain is a subjective expression, objective quantification of pain and its intensity has been one of the greatest challenges faced by healthcare professionals.
- Pain intensity or severity varies considerably among populations and is affected by various factors.
- The intensity of pain can be expressed verbally or nonverbally and that adds to the complexity of its measurement.
- Assessment is best performed using reliable and valid pain assessment scales and tools. Most of the tools used in the assessment of pain are single-dimensional scales that measure only the pain intensity.
- Examples of these unidimensional scales include:
  - Numerical Pain Rating Scale (NPRS)
  - Visual Analog Scale (VAS)
  - The Verbal Rating Scales (VRS)
  - Wong–Baker FACES pain rating scale.
- Multidimensional scales are more complex and time-consuming but may measure the intensity, nature, and location of the pain, and impact the pain is having on activity or mood. These are useful in complex or persistent acute or chronic pain cases when intensity needs to be assessed as well as social support, interference with ADL, and depression are present. There are several multidimensional pain scales that are used to assess patients with pain.
- The two pain scales that are most commonly used are:
  1. The Brief Pain Inventory (BPI) and
  2. The Short-Form McGill Pain Questionnaire (SF-MPQ).

Table 3.5 describes the advantages and disadvantages of the various pain assessment scales.

Aggravating and Relieving Factors

Aggravating and relieving factors can be assessed as follows:
- The factors which alter the perception of pain may give a clue to the nature of the pain.
- It also provides information as to whether the patient has tried to relieve pain and various treatment modalities are used for the same.
- Aggravating factors include those that precipitate or worsen the pain.
- Relieving factors are those that alleviate, reduce, or abolish the pain.
- People who say that nothing eases the pain can be asked about the posture in which they are least uncomfortable.
- For example, specific ADL such as bending forward or lifting objects, walking a few meters, or standing for long may be some of the pain aggravating or provocative factors. In contrast, pain-relieving factors should also be considered and interviewed. For example, about completely resting or avoiding specific movements producing pain, taking medications, and application

Table 3.5: Advantages and disadvantages of pain assessment scales.

Assessment tool	Advantages	Disadvantages
NPRS	• Validated scale for acutely ill patients • Easy to use • Results are simple to record • Good evidence for construct validity	• Patients may have difficulty relating pain to numbers • Scores cannot necessarily be treated as ratio data
VAS	• Can measure pain state and changes in the clinical situation • Validated tool for measuring acute and chronic pain • Validated tool for research • Can also be used to measure mood, distress, and nausea • Scores can be treated as ratio data • Good evidence for construct validity	• Cannot measure all aspects of pain • Can take more time • Patients may find it difficult to relate their pain on a line • Difficult to use in the immediate postoperative period because of impaired cognition
VRS	• Can quantify sensory involvement • Can assess affective aspects of pain • Better for distinguishing between intensity and unpleasantness • Easy to administer • Easy to score • Good evidence for construct validity	• Can be difficult for persons with limited vocabulary • Variability in expression of pain • People are forced to choose one word, even if no word on the scale adequately describes their pain intensity • Scale is noncontinuous, so it has limitations for research purposes
FACES	• Validated and reliable in children • Can be used in adults having cognitive disabilities • Simple to use	• No evidence regarding relative compliance rates • Limited number of response categories • Scores cannot necessarily be treated as ratio data • Emotions may confound the assessment • Pain assessment may vary because of cultural variations

(NPRS: Numerical Pain Rating Scale; VAS: Visual Analog Scale; VRS: Verbal Rating Scales)

of heat or cold might be pain-relieving maneuvers recorded from the patient.

Functional Impairment due to Pain

Functional impairment due to pain has the following characteristics:

- The effects of pain on ADL determine associated disabilities and handicaps. Interference with the normal daily activities of life will give a clue about the severity of the pain. Walking, performing domestic chores, or continuing to work in their occupation may all be affected.
- Special attention should be paid to the different ways patients compensate for their inability to perform their day-to-day tasks.
- Interference with sleep and inability to take care of themselves can give an indication of the disability.
- Biopsychosocial issues should be assessed in the history to assess attitudes and beliefs about pain, behavior toward pain, any compensation issues, and any treatment or diagnosis issues. It also gives an indication of the state of emotions of the patient, his or her family environment, and factors at work contributing to the pain.
- Functional Activity Scale can be used to measure the level of independence or the limitation in activity encountered by patients.

OBJECTIVE EXAMINATION

Objective examination begins with observation of the patient which includes general observation as in observing the patient as they enter the clinic and local observation related to the complaints of the patient. General observation provides insight into the probable symptoms the patient might complain, and it includes the observation of gait, posture, and abnormal limb positions in general. A proper observation paves way for a better physical examination and saves time for the therapists and patients. Needless to say, it avoids and limits unnecessary components that can be eliminated from the examination aspect. Most parameters that are observed qualitatively need to be measured quantitatively during physical examination. For instance, specific postural deviations observed can be measured for the amount of deviations in degrees and can be used as a measure to compare the improvements gained and find out the efficacy of a treatment.

Observation

Local observation refers to looking for abnormalities or deviations in specific segments of the body or joints in relation to the symptoms as provided by the patient. It includes but is not limited to the following:

- Changes in skin color, obvious texture differences over the affected limb segments.

- Presence of scars indicative of recent or past injury or surgery, type of scar, any skin lesions.
- Attitude of the limb with functional movements or activities.
- Symmetry of segments of the body in relation to its proximal and distal alignments.
- Presence of localized swelling or edema.
- Presence of muscle wasting, atrophy, or hypertrophy.
- Presence of any obvious deformity:
  - *Structural:* Deformities that can be observed even at rest or in resting position of the limb or segment. For example, tibial varus, which is observed in both weight- and nonweight-bearing positions.
  - *Functional:* Deformities that are observed only during change in positions or during functional activities. For example, flexible flat foot is observed in weight-bearing position, which disappears as soon as the limb goes into nonweight-bearing.

At the end of observation, the therapists need to correlate the findings with the complaints received from the patient during the history-taking phase. This will provide a firm background for the therapists to proceed in the right direction of physical examination.

Posture Assessment

Posture assessment involves the following:
- Posture assessment refers to analysis of body segments in any weight-bearing static position such as standing, sitting, and lying.
- It helps in identifying the defects in segments of the body that may lead to various musculoskeletal problems.
- Postural compensations or adaptations can be both a cause and an effect of a clinical condition. Musculoskeletal problems frequently lead to postural changes which in turn worsen the musculoskeletal problem leading to a cascade of compensating causes and effects. Similarly, asymptomatic postural adaptations can lead to undue mechanical stress, predisposing a person to either acute injury or chronic mechanical distress.
- The most common method used to assess posture in clinical practice is the **visual observation** method.
- The ability to perform a visual postural assessment accurately and thoroughly requires many skills on the part of the therapist.
- The therapist must be able to visualize the parts of the body as a whole and in turn assess them in reference to their interaction in the entire anatomical structure. In correct posture, the line of gravity (LoG) passes through the axes of almost all the joints, with the body segments aligned vertically. The LoG is represented by a vertical line drawn through the body's center of gravity, located at the second sacral vertebra (S2). The LoG is an ever-changing reference line that responds to the constantly altering body position during upright posture.

- It is very difficult to define or term a "normal" posture as people come in various sizes and shapes. Hence, terms such as "optimal" or "ideal" posture can be used since it is difficult to have a perfect posture. The only advantage of this method is that it does not require any specialized equipment to assess posture. Disadvantages of this method are that quantitative data cannot be obtained and there is poor interrater agreement.

The other common and one of the conventional methods described in the literature is **plumb line method** and is commonly used in conjunction with a **postural grid**. This method measures postural deviations and was used commonly owing to its low cost and simplicity. However, the disadvantage is that this method too cannot be used to produce quantifiable data **(Figs. 3.1A to C)**.

Goniometric Measurement of Postural Angles

Goniometric measurement of postural angles of the body is another way to assess posture. Some of the angles commonly measured are:
- Craniovertebral angle
- Cranial rotation angle for head-neck posture.

However, the reliability of these measurements varies from poor to good to excellent according to various literature, especially a poor interrater reliability.

Radiographic Method

Radiographic method is considered to be a gold standard procedure for measuring postural deviations; however, the cost and the risk of exposure of patients to harmful radiations are the drawbacks **(Fig. 3.2)**.

Other recent advances in postural assessment include **photographic and digitization method,** where photographic images are obtained and analyzed for any

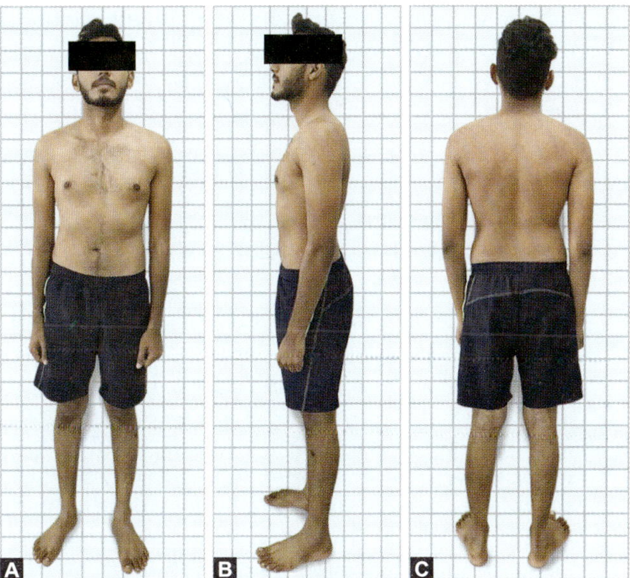

Figs. 3.1A to C: Postural analysis: (A) Anterior view; (B) Lateral view; (C) Posterior view.

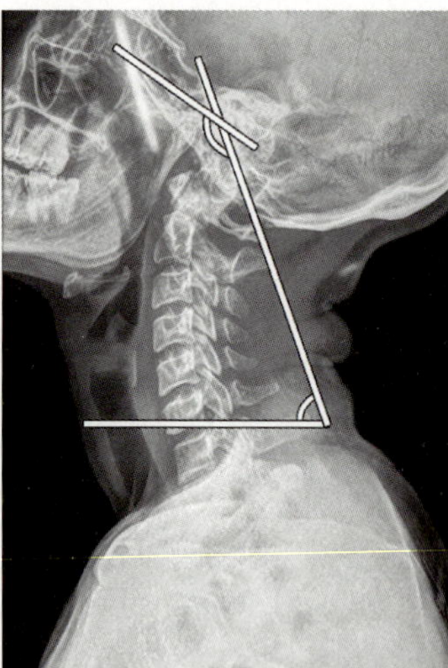

Fig. 3.2: Craniovertebral angle from a radiographic film.

deviations. Markers are placed on anatomical landmarks for identification and processed for analysis.

An improvised version of the photographic method is the **photogrammetric method,** where images obtained from digital camera in frontal and sagittal views are analyzed using postural analysis software to objectively identify postural deviations. Data obtained from this method is quantifiable and reliable.

Apart from the above-mentioned procedures to analyze posture, various other methods exist, which include but are not limited to **posturometer, flexiruler, and Moir**é **topography**. Some of these methods are least used owing to their cost.

Gait Assessment

Gait assessment mainly consists of two areas: qualitative observation such as visual inspection, also termed as observational gait analysis, and quantitative approaches that examine gait behaviors using laboratory measurements. Both methods are explained in detail in Chapter 6: Assessment of Gait.

To summarize observational gait assessment in nutshell, therapist may need to look for the following:
- Inappropriate width of the base of support while walking.
- High stepping of the affected limb to clear the ground.
- Asymmetrical stance to swing ratio, limp (antalgic).
- Reduced arm swing
- Reduced trunk rotation
- Asymmetrical leaning of the body to one side.
- Inappropriate weight shift and loading.

Physical Assessment

Based on the history obtained and observations made, therapists can use appropriate physical assessment methods to confirm the diagnosis. This requires a systematic examination process conducted in line with the symptoms expressed by the patients, to elicit the signs leading to the diagnosis.

It is important to monitor the **vital signs** before beginning the physical assessment. The four vital signs considered primary in a standard medical setting are:
1. Heart or pulse rate
2. Blood pressure
3. Respiratory rate
4. Body temperature

These are taken to assess the general health status of the person and provide clues to the presence of possible systemic diseases. The values of vital signs vary with gender, age, weight, height, and activity levels of the individual.

Palpation

Palpation can be described as follows:
- In the case of history of pain, palpation of the local area of pain for tenderness is important in understanding the structure that might be involved in the pathology. Grading tenderness on palpation objectifies the patient's subjective representation **(Box 3.3)**.
- It helps the therapist to differentiate the tensile characteristics of the structures, e.g., increased spasm in a particular muscle or changes in muscle tone (increased or decreased).
- It also helps to identify the presence of nodules or fibrous bands as may be the case with myalgic pain syndromes.
- Palpation can be used to confirm the suspected changes in bone or joint structures that were identified during observation.
- Temperature variations can be palpated locally to identify the early warning of inflammation, impending infection, and possible foot ulceration. Temperature differences of four or more degrees between the right and left foot are a predictive risk factor for foot ulcers. Other signs and symptoms of vascular changes of an affected extremity may include paresthesia, muscle fatigue and discomfort, or cyanosis with numbness, pain, and loss of hair from a reduced blood supply.
- Capillary filling of the fingers and toes is an indicator of peripheral circulation. Capillary refill test is to be performed by pressing down on the nail bed followed by release and is observed first for blanching (whitening) followed by return of color within 3 seconds after release of pressure (normal response).

Observation of **surgical scars** will refocus the therapist's attention to previous medical or surgical condition even though most of them might not be relevant to the patient's present complaints. Type of scar in terms of

BOX 3.3: Grades of tenderness.
Grade 1: Patient complains of pain
Grade 2: Patient winces with pain along with complaints
Grade 3: Patient withdraws the segment or limb along with wincing
Grade 4: Patient denies palpation of site of tenderness.

its mobility and adherence, length of scar, and its location are all vital especially if the scar is localized to the area of chief complaints of the patient.

Similar to scar assessment is the assessment of **edema** where the presence of it on observation leads to its palpation and quantitative measurement.

Types of Edema/Swelling

- Palpable swelling caused by an increase in interstitial fluid volume is observed as edema. Other than localized edema, it is difficult to clinically observe unless the interstitial volume increases by 2.5–3 L. Edema can be of different types:
  1. Peripheral edema
  2. Pedal edema
  3. Lymphedema
  4. Dependent edema
  5. Pitting and nonpitting edema
- The common site of edema is the legs and the most likely cause, especially in patients over the age group of 50, is venous insufficiency.
- Onset of edema is a key element in identifying the chronicity, as an acute onset of less than 72 hours mostly relates to deep vein thrombosis.
- Similarly, edema from deep vein thrombosis and reflex sympathetic dystrophy are mostly painful, and chronic venous insufficiency causes a low-grade aching. Edema as observed in lymphedema is usually painless.
- In the presence of edema, history of any systemic disease, history of neoplasm, and or radiation should always be suspected. If the patient's history suggests an improvement in edema overnight, it is suggestive of venous edema. Distribution of edema is also important: unilateral leg edema is generally suggestive of a local cause such as deep vein thrombosis, venous insufficiency, or lymphedema; bilateral edema is suggestive of local cause or systemic diseases such as kidney disease, and generalized edema is suggestive of systemic disease.
- Edema can be quantitatively measured using various methods; however, the procedure differs for pitting and nonpitting edema.
  - The most commonly used method for measuring nonpitting edema is the circumference measurement of the edematous limb.
  - The second method is assessing edema by measuring leg volume using water displacement volumetry.
  - Other expensive methods such as optoelectronic procedure, computerized tomography (CT) scan, high-resolution magnetic resonance imaging (MRI), and dual X-ray absorptiometry are also used. (This is described in detail in Chapter 16: Peripheral Vascular Diseases).
- Pitting edema is assessed on observation of the presence of depression in areas where pressure is applied and

Table 3.6: Scoring system for pitting edema.	
Grade 0	No edema
Grade 1+	• Slight pitting • ≤2 mm indentation • No visual distortion • Disappears rapidly
Grade 2+	• 2–4 mm indentation • Somewhat deeper pitting • No readably detectable distortion • Disappears in 10–15 s
Grade 3+	• 4–6 mm indentation • Pit is noticeably deep • May last >1 min • Dependent extremity looks fuller and swollen
Grade 4+	• 6–8 mm indentation • Pit is very deep • Last as long as 2–5 min • Dependent extremity is grossly distorted

the indentation is measured and recorded. **Table 3.6** provides the scoring system for pitting edema.

Sensory Examination and Reflexes

In specific musculoskeletal conditions, the involvement of neurological structures cannot be overlooked upon. This introduces the need for the therapist to go for a thorough sensory examination. For example, muscular weakness if associated with the patient's symptoms may be due to a spinal nerve problem or peripheral nerve pathology. Examining the reflexes and the sensory system helps to differentiate neuronal damage from musculoskeletal pathology. Weakness associated with reflexive changes and discrepancies within the sensory system may indicate the nervous system as the culprit that is causing the disease. Furthermore, evidence gathered from the neurological examination can determine if a lesion originates in the central nervous system versus the peripheral nervous system. Testing strength, reflexes, and sensory systems are part of a neurological examination, but it is also part of a complete musculoskeletal examination (Described in detail in Chapter 4: Neurological Assessment).

Motor Examination

Motor examination refers to assessment of movements through the integrity of the hard and soft tissues including the inert and contractile structures. Inert structures are those soft tissue structures that lack the capacity to contract and relax, such as capsule, ligament, fascia, and bursae. Muscles and tendons form the contractile unit because of their ability to contract and relax.

Based on this, motor examination primarily includes assessing passive movements, active movements, resisted isometric movements, and, in some cases, combined movements.

Anatomical and Physiological Barriers

It is imperative to keep in mind that every movement has an anatomical barrier and a physiological barrier. The anatomical barrier marks the end of passive movement and the physiological barrier marks the end of active movement. Since in a normal joint, the physiological barrier occurs before the anatomical barrier, the range of passive movement is normally always slightly greater than the active movement.

Active Movements

Active movements testing helps in the following:
- Active movement testing provides information on both the contractile and noncontractile structures and can be used to assess the quality and quantity of movement.
- It also provides information on the patient's willingness to move the limb segment, the patient's ability to follow instructions, the active ROM (AROM) of the joint tested and in turn the ability of the patient to perform functional activities.
- It also provides the clinician with information regarding the degree of the patient's flexibility, mobility, and strength.
- Bilateral and symmetrical movement allows comparison of the AROM with the unaffected side, if available.
- When the patient actively moves through the range, emphasize the exactness of the movement to the patient so that substitute motion at other joints is avoided.

The common reasons for abnormal findings during AROM testing can be multifactorial including:
- Pain
- Muscle weakness
- Tightness
- Spasm
- Other pathomechanical factors such as altered joint–muscle interaction or length–muscle relationship.

When there is restriction of AROM recorded during the testing, passive range of motion (PROM) needs to be measured and recorded. If the patient exhibits pain-free full AROM, therapist should proceed to resisted movement test.

Passive Movements

Passive movements test the inert structures that include the:
- Joint capsule
- Joint menisci
- Ligaments
- Fascia
- Bursae
- Dura mater
- The dural nerve root sleeve
- Relaxed muscle and tendon can act as inert structures when they are stretched by their opposite passive movement.

Passive movements principally give information on:
- Pain
- Range
- End-feel

If the patient does not achieve full anatomical range, the end of the available motion is referred to as the **pathological limit**.
- If pain is present before a sense of structural resistance is felt, the condition can be considered to be acute. Because of the pain, the patient will prevent the movement well before the anatomical structures limit the range.
- If resistance is noted before the onset of pain, the condition can be considered to be chronic. The structures being stretched at the end of the range will cause the discomfort.
- In general, pain during passive movement reflects damage or injury to inert structures. Pain during PROM of all movements of a joint might be due to injury or involvement of joint capsule and pain during extremes of ROM in the contralateral direction might be due to ligament sprains.

For example, pain perceived by the patient on passive ROM of more than one movement in shoulder (commonly abduction, external rotation, and internal rotation) is considered a pathological representation of capsule and pain during forceful or extreme plantar flexion and/or inversion is a pathology related to the lateral ligament of the ankle.
- Quantification of joint's PROM is necessary and always should be performed first on the unaffected side and compared with the affected side, as individual variations exist in normal ROM of every joint. Both hypomobility and hypermobility need to be measured and recorded.
- As the terminology suggests, end feel refers to the quality of resistance felt at the end of PROM and is elicited by applying overpressure at the end of PROM. End feel can be normal or abnormal. Normal end feel is again divided into three subcategories:
  1. Hard
  2. Soft
  3. Elastic
- Abnormal end feel represents the early limitation of ROM and is classified into:
  - Hard
  - Springy
  - Spasm
  - Empty

Description of normal and abnormal end feel is provided in **Table 3.7**.

The pattern of resistance provided during a passive movement test along with end feel provides insight related to the capsule involvement in the injury or pathology. The **capsular pattern** is a limitation of movement in a defined pattern which is specific to each joint and indicates the presence of arthritis. The pattern varies from joint to joint

Table 3.7: Types of end feel and its description with examples.

Type of end feel	Description	Example
Normal		
Hard	Bone to bone	Elbow extension, knee extension
Soft	Soft tissue approximation	Knee flexion, elbow flexion (muscular individual)
Elastic	Tissue stretch	Shoulder external rotation, ankle dorsiflexion, forearm pronation
Abnormal		
Hard	Bone to bone before the end of anatomical barrier	Frozen shoulder, arthritis
Springy	Mechanical joint displacement (loose body)	Meniscal tear
Spasm	Resistance to passive ROM associated with pain	Acute injury leading to protective spasm
Empty	Premature halt of ROM by the patient who does not allow the therapist to examine because of pain	Fracture, neoplasm, or septic arthritis

Table 3.8: Capsular pattern in joints.

Joint	Capsular pattern
Cervical	Side flexion → rotation
Shoulder	Lateral rotation → abduction → medial rotation
Elbow	Flexion → extension
Humeroulnar	Flexion → extension
Humeroradial	Flexion → extension → supination → pronation
Proximal radioulnar	Supination → pronation
Distal radioulnar	Extremes of rotation (normally painful)
Wrist	Flexion → extension
Hip	Flexion → abduction → medial rotation
Knee	Flexion → extension
Ankle	Plantar flexion → dorsiflexion (in conditions where muscle length is normal)

and is characterized by the limitation of movement in a fixed proportion. It should be noted that only joints that are controlled by muscles exhibit a capsular pattern, e.g., the distal tibiofibular joint or the sacroiliac joint does not have any capsular pattern. **Table 3.8** describes the capsular pattern of major joints in the body.

AROM and PROM can be an effective tool to measure both hypo- and hypermobility of joints.

Muscle Strength Testing

Muscle strength testing can be described as:
- Manual muscle testing (MMT) is a procedure used to evaluate the strength of individual muscles and muscle groups based on the ability of the muscle(s) to move a joint in relation to forces of gravity and or manual resistance.
- It is imperative to understand that this testing method is limited in neurological disorders where there is alteration in muscle tone especially hypertonia with alteration in reflex activity, or in case of loss of cortical control due to lesions in the central nervous system.
- MMT is best performed in loose-packed position of joints as close-packed position will enable the patient to lock the joint and hold the joint against resistance even with a weak agonist muscle. This will lead to inaccurate assessment of muscle strength. Loose-packed position is also advantageous in measuring isometric strength of muscles in patients because of decreased tension

in joint capsule and ligaments and decreased intra-articular pressure in loose-packed position.

Table 3.9 represents the close-packed and loose-packed position of joints.

The basics of performing MMT procedures usually require the examiner to first isolate a muscle group so that gravity has no impact on the test, then the application of external force and measurement of the results. Results of the test vary depending upon the testing procedures being used. Various methods assess muscle strength, the popular methods being Medical Research Council (MRC) grading, Daniel and Worthingham grading system, and the Kendall and McCreary approach. Comparison of all three methods is provided in **Table 3.10.**

It should be noted that some literature report three and four grades that relate to 2+ and 3+, respectively. It must also be remembered that the grades obtained with MMT are largely subjective and depend on a number of factors including:
- The effect of gravity
- The manual force used by the clinician
- The patient's age
- The extent of the injury
- Cognitive and emotional factors of both patient and clinician.

Muscle strength can also be quantitatively measured using other sophisticated strength measuring devices to produce accurate, reliable evaluations.

The following may give objective, valid, and reliable measures of muscle strength:
- The hand-held dynamometer
- Free weights
- The use of the cable tensiometer
- The handgrip dynamometer
- The pinch gauge
- Isokinetic dynamometers

Table 3.9: Close packed and loose-packed position of joints.

Joints	Close packed	Loose packed
Temporomandibular	Clenched teeth	Mouth slightly open
Glenohumeral (shoulder)	Abduction and external rotation	55–70° abduction, 30° horizontal adduction, rotated so that the forearm is in the transverse plane
Acromioclavicular	Arm abducted to 90°	Arm resting by side, shoulder girdle in the resting position
Sternoclavicular	Maximum shoulder elevation	Arm resting by side, shoulder girdle in the resting position
Elbow	Extension	70° elbow flexion, 10° forearm supination
Radiohumeral	Elbow flexed 90° forearm supinated 5°	Full extension, full supination
Proximal radioulnar	5° supination	70° elbow flexion, 35° forearm supination
Distal radioulnar	5° supination	10° forearm supination
Radiocarpal (wrist)	Extension with radial deviation	Midway between flexion–extension with slight ulnar deviation
Trapeziometacarpal	Full opposition	Midway between abduction–adduction and flexion–extension
Metacarpophalangeal (thumb)	Full opposition	Slight flexion
Metacarpophalangeal (fingers)	Full flexion	Slight flexion with slight ulnar deviation
Interphalangeal	Full extension	Slight flexion
Hip	Full extension, internal rotation, and abduction	30° flexion, 30° abduction, and slight external rotation
Knee	Full extension and external rotation of the tibia	25° flexion
Talocrural (ankle)	Maximum dorsiflexion	10° plantar flexion, midway between maximum inversion and eversion
Subtalar	Full supination	Midway between extremes of inversion and eversion
Midtarsal	Full supination	Midway between extremes of ROM
Tarsometatarsal	Full supination	Midway between extremes of ROM
Metatarsophalangeal	Full extension	Neutral
Interphalangeal	Full extension	Slight flexion
Facet (spine)	Extension	Midway between flexion and extension

Table 3.10: Comparison of MMT grading systems.

MRC grading	Daniel and Worthingham grading	Kendall and McCreary (%)	Explanation
0	0	0	No palpable or observable muscle contraction
1	Trace	5	Flicker of contraction without any visible movement
2–	Poor –		Partial range of motion possible with elimination of gravity (horizontal plane)
2	Poor	20	Full range of motion with elimination of gravity (horizontal plane)
2+	Poor +		Partial range of motion against gravity
3	Fair	50	Full range of motion against gravity
3+	Fair +		Partial range of motion against gravity and against minimal resistance
4	Good	80	Full range of motion against gravity and against minimal resistance
4+	Good +		Partial range of motion against gravity and against submaximal resistance
5	Normal	100	Full range of motion against gravity and against submaximal resistance

(MMT: manual muscle testing; MRC: Medical Research Council)

Muscle strength can also be measured using repetition maximum (RM), and the method used here is 1 RM for strength. This refers to the maximum amount of weight that can be lifted by a person only once without any compensatory mechanism. It is a common method used in physiotherapy to identify the strength of a muscle and is widely used as a procedure to progress the resistance required in rehabilitation to improve muscle strength.

A variation in MMT to test the maximum isometric contraction is invariably used in clinical practice where the therapists instruct the patient to hold the position of joint and apply sufficient force to "Break" the position. It is also called the Break test and is administered where the muscle strength is in the grade range of 3–5. It is impractical to apply this method when the muscle strength has a grade less than 3.

PROM should be assessed before evaluating muscle strength, as the available PROM will be considered the range muscles can be expected to move the segment of the body for muscle strength assessment.

Muscle Power Testing

Brief description of muscle power testing is given below:
- Muscle power is different from strength as it is a product of dynamic muscular force and muscle contraction velocity.
- Power is a direct functional representation of muscle strength and is of greater importance than muscle strength in the assessment.
- Most power activities involve shorter duration, higher intensity, and explosive type contractions.
  - The commonly used power test for lower extremity is the vertical jump test that measures the lower extremity power output, and the jump height is usually recorded as the distance score either in centimeter or inches **(Figs. 3.3A to C)**.

Muscular Endurance Testing

Muscular endurance testing is described as follows:
- Endurance of muscle refers to the ability of a muscle or group of muscles to sustain contractions at a constant yet-reduced load.
- In contrast to muscle strength, the load used here is minimal and the repetitions maximum.
- When the objective of the therapist is to increase the tone of the muscle, endurance training should be the option.
- To assess muscle endurance 10 RM is evaluated, which refers to the maximal weight that can be lifted 10 times without any compensatory mechanism.
- Muscular endurance can also be assessed quadrant wise—upper, lower, and mid.
  - Upper quadrant test includes the push-up test which is one of the best ways to assess upper-body

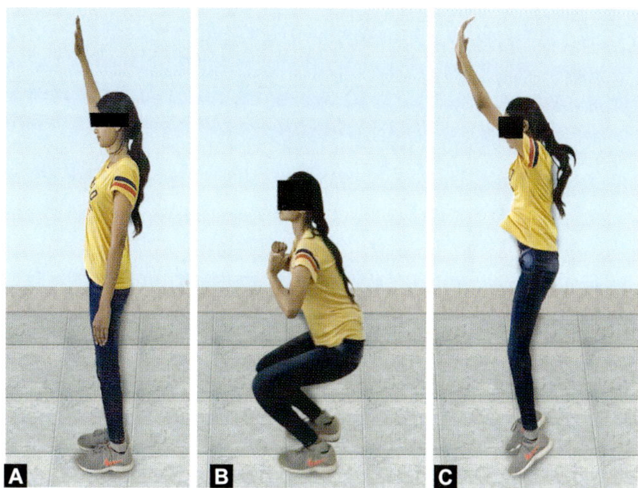

Figs. 3.3A to C: Vertical jump test.

endurance especially in the muscles of the chest and shoulder. This technique can be modified as knee push-up when the patient feels the push up difficult to perform. The common version of the push-up test is to measure the maximum number of push-ups in a set time mostly for a minute. It can also be conducted as an untimed maximum push-up test **(Figs. 3.4A and B)**.
- The plank test measures the endurance of the mid-quadrant of the body that includes abdominals, hips, and lower back. This test measures the total time, the person holds the plank position. It can be graded as excellent or good or poor based on the hold time. For example, if a person holds the position for more than 6 minutes, it is considered as excellent **(Fig. 3.5)**.
- Squat test measures muscular endurance of lower body specifically hip, knee, and lower back muscles and it measures the number of repetitions completed before fatigue. A proper observation of the accuracy of the squat performed is essential during the entire test **(Fig. 3.6)**.

Test results for all the above-mentioned tests need to be carefully evaluated as there are variations in the test performances based on age, gender, and previous fitness levels.

Resisted Isometric Testing

Characteristics of resisted isometric testing are given below:
- This testing procedure is used to identify the pathology in the contractile tissue structures, by allowing the patient to isometrically contract against maximal resistance of the therapist.
- By modifying the resistance appropriately, therapist can hold the joint in a position of stillness so that the stress on the noncontractile structures is minimized. This testing helps to isolate the musculotendinous unit as the cause of pain.

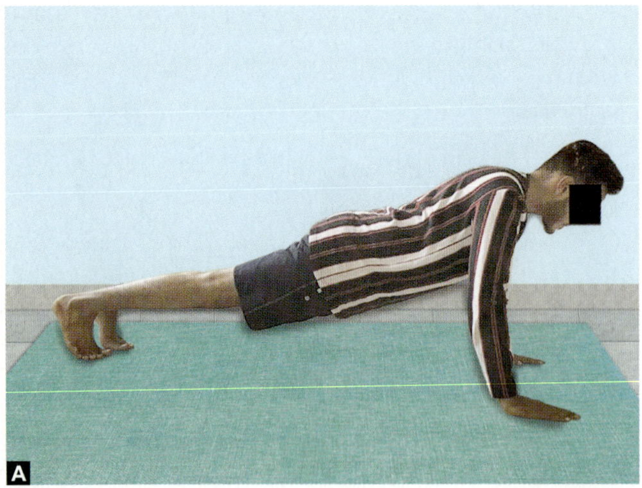 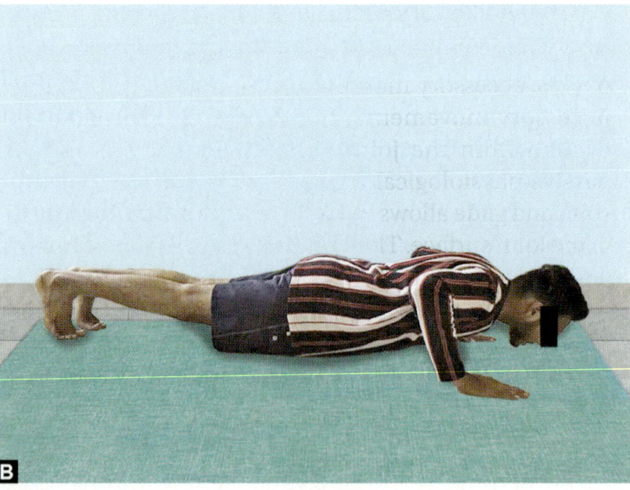

Figs. 3.4A and B: Push-up test.

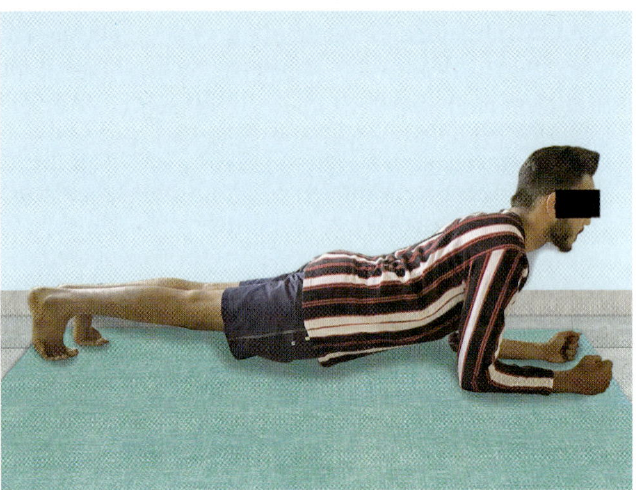

Fig. 3.5: Plank test.

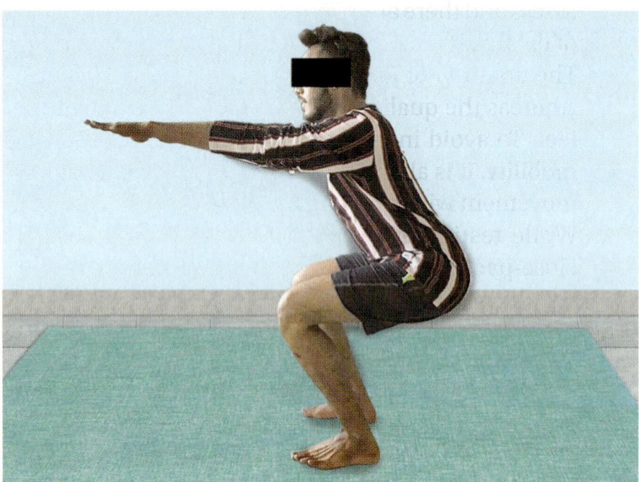

Fig. 3.6: Squat test.

- Response to the resistance offered by the therapist can be:
  - Strong or weak
  - Painless or painful
- Grading of resisted isometric testing is a combination of strength of contraction and pain. It can be:
  - Strong and painless
  - Strong and painful
  - Weak and painless
  - Weak and painful

If the movement is painful it reveals a musculoskeletal dysfunction and if it is weak and painless it is possible that the etiology is neurological. **Table 3.11** represents the grading of resisted isometric testing and its interpretation.

Table 3.11: Grading of resisted isometric testing.		
Grades	*Response*	*Interpretation*
Strong and painless	Patient can maintain a contraction against the resistance of the therapist	Normal musculotendinous structures
Strong and painful	Patient is able to generate force against the resistance of the therapist but pain response of the patient increases with an increase in resistance of the therapist	Injury to some part of the muscle or tendon
Weak and painless	Patient is not able to generate enough force against the resistance of the therapist but pain level remains unchanged	Either full rupture of muscle or interruption of nervous innervation to the muscle
Weak and painful	Patient is not able to generate force against the resistance of the therapist, and pain response of the patient increases with an increase in resistance of the therapist	Gross lesion probably a fracture or metastatic lesion

Passive Accessory Movement Testing (Joint Play)

While physiological motion is controlled by contractile tissues, accessory motions are controlled by inert tissues. Accessory movements (joint play) are movements that occur within the joint simultaneously with active or passive physiological movements. A combination of roll, spin, and glide allows the joint to move following the shape of the joint surface. The former is termed **osteokinematics** and the later **arthrokinematics**. These movements are not under the volitional control of the patient and are totally independent from muscle contraction. To obtain full, pain-free physiological ROM, the accessory movements must be present and full. When the therapist observes hypomobility in joint during AROM and/or PROM testing, joint play is tested. This indirectly provides inputs on the joint mobility.

- Joint mobility testing using joint play is difficult to assess and there are poor intra- and interrater reliability of the test.
- The quantity of joint play is measured in millimeters, whereas the quality of the movement is graded as end feel. To avoid individual differences in joint play and mobility, it is always advised to compare the quality of movement with the uninvolved side.
- While testing for joint play, it is advisable to avoid close-packed position and use loose-packed position.
- If pain or restriction in ROM is encountered, which prevents the joint to be placed in resting position, then a position closer to the resting position and comfortable to the patient should be used.
- Joint play is assessed by moving one of the articular surfaces of a joint against the other stable articular surface according to the concavo-convex rule and the amount of excursion occurring in that particular direction is evaluated.
- Joint excursion is determined by either performing a glide or a distraction and moving the bone to the end of ROM. Presence of pain and/or type of resistance felt at the end of ROM indicates dysfunction.

Table 3.12 represents the classification and grading of joint mobility assessed using PAM testing, based on which the possible treatment options are decided by the therapist.

Muscle Length Testing

With biomechanical principles of muscle insufficiency (both active and passive), muscle length testing has been one of the valuable tools to assess the extensibility of muscle over joints it acts on. It is equally important to assess the length of both one joint and multi-joint muscles and the test procedure marginally varies for muscles of one joint and multi-joints. It consists of movements in the opposite direction of the action of agonistic muscle being tested by fixing the bone of origin, thereby increasing the distance between the origin and insertion of that particular muscle. Muscle length test uses passive or active-assisted movements to determine the extensibility of the muscle. For example, one joint hip adductor is tested by passively abducting the hip to the limit of range of maximum stretch of hip adductors. With a firm end feel, the limit of hip abduction can be felt, and at that point, the PROM of hip abduction is measured using a goniometer. The difference between the actual PROM and the measured PROM indirectly provides the measurement of the length of the shortened hip adductors.

For measuring the length of two joint muscles, for example triceps brachii, the shoulder of the patient is placed in full forward elevation so as to stretch the triceps at shoulder joint. The extended elbow is then flexed to the point till a firm end feel is felt. Measurement of PROM of elbow flexion represents the length of triceps **(Fig. 3.7)**.

In the case of multi-joint muscles, e.g., long finger flexors of the upper limb, elbow, and fingers are placed in full extension to stretch these muscles at the forearm and fingers. This is followed by extension of the wrist passively and at the point of firm end feel in case of shortening of the finger flexors, PROM of wrist extension is measured which represents the length of long finger flexors. **Table 3.13**

Table 3.12: Joint mobility grading.		
Grades	Description	Treatment options
0	No motion between the articulating surfaces, joint ankylosed	Surgery
1	Considerable limitation between articulating surfaces, extremely hypomobile	Mobilization and manipulation
2	Slight limitation between the two articulating surfaces, slightly hypomobile	Mobilization and manipulation
3	Amount of movement between the articulating surfaces is normal	No dysfunction, hence no treatment required
4	Slight increase in excursion between the articulating surfaces, slightly hypermobile	Stability exercises, taping or stability positions, and postural correction
5	Considerable increase in excursion between the articulating surfaces, extremely hypermobile	Stability exercises, taping or stability positions, and postural correction
6	Unstable joint	Bracing, taping, splinting, surgical stabilization

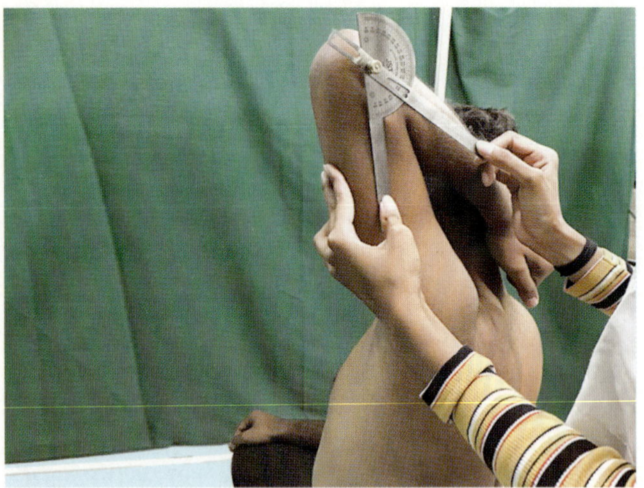

Fig. 3.7: Length testing for triceps.

consists of a list of some of the commonly used muscle length testing procedures.

Functional Assessment

(Described in detail in Chapter 8: Assessment of Function).

The aforementioned components cover the assessment of the physical aspects of a condition or a disorder. However, physiotherapists not only deal with the physical component but the main goal of rehabilitation is to also get back the functional status of the patient to predisease or preinjury levels. Hence, functional assessment should focus on the evaluation of disability based on the physical impairments and should cover all domains including ADL not limited to mobility, transfers, and ambulation; basic self-care activities, ability to maintain personal hygiene, added complex activities in day-to-day life also termed as instrumental ADL, ability to function independently at work and other recreational activities.

- The main purpose of conducting a functional assessment is to identify the individual's physical capabilities related to specific functions of interest.
- Its objective is to identify the unique obstacles to goal attainment for an individual with disability.

It should span the entire rehabilitation process of the patient. Various functional scales in the form of self-reported perception-based questionnaires for indirect analysis or performance-based outcome measurements for direct analysis can be used for functional evaluation. The choice of functional evaluation should be based on the ability of the scale to provide scope for the physiotherapist to assess the baseline function of the individual, to establish goals, and to develop appropriate plan of care and rehabilitation measures.

- Self-reported measures require an individual being assessed to complete a questionnaire asking about the overall ability of the individual to perform a specific set of functional tasks. Examples of these type of functional measures Katz index for ADL, Roland–Morris Disability: Questionnaire, Western Ontario McMasters University's (WOMAC) Arthritis Index, Knee injury and Osteoarthritis Outcome Score (KOOS), Disabilities of Arm, and Shoulder and Hand (DASH).
- Performance-based measures require that the individual being assessed perform a set of functional tasks so that his/her ability to execute them can be ascertained. A number of instruments are available for integrated assessment of physical and mental function. Performance-based measurement requires formal and substantial control of assessment conditions and the information as it is collected. This involves testing relevant stereotyped tasks performed by patients in day-to-day activities including their occupation, in the outpatient or rehabilitation setting. It can also be significant to monitor functional increments or

Test	Description
Table 3.13: Commonly used muscle length test and muscle(s) being tested.	
Test	*Description*
Apley's Scratch test	Test for upper extremity flexibility; actual muscles being evaluated are poorly defined and interpretation is variable
Shoulder and wrist elevation test	Test for shoulder flexibility; strength of shoulder and trunk muscles may affect this length test procedure
Latissimus dorsi test	Test for length of latissimus dorsi
Pectoralis major/minor test	Test for length of pectorals
Triceps test	Test for length of triceps
Schober test	Test for lumbar flexion ROM and indirectly extensibility of extensors; it is not a pure muscle length test unless joint involvement, such as ankylosing spondylitis is ruled out
Finger to floor test	Test for length of back extensors
Thomas test	Test for length of iliopsoas and rectus femoris
SLR test, active/passive knee extension test, sit and reach test	Test for length of hamstrings
Ober/modified Ober test	Test for length of ITB and TFL

(ITB: iliotibial band; SLR: straight leg raise; TFL: tensor fascia lata)

> **BOX 3.4:** Commonly used functional scales for evaluation.
>
> Self-reported measures:
> - Barthel Index
> - Disabilities of Arm, Shoulder, and Hand (DASH)
> - Fatigue Severity Scale
> - Foot Function Index (FFI)
> - Functional Independent Measure (FIM)—clinician reported
> - Katz ADL Index
> - Knee injury and Osteoarthritis Outcome Score (KOOS)
> - Lower Extremity Functional Scale (LEFS)
> - McGill Pain Questionnaire
> - Neck Disability Index (NDI)
> - Numerical Pain Rating Scale (NPRS)
> - Oswestry Disability Index
> - Patient-specific Functional Scale
> - Roland–Morris Disability Questionnaire
> - Western Ontario McMasters University's (WOMAC) Arthritis Index.
>
> Performance-based measures:
> - 30 seconds sit-to-stand test
> - 6-minute walk test
> - Dynamic Gait Index (DGI)
> - Action Research Arm Test (ARAT)
> - Balance Error Scoring System (BESS)
> - Berg Balance Scale (BBS)
> - Foot Posture Index (FPI)
> - Fugl–Meyer Assessment of Motor Recovery after Stroke
> - Functional Movement Screen (FMS)
> - Functional Reach Test
> - Gross Motor Function Measure (GMFM)
> - National Institute of Health Stroke Scale (NIHSS)
> - Stroke Rehabilitation Assessment of Movement (STREAM)
> - Timed Up and Go test (TUG)
> - Y Balance Test

decrements over time. However, the challenges of performance-based testing include observer bias or incompetency, availability of substantial resources to create a simulated work environment, and time-specific variations. Examples include Dynamic Gait Index (DGI), Berg Balance Scale (BBS), and Action Research Arm Test (ARAT).

The self-reported and performance-based functional tests can be region-specific or function-specific. **Box 3.4** provides some of the commonly used scales or tests in functional evaluation.

Every functional test or scale that is performed to evaluate the functional capability of the individual should be interpreted with either grades or scores. Some scales define the ranges of scores as measures of ability or disability, whereas some scores are merely used as comparative outcomes for determining whether the rehabilitation has any impact in improving the symptoms or signs in the patient.

Scales that provide normative data for comparison (which can be age defined or gender defined) can be used to determine the point whether the patient is falling within the normal values or is deviant from the normal values.

For example, in Berg Balance Scale, the total score of the observation is calculated out of 56 possible points. A score of 50–56 represents normal balance or no risk of fall, 33–49 represents mild balance impairment or low risk of fall, 15–32 represents moderate balance impairment and risk of fall, and 0–14 represents severe balance impairment or high risk of fall.

Roland–Morris Questionnaire measures disability due to back pain in which scores range from 0 to 24. In this, the questionnaire is administered before the rehabilitation and the scores compared after a specific duration of rehabilitation. Minimum Detectable Change of four points as compared to prerehabilitation scores suggests improvements in the functioning after the rehabilitation and is used as a measure to determine the efficacy of the treatment.

Special Tests

David Magee describes special tests as:
- Clinical accessory
- Provocative
- Motion
- Palpation
- Structural tests

Special tests are procedures that can be of significance to identify and differentiate structures that are involved in the pathology, to identify unusual signs that are sometimes unrelated to the symptoms, to make a differential diagnosis and probably to make a tentative diagnosis.

When a positive result is obtained from a special test, it may be suggestive of a particular condition; however, that does not necessarily rule out the condition if the test is negative. Also, the findings of these tests are dependent on the patient's ability to relax, while the test is being performed and the ability of the therapist to skillfully perform the test and interpret the results appropriately.

- Therapists should understand the basic statistical significance of using special test(s) as the accuracy of these tests is represented statistically—sensitivity, specificity, and likelihood ratio (LR).

Clinical Pearl

Special tests should be carried out only when there is an indication suggestive from the history or previous objective examination which is clearly based on the skill sets of the physiotherapists.

Clinical Pearl

Similar to any investigative procedure available in musculo-skeletal conditions, special tests should not be used in isolation and results from these tests should always be correlated clinically.

- To keep it simple, the value of a highly sensitive test is that, if negative, the therapist can effectively rule out the condition. For example, Neer's impingement test with a sensitivity of 0.93, if found negative, strongly suggest the patient does not have impingement.
- A highly specific test if found positive suggests the presence of the condition; however, a negative test does not necessarily rule out the condition. For example, McMurray test for meniscal tear has a specificity of 0.71 and if results are positive it is highly suggestive of the presence of meniscal tear.
- LRs are the best statistics to assess the clinical usefulness of a diagnostic test as they combine the sensitivity and specificity into a ratio that quantifies a shift in the probability of a condition being present or absent in the event of a negative or positive test. The LR+ indicates the increase in odds favoring the target condition being present when the test result is positive. A large LR+ indicates that the condition is more likely to be present. The LR– is the probability of the target condition being present given a negative test result. A small LR– indicates that the condition is less likely to be present.

Box 3.5 represents the diagnostic characteristics of Hawkins–Kennedy impingement sign in terms of its sensitivity, specificity, and LR.

In most cases, special tests should be tested in clusters as that increases the LR for diagnosis. For example, Hawkins–Kennedy impingement sign when clustered with painful arc sign and the infraspinatus test, and with all three tests showing positive results, the positive LR increases from 3.33 to 10.56. In the case of any two of the three tests are positive, the positive LR is 5.03 which is again better as compared to the positive LR when the test is used in isolation.

Musculoskeletal Imaging

Many investigative procedures related to imaging are available nowadays, and a basic understanding of how to observe and interpret is essential for better correlation of the physical findings.

Musculoskeletal imaging is not always required, especially when the clinical examination has narrowed down the diagnosis. However, in situations where the clinical examination has further opened up the possibilities of more differential diagnoses, additional screening procedures might allow the therapist to confirm a firm diagnosis. These imaging techniques are mostly regional and include:

- X-ray
- CT scans
- MRI scans
- Ultrasound imaging
- Bone scans
- Single-photon emission controlled tomography or positron emission tomography scans.

Table 3.14 provides the basic information on the imaging techniques.

Table 3.14: Basic interpretation of commonly used musculoskeletal imaging techniques.

Imaging technique	Structure imaged for	Look out for
Radiography (X-ray)	Skeletal, joint, and soft tissue structures	Fracture, subluxation, dislocation, spurs, osteophytes, bone density, sclerosis, joint spaces, gross wasting, or swelling
CT scans	Skeletal, joint, and soft tissue structures	Subtle or complex fractures, degenerative changes, multiple injuries to both osseous and soft tissue structures, spinal stenosis (if performed as CT myelography), intervertebral disc lesions (combined with discogram), loose bodies, osseous alignment in any plane
MRI	Skeletal, joint, and soft tissue structures	Changes in bone marrow (tumors), stress fractures, avascular necrosis, sports injuries (specially to distinguish partial and complete tears of tendons and ligaments), meniscal injuries, nerve root impingement
Ultrasound	Good to identify soft tissue structures and limited ability on skeletal, joint structures	Internal architecture of muscles, tendons, degenerative changes of tendons and ligaments, inflammation of nerve and changes in nerve diameter, cysts, and bursae

(CT: computerized tomography; MRI: magnetic resonance imaging)

BOX 3.5: Diagnostic characteristics of Hawkins–Kennedy impingement sign.

- *Sensitivity:* 0.62–0.92
- *Specificity:* 0.25–1.00
- *Positive likelihood ratio:* 1.20–3.33
- *Negative likelihood ratio:* 0.21–0.55

Electrodiagnosis

This is described in detail in Chapter 7: Electrodiagnosis.

Significance of Red Flags in Diagnosis

Looking for red flags as a part of differential diagnosis not only saves patients potentially from getting damaged, it also helps in precluding inappropriate patients from treatment.

BRIEF NOTE ON DIFFERENTIAL DIAGNOSIS

Since most of the symptoms are commonly presented in most diagnostic conditions, differential diagnosis has become an integral component in screening process for physiotherapists, which enables them to identify inappropriate referrals, to identify concurrent inappropriate conditions accompanying the patient's symptoms and signs, to generate a working diagnosis and in turn to make the rehabilitation protocol a more functional one.

The clinical differential diagnosis is provisional most of the time and is subject to change as the therapist gains further information from more objective examination.

For example, neck pain may be caused by various diagnostic conditions such as degenerative changes (spondylosis), discogenic disorders, infection of bone, myofascial issues, whiplash injury, muscle spasm, tumors or even referred from viscera. To arrive at an appropriate differential diagnosis, therapist should use a patient-centered model of clinical reasoning that should include and be based upon the subjective information gathered from the patient or the relative, objective data obtained from the clinical examination and interpretation of results obtained from other tools such as special tests and diagnostic imaging. This leads the therapist to a consolidated diagnosis and in turn a patient-centered rehabilitation approach which is more functional than physical.

SUMMARY

The many musculoskeletal dilemmas faced by the therapist on a daily basis challenge the caregiver to provide the most appropriate therapeutic intervention. The purpose of examination and/or testing procedures in musculoskeletal conditions is to examine the function of the different tissues of the moving parts. Each tissue of the body has its particular function. It acts either as an isolated structure or as part of a group of structures. Function differs, depending on whether a tissue is built to make other tissues move (musculotendinous structures), to control range of movement (capsulo-ligamentous structures), to facilitate movement (bursae), or to activate movement (nerve structures). Hence, an accurate examination of the musculoskeletal system is a critical component of physiotherapy assessment and diagnosis in musculoskeletal problems. This can be best accomplished by the therapist when he/she possesses a thorough knowledge of anatomy, biomechanics, kinesiology, pathomechanics as well as an understanding of the structure, and response of various tissues of the body to any pathology or injury. With this basic knowledge therapist can perform a well-organized, systematic and specific examination which includes subjective and objective components. It is essential for the therapist to master the skill of utilizing a set of sequences in logical order so that no information is missed out. This will enable the therapist to focus on specific diagnosis and enhance the patient's recovery by means of targeted functional goals leading to functional rehabilitation.

Review Questions

1. Recall Goodman's screening model and identify key factors.
2. Identify components of SOAP format of documentation in assessment and evaluation.
3. Differentiate assessment and evaluation with a clinical case example.
4. Differentiate signs and symptoms with a clinical case example.
5. Recall and enlist components of subjective examination.
6. Enlist various dimensions of pain and its assessment parameters.
7. Correlate line of gravity and its relation to assessment of posture using posture grid analysis.
8. Correlate the significance of sensory assessment in musculoskeletal examination.
9. Differentiate between muscle strength, power, and endurance.
10. Identify tests used to measure power and endurance and its normative values.
11. Identify sensitivity, specificity, and likelihood ratio for most commonly used special tests.
12. Identify the significance of differential diagnosis in musculoskeletal examination.
13. Enlist the commonly identifiable red flags in musculoskeletal examination.

BIBLIOGRAPHY

1. Fink R. Pain assessment: the cornerstone to optimal pain management. Proc (Bayl Univ Med Cent). 2000;13:236-9.
2. Goodman CC, Snyder. Differential diagnosis for physical therapists—screening for referral. USA: Elsevier; 2013.
3. Harrison AL, Barry-Greb T, Wojtowicz G. Clinical measurement of head and shoulder posture variables. J Orthop Sports Phys Ther. 1996;23:353-61.
4. Iunes DH, Bevilaqua-Grossi D, Oliveira AS, et al. Comparative analysis between visual and computerized photogrammetry postural assessment. Rev Bras Fisiotcr. 2009;13:308 15.
5. James H, Cyriax PJC. Cyriax's illustrated manual of orthopaedic medicine. Oxford: Butterworth Heinemann; 1993.

6. Kilinç F, Yaman H, Atay E. Investigation of the effects of intensive one-sided and double-sided training drills on the postures of basketball playing children. J Phys Ther Sci. 2009;21:23-8.

7. Magee DJ. Orthopedic physical assessment. Missouri: Saunders Elsevier; 2006.

8. Mathers JJ. Differential diagnosis of a patient referred to physical therapy with neck pain: a case study of a patient with an atypical presentation of angina. J Man Manip Ther. 2012;20:214-8.

9. Radaš J, Bobić TT. Posture in top-level Croatian rhythmic gymnasts and non-trainees. Kinesiology. 2011;43:64-73.

10. Sacco ICN, Alibert S, Queiroz BWC, et al. Reliability of photogrammetry in relation to goniometry for postural lower limb assessment. Rev Bras Fisioter. 2007;11:411-7.

11. Santos MM, Silva MPC, Sanada LS, et al. Photogrammetric postural analysis on healthy seven to ten-year-old children: interrater reliability. Rev Bras Fisioter. 2009;13:350-5.

12. Singla D, Veqar Z. Methods of postural assessment used for sports persons. J Clin Diagn Res. 2014;8:LE01-4.

13. Souza JA, Pasinato F, Basso D, et al. Biophotogrammetry: reliability of measurements obtained with a posture assessment software (SAPO). Rev Bras Cineantropom Desempenho Hum. 2011;13:299-305.

Neurological Assessment

Suvarna Ganvir

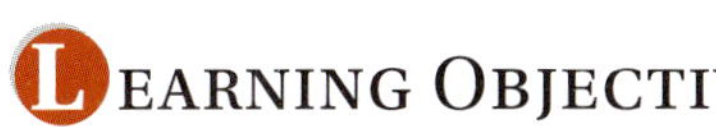 LEARNING OBJECTIVES

After reading this chapter, the readers should be able to:

♦ Understand how to assess patients with neurological dysfunction theoretically and practically
♦ Perform the neurological assessment in a less time-consuming and more effective manner
♦ Understand intricacies involved in assessment with more emphasis on practical aspect
♦ Learn techniques that minimize discomfort caused to the patient and maximize cooperation from them

CHAPTER OUTLINE

- Patient history
- General examination
- Systems review
- Observation and palpation
  - Posture assessment
- Neurological examination
  - Higher mental functions
  - Level of consciousness/arousal
  - Cognition
  - Speech
  - Perception
- Cranial nerve examination
- Sensory assessment
  - Superficial sensations
  - Deep sensations
  - Combined cortical sensations
- Motor examination
  - Tone
  - Reflex integrity
  - Range of motion
  - Muscle performance
- Coordination assessment
- Assessment of balance
  - Sensory organization test
  - Clinical test for sensory interaction on balance
  - Movement strategies for balance
  - Functional balance grades
- Performance-based measures
- Self-report measures
- Assessment of gait
- Hand evaluation
  - Observation
  - Physical evaluation
  - Edema assessment
  - Mapping
  - Categories of tests
  - Grips and pinch strength
  - Michigan hand outcomes questionnaire
  - Electrodiagnosis
- Functional assessment

INTRODUCTION

Assessment of patients with neurological dysfunction often poses four major questions in the mind of therapist.

1. Whether it is an upper motor neuron lesion or lower motor neuron lesion?
2. What is the most appropriate way of assessment?
3. Should specific steps be followed or should patient discomfort during the process be addressed on a priority basis?
4. How to write the physical and functional diagnosis of patient?

Most of the questions can be answered by careful history taking and accurate physical examination. Each step taken in the examination of the patient, from the first visual impression to history taking to physical examination, should aim toward answering these questions.

Neurological assessment is a time-consuming process at the beginning but with practice it becomes simpler and time management comes handy.

- Patient's comfort is of utmost important during the assessment.

Clinical Pearl

A therapist should carefully examine **the patient by following all the steps and should not assume certain findings without assessing them.**

- Patient should not be made to change the position quite often. Instead all assessments in one position should be completed at one go and then other position should be given.
- Many a times the patient is not cooperative or is in a semiconscious state, when he is not able to answer the questions. In such cases, a caregiver should be approached for some part of assessment.
- Patient's cooperation is of utmost importance for the accurate findings. This can be achieved by simple one-sentence commands or instructions to the patient in their language. This will help the patient to understand what is expected of them during the assessment process and they will act accordingly.
- One should not show hesitation while asking some personal questions such as bladder or bowel problems, and addictions. But, at the same time, a therapist should be careful enough to frame appropriate words in the presence of a caregiver who may answer some questions on the behalf of patient.
- Sometimes it is frustrating for the patient that they are not able to move a part of the body due to weakness. In this case, patient should not be asked to repeat the same movement again and again.
- The assessment performa should be handy so that all points of assessment are covered at one time, with due consideration of the patient's physical and mental condition.
- It is the responsibility of the therapist that the patient is safe and does not experience any adverse event during the assessment such as a fall in standing position due to poor balance. If it happens, apart from getting injured, patient may also lose confidence in the assessor and hence may not cooperate further.

As with any systemic examination, neurological examination starts with collecting demographic information in the form of name, age, gender, residence, occupation (including the nature of work), and hand dominance.

PATIENT HISTORY

It is the first information about patient condition, which the therapist should obtain very carefully. Patient should be allowed to describe the complaints with the utmost detail. The therapist may decide the relevance of the information obtained from the patient and note down the relevant points. If the patient is not able to describe their condition, a close family member who is well acquainted with patient's condition should describe the complaints to the therapist.

- Patient's **present complaints** should be written in the chronological order, i.e., the complaint with the longest duration should be written first and then other complaints should follow the same sequence. While writing the **chief complaints**, duration of complaint must be mentioned along with it. Complaints that are not associated with the present disease can be written as **associated complaints** after chief complaints.
- Chief complaints are explained in detail under the title ***"History of Present Illness (HOPI)."*** While writing HOPI in patients with neurological dysfunction, it is necessary to describe course of neurological complaints right from the onset till the day when the patient is being examined. The progress of the disease should be described in terms of changes in the symptoms over a period of time. For example, weakness may increase and spread from one part to another or it may reduce so that a specific part of the body regains function. Since the complaints need to be mentioned in patient's words, the progress of the disease is usually described in terms of functional abilities by the patient.
- Hence, the effect of symptoms on activities of daily living (ADLs) or occupation needs to be described here. This would also help to determine the effectiveness of treatment at a later stage. Any difficulty in performing the ADLs should be mentioned in detail.
- Also it is necessary to incorporate information regarding consultation with other health-care professionals and any investigations done during this time (though the detailed report should not be mentioned here). A detailed note should be made of the investigations done till date along with findings and exact date of investigation. This helps to understand the extent of lesion.
- Personal history, including sexual issues.
- Past history, including medical and surgical conditions. History of previous and current medications along with duration and dosages must be asked. One should be aware about effect of such medications on the body. For example, the drug for patients with Parkinsonism, Safinamide, has ON and OFF times when the symptoms may change considerably.
- Family history should be taken to identify hereditary disease in the family and also to assess the health of people in the patient's home support system. Knowledge of the health and fitness of the spouse and other family members can be useful in deciding certain discharge parameters.
- Socioeconomic status maybe using Kuppuswamy socioeconomic scale should be taken.
- Occupational history: Details of occupation-related information specifically the kind of work an individual has to perform should be asked for.
- Psychological history.
- Information should be asked regarding the status of bladder and bowel functioning in terms of sensation of

fullness of bladder or bowel, control over the movement of urine or feces, any history of episodes of involuntary passing of urine or feces. Neurogenic bladder refers to dysfunction of the urinary bladder due to disease of the central nervous system or peripheral nerves involved in micturition. There are two major types of bladder control problems that are associated with a neurogenic bladder. Depending on the nerves involved and nature of the damage, the bladder becomes either overactive (spastic or hyperreflexive) or underactive (flaccid or hypotonic). Bladder fullness sensation is usually present in overactive bladder but due to spastic muscles patient is not able to control the passing of urine; hence, there is urge incontinence (inability to control passage of urine once the fullness sensation is perceived). In flaccid bladder, patient does not have sensation of bladder fullness and flaccid muscles cannot contract to void the urine once the capacity is full. Hence, the capacity of bladder and residual urine is increased. There is overflow incontinence but no urgency.

Before proceeding to the examination of the patient, the above information should be sought to understand the course of disease and the influence that it has on the functioning of individual.

GENERAL EXAMINATION

The routine general examination in the form of the following should be done.
- Temperature
- Respiratory rate
- Pulse rate
- Pallor
- Icterus
- Cyanosis

Careful inspection should be done for the presence of any pressure sores or callosities or ulcer. Use of any external aids should also be noted, such as any drains, catheter, and splints.

SYSTEMS REVIEW

A careful review of the systems should be done thoroughly to identify clues to diseases not otherwise identified in history. This should mainly focus on head and neck, respiratory, cardiovascular, gastrointestinal, genitourinary, musculoskeletal, neurologic, psychiatric, endocrine, dermatologic, and other constitutional symptoms. Details on investigatory findings as well as drug chart should also be made while reviewing other systems.

OBSERVATION AND PALPATION

This aspect of neurological assessment mainly focuses on posture assessment, attitude of limb, observation of few vital signs, and careful inspection of presence of any external aids.

Posture Assessment

The routine principles regarding posture assessment need to be followed for patients with neurological dysfunction. The patient should be evaluated in static positions of sitting and standing in frontal and sagittal view. A postural grid may be used for better evaluation of posture. Postural symmetry should be determined by using an imaginary vertical line of gravity. In standing, this line of gravity is expected to fall close to most of the joint axis and divides the body into right and left halves or anterior and posterior halves in frontal and sagittal view, respectively.

Clinically, posture assessment includes relative position of different parts of the body with respect to this imaginary line. Ability to maintain a static posture without any support or assistance is a pre-requisite for posture assessment. This means that if the patient is not able to maintain static sitting or standing position with or without support, then the posture cannot be checked in that position.

During static erect sitting position, posture can be assessed from head to toes. First observation should be made of the position of the hands. Similarly, static erect standing can also be checked noting any assistance required for standing and position of the relative parts of the body. Patient should be adequately exposed with special emphasis on the expected areas of deviation. During erect standing posture, antero-posterior sway can be measured with the help of specific devices. Postural sway should not exceed more than 7–12° in antero-posterior direction and 5–7° on medial lateral direction.

NEUROLOGICAL EXAMINATION

Higher Mental Functions

Assessment of higher mental functions is an integral and most important part of the assessment in neurological examination. It is an essential first step in the assessment of neurological examination. It makes the rest of the assessment more valid; hence, appropriate interpretations can be made.

Level of Consciousness/Arousal

First thing that the therapist needs to ascertain is that the patient is conscious so that he will respond to the rest of the assessment in the most effective manner. Consciousness is defined as the state of full awareness and being fully oriented to time place and person and responding to the given stimuli in the most appropriate manner. It depends on the brainstem and cortical functioning.

When examining patients with reduced levels of consciousness, noting the type of stimulus needed to arouse the patient and the degree to which the patient can respond when aroused is a useful way of recording this information **(Box 4.1)**. Glasgow Coma Scale and RLA scale used to assess levels of cognitive functioning is described in Chapter 35: "Head Injury."

> **BOX 4.1:** Five stages of consciousness.
>
> Full consciousness, lethargy, obtundation, stupor, and coma.
> 1. **A full or normal level of consciousness** is one in which the patient is fully awake and is able to respond to stimuli at the same lower level of strength as most people who are functioning without neurologic abnormality.
> 2. **Lethargy** or clouded consciousness is a state of reduced awareness, main deficit of which is one of inattention. Stimuli may be perceived at a conscious level but are easily ignored or misinterpreted.
> 3. **Delirium** is an acute or subacute (hours to days) onset of a grossly abnormal mental state often exhibiting fluctuating consciousness, disorientation, heightened irritability, and hallucinations. It is often associated with toxic, infectious, or metabolic disorders of the central nervous system.
> 4. **Obtundation** refers to moderate reduction in the patient's level of awareness such that stimuli of mild-to-moderate intensity fail to arouse; when arousal does occur, the patient is slow to respond.
> 5. **Stupor** may be defined as unresponsiveness to all but the most vigorous of stimuli. The patient quickly drifts back into a deep sleep-like state on cessation of the stimulation. Coma is unarousable unresponsiveness. The most intense or vigorous of noxious stimuli may or may not elicit reflex motor responses.

Cognition

Cognition is the act or process of knowing, including awareness, reasoning, judgment, intuition, and memory. A screening of cognitive abilities includes orientation, attention, and memory; communication; and executive or higher order cognition (e.g., calculating abilities, abstract thinking, and constructional ability).

Orientation

Orientation is assessed with respect to time, place, and person.
- Simple questions are asked related to time such as "what time of the day is it now?" or "what is the season at present?"
- For place-related orientation, patient may be asked about the name of hospital "where he is right now? Name of the city or place of his residence."
- Orientation regarding person can be checked with the questions about himself or about family members and friends.
- Additionally, another domain circumstance can be examined by asking what happened with them, what kind of place are they in, and why do people come to such places. The patient must be able to receive, store in, and recall new information when asked these questions. Patients with delirium or advanced dementia are commonly disoriented.

Attention

Attention is the directing of consciousness to a person, thing, perception, or thought. It is mainly of four types:

selective, divided, sustained, and alternating. Patients with attention deficit may not be able to concentrate during the exercise program and may not contribute actively, which will delay the recovery.
1. *Selective attention* can be assessed by asking the patient to attend to a particular task, e.g., asking them to repeat a short list of numbers forward and backward, i.e., the digit span test. Normally, individuals can recall seven forward and five backward numbers. Those having communication impairments can be read to a list of items by the therapist, and they should signal each time a particular item is mentioned.
2. *Sustained attention* is tested by determining how long the patient is able to maintain attention on a particular task (time on task).
3. *Alternating attention* (attention flexibility) is examined by requesting the patient to alternate back and forth between two different tasks (e.g., add the first two pairs of numbers, then subtract the next two pairs).
4. The patient is asked to perform two tasks simultaneously in order to determine *divided attention*.

Memory

Memory includes:
- Immediate memory
- Short-term memory (STM)
- Long-term memory (LTM)
- Motor memory

Immediate memory is assessed by asking the patient to repeat immediately a list of familiar items or a simple sentence said by the therapist.

STM is checked by asking the patient to recall the events that happened during that day.

LTM is related to recall of facts or events, which happened in recent years.

Motor memory is related to the performance of a task, which can be assessed by asking the patient to describe the steps of a particular activity that he used to do before the current episode. **Table 4.1** describes the different types of memory disorders.

Mini-Mental State Examination (MMSE) scale is used for assessing the overall cognitive impairment. It is a 30-point questionnaire with simple questions. The Mini-Mental State Examination is scored on a scale of 0–30

Table 4.1: Types of memory disorders.	
Name	*Description*
Amnesia	Pronounced memory loss
Anterograde amnesia	Inability to learn new material acquired after a UMN lesion
Retrograde amnesia	Inability to remember previous learning acquired before the injury
Delirium	Impairments in immediate and STM
Dementia	Broad-based memory impairments and learning

(STM: short-term memory; UMN: upper motor neuron)

> **BOX 4.2:** Interpretation of Mini-Mental State Examination scale.
>
> - Severe cognitive impairment: 0–17
> - Mild cognitive impairment: 18–23
> - No cognitive impairment: 24–30

as shown in **Box 4.2** with scores >24 interpreted as normal cognitive status. A score of 23 and below indicates borderline cognitive impairment.

According to Faber's interpretation of the mental status, examination must take into account the patient's native language, education level, and culture as these factors can affect performance. For detailed cognitive examination, the following are assessed:

- Calculating ability
- Abstract thinking
- Constructional ability

Calculating ability is tested by simple arithmetic calculations or serial seven test (subtracting 7 from 100 consecutively). Abstract thinking is tested by asking interpretation of common proverbs. Constructional ability is assessed by the ability to copy the figures.

Higher order executive functions to be assessed also consist of *volition*, *planning*, *purposive action*, and *effective performance*. They have traditionally been associated with the frontal and prefrontal cortex, but the current view is that they are mediated by reciprocal connections with other cortical and subcortical regions via the dorsolateral prefrontal-subcortical circuit.

Speech

Speech should be assessed for articulation problems (dysarthria), which are seen as speech errors, vocal quality, pitch and volume difficulties in timing. Fluent (Wernicke's) aphasia is evident by smooth speech but full of errors with respect to neologisms (nonsense words), paraphasias (misuse of words), and circumlocutions (word substitution). Non-fluent (Broca's) aphasia is characterized by slow speech with hesitancy, limited vocabulary, and impaired syntax. This is discussed in depth in the chapter "Disorders of Speech."

Perception

Perception is the integration of sensory impressions into information that is psychologically meaningful. It is the ability to:

- Select those stimuli that require attention and action.
- Integrate those stimuli with each other and with prior information.
- Finally interpret them.

It consists of body scheme and body image impairments, spatial relation impairments, agnosia, and apraxia **(Table 4.2)**.

Table 4.2: Perceptual deficits to be tested in neurological assessment.

Body scheme, body image impairments

Unilateral neglect, anosognosia, somatoagnosia, right–left discrimination, finger agnosia

Spatial relation impairments (complex perception)

Figure-ground discrimination, form discrimination, spatial relations, position in space, topographical disorientation, depth and distance perception, vertical disorientation

Agnosia

Visual agnosia, auditory agnosia, tactile agnosia

Apraxia

Ideomotor apraxia, ideational apraxia, buccofacial apraxia

Body Scheme and Body Image Impairments

Following are the body scheme and body image impairments:

1. **Unilateral neglect:** Unilateral neglect is the inability to register and integrate stimuli and perceptions from one side of the body (body neglect) and the environment or hemispace (spatial neglect of the area surrounding one side of the body), which is not due to a sensory loss. This may occur despite intact visual fields, or concomitantly with right or left homonymous hemianopia; however, it is not caused by homonymous hemianopia.
   Lesion area: Inferior–posterior regions of the right parietal lobe.
   Clinical example: Patient may ignore the left half of the body when dressing and forget to put on the left sleeve or left pants leg. Often a male patient will forget to shave the left half of his face. A female patient may neglect to put makeup on the left side of her face or wear accessory on one side of the body.
   Testing: The Behavioral Inattention Test, which consists of nine activity-based subtests and six pen and paper subtests **(Fig. 4.1)**.

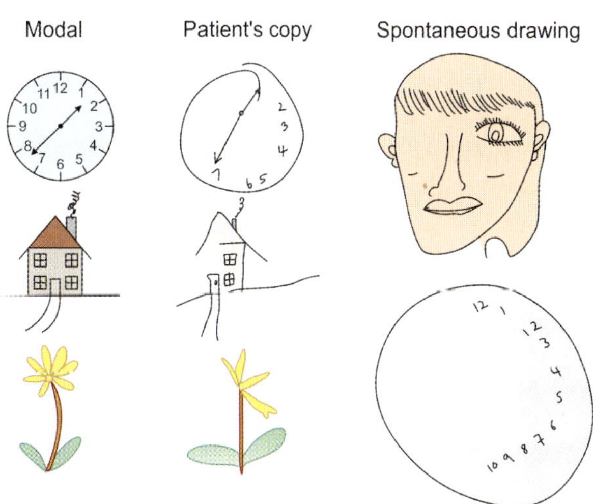

Fig. 4.1: Example of drawing from a patient with left neglect following stroke.

2. **Anosognosia:** Anosognosia is a severe condition, including denial and lack of awareness of the presence or severity of one's paralysis. It is defined as a lack of awareness, or denial, of a paretic extremity as belonging to the person, or a lack of insight concerning, or denial of, paralysis.
   Lesion area: Pathogenesis is slightly unclear, and region of the supramarginal gyrus is mostly involved.
   Clinical example: Patient believes nothing is wrong with them and may disown paralyzed limbs or refuse to accept responsibility. They may describe that limb has its own mind or it was left behind at home.
   Testing: Patient is asked what happened to the arm or leg, whether they are paralyzed, how the limb feels, and why it cannot be moved. A patient with anosognosia may deny the paralysis, say that it is of no concern, and fabricate reasons why a limb does not move the way it should.

3. **Somatoagnosia:** Somatoagnosia, or impairment in body scheme, is a lack of awareness of the body structure and the relationship of body parts to oneself or to others. Somatoagnosia is also referred to as autopagnosia or simply body agnosia.
   Lesion area: Dominant parietal lobe.
   Clinical example: Patient is unable to perceive the relations between body parts and, thus, may have difficulty in performing transfer activities. Commands such as "move your left shoulder toward right hip" or "bring your right hand across the chest and reach the left ear."
   Testing: Patient is asked to point to body parts on themselves, as directed by the therapist, and on a picture of a human figure. Patient may be asked to mimic movements as done by the therapist. Questions relating to relationship between body parts such as "is your leg below your head?" may be posed.

4. **Right-left discrimination:** Inability to identify the right and left sides of one's own body or of that of the examiner is referred to as right–left discrimination. Movements in response to verbal commands comprising right and left terms and imitating movements may be a problem.
   Lesion area: Parietal lobe of either hemisphere.
   Clinical example: Patients with this impairment fail to distinguish right and left arm or leg. They may be unable to discern right and left shoe or follow commands such as "bend your right leg" or "move to the left from the center." They also fail to differentiate the left and right side of the therapist.
   Testing: Patient is asked to point to body parts on command, such as right ear, left foot, and right arm. Six responses are elicited on either the patient's own body, on that of the therapist, or on a model or picture of the human figure. It is important to rule out somatoagnosia by testing the patient first without using the words "right" and "left."

5. **Finger agnosia:** Inability to identify the fingers of one's own hands or of the hands of the examiner is referred to as finger agnosia.
   Lesion area: Lesion is usually located in either parietal lobe, in the region of angular gyrus of the left hemisphere.
   Clinical example: Difficulty in naming fingers on command, mimicking finger movements or identifying which finger was touched.
   Testing: *Sauguet's test*, where the patient is asked to move or point to his or her finger when named by the therapist is generally used, 5–10 commands from the therapist are usually adequate. It is not a standardized tool and consists of the following:
   - Patient is asked to name the fingers touched by the therapist, with the eyes open (EO) (five times) and if successful, with vision occluded (five times).
   - Patient is asked to point to the fingers named by the therapist on the patient's own hands (10 times), on the therapist's hands (10 times), and on a schematic model (10 times).
   - Patient is asked to point to the equivalent finger on a life-sized picture when the therapist touches each finger.
   - Patient is asked to imitate finger movements, e.g., curl the index finger and touch the thumb to the middle finger.

Spatial Relation Impairments (Complex Perception)

The spatial relation impairments include:

1. **Figure-ground discrimination:** Figure-ground discrimination or perception refers to the ability to separate the elements of a visual image on the basis of contrast (e.g., light, dark), to perceive an object (figure) against a background (ground).
   Lesion area: Parieto-occipital lesions of the right hemisphere and less frequently the left hemisphere.
   Clinical example: Patient may be unable to locate objects from a closet or locate buttons on a shirt, or distinguish button holes in a monochrome shirt.
   Testing: Functional-based tests, or Ayres Figure–Ground test can be used.

2. **Form discrimination:** Inability to perceive or attend to subtle differences in form and shape, comprise impairments in form discrimination.
   Lesion area: Parieto-temporooccipital region (posterior association areas) of the non-dominant lobe.
   Clinical example: Patient may fail to distinguish between similar forms such as pen and toothbrush or between a vase with water jug and may get confused between them.
   Testing: A number of items similar in shape and different in size are presented in front of the patient to identify and each is presented several times in a variety of different positions. It is important to distinguish this from visual agnosia.

3. **Spatial relations:** A spatial relation disorder, or spatial disorientation, is the inability to perceive the relationship of one object in space to another object, or to oneself.

   Lesion area: Inferior parietal lobe or parieto-occipital-temporal junction, usually of the right side.

   Clinical example: Patient may find it difficult to set a table for dinner with placing of fork, spoon, plates in appropriate place, or to tell the time from a clock because of difficulty in perceiving the relative positions of the hands.

   Testing: Valid and reliable tests such as Rivermead Perceptual Assessment Battery and the Arnadottir OT-ADL Neurobehavioral Evaluation.

4. **Position in space:** Position in space impairment is the inability to perceive and to interpret spatial concepts such as up, down, under, over, in, out, in front of, and behind.

   Lesion area: Non-dominant parietal lobe.

   Clinical example: Patient finds it difficult when asked to place foot on floor, hand over the table, and back against the wall. They may not know what to do.

   Testing: A toothbrush can be placed in a cup and under a cup, and the patient is then asked to indicate the location of the toothbrush. This can be tested with use of various other instruments or devices.

5. **Topographical disorientation:** Difficulty in understanding and remembering the relationship of one location to another is referred to as topographical disorientation.

   Lesion area: Right retrosplenial cortex, with Brodmann's area 30 or bilateral parietal lesions.

   Clinical example: Difficulty in finding way back home or places which are familiar, and also in describing spatial characteristics of familiar surroundings, such as the layout of their bedroom at their home.

   Testing: Patient is asked to describe or to draw a familiar route, such as the block on which he or she lives, the layout of his or her home, or a major neighborhood intersection.

6. **Depth and distance perception:** Inaccurate judgment of direction, distance, and depth underlies depth and distance perception.

   Lesion area: Posterior right hemisphere in the superior visual association cortices.

   Clinical example: Missing chair while attempting to sit, missing pouring water in glass, or overfilling when it reaches fill.

   Testing: Patient is asked to take or to grasp an object that has been placed on a table for distance perception. Patient can be asked to fill a glass of water for depth perception.

7. **Vertical disorientation:** A distorted perception of what is vertical is referred to as vertical disorientation.

   Lesion area: Non-dominant parietal lobe.

Clinical example: A person with distorted verticality views the world differently and this may affect their upright posture.

Testing: The therapist holds a cane vertically and then turns it sideways to a horizontal plane and asks patient to turn it back to original position. This can be done in a dark room with the aid of a luminous rod handed to patient to reposition in vertical plane.

Agnosias (Simple Perception)

Agnosia is the inability to recognize or make sense of incoming information despite intact sensory capacities. The following types are commonly seen:

1. **Visual agnosia:** Visual object agnosia is the most common form of agnosia. It is defined as the inability to recognize familiar objects despite normal function of the eyes and optic tracts.

   Lesion area: Occipito-temporo-parietal association areas of either hemisphere.

   Clinical example: Inability to find the razor on the sink despite adequate scanning abilities. The razor can only be located by touch.

   Testing: Several common objects are placed in front of the patient, and they are asked to name the objects, to point to an object named by the therapist, or to demonstrate its use.

2. **Auditory agnosia:** Auditory agnosia was defined originally as a selective disorder of sound recognition.

   Lesion area: Dominant temporal lobe.

   Clinical example: Patients may often say "I can hear you, but cannot translate it," or inability to discriminate between verbal and nonverbal sounds, particularly environmental sounds such as dog barking, tree leaves rumbling or door bell, thunder sound.

   Testing: Usually done by speech language therapist, with closed eyes, patient is asked to identify the source of various sounds, either verbally or by pointing on a picture.

3. **Tactile agnosia/astereognosis:** Tactile agnosia, or astereognosis, is the inability to recognize forms by handling them, although tactile, proprioceptive, and thermal sensations may be intact.

   Lesion area: Parieto-temporo-occipital lobe (posterior association areas) of either hemisphere.

   Clinical example: Patient may be unable to identify a familiar object with eyes closed (EC). Difficulty with clothing fasteners despite intact motor function. Inability to recognize objects that are in one's pockets unless vision is also used.

   Testing: Patient is asked to identify objects placed in the hand by examining them manually without visual cues.

Apraxia

Apraxia is characterized by an inability to perform purposeful movements, which cannot be accounted for by inadequate strength, loss of coordination, impaired sensation, attentional difficulties, abnormal tone, movement disorders, intellectual deterioration, poor comprehension, or uncooperativeness. They can be of three types, described as follows:

1. **Ideomotor apraxia:** Ideomotor apraxia refers to a breakdown between concept and performance due to a disconnection between the idea of a movement and its motor execution.

   Lesion area: Left dominant hemisphere.

   Clinical example: Patient may be unable to follow a command such as opening a lock using a key but will do so spontaneously on seeing it. A male patient may be able to identify a comb and its use, but when asked to do so on command, they may fail.

   Testing: Goodglass and Kaplan test for apraxia, composed of universally known movements, such as blowing, brushing teeth, hammering, and shaving, is used. First, the patient is asked, "Show me how you would bang a nail with a hammer." If the patient fails to do this or uses his or her fist as if it were a hammer, the patient is told, "Pretend to hold the hammer." If the patient fails following this instruction, the therapist demonstrates the act and asks the patient to imitate it. The patient with apraxia typically will not improve after demonstration but will improve with use of the actual implements.

2. **Ideational apraxia:** Ideational apraxia is a failure in the conceptualization of the task. It is an inability to perform a purposeful motor act, either automatically or on command, because the patient no longer understands the overall concept of the act, cannot retain the idea of the task, or cannot formulate the motor patterns required.

   Lesion area: Dominant parietal hemisphere.

   Clinical example: Patients may misuse objects, have difficulty matching objects and actions, be unaware of the mechanical advantage afforded by tools, or be unable to judge whether a gesture is well- or ill-formed, such as when presented with toothbrush and toothpaste and asked to brush teeth, they may put toothpaste tube in mouth and may fail to describe the task even when asked to do so verbally.

   Testing: Similar to ideomotor apraxia.

3. **Buccofacial apraxia:** It is characterized by an impairment of skilled movements involving the face, mouth, tongue, larynx, and pharynx on command.

   Lesion area: Due to lesions in the frontal and central opercula, anterior insula, and a small area of the first temporal gyrus (adjacent to the frontal and central opercula).

   Clinical example: Blowing a candle or a kiss, on verbal command, may be difficult for the patient. However, they may be able to do so spontaneously.

   Testing: Usually done by speech language therapist.

CRANIAL NERVE EXAMINATION

It is used to identify any lesion in the cranial nerves by physical examination. It has nine components. Each test is designed to assess the status of one or more of the 12 cranial nerves (I–XII) as described in **Table 4.3.** These components correspond to testing the sense of smell (I), visual fields and acuity (II), eye movements (III, IV, VI) and pupils (III, sympathetic and parasympathetic), sensory function of face (V), strength of facial (VII) and shoulder girdle muscles (XI), hearing (VII, VIII), taste (VII, IX, X), pharyngeal movement and reflex (IX, X), and tongue movements (XII).

Table 4.3: Cranial nerve examination.

Nerves	Function	Test	Possible abnormal findings
I Olfactory nerve	Sense of smell	• Smell is tested in each nostril separately by placing stimuli under one nostril and occluding the opposing nostril • The stimuli used should be nonirritating and identifiable • Some examples of stimuli include cinnamon, cloves, camphor, and eucalyptus	Anosmia (inability to detect smells), seen with frontal lobe lesion
II Optic	Visual fields and acuity	Test visual acuity Central: Snellen eye chart; test each eye separately (covering the other eye); test at a distance of 20 ft	Blindness, myopia (impaired far vision), presbyopia (impaired near vision)
		Test peripheral vision (visual fields) by asking the patient to cover one eye while the examiner tests the opposite eye. The examiner wiggles a finger in each of the four quadrants and asks the patient to state when the finger is seen in the periphery	Field defects: Homonymous Hemianopia

(Contd...)

(Contd...)

Nerves	Function	Test	Possible abnormal findings
II and III Optic and oculomotor	Pupillary reflexes	• Pupillary light reflex is tested by having the patient stare into the distance as the examiner shines the penlight obliquely into each pupil • Pupillary constriction is tested for the examined eye (direct response) and the opposite eye (consensual response)	Absence of pupillary constriction
		• Examine pupillary size/shape	• Anisocoria (unequal pupils) • Horner's syndrome, CN III paralysis
III, IV, and VI Oculomotor, trochlear, and abducens	Extraocular Movements	Tested by standing 1 m in front of the patient and asking the patient to follow a target with eyes only, and not the head (patient is asked to look in each direction) and pursuit eye movements (patient follows moving finger)	• Strabismus (eye deviates from normal conjugate position) • Impaired eye movements • Double vision
III Oculomotor	• Medial, superior, and inferior rectus • Inferior oblique: turns eye up, down, and in • Elevates eyelid	• Observe position of eye • Test eye movements	• Strabismus: eye pulled outward by CN VI • Eye cannot look upward, downward, and inward movements • May see ptosis, pupillary dilation
IV Trochlear	Superior oblique: turns eye down when adducted	Test eye movements	• Cannot look down when eye is adducted
VI Abducens	Lateral rectus: turns eye out	• Observe position of eye • Test eye movements	• Esotropia (eye pulled inward) • Eye cannot look out
V Trigeminal Ophthalmic maxillary mandibular divisions	Sensory: face	• Light touch is tested in each of the three divisions of the trigeminal nerve and on each side of the face using a cotton wisp or tissue paper • The ophthalmic division is tested by touching the forehead, the maxillary division is tested by touching the cheeks, and the mandibular division is tested by touching the chin • For pain and temperature repeat the same steps as light touch but use a sharp object and a cold tuning fork, respectively	• Loss of facial sensations, numbness with CN V lesion • Trigger area with trigeminal neuralgia
	Sensory: cornea	• Test corneal reflex: touch lightly with wisp of cotton	• Loss of corneal reflex ipsilaterally (blinking in response to corneal touch)
	Motor: muscles of mastication	• Palpate temporal and masseter muscles • Observe spontaneous movements • Have patient clench teeth, hold against resistance	Weakness, wasting of muscles when opened, deviation of jaw to ipsilateral side

VII Facial	Facial expression	• Test motor function of facial muscles
		• Raise eyebrows, frown
		• Show teeth, smile
		• Close eyes tightly
		• Puff out both cheeks
			• Paralysis:
			  – Inability to close eye
			  – Drooping corner of mouth
			  – Difficulty with speech articulation
			• Unilateral LMN: Bell's palsy (PNI)
			• Bilateral LMN: Guillain-Barré syndrome
			• Unilateral UMN: stroke

(Contd...)

(Contd...)

Nerves	Function	Test	Possible abnormal findings
	Sensory: taste to anterior two-thirds of tongue	Apply saline solution and sugar solution using a cotton swab	Incorrectly identifies solution
VIII Vestibulocochlear (acoustic)	Vestibular function	Test balance: VSR Test eye–head coordination: VOR	Vertigo, dysequilibrium Gaze instability with head rotations, nystagmus (constant, involuntary cyclical movement of the eyeball)
	Cochlear function	• Test auditory acuity • Test for lateralization (Weber test): place vibrating tuning fork on top of head, midposition; check if sound heard in one ear, or equally in both • Compare air and bone • conduction (Rinne test): place • Vibrating tuning fork on mastoid bone, then close to ear canal; sound heard longer through air than bone	Deafness, impaired hearing, and tinnitus Unilateral conductive loss: sound lateralized to impaired ear Sensorineural loss: sound heard in good ear Conductive loss: sound heard through bone is equal to or longer than air Sensorineural loss: sound heard longer through air
IX Glossopharyngeal	Sensory to posterior one-third of tongue, pharynx, and middle ear	• Apply saline solution and sugar solution to the tongue • Not typically tested	Incorrectly identifies solution
IX, X Glossopharyngeal and vagus	Phonation	Listen to voice quality	Dysphonia: hoarseness denotes vocal cord weakness: nasal quality denotes palatal weakness
	Swallowing	Examine for difficulty in swallowing glass of water	Dysphagia
	Palatal pharynx control	Have patient say ~AH~- observe motion of soft palate (elevates) and position of uvula (remains midline)	Paralysis: Palate fails to elevate (lesion of CN X); asymmetrical elevation with unilateral paralysis
	Gag reflex	Stimulate back of throat lightly on each side	Absent reflex: lesion of CN IX possibly CN X
XI Spinal accessory	Motor function	Examine bulk, strength	• LMN: Atrophy, fasciculations, ipsilateral weakness
	Trapezius muscle	Shrug both shoulders upward against resistance	• Inability to shrug ipsilateral shoulder, shoulder droops
	Sternocleidomastoid	Turn head to each side against resistance	• Inability to turn head to opposite side • UMN lesion: weakness of ipsilateral sternocleidomastoid and contralateral trapezius
XII Hypoglossal	Tongue movements	Listen to patient's articulation Examine resting position of tongue Examine tongue movement: ask patient to protrude tongue, move side to side	• Dysarthria (seen with lesions of CN X or CN XII also V, VII) • Atrophy or fasciculations of tongue (LMN, ALS) • Impaired movements • Deviation to weak side • UMN lesion: tongue deviates away from side of cortical lesion

(LMN: lower motor neuron; UMN: upper motor neuron; VOR: vestibular ocular reflex; VSR: vestibulospinal reflex; CN: cranial nerve; ALS: amyotrophic lateral sclerosis; PNI: peripheral nerve injury)

SENSORY ASSESSMENT

Sensory assessment is the subjective assessment in which cooperation, alertness, and understanding of the patient are the most important factors.

- Hence, the patient needs to be prepared before testing the sensations.
- A full explanation of the purpose of testing should be given to the patient in the language they understand.
- Patient should be informed that they should not guess in case if they are not certain about the response.
- Patient should be in a comfortable position during the testing.
- Proper demonstration should be given about the entire process of testing before the actual administration of test. While demonstrating, the vision should not be occluded, whereas during the actual testing the patient is asked to keep their EC or a fabric blindfold is used. A small screen can also be placed in between the eyes and the part where testing is done. Patient may become uncomfortable if they are blindfolded for a long time. So the patient should be enquired about their well-being from time to time.
- The environment should be quiet and well lighted.

Sensations are checked in the order of superficial, then deep and then cortical. In case the superficial sensations are affected, some deep and cortical sensations cannot be examined. For example, if superficial touch sensation is affected, graphesthesia cannot be checked over the same area. In a way it can be said that the superficial sensations are primitive in nature. The stimuli should be applied in a random, unpredictable manner. Patient should not be able to guess the location of next stimulus. Patient needs to reply verbally to the stimulus provided. In case a patient is having speech affection, hand or neck gesture can be used. Patient should be trained for this before beginning the actual testing. Skin area with scar, callused area, or rough thick skin may have greater threshold. Instruments used for one patient should be cleaned thoroughly before using it for the next patient to prevent transmission of pathogens. For the very same reason, hands should be washed appropriately.

Thorough knowledge of sensory supply and structures responsible for it is necessary for proper interpretation and possible differential diagnosis. Sensory testing may begin from distal to proximal area. Segment with sensory deficit must be checked in detail so as to ascertain the boundaries of sensory deficit. This will help to localize the lesion. A skin pencil may be used with permission of the patient to draw the exact location and extent of sensory loss. Dermatome diagram can be used to mark the area of affection (**Fig. 4.2** and **Box 4.3**).

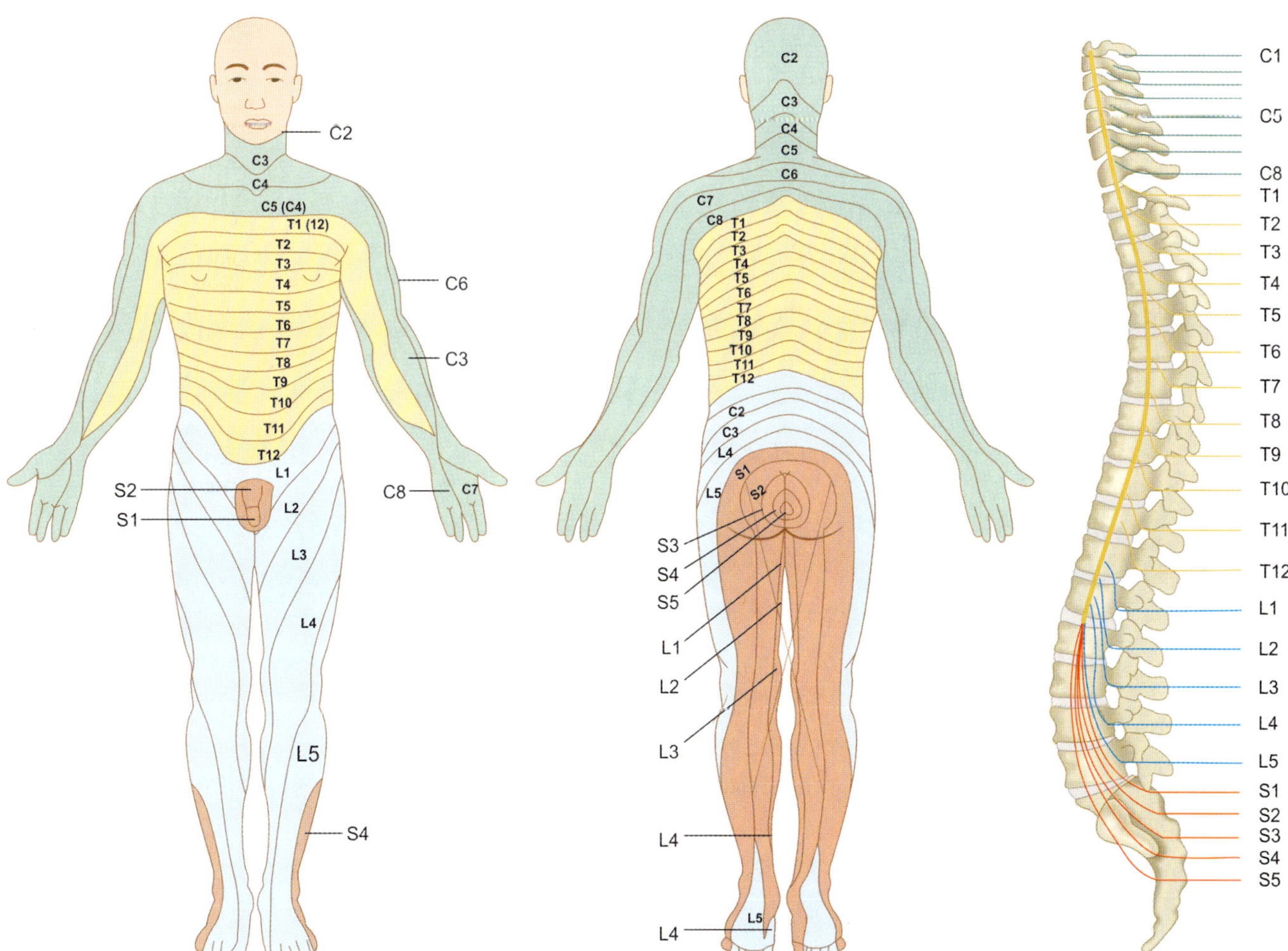

Fig. 4.2: Body chart for dermatomal distribution.

> **BOX 4.3:** A grading scale can be used to note the extent of affection for each deficit area.
>
> - 0 stands for absent
> - 1 indicates impaired
> - 2 indicates normal
> - NT indicates not testable

Superficial Sensations

There are four types of superficial sensations—pain, temperature, touch, and pressure. Eyes should be closed while checking the sensations.

Pain Perception (Sharp/Dull Discrimination)

Pain perception involves the following:

- The sharp and dull ends of the large headed safety pin are randomly applied perpendicular to the skin.
- Care should be to taken to avoid overlapping of the stimuli by successive application at the same area or too close to each other.
- Pressure applied at each area should be similar.
- Patient should immediately verbally reply "sharp" or "dull" when the stimulus is applied or may use gesture in the case of speech affection.

Temperature Awareness

Temperature awareness includes the below:

- It is the ability to distinguish between warm and cool stimuli.
- It is assessed with two test tubes filled with warm water and other is filled with crushed ice. Ideal temperature for cold sensation testing is 5–10°C and for warm sensation testing is 40–45°C. Side of the test tube is kept in contact with the skin rather than only the distal ends.
- Care should be taken not to tilt the tube excessively to avoid spillage.
- Tubes should be applied randomly over different parts in order to avoid guessing by the patient.
- Temperature in the tubes should not exceed the prescribed limit as it would create a pain sensation.
- The patient should reply "hot" or "cold" in response to the application of the said test tube.

Touch Sensation

Touch sensation is checked as below:

- For this, the area to be tested is lightly touched or stroked with piece of cotton or camel hair brush. While stroking, it should not create a tickling sensation.
- It should be applied randomly over different areas but therapist should be cautious to cover all the dermatomes or all areas of peripheral nerve supply.
- The patient is asked to respond "yes" or "no" when the stimulus is applied.

Pressure Sensation

Below are the techniques used for pressure sensation:

- In this, a firm pressure is applied on the patient's body part with the help of therapist's fingertip. Pressure should be enough to indent the skin so that the receptors are stimulated.
- It should not cause discomfort to the patient.
- Similar care as that of touch sensation should be taken during the administration of test.

Deep Sensations

It includes kinesthesia, proprioception, and vibration.

Kinesthesia

Kinesthesia includes the below:

- In this test, the extremity or joints are moved through a small range of movement.
- Care should be taken so that the excessive pressure is not applied during movement, which will help the patient to guess the direction of movement.
- A field test or trial run should be conducted prior to actual test. Therapist should explain to the patient the direction of movement in their local language so that they are able to respond appropriately. During the test, patient should respond verbally the direction of movement while the extremity is in motion. The patient may also respond by simultaneously duplicating the movement on the other side. When moving the limb, it should be held in such a way so as not to provide direction of movement, e g., the toe or thumb should be held on either side and moved into flexion or extension.

Proprioception Awareness

Proprioception awareness is tested as described below:

- This test is related to joint position and awareness of joints at rest.
- The joint is moved through a range and held in a static position.
- Care should be taken that there is no pain or discomfort caused to the patient during movement. In the case of flaccidity, the joint should be moved with extra care, avoiding any jerk especially toward the end of range of movement.
- Hand pressure or grip should be gentle, which does not cause discomfort or does not provide clue to the position.
- Patient should respond verbally the exact position of joint or replicate the positioning done by the therapist on the other side.

Vibration Perception

Vibration perception is checked as below:

- With a tuning fork of 128 Hz, the tines are hit against the palm and the base of fork is placed on the superficial bony prominences such as mastoid process, olecranon process, radial styloid process, and lateral malleolus.
- Before actual testing, a trial run over relatively non-affected area should be given to the patient so that they understand the vibration sensation to be felt during the testing.
- Patient's eyes are closed during the test.
- Vibrating and non-vibrating stimuli should be given randomly so that there is less guess work by the patient.

- Patient is asked to respond verbally regarding the sensation felt or they may indicate by predefined body gesture.

Combined Cortical Sensations

Superficial sensations must be intact for testing the cortical sensations. In the absence of superficial sensation, cortical sensations cannot be tested and this should be documented.

Tactile Localization

Tactile localization test is done as shown below:
- In this test, the stimulus is applied in the form of gentle touch to the specific area of the body with the help of a cotton, wool, or therapist's finger.
- Patient is asked to respond by localizing the area where they felt the stimulus. They may actually show area with their hands or may describe the area such as outer side, below the knee joint.
- Random application of the stimulus should avoid guessing by the patient.

Two-point Discrimination

Two-point discrimination includes the following:
- In this test, two sharp stimuli are applied at the same time at some definite distance from each other with EC.
- Patient is asked to respond whether they are feeling one or two stimuli. If the patient answers as two stimuli, the distance is reduced till patient feels only one stimulus. The distance at which they had felt two stimuli is noted.
- An aesthesiometer or two pens can be used for this test **(Fig. 4.3)**. However, when using pens for the test, care should be taken to apply similar pressure with both pens.
- It is important to note that different body areas have different normal values of two-point discrimination, with the distance being least at tip of fingers and maximum in the back.

Double Simultaneous Stimulation

Double simultaneous stimulation is described as:
- The ability to perceive simultaneous touch stimuli is referred to as double simultaneous stimulation (DSS). With equal pressure, the therapist at the same time touches:
  - Identical locations on opposite sides of the body
  - Proximally and distally on the opposite sides of the body
  - Proximal and distal locations on the same side of the body
- The patient states when they perceive a stimuli and the number of stimuli they perceive, verbally.
- DSS is a method of testing afferent visual, somatosensory, and auditory pathways for signs of unilateral brain damage. A patient with unilateral damage will typically detect a single stimulation on the contralateral side but identify only ipsilateral stimulation during bilateral simultaneous stimulation. This tendency to suppress (or neglect) the contralateral stimulation is also referred to as "extinction." While unilateral damage may result in decreased or weakened registration of single, contralateral stimuli, these contralateral stimuli are not detected when in competition with stronger, ipsilateral stimuli.

Stereognosis

Stereognosis is described as follows:
- It is the ability to identify the object placed in the hand with EC.
- Two or three small easily identifiable objects are used for this test. These objects are shown to the patient first to confirm that the patient knows the names of these objects. Then each object is placed one by one in either hand of patient with their EC, they are allowed to handle the object and then they are asked to name the object.

Graphesthesia

Graphesthesia is described as follows:
- It is the ability to identify the shape or numbers written on the skin.
- In this test, some familiar shapes, alphabets, or numbers are written on the skin. A demonstration in the form of these shapes on a sheet of paper should be done prior to actual testing so that patient is aware about the tracing to be done on their body.
- Patient is asked to close their eyes and these drawings are traced on patient's body preferably on the palm region by the therapist's fingers. Patient is asked to identify the exact tracing done on their body. A brief time is allowed for them to respond and once they answer it then the next tracing is done.
- Tracing should not be done in quick succession otherwise it will confuse the patient. Also care should be taken that tickling sensation is not felt by the patient.

Barognosis

Barognosis is described as follows:
- It is the ability of an individual to differentiate between two similar objects based on their weights.
- In this test, two similar objects are placed in the hands with EC. The patient needs to identify which one of the

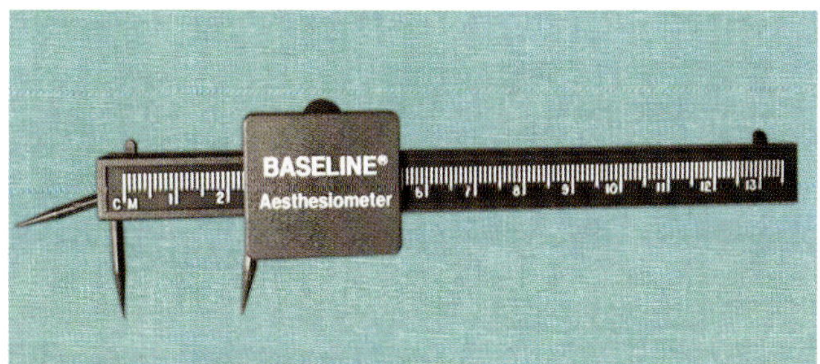

Fig. 4.3: Aesthesiometer for testing two-point discrimination.

> **BOX 4.4:** Special instruments to assess sensations.
>
> - TSA-II Thermal Sensory Analyzer+VSA3000 (Medoc, Ltd., Durham, NC)
> - von Frey Aesthesiometer (Somedic Sales AB, Hörby, Sweden)
> - Touch-Test Sensory Evaluator (North Coast Medical, Inc., Morgan Hill, CA)
> - Rydel-Seiffer 64/128 Hz Graduated Tuning Fork (US Neurologicals, Kirkland, WA)
> - Rolltemp (Somedic Sales AB, Hörby, Sweden)
> - Bio-thesiometer (Bio-Medical Instrument Co, Newbury, OH)
> - Vibrameter (Somedic Sales AB, Hörby, Sweden)
> - SENSEBox (Somedic Sales AB, Hörby, Sweden)
> - MSA (Modular Sensory Analyzer) thermotest

two is heavier or lighter. Patient may manipulate the object with their hands so as to judge the weight. So it is necessary that both objects are of similar shape.

Recognition of Texture

Recognition of texture is described as follows:

- It is the ability to identify different textures applied on patient's body. These textures include soft, smooth, coarse, and hard.
- They are applied randomly on various parts of the body and the patient is asked to identify the texture.

Apart from the traditional ways to test sensations, specialized testing systems and instruments have now become available with the advent of various technological advancements **(Box 4.4)**.

MOTOR EXAMINATION

It starts with examination of tone followed by range of motion (ROM) and manual muscle testing. Reflex integrity, muscle performance, strength, power, and endurance are also important components in motor function assessment.

Tone

Tone is defined as a state of preparedness of a muscle for contraction. It is also defined as resistance of muscle to passive elongation or stretch when an individual attempts to maintain muscle relaxation. There are various factors that may affect the tone such as:

- Position of body
- Interaction of neck reflexes
- Voluntary effort
- Stress
- Febrile state
- Pain
- Medical status
- Medication
- Central nervous system (CNS) arousal
- Degree of volitional movement

There are three types of tonal abnormalities:

1. Hypertonia (increase in tone)
2. Hypotonia (decrease in tone)
3. Dystonia (impaired or disordered tone)

- **Hypertonia** is of two types, i.e., **spasticity** and rigidity.
  - Spasticity is seen in patients with injury to pyramidal tracts or upper motor neuron (UMN) lesion. It is typically characterized by velocity-dependent resistance to passive stretch to a muscle. With the increase in velocity of passive movement, resistance felt by therapist also increases. At times, initial high resistance is followed by a sudden inhibition or relaxation, i.e., letting go of the limb. This is termed **clasp-knife** response. Chronic spasticity is sometimes associated with clonus. It is checked by giving a sudden stretch to a spastic muscle. In response, there is cyclical, spasmodic alteration of muscular contraction and relaxation of the stretched spastic muscle. It is commonly seen in plantar flexors but can also be seen in wrist joint flexors.
  - **Rigidity** is seen in patients with basal ganglia lesion, typically associated with Parkinson's disease. Resistance felt is independent of the velocity of passive movement. When resistance is felt throughout the ROM, it is called **lead pipe** rigidity, whereas when ratchet-like jerkiness is felt during parts of the passive movement, it is called **cogwheel** rigidity. There is increased tone in flexors and extensors. Tremors can also be seen along with rigidity. It is usually seen in upper extremity movements.
- **Hypotonia** or flaccidity occurs when resistance to the passive movement is reduced or absent. It is caused due to lower motor neuron (LMN) lesion. In patients with cerebellar lesion, mild reduction in tone is seen. Also in the acute stages of spinal cord injury or cerebral dysfunction such as spinal shock and cerebral shock, respectively, muscles lose their tone. Muscles feel flabby to touch and the extremity becomes floppy.
- **Dystonia** is a disordered tonal abnormality, a type of hyperkinetic disorder, which is associated with involuntary movements involving large portions of the body. It is seen in lesions of basal ganglia or it may sometimes be inherited. It may be restricted to one part of the body as in the case of torticollis or it may involve more than one segment, i.e., dystonic posturing or movements of the entire upper limb.
  - **Decorticate and decerebrate rigidity**: Sustained contraction and posturing of the upper limbs in flexion and lower limbs in extension is seen in decorticate rigidity. Lesion of corticospinal tract at the level of diencephalon causes this **decorticate rigidity**. On the other hand, sustained contraction and posturing of trunk and both upper and lower limbs in extension is called **decerebrate rigidity**. Lesion of corticospinal tracts and brainstem

between the superior colliculus and vestibular nucleus causes decerebrate rigidity. **Opisthotonus** is a rigid hyperextended position due to strong and sustained contraction of neck and trunk muscles.

Tone Assessment

Tone assessment can be done by observation, passive motion testing, and active motion testing.

- **Initial observation:** Patient's limbs should be carefully observed for the presence of any specific posturing. In the case of low tone or flaccidity, lower limbs are usually seen in externally rotated position with foot in plantarflexed position. Muscles appear to be flabby and soft. In the case of hypertonicity, muscles appear to be stiff and the extremities are in extended position. However, palpation should be done to confirm the findings.
- **Passive motion testing:** This is the most ideal way of checking the tone of muscles. In this, resistance to the passive stretch to a muscle is assessed. Patient should be fully relaxed and should not hold the joint voluntarily. Patient should be instructed to let therapist know about any pain or discomfort during the movement. Therapist should keep a watch on patient's face to note any signs of pain and discomfort. Testing should not be done in a painful range as patient may hold the extremity so as to guard against the pain. The extremity should be held properly and supported adequately so that any mishap can be avoided. In the case of normal tone, the limb can be moved easily in the direction desired. Sometimes patients are not able to relax during the testing and false resistance may be felt. In this case, patient's attention is diverted from the testing, which may allow the muscles to relax. Jendrassik maneuver can be used in which the patient clenches the teeth, flexes both sets of fingers into a hook-like form, and interlocks those set of fingers together. In case the resistance is felt during the movement, increasing the velocity of passive movement will help to determine the presence of spasticity. If the resistance increases with increasing velocity, then it indicates spasticity. If the resistance remains the same, it probably indicates tightness or rigidity of a muscle. While testing comparison should be made between right and left extremities, upper and lower extremity, affected and unaffected side. Preferably the testing should be done in one position as change of position may alter the tone of muscles (postural tone). Care should be taken to test muscles in the same position during reassessment. Tone can be graded on 0–4+ scale as shown in **Box 4.5**.

Once it is established that there is spasticity in muscles, it can be further graded with the gold standard scale, i.e., Modified Ashworth Scale. It is a subjective 5-point ordinal scale as shown in **Box 4.6**.

Modified Tardieu Scale (MTS): It considers R2, R1, and R2–R1 to measure spasticity. The R2 is the passive ROM

<table><tr><td colspan="2">BOX 4.5: Grading of tone.</td></tr><tr><td colspan="2">0 – stands for no response
1+ – indicates decreased muscle tone
2+ – indicates normal tone
3+ – indicates exaggerated response (hypertonia)
4+ – indicates sustained response (severe hypertonia)</td></tr></table>

<table><tr><td colspan="2">BOX 4.6: Modified Ashworth scale for grading spasticity.</td></tr><tr><td>0 –</td><td>indicates no increase in muscle tone.</td></tr><tr><td>1 –</td><td>indicates slight increase in muscle tone, manifested by a catch and release or by minimal resistance at the end of range of motion (ROM).</td></tr><tr><td>1+ –</td><td>shows slight increase in muscle tone manifested by a catch, followed by minimal resistance throughout the remainder (less than half) of the ROM.</td></tr><tr><td>2 –</td><td>shows more marked increase in tone through most of the ROM, but affected part easily moved.</td></tr><tr><td>3 –</td><td>indicates considerable increase in muscle tone, passive movement is difficult.</td></tr><tr><td>4 –</td><td>indicates affected part rigid in flexion or extension.</td></tr></table>

<table><tr><td colspan="2">BOX 4.7: Modified Tardieu scale.</td></tr><tr><td>0 –</td><td>shows no resistance throughout passive movement.</td></tr><tr><td>1 –</td><td>indicates slight resistance throughout, with no clear catch at a precise angle.</td></tr><tr><td>2 –</td><td>indicates clear catch at a precise angle followed by release.</td></tr><tr><td>3</td><td>shows fatigable clonus (<10 seconds) occurring at a precise angle.</td></tr><tr><td>4 –</td><td>shows unfatigable clonus (>10 seconds) occurring at a precise angle.</td></tr></table>

(PROM) measured during slow passive stretch. The R1 is the angle of muscle reaction measured during fast passive stretch and occurs in a particular angle of "catch" from hyperactive stretch reflex. Large and small differences between R2 and R1 indicate spasticity and muscle contracture, respectively. Quality of muscle reaction during fast passive stretch is also graded based on 0–4 scores and is defined as the MTS scores shown in **Box 4.7**.

Active motion testing: Another way of testing tone is with "pendulum test." With knees flexed at the end of table, patient's knee is fully extended and then it allowed to drop gently so that it swings. Normally, the leg swings for several oscillations, whereas hypertonic leg is resistant to the swing and will quickly return to the resting position.

Reflex Integrity

Deep tendon reflexes: The deep tendon reflex (DTR) results from stimulation of the stretch-sensitive IA afferents of the neuromuscular spindle producing muscle contraction via a monosynaptic pathway. DTRs are tested by tapping sharply (but not painfully) over the muscle tendon with a standard reflex hammer or with the tips of the therapist's fingers. Patient is instructed to relax, and

<table>
<tr><td colspan="2" style="text-align:center">BOX 4.8: Grades of deep tendon reflex testing.</td></tr>
<tr><td>0 –</td><td>indicates absent, no response.</td></tr>
<tr><td>1+ –</td><td>indicates slight reflex, present but depressed, low normal.</td></tr>
<tr><td>2+ –</td><td>indicates normal, typical reflex.</td></tr>
<tr><td>3+ –</td><td>indicates brisk reflex, possibly but not necessarily abnormal.</td></tr>
<tr><td>4+ –</td><td>indicates very brisk reflex, abnormal, clonus.</td></tr>
</table>

muscle is placed in midrange to elicit an appropriate response. Reflexes are graded on a 0 to 4+ scale **(Box 4.8)**. An abnormally brisk reflex grade of 4 occurs when repetitive muscle contractions persist while the tendon is being stretched. This is called *clonus* and is best demonstrated at Achilles tendon.

DTRs are increased in UMN syndrome (*hyperreflexia*) and decreased in LMN syndromes (*hyporeflexia*). Valid test results are obtained when the patient is relaxed and not thinking about what the therapist is doing. *Jendrassik maneuver* can be used in which the patient clenches the teeth, flexes both sets of fingers into a hook-like form, and interlocks those set of fingers together. Routinely tested DTRs in clinical practice are described in **Table 4.4.**

Superficial cutaneous reflexes: Most superficial reflexes are cutaneous, provoked by tactile stimuli to a localized area of skin. An exception to this is, pupillary light reflex, which is cranial nerve mediated superficial reflex and involves stimulation with shining light into the pupil of the eye. Other cutaneous reflexes do not involve cranial nerves and may be diminished or absent due to an interrupted reflex arc at LMN level or from UMN lesion. Abdominal and plantar reflex are the commonly tested superficial reflexes listed in **Table 4.5.**

Pathological reflexes

Babinski sign: An abnormal response (positive Babinski sign) consists of extension dorsiflexion (upgoing) of the big toe, with fanning of the lateral four toes. It is indicative of a corticospinal (UMN) lesion.

Chaddock's sign: Chaddock's reflex (or sign) is elicited by stroking around the lateral ankle and up the lateral dorsal aspect of the foot. It also produces extension dorsiflexion of the big toe and is considered a confirmatory toe sign.

Documenting Reflex Integrity

Reflex integrity is evaluated according to:
- Amount (i.e., size, magnitude) of motor response
- Latency (i.e., time taken to elicit) of motor response.

Documentation of reflex abnormalities should also include:
- What specific reflexes were tested?
- The degree of abnormality observed?
- Associated signs (e.g., UMN syndrome)
- Factors that modify reflexes (such as emotion).

Primitive and Tonic Reflexes

In the case of pediatric patients, it is necessary to check any abnormal persistence of primitive reflexes beyond a specific age. **Tables 4.6** and **4.7** show the composite list of reflexes that should be examined.

Table 4.4: Examination of deep tendon reflexes.		
Reflex	*Stimulus*	*Response*
Biceps (C5, C6)	Support the forearm in therapist's forearm. Therapist places the thumb on the biceps tendon, and taps on it to stimulate a response	Slight contraction of elbow flexors
Brachioradialis (C5, C6)	Therapist holds the patient's thumb to relax the forearm. Tapping on the forearm, 2–3 cm above the radial styloid process	Forearm flexes and supinates slightly
Triceps (C7–C8)	Shoulder abducted, elbow flexed 90°, supporting the upper arm, the therapist palpates the triceps tendon and taps on it	Slight contraction of elbow extensors
Finger flexors (C6–T1)	Holding the hand in neutral position, and placing finger across palmar surface of distal phalanges of four fingers, therapist taps	Slight contraction of finger flexors
Quadriceps (L2–L4)	High sitting position, allowing leg to suspend freely, tapping below the knee cap	Slight contraction of knee extensors
Achilles (S1–S2)	In prone, knee flexed, hip externally rotated, foot is dorsiflexed and Achilles tendon is tapped above calcaneal insertion	Slight contraction of plantarflexors
Jaw jerks (CN 5)	Sitting, jaw relaxed and slightly open, therapist places finger on chin, taps downward in jaw opening direction	Jaw rebounds and closes

Table 4.5: Examination of superficial cutaneous reflexes.		
Reflex	*Stimulus*	*Response*
Plantar (S1, S2)	With blunt object, stroke the lateral aspect of the sole, moving from the heel to the ball of the foot, curving medially across the ball of the foot	Flexion (plantarflexion) of the great toe, and sometimes the other toes
Abdominal (T8–T12)	In supine, relaxed position, brisk, light strokes are made over each quadrant of the abdominals from the periphery to the umbilicus	Localized contraction under the stimulus, causing the umbilicus to move toward the stimulus

Table 4.6: Primitive reflexes (spinal level).

Reflex	Stimulus	Response
Flexor withdrawal	Noxious stimulus (pinprick) to sole of foot. Tested in supine or sitting position	Toes extend, foot dorsiflexes, entire LE flexes uncontrollably Onset: 28 weeks of gestation Integrated: 1–2 months
Crossed extension	Noxious stimulus to ball of foot of LE fixed in extension; tested in supine position	Opposite LE flexes, then adducts and extends Onset: 28 weeks of gestation Integrated: 1–2 months
Traction	Grasp forearm and pull up from supine into sitting position	Grasp and total flexion of the UE Onset: 28 weeks of gestation Integrated: 2–5 months
Moro	Sudden change in position of head in relation to trunk; drop patient backward from sitting position	Extension, abduction of UEs, hand opening, and crying followed by flexion, adduction of arms across chest Onset: 28 weeks of gestation Integrated: 5–6 months
Startle	Sudden loud or harsh noise	Sudden extension or abduction of UEs, crying Onset: birth Integrated: persists
Grasp	Maintained pressure to palm of hand (palmar grasp) or to ball of foot under toes (plantar grasp)	Maintained flexion of fingers or toes Onset: palmar, birth; plantar, 28 weeks of gestation Integrated: palmer, 4–6 months; plantar, 9 months

(LE: lower extremity; UE: upper extremity)

Table 4.7: Tonic/brainstem reflexes.

Reflex	Stimulus	Response
ATNR	Rotation of head to one side	Flexion of skull limbs, extension of jaw limbs, "bow and arrow" or "fencing" posture Onset: Birth Integration: 4–6 months
STNR	Flexion or extension of head	With head flexion: flexion of UEs, extension of LEs, with head extension: extension of UEs, flexion of LEs Onset: 4–6 months Integration: 8–12 months
TLR or STLR	Prone or supine position	With prone position: increased flexor tone, flexion of all limbs; with supine position: increased extensor tone or extension of all limbs Onset: birth Integration: 6 months
Positive supporting	Contact to the ball of the foot in upright standing position	Rigid extension (co-contraction) of LEs Onset: birth Integration: 6 months
Associated reactions	Resisted voluntary movement in any part of the body	Involuntary movement of the resting extremity Onset: birth–3 months Integration: 8–9 years

(ATNR: asymmetrical tonic neck reflex; STNR: symmetrical tonic neck reflex; TLR or STLR: symmetrical tonic labyrinthine reflex; LE: lower extremity; UE: upper extremity)

Range of Motion

The features of ROM are as follows:

- ROM can be tested by performing active and passive joint motions.
- PROM is performed by the therapist without the assistance of the patient.
- Universal goniometers are used for this examination, and joint mobility is assessed which can be hypomobility or hypermobility. In neurological assessment, PROM precedes active ROM (AROM) testing, since voluntary control gradation is a prerequisite for AROM testing, especially in UMN lesions. On the other hand, in LMN lesions, AROM testing may serve as a useful means of assessing and comparing joint mobility on both sides.
- Contractures, tightness, and deformities are noted with ROM test and also, variations in quality and pattern of joint motion to identify the underlying etiology may enable effective treatment.
- However, it is important to note that ROM is an effective screening procedure, and the presence of positive

findings may also require a variety of additional tests for musculoskeletal structures.

Muscle Performance

Muscle performance differs from muscle strength, power and endurance as follows:

- Muscle performance is "the capacity of a muscle or a group of muscles to generate forces."
- Muscle strength is "the muscle force exerted by a muscle or a group of muscles to overcome a resistance under a specific set of circumstances."
- Muscle power is "work produced per unit of time or the product of strength and speed."
- Muscle endurance is "the ability to sustain forces repeatedly or to generate forces over a period of time."

Examination of Muscle Strength, Power, and Endurance

Standardized methods and protocols are required for testing of muscle strength such as manual muscle testing, and use of advanced tools such as:

- Handheld dynamometers
- Isokinetic systems
- Use of EMG instrumentation in the form of analysis of muscle timing, including amplitude, duration, waveform, and frequency.

Manual muscle testing: Strength of the muscles should be checked according to the principles of manual muscle testing as described by Kendall. Muscles should be graded according to the 0–5 grading system as shown in **Box 4.9**.

- The patient should be positioned in such a way that the proximal part of the joint over which the muscle acts is completely supported and the distal part is free to move.
- The desired action of the muscle should be in the antigravity position.
- Patient should be instructed to perform as much movement as possible with minimal effort and should not hold the breath to gain the desired action.
- The muscles should be tested in a definite sequence but there should not be too much frequent change in the position of the patient, which otherwise might lead to fatigue and thereby uncooperation. For example, with the patient in supine lying position, shoulder flexors can be checked for grade 3, abductors for grade 2, elbow flexors for grade 3, hip abductors for grade 2,

0 – stands for no contraction.
1 – indicates flicker contraction.
2 – indicates movement in gravity-eliminated position.
3 – indicates ability to hold test position against gravity.
4 – indicates ability to hold position against gravity with minimal resistance.
5 – indicates ability to hold test position against gravity with maximal resistance.

- Good indicates normal.
- Fair indicates around half the range of motion or minimal movement.
- Poor indicates flicker of contraction.
- Absent indicates no muscle contraction.

hip flexors for grade 3, and so on. Similarly, different muscle groups can be checked in both side lying position and prone lying position, in patients with extensive neurological affection, such as quadriplegic patients it may not be possible to assess the strength of all muscles at one time; hence, it can be checked in one or two more sittings.

- In some cases, the standard position for testing particular muscle strength cannot be assumed by the patient. In such a case, an alternate position can be given and it should be documented accordingly. If there is any substitution by other muscles or there is a presence of trick movement, it should also be noted and documented for further use. Facial muscles can be graded according to functional grades as shown in **Box 4.10**.

Fatigue

Following are the features of fatigue:

- Fatigue is a sustained sense of exhaustion and decreased capacity for physical and mental work at the usual level.
- Fatigue can result from either excessive activity caused by an accumulation of metabolic waste products (e.g. lactic acid); malnutrition (i.e. deficiency of nutrients); cardiorespiratory disturbances (i.e. inadequate oxygen and nutrients to the tissues); emotional stress; and other factors.
- Fatigue is usually protective and guards against overwork and injury, but in some conditions such as post-polio syndrome or chronic fatigue syndrome, it is a serious problem, since it can cause significant restrictions in their functional activities and work.

Assessment of fatigue begins with the initial interview, where the patient is asked to identify those activities that are fatiguing, the frequency and severity of fatigue episodes, and the circumstances causing the onset of fatigue. It is important to identify the fatigue threshold, defined as "that level of exercise that cannot be sustained indefinitely." Assessment of fatigue can be done using self-reported questionnaires such as Fatigue Severity Scale, or performance-based measures such as Borg Scale for Rating of Perceived Exertion.

Voluntary Control

Voluntary control can be described as follows:

- **Synergies** occur due to functionally linked muscles that are controlled by the CNS to act together to produce a desired motor action.

- **Degree of freedom** refers to the number of separate independent dimensions of movement that must be controlled by engaging these cooperative units of muscle action.
- In individuals with normal motor control, voluntary movement patterns are functional, task specific, highly variable and timed, depending on the task purpose and environment.
- The CNS controls patterns of single limb and multiple limb movements, bilateral (bimanual) symmetrical and asymmetrical movements, reciprocal movements, patterns of proximal stabilization and postural support.

Abnormal synergistic patterns: Lesions of the corticospinal tracts can produce abnormal **obligatory synergies**, defined as movements that are primitive and highly stereotyped. **Table 4.8** shows the common synergy patterns following stroke.

Examination of voluntary movements should be done on the following aspects:

- Whether voluntary movement can be initiated, whether it can be completed?
- How the movement is carried out?
- Which muscle groups are linked together?
- Are there associated reactions: linkages between upper and lower limbs or one side to another?
- When do these patterns occur, under what circumstances, and what variations are possible?

As CNS recovery progresses, the synergy patterns become less dominant and reemerge only under conditions of stress or fatigue. Lessening of synergy dominance and emergence of selective movement control are evidence of sequential recovery in patients with stroke.

Following things should be documented during first assessment and reassessment as well:

- What abnormal synergies are present?
- The overall strength of the synergies present.

- The strongest components in each synergy.
- The influence of other UMN signs on synergies.
- What variations in movement from the typical synergies are possible?
- The effect of obligatory synergies on function.

Associated reactions: Associated reactions are automatic responses of the involved limb resulting from action occurring in some other part of the body, either by voluntary or reflex stimulation (e.g., resistance or asymmetrical tonic neck reflex). They are commonly elicited when some degree of spasticity is present and are infrequently seen in a limb exhibiting minimal muscle tone. Generally speaking, although not true in every case, associated reactions elicit the same direction of movement (i.e., flexion evokes flexion) and the opposite direction (i.e., flexion evokes extension) in the lower extremity. Brunnstrom classified stages of recovery into six stages as shown in **Box 4.11**. Bobath's stage of motor recovery is described in **Box 4.12**. **Table 4.9** shows difference between upper motor neuron and lower motor neuron syndrome.

CO-ORDINATION ASSESSMENT

Co-ordination assessment should be as follows:

- It is performed under two categories, i.e., non-equilibrium test and equilibrium tests.
- The non-equilibrium coordination tests deal with the components of limb movement in terms of alternate or reciprocal motion, movement composition and movement accuracy.

Table 4.8: Synergy patterns following stroke.

	Flexion synergy components	Extension synergy components
Upper extremity	• Scapular retraction/ elevation or hyperextension • Shoulder abduction, external rotation • Elbow flexion, forearm supination • Wrist and finger flexion	• Scapular protraction, shoulder adduction, internal rotation • Elbow extension, forearm pronation • Wrist and finger flexion
Lower extremity	• Hip flexion, abduction, external rotation • Knee flexion, ankle dorsiflexion, inversion, toe dorsiflexion	• Hip extension, adduction, internal rotation • Knee extension, ankle plantarflexion, inversion, toe plantarflexion

BOX 4.11: Brunnstrom grading of voluntary control.

- **Stage 1:** The patient is completely flaccid, no voluntary movement, and patient is confined to bed.
- **Stage 2:** Basic limb synergy develops, no voluntary movement can be done as spasticity appears but is not marked.
- **Stage 3:** Basic limb synergy develops voluntarily and is marked, spasticity is marked. (This is the stage of maximal spasticity.)
- **Stage 4:** Spasticity begins to decrease, four movement combinations deviate from basic limb synergies and become available, which are placing the hand behind the body, alternative pronation–supination with the elbow at 90° flexion and elevation of the arm to a forward horizontal position.
- **Stage 5:** There is relative independence of the basic limb synergies. Spasticity is waning, and movements can be performed as arm raising to a side horizontal position, alternative pronation–supination with the elbow extended and bringing hand over the head.
- **Stage 6:** There are isolated joint movements.

BOX 4.12: Bobath grades of motor recovery.

1. Flaccid
2. Spastic
3. Stage of spontaneous recovery

Table 4.9: Comparison of upper motor neuron (UMN) and lower motor neuron (LMN) syndromes.

Signs	UMN lesion	LMN lesion
Structures involved	Central nervous system cortex, brainstem, corticospinal tracts, spinal cord	Cranial nerve nuclei/nerves, peripheral nerve, spinal cord: anterior horn cell, spinal roots
Pathology	Stroke, traumatic brain injury, spinal cord injury	Polio, Guillain–Barré syndrome, peripheral nerve injury, peripheral neuropathy, radiculopathy
Tone	Hypertonicity	Hypotonicity, flaccidity
Deep tendon reflexes	Hyperreflexia, clonus, positive Babinski sign	Hyporeflexia
Superficial reflexes	Exaggerated	Decreased or absent
Muscle bulk	Disuse atrophy	Neurogenic atrophy, severe wasting
Voluntary movements	Impaired or absent (obligatory mass synergy)	Weak or absent

- The equilibrium tests consider the ability to maintain the body in equilibrium against gravity in a static and dynamic fashion.
- The routine sequence of coordination test starts from non-equilibrium test in form of unilateral to bilateral and then moving to symmetrical task. It is then further progressed to equilibrium test.
- A full explanation of the purpose of the testing should be given to the patient before starting the test.
- If needed a demonstration of the test can be given, but not mentioning the ideal response.
- Patient should be given a suitable position so that they can comfortably perform the desired movement.
- Any restriction in form of clothing, a brace or splint should be removed.
- Once the patient starts doing the movement, the therapist should carefully observe the performance in terms of the smoothness of the movement, accuracy of the movement and any deviation from the normal movement.
- The non-equilibrium tests should be graded on a 0–4 grading system as shown in **Box 4.13**. A list of non-equilibrium tests with a brief description is shown in **Table 4.10**. Similarly, equilibrium tests can also be graded as shown in **Box 4.14**. A list of equilibrium tests is shown in **Table 4.11**.

While testing these positions, care should be taken that the therapist is near the patient to support him in case the patient falls. To avoid any untoward incidence, patient should be instructed to inform in case they are not comfortable or confident in performing the test.

BOX 4.13: Grading of non-equilibrium tests.

- 0 – is no activity possible.
- 1 – is severe impairment in terms of initiation of the activity.
- 2 – is moderate impairment in terms of complete movement but in a slow, awkward, and unstable fashion.
- 3 – shows minimal impairment in which free movement is possible but with less than normal control, speed, and steadiness.
- 4 – is normal performance.

ASSESSMENT OF BALANCE

A body is said to be in balance when all the forces acting on the body are balanced in such way that the net resultant force is zero and the center of mass is within the stability limits and base of support. Following are the primary purposes of clinical balance assessments:

1. To identify whether or not a balance problem exists.
2. To determine the underlying cause of the balance problem.

- Balance should be assessed in the static and dynamic positions during sitting and standing.
- Patient should be instructed to sit in a high sitting position so that feet are not touching the ground with hands crossed across the chest. If the patient is able to maintain this position for 20 seconds, their static balance is said to be intact. Further dynamic balance is checked in the same position. Patient is given small range perturbations in all directions against which patient needs to maintain their position which assesses reactive balance. Anticipatory balance can be checked by asking the patient to reach their hands in different directions.
- Care should be taken to increase the range of perturbations or reach in a gradual way so that patient gets time to accommodate strategies to maintain balance. It is advisable for a fresh therapist to ask caregiver or colleague to be near the patient so that in case the patient loses balance, they can be saved from a fall.

Sensory Organization Test

Sensory organization test (SOT) is a form of posturography, which quantitatively assesses an individual's ability to use and integrate different sensory inputs. Subjects stand on dual-force plates in a three sides surround posturography system **(Fig. 4.4)**. Degree of anterior–posterior sway is recorded. Six independent sensory conditions are tested, with each condition consisting of three 20-second trials.

The six conditions include:

1. EO on firm surface
2. EC on firm surface
3. EO with sway referenced visual surround (altered vision)
4. EO on sway referenced support surface (unsteady surface)

Table 4.10: Non-equilibrium tests.

Name of the test	Description
1. Finger to nose	The shoulder is abducted to 90° with elbows extended. The patient is asked to bring the tip of index finger to the tip of their nose. Alterations may be made in initial starting position to observe the performance from different planes of motion
2. Finger to therapist finger	The patient and therapist sit opposite each other. The therapist's index finger is held in front of the patient. The patient is asked to touch his/her index finger to tip of therapist index finger. Position of therapist finger may be altered during testing to observe ability to change distance, direction and force of movement
3. Finger to finger	Both shoulders abducted to 90° with elbows extended. Patient is asked to bring both the hands toward midline and approximate the index fingers from opposing hands
4. Pronation and supination—dys-diadochokinesia	With elbows flexed to 90° and held close to the body the patient alternately turns the palms up and down. This test also may be performed with shoulders flexed to 90° and elbows extended. Speed may be gradually increased. The ability to reverse movements between opposing muscle groups can be examined at many joints. Examples include active alternation between flexion and extension of the knee, ankle, elbow, and fingers
5. Rebound test	The patient is positioned with the elbow flexed. The therapist applies sufficient manual resistance to produce an Isometric contraction of biceps. Resistance is suddenly released. Normally, the opposing muscle group (triceps) will contract and check movement of the limb. Many other muscle groups can be tested for this phenomenon, such as the shoulder abductors or flexors and elbow extensors
6. Pointing and past pointing	The patient and therapist are opposite each other, either sitting or standing. Both patient and therapist bring shoulders to a horizontal position of 90° of flexion with elbows extended. Index fingers are touching or the patient's finger may rest lightly on the therapist's. The patient is asked to fully flex the shoulder (fingers will be pointing toward ceiling) and then return to the horizontal position such that index fingers will again approximate. Both arms should be tested, either separately or simultaneously. A normal response consists of an accurate return to the starting position. In an abnormal response, there is typically a "past pointing," or movement beyond the target. Several variations to this test include movements in other directions such as toward 90° of shoulder abduction or toward 0° of shoulder flexion (finger will point toward floor). Following each movement, the patient is asked to return to the initial horizontal starting position
7. Alternate heel to knee, heel to toe	From a supine position, the patient is asked to touch the knee and big toe alternately with the heel of the opposite extremity
8. Heel on shin	From a supine position, the heel of one foot is slid up and down the shin of opposite lower extremity (LE)

BOX 4.14: Grading of equilibrium tests.

0 – means unable to maintain balance.
1 – shows moderate-to-maximal assistance to maintain positions.
2 – is minimal assistance to maintain position.
3 – is able to maintain balance without assistance or support but with limited postural sway.
4 – is considered as normal in which the patient is able to maintain steady balance without support.

Table 4.11: Equilibrium tests.

1. Sitting in a normal comfortable posture
2. Sitting weight shifting in all directions
3. Standing in a normal comfortable posture
4. Standing feet together (narrow base of support)
5. Standing on one foot
6. Standing with one foot directly in front of the other in tandem position (toe of one foot touching heel of opposite foot)
7. Standing: EO to EC (Romberg test)
8. Standing in tandem position: EO to EC (Sharpened Romberg test)

(EC: eyes closed; EO: eyes open)

5. EC on sway referenced support surface
6. EO on sway referenced support surface and surround (unsteady surface and altered vision).

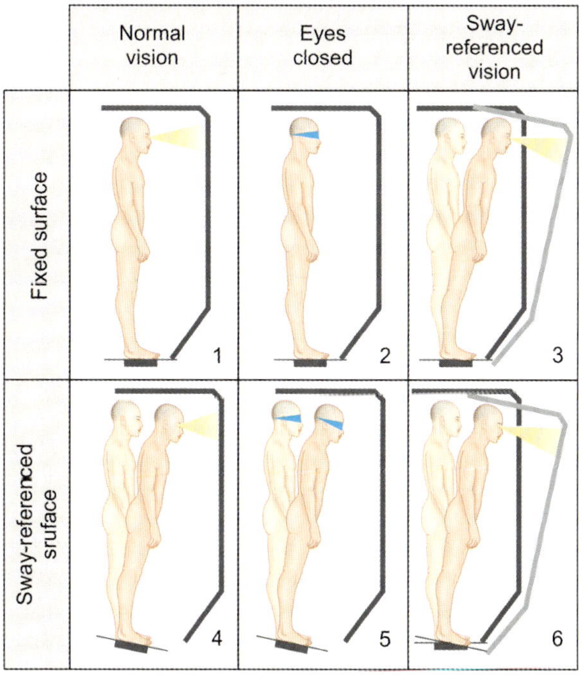

Fig. 4.4: Sensory organization test.

The scoring system consists of:

- **Equilibrium scoring:** Center of gravity (COG) and postural sway is measured under each condition, and a composite equilibrium score is computed from the weighted average of the sway measured with each of the sensory conditions. Sway and equilibrium scores are calculated as a percentage based on degree of sway from vertical (100% perfect equilibrium and 0% results in a fall).
- Sensory analysis is used to determine how much the patient relies on each of the systems contributing to balance (somatosensory, visual, and vestibular systems). This is analyzed through ratios of individual equilibrium scores (i.e., condition 2 score/condition 1 score).
- **COG alignment:** reflection of the patient's COG position relative to center of base of support (BOS) at start of each trial of the sensory organization test (SOT).
- A strategy analysis produces quantitative data about relative amount of movement about the ankles and the hips that the patients used to maintain balance during each trial. This determines how much of an "ankle strategy" and "hip strategy" is used and can be compared to the type of condition in which one strategy predominantly occurs over the other (i.e., ankle strategy is used more often with unsteady surface).

Clinical Test for Sensory Interaction on Balance

The clinical test for sensory interaction on balance can be described as follows:

- When sophisticated equipment such as posturography are not available or feasible to use, a modified version which can be performed in clinical or home setup is Clinical Test for Sensory Interaction on Balance (CTSIB).
- It is a low-tech version of SOT developed by Shumway Cook and Horak, which utilizes medium-density foam to substitute for a moving platform and a modified visual dome (Japanese lantern affixed to the subject's head) to substitute for a moving visual surrounding.
- The six testing conditions are similar to SOT, and a newer version of CTSIB has also been developed—modified CTSIB, which utilizes four different sensory test conditions (EO and EC on flat surface and on foam). This version is more commonly used currently, and the same posture is adopted in both versions (i.e., feet shoulder-width apart). Three 30-second trials are used and times in balance and increased sway or loss of balance are recorded.

Movement Strategies for Balance

Humans have evolved methods to take in order to preserve their bodies to the best of their abilities. One of these remarkable mechanisms is how one maintains balance as a bipedal (two-legged) species. It is body's very own unconscious defense mechanism that helps to

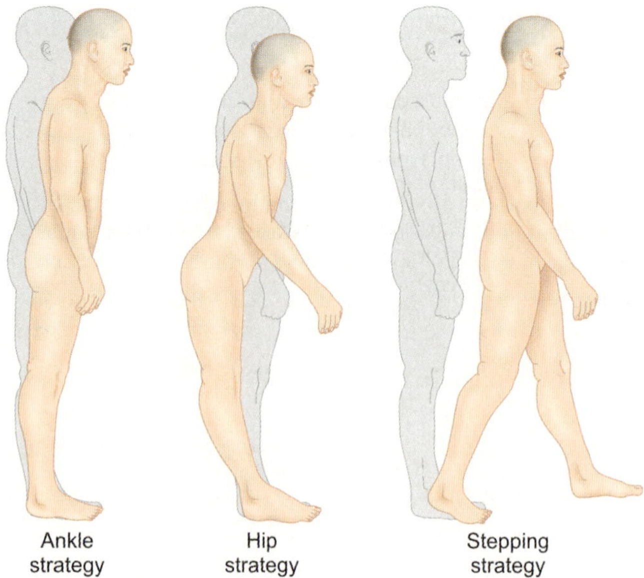

Fig. 4.5: Strategies for maintaining balance.

prevent against falls when the surfaces or situations are challenging. The following are some of the strategies employed **(Fig. 4.5)**:

1. Ankle strategies
2. Hip strategies
3. Stepping/grasping strategies
4. Head stabilization in space (HSS) strategies
5. Head stabilization on trunk (HST) strategies

- Strategies that refer to those movement strategies used to control the center of mass (COM) over a fixed BOS are referred to as *in-place or fixed support strategies* such as ankle and hip strategy.
- *Change-in-support strategies* are defined as movements of the lower or upper limbs to make a new contact with the support surface such as stepping or grasping strategy.
- Two *head-stabilizing strategies* have also been described, which are proactive strategies and differ greatly from reactive strategies because head-stabilizing strategies occur in anticipation of the initiation of internally generated forces caused by changes in position from sitting to standing. HSS and HST are a part of these head-stabilizing strategies.

Functional Balance Grades

For documentation, functional balance grades can be used, which consist of descriptors that can be used to define both static and dynamic control in sitting and standing **(Table 4.12)**.

Performance-based Measures

Berg Balance Scale

The Berg Balance Scale (BBS) is an objective measure of static and dynamic balance abilities. The scale consists of 14 functional tasks performed in everyday life. The scoring

Table 4.12: Functional balance grades.

Grade	Description
4 normal	In static, patient able to maintain steady balance without handhold support. In dynamic, patient accepts maximal challenge and can shift weight easily within full range in all directions
3 good	In static, patient is able to maintain balance without handhold support, limited postural sway. In dynamic, patient accepts moderate challenge and is able to maintain balance while picking up object off floor
2 fair	In static, patient is able to maintain balance with handhold support and may require occasional minimal assistance. In dynamic, patient accepts minimal challenge and is able to maintain balance while turning head/trunk
1 poor	In static, patient requires handhold support and moderate to maximal assistance to maintain position. In dynamic, patient is unable to accept challenge or move without loss of balance
0 absent	Patient is unable to maintain balance

uses a 5-point ordinal scale, with scoring range from 0 to 4, where 0 indicates that the patient is "unable to perform" and 4 indicates that the patient "performs independently and meets time and distance criteria." A maximum score of 56 points is possible.

Components of BBS are:

- Sitting to standing
- Standing unsupported
- Sitting with back unsupported but feet supported on floor or a stool
- Standing to sitting
- Transfers
- Standing unsupported with EC
- Standing unsupported with feet together
- Reaching forward with outstretched arm while standing
- Picking up object from the floor from a standing position
- Turning to look behind over your left and right shoulder while standing
- Turning 360
- Placing alternate foot on step or stool while standing unsupported
- Standing unsupported one foot in front
- Standing on one leg

Functional Reach Test

Functional reach test is explained as follows:

- Functional reach test is a clinical outcome measure and assessment tool for ascertaining dynamic balance in one simple task.
- It was developed by Pamela Duncan et al., in 1990. They defined functional reach as "the maximal distance one can reach forward beyond arm's length, while maintaining a fixed base of support in the standing position."
- This test measures the distance between the lengths of an outstretched arm in a maximal forward reach from a standing position, while maintaining a fixed base of support.
- Scores < 15 or 18 cm indicate limited functional balance. Most healthy individuals with adequate functional balance can reach 25 cm or more.

Timed "Up and Go" Test

Timed "Up and Go" test can be described as follows:

- It is developed by Podsiadlo and Richardson in 1991 and measures, in seconds, the time taken by an individual to stand up from a standard arm chair (approximate seat height of 46 cm, arm height 65 cm), walk a distance of 3 m (approximately 10 feet), turn, walk back to the chair, and sit down.
- This clinical test, developed in a medical setting, asks subjects to wear their regular footwear and use their customary walking aid (none, cane, walker). No physical assistance is given.
- Patient start with their back against the chair, their arms resting on the armrests and their walking aid at hand. Patient is instructed that, on the word "go" they are to get up and walk at a comfortable and safe pace to a line on the floor 3 m away, turn, return to the chair and sit down again. Patient walks through the test once before being timed in order to become familiar with the test. Either a stopwatch or a wristwatch with a second hand can be used to time the trial.
- A cutoff score of ≥13.5 seconds was shown to predict falls in community-dwelling frail elders. Scores of ≥30 seconds correspond with functional dependence in people with pathology.

Performance-oriented Mobility Assessment

Performance-oriented mobility assessment (POMA) is described as follows:

- Tinetti et al., developed a scaled called Performance Oriented Mobility Assessment, which provides a brief and reliable measure of both static and dynamic balance.
- This test has two subscales of balance and gait with 13 maneuvers in the balance portion and 9 maneuvers in the gait portion, and the balance subscale, the performance-oriented assessment of balance, can be used individually as a separate test of balance.
- The balance maneuvers are graded on an ordinal scale as normal (2 points), adaptive (1 point), or abnormal (0 points). The gait maneuvers are graded as normal or abnormal, with the exception of a few items. A combination of the total points for the balance and gait portions are summed together to determine the final score. Scores less than 18 imply high fall risk, between

19 and 23 imply moderate fall risk, and greater or equal to 24 imply low fall risk.

Dynamic Gait Index

Following are the features of dynamic gait index:
- The dynamic gait index was developed as a clinical tool to assess gait, balance, and fall risk.
- It evaluates not only usual steady-state walking but also walking during more challenging tasks. It assesses the individual's ability to modify balance while walking in the presence of external demands.
- Eight functional walking tests are performed by the subject and marked out of three according to the lowest category which applies. 24 is the total individual score possible. Scores of 19 or less have been related to increase incidence of falls.

Walking While Talking

Features of walking while talking (WWT) are the following:
- Considered to be a dual-task test, WWT, also known as walkie-talkie test, is used to determine the effects of attentional demands by introducing a secondary task, talking, while walking.
- Individual is asked to walk 20 ft, turn 180°, and return 20 ft while either reciting the alphabet (simple) or reciting alternate letters of alphabet (complex).
- 20 seconds or longer for WWT-simple, and in WWT-complex, 33 seconds or longer are indicative of fall risk.

Self-report Measures

Balance Efficacy Scale Test

Balance efficacy scale test is described as follows:
- Another scale developed by Tinetti et al., which is a self-reported measure that examines how confident an individual feels while performing 10 items of ADL and functional mobility.
- Individuals are asked to consider how confident they feel in doing each of the activities listed without falling. The individual is asked to rate his or her confidence level on a 0 (not at all) to 10 (completely confident) scale. The highest score is 100 (completely confident on all 10 items) and represents high self-efficacy, whereas the bottom score of 0 represents low self-efficacy.

Activities of Balance Confidence

Following are the features of activities of balance confidence (ABC):
- ABC is a useful questionnaire that evaluates self-perceived balance confidence while attempting 16 different ADLs.
- However, it has been shown to relate better to what activities people actually avoid than to future falls.
- Ratings consist of whole numbers (0–100) for each item, where 0 implies no confidence and 100 implies complete confidence in performing a particular activity.

Fall Efficacy Scale

Listed below are the features of fall efficacy scale (FES):
- The FES was one of the first scales to assess the perceptions of older adults themselves. A well-known and widely used scale, the FES and, now, the modified-FES attend to the role of confidence and how confidence (or its opposite, fear) is implicated in falls.
- A total score of greater than 70 indicates that the person has a fear of falling. The FES is a 10-item test rated on a 10-point scale from not confident at all to completely confident. It is correlated with difficulty getting up from a fall and level of anxiety.

ASSESSMENT OF GAIT

To assess gait, the following are to be considered:
- Patients with neurological affection exhibit variety of gait abnormalities. While sophisticated measures are available for assessment of gait, visual observation has its own place during busy clinical hours.
- A therapist should develop an eye for quick observation of different phases of gait.
- A level ground area of minimum 4–5 m should be chosen. Patient should be instructed that they have to walk a defined area with or without support, in case they feel any discomfort, they should immediately inform, walk in a normal casual way, and keep looking straight ahead.
- Patient should be adequately exposed to examine the lower extremity joints, with due consent from them. In the case of female patients, a curtain should be used. A caregiver should accompany the patient throughout the walkway.
- In case the patient needs any assistive device to walk, they should be allowed to use it during assessment.
- They should walk barefoot so that ankle and toes can be examined properly.
- Therapist should carefully walk with the patient noting down movements of hip, knee, ankle, and trunk during different subphases of gait from sagittal and frontal view. Hand movement and trunk position should also be noted.

Documentation of gait analysis should include overall status of gait, to begin with. It should start with if the patient is walking independently or with some support. Description of support should be given next in the form of manual assistance, assistive device, walking aid (walker, cane in the right/left hand, crutches), etc. Further, quality of walk should be described in terms of base of support, position of hands, any break taken in between, smoothness of movement, etc. Subphase analysis should be described next for both sides. A tabular form may be used for the detailed description **(Table 4.13)**. Detailed description

Table 4.13: Observational gait analysis form.

Rt/Lt	Heel strike	Foot flat	Mid stance	Heel off	Toe off	Acceleration	Mid swing	Deceleration
Ankle	0°	10–15°PF	5°DF	10°DF	20°PF	10°PF	0°	0°
Knee	0°	15°F	0°	0°	40°F	60°F	25°F	0°
Hip	25°F	20°F	0°	5°E	0°	15°F	25°F	25°F
Trunk*								

Separate table should be used for right and left side.
*Position of trunk should be mentioned at each subphase. Ideally it should be in neutral position. In patients with hip abductor weakness, there may be side bending of the trunk.

BOX 4.15: Spatial parameters (distance parameters).

- **Step length:** This is the distance between corresponding successive points of heel contact of the opposite feet. If the gait is normal the right step length is equal to left step length. This parameter can give a great insight into a patient's problem.
- **Stride length:** This is the distance between successive points of heel contact of the same foot. In normal gait this is equal to double the step length.

BOX 4.16: Temporal parameters (time parameters).

- **Stance time:** It is the amount of time that elapses during the stance phase of one extremity in gait cycle.
- **Single support time:** It is the amount of time for which only one extremity is in contact with the ground.
- **Double support time:** It is time for which both extremities are in contact with the ground.
- **Stride duration:** It is the time required to complete one stride and it is normally twice that of step duration.
- **Cadence:** This is the number of steps per unit time measured in steps per minute.
- **Speed (velocity):** This is the distance covered by the body per unit time, usually measured in m/s. Patients with problems tend to walk at a slower velocity in order to decrease the forces and moments they have to cope with in gait. If the patient's condition is improved the velocity should go up.
- **Single limb support:** This is the amount of time spent on a limb expressed as a percentage of the gait cycle.

---

of gait analysis is discussed in the chapter "Assessment of Gait" **(Boxes 4.15 and 4.16)**.

HAND EVALUATION

The purposes of hand evaluation are to identify:
- Physical limitations such as loss of ROM
- Functional limitations such as inability to perform daily tasks
- Substitution patterns to compensate for loss of sensation or motor function

- Established deformities such as joint or muscle contracture.

The movement of arm and hand must be coordinated for movement function. Shoulder motion is necessary for positioning the hand and elbow for daily activities. The wrist is the key point in the position of function. Skilled hand performance depends on wrist stability. Function also depends on arm and shoulder stability and mobility for fixing or positioning the hand for functional use. The thumb is of greater importance than any other digit. Effective pinch is almost impossible without a thumb. Within the hand, the proximal interphalangeal joint is critical for grasp and is considered to be the important small joint.

Observation

The therapist should observe the appearance of arm and hand on the following points:
- Position of arm and hand at rest and the carrying posture
- How does the patient treat the injured hand—overprotected or ignored
- Skin condition
- Any laceration sutures/scars
- Swelling
- Apparent contractures of web space

The therapist should ask the patient to perform some simple bilateral ADL such as:
- Buttoning and unbuttoning
- Putting on shirt
- Opening a jar
- Threading a needle

One can observe the appearance of spontaneous movement and use of affected hand and arm.

Physical Evaluation

Physical evaluation includes the following:
- Joints must be assessed for active and passive mobility or fixed deformities and any other tendency to assume a position of deformity. **Figure 4.6** shows a smaller finger goniometer.

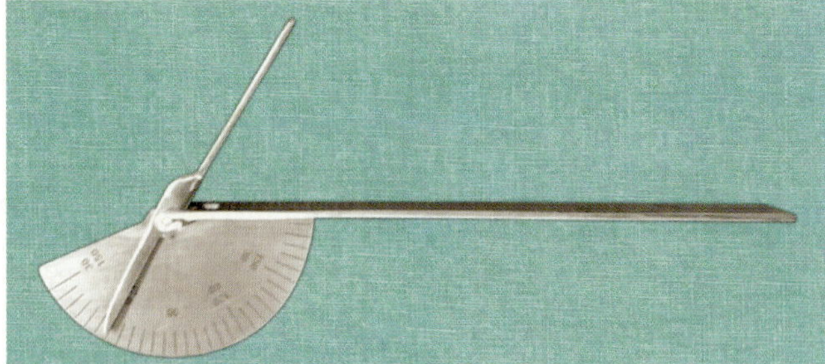

Fig. 4.6: Finger goniometer.

- Ligaments must be evaluated for laxity or contracture and their ability to maintain joint stability.
- Tendons must be assessed for integrity—contractures or overstretching.
- Muscles are tested for strength and function.

Edema Assessment

Hand volume is measured to assess the presence of extracellular and intracellular edema. Volume measurement is usually done to determine the effect of treatment. A commercial volume meter is used to assess hand edema. The device can be used to assess the change in hand size resulting from localized swelling or generalized edema or atrophy. There is often a normal 10-mL difference between right and left hands, between dominant and non-dominant hands. If swelling is a problem, difference of 30–50 mL can be noted. A method of assessing edema of an individual finger or joint is circumferential method using either a circumference tape or jewelers' ring size standards.

Mapping

The hand is assessed for any abnormal sensations from proximal to distal and from radial to ulnar directions. The areas of change of sensations are carefully marked. Mapping should be repeated at monthly intervals during nerve regeneration.

Categories of Tests

A variety of evaluations may be required to assess sensations adequately. These tests can be divided into three categories:
1. Modality test for pain, heat, cold, and touch, pressure
2. Functional tests to assess the quality of sensations, (tactile gnosis) by Moberg stationary and moving two-point discrimination and Moberg pick up tests.
3. Objective tests that do not require active participation by the patient such as wrinkle test and ninhydrine test for sympathetic dysfunction.

Grips and Pinch Strength

A standard adjustable hand dynamometer is recommended for assessing grip strength. The subject should be seated with shoulder adducted and neutrally rotated, the elbow flexed at 90°, forearm in neutral position, the wrist

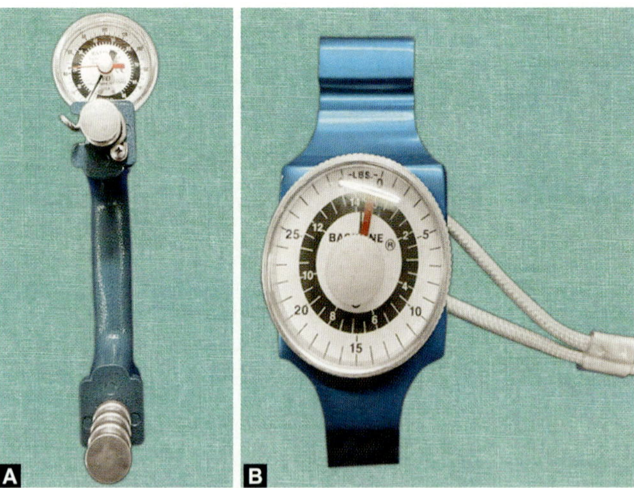

Figs. 4.7A and B: (A) Dynamometer; (B) Pinch gauge.

between 0–30° extension and 0–15° ulnar deviation. Three trials are taken for each hand with the dynamometer. The patient squeezes the dynamometer with as much force as he can, two separate times with a 2–3-minute rest period in between **(Fig. 4.7A)**. The pinch gauge measures the strength of a pinch in pounds **(Fig. 4.7B)**.

The following grips and pinch should be evaluated:
- Two-point pinch or tip pinch—thumb pinch to index finger
- Lateral or key pinch—thumb pulp to lateral aspect of middle phalanx of index finger
- Three-point pinch—thumb tip to tips of index and long fingers.

Types of grips include:
1. Cylindrical grip
2. Spherical grip
3. Hook grip
4. Lateral prehension

Extensor musculature predominates in the maintenance of lateral prehension, whereas in other, three flexor muscles predominate the activity.

Further, clinical tests can be performed for specific dysfunction in peripheral neuropathic conditions. A patient with particular nerve lesion will not be able to perform the given activity.
- Ulnar nerve—ask the patient to pinch with the thumb and index finger and palpate the first dorsal interosseous muscle.
- Radial nerve—ask the patients to extend the fingers and wrist.

Clinical Pearl

Clinically, hand function should be assessed with the help of common objects with different shapes such as ball, bottle, small hand bag, and key. Note should be made of the position of fingers and thumbs at the time of grasping an object. In patients with stroke, ability of release by extensor muscles also needs to be assessed.

- Median nerve—ask the patient to oppose the thumb with finger flexion.
- Patients may also develop compression syndrome of ulnar and radial nerves, which will be indicated by paresthesia along the course of those nerves.

Michigan Hand Outcomes Questionnaire

The Michigan Hand Outcomes Questionnaire (MHQ) is a hand-specific outcomes instrument that measures outcomes of patients with conditions of, or injury to, the hand or wrist. The MHQ contains six distinct scales:

1. Overall hand function
2. ADLs
3. Pain
4. Work performance
5. Esthetics
6. Patient satisfaction with hand function

The MHQ has 37 core questions, takes approximately 15 minutes to complete, and can be self-administered or administered by research personnel. It can be used to assess a patient's general hand function or if administered several times (i.e., pre- and postoperatively), it can be used to assess changes in hand function. However, it needs specific training and permission to use for research purposes.

Electrodiagnosis

This can be used as a special investigation to confirm a diagnosis. This is described in detail in the chapter "Electrodiagnosis."

FUNCTIONAL ASSESSMENT

Functional assessment measures an individual's level of function and ability to perform functional or work-related tasks on a safe and dependable basis over a defined period of time. It evaluates specific things, such as grooming, bathing, dressing or more general aspect such as quality of life. It consists of the assessment of ADLs, which measure the performance of basic functional skills needed to care for oneself independently. They are an essential component in rehabilitation medicine assisting with quality assurance, ongoing quality improvement, cost/benefit analysis, education, and research and have been described in the chapter "Assessment of Function" in detail.

SUMMARY

Assessment of patients with neurological dysfunction is a time-consuming process but once the assessment is done properly, goal setting becomes easier. It takes time for a therapist to develop the expertise in the assessment process but can be achieved with continuous practice. A perfect assessment cannot be done without cooperation from the patient; hence, proper communication with the patient is a key. Last but not the least, documenting the findings helps to review and track the progress of patient and hence should be done meticulously.

Case Scenario

A 31-year-old male businessman met with an accident 5 months back. His MRI findings revealed spinal cord injury at T8 level. He underwent surgery to stabilize fracture site by internal fixation and decompression. After ICU stay for 10 days, he was transferred to general ward for long-term care. He was dependent in his bed mobility and had poor control over his upper extremity due to pain at operation site; however, PROM was full. He needed maximum support for supine-to-sit activity. His both lower extremities were hypotonic and did not have any active movement. Now he is 5 months post spinal cord injury (SCI) and under regular physiotherapy management.

Physical Therapy Examination

- **Communication/cognition:** Alert, oriented to time, place and person, able to follow multistep commands.
- **Cranial nerve integrity:** All cranial nerves are intact.
- **Sensory integrity:**
  - Intact pin prick and light touch up to T12
  - Proprioception intact in bilateral UEs, absent below T12
- **Intact anal sensations.**
- **Joint integrity and mobility:**
  - ROM of bilateral upper extremity is complete and pain free actively and passively.
  - PROM of lower extremity is complete and pain free.
- **Tone:** Bilateral lower extremity tone is reduced.
- **Reflex integrity:**
  - Bilateral ankle and plantar reflex are diminished
  - Bilateral knee reflex is absent
  - Abdominal reflex is absent in every quadrant.
- **Muscle performance:**
  - Bilateral upper extremity grade 5
  - Bilateral hip flexors, knee extensors grade 2
  - Bilateral hip extensors, knee flexors grade 1
  - Bilateral dorsiflexors and plantar flexors grade 0.
- **Postural control and balance:**
  - Head and pelvic control—good
  - Pelvic control—fair
  - Able to sit independently for prolong period
  - Able to maintain balance in sitting at the edge of the bed in weight-bearing position
  - Able to reach in all three planes in sitting
  - Able to stand with normal base of support, AFO and walker up to minutes.
- **Functional mobility:**
  - Rolling on either sides—minimal assistance
  - Supine to prone—minimal assistance
  - Supine to long sitting—minimal assistance
  - Kneel sitting to kneeling—moderate assistance
- **Locomotion:**
  - Unable to ambulate
  - Able to propel on wheelchair on level surface with minimal assistance.

Contd...

Contd...

- **Wheelchair skills:**
  - Require assistance with locking wheel locks and removing foot rest.
  - ASIA Scale
    - » Neurological level—T12
    - » Incomplete injury—score C

Guiding Questions:
1. What is the change in patient's functional status in the last 6 months?
2. Develop problem list in terms of direct impairments, indirect impairments, and functional limitations.
3. Determine physical therapy diagnosis.

Review Questions

1. Describe the types of memory along with their disorders.
2. Describe the five terms used to document a patient's level of consciousness.
3. What are the typical patterns of spasticity in upper motor neuron syndrome?
4. Explain the purposes of screening the sensory system along with any three pathologies that indicate the need for sensory examination.
5. Describe in detail preparation of patient for checking sensations.
6. Describe the procedure of testing trigeminal nerve.
7. Enumerate abnormal tonal abnormalities along with conditions in which it is seen.
8. Describe the procedure of checking the strength of muscles along with its significance.
9. Describe the purposes of performing coordination tests.
10. Name the standardized tests available to examine balance? Explain interpretation of each test along with its procedure.
11. Describe basic terminology used in the description of ICF for a neurological dysfunction.

BIBLIOGRAPHY

1. Alexander EK. Perspective: moving therapist beyond an organ-based approach when teaching medical interviewing and physical examination skills. Acad Med. 2008;83(10):906-9.
2. Arnadottir G. The brain and behavior: assessing cortical dysfunction through activities of daily living. St. Louis, MO: Mosby; 1990.
3. Bigler ED, Tucker DM. Clinical assessment of tactile extinction: traditional double simultaneous stimulation versus quality extinction test. Arch Clin Neuropsychol. 1989;4:283-96.
4. Blatchly CA, Gombash LL. A study of CTSIB. Phys Ther. 1993; 73:346.
5. Campbell WW, DeJong RN. De Jong's the neurologic examination, 6th Indian edition. Wolters Kluwer. Philadelphia. USA Lippincott Williams & Wilkins; 2005.
6. Camp CJ, Skrajner MJ, Lee MM, Judgej KS. Cognitive Assessment in Late Stage Dementia. In: Lichtenberg PA (ed). Handbook of Assessment in Clinical Gerontology, 2nd edition. Academic Press; 2010;531-55.
7. Clendaniel RA. Outcome measures for assessment of treatment of the dizzy and balance disorder patient. Otolaryngol Clin North Am. 2000;33(3):519-33.
8. Gassel MM, Diamantopoulos E. The Jendrassik maneuver. Neurology. 1964;14:555-60, 640-42.
9. Henderson VW. Chapter 17: Cognitive assessment in neurology. In: Handbook of clinical neurology. 2009. https://doi.org/10.1016/S0072-9752(08)02117-9.
10. Herman T, Inbar-Borovsky N, Brozgol M, et al. The Dynamic Gait Index in healthy older adults: the role of stair climbing, fear of falling and gender. Gait Posture. 2009;29(2):237-41. Epub 2008 Oct 8.
11. Johnston SC, Hauser SL. The beautiful and ethereal neurological exam: an appeal for research. Ann Neurol. 2011;70:A9-10.
12. Kendall FP, McCreary EK, Provance PG. Muscles: testing and function. Baltimore, MD: Williams &Wilkins; 1993
13. Meyers AM, Fletcher PC, Myers AH, et al. Discriminative and evaluative properties of the activities-specific balance confidence (ABC) scale. J Gerontol A Biol Sci Med Sci. 1998;53:M287-94.
14. Nakamura DM, Holm MB, Wilson A. Measures of balance and fear of falling in the elderly: a review. Phys Occup Ther Geriatr. 1998;15(4):17-32.
15. O'Sullivan SB, Schmitz TJ. Physical rehabilitation, 5th edition. Philadelphia, PA: FA Davis; 2007.
16. Pedalini ME, Cruz OL, Bittar RS, Grazel SS. Sensory organization test in elderly patients with and without vestibular dysfunction. Acta Otolaryngol. 2009;129(9):962-5.
17. Pedretti LW. C V A in occupational therapy practice skill for physical dysfunction, 3rd edition. 1990. pp. 603-22.
18. Quintana LA. Evaluation of perception and cognition in occupational therapy. Occupational therapy for physical dysfunction. 3rd edition. Baltimore. Williams and Wilkins; 1989.
19. Shumway-Cook A, Horak F. Assessing the influence of sensory interaction on balance: Suggestion from the field. Phys Ther. 1986;66:1548.
20. Shumway-Cook A, Woollacott M. Motor control—translating research into clinical practice, 3rd edition. Philadelphia, PA: Lippincott Williams & Wilkins; 2007.
21. Tate R, McDonald S. What is apraxia? The clinician's dilemma. Neuropsychol Rehabil. 1995;5:273.
22. Tinetti M, Richman D, Powell L. Falls efficacy as a measure of fear of falling. J Gerontol. 1990;45:P239-43.
23. Tinetti ME. Performance-oriented assessment of mobility problems in elderly patients. JAGS. 1986;34:119-26. Scoring description: PT Bulletin Feb. 10, 1993.
24. Verghese J, Kuslansky G, Holtzer R, et al. Walking while talking: effect of task prioritization in the elderly. Arch Phys Med Rehabil. 2007;88(1):50-3.
25. Whiting SE, Uncoln NB, Bhavnani G, Cockburn J. The Rivermead Perceptual Assessment Battery. Windsor: NFER-Nelson; 1985.
26. Wiles CM. Introducing neurological examination for medical undergraduates—how I do it. Pract Neurol. 2013;13(01):49-50.
27. Zoltan B. Vision, perception and cognition: a manual for evaluation and treatment of the neurologically impaired adult, 3rd edition rev. Thorofare, NJ: Charles B. Slack; 1996.
28. Árnadóttir G. The brain and behavior: assessing cortical dysfunction through activities of daily living. St Louis, MO: Mosby; 1999.

Cardiorespiratory Assessment

Dipali Rana, Neeta J Vyas

LEARNING OBJECTIVES

After reading this chapter, the readers should be able to:

- Understand how anatomy and physiology of the cardiopulmonary system influence the assessment process
- Understand the nuances of history taking and develop keen observation
- Develop a thorough knowledge of pathophysiology of the cardiopulmonary system and understand their influence on the assessment process
- Gain knowledge about an easy approach to detailed and comprehensive cardiopulmonary examination
- Understand the interpretation of various investigative procedures used for cardiopulmonary assessment
- Understand the process of differential diagnoses

CHAPTER OUTLINE

- Problem-oriented medical records
  - First step
- Demographic details
- History
- Subjective assessment
  - Breathlessness (dyspnea)
  - Cough
- Sputum and hemoptysis
  - Wheeze
  - Chest pain
  - Other symptoms
- Objective assessment
  - Airway
  - Breathing
  - Circulation
  - Disability
  - Exposure
- International Classification of Functioning Disability and Health Assessment

INTRODUCTION

Clinical assessment forms a vital part of the clinical reasoning process and involves the detailed process of identifying problem areas through recognition and interpretation of abnormal and normal signs and symptoms and clinically assessing these signs and symptoms to form a diagnosis. Assessment involves information gathering through interview and referring to medical files and performing a subjective and objective examination.

Documentation forms a critical component of the patient care. Documentation is important for recording patient data for current as well as the future reference, for comparison during follow-up visits, to analyze and decide the prognosis of the patient, to decide whether the intervention is helpful or not, for communication between various disciplines of medical care and for reimbursement purposes. Documentation should be as objective as possible to minimize discrepancies between the referring people. It should be well written and legible (if written) or in the digital form (more convenient), precise and concise. The records usually contain the details of patient assessment, examination details, results of the various tests performed, and plan of future care.

PROBLEM-ORIENTED MEDICAL RECORDS

Problem-oriented medical record (POMR) is used as the method of recording the assessment, management, and progress of a patient.

It can be divided into five sections:

1. Database
2. Problem list
3. Initial plan and goal
4. Progress notes
5. Discharge summary

The approach to all patients is the same. The underlying principles are:

- Use the airway, breathing, circulation, disability, and exposure (**ABCDE**) approach to assess and treat the patient.
- Do a complete initial assessment and reassess regularly.
- Treat life-threatening problems before moving to the next part of assessment.
- Assess the effects of treatment.
- Communicate effectively—use the situation, background, assessment, recommendation or reason, story, vital signs, plan approach.

Remember: It can take a few minutes for treatments to work, so wait a short while before reassessing the patient after an intervention.

First Step

Following steps need to be taken:

1. Ensure personal safety. Wear apron, mask, and gloves as appropriate.
2. First look at the patient in general to see if the patient appears unwell.
3. If the patient is awake, ask "How are you?" If the patient appears unconscious or has collapsed, shake him and ask "Are you alright?" If he responds normally he has a patent airway, is breathing and has brain perfusion. If he speaks only in short sentences, he may have breathing problems. Failure of the patient to respond is a clear marker of critical illness.
4. This first rapid "look, listen, and feel" of the patient should take about 30 seconds and will often indicate a patient is critically ill or not.

DEMOGRAPHIC DETAILS

Demographic details are as follows:

Name: For identification and communication

Age: For identification of age-specific disease—children, adult, geriatric group

Gender: For identification of gender-specific disease—male and female

Weight and height: For body mass index (BMI) calculation

Obesity or malnourishment can compromise respiratory functions. BMI should be checked **(Table 5.1)**.

Lifestyle: For identification of lifestyle-specific disease—sedentary, active

Occupation: For identification of occupation-specific disease and also helps in vocational guidance

Residence: For identification of area-specific disease—slums, urban, rural, and emphasis on stairs and slopes

Referred by: Either themselves or doctor name—to communicate with doctor as a team work

Table 5.1: BMI classification as per WHO for Asian and general population

Category	Asian population (kg/m^2)	General population (kg/m^2)
Underweight	Below 18.5	Below 18.5
Normal	18.5 – 22.9	18.5 – 24.9
Overweight	23 – 27.5	25 – 29.9
Obese	>27.5	> 30

Provisional diagnosis: From doctor's note

Chief complaint: Pertaining to present condition and which most affect the patient in their activity of daily living.

HISTORY

History forms a vital component of the assessment process. It is the skill of the interviewer to gain information from the patient's history in order to recognize symptoms that may direct them to a cardiac or pulmonary pathology. History taking also helps develop a good patient–therapist rapport. It is always a good choice to allow the patient narrate details of history in their own words and at their own pace. The therapist should not hurry or interrupt the patient and should try to be a patient listener. History can be divided into the following components:

- **Chief complaint:** The therapist should question the patient at depth about the reason they (the patient) have sought medical care.
- **History of present condition:** Questions exploring the details about the chief complaint can be asked but they should be non-leading and in words that are comprehensible to the patient. The interviewer should try to gain information about the onset, duration, and progression of the symptoms along with any associated factors that might be present. Various medical facilities have their own questionnaires that can aid the novice health-care provider in history taking. Questionnaires in spite of being helpful and time saving depersonalize the history-taking process and reduce the level of patient satisfaction and negatively impact the patient–therapist relationship.
- **History of previous medical/surgical conditions:** The therapist needs to inquire about and create the entire list of medical (comorbidities such as diabetes and hypertension) and surgical problems that the patient had in the past written in disease-specific grouping or chronological account. It is also important to note the current status of the medical or surgical condition. This helps in narrowing down any associated pathologies, e.g., an individual suffering from dyslipidemia becomes susceptible to an angina episode.
- **Drug history:** A list of patient's current medication (with dosage and timings) and drug allergies should also be noted.
- **Family history:** A list of any major diseases suffered by members of immediate family should be documented.

This helps in cases of inherent or genetic disorders, e.g., a family history of myocardial infarction (MI) increases the risk of sustaining an MI or diabetes.

- **Socio-economic history:** Questions pertaining to the family and social life of the individual give an insight into the psychology of the patient. It also allows the therapist to know the financial burdens the family may sustain in case of any expensive intervention if required.
- **Personal history:** History of sleep, appetite, bowel/bladder function, nutrition, smoking, and alcohol use should be noted. The number of pack years may be calculated as relative risk of chronic obstructive pulmonary disorders (COPD), i.e. (average number of packs/day) (number of years smoked).

SUBJECTIVE ASSESSMENT

It is based on an interview with patient and starts with open-ended questions. Five main symptoms of respiratory diseases need to be assessed:

1. Breathlessness
2. Cough
3. Sputum and hemoptysis
4. Wheeze
5. Chest pain

For each of these symptoms, ask about:

- **Duration:** Both absolute time since first recognition (months, years) and duration of present symptoms (days, weeks)
- **Severity:** In absolute terms and relative to recent and distant past
- **Pattern:** Seasonal or daily variation
- Aggravating and relieving factors.

Breathlessness (Dyspnea)

Dyspnea is the subjective awareness of an increased work of breathing and a major symptom of cardiac and respiratory diseases. Dyspnea may be normal in certain circumstances such as high altitude or after vigorous exercise. Dyspnea occurs when the demand for oxygen by the body exceeds the supply.

There are three causes of dyspnea:

1. Increased awareness of normal breathing by the subject
2. Increased work of breathing
3. Abnormal ventilatory system

Increased awareness of normal breathing occurs usually due to anxiety. This may be called **psychogenic dyspnea**. The breathing pattern is irregular with frequent sighing by the individual. It may occasionally be accompanied by tingling and numbness in the hands and feet and numbness around the mouth and lightheadedness.

Lung dysfunction may lead to a compensatory increased activity of the respiratory muscles (increased work of breathing), causing dyspnea. This may be seen

Table 5.2: Pathologies presenting with acute and subacute dyspnea.

Acute dyspnea	Subacute dyspnea
• Pulmonary embolism	• Emphysema
• Pneumothorax	• Pulmonary fibrosis
• Acute asthma	• Chest wall deformities
• Pulmonary congestion (secondary to congestive cardiac failure)	• Respiratory muscle dysfunction
	• Occupational lung diseases
• Pneumonia	• Chronic congestive cardiac failure
• Upper airways obstruction	
	• Severe pleural effusion

in inflammatory or fibrotic lung pathologies, increased cardiac output due to anemia, obstructive disorders of the lung, etc.

The ventilatory apparatus comprises the respiratory muscles, nerves supplying the respiratory muscles, and the thoracic cage. Any abnormality in the ventilatory apparatus also causes dyspnea due to abnormal length–tension relationships and abnormal biomechanics of the chest cavity. This may be seen in kyphoscoliosis, extreme obesity, severe pleural effusion, muscular dystrophy, myasthenia gravis, spinal cord and peripheral nerve injuries, poliomyelitis, etc.

The interviewer needs to ask about the onset and progression of the dyspnea. Dyspnea can be acute or subacute in onset and character. Acute onset of dyspnea usually indicates cardiac failure than chronic respiratory diseases. **Table 5.2** presents different conditions related to acute and subacute dyspnea.

Various outcome measures such as New York Heart Association (NYHA) grading, Borg's scale (RPE), American Thoracic Society (ATS) dyspnea scale, and Visual Analog Scale can be used for the assessment of dyspnea **(Box 5.1)**.

A. NYHA grades of dyspnea:

Grade 1: No symptoms and limitation in ordinary physical activity

Grade 2: Mild symptoms, angina, and slight limitation in ordinary activities

Grade 3: Marked limitation in activity due to symptom, even during less than ordinary activity.

Grade 4: Severe limitation, experience symptoms even at rest mostly bed-bound patient

B. MMRC (Modified Medical Research Council):

Grade 0: No dyspnea except with strenuous exercise

Grade 1: Dyspnea when walking up on the hill or hurrying on the level

Grade 2: Walks slower than most on the level or stops after 15 minutes of walking on the level

Grade 3: Stops after a few minutes of walking on the level

Grade 4: Dyspnea with minimal activity such as getting dressed or too dyspneic to leave the house

C. ATS grades of dyspnea (Table 5.3):

BOX 5.1: Patterns of dyspnea.

- **Acute dyspnea:** If shortness of breath starts suddenly, it is called an acute dyspnea. Acute dyspnea might be secondary to an acute problem.
- **Subacute dyspnea:** It is a chronic progressive pattern of dyspnea that gradually becomes increasingly severe with exertion.
- **Exertional dyspnea:** Dyspnea provoked by physical effort or exertion.
- **Orthopnea:** Shortness of breath occurs when lying flat, causing the person to have to sleep propped up in bed or sitting in a chair.
- **Platypnea:** Shortness of breath is relieved when lying down and worsens when sitting or standing.
- **Trepopnea:** Dyspnea is sensed while lying on one side but not on the other.
- **Paroxysmal nocturnal dyspnea (PND):** PND refers to attacks of severe shortness of breath and coughing that generally occur at night. It usually awakens the person from sleep.
- **Functional dyspnea:** Shortness of breath without apparent underlying disease.

Table 5.3: American Thoracic Society grades of dyspnea.

Grade	Degree	Description
Grade 0	None	No trouble of dyspnea on level/uphill
Grade 1	Mild	Dyspnea on at level/uphill
Grade 2	Moderate	Walks slower than the person of same age
Grade 3	Severe	Tops after 100 yards
Grade 4	Very severe	Breathlessness at rest

Cough

Coughing is a common reflex action that clears the throat of mucus or foreign irritants. Important features are its effectiveness and whether it is productive or dry. Severity ranges from occasional disturbance to continual trouble. Cough can be acute (<3 weeks) or chronic (>8 weeks).

Details pertaining to the coughing need to be asked **(Tables 5.4 and 5.5):**

- Onset of cough—sudden or insidious; association with other symptoms
- Duration of cough and frequency—episodic or persistent, seasonal or perennial
- Severity of cough—duration of each coughing spell and its impact on routine activities and rest
- Productive or dry
- Aggravating and relieving factors
- Change in the pattern of cough in the recent past **(Box 5.2).**

Cough can also be habitual or psychogenic (associated with a throat-clearing sound and disappearing at rest). Diagnosis of psychogenic cough can be made only after an extensive evaluation ruling out all other possible pathologies.

Table 5.4: Characteristics of cough related to pulmonary causes.

Pathology	Characteristics
Pharyngeal infections	Hacking cough associated with soreness of throat and frequent throat clearing
Laryngeal infections	Barking cough with hoarseness of voice and stridor during inspiration
Acute tracheo-bronchitis	Acute self-limited cough associated with runny nose and eyes and soreness of the throat
Pertussis	Paroxysmal productive cough ending with a whooping sound
Chronic bronchitis	Chronic productive cough on most days for <3 consecutive months and for <2 successive years; worse in the morning
Bronchiectasis	Productive cough (copious in amount) with foul-smelling sputum expectoration and occasional hemoptysis
Cystic fibrosis	Chronic cough since early childhood associated with dyspnea and hemoptysis
Tracheal neoplasms	Change in the pattern of cough in a chronic smoker along with hemoptysis
Bronchogenic carcinoma	Nonproductive to productive cough persisting weeks to months; frequent hemoptysis
Alveolar cell carcinoma	Similar to bronchogenic carcinoma
Bronchial asthma	Chronic or recurrent cough; may be associated with wheezing and/or dyspnea
Aspiration	Cough at night with heartburn and difficulty in swallowing
Foreign body	Nonproductive cough with wheezing or evidence of asphyxiation; history of foreign body ingestion
Lobar pneumonia	Dry painful cough in the initial period (preceded by symptoms of upper respiratory tract infections), progressing to productive cough
Bronchopneumonia	Dry or productive cough beginning as acute bronchitis
Viral pneumonia	Paroxysmal cough with mucoid or blood-stained sputum expectoration; flu-like symptoms may be seen
Lung abscess	Sudden onset of cough or change in amount of expectoration (foul-smelling purulent sputum)
TB	Chronic productive cough with occasional hemoptysis; persistent for weeks to months
Pulmonary edema	Acute cough associated with severe dyspnea
Pulmonary thromboembolism	Acute cough associated with dyspnea and hemoptysis
Pleural effusion	Dry cough associated with dyspnea and chest pain
Smoking	Persistent cough marked during morning; slightly productive
Pulmonary infarction	Cough usually associated with hemoptysis and pleural effusion

Table 5.5: Characteristics of cough related to extrapulmonary causes.

Pathology	Characteristics
Drug-induced cough	Dry, annoying, incessant cough; positive drug history of ACE inhibitors, and β blockers
Post-nasal drip syndrome	Chronic cough with associated symptoms such as frequent throat clearing, nasal congestion, hoarseness, and feeling of something dripping at the back of throat
Vocal cord dysfunction	Chronic cough with severe acute dyspnea not responsive to asthma therapy (features mimic asthma)
GERD	Dry or productive cough since 2 months in nonsmokers or those not having environmental irritant exposure with normal or near-normal chest radiograph with a complaint of heartburn; coughing aggravated while lying down and at night
LPR or reflux-induced laryngitis	Dry cough with no exposure to environmental irritants; frequent throat clearing and voice change; coughing aggravated on standing and while eating
CHF	Dry irritating cough, particularly nocturnal (may be confused with asthma or bronchitis); coughing and dyspnea aggravated with supine lying
Acute pericarditis	Non-productive cough with shortness of breath
Aortic aneurysm	Brassy non-productive cough, occasionally associated with chest pain or tenderness, hoarseness of voice or back pain
Mediastinal tumors	Brassy non-productive cough; may be associated with body positions

(ACE: angiotensin-converting enzyme; CHF: chronic heart failure; GERD: gastroesophageal reflux disease; LPR: laryngopharyngeal reflux)

Clinical Pearl

Postoperative strength and effectiveness of cough are important to assess.

Cough complications:
- Chronic cough—fractured ribs (cough fractures), hernias
- Stress incontinence (especially in women)
- Syncope (men, smokers > women, nonsmokers)
- Headache, back pain, muscular tears, hematomas.

Sputum and Hemoptysis

Sputum is the material that is coughed up from the respiratory tract. Small amounts of tracheobronchial secretions that are produced every day are cleared out by the mucociliary clearance mechanism. Approximately 100 mL of tracheobronchial secretions are produced daily and cleared subconsciously. In pathological states, the mucociliary clearance mechanism is inadequate to clear out the secretions due to a change in the quantity or physical characteristics of the secretions.

Sputum consists of two distinct components:
1. Thick mucus material—consisting of mucus, cells, and other cellular material
2. Serous fluid—not containing any cells or cellular material; containing saliva.

The sputum can also contain necrotic tissue, vomitus or other aspirated fluid, foreign particles, and microorganisms. Color, consistency, and quantity of the sputum produced should be determined. It clarifies the diagnosis and severity of disease.

Sputum analysis consists of macroscopic and microscopic assessment as described in **Box 5.2** and **Box 5.3** respectively. **Table 5.6** shows the causes of different sputum findings.

BOX 5.2: Macroscopic assessment of sputum.

Color:
- Normal sputum—mucoid and clear
- Bacterial infections—purulent sputum containing pus
- Inflammation—yellow sputum
- Pneumococcal pneumonia—uniformly rusty appearing purulent sputum
- *Klebsiella pneumoniae* pneumonia—bright red streaks in viscid sputum
- Gram-negative bacilli infections—greenish black sputum.

Odor:
- Normal sputum—odorless
- Bacterial infection—foul smelling sputum

Viscosity:
- Normal sputum—thin and watery
- Asthma—thick, stick, and tenacious sputum

Volume (can be estimated as 1 teaspoon, 1 egg cup, 1/2 cup, 1 cup)
- Normal sputum—less in volume
- Bronchitis, tuberculosis, pneumonia—increased volume of sputum

---

BOX 5.3: Microscopic assessment of sputum.

Charcot–Leyden crystals:
- Double pyramid shaped, elongated mass of eosinophil
- Associated with asthma

Curschmann's spirals:
- Small bronchi casts
- Associated with bronchial obstruction, viz. asthma

Eosinophils: Associated with asthma and similar hypersensitivity disorders.

Neutrophils: Associated with fungal and bacterial pneumonia and chronic bronchitis

Table 5.6: Sputum analysis.

Description	Causes
Green or greenish colored infection	Pneumonia, cystic fibrosis (green from degenerative changes in cell debris)
Rust colored	Pneumococcal bacteria, pulmonary TB
Brownish	Chronic bronchitis (greenish/yellowish/brown), chronic pneumonia (whitish—brown)
Yellowish purulent	Pus—hemophilus
Yellowish-green (mucopurulent)	Treatment with antibiotics that reduce symptoms—bronchiectasis, cystic fibrosis, pneumonia
Whitish gray	Chronic allergic bronchitis
White, milky, or opaque (mucoid)	Viral infection or allergy (asthma)
Foamy white	Earlier phase—pulmonary edema
Frothy pink	Severe pulmonary edema
Black	Black specks in mucoid secretions—smoke inhalation (fires, tobacco, heroin), coal dust

(TB: tuberculosis)

Sputum can be graded macroscopically according to Miller and Jones classification (1963):

- M1: mucoid with no suspicion of pus
- M2: predominantly mucoid, suspicion of pus
- P1: 1/3 purulent, 2/3 mucoid
- P2: 2/3 purulent, 1/3 mucoid
- P3: >2/3 purulent

In clinical practice, it is classified as mucoid, mucopurulent, and purulent.

Hemoptysis is defined as the presence of blood in sputum. The amount of blood may range from little specks to frank blood which may be life threatening. Frank blood in sputum may require bronchial artery embolization or surgery. The timing and frequency of hemoptysis can be used to know the cause.

- Isolated hemoptysis may be the first sign of bronchogenic carcinoma in some patients.
- If the hemoptysis is recurrent, it may be an indication of chronic infective lung diseases, viz. bronchiectasis, tuberculosis (TB), and fungal infection.

The examiner should also inquire about a history of nosebleeds, since nocturnal nose bleed may cause aspiration of the blood at night and expectoration in morning.

The amount of bleeding is also useful in the process of diagnosis.

- Massive hemoptysis is usually seen in lung cancer, TB, bleeding diathesis (during chemotherapy, anticoagulation), and cystic fibrosis.
- Bronchitis and pneumonia are common causes of hemoptysis but usually in small amounts.

Table 5.7: Distinguishing features of stridor and wheeze.

Stridor	Wheeze
Inspiratory	Expiratory
Due to upper airway obstruction	Due to lower airway obstruction
May be caused due to foreign body	May be caused due to asthma, COPD, etc.

(COPD: chronic obstructive pulmonary disorders)

Wheeze

Wheeze is the whistling or musical sound produced by turbulent airflow through narrowed airways. Sometimes, stridor is mistakenly called wheeze **(Table 5.7)**. Wheezing associated with dyspnea usually indicates cardiac or pulmonary pathology.

Adult onset wheezing (>40 years of age) usually points towards heart failure. A childhood onset of wheezing indicates asthma.

Chest Pain

A definitive cause of chest pain cannot be fully established without diagnostic medical tests, but origin can be determined by careful history taking. Chest pain can be of two types:

1. Chest wall pain (superficial, well-localized pain arising from thoracic cage structures)
2. Visceral pain (deep, poorly localized pain arising from visceral structures such as heart, aorta, lungs, pericardium, and mediastinum) **(Table 5.8)**.

Chest wall pain is characterized by local tenderness and pain that varies in intensity and is intermittent. It usually occurs after exertion, unlike cardiac pain that occurs during exertion. Chest wall pain may indicate trauma or fracture of ribs, degenerative disk disease in cervical or thoracic spine, kyphoscoliosis, Pancoast's tumor, herpes zoster or rarely thromboembolism of vein draining the chest wall.

Table 5.8 presents various visceral chest pains that may occur.

Other Symptoms

Apart from the above, following is the list of other symptoms:

- **Incontinence:** It is due to chronic cough. When intra-abdominal pressure increases with coughing, it causes urine leakage. Sometimes due to fear of this, subject will try to suppress cough or not be able to perform strong and effective coughing which may interfere in physiotherapy treatment. So, it should be ruled out and treated if present.
- **Fever:** It is usually due to infection. Low-grade fever is common in pneumonia, malignancy, and bronchitis. Evening fever with sweating occurs in TB.

Table 5.8: Characteristics of various visceral chest pains.

Visceral pain	Characteristics
Pleuritic pain	• Originates from parietal pleura or endothoracic fascia • Sharp, stabbing kind of pain • Aggravated by inspiration (deep breathing, coughing, or laughing)
Tracheitis	• Constant burning pain in center of chest • Aggravated by breathing
Cardiac chest pain	• Build up or escalation of pain • Pain cannot be demonstrated by a single pointing finger but a whole fist or hand (angina sign) • Has a deep component; may be referred superficially
Pulmonary hypertension	• Mimics angina pectoris • Chest pain absent at rest, occurring during exertion; not relieved by sublingual nitrates • Associated with dyspnea
Pericardial pain	• Midline chest pain mimicking pleural involvement • Aggravated with coughing, deep breathing, swallowing, lying down, and movements • Occasional referral of pain to left shoulder or scapula • Relieved by sitting, leaning forward or right side lying
Esophageal pain	• Substernal chest pain, aching or squeezing in character, may radiate to one or both arms, or may radiate to the back • Relieved by sublingual nitrates, antacids or change in position from supine to sitting • Associated with odynophagia, dysphagia, and regurgitation • Precipitated by ingestion of hot or cold fluids, spicy food, or emotional distress

Fever can occur in certain cardiac conditions such as endocarditis.

■ **Headache:** Occurs due to lack of oxygen combined with CO_2 retention. Found in COPD and severe respiratory failure.

■ **Fatigue and weakness**: May be related to physical inactivity, decreased muscle strength, depression, anxiety, emotional distress, anemia, insufficient cardiac output [e.g., in chronic heart failure (CHF)], potassium depletion or hypokalemia (due to ingestion of diuretics), or postural hypotension (caused due to antihypertensives).

■ **Pedal edema:** CHF may lead to bilateral pedal edema. It is also common among patients having renal disorders, liver diseases, and anemia. Thrombophlebitis or varicose veins may lead to unilateral pedal edema.

■ **Hoarseness of voice:** Usually a symptom of laryngeal dysfunction. Possible causes include trauma during

BOX 5.4: Rating of perceived exertion.

Rating of perceived exertion (RPE) is a measure used to assess the extent of exertion felt during exercising or any other activity. It is a subjective measure assessed using the Borg or the modified Borg scale **(Figs. 5.1 and 5.2)**.

RPE scale

6	
7	Very, very light
8	
9	Very light
10	
11	Fairly light
12	
13	Somewhat hard
14	
15	Hard
16	
17	Very hard
18	
19	Very, very hard
20	

Fig. 5.1: Borg scale.

0	Nothing at all
0.5	Very, very slight (just noticeable)
1	Very slight
2	Slight
3	Moderate
4	Somewhat severe
5	Severe
6	
7	Very severe
8	
9	Very, very severe (almost maximal)
10	Maximal

Fig. 5.2: Modified Borg scale.

intubation, laryngeal polyps or tumors, recurrent laryngeal nerve damage due to mediastinal or lung tumors, enlarged mediastinal lymph nodes, aortic aneurysm, or pulmonary artery dilation. **Box 5.4** shows the rating of perceived exertion (RPE) which often accompanies subjective assessment.

OBJECTIVE ASSESSMENT

Each component of the objective assessment can be thought of being divided into four subcomponents:

1. Look
2. Feel
3. Listen
4. Examination

It makes the assessment more organized and time saving and easy to understand. Some important anatomical landmarks for objective assessment are shown in **Box 5.5**.

> **BOX 5.5:** Topographical anatomic landmarks **(Figs. 5.3A to C)**.
> - Midsternal line: vertical line bisecting the sternum
> - Midclavicular lines: vertical lines bisecting the clavicle, lies parallel to the MSL; one for each side—left and right
> - Anterior axillary lines: lines through the anterior axillary fold
> - Midaxillary lines: lines through the midaxillary fold
> - Posterior axillary lines: lines through the posterior axillary fold
> - Midspinal or vertebral line: line passing through the spinous processes of the vertebrae
> - Midscapular lines: lines bisecting inferior angles of scapulae; parallel to midspinal line

Airway

The term "airway" in its day-to-day usage refers to the upper airway which may be defined as the extrapulmonary air passage, consisting of the nasal and oral cavities, pharynx, larynx, trachea and large bronchi **(Fig. 5.4)**. The purpose of the airway component of the objective assessment is to establish the patency of the upper airway. Any deviations or obstruction in the upper airways should be checked.

Maintaining a patent airway is essential for adequate oxygenation and ventilation and failure to do so, even for a brief period of time, can be life-threatening due to hypoxia and subsequent death. **Box 5.6** shows the common causes of airway obstruction.

Airway—Look

Check whether the patient is self-ventilating or using any artificial airways. If the patient is using artificial airway, note the form of artificial airway—nasopharyngeal airway, oropharyngeal airway, endotracheal tube, tracheostomy tube, high flow oxygen mask, oxygen mask, and nasal cannula. Check the following:
- Position of artificial airway
- Patency of artificial airway
- Swelling of mouth and neck
- Other abnormalities in the oral cavity—mouth, teeth, and tongue
- The color of the face, oral mucosa, and lips (central cyanosis—cyanosis of tongue and mouth; caused by hypoxia; may be a late sign of airway obstruction).

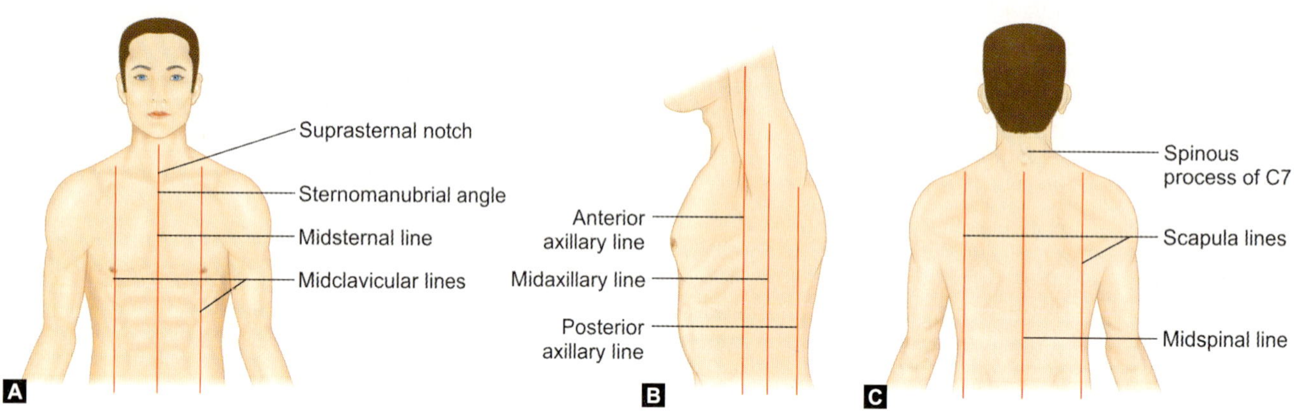

Figs. 5.3A to C: Topographic landmarks of the chest: (A) Anterior; (B) Lateral; (C) Posterior.

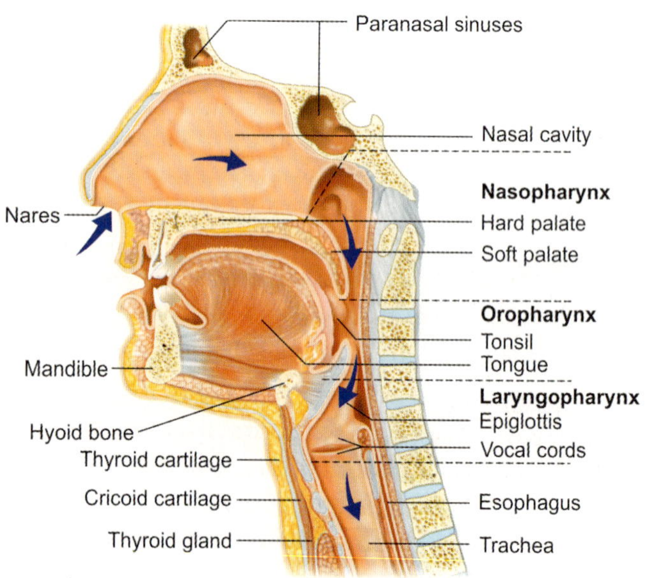

Fig. 5.4: Airway.

> **BOX 5.6:** Common causes of airway obstruction.
> - Altered level of consciousness (LOC) causing pharyngeal obstruction by tongue
> - Inhalation of foreign objects
> - Excessive pulmonary secretions
> - Swelling
> - Invasive tumors

Airway—Feel

Movement of air in and out of airways should be checked by placing hand against airway to feel the flow of air out during expiration. Further, the rise and fall of the chest should be noted.

Tracheal Position

The tracheal position needs to be palpated, as a deviated trachea can obstruct the airflow. Tracheal deviation can be using the following techniques:

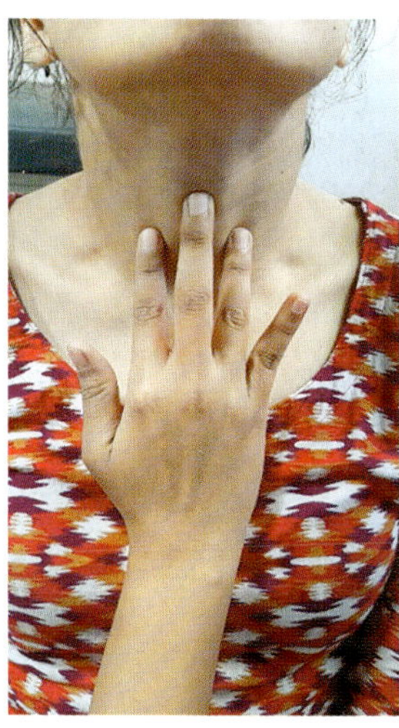

Fig. 5.5: Tracheal position assessment.

- Gently bend the head to relax the sternocleidomastoid (SCM) muscle. By inserting your finger between the trachea and sternomastoid, assess and compare the space on either side. You can measure it with three fingers **(Fig. 5.5)**. Assess and compare the space between the trachea and sternomastoid on either side. Keep the tips of your index and ring fingers over the medial end of the clavicles. Then, with the middle finger, assess the space between the trachea and sternomastoid. Tracheal deviation is a clinical sign and it presents unequal intrathoracic pressure within the chest cavity.
- The physiotherapist places index finger in medial aspect of suprasternal notch and this is repeated on the opposite side. An equal distance between clavicle and trachea should exist bilaterally.

Tracheal deviation indicates mediastinal shift.

- Contralateral deviation: Pneumothorax and pleural effusion
- Ipsilateral deviation: Fibrosis, collapse, and atelectasis.

Airway—Listen

Usually, normal quiet breathing is inaudible at mouth. Airflow sounds differently when airways are blocked, narrowed, or filled with fluid. Several abnormal sounds can be heard at the mouth:

- Gurgling—indicates presence of fluid in upper airway
- Wheezing—indicates presence of obstruction in the lower airway
- Stridor—indicates presence of obstruction in upper airway
- Crowing—indicates laryngeal spasm
- Grunting—indicates flail chest
- Snoring—indicates pharyngeal obstruction by the tongue.

Wheezes are usually louder than the underlying breath sounds and are often audible at the patient's open mouth and occasionally at some distance from the patient. The normal sound of the patient should also be noted by asking the patient some questions, provided the patient is conscious. If the airway is found to be not patent, artificial airway should be inserted taking care of all the necessary precautions.

Breathing

The breathing component includes the assessment of the anatomical and physiological structures related to breathing. Features such as shortness of breath, inability to speak at all or speak in long sentences, and distress during any physical activity should be noted. In critically ill patients, the level of ventilatory support, mode of ventilation, drains (presence and patency), lines and tubes, and presence of any wounds should be noted.

Breathing—Look

Chest Shape

It should be symmetrical with the ribs, in adults, descending at approximately 45° from spine. The ratio of the transverse to anteroposterior (AP) diameter should be noted (normally transverse diameter >AP diameter). The normal transverse to anteroposterior diameter ratio is 7:5. The presence of thoracic kyphosis should be observed.

Common abnormalities:

- Barrel chest (hyperinflation): Increased AP diameter, ribs less oblique, prominent sternal angle, arched sternum; seen in association with kyphosis due to aging or hyperinflation due to pulmonary emphysema **(Fig. 5.6)**.
- Funnel chest (Cobbler's chest, pectus excavatum): Depression in lower part of sternum that may be congenital, following rickets in childhood or occupational deformity in cobblers; due to sternal depression, normal cardiac shadow may appear enlarged on chest X-ray **(Fig. 5.6)**.
- Pigeon chest (pectus carinatum, keeled chest): Sternum displaced anteriorly, depression on either side of sternum associated with bead such as enlargement at costochondral junction (rickety rosary), transverse groove seen passing outward from xiphisternum to midaxillary line (Harrison's sulcus) **(Fig. 5.6)**.
- Thoracic kyphoscoliosis: Spine is curved and thorax shows corresponding deformities; Distortion of underlying lungs—make interpretation of lung findings very difficult **(Fig. 5.7)**.
- Bulging: One side may bulge in pleural effusion, pneumothorax, tumors, aneurysm, empyema, cardiomegaly, or scoliosis.
  Localized bulging: Aortic aneurysm, pericardial effusion, liver abscess, chest wall tumors
- Depression or flattening:
  Localized: One side or any area of chest wall may be depressed or flattened. This is seen in fibrosis, collapse, pleural adhesions, and unilateral muscle wasting due to polio or congenital absence of pectorals.
- Flat chest (phthinoid chest): AP diameter is reduced in chronic nasal obstruction, bilateral TB, or childhood rickets. In advanced TB, scapula is winged and is called alar chest.

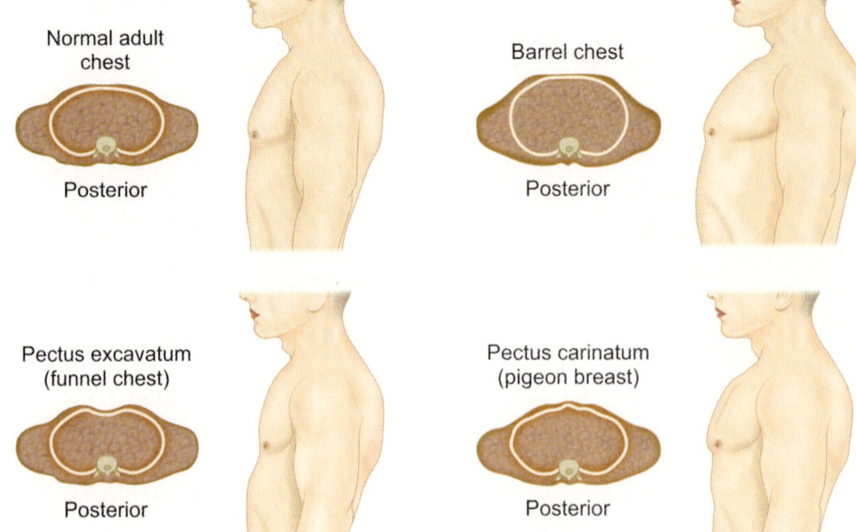

Fig. 5.6: Abnormal shapes of the chest.

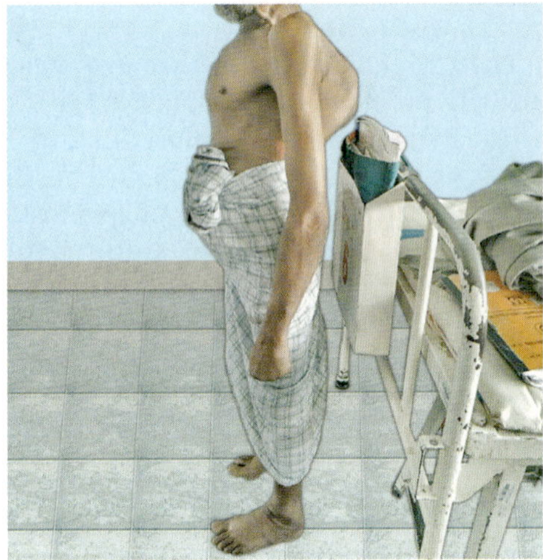

Fig. 5.7: Thoracic kyphoscoliosis.

Chest and Abdominal Movement

Normally, both sides move uniformly and there is no bulging or indrawing. There is uniform and symmetrical increase in the transverse, AP, and vertical diameters.

Abnormalities include:

- Unilateral diminished movement: Obstruction of main bronchus, consolidation, fibrosis of lung, pleural adhesions, massive collapse, hydropneumothorax, pleural effusion
- Bilateral diminished movements: Emphysema, bilateral fibrosis, collapse, consolidation, hydropneumothorax, bronchial asthma, paradoxical breathing
- Abdominal distension: Obesity, ascites, abdominal surgeries, pregnancy
- Intercostal indrawing (intercostal space drawn in during inspiration): Severe inspiratory airflow resistance
- Flail chest (reverse movement of the chest during breathing): Multiple rib fractures

- Hoover sign (paradoxical movement of the lower chest wall): Severe chronic airflow limitation (severe hyperinflation)
- Paradoxical breathing (paradoxical movement of entire chest wall): Bilateral diaphragm weakness or paralysis, e.g., in high cervical spinal cord injury
- Supraclavicular indrawing: Acute asthma.

Breathing Pattern

- Normal breathing should have a regular rate and rhythm.
- The normal respiratory rate (RR) is 12–16 breaths/min.
- The normal inspiratory:expiratory (I:E) ratio lies within a range of 1:1.5–1:2.
- Accessory muscles of respiration should not be used, and there should be no increased work of breathing (observable effort required for respiration).

Types of breathing pattern:

- Males: abdominothoracic
- Females: thoracoabdominal
- Thoracic: diaphragmatic paralysis, peritonitis, ascites
- Abdominal: pleurisy, collapse of lung

Abnormalities in breathing patterns include the ones shown in **Table 5.9**.

Other abnormalities include:

- Sighing respiration: Breathing punctuated by frequent sighs. Occasional sighs are normal.
- Obstructive breathing: I:E = 1:3 or 1:4, prolonged expiration due to increased airway resistance. If RR increases, patient lacks sufficient time for full expiration and air trapping occurs.

Presence of Chest Tubes/Intercostal Drainage Tube

An intercostal drainage (ICD) tube is placed between two ribs into the pleural space to remove air, fluid, or pus. They are used routinely after any cardiothoracic surgery as

Table 5.9: Abnormal breathing patterns.

Breathing pattern	Characteristics	Causes
Tachypnea	Rapid shallow breathing	Restrictive lung diseases, pleuritic chest pain, elevated diaphragm
Hyperpnea, hyperventilation	Rapid deep breathing	Exercise, anxiety, metabolic acidosis in comatose patients, infarction, hypoxia, or hypoglycemia affecting midbrain or pons
Kussmaul breathing	Air hunger	Diabetic ketoacidosis, alcoholic or starvation ketoacidosis and in uremia
Bradypnea	Slow breathing	Secondary to diabetic coma, drug-induced respiratory depression, increased intracranial pressure (ICP)
Cheyne–Stokes breathing	Respiration waxes and wanes cyclically, periods of deep breathing alternate with periods of apnea	Children and aging people show this in sleep, heart failure, uremia, drug-induced respiratory depression, brain damage
Ataxic breathing; also called Biot's breathing	Unpredictable irregularity	Respiratory depression, brain damage, meningitis, increased ICP
Apneustic breathing	Prolonged inspiration and respiration or apnea	Damage to upper portion of pons

postoperative drainage tube. Observation must be made of fluid level within the tube, which should oscillate or swing with every breath.

If it does not swing:

- The tube is not patent or
- Not in proper place or
- No more fluid within pleural place.

If there is continuous suction attached to the tube, it dampens fluid swing.

Breathing—Feel

Chest Expansion

A note of the amount and symmetry of the chest expansion should be made. The chest expansion is normally symmetrical on both sides.

Measurement Technique

Chest expansion is measured by placing thumbs posteriorly about at the level of and parallel to 10th ribs, with hands grasping lateral rib cage. Slide hands medially a bit, to raise loose skin folds between thumbs and spine. Ask patient to inhale deeply. Watch divergence of thumbs during inspiration and feel for range and symmetry. Both sides should move equally—3–5 cm. Similar technique may be used anteriorly to measure basal movements. Measurement of apical movement is more difficult. It is done by placing the hand over upper chest anteriorly and a qualitative comparison of two sides can be made. Additionally, chest expansion can be examined using measure tape technique. This can be done at three levels—axilla, nipple, and xiphisternum—to assess all the three zones **(Figs. 5.8A to C).**

Diaphragmatic Excursion

Diaphragmatic movement during breathing can be assessed using mediate percussion.

Technique: The patient is asked to take a deep breath and hold. Percussion is performed—the lowest point of resonant note on percussion is the lowest level of diaphragm. The patient then exhales out and percussion is repeated. The lowest level of resonant note is again noted. The level of diaphragm moves up. The distance between these two points denotes the diaphragmatic excursion (normal 3–5 cm).

Tenderness

Areas of tenderness can be assessed for degree of discomfort and reproducibility. Differentiation of chest pain either due to angina or musculoskeletal origin can be made.

Subcutaneous Air

Air in subcutaneous tissues of chest, neck, or face produces crackling in skin on palpation. It may be due to an air leak from a chest tube.

Tactile Vocal Fremitus (TVF)

Fremitus refers to palpable vibrations transmitted through bronchopulmonary system to the chest wall when patient speaks. Ask patient to repeat words "99" or "one-one-one." If fremitus is faint, ask to speak more loudly. Palpate and compare symmetrical areas of lungs, using either ball of hand (bony part of palms at base of fingers) or ulnar surface of hand. Identify, describe, and localize areas of increased or decreased fremitus.

It is typically more prominent in interscapular area than in lower lung fields. It is more prominent on the right side than the left side.

- Disappears below diaphragm
- Reduced or absent over precordium
- Reduced or absent when voice is soft
- Pathological reduced or absent fremitus: When transmission of vibration from larynx to surface of chest is impeded.
  Causes: Obstructed bronchus, COPD, pleural effusion, fibrosis, pneumothorax, infiltrating tumors, thick chest wall.
- Pathological increased fremitus: when increased transmission.
  Causes: Consolidated lung.

Box 5.7 shows palpation to examine breathing.

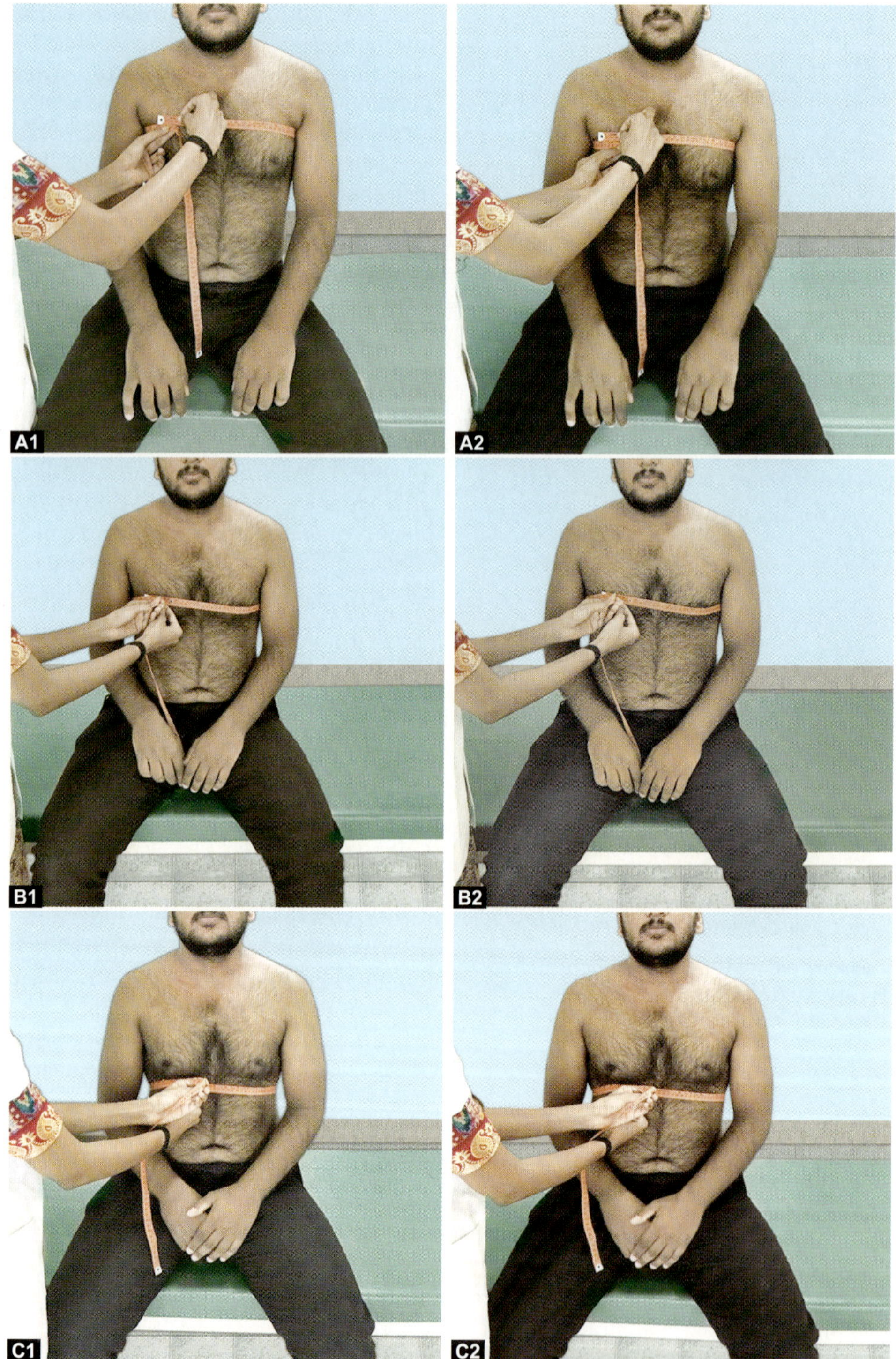

Figs. 5.8A to C: Measurement of chest expansion: (A) At axilla; (B) At nipple level; (C) At xiphisternum—(A1, B1, C1) inspiration and (A2, B2, C2) expiration.

BOX 5.7: Palpation to examine breathing.

- **Pleural fremitus**—palpable vibration of the chest caused due to rubbing of the two pleural layers
- **Tussive fremitus**—palpable vibration of the chest during coughing
- **Rhonchal or bronchial fremitus**—palpable vibration of the chest caused due to movement of air through large partially obstructed airways.

Breathing—Listen

Speech

It should be noted that whether the speech is fluent or the subject needs to take frequent breaks when speaking due to breathlessness.

Cough

Coughing is a forceful expiratory act. The quality of cough (strong, weak, painful, etc.) needs to be assessed.

It can even signify the location of irritant—depending on whether it is a repetitive small cough, 2–3 bouts of large coughs or a single bout of strong cough.

Percussion

Percussion is the method of tapping against the chest wall to assess the underlying structures. It sets the chest wall and underlying tissues into motion, producing audible sounds and palpable vibrations. The normal percussion note of the chest is due to the underlying lung tissue containing normal amount of air in the lung tissues. It has distinct clear character with low pitch.

Technique for right-handed person:

- Hyperextend the middle finger of left hand—pleximeter finger
- Press its distal interphalangeal joint (DIP) firmly on surface to be percussed
- Avoid contact by any other part of hand, it would damp vibrations
- Position right forearm quite close to the surface with hand cocked upward
- Right middle finger should be partially flexed, relaxed and poised to strike—plexor
- With a quick, sharp but relaxed wrist motion, strike pleximeter finger with plexor (right). Aim at DIP joint.

Use the lightest percussion that will produce a clear note. A thick chest wall requires heavier percussion. Thump about twice in one location and then move on. Sounds will be better perceived by comparing one area with another than repetitive thumping. Posterior thorax can be percussed, while patient keeps both arms crossed in front of chest. While percussing lower posterior chest, stand somewhat to side rather than directly behind patient.

The front of the chest yields a more resonant note than back because of lesser bulk of musculature in front than at back.

Different notes can be heard on percussion.

- Impaired note: When the amount of air in alveoli decreases as in consolidation, infiltration, fibrosis, and collapse of lung, the lungs fail to vibrate sufficiently to the percussion stroke. Loss of resonance results in an impaired note.
- Dull note: An impaired note of greater degree is a dull note. It is found in consolidation, infiltration, fibrosis, collapse, and plural thickening.
- Stony dull note: A percussion note completely devoid of resonance or displaying extreme dullness is a stony dull note. It is classically found in pleural effusion because

Clinical Pearl

Vibrations transmit through the bones of this joint to underlying chest wall. Use tip of plexor, not pad. Plexor should be right angle to pleximeter. Withdraw the plexor quickly to avoid damping the vibrations that are created. Movement should be at wrist—it should be direct, brisk yet relaxed, and little bouncy.

fluid dampens the vibration of both the chest wall and underlying lung. It may also occur in lung fibrosis with pleural thickening or with solid intrathoracic tumor.

- Tympany: This is a drum-like resonance that is normally encountered over stomach, intestines, larynx, and trachea. When it occurs over chest wall, it may be due to pneumothorax, superficial empty cavity, and emphysema.
- Subtympany: A hyperresonant note with a boxy quality that occurs due to relaxed lung just above level of pleural effusion.
- Hyperresonance: A note in between normal resonance and tympany can be elicited over normal lung tissue by keeping the chest wall in full inspiration during percussion. It occurs in pneumothorax, emphysema, large cavity, congenital lung cyst, and emphysematous bullae.
- Bell tympany: This is a high-pitched tympanic sound, heard over the chest in case of massive pneumothorax. When a silver coin is placed on the affected side and percussed with a second silver coin, the ear or stethoscope applied over the opposite side of chest may detect a clear bell-like sound.
- Kronig's isthmus: This is a band of resonance 5–7 cm in width, connecting lung resonance over the anterior and posterior aspects of each side of chest. It is bounded medially by dullness of neck muscle and laterally by dullness of shoulder muscles.

  Abnormalities:
  - Absence on either side suggests pulmonary fibrosis due to TB
  - Increased width of resonance suggests emphysema.
- Normal dullness:

Liver dullness and span: It is over right side, 5th intercostal space in midclavicular, seventh space in midaxillary and ninth space in midscapular line. It may be present in fourth intercostal space at midclavicular line in pyogenic abscess of liver, diaphragmatic paralysis, collapse of lower lobe of lung. It may be pushed down to sixth intercostal space in midclavicular line in emphysema, right-sided pneumothorax, air in peritoneal cavity, terminal cirrhosis.

Cardiac dullness: On the left side of chest wall, the lung resonance is encroached by an area of cardiac dullness. Normal cardiac dullness is in third and fourth left parasternal line, fifth left midclavicular line. This area of dullness may be decreased in emphysema, left-sided pneumothorax. It may be increased with cardiomegaly and shifting of heart to left side.

Tidal percussion: Percussion of upper border of liver dullness on right side anteriorly on inspiration and expiration serves to determine the range of lung expansion. It is restricted in pulmonary diseases at lungs bases, empyema, and subdiaphragmatic abscess.

Shifting dullness: In the case of hydropneumothorax in sitting position, there is a hyperresonant note above followed by dullness below. On changing the posture to supine, this area of dullness of fluid changed as air and fluid will shift. This is shifting dullness and signifies presence of both air and fluid.

Percussion myokymia: In a chronically wasted individual as in pulmonary TB, a percussion stroke over the front of chest close to sternum may cause transient twitching of muscles that is more marked on side of pulmonary affection.

Limitation of percussion:

- It is not possible to percuss deeper than 5 cm; hence, it is not possible to detect a lung lesion covered by a layer of air or fluid > 5 cm thick.
- A lesion < 2 cm in diameter does not cause any change in percussion note.
- Free fluid < 200 mL in pleural cavity may not be detected on percussion.

Auscultation (Box 5.8)

> **BOX 5.8:** Auscultation.
>
> Auscultation is the art of listening to sound produced by the body with the help of stethoscope. Auscultation can be performed for:
> - **Breath sounds**—normal, abnormal, adventitious
> - **Voice sounds**—egophony, bronchophony, whispered pectoriloquy
> - **Extrapulmonary sounds**—pleural rub
> - **Heart sounds**

Breath Sounds

Breath sounds can be heard using auscultation. There are 10 and 9 sites, respectively, for posterior and anterior chest walls for auscultation. The auscultatory sequence should be followed for better examination of the breath sounds. Three kinds of breath sounds can be heard during auscultation—normal, abnormal (including voice sounds), and adventitious sounds.

Technique: The subject should be sitting, leaning forward slightly. They should be asked to breathe deeper than normal for several respiratory cycles through the mouth. The breath sounds should then be heard using the stethoscope following the auscultatory sequence **(Figs. 5.9A and B)**. Each site should be auscultated for one complete breath, and comparison should be made with the same site on the other side. Start with the lung apex on the posterior chest wall and sequentially move caudally. Next, move to the lateral and anterior chest walls. Auscultation should also be done over the mouth, sternum, and larynx for better evaluation of the tracheal sounds **(Box 5.9)**.

Normal breath sounds: Normal breath sounds can be classified as tracheal, bronchial, vesicular, and bronchovesicular **(Table 5.10)**.

As therapist auscultates from top to bottom, the breath sound is quieter at the bases than at the apices. Infants and children have louder, harsher breath sounds as a result of thinness of chest wall and the airways being closer to its surface.

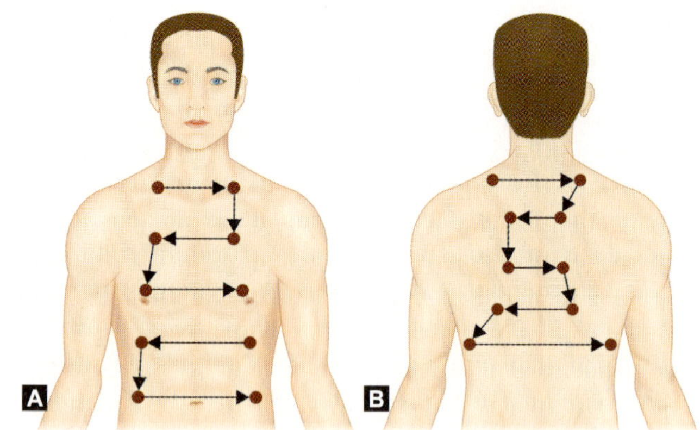

Figs. 5.9A and B: Auscultation of breath sounds. (A) Anterior view; (B) Posterior view.

> **BOX 5.9:** Auscultation of bed-ridden patients.
>
> Debilitated, comatose, or bed-ridden patients can be auscultated by turning them on their sides. In such patients, auscultation should be done first over the dependent regions of the lung, as secretions or fluids tend to collect in the gravity-dependent areas, producing abnormal sounds in these regions, which may disappear when the patient is turned to the other side.

Table 5.10: Normal breath sounds.

Breath sounds	Characteristics
Tracheal and bronchial sounds	High-pitched sounds produced by turbulent flow over the trachea and bronchi throughout inspiration and expiration; pause exists between inspiration and expiration phase
Vesicular breath sounds	Faint sound heard over remaining peripheral lung fields having primarily an inspiratory component with only initial one-third of expiratory phase audible; intensity is softer because of dampening caused by spongy lung tissue
Bronchovesicular breath sounds	High-pitched sound (pitch midway between bronchial and vesicular sounds) heard in areas between the bronchi and smaller airways; equal inspiratory and expiratory cycles, differentiating feature is lack of pause; heard best where bronchi or central lung tissue is close to the surface (superior to clavicle, suprascapular, parasternal, and interscapular areas)

Abnormal breath sounds: Abnormal breath sounds can be described as when sound transmission changes as a result of underlying pathologic process. Sound transmission is enhanced when liquid or solid is the medium.

Abnormal breath sounds can be divided into:

- Bronchial
- Decreased
- Absent

Bronchial sounds: Bronchial sounds are normally heard over the bronchi. However, in pathological processes, these sounds can be considered abnormal when they are heard over the chest wall through the peripheral lung tissues when it becomes airless (due to accumulation of fluid, secretions, etc.). In consolidation type of pneumonia where the lung tissue is airless, sound from adjacent bronchi is enhanced and becomes higher pitched and expiratory component becomes louder and more pronounced. A consolidated lung provides a better medium for transmission of sounds, and hence, they can be heard louder over the lung fields. Compression of lung tissue from extrapulmonary source also produces bronchial sounds, e.g., compression due to increased pleural fluid (pleural effusion), tumor. The I:E ratio changes to 1:1–1:2.

Pathological conditions: Atelectasis, fibrosis, pleural effusion, consolidation, lung collapse.

Decreased or absent breath sounds: Decreased breath sounds are normal vesicular sounds which are further diminished. Absent breath sounds are when no sounds are audible. Breath sounds can be reduced or absent when transmission of sound is diminished or abolished. It occurs in conditions where the transmission of airflow into lungs is limited or in pathologies affecting the pleurae or obese individuals where there may be a reflection of the breath sounds at the parietal or visceral pleura. Decreased or absent breath sounds can be caused by internal pulmonary pathology or can be secondary to nonpulmonary pathology. Hyperinflation caused by emphysema causes decreased sound transmission as a result of loss of normal structure.

Pathological conditions:
- Diaphragmatic paralysis
- Airway obstruction
- Pneumothorax
- Pleural effusion
- Pulmonary fibrosis
- Flung hyperinflation
- Use of positive end-expiratory pressure (PEEP) during assisted ventilation

Extra-pulmonary causes include:
- Tumors
- Obesity
- Neuromuscular weakness (muscular dystrophy)
- Musculoskeletal deformity (kyphoscoliosis)
- Pain

Adventitious breath sounds: They are extraneous sounds produced over the bronchopulmonary tree. The classification of adventitious sounds is rather a tricky one. It is difficult to classify the sound heard into any specific category; however, the classification suggested by the International Lung Sound Association (ILSA) can guide the novice examiner through the process. The adventitious sounds were previously classified into continuous and discontinuous or interrupted sounds. Continuous sounds were further classified as high- and low-pitched wheezes; discontinuous sounds were classified as coarse, medium, and fine crackles. The ILSA simplified the process and classified the continuous sounds into wheeze and rhonchi and the discontinuous sounds into fine and coarse crackles **(Fig. 5.10 and Table 5.11)**.

Continuous adventitious sounds: These are abnormal sounds superimposed over normal breath sounds. They possess a duration of >250 ms. They can be further divided as—high pitched (wheeze, stridor, and gasp) and low pitched (rhonchi and squawk).

Features of high-pitched continuous adventitious sounds are:

Wheeze:
- Continuous, high pitched musical tone.
- Dominant frequency of 400 Hz or more.
- Hissing or whistling quality.
- Heard during expiration; occasionally may occur during inspiration or may be biphasic.
- Caused due to air vibrating in a narrowed airway.
- Occasionally heard at patient's mouth.
- Can be classified as high or low pitched, monophonic (single pitch) or polyphonic (multiple pitch), localized or widespread.
- Monophonic wheeze indicates single obstructed airway; polyphonic wheeze indicates widespread airway narrowing.
- It is an indication of bronchospasm, foreign bodies, airway thickening caused by mucosal edema or muscle hypertrophy and sputum accumulation.

Stridor:
- Has a hissing and musical quality.
- High pitch—500 Hz or more.
- Heard during inspiration, occasionally may occur during expiration, or may be biphasic.
- Unlike wheeze, stridor is generated due to turbulent airflow in the larynx or bronchial tree.
- Suggestive of upper airway obstruction.
- Indication of croup, epiglottis or laryngeal edema or foreign body in upper airway tract.

Gasp:
- Inspiratory gasps occur post coughing when the patient tries to breathe in.
- Whoop sound of inspiratory gasp may be created when air moves rapidly into the respiratory tract.
- High pitch, long duration.
- Whoop sound pathognomonic of whooping cough (pertussis).

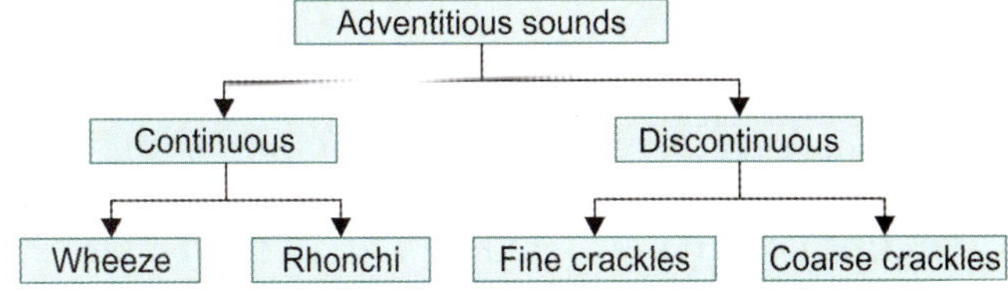

Fig. 5.10: Types of adventitious breath sounds.

Table 5.11: Adventitious breath sounds.

Adventitious breath sound	Phase	Quality	Causes	Pathologies
Wheeze	Inspiratory, mostly expiratory, biphasic	Sibilant, musical	Airflow limitation, airway narrowing	Asthma, foreign body, COPD
Rhonchi	Inspiratory, mostly expiratory, biphasic	Sibilant, musical	Bronchial secretion, mucosal thickening	COPD, bronchitis
Stridor	Inspiratory	Sibilant, musical	Upper airway obstruction, turbulent airflow in laryngeal or lower bronchial tree	Epiglottis, foreign body, croup, laryngeal edema
Fine crackle	Late inspiration	Nonmusical, explosive	Explosive opening of small airways	Pneumonia, lung fibrosis, congestive heart failure
Coarse crackle	Early inspiration, expiration or both	Nonmusical, explosive	Air bubble in large bronchial segments	COPD, chronic bronchitis, bronchiectasis
Pleural rub	Biphasic	Nonmusical, rhythmic	Rubbing of pleurae against each other	Pleuritis, pleural tumor
Gasp	Inspiratory	Whoop	Gasping for breath	Whooping cough
Squawk	Inspiratory	Short musical, nonmusical	Oscillation of peripheral airways	Hypersensitivity pneumonia, common pneumonia

(COPD: chronic obstructive pulmonary disorder)

Rhonchi:
- Low-pitched wheezes
- Dominant frequency of 200 Hz or less
- Heard both during inspiration and expiration
- Has a snoring quality
- Attributed to obstructive process in the larger more central airways, e.g., COPD and asthma.

Squawk:
- Heard during inspiratory phase
- Mix of musical and nonmusical sound
- 200–300 Hz pitch
- Suggestive of hypersensitivity pneumonia, or sometimes common pneumonia.

Discontinuous adventitious sounds: Adventitious sounds with duration <25 ms. They can be further classified based on the source of generation as fine and coarse crackles and pleural rub.

Crackles:
- Discontinuous, intermittent, explosive popping or clicking, nonmusical sounds
- Low-pitched sound
- Heard predominantly on inspiration
- Similar to sound of rubbing hair between fingers or Velcro popping
- Can be classified as fine or coarse; localized or widespread; early or late
- Fine crackles are brief, soft, and high pitched
- Coarse crackles are brief (although slightly longer than fine crackles), loud, and low pitched **(Table 5.12)**
- Localized crackles may occur in dependent alveoli.
- Pathological mechanism: air bubbling through secretions and sudden opening of closed small airways during inspiration leading to a transient airway vibration.
- Indicate a peripheral airway process.

Table 5.12: Distinguishing features between fine and coarse crackles.

Fine crackles	Coarse crackles
Explosive opening of small airways	Generated by air bubbles in large bronchi
Nonmusical, high pitch around 650 Hz	Low pitch around 350 Hz
Heard only during late inspiration	Heard during early inspiration or during expiration
Not heard at mouth	Heard at mouth
Altered by body position change; unaltered by coughing	Altered by coughing; unaltered by body position change
Associated with pneumonia, congestive heart failure, and lung fibrosis	Associated with chronic bronchitis, COPD and bronchiectasis

(COPD: chronic obstructive pulmonary disorder)

Pleural rub **(Table 5.13)**:
- Non-musical short grating, rubbing, creaky sounds
- Low pitch below 350 Hz
- Present during both phases of respiration
- Caused due to friction between both the pleural surfaces
- Suggestive of pleural inflammation or tumor.

Voice Sounds

These are vibrations produced during speech; they are transmitted to the chest wall through the tracheobronchial tree **(Table 5.14 and Box 5.10)**.

Breathing—Examination

Respiratory Rate

Respiratory rate (RR) is the number of respiratory cycles in 1 minute; 12–16 breaths/min are measured with patient

Table 5.13: Distinguishing features between pleural rub and crackles.

Pleural rub	Crackles
Biphasic	Inspiratory or expiratory or biphasic
Localized to small area	Widespread
Palpable	Nonpalpable
Unaltered by coughing	Altered by coughing
Sound intensified by pressure of stethoscope	No effect by pressure of stethoscope
Associated with pleuritic chest pain or tenderness	Not associated with tenderness or pain

Table 5.14: Voice sounds.

Voice sounds	Characteristics
Bronchophony	Voice sounds auscultated over chest wall Normal—same as the sound heard through the neck
Egophony	Voice sounds having slightly higher pitch than bronchophony; auscultated over the chest wall
Whispered pectoriloquy	High-pitched whispers transmitted through airless, consolidated lung

BOX 5.10: Techniques to auscultate voice sounds.

Bronchophony
- Patient is asked to repeat words "ninety nine"
- Normal lung tissue—words are unintelligible
- Consolidated lung—words easily understood

Egophony
- Patient is asked to say "E"
- Normal lung tissue—"e" heard as "e"
- Consolidated lung—"e" heard as "A-aay"

Whispered pectoriloquy
- Patient is asked to whisper words "1-2-3"
- Normal lung tissue—words are unintelligible
- Consolidated lung-sounds become distinct and clear

seated comfortably. RR may be affected due to several factors such as age, body size, stature, body position, and exercise **(Table 5.15)**.

- Tachypnea: RR>20, seen in lung diseases, metabolic acidosis, anxiety
- Bradypnea: RR<10, CNS depression by narcotics or trauma

Along with the rate, the depth and rhythm of respiration should also be noted.

Oxygen Saturation (SaO_2 and SpO_2)

It is the percentage of oxygenated hemoglobin compared to the total amount of hemoglobin in the blood. Normal values range from 96 to 99%. It can be measured invasively with arterial blood gas (ABG) analysis (called SaO_2) and noninvasively with pulse oximeter (called SpO_2). Oxygen saturation does not reflect the oxygenation of tissues or the patient's ability to ventilate.

Table 5.15: Factors affecting respiratory rate (RR).

Factor	Characteristics
Age	• Newborn—30–90 breaths/min • Adults—12–16 breaths/min • Increases in elderly individuals due to loss of elasticity, weakness of respiratory muscles, reduced thoracic mobility, and reduced lung volume
Body size and stature	Men have lower RR than women; adults have lower RR than children
Exercise	RR increases with exercise
Body position	Increased RR in recumbent position
Stress/emotional status	Increased RR during stressful and emotional states
Environment	Increased RR at high altitudes, with exposure to pollutants, certain gases, etc.
Drugs	• Decreased RR with central nervous system (CNS) depressing drugs, e.g., narcotics and barbiturates • Increased RR with bronchodilators

Pulse Oximetry

Pulse oximetry is used to determine the oxygenation level of the arterial blood with each pulse non-invasively using a pulse oximeter. Beurer's high quality ECG device and pulse oximeter are more reliable than portable devices as shown in **Figures 5.11A and B** for monitoring the values. Normal levels lie in the range of 96–100%. Values lower than 90% are considered significant and warrant urgent attention.

- Hypoxemia—deficient oxygenation of blood
- Hypoxia—deficient oxygenation of tissues
- Anoxia—complete lack of oxygen.

Pulse oximetry can be used to:

- Identify hypoxemia
- Monitor the patient during activity
- Evaluate patient response to treatment.

Arterial Blood Gases

It is an invasive technique that determines the pH, partial pressure of oxygen (PaO_2), partial pressure of carbon

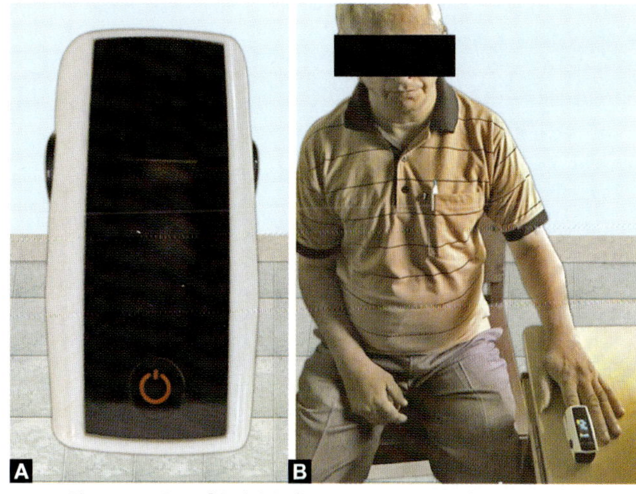

Figs. 5.11A and B: (A) Pulse oximeter; (B) Pulse oximetry.

Table 5.16: Normal arterial blood gases (ABG) parameters.

ABG parameters	Normal values
pH	7.35–7.45
$PaCO_2$	35–45 mm Hg
PaO_2	80–100 mm Hg
HCO_3^-	22–26 mmol/L
Base excess	−2 to +2

dioxide ($PaCO_2$), bicarbonate concentration (HCO_3), and base excess (BE) values. Blood is drawn from any of the major arteries and the following values are determined **(Table 5.16)**.

Pulmonary Function Tests

It helps in the evaluation of the mechanical function of the lungs **(Fig. 5.12)**. They are based on research norms such as gender, height, and age.

Predicted values → compare with actual values → result → normal/obstructive/restrictive components

Pulmonary function tests (PFTs) are categorized as volume, flow, or diffusion studies (helium dilution, nitrogen washout, plethysmography, spirometry). By interpreting a patient's pulmonary function test diagnosis of pulmonary disease, dysfunction and improvement with treatment will be evaluated.

Respiratory Muscle Strength

Respiratory muscle strength can be assessed by measuring the maximal inspiratory pressure (MIP or $P_i$max), and the maximal expiratory pressure (MEP or $P_e$max). The MIP reflects the strength of the diaphragm and other inspiratory muscles, while the MEP reflects the strength of the abdominal muscles and other expiratory muscles. A well-validated alternative or additional test of inspiratory muscle strength is maximal sniff nasal inspiratory pressure (SNIP). Common indications for measurement of the MIP, SNIP, and MEP include:

- Respiratory muscle weakness is suspected, such as in a patient with known neuromuscular disease, a weak cough, or unexplained dyspnea (particularly orthopnea).
- Lung function tests show reduced vital capacity or an increased diffusion capacity of unknown etiology.
- Evaluation of whether known respiratory muscle weakness has improved, remained stable, or worsened.

Thoracic Imaging

Chest radiographs, high-resolution computed tomography, ultrasonography help in finding out extent and severity of disease.

Bronchoscopy

Bronchoscopy is a procedure to look at the lungs and air passages. It is usually performed by a doctor who specializes in lung disorders (a pulmonologist). During bronchoscopy, a thin tube (bronchoscope) is passed through the nose or mouth, down to throat and into the lungs. By visualization of air passages and by taking **bronchoalveolar lavage**, it will help to diagnose lung diseases.

Circulation

This section includes the assessment of the anatomical and physiological components related to cardiovascular system.

Circulation—Look

Skin Color

Check for skin color changes such as pale or blue discoloration. This may be due to anemia or cyanosis. Usually, central cyanosis is seen over tongue and eyes while peripheral cyanosis over distal extremities.

Skin Turgor

It is skin's ability to deform and return to its normal elastic state. It is assessed by pinching the skin at the back of hand and observing how quickly it returns to normal. Prolonged skin tenting is suggestive of dehydration.

Jugular Venous Pressure

On the side of neck, it is seen as flickering impulse in jugular vein. It is normally seen at base of neck when

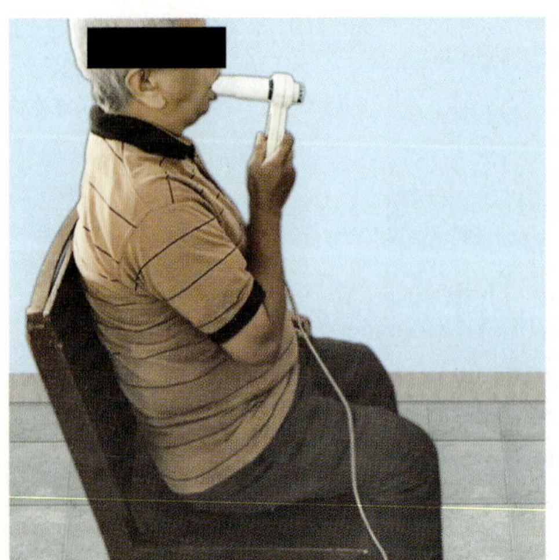

Fig. 5.12: Pulmonary function testing (PFT) with spirometry.

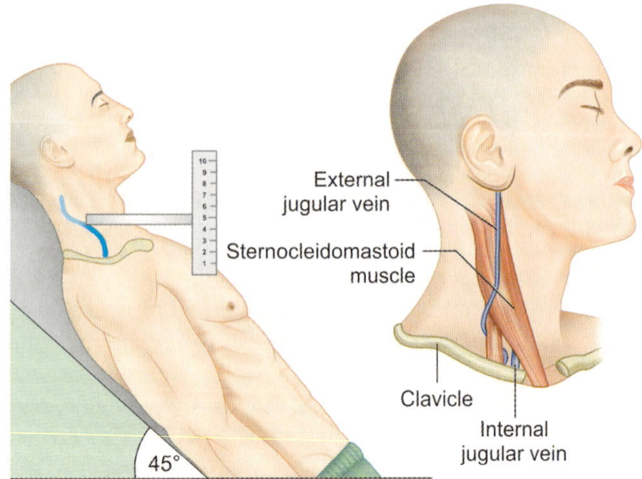

Fig. 5.13: Jugular venous pressure.

lying back at 45° (**Fig. 5.13**). It is measured in relation to sternal angle. Normal jugular venous pressure at the base of neck corresponds to a vertical height approximately 3–4 cm above sternal angle. It provides a quick assessment of volume of blood in great vessel entering the heart.

It is elevated in right heart failure, constrictive pericarditis, superior vena cava obstruction, and chronic lung diseases, complicated by cor pulmonale.

Peripheral Edema

It is usually a sign of chronic cardiac failure. But also found in low albumin, impaired lymphatic function or drug side effects.

Circulation—Feel

Temperature

Local as well as body temperature should be determined.

- **Body temperature:** Body temperature presents as a balance between the heats produced and lost.
  - The normal body temperature is 98.6°F or 37°C.
  - Fever or pyrexia refers to an increase in body temperature. Unusually high temperatures (>106°F) are termed hyperthermia or hyperpyrexia. For every 0.6° rise in temperature—10% increase in O_2 consumption and CO_2 production. This places extra demand on CV system and so compensatory rise in HR and RR.
  - Lowered body temperatures are referred to as hypothermia.

  Body temperature is influenced by several factors—time of the day, age, menstrual cycle, stress, emotional status, external environment, pregnancy, measurement site, etc. The instrument used to measure the temperature is called a thermometer. Body temperature can be measured at various sites—oral, rectal, tympanic, axillary, etc. (**Fig. 5.14**).
- **Local temperature:** Palpate the extremities to evaluate the local temperature. Cold and pale limbs are suggestive of poor peripheral perfusion and cardiovascular affection, while warm extremities are seen in febrile septic patients.

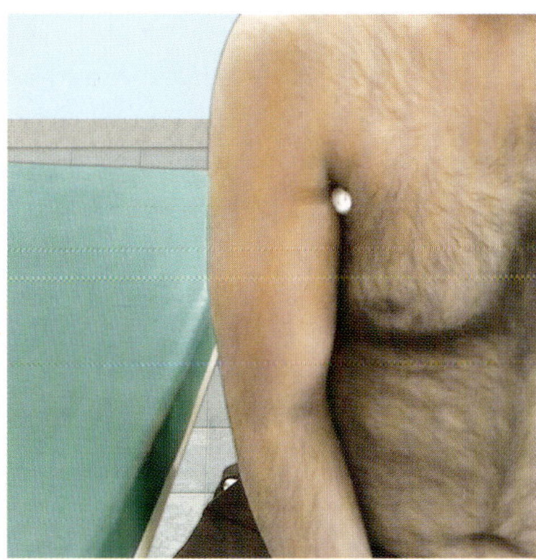

Fig. 5.14: Measurement of axillary temperature.

Peripheral Pulses

The superficial artery can be checked to feel for pulsation such as radial, brachial, carotid, and femoral. Reduced pulse suggests poor cardiac output. Right and left pulses should be checked and compared to determine coarctation of aorta or obstructive arterial disease. Dorsalis pedis artery should palpate to determine the integrity of distal blood flow. It should be palpated on the superior surface of the foot lateral to the tendon of the great toe.

Pulse Rate

When the radial pulse is used to count the heart rate (HR) the three-finger method should be used. Place the pads of three middle fingers over the artery. Where proximal (index) finger obliterates, distal (ring) finger empties the vessel (milking) and middle finger palpates, feel the vessel wall. If rhythm—regular, rate—normal, count for 15 seconds. If rate—unusually fast or slow, count for 60 seconds. The normal rate is 60–100 beats/min.

Tachycardia: HR>100 beats/min at rest. It is seen in:

- Anxiety
- Exercise
- Fever
- Anemia
- Hypoxia
- Cardiac diseases
- Even with bronchodilators and some cardiac drugs.

Bradycardia: HR<60 beats/min. Normal finding in athletes. Some cardiac drugs, e.g. beta-blockers cause bradycardia.

Palpitation: Feeling of irregular or rapid HR perceived by the patient without palpating the pulse.

Pulse Rhythm and Quality

The pulse should be assessed for rhythm and quality. In rhythm check either the rhythm is regular or irregular. Any additional or missed beat should be noted. In quality either the pulse is strong enough or it is feeble pulse.

- A significant decrease in pulse amplitude during inspiration known as *pulsus paradoxus* occurs in pericarditis or cardiac tamponade.
- A large volume pulse followed by a small volume pulse in repeating order known as *pulsus alternans* which is sign of severe cardiac failure.
- A collapsing pulse with an early peak is a sign of aortic regurgitation.

Circulation—Listen

Auscultation of the heart requires excellent hearing and the ability to distinguish subtle differences in pitch and timing with the help of stethoscope. High-pitched sounds are best heard with the diaphragm of the stethoscope. Low-pitched sounds are best heard with the bell. Major auscultatory findings include heart sounds and murmurs.

Heart sounds are brief, transient sounds produced by valve opening and closure; they are divided into systolic and diastolic sounds.

> **BOX 5.11:** Heart sounds.
> - S1 is caused by the closure of the mitral and tricuspid valves.
> - S2 is caused by the closure of the aortic and pulmonic valves.
> - The third heart sound (S3), when audible, occurs early in ventricular filling. This sound is normal in children, but when heard in adults, it is often associated with ventricular dilation as occurs in systolic ventricular failure.
> - The fourth heart sound (S4), when audible, is caused by vibration of the ventricular wall during atrial contraction. This sound is heard in patients with ventricular hypertrophy, myocardial ischemia, or in older adults.

There are four discrete positions to listen to heart sounds **(Box 5.11)**:

1. First position (aortic) is between the second and third intercostal space at the right sternal border (S1).
2. The second (pulmonic) is between the second and third intercostal space at the left sternal border (S2).
3. Mitral sound at the fifth left intercostal space over the midclavicular line (S3).
4. Tricuspid sound at the fourth left intercostal space lateral to the sternum (S4).

Murmurs are produced by blood flow turbulence and are more prolonged than heart sounds. They may be systolic, diastolic, or continuous.

Intensity describes the loudness of the murmur on a scale of 1–6, as indicated by Levine's six-point grading scale **(Table 5.17)**.

Circulation—Examination

Blood Pressure

Contraction of the heart (systole) increases the mean arterial blood pressure (systolic BP) and relaxation of the heart causes a fall in the mean arterial BP (diastolic BP).

Normal BP: 119/79 mm Hg. Measured using sphygmo-manometer (mercury).

Technique of measurement:

- Patient should be comfortable, relaxed, arm free of clothing. Center inflatable bag over brachial artery. Lower border—2.5 cm above antecubital crease. Secure cuff snugly.
- Loose cuff gives falsely high readings. Position patient's arm slightly flexed at elbow.
- Support it manually or rest it on a pillow or table (sustained muscle contraction raise diastolic BP 10%). Cuff should lie at heart level, if difference of 13.6 cm—error 10 mm Hg.
- Brachial artery below heart level—high BP
- Brachial artery above heart level—low BP

Find brachial artery medial to biceps tendon. With thumb or fingers of one hand on brachial artery, rapidly inflate cuff to about 30 mm Hg above level of pulse disappearance. Deflate cuff slowly until feeling of pulse. Deflate completely. This palpatory systolic pressure helps to avoid being misled by an auscultatory gap.

Auscultatory method:

- Inflate cuff again to about 30 mm Hg above palpatory systolic pressure **(Fig. 5.15)**
- Deflate slowly—2–3 mm Hg/s
- Rapid deflation
  - Underestimation of systolic pressure
  - Overestimation of diastolic pressure Note level at which sounds heard—at least two consecutive beats, its systolic pressure.
- Continue to lower pressure slowly until sounds become muffled and then disappear.
- Disappearance point—diastolic pressure. Avoid slow, repetitive inflation of cuff—resulting venous congestion can cause artifactually low-systolic and high-diastolic pressure.

Hypertension: On at least two consecutive visits, two or more readings with diastolic pressure averages ≥90 mm Hg, systolic pressure>140 mm Hg. It is generally due to the change in vascular tone or aortic valve diseases.

Hypotension: <90/60 mm Hg, normal finding in sleep

Daytime hypotension—heart failure, blood loss, reduced vascular tone

Normally from sitting to standing systolic pressure fall or unchanged, diastolic pressure rises.

Substantial fall in systolic pressure, ≥20 mm Hg, with symptoms indicate orthostatic or postural hypotension.

Table 5.17: Grades of murmurs.	
Grade	**Intensity**
1.	Very faint—easily missed
2.	Quiet—barely audible
3.	Moderately loud—but easily heard—same intensity as S1 or S2
4.	Loud, but usually no thrill present
5.	Very loud, thrill present
6.	Heard with stethoscope off chest—thrill present

Source: Lippincott, Williams and Wilkins, 2005.

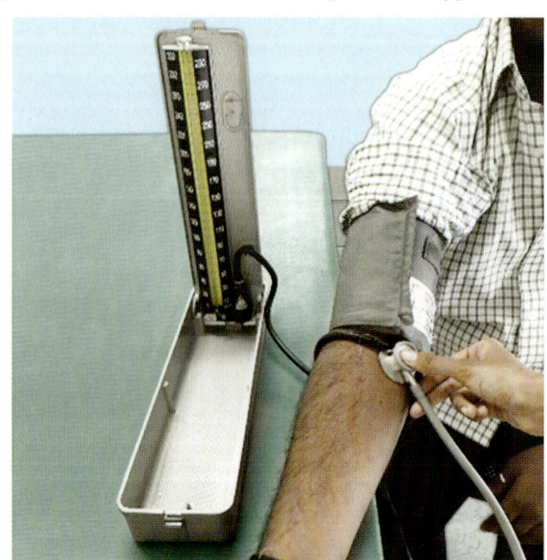

Fig. 5.15: Blood pressure measurement.

Electrocardiogram

An electrocardiogram (ECG) is a test to measure the electrical activity of the heartbeat. With each beat, an electrical impulse travels through the heart. It is measured by placing 12 electrodes in standardized position around the chest.

An ECG gives two major kinds of information.

1. By measuring time intervals on the ECG, a doctor can determine how long the electrical wave takes to pass through the heart. Finding out how long a wave takes to travel from one part of the heart to the next shows if the electrical activity is normal or slow, fast, or irregular.
2. By measuring the amount of electrical activity passing through the heart muscle, a cardiologist may be able to find out if parts of the heart are too large or are overworked.

Central Venous Pressure

It is the pressure at the tip of an indwelling central venous catheter in the vena cava close to the right atrium of the heart. It closely reflects pressure within the right atrium. Normal value: 2–6 mm Hg. It increases in heart failure and decreases in dehydration.

Cardiopulmonary Exercise Testing

It is important to perform this test to determine cardiopulmonary fitness. It can be an incremental graded exercise test to measure maximum oxygen uptake or simple walk test such as 6-minute walk test and shuttle walk test **(Box 5.12)**.

Disability

This component includes the evaluation of neuromuscular functions. Any neuromuscular conditions can compromise cardiopulmonary function, and vice versa.

Disability—Look

Level of consciousness of the patient should be noted. It can be measured using the Glasgow Coma Scale (GCS).

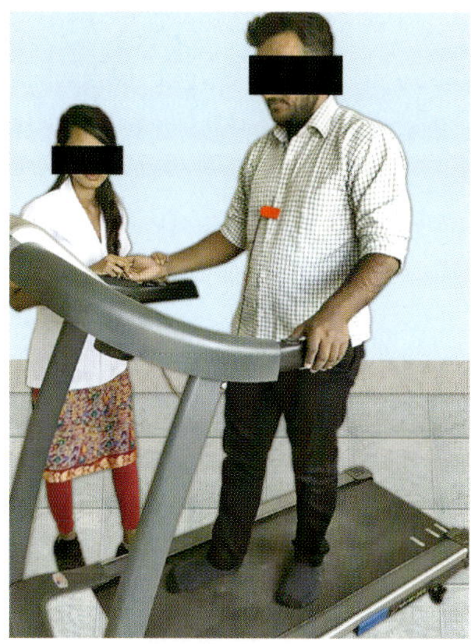

Fig. 5.16: Treadmill test.

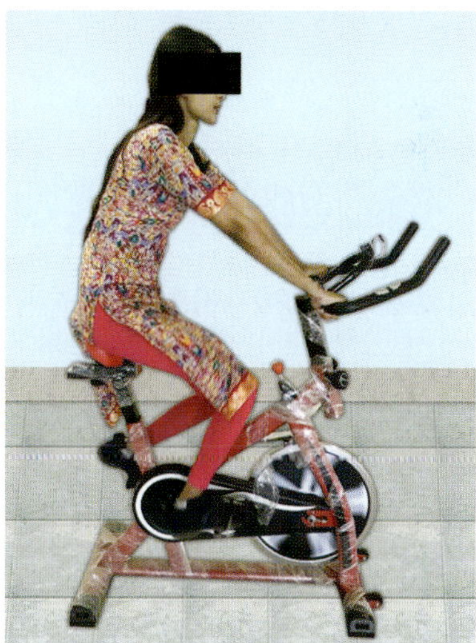

Fig. 5.17: Bicycle test.

If consciousness is impaired, then the risk of aspiration and retention of secretions increase. Check the presence or absence of:

- Nasogastric tube
- Intravenous line
- Central venous pressure line etc.
- Level of cardiovascular support including drugs to control BP and cardiac output
- Pacemaker
- Mode and route of ventilation and other mechanical devices.

Glasgow Coma Scale

The GCS rates the patient from 3 to 15 based on their best observed motor, verbal and eye responses **(Fig. 5.18)**.

Disability—Feel

Examine the tone of the muscles. During limb movement, the resistance should be determined by feel. Either tone is flaccid, spastic, or rigid. From this component, one can get an idea of what to measure in the next component.

BOX 5.12: Exercise tolerance testing (ETT).

- **Maximal tests**
  - Treadmill tests **(Fig. 5.16)**
    - » Balke treadmill test
    - » Bruce treadmill test.
  - Field tests
    - » Incremental Shuttle walk test
- **Submaximal tests**
  - Bicycle tests **(Fig. 5.17)**
    - » Astrand-Rhyming bicycle test
  - Field tests
    - » 6-minute walk test
    - » 12-minute walk test (Cooper VO_{2max} test)
    - » Endurance shuttle test
  - Step tests
    - » Harvard step test
    - » Canadian step test
    - » Queen's college step test

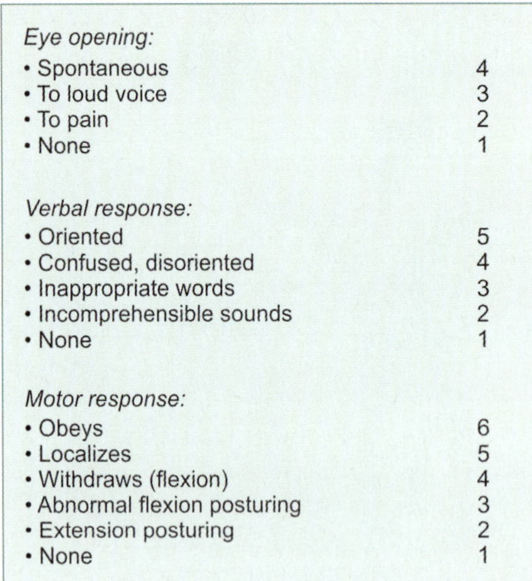

Fig. 5.18: Glasgow Coma Scale.

Eye opening:
- Spontaneous — 4
- To loud voice — 3
- To pain — 2
- None — 1

Verbal response:
- Oriented — 5
- Confused, disoriented — 4
- Inappropriate words — 3
- Incomprehensible sounds — 2
- None — 1

Motor response:
- Obeys — 6
- Localizes — 5
- Withdraws (flexion) — 4
- Abnormal flexion posturing — 3
- Extension posturing — 2
- None — 1

Disability—Listen

- Airway patency should be checked.
- Listen to the speech. It will provide information regarding cognitive function. Check whether there is any speech abnormality—dysarthria, dysphagia (impaired swallowing), expressive aphasia (difficulty to create speech), or receptive aphasia (difficulty to understand speech).
- Check whether the patient is oriented in the form of time, place, and person.

Disability—Examination

In some patients, it is important to complete the full neurological or musculoskeletal assessment at this point. For example, the patients who have experienced a prolonged stay in critical care due to any condition may develop reduced sensation, muscle strength, range of motion, and impaired functional ability. If a proper neuro-musculoskeletal assessment has been done, then it will help in making sensible treatment goals for patient's fully recovery.

Manual muscle testing, range of motion, sensations, and reflexes should be checked according to standard methods.

Functional Ability

It should be checked by the standard validated scales and measurement tools depending on impairment and activity limitation. The scales include assessment of balance, walk distance, shoulder or leg disability, etc.

Quality of Life

It is important to assess the quality of life as it will provide information that how much the disease actually affects patients pertaining to their daily routine. It is used as a measure of response to treatment also. For example, SF-36 and many disease-specific scales are available which check patient's quality of life. Scales such as Coronary Revascularization Outcome Questionnaire can be used for patients undergoing and underwent cardiac procedures such as coronary artery bypass grafting or angioplasty, St. George's Respiratory Questionnaire can be used for respiratory disorders, etc.

Exposure

This is the final component. It includes the assessment of full areas of body. Patient should be treated as a whole and so assessment should be as a whole. This component involves exposure to assess the areas not included in A-B-C-D.

Exposure—Look

Skin Color and Condition

Check face, chest, and extremities. Is the skin dry or peeling? See for any rashes, patches, scare. Check for pressure sore, if present pressure sores can limit patient's activity.

Eyes

It should be examined for pallor (anemia), plethora (increased Hb), or jaundice (yellow color due to liver or blood disturbances). Drooping of one eyelid with enlargement of that pupil suggests—Horner's syndrome (disturbance in sympathetic nerve supply to that side of head).

Limb Exposure

Check for any contracture, deformity, amputation, and muscle mass. Is muscle wasting, muscle twitching present?

Hands

Fine tremor will be seen with high dose bronchodilators. Sweaty hands with irregular flapping tremor—acute CO_2 retention. Weakness and wasting of small muscles in hand are suggestive of early signs of upper lobe tumor involving brachial plexus (Pancoast tumor). Fingers may show nicotine staining from smoking. Check for clubbing of fingers.

Clubbing: Loss of angle between nail bed and nail itself. It is a sign of chronic hypoxia. Exact cause is unknown **(Fig. 5.19)**.

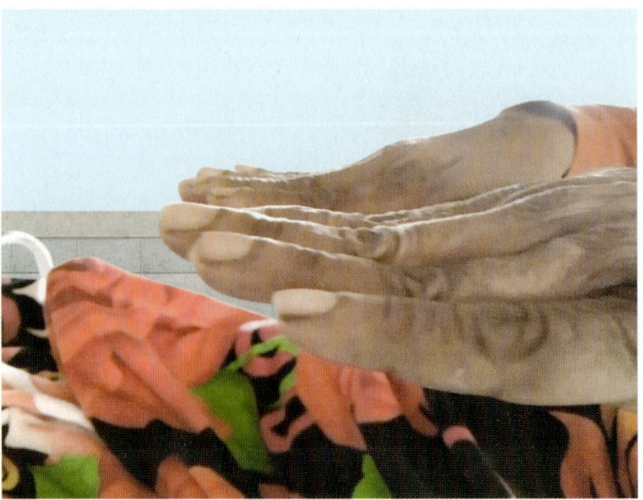

Fig. 5.19: Clubbing.

Causes of clubbing:

- Lung diseases: Infective (bronchiectasis, lung abscess, empyema), fibrotic, malignant (bronchogenic carcinoma, mesothelioma)
- Cardiac diseases: Congenital cyanotic heart diseases, bacterial endocarditis
- Others: Familial, cirrhosis, GI diseases.

Grades of clubbing:

- Grade 1: Softening of nail bed
- Grade 2: Obliteration of angle of nail bed
- Grade 3: Overlying skin becomes tense, shiny, wet and increasing curvature of nail, parrot beak, and drum stick appearance
- Grade 4: Swelling of fingers in all directions associated with hypertrophic pulmonary osteoarthropathy causing pain and swelling of hand, wrist, etc. and X-ray shows subperiosteal new bone formation.

Schamroth's sign: Normally when two fingers are held together with nails facing each other, a space is seen at the level of approximately nail fold. This is lost in case of clubbing **(Fig. 5.20)**.

Abdomen

Any localized protrusion is suggestive of hernias. Generalized distention may be due to ascites. Check for any incision (postoperative), tubes, or stoma. Sometimes, these factors can prevent active strong coughing.

Exposure—Feel

Palpate abdomen especially the four quadrants of abdomen—right and left upper quadrant, right and left lower quadrant. Check for any tenderness. Check for **diastasis recti** (separation of rectus abdominis muscle). A hard, painful, distended abdomen will hamper descent of diaphragm and so respiratory function.

Exposure—Listen

Bowel sounds should be checked with stethoscope in right lower quadrant. Normal bowel sounds are gurgles.

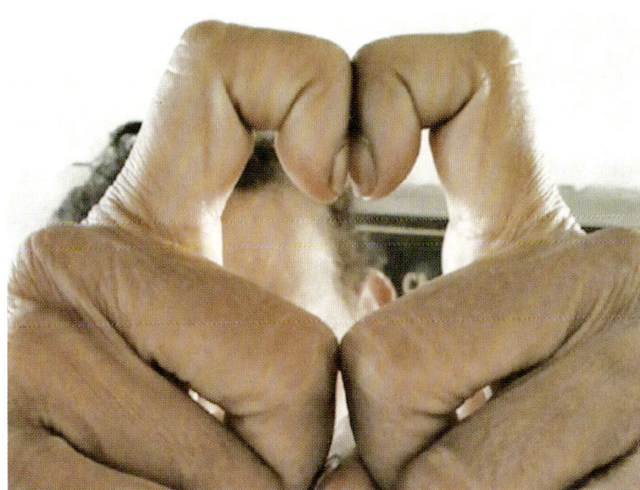

Fig. 5.20: Schamroth's sign.

Absent sounds are suggestive of constipation or paralytic ileus. High-pitched tinkling sounds are present in bowel distention.

Exposure—Examination

Laboratory Investigations

It includes sputum, blood, and urine examination. It is important to know the biochemical markers as certain physiotherapy treatments need to be based on the concerned findings. For example, patient with very low platelets are at higher risk of bleeding. A very careful physiotherapy intervention would be required for such a patient. Similarly, certain bronchodilators decrease the potassium level and so are not recommended in hypokalemia. It is considered unsafe to let cardiac disease patients who have a very low level of hemoglobin exercise vigorously. Sputum examination will reveal the bacterial species that cause chest infection.

INTERNATIONAL CLASSIFICATION OF FUNCTIONING, DISABILITY AND HEALTH ASSESSMENT

Finally from the above data, make a note of patient's health condition according to ICIDH-2 or ICF model in brief. It includes body structure and function, activity limitation, participation, environmental factors, and personnel factors.

SUMMARY

Cardiopulmonary diseases form a huge proportion of the diseases found in the modern world. It is imperative to note the finer nuances in such delicate cases as these pathologies deal directly with the respiration and circulation of the body—two functions that are vital for each living cell of the body to keep living. The cardiopulmonary assessment entails a detailed history, subjective examination, and objective examination that include assessment of ABCDE. Along with these findings, it is important to assess the functional levels of the patient. A detailed assessment helps in the formulation of a detailed and specific management plan for each individual, thus helping the individual gain a better physical, physiological, and functional outcome.

Review Questions

1. Write a detailed assessment of a 65-year-old patient with chronic bronchitis.
2. Explain the grades of clubbing.
3. How will you assess the history of a patient presenting with complaint of chest pain?
4. Explain the different breath sounds in detail.
5. Write short notes on:
   a. Dyspnea
   b. Sputum analysis
   c. Cough

BIBLIOGRAPHY

1. Australian Resuscitation Council. ANZCOR guidelines. 2016.
2. Farzan S. Chapter 38: Cough and sputum production. In: Walker HK, Hall WD, Hurst JW (Eds). Clinical methods: the history, physical, and laboratory examinations, 3rd edition. Boston, MA: Butterworths; 1990. Available from https://www.ncbi.nlm.nih.gov/books/NBK359.
3. Frownfelter D, Dean E. Cardiovascular and pulmonary physical therapy: evidence to practice, 5th edition. Mosby Inc; 2012.
4. Gupta S, Sharma R, Jain D. Airway assessment: predictors of difficult airway. Indian J Anaesth. 2005;49(4):257-62.
5. Lacy P, Lee JL, Vethanayagam D. Sputum analysis in diagnosis and management of obstructive airway diseases. Ther Clin Risk Manag. 2005;1(3):169-79.
6. Pramono R, Bowyer S, Rodriguez-Villegas E. Automatic adventitious respiratory sound analysis: a systematic review. PLoS One. 2017;12(5):e0177926. doi:10.1371/journal.pone.0177926.
7. Pryor J, Prasad A. Physiotherapy for respiratory and cardiac problems: adults and pediatrics, 3rd edition. Churchill Livingstone; 2002.
8. Pryor J, Prasad A. Physiotherapy for respiratory and cardiac problems: adults and pediatrics, 5th edition. Churchill Livingstone; 2008.
9. Rao KMN. Diagnosis and management of chronic cough due to extrapulmonary etiologies. Indian J Clin Prac. 2014;25(5):437-42.
10. Resuscitation Council (UK). Resuscitation guidelines. 2015.
11. Sarkar M, Madabhavi I, Niranjan N, et al. Auscultation of the respiratory system. Ann Thorac Med. 2015;10(3):158-68. doi:10.4103/1817-1737.160831.
12. Tietze KJ. Review of laboratory and diagnostic tests. In: Clinical skills for pharmacists, 3rd edition. 2012. pp. 86-122.

Assessment of Gait

Saravanan M

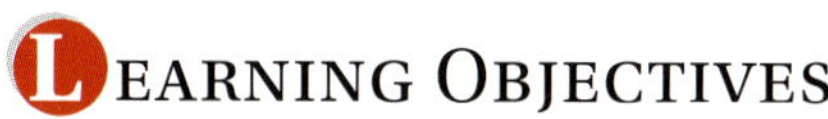LEARNING OBJECTIVES

After reading this chapter, the readers should be able to:

♦ Understand the phases of gait cycle and the interaction of various body segments and joints during the phases
♦ Gain an in-depth knowledge of functional goals of gait in humans
♦ List measurable parameters in gait such as distance and time measurements of gait and the methods to analyze and record these variables using the available options for physiotherapists
♦ Know about the importance of gait assessment in rehabilitation and various methods that can be effectively used in gait analysis
♦ Understand that normal walking and gait biomechanics explains the remarkable efficiency of human walking process and also understand some pathological gait patterns and how it affects normal gait.

CHAPTER OUTLINE

- Purpose of gait analysis
- Gait mechanics
  - Gait cycle
  - Functional goals of gait
  - Stance phase
  - Swing phase
  - Temporal-spatial parameters of gait
  - Determinants of gait
  - Joint kinematics
  - Muscle activation during gait
  - Ground reaction forces
- Gait assessment/analysis
  - Observational gait analysis
  - Instrumented gait analysis
  - Muscle activity during stance phase
  - Muscle activity during swing phase
- Clinical application of instrumented gait analysis

INTRODUCTION

Human gait is defined as bipedal, biphasic forward propulsion of center of gravity of the human body, in which there are alternate sinuous movements of different segments of the body with least expenditure of energy. Human gait is a complex phenomenon and owing to the functional versatility of the lower limbs included in walking, which again can vary depending on the surface walked, such as walking on a flat surface, stair climbing (ascending or descending), or on a resilience surface. Different gait patterns are characterized by differences in limb movement patterns, overall velocity, forces, kinetic and potential energy cycles, and changes in the contact with the surface.

The systematic study of propulsion of human body through means of observation and augmented measurement is termed "gait assessment or analysis." Gait assessment becomes imperative in individuals where the ability to walk is affected due to musculoskeletal or neurological symptoms. It is a tool that every clinician should be an expert in, especially while dealing with individuals with such walking disabilities. Over the past few decades, gait assessment has evolved exponentially in providing the best possible diagnostic and in turn treatment care, especially in the field of rehabilitation. From the basic idea of observing the human movement pattern subjectively to measuring specific variables of the different subphases of gait, the evolution of gait assessment and analysis has improved by far and made interpretation of changes in gait patterns easy, quick, and precise.

PURPOSE OF GAIT ANALYSIS

The purpose of gait analysis is as follows:

- Gait analysis is one of the most fundamental steps commonly used in neuro and musculoskeletal examination.

- The application of gait dynamics to healthcare field is increasing as research in this area is ever expanding and newer equipment are readily available. Therapeutic recommendations on functionality of gait improvisation are most commonly based on the clinical examination, including gait analysis of various forms.
- Normative gait data is very essential for diagnosing and managing abnormal gait patterns.
- This quantitative analysis will improve the ability of the therapist to not only diagnose and treat disability pertaining to gait but also measure the effectiveness of assistive devices used for ambulation.
- Another area where gait and motion analysis is widely used is in sports where it is used to help athletes run efficiently and thereby increase their performance.
- Last, but not the least, analysis of gait can be used as a biometric measure in forensics to recognize people by the way they walk.

GAIT MECHANICS

Understanding a "normal" gait pattern and its basic mechanics forms the foundation for any assessment method involved in diagnosis of gait abnormality. Since "normal" covers both genders, a wide range of population in any age-groups and population with a still wider range of body shapes and geometry, it becomes difficult to set a standard "normal" as reference while assessing gait and should be dealt with utmost care. **Table 6.1** describes the common terminologies used, when addressing gait and its associated deviations.

Gait Cycle

The gait cycle (GC) can be termed the time interval or cyclical sequence of movement patterns occurring from the moment the heel of one foot strikes the ground to the heel of the same foot striking the ground again. Although there are variations in the definition of different phases involving GC, it has been broadly divided into two phases: stance phase and swing phase. The stance phase contributes to 60% of the GC and can be subdivided into double-limb support and single-limb support. In double-limb support, which occurs twice in a GC, both feet remain contacted with the ground. Double-limb support phase represents 10% of the entire GC but decreases with increased walking speed and ultimately disappears as one begins to run. At slower walking velocities, the double-limb support times are greater. Single-limb supported stance comprises up to 40% of the normal GC and occurs once in a cycle. With increases in walking speed, the duration of double-limb support decreases until it becomes zero for running.

Further in-depth analysis of GC involves classification of gait into phases as per the traditional gait nomenclature

or as per the Rancho Los Amigos (RLA) nomenclature. **Figure 6.1** shows the phases of GC as per traditional and RLA nomenclatures. Traditional nomenclature is used to describe the gait of subjects considered normal as all the subphases readily correlate with normal pattern of walking. However, this traditional nomenclature falls short while describing pathological deviations in gait involving the lower extremity in some conditions. RLA nomenclature generally covers these short comings and can be applied to any type of gait. **Table 6.2** summarizes the phases of GC as per traditional and RLA nomenclature.

Functional Goals of Gait

As identified by Perry, each of these phases has a functional goal that is accomplished by synergistic motions of various segments of the body in selective patterns. These sequential motion patterns enable the body to accomplish the following three basic tasks, which are vital for balanced propulsion of the body:

1. Weight acceptance
2. Single-limb support
3. Limb advancement

Weight Acceptance

This is considered to be the most demanding task of all three as there is abrupt transfer of body weight onto a relatively unstable limb, which has just completed its forward swing. It begins with the initiation of stance phase (initial contact) and ends with the loading response. Shock absorption, initial limb stability, and preservation of progression are the three functional patterns needed to accomplish this task. It occupies 0–12% of the GC **(Fig. 6.2)**.

Single-Limb Support

This task begins with the next two phases of GC (midstance and terminal stance), when the stance limb takes the responsibility of supporting the body weight allowing the initial and terminal swing to occur in the opposite limb. It ends once the swinging foot contacts the ground. Progression of the center of gravity over the stationary foot followed by progression beyond the supporting foot and stability of limb and trunk are the functional patterns needed to accomplish this task. It occupies 12–50% of the GC **(Fig. 6.2)**.

Limb Advancement

This task concentrates on preparing the body segments to meet the high demands placed on the advancing limb as it enters into the stance phase completing the swing phase. It involves all the four subphases of the swing phase, namely preswing, initial swing, midswing, and terminal swing. Positioning the limb for swing, foot clearance, progression of the trailing limb, and preparation of stance

Table 6.1: Terminologies used in gait.

Terminology	Description
Gait cycle	The period of time from one event (usually initial contact) of one foot to the following occurrence of the same event with the same foot
Stance phase	The period of time when the foot is in contact with the ground. Approximately 62% of the GC
Swing phase	The period of time when the foot is not in contact with the ground. In those cases where the foot never leaves the ground (foot drag), it can be defined as the phase when all portions of the foot are in forward motion. Approximately 39% of GC
Double support	The period of time when both feet are in contact with the ground. This occurs twice in the GC, at the beginning and end of stance phase. Also referred to as left and right double-limb stance or LDLS and RDLS, respectively
Single support	The period of time when only one foot is in contact with the ground. In walking, this is equal to the swing phase of the other limb
Observational gait assessment	A qualitative visual description of an individual's upper and lower extremities, pelvis, and trunk motion during ambulation
Motion analysis	Interpretation of computerized data that documents an individual's lower and upper extremities, pelvis, trunk, and head motion during ambulation
Markers	Active or passive objects (balls, hemispheres, or disks—see below) aligned with respect to specific bony landmarks used to help determine segment and joint position in motion analysis
Active markers	Joint and segment markers used during motion analysis that emit a signal
Passive markers	Joint and segment markers used during motion analysis that reflect visible or infrared light
Electrogoniometer	An electrical transducer that can be attached to adjacent segments to measure a joint angle. Different designs accommodate changes in joint center of rotation location and three-dimensional motion
Step length	The distance from a point of contact with the ground of one foot to the following occurrence of the same point of contact with the other foot. The right step length is the distance from the left heel to the right heel when both feet are in contact with the ground, expressed in meters (m)
Stride length	The distance from initial contact of one foot to the following initial contact of the same foot. Sometimes referred to as cycle length, expressed in meters (m)
Cadence	The rate at which a person walks, expressed in steps per minute
Stance/swing ratio	The ratio of the stance period to the swing period
Walking base (or stride width)	The side-to-side distance between the feet, which is typically measured from the ankle joint center
Foot switch	A device that measures the duration of foot contact of a designated part of the foot
Instrumented walkway	A pathway that either contains sensors in the floor or sensors around the walkway that monitor gait
Reaction force	The force a body A exerts on a second body B in response to a force exerted by body B on the body A. The reaction force has equal magnitude but opposite direction relative to the force exerted on the body A by body B, expressed in Newton (N)
Resultant GRFs	The vector summation of the three reaction forces resulting from the interaction between the foot and ground. The resultant GRF has three vector components, i.e., the vertical, mediolateral and anteroposterior
Force plate	A transducer that is set in the floor to measure, about some specified point, the force and torque applied by the foot to the ground. These devices provide measures of the three components of the resultant GRF vector and the three components of the resultant torque vector
Center of pressure	A point on the ground where the resultant GRF can be assumed to act. The center of pressure is typically calculated from the force and torque measured by a force plate. In a two-dimensional case, the center of pressure is the point where the resultant GRF alone (with no torque) can act and have an effect equivalent to the measured GRF and torque. In three dimensions, however, there is generally no point where the force and torque can be replaced by just an equivalent force. Thus the center of pressure is taken to be the point where either (1) the resultant GRF and a vertical torque or (2) the resultant GRF and a torque parallel to the resultant ground reaction (i.e., the torque with minimum magnitude) can act and have an effect equivalent to the measured GRF and torque

(GC: gait cycle; GRFs: ground reaction forces; LDLS: left double limb support, RDLS: right double limb support)

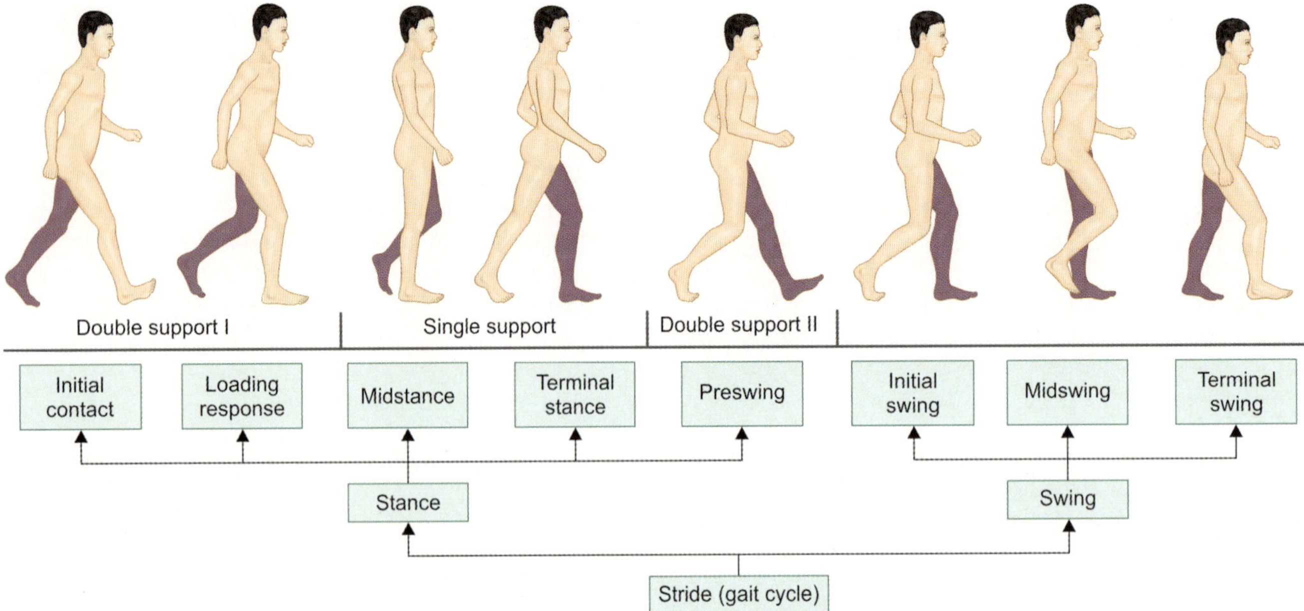

Fig. 6.1: Gait cycle including stance and swing phases.

Table 6.2: Gait cycle and its phases.	
Classic gait terms	*RLA gait terms*
Stance phase	
Heel strike	Initial contact
Foot flat	Loading response
Midstance	Midstance
Heel off	Terminal stance
Toe off	Preswing
Swing phase	
Acceleration	Initial swing
Midswing	Midswing
Deceleration	Terminal swing

(RLA: Rancho Los Amigos)

are the functional patterns needed to accomplish this task. It occupies 12–50% of the GC **(Fig. 6.2)**.

Stance Phase

The period during which the foot is in contact with the ground is termed "stance phase." It begins as soon as the heel strikes the ground and ends when the same foot leaves the ground. It is further subdivided into five phases **(Fig. 6.3)**:

1. **Initial contact** (0%) marks the beginning of stance phase when the foot first contacts the ground. Normally, there is a pattern of heel striking the ground first in normal individuals; hence, the traditional term "heel strike" is used to describe this phase. Abnormal patterns of initial contact include lack of heel strike, foot placed flat directly on initial contact or toes placed directly.

2. **Loading response** (0–10%) begins immediately after initial contact and is followed by the entire plantar surface of the foot coming into contact with the ground and the body weight being transferred onto the stance limb. It ends when the opposite foot leaves the ground. This marks the first period of double-limb support.

3. **Midstance** (10–30%) begins once the opposite foot leaves the ground and the center of gravity is directly over the stance limb.

4. **Terminal stance** (30–50%) begins when the heel of the stance limb rises to leave the ground and the weight is shifted to the forefoot over the ball of the foot. The body moves forward taking the weight off the stance limb.

5. **Preswing** (50–60%) begins when the weight of the body is shifted from the toe of the stance limb and is prepared to enter the swing phase. This also refers to initial contact of the opposite limb and a phase of second double-limb support.

Swing Phase

This phase occurs when the foot is not in contact with the ground. It begins as soon as the foot leaves the ground and ends when the heel of the same foot contacts the floor during initial contact. It is further subdivided into three phases **(Figs. 6.3A to C)**:

1. **Initial swing** (60–70%) marks the beginning of swing phase where the toes of the foot leaves the ground and ends when the swinging foot is directly under the body.

2. **Midswing** (70–85%) marks the presence of swinging foot opposite to the weight-bearing stance limb with maximum knee flexion. During this phase, the swing limb passes directly beneath the body.

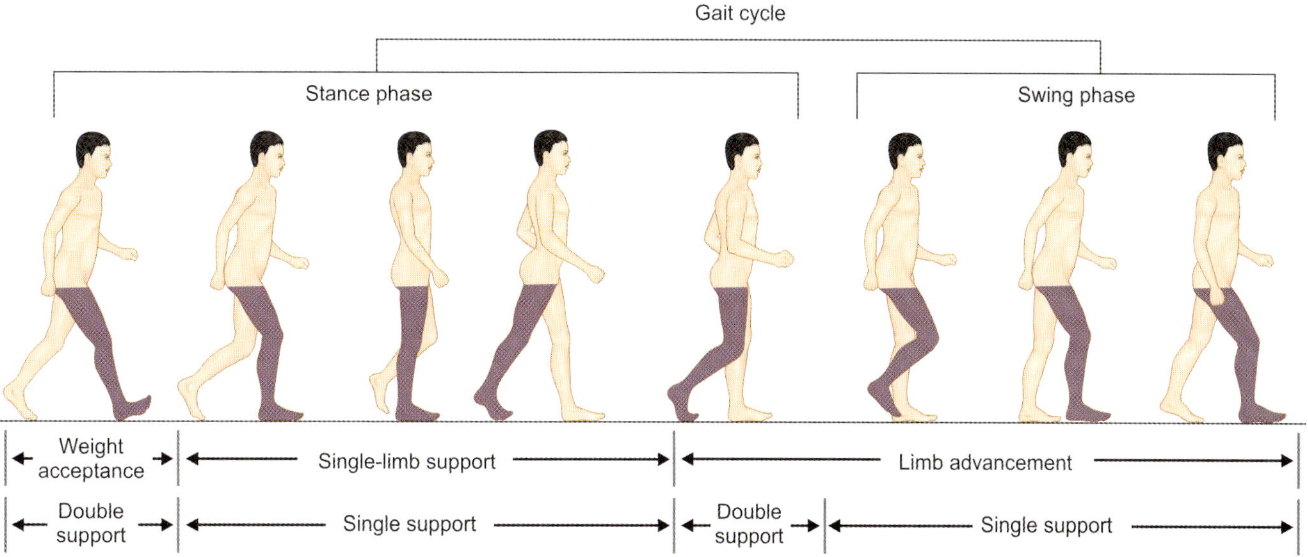

Fig. 6.2: Sequential motion patterns—weight acceptance, single-limb support, and limb advancement.

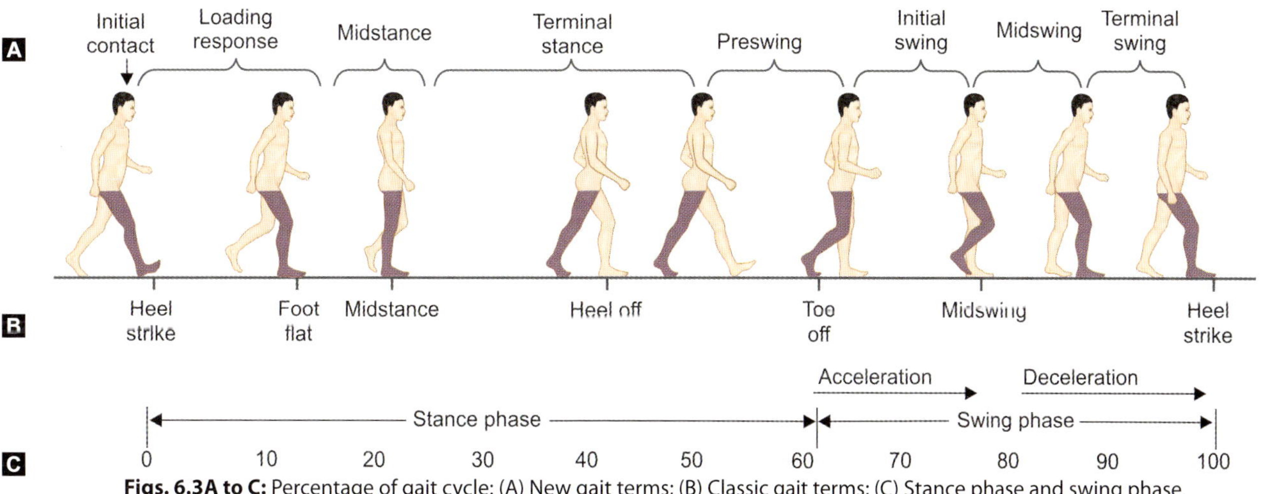

Figs. 6.3A to C: Percentage of gait cycle: (A) New gait terms; (B) Classic gait terms; (C) Stance phase and swing phase.

3. **Terminal swing** (85–100%) marks the completion of a GC and prepares the limb for the next cycle. It ends just prior to initial contact of the same foot.

Thus gait includes simultaneous cyclic pattern involving both the lower limbs, when one limb is in stance phase, the other is in swing phase.

Temporal-Spatial Parameters of Gait

The temporal and spatial parameters of walking are widely used to describe normal and pathological gait. This includes step length, stride length, step width, stride width, base of support, stride length to lower extremity ratio, step time, stride time, stance duration, stride duration, swing-to-stance ratio, speed, and cadence. These parameters are based on a constant direct progression and can be applied to straight or linear walking only.

The temporal and spatial parameters are normally termed the "vital signs of gait" **(Table 6.3)**. Measurement of these parameters are vital in detecting pathological functions, for instance, risk of falls in elderly, or it can function as a means of comparison of values under different circumstances or as a functional measure to evaluate the ability or disability of an individual.

However, it is imperative to bear in mind that there exists biological variability while measuring any parameter over a period of time. These variations can be intrapersonal owing to the differences in gait over a period of time or interpersonal owing to anatomical and physiological differences observed among populations. Interrater and intrarater variabilities are also common as the methods used to analyze gait may vary and it also depends on the skill levels of the person analyzing gait. Therapists should be aware of these variabilities beforehand to avoid error in gait analysis.

Stride refers to the sequence of events between the contact of one foot with the ground and the next contact of the same foot with the ground. **Step** refers to the sequence

Table 6.3: Gait variables: Quantitative gait analysis.	
Gait	*Description*
Speed	A scalar quantity that has magnitude but no direction
Cadence	The number of steps taken per unit of time (e.g., steps/min)
Velocity	Measure of body's motion in a given direction
Linear velocity	Rate at which a body moves in a straight line
Angular velocity	Rate of rotation of a body segment around an axis
Walking velocity	Rate of linear forward motion of the body (cm/s or m/s)
Acceleration	Rate of change of velocity of a body with respect to time
Angular acceleration	Rate of change of angular velocity of a body with respect to time
Stride time	Amount of time that elapses during one stride
Step time	Amount of time that elapses during one step
Stride length	Linear distance between two successive points of contact of the same foot
Swing time	Amount of time during gait cycle that one foot is off the ground
Double support time	Amount of time spent in gait cycle when both the lower extremities are in contact with supporting surface
Cycle time	Amount of time required to complete a gait cycle
Step length	Linear distance between two successive points of contact of the right and left lower extremity

of events between the contact of one foot with the ground and the next contact of the opposite foot with the ground. A step is basically half of a stride and it takes one left step and one right step to complete a stride.

Spatial (Distance) Measures

Spatial parameters in gait refer to measurements related to distance variables and it includes:
- Step length
- Stride length
- Stride length to lower extremity length ratio
- Step or stride width
- Foot angle (degree of toe-out).

Step length: Step length is the distance between the heel strike of one foot and the heel strike of the opposite foot.

Since step length should be same for each leg, comparative analysis of right and left step lengths would provide an insight into gait symmetry. Step length is directly proportional to walking speed, which means an increase or decrease in walking speed increases or decreases step length, respectively.

Stride length: Stride length is the distance between the heel strike of one foot and the heel strike of the same foot. The length of one stride covers all the events of a GC.

Stride length/lower extremity length ratio: It is the ratio between stride length and lower extremity length. Stride length can be normalized by dividing stride length by leg length or by total body height, so people of different sizes can be compared.

Step or stride width: The step or stride width is also referred to as width of walking base in gait analysis. The perpendicular distance between the most medial point of the inner border of each foot provides the step width of an individual.

Foot angle (degree of toe-out): The angle formed by the line of progression of the foot with a line intersecting the center of heel and the second toe is termed "foot angle or degree of toe-out." This represents the angle of foot placement.

Figure 6.4 describes the diagrammatic representation of spatial parameters of gait.

Temporal (Time) Measures

Temporal parameters in gait refer to measurements related to time variables and it includes:
- Stance time
- Swing time
- Stride time
- Swing-to-stance ratio
- Cadence
- Walking speed

Stance time: It is the amount of time that elapses during the stance phase of one extremity in a GC. It can be a measure of percentage (60%) or can be measured in seconds.

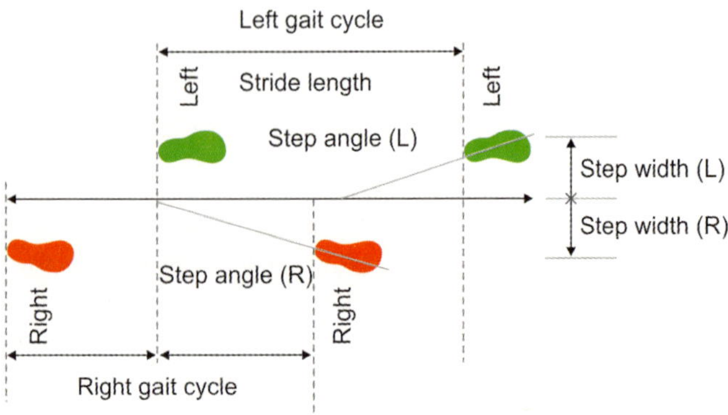

Fig. 6.4: Spatial measures of gait.

Swing time: This refers to the time in seconds that the reference foot is off the ground during a GC. Similar to stance time, this also is measured either in percentage (40%) or in seconds.

Stride time: It is the time taken in seconds from ground contact of one foot to ground contact of the same foot. It refers to the time taken to perform a single stride.

Swing-to-stance ratio: It is the ratio between the swing time and the stance time.

Cadence: Cadence is defined as the number of steps taken by any person per minute or per second.

Walking speed: Walking speed is determined and affected by step length and cadence. Walking speed is directly proportional to cadence and step length. It can be calculated from the equation:

$$\text{Speed} = \frac{\text{Distance}}{\text{Time}}$$

Based on various studies in the past, the ranges of normative values for some of the spatial and temporal parameters are provided in **Table 6.4**.

Determinants of Gait

Since walking is considered a series of losses and recoveries of balance, there is always a forward momentum of the body carrying the Center of Mass (CoM) beyond the foot moving forward. Alternative relocations of the foot to new positions thus carry the body forward preventing any fall. This process continues until the foot placement stops the forward momentum of the body and the body retains balance over its base of support. The amount of energy consumed for walking would be less if the deviation of the CoM is at its minimum. Hypothetically, this is possible if the body is moving along a straight line as if moving on a wheel not on foot. From its position just anterior to the second sacral vertebra, the CoM shows notable displacement in the forward direction during gait, along with two sinusoidal movement patterns in the vertical and side-to-side directions. At about 5% and 55% of the GC (at the midpoint of both periods of double-limb support), the CoM is at its minimal height. Conversely, the CoM is at its maximal height during the midpoint of both periods of single-limb support (at 30% and 80% of GC).

Midpoint of stance phase on the stance leg is the position in which there is maximum displacement of CoM to the side. For example, the CoM is displaced maximally on to the left side during midpoint of stance phase on the left leg (30% of GC) and there is maximal sideways displacement to the right at midpoint of stance phase of the right leg (80% of GC). An average aged adult shows a total displacement of 5 cm of CoM in the vertical direction and a total displacement of 4 cm of CoM in the side-to-side directions.

Inman described several factors responsible to flatten the arc in the vertical and horizontal planes, thereby reducing the displacement of CoM which in turn decreases the energy expenditure during gait. This would result in a smooth sinusoidal translation of the CoM along a path that would require the least amount of energy. Any increase in the vertical or horizontal displacement would thereby increase the cost of walking. These were described by Inman as the components of gait, which he referred to as the six determinants of gait.

First determinant—pelvic rotation in horizontal plane: There is anterior rotation of pelvis on the swing leg and posterior rotation during midstance. A total rotation of 3–5° occurs on each side and it is maximum just before heel strike. It facilitates longer stride length with same amount of hip flexion of the advancing leg and hip extension of the retreating leg. This does not change the displacement of CoM significantly.

Second determinant—pelvic tilt in frontal plane: This refers to hike and drop in pelvis during normal walking. During normal gait, the pelvis drops 4–5° away from the stance leg and toward the swing leg. As the pelvis on the swing leg is dropped, the hip abductors of the stance hip control pelvic tilt.

Third determinant—knee flexion: Eccentric contraction of quadriceps facilitates approximately 15° of knee

	Parameters	Range of values available in research literature
Spatial	Step length	0.70 ± 0.01 to 0.81 ± 0.05 (in m)
	Stride length	1.33 ± 0.09 to 1.63 ± 0.11 (in m)
	Step width	0.61 ± 0.22 to 9.0 ± 3.5 (in cm)
	Foot angle	5.1 ± 5.7 to 6.8 ± 5.6 (in °)
Temporal	Stance time	0.63 ± 0.07 to 0.67 ± 0.04 (in sec)
	Swing time	0.39 ± 0.02 to 0.40 ± 0.04 (in sec)
	Stride time	1.00 ± 0.23 to 1.12 ± 0.07 (in sec)
	Swing-to-stance ratio	0.63–0.64
	Cadence	100–131 (steps/min)
	Walking speed	0.82 ± 0.16 to 1.60 ± 0.16 (in m/s)

Table 6.4: Normative values of spatiotemporal variables from various literature.

flexion during midstance and this decreases the vertical displacement of CoM.

The above-mentioned first three determinants reduce 2.5 cm of vertical displacement with each stride thereby facilitating energy conservation during walking.

Fourth and fifth determinants—knee ankle and foot motion: These combined motions of knee, ankle, and foot occur as a synchronized movement pattern as a result of eccentric contraction of dorsal flexors and knee extensors controlling plantar flexion and knee flexion, respectively, during the first part of the stance phase. They prevent sudden changes in the displacement of CoM thus facilitating a smooth sinusoidal curve.

Sixth determinant—lateral pelvic movement: This refers to the side-to-side movement or lateral sway of pelvis occurring with each step. Pelvic shift to left or right occurs over the weight-bearing limb to provide stability during the stance phase. The amount of lateral sway depends on the base of support. Also, the normal physiologic valgus of knee, which is the angle formed between the tibia and femur, helps to reduce the amount of pelvic shift required for stability, thereby reducing the energy consumed and this also allows the feet to remain closer during forward progression of gait.

Joint Kinematics

Apart from the above-mentioned parameters, range of motion (ROM) of joints and appropriate muscle activity during walking also determines the efficiency of gait. ROM is observed during gait analysis and is again measured to correlate with the possible skeletal and joint pathology. **Table 6.5** summarizes some kinetic gait variables used in gait analysis.

As proposed by Perry, the optimal ROM of the lower extremity required for walking is provided in **Table 6.6.**

Ankle remains in neutral during initial contact with variations, including minimal plantar flexion amounting to 3–5°. Loading response requires 7° of plantar flexion, which is followed by the ankle changing its direction toward dorsiflexion where the tibia moves over the stationery foot. Dorsiflexion is at its maximum (10°) during midstance, which is maintained until the end of the single-limb support period. There is rapid ankle plantar flexion at the end of stance phase, where it reaches its maximum (30°). Final range of dorsiflexion occurs with the initiation of preswing and a neutral ankle is maintained during the rest of the GC.

Optimal joint angles and muscle activity of the lower limb during gait and its various phases are summarized in **Figure 6.5.**

There are variations in the range of knee motion during initial contact, which ranges from a slight hyperextension (−2°) to flexion 5°. The stance knee is under maximal weight-bearing load as it moves from loading response to midstance with a flexion angle of about 18°. From this

Table 6.5: Gait analysis: Kinetic gait variables.

Variables	Description
Ground reaction forces	Vertical, anterior–posterior and medial–lateral forces created as a result of foot contact with the supporting surface
Pressure	Force per unit area, peak pressure, pressure time integral, and overall pattern of pressure distribution under the foot are measured in gait analysis
CoP	Point of application of resultant force. It is used as a measure of stability of a subject who is either standing or walking on foot plate
Torque	Force X perpendicular distance or moment arm. Rotational effect produced by the application of a force

(CoP: Center of Pressure)

Table 6.6: Optimal range of motion of lower extremity required for normal gait.

Joint	Motion	Occurrence in gait cycle (%)
Ankle	Plantar flexion to 7°	0–12
	Dorsiflexion to 10°	12–48
	20° Plantar flexion	48–62
	Dorsiflexion to neutral	62–100
Knee	Flexion to 18°	0–15
	Extension to 5°	15–40
	Flexion to 65°	40–70
	Extension to 2°	70–97
Hip	Flexion 30°	0
	Flexion 35°	85
	Extension 10°	50

maximum flexion, the knee starts extending and reaches 3° flexion as terminal stance begins. Preswing and initial swing record the maximum of knee flexion angle, which varies between 60 and 70°. With the onset of midswing, there is rapid recovery of knee motion into extension until terminal swing where knee extension reaches 3°.

Hip is flexed to about 20° during initial contact and starts losing around 3–5° of hip flexion with loading response. There is progressive extension of hip as the limb approaches midstance, which reaches the neutral position at terminal stance. With the GC approaching preswing, it marks the peak extension in hip (10°), and with progression of gait, there is reversal of hip extension to flexion. Once again, neutral hip position is attained at the end of stance phase, which is followed by 10° of flexion during initial swing progressing to maximum hip flexion of 25° at terminal swing.

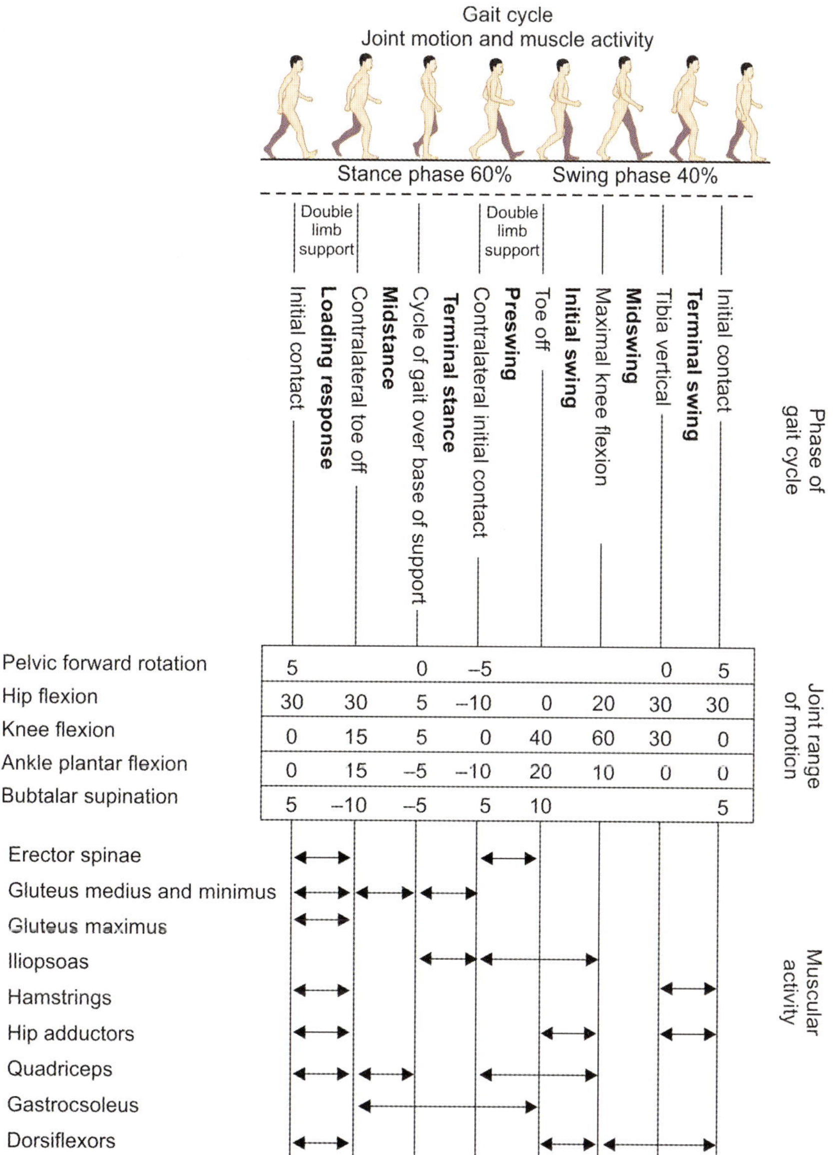

	Initial contact	Loading response	Contralateral toe off / Midstance	Terminal stance	Contralateral initial contact / Preswing	Toe off / Initial swing	Maximal knee flexion / Midswing	Terminal swing	Initial contact
Pelvic forward rotation	5		0	−5				0	5
Hip flexion	30	30	5	−10	0	20	30		30
Knee flexion	0	15	5	0	40	60	30		0
Ankle plantar flexion	0	15	−5	−10	20	10	0		0
Bubtalar supination	5	−10	−5	5	10				5

Fig. 6.5: Joint angles and muscle activity of lower limb during gait.

Overall the ROM required in lower extremity joints for an optimal gait pattern can be summarized as follows:

- Hip—20° of extension to 20° of flexion
- Knee—neutral (0°) to 60° flexion
- Ankle—30° plantar flexion to 10° dorsiflexion

Other than the analysis of ROM of lower extremity, the movement pattern of head, arm, and trunk (HAT) also requires special mention in gait analysis **(Fig. 6.6)**. A normal gait observation shows head and trunk progressing as a single unit except mild vertical displacements as observed during instrumented analysis of gait. With reference to head height during gait, HAT shows both vertical and lateral displacements.

The vertical displacement is lowest during loading response and preswing (double-limb support) and

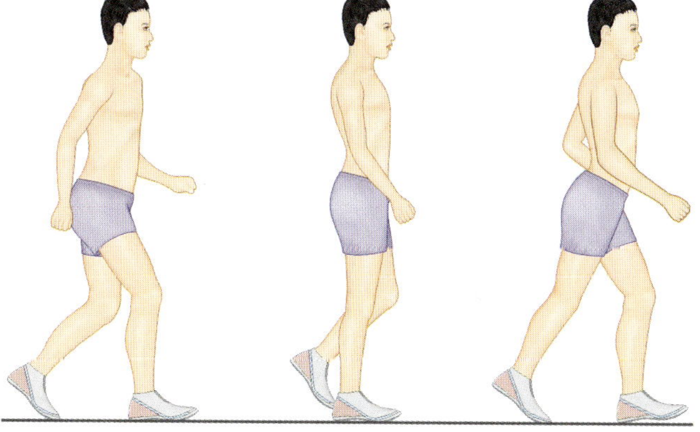

Fig. 6.6: Simultaneous linear and angular motions of arms and legs in relation to a linear head and trunk motion.

is highest during midstance. The range of vertical displacement is 2.5–4 cm upward and equally downward.

With reference to head location or deviation from midline, HAT is in midline during double-limb support period and is displaced to right with right side single-limb stance and to left with left side single-limb stance. An average of 4.5 cm total arc of deviation is expected in both left and right directions.

Pelvis motion occurs in all three planes during gait with an observed anterior/posterior tilt of 4° in sagittal plane, contralateral drop/hike of 4° in coronal plane, and posterior/anterior rotation of 10° in transverse plane.

Reciprocal arm movement of flexion and extension is observed with a total displacement of 30–40°. There is maximum backward swing of the arm with the initiation of GC (initial contact) and maximum forward swing of the arm at the end of the stance period (terminal stance).

Muscle Activation During Gait

About 10–40% of GC records some or other electrical activity of almost all muscles of the lower extremity measured electromyographically. Basic knowledge of the phases of activation of these musculatures provides insight into their kinetic functions and thereby allows gait deviations to be easily understood.

Muscle activation during gait is discussed under different heading in this chapter, where the activation is studied extensively using electromyography (EMG). Various lower limb muscles that are active during the different phases of gait are presented in **Figure 6.7**.

Any reductions in joint ranges, due to stiff joints or muscle weakness, would result in considerable deviation from the optimal gait pattern. Joint ROM assessment alongside muscle strength assessment prior to or after a gait assessment provides an insight of possible musculoskeletal factors responsible for restriction in an optimal gait pattern.

An efficient gait pattern is the one in which the body strives to minimize energy cost while walking. During ambulation, the energy efficiency is at its greatest when the speed of walking is approximately 1.33 m/s, which is the speed most commonly adopted by individuals across the globe. There is an increase in energy consumption with an increase or decrease in this walking speed. As mentioned

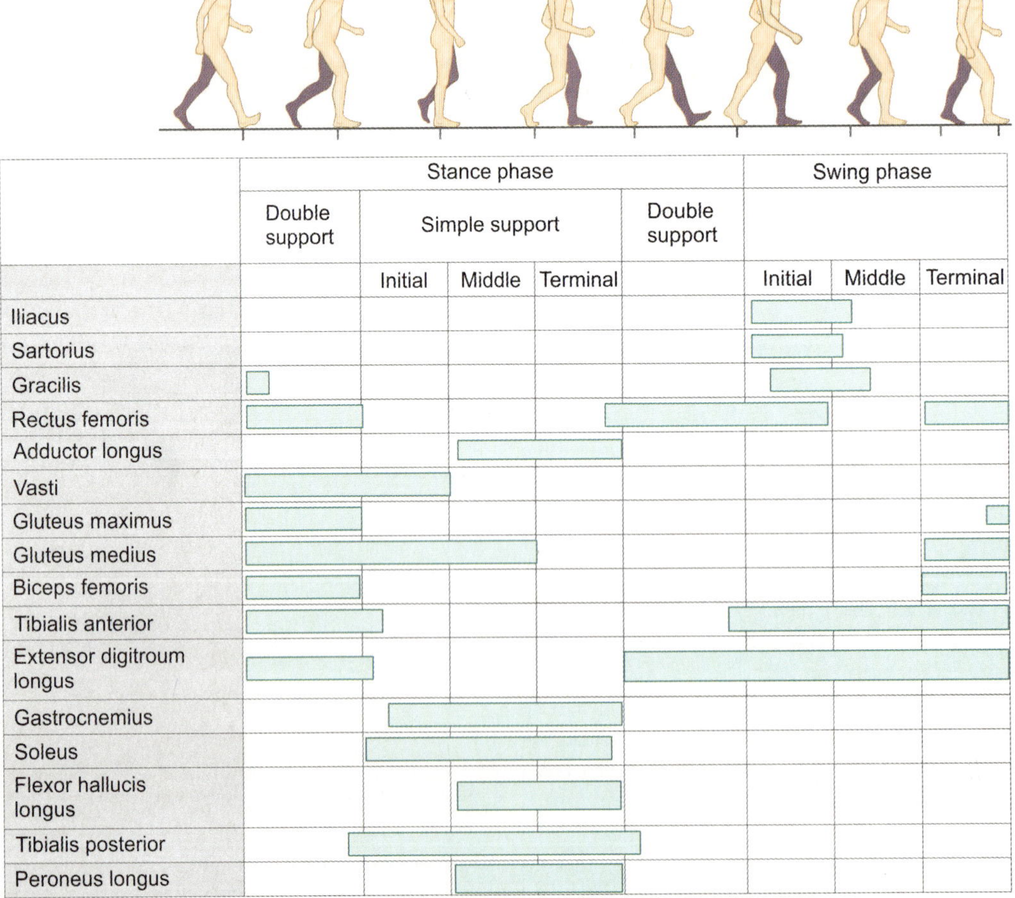

Muscle	Stance phase — Double support	Stance phase — Simple support: Initial	Stance phase — Simple support: Middle	Stance phase — Simple support: Terminal	Stance phase — Double support	Swing phase: Initial	Swing phase: Middle	Swing phase: Terminal
Iliacus						■		
Sartorius						■		
Gracilis	■					■		
Rectus femoris	■				■	■		■
Adductor longus			■	■				
Vasti	■	■						
Gluteus maximus	■	■						■
Gluteus medius	■	■	■	■				■
Biceps femoris	■	■						■
Tibialis anterior	■	■				■	■	■
Extensor digitroum longus	■	■			■	■	■	■
Gastrocnemius		■	■	■				
Soleus		■	■	■				
Flexor hallucis longus			■	■				
Tibialis posterior		■	■	■				
Peroneus longus			■	■				

Fig. 6.7: Muscle activation during gait cycle measured using EMG. (EMG: electromyography)

earlier in the determinants of gait section, five kinematic strategies provide support to reduce the displacement of CoM and thereby reduce the energy cost of walking.

In the absence of an optimal gait pattern, the common mechanism is that individuals with such gait walk slowly to keep the rate of energy consumption at comfortable and optimal level as a means to conserve energy.

A comprehensive understanding of kinematics and kinetics of gait is essential for assessing and interpreting patterns and pathology in gait. Although kinetics of gait cannot be observed visually, they are an integral part of observed kinematics.

Ground Reaction Forces

Foot forces are the forces exerted by the foot on the ground when they make contact with the ground during walking. Conversely, according to Newton's third law, a force equal in magnitude and in the opposite direction is exerted on the foot from the ground, which is termed "ground reaction forces" (GRFs). These GRFs are expressed in three axes, namely vertical, anteroposterior, and mediolateral. Peak GRFs in the vertical axis occur at the time of loading response and terminal stance where the force is about 120% of the body weight. Anteroposterior direction of GRFs correlates to the shear forces applied parallel to the supporting surface. During initial contact, the GRF is in the posterior direction, and during terminal stance and preswing, it is in the anterior direction. The peak anteroposterior GRF is about 20% of body weight during the above-mentioned phases of GC.

The components of GRFs on the human body during walking are presented in **Figure 6.8.**

These shear forces increase with larger step length as the angle between the lower extremity and the floor increases. There is relatively a small magnitude of GRFs in the mediolateral direction, which is less than 5% of body weight and it depends on the relationship between the position of the body's CoM and the location of the

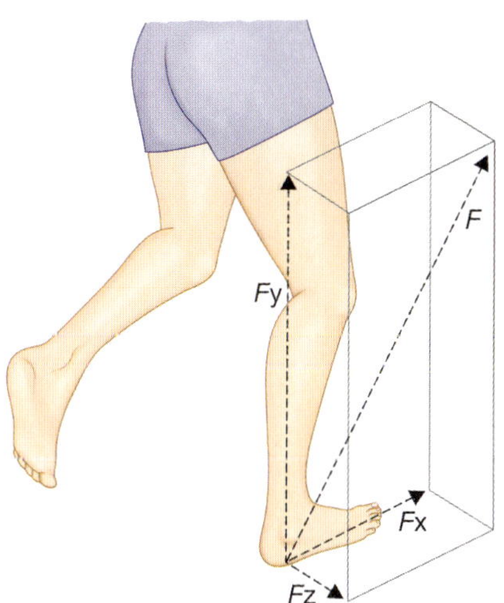

Fig. 6.8: Components of ground reaction forces (F)—F_X (anteroposterior), F_Y (vertical), and F_Z (mediolateral) forces.

foot. An increase in these shear forces can be observed in individuals with wider step widths and is less as the body's CoM is kept directly over the feet.

GAIT ASSESSMENT/ANALYSIS

Gait analysis is the systematic evaluation of the dynamics of gait. It is a process of measuring and evaluating the walking patterns of patients with specific gait-related problems. Gait analysis is also referred to as motion analysis.

The purpose of gait analysis is to diagnose and discover underlying pathologies of gait impairment and develop rehabilitation programs relevant to the diagnosis. This can be accomplished by quantifying and interpreting human movement patterns during gait, which is possible only with better understanding of human gait patterns. Deviations from normative movement patterns can be an indicator of nerve damage, injuries, anatomical abnormalities, and other neurological or musculoskeletal problems. The basis of gait analysis is the assumption that gait abnormality is due to underlying neurological or musculoskeletal disorders. In addition, environmental hazard or heavy clothing can affect gait behavior, which results in abnormal gait patterns. Thus quantitatively assessing deviation from normative gait patterns can indirectly provide insight into the mechanisms behind neurological and/or musculoskeletal diseases and adaptation of challenged environment that affect joint movements during gait.

Baker had identified the following four reasons for performing a clinical gait analysis:
1. Assessment: Extent, severity, or nature of the disease or injury.
2. Diagnosis: To diagnose between disease entities.
3. Monitor: The progress in the absence or presence of intervention.
4. Prediction: Outcome of the intervention.

The most common use is for the assessment of patients with a known condition prior to planning treatment.

Gait assessment mainly consists of two areas: qualitative observation such as visual inspection, also termed "observational gait analysis" (OGA), and quantitative approaches that examine gait behaviors using laboratory measurements.

Observational Gait Analysis

Observational gait analysis (OGA) refers to the visual assessment of a patient's gait, where the therapist focuses on movement patterns of the hips, knees, and ankles. This does not require any specialized equipment and is performed in a clinical setting to observe gross gait abnormalities. It requires a good clinical expertise especially in the area of theoretical biomechanics to assess gait through observation. The human eye is highly sensitive to detecting deviations from normal gait but not necessarily to identifying primary problems or compensatory strategies. Despite these facts, the obvious limitations of OGA are: it is relatively subjective in nature leading to poor reliability, validity, sensitivity, and specificity. It is also difficult for the therapist to observe multiple events and body segments concurrently, leading to errors in observation **(Box 6.1)**.

A thorough OGA involves watching the individual while he/she makes a number of walks and the observation should be covering all the directions—anterior, posterior, and lateral (right and left) **(Table 6.7)**. A logical order is essential to visualize gait or its abnormalities and a walkway free of obstacles with a distance of at least 10–12 m.

OGA is best performed with the initiation of a general assessment that includes observation of symmetry and smoothness of movement of body as a whole and as segments. Wherever required, measurements can be taken to consolidate the presence or absence of any abnormality. Observation of an individual during ambulation includes but is not limited to the following:

- Symmetrical orientation of the head and neck over the trunk
- Position of segments of the upper limb in relation to trunk
- Categorization of amount of arm swing during ambulation as:
  - Optimal
  - Decreased
  - Increased

BOX 6.1: Four limitations of OGA.

1. It is transitory, no permanent record can be made available.
2. Human eye cannot observe high-speed events occurring in gait.
3. Forces involved in gait cannot be observed, only movements are observed.
4. It depends entirely on the skills of the observer.

(OGA: observational gait analysis)

Table 6.7: Direction of observation by clinician and gait abnormalities.

Gait abnormalities	Direction of observation
Circumduction	Anteroposterior
Hip hiking	Anteroposterior
Excessive or reduced hip rotation	Anteroposterior
Abnormal foot contact	Anteroposterior
Abnormal foot rotation	Anteroposterior
Lateral trunk bending	Lateral (right or left)
Increased lumbar lordosis	Lateral (right or left)
High steppage	Lateral (right or left)
Vaulting	Lateral (right or left)
Excessive knee flexion/extension	Lateral (right or left)
Inadequate push off	Lateral (right or left)

- Symmetrical midline orientation of lower trunk in relation to upper trunk
- Changes in position of pelvis and hip
- Amount of knee flexion and extension
- Amount of ankle plantar flexion and dorsiflexion
- Categorization of foot supination and pronation as:
  - Optimal
  - Excessive

Optimal gait requires sufficient ROM and muscle strength at each of the participating joint and a sophisticated control of the central nervous system. Any deviation observed during OGA can be the result of direct reflection of an impairment or may be a biomechanical compensation of an impairment present elsewhere. Hence, a comprehensive examination should always precede a gait analysis, which includes the presence of any neurological or musculoskeletal abnormality.

Perry identifies various factors that can predispose to deviations in gait patterns, which include but are not limited to functional deformities as a result of tissue stiffness, muscle weakness, proprioceptive impairment, pain, and impaired motor control like increased tone (spasticity, rigidity).

OGA can be complimented by **recording forms** used to record gait components, which can range from self-reported measures to performance-based measures. One example of the self-reported measure is the Established Populations for the Epidemiological Study of the Elderly (EPESE) self-report battery, a global self-reported measure of mobility derived from Katz Activity of Daily Living (ADL), Rosow–Breslau scale of mobility disability, and Nagi index of basic physical activities. Performance-based measures include but are not limited to assessment of gait speed, response to changing task demands, simulation of functional mobility and self-reported or measured risk of falls. Examples include measurement of gait speed over a 5 m walkway at either comfortable walk speed or fast walk speed or the Timed Up and Go (TUG) test. Dynamic Gait Index (DGI) evaluates gait alterations in response to changing demands, including gait speed changes, head turns, clearing an obstacle, and stair climbing. The Emory Functional Ambulation Profile measures the time taken to complete the walking task under five environmental circumstances with or without assistive devices. This profile is used commonly in stroke patients. Established Populations for the EPESE Short Physical Performance Battery measures the ability to maintain tandem stance and the time taken to walk 8 ft at normal speed of walking and the time taken to rise from a chair. Functional Ambulation Classification uses a scale to rate the extent of assistance needed (stand by, intermittent support, continuous support) to walk on varying surfaces (level, nonlevel, inclined, stairs). Functional obstacle course uses a series of 12 functional simulations involving mobility tasks commonly encountered in and around home environments. Different textures of flooring are used along with up and down ramps and stairs, over and around small obstacles. The time taken to complete the task as well as the quality of the movement is measured. This can be either observed and quantified or recorded on a video tape for further analysis.

Some examples of self-reported and performance-based measures used in gait assessment are mentioned in **Table 6.8**.

Rivermead Visual Gait Assessment that was developed to evaluate gait of individuals with neurological disorders measures joints of the body (both upper and lower limbs with trunk) in stance and swing phases. A four-point Likert scale is used to grade segmental joint positions as normal (0), mild (1), moderate (2), or severe (3) including the direction of deviation if any.

Another more comprehensive OGA system that is widely reported in literature is the RLA system of OGA pioneered by Ranchos Los Amigos Hospital **(Fig. 6.9)**. It has the advantage of being simple to use in a clinical set up and its low cost other than the less time it takes to administer. It combines observation of temporal parameters of gait with kinematics. Since it is not pathology specific, it can be widely used for a range of population. However, therapist administering this system needs specialized training to use it effectively and should have a complete understanding and knowledge of kinetic and kinematic terminologies related to gait.

Diagnosis of gait abnormalities depends on three separate sets of information, which should be readily available. First, comprehensive knowledge of functional gait problems is induced by the type of pathology such as weakness, tightness or stiffness, and pain and second, thorough understanding of normal gait pattern, which can be used as a template for comparison with pathological states. The third set is skilled observation from the observer

failing which the need for an advanced gait analysis system to identify gait abnormalities becomes inevitable.

Instrumented Gait Analysis

Objective assessment of gait implies quantitative measurement using some sort of tools to get a number of a measured parameter. For example, a pedometer is used to count the number of steps (cadence) taken over a period of time by means of activity monitoring.

The technologies commonly used in clinical gait analysis include specialized computer–interfaced video cameras, passive reflective markers, multicomponent force platforms, and dynamic EMG.

The advance of three-dimensional (3D) quantitative gait analysis includes kinematic, kinetic, and dynamic electromyographic assessment, enabling therapists to measure and differentiate gait deviations objectively and understand the primary problem behind a complex disorder more accurately than observational analysis.

A 3D quantitative analysis consists of three components: kinematics, kinetics, and dynamic EMG assessment. Measurements of gait kinematics are taken using electrogoniometers, gait mats, magnetic and optical systems. Electrogoniometers are probably the simplest method and are an electronic version of the conventional goniometer used in clinics. Electrogoniometers can be used to measure 2D or 3D joint motions. Despite the fact that this can be used to derive 3D data, it is mainly used for 2D measurements.

The more efficient and accurate techniques in instrumented gait analysis include placing the markers, also called sensors, on human joints and then capturing them using image processing. Gait analysis uses different types of motion sensors and systems and can be broadly classified as wearable and nonwearable sensors for easy understanding, which are briefly explained below:

Wearable sensors include motion sensors that are worn or attached to various joints of interest of the human body such as the hip, knee, ankle, and foot or shoulder. The movement signal recorded by these sensors can be used to perform gait analysis quantitatively. These markers can be recognized using image processing techniques. Markers can be active as well as passive.

- Active markers specifically consist of light emitting diodes, which emit light of their own to the capturing source (camera).
- Passive markers are made of Scotchlite or radium, which is light reflecting materials. These passive markers reflect the incident light directly back to the capturing source (camera).

Wearable sensor-based systems can measure kinematic variables of a single or multiple body segments of the subject during motion. Some examples of wearable sensors include:

- Accelerometer
- Gyroscope

Table 6.8: Examples of self-reported and performance-based measures of gait assessment.	
Self-reported measures	*Performance-based measures*
EPESE self-report battery	EPESE Short Physical Performance Battery
Katz activities of daily living	Gait speed
Rosow–Breslau scale of mobility disability	Six-minute walk test
Nagi Disability Index	• Dynamic Gait Index • Timed Up and Go test • Long-Distance Corridor Walk • Emory Functional Ambulation Profile • Gait Abnormality Rating Scale • POMA/Tinetti Balance and Gait Scale

(EPESE: Established Populations for the Epidemiological Study of the Elderly; POMA: Performance-Oriented Mobility Assessment)

Gait analysis: Full body

Rancho Los Amigos Medical Center
Physical Therapy Department

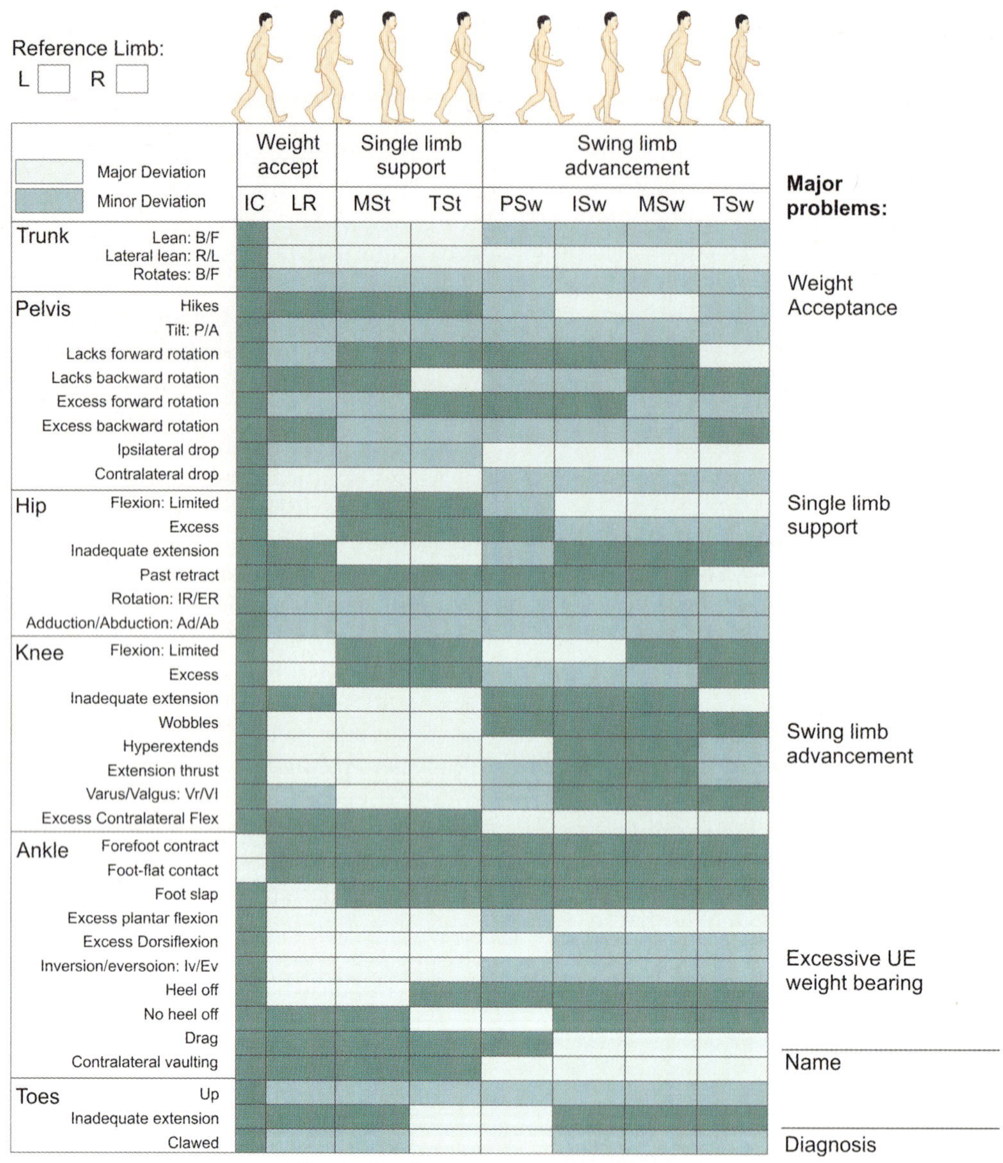

Fig. 6.9: Rancho Los Amigos gait analysis form.
Source: LAREI, Rancho Los Amigos Medical Center, Downey, CA, 1996

- Electrogoniometer (flexible)
- Force sensors
- Sensors for EMG

Three common types of accelerometers are used commonly in gait analysis. They are piezoelectric, piezoresistive, and capacitive accelerometers. Piezoresistive and capacitive accelerometers can provide dual acceleration components and have higher stability. Thus these types of accelerometers are suitable for measuring the motion status in the human gait. By attaching these accelerometers to the feet or legs, the acceleration/velocity of the feet or legs in the gait can be determined to perform the gait analysis.

A gyroscope is an angular velocity sensor, which can be applied for the measurement of the motion and posture of the human segment in gait analysis by measuring the angular rate. A gyroscope is normally used in combination with accelerometer in gait analysis to record the reorganization of various gait phases. Some other advanced wearable sensors include electromagnetic tracking system, sensing fabric, and force sensors (embedded into footwear of patient).

Nonwearable sensors provide accurate data and are highly sensitive. They are expensive as compared to wearable devices and require a dedicated laboratory. Sensors in this category include optical motion capture based on optoelectronic stereophotogrammetry, force platforms, balance boards for dynamic gait testing (with induced perturbations), and instrumented walkway mats. Most of the abovementioned devices are combined to collect and record multiple outcome measures in gait analysis. Force platforms are used to measure GRF and are embedded to walkways or in treadmills and they measure cyclic recordings of GC. It can also measure Center of Pressure, which is a measure of the distribution of weight and forces from stance till completion of the entire GC. It requires skills to interpret the data that is obtained from force platform and is normally expensive. When combined with EMG, it can provide extended information on the kinetics of gait. Instrumented walkway mats include a portable mat embedded with sensors to identify the foot contacts. It is helpful in measuring spatiotemporal parameters of gait and is highly sensitive to changes **(Table 6.9)**.

Kinetics refers to measurement of joint moments and power, which is calculated using GRF data obtained using force plates. Joint moments, GRF are further calculated by combining the information obtained from kinematic analysis such as joint position, speed, and cadence. Dynamic EMG recordings provide information about the timing of muscle activity, its duration and type of muscle work during specific phases of GC.

Muscle Activity During Stance Phase

At initial contact, a deceleration of the limb begins by simultaneously activating the knee extensor and flexor muscles to correctly position the knee before it accepts weight. The hip extensors slow the forward movement of the leg down by contracting eccentrically. During loading response, the ankle dorsiflexors eccentrically contract as the foot reaches the ground. The knee extensors also contract eccentrically as the knee bends, but as the knee extends the contraction changes to concentric. The gluteus medius muscle isometrically contracts in order to stabilize the pelvis. The erector spinae is also active during loading response, which is characterized classically as a mechanism to stabilize the trunk during weight transfer and to prevent its forward flexion during the rapid slowing of forward movement, which occurs in initial contact. The body's center of gravity reaches its highest point during midstance. As the body moves over the stance limb, the intrinsic foot muscles are activated to convert the foot into an increasingly rigid structure. This supination force is augmented by the activity of ankle plantar flexors, which act eccentrically to control dorsiflexion. The quadriceps contracts concentrically to initiate knee extension. Along with momentum and passive resistance from bones and ligaments to gravity, nearly all the support is provided by the anterior and posterior parts of the gluteus medius/minimus muscles in an isometric contraction to eccentrically control pelvic drop against gravity in unilateral stance during walking. At terminal stance, the body accelerates forward and nearly all the muscle work is

Table 6.9: Advantages and disadvantages of wearable and non-wearable sensors.

Advantages	Disadvantages
Wearable sensors	
Can measure gait of patient in everyday environment	Number of variables that can be measured is limited as compared to nonwearable sensors
Can be used for extended period of times	Placement of sensors on body parts might impair certain movement and daily activities
Advanced wireless sensors can remotely send signals to the laboratory	Measurement error is high as compared to nonwearable sensors
Connectible to various systems such as smart phone and watches	More susceptible to signal noise and artifacts, which might affect the data recorded
Low cost	
Patient is engaged actively in the assessment process of providing real-time information	
Patient's clinical visit to laboratory is minimal	
Nonwearable sensors	
Provide the most comprehensive measurements	Costly and expensive
Highly accurate, reliable, and sensitive to minor changes	Normal subject gait can be altered due to walking space restrictions required by the measurement system
Allows simultaneous analysis of multiple gait parameters captured from different approaches	Difficult to employ and record everyday activity
Complex analysis systems allow more precision and have more measurement capacity	
Measurement process controlled in real time by the specialist	

generated by a shortening contraction of the ankle plantar flexors. Just before preswing, hip flexors concentrically contract in order to prepare the leg for swing phase and therefore unloading. The quadriceps is inactive during this phase, as GRFs and activity of plantar flexors maintain knee extension. Preswing is a period of widespread muscle activity where plantar flexors contract concentrically producing a propulsive "push off." Hip flexors shift from eccentric to concentric activity to advance the extremity to swing phase. The erector spinae are active during preswing with greater EMG activity than in loading response.

A comprehensive diagrammatic representation of muscle activity of lower limb during stance phase of a GC is provided in **Figure 6.10.**

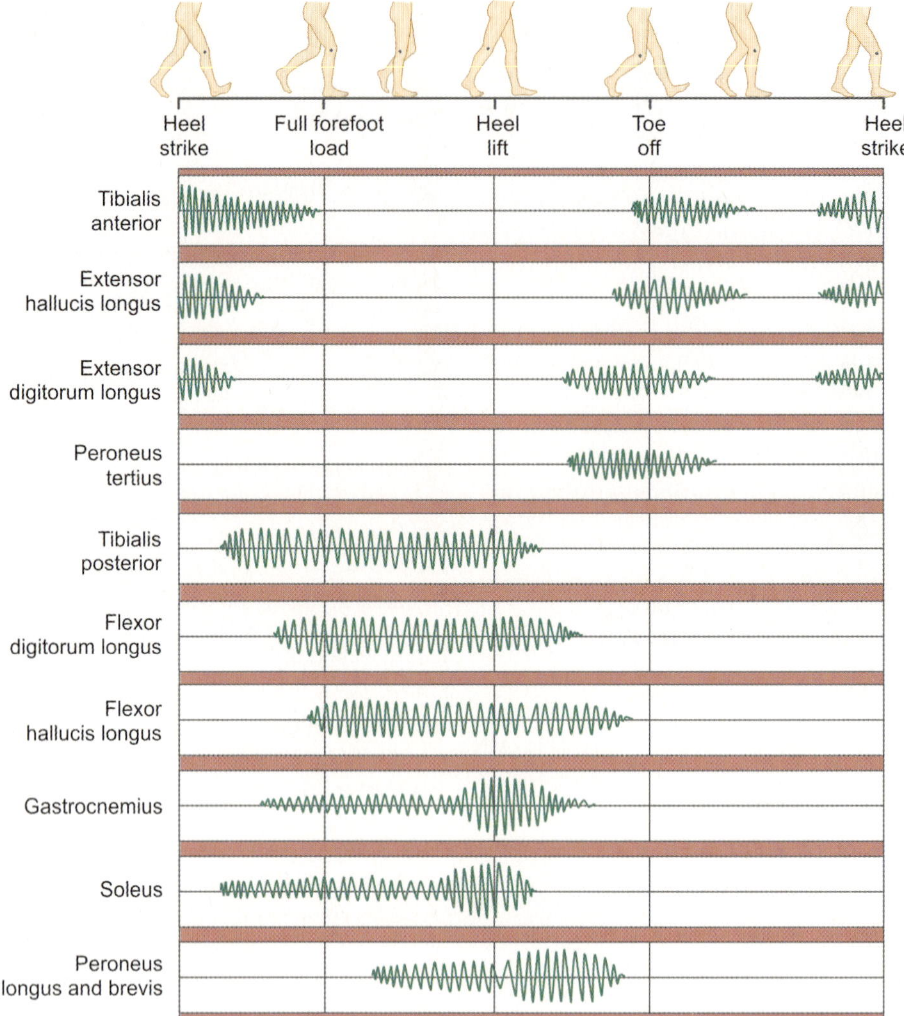

Fig. 6.10: Muscle activity in the lower limb during stance phase of a single gait cycle.

Muscle Activity During Swing Phase

At the beginning of swing, the ankle dorsiflexors contract concentrically to allow the foot to clear off the ground and remain contracted throughout the whole swing phase. Hip flexors and knee extensors primarily rectus femoris continue their preswing activity. During midswing, all muscle activities virtually cease except for the dorsiflexors as the extremity's inertia carries it through swing like a pendulum. At terminal swing, the goal is to decelerate the leg and prepare it for weight acceptance and the hamstrings contract either isometrically or eccentrically in order to slow both hip flexion and knee extension. The contraction in the ankle dorsiflexors changes from concentric to isometric or eccentric.

A comprehensive diagrammatic representation of muscle activity of lower limb during stance phase and swing phase of a GC is provided in **Figure 6.11**.

Limitations of quantitative gait analysis include artificiality of walking due to attachment of electrodes to the body, high cost, the need for a well-trained team, and potential errors. The potential source of errors includes type, size and placement of electrodes and markers, errors during analysis of the obtained data or during interpretation of data, artifacts and calibration errors, system errors, and poor training.

CLINICAL APPLICATION OF INSTRUMENTED GAIT ANALYSIS

Clinical application of any gait analysis depends on the identification of impairment present, which is obtained from careful interpretation of data obtained from the analysis. The significant role of gait analysis in clinical application primarily falls into three basic purposes: diagnostic, monitoring, and research.

Since it is beyond the scope of this chapter to discuss all the possible gait deviations, some common deviations and their possible interpretation in relation to OGA and instrumented gait analysis is considered here. As mentioned earlier, the features of a pathologic gait depend on the nature of the impairment and the ability of the individual to compensate for that impairment, which may vary with individuals.

Classic gait terminology:	Heel strike	Foot flat	Midstance	Heel off	Toe-off	Acceleration	Midswing	Deceleration
Rancho Los Amigos terms New terminology	Initial contact	Loading response	Midstance	Terminal stance	Preswing	Initial swing	Midswing	Terminal swing
	Stance phase 60%					Swing phase 40%		
% of total phase	0–2%	0–10%	10–30%	30–50%	50–60%	60–73%	73–87%	87–100%
Iliopsoas	Inactive	Inactive	Inactive	Concentric	Concentric	Concentric	Concentric	Inactive
Gluteus maximus	Eccentric	Inactive	Inactive	Inactive	Inactive	Inactive	Inactive	Inactive
Gluteus medius	Eccentric	Eccentric	Eccentric	Eccentric	Inactive	Inactive	Inactive	Inactive
Hamstrings	Eccentric	Eccentric	Inactive	Inactive	Inactive	Eccentric	Eccentric	Eccentric
Quadriceps	Eccentric	Eccentric	Inactive	Inactive	Eccentric	Eccentric	Inactive	Inactive
Pretibial muscles	Eccentric	Eccentric	Inactive	Inactive	Inactive	Concentric	Concentric	Concentric
Calf muscles	Inactive	Inactive	Eccentric	Concentric	Concentric	Inactive	Inactive	Inactive

Key: ☐ Inactive ▨ Concentric ▩ Eccentric

Fig. 6.11: Muscle activity in the lower limb during a single gait cycle.

Pain is considered an important factor in deviating an optimal gait, which is referred to as antalgic gait, commonly referred to the suspected joint producing pain, as antalgic hip gait or antalgic knee gait. Pain prevents the individual to avoid weight bearing on the painful side leading to typical characteristic features such as shorter step length and decreased stance time. This is also associated with a lateral lean of the trunk toward the swing leg (pain-free side) in an attempt to alleviate weight bearing on the painful side.

Neurological patterns of pathological gait can be observed in neurological conditions such as stroke, Parkinson's disease, cerebellar dysfunction (ataxia), and cerebral palsy. Increased tonicity (spasticity) affecting the extensor musculatures (decreased knee flexion and ankle dorsiflexion) commonly results in stiff legged gait pattern in which the individual circumduct and progress forward. If there is a foot drop, there is a pattern of high stepping with increased knee flexion to compensate for the weak dorsiflexors, which facilitate ground clearance during walking. A short, accelerated stepping pattern with reduced or absence of arm swing and a stiff flexed trunk is observed in individuals with Parkinson's disease, termed "Festinating gait."

Cerebellar ataxia has its own distinguished characteristics of abnormal gait pattern in which there is reduced gait velocity and stride length and irregular stepping both in direction and distance (Drunken gait).

Kinetic studies of GRFs demonstrated a reduced peak at weight acceptance, reflecting a difficulty planting the foot soundly. A greater degree of imbalance is observed when the patient is given the task to turn while walking and irregular foot placements are evident when the patient walks in a straight path **(Fig. 6.12)**.

Imbalance in static and dynamic position is evident in tandem stance and during attempts to walk in tandem. These deficits are masked when the patient walks briskly and hence is observed during assessment while the patient is asked to walk at a slower pace than normal.

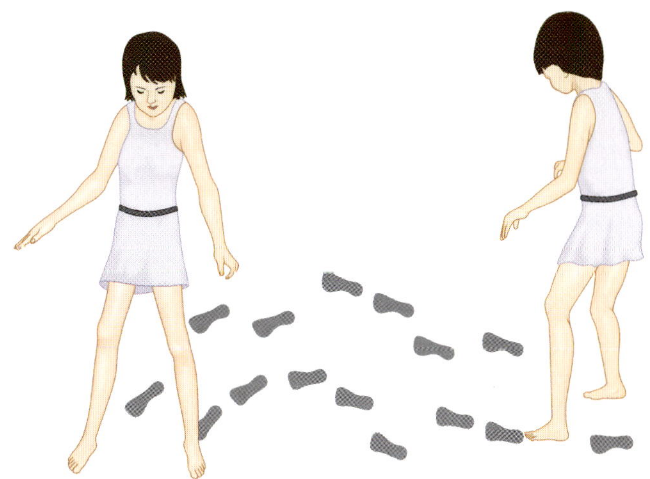

Fig. 6.12: Cerebellar gait.

Musculoskeletal deficits either due to excessive or limited ROM or due to ineffective muscle strength lead to various gait deviations. Tightness of muscle or muscle groups, weakness of muscles, joint instability, or tissue laxity may contribute to deviations. In the presence of plantar flexors contracture, during initial contact, forefoot makes contact with the ground due to decreased dorsiflexion. During midstance, knee hyperextension compensates for the decreased dorsiflexion and during terminal stance forward leaning of the trunk is used as a strategy to maintain forward progression of CoM. Knee flexion contracture leads to crouching of the stance leg, which in turn results in excessive hip and knee flexion of the contralateral limb to facilitate toe clearance during swing.

One of the common musculoskeletal disorders encountered by therapists in their day-to-day practice is osteoarthritis (OA) of the knee joint, which frequently leads to gait impairment. Secondary complications of knee joint OA is joint deformity where tibial varum is common. The foremost sign observable as an outcome measure in patients with knee OA is the slower walking speed. Depending on various factors such as severity of pain and overall weight of the body, antalgic gait pattern can be present. Clinical gait analysis can be used to identify the pathological representation ranging from as simple as observing and recording the decreased weight bearing in stance phase on the affected side, to quantitatively measure and record the joint moment forces during different phases. In summary, patients with OA knee tend to keep their knee in extension to reduce the need for quadriceps activity and associated compressive forces. It may be accompanied by an antalgic gait pattern characterized by a reduced stance time and shorter step length.

It is a common observation among therapists that circumduction gait is typical of patients with hemiplegia. Hence, circumduction gait is used synonymously as hemiplegic gait, which is a misnomer. Hip circumduction during swing phase of GC can occur due to lack of shortening of the swinging extremity failing to facilitate ground clearance, which can be a result of reduced hip flexion, reduced knee flexion, and or lack of ankle dorsiflexion.

Apart from these pathological conditions, gait assessment is also very important in conditions where patients use any sort of assistive devices for ambulation (Gait with assistive devices is described in Chapter 11).

SUMMARY

Walking is considered a complex function as it integrates all the joints of the lower extremity. A thorough understanding of the kinesiology of locomotion serves a prerequisite to any expert in healthcare profession to assess and evaluate individuals with gait abnormalities. A comprehensive knowledge of kinetic and kinematics

of gait makes understanding of gait analysis easy. Any limitation of motion in one joint can have a profound effect on the quality and quantity of movement during gait. Neuromusculoskeletal factors can contribute to deviations in gait, which is often minimized through biomechanical compensations naturally adopted by individuals. When this fails, the role of clinician comes up to device strategies to compensate and correct the deviations. These strategies not only include exercise to improve muscle strength, ROM, and flexibility but also activities targeting functional improvement and patient education.

Review Questions

1. Identify gait cycle based on subphases of stance and swing.
2. Differentiate traditional and RLA nomenclature of gait cycle.
3. Discuss the functional goals of gait.
4. Enlist the percentage of phases of gait cycle.
5. Enlist the spatial parameters of gait assessment.
6. Enlist the temporal parameters of gait assessment.
7. What are the methods to measure spatial and temporal parameters of gait?
8. List and discuss the determinants of gait.
9. What is the significance of each determinant of gait?
10. What is the optimal ROM required from various lower extremity joints for walking?
11. Discuss the components of ground reaction forces?
12. Brief out the reasoning for performing clinical gait analysis?
13. Discuss the disadvantages and limitations of observational gait analysis.
14. Differentiate wearable and nonwearable sensors in gait analysis.
15. What is the pathology behind hemiplegic gait, cerebellar gait, Parkinson's gait? Differentiate the deviations.
16. What is the pathomechanics behind antalgic hip gait, antalgic knee gait, and knee-to-hand gait?

BIBLIOGRAPHY

1. Alexander NB, Guire KE, Thelen DG, et al. Self-reported walking ability predicts functional mobility performance in frail older adults. J Am Geriatr Soc. 2000;48:1408-13.
2. Anderson FC, Pandy MG. Individual muscle contributions to support in normal walking. Gait Posture. 2003;17:159-69.
3. Andriacchi TP, Ogle JA, Galante JO. Walking speed as a basis for normal and abnormal gait measurements. J Biomech. 1977;10:261-8.
4. Baker R. Gait analysis methods in rehabilitation. J Neuroeng Rehabil. 2006;3:4.
5. Baokes JL, Rab GT. Human walking. Philadelphia, PA: Lippincott; 2006.
6. Blanc Y, Balmer C, Landis T, et al. Temporal parameters and patterns of the foot roll over during walking: normative data for healthy adults. Gait Posture. 1999;10:97-108.
7. Bouten CV, Koekkoek KT, Verduin M, et al. A triaxial accelerometer and portable data processing unit for the assessment of daily physical activity. IEEE Trans Biomed Eng. 1997;44:136-47.

8. Chang RW, Dunlop D, Gibbs J, et al. The determinants of walking velocity in the elderly. An evaluation using regression trees. Arthritis Rheum. 1995;38:343-50.

9. Chen CP, Chen MJ, Pei YC, et al. Sagittal plane loading response during gait in different age groups and in people with knee osteoarthritis. Am J Phys Med Rehabil. 2003a;82:307-12.

10. Chen WL, O'connor JJ, Radin EL. A comparison of the gaits of Chinese and Caucasian women with particular reference to their heel strike transients. Clin Biomech (Bristol, Avon). 2003b;18:207-13.

11. Chris K. Clinical gait analysis. Washington, DC: Churchill Livingstone; 2004.

12. Craik RL, Oatis CA. Gait analysis: theory and application. St. Louis, MO: Mosby; 1995.

13. Cunningham DA, Rechnitzer PA, Pearce ME, et al. Determinants of self-selected walking pace across ages 19 to 66. J Gerontol. 1982;37:560-4.

14. Eastlack ME, Arvidson J, Snyder-Mackler L, et al. Interrater reliability of videotaped observational gait-analysis assessments. Phys Ther. 1991;71:465-72.

15. Goodkin R, Diller L. Reliability among physical therapists in diagnosis and treatment of gait deviations in hemiplegics. Percept Mot Skills. 1973;37:727-34.

16. Himann JE, Cunningham DA, Rechnitzer PA, et al. Age-related changes in speed of walking. Med Sci Sports Exerc. 1988;20:161-6.

17. Isacson J, Gransberg L, Knutsson E. Three-dimensional electrogoniometric gait recording. J Biomech. 1986;19:627-35.

18. Johnston RC, Smidt GL. Measurement of hip-joint motion during walking. Evaluation of an electrogoniometric method. J Bone Joint Surg Am. 1969;51:1082-94.

19. Kadaba MP, Ramakrishnan HK, Wootten ME, et al. Repeatability of kinematic, kinetic, and electromyographic data in normal adult gait. J Orthop Res. 1989;7:849-60.

20. Katoh Y, Chao EY, Laughman RK, et al. Biomechanical analysis of foot function during gait and clinical applications. Clin Orthop Relat Res. 1983;177:23-33.

21. Krebs DE, Edelstein JE, Fishman S. Reliability of observational kinematic gait analysis. Phys Ther. 1985;65:1027-33.

22. Kuo AD. The six determinants of gait and the inverted pendulum analogy: a dynamic walking perspective. Hum Mov Sci. 2007;26:617-56.

23. Larsson LE, Odenrick P, Sandlund B, et al. The phases of the stride and their interaction in human gait. Scand J Rehabil Med. 1980;12:107-12.

24. Lehmann JF, de Lateur BJ, Price R. Biomechanics of abnormal gait. Phys Med Rehabil Clin N Am. 1992;3:125-38.

25. Lord SE, Halligan PW, Wade DT. Visual gait analysis: the development of a clinical assessment and scale. Clin Rehabil. 1998;12:107-19.

26. Muro-de-la-Herran A, Garcia-Zapirain B, Mendez-Zorrilla A. Gait analysis methods: an overview of wearable and non-wearable systems, highlighting clinical applications. Sensors (Basel). 2014;14:3362-94.

27. Ostrosky KM, Vanswearingen JM, Burdett RG, et al. A comparison of gait characteristics in young and old subjects. Phys Ther. 1994;74:637-44; discussion 644-6.

28. Palliyath S, Hallett M, Thomas SL, et al. Gait in patients with cerebellar ataxia. Mov Disord. 1998;13:958-64.

29. Perry J. Gait analysis normal and pathological function. New York, NY: SLACK; 1992.

30. Pietraszewski B, Winiarski S, Jaroszczuk S. Three-dimensional human gait pattern—reference data for normal men. Acta Bioeng Biomech. 2012;14:9-16.

31. Saleh M, Murdoch G. In defence of gait analysis. Observation and measurement in gait assessment. J Bone Joint Surg Br. 1985;67:237-41.

32. Saunders JB, Inman VT, Eberhart HD. The major determinants in normal and pathological gait. J Bone Joint Surg Am. 1953;35-A:543-58.

33. Schache AG, Baker R, Lamoreux LW. Defining the knee joint flexion-extension axis for purposes of quantitative gait analysis: an evaluation of methods. Gait Posture. 2006;24:100-9.

34. Shanahan CJ, Boonstra FMC, Cofre lizama LE, et al. Technologies for advanced gait and balance assessments in people with multiple sclerosis. Front Neurol. 2017;8:708.

35. Tao W, Liu T, Zheng R, et al. Gait analysis using wearable sensors. Sensors (Basel). 2012;12:2255-83.

36. Toro B, Nester C, Farren P. A review of observational gait assessment in clinical practice. Physiother Theory Pract. 2003;19:137-49.

37. Toro B, Nester CJ, Farren PC. The status of gait assessment among physiotherapists in the United Kingdom. Arch Phys Med Rehabil. 2003;84:1878-84.

38. Wallmann HW. Introduction to observational gait analysis. Home Health Care Manage Pract. 2009;22:66-68.

39. Yavuzer G. Three-dimensional quantitative gait analysis. Acta Orthop Traumatol Turc. 2009;43:94-101.

40. Zeng H, Zhao Y. Sensing movement: microsensors for body motion measurement. Sensors (Basel). 2011;11:638-60.

Electrodiagnosis

Megha S Sheth, Priyasingh Rangey

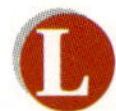

LEARNING OBJECTIVES

After reading this chapter, the readers should be able to:
- Understand the concept of electrodiagnostic medicine
- Learn the different tests involved in electrodiagnostic medicine
- Learn about strength–duration curves, faradic, and galvanic test and other tests used to evaluate degeneration of a nerve
- Understand the process of electroneurological testing using electromyography (EMG) and nerve conduction studies
- Learn to perform EMG and nerve conduction velocity testing
- Discuss H reflex and F wave.

CHAPTER OUTLINE

- Introduction
  - Effects of peripheral nerve damage
  - Changes in electrical reactions
  - Causes of decreased voluntary muscle power
  - Parts of the human body accessible for electrical stimulation and testing
  - Types of electrical currents used in electrodiagnosis
- Faradic–galvanic test/F and G test/faradic and interrupted direct current test
  - Parameters
  - Technique
  - Interpretation
  - Advantages
  - Disadvantages
- Reaction of degeneration test
  - Parameters
  - Technique
  - Interpretation
- Strength-duration curve
  - Purpose of strength–duration curve
  - Electrical parameters of SDC
  - Technique
  - Parameters for evaluating strength–duration curve
  - Characteristics of strength–duration curve
  - Signs of restoration of nerve supply
  - Signs of progressive denervation
  - Advantages
  - Disadvantages
- Galvanic twitch/tetanus ratio
  - Parameters
  - Technique
  - Disadvantages
- Nerve conduction studies
  - Factors affecting nerve conduction velocity
  - Motor nerve conduction studies
  - Sensory nerve conduction studies
  - Pathophysiology
  - Techniques of application for commonly evaluated nerves
- Electromyography
  - Uses of electromyography
  - Instrumentation
  - Factors
  - Recording parameters
  - Recording procedure
  - Recording of activity
- H reflex
  - Technique
  - H:M ratio
  - Clinical implication
- F wave
  - Characteristics of F wave
  - Uses of F waves
  - Physiology
  - Technique
  - Limitations
- Documentation and reporting
- Other electrodiagnostic tests

INTRODUCTION

Electrodiagnosis is the detection of electrical reactions of muscles and nerves for diagnosis or prognosis by the use of electrotherapeutic current or electrodes. It is basically the study of the electrophysiological properties and characteristics of various biological tissues for diagnostic purposes. It includes, but is not limited to:

- Electromyography (EMG)
- Nerve conduction studies (NCS)
- Electroencephalography
- Electrogastrography
- Electroretinography
- Evoked potential studies
- Strength–duration curve (SDC)
- Reaction of degeneration test (RD test), etc.

BOX 7.1: Definition of electrodiagnosis and electrodiagnostic medicine.

The American Association of Neuromuscular and Electrodiagnostic Medicine (AANEM) defines electrodiagnosis as *"The scientific methods of recording and analyzing biologic electrical potentials from the central, peripheral, and autonomic nervous systems and muscles."*
Electrodiagnostic medicine is *"A specific area of medical practice in which a physician integrates information obtained from the clinical history, observations from physical examination, and scientific data acquired by recording electrical potentials from the nervous system and muscle to diagnose, or diagnose and treat diseases of the central, peripheral, and autonomic nervous systems, neuromuscular junctions, and muscle."*

Clinical electrodiagnosis involves the recording, display, measurement, and interpretation of action potential arising from the central nervous system (evoked potentials), peripheral nerves (NCS), and muscles (EMG) **(Box 7.1)**.

Effects of Peripheral Nerve Damage

Changes that take place at the tissue level following a nerve lesion are shown in **Figures 7.1 and 7.2**.

When there is peripheral nerve injury, one or more of the following are seen:

- Muscle weakness or paralysis and loss of sensation—immediately after lesion.
- Muscle atrophy—this is seen over 3 months after injury stabilizing at around 6–9 months where the muscle loses bulk and becomes thinner.
- Increased sensitivity to acetylcholine (ACh).
- Spontaneous muscle twitches known as "fibrillations."

If a muscle gets reinnervated in sufficient time some of these changes can be reversed.

Changes in Electrical Reactions

- Because of axonal degeneration the muscle loses its capacity to respond to a short pulse duration electrical impulse **(Fig. 7.3)**. (Does not respond to surged faradic (SF) current.)
- It becomes more excitable because of hyperreactivity to ACh and so a response to long pulse duration current (LPDC) is seen at a lower intensity.
- There is a reversal of polarity and so anode becomes more stimulating than the cathode.
- Ability to accommodate slow-rising pulses decreases.

Causes of Decreased Voluntary Muscle Power

When a person is unable to voluntarily contract a muscle or use a limb, the following possibilities exist:

1. An upper motor neuron (UMN) lesion
2. A lower motor neuron (LMN) lesion that includes the peripheral nerve, anterior horn cell (AHC), and nerve root.
3. Muscle damage by disease or a tendon injury
4. Neuromuscular (NM) junction abnormalities
5. Functional disorder

Parts of the Human Body Accessible for Electrical Stimulation and Testing

Human body parts accessible for electrical stimulation (ES) and testing are as follows:

- LMN below its exit from vertebral canal
- Muscle

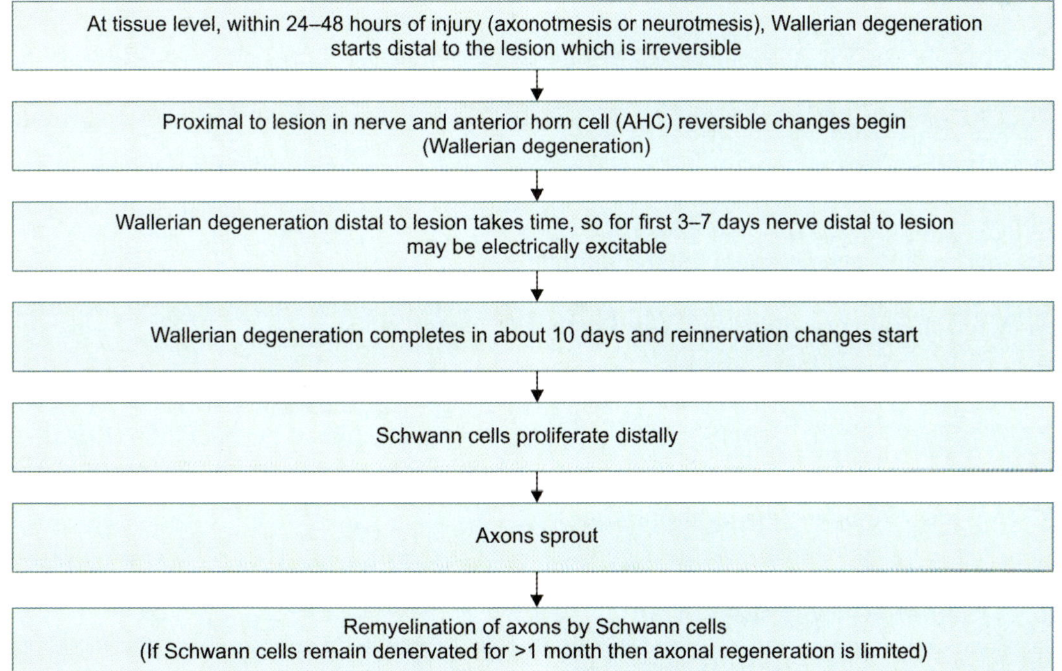

Fig. 7.1: Changes taking place at the tissue level following a nerve lesion.

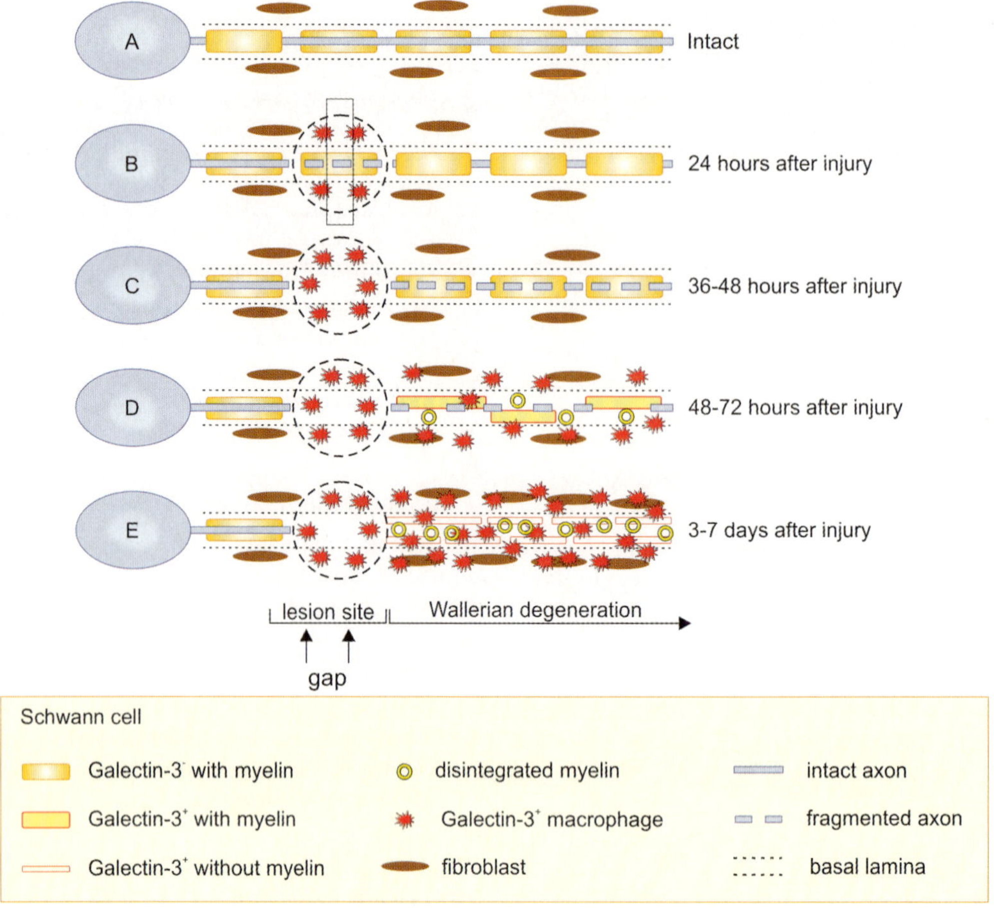

Fig. 7.2: Wallerian degeneration.

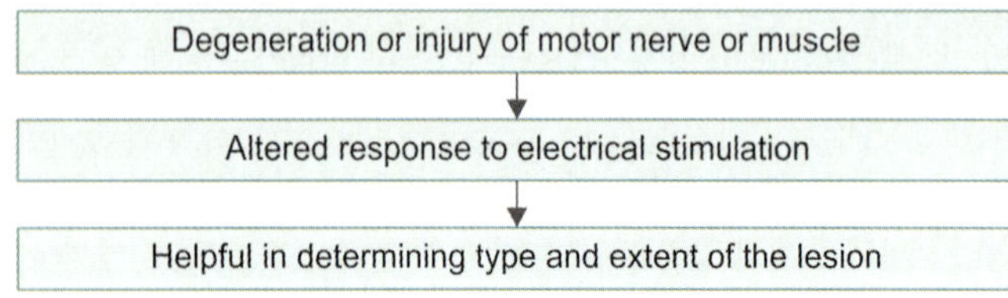

Fig. 7.3: Changes in electrical reactions.

In the presence of a UMN lesion:
- There are no changes in LMN or muscle.
- There are no changes in response to electrical stimulation.
- Sometimes, nerves and muscles are hyperexcitable and react to lower intensity of current.

Classification of peripheral nerve injuries according to Seddon:
1. Neurapraxia:
   - There is demyelination of the nerve, either of a segment or of the complete nerve.
   - Normal response to electrical reactions is seen of the affected muscles below the level of lesion if there is a conduction block.
   - There is a loss of response to stimulus given to nerve trunk above the site of lesion.
2. Axonotmesis and neurotmesis:
   - There is an altered response to electrical stimuli.
   - If all nerve fibers supplying a muscle degenerate, complete reaction of degeneration (CRD) is seen.

- If some fibers degenerate, partial reaction of degeneration (PRD) is seen.

AHC lesion:
- Depends on the extent of damage
- If degeneration of nerve fibers present → reaction of degeneration is seen
- Less severe lesion of AHC → no reaction of degeneration is seen.

Neuromuscular (NM) junction defects: Methods other than simple electrical stimulation are needed for diagnosis. Response to repeated stimuli is altered.

Muscle lesions:
- No degeneration of motor nerve → normal reaction to ES is seen → decrease in strength of contraction may be seen
- If complete loss of muscle tissue → no response to ES or no reaction of degeneration (RD) is seen which is known as absolute reaction of degeneration (ARD).

Functional disorders: No alteration to ES response.

Types of Electrical Currents Used in Electrodiagnosis

Two types of electrical currents are used in electrodiagnosis:
1. Short pulse duration current—SPDC/SF current
2. LPDC/interrupted galvanic (IG)/interrupted direct current (IDC).

FARADIC–GALVANIC TEST/F AND G TEST/FARADIC AND INTERRUPTED DIRECT CURRENT TEST

This test uses the IG and faradic current for diagnosis of a nerve injury or a tendon cut.

Parameters

Parameters of faradic-galvanic test are as follows:
- Faradic current:
  - Pulse duration—0.1–1 ms
  - Pulse frequency—50–100 Hz
  - Surge duration on and off so as to produce a tetanic contraction of innervated muscle
  - Intensity—to produce a minimal contraction
- IG current:
  - Pulse duration—100 ms or longer
  - Pulse frequency—1 Hz, to get 1 twitch contraction per second
  - Intensity—to produce a minimal contraction.

Techniques

F and G test is performed using the following techniques:
- The nerve is stimulated using first an LPDC (IG) and then an SPDC (SF), and the response to both are seen.
- Find the motor point of a muscle using the IG current and check the response.
- Keeping the motor point the same check the response to the SF current.

Interpretation

F and G test can be interpreted as follows:

Response to IG current can be:
- Brisk contraction = innervated muscle or a neurapraxia injury
- Sluggish contraction = denervated muscle
- No contraction = fibrosis of muscle

Response to SF current can be:
- Brisk contraction = innervated muscle or a neurapraxia injury
- No contraction = denervated muscle

  The principle of this test is that a denervated muscle loses its property to respond to an SPDC.

  If a muscle contraction is seen and a related joint movement is seen, it implies tendon continuity.

Advantages

Advantages of faradic and IDC test are as follows:
- Simple
- Easy
- Cheap
- Quick
- Gives an idea whether nerve degeneration is present or not especially in the early stages.

Disadvantages

Following are the disadvantages of Faradic and IDC test:
- Does not give the exact site of nerve injury
- Does not describe the severity or extent of injury
- Does not show a change with regeneration.

REACTION OF DEGENERATION TEST

This is similar to the F and G test except for the fact that only SF current is used and response is checked.
- Used to assess the level of innervation of skeletal muscle
- Provide information on integrity of alpha motor neurons innervating skeletal muscle.

Parameters

Parameters of RD test are as follows:
- Monophasic or biphasic—SF current
- Pulse duration—0.1 ms
- Frequency—20–50 Hz

Technique

Following is the technique used for RD test:
A muscle is stimulated along the course of a nerve using an SPDC and the response is observed. One begins with a proximal muscle and proceeds distally till response to electrical stimulation stops.

Interpretation

The test can be interpreted as follows:
- Normal muscle → smooth tetanic contraction
- Denervated muscle → no muscle contraction → "reaction of degeneration" → loss of innervation to muscle
- Partial denervation → some fibers lost → elicits contraction but force decreased → "PRD."

  This is a quick way to find the level of injury as a response to SPDC below that is lost.

STRENGTH–DURATION CURVE

It is an electrodiagnostic procedure that plots in a graphic form the strength required of a stimulating current against a series of decreasing pulse durations. Selected pulse durations in milliseconds and fractions of milliseconds are used to stimulate a muscle through the nerve at their motor points. The intensity of current required for each pulse is noted. A graph is plotted with pulse duration on the X-axis and the intensity of current on the Y-axis. The curve is then compared with the characteristics described below for interpretation. Repeated strength–duration curves (SDCs) show a shift in the curve which implies worsening or improvement of the condition.

Purpose of Strength–Duration Curve

The purpose of SDC is to:
- Determine the level of innervation of skeletal muscle by a motor neuron after nerve injury or disease.

- Reflect the ratio of innervated to denervated muscle fibers.
- Assess the progress or deterioration of motor innervation.

Electrical Parameters of SDC

Following parameters are used to evaluate SDC:
- Rectangular, monophasic pulsed current
- Frequency of 1 Hz
- Pulse duration ranges from 0.01 to 300 ms
- Constant current (CC) (more accurate) or constant voltage (CV) (more comfortable) stimulator
- Cathode: At motor point of muscle
- Anode: Over the muscle few cm away from the motor point or other convenient areas
- Response: Minimally detectable (visible) twitch contraction.
  - Response of usually, two muscles supplied by the nerve distal to damaged area are examined, one proximal and one distal usually starting 7–10 days after injury
  - Tests repeated every 2 weeks (depending on site of injury and muscle tested).

Techniques

SDC is performed using the following techniques:
- Patient is explained the procedure and placed in comfortable position.
- The part to be tested is exposed and kept well supported.
- The room should be well lighted.
- Check contraindications if any.
- Cover the abrasions, decrease skin resistance.
- Therapist should be in a comfortable position with hand stable throughout the procedure.
- Active electrode should be as small as possible to avoid spreading the current.
- Set the parameters as described above with intensity on zero, pulse duration at 300 ms, and electrodes in position.
- Stimulate with an active electrode at or around the motor point area to get a minimal visible contraction. Find the best point and note the intensity of current needed. Successively decrease the pulse durations, increase the intensity of current if needed, and make a note of the intensity for the particular pulse duration. Repeat for all pulse durations up to 0.01 ms.
- Maintain the same position, angle, and pressure for the active electrode.
- Plot the graph of the strength of the current (*Y*-axis) versus the pulse duration (*X*-axis).
- Note the name, age, gender, date of injury, and date of performing the test along with the diagnosis and interpretation.

Parameters for Evaluating Strength–Duration Curve

SDC is evaluated based on:
- Shape of curve
- Rheobase
- Chronaxie
- Rise time
- Utilization time
- Pulse ratio

Shape of Curve

The SDC of any muscle whether innervated or denervated (completely or partially) has a characteristic shape. The details of the shape of SDC are described in the following segment on characteristics of SDC.

Rheobase

It is the minimum intensity of current (V or mA) required to produce a threshold motor (or sensory or pain) response to an infinitely long pulse. Rheobase is usually the intensity of current needed to produce a minimum contraction at 100 or 300 ms.

Factors influencing rheobase:
- Muscle being tested
- Temperature
- Blood supply
- Edema
- Electrode size, position, and pressure
- Skin resistance—texture and moisture
  (Threshold increased with decreased temperature, decreased blood supply, increased edema, or poor localization of motor point).
- Innervated: 2–18 mA or 3–40 V
- Denervated: Lower than normal

Chronaxie

It is the pulse duration necessary to obtain a threshold response using a pulse with intensity twice the rheobase intensity.
- Innervated   : <1 ms for CC
                  : <0.1 ms for CV
- Denervated   : >10 ms for both CC and CV

Rise Time

It is the pulse duration at which one needs to increase the intensity of current more than the rheobase intensity. It is late in normal innervation and early with denervation.

Utilization Time

It is the shortest pulse duration at which you get a minimal stimulation with intensity of current equal to rheobase current. It is the pulse duration that should be used for treatment purposes.

Pulse Ratio

It is the ratio of intensity of current required to produce a minimum contraction at 1 ms to the intensity of current required to produce a minimum contraction at 100 ms.

$$\text{Pulse ratio} = \frac{\text{Intensity at 1 ms}}{\text{Intensity at 100 ms}}$$

Characteristics of Strength–Duration Curve

Following are the characteristics of SDC:
1. **Normal innervation (Fig. 7.4):**
   - Shape—straight line, parallel to the X-axis, rising for the last few pulse durations. Same strength of stimulus is required to produce the response with all impulses of longer duration.
   - Shorter duration requires increase in amplitude.
   - It is a complete curve with the response seen to all pulse durations.
   - No kink is seen
   - Rise time—point at which the curve begins to rise is variable, but usually 1 ms with CC stimulation and 0.1 ms with CV stimulator.
   - Utilization time—it is shorter pulse duration usually 3 or 0.3 ms.
   - Pulse ratio—it is <2.2.
2. **Complete denervation (Fig. 7.5):**
   - Increase in intensity of current required for successively decreasing pulses. For all impulses of 100 ms or lesser duration → stimulus increased for each pulse duration.
   - Very short duration → no response.
   - Incomplete curve
   - Curve rises steeply
   - Shifted to right
   - No kink seen
   - Rise time is early, usually 30 or 100 ms.
   - Utilization time—it is larger pulse duration usually 100 ms.
   - Pulse ratio—it is >2.5.
3. **Partial denervation (Fig. 7.6):**
   - Some fibers degenerated, some intact

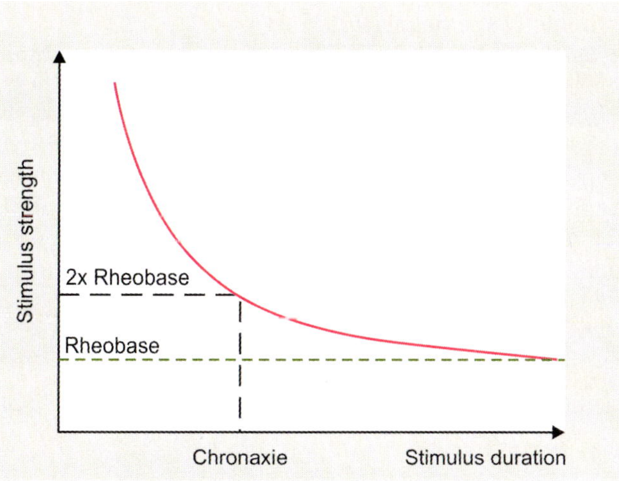

Fig. 7.4: Normal strength–duration (SDC) curve.

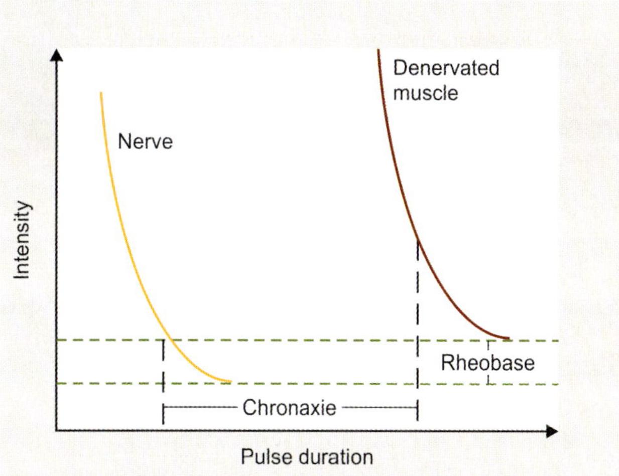

Fig. 7.5: Complete reaction of degeneration (CRD) in strength–duration curve (SD).

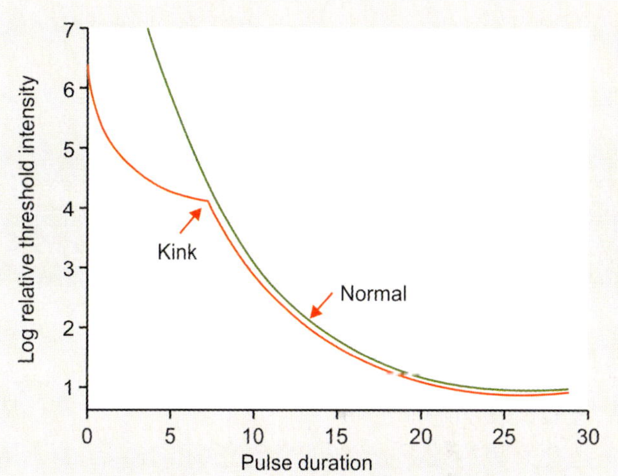

Fig. 7.6: Comparison of normal and partial reaction of degeneration (PRD) curves.

- Long pulse duration impulse → stimulates both denervated and innervated fibers
  ↓
  Contraction produced with low intensity
- Short pulse duration impulse → denervated fibers respond less readily → stronger stimulus required to produce perceptible contraction → curve rises steeply like denervated muscle
- Very short impulse → few innervated fibers respond to higher stimulus, contraction of denervated fibers not obtained → curve similar to innervated muscle
- Therefore right-hand part of curve similar to denervated muscle, left-hand part similar to innervated muscle
  ↓
  "kink" seen where two parts meet
- Shape of curve indicates proportion of denervation
  ↓
  Large number of fibers denervated → curve more similar to denervated muscle

↓

Majority of fibers innervated → curve resembles more to that of an innervated muscle

- Rheobase and chronaxie depend on the amount of denervation present.

Signs of Restoration of Nerve Supply

Signs of restoration of nerve supply are:
1. Kink appears in curve and moves to the right
2. Curve moves down and to the left.

Signs of Progressive Denervation

Signs of progressive denervation are:
1. Appearance of kink which shifts to the left
2. Increase in slope and curve shifts to right.

Advantages

Following are the advantages of SDC:
- Most satisfactory method at present available for routine testing of electrical response in peripheral nerve injury (PNI)
- Simple, quick
- Indicates proportion of denervation
- Series of tests gives changes in condition
- Noninvasive
- Inexpensive.

Disadvantages

The disadvantages of SDC are as follows:
- In large muscles, full picture not clearly shown (as only few fibers respond)
- Does not indicate site of nerve lesion
- Low reliability (intertester).

GALVANIC TWITCH-TETANUS RATIO

It determines the relationship between intensity of current required to obtain a single twitch contraction to the intensity needed to elicit a sustained tetanic contraction.

Parameters

Following are the parameters of galvanic twitch-tetanus ratio test:
- Direct current (DC) (monophasic pulsed current with long duration)
- Frequency—1/s and 50/s.

Technique

The technique of performing galvanic twitch-tetanus ratio is as follows:
- Motor point stimulation with cathode

↓

With frequency of current at 1 Hz, intensity increased gradually till twitch contraction

↓

Intensity recorded

With frequency of current at 50 Hz, intensity increased to produce a sustained tetanic like contraction

↓

Intensity recorded

$$\text{Galvanic twitch-tetanus ratio} = \frac{\text{Intensity at freq 1/s}}{\text{Intensity at freq 50/s}}$$

- Partially innervated muscle ratio 1:3.5–1:6.5
- Completely denervated muscle ratio 1:1–1:1.5.

Disadvantages

The disadvantages of galvanic twitch-tetanus ratio test are:
- Procedure extremely uncomfortable to subject
- Rarely used.

NERVE CONDUCTION STUDIES

The AANEM defines NCS as "recording and analysis of electric waveforms of biologic origin elicited in response to electric or physiologic stimuli." They are also termed nerve conduction velocity (NCV) tests since this particular group of tests records and analyzes the waveforms generated by peripheral nerves (motor or sensory) by measuring their conduction velocities. The waveforms studied are termed compound sensory nerve action potential (SNAP) (for sensory nerves), compound motor nerve action potential (for motor nerves), and mixed nerve action potential (for mixed nerves). NCS are extremely helpful in the evaluation of NM disorders, particularly the pathologies involving peripheral nerves. The NCS help in evaluating the muscle, NM junction, peripheral nerve, dorsal root ganglion, and the AHC.

NCS can be used to:
- Confirm a diagnosis
- Rule out other differential diagnoses
- Identify a subclinical pathology
- Localize the point of lesion along a nerve
- Objectively define the severity of a pathology along with the character of the abnormality, e.g., conduction block or demyelination
- Distinguish the peripheral nerve disorders from disorders involving the AHC, muscle, NM junction, or the central nervous system
- Identify anomalous innervation
- Assist in establishing anticipated goals and outcomes for patient with musculoskeletal and NM disorders.

NCS involve direct stimulation of the peripheral nerve (sensory or motor or mixed) through the skin to initiate an impulse. It can be performed for any peripheral nerve that lies superficial enough to be stimulated at two distinct points along its course through the skin. The ulnar, median, radial, common peroneal, tibial, femoral, and sciatic nerves are the common nerves tested for motor NCV (MNCV). The median, ulnar, radial, sural, and the superficial peroneal nerves are the common nerves tested for sensory NCV (SNCV). Since most of the peripheral nerves in the human body are of the mixed type, it is impossible to get isolated monitoring of the motor or sensory nerves. Hence, to isolate the impulses conducted by the motor axons of the mixed nerve, an appropriate distal muscle is selected and evoked potentials are recorded from it. And for the recording of SNCV, impulses are received or stimulation is applied at digital sensory nerves.

Factors Affecting Nerve Conduction Velocity

Physiological Factors

Physiological factors affecting NCV are as follows:

1. **Age:**
   - NCV in a full-term infant is half of that measured in an adult.
   - It keeps on increasing till the age of 3.5 years when it reaches equivalent to that of an adult as the process of myelination is completed.
   - It again starts declining by the age of 35–40 years, but the changes are minor and in most cases, insignificant.
   - The decline in NCV is <10 m/s at the sixth or even in the eighth decade of life.
2. **Gender:**
   - Females tend to have higher NCV than males along with having shorter latencies.
   - In antidromic conduction, the SNAP amplitude is higher in females; may be due to lower digital circumference in females which creates a lower subcutaneous tissue to nerve tissue ratio.
   - In orthodromic conduction, the SNAP amplitude tends to be the same for males and females.
3. **Body mass index (BMI):** In individuals with higher BMI, the SNAP tends to remain the same for the lower extremity nerves, but there is a reduction in the SNAP in the upper extremity nerves.
4. **Upper extremity and lower extremity:**
   - The upper extremity nerves (median and ulnar) tend to conduct impulses faster than the lower extremity (tibial and peroneal) nerves.
   - The height of an individual too seems to play an important role in this. An increase in height reduces the NCV. The longer the nerves, the slower the conduction.
   - Also, there is faster conduction in proximal muscles compared to their distal counterparts.
5. **Temperature:**
   - A reduction in temperature causes a slowing of the NCV and an increase in the amplitude.
   - Each 1°C reduction in the temperature causes an increase in the latency by 0.3 ms due to cooling of the sodium channels.
   - An increase in temperature in the range of 29–38°C causes an increase in the velocity by 5% for every 1°C rise **(Box 7.2)**.

Technical Factors

Technical factors affecting NCV are as follows:

1. **Stimulating system**
   - Failure of the stimulating system causes submaximal stimulation and hence, produces small responses or no response at all.

> **BOX 7.2:** Temperature settings of the electrodiagnostic laboratory.
>
> The temperature of the electrodiagnostic laboratory should be set between 21 and 23°C and the skin temperature should be below 34°C. In case the limb is cool, it should be warmed before the test using an infrared radiation therapy or warm water immersion. In case the limb is warm, the body temperature should be checked, and if it is found to be raised, further evaluation should be postponed until the temperature normalizes.

   - The current may also be shunted between the anode and cathode due to sweat or by the formation of a bridge by the conducting jelly.
2. **Recording system:** Faulty connection in the recording system leads to errors. A break in the electrode wire; a connection to the wrong amplifier; or an incorrect oscilloscope setting of filter, gain, or sweep are the common errors that may occur.
3. **Spreading of current:** Spreading of the stimulation current to adjacent nerves or nerve roots may occur due to incorrect amplitude of stimulating current or some pathological features.
4. **Anomalous innervation:** An anomalous crossover between muscles also can affect the NCV.
   - Median to ulnar nerve communication
   - Ulnar to median nerve communication
   - Tibal to peroneal nerve communication
   - Variations in the innervations of the intrinsic muscles of hand
   - Presence of an accessory deep peroneal nerve.

Motor Nerve Conduction Studies

Motor NCS (MNCS) can be performed for any nerve that can be stimulated at two distinct points along its course, and the electrical activities can be recorded from the somatic muscles innervated by that particular nerve. As mentioned earlier, the common nerves tested for MNCV are the ulnar and median nerves for the upper extremities and tibial and peroneal nerves for the lower extremities, MNCV can also be measured for the musculocutaneous, facial, spinal accessory, femoral, and phrenic nerves, but it requires a lot of technical expertise and professional experience. Suprascapular, axillary, and intercostal nerves are rarely studied.

Stimulation of a purely motor or mixed nerve causes a mechanical and an electrical response in the innervated muscle. The mechanical response is the muscle twitch or contraction that occurs (not clinically recorded). The electrical response [called the compound muscle action potential (CMAP)] is the summated electrical activity of the muscle fibers supplied by the stimulated nerve and lying in the vicinity of the recording electrode **(Box 7.3)**.

Principles of Motor Nerve Conduction Velocity

Stimulation

Stimulation, as mentioned earlier, is applied at two distinct points along the course of the nerve. The nerve should be

BOX 7.3: Definition of compound muscle action potential by the American Association of Neuromuscular and Electrodiagnostic Medicine.

"The summation of nearly synchronous muscle fiber action potentials (MFAPs) recorded from a muscle, commonly produced by stimulation of the nerve supplying the muscle either directly or indirectly." (MFAP is the action potential recorded from a single muscle fiber).

stimulated at a place where it lies superficial in order to avoid dissipation of current and inadvertent stimulation of surrounding structures, e.g., ulnar nerve at wrist and elbow.

- Electrodes used—usually surface electrodes; occasionally in the case of edema or fatty tissues, needle electrode may be used but it carries risk of trauma to the underlying structures.
- Stimulus strength—supramaximal stimulus (supramaximal stimulus intensity can be selected as one third greater than the intensity required to produce a maximal response).
- Electrode placement—cathode should lie closer to the recording electrode as cathode causes activation, i.e., depolarization and the anode, if used, may sometimes block the conduction due to hyperpolarization.
- Stimulus parameters—square wave pulse of 0.1 ms duration; intensity used can vary in the range of 5–40 mA, but 25 mA intensity is adequate in most cases (higher intensity of stimulus may be required in a diseased or deep nerve).

Recording

Placement of electrodes
- Recording electrodes—over the belly tendon montage with the active electrode closer to the motor point and the reference electrode over the tendon
- Ground electrode—between the stimulating and recording electrode.

Since the recordings are done only from a selected subset of muscles innervated by the studied nerve, they assess only the axons supplying that particular muscle.

Recording of the response can be done using surface or needle electrodes **(Table 7.1)**.

Measurement

"A CMAP evoked from a muscle by an electric stimulus to its motor nerve is called the M wave." Convention dictates recording of M wave generated by a supramaximal stimulus for MNCS. This is due to the fact that with a supramaximal

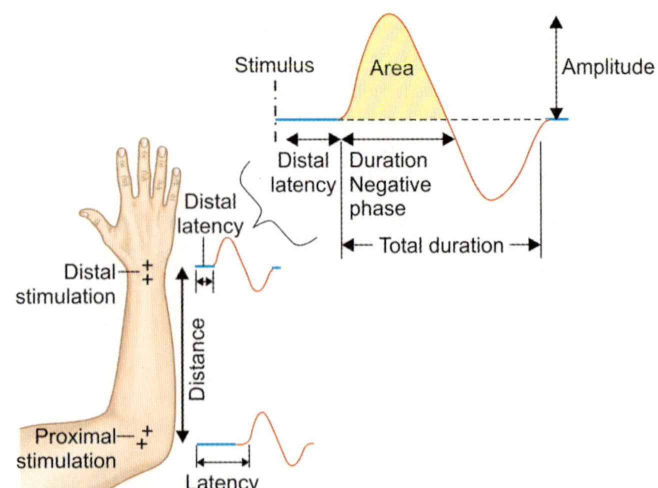

Fig. 7.7: Parameters of compound muscle action potential (CMAP).

Table 7.2: Parameters describing the M wave.

Parameter	Characteristics
Onset latency	• Time elapsed from stimulus artifact (point of stimulation) to the initial deflection (either positive or negative) from the baseline • Time required by the fastest conducting nerve fibers to conduct the impulse to the nerve terminals and finally to the muscle fibers • Includes time required for neuromuscular transmission and propagation along the muscle membrane—residual latency • Measured in milliseconds (ms)
Duration	• Time elapsed from onset to end of negative deflection • Occasionally time elapsed from onset to negative peak, positive peak, or subsequent return to baseline may also be measured • Measured in milliseconds (ms)
Amplitude	• Height from baseline to negative peak • Occasionally, the height from negative to positive peak may also be measured • Measured in millivolts (mV)
Area	• It is the area of the negative phase of the M wave or the total area under the M wave • Measured in ms–mV
NCV	• Ratio of the distance between the two points of stimulation to the difference of latencies for the two points • Measured in meters/second (m/s)

stimulus, all the fibers within a muscle innervated by the concerned nerve contribute to the potential. The earliest component of the M wave reflects the fastest conducting fibers of the nerve.

The M wave is described based on the following parameters **(Fig. 7.7 and Table 7.2)**:
- Onset latency
- Duration
- Amplitude

Table 7.1: Characteristics of surface and needle electrodes.

Surface electrode	Needle electrode
• Noninvasive • Lesser risk of infection • Can be easily repositioned to get maximal response	• Have higher impedance • Can be fixed, hence more stable • More accurate, if positioned correctly (in subcutaneous tissue immediately adjacent to the muscle) • Assess only a limited area

- Area
- NCV
- Configuration

The onset latency is the sum of the conduction in the fastest fibers, the NM transmission, and the propagation along the muscle membrane. It is the time taken by the action potential to travel from the site of stimulation to the nerve terminal along with the NM transmission and the time required to activate the underlying nerve. Hence, it is not possible to calculate an NCV for the distal segment of the nerve. But rather an estimate can be made by means of the residual latency which compares the expected latency (calculated based on the proximal NCV) with the actual latency. This is vital for evaluating distal demyelinating processes. For accurate measurements of MNCV, the minimum distance between the two sites of stimulation should be 10 cm as this reduces the errors due to faulty measurement of distance. Latency is directly proportional to the distance between the stimulating electrode and the muscle. Peak latencies are hence, less reliable for the calculation of NCV, since they represent activation of different axons at the proximal and distal sites of stimulation.

$$NCV = \frac{\text{Distance between proximal and distal stimulation points}}{\text{Difference between the proximal and distal latencies}}$$

Since the calculation of NCV is based on the distance between the stimulation points, the longer the distance the more reliable the velocity calculation. By comparing the conduction in a particular segment of the nerve to the conduction in the other segments or to the normal values, one can determine the affected segment of the nerve and localize the lesion along the length of the nerve **(Box 7.4)**.

Area of the negative phase of the CMAP is suggestive of the total number of muscle fibers recruited. The area of the CMAP will be dependent on the positioning of the recording electrodes rather than the stimulating electrodes. The measurement of the area requires complex computerized analysis, and hence, it is easier to determine the amplitude of the CMAP rather than the area. The normal amplitude lies somewhere between 2 and 20 mV; it can be lower for some nerves in case of proximal stimulation. The area and the amplitude both provide an idea about the number of muscle fibers being recruited. They both are most affected by the distance between the muscle and the recording electrode, and therefore, any change in the distance between the muscle and recording electrode, e.g., excess fat or edema, alters the area and amplitude.

Temporal dispersion is the dispersion of the CMAP due to phase cancelation which is seen in acquired demyelinating neuropathies because of the varying amounts of demyelination. Phase cancelation occurs due to the overlapping of the negative and positive phases. This occurs because of the varied conduction velocities of the demyelinating fibers.

An increase of >20% on proximal stimulation compared to distal stimulation is suggestive of temporal dispersion.

The normal configuration of the CMAP, when the recording is done at the end-plate region, is biphasic with initial negativity and following positivity. If the active electrode is not placed over the end-plate region, the configuration is triphasic with initial positivity, making the measurements for latency less accurate. In the case of stimulation of peroneal nerve, proximal stimulation may cause a potential with initial positivity due to volume conduction by the large proximal muscles. This initial positivity should be disregarded while making measurements for latencies.

The amplitude, area, and latency of the CMAP vary with the site of stimulation. With more proximal stimulations, the distance between the stimulation point and the muscle increases leading to an increase in the latency. Also, activation of the motor units (MUs) is not synchronized, causing a longer and lower CMAP. A reduced area and amplitude of the CMAP compared to normal values suggest the presence of a disease. If the reduction is in a localized segment of the nerve, the disease is focal (most likely, acute compression neuropathy). Whereas if the reduction occurs gradually along the length of the nerve, the pathology is more diffuse.

Breaking of the CMAP into irregular waveform with spike components or relative desynchronization, due to isolation of the action potentials of individual MUs due to dispersion is termed as *temporal dispersion* (**Box 7.5 and Fig. 7.8**). It can be normal in the case of stimulation over a long nerve or it may be indicative of demyelination or reinnervation. Here, particularly the duration of the negative phase of the CMAP is increased. There might be some other waveforms that might be seen during the procedure in addition to the M wave **(Box 7.6)**.

- For upper extremity—40–55 m/s
- For lower extremities—50–70 m/s.
- Faster conduction in the proximal segments of the nerves

- *M wave satellite:* A small wave seen post the M wave; due to conduction in the slow fibers
- *A wave:* Similar to the F wave; occurs due to branching of axon in the peripheral nerve or backfiring of axon along its length or ephaptic transmission between adjacent axons
- *Late response similar to F wave:* Occurs in peripheral nerve diseases with high irritability, electrical stimulation distal to a branching produces an antidromic potential that becomes orthodromic at the branching site and produces a potential similar to F wave with shorter latency

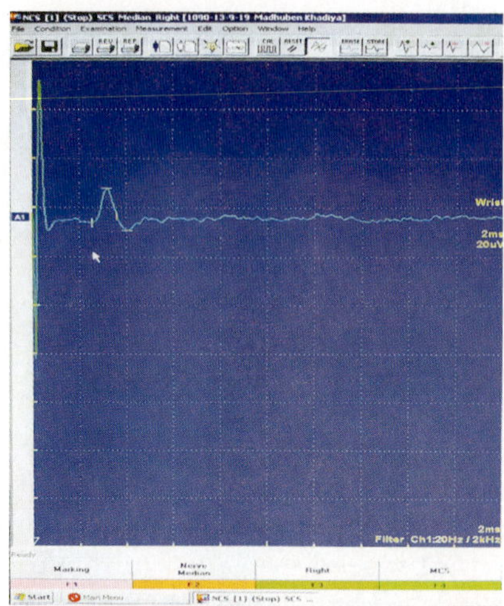

Fig. 7.8: Normal median sensory nerve action potential (SNAP).

Sensory Nerve Conduction Studies

Sensory NCS (SNCS) is used to evaluate sensory axons. Evaluation of sensory axons can be done:

- Stimulating and recording from a cutaneous nerve
- Stimulating a mixed nerve and recording from a cutaneous nerve
- Stimulating a cutaneous nerve and recording from a mixed nerve
- Stimulating a cutaneous or mixed nerve and recording from the spinal column or the cerebral hemispheres [somatosensory evoked potentials (SSEPs)].

The SNAP is much less in amplitude than the CMAP and hence, may be often obscured by the artifacts. To produce reliable results, averaging of several potentials may be required.

Commonly studied nerves include (but are not limited to)—ulnar, median, radial, sural, peroneal and plantar nerves. SNCV can be measured antidromically or orthodromically **(Table 7.3)**:

- Orthodromic conduction—propagation of a nerve impulse in the direction same as physiologic conduction, i.e., toward the muscle for motor fibers and toward the spinal cord for sensory fibers **(Fig. 7.9)**.
- Antidromic conduction—propagation of a nerve impulse in the direction opposite to the physiologic conduction, i.e., away from the muscle for motor fibers and away from the spinal cord for sensory fibers **(Fig. 7.10)**.

Uses of Sensory Nerve Conduction Studies

Sensory nerve conduction study is used for the following:

- Identification of diffuse sensory fiber involvement
- Focal lesions involving cutaneous nerves
- Disorders involving only the sensory fibers of a mixed nerve
- More sensitive than MNCS in identifying mild or early disorders.

Table 7.3: Orthodromic and antidromic recording of sensory nerve action potential (SNAP).

Orthodromic conduction	Antidromic conduction
Distal part of nerve stimulated	Proximal part of nerve stimulated
SNAP recorded at proximal part	SNAP recorded at distal part
Ring electrodes used for stimulation	Surface electrodes used for stimulation
Surface or needle electrodes used for recording	Surface or needle electrodes used for recording

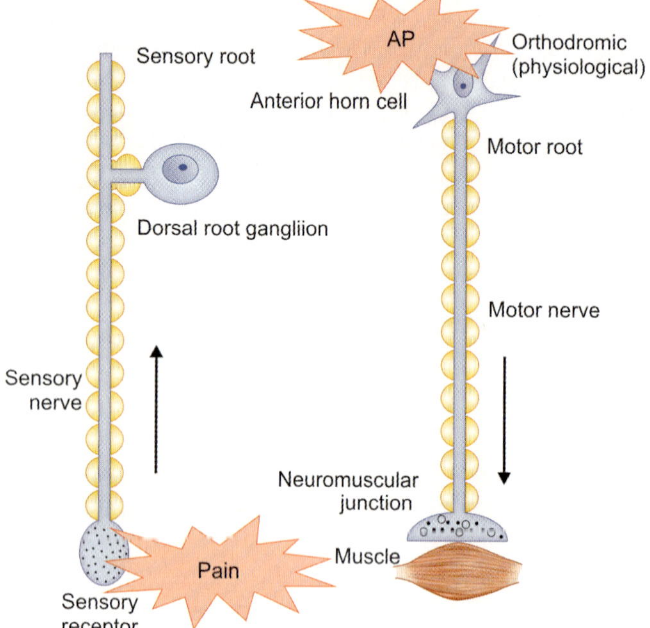

Fig. 7.9: Orthodromic conduction.

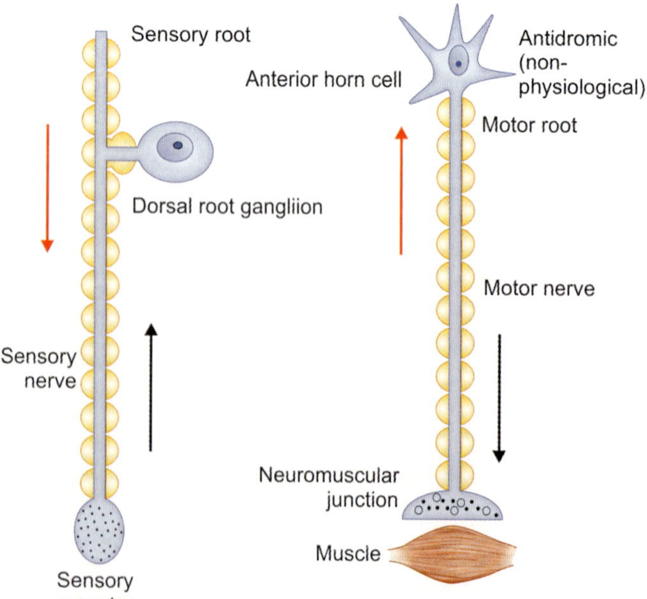

Fig. 7.10: Antidromic conduction.

Principles of Sensory Nerve Conduction Studies

Stimulation

Stimulation can be provided in any direction along the course of the nerve, since the conduction velocity remains the same with either orthodromic or antidromic conduction. Stimulation along orthodromic conduction may give a small SNAP and stimulation along antidromic conduction may produce a larger SNAP but also produce a motor response that may interfere with the recording of the sensory response. Stimulation parameters for SNCV are similar to those used for MNCV.

Recording

Recording of compound SNAPs is difficult than CMAP due to the smaller size. Ring electrodes are usually used for recording SNAPs since they are more comfortable, but needle electrodes, if used, are more accurate and can amplify the potential fivefold.

Parameters of the Sensory Nerve Action Potential

The parameters of the SNAP are as follows:
- Configuration—triphasic with initial positivity **(Fig. 7.11)**
- Latency—corresponding to distance from the stimulating electrode.
- Amplitude—proportional to number of active axons, synchrony of axonal firing, and distance between the nerve and recording electrode (estimated based on the rise time).

Since the SNAP requires a high amplification, artifacts always remain an issue with the recording. The examiner needs to take care of:
- Placement of ground electrodes
- Elimination of conducting bridges between ground and stimulating electrodes
- Orientation of ground and stimulating electrodes
- Reduction of ground muscle activity by gentle manipulation or auditory feedback about the muscle contraction to the subject
- Setting the temperature accurately.

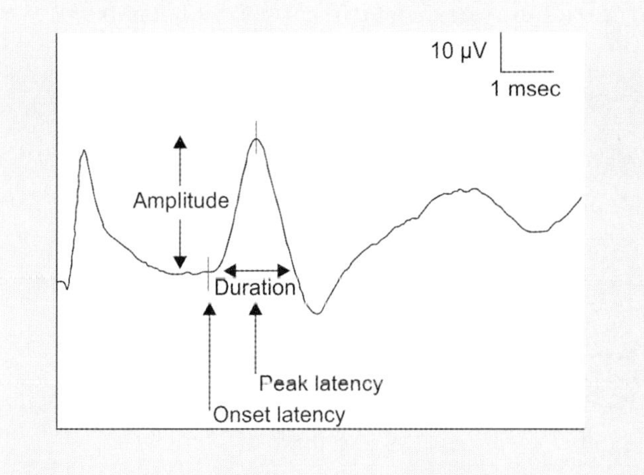

Fig. 7.11: Parameters of sensory nerve action potential (SNAP).

Orthodromic activation is preferred for ulnar and median nerves, whereas antidromic activation is preferred for radial and sural nerves. The active electrode immediately adjacent to the nerve and the reference electrode as far away as possible is the ideal placement of electrodes for recording SNAP. However, with the reference electrode as far away as possible, there is a great increase in the artifacts recorded from the tissues lying between the two electrodes. Due to this, a compromise is met with having the reference electrode placed 4 cm away from the active electrode to get a good SNAP with minimum noise. The reference electrode can be placed laterally away or along the course of the nerve. If it is placed along the course of the nerve, it leads to an inverted SNAP. Since the active electrode potential (near field potential) also lies in the same direction, both these potentials get summated which may be seen as an increase in the size of the potential in the graph. With the lateral placement of the reference electrode, there is the risk of recording the near field potential. For such problems, a needle electrode may be used which produces a small size near field potential, causing lesser distortion.

Measurement

The parameters of measuring SNCS are the same as that for MNCS but are rather a little challenging task due to smaller size and different configuration. With SNCS, the amplitude varies from few microvolts to 200 μV and the SNCV is higher than MNCV. But since the potentials are small, there may sometimes be a lot of confusion regarding the waveform. A significant portion of the waveform may be noise. Hence, a SNCV of a single nerve is unreliable and averaging needs to be done.

The averaged SNAP waveform is triphasic with initial positivity due to the current moving closer to the active electrode and later positivity due to the current moving away from the electrode.

Latency is measured up to the onset of negativity regardless of there being an initial positivity (in which case onset of negativity is taken as the peak of the preceding positivity).

SNCV is measured using the same technique as for MNCV. But, for a sensory nerve, there is no NM junction, and therefore, no time is consumed for NM transmission. So, the SNCV can be measured using stimulation of a single site. Better outcomes can be obtained using the "inching" technique especially for ulnar nerve **(Boxes 7.7 and 7.8)**.

The amplitude and area of the SNAP provide information regarding the number of axons and their sizes. A reduction in the area and amplitude of the SNAP occur as the range of the conduction velocities of sensory nerves is large and cancelation of the negative phases of the waveform occurs due to the initial and late positivity. This especially occurs over long distances **(Fig. 7.8)**.

> **BOX 7.7:** Inching technique.
>
> Analysis of waveform after stimulation of a nerve at consecutive short segments of a fixed length is known as the "inching" technique. The segments are usually 1–2 cm long, but there has been a lot of discrepancy in the literature regarding this. Shorter segments (1–2 cm) are more sensitive but they are more time-consuming, complex, and lead to several experimental errors, whereas longer segments (10 cm) lead to lesser experimental errors and false positives but are less sensitive. Studies have reported 81% sensitivity using shorter 1–2 cm segments (inching technique).
>
> The inching technique using across elbow segments has been found essential in the diagnosis of mild to moderate ulnar neuropathy at the elbow.

> **BOX 7.8:** The collision method.
>
> The collision method involves applying stimulation at two sites along the length of the same nerve simultaneously. This helps in examining the slow conducting fibers of a nerve.

Pathophysiology

Three types of alterations occur in the peripheral nerve disorders **(Table 7.4)**:

1. Conduction slowing
2. Conduction block
3. Reduced or absent motor or sensory potentials.

Conduction Slowing

It is seen as a prolonged latency. It occurs with segmental demyelination or narrowing of axons. It is seen more often in chronic disorders.

Conduction Block

Conduction block is a 20–50% reduction in the amplitude or area of the negative peak of CMAP on proximal stimulation compared to distal stimulation. It occurs with metabolic alteration in the membrane of the nerve, e.g., application of local anesthesia or with structural alteration of the myelin sheath, viz. telescoping and segmental demyelination. It is seen more often in rapidly developing disorders.

Both duration and amplitude need to be considered while making a diagnosis of conduction block. A reduction of 20% (possible conduction block) of the amplitude of CMAP with a normal duration and a reduction of 30% (probable conduction block) with increased duration are suggestive of conduction block **(Box 7.9)**.

Reduced or Absent Motor or Sensory Potentials

Axonal degeneration is predominantly seen in the following pathologies **(Table 7.5)**:

- Guillain-Barré syndrome (GBS) (selected patients)
- Diabetes (selected patients)
- Alcoholic neuropathy
- Toxic neuropathy
- Carcinoma
- Uremia
- Collagen and vascular pathologs

Segmental demyelination is predominantly seen in the following pathologies **(Table 7.5)**:

- Guillain-Barré syndrome (selected patients)
- Diabetes (selected patients)
- Chronic inflammatory neuropathy
- Diphtheric neuropathy
- Refsum disease
- Leukodystrophies

Techniques of Application for Commonly Evaluated Nerves

Median Nerve

MNCS (Figs. 7.12 and 7.13):

- Recording electrode—close to motor point of abductor pollicis brevis
- Reference electrode—3 cm distal to first metacarpophalangeal joint
- Stimulation sites:
  1. Wrist—3 cm proximal to distal wrist crease
  2. Elbow—near volar crease of brachial pulse

Table 7.4: Nerve conduction studies in common neuromuscular (NM) disorders.

	MNCS			SNCS		
	Duration	Amplitude	MNCV	Duration	Amplitude	SNCV
Regenerating nerve	Increased	Decreased	Decreased	Decreased	Decreased	Decreased
Axonal neuropathy	Normal	Decreased	>70%	Normal	Greater decrease	>70%
Demyelinating neuropathy	Increased proximally	Decreased proximally	<50%	Increased proximally	Decreased	<50%
Mononeuropathy	Increased	Decreased	Decreased	Increased	Greater decrease	Decreased
Myopathy	Normal	Occasionally decreased	Normal	Normal	Normal	Normal
Motor neuron disease	Normal	Greater decrease	>70%	Normal	Normal	Normal
NM disorders	Normal	Occasionally decreased	Normal	Normal	Normal	Normal

(MNCS: motor nerve conduction studies; MNCV: motor nerve conduction velocity; SNCS: sensory nerve conduction studies; SNCV: sensory nerve conduction velocity)

BOX 7.9: Hallmark of conduction block.

Reduction of amplitude of potential on stimulation proximal to the site of block.

Table 7.5: Features of axonal degeneration and segmental demyelination.

Axonal degeneration	Segmental demyelination
Reduced amplitudes of CMAP	Prolonged distal latency
Reduced amplitudes of SNAP	Conduction slowing across affected segment
Normal or near-normal NCV	Conduction block
	Temporal dispersion

(CMAP: compound muscle action potential; NCV: nerve conduction velocity; SNAP: sensory nerve action potential)

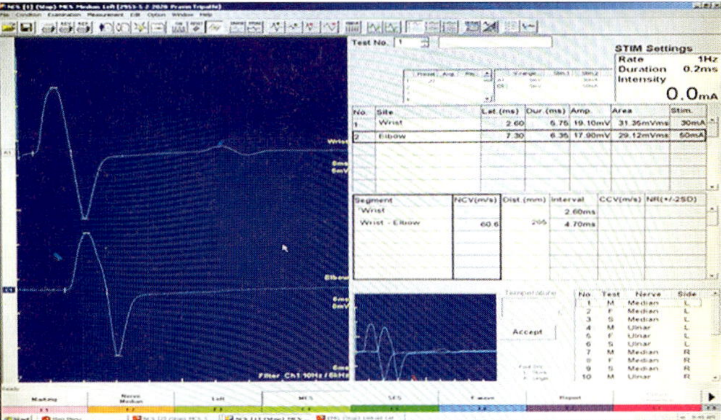

Fig. 7.12: Normal compound muscle action potential (CMAP) of median nerve.

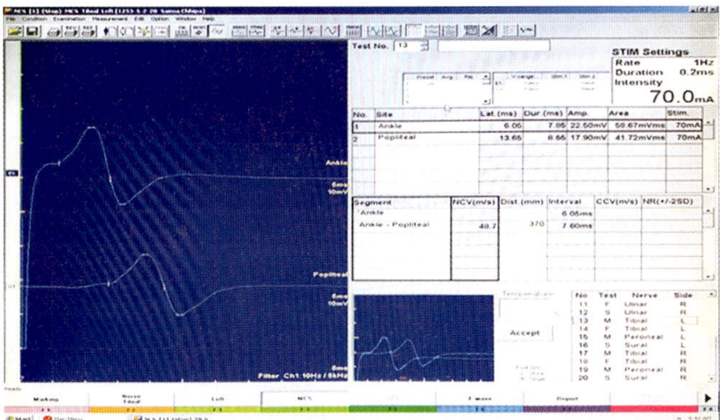

Fig. 7.13: Prolonged distal latency for median nerve motor nerve conduction studies (MNCS).

3. Axilla
4. Erb's point

SNCS:
- Measured orthodromically or antidromically
- **Orthodromic conduction:**
  - Recording electrode—3 cm proximal to distal wrist crease
  - Reference electrode—3 cm proximal to recording electrode
  - Stimulation—second or third finger (cathode at the first interphalangeal (IP) joint and anode 3 cm distal to cathode).

- **Antidromic conduction:** Location of stimulating and recording electrodes is reversed. Reference electrode is placed at the same location.

Ulnar Nerve

MNCS:
- Since the ulnar nerve slides with elbow flexion and extension, a standard position is used to evaluate it. The elbow should be placed between 90 and 135° of flexion throughout the procedure.
- Recording electrode—over abductor digiti minimi
- Reference electrode—3 cm distal to the distal wrist crease on the lateral aspect of the palm.
- Stimulation sites:
  1. Wrist—3 cm proximal to the proximal wrist crease.
  2. Elbow—4 cm distal to the olecranon process.
  3. Elbow—10 cm proximal to the olecranon process.
  4. Axilla
  5. Erb's point

SNCS:
- Measured orthodromically or antidromically
- **Orthodromic conduction:**
  - Stimulation at IP joint of fifth finger
  - Recording can be done at various sites along the course of the nerve.
- **Antidromic conduction:**
  - Stimulation placing cathode 3 cm proximal to distal crease of wrist
  - Recording from fourth or fifth digit.

Radial Nerve

MNCS:
- **Stimulation sites:**
  - At the elbow between triceps and brachioradialis muscle
  - Proximal and distal to the spiral groove
  - At the Erb's point
- Recording electrode—extensor pollicis longus and abductor pollicis longus
- Reference electrode—styloid process.

SNCS:
- **Antidromic conduction:**
  - Recording electrode—first web space
  - Reference electrode—3 cm distal to recording electrode
  - Stimulation site:
    - 10–14 cm proximal to recording electrode at lateral edge of radius
    - Proximal stimulation at elbow between biceps and brachioradialis
- **Orthodromic conduction:**
  - Stimulation site—thumb
  - Recording at wrist, elbow, and axilla.

Sciatic Nerve

MNCS:
- Recording electrode—distal muscle innervated by peroneal nerve, e.g., extensor digitorum brevis (EDB)

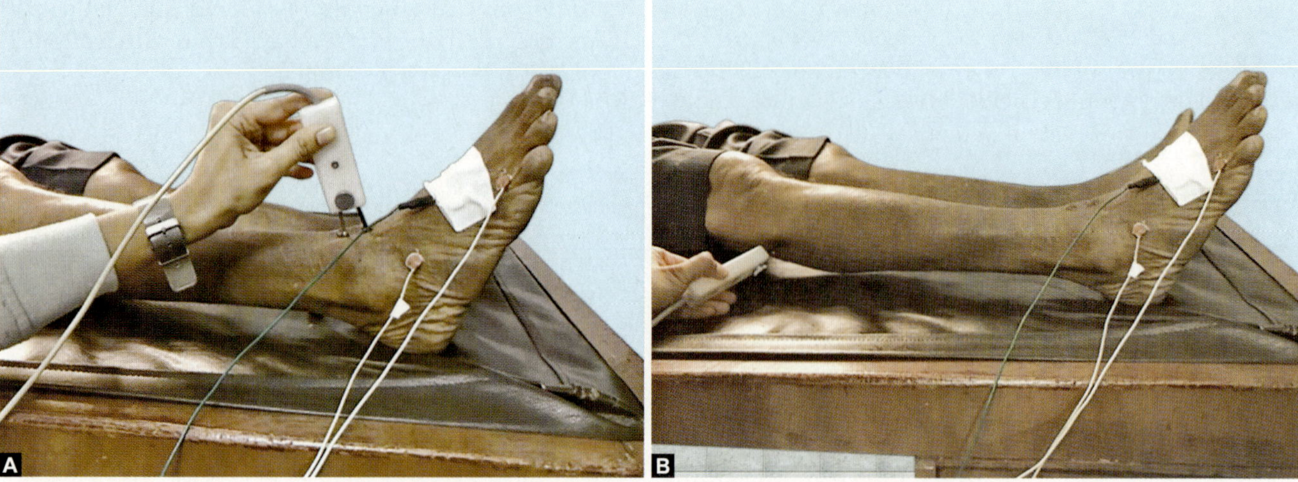

Figs. 7.14A and B: (A) Distal; (B) Proximal stimulation for peroneal nerve.

or muscle innervated by tibial nerve, e.g., abductor halluces

- Stimulation sites:
  - Lateral trunk at head of fibula
  - Medial trunk at apex of popliteal fossa
  - Below gluteal fold.

SNCS: Not possible due to deep-seated location of the nerve.

Common Peroneal Nerve

Common peroneal nerve can be commonly evaluated by:
- Recording electrode—over EDB
- Stimulation sites **(Figs. 7.14A and B)**:
  - At ankle
  - 2 cm distal to neck of fibula
  - 5–8 cm above the neck of fibula.

Sural Nerve

Sural nerve can be commonly evaluated by:
- Position—leg in lateral and relaxed position
- Antidromic conduction:
  - Recording electrode—between lateral malleolus and tendo-Achilles
  - Stimulation sites:
    - 10–16 cm proximal to recording electrode
    - Distal to lower border of gastrocnemius at the junction of middle and lower third of leg.

Tibial Nerve

Tibial nerve can be commonly evaluated by:
- Recording electrode—over abductor hallucis or abductor digiti quinti slightly below and anterior to navicular tuberosity **(Fig. 7.15)**
- Stimulation sites:
  - Behind and proximal to medial malleolus
  - Popliteal fossa along flexor crease of knee slightly lateral to midline.

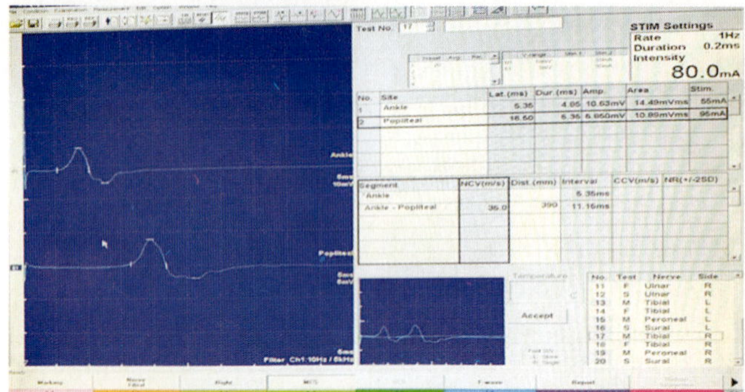

Fig. 7.15: Prolonged distal latency with reduced motor nerve conduction velocity (MNCV) for tibial nerve.

ELECTROMYOGRAPHY

Electromyography (EMG) is the recording of the electrical activity of muscles **(Box 7.10)**. It deals with the development, recording, and analysis of myoelectric signals. EMG can be thought of being two faced—one that deals with the scope of NM diseases or trauma (clinical EMG) and another that deals with study of muscle function (kinesiological EMG).

Clinical EMG deals with identifying and recording myoelectric potentials from skeletal muscle fibers. Kinesiological EMG deals with the study of muscle activity during movements. Discussion of kinesiological EMG is out of the scope of this chapter, only clinical EMG will be discussed henceforth.

EMG evaluates the motor unit (MU) activity. The MU comprises of the AHC, axon, NM junction, and the muscle fibers it supplies. When the impulse is conducted

> **BOX 7.10:** Definition of electromyography (EMG).
>
> *AANEM defines EMG as:*
> "The recording and study of insertion, spontaneous, and voluntary activity of muscle with a recording electrode (either a needle electrode for invasive EMG or a surface electrode for kinesiologic studies)."

by the axon, it causes depolarization of the muscle fibers it supplies. This causes an electrical potential to be generated that manifests as an MU action potential (MUAP). The potential generated by a single muscle fiber is called muscle fiber action potential (MFAP).

Uses of Electromyography

EMG can be used for the following:
- Helps look into the activity of a muscle
- Helps in localizing the lesion to neural, muscular, or junctional component of the MU
- Helps establish a diagnosis and a prognosis (when used in conjunction with other tests)
- Measures muscle performance
- Aids decision-making process pre- and postoperatively
- Helps in documenting interventional and training regimes
- Can be used as a form of biofeedback
- Aids in improving sports performance
- Detects muscle response in ergonomic evaluation.

Instrumentation

The instrumentation in EMG is a phase system—input, processor, and output.

There are three phases involved in the instrumentation of EMG.
1. **Input phase:** Electrodes
2. **Processor phase:** Amplifier, signal averagers, integrators, filters
3. **Output phase:** Oscilloscope, recorders

Input Phase

Electrodes

An electrode is a transducer that helps in transforming one form of energy into another. Various types of electrodes exist—surface, invasive, implanted, etc. In clinical EMG, only surface and invasive electrodes are used. Surface electrodes **(Fig. 7.16)** are not commonly used as they do not allow localization **(Table 7.6)**. Fine-wire indwelling electrodes are used for kinesiological studies.

Needle electrodes

Needle electrodes resemble a needle and hence, are named so. Four different types of needle electrodes can be used for EMG recording:

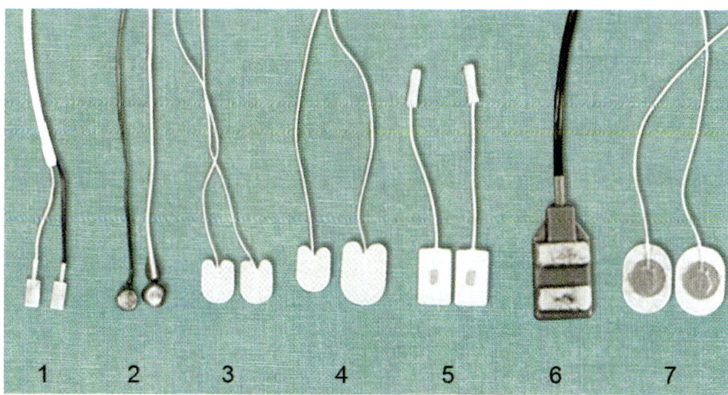

Fig. 7.16: Types of surface electrodes.

Table 7.6: Differences between surface and needle electrodes.	
Surface electrode	*Needle electrode*
Noninvasive	Invasive
Comfortable for the subject	Uncomfortable for the subject
Difficult to stabilize, hence leads to a lot of noise	Easy to stabilize, so less noise is recorded
Records activity from a large area, hence localization is difficult	Records activity from a specific area—only a few fibers, hence precise
Gives information about more number of fibers	Give information about only selected muscle fibers

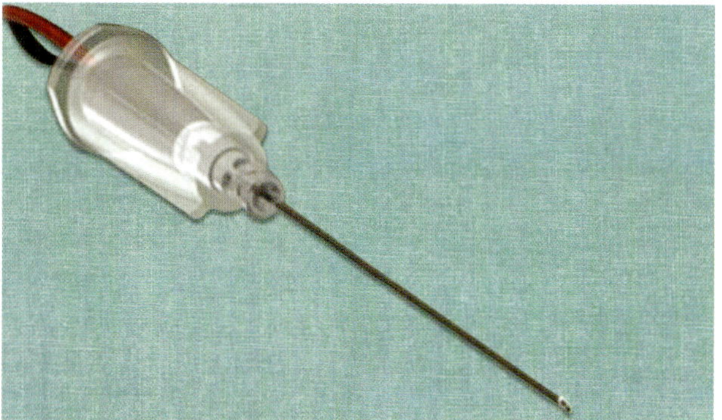

Fig. 7.17: Concentric needle electrode.

1. **Concentric needle electrodes (Fig. 7.17):**
   - Most commonly used
   - 24–26 gauge needle with fine wire in the lumen
   - Tip is beveled to give a larger surface area of 125 × 580 µm
   - Records minimal surrounding noise.
2. **Monopolar needle electrodes (Fig. 7.18):**
   - 22–30 gauge needle with Teflon coating
   - Tip—approximately 500 µm in diameter
   - Less painful and cheaper compared to concentric needle electrode
   - Requires an additional reference electrode which needs to be placed near the active electrode, hence requiring a change with each changing evaluated muscle
   - Leads to greater electrical noise.
3. **Single fiber needle electrodes (Fig. 7.19):**
   - Steel cannula of 0.5–0.6 mm diameter covering 1–14 insulated platinum or silver wires
   - Record from an extremely small area, hence cannot be used for MU size estimation
   - Used for study of NM transmission and fiber density.
4. **Macroelectrodes (Fig. 7.20):**
   - 50-mm steel cannula with 25 µm diameter platinum wire
   - Records from a large number of muscle fibers.

The EMG instrumentation requires three electrodes:
1. Recording electrode—electrode recording the action potential or electrical activity

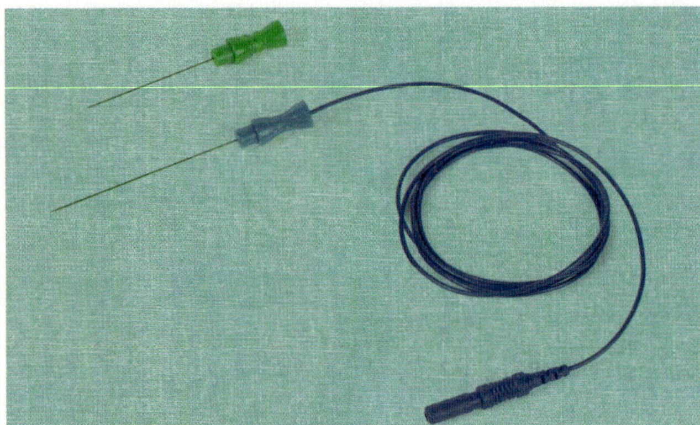

Fig. 7.18: Monopolar electrode.

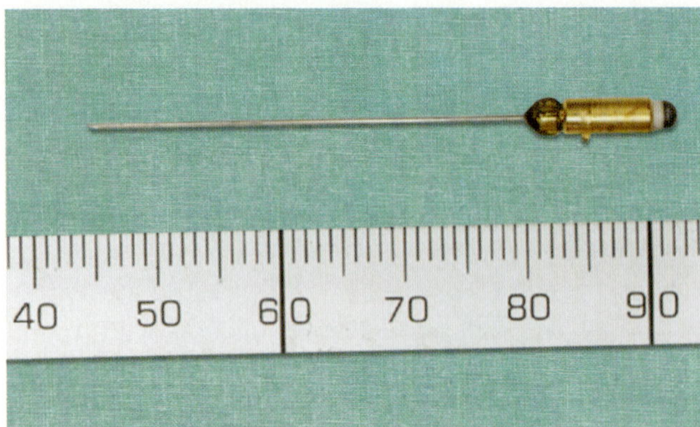

Fig. 7.19: Single fiber electrode.

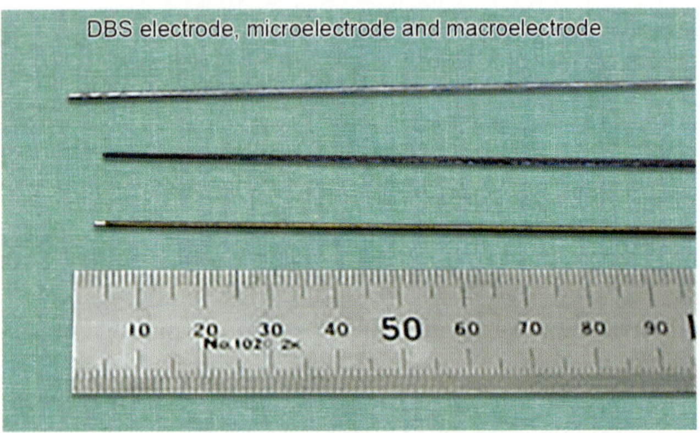

Fig. 7.20: Macroelectrode.

2. Ground electrode—used to cancel the external noise interference effect
3. Reference electrode—to record activity to compare with the activity recorded by recording electrode.

Recording and reference electrodes are placed near each other to receive a bipolar reading. The difference in the potentials recorded by both these electrodes is processed.

Processor Phase

Cross Talk

Electrical activity from other surrounding muscles may also be recorded by the recording electrode due to volume conduction. This unwanted activity arising from inside the tissues is called cross talk. Double differentiation using a 3-bar electrode can help eliminate cross talk.

Artifact

Any unwanted electrical activity arising from outside of the body tissues that are being examined is called artifact. To reduce the noise, artifact, and interference, the examiner should prepare the skin appropriately and arrange the instrumentation accurately. Signal processing techniques can be used for noise reduction, e.g., band-pass filters, wavelet transform filters, and adaptive noise cancelation filters.

Movement artifact

The electrode is a metallic surface that is surrounded by electrolyte (oil or moisture of the skin, conducting gel, or tissue fluids). An ion exchange takes place between the electrode and electrolyte, resulting in a potential difference between the two electrodes during any activity, which is recorded as a bioelectric event. During rest or when there is no muscle activity, there is no potential difference between the two electrodes. But during activity, there is a difference of potential which may be recorded as a low-frequency signal called movement artifact. This may be reduced by the use of conducting gel between the metal and skin or use of silver/silver chloride electrodes. Most of the movement artifacts lie below 10–20 Hz and do not cause any change in the amplitude but can cause a wavy baseline. They can be eliminated by properly fixing the electrodes or using high-pass filters above 20 Hz.

Power Line Interference

Artifacts produced by power lines and electrical equipment, e.g., electrical modalities, cellphones, lights, vibrators, fans, and radios, are called power line interferences. They produce a constant hum in the recorded signal and can be eliminated using notch filters of 60 Hz signals.

Electrocardiogram

Electrocardiogram can cause artifacts when electrodes are placed over the trunk, upper thigh, or arm. Use of an amplifier with appropriate calibrations and correct placement of ground electrode can help in reducing ECG signal but they cannot be completely eliminated.

Amplifiers

Amplifiers are used to amplify the received signal (**Fig. 7.21**). The frequency response should be in the spectrum of 2 or 20–10,000 Hz to allow uniform amplification without distortion. The frequency response can be altered using filters, to allow attenuation of noise or other interference signals.

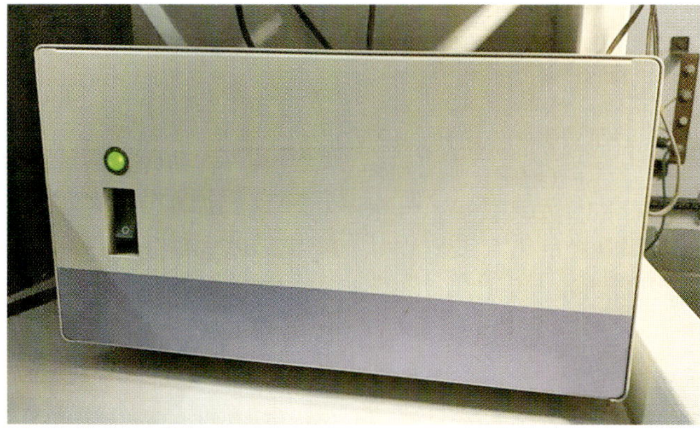

Fig. 7.21: Amplifier.

Differential amplifiers

Differential amplifiers are used to amplify the recorded signals since biologic signals are very small. They convert the electrical potential into a voltage signal and amplify it. Since the recorded potential also contains unwanted noise, the electrodes transmit their signals to two different sides of the amplifier. The difference between these signals is then processed and amplified. Noise being a common signal on both sides is canceled out.

Signal Averagers

Averaging involves extraction of extremely small signals embedded in larger noise, e.g., SNAP in EMG signals. The time-locked signals are made prominent and noise, being random is canceled out. These time locked sequential responses are summated, averaged, and then displayed on the screen. The signal-to-noise ratio (SNR) is dependent on the number of responses averaged.

$$\text{SNR} = \frac{\text{Signal amplitude} \times \sqrt{\text{number of sweeps}}}{\text{Noise amplitude}}$$

Common Mode Rejection Ratio

It is a measure of the proportion of amplification of the desired signal voltage to the unwanted signal. The higher the common mode rejection ratio (CMRR), the better. The CMRR of a good differential amplifier should be > 100,000:1.

Gain

Gain is the ability of the amplifier to amplify signals. It is the ratio of the output signal to input signal level. Higher signal causes a small signal to appear large.

Sweep

Latency and duration measurements depend on the gain and sweep speed. With higher gain and increased sweep speed, the latency is shorter.

Frequency Bandwidth

The frequency bandwidth outlines the maximum and minimum frequency that will be processed. The frequency spectrum of the EMG signal is inversely proportional to the distance between the two electrodes. The spectrum ranges from 10 to 500 Hz for surface electrodes and 10 to 1,000 Hz for fine-wire electrodes. The use of a frequency bandwidth helps reduce and eliminate high- and low-frequency artifacts.

Filters

Filter is an electronic device used to electronically remove unwanted signals or noise.

Four types of filters are used:
1. Notch filter—removes direct current (DC) and 60-Hz alternating current (AC) line noise
2. High-pass filter—removes low-frequency signals (low cut filters)
3. Low-pass filter—removes high-frequency signals (high cut filters)
4. Band-pass filter—allows passage of only specific frequency ranges; often set between 20 and 300 Hz.

Output Phase

Display

Two types of waveform displays used:
1. Analog oscilloscope display
2. Computer-based digital video display

The type of display used is based on the type of information that is desired and the instrumentation that is available.

1. **Analog oscilloscope display (Fig. 7.22):** The display unit is a cathode ray tube. The waveform is displayed directly after amplification and filtering.
   Advantages:
   - There is no mechanical limitation in the dynamic high-frequency response as there is no fixed frequency range.
   - Details of the waveform can be reproduced.
   - It is an optimal means of displaying the changing amplitude against time.
   Disadvantages: Does not quantify waveforms.
2. **Computer-based digital video display (Fig. 7.23):** It provides a digital display, by incorporating an analog-to-digital converter and digital processing techniques. The signals are sampled at discrete time intervals and the amplitude is quantified after amplification and filtering.

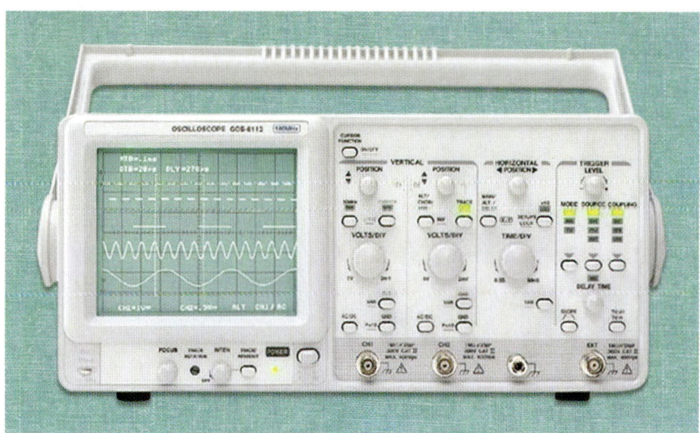

Fig. 7.22: Analog oscilloscope.

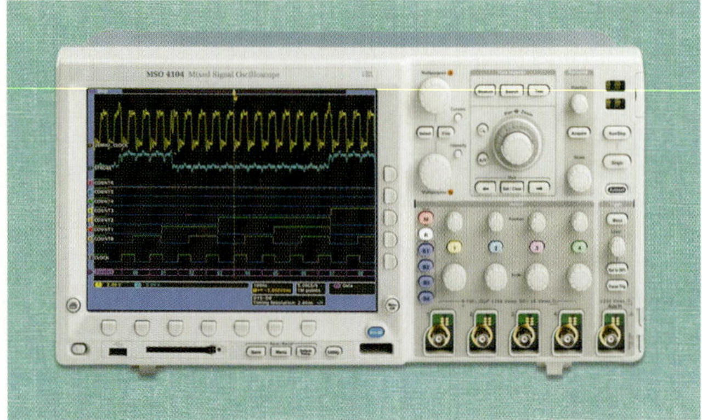

Fig. 7.23: Digital oscilloscope.

Advantages: Signals can be redisplayed with greater sensitivity without losing waveform accuracy.

Disadvantages: There are only a limited number of pixels available for display, resulting in loss of certain details of the waveform.

Recorders

The use of recorders is greater in kinesiological studies. Graphic recorders, digital recorders, etc. can be used to record and store the data extracted during the study.

A setup of EMG and NCV equipment is shown in **Figure 7.24**.

Factors

Factors that affect EMG signal are:

- Tissue characteristics—tissue type, thickness, temperature, and physiological changes lead to variations in the EMG signal.
- Physiological cross talk
- Change in the distance between the electrode and the signal origin site.
- External noise
- Electrodes
- Amplifiers

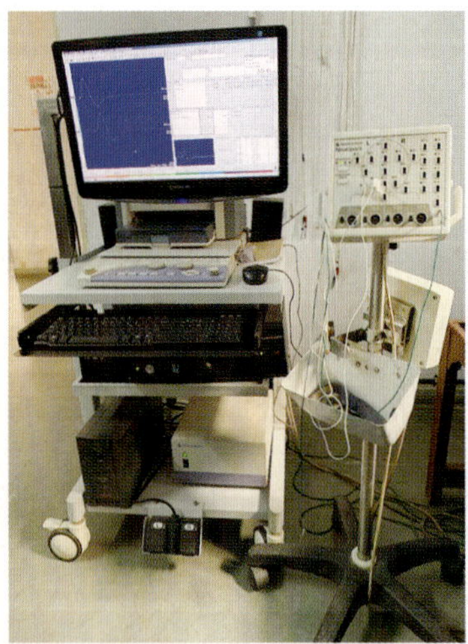

Fig. 7.24: EMG–NCV equipment setup.
(EMG: electromyography; NCV: nerve conduction velocity)

Recording Parameters

Recording parameters are:

- Sweep speed—5–10 ms/division for spontaneous activity, 5 ms/division
- Amplification—50 µV/division for spontaneous activity, 200 mV/division for MUAP
- Filter setting—20–10,000 Hz for spontaneous activity, low filter at 2–3 Hz for MUAP
- Gain—100 mV/division for MUAP.

Recording Procedure

The recording procedure requires the following steps:

- A thorough evaluation of the patient to exclude or reach a diagnosis so as to evaluate only the required muscles as the procedure can be uncomfortable for the patient.
- The patient should be explained the procedure of the test.
- Selection of the muscle based on the suspected diagnosis.
- Instruction to the patient about the maneuver of contraction and relaxation of the muscle.
- Identifying the muscle through contraction and relaxation.
- Locating the needle insertion point a little farther from the motor point to avoid end-plate noise.
- Insertion of the needle quickly and precisely in a relaxed muscle.
- Confirming the position of the electrode by observing sharp MUAPs on minimal contraction (reposition needle if MUAPs are not sharp).

Recording of Activity

Three types of activities are recorded in EMG.

1. Insertional activity
2. Spontaneous activity
3. Voluntary activity

Insertional activity: Electrical activity on the insertion of needle electrode into the muscle is called insertional activity. The insertion of the needle causes mechanical damage producing a brief burst of electrical activity which lasts a little longer than the needle movement. These are high-frequency positive or negative spikes that appear in a cluster. The duration of the insertional activity also depends on the examiner's skills but usually lasts only 300 ms. At least 4–6 brief needle movements need to be made in all the four quadrants of a muscle to evaluate insertional activity. Insertional activity can be normal, decreased, absent, increased, or prolonged **(Table 7.7)**.

Spontaneous activity: No electrical activity is recorded from a healthy muscle at rest other than at the end-plate region. Insertion at the end plate causes activity as there are a higher number of NM junctions. This activity can be in the form of end-plate noise or end-plate spikes.

End-plate noise
Features of end-plate noise are:

- Irregular, monophasic negative potentials **(Fig. 7.25)**
- Amplitude <100 µV

Table 7.7: Abnormal insertional activity.

Abnormalities	Characteristics
Increased or prolonged	• Any activity other than the end-plate potential (EPP) lasting >300 ms after the needle movement • Occurs due to irritated muscle membrane • Seen in denervated muscles (early denervation), some inherited syndromes and myotonia
Decreased	• Reduced amplitude of the insertional activity • Seen in muscle fibrosis (long-term denervation), myopathies where fat replaces connective tissue, periodic paralysis (during attack), muscle necrosis (in compartment syndrome), or if the needle has been placed in tissue other than muscle • It may be physiologically reduced in muscular individuals particularly in calf muscles

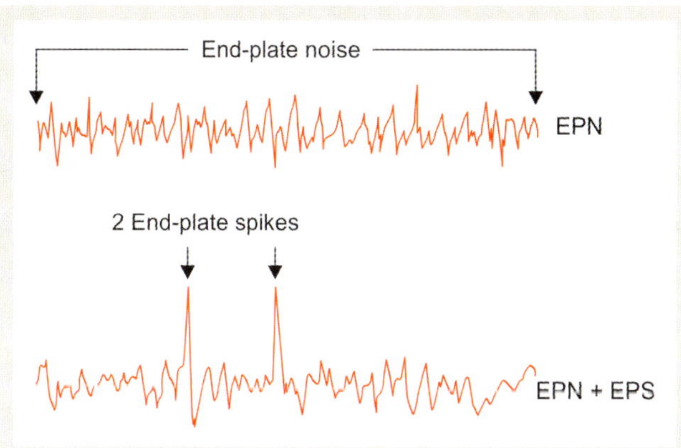

Fig. 7.25: End-plate noise and spikes.

- Duration of 0.5–2 ms
- Seashell-like sound
- Occur due to spontaneously released vesicles of ACh
- Called miniature end-plate potentials (MEPPs).

End-plate spikes
Features of end-plate spikes are:
- Biphasic with an initial negative deflection, brief, rapid occurring, spiky, and irregular **(Fig. 7.25)**
- Amplitude <1,000 µV or 1 mV
- Duration of 2–4 ms
- Sound similar to fat sputtering in a frying pan
- Result from the summation of MEPPs to produce localized EPPs.

To avoid these activities, the needle should be inserted slightly farther than the muscle end-plate near the center of the belly of the muscle.

End-plate noise and spikes are normal spontaneous activities. There are abnormal spontaneous activities as well which can be categorized into two categories:
1. Abnormal spontaneous activities originating from the muscle fiber:
   - Fibrillations
   - Positive sharp waves (PSWs)
   - Myotonic discharges
   - Complex repetitive discharges
2. Abnormal spontaneous activities originating from the motor neuron or axon:
   - Fasciculations
   - Doublets, triplets, and multiplets
   - Myokymia
   - Neuromyotonia
   - Cramps

Abnormal spontaneous activities originating from the muscle fiber: Abnormal spontaneous activity originating from a muscle fiber represents lack of innervation that makes the resting membrane potential (RMP) less negative and unstable. This causes the RMP to approach the threshold required to generate an action potential, making it fire independently in absence of external stimulation or induced by the needle movement.

1. **Fibrillation potentials (FPs) and PSWs:** FPs and PSWs are single muscle fiber discharges seen in LMN or muscular lesions. Infrequently, UMN lesions (stroke, spinal cord injury, and traumatic brain injury) may also show FPs and PSWs. They can be identified by their characteristic sound of the clicking of a clock **(Box 7.11)**.

Characteristics of FPs **(Fig. 7.26)**:
- Biphasic or triphasic with initial positivity
- Firing rate—0.5–15 Hz
- Amplitude—20–200 µV
- Duration—1–5 ms
- Sound similar to rain drop on roof
- Characteristic finding—regularity

Characteristics of PSWs **(Fig. 7.27)**:
- Regular long-duration biphasic potentials with initial sharp positivity followed by long-duration negative phase causing a saw tooth appearance

BOX 7.11: Grading of fibrillation potentials and positive sharp waves.

0: None
+1: Persistent single train (>1 s) of potential in at least two areas
+2: Moderate number of potentials in three or more areas
+3: Many discharges in most muscle areas
+4: Full interference pattern of FPs or PSWs; obscuring the baseline

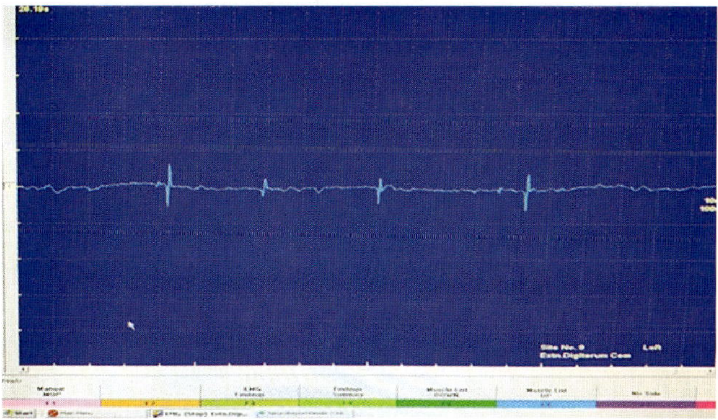

Fig. 7.26: Fibrillation potentials.

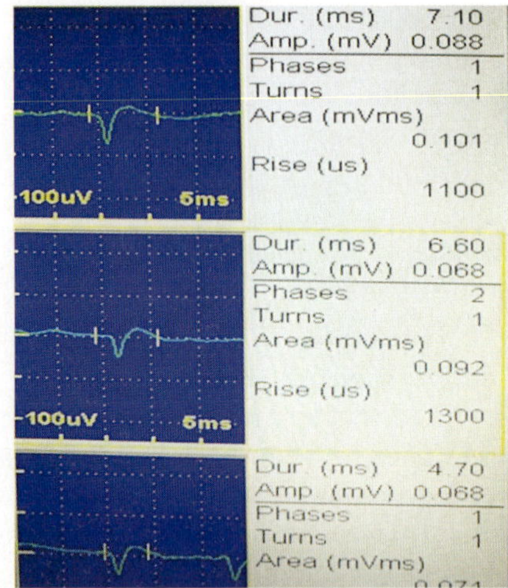

Fig. 7.27: Positive sharp waves.

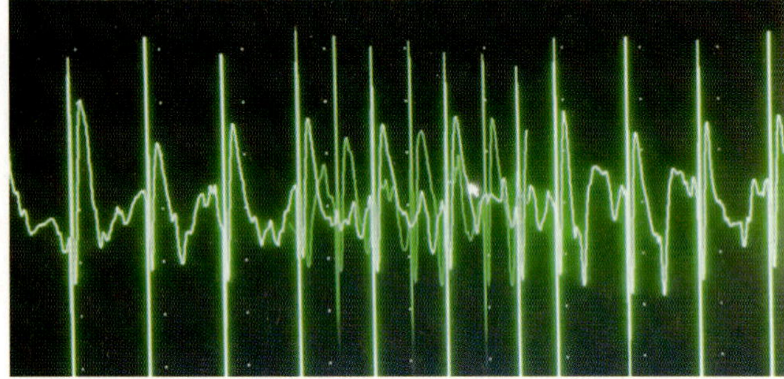

Fig. 7.28: Myotonic discharges.

- Amplitude—20–200 μV
- Duration—10–30 ms
- Sound similar to dull pop
- Recorded from injured muscle fibers.

Causes of FPs and PSWs:
- Neurogenic causes:
  a. AHC disorders
  b. Axonal neuropathy
  c. Radiculopathy
  d. Plexopathy
- NM junction disorders:
  a. Myasthenia gravis
  b. Botulism.
- Myogenic causes:
  a. Muscular dystrophy
  b. Muscle trauma
  c. Myositis
  d. Hyperkalemic periodic paralysis.

2. **Myotonic discharges (Fig. 7.28):**
   - Single muscle fiber potentials triggered by needle movement, voluntary contraction, or percussion
   - Caused by alteration of ion channels in the membrane of the muscle
   - May be seen with or without clinical myotonia
   - Characteristic finding—smooth change of rate and amplitude; waxing and waning nature

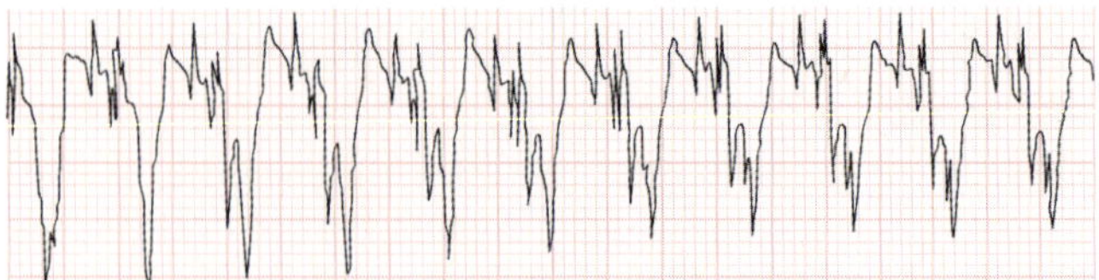

Fig. 7.29: Complex repetitive discharges.

- Frequency—20–150 Hz
- Sound similar to dive bomber
- Can be classified as positive waves and brief spikes depending on the location of the needle electrode
- Positive waves resemble PSWs and brief spikes resemble FPs; but can be distinguished by the waxing and waning nature.
- Causes:
  - Paramyotonia
  - Myotonia congenital
  - Myotonia dystrophica
  - Polymyositis
  - Hyperkalemic periodic paralysis

3. **Complex repetitive discharges (Fig. 7.29)**
   - Complex repetitive discharges occur due to repetitive and synchronous firing of a group of muscle fibers either spontaneously or by needle movement
   - At least 10 distinct potentials with interval of <0.5 to >200 ms
   - Sound similar to a machine
   - Caused by depolarization of a single muscle fiber followed by ephaptic transmission to surrounding denervated muscle fibers.
   - Causes:
     - Myogenic causes:
       - Polymyositis
       - Myxedema
       - Muscular dystrophy
     - Neurogenic causes:
       - Poliomyelitis
       - Spinal muscular dystrophy
       - Chronic radiculopathies
       - Amyotrophic lateral sclerosis
       - Chronic neuropathies

Abnormal spontaneous activities originating from motor neuron or axon: Abnormal spontaneous activities are:

1. **Fasciculation potentials (Figs. 7.30A and B):**
   - Spontaneous contractions of a group of muscle fibers which may be part of or a whole MU
   - Random and irregular
   - Firing rate—0.1–10 Hz
   - Variable size and shape dependent on the MU and distance from recording electrode
   - Appearance may resemble normal or abnormal MUAP

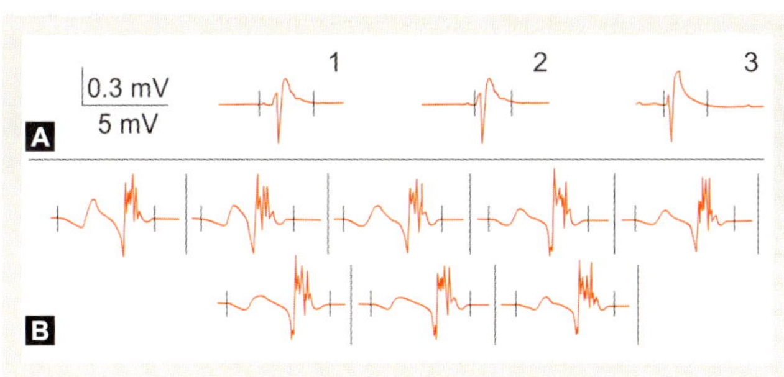

Figs. 7.30A and B: Fasciculation potentials.

- Can occur in normal individuals as well (Benign fasciculations)—will not be accompanied by weakness, reflex changes, and wasting
- Causes:
  a. Neurogenic causes:
     - Spinal muscular atrophy
     - Muscular dystrophy
     - Syringomyelia
     - Chronic radiculopathies
     - Peripheral neuropathies
  b. Metabolic disorders:
     - Uremia
     - Tetany
     - Thyrotoxicosis

2. **Myokymia:**
   - Grouped fasciculations
   - Spontaneous bursting, repetitive discharges
   - Associated with fine, quivering of the muscle
   - Firing rate—40–60 Hz
   - Bursts of 2–10 potentials with intervals of 0.1–1.0 second duration
   - Sound similar to a marching soldiers
   - Result from ephaptic transmission along demyelinated nerve
   - Facial myokymia—multiple sclerosis, pontine gliomas, polyradiculopathy, etc.
   - Limb myokymia—chronic nerve compression and radiation plexopathy.

3. **Doublets, triplets, and multiplets:**
   - Spontaneous potentials firing in two, three, or multiple groups
   - Occur due to spontaneous depolarization of the MU or its axon
   - Seen in hyperventilation, motor neuron disease, tetany, and other metabolic disorders.

4. **Neuromyotonia:**
   - Firing of single potential at 150–250 Hz
   - Not influenced by voluntary activity
   - Wax and wane in amplitude and frequency
   - Can be familial or autoimmune
   - Also seen in tetany, spinal muscular atrophy, pseudomyotonia, neuromyotonia, chronic demyelinating neuropathy, etc.

5. **Cramp potentials:**
   - Spontaneous potentials with abrupt onset and cessation
   - Firing rate—40–60 Hz
   - Seen in salt depletion, myxedema, pregnancy, uremia, and also in normal.

Voluntary activity: MUAPs recorded in routine EMG are small and low threshold, indicating origin from type I muscle fibers. The MUAP represents the sum of the individual MFAPs. MUAPs should be assessed based on their morphology, stability, and firing pattern.

1. **Morphology:** The morphology of the MUAP is described based on the amplitude, duration, rise time, and number of turns **(Fig. 7.31 and Box 7.12)**.
   Duration:
   - Measured from initial deflection to return to baseline
   - Varies from 5 to 15 ms depending on muscle temperature, age, and muscle examined
   - Duration of proximal muscle MUAP shorter than distal.

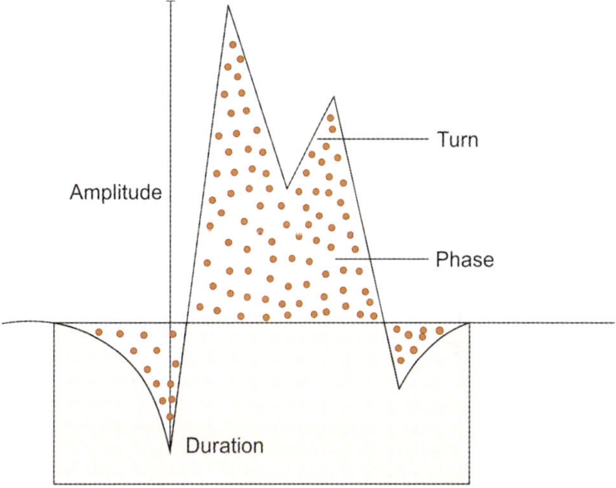

Fig. 7.31: Parameters of a normal motor unit action potential (MUAP).

BOX 7.12: Factors affecting motor unit action potential.

- Technical variables:
  - Type of needle electrode
  - Characteristics of recording surface, cable, preamplifier, amplifier, and method of recording
- Physiological variables:
  - Age
  - Muscle
  - Location of needle
  - Muscle temperature
  - Activation procedure
  - Number of muscle fibers in the MU
  - Fiber density
  - Location of end plate
  - Surrounding tissues—fat, muscles, blood vessels, etc.

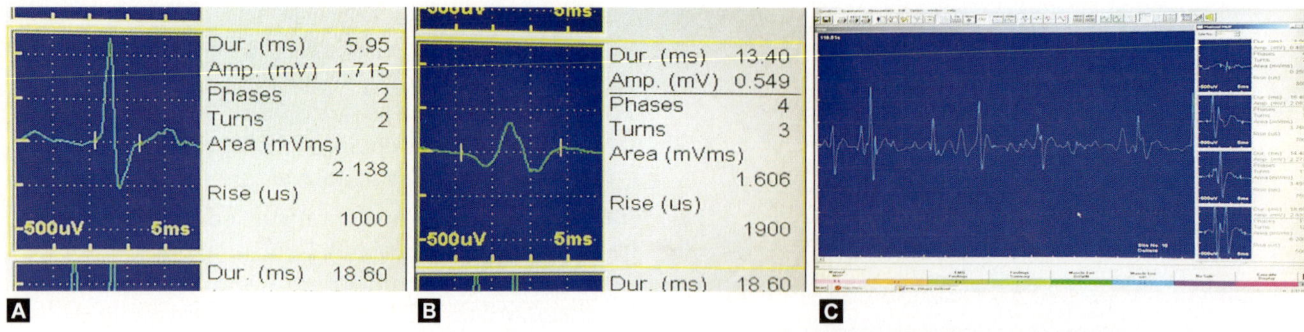

Figs. 7.32A to C: Phases in motor unit action potential (MUAP): (A) Biphasic; (B) Triphasic; (C) Polyphasic.

Rise time:
- Duration from initial positive to subsequent negative peak
- Indicates distance between needle electrode and muscle fiber
- <500 μs duration acceptable
- Slower rise time signifies the need to reposition the electrode.

Amplitude:
- Measured from peak to peak
- 0.1–2.0 mV
- A measure of muscle fibers nearer to recording electrode
- Depends on age, fiber density, synchrony of firing, muscle temperature, etc.

Phases (**Figs. 7.32A to C**):
- Inverted triphasic potential with initial positivity
- Measure of synchrony of firing
- Polyphasic potential—potential having more than four phases; have a high-frequency clicking sound.

2. **Stability:**
   - Variation in MUAP is indicative of abnormal NM transmission.
   - Unstable potential—changes morphology from potential to potential.

3. **Firing pattern:**
   - Firing rate of a normal muscle is fixed.
   - According to **Henneman's size principle**, the MUs are recruited from the smallest to the largest in size.
   - As the strength of contraction increases, there is an increase in the firing rate till a point is reached where the MUAP can no longer be individually analyzed (interference pattern) (**Fig. 7.33**).
   - Activation signifies the firing rate while recruitment signifies the ability to recruit new MUs with increasing firing rate—these features need to be analyzed for the study of firing pattern.
   - Early recruitment is a characteristic feature of myopathy.

Abnormalities of motor unit action potentials

Short-duration motor unit action potentials: Following are characteristics of short-duration motor unit action potentials:

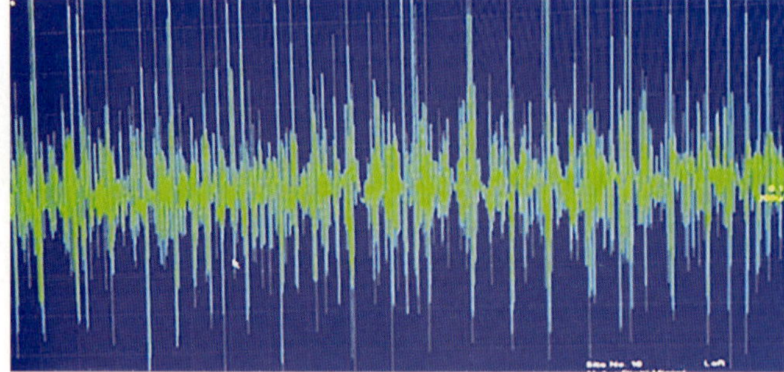

Fig. 7.33: Good recruitment pattern.

- Duration is shorter than the normal range for that age and gender
- Indicative of loss or segmentation of muscle fibers
- Causes—(1) myopathies and NM junction disorders and (2) early sign of reinnervation.

Long-duration motor unit action potentials: Following are characteristics of long-duration motor unit action potentials:
- Duration is longer than the normal range for that age and gender
- Seen in motor neuron diseases, chronic radiculopathy, axonal neuropathy with collateral sprouting, later stages of polymyositis
- Caused by an increase in fiber density, loss of synchrony, or increase in muscle fibers in a MU.

Polyphasic motor unit action potentials: Following are characteristics of polyphasic motor unit action potentials:
- Indicative of increased fiber density
- Seen in myopathies
- Satellite potentials (**Box 7.13**).

BOX 7.13: Satellite potentials.

- Late potentials time locked to main motor unit action potential.
- Seen in early reinnervation
- Formation of new collateral sprouts from adjacent normal innervated muscles to reinnervate denervated muscle fibers leads to delayed conduction and excitation of the muscle fiber, resulting in satellite potentials

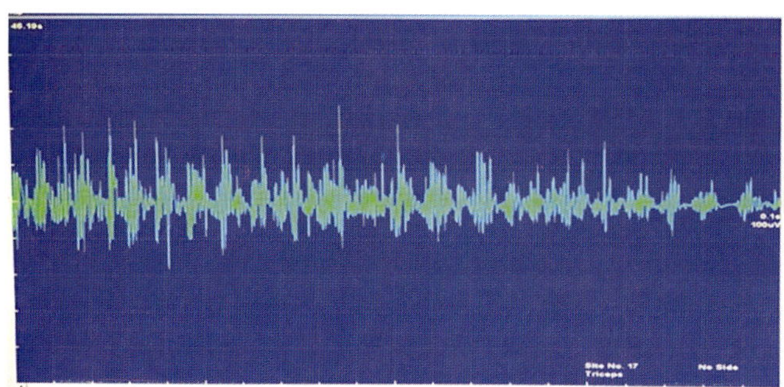

Fig. 7.34: Recruitment pattern in neurogenic disorder.

Mixed pattern: Following are abnormalities in the mixed pattern:

- Mixed pattern comprising polyphasic, short and long MUAPs
- Cause—both neurogenic disorders and myopathies.

Abnormal recruitment of motor unit action potentials

Abnormal recruitment of motor unit action potentials is of two types:

1. Reduced recruitment—found in all neurogenic disorders **(Fig. 7.34)**
2. Rapid recruitment—found in myopathies.

Interference pattern: Interference pattern is a less dense pattern indicative of poor effort, loss of MUs, or UMN lesions.

H REFLEX

H reflex or the Hoffman reflex is a late response. Late responses are responses or potentials that appear after the motor response or the M wave (main wave) due to the stimulation of a mixed nerve. F wave and axon reflex are other types of late responses **(Box 7.14)**.

> **BOX 7.14:** Definition by American Association of Neuromuscular and Electrodiagnostic Medicine (AANEM).
>
> *AANEM defines H reflex or H wave as:*
> "A compound muscle action potential with a consistent latency recorded from muscles after stimulation of the nerve."

The H reflex was described by Paul Hoffman in 1910 and 1918. Later, Magladery and McDougal recognized it as the "H reflex" for the original contribution made by Hoffman. The H reflex is a monosynaptic reflex elicited on submaximal stimulation and recorded from a selected group of physiologic extensors, particularly the calf muscles on stimulation of the tibial nerve. It cannot be recorded from the small muscles of hands and feet in adults but can be recorded from the same in children <2 years of age.

The H reflex allows the evaluation of the proximal segments of the nerve, i.e., the roots and plexuses. Compared to F wave and SSEPs, they are better as F waves only analyze the motor fibers of the nerve and SSEPs only evaluate the sensory fibers.

Reflex arc for H reflex **(Fig. 7.35)**:

- Fast conducting group Ia fibers act as afferents
- Spinal cord—site for synapsing of afferent fibers with alpha motor neurons
- Efferent fibers supplying the muscle.

H reflex is elicited on submaximal stimulation but is inhibited by a stronger stimulus due to:

1. Collision of orthodromic impulses with the antidromic conduction by motor axons
2. Renshaw cell inhibition
3. Inhibition by adjoining motor neurons
4. Supraspinal inhibition.

Throughout literature, H reflex has been likened to the tendon reflex, the only difference being the bypassing of muscle spindle mechanisms by the H reflex **(Table 7.8)**. However, there are several differences between them.

Techniques

The most commonly recorded H reflex is that of the soleus muscle, which is explained below:

Position: Semireclining or prone lying with thigh and leg supported, foot at right angle with the tibia.

Recording:

- For soleus muscle:

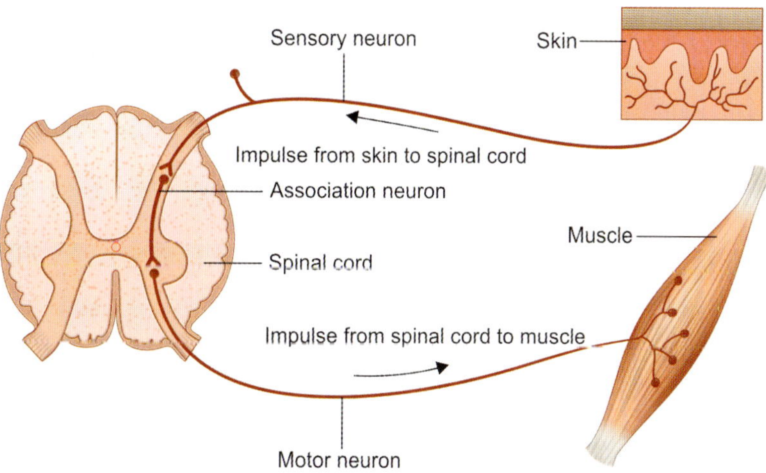

Fig. 7.35: H reflex.

Table 7.8: Difference between H reflex and tendon reflex.

H reflex	Tendon reflex
Bypasses the muscle spindle, hence less affected by fusimotor drive	
One impulse/axon	Multiple impulses with percussion
Electrical stimulus recruits Ia and Ib fibers equally, produces single discharge in each afferent fiber	Excites Ia fibers more intensely, causing high-frequency repetitive discharges in afferent fibers
Electric stimulus recruits afferents from all calf muscles and intrinsic muscles	Percussion causes wider excitation, exciting muscle spindles in the thigh muscles as well
EPSP shorter	EPSP longer
More affected by presynaptic inhibition	Less affected by presynaptic inhibition

(EPSP: excitatory postsynaptic potential)

- Recording electrode—distal edge of calf muscle, medial to tibia half way between stimulation point and medial malleolus
- Reference electrode—Achilles tendon
- For flexor carpi radialis: Recording electrode—junction of upper one-third and lower two-third of line joining medial epicondyle and radial styloid.

Stimulation:
- Square wave pulse of 1 ms duration for sensory fibers
- Stimulus frequency—0.2 Hz or less to allow recovery from previous stimulus
- Intensity may be adjusted to avail maximum H response amplitude
- For soleus—stimulation of posterior tibial nerve in the popliteal fossa
- For flexor carpi radialis—stimulation at cubital fossa
- At least five responses to be studied.

Measurement:
- Latency—stimulus artifact to the first deflection from baseline
- Amplitude—base to negative peak or peak to peak.

Normal values: Normal values of soleus H reflex in adults:
- Mean latency: 30.0 ± 2.1 ms
- Right/left difference (i.e., symmetry): 0.09 ± 0.70 ms
- Soleus H reflex = 3.00 + 0.1419 × height (cm) + 0.0643 × age (years) ± 1.47.

Normal values for flexor carpi radialis H reflex in adults:
- Mean latency: 16.84 ± 1.33 ms
- Right/Left difference: 0.002 ± 0.42 ms
- Flexor carpi radialis (FCR) H reflex = 0.44 + 0.0925 × height (cm) + 0.0316 × age (years) ± 0.83.

  A normal response should lie within ±5.5 ms of the calculated latency.

H:M Ratio

It is the ratio of the peak to peak amplitude of the maximum H reflex to the peak to peak amplitude of the maximum M wave. It provides a measure of the proportion of motor neuron pool activation during H response. Normal soleus H:M ratio is <0.7.

Clinical Implications

Clinical implications are:
- Evaluates proximal motor and sensory pathways
- Helps in evaluating plexopathies and radiculopathies
- GBS—H reflex may be absent or dispersed or delayed
- S1 radiculopathy—soleus H reflex may be absent
- C6–C7 radiculopathy—flexor carpi radialis H reflex may be abnormal
- Identifies nerve root involvement before any EMG changes
- Slowed latency—abnormal dorsal root function due to disc herniation or impingement.

F WAVE

F waves are forms of NCS used to evaluate the proximal segment of a nerve that is inaccessible for routine NCS **(Box 7.15)**. They were first recorded from the foot muscles by Magladery and McDougal in 1950, hence named "F wave." They are late responses **(Fig. 7.36)** that result from antidromic activation of the motor neurons. They involve the spinal cord as conduction occurs through the spinal cord at the interface between peripheral nervous system and central nervous system.

Characteristics of F Wave

Following are the characteristics of F wave:
- Smaller compared to the main wave (M wave)

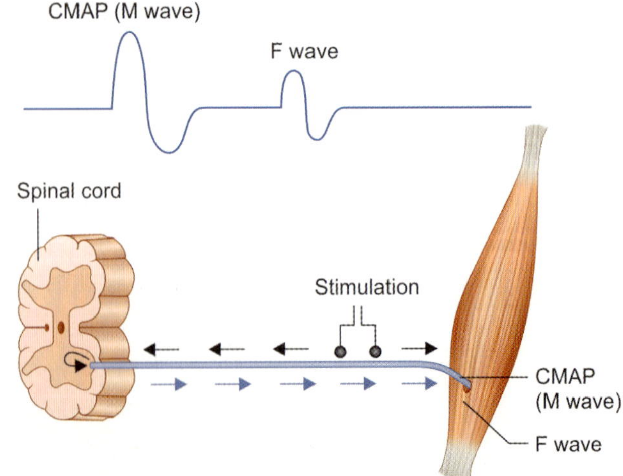

Fig. 7.36: F wave.

BOX 7.15: Definition of F wave by the American Association of Neuromuscular and Electrodiagnostic Medicine (AANEM).

The AANEM defines F wave as:
"An action potential evoked intermittently from a muscle by a supramaximal electric stimulus to the nerve due to antidromic activation of motor neurons."

- The amplitude of F wave is 1–5% of the M wave—more than 20 mV
- Has a variable configuration
- Latency longer than M wave
- Latency longer with more distal sites of stimulation
- Latency in upper limb—approximately 30 seconds; latency in lower limb—approximately 60 seconds
- The F wave is an inconsistent response, hence needs at least 10 consecutive trials for calculation
- Easy to elicit using supramaximal stimulus, unlike H reflex **(Table 7.9)**.

Uses of F Waves

F waves are used to:
- Evaluate the proximal segment of a nerve
- Compare the conduction in the proximal and distal segments of a nerve
- Determine site of conduction slowing, e.g., to differentiate a root lesion from a distal neuropathy
- Most useful in conditions involving the most proximal segment of a nerve, e.g., thoracic outlet syndrome, Guillain-Barré syndrome, radiculopathies with multiple root involvement, brachial plexus injuries, etc.
- Evaluate effectiveness of therapeutic interventions used for spasticity.

Physiology

The alpha motor neuron forms both the afferent and the efferent pathway for F wave **(Fig. 7.37)**. Since there is no synapse involve, the F wave is not a reflex but only a measure of motor conduction. Also, since there is reactivation of only a few AHC axon hillocks and orthodromic action potentials are generated only in a few motor axons, the amplitude of F wave is much smaller than the M wave.

Technique

F wave can be recorded using the following technique:
- **Stimulation:**
  - Recording from any distal muscle by stimulating the appropriate nerve
  - Intensity—supramaximal (20–25% higher than that required to generate M wave)
  - Rate of stimulation—≤5 Hz

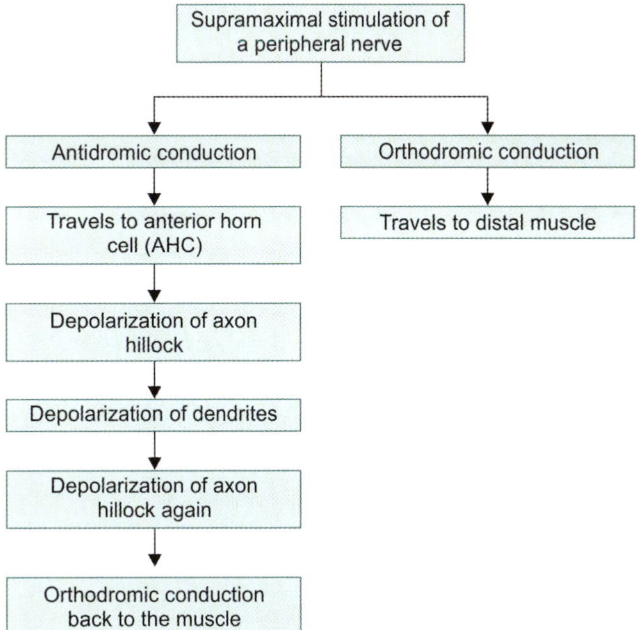

Fig. 7.37: Physiology of F wave.

- Cathode placed proximal to anode, to prevent anodal block.
- **Recording**
  - Recording electrode—in a belly tendon montage
  - Amplitude gain—200–500 µV/division
  - Filter settings—30–10 kHz
  - Sweep speed—5–10 ms/division
  - Muscle needs to be completely relaxed, as a contracted state can enhance F waves or produce an H reflex.
- **Measurement:** Parameters used for measurement of F wave are presented in **Table 7.10**.

Limitations

Following are the limitations of F wave:
- Changes in F response should also be clinically correlated. In the case of partial or incomplete lesions, there may be few fibers left that may allow faster conduction, leading to a normal F wave.
- Parameters, such as chronodispersion and repeater F waves require >100 stimuli that make the process uncomfortable for the subject and tedious for the examiner.
- They may be difficult to interpret in proximal muscles as they lie close together and may sometimes, overlap.
- Utility of F waves for diagnosis of radiculopathy is limited since only median, ulnar, and tibial nerves are routinely evaluated which allow evaluation of C8, T1 and L5, S1 roots only.

DOCUMENTATION AND REPORTING

Documentation and reporting of the electrodiagnosis (EDX) examination need to be detailed and precise. The following elements should be incorporated in the report:
- Demographics and identification information of the subject—name, age, gender, contact number, medical

Table 7.9: Distinguishing features of F wave and H reflex.

Parameter	F wave	H reflex
Stimulus	Supramaximal	Submaximal
Increase in stimulus	Facilitatory	Inhibitory
Morphology	Variable	Fixed
Motor units recruited in M wave	Different	Same
Amplitude	1–5% of M wave	50–100% of M wave
Recorded in	Distal muscles	Soleus, vastus medialis, flexor carpi radialis
Clinical importance	Polyneuropathy and radiculopathy	Polyneuropathy and radiculopathy

Table 7.10: Parameters of F wave.

Parameter	Description
F latency	• Minimal latency usually recorded • Related to age, limb length and height • Upper limit in normal individuals—31 ms for hands and 61 ms for foot muscles • Marked prolongation of F wave latency—suggestive of demyelinating neuropathy • Comparison with distal latency helps comparison of proximal and distal nerve involvement • F wave latency may also be prolonged in radiculopathy
Chronodispersion	• Difference between minimal and maximal latencies • Measure of range of conduction of F waves • Requires large number of F waves to be studied (at least 50–60 waves) • Higher sensitivity in demyelinating neuropathy
Amplitude (F:M ratio)	• Mean amplitude of F wave usually recorded • Peak to peak amplitudes used • Measure of amount of motor neuron pool activated through antidromic stimulation
Persistence	• Ratio of number of responses to number of stimuli • Requires only 10 stimuli to be studied • Extensors of leg and flexors of arm have higher persistence (80%) compared to antigravity muscles (30%) • Persistence may be reduced in axonal injuries • Absent F waves with normal M waves characteristic of peripheral nerve demyelination
Repeater F waves	• Number of similar appearing F waves among a series of F waves • Documented as number of repeater waves out of total F waves analyzed • Indicative of selectivity of motor unit discharges amongst a series of F waves • Increases in axonal neuropathy and anterior horn cell (AHC) disorders • Requires 100–200 F waves to be analyzed, making the use of computer essential

record number, date of birth, name and contact details of referring physician, name of the examiner, date of examination, the test being performed, site of examination (left or right side, upper or lower extremity, segment of body evaluated, nerve or muscle evaluated), etc.

- History and physical examination related to the presenting pathology—needs to be assessment based and progressive
- Electrodiagnostic findings—presented in graphical and tabular forms along with all the waveforms and quantitative values
- Clinical summary or interpretation—findings made by the examiner after correlating the EDX findings with clinical findings

- Conclusion—should be succinct and address the need of the referring physician for the EDX test; should include the side evaluated (left or right), whether the study was normal or abnormal, final diagnosis of the examiner, other differential diagnoses that were ruled out and the reasons for the same, pathophysiology and the prognosis, if applicable.

OTHER ELECTRODIAGNOSTIC TESTS

Several other tests may also be used for the electrodiagnostic purpose in addition to those mentioned above. **Table 7.11** shows other commonly used electrodiagnostic tests.

Table 7.11: Other commonly used electrodiagnostic tests.

Test	Characteristics
Evoked potentials	• Electric waveform elicited by and temporally related to a stimulus, most commonly an electric stimulus delivered to a sensory receptor or nerve, or applied directly to a discrete area of the brain, spinal cord, or muscle • For example, auditory evoked potentials, somatosensory evoked potentials, and visual evoked potentials
EEG	• Noninvasive electrophysiological method to record electrical activity of the brain from the surface of the skull
ECoG	• Also called intracranial EEG as it is invasive • Intraoperative recording of electrical activity of the brain directly from an exposed cerebral cortex
ECG	• Electrophysiological technique of measuring electrical activity of the heart
EGG	• Measures gastric myoelectric activity
Blink response	• Compound muscle action potentials evoked from orbicularis oculi muscles as a result of brief electric or mechanical stimuli applied to the cutaneous area innervated by the supraorbital (or less commonly, the infraorbital) branch of the trigeminal nerve
RNS	• The technique of repeated supramaximal stimulation of a nerve while recording successive M waves from a muscle innervated by the nerve

(ECG: electrocardiography; ECoG: electrocorticography; EEG: electroencephalography; EGG: electrogastrography; RNS: repetitive nerve stimulation)

SUMMARY

Electrodiagnosis forms a vital part of the diagnostic and decision-making process. It involves a string of tests that can be used to evaluate the various systems of the body. Though the testing procedure is extensive and often cumbersome for the therapist and subjects both, the results availed help a huge amount in establishing a diagnosis, formulate a management plan and monitor it, and assess the prognosis of the pathology. It should be remembered by the examiner that a diagnosis cannot be formulated solely based on the findings of the electrodiagnostic tests and these results need to be correlated clinically.

Review Questions

1. What is electrodiagnosis? Which different tests are included in it?
2. Describe the strength–duration curve in detail along with the technique of application.
3. Explain the faradic–galvanic test in detail.
4. What is electromyography? Describe the various abnormal spontaneous potentials seen in EMG.
5. What is nerve conduction test? How will you perform NCV for median nerve and tibial nerve?
6. Write short notes on:
   a. Reaction of degeneration
   b. Normal CRD and PRD strength–duration curve
   c. H reflex
   d. F wave
   e. Insertional activity
   f. Characteristics of a normal MUAP
   g. Temporal dispersion and conduction block.

BIBLIOGRAPHY

1. AANEM (American Association of Neuromuscular and Electrodiagnostic Medicine). Glossary of terms in Neuromuscular and electrodiagnostic medicine. In: Muscle and nerve supplement, 3rd edition; 2015.
2. Aminoff AJ. Electrodiagnosis in clinical neurology, 5th edition. Philadelphia, PA: Elsevier Churchill Livingstone Publications; 1999.
3. Azrieli Y, Weimer L, Lovelace R, et al. The utility of segmental nerve conduction studies in ulnar mononeuropathy at the elbow. Muscle Nerve. 2003;27:46-50.
4. Burke D. Clinical uses of H reflexes of upper and lower limb muscles. Clin Neurophysiol Pract. 2016;1:9-17.
5. Forster A, Palastanga N. Clayton's electrotherapy—theory and practice, 8th edition. London, UK: CBS Publications Ltd; 2005.
6. Frontera WR, DeLisa JA. DeLisa's physical medicine & rehabilitation: principles and practice, 5th edition. Philadelphia, PA: Lippincott Williams and Wilkins; 2010.
7. Misra UK, Kalita J. Clinical neurophysiology, 3rd edition. New Delhi, India: Elsevier Publications; 2017.
8. Nanda BK. Electrotherapy explained, 2nd edition. New Delhi, India: Jaypee Publications; 2014.
9. O'Sullivan SB, Schmitz TJ, Fulk GD. Physical rehabilitation, 6th edition. Philadelphia, PA: F.A. Davis Company Publications; 2014.
10. Robertson V, Ward A, Low J, et al. Electrotherapy explained—principles and practice, 4th edition. Philadelphia, PA: Elsevier Publications; 2006.
11. Robinson AJ, Snyder-Mackler L. Clinical electrophysiology: electrotherapy and electrophysiologic testing. Baltimore, MD: Lippincott Williams and Wilkins; 1989.

8

CHAPTER

Assessment of Function

Amit V Nagrale

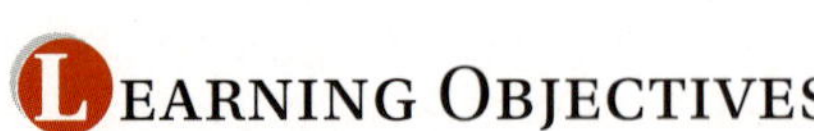

LEARNING OBJECTIVES

After reading this chapter, the readers should be able to:

♦ Understand the concepts of health, function, activity, and participation
♦ Understand the concepts of impairment, activity limitation, participation restriction, functional limitation, and disability
♦ Gain an introduction to International Classification of Functioning, Disability and Health (ICF) with classification and uses
♦ Examine and measure the functions by three levels
♦ Compare the characteristics of various formal tests of function, including physical function tests and multidimensional functional assessment instruments
♦ Identify factors to be considered in the selection of instruments for testing function
♦ Compare and contrast various scoring methods used in functional instruments
♦ Gain knowledge regarding issues of reliability and validity as they relate to functional instruments
♦ Develop a functional plan when presented with a clinical case study.

CHAPTER OUTLINE

- International Classification of Functioning, Disability and Health
  - What is ICF?
  - Components of the ICF
  - Classification of ICF with definitions
  - Uses of ICF
- Examination of function
  - Purpose of functional assessment
- Measures of functional assessment
  - Impairment-based measures
  - Self-reported measures
  - Physical performance measures
- Functional instruments
- Selected instruments for assesing function
  - Barthel index
  - The Katz index of ADL
- The Lawton instrumental activities of daily living scale
- Functional independence measure
- Sickness impact profile
- Outcomes and assessment information set
- The short form-36
- Considerations in selection of instruments

INTRODUCTION

The main purpose of rehabilitation is to return the individual to a lifestyle as close to the previous function as possible or to increase the current potential for function and maintain it throughout life.

The quality of life is a generally leveled concept, deeply influenced by **(Box 8.1)**:

- **Physical** health of the person
- Their **psychological** status
- The level of **independence**
- **Social** relations
- Their relation toward the main characteristics of their **environment**.

A health system aims to improve the health of the people.

Normal aging changes and health problems are often reflected in declines in the physical abilities, which can render them less independent, less safe and can make daily tasks much harder for them. One of the methods to evaluate the physical health status is through functional

---

> **BOX 8.1:** Definition of Quality of Life (QoL).
>
> The World Health Organization (WHO) defines quality of life as individual's perception of their position in life in the context of the culture and value systems in which they live and in relation to their goals, expectations, standards, and concerns.

BOX 8.2: Definition of health.

In 1948, World Health Organization (WHO) constitution has defined health as "A state of complete physical, mental and social well-being, and not merely the absence of disease and infirmity".

assessment, which provides data that may indicate decline or improvement in health, allowing the health-care provider to intervene.

Function is usually classified into two types: instrumental activities of daily living (IADLs) and basic activities of daily living (ADLs). Functional assessment in this chapter is conceptualized as a comprehensive evaluation of the physical abilities required to maintain independence.

A broad conceptual framework is necessary to fully understand the concept of health and its relationship to functional disability. Terms such as "well-being," "health-related quality of life," and "functional status" are often used interchangeably to describe health status (**Box 8.2**).

Nagi developed a model that explicates health status and the relationship among the various terms used to describe health status (**Fig. 8.1**). This model has been found throughout the American literature. The model used in this chapter to clear the concept of health status and the processes by which individual becomes disabled begins with pathology or disease process that utilizes the body's defenses and response mechanisms.

INTERNATIONAL CLASSIFICATION OF FUNCTIONING, DISABILITY AND HEALTH

What is ICF?

The ICF (*International Classification of Functioning, Disability and Health*) is World Health Organization's (WHO's) framework for measuring health and disability at both the individual and population levels. "ICF is the ruler that can be used for precise measurement of health and disability" (Brundtland, 2002). ICF belongs to the "family" of international classifications developed by the WHO for application to various aspects of health. The overall aim of the ICF classification is to provide a unified and standard language and framework for the description of health and health-related states. It defines components of health and some health-related components of well-being (such as education and labor). The domains contained in ICF can, therefore, be seen as *health domains* and *health-related domains*.

Components of the ICF

These domains are described from the perspective of the body, the individual and society in two basic lists:
1. Body functions and structures
2. Activities and participation.

Functioning is an umbrella term encompassing all body functions, activities, and participation; similarly, *disability* serves as an umbrella term for impairments, activity limitations, or participation restrictions. Functioning and disability associated with health conditions are classified in ICF (**Box 8.3**).

Classification of ICF with Definitions

ICF has two *parts*, each with two *components* (**Fig. 8.2**):
1. Part 1: Functioning and disability
   a. Body functions and structures
   b. Activities and participation
2. Part 2: Contextual factors
   a. Environmental factors
   b. Personal factors

Uses of International Classification of Functioning, Disability and Health

ICF is a classification of human functioning and disability. It is used to (**Table 8.1**):
1. Offer an excellent conceptual framework for envisioning the consequences of health condition or pathology on the function of individuals.

BOX 8.3: Terminology related to ICF structure.

- Body functions are the physiological functions of body systems (including psychological functions).
- Body structures are anatomical parts of the body such as organs, limbs and their components.
- Impairments are problems in body function or structure such as a significant deviation or loss.
- Activity is the execution of a task or action by an individual.
- Participation is involvement in a life situation.
- Activity limitations are difficulties an individual may have in executing activities.
- Participation restrictions are problems an individual may experience in involvement in life situations.
- Environmental factors make up the physical, social, and attitudinal environment in which people live and conduct their lives.

(ICF: International Classification of Functioning, Disability and Health)

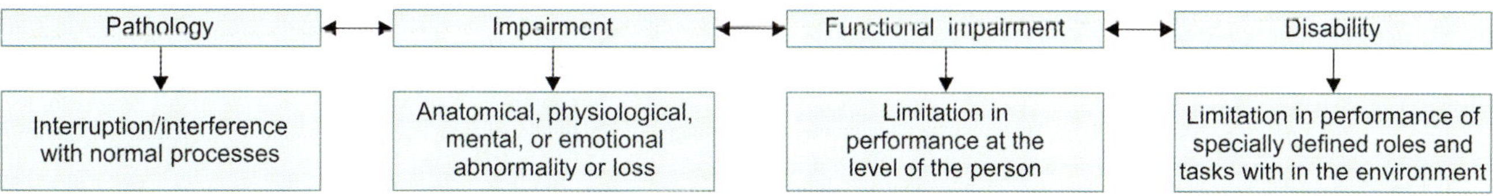

Fig. 8.1: Nagi's model of the process of disablement.

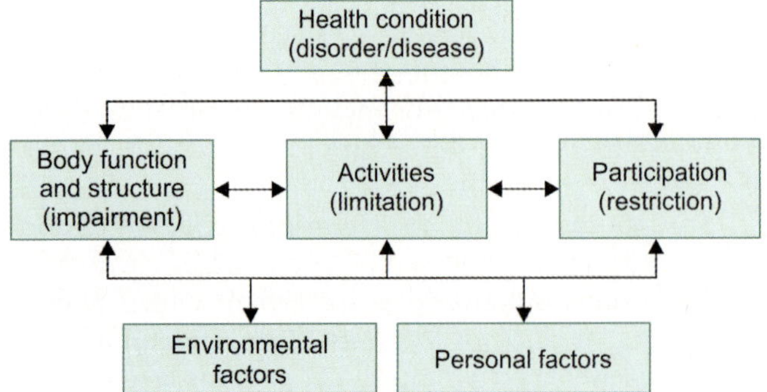

Fig. 8.2: The ICF model: interaction between ICF components.

(ICF: International Classification of Functioning, Disability and Health)

Source: Permission from World Health Organization: International Classification of Functioning, Disability and Health: ICF short version. Geneva: World Health Organization; 2001.

2. Select appropriate interventions, follow the patient's recovery, and assess treatment outcomes.
3. Monitor progress of the patients and their responsiveness.
4. Evaluate the psychometric quality of measures to determine if they are meaningful for diagnosis or for evaluation of the progress.

Table 8.1: Examples of classification of clinical observations or measurements using the components of ICF.

ICF components	Examples
Health condition	• Infarction of neurons in precentral gyrus of cerebral cortex • Fracture of distal tibia • Transtibial amputation of left leg • Tear of anterior cruciate ligament • Deep vein thrombosis
Impairments	• Paralysis • Weakness • Sensory loss • Restriction in ROM • Inadequate balance • Impaired gait • Poor coordination • Inability to cough
Activity limitations	• Inability to walk on level surface • Inability to dress or undress oneself • Inability to make a meal • Inability to lift a heavy object • Inability to walk up and down a flight of stairs
Participation restriction	• Inability to care for oneself without assistance • Inability to work at normal occupation • Inability to fulfill role as a parent • Inability to play regular recreational activity

(ICF: International Classification of Functioning, Disability and Health; ROM: range-of-motion).

EXAMINATION OF FUNCTION

Analysis of the function mainly focuses on the functional activities and measurement of the individual's ability to do all activities successfully. Functional testing measures how a person does certain tasks or fulfills certain roles in the various dimensions of living. Application of selected measures yields data that can be used as:

- Baseline information for setting function related goals and outcomes of intervention
- Indicators of a patient's abilities and progression toward complex functional activities
- Set criteria for rehabilitation
- Monitoring individual's level of safety in performing a specific task and risk of injury while performance
- Evidence of the effectiveness of a specific intervention.

Purpose of Functional Assessment

The purpose of functional assessment is to:
- Indicate presence and severity of disease
- Measure a person's need for care
- Monitor change over time
- Maintain an optimally cost-effective clinical operation
- Identify the problems and needs of individuals, defining therapy goals, planning, and implementing interventions, and assessing the effect of interventions using different measurement tools.
- Cover the body dimension and activities dimension of the ICF.

MEASURES OF FUNCTIONAL ASSESSMENT

Function is measured in a number of different ways, including:
- Impairment-based measures
- Self-reported measures
- Physical performance measures (PPM) **(Fig. 8.3)**.

Impairment-based Measures

Impairment-based measures are as follows:
- Impairments are defined as a dysfunction or a significant structural abnormality in a specific body part or system.
- Findings of impaired joint mobility, motor function, muscle performance, range-of-motion (ROM), and sensation are considered problems that are limited to the impairment level.

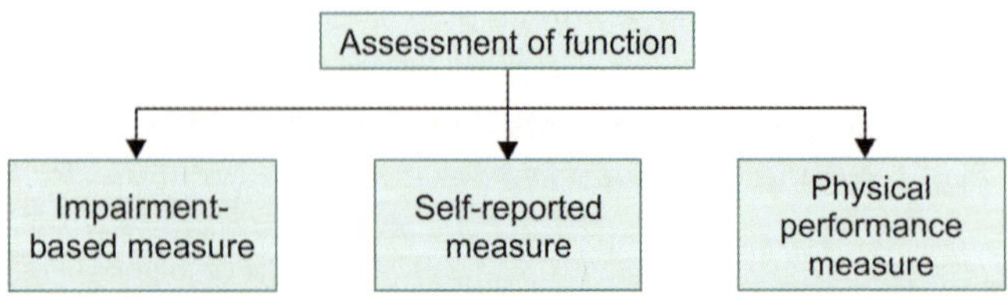

Fig. 8.3: Conceptual model of comprehensive assessment of function.

- These impairments, alone or in combination, can contribute to limited function and ultimately may have consequences over physical functioning.
- For example, an impaired humeral head inferior translation can contribute to the inability of a person to comb their hair due to mechanical shoulder impingement pain. Restricted ROM at the hip may lead to a limp during gait.
- Clinical special tests are used to determine the tissue that may be the source of the symptoms and are impairment-based assessments.
- A clinical examination finding of impairment does not always correspond to a functional loss.
- Using the previous examples of restricted inferior glide and a limp originating from a lack of ROM of the hip helps represent the precarious relationship. Limited humeral head inferior glide may not always directly correlate with the actual concept of physical function (combing hair), as the patient may compensate by side-bending their head toward the involved extremity or through use of the opposite extremity. Poor ROM and a limp may be subthreshold for patients whose activity levels are low, thus they do not compromise the individual to the point where their expectations are altered.

Self-reported Measures

Self-reported measures are as follows:
- Self-reported measures are common measures where respondents are asked to report directly on their own behaviors, beliefs, attitudes, or intentions. They are subject-completed, relying on self-perception of mobility status, and performance of daily activities.
- They typically assess the subject's performance difficulties, restrictions, or need for assistance associated with functional activity.
- They are typically in form of questionnaire, which may seem subjective in nature but objectifies a person's perception. Use of self-reported measures should be preceded by careful evaluation of instrument reliability, responsiveness, and validity. Much work has been dedicated towards the development of these tools. Nearly all body regions or conditions have dedicated self-reported functional measures. For example, Short Form-36 (SF-36) is a self-reported measurement tool.
- The questionnaires where the patient reports on health or physical function are known as patient-reported outcomes (PROs). PROs can be categorized as disease specific or generic. PROs have been defined as "any report of the status of a patient's health condition that comes directly from the patient, without interpretation of the patient's response by a clinician or anyone else" (Kyte et al., 2015). For example, Geriatric Depression Scale is a self-rating scale used as a screening test to detect depression in elderly individuals, and it is not generic but disease specific.

Physical Performance Measures

Physical performance measures (PPM) are as follows:
- PPM have become increasingly popular methods of measuring specific characteristics of function, especially in postinjury assessment, determining fall risks and sports performance/injury prediction. Although several authors have described these tests as functional tests, a more accurate depiction of these testing methods is that they are measures of physical performance.
- While some of these tests have demonstrated causal relationships for both postinjury and preinjury risk assessments, they are often just one test and measure just one parameter of function.
- Additionally, the depth of investigation into these relationships is lacking.
- Examples of PPM include, Timed Up and Go test, 6-minute walk test, where a person is given a task and is asked to perform it, based on which an inference of their level of either functional status or impairments, directly or by observation is made.

FUNCTIONAL INSTRUMENTS

Functional instruments are as follows:
- Functional ability refers to a person's ability to perform tasks that are required for living.
- Dependency is defined as the inability to carry out ADLs without regular help from another person.
- Functional status can be assessed by direct examination of the patient or knowledgeable informant.
- An assessment of functional status should include, at minimum, an evaluation of the patient's ability to perform IADLs and ADLs. ADLs are activities in which people engage on a day-to-day basis, including personal care activities that are fundamental to caring for oneself and maintaining independence. IADLs are defined as those activities, accomplishment of which is necessary for continued independent residence in the community as they are more sensitive for subtle functional deficiencies than the ADLs.
- Functional status refers to the ability to perform daily activities required to meet basic self-care needs and to maintain health and well-being. Functional status reflects both functional capacity, what an individual is capable of doing, and functional performance, what an individual actually does in daily life.
- Functional status may be affected by impairments in physical, cognitive, sensory, or social function.
- Approximately 75% people over the age of 75 years limit their activities due to functional impairments each year; 40% experience restricted activity in two consecutive months. Almost 50% of people of 85 years of age and older require assistance in one or more ADLs. As many as 25% of older community-dwelling adults have at least one impairment in IADLs.

Among patients admitted to general medical hospital units, almost 40% have at least one ADL impairment, 65% have one or more IADL impairments, and 30% have mobility impairments.

- Functional status can also be assessed using one of the several available valid and reliable instruments.
- Functional status is typically described in terms of the patient's ability to perform IADL and ADL.
- Conducting and documenting an assessment and monitoring changes in daily functioning is crucial.
- Functional assessment includes evaluation of physical, psychological, and socioeconomic domains.
- Physical functioning may focus on ADLs that include feeding, bathing, dressing, mobility, and toileting independently. Assessment of IADLs addresses more advanced self-care activities, such as shopping, cooking, and managing finances and medications.
- Standardized assessment instruments such as the Barthel or Katz indices can provide information on the patient's capacity for self-care and independent living.

SELECTED INSTRUMENTS FOR ASSESSING FUNCTION

Barthel Index (Appendix A)

The Barthel index can be described as follows:

- The Barthel index/scale is used to measure performance in ADLs.
- This scale measures the degree of assistance required by an individual on 10 items of mobility and self-care ADL, a higher score reflects greater ability to function independently following hospital discharge. The Barthel index includes 10 personal activities such as toileting, bathing, and dressing.
- Levels of measurement are limited to either complete independence or needing assistance. Each activity is scored in ordinal scale.
- The Barthel index was found to have a test–retest reliability of 0.89. The use of the Barthel index to document progress in medical rehabilitation began even before its publication and has continued to the present.
- The potential value of this instrument in stroke population is known and is a useful means in predicting functional prognosis in rehabilitation of stroke patients. Higher admission scores indicate greater overall improvement, thus providing a valid measure of the degree of disability.

The Katz Index of ADL (Appendix B)

The Katz index of ADL can be described as follows:

- In 1969, a medical doctor Sidney Katz realized the need for improving functional assessment in the aged because he needed a better means of evaluating interventions.
- The Katz ADL index was first developed in an effort to find a way to assess function and how it changed over time in the elderly.

- Katz et al. assessed the interrater reliability, reporting that differences between observers scoring decisions occurred once in 20 evaluations. In terms of cultural validity, the Katz ADL index demonstrated good internal consistencies for each ethnic group (Cronbach's alphas: 0.84–0.94) in Dutch, Turkish, and Moroccans. This indicated that the Katz index of ADL is valid to assess functional performance of these culturally diverse elderly. With regard to content validity, Katz presented some theoretical justification for the selection and inclusion of items on the scale.
- The Katz ADLs scale was developed to measure functional status in the elderly and in those with chronic disease.
- The observer determines the level of independence on a 3-point scale ranging from independent to dependent in each of the following six activities:
  1. Bathing
  2. Dressing
  3. Toileting
  4. Transferring
  5. Continence
  6. Feeding
- It was initially designed for use by direct observation over a period of weeks but has been adapted for use in an interview setting. Because it was used to identify impairments in basic skills, it may be most useful in populations with pre-existing impairments (such as a nursing home setting) or to identify care needs after acute events such as hospitalization.

The Lawton Instrumental Activities of Daily Living Scale (Appendix C)

The Lawton IADLs scale can be described as follows:

- The Lawton IADLs scale is an instrument developed to assess independent living skills. It differentiates among task performances, including the amount of help and amount of time needed to accomplish each task.
- There are eight domains of function, which may be assessed by the Lawton IADL scale.
- The Lawton Brody IADL scale was developed to assess performance in everyday tasks among community-dwelling elderly and is commonly used in conjunction with the ADL scale.
- The IADL scale evaluates skills necessary to live independently, including:
  - Using the telephone
  - Food preparation
  - Handling finances
  - Taking medications
- Compared with Katz's ADL scale, which assesses basic functions, it is probably more sensitive to early changes in functional status. It provides self-reported information about functional skills necessary to live in the community. It can also be a good assessment in identifying specific problem areas in the elderly, which can lead to better patient-centered care and a

more in-depth care plan for the community supports that need to be in place to help the individual remain independent.

- The Lawton IADL was originally tested concurrently with the Physical Self-Maintenance Scale (PSMS). Reliability was established with 12 subjects interviewed by one interviewer with the second rater present but not participating in the interview process. Interrater reliability was established at 0.85. The validity of the Lawton IADL was tested by determining the correlation of the Lawton IADL with four scales that assessed domains of functional status, the Physical Classification (6-point rating of physical health), Mental Status Questionnaire (10-point test of orientation and memory), Behavior and Adjustment rating scales (4–6-point measure of intellectual, personal, behavioral and social adjustment), and the PSMS. All correlations were significant at the 0.01 or 0.05 level, indicating that the instrument had validity and that the degree to which the tool actually assesses what it is intended to assess is valid.

Functional Independence Measure

The Functional Independence Measure (FIM) can be described as follows:

- The FIM scale assesses physical and cognitive disability.
- This scale focuses on the burden of care—that is the level of disability indicating the burden of caring for them.
- The FIM scale is used to measure the patient's progress and assess rehabilitation outcomes. This scale is useful in clinical settings of rehabilitation. The FIM has been used extensively in rehabilitation, including that for stroke and multiple sclerosis. Scores are responsive to change and also reflect the patient's discharge destination.
- Its items are scored on the level of assistance required by an individual to perform ADL. The scale includes 18 items, of which 13 items are physical domains based on the Barthel index and 5 items are cognition items. Each item is scored from 1 to 7 based on level of independence, where 1 represents total dependence and 7 indicates complete independence. The scale can be administered by a physician, nurse, therapist, or layperson. Possible scores range from 18 to 126, with higher scores indicating more independence. Alternatively, 13 physical items could be scored separately from 5 cognitive items.

Sickness Impact Profile

The Sickness Impact Profile (SIP) can be described as follows:

- The SIP-136 is a generic measure of the impact of disability on physical status and emotional well-being. It is administered via a 136-item questionnaire which requires "yes" or "no" responses.

- It has 12 domains, including mobility and ambulation items. A shorter version (68 items) is also available. It has three main domains, including a physical domain that assesses ambulation, mobility, and body care.
- SIP questionnaire is designed to measure patients' dysfunction through his everyday behavior, and generally related to the disease. Since it measures general health status, it is appropriate in large number of diseases and also in trauma patients.
- Each item has its value as well as total values of categories and dimensions. The general score of SIP categories or dimensions is multiplied by hundred obtaining the result in percentages, where 0% represents completely healthy patients, and 100% represents very difficult patients with a 100% dysfunction, completely dependent on another person in all aspects of life. Reliability ranges from r = 0.88 to 0.92 for overall SIP score and 0.50 to 0.56 for category items.

Outcomes and Assessment Information Set

The Outcomes and Assessment Information Set (OASIS) can be described as follows:

- The assessment tool containing standardized data elements is known as the OASIS.
- The OASIS addresses six major domains:
  1. Sociodemographic
  2. Environment
  3. Support system
  4. Health status
  5. Functional status
  6. Behavioral status
- Medical professionals collect OASIS on:
  - Admission to home health-care services
  - Transfer to another site of care (e.g., hospital)
  - Resumption of care (following a hospital stay)
  - Follow-up (at least 60 days)
  - Discharge from home healthcare
  - Death
- OASIS items used in the comprehensive assessment of patients serve as a source of data for practitioners when developing a plan of care for the patient.
- In the OASIS tool, each ADL and IADL item is organized conceptually according to the following:
  - Whether a person can conduct the activity independently
  - With the use of an assistive device or human supervision
  - With the help of another person
  - Cannot do the activity at all

This is in contrast to some measurement approaches in which a person is asked about the level of difficulty with which they can conduct ADLs or IADLs.

The OASIS ADL items are:
  - Grooming
  - Dressing upper body
  - Dressing lower body
  - Bathing
  - Toileting

- Transferring
- Ambulating
- Eating

OASIS IADLs include:

- Meal preparation
- Transportation
- Laundry
- Housekeeping
- Shopping
- Telephone

- Interrater reliability for ADL and IADL items (except for transportation) were found to be highly adequate (kappa scores ≥0.60) with all but one item scored higher than 0.70.

The Short Form-36 (Appendix D)

The SF-36 can be described as follows:

- The SF-36 health survey is a 36-item, patient-reported survey of patient health. The SF-36 is a measure of health status and it is commonly used in health economics as a variable in the quality of life calculation to determine the cost-effectiveness of health treatment.
- The SF-36 contains 36 items based on questions used in the RAND Health Insurance Study. It was named the SF-36, because it was a short form of the Medical Outcome Study instrument, which originally had 113 items with only 36 questions from the original version.
- The SF-36 demonstrates high reliability and validity (correlation coefficient ranging from 0.81 to 0.88).
- The SF-36 questionnaire provides score in two components:
  1. The physical component summary scores
  2. The mental component summary scores.
- It covers eight health domains:
  1. Physical functioning (10 items)
  2. Bodily pain (2 items)
  3. Role limitations due to physical health problems (4 items)
  4. Emotional well-being (5 items)
  5. Social functioning (2 items)
  6. Vitality (4 items)
  7. Mental health (4 items)
  8. General health perceptions (5 items)
- Scores of each domain range from 0 to 100, with higher score denoting a more favorable health status or better health-related quality of life.

Considerations in Selection of Instruments

A large number of instruments have been developed to assess and to classify function. It is important to remember that no instrument is perfect for all patients or all situations. No instrument can measure all the items potentially relevant to a particular individual and provide the perfect composite picture. For example, one instrument may provide an extensive measure of ADL but not deal with psychological or social dimensions

---

> **BOX 8.4:** Critical questions to ask when selecting an instrument.
>
> 1. What are the domains or categories that the assessment instrument focuses on?
> 2. How adequately does the instrument measure the domain or domains being sampled?
> 3. What areas of physical function are included? Does the instrument measure activity of daily living (ADL)? Does the instrument measure instrumental ADLs?
> 4. What type of scoring system is used?
> 5. Are multiple instruments necessary to provide a more complete picture of functional status?
> 6. Who completes the instrument—the clinician, the patient (self-report), or family member?
> 7. How long does the instrument take to complete?

of function. Another instrument may investigate social functioning while omitting some ADL tasks. Many items overlap from instrument to instrument. For example, a question on the ability to ambulate is a common item found in most physical function instruments.

Although instruments may cover the same kind of activity, the questions posed about the performance of the same activity may be quite different. For example, one instrument may investigate the degree of difficulty and of human assistance required to "dress yourself, including handling of closures, buttons, zippers, snaps." Another may ask, "How much help do you need in getting dressed?" As discussed, differences also may exist in the time frames sampled in the various instruments.

Critical questions to ask in selecting an instrument are presented in **Box 8.4**.

Variety of instruments may provide the kind of data desired but should be considered for use with regards to reliability or validity of the measurements. Factors such as orientation of the user, the purpose for using the instrument, and the relevance of particular functional items all enter into the decision-making process. At the end, the choice of instrument may be dictated by practical considerations. For example, self-reported instruments, which rely on information from the patient, are limited in use to mentally competent individuals.

SUMMARY

This chapter has presented a conceptual framework for a specific terminology of health, impairment, participation restriction, and disability and the functional assessment.

Disablement describes the consequences of disease in terms of its effects on body structures and functions (i.e., impairments), the ability of the individual to perform meaningful tasks (i.e., activity limitations), and the ability to fulfill one's roles in life (i.e., participation restrictions).

Function can be assessed in various ways, and capturing this is a multidimensional approach consisting of impairment-based, self-reported as well as performance-based measures. Functional assessment is particularly important because the primary goal of medical rehabilitation is to enhance physical function and independence. Hence, formalized functional assessment is desirable not only for assessing a person's activity status but also for objective and explicit documentation of functional improvement. This chapter provides an understanding of commonly used outcome measures of function, which will facilitate professional education, knowledge, and understanding the individual goal setting for patients.

Review Questions

1. What is ICF? What are the components of ICF? What is the relation between the components?
2. What are the criteria to select an instrument in assessment?
3. What are the factors affecting function and how can they be controlled?
4. How does functional status relate to health?
5. What are the types of measures for function? How are they different from each other?
6. Write a short note on the following:
   a. SF-36
   b. Barthel index
   c. Instrumental activities of daily living
   d. Functional Independence Measure
7. A 35-year-old computer worker has low back pain radiating to right lower limb. What is the ICF framework for impairments, activity limitations and participation restriction and environmental factors?

BIBLIOGRAPHY

1. Bergner M, Bobbitt R, Carter W, et al. The Sickness Impact Profile: development and final revision of a health status measure. Medical Care. 1981;19(8):787-805.
2. Brundtland G. World summit on sustainable development. BMJ. 2002;325(7361):399-400.
3. Cook C. The lost art of the clinical examination: an overemphasis on clinical special tests. J Man Manipulative Ther. 2010;18(1):3-4.
4. Denzin N, Nagi S. Disability and rehabilitation: legal, clinical, and self-concepts and measurement. Am Soc Rev. 1971;36(3):575.
5. Graf C. The Lawton Instrumental Activities of Daily Living Scale. Am J Nurs. 2008;108(4):52-62.
6. Granger C, Hamilton B, Keith R, et al. Advances in functional assessment for medical rehabilitation. Top Geriatr Rehabil. 1986;1(3):59-74.
7. Granger C, Hamilton B, Linacre J, et al. Performance profiles of the functional independence measure. Am J Phys Med Rehabil. 1993;72(2):84-9.
8. Herrman H, Metelko Z, Szabo S, et al. Study protocol for the World Health Organization project to develop a Quality of Life assessment instrument (WHOQOL). Qual Life Res. 1993;2(2):153-9.
9. Jette A. Physical disablement concepts for physical therapy research and practice. Phys Ther. 1994;74(5):380-6.
10. Jurkovich G, Mock C, MacKenzie E, et al. The sickness impact profile as a tool to evaluate functional outcome in trauma patients. J Trauma. 1995;39(4):625-31.
11. Katz S, Ford AB, Moskowitz RW, et al. Studies of illness in the aged: the index of ADL: a standardized measure of biological and psychosocial function. JAMA. 1963;185(12):914-19.
12. Katz S. Assessing self-maintenance: activities of daily living, mobility and instrumental activities of daily living. JAGS. 1983;31(12):721-6.
13. Kyte D, Calvert M, van der Wees P, et al. An introduction to patient-reported outcome measures (PROMs) in physiotherapy. Physiotherapy. 2015;101(2):119-25.
14. Lawton MP, Brody EM. Assessment of older people: self-maintaining and instrumental activities of daily living. Gerontologist. 1969;9(3):179-86.
15. Madigan E, Fortinsky R. Additional psychometric evaluation of the Outcomes and Assessment Information Set (OASIS). Home Health Care Serv Q. 2001;18(4):49-62.
16. McDowell I, Newell C. Measuring health: a guide to rating scales and questionnaires. OUP; 1996.
17. Reijneveld S, Spijker J, Dijkshoorn H. Katz' ADL index assessed functional performance of Turkish, Moroccan, and Dutch elderly. J Clin Epidemiol. 2007;60(4):382-8.
18. Reiman M, Manske R. The assessment of function. How is it measured? A clinical perspective. J Man Manipulative Ther. 2011;19(2):91-9.
19. Reuben D, Siu A, Kimpau S. The predictive validity of self-report and performance-based measures of function and health. J Gerontol. 1992;47(4):M106-10.
20. Shaughnessy P, Crisler K, Schlenker R. Outcome-based quality improvement in home health care. Qual Manage Health Care. 1998;7(6):58.
21. Verbrugge L, Jette A. The disablement process. Soc Sci Med. 1994;38(1):1-14.
22. Weich KN. A review of functional assessment instruments. Physical Therapy Scholarly Projects; 1993. p. 465.
23. World Health Organization. Bull World Health Organ. 1948;1(1):5.
24. Wylie C. Measuring end results of rehabilitation of patients with stroke. Public Health Rep (1896-1970). 1967;82(10):893.

APPENDIX A: THE BARTHEL INDEX

Patient Name :________________________________

Rater Name :________________________________

Date:________________________

Activity	Score

Feeding
 0 = unable
 5 = needs help cutting, spreading butter, etc., or requires modified diet
10 = independent   ______

Bathing
0 = dependent
5 = independent (or in shower)   ______

Grooming
0 = needs to help with personal care
5 = independent face/hair/teeth/shaving (implements provided)   ______

Dressing
 0 = dependent
 5 = needs help but can do about half unaided
10 = independent (including buttons, zips, laces, etc.)   ______

Bowels
 0 = incontinent (or needs to be given enemas)
 5 = occasional accident
10 = continent   ______

Bladder
 0 = incontinent, or catheterized and unable to manage alone
 5 = occasional accident
10 = continent   ______

Toilet Use
 0 = dependent
 5 = needs some help, but can do something alone
10 = independent (on and off, dressing, wiping)   ______

Transfers (Bed to Chair and Back)
 0 = unable, no sitting balance
 5 = major help (one or two people, physical), can sit
10 = minor help (verbal or physical)
15 = independent   ______

Mobility (On Level Surfaces)
  0 = immobile or <50 yards

  5 = wheelchair independent, including corners, >50 yards

10 = walks with help of one person (verbal or physical) >50 yards

15 = independent (but may use any aid; for example, stick) >50 yards   ______

Stairs
  0 = unable

  5 = needs help (verbal, physical, carrying aid)

10 = independent   ______

Total (0–100): ______

Source: Mahoney FI, Barthel D. "Functional evaluation: the Barthel Index."

APPENDIX B: KATZ INDEX OF INDEPENDENCE IN ACTIVITIES OF DAILY LIVING

Patient Name :_______________________________

Patient ID :_______________________________

Date:_______________________

Activities Points (1 or 0)	Independence (1 Point) **No** supervision, direction or personal assistance	Dependence (0 Points) **With** supervision, direction, personal assistance or total care
Bathing Points: __________	**(1 Point)** Bathes self completely or needs help in bathing only a single part of the body such as the back, genital area or disabled extremity	**(0 Points)** Need help with bathing more than one part of the body, getting in or out of the tub or shower. Requires total bathing
Dressing Points: __________	**(1 Point)** Get clothes from closets and drawers and puts on clothes and outer garments complete with fasteners. May have help tying shoes	**(0 Points)** Needs help with dressing self or needs to be completely dressed
Toileting Points: __________	**(1 Point)** Goes to toilet, gets on and off, arranges clothes, cleans genital area without help	**(0 Points)** Needs help transferring to the toilet, cleaning self or uses bedpan or commode
Transferring Points: __________	**(1 Point)** Moves in and out of bed or chair unassisted. Mechanical transfer aids are acceptable	**(0 Points)** Needs help in moving from bed to chair or requires a complete transfer
Continence Points: __________	**(1 Point)** Exercises complete self-control over urination and defecation	**(0 Points)** Is partially or totally incontinent of bowel or bladder
Feeding Points: __________	**(1 Point)** Gets food from plate into mouth without help. Preparation of food may be done by another person	**(0 Points)** Needs partial or total help with feeding or requires parenteral feeding
Total points: ________	**Scoring:** 6 = High (*patient independent*) 0 = Low (*patient very dependent*	

Source: *try this:* Best Practices in Nursing Care to Older Adults, The Hartford Institute for Geriatric Nursing, New York University, College of Nursing, www.hartfordign.org.

APPENDIX C: LAWTON–BRODY INSTRUMENTAL ACTIVITIES OF DAILY LIVING (IADL) SCALE

Patient Name :_______________________________

Patient ID :_______________________________

Date:_______________________

Scoring: For each category, circle the item description that most closely resembles the client's highest functional level (either 0 or 1)

A. Ability to Use Telephone		E. Laundry	
1. Operates telephone on own initiative—looks up and dials numbers, etc.	1	1. Does personal laundry completely	1
2. Dials a few well-known numbers	1	2. Launders small items—rinses, stockings, etc.	1
3. Answers telephone but does not dial	1	3. All laundry must be done by others	0
4. Does not use telephone at all	0		
B. Shopping		**F. Mode of Transportation**	
1. Takes care of all shopping needs independently	1	1. Travels independently on public transportation or drives own car	1
2. Shops independently for small purchases	0	2. Arranges own travel via taxi, but does not otherwise use public transportation	1
3. Needs to be accompanied on any shopping trip	0	3. Travels on public transportation when accompanied by another	1
4. Completely unable to shop	0	4. Travel limited to taxi or automobile with assistance of another	0
		5. Does not travel at all	0
C. Food Preparation		**G. Responsibility for Own Medications**	
1. Plans, prepares and serves adequate meals independently	1	1. Is responsible for taking medication in correct dosages at correct time	1
2. Prepares adequate meals if supplied with ingredients	0	2. Takes responsibility if medication is prepared in advance in separate dosage	0
3. Heats, serves and prepares meals, or prepares meals, or prepares meals but does not maintain adequate diet	0	3. Is not capable of dispensing own medication	0
4. Needs to have meals prepared and served	0		
D. Housekeeping		**H. Ability to Handle Finances**	
1. Maintains house alone or with occasional assistance (e.g., "heavy work domestic help")	1	1. Manages financial matters independently (budgets, writes checks, pays rent, bills, goes to bank), collects and keeps track of income	1
2. Performs light daily tasks such as dish washing, bed making	1	2. Manages day-to-day purchases, but needs help with banking, major purchases, etc.	1
3. Performs light daily tasks but cannot maintain acceptable level of cleanliness	1	3. Incapable of handling money	0
4. Needs help with all home maintenance tasks	1		
5. Does not participate in any housekeeping tasks	0		
Score		**Score**	
		Total score_________________	

A summary score ranges from 0 (low function, dependent) to 8 (high function, independent) for women and 0 through 5 for men to avoid potential gender bias.

Source: *try this:* Best Practices in Nursing Care to Older Adults, The Hartford Institute for Geriatric Nursing, New York University, College of Nursing, www.hartfordign.org.

APPENDIX D: MEDICAL OUTCOMES STUDY: 36-ITEM SHORT FORM SURVEY INSTRUMENT

RAND 36-Item Health Survey 1.0 Questionnaire Items

1. **In general, would you say your health is:**

Excellent	1
Very good	2
Good	3
Fair	4
Poor	5

2. **Compared to one year ago, how would your rate your health in general now?**

Much better now than one year ago	1
Somewhat better now than one year ago	2
About the same	3
Somewhat worse now than one year ago	4
Much worse now than one year ago	5

The following items are about activities you might do during a typical day. Does **your health now limit you** in these activities? If so, how much?

(Circle One Number on Each Line)

	Yes, limited a lot	Yes, limited a little	No, Not limited at all
3. **Vigorous activities,** such as running, lifting heavy objects, participating in strenuous sports	1	2	3
4. **Moderate activities,** such as moving a table, pushing a vacuum cleaner, bowling, or playing golf	1	2	3
5. Lifting or carrying groceries	1	2	3
6. Climbing **several flights** of stairs	1	2	3
7. Climbing **one flight** of stairs	1	2	3
8. Bending, kneeling, or stooping	1	2	3
9. Walking **more than a mile**	1	2	3
10. Walking **several blocks**	1	2	3
11. Walking **one block**	1	2	3
12. Bathing or dressing yourself	1	2	3

During the **past 4 weeks**, have you had any of the following problems with your work or other regular daily activities **as a result of your physical health?**

(Circle One Number on Each Line)

	Yes	No
13. Cut down the amount of time you spent on work or other activities	1	2
14. **Accomplished less** than you would like	1	2
15. Were limited in the **kind** of work or other activities	1	2
16. Had **difficulty** performing the work or other activities (for example, it took extra effort)	1	2

During the **past 4 weeks**, have you had any of the following problems with your work or other regular daily activities **as a result of any emotional problems** (such as feeling depressed or anxious)?

(Circle One Number on Each Line)

	Yes	No
17. Cut down the **amount of time** you spent on work or other activities	1	2
18. **Accomplished less** than you would like	1	2
19. Did not do work or other activities as **carefully** as usual	1	2

20. During the **past 4 weeks**, to what extent has your physical health or emotional problems interfered with your normal social activities with family, friends, neighbors, or groups?

(Circle One Number)

Not at all	1
Slightly	2
Moderately	3
Quite a bit	4
Extremely	5

21. How much **bodily** pain have you had during the **past 4 weeks?**

(Circle One Number)

None	1
Very mild	2
Mild	3
Moderate	4
Severe	5
Very severe	6

22. During the **past 4 weeks**, how much did pain interfere with your normal work (including both work outside the home and housework)?

(Circle One Number)

Not at all	1
A little bit	2
Moderately	3
Quite a bit	4
Extremely	5

These questions are about how you feel and how things have been with you **during the past 4 weeks**. For each question, please give the one answer that comes closest to the way you have been feeling.

How much of the time during the **past 4 weeks** . . .

(Circle One Number on Each Line)

	All of the time	Most of the time	A good bit of the time	Some of the time	A little of the time	None of the time
23. Did you feel full of pep?	1	2	3	4	5	6
24. Have you been a very nervous person?	1	2	3	4	5	6
25. Have you felt so down in the dumps that nothing could cheer you up?	1	2	3	4	5	6
26. Have you felt calm and peaceful?	1	2	3	4	5	6
27. Did you have a lot of energy?	1	2	3	4	5	6

	All of the time	Most of the time	A good bit of the time	Some of the time	A little of the time	None of the time
28. Have you felt downhearted and blue?	1	2	3	4	5	6
29. Did you feel worn out?	1	2	3	4	5	6
30. Have you been a happy person?	1	2	3	4	5	6
31. Did you feel tired?	1	2	3	4	5	6

32. During the past 4 weeks, how much of the time has your physical health or emotional problems interfered with your social activities (such as visiting with friends, relatives, etc.)?

(Circle One Number)

All of the time	1
Most of the time	2
Some of the time	3
A little of the time	4
None of the time	5

How **True** or **False** is each of the following statements for you.

(Circle One Number on Each Line)

	Definitely true	Mostly true	Do not know	Mostly false	Definitely false
33. I seem to get sick a little easier than other people	1	2	3	4	5
34. I am as healthy as anybody I know	1	2	3	4	5
35. I expect my health to get worse	1	2	3	4	5
36. My health is excellent	1	2	3	4	5

Assessment of Environment

Amit V Nagrale

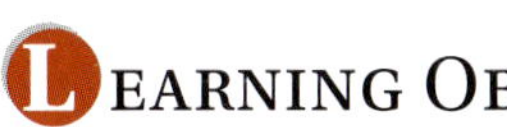 LEARNING OBJECTIVES

After reading this chapter, the readers should be able to:

- Understand environmental attributes and barriers that induce fall risks or injuries in adults
- Understand how environmental factors interact with patient factors during fall events
- Understand the purpose and benefits of environment assessment
- Become familiar with the different tools to carry out comprehensive evaluation of home and work environment
- Understand the role of physical therapist in examination of physical environment
- Gain knowledge of the strategies to examine environmental impact on patient functions
- Understand the benefits of environmental modifications on patient function
- Get acquainted with the guidelines and considerations for the worksite assessment
- Gain knowledge the checklist for employer's health and safety.

CHAPTER OUTLINE

- Community design, physical activity, and health: a conceptual model
  - Purpose
- Home environment
  - Benefits of home environment assessment
  - Measuring tools for home assessment
  - Home modification strategies
  - Case scenario
- Work environment
  - What is a workplace assessment?
  - Benefits of a workplace assessment
  - Workplace assessment
  - Tools for workplace assessment
- Legislations
  - Workmen's Compensation Act or Employee's Compensation Act, 1923
  - The Indian Factories Act, 1948
  - Employees State Insurance Act, 1948

INTRODUCTION

A physical environment can be described as anything we can physically experience through our senses such as touch, smell, sight, hearing, and/or taste. The physical environment includes both the natural and human-made environment. For example, the physical environment of house can include the human-made structures such as the walls, the pipes, floors, appliances as well as the natural environment such as the air circulating in the house. A concept of physical environment is quite enormous in scope, ranging from the physical to biophysical and from natural to the social environments.

The environment encompasses a substantial range of components that impact human function and includes the individual's home, neighborhood, community, and methods of transportation, in addition to the individual's educational, workplace, entertainment, commercial, and natural settings. Environmental barriers are defined as physical impediments that prevent individuals from functioning optimally in their surroundings and include safety hazards, access problems, and home or workplace design difficulties. Accessibility is the degree to which an environment affords use of its resources with respect to an individual's level of function **(Boxes 9.1 and 9.2)**.

> **BOX 9.1:** Definition of universal design.
>
> Universal design refers to the design of products and environments to be used by all people, to the greatest extent possible, without the need for adaptation or specialized design.

> **BOX 9.2:** Seven principles of universal design developed at the center for universal design.
>
> 1. **Equitable use:** The design is useful and marketable to people with diverse abilities.
> 2. **Flexibility in use:** The design accommodates a wide range of individual's preferences and abilities.
> 3. **Simple and intuitive use:** Use of the design is easy to understand, regardless of the user's experience, knowledge, language skills, or current concentration level.
> 4. **Perceptible information:** The design communicates necessary information effectively to the user, regardless of ambient conditions or the user's sensory abilities.
> 5. **Tolerance for error:** The design minimizes hazards and the adverse consequences of accidental or intended actions.
> 6. **Low physical effort:** The design can be used efficiently, comfortably, and with minimum fatigue.
> 7. **Size and shape for approach and use:** Appropriate size and shape is provided for approach, reach, manipulation, and use regardless of user's body size, posture, or mobility.

Several examples of universal design elements include:

- Stepless entrance
- Wide hallway and doorways
- No doorway thresholds
- Use of nonslip floors
- Lever door handles
- Rocker light switches
- Single handle sink faucets
- No-step shower access.

The impact of the physical environment on health and well-being is well established, and the World Health Organization has conceptualized the physical environment as one important component of the quality of life. The ability to walk safely and independently, referred to as "mobility," is a fundamental part of both basic activities of daily living (BADL) and instrumental activities of daily living. Community design influences human behavior.

COMMUNITY DESIGN, PHYSICAL ACTIVITY, AND HEALTH: A CONCEPTUAL MODEL

It provides a simple model of the relationships between physical activity, health, and the environments in which people live and work **(Fig. 9.1)**. The built environment denotes the form and character of communities. It is made of countless specific places—homes, offices, parks, parking lots, community, etc. This model utilizes three broad categories—transportation systems, land use patterns, and urban design characteristics. Transportation systems connect places to each other, determining how feasible it is to use different types of transportation, including walking and bicycling, wheelchair, to get from one place to another.

The Americans with Disabilities Act in 1990 expanded accessibility to the private sector to improve employment opportunities as well as environmental access to retail business, cultural events, movie theaters, restaurants, travel, etc. Other access symbols identify the availability of assistive listening devices, telephones, which allow the user to communicate using a keyboard and visual display, volume-controlled telephones, or availability of sign language interpretation. These symbols are presented in **Table 9.1** to identify and make public availability of accessible services.

Purpose

The purposes of an environmental examination are to:

- Determine the degree of patient safety and level of function in the physical environment.
- Identify environmental barriers that may impact physical functions.
- Make realistic recommendations regarding environmental accessibility and accommodations to the patient, support network (family, friends, caregivers, coworkers, professional colleagues, and neighbors), employer, government agencies or the potential funding sources, and third-party payers.
- Determine the need for adaptive equipment or assistive technology to support and promote function.
- Assist in preparing the patient and support network for the patient's return to a former environment and to help determine whether further services may be required (i.e., outpatient treatment and home care services).

HOME ENVIRONMENT

Introduction

Home environment assessments are performed to ensure that patients can safely return and/or reintegrate into their home environment. It allows patients who have physical illness or impairments to regain functional mobility within their home environment. It helps to identify potential environmental barriers and mitigate these potential hazards, before the patient incurs further injury. Home assessment helps to identify potential barriers within the patient's home (interior) and around the patient's home (exterior) (e.g., yard, carpet, and sidewalks). It has been clinically and statistically proven that discharged patients who get readmitted to an acute care hospital are because of falls that occur at their homes.

The interaction of environmental factors with the patient-related factors often contributes to a fall. Knowing the circumstances surrounding falls is essential

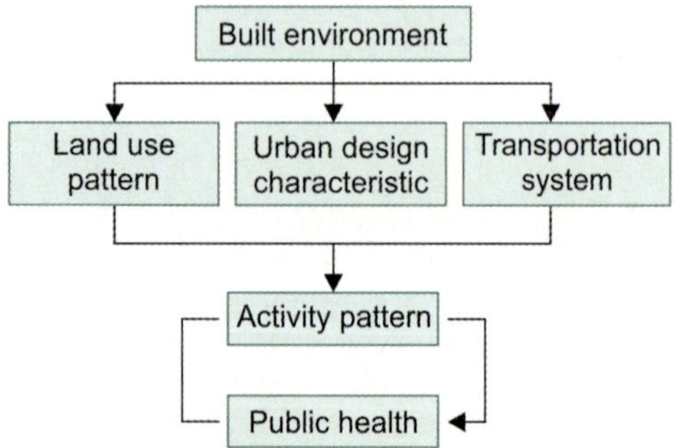

Fig. 9.1: Conceptual model of community design.

Table 9.1: Disability access symbols.		
	Access (other than print or Braille) for individuals who are blind or have low vision	This symbol indicates access for people who are blind or have low vision, best used in places such as a guided tour, a path to a nature trail or a scent garden in a park; and a tactile tour or a museum exhibition that may be touched
	Symbol for wheelchair accessibility	The wheelchair symbol indicates access for individuals with limited mobility, including wheelchair users. Remember that a ramped entrance is not completely accessible if there are no curb cuts, and an elevator is not accessible if it can only be reached via steps
	Audio description	Blind or low-vision people may enjoy performing arts, visual arts, television, video, and film that offers live commentary or narration (via headphones and a small transmitter) of visual elements provided by a trained audio describer. An adapter for nonstereo TVs may also be available
	TTY	This device is also known as a text telephone or telecommunications device for the deaf. TTY indicates the presence of a device used with the telephone for communication with and between deaf, hard of hearing, speech impaired and/or hearing persons
	Volume control telephone	This symbol indicates the presence of telephones that have handsets with amplified sound and/or adjustable volume controls
	Assistive listening systems	These systems transmit amplified sound via hearing aids, headsets, or other devices
	Sign language interpretation	The symbol indicates that sign language interpretation is provided for a lecture, tour, film, performance, conference, or other program
Large Print	**Accessible print (18 pt. or larger)**	Large print is indicated by the words: "Large Print," printed in 18 pt. or larger text. In addition to identifying large print versions of books, pamphlets, museum guides, and theater programs, one may use the symbol on conference or membership forms with large print. Sans serif or modified serif print with high contrast is important, and special attention should be paid to letter and word spacing

Contd...

Contd...

![information symbol]	**The information symbol**	Knowing where to find what one needs is almost as valuable as finding it. The information symbol indicates the location for specific information or materials concerning access, such as "LARGE PRINT" materials, audio cassette recordings of materials, or sign interpreted tours
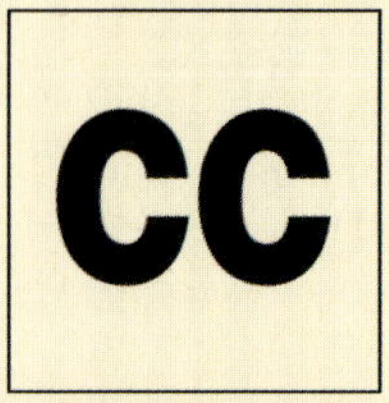 **CC**	CC	CC (commonly known as subtitles) enables people who are deaf or hard of hearing to read a transcript of the audio portion of a video, film, exhibition, or other presentation. As the video plays, text captions transcribe (although not always verbatim) speech and other relevant sounds
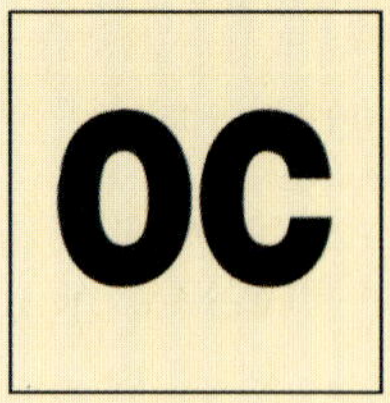 **OC**	OC	This symbol indicates that captions, which translate dialogue and other sounds in print, are displayed on the videotape, movie, television program or exhibit audio. OC is preferred by many, including deaf and hard-of-hearing individuals, and people whose second language is English. It also helps teach children how to read and keep sound levels to a minimum in museums and restaurants
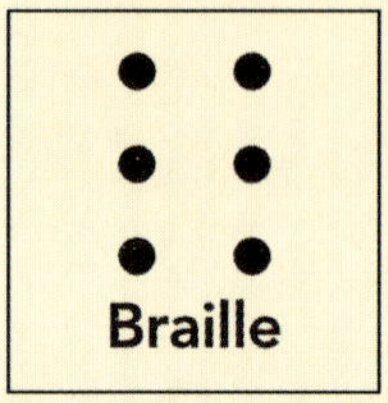 **Braille**	**Braille symbol**	This symbol indicates that printed material is available in Braille, including exhibition labeling, publications, and signage

(CC: closed captioning; OC: opened captioning; TTY: telephone typewriter)

for understanding how behavioral and environmental factors interact in fall events. The environmental hazards remain unnoticed as the clinicians seldom observe the environmental hazards present in the patient's home, where most falls occur. The World Health Organization in 2012 listed home assessment and environmental modification for people with known fall risk factors or a history of falling, as one of five important strategies to prevent falls. Out of multiple risk factors, about 10% of the falls have been reported during acute illness, 5% during hazardous activity, and 44% in the presence of environmental hazards. Most of the falls have been reported inside the home (66.8%) as compared to outside (26.4%), which necessitates the assessment of home environment as a need of the hour.

Regardless of whether an injury occurred, the largest proportion of falls happened in the living room and bedroom. However, 41 of 528 (7.8%) of falls with no injury and 44 of 255 (17.3%) of falls with any injury occurred in the bathroom. These results support the need to promote safety modifications such as grab bars and may indicate a need for assistance with bathing. There is diversity in assessment methods for the home environment from the health-care providers.

Home environment assessment is a crucial factor when understanding fall risk and safety in older adults. Other than intrinsic factors such as muscle strength, balance, proprioception, attention, and vision; extrinsic factors such as floors, rugs or carpets, lighting, and assistive devices also pose a significant risk in the home environment assessment and intervention. **Figures 9.2 to 9.5** describe the need for tools to assess home environment.

Following information should be gathered while examining environment:

- Information about the patients' current level of function (such as communication skills, bed mobility, transfers, and locomotion) should be obtained.

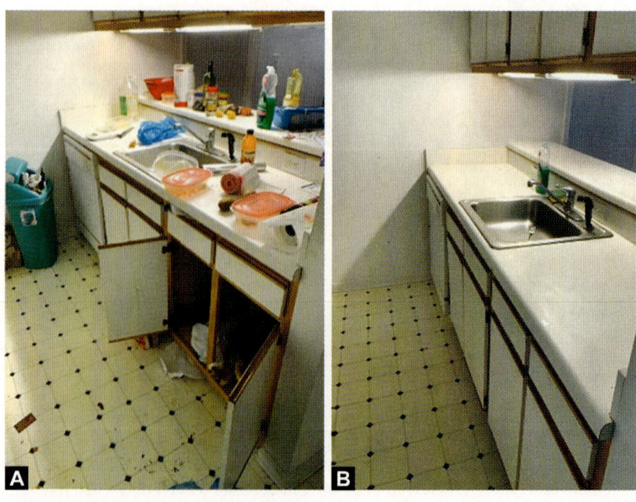

Figs. 9.2A and B: Are we comparing one patient's home to another?

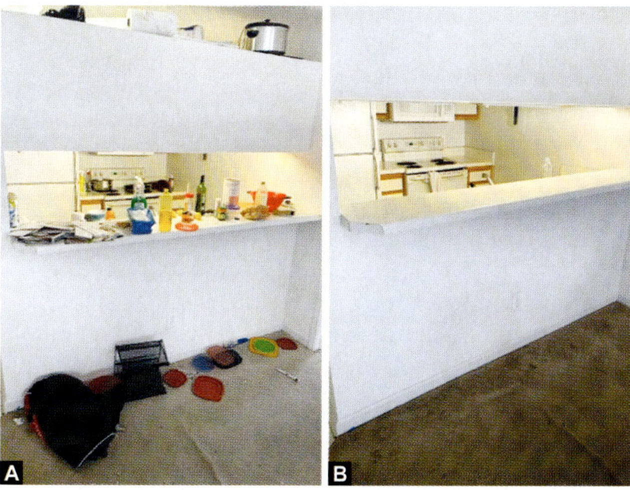

Figs. 9.3A and B: Are we REALLY looking at the risk areas present in any home?

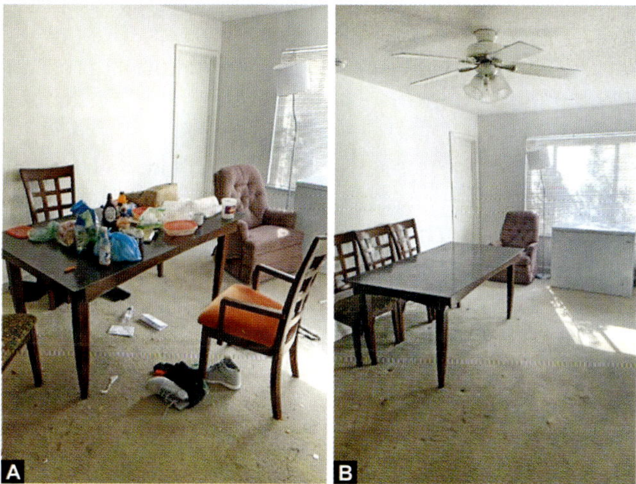

Figs. 9.4A and B: Are we using a standardized approach?

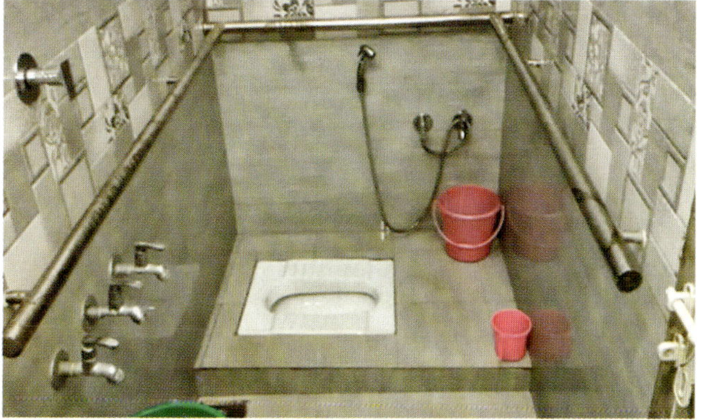

Fig. 9.5: Grab bars installed in Indian toilet (*Note:* Appropriate height of grab bars should be provided).

- Data from all involved disciplines (occupational therapist, physical therapist, speech-language pathologist, and so forth) should be gathered.
- Information regarding physical assistance or verbal cueing required for performance of functional activities should be taken.

- Characteristics and dimensions of required adaptive or assistive devices and equipment (e.g., walker, crutches, raised toilet seat, commode, and hospital bed).
- Information about predicted level of function or improvement (expected outcomes).
- Nature of the activity limitations or participation restriction (i.e., static or progressive).
- Insurance coverage, financial resources, and availability of potential funding sources (in terms of capacity to modify environment or obtain needed adaptive and assistive devices or assistive technology).
- Knowledge of the patient's future plans (household management, family care, employment outside the home, school, and vocational training).
- Knowledge of whether the house is owned or rented; the type and ownership of the home can affect or even preclude the type of modifications the patient may require.
- Information about the relative permanence of the dwelling; if the patient has plans to move in the near future, it will influence the type of modifications recommended (e.g., installing permanent ramps versus removable ones or paving gravel driveway).

Benefits of Home Environment Assessment

Benefits of home environment assessment are:
- To alleviate the fall risk
- To support the caregivers of patients with cognitive disorders
- To assist in recovery and recuperation
- To support aging in place
- To compensate for the visual impairment

Measuring Tools for Home Assessment

Many older adults need to improve their home environment to prevent falls, and they may be able to do so if support is available. There are various tools which are developed for the evaluation of home environment **(Box 9.3)**.

The Center for Disease Control and Prevention (CDC) has developed a tool kit—**Check for Safety:** A Home Fall Prevention Checklist for Older Adults—to help healthcare professionals prevent falls in older adults. The CDC's key strategy is home safety, and the agency's checklist

---

BOX 9.3: Other comprehensive tools.

- The safe at home: A quick home safety assessment
- The falls risk assessment
- The safe living guide: A guide to home safety for seniors
- The home safety self-assessment tool
- The home falls and accidents screening tool
- Home environmental assessment protocol
- The home environment assessment for the visually impaired
- The safety assessment of function and environment for rehabilitation
- Safety assessment scale

includes 17 items that older adults can use to make their homes safer. The checklist addresses whether a problem exists and offers potential solutions. Online and hard copy versions are available free of charge.

The safe at home is a screening tool to determine whether a person can identify common home safety issues and fix the problems independently by following a few specific directions.

The falls risk assessment is a comprehensive fall risk assessment instrument listing many fall risk factors, but home fall risk is limited to one item, "environmental hazards."

The safe living guide offers checklists in nine areas (outside, inside, stairs, fire and hazardous materials, bathroom, kitchen, bedroom, garage/basement/workroom, and childproofing) and is aimed at all populations, but it does not offer solutions for home risk factors. The Safe Living Guide is not targeted for use by older adults.

The Home Safety Self-Assessment Tool (HSSAT) is formulated for community-dwelling older adults and their informal caregivers, such as families and friends, as a guide to prevent home falls. It is an instrument to identify fall risk factors inside the home. By exposing these risk factors, it appears that older adults raise their awareness for fall risk factors in general. The risk factor section is comprehensive, covering 64-risk items in nine areas of the home (front and back entrances, hallway or foyer, living room, kitchen, bedroom, bathroom, staircases, and laundry room/basement) and offering solutions and advice for each item on the list.

It includes information regarding ways to improve the home environment, tips for fall prevention. The exclusiveness of the HSSAT is characterized by pictures drawn for nine home areas that depict problems as well as solutions, numbered to coincide with the item number in the fall risk factor section and for each solution. Risks can be summed for each area and a grand total generated for all areas within the home.

The HSSAT acts as an instrument to assess fall risk factors. In the HSSAT, risk factors in each home area are listed to raise awareness for current and possible future falls. For example, some people may not be aware that clutter is a fall risk until they see it on the list. By reviewing each risk item, users may be able to match the risks listed in the HSSAT with identified risks in their own home environment. The booklet includes sections to help users modify their own fall risks. For example, after finding grab bars a necessity in the bathroom, older adults may not know what kind of grab bars are available.

Content validity, test–retest reliability, interrater reliability, construct validity, and responsiveness to change have been established for the HSSAT. The HSSAT booklet can be used to identify fall risks and facilitate fall hazard reduction in a home environment for community-dwelling older adults. The HSSAT has been found more effective in identifying risk factors than the CDC's checklist, possibly because the HSSAT lists recurring risk factors in each area of the home, whereas the CDC checklist only has broad categories such as floors, stairs and steps, kitchen, and bedroom. Older adults may not remember general risk items when they go to different areas in the home to assess risk factors.

Use of the HSSAT hastens the older adults' awareness of safety hazards in their home environment by returning locus of control to residents when identifying environmental hazards and plans for correction within their home and providing an opportunity to analyze the activity and environment interface for safe engagement in home-based occupations.

The home falls and accidents screening tool (HOME FAST) is designed as part of a comprehensive health assessment instrument to measure fall risk for older people within their home environment. It has demonstrated fair-to-good level of agreement between raters (kappa = 0.62) while "Hazardous outside paths" was the only item that demonstrated poor agreement (kappa = 0.30).

HOME FAST is psychometrically sound, sensitive to change, detects fall risk, and requires a short time to administer. The HOME FAST includes items about the physical features of the home as well as the functional capacity of an individual within their home, and hazards are scored as being present or not. The HOME FAST has established interreliability and content validity.

Home environmental assessment protocol (HEAP), developed in 2002, is reported as valid and reliable measure. It consists of 192 items that are summed into separate indices representing the number of hazards, adaptations, and level of clutter and comfort in eight areas of the home **(Box 9.4)**. These items are rated through caregiver interview, direct observation with caregiver clarification, and direct observation; the presence or absence of safety hazards, adaptations, visual cues, and comfort are scored as present or not.

There are many opportunities for information technology to be integrated into the assessment and management of fall risk in older adults.

BOX 9.4: Various environmental attributes should be measured to reduce the fall risk in older adults.

- Inadequate task lighting in the kitchen or bathroom
- Poor ambient lighting in the living room
- Lack of visual clarity in hallways
- Trip hazards in the entry or stairs
- Slippery floors in kitchens and bathrooms (especially when wet)
- Inappropriate furnishing in living areas
- Poorly specified equipment or adaptive devices in the home
- Anthropometric factors (e.g., a person's height, upper or lower reach range, and use of assistive devices)

The home environment assessment for the visually impaired (HEAVI) is a novel tool, designed to identify specific hazardous items that may contribute to fall risk in persons with poor vision. This home assessment tool has adapted many items from the HEAP but excluded items specific to individuals with dementia and caregivers (e.g., lack of safety latches on cabinet doors and lack of safety adaptations to oven/stove).

The HEAVI tool includes 10 items assessing lighting and 2 items assessing contrast between objects. Both are particularly important for those with vision loss, and lack of appropriate lighting and contrast, it places those with visual impairment at greater risk of falling. Additionally, this tool includes a greater emphasis on objective measurements, which are typically not evaluated in existing home assessments. Lastly, this instrument is intended to grade the home, and not the person within the home. To that extent, it may be relevant when setting up residences for older adults (where the person living there may not be known) and for common spaces where multiple people will be living.

The safety assessment of function and environment for rehabilitation (SAFER) tool assesses an individual's abilities to safely manage functional activities within their home. This assessment considers both the environmental features along with client's capabilities. It consists of 97 items with 14 sections (living situation, mobility, kitchen, fire hazards, eating, household, dressing, grooming, bathroom, medication, communication, wandering, memory aids, and general). It is designed for older adults (who may or may not have cognitive impairments) but can also be used for other age-groups. This tool is comprehensive, valid, and reliable [intraclass coefficient (ICC 0.83)], covering multiple areas, but it is not a quick screening tool.

Safety assessment scale (SAS) was developed in 2001 in Canada to assess and decrease the risk of accidents for individuals with dementia living at home. The assessment focuses not only on environmental factors but also on behaviors in the home, which may put an individual at risk. There is a short form and long form available. The short form has 7 sections and 19 questions with a maximum score of 47. The long form has 9 sections and 32 questions with a maximum score of 72. Short form can be used as a screening tool to identify level of risk for many different types of accidents. The long form can be used to guide intervention. It has excellent interrater reliability for the long form: 0.88. Individuals with a score of 12+ should be under close attention of health-care professionals (based on sensitivity). A score of 15+ suggests the individual is at serious risk of injury (based on specificity of the tool).

Home Modification Strategies

The following areas can be assessed and modified per the needs of the patient **(Box 9.5)**:

BOX 9.5: Areas to be assessed and modified.

- Bathroom
- Steps
- Ramps
- Handrails
- Doors
- Bathtub/shower
- Bed
- Kitchen

Safety and Convenience

Convenience issues are safety issues. One must be able to move easily and safely to each part of the facilities, and one needs to be able to do it conveniently enough so that one is not tempted to do unsafe things. If the current bathroom is not safe, or it is not found convenient, one can look at a remodel.

Lower Level Accessible Bathroom

If the house has stairs, one of the best ways to reduce risk is to have a bathroom on the lower level floor. Chair lifts can help with this, but a bathroom on the ground floor is very important with aging. The bathroom must be accessible, which means a bigger space that can accommodate a walker or a wheelchair. With a larger space, the bathroom will be much safer and easier to use as one ages **(Boxes 9.6 and 9.7)**.

Steps

Steps in entryways pose a risk of tripping or falling for everyone, but they are especially dangerous to seniors. Steps should be at least 3-ft wide, although a greater width is preferred **(Fig. 9.6)**. Handrails should extend beyond the bottom and top of the stairs to provide solid footing for their entire length. Handrails should also be round so they are easy to grip. Exterior steps should have non slip rubber treads or tape as a minimum preventative measure against slipping. Steps also require adequate lighting to ensure the steps are clearly visible.

BOX 9.6: Toilet modifications.

If it is Indian toilet, toilet converter can be used to convert into the Western toilet. It is used to make the sitting position comfortable while toileting and changes the squatting position to chair sitting. Toilet converter helps in reducing the cost of installing a western commode and also saves time. Also Grab bars or ropes can be added for easy sit to stand.

BOX 9.7: Slope modifications.

Slope is usually expressed as the ratio of the ramp's height, or rise, to its length, or run. For example, a slope of 1:12 means that the ramp rises 1 inch for every 12 inch of its run. The length of each ramp segment is determined by its rise, which should never exceed 30 inch. In the case of a 1:12 slope, this requirement means that the length of each ramp segment should be no more than 30 feet.

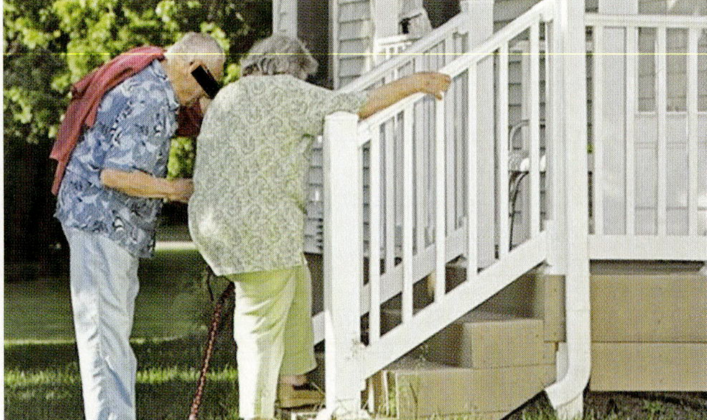

Fig. 9.6: Ideal steps.

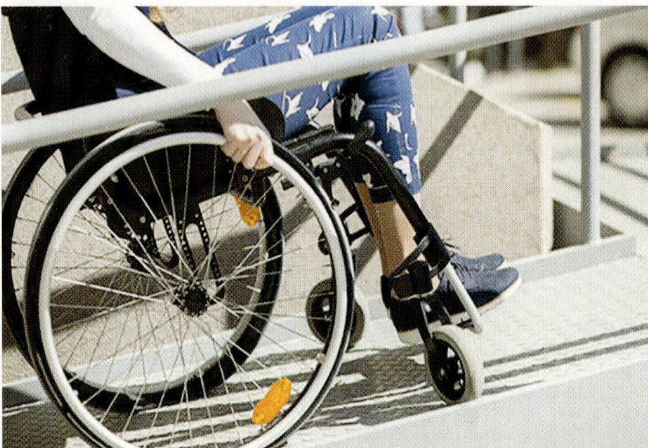

Fig. 9.7: Wheelchair ramp.

Wheelchair Ramps

A wheelchair ramp **(Fig. 9.7)** can be one of the most effective ways of improving accessibility at the entrances to a home. Ramps are a boon not only to people who are actually confined to a wheelchair but also to those who simply need a less stressful way of leaving and entering the home. The Americans with Disabilities Act (ADA) of 1990 establishes design standards for commercial wheelchair ramps that may be useful for constructing a ramp for private use. (An U-shaped ramp, for example, is often a better choice for entryway with limited space on the outside).

Handrails

A wheelchair ramp should have handrails **(Figs. 9.8A and B)** on both sides of the ramp if its run is longer than 6 feet or its rise is greater than 6 in. The height of the handrail above the ramp should be between 34 and 38 inch, with a minimum of 1.5 inch between the rail and any solid surface outside the ramp. The ramp should also have a curb on both sides to prevent the wheelchair from rolling off the ramp. The opposing handrails must be at least 36 inch apart to ensure the ramp can accommodate a wheelchair. Since each hand rail is 1.5 inch wide and requires 1.5 inch of clearance on the outside of the ramp, this means that any ramp must be at least 42 inch wide.

Doors

Traditional handles are usually not very convenient for aging homeowners. A D-shaped handle, known as a **D handle or a loop handle (Fig. 9.9)**, gives a better grip and should be used on all doors.

Case Scenario

A lady with multiple sclerosis may want to modify the following areas of her home in the given manner:

1. Stairs
   - **Steps:** Paint the edges so they are easier to spot.
   - **Handrails:** Put sturdy ones on both sides of stairs.
   - **Ramps:** One can avoid stair climbing by putting in a ramp. It should not rise more than 1 inch/feat and should be between 30 and 40 inch wide.
2. Doors
   - **Outside doors**: If a wheelchair or scooter is being used, the outside doors should be 36 inch across so it can fit through. Sometimes just changing hinges makes the difference.
   - **Inside doors**: In order to be able to enter when in a wheelchair, the bedroom, bathroom, and closet doors should be at least 32 inch wide. If changing

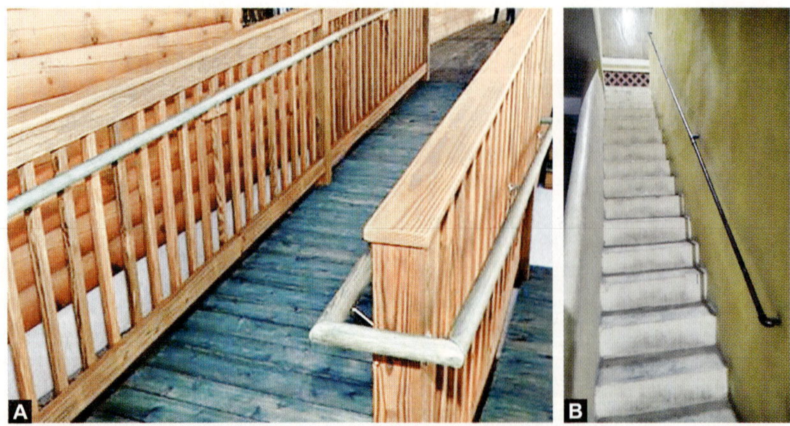

Figs. 9.8A and B: (A) Ramp with handrails. (B) Handrails installed in a stepway.

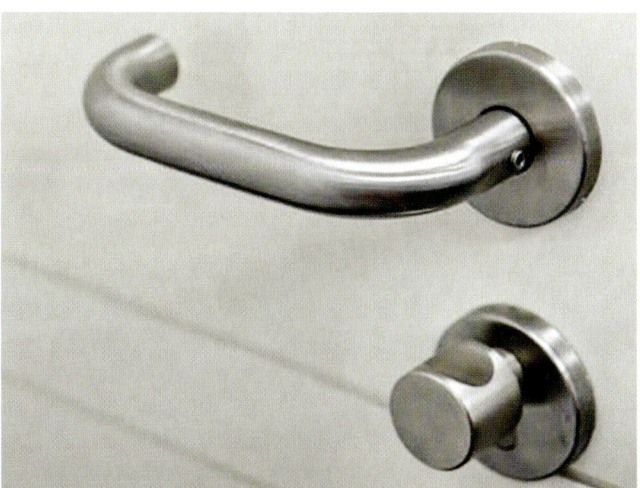

Fig. 9.9: Doors and handles.

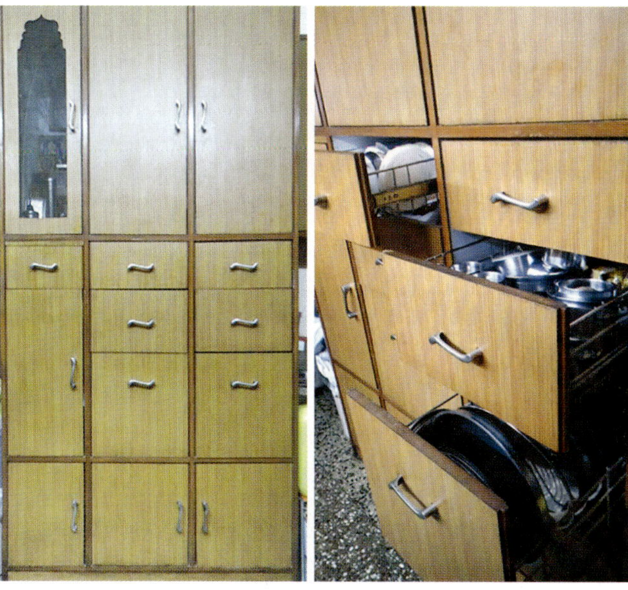

Fig. 9.10: Kitchen areas can be organized with use of appropriate shelves.

the hinges does not work, one can take off the door entirely and replace it with curtains.

- **Threshold to doors:** One may want to remove any piece of wood or metal in front of or underneath a door frame.
- **Handles:** Traditional doorknobs can be replaced with lever-style handles that are easier to open.

3. Bathroom
   - **Toilet seats:** It is easier to sit down and stand up when seats are higher. If one uses a wheelchair, seats should be at the same height as the chair.
   - **Grab bars:** These should be put near the toilet and shower. A rehabilitation or occupational therapist can make sure that the place is safe and useful.
   - **Bathtubs and showers:** A shower chair or bench is helpful. Remodeling a bathroom can be considered by adding a wheelchair-accessible shower with curtains so one does not have to step over the tub edge. Add a nonstick mat, and swap an overhead showerhead for one with a long hose.
   - **Sinks:** Look into getting a wall-mounted sink. Because there is extra space below, one can roll up closer in a wheelchair.

4. Bedroom
   - **Bed:** Consider buying a hospital bed. It can be raised to change the sheets more easily. Also, the height can be adjusted to make it easier get in and out of a wheelchair. Place the bed 4.5 feet away from the walls on each side so it is easier to make the bed in the morning. If the individual is ambulatory, carpets can be removed to prevent falls.
   - **Blinds:** Replace short strings or rods with longer ones.

5. Kitchen **(Fig. 9.10)**
   - **Cabinets:** The cabinet can be removed from them under the sink, but the cabinet base can be left in place to use as a footrest if one uses a scooter. Insulation should be added to the pipes to avoid burns.

- **Countertops:** Plan a work center with all of the cooking gear handy. Lower at least one countertop to make it easier to reach from a chair. Swap manual for electric can openers and install slide-out drawers.
- **Appliances:** Choose electric ones with controls on the front or center.

Specialized arrangement and modifications need to be incorporated based on individualized needs of a certain population. An example in **Box 9.8** shows the set of modifications applicable to obese group of individuals.

> **BOX 9.8:** Bariatric considerations.
>
> - *Patient family and caregiver training:* Training and patient handling for obese patients is critical. Obese patients may require assistance in routine self-care activities. Safety and injury prevention for patient and caregivers should be promoted.
> - *Physical assistance:* Assistance may be required by more than one individual. Often two or three individuals are needed for transfer and handling.
> - *Bariatric equipment:* Oversized, highly durable, heavier equipment with increased weight capacity may be needed. Bariatric aids may include lift recline chairs and lifting devices for seating and lifting assistance to users, heavy duty and adjustable beds, bed transfer boards, hoists and slings, patient lifters, pressure care mattresses as bedroom equipments, heavy duty bath transfers, bathroom chairs and benches, mobile shower and commode chairs, grab bars and handles for bathrooms, and bariatric rollators, wheelchairs and walking aids for mobility assistance.
> - *Risk of ulceration:* Developing pressure ulcers is common in obese individuals due to bodyweight and immobility. Due to inability to change positions frequently, creating excess pressure on susceptible areas for longer duration may contribute to ulcers. Moisture and perspiration may aggravate the problem. Specialized mattresses such as pneumatic, low air loss with alternating pressure can help.

Contd...

Contd...

- *Care environment:* Bariatric equipment facilitates the need of larger spaced rooms, with wide passages, door widths, and windows. Environmental control unit is important to consider.
- *Bathroom:* Floor mounting toilets and sinks are required. Longer grab bars with sufficient weight capacity should be installed on reinforced walls. Bariatric seat and shower hand sprayers will assist along with a shower stall.

WORK ENVIRONMENT

Introduction

Each year around 140–150 million working days are lost due to workplace sickness leave in the short-term, while one-fifth are lost in the long-term and can lead to people falling out of work. Over 300,000 people move from work to claiming incapacity benefits each year. Environmental assessment can be defined as identifying, estimating, and evaluating the environmental impacts of existing and proposed projects, by conducting environmental studies, to mitigate the relevant negative effects prior to making decisions and commitments.

It is an opportunity to tour and observe the workplace to understand more about the setting employees work in and the physical factors at and nearby the worksite that support or hinder employee health and evaluate the physical and organizational work environment for health hazards and risks. The built environment includes all the physical parts of the worksite (e.g., building, open spaces, streets, and infrastructure), which can influence employee health. It considers components such as land use patterns, transportation systems, and design features.

- Land use patterns refer to the spatial distribution of human activities.
- Transportation systems refer to the physical infrastructure and services that provide the spatial links or connectivity among activities.
- Design refers to the esthetic, physical, and functional qualities of the built work environment, such as the design of buildings and streetscapes, and relates to both land use patterns and the transportation system.

An assessment of the physical work environment can identify a number of opportunities for employers to create access and opportunity for employees to practice healthy behaviors, such as physical activity, or discourage unhealthy behaviors, such as creating a tobacco-free work environment.

To properly identify health risks and hazards from the work environment that may cause occupational disease or injury and institute prevention and control measures for these risks, employers can implement a system that involves collecting data from many sources, including workplace inspections, measurement and evaluation of exposure, examination of workers, record keeping, and reporting of health effects and exposures for acute (when the time between exposure and disease or injury is short) or chronic conditions (e.g., resulting from repeated exposure).

Direct observation of the work environment through a workplace inspection is an important source of data. Inspections can be conducted:

- On a regular and routine basis to identify hazards
- Following an incident or accident resulting in injury to identify cause(s)
- When someone at the workplace requests an inspection due to a suspicion of a health or safety hazard.

Because of their familiarity with the worksite and work environment, workers are good sources of environmental health and safety risk information and may provide information not found in formal records, e.g., Occupational Safety and Health Administration (OSHA) or worker's compensation claims. However, the information workers provide should not substitute for a professional evaluation of the workplace practices and the work environment by an industrial hygienist or ergonomist.

An environmental assessment should include the following aspects:

- Setting
  - Overall site layout—number of buildings (freestanding or connected), square footage (internal), acreage (external—how big is the campus for things like walkability), and traffic patterns
  - Meeting and multipurpose rooms
  - Grounds and parking lot
  - Stairs/elevators
  - Appropriate noise level, lighting, ventilation, ergonomics, and safeguards for machines and equipment.
- Communication about health and wellness
  - Signs/bulletin board postings about health and wellness **(Fig. 9.11)**
  - Information kiosks
  - Computer and internet

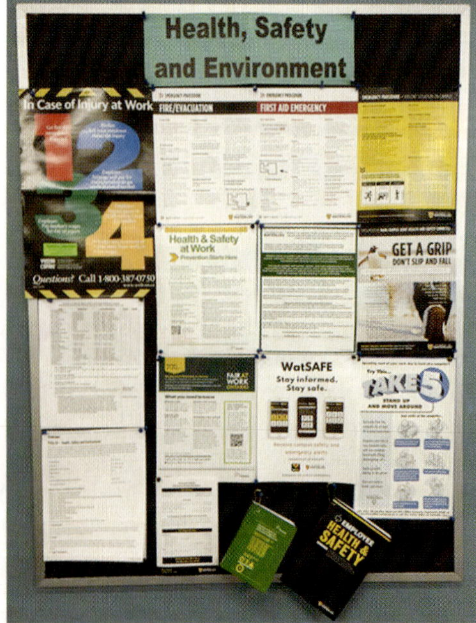

Fig. 9.11: Bulletin boards at workplace.

- Fitness environment
  - On-site fitness center, including types of equipment and their condition
  - Accessibility for bikes/other forms of transportation (e.g., bike racks)
  - Outdoor physical activity options (e.g., walking paths and running trails)
  - Nearby community fitness facilities
  - Shower/changing room facilities
- Occupational health clinic
  - Staffing
  - Hours of operation
  - Facilities
- Nutritional environment
  - Cafeteria hours, selections, including nutritional value and hygiene of food
  - Vending machine location(s) and selections, including price
  - Break rooms/eating areas
  - Nearby restaurants and food retailers
- Safety Environment Review of Material Safety Data Sheets
  - Hazards inventory includes physical (e.g., noise, extreme heat or cold), ergonomic (e.g., repetitive motion), chemical (e.g., gases and vapors), biological (e.g., animals and plants), and psychosocial (workload; hours worked) hazards.
  - Job-specific safety training
- Safety equipment (e.g., fire extinguishers and automated external defibrillators)
  - Availability and maintenance of personal protective equipment
  - Training in the use of personal protective or other safety equipment
- Community resources (presence/absence of these in close proximity to the worksite)
  - Sidewalks
  - Hospitals/pharmacies
  - Parks and recreational areas
  - Cleanliness and hygiene of the workplace
  - Assessment of psychological environment

A final component of work environment assessment includes direct observations of employees in their normal working environment going about their normal routines. These direct observations are important to understand the following:

- How employees operate within the physical and social environment? The team may observe issues that went unreported during interviews because employees are too close to their situations.
- How workers interact with managers and each other?
- Where the organization's social norms (e.g., acceptable standards of behavior) are generated and where social support networks exist?
- The level of trust, confidence, and level of employee engagement in the organizational mission and work processes.

- For worksites with established health promotion opportunities, the team can arrange to have the opportunity to see these programs in action (**Figs. 9.12 and 9.13**).

Key things to consider when conducting direct observations:

- Vary observation days and times so that they are a more representative sample of employees (e.g., multiple shifts).
- Explain to employees the purpose for observing and get their permission before doing so. Remember that employees may alter their normal routines in the presence of an observer.
- Make a list prior to observing key health behaviors of interest such as posture at the workstation, physical intensity of the work, perceived stress levels, or interactions with coworkers and record observations.

Key things to think about when conducting an environmental assessment include the following:

- It is often helpful to have an employee/liaison accompany the team to provide insights into their workplace (e.g., information about how often bulletin boards are updated and snack and drink machine vendors).
- In most cases, it will be necessary for an employee/liaison to accompany the team for safety purposes. Depending on the workplace, the team will need to comply with all safety regulations (e.g., wearing protective clothing and equipment).
- In unionized workplaces, union representatives should be part of the environmental assessment team and engage in all the activities related to the assessment.
- If the team is assessing a workplace that operates multiple shifts, it may be helpful to conduct the environment assessment at different times throughout the working day. The environment may be different at night than during the daytime shifts.
- Take pictures if allowed to emphasize a point or provide visual detail in a report. Make sure to ask for approval from the company before taking any pictures.

What is a Workplace Assessment?

Workplace-based assessment is one of the modalities, which assesses the trainee in authentic settings. Workplace assessments are participatory assessments of a workplace as a whole or one particular section of it. They may be conducted to examine the safety and health conditions in the workplace or causes of unresolved conflict. The discoveries about the strengths, needs, opportunities, and threats in the workplace give managers and human resource personnel a clear idea of what is needed to improve harmony, meet objectives, and ensure a culture that demonstrates the delineated values. The key feature of a workplace assessment is that it focuses on circumstances and the impacts of those circumstances on employees.

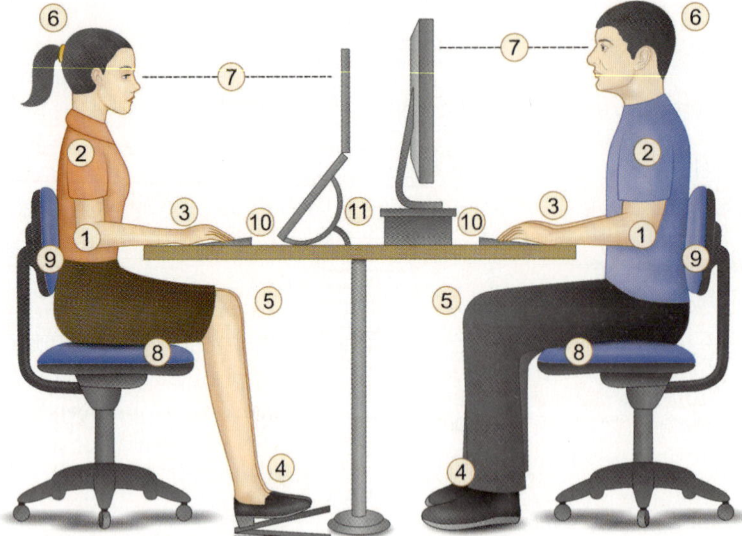

Fig. 9.12: Ideal work site setting for computer operator.

Benefits of a Workplace Assessment

Benefits for the Organization

Benefits for the organization are as follows:

- A healthier and happier workforce
- Elimination of reasons that are causing conflict in the workplace
- Fulfillment of legal requirements and reduction in the number of lawsuits
- Improvement in employee morale
- Increased understanding of each other's mind styles and what works and does not work for each person
- Increased understanding of policies and rules
- Protection for the workforce from both immediate and potential dangers
- Reduction in absenteeism rates
- Reduction in employee turnover
- Reduction in the number of formal complaints made by employees

Benefits for Employees

Benefits for employees are as follows:

- Better working conditions that result when coworkers are present and productive and others do not have to compensate for their inability to fulfill their roles.
- Comfort that this process is less confrontational than other methods, which could be used, such as town halls or face-to-face mediation.
- Confidence that action will be taken to improve working conditions or solve conflict
- Improvement in morale when management tangibly demonstrates its commitment meaningful discussions and action to resolve difficult issues
- Knowledge that issues which could result in work-related illness and conflict are resolved
- Knowledge that timely, relevant information is gathered that provides insight into current workplace dynamics and enables realistic opportune decisions to be made.
- Opportunity to voice concerns and know they are heard.

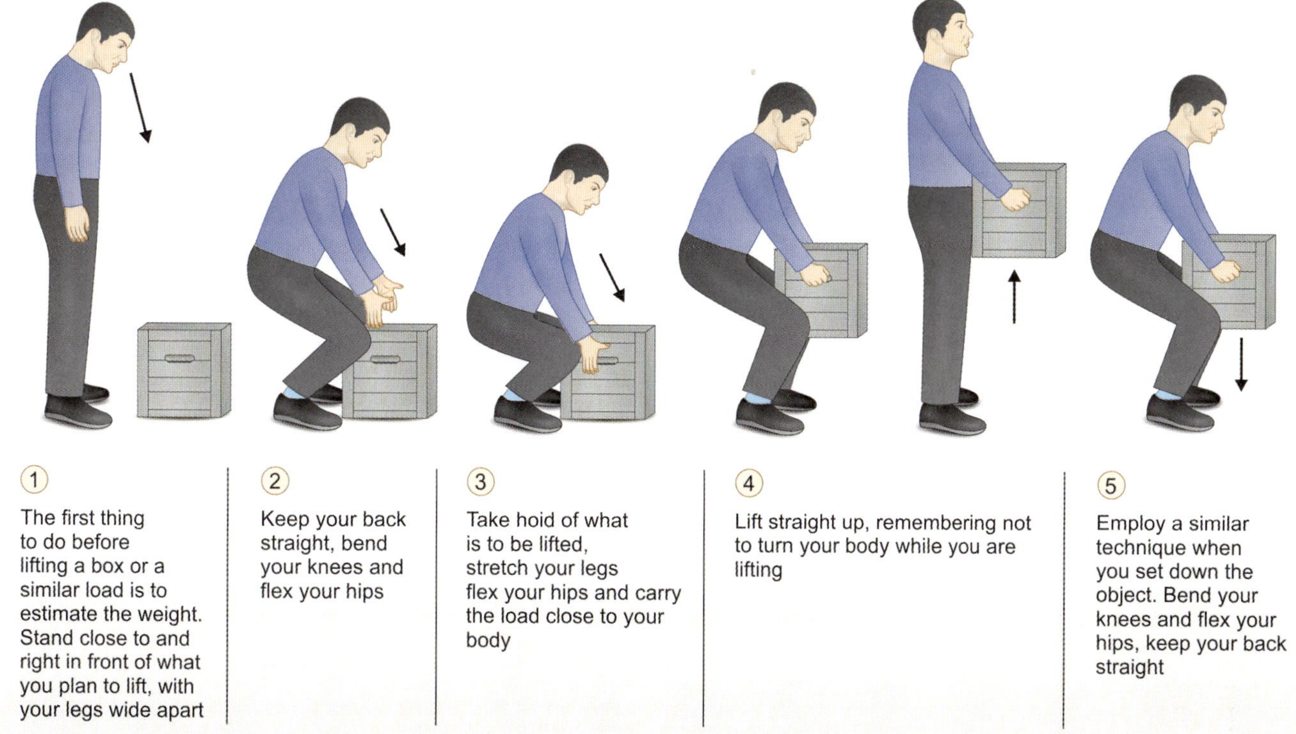

Fig. 9.13: Ideal weight-lifting techniques for laborers.

Workplace Assessment

Risks exist in all working environments. Risks, whether they are serious and life-threatening or not, must be identified in order for the organization to provide solutions designed to protect the health and well-being of the workforce.

Industrial environments usually possess obvious risks to employee safety. However, office environments also possess risks and stressors. Therefore precautions and preventative measures are implemented in these industries as well. In office environments, employees may suffer from migraines, back pain, strain injuries, psychological problems, and stress due to conflict. Discerning even the smallest risk is the fundamental purpose of a workplace assessment.

Workplace Assessment Process

Workplace assessment process includes:
- Engaging in a discussion with the client to determine the issue leading to the symptoms and absenteeism.
- Identifying the best method to assess the facts or stories surrounding the issue, such as individual interviews or focus groups, or town hall meetings.
- Utilizing direct or open-ended questions to find specific facts or elicit stories and perceptions.
- Delivering a report that includes analysis and suggestions/recommendations. Recommendations often include the need for workplace mediation, executive coaching, or workshops on specific topics
- Providing direct services to resolve situations where the organization is unable to offer those services at this time or where the organization lacks the required expertise.

How to Ensure a Good Workplace Assessment?

To ensure a good workplace assessment, the following should be monitored:
- It is important to provide all necessary support to ensure that the consultant can identify the source of the problems as well as what can be done to resolve them. Resolutions rarely work if the focus is placed on the symptom, there is fear associated with naming the issue, or the root cause is ignored or remains unidentified.
- It is imperative to outline for the consultant policies, procedures, or formal and informal practices, which are common in the organization.
- Management needs to make it easy for employees who are experiencing issues to contribute their own stories and knowledge about the situation and offer their resolutions.
- Ensure the assessment is documented providing a reference when making alterations or changes to physical conditions, policies or practices.
- After the assessment has been completed and issues have been prioritized and resolution implemented to conduct a follow-up evaluation to determine whether the selected solutions improved working conditions or resolved the conflict.

Tools for Workplace Assessment

The employee-level **health needs assessment (HNA)** survey provides a systematic way to plan workplace health initiatives while also giving an opportunity to engage staff and helping to emphasize employer's commitment. The questions recommended are questions that have been validated and piloted. They are aimed at providing information on staff's reported behavior that matches their actual behavior well, and which can be compared with national data, so one knows how the workforce compares. The section at the end provides the employer with an opportunity to seek staff's views on their "offer": the action employers are proposing to take. The length of a questionnaire is a key factor influencing response rates, with shorter questionnaires tending to obtain better response rates.

The **Employer Checklist on Workplace Environment and Satisfaction** is a self-assessment tool for employers to evaluate their workplace on:

- Satisfaction and engagement
- Quality of work–life balance
- Personal and professional growth
- Compensation and recognition
- Workplace health and safety.

The checklist is designed to evaluate the workplace environment and satisfaction level. The more statements that you check off, the closer you are to achieving a more positive and productive workplace. A positive workplace means less absenteeism and turnover and more productivity **(Appendix)**.

The Safety and Health Program Assessment Worksheet developed by **Occupational Safety and Health Administration (OSHA)**, the United States, is an evaluation tool to assess the employer's safety and health management system. Further, it can be used to provide information to an employer on the safety and health management system at one establishment and how it stacks up vis-à-vis other establishments in the same industry. The worksheet is based on the 1989 Safety and Health Management Guidelines and consists of those elements used to evaluate a company's measures for health and safety.

The purpose of this worksheet is to ensure precise safety and empower the consultants and give them a more confident voice in advising employers on how to prioritize their safety and health expenditures in an effort to receive the greatest benefit for the amount spent. Revised OSHA Form-33 has found to be valid and reliable tool for assessing and communicating the occupational injuries and illness to the employers.

Scoring method: Out of total 58 attributes, 8–12 is considered average, while 3–6 is taken up as low score. This scoring method is based on the data collected by the consultant. Only those attributes for which data has been collected during the visits may be scored. A quick summary of the scoring method for the attributes is shown in **Box 9.9.**

The American Association of Critical-Care Nurses (AACN) Healthy Work Environment Assessment Tool (HWEAT) evaluates a work environment based on each

BOX 9.9: Scoring and recommendation of OSHA.

Zero: No safety or health procedures/policies are even partially present to correct this hazard. (No activity)
One: Some safety or health procedures/policies are present although major improvements are needed. (Little activity)
Two: Considerable safety or health procedures/policies are present with only minor improvements needed. (Most activity completed)
Three: No additional safety or health procedures/policies are needed at this time. (No additional activity needed)

Source: Consultation Policies and Procedures Manual Chapter 4, OSHA 2004.

of the standards but does not diagnose specific challenges within a standard. This tool is used to identify problems and evaluate progress, not to diagnose specific causes. This is a screening tool, not a diagnostic test.

For example, most standards require support and collaboration among administrators, nurse managers, physicians, nurses, and other staff. Creating a healthy work environment is more than a thing to do. It is a way of being that relies on the strength of the entire team. The culture becomes compromised when any part of the team fails to support a standard.

It consists of 18-question assessment that should take no more than 10 minutes to complete. This tool evaluates the environment based on the standards and not individual groups within a team. It isn't designed to place blame or to isolate specific factors. The psychometric characteristics of this tool showed internal consistency with identical factor structures and Cronbach's alpha scores of 0.80 or better.

Tool for Observing Worksite Environments

Guidelines for assessment are as follows:

1. Obtain permission from manager to inspect the building and the grounds. Make observations in the daylight. It would be desirable to have an escort to make sure one covers all the stairwells, lunch rooms, vending machines, etc. However, do all observations independently.
2. If there is no one to accompany, it would be useful to check with someone (e.g., the manager's secretary) to make sure one does not miss the fitness center, cafeteria, showers, etc. Go through the major points of the assessment with them.
3. If possible, walk down all corridors on every floor, so one does not miss any of the items. Go into the target areas, such as the lunch room, cafeteria, and fitness center; only write down what you actually observe.
4. There are three environments that are evaluated. The first is the "worksite," which is the area of the building that is under one management. The second is the "grounds," which is the area around the worksite building. The third is the "community," which is the area just beyond the grounds.

If the worksite is in its own building that is not shared, that plot of land, including parking, will be the grounds. If the building or plot of land is shared with other tenants, the entire plot of land is considered the grounds. Thus the cafeteria, showers, fitness centers, or parking may be shared with other companies. However, only assess the stairways, elevators, and vending machines that are in the parts of the building owned or leased by the target company or in shared areas.

If the workplace is in a large commercial or industrial complex, the complex may be too large to consider the workplace grounds. In this case, define grounds as you see fit and ask employees what they consider part of their worksite. Examine the bulletin boards as you go around the worksite. At each bulletin board, examine postings for target notices. Only evaluate the first page or first layer of postings. For dietary information, do not evaluate postings of menus. For physical activity, do not assess signs related to movement safety at work; only those that are related to promotion of physical activity. Signs and posters can be posted anywhere. There is not a distinction whether signs are on bulletin boards or posted elsewhere.

5. For dining areas look for labeling that is visible on a casual inspection of the area. Record what you can see standing where you would stand if you were ordering or going through a cafeteria line. It is not necessary to examine every package. The only thing to specifically look for is whether low-fat milk and yogurt are available. For these, you will need to look at the labels.

6. Labeling of low-fat items should be easily visible, such as on separate signs or placards. Nutrition information signs may be in front of items on a cafeteria line, and they should show content of fat, cholesterol, calories, or sodium. For food areas, if salad or fruit is listed on the menu, it is available.

7. Under Grounds Assessment, examiner is interested in open space/grassy areas that are large enough to use for physical activities such as football, volleyball, walking, or lead to places where one could walk or run.

8. The Community Assessment does not need to be completed as part of the tour. It can be completed at a time separate from the site visit with the employees, thereby limiting employee burden. When conducting the scan of the community environment within the 0.5-mile radius (5 blocks) of the worksite, cover main streets predominantly. To further focus the scan, get suggestions from staff regarding where people typically go to eat, shop, or engage in physical activity.

The other tools for work environment evaluation include **Occupational Hazard Questionnaire** devised by the status of occupational health in India through a collaborative project of Indian Association of Occupational Health and National Institute of Occupational Health, Ahmedabad. However, its reliability and validity have not been yet established.

Similarly, **Individual Stress Identification Tool** developed by the University of Cambridge is also an optimal measure to measure the work stress at individual level; however, the psychometric properties are still not available.

Funding for Environmental Modifications

The patient/client to achieve environmental accessibility information on resource organizations can also be obtained from the National Council on Disabilities. Potential sources of funding include private medical insurance companies, home equity or other types of bank loans, Veterans Administration, the Division of Vocational Rehabilitation (DVR), and the Workers' Compensation Commission.

An important consideration is that not all patients will have current housing that is amenable to modification (e.g., an individual who previously lived in a third floor walk-up apartment and now uses a wheelchair). In such instances, the local Housing and Urban Development (HUD) office will be an important resource. Finally, creative funding for specific items (such as specialized adaptive equipment not covered by other resources) may be available through private organizations or foundations.

LEGISLATIONS

Legislations include the following:

- The *American Disability Act (ADA) of 1999:* The law ensures rights protection and equal opportunity in the areas of government services, employment, public transportation, privately owned transportation available to the public, telephone service, and public accommodations.

- The *Fair Housing Amendment Act of 1988:* The law prohibits discrimination in housing on the basis of race, color, religion, gender, disability, familial status, and national origin. The Act includes private housing, state and local government housing, and any housing that receives federal financial support.

- The *Rehabilitation Act of 1973:* The law prohibits discrimination in federal employment, stipulates accessibility within federal buildings, and establishes the Architectural Transportation Barriers and Compliance Board.

- The *Architectural Barrier Act of 1968*: The law provided that certain buildings that were financed by federal funds be designed and constructed "to insure that physically handicapped persons will have ready access to, and use of, such buildings."

- The *Telecommunications Act of 1996:* It stipulates that manufacturers of "telecommunications equipment or customer premises equipment shall ensure that the equipment is designed, developed, and fabricated to be accessible to and usable by individuals with disabilities, if readily achievable."

Various acts formed by the Indian government include:
- Workman's Compensation Act
- The Indian Factories Act
- Employees State Insurance Act

Workmen's Compensation Act or Employee's Compensation Act, 1923

This act provides for the payment by certain classes of employers to their employees of compensation for injury by accident. Disability can be partial or total. In both situations, the employee has a reduced working capacity due to the accident that occurred at the workplace.

"Partial disablement" and "Total disablement" can be temporary or permanent.

Employer's liability for compensation:
1. If personal injury is caused to an employee by accident arising out of and in the course of his employment, his employer shall be liable to pay compensation.
2. If the employee contracts any disease from place of employment, the amount of compensation for deaths, permanent total disablement, permanent partial disablement, temporary disablement, whether total or partial, depends on the wages of the employee.

The Indian Factories Act, 1948

This lays down the precautions for safety of workers:
- Who work with machinery?
- Who work with lifting devices and weights?
- For protection of eyes of workers who work with flames, etc.
- Precaution against fumes, etc.
- Specifications for age, hours of work
- Occupational disease notification (accidents, ergonomics).

Employees State Insurance Act, 1948

Employees State Insurance Act, 1948 can be described as follows:
- An Act to provide for certain benefits to employees in the case of sickness, maternity and "employment injury."
- "Employment injury" means a personal injury to an employee caused by accident or an occupational disease arising out of and in the course of his employment, being an insurable employment, whether the accident occurs or the occupational disease is contracted within or outside the territorial limits of India.

The insured person shall be entitled to periodical payments:
- To the insured person in the case of sickness certified by duly appointed medical practitioner or suffering from disablement.
- To the insured woman in the case of confinement or miscarriage or sickness arising out of pregnancy, confinement, premature birth of child, or miscarriage.
- To dependent of insured person in the case of their death.
- To medical treatment for insured persons
- To rehabilitation allowance

SUMMARY

Most of the Indian population still continues traditional practices of squatting such as when using Indian toilet and sitting cross-legged for most day-to-day activities such as eating or doing household activities. Such home environment enables the need of modifications in the toilet seat, especially in the older adults. Modifying the seat to western commode will reduce the impact of forces occurring with increased and sustained knee flexion as in Indian toilets. Also, advises on utilizing ergonomically sound furniture for avoiding cross-legged sitting will not only minimize the forces acting across the knee joint but also lessen the possibility of falls in older adults, which occurs commonly when rising from cross-legged sitting from the floor. Older adults in India often use streets and roads for daily walking, due to which active individuals tend to fall outside the home, and frail ones fall inside the home. Hence, making the outdoor environment suitable, accessible, and safe is equally imperative while addressing this as a public health problem.

Home safety assessment and modifications may be helpful in reducing falls and related injuries. The vulnerable population should be examined from the aspect of physical as well as social infrastructure so as to avoid missed findings and address the associated attributes. The barrier-free environment will ultimately assist the older individuals to achieve functional independence and ensure safe environment for survival too.

Good work is good for health and better employee health is good for business. It is warranted that protecting and improving the health of workforce can yield their business, recognizing that employees are their most valuable asset. In order to improve and protect the health of the employees and maximize the benefit to the organization, thorough evaluation of the workplace environment is mandatory. It is claimed that healthy workplaces are crucial to protect the optimal health and bear a vital role in preventing illness and facilitating the employers to reduce absenteeism from the work.

Review Questions

1. Explain the concept of universal design.
2. What are the purposes for performing an examination of the environment?
3. What data collection or measuring tools are used for examination of the home environment?
4. What data collection or measuring tools are used for examination of the work environment?

BIBLIOGRAPHY

1. American Academy of Orthopaedic Surgeons, Fall and Hip fractures 2007. https://aaos.org/globalassets/quality-and-practice-resources/hip-fractures-inthe-elderly/hip-fx-timing-measure-technical-report.pdf Last Accessed on January 10,2020.

2. Asadi-Lari M, Gray D. Health needs assessment tools: progress and potential. Int J Technol Assess Health Care. 2005 Summer;21(3):288-97.

3. Autenrieth DA, Brazile WA, Gilkey DP, et al. Client perceptions of occupational health and safety management system assistance provided by OSHA on-site consultation: results of a Survey of Colorado Small Business consultation clients. J Occup Environ Hyg. 2015;12(11):804-17.

4. Balaman SY. Chapter 4—Sustainability issues in biomass-based production chains decision-making for biomass-based production chains. In: The basic concepts and methodologies. Elsevier;2019. pp. 77-112.

5. Barstow BA, Bennett DK, Vogtle LK. Perspectives on home safety: do home safety assessments address the concerns of clients with vision loss?. Am J Occup Ther. 2011;65(6):635-42.

6. Becker F. Improving organizational performance by exploiting workplace flexibility. J Fac Manage. 2002;1:154-62.

7. Becker FO. Workspace creating environments in organization. New York: Praeger; 1981.

8. Carroll NV, Slattum PW, Cox FM. The cost of falls among the community dwelling elderly. J Manag Care Pharm. 2005;11:307-16.

9. Centers for Disease Control and Prevention. Check for safety: a home fall prevention checklist for older adults. 2005.

10. Centers for Disease Control and Prevention and The Merck Company Foundation. The state of aging and health in America. Whitehouse Station, NJ: The Merck Company Foundation; 2007.

11. Chandrasekar K. Workplace environment and its impact on organizational performance in public sector organizations. IJECBS. 2011;1:1-20.

12. Chapins A. Workplace and the performance of workers. Reston: USA; 1995.

13. CHEW. The enhanced SWAT Tool for Observing Worksite Environments (TOWE) adapted from RTI for CDC from the Checklist of Health Promotion Environments at Worksites. Oldenburg: CHEW; 2002.

14. Connor JA, Ziniel SI, Porter C, et al. Interprofessional use and validation of the AACN Healthy Work Environment Assessment Tool. Am J Crit Care. 2018;27(5):363-71.

15. Consultation Policies and Procedures Manual. Chapter 4—OSHA. 2004.https://www.osha.gov/enforcement/directives/04-06-csp-02.

16. Cornetti D, Sondrup R. Evidence-Based Home Assessment Tools and resources for PTs and PTAs. Home Health Section of the American Physical Therapy Association, 27. 2016.

17. Dhar HL. Gender, aging, health and society. J Assoc Physicians India. 2001;49:1012-20.

18. Dilani A. Design and health III: Health promotion through environmental design. IADH; 2004.

19. Donoghue OA, Ryan H, Duggan E, et al. Relationship between fear of falling and mobility varies with visual function among older adults. Geriatr Gerontol Int. 2014;14(4):827-36.

20. Drennan F. Making the safety/fitness connection. ISHN. Aug 2002.

21. Flemming PJ. Utilization of a screening tool to identify homebound older adults at risk for falls: validity and reliability. Home Health Care Serv Q. 2006;25:1-26. http://dx.doi.org/10.1300/J027v25n03_01.

22. Frank LD, Engelke PO. The impact of the built environment on physical activity. J Plan Lit. 2001;16(2):202-18.

23. Freeman EE, Munoz B, Rubin G, et al. Visual field loss increases the risk of falls in older adults: the Salisbury Eye evaluation. Invest Ophthalmol Vis Sci. 2007;48(10):4445-50.

24. Gitlin LN, Schinfeld S, Winter L, et al. Evaluating home environments of persons with dementia: interrater reliability and validity of the Home Environmental Assessment Protocol (HEAP). Disabil Rehabil. 2002;24(1-3):59-71.

25. Grawitch MJ, Ballard DW. The Psychologically Healthy Workplace: Building a Win–Win Environment for Organizations and Employees, Available from https://www.apa.org/pubs/books/The-Psychologically-Healthy-Workplace-Intro-Sample.pdf.Last accessed February 5, 2020.

26. Johnson SJ. Frequency and nature of falls among older women in India. Asia Pac J Public Health. 2006;18(1):56-61.

27. Josephson KR, Fabacher DA, Rubenstein LZ. Home safety and fall prevention. Clin Geriatr Med. 1991;7:707-32.

28. Mackenzie L, Byles J, Higginbotham N. Professional perceptions about home safety: cross-national validation of the Home Falls and Accidents Screening Tool (HOME FAST). J Allied Health. 2002;31:22-8.

29. Mackenzie L, Byles J, Higginbotham N. Reliability of the Home Falls and Accidents Screening Tool (HOME FAST) for identifying older people at increased risk of falls. Disabil Rehabil. 2002;24(5):266-74.

30. Mann WC, Locher S, Justiss MD, et al. A comparison of fallers and non-fallers in the frail elderly. Technol Disabil. 2005;14:1-8.

31. Mehraban HA, Mackenzie LA, Byles JE. A self-report home environment screening tool identified older women at risk of falls. J Clin Epidemiol. 2011;64:191-9.

32. Mike A. Visual workplace: how you see performance in the planet and in the office. Int J Financ Trade. 2010;11:250-60.

33. Moylan KC, Binder EF. Falls in older adults: risk assessment, management and prevention. Am J Med. 2007;120:493-7.

34. Oliver R, Blathwayt J, Brackley C, et al. Development of the Safety Assessment of Function and the Environment for Rehabilitation (SAFER) tool. Can J Occup Ther. 1993;60(2):78-82.

35. Poulin de Courval L, Gelinas I, Gauthier S, et al. Reliability and validity of the safety assessment scale for people with dementia living at home. Can J Occup Ther. 2006;73(2):67-75.

36. Public Health Agency of Canada. The safe living guide: aguide to home safety for seniors. Ottawa, ON; 2011. Available from https://www.canada.ca/en/public-health/services/health-promotion/aging-seniors/publications/publications-general-public/safe-living-guide-a-guide-home-safety-seniors.html Last Accessed on January 10, 2020.

37. Romli MH, Mackenzie L, Lovarini M, et al. Pilot study to investigate the feasibility of the Home Falls and Accidents Screening Tool (HOME FAST) to identify older Malaysian people at risk of falls. BMJ Open. 2016;6:e012048.

38. Rubenstein LZ. The importance of including the home environment in assessment of frail older persons. JAGS. 1999;47:111-2.

39. Schmitz TJ. Chapter on examination of the environment. Textbook of physical rehabilitation, 5th edition. FA Davis Co. Ltd. USA; 2007. pp.401-67.

40. Stevens JA, Mahoney JE, Ehrenreich H. Circumstances and outcomes of falls among high risk community-dwelling older adults. Inj Epidemiol. 2014;1:5.

41. Swenor BK, Yonge AV, Goldhammer V, et al. Evaluation of the Home Environment Assessment for the Visually Impaired (HEAVI): an instrument designed to quantify fall-related hazards in the visually impaired. BMC Geriatr. 2016;16:214.

42. Tinetti ME, Speechley M, Ginter SF. Risk factors for falls among elderly persons living in the community. N Engl J Med. 1998;319:1701-7.

43. Tomita MR, Saharan S, Rajendran S, et al. Schweitzer psychometrics of the Home Safety Self-Assessment Tool (HSSAT) to prevent falls in community-dwelling older adults. Am J Occup Ther. 2014;68:(6). 711-8.

44. Veitch JA, Charles KE, Newsham GR, et al. Workstation characteristics and environmental satisfaction in open-plan offices. In: COPE field findings (NRCC-47629). National Research Council; 2004.

45. World Health Organization Quality of Life Group. Development of the WHOQOL: rationale and current status. Int J Ment Health. 1994;23:24-56.

APPENDIX: EMPLOYER CHECKLIST ON WORKPLACE ENVIRONMENT AND SATISFACTION

The Employer Checklist on Workplace Environment and Satisfaction is a self-assessment tool for employers to use to evaluate their workplace on:

- Satisfaction and Engagement
- Quality of Work-Life Balance
- Personal and Professional Growth
- Compensation and Recognition
- Workplace Health and Safety

The checklist is designed to evaluate the workplace environment and satisfaction level. The more statements that you check off, the closer you are to achieving a more positive and productive workplace. A positive workplace means less absenteeism and turnover. This means increased productivity. How does this affect the wage gap? Research has shown that factors that cause absenteeism and turnover are also key causes of the wage gap. Therefore, addressing these factors not only increases productivity, but also contributes to closing the wage gap.

EMPLOYER CHECKLIST ON WORKPLACE ENVIRONMENT AND SATISFACTION

Satisfaction and Engagement

1. Our workplace inspires our employees to be the best workers that they can be.
2. Our workplace allows workers to do interesting and challenging work.
3. Managers encourage employees to work in a way that allows employees to get a sense of personal accomplishments.
4. Our workplace is a positive place to work.
5. Our workplace is a good place to work.
6. Our workplace is able to attract and retain skilled workers.

Quality of Work-life Balance

7. Managers encourage employees to balance their work and personal/family life.
8. Our workplace allows employees to balance their work and personal/family life by offering them the support that they need when they need it.
9. Our workplace allows employees enough time to complete their work without requiring them to do overtime.
10. Our workplace provides employees with the resources, tools and support that they need to do their jobs to the best of their abilities.
11. Our workplace helps employees manage any stress that may arise at work.

Personal and Professional Growth

12. Our workplace enables all of our employees to fully apply their knowledge and skills to their jobs.
13. Our workplace provides our employees with opportunities for training and professional development.
14. Our workplace provides our employees with opportunities for advancement and growth in their careers.
15. Our work environment enables our employees to feel fully productive.
16. Career opportunities in our workplace go to those who deserve them (merit).

Compensation and Recognition

17. Our workplace communicates clearly how each employee's work contributes to the overall goals of the workplace.
18. Managers give employees sincere and effective feedback about their work performance.
19. Managers are encouraged to recognize employees for the work that they do.
20. Managers are encouraged to make their employees feel valued and appreciated at the workplace.
21. Our workplace offers our employees an appropriate wage/salary for their work.
22. Our workplace offers equitable compensation.

Workplace Health and Safety

23. Our workplace provides a safe workplace.
24. Our workplace discourages and does not tolerate any harassment and discrimination (age, gender, sexual, racial, etc.).
25. Our workplace discourages and does not tolerate workplace bullying (verbal, emotional, physical).
26. Our workplace knows how to deal with workplace safety, health, harassment and discrimination issues.
27. Employees are comfortable discussing any workplace concerns with their supervisor/managers without fear of reprisal.
28. Our workplace is committed to responding to any concerns raised from our employees.

10

CHAPTER

Pain Assessment and Management

Megha S Sheth, Priyasingh Rangey, Srishti S Sharma

LEARNING OBJECTIVES

After reading this chapter, the readers should be able to:

♦ Understand the concept of "pain" and "chronic pain"
♦ Understand the theories of pain and the types of pain in relation to clinical variance of patients with pain
♦ Understand the physiology of pain and chronic pain, the pathways, and the relation of pain physiology to physiotherapy interventions
♦ Gain knowledge of the psychosocial aspects in the development and management of pain and chronic pain
♦ Evaluate pain and use various pain assessment tools
♦ Describe the management options available, including medical, interventional, and surgical
♦ Formulate a physiotherapy intervention plan based on the assessment.

CHAPTER OUTLINE

- Theories of pain
  - The specificity theory
  - Pattern theory
  - Gate control theory
  - Peripheral and central sensitization
- What is pain?
- Physiology of pain
  - Pain pathway
  - Neuromodulation of pain
  - Neurophysiologic explanations of pain control
  - Biopsychosocial model in chronic pain
- Classification of pain
  - Based on duration
  - Based on underlying pathophysiology
  - Based on origin
  - Classification of chronic pain

- Psychosocial implications of pain
  - Fear–avoidance behavior
  - Coping, catastrophizing, and acceptance
  - Depression and anxiety
  - Psychosocial factors associated with chronic pain
  - Pain behavior clusters
- Pain assessment
  - History and examination
  - Diagnosis and physical examination
  - Tools specific for the assessment of chronic pain
- Pain management
  - Pharmacological management of pain
  - Interventional management of pain
  - Physical therapy management of pain
  - Alternative therapies
  - Cognitive behavioral therapy
  - Pain neuroscience education

INTRODUCTION

The attempt to understand pain represents one of the oldest challenges in the history of medicine. Pain has a valuable role in medical action, as the symptom par excellence and, therefore, as a precious and meaningful tool. In Greek, the word "pain" means penalty. Plato said that pain arises from within the body indicating that pain is more of an emotional experience. In 1995, Dr Campbell presented the idea of evaluating pain as a vital sign, in order to reduce the burden of under assessment and inadequate treatment of pain. This stimulated the concept of "pain as the fifth vital sign." According to a 2014 study on the global burden of chronic pain, at least 10% of the world's population is affected by a chronic pain condition and every year, an additional 1 in 10 people develops chronic pain.

Pain is common and inadequately managed pain results into many adverse consequences. This not only affects the patients, but also their families, and society as a whole and can be broadly categorized as physiological, psychosocial [quality of life (QOL)], and financial consequences. Pain is the most common symptom of disease, which accompanies one from an early age. As a part of aging, the number of people who require management of pain from back disorders, degenerative joint conditions, visceral diseases, and cancer increases. However, pain in children and adolescents has also become quite common; hence, a focus is given to a lot of research these days. Since this may disrupt their school and social activities, it increases their risk for the development of negative health behaviors such as physical inactivity.

THEORIES OF PAIN

A number of theories have been postulated to describe mechanisms underlying pain perception. The existing theories of pain may be appropriate for the interpretation of some aspects of pain but are not yet comprehensive. The history of pain problems is as old as that of human beings; however, the understanding of pain mechanisms is still far from sufficient. The main focus of this section is theories postulated since the 17th century and to then provide an overview of current thinking **(Box 10.1)**. Among all theories proposed such as Strong's Theory (1895), Central Summation Theory (Livingston, 1943), the Fourth Theory of Pain (Hardy, Wolff, Goodell, 1940), the most influential theories of pain perception include the specificity theory, pattern theories, and gate control theory of pain.

The Specificity Theory

The specificity theory was one of the most influential theories of pain in history **(Fig. 10.1)**. In 1811, Charles Bell (1774–1842), a Scottish physician and anatomist, described in his privately circulated book "An Idea of a New Anatomy of the Brain" that the dorsal and ventral roots of the spinal nerves served different functions. He emphasized the involvement of the ventral roots in control of muscle contraction, but without a clear description of the functions of the dorsal roots.

Eleven years later in 1822, François Magendie (1783–1855), a French physiologist, verified the sensory characteristic of the dorsal root. This was finally referred to as the Bell–Magendie law, stating that the anterior branches of spinal nerve roots contain only motor fibers and that the posterior roots contain only sensory fibers. These discoveries provided a fundamental basis for the scientific study of pain issues. Based largely on this law, the German physiologist Johannes P Müller (1801–1858) developed the concept of "sensory nerve specificity," the "law of specific nerve energies." This theory states that different sets of nerve fibers, when stimulated, elicit different sensations by virtue of their central connections.

BOX 10.1: Theories of pain: History and overview.

Intensive Summation Theory (Erb, 1874): This theory, built on Aristotle's concept that pain resulted from excessive stimulation of the sense of touch, was described by several authors. In the 1840s, Erb maintained that every stimulus was capable of producing pain if it reached sufficient intensity. The theory was further developed by Goldscheider in 1894, who described both stimulus intensity and central summation as critical determinants of pain. It was implied that the summation occurred in the dorsal horn cells.

Specificity Theory (Von Frey, 1895): This theory is based on the assumption that the free nerve endings are pain receptors, and that the other three types of receptors are also specific to a sensory experience. Pain perception was viewed as a function of the amount of physical damage alone.

Strong's Theory (Strong, 1895): Strong believed that pain was an experience based on both the noxious stimulus and the psychic reaction or displeasure provoked by the sensation.

Pattern Theories (Nafe, 1934): Early pattern theories suggested that all cutaneous qualities are produced by spatial and temporal patterns of nerve impulses rather than by separate, modality-specific transmission routes.

Central Summation Theory (Livingston, 1943): This theory proposed that the intense stimulation resulting from nerve and tissue damage activated fibers that projected to internuncial neuron pools within the spinal cord. Abnormal reverberating circuits were created, with self-activating neurons. Prolonged abnormal activity bombarded cells in the spinal cord, and information was projected to the brain for pain perception.

The Fourth Theory of Pain (Hardy, Wolff, and Goodell, 1940s): This theory expanded on Strong's theory and stated that pain was composed of two components: the perception of pain and the reaction one has to it. The reaction was described as a complex physiopsychological process involving cognitive functions of the individual, and influenced by past experiences, culture, and various psychological factors that produce great variation in the "reaction pain threshold."

Sensory Interaction Theory (Noordenbos, 1959): This is a description of two systems involving transmission of pain and other sensory information with a fast and slow system. The slow system, composed of unmyelinated small-diameter fibers, was presumed to conduct somatic and visceral afferents. The fast system, composed of large fibers, was said to inhibit transmission of the small fibers.

Gate Control Theory (Melzack and Wall, 1965): This theory proposed that the neural mechanisms in the dorsal horns of the spinal cord act like a gate that can increase or decrease the flow of nerve impulses from peripheral fibers to the spinal cord cells that project to the brain. The somatic input is therefore subjected to the modulating influence of the gate before it evokes pain perception and response. It is suggested that large fiber inputs tend to close the gate, whereas small fiber inputs generally open it. Descending controls from the brain also influence what is experienced.

Muller proposed that specific receptors have a low threshold for a particular stimulus (adequate stimulus) but could respond to other forms of stimuli if these were of higher intensity. Von Frey expanded the Muller's concept;

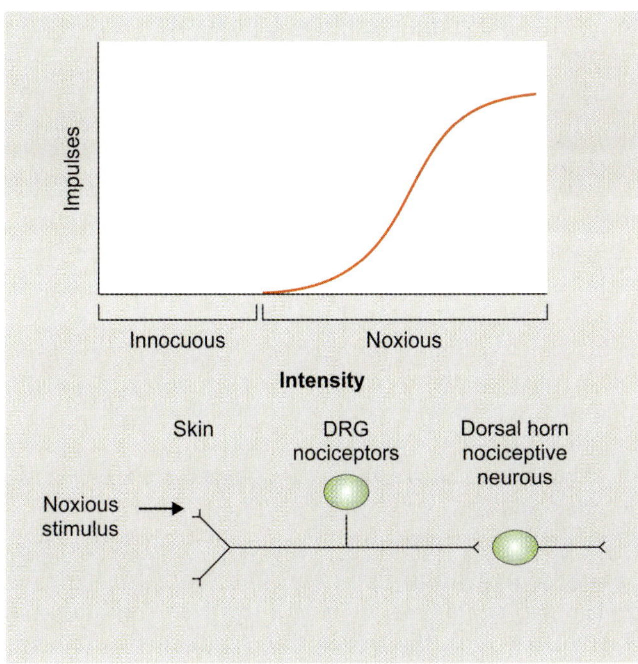

Fig. 10.1: Specificity theory.

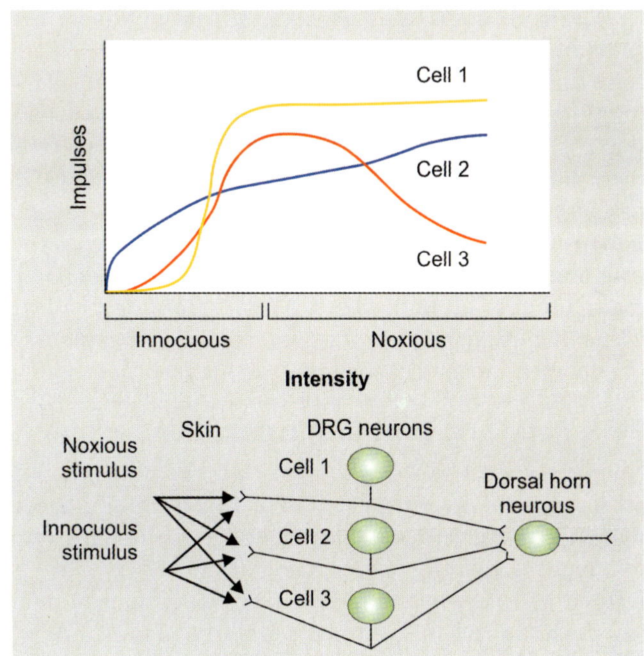

Fig. 10.2: Pattern theory.

however, his evidence of four basic receptors is inadequate to account for variety of painful stimuli. This difficulty led to a different interpretation of pain perception—that of pattern theory.

Pattern Theory

This theory **(Fig. 10.2)**, also known as intensity theory formalized by Goldscheider in 1894, states that the absence of specific pain receptors, pathways, or groups of neurons dedicated to the transmission of painful stimuli is its basic assumption. This theory attributes the sensation of pain to the pattern or frequency and intensity of stimulation applied that excite touch, pressure, or temperature receptors in the skin. If stimulus is of sufficient frequency and intensity, regardless of the energy form, the sensation is perceived as painful. The temporal and spatial summation of impulses is thought to be the basic mechanism underlying this theory. Goldscheider suggested a neurophysiological model to describe this summation effect: repeated subthreshold stimulation or suprathreshold hyperintensive stimulation could cause pain. He suggested further that the increased sensory input would converge and summate in the gray matter of the spinal cord.

Gate Control Theory

Melzack and Wall (1965) carefully discussed the shortcomings of the specificity and pattern theories—the two dominant theories of the era—and attempted to bridge the gap between these theories with a framework based on the aspects of each theory that had been corroborated by physiological data **(Fig. 10.3)**. Information concerned with

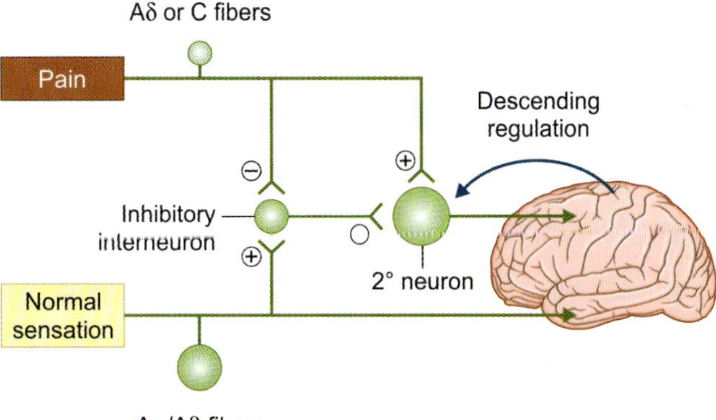

Fig. 10.3: Pain theory by Melzack and Wall.

the pain impulses transmitted from first centrally located cells in the spinal cord depends on the three factors:

1. The arrival of nociceptive impulses at the level of spinal cord.
2. The convergent effect of other peripheral afferent impulses, which may enhance or diminish the pain message.
3. The presence of control mechanisms within the central nervous system (CNS) that can influence the activity of dorsal horn cells of the spinal cord.

This system consists of four components, namely:

1. Afferent neurons
2. Mural interactions within the dorsal horn of spinal cord
3. Transmission cells or T cells
4. Descending controls from higher brain centers.

The gate consists of small inhibitory cells in the substantia gelatinosa of dorsal horn and T cells, which relay the information to higher centers. Input from small-diameter afferents will activate the T cells and when nociceptive information reaches a threshold that exceeds the inhibition elicited, it "opens the gate" and activates pathways that lead to the experience of pain and its related behaviors. Input from large-diameter afferents closes the gate and blocks the transmission of impulses from small diameter afferent pain fibers. Activity from descending fibers that originate in supraspinal regions and project to the dorsal horn could also modulate this gate.

Peripheral and Central Sensitization

Neuronal excitation in nociception is a dynamic process, allodynia and hyperalgesia **(Box 10.2)** amplify these dynamic changes. Hyperalgesia/allodynia is divided into two types. Hyperalgesia occurring at the site of injury is termed "primary hyperalgesia," whereas enhanced pain sensitivity in the surrounding uninjured area is termed "secondary hyperalgesia." Peripheral sensitization occurs due to sensitization of peripheral nerve endings as a result of primary hyperalgesia. Central sensitization occurs due to changes in the spinal cord and higher brain areas as a result of secondary hyperalgesia **(Fig. 10.4)**.

Peripheral sensitization is a decrease in threshold, an increase in responsiveness and occasionally a spontaneous activity of peripheral ends of nociceptors. It occurs following tissue damage and inflammation and arises due to the action of inflammatory chemicals released at the affected site by both sensory nerve fibers and inflammatory cells. Some of these compounds can directly activate peripheral nociceptors (such as protons, ATP, and serotonin), while others have a more modulating role leading to enhanced responsiveness of nerve endings. Increased sensitivity occurs due to two processes:

1. Early post-translational changes in the peripheral terminals of nociceptors, e.g., phosphorylation of ion channels.
2. Altered gene expression

Central sensitization differs from peripheral sensitization. Peripheral sensitization is due to post-translational and transcription changes in the terminal ends of high-threshold nociceptors resulting in primary hyperalgesia. Central sensitization in contrast typically manifests in tactile allodynia and secondary hyperalgesia (in tissue not affected by any harmful condition). Pain is generated as a consequence of changes within the CNS that lead to alterations of how to interpret sensory inputs, rather than reflecting the presence of peripheral noxious stimuli. The newly proposed definition by the International Association for the Study of Pain (IASP) describes "central sensitization" as the "increased responsiveness of nociceptive neurons in the CNS to their normal or subthreshold afferent input. Mechanism governing these central changes are shorter lasting, activity triggered mechanisms include windup and heterosynaptic potentiation, whereas long-lasting effects are due to alterations in microglia, astrocytes, gap junctions, membrane excitability, and gene transcription, all of which can contribute to the maintenance of central sensitization.

BOX 10.2: Common terms associated with pain.	
Allodynia	Pain due to a stimulus that does not normally provoke pain
Analgesia	Absence of pain in response to stimulation that would normally be painful
Causalgia	A syndrome of sustained burning pain, allodynia, and hyperpathia after a traumatic nerve lesion, often combined with vasomotor and sudomotor dysfunction (such as diabetic autonomic neuropathy) and later trophic changes
Hyperalgesia	An increased response to a stimulus that is normally painful
Hypalgesia	Decreased response to pain
Hyperpathia	A painful syndrome characterized by an abnormally painful reaction to a stimulus, especially a repetitive stimulus, as well as an increased threshold
Placebo	A placebo is an inert treatment, such as a sugar pill or fake treatment, that is beneficial because the patient believes it will be beneficial
Nocebo	Opposite of placebo. A nocebo is an inert treatment or event that increases symptoms because the patient believes it will increase symptoms
Paresthesia	An abnormal sensation, whether spontaneous or evoked
Hyperesthesia	Increased sensitivity to stimulation, excluding the special senses
Dysesthesia	An unpleasant abnormal sensation, whether spontaneous or evoked

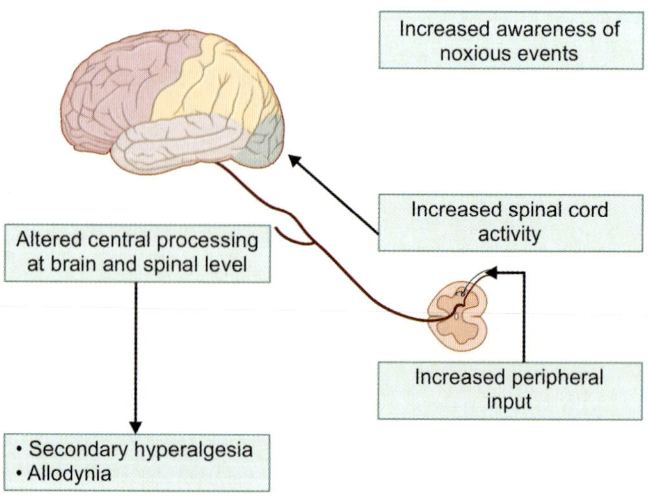

Fig. 10.4: Central sensitization of pain.

- *Windup or homosynaptic potentiation* describes a phenomenon of increasing action potential output from dorsal horn neurons during a train of low-frequency firing of C fibers. By this repetitive C fiber stimulus, higher calcium levels are achieved in the C fiber central presynaptic terminal, which leads to release of increasing glutamate and peptides (such as SP and CGRP), resulting in increasing postsynaptic depolarization. This process results in progressively increasing output of the dorsal horn neuron during a train of identical incoming C fiber stimuli. The temporary plasticity created by windup is dependent on constant incoming activity and thus does not outlast the stimulus.
- *Heterosynaptic potentiation* in the spinal cord differs from the windup phenomemon in two ways: the increased responsiveness of the dorsal horn neuron outlasts the primary stimulus by hours; these changes affect the response triggered by the primary stimulus, and the response to stimuli from other afferents converging on the same dorsal horn neuron. Ultimately, subthreshold incoming stimuli from converging nociceptors as well as high-threshold Aβ fibers are converted to suprathreshold action potentials due to the changes at the dorsal horn neuron. This manifests clinically as hyperalgesia (stimuli originating from C and A-delta nociceptors), allodynia (stimuli originating from Aβ fibers) as well as secondary hyperalgesia due to recruitment of fibers supplying sensation to areas outside the primarily injured area.

WHAT IS PAIN?

In 1968, McCaffery defined pain as "whatever the experiencing person says it is, existing whenever she/he says it does." This definition emphasizes that pain is a subjective experience with no objective measures. It also stresses that the patient, not clinician, is the authority on the pain and that his or her self-report is the most reliable indicator of pain. In 1979, the IASP introduced the most widely used definition of pain. The IASP defined pain as an "unpleasant sensory and emotional experience associated with actual or potential tissue damage, or described in terms of such damage." This definition emphasizes that pain is a complex experience that includes multiple dimensions.

Pain is a cardinal symptom of inflammation and is valuable in the diagnosis of many disorders and conditions. It may be:

- Mild or severe
- Chronic or acute
- Lancinating
- Burning
- Dull or sharp
- Precisely or poorly localized
- Referred

Experiencing pain is influenced by the following factors:

- Physical
- Mental
- Biochemical
- Psychological
- Physiologic
- Social
- Cultural
- Emotional

It is subject to a wide range of influences and therefore there is considerable variation in the perception of pain between individuals. Pain should not be viewed exclusively as either a sensation or an emotion, since either assumption precludes particular characteristic necessary to the painful experience. Factors such as memory of previous experiences, psychological influences and pain tolerance variation cannot be accounted for by an isolated definition. In recent times, the concept of "pain" has evolved from one-dimensional to a multidimensional entity involving sensory, cognitive, motivational, and affective qualities.

The primary purpose of pain is to protect the body. It occurs whenever there is tissue damage, and it causes the individual to react to remove the painful stimulus. Pain is also a sensation with more than one dimension. To the individual, pain is both an objective and a subjective experience. The objective dimension is the physiological tissue damage causing the pain. The subjective dimensions include the following:

- *A perceptual component: The client's awareness of the location, quality, intensity, and duration of the pain stimulus.*
- *An affective component: The psychological factors surrounding the client's pain experience, including the client's personality and emotional state.*
- *A cognitive component: What the client knows and believes about the pain resulting from his or her cultural background and past pain experiences (both personal pain experiences and those of others).*
- *A behavioral component: How the client expresses the pain to others through communication and behavior.*

  These together constitute pain experience to a person. Hence, each component needs to be addressed for an overall successful management of a person's pain. Subjective components, if ignored can result in correction of underlying tissue damage, without curing their pain perception.

Nociception refers to the process by which information about tissue damage is conveyed to the CNS. Exactly how this information is ultimately perceived as painful is unclear. In addition, there can be pain without nociception (e.g., phantom limb pain) and nociception without pain. But classic descriptions of pain typically include four processes **(Fig. 10.5)**:

1. Transduction
2. Transmission
3. Perception
4. Modulation

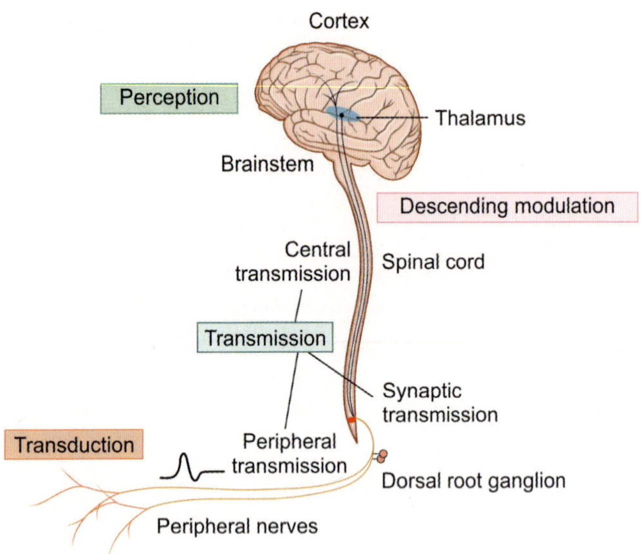

Fig. 10.5: Processes of pain.

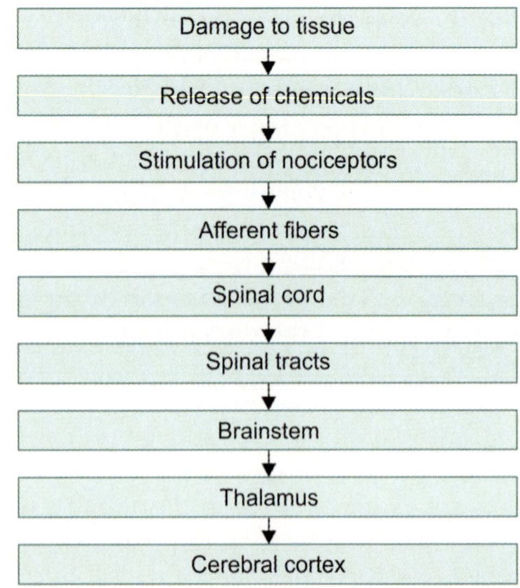

Fig. 10.6: Flowchart showing the pain pathway.

Transduction refers to the conversion of the energy from a noxious thermal, mechanical, or chemical stimulus into electrical energy (nerve impulses) by sensory receptors called nociceptors.

Transmission refers to the transmission of these neural signals from the site of transduction (periphery) to the spinal cord and brain.

Perception refers to the appreciation of signals arriving in higher structures as pain.

Modulation consists of descending inhibitory and facilitatory inputs from the brain that influence (modulate) nociceptive transmission at the level of the spinal cord.

PHYSIOLOGY OF PAIN

Pain is a physiological response to a noxious stimulus. The pathway that it follows is a multidimensional system comprising of the central as well as the peripheral nervous system (PNS).

The pain pathway has the following components **(Figs. 10.6 and 10.7)**:

- PNS—nociceptors and afferent fibers (A-delta and C fibers)
- Spinal cord—dorsal and ventral horn
- Spinal tracts—lateral spinothalamic tract (LST) and medial spinothalamic tract (MST)
- Brainstem—reticular formation (RF), periaqueductal gray (PAG) matter, and nucleus raphe magnus (NRM)
- Thalamus—medial and lateral
- Cerebral cortex—somatosensory cortex and limbic system

There are three different orders of neurons:

1. First-order neurons: Peripheral receptor to dorsal horn of spinal cord
2. Second-order neurons: Dorsal horn of spinal cord to thalamus
3. Third-order neurons: Thalamus to cerebral cortex

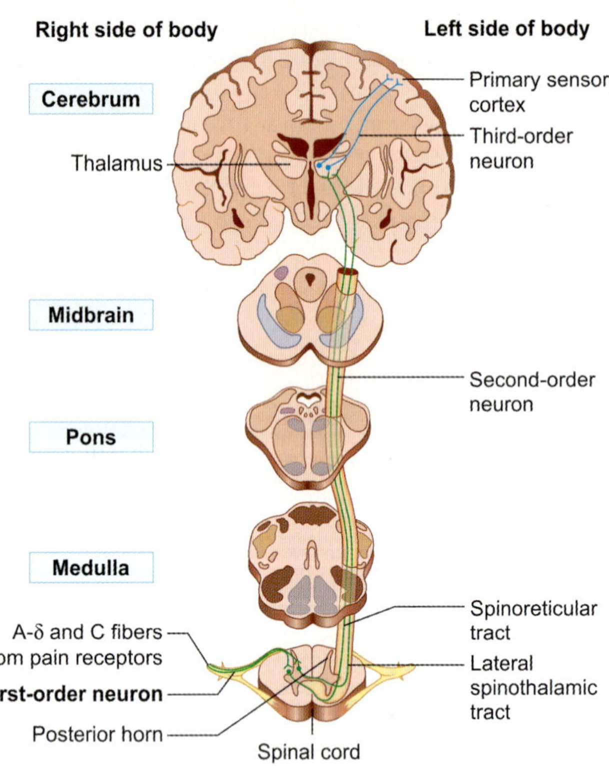

Fig. 10.7: Pain pathway.

Pain Pathway

Peripheral Nervous System

PNS can be described as follows:

- Nociceptors: These are specialized sensory receptors that respond to noxious stimuli **(Fig. 10.8)**.
- Nociceptors can be stimulated using four different mechanisms:
  a. Mechanical—direct force or pressure
  b. Chemical—release of specific chemicals in response to inflammatory agents or injury

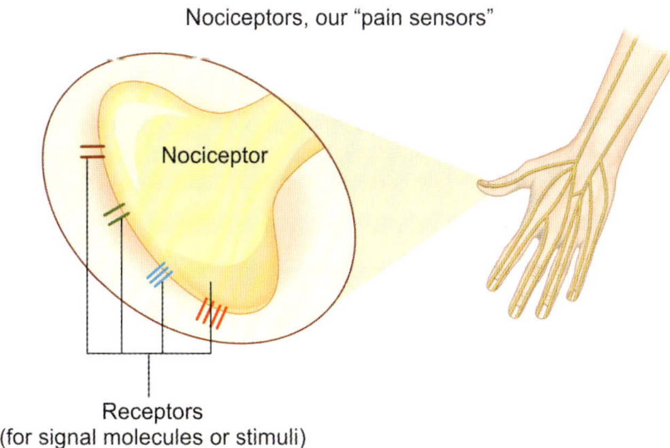

Fig. 10.8: Structure of nociceptor.

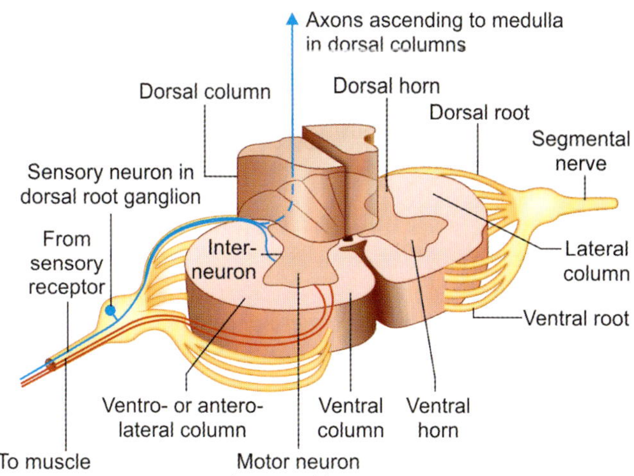

Fig. 10.9: Transverse section of spinal cord.

c. Thermal—extreme temperature changes, including both hot and cold

d. Polymodal stimulation—a combination of the above three types of stimuli

These nociceptors are present in almost all the tissues of the body. Nociceptors follow the property of sensitization like other receptors. Sensitization means that if a stimulus is maintained for longer than a certain amount of period, the threshold for activation of the concerned receptor is lowered and it fires more rapidly.

- Afferent fibers: These are A-delta and C fibers. Some nociceptors transmit information to the A-delta fibers, whereas others do so via the C fibers (**Table 10.1**).

Dorsal Horn of Spinal Cord

All the A-delta and C fibers have their cell bodies in the dorsal root ganglion (**Fig. 10.9**). Of these, all the A-delta fibers and almost 70–85% of the C fibers have their central connections entering the dorsal horn through the dorsal root. The remaining 15–30% C fibers return to their respective peripheral nerve and enter through the ventral root and then move toward the dorsal horn.

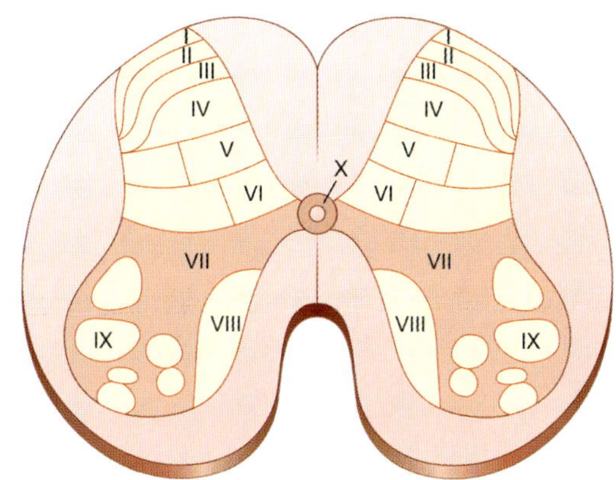
Fig. 10.10: Arrangement of laminae in dorsal and ventral horn of spinal cord.

Rexed B in 1952 gave the cytoarchitectonic organization of the spinal cord in the cat. He explained that the spinal cord comprises 10 different segments or laminae. Laminae I–VI form the dorsal horn of the spinal cord (**Fig. 10.10**).

- Lamina I—marginal zone
- Lamina II—substantia gelatinosa
- Laminae III and IV—nucleus proprius
- Lamina V—neck of dorsal horn
- Lamina VI—base of dorsal horn

These laminae, especially laminae I, II, III, and V, receive the incoming central connections of the afferent fibers. Here, the fibers synapse with central nociceptive transmission cells. The neurotransmitter involved here is substance P.

The central nociceptive transmission cells are of two types—nociceptive-specific (NS) neurons and wide dynamic range (WDR) neurons. NS neurons are located primarily in Lamina I and respond only to nociceptive fibers, whereas Lamina V contains the WDR neurons and responds to nociceptive as well as other large-diameter fibers.

After synapsing, the fibers from the central nociceptive transmission cells cross to the opposite side of the spinal cord and transmit the incoming pain signals through one of the tracts.

Table 10.1: Difference between A-delta and C nerve fibers.	
A-delta fibers	*C fibers*
A-delta nociceptors respond to mechanical stimuli and hence convey sharp, pricking kind of pain	C nociceptors are polymodal and hence carry deep, aching pain
Thinly myelinated	Nonmyelinated
Comparatively faster conducting; around 15 m/s	Slow conducting; around 1 m/s
Conduct fast pain	Conduct slow pain
Comparatively large diameter	Small diameter
Innervate skin and underlying tissues	Innervate all body tissues except CNS
Transmit detailed information about localization of pain	Transmit diffuse information related to affective response of pain

(CNS: central nervous system)

Spinal Tracts

The two main tracts carrying the nociceptive information are the LST and the MST.

1. *LST:* Information from A-delta fibers is carried by this tract. Thus the fast traveling sharp pain is conducted by this tract. It has fewer relays, synapses, or collaterals and hence ends directly in the thalamus with a few fibers terminating in RF.
2. *MST:* This tract is a system of different relays and several collaterals and hence slowly and indirectly conducts information to the thalamus. Slow, dull-aching pain information from the C fibers is carried by this tract. About 10–25% fibers reach the thalamus, while the rest of the fibers terminate in the RF, tectal area of the mesencephalon and the PAG matter.

Brainstem

The brainstem receives more collaterals from the MST than the LST. The RF, PAG matter, and NRM are the brainstem structures that are essential in the pain pathway.

- The RF spans from the medulla to the thalamus. It relays information to the various parts of cerebral cortex and also sends information to the descending motor pathways.
- The PAG and NRM play an essential role in the descending pain suppression system and opioid analgesia.

Thalamus

The thalamus acts as a hub from where all information is relayed **(Fig. 10.11)**. It consists of a group of nuclei but only two nuclei are important for the transmission of pain—the ventrobasal complex and the medial and interlaminar group of nuclei.

- The ventrobasal complex receives the pain signals from the LST. Since here the nuclei are arranged topographically, the pain received here can be localized. From here, the information is transmitted further to the primary sensory cortex.
- The MST sends impulses to the medial and interlaminar group of nuclei. The nuclei here do not

have a topographic arrangement; hence, the pain is not well localized. From here, the impulse travels to the cerebral cortex, basal ganglia, and limbic system.

Cerebral Cortex

The final and most important structure is the somatosensory cortex **(Fig. 10.12)**. It is responsible for the perception and interpretation of pain. It perceives the intensity, location, and kind of pain. The somatosensory cortex contains the sensory homunculus. Due to this spatial representation of the body based on the receptors present in each body part (sensory homunculus), there is a difference between the pain perceived in different parts of the body by the same kind and intensity of stimulus.

The somatosensory cortex has another area closely related to it—the association cortex. The association cortex is responsible for associating pain with past experiences and memories **(Fig. 10.13)**.

The limbic system has connections to the hypothalamus and the cerebral cortex. It plays an important role in the emotional aspect of pain.

Neuromodulation of Pain

The passage of nociceptive information may be interrupted at several stages along the ascending nociceptive pathways to produce neuromodulation of pain. Four anatomical levels, which make up the ascending pathways, are as follows:

1. Peripheral
2. Spinal segmental
3. Segmental
4. Cortical

Peripheral Level

This involves a reduction of the amount of those chemicals released in response to tissue damage, which are responsible for nociceptor activation. It also consists of modalities that affect cell permeability and thus reduce the amount of exudate formed in an inflammatory reaction.

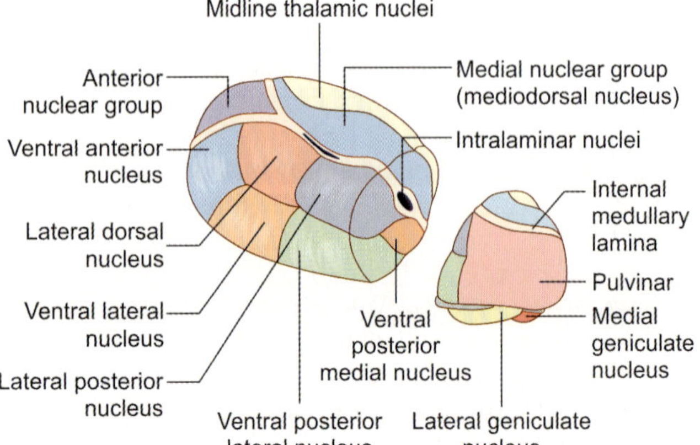

Fig. 10.11: Structure of thalamus.

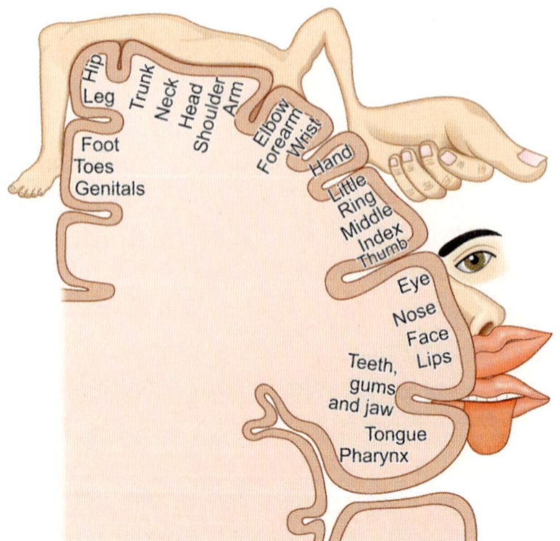

Fig. 10.12: Sensory homunculus.

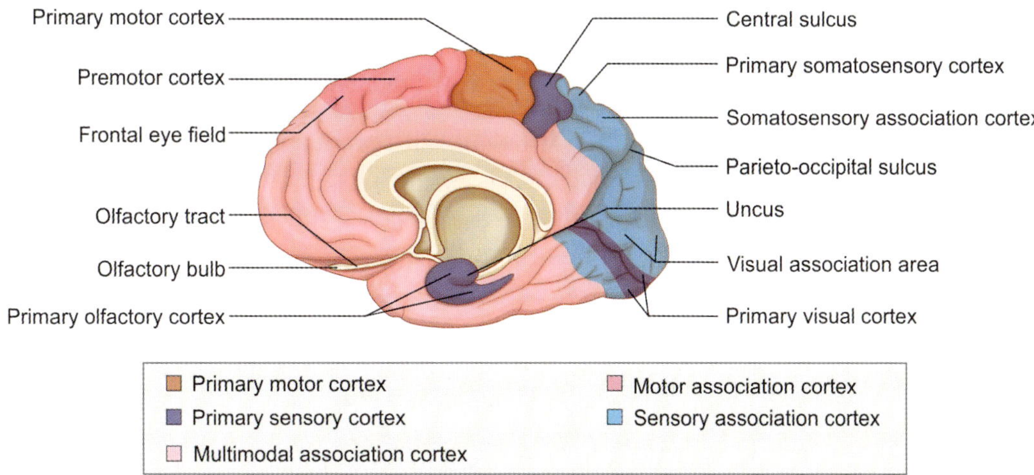

Fig. 10.13: Sensory cortex.

Pressure exerted by the exudates upon the nociceptors can initiate activity in the nociceptive pathways.

Spinal Segmental Level

This involves inhibition of activity in the small-diameter Group III and IV fibers before the incoming information ascends further up the neural axis. Segmental inhibition and physiological blocking are the two mechanisms that occur at this level.

Supraspinal Level

The ascending pathway makes important synaptic connections with several brainstem structures involved with descending pain modulation systems. Placebo and counterirritation also operate at this level.

Cortical Level

This involves interventions that modify the individual's perception and interpretation of pain. Behavior modification and cognitive strategies are examples of psychological approaches operating at this level.

A broad spectrum of interventions and physio-therapeutic modalities and techniques, which activate the pain modulating mechanism at each of these levels, are described in **Table 10.2**.

Neurophysiologic Explanations of Pain Control

Three analgesic mechanisms have been presented by the models as proposed by Melzack and Wall.

1. Stimulation from ascending A-beta afferents results in the blocking of impulses carried along A-delta and C afferent fibers.
2. Stimulation from descending pathways in the dorsolateral tract of spinal cord by A-delta and C afferent fibers.
3. The stimulation of A-delta and C afferent fibers causes the release of endogenous opioids [beta endorphin

Table 10.2: Pain modulation at different levels using physiotherapy techniques and agents.

Peripheral level	
• Removal of chemical irritants	• Therapeutic exercise • Manual therapy • PEMF • Ultrasound • Heat • Compression unit
• Alteration of cell permeability	• Cold • Ultrasound
Spinal segmental level	
• Segmental inhibition	• Manual therapy • Heat and cold • High-frequency/low-intensity TENS
• Physiological blocking mechanism	• IFC • Brief, intense TENS
Supraspinal level	
• Descending pain suppression system	• Acupuncture • Low-frequency/high-intensity TENS
• Counterirritation	• UVR • Heat and cold • IFC • Diadynamic currents
• Placebo	• TENS
Cortical level	
• Behavior modification	• Neutral response to pain behavior • Positive response to wellness behavior
• Cognitive strategies	• Cognitive behavior therapy • Therapist–patient communication

(IFC: interferential currents; PEMF: pulsed electromagnetic frequency; TENS: transcutaneous electrical nerve stimulation; UVR: ultraviolet radiation)

(BEP)], resulting in prolonged activation of descending analgesic pathways.

Blocking Pain Impulses with Ascending A-beta Input

Pain modulation caused by sensory stimulation and the resultant increase in impulses in the large-diameter (A-beta) afferent fibers was proposed by the gate control theory of pain. As described earlier, impulses ascending on these fibers stimulate the substantia gelatinosa in the dorsal horn of the spinal cord. This in turn inhibits the synaptic transmission in the large and small-diameter afferent pathways. The balance between input from the small- and large-diameter afferents determines how much of the pain message is blocked or gated. This theory also proposes that A-delta and C fiber impulses inhibit substantia gelatinosa facilitating the perception of pain. The pain sensation does not diminish rapidly because free nerve endings do not accommodate and the afferent impulses from them "open the gate" to further the transmission of pain message.

Castel introduced an endogenous opioid analogous to the gate control theory and his theory proposed that increased neural activity in A-alpha and A-beta primary afferent pathways triggers a release of enkephalin from enkephalin interneurons in the dorsal horn. These neuroactive amines inhibit the synaptic transmission in the A-delta and C fiber afferent pathways. The end result, as in gate control theory, is that the pain message is blocked before it reaches sensory levels. This is presynaptic inhibition of dorsal horn synapse transmission owing to A-beta fiber stimulation at enkephalin interneurons **(Fig. 10.14)**.

Descending Pain Control Mechanisms

The central control originating in higher centers of the CNS could affect the dorsal horn gating process. Impulses from the thalamus and brainstem **(central biasing)** are carried into the dorsal horn on efferent fibers in the dorsal and dorsal lateral paths. Impulses from the higher centers act to close the gate and block the transmission of pain message at the dorsal horn synapse. Castel offers an endogenous opioid model of descending influence over dorsal horn synapse activity. Stimulation of PAG region of the midbrain and raphe nucleus in the pons and medulla by ascending neural input, especially from A-delta and C fiber afferents, and possibly central biasing, activates the descending mechanism.

The PAG stimulates the raphe nucleus. The raphe nucleus in turn sends impulses along serotonergic efferent fibers in the dorsal lateral tract, which synapse with enkephalin interneurons. The interneurons release enkephalin into the dorsal horn, inhibiting the synaptic transmission of impulses to the second-order afferent neurons **(Fig. 10.15)**.

A second descending, noradrenergic pathway projecting from the pons to the dorsal horn has also been identified. This model provides a physiologic explanation for the analgesic response to brief, intense stimulation. The analgesia following acupressure and use of some transcutaneous electrical nerve stimulators (TENS), etc. is attributed to this descending pain control mechanism.

Beta Endorphin and Dynorphin

There is sufficient evidence that stimulation of small diameter afferents (A-delta and C) can stimulate the release of other endogenous opioids. BEP and dynorphin are neuroactive peptides with potent analgesic effects. The term **endorphin** refers to an opiate-like substance produced by the body. It is apparent that these large endogenous substances play a significant role in pain relief of patients.

One of the sources of BEP is anterior pituitary. It shares the prohormone pro-opiomelanocortin with

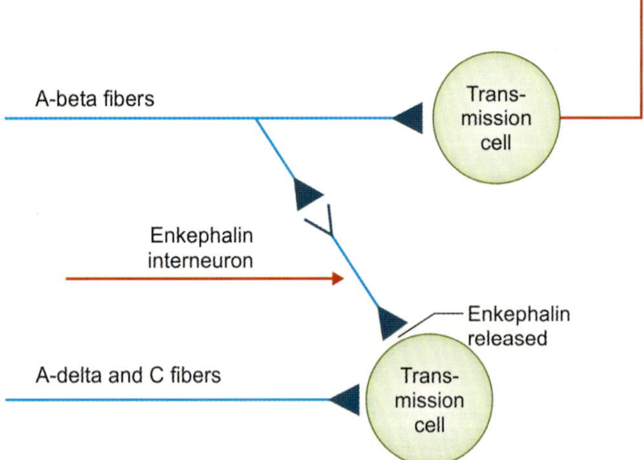

Fig. 10.14: Presynaptic inhibition of dorsal horn synapse transmission.

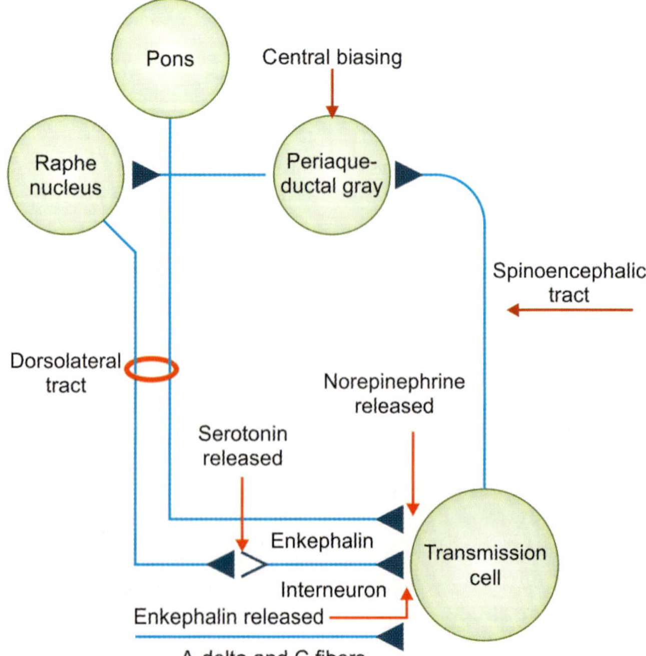

Fig. 10.15: Stimulation of PAG in the midbrain and the raphe nucleus. (PAG: periaqueductal gray)

adrenocorticotropin. Prolonged (20–40 minutes) small diameter afferent fiber stimulation has been thought to trigger the release of BEP from anterior pituitary gland. Electroacupuncture and possibly TENS with long phase durations and low pulse rates (1–5 pulses/s) will cause small-diameter afferent fiber depolarization necessary for BEP release. BEP does not readily cross the blood-brain barrier, suggesting that if BEP or other endogenous opioids are active analgesic agents within the CNS, they are released from areas within the brain.

The neurons in the hypothalamus that send the projections to PAG and noradrenergic nuclei in the brainstem contain BEP. It is possible that BEP released from these neurons by stimulation of hypothalamus is responsible for the analgesic response to the treatments. Dynorphin, a more recently isolated endogenous opioid, is found in PAG, rostroventral medulla, and the dorsal horn. It has been noted that dynorphin is released during electroacupuncture. It may be responsible for suppressing the response to noxious mechanical stimulation.

Biopsychosocial Model in Chronic Pain

- Compared to the earlier dualistic approaches to understanding pain, the **gate control theory** can be viewed as the first mind–body perspective to introduce the integration of the CNS with cognitive processes. An extension to this theory, termed the **Neuromatrix Model of Pain**, was proposed by Melzack in 1999. This theory incorporates the stress component with pain. As per the original work of Selye, stress serves as a mechanism of adaptation, such that the body will respond to challenging or dangerous situations in an attempt to lessen any problematic consequences. The two neuroendocrine systems, the sympathetic-adrenomedullary system and the hypothalamic-pituitary–adrenocortical (HPA) axis, serve to activate this fight or flight system. However, hyperactivity of the HPA system can be seen to intensify the pain condition. When dealing with chronic pain, individuals experiencing elevated levels of stress may actually exacerbate the pain experience. As stress intensifies pain, the increased level of pain, in turn, inevitably becomes a stressor that continues to threaten homeostasis. Based on the theory provided by Melzack, each individual's distinct neuromatrix—comprised genetics, sensory modalities, and memory—determines the overall interpretation of the experience of pain.
- The biopsychosocial model of pain has become the most heuristic approach to truly understanding the concept of "pain." This approach views a physical disorder as the result of an intricate and dynamic interaction among biological, psychological, and social factors that can often antagonize the pain condition. Individuals tend to express variability in their pain experiences due to the range and interaction of these factors that modulate the interpretation of symptoms. It was first introduced in medicine by Engel who described that, as

a medical illness became more chronic in nature, then psychosocial "layers" (e.g., distress, illness behavior, and the sick role) emerged to complicate assessment and treatment. Subsequently, Loeser, applied this model to pain, and from this perspective, there were four dimensions related to the idea of pain: nociception, pain, suffering, and pain behavior.

- Chronic pain is viewed as an illness that cannot be cured but only managed. Therefore, the biopsychosocial perspective is directed at the illness, rather than the disease, and this approach focuses on the diversity and the individual differences in the overall pain experience. The interwoven connection of the biological, psychological, and social elements unique to each chronic pain patient must be attended to, for a full understanding of the patient's condition. Standard treatment protocols prove to be deficient if any one of these components is ignored. Because patients with the same diagnosis can respond differently to a standard treatment protocol, the goal in the biopsychosocial approach to assessment and management is to tailor the treatment to the specific needs of the individual.
- A recent advance in this model outlines how the neuroendocrine system affects the chronic pain condition. In addition to the impact of general emotional distress, elevations of stress hormones produced by the HPA system, such as cortisol, have been found to exacerbate pain conditions. Several recent studies have associated HPA dysfunction with chronic pain conditions, such as fibromyalgia, chronic fatigue syndrome, chronic pelvic pain, temporomandibular pain disorder, rheumatoid arthritis, and multiple sclerosis.
- Overall, these pain models are useful in conceptualizing the perception of pain and pain relief. These models will help the therapist understand the effects of therapeutic modalities and form a sound rationale for modality application. The therapist should adapt these models to fit new development.

CLASSIFICATION OF PAIN

Pain classification does not necessarily define the diagnosis; however, it usually helps in guiding the treatment. Careful characterization of the pain facilitates prompt diagnosis and treatment. Multitude of systems exist for classifying pain, which include multidimensional classification system, such as IASP classification of chronic pain, and a variety of systems based on a single dimension of pain experience, such as those based on pain duration, underlying pathophysiology, and origin/source of pain, which are most commonly used.

Based on Duration

Traditionally, pain has been categorized as either acute or chronic. More recently, the term "persistent pain" has been used to differentiate chronic pain that defies intervention from conditions, where continuing (persistent) pain is

> **BOX 10.3:** Key features of acute and chronic pain.
>
> **Acute pain**
> - Pain usually concordant with degree of tissue damage, which remits with resolution of the injury
> - Reflects activation of nociceptors and/or sensitized central neurons
> - Often associated with autonomic nervous system and other protective reflex responses (e.g., muscle spasm, "splinting").
>
> **Chronic pain**
> - Low levels of identified underlying pathology that do not explain the presence and/or extent of the pain
> - Perpetuated by factors remote from the cause
> - Continuous or intermittent with or without acute exacerbations
> - Symptoms of ANS hyperactivity less common
> - Irritability, social withdrawal, depressed mood and vegetative symptoms (e.g., changes in sleep, appetite, and libido), disruption of work, and social relationships may be seen

a symptom of a treatable condition. More research has been devoted to chronic pain and its treatment, but acute and persistent pain confront the therapist most often. Recurrent pain includes repeated episodes of acute pain, such as recurrent low back strain, or chronic pain in which the symptoms are intermittent, such as a migraine headache. **Box 10.3** shows the key features of acute and chronic pain.

Acute Pain

Acute pain was once defined simply in terms of duration. It is now viewed as a "complex, unpleasant experience with emotional and cognitive, as well as sensory features that occur in response to tissue trauma." Earlier definitions state it is localized, occurs in the proportion of intensity of the stimuli, and lasts only as long as the stimuli or the tissue damage exists. In contrast to chronic pain, relatively high levels of pathology usually accompany acute pain and the pain resolves with healing of the underlying injury. Acute pain is usually nociceptive but may be neuropathic. Common sources of acute pain include trauma, surgery, labor, medical procedures, and acute disease states. Acute pain serves an important biological function, as it warns of the potential for or extent of injury. A host of protective reflexes (e.g., withdrawal of a damaged limb, muscle spasm, and autonomic responses) often accompany it. Usually it is relieved by interventions directed at correcting the injury.

Chronic Pain

Chronic pain was once defined as pain that extends 3 or 6 months beyond onset or beyond the expected period of healing. Sometimes, referred to as intractable pain, it is defined as pain that continues after the stimulus has been removed or the tissue damage heals. However, new definitions differentiate chronic pain from acute pain based on more than just time. Chronic pain is now

recognized as pain that extends beyond the period of healing, with levels of identified pathology that are often low and insufficient to explain the presence and/or extent of the pain. Chronic pain is also defined as a persistent pain that "disrupts sleep and normal living, ceases to serve a protective function, and instead degrades health and functional capability." Thus, unlike acute pain, chronic pain serves no adaptive purpose. Chronic pain may be nociceptive, neuropathic, or both and caused by injury (e.g., trauma and surgery), malignant conditions, or a variety of chronic non–life-threatening conditions (e.g., arthritis, fibromyalgia, and neuropathy). In some cases, chronic pain exists de novo with no apparent cause. Although injury often initiates chronic pain, factors pathogenetically and physically remote from its cause may perpetuate it. Environmental and affective factors also can exacerbate and perpetuate chronic pain, leading to disability and maladaptive behavior.

Based on Underlying Pathophysiology

Neuropathic Pain

Pain initiated or caused by a primary lesion or dysfunction of the CNS is referred to as central neuropathic pain. It is caused by abnormal signals in the CNS or PNS, demonstrating injury or impairment. Causes of neuropathic pain may include inflammation, trauma, infections, tumors, metabolic diseases, toxins, or neurological disease.

Dermatomal: peripheral neuropathic pain

Nondermatomal: central neuropathic pain, fibromyalgia.

Peripheral/Nociceptive Pain

It results from noxious irritation of the nociceptors. The character of peripheral pain depends on the location and intensity of the noxious stimulation, as well as which fibers carry the information into the dorsal gray matter. Information carried on A-delta fibers is sharp and well localized, begins rapidly, and lasts only as long as the stimulus is present, whereas information carried on C fibers is dull and diffuse, has a delayed onset, and lasts longer than the duration of the stimulus, resulting in sharp fast pain and slow dull pain, respectively. In nociceptive pain, the CNS is functioning appropriately. There is a close association between the intensity of the stimulus and the perception of pain, indicating real or potential tissue damage.

Inflammatory Pain

It increases sensory sensitivity after tissue damage, discouraging use and further damage, allowing for tissue repair; the pain is due to hypersensitivity resulting from peripheral injury, pathology, or other inflammatory process. Inflammatory pain is generally a beneficial mechanism for encouraging rest of the involved tissues; however, it becomes counterproductive when severe or ongoing.

Based on Origin

Visceral pain arises from visceral organs, while pain coming from tissues is called somatic pain.

Visceral Pain

It is diffuse, difficult to localize and often referred to a distant, usually superficial, structure. It may be accompanied by symptoms such as nausea, vomiting, changes in vital signs as well as emotional manifestations. The pain may be described as sickening, deep, squeezing, and dull.

Somatic

It is a severe chronic or aching pain that is inconsistent with injury or pathology to specific anatomical structures and cannot be explained by any physical cause because the sensory input can come from so many different structures supplied by the same nerve root. Superficial somatic pain may be localized, but deep somatic pain is more diffuse and may be referred.

On examination, somatic pain may be reproduced, but visceral pain is not reproduced by movement.

Localized Pain

Pain confined to the site of distribution origin (e.g., cutaneous pain, some visceral pain, arthritis, and tendonitis).

Referred Pain

Pain that is referred to a distant structure is known as referred pain (e.g., visceral pain such as angina, pancreatitis, appendicitis, and acute cholecystitis). It is felt at a point other than its origin and usually follows a specific pattern. It is the result of a convergence of the primary afferent neurons from deep structures and muscles to secondary neurons that also have a cutaneous receptive field.

Projected Pain

Pain transferred along the course of a nerve with a segmental distribution (e.g., herpes zoster) or a peripheral distribution (e.g., trigeminal neuralgia).

Classification of Chronic Pain

Apart from those mentioned above, the 11th edition of International Classification of Disease (ICD-11) has classified chronic pain into subtypes **(Box 10.4)**. Chronic pain is a frequent condition, affecting an estimated 20% of people worldwide, and this code should be used if a pain condition persists or recurs for longer than 3 months.

Chronic primary pain is chronic pain in one or more anatomical regions that is characterized by significant emotional distress (anxiety, anger/frustration, or depressed mood) and functional disability (interference in daily life activities and reduced participation in social

> **BOX 10.4:** ICD-11 classification of chronic pain.
> - Chronic primary pain
> - Chronic cancer-related pain
> - Chronic postsurgical and post-traumatic pain
> - Chronic neuropathic pain
> - Chronic secondary headache and/or orofacial pain
> - Chronic secondary visceral pain
> - Chronic secondary musculoskeletal pain

roles). Chronic primary pain is multifactorial: biological, psychological, and social factors contribute to the pain syndrome. Patients with chronic primary pain often report increased depressed and anxious mood, as well as anger and frustration. In addition, the pain significantly interferes with daily life activities and participation in social roles. Chronic primary pain is a frequent condition, and treatment should be geared toward the reduction of pain-related distress and disability.

Chronic cancer-related pain is a new diagnosis, since cancer pain has not been represented in the ICD earlier. It is caused by the cancer (primary tumor or metastases) or cancer treatment. Chronic postsurgical and post-traumatic pain is frequent after multiple trauma (46–85%) and is now represented in ICD. It develops after a surgical procedure or tissue injury and persists at least 3 months after surgery or tissue trauma. It excludes cancer-related pain but may include neuropathic pain. Due to the different causality/medicolegal aspects, postsurgical pain and pain after all other trauma are differentiated.

Both primary and secondary headaches or orofacial pains (OFP), including temporomandibular disorders that occur at least on 50% of the days in the last 3 months, comprise chronic headache or OFP. **Chronic secondary pain** following involvement of visceral and systemic structures is also included in this code. Persistent recurrent pain originating from the internal organs of the head, neck, thorax, abdomen, or pelvic cavity comprises chronic visceral pain. Chronic musculoskeletal pain syndromes with a direct involvement of bone, joint, muscle, spine, or related soft tissue are also included in ICD-11. This is limited to nociceptive pain from these tissues and thus excludes referred pain and neuropathies but includes muscle pain due to spasticity. Whereas conditions with causes that are incompletely understood, such as chronic widespread pain, nonspecific pain, chronic pelvic pain should be categorized into chronic primary pain.

PSYCHOSOCIAL IMPLICATIONS OF PAIN

Pain is an individual, multifactorial experience influenced by culture, previous pain events, beliefs, moods, and ability to cope. As defined earlier, pain is a psychological phenomenon. Pain-related disability is generally related to psychological factors. A soldier wounded with a gunshot is still capable of continuing the war, whereas a regular citizen may perceive an injection to be painful.

Psychosocial issues include factors that affect patient's ability to cope with pain and thus impact the treatment planning. They are as follows:

- Fear–avoidance behavior (FAB)
- Coping, catastrophizing, and acceptance
- Depression and anxiety
- Psychosocial factors associated with chronic pain
- Pain behavior clusters

Cognitive development and individual understanding of pain are factors to be considered too.

Fear–Avoidance Behavior

Chronic pain involves the limbic system along with the CNS pathways. Therefore, it elicits emotional responses on recognizing pain intensity and localization. Patients own experiences of the past of not getting better or recurrence of pain makes them avoid certain maneuvers and activities. This is the beginning of a vicious cycle of an activity causing pain, which increases fear, leading to a decrease in physical activity. This further leads to complications of inactivity, disuse and deconditioning, muscle atrophy, and joint stiffness. FAB should not be confused with nonadherence or noncompliance. "Kinesiophobia" is a term used to describe fear of movement as movement may cause pain.

Clinical Pearl

Fear–avoidance behavior in a patient needs to be recognized and tackled for complete rehabilitation.

Coping, Catastrophizing, and Acceptance

As pain becomes chronic, there is less correlation of findings of pain assessment by the therapist with the impairments or functional limitations that the patient complains about. One of the risk factors extensively studied is "coping," i.e., the individual's ability to manage his/her pain or distress. This suggests the need for biopsychosocial-based rehabilitation in the management of chronic pain.

Catastrophizing behavior is one that describes the pain as being terrible, incapacitating, or unbearable. Catastrophizing is currently defined as: "an exaggerated negative mental set brought to bear during actual or anticipated painful experience." It has been found to be correlated with increased pain perception, depression, and pain severity in chronic pain. In other words, catastrophizing not only contributes to heightened levels of pain and emotional distress but also increases the probability that the pain condition will persist over an extended period of time. Preoperative fear of pain is associated with higher pain levels postoperatively.

Acceptance of the pain situation has been found to improve physical and psychological functioning in individuals with chronic pain. It involves a shift away from finding a cure to doing tasks that are pain free.

Clinical Pearl

It is becoming increasingly clear that catastrophic thinking in relation to pain might be a risk factor for chronicity. Negative emotions can be a hindrance in management of pain.

Depression and Anxiety

Depression and pain have been found to be interrelated. Chronic pain can lead to depression and depression can lead to increased perception of pain. It is a linear relation, with increased pain intensity associated with higher risk of depression. Stress, anxiety, and depression need to be recognized and the patient should be referred for further care.

Psychosocial Factors Associated with Chronic Pain

Personal habits of addiction describe the emotional level of the patient. History of physical abuse and previous **pain and trauma** has been shown to influence intervention in chronic pain. **Social reinforcement** can be a powerful tool in shaping pain behavior. **Rapport building and relationship and compliance** of patients are also affected with chronic pain, which may be a reason for unsatisfactory results.

Alert flags to chronic pain need to be analyzed appropriately. Yellow flags have been defined as psychosocial factors that increase the likelihood that acute pain will progress into chronic pain and disability. As per a terminology proposed by Nicholas et al., yellow flags include beliefs, emotional responses, and pain behavior; orange flags represent frank psychiatric symptoms; and blue flags reflect the interaction between work and health perceptions. **Table 10.3** outlines these terminologies.

Table 10.3: Flags for chronic pain.

Flag	Underlying problem	Clinical examples
Red	Serious physical pathology	Fracture, tumor, and cauda equina
Orange	Psychiatric problem	Depression, post-traumatic stress disorder, and personality disorders
Yellow	Beliefs, appraisals, and judgment	Negative pain beliefs and expectation of poor outcome
	Emotional responses	Fear, anxiety, catastrophization, and distress
	Pain behavior, including pain coping strategies	Fear–avoidance behavior and dependence on passive interventions
Blue	Perceptions about relationship between work and pain	Beliefs such as work will cause further injury and pain, supervisor and coworkers are unsupportive
Black	System or contextual obstacles	

Table 10.4: Pain behavior clusters.

Classification	Characteristics	Management approaches recommended
Well-adapted	Low levels of pain, distress and interference with life, high self-efficacy, and physically active	Pain education, coping skills, and CBT
Dysfunctional	Highly intense pain, interferes with activity, pain behavior, social support and solicitousness, and negative pain self-talk	CBT and operant restructuring
Distressed with little social support	Low self-efficacy, social support, solicitousness of others, distress, and daily perceived stress	CBT, including stress and pain management
Psychophysi-ologically highly reactive	High stress reactivity, muscle tension, daily stress, low social support, low activity, and little reinforcement for pain behavior	Relaxation, BFB, and CBT

(BFB: biofeedback; CBT: cognitive behavioral therapy.)

Pain Behavior Clusters

Pain behavior refers to the various actions or postural displays that are enacted during the experience of pain. FAB has been discussed, other upcoming concepts are discussed in this segment. Pain persistence behavior is when individual ignores or denies pain, and continues activity in spite of pain, sets unrealistic goals, ignores physical limits, and has low social support **(Table 10.4)**.

PAIN ASSESSMENT

Pain assessment is the key to effective pain management. A comprehensive pain assessment is needed to generate appropriate differential diagnosis. Measurement of pain is an important component of clinical practice. Studies have found that two of the chief barriers for healthcare professionals are poor pain assessment and lack of knowledge about pain.

Clinical Pearl

Pain assessment has three **keystones**—history, examination, and special tests or investigations.

Additionally, clinicians' personal belief systems, attitudes, and fears can directly influence the manner in which they and their patients respond to the varied dimensions of pain management. Its importance is evident in the frequency with which it drives healthcare utilization and its impact on the QOL. Careful hearing of patient's symptoms will help direct the examination and will be useful in narrowing the differential diagnosis. The purpose of assessment is to get information regarding the origin of pain and the problems caused because of or related to pain so appropriate treatment can be given. Therefore, examination needs to be very precise. The subjective and objective dimensions of pain as described earlier need to be documented.

Assessments used in chronic pain that focus only on biological and physiological aspects may not be valid in predicting impairment or disability. It is therefore important to consider measures that may be able to identify how the various tools assimilate into a complete analysis of the individual's pain condition. A step-wise approach to assessment has been advised, beginning with a general evaluation of the factors under consideration and leading up to a more definitive diagnosis. By taking this multidimensional view, the biopsychosocial approach to assessment will lead to a better understanding of the patient's pain condition and, ultimately, to a comprehensive treatment protocol customized to the individual's unique situation.

Clinical Pearl

History is most important and requires time, patience and effort. Examination confirms what history implies.

History and Examination

History reveals how the problem started, the site of the problem, and why the problem occurred. History should look for red flags too **(Box 10.5)**. It should include all the following **(Box 10.6)**:

A. **Site, location, body maps:**
- Where is the pain?
- Is it a localized pain or is it generalized or does it radiate down to any limb?
- Can the site be shown on a body map?
- Has the pain moved or spread?
- Are there trigger points?
- Is the pain neuropathic in origin? Does it have a dermatomal pattern? or Is it peripheral, visceral, or somatic?

BOX 10.5: Red flags for pain assessment.

Red flags: Night pains are indicative of severe conditions such as malignancies. They are usually seen because the protective muscle spasm relaxes and uncontrolled movement causes excruciating pain because of which patient gets up in the middle of the night.

Pain not related to movement may not have a musculoskeletal etiology but could be because of a systemic cause that needs to be ruled out. An example is low back pain not changing with body position or having diurnal variations could be because of kidney problems, left arm pain could be because of cardiac problems.

> **BOX 10.6:** The pneumonic QISS TAPED can be used to remember elements of assessment.
>
> **Q**uality of pain
> **I**mpact of pain on activities of daily living, function and quality of life
> **S**ite and location
> **S**everity and intensity
> **T**emporal characteristics
> **A**ggravating and alleviating factors
> **P**ast responses and preferences
> **E**xpectations and goals
> **D**iagnosis and physical examination

Referred pain may be perceived as originating from a structure innervated by the same spinal segmental level or from the same sclerotome or dermatome. It is generally felt deep with indistinct boundaries. The areas of pain may be marked on a body chart **(Fig. 10.16)**.

B. Temporal characteristics or diurnal variations: The onset, duration, and progression of pain is to be asked.

- When did it start, since when is it paining?
- Mode of onset—sudden onset or gradual.
- How has it progressed over time—Is it the same, or has it worsened?
- Duration—What is the chronicity and frequency of pain? It is important to differentiate whether the pain is acute pain or chronic pain as described earlier.
- Is the pain constant, periodic, episodic, or occasional? Constant pain is suggestive of chemical irritation, tumors, or possible visceral lesions.
- Timing of pain—In the morning, for a short period and better with activity is indicative of degenerative arthropathy. If it continues for more hours, it is indicative of inflammatory arthropathy.
- Congenital—Is the problem since birth?

Clinical Pearl

The more acute the pain, the more careful should an examiner be in examination.

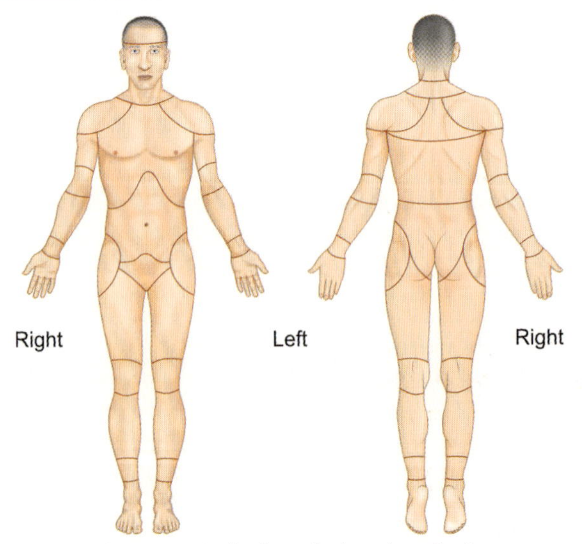

Fig. 10.16: Body charts for location of pain.

C. Aggravating and alleviating factors or provocative and relieving factors:

- What makes it better or worse?—Rest or activity
- Has there been a change with treatment?
- What are the present medications? Is the pain decreasing after pain medications?
- Related to movement—Does it change with movement? This indicates irritability of the tissue. It also indicates mechanical pain. Does the pain occur at the beginning of the movement, in the middle or at the end of a movement?
- Relation to posture or position—pain on sitting cross legged suggestive of piriformis syndrome.
- Is there a repetitive stress that is leading to the injury and pain? Any occupation-related factors that may be responsible for the pain?
- How is the sleep of the patient?

D. Quality of pain:

- Characteristics of pain can be another means of identifying the cause of pain.
- Does the client use words indicating mechanical (pressing, bursting, stabbing), chemical (burning), neural (numb, "pins and needles"), or vascular (throbbing) origin?
- Sharp, burning pain is associated with nerve and runs in the distribution of specific nerves. Deep boring and localized pain indicates origin in the bone. Diffuse aching and poorly localized tends to be vascular and may be referred to other areas of the body. Muscle pain is usually hard to localize, is dull and aching, is often aggravated by injury, and may be referred to other areas **(Table 10.5)**.

E. Severity, quantity or intensity of pain: There are many scales to measure the severity or intensity of pain and to quantify the amount of pain. The rating describes the patient's interpretation and is a combination of physical, psychological, and emotional variations. Pain assessment can be performed under static and dynamic conditions depending on patient's complaint.

Unidimensional scales: These scales only assess pain and no other dimension. Patients' self-report is the gold standard of pain assessment.

Table 10.5: Type of pain and its origin.	
Type of pain	*Structure*
Cramping dull aching	Muscle
Dull aching	Ligament, joint capsule
Sharp shooting	Nerve root
Sharp bright lightning like	Nerve
Sharp severe intolerable	Fracture
Burning pressure such as stinging aching	Sympathetic
Deep dull	Bone
Throbbing diffused	Vascular

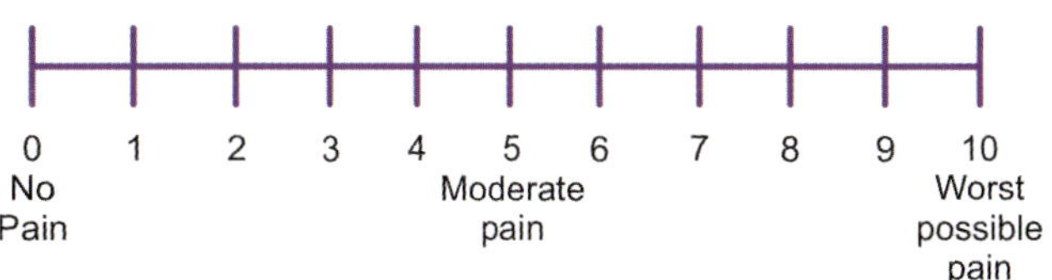

Fig. 10.18: Numerical pain rating scale.

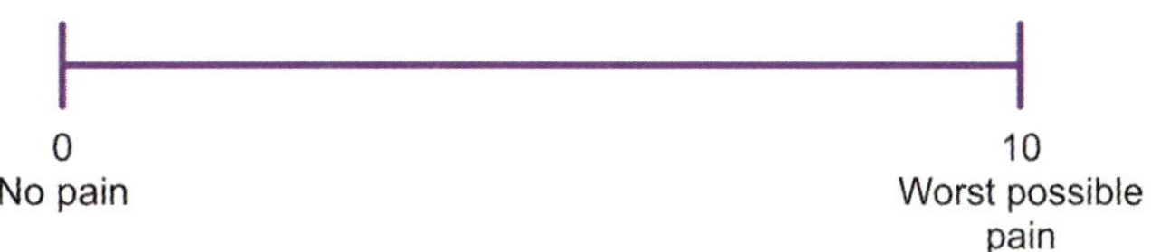

Fig. 10.19: Visual analog scale.

Clinical Pearl

Pain is a subjective experience. The experience, tolerance, and meaning of the sensation are unique for each individual.

Clinical Pearl

The pain measurement tool should be appropriate to the individual according to his age, cognitive and emotional level, and culture.

1. **Verbal rating scale:** The patient is asked about the severity of pain. Response is noted as no pain, mild, moderate, and severe. The advantage of this scale is that it is easy to express and understand especially in illiterate population and elderly and not time-consuming. The disadvantage is lack of reproducibility. Also the difference in pain may not be assessable.
2. **Binary scales:** There are only two answers possible to the question, "Do you have pain?"—"yes" or "no," "Has the pain reduced?"—"yes" or "no." This is again easy to understand but not reproducible.
3. **Faces rating scale (Wong–Baker scale):** The patient is presented with pictures of various facial expressions ranging from a smiling face to an extremely unhappy one. The patient is asked to point to the face that is closest to his/her feelings. The advantage is that it is easy to understand and can be used in conditions where there are language and communication issues as in deaf and dumb patients or in neurological conditions where patient may have aphasia **(Fig. 10.17)**.
4. **Numeric pain rating scale (NPRS) (Fig. 10.18):** This is one of the commonly used scales. It is a straight line marked from 0 to 10 with equal divisions. It has good validity and reliability. A change in 2 points from baseline scores is considered to be the minimal clinically important difference to consider a positive response for treatment. This is an ordinal scale but because of its high validity the scale can be considered equivalent to interval scales. The patient is asked to make three pain ratings, corresponding to current, best, and worst pain experienced over the past 24

hours. The average of the three ratings can be used to represent the patient's level of pain over the previous 24 hours. A rating of 0–3 is indicative of mild pain, 4–7 is moderate pain, and 8–10 is severe pain [minimal detectable change (MDC) over 24 hours—31.8% or 3.5 points; test–retest reliability—0.63].

5. **Visual analog scale (VAS) (Fig. 10.19):** It is a 10-cm horizontal line with markings at both ends, one end has no pain and the other has worst pain imaginable. The patient has to mark a point on the line to indicate the severity of pain. This is a simple and efficient measure of pain. It may be difficult to understand compared to the other scales but has good reliability and validity **(Box 10.7)**.
6. **4-item pain intensity measure (P4 scale) (Fig. 10.20):** The P4 consists of four items that address pain intensity in the morning, afternoon, evening, and with activity over the past 2 days. Each item is scored on a 0-to-10 NPRS, therefore the total P4 scores can vary from 0 (no pain) to 40 (the highest possible pain level). Most patients can complete the P4 in less than a minute and clinicians can score the measure in 5 seconds without the use of computational aids (test–retest reliability—0.78; MDC—22%).
7. **WILDA approach to pain assessment:** This method incorporates five components of pain assessment—**W**ords to describe pain (there are 21 words), **I**ntensity, **L**ocation, **D**uration, and **A**ggravating and alleviating factors. It is presented as a pocket card that can be used by healthcare providers to summarize their assessment. The other side of the card has a VAS to measure the intensity of pain **(Box 10.8)**.

F. Impact of pain on ADL, function and QOL/ multidimensional scales: Multidimensional scales are

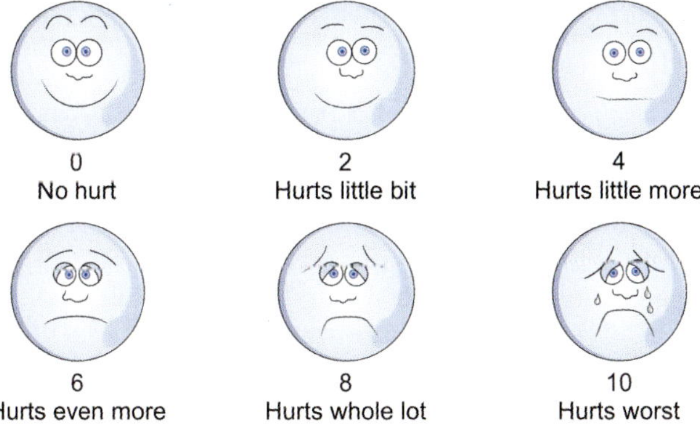

Fig. 10.17: Wong–Baker scale of pain.

BOX 10.7: NPRS and VAS.

There is a moderate association between numeric pain rating scale (NPRS) and visual analog scale (VAS). Majority of patients of all ages and both genders prefer NRS. Self-reporting of pain should be used when possible as pain by definition is a subjective experience. Verbal rating scale, NPRS, and VAS have excellent test–retest reliability. VAS is most reliable.

On average, how bad has your pain been...											
	No pain										Pain as bad as it can be
In the *morning* over the past 2 days?	0	1	2	3	4	5	6	7	8	9	10
In the *afternoon* over the past 2 days?	0	1	2	3	4	5	6	7	8	9	10
In the *evening* over the past 2 days?	0	1	2	3	4	5	6	7	8	9	10
With *activity* over the past 2 days?	0	1	2	3	4	5	6	7	8	9	10

Fig. 10.20: P4 scale.

BOX 10.8: OPQRST Pneumonic.

O – onset
P – provocation/palliation/aggravating and alleviating factors
Q – quality/quantity
R – region
S – severity
T – timing

---

used to assess pain and the effect that pain has on physical and psychological functioning. What is the impact of pain in patient's life? Does it not allow doing something that they should be or want to do?

Clinical Pearl

It is important to understand that pain can adversely affect patient's function, quality of life, emotional state, social and vocational function, and general well-being. Therefore, pain assessment should be multidimensional when required. Even if psychological components do exist it is necessary to examine and rule out physical components for a better treatment plan.

1. **McGill pain questionnaire:** It was formed by Melzack and Torgerson in 1971. It consists of 20 descriptive words, which can be divided into three major dimensions. 10 sets describe sensory-discriminative (nociceptive pathway), 5 sets describe motivational-affective (reticular and limbic structure), 1 set describes cognitive evaluation, and 4 sets describe miscellaneous dimensions. The scale is very descriptive with words that characterize pain and correlate well with pain syndromes. The person needs to be able to describe the pain that may be difficult under high level of anxiety and with people who are less educated. This scale may be culturally inappropriate for many countries because of language barriers.

2. **Brief pain inventory:** It has two parts, one measuring the intensity of pain (sensory dimension) and the other measuring its interference with the patient's life (reactive dimension). This scale is valid in measuring cancer pain and shows good sensitivity to treatment. It is now also used as a generic pain questionnaire for other chronic pain conditions. It is available in a short (9 items) form and long (17 items) form (internal consistency—0.85–0.88).

3. **West Haven–Yale Multidimensional Pain Inventory (WHYMPI/MPI):** The WHYMPI assesses chronic pain in individuals. It is based on the cognitive behavioral theory of pain. Advantages are its brevity and clarity, multidimensional focus, and its strong psychometric properties. Three parts of the inventory, comprised 12 subscales, examine the impact of pain on the patient's lives, the responses of others to patient's communications of pain, and the extent to which patient's participate in common daily activities.

4. **Medical outcomes study 36-item health survey (SF36):** The QOL questionnaire has two questions related to intensity of pain and interference in the last 4 weeks.

5. **Memorial pain assessment card:** This consists of three separate VASs to assess pain, pain relief, and mood. Card includes a set of adjectives to describe pain intensity.

6. **Global pain questionnaire:** This scale has subsets of questions about clinical pain intensity, feelings about pain, clinical outcomes of pain, and activities affected because of pain. Each subset has a score of 25 with a total of 100.

7. **The Pain Disability Index (PDI):** PDI is a simple and rapid instrument for measuring the impact that pain has on the ability of a person to participate in essential life activities. This can be used to evaluate patients initially to monitor them over time and to judge the effectiveness of interventions. It has modest test–retest reliability and discriminates between patients with low and high levels of disability (intraclass correlation coefficient for test–retest reliability—0.91).

G. Quality or nature of pain: Screening tools for neuropathic pain, i.e., sharp, burning type.

Interview and physical tests:

1. **Leeds assessment of neuropathic symptoms and signs:** It consists of two components in the form of symptoms and signs. Each item has two possible answers, "yes" or "no." Score > or equal to 12/24 indicates pain to be neuropathic. There is a need for confirmation by clinical examination and pin prick test.

2. **Douleur Neuropathique en 4 Questions (DN4):** It is a screening tool for neuropathic pain consisting of interview questions (DN4-interview) and physical tests. It has a total score of 10.

Interview based questionnaire:

1. **Neuropathic pain:** It is a self-questionnaire consisting of 12 items of which 10 are related to sensations or sensory response and 2 are related to affective component. Each item is scored on a Likert scale of 0 (no pain) to 100 (worst possible pain) (sensitivity—66.6%, specificity—74.4%).

2. **Pain DETECT:** It is a patient-based self-report questionnaire consisting of nine items. There are 7 sensory descriptions that are scored on a scale of 0 (no) to 5 (strongly) and 2 related to the spatial (radiating) and temporal characteristics that are scored as 1 (yes) or 0 (no). A score of >19 indicates neuropathic pain is likely and <12 is indicative of the pain less likely to be neuropathic. No clinical examination is needed with this scale.

3. **ID pain—a neuropathic pain screen:** It is a self-reported questionnaire consisting of 5 sensory descriptions and one item regarding pain located in the joints. Higher scores indicate neuropathic pain. It is used in the geriatric population.

H. Past responses and preferences:
- Did the patient have pain in the past?
- What did he/she do at that time?
- Information regarding other past, personal, and family history should also be collected.

I. Expectations and goals: Patient has an important role in the practice of evidence-based physiotherapy. Patients' knowledge and beliefs about pain are assumed to play a role in pain perception, function, and response to treatment. Patients may be reluctant to tell their healthcare providers when they have pain, may attempt to minimize its severity, may not know they can expect pain relief, and may be concerned about taking pain medications for fear of deleterious effects. A comprehensive approach to pain assessment includes evaluating patients' knowledge and beliefs about pain and its management and reviewing common misconceptions about analgesia.

Diagnosis and Physical Examination

Following the assessment of pain, a thorough musculoskeletal or neurological examination needs to be done followed by special tests such as electrodiagnostic testing and imaging or laboratory findings to confirm the diagnosis. Other special tests can be performed to reproduce the pain.

Algometry Testing

Pressure pain threshold (PPT) is defined as the minimum force applied, which induces pain. This measure has proven to be commonly useful in evaluating tenderness symptoms. Both thermal and PPT **(Fig. 10.21)** digital algometer are available.

Nonverbal Assessment

Subjects who are unconscious or cannot respond to commands must be assessed by observational means such as body language, movement, and nonverbal pain

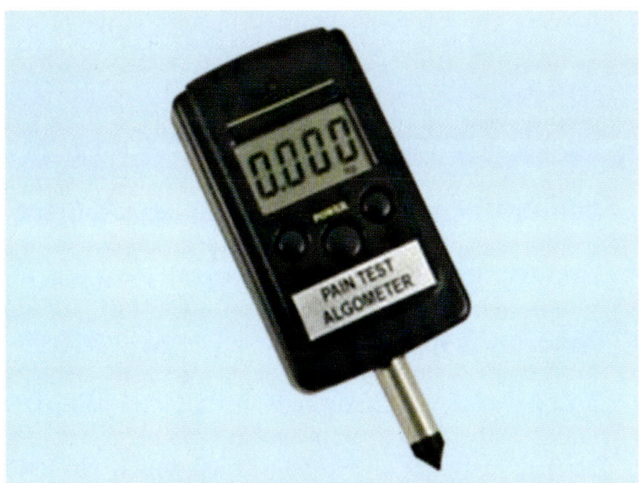

Fig. 10.21: Digital pressure algometer.

behavior. Reliance on nonverbal cues, e.g., changes in vital signs, moaning, facial grimacing, or muscle tenseness—is not practical or reliable. Diverse responses to pain atypical of conventional pain behaviors have been noted in patients. For example, a patient who may normally rock and moan may become quiet and be withdrawn when experiencing pain.

Observation of posture and gait along with assistive devices can also add information to help diagnose.

Observation of overt pain behavior may contribute to information regarding the physical and psychological aspects of pain. Overt behavior includes guarding, bracing, rubbing, grimacing, and sighing.

Pain Assessment Tools for Children

1. **FLACC scale:** The acronym stands for Face, Legs, Activity, Cry, and Consolability. Each category is scored on a 0–2 scale, which results in a total pain score of 0–10. The person assessing the child should observe the child briefly and then score according to the description supplied. It has a high degree of usefulness for cognitively impaired and critically ill children.

2. **Wong–Baker FACES pain scale**
3. **VAS—8 years and older**
4. **Physiological considerations.**

With the presence of pain, vitals such as heart rate and blood pressure may increase, respiratory rate may shift from normal, i.e., increase, decrease, or change pattern, and oxygen saturation may decrease. These cannot be used in isolation.

Psychological Assessment Tools

Patients in pain may have some psychological disorders such as anxiety, depression, and behavior modifications. Following scales can be used for the assessment of psychological aspects in the patient.

- **Pain Catastrophizing Scale (PCS):** The PCS comprises of 13 items. The participants are asked to rate the 13 feelings or thoughts when in pain while recalling the past painful experiences, on a 5-point scale with 0 being not at all and 4 being all the time. Three subscale scores that assess rumination, magnification and helplessness, and a total score are obtained. Total score is calculated by adding all the individual item scores. The minimum score is 0 and maximum score is 52. The PCS has adequate to excellent internal consistency (coefficient alphas: total PCS = 0.87, rumination = 0.87, magnification = 0.66, and helplessness = 0.78).

- **The Pain Self-Efficacy Questionnaire (PSEQ):** The PSEQ is a 10-item questionnaire that was developed to assess the confidence that people with ongoing pain have in performing activities when in pain. The PSEQ can be used in all persisting pain presentations. It covers a range of functions, including household work, socializing, work, as well as how the person can cope with pain without medication. It takes only 2 minutes to complete. Internal consistency is high (0.92 Cronbach's alpha) and test–retest reliability of a 3-month period is high. Validity is reflected in high correlations with measures of pain-related disability, coping strategies, and other more activity-specific measure of self-efficacy beliefs, the Self-Efficacy Scale. The PSEQ-2 appears to be a robust measure of pain self-efficacy.

- **Dallas Pain Questionnaire (DPQ):** The DPQ assesses the amount of chronic spinal pain that affects four aspects of the patients' lives, including daily and work–leisure activities, anxiety–depression, and social interest. The DPQ is both an externally reliable and internally consistent instrument. DPQ can be used for clinical and research purposes.

- **The Tampa Scale of Kinesiophobia (TSK-11):** The TSK is a 17-item questionnaire, which can be used to assess the subjective rating of kinesiophobia or fear of movement. The TSK is a self-completed questionnaire. The minimum score is 17 and maximum score is 68. A higher score indicates higher degree of kinesiophobia, whereas a lower score indicates lesser degree of kinesiophobia.

  TSK-11 scales have been proved to be reliable and valid as demonstrated by acceptable levels of internal consistency, as well as evidence of discriminant, concurrent criterion-related, and incremental validity. The items have been found to be adequately competent in predicting the desired variables. Somatic focus uniquely predicts perceived disability, while activity avoidance uniquely predicts actual physical performance, controlling for pain severity. The 2-factor structure of the TSK-11 has been found to be a brief, reliable, and valid measure of kinesiophobia for chronic pain patients. The TSK-11 can be used in future research and in clinical settings.

- **FAB Questionnaire (FABQ):** Fear-avoidance beliefs about physical activity and work might be responsible for certain behavior in relation to low back pain and disability. The Fear-Avoidance Beliefs Questionnaire (FABQ) is based on the theories of FAB. It addresses the patient's beliefs regarding the affection of low back pain by physical activity and work. It has two components—physical activity (FAB-PA) and work (FAB-W).

- **Patient Health Questionnaire (PHQ-9):** The PHQ is a self-administered version of the PRIME-MD diagnostic instrument for common mental disorders. The PHQ-9 is the depression module based on the DSM-IV criteria. It scores each DSM-IV criteria on a 4-point scale where 0 is not at all and 3 is nearly every day. It has been validated for use in primary care as a tool to monitor the severity of depression and response to treatment. It cannot be used as screening tool for depression. PHQ-9 score ≥10 had a sensitivity of 88% and a specificity of 88% for major depression. In addition to making criteria-based diagnoses of depressive disorders, the PHQ-9 is also a reliable and valid measure of depression severity. These characteristics plus its brevity make the PHQ-9 a useful clinical and research tool.

- **Beck Depression Inventory (BDI):** The BDI is a 21-item, self-report rating inventory that measures characteristic attitudes and symptoms of depression. The BDI demonstrates high internal consistency, with alpha coefficients of 0.86 and 0.81 for psychiatric and nonpsychiatric populations, respectively.

- **Hamilton Depression Rating Scale (HAM-D):** The HAM-D form also lists 21 items, the scoring of which is based on the first 17. It generally takes about 15–20 minutes to complete the interview and to score the results. Eight items are scored on a 5-point scale, ranging from 0 = not present to 4 = severe. Nine items are scored from 0 to 2. The sensitivity of the scale was found to be 86.4% and the specificity was 92.2%.

- **Hospital Anxiety and Depression Scale (HADS):** HADS was originally developed by Zigmond and Snaith (1983) and is commonly used by doctors to determine the levels of anxiety and depression that a person is experiencing. The HADS is a 14-item scale that generates ordinal data.

- **Depression, Anxiety, and Stress Scale (DASS):** The DASS is a 42-item self-report instrument designed to measure the three related negative emotional states of depression, anxiety, and tension/stress. The DASS is a set of three self-report scales, which can measure the negative emotional states of depression, anxiety, and stress. In addition to the basic 42-item questionnaire, a short version, the DASS21, is also available with seven items per scale.

Clinical Pearl

A prerequisite to proper diagnosis is thorough knowledge of functional anatomy. Conclusion of examination must reveal what tissue has been impaired and what needs to be done.

Assessing Psychosocial Factors Affecting Chronic Pain

The SCEBS model addresses somatic/biological, psychological (cognitive, emotional, and behavioral), and social domains of chronic pain **(Box 10.9)**. Similarly, PSCEBSM model was adapted from SCEBS model, which includes pain type, somatic and medical factors, and psychological, social domains are similar to previous one. Last component motivation is assessed in this model, which consists of patients' perception of source of pain, expectations, and readiness to change **(Box 10.10)**.

BOX 10.9: SCEBS model of chronic pain assessment.	
1. Somatic	Symptoms, duration, nature, location, intensity, temporal variation, and diagnostic test results
2. Psychological	
2a. Cognition	• Expectation regarding PT • Attribution: Patients' explanation for the complaints • Catastrophizing: Thoughts and reactions to symptoms/complaints • Self-efficacy: Feeling of control over symptoms, ability to do things to decrease complaints
2b. Emotional	Feeling about the symptoms, emotional balance, insecurity, depression, anxiety, feeling overwhelmed
2c. Behavioral	• Dealing with the complaint: How the patient responds to symptoms, attempts to decrease symptoms, and success of the strategies • Functional limitation: Activities and extent to which they are limited by these complaints • Avoidance: Activities discontinued during or because of symptoms, anxiety about activities, what other people notice about your behavior during symptoms • Talking about complaints: With whom? How often? What do they say?
3. Social	Do others notice when you have complaints? What do they notice or think how do others react? What does your partner think causes your complaints? How do you feel about this? Do the complaints affect your social life, work/hobby/sports?

BOX 10.10: PSCEBSM model of chronic pain assessment.	
1. Pain type	Distinguish between nociceptive, neuropathic, and central sensitization
2. Somatic and medical factors	Comorbidities changed movement patterns, exercise capacity, strength:medications
3. Cognitive factors	Cognitions and perceptions about the physical and mental aspects of pain, expectations regarding care, prognosis, and emotional representation of pain. Catastrophizing, perceived injustice or harm
4. Emotional factors	Anger, anxiety, fear, depression, and post-traumatic stress. Fear of movement, avoidance behaviors, psychological issues related to work, family, finances, or social issues
5. Behavioral factors	Behavioral adaptations to pain: healthy response, fear-avoidance, pain persistence
6. Social factors	Housing/living situation, social environment, work, relationships. Prior treatments and attitudes toward prior/other healthcare providers. Social support
7. Motivation	Readiness to change, perceptions about the cause of pain and treatment expectations. Psychological flexibility, stage of change

Tools Specific for the Assessment of Chronic Pain (Table 10.6)

Table 10.6: Tools for assessing chronic pain.		
Scale	*Items*	*Properties*
BPI	Severity of pain, impact of pain on daily function, location of pain, pain medications, and amount of pain relief in the past 24 h or the past week	Cronbach's alpha reliability ranges from 0.77 to 0.91
CPG	Assesses two dimensions of overall chronic pain severity: pain intensity and pain-related disability	Cronbach's alpha = 0.74
PDQ	Measures disability caused by pain, with two main domains: functional condition, psychosocial component	Cronbach's alpha = 0.96
PEGA	Consists of intensity and interference domains, with overall score of 10	Cronbach's alpha = 0.73
Central sensitivity inventory	Two parts: Part A includes 25 questions related to common CSS symptoms. Part B determines if the patient has been diagnosed with certain CSS disorders or related disorders, such as anxiety and depression	Test–retest reliability = 0.817; Cronbach's alpha = 0.879

(BPI: brief pain inventory; CPG: chronic pain grade questionnaire; PDQ: pain disability questionnaire; PEGA: pain, enjoyment, and general activity)

PAIN MANAGEMENT

The WHO in 1986 developed the WHO analgesia ladder for guiding the physicians to deal with complaints of pain in cancer patients. Over the years, this analgesia ladder has been modified and revised. The WHO analgesia ladder is based on five basic principles that can be applied to patients with acute pain or chronic pain not having cancer (**Fig. 10.22**).

1. Administration of the analgesics via oral route
2. Proper timing of the analgesics
3. Dose of the analgesics should be decided based on the intensity of pain measured on a pain rating scale.
4. Doses of the analgesics should be tailor-made for the patient.
5. Prescription for the analgesic should be detailed.

The WHO ladder advises to prescribe analgesics in a step-wise fashion starting with nonopioid medications such as NSAIDs. The medications are then increased to weak opioids and later strong opioids if the pain persists or increases. There have been other revisions and modifications that have suggested the addition of neurosurgical procedures as a fourth step.

The American Pain Society has also given recommendations for the management of acute pain, chronic cancer and noncancer pain.

- The patients should be regularly screened for any pain-related symptoms, as the patients sometimes tend to withhold pain thinking it of as a normal phenomenon. Any pain should be identified and managed as promptly as possible.
- Any decision about the management of pain should be made after a detailed discussion between the healthcare provider, the patient, and the family. The management plan should be made according to the needs of the patient and the evidences available regarding each individual case.
- The treatment patterns should be improved so that the regular use of the analgesics is removed and a pattern

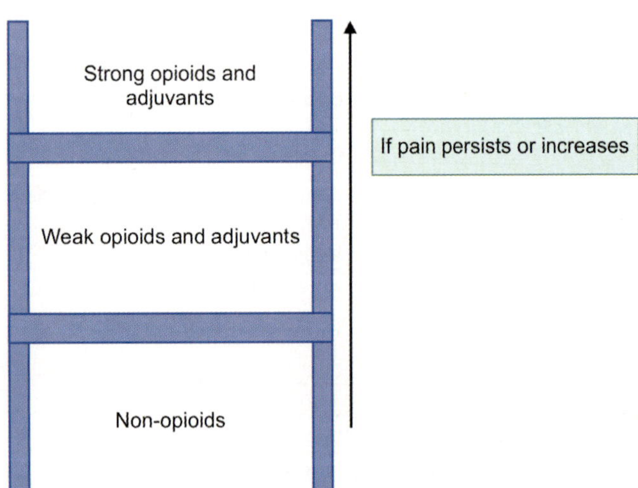

Fig. 10.22: WHO analgesia ladder.

> **BOX 10.11:** Pain can be managed by different means.
>
> Management of pain can be undertaken using:
> - Pharmacologic drugs
> - Interventions
> - Other nonpharmacologic treatment, including physiotherapy.

can be formulated where there is a combination of both scheduled and provided-as-needed doses of analgesia.

- Regular reassessment of pain and follow-up should be taken. The management plan should be modified according to any changes in the pain intensity, pain frequency, functional status of the individual, and any side effects.
- Regular monitoring of the treatment processes and the outcomes should be done (**Box 10.11**).

Pharmacological Management of Pain

This includes administration of analgesic drugs usually by the oral route (**Fig. 10.23**).

Non-opioids

These are weak analgesics having a combined use for pain relief, anti-inflammation and against pyrexia. They are not capable of depressing the CNS and are not likely to cause a physical dependence. Their primary action is on the peripheral mechanisms of pain while having a secondary impact of raising the pain pressure threshold.

Weak Opioids

These are less effective in relieving pain than the strong opioids but better than nonopioids. They are usually used for mild-to-moderate pain. Both codeine and dihydrocodeine have antitussive action. They can be used for treating dyspnea too.

Strong Opioids

These have a strong analgesic effect. However, they also cause CNS depression leading to drowsiness and sleep. Morphine has a soothing effect over the mood and it gives a sense of detachment from the surrounding environment. It also depresses the respiratory center, cough center, and temperature controlling centers. Hence, it has a high abuse rate. Methadone, on the other hand, has almost similar analgesic properties to morphine, but it has less intense subjective effects, leading to lower abuse rate than morphine. These are indicated for severe intense pain.

Methadone has become an important analgesic due to its strong analgesic effect and comparatively lesser side effects. It is now commonly used in the treatment of cancer pain, chronic pain not related to cancer, and neuropathic pain.

Table 10.7 describes some analgesic drugs with their adverse effects and contraindications.

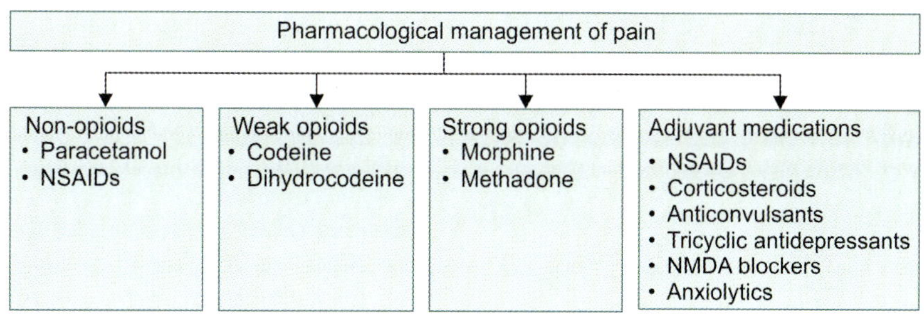

Fig. 10.23: Pharmacological management of pain.

Table 10.7: Analgesics.

Group	Name of the drug	Indications	Adverse effects	Precautions/contraindications
Nonopioids	NSAIDs and paracetamol	Mild pain	Peptic ulcers, gastric bleeding, chronic renal failure, and hepatic failure	Sensitivity to NSAIDs, children, liver disorders, diabetes, and some drugs during pregnancy
Weak opioids	Codeine and dihydrocodeine	Mild-to-moderate pain	Constipation	Respiratory distress, liver disease, infants, head injury, and patients at risk of paralytic ileus
Strong opioids	Morphine	Severe pain	Sedation, lethargy, hypotension, allergic reactions, morphine poisoning, and drug tolerance and dependence	Infants and elderly, patients having respiratory insufficiency, bronchial asthma, head injury, and liver and kidney disorders
	Methadone	Severe pain	Constipation, sweating, and loss of libido	Infants, alcoholism, hypersensitivity, head injury, liver or kidney disease, and respiratory distress

Adjuvant Analgesics

Adjuvant analgesics **(Table 10.8)** are drugs having some other primary indication but having pain relief as a secondary indication. Adjuvant analgesics should be considered along with the primary analgesics for better pain relief and QOL. N-methyl-D-aspartate (NMDA) receptor antagonists have shown preventive analgesic effects.

Acute pain: In the acute stage, a step-down approach on the ladder is used. When the patient is in intense pain, one can start directly at the third step and then descend down the ladder gradually as the pain is controlled. NSAIDs, paracetamol, and COX-2 inhibitors have been proven to be effective in providing analgesia for acute pain but their use is limited due to their multiple adverse effects. Patient-controlled analgesia

Table 10.8: Adjuvant analgesics.

Drug group	Name of the drug	Indications	Adverse effects
NSAIDs	Diclofenac	Soft tissue pain, liver pain, joint pains, rheumatoid arthritis, and rheumatic fever	Sensitivity to NSAIDs, children, liver disorders, diabetes, and some drugs during pregnancy
Corticosteroids	Dexamethasone and methylprednisolone	Rheumatoid arthritis, renal disorders, liver pain, and nerve compression	Cushing-like appearance, osteoporosis, peptic ulcers, diabetes mellitus, epilepsy, and renal failure
Anticonvulsants	Gabapentin and pregabalin	Neuralgic pain due to diabetic neuropathy and postherpetic neuralgia, migraine, complex regional pain syndrome	Sedation, tiredness, rashes and allergic reactions
Tricyclic antidepressants	Amitriptyline and nortriptyline	Neuropathic pain, and cancer pain	Sedation, confusion, seizures, and sexual problems, rashes
NMDA blockers	Ketamine and nitrous oxide	Dental and obstetric analgesia and neuromuscular pain	Peripheral neuropathy, bone marrow depression, and hypertension
Anxiolytics	Diazepam and alprazolam	Muscle spasm, neuropathic pain	Dizziness, vertigo, amnesia, and drug tolerance

is a safer option when drug dependence is believed to be low. In patients, who are unresponsive to opioids, ketamine has been proven to be of help.

Chronic pain: An upward movement or step-up approach is considered for the chronic pain or cancer pain. One should start at the first step and then gradually move up the ladder if the patient's pain persists or is aggravated. Chronic pain is usually treated with NSAIDs and opioids. However, the side effects of long-term use of NSAIDs are many. Cannabinoids have been proven to be mildly effective for the treatment of neuropathic pain, e.g., pain related to multiple sclerosis.

Interventional Management of Pain

Interventional management includes any injections given for pain relief, any surgical procedures done, or any implanted devices **(Table 10.9)**. Such management options should always be looked for before moving on to surgical options. Interventional therapies are most effective for uncontrollable and unremitting pain. Pain that is unresponsive to conventional analgesics or leads to major side effects can be treated with interventional therapies.

Guidelines for the use of interventional therapies:
- Pain should be tried to be managed using the traditional analgesics according to the WHO analgesia ladder, and only when those options fail or intolerable side effects develop, should interventional therapies be considered.
- Detailed assessment of the pain should be done related to all aspects. Pain intensity, site, frequency and its implications on the function and QOL should be documented.
- Inspection of the site where the intervention would be done for the presence of any contraindications or precautionary measures. The presence of any infection, neurological deficit, wound, allergies, etc., should be documented.
- The patient should always be given a trial before performing the actual procedure to see the effectiveness of the intervention and know about any reactions or side effects and the comfort of the patient with the device.

Physical Therapy Management of Pain

Physical therapy has an array of different modalities, exercises, and physical agents that can be used for analgesia **(Fig. 10.24)**. The choice of the treatment that is used should be purely based on the assessment findings, patient convenience, and evidences supporting the treatment. Each patient is a different individual. Hence, the treatment plan for each patient should be tailor-made according to the symptoms and requirements.

Table 10.9: Interventional Pain Management Therapies.

Procedure		Features	Indications
Injections		Injections of corticosteroids, anesthetics, anti-inflammatory agents, botulinum toxin, or analgesics are given within joint cavities, over trigger points, or in the muscle belly or tendon, nerves or within the epidural space or intrathecal	Myofascial pain syndrome, arthritis, fibromyalgia, radiculopathies, joint pains such as low back pain, sacroiliac joint pain, and chronic neuropathic pain
Percutaneous ablative techniques	Continuous or pulsed radio-frequency	Application of pulsed or continuous radio-frequencies to the neural tissue	Peripheral neuropathies, radiculopathies, arthrogenic pain, postsurgical pain, trigger points, and cancer pain
	Microwave ablation	Application of microwaves to the neural tissue	Peripheral neuropathies, radiculopathies, and cancer pain
	Cryoneuroablation	Application of cold using N_2O or CO_2 to tissues	Trigeminal neuralgia, postoperative pain, low back pain, facet arthropathy, peripheral neuropathies, and cancer pain
	MR guided HIFU	Application of high-intensity ultrasonic waves under MR guidance over local tissues	Cancer pain and neuropathies
Percutaneous disk decompression		Minimally invasive procedure that decompresses the IV disk percutaneously	Prolapsed intervertebral disk
Implantable electrical stimulator		Subcutaneous stimulation of peripheral nerves or spinal cord	Peripheral neuropathies, radiculopathies and postoperative pain
Implantable drug delivery systems		Controlled infusion of drugs into the body using implanted devices	Cancer pain and spinal cord injury

(HIFU: high-intensity focused ultrasound; MR: magnetic resonance)

Clinical Pearl

Physical therapy may not be the mainstay for any pain management program but it forms a key component of it.

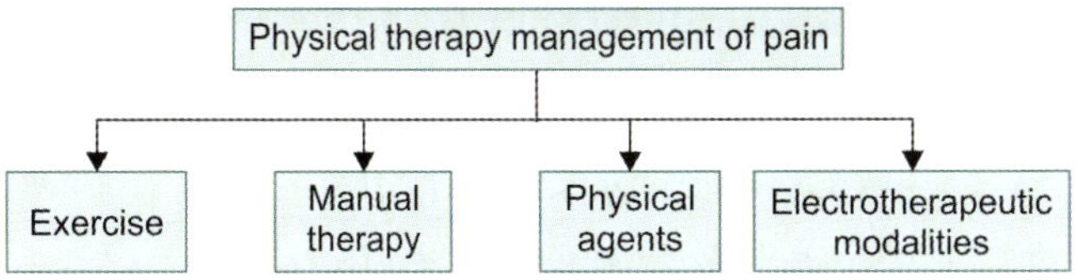

Physical therapy management of pain

Exercise | Manual therapy | Physical agents | Electrotherapeutic modalities

Fig. 10.24: Physical therapy management of pain.

Therapeutic Exercise

Therapeutic exercise forms a foundational component of the physical therapy management. Exercise works in various ways to relieve pain.

- It helps to strengthen the muscles and hence effectively increases the support being applied to the anatomical structure and also unloading the painful structure.
- It releases endorphins that help in modulating the pain.
- It improves the psychological profile of the patient by restoring function, making them more independent, and decreasing the fear associated with loss of balance or dependence.
- It reduces impairments and thereby reduces the pain associated with them.
- It reduces peripheral edema or local swelling, relieving the pressure on the nerve fibers.
- It causes an increase in the local temperature leading to increase in blood flow, which reduces spasm and washes out local irritants.

Therapeutic exercise may include exercises for improving balance, cardiopulmonary and muscular fitness, neuromuscular coordination, strength and flexibility. Exercise programs such as back school program and McKenzie exercises have been very effective in reducing back pain and disability in low back pain patients.

- Aerobic exercises have been proven to reduce pain perception in both patient and nonpatient populations.

- Aquatic exercises help in relieving pain through their warming or buoyancy-related blocking of nociception by stimulation of thermal and mechanoreceptors. The warmth also causes increase in blood supply to the affected area, leading to wash out of chemicals causing the nociception. Aquatic exercises are extremely helpful in conditions where weight-bearing is limited, e.g., bone fractures.
- Strengthening, stretching, and coordination and proprioceptive exercises stimulate the mechanoreceptors and proprioceptors, activating the pain gate control system and ultimately causing pain relief.

Manual Therapy

Manual therapy is any treatment provided by the therapist, in direct physical contact with the patient. The purpose of manual therapy is to relieve pain along with improving tissue extensibility, joint range of motion, manipulating the soft tissues and bones forming the joint, relaxation and relieving swelling. Manual therapy includes various techniques such as manipulation, mobilization, relaxation techniques, and massage therapy.

- Massage therapy is the scientific manipulation of soft tissues at correct depth and speed. Massage therapy has been known to induce relaxation and thereby releasing endorphins, which raises the pain threshold. It also increases local blood flow, which clears up the accumulated pain causing metabolites.
- Joint and soft-tissue manipulation and mobilization focus on the correction of the normal structural alignment. These techniques have a better effect when used along with therapeutic exercise. Mobilization given along with the exercises has showed a moderate effect size on pain in knee osteoarthritis subjects.
- Relaxation techniques tend to have weak improvement in acute pain. However, since they have no possible side effects, there is no harm in using them.

Electrophysical Agents

Physical agents are the materials used in rehabilitation **(Tables 10.10 and 10.11)**. They aid in the process of

Table 10.10: Physical agents used in physical therapy management.		
Physical agent	*Description*	*Physiological effects*
Heat therapy **(Fig. 10.25)**	Application of warmth to the tissues increasing the local temperature, e.g., hot packs and paraffin wax bath	• Increased metabolic activity • Vasodilation • Stimulation of thermoreceptors
Cold therapy **(Fig. 10.26)**	Application of cold to the tissues decreasing the local temperature, e.g., cold packs and vapocoolant sprays	• Decreased metabolic activity • Vasoconstriction followed by vasodilation • Stimulation of thermoreceptors
Hydrotherapy	Using water to get therapeutic benefits, e.g., whirlpool bath and Hubbard tank	• Increased metabolic activity • Vasodilation • Stimulation of thermoreceptors and mechanoreceptors • Debridement • Gentle massaging effect
Traction	Application of a force that causes pulls apart the underlying structures	• Joint distraction • Relieves pressure over nerves, nerve roots and disk • Elongates muscle and surrounding structures

Table 10.11: Electrotherapeutic modalities used in physical therapy management.

Electrotherapeutic modality	Description	Physiological effects
Ultrasound therapy (Fig. 10.27)	Ultrasonic waves of specific frequency transmitted into tissues—increasing the rate of healing, relieving pain, increasing tissue extensibility, and relieving edema. Phonophoresis can be used with drugs	• Increased local temperature • Increased metabolic activity • Vasodilation • Cavitation • Massaging effect • Increased cell permeability and membrane transport
Low-level laser therapy	Application of amplified electromagnetic energy concentrated over a specific area	• Promotes collagen formation • Promotes ATP production • Inhibits microbial growth • Reduces inflammation
Electrical stimulation—Galvanic or Faradic	Application of different waveforms of low-frequency electrical currents for varying durations or constant current as in iontophoresis with drugs	• Stimulation of nerve and muscle fibers • Stimulation of mechanoreceptors • Production of muscle contraction • Increased local blood flow • Reduction of muscle spasm
TENS **(Fig. 10.28)**	Application of low-frequency electrical currents of a specific waveform, intensity, and duration	• Stimulation of nerve fibers • Release of endogenous opioids
PEMF	Application of pulsed waveforms of varying wavelengths of electromagnetic fields	• Altered cell membrane permeability
Biofeedback	Works on motor control and learning and feed-forward and feedback mechanisms	• Muscle relaxation • Muscle facilitation • Relaxation of CNS • Release of endorphins
IFC **(Fig. 10.29)**	Application of medium frequency currents to produce low-frequency current within the tissues	• Stimulation of Aα and Aβ nerve fibers • Other mechanisms
Diadynamic currents	Application of half or full wave rectified sinusoidal currents	• Stimulation of nerve fibers

(CNS: central nervous system; IFC: interferential currents; PEMF: pulsed electromagnetic frequency; TENS: transcutaneous electrical nerve stimulation)

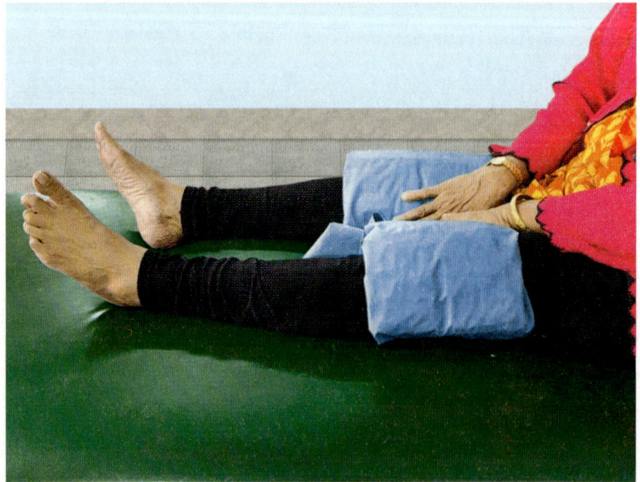

Fig. 10.25: Hot packs for knee.

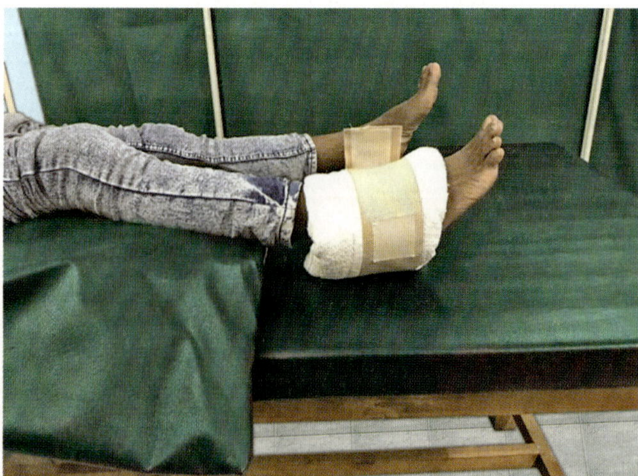

Fig. 10.26: Ice pack for ankle sprain.

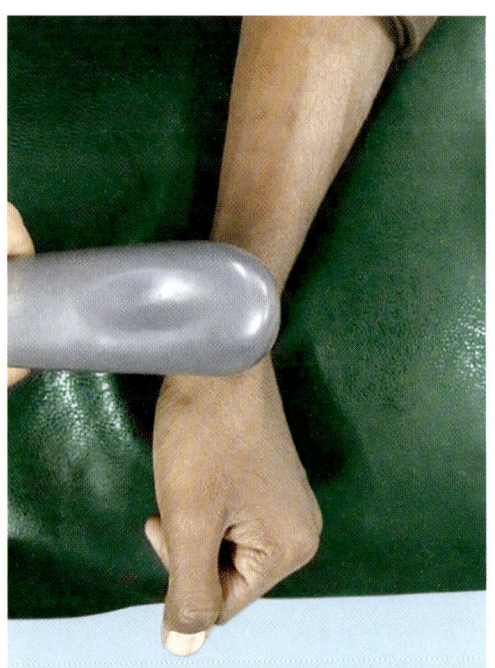

Fig. 10.27: Ultrasound therapy for De Quervain tenosynovitis.

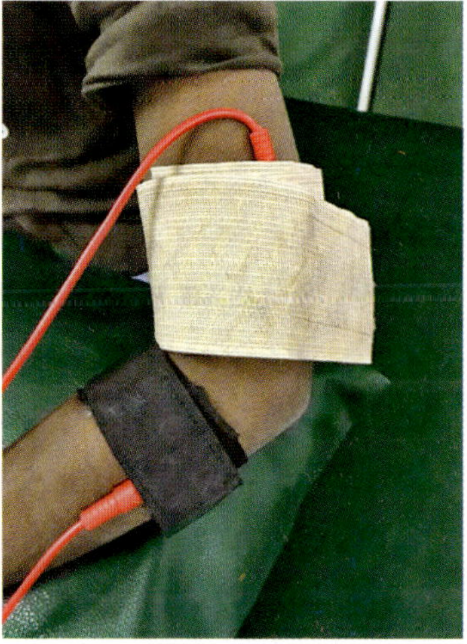

Fig. 10.28: TENS for tennis elbow.
(TENS: transcutaneous electrical nerve stimulation)

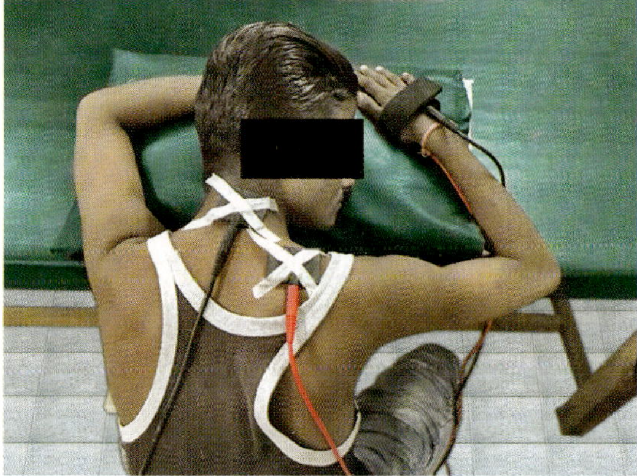

Fig. 10.29: IFC for trapezitis with pain radiating to hand.
(IFC: interferential currents.)

rehabilitation. These include heat, cold, water, or pressure. Electrotherapeutic modalities are electrical agents that use electromagnetic radiations or electrical currents of various frequencies to produce therapeutic benefits. With advancing technologies, new modalities are coming up every day.

Research has shown that there is insufficient, weak, or inconclusive evidence related to most of the physical agents and electrotherapeutic modalities for pain relief when used alone. But when these are used along with exercises or in combination with other modalities, they cause effective pain relief.

- In 2014, the Cochrane Database of Systematic Review found unclear evidence of the effectiveness of PEMF in reducing pain alone in subjects with adhesive capsulitis. They also concluded that Low Level LASER therapy (LLLT) when used alone or in adjunct to exercises produces pain relief significantly.
- A meta-analysis in 2017 found moderate evidence that electrotherapy, including TENS and pulsed electromagnetic fields improved the postsurgical pain and reduced the consumption of opioids after a total knee arthroplasty surgery.
- A randomized, double-blind, placebo-controlled trial in 2017 concluded that PEMF decreased edema, analgesic use, and postsurgical pain significantly in women undergone cesarean section.
- A systematic review in 2019 concluded that therapeutic ultrasound may be considered in the management of chronic low back pain and neck pain as it relieves pain for the short term. However, they could not make any recommendations for the same.
- Improvements in pain, function and the physical component of SF-36 (QOL) were observed after application of ultrasound, IFT, and TENS in subjects with shoulder impingement syndrome in a prospective randomized controlled trial.

Alternative Therapies

There are several alternative therapies that also have an impact on pain perception. Some of these are yoga, tai chi, cognitive behavioral therapy (CBT), acupuncture, dry needling, chiropractic, meditation, and hypnosis.

Tai chi has been recommended by the California Guidelines for patients with arthritis and fibromyalgia when requested by the patients themselves. **Acupuncture** and **dry needling** have several reported adverse effects; hence, they should be used with caution. **Yoga** has been found to have beneficial effects on pain coping mechanisms and disability. Also, there are little-to-no adverse effects. CBT also is very effective in reducing pain experiences and improving coping strategies in patients with chronic pain.

Physical therapy may be advised to patients who have inadequate pain relief with traditional analgesics. It is used as an allied therapy to achieve greater pain relief. It is very important for the physical therapist to realize their limitations whenever the pain cannot be controlled by physical therapy along with the medications. At this point, the therapist should be aware enough to refer the patient back to the physician or the surgeon for other options. It should also be realized that before going for any surgical or invasive alternatives, the doctor should have tried all other options. The use of alternative therapies should be considered when all other therapies fail or the patient is intent upon or motivated to try them. A multidisciplinary approach to pain always works better than a single-disciplinary approach since pain is a multifaceted symptom.

Cognitive Behavioral Therapy

Cognitive behavioral therapy is a psychosocial therapeutic approach, pioneered by Aaron Beck. CBT is based on the theory that all individuals have two levels of thought—automatic thoughts and maladaptive thoughts. The maladaptive or irrational thoughts lead to a maladaptive behavior, which needs to be changed by the individual.

Cognitive behavioral therapy has six phases:

1. Assessment
2. Reconceptualization
3. Skills acquisition
4. Skills consolidation and application training
5. Generalization and maintenance
6. Post-treatment assessment and follow-up

Assessment involves interviewing the patient and their family and administration of self-report measures that may guide toward the apt therapeutic approach. The psychosocial and behavioral factors affecting disability are evaluated.

The CBT approach is based on the theory that most of the patient's pain arises from irrational and maladaptive thoughts such as "I cannot get better" or "I am in so much of pain." The distorted cognition due to pain creates faulty emotions, which give rise to maladaptive behavior **(Fig. 10.30)**.

- The **reconceptualization phase** is a central feature of CBT that helps the patient to challenge these irrational and maladaptive thoughts and question their rationality. Pain is viewed as an addressable problem rather than being thought of something that is vague and an overwhelming experience. The patient is prepared for the interventional approaches in order to reduce anxiety related to the intervention and increase patient adherence. On first contact with the patient, pain questionnaires related to the patient's beliefs and thoughts about the pain, their ability to control pain and impact of pain on their lives are administered. The patient is introduced to the concept of "pain behavior" and "operant pain." They may be asked to manage a "pain diary" that records all the information (intensity, frequency, impact on the psychology of the patient, etc.) about pain episodes over the period of 1–2 weeks. Evaluation of the patient's strength and capabilities is also made. Preliminary goals are made on the basis of the information availed through assessment. Patients are asked to give up a sedentary lifestyle and accept a more physically active lifestyle instead. Use of analgesics is gradually reduced and ultimately eliminated. The reconceptualization phase focuses on building a psycho-physiological model of pain based on the theory given by Melzack and Wall in contrast to the sensory-physiological model of pain believed by the patient. The patient is educated that chronic pain might not just be related to a damaged tissue and that chronic pain has cognitive, emotional, and behavioral aspects as well. The importance of self-management is explained to the patient.

- The **skills acquisition phase** is focused on teaching the patient how to steer clear of irrational thoughts and how to deal with everyday obstacles in life. A variety of cognitive and behavioral coping strategies (diversion of attention, relaxation, and controlled breathing) are taught to the patient. The treatment plan would include lifestyle modification, communication skills training, problem-solving, and relaxation strategies. Activity pacing, biofeedback, and scheduling activities that give pleasure, graded activity, etc., are taught to the patient to overcome the behavior and fear associated with pain.

- The **skills consolidation and application training phase** attempts to reinforce the skills learned in skills acquisition phase through giving tasks and homework. The patient is given imaginary situations and asked how they will manage their pain in those situations. They are given homework assignments too.

- **Generalization and maintenance phase** prepares the patient to cope after the termination of the treatment.

- **Post-treatment assessment and follow-up** is to monitor and evaluate the patient's skills in coping with their life.

CBT does not work on the physiological aspect of pain, but rather the psychological aspect of it. The reframing of maladaptive thoughts and coping strategies cause a decrease in the distress of the individual, reducing the pain to some extent. The plan of care developed by a physical therapist already incorporates several of the pain coping mechanisms such as graded activity, pacing, and problem-solving. With the increasing prevalence of musculoskeletal

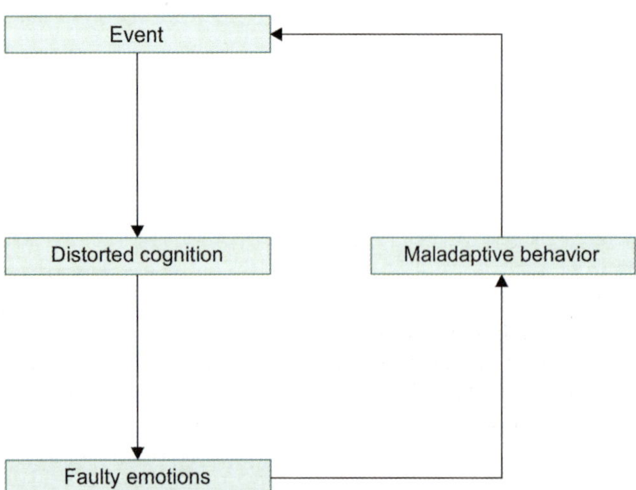

Fig. 10.30: Psychosocial development of pain.
Source: Adapted from Bhattacharya et al. (2013).

injuries and cancer, chronic pain has now become quite common. CBT has proven to be a beneficial tool in the management of chronic pain associated with pathologies such as fibromyalgia, low back pain, headaches and migraines, and arthritis.

Pain Neuroscience Education

Pain neuroscience education (PNE) is a new strategy for dealing with chronic pain.

- It is an educational strategy that incorporates the multidimensionality of a pain experience and helps patients reconceptualize pain through understanding the multiple neurophysiological, neurobiological, sociological, and physical components that may be involved in their individual pain experience.
- It utilizes various metaphors and analogies to explain the neurophysiological processes of pain occurring within the patient, along with the various other multidimensional aspects that may contribute to the patient's pain experience.
- It is an intervention used in the management of chronic pain, which aims to reconceptualize an individual's understanding of their pain as less threatening. Alternative names for PNE include explain pain, therapeutic neuroscience education, pain biology education, and pain neurophysiology education.

Pain biology education is a relatively new intervention for the management of CLBP.

- It is a cognitive behavioral-based intervention that attempts to reduce pain and disability by explaining the biology of the pain to the patient.
- The basic difference between CBT and PNE is that it does not work on pain coping strategies, rather it shifts an individual's attention toward understanding the process of pain.
- Current best evidence provides strong support for PNE to positively influence pain ratings, dysfunctions, fear-avoidance, and pain catastrophization, limitations in movement, pain knowledge, and healthcare utilization.

Explaining pain (EP) refers to a range of educational interventions that aim to change one's understanding of the biological processes that are thought to underpin pain as a mechanism to reduce pain itself. It draws on educational psychology, in particular conceptual change strategies, to help patients understand current thought in pain biology.

- The core objective of the EP approach to treatment is to shift one's conceptualization of pain from that of a marker of tissue damage or disease to that of a marker of the perceived need to protect body tissue.
- It increases knowledge of pain-related biology, decreases catastrophizing, and imparts short-term reductions in pain and disability.
- It presents the biological information that justifies a biopsychosocial approach to rehabilitation **(Box 10.12)**.

BOX 10.12: Key features of Explaining Pain (EP).

- EP is not a technique but a range of educational interventions
- EP aims to change understanding of the biological processes that underpin pain
- EP emphasizes the distinction between nociception and pain
- EP emphasizes that pain is a protective mechanism, not an indicator of tissue damage
- EP increases pain-related biological knowledge and decreases catastrophizing
- EP presents biology of pain that underpins a biopsychosocial approach

SUMMARY

Pain is common, and yet a complex experience that includes not only physiological mechanisms but also multiple dimensions, especially when dealing with chronic pain. Various classification systems of pain exist, and the one based on duration is most commonly discussed. Underassessment of pain is a major cause of inadequate pain management. Assessment tools play an important role in this process, where both choice of tool and the general approach to assessment should reflect the needs of the patient. Diagnostic tools may aid, but they are meant not to replace but supplement comprehensive history and physical examination. Pharmacological as well nonpharmacological treatments in the form of psychological and physical rehabilitation constitute the mainstay of pain management. In rare cases, surgical treatment strategies are also employed. In addition to relieving pain, physical rehabilitative methods can reduce fear and anxiety, improve physical function, and alter physiological responses to pain. Chronic pain may lead to various psychological implications, and adequate attention should be directed at addressing social and psychological consequences of the pain as well as any physical pathology, with measures such as patient education, regular assessment, management of contributing illnesses, acceptance, motivation, and coping strategies. Successful management of pain entails multimodal therapy, and this in turn improves the overall quality of healthcare systems.

Review Questions

1. Explain Gate control theory of pain.
2. Define and classify pain. What are neuro-modulation of pain?
3. What are the psychosocial implications of pain?
4. Explain: peripheral and central sensitization of pain.
5. Describe biopsychosocial model of pain.
6. Describe tools of assessment of pain.
7. What are the psychosocial factors associated with chronic pain?
8. Write a note on various management approaches of pain.
9. Explain: cognitive behavioral therapy for pain management.
10. Enlist the flags for chronic pain.

BIBLIOGRAPHY

1. Alghadir AH, Anwer S, Iqbal A, et al. Test–retest reliability, validity, and minimum detectable change of visual analog, numerical rating, and verbal rating scales for measurement of osteoarthritic knee pain. J Pain Res. 2018;11:851-6.

2. Asghari A, Nicholas MK. Pain self-efficacy beliefs and pain behaviour. A prospective study. Pain. 2001;94:85-100.

3. Ballantyne JC, Fishman SM, Rathmell JP. Bonica's management of pain. 5th edition. Wolters Kluwer publication; 2018.

4. Basbaum A. Specificity versus patterning theory: continuing the debate. In: McCaffrey P, Andrews N (Eds). Pain research forum. Available from http://www.painresearchforum.org/forums/discussion/7347-specificity-versuspatterning-theory continuing-debate.

5. Beck AT, Steer RA, Garbin MG. Psychometric properties of the Beck Depression Inventory: Twenty-five years of evaluation. Clin Psychol Rev. 1988;8(1):77-100.

6. Beck AT, Ward CH, Mendelson M, et al. An inventory for measuring depression. Arch Gen Psychiatry. 1961;4:561-71.

7. Bennett M. The LANSS Pain Scale: the Leeds assessment of neuropathic symptoms and signs. Pain. 2001;92:147-57.

8. Bhatnagar S, Gupta M. Evidence-based clinical practice guidelines for interventional pain management in cancer pain. Indian J Palliat Care. 2015;21(2):137-47.

9. Bhattacharya L, Chaudhari B, Saldanha D, et al. Cognitive behavior therapy. Med J Dr DY Patil Vidyapeeth. 2013;6(2):132-8.

10. Campbell J. APS 1995 Presidential address. Pain Forum. 1996;5(1):85-8.

11. Chapman C, Nakamura Y. A Passion of the soul: an introduction to pain for consciousness researchers. Conscious Cogn. 1999;8(4):391-422.

12. Cleeland CS, Ryan KM. Pain assessment: global use of the brief pain inventory. Ann Acad Med Singapore 1994;23(2):129-38.

13. Cruccu G, Truini A. Tools for assessing neuropathic pain. PLoS Med. 2009;6(4):e1000045.

14. Engel GL. The need for a new medical model: a challenge for biomedicine. Science. 1977;196(4286):129-36.

15. Fink R. Pain assessment: the cornerstone to optimal pain management. Proc (Bayl Univ Med Cent). 2000;13(3):236-9.

16. Fishman B, Pasternak S, Wallenstein SL, et al. The memorial pain assessment card: a valid instrument for the evaluation of cancer pain. Cancer. 1987;60:1151-8.

17. Freynhagen R, Baron R, Gockel U, et al. painDETECT: a new screening questionnaire to identify neuropathic components in patients with back pain. Curr Med Res Opin. 2006;22(10):1911-20.

18. Gatchel RJ, Rollings KH. Evidence-informed management of chronic low back pain with cognitive behavioral therapy. Spine J. 2008;8(1):40-4. doi:10.1016/j.spinee.2007.10.007.

19. Giordano PCM, Alexandre NMC, Rodrigues RCM, et al. The Pain Disability Questionnaire: a reliability and validity study. Rev Lat Am Enfermagem. 2012;20(1):76-83. https://dx.doi.org/10.1590/S0104-11692012000100011.

20. Gordon DB, Dahl JL, Miaskowski C. et al. American pain society recommendations for improving the quality of acute and cancer pain management: American pain society quality of care task force. Arch Intern Med. 2005;165(14):1574-80.

21. Grove G. Acute Pain Management: Operative or Medical Procedures and Trauma, Acute Pain Management in Children: Operative or Medical Procedures. J Nur Care Qual. 1995;10(1):87-8.

22. Grönblad M, Hupli M, Wennerstrand P, et al. Intercorrelation and test-retest reliability of the Pain Disability Index (PDI) and the Oswestry Disability Questionnaire (ODQ) and their correlation with pain intensity in low back pain patients. Clin J Pain. 1993;9(3):189-95.

23. Haefeli M, Elfering A. Pain assessment. Eur Spine J. 2006;15(Suppl. 1):S17-24.

24. Hulla R, Brecht D, Stephens J, et al. The biopsychosocial approach and considerations involved in chronic pain. Healthy Aging Res. 2019;08(01):581-624.

25. Innes JA, Maxwell SRJ. Davidson's Essentials of Medicine, 2nd edition. Edinburgh, NY: Churchill Livingstone Elsevier; 2016. pp. 279-84.

26. International Association for the Study of Pain (IASP). IASP Taxonomy: Part III: Pain Terms, A Current List with Definitions and Notes on Usage" (pp 209-214). In: Merskey H, Bogduck N (Eds). Classification of Chronic Pain, Second Edition, IASP Task Force on Taxonomy, IASP Press, Seattle; 1994.

27. Jansen MJ, Viechtbauer W, Lenssen AF, et al. Strength training alone, exercise therapy alone, and exercise therapy with passive manual mobilisation each reduce pain and disability in people with knee osteoarthritis: a systematic review. J Physiother. 2011;57(1):11-20.

28. Keefe FJ. Cognitive behavioral therapy for managing pain. Clin Psychol. 1996;49(3):4-5.

29. Keller S, Bann CM, Dodd SL, et al. Validity of the brief pain inventory for use in documenting the outcomes of patients with noncancer pain. Clin J Pain. 2004;20(5):309-18.

30. Kerns RD, Turk DC, Rudy TE. The West Haven-Yale Multidimensional Pain Inventory (WHYMPI). Pain. 1985;23(4):345-56.

31. Khooshideh M, Latifi Rostami SS, Sheikh M, et al. Pulsed electromagnetic fields for postsurgical pain management in women undergoing cesarean section: a randomized, double-blind, placebo-controlled trial. Clin J Pain. 2017;33(2):142-7.

32. Kraus SJ, Backonja M. Development of a neuropathic pain questionnaire. Clin J Pain. 2003;19(5):306-14.

33. Krebs EE, Lorenz KA, Bair MJ, et al. Development and initial validation of the PEG, a three-item scale assessing pain intensity and interference. J Gen Intern Med. 2009;24(6):733-8. doi:10.1007/s11606-009-0981-1.

34. Kroeling P, Gross A, Graham N, et al. Electrotherapy for neck pain (review). Cochrane Database Syst Rev. 2013;26(8):CD004251.

35. Kroenke K, Spitzer RL, Williams JBW. The PHQ-9: validity of a brief depression severity measure. J Gen Intern Med. 2001;16(9):606-13.

36. Lawlis GF, Cuencas R, Selby D, et al. The development of the Dallas Pain Questionnaire. An assessment of the impact of spinal pain on behavior. Spine. 1989;14(5):511-6.

37. Loeser JD. Concepts of pain. In: Stanton-Hicks J, Boaz R (Eds). Chronic low back pain. New York, NY: Raven Press; 1982.

38. Macintyre PE, Walker S, Power I, et al. Acute pain management: scientific evidence revisited. BJA. 2006;96(1):1-4.

39. Macintyre PE, Walker S, Power I, et al. Acute pain management: scientific evidence revisited. BJA: British Journal of Anaesthesia. 2006;96(1):1-4.

40. Manworren RCB, Hynan LS. Clinical validation of FLACC: preverbal patient pain scale. Pediatr Nurs. 2003;29(2):140-6.

41. Mariano A. Chronic pain and spinal cord injury. Clin J Pain. 1992;8(2):87-92.

42. Mayer TG, Neblett R, Cohen H, et al. The development and psychometric validation of the central sensitization inventory (CSI). Pain Pract. 2012;12(4):276-85.

43. McCaffery M, Moss F. Nursing intervention for bodily pain. Am J Nurs. 1967;67(6):1224.

44. Melzack R, Wall P. Pain mechanisms: a new theory. Science. 1965;150(3699):971-8.

45. Melzack R. The McGill Pain Questionnaire. Pain measurement and assessment. New York, NY: Raven Press; 1983.

46. Merskey H. Pain specialists and pain terms. Pain. 1996;64(1):205.

47. Moayedi M, Davis K. Theories of pain: from specificity to gate control. J Neurophysiol. 2013;109(1):5-12.

48. Moseley GL, Butler DS. Explain pain supercharged. Adelaide, SA: Noigroup Publications; 2017.

49. Moseley GL, Butler DS. Fifteen years of explaining pain: the past, present, and future. J Pain. 2015;16:807-13.

50. Moseley GL, Nicholas MK, Hodges PW. A randomized controlled trial of intensive neurophysiology education in chronic low back pain. Clin J Pain. 2004;20:324-30.

51. Nichols DS, Glenn TM. Effects of aerobic exercise on pain perception, affect, and level of disability in individuals with fibromyalgia. Phys Ther. 1994;74:327-32.

52. Noori SA, Rasheed A, Aiyer R, et al. Therapeutic ultrasound for pain management in chronic low back pain and chronic neck pain: a systematic review. Pain Med. 2019;pny287. https://doi.org/10.1093/pm/pny287.

53. Page MJ, Green S, Kramer S, et al. Electrotherapy modalities for adhesive capsulitis (frozen shoulder). Cochrane Database Syst Rev. 2014;(10):CD011324.

54. Pieber K, Herceg M, Paternostro-Sluga T. Electrotherapy for the treatment of painful diabetic peripheral neuropathy: a review. J Rehabil Med. 2010;42(4):289-95.

55. Portenoy R. Development and testing of a neuropathic pain screening questionnaire: ID Pain. Curr Med Res Opin. 2006;22(8):1555-65.

56. Portenoy RK, Kanner RM. Definition and assessment of pain. In: Portenoy RK, Kanner RM (Eds). Pain management: theory and practice. Philadelphia, PA: FD Davis; 1996. pp. 18-3.

57. Price DD, Mao J, Mayer DJ. Central mechanisms of normal and abnormal pain sates. In: Fields HL, Liebeskind JC (Eds). Progress in pain research and management Vol. 1. Seattle, WA: IASP Press; 1994. pp. 61-84.

58. Rothaug J, Weiss T, Meissner W. How simple can it get? Measuring pain with Numerical Rating Scale (NRS) items or binary items. Clin J Pain. 2013;29(3):224-32.

59. Ryan CG, Gray HG, Newton M, et al. Pain biology education and exercise classes compared to pain biology education alone for individuals with chronic low back pain: a pilot randomised controlled trial. Man Ther. 2010;15:382-7.

60. Salaffi F, Stancati A, Silvestri CA, et al. Minimal clinically important changes in chronic musculoskeletal pain intensity measured on a numerical rating scale. Eur J Pain. 2004;8:283-91.

61. Seers K, Carroll D. Relaxation techniques for acute pain management: a systematic review. J Adv Nurs. 1998;27(3):466-75.

62. Spadoni GF, Stratford PW, Solomon PE, et al. The evaluation of change in pain intensity: a comparison of the P4 and single-item numeric pain rating scales. J Orthop Sports Phys Ther. 2004;34(4):187-93.

63. Speckens AEM, van Hemert AM, Spinhoven P, et al. Cognitive behavioural therapy for medically unexplained physical symptoms: a randomised controlled trial. BMJ (Clinical Research Ed). 1995;311(7016):1328–32.

64. Stafleu Van Loghum H, Netherlands Strik JJ, Honig A, et al. Sensitivity and specificity of observer and self-report questionnaires in major and minor depression following myocardial infarction. Psychosomatics. 2001;42(5):423-8.

65. Swinkels-Meewisse EJCM, Swinkels RAHM, Verbeek ALM, et al. Psychometric properties of the Tampa Scale for kinesiophobia and the fear-avoidance beliefs questionnaire in acute low back pain. Man Ther. 2003;8(1):29-36.

66. Tan G, Jensen MP, Thornby JI, et al. Validation of the brief pain inventory for chronic nonmalignant pain. J Pain. 2004;5(2):133-7.

67. Tedesco D, Gori D, Desai KR, et al. Drug-free interventions to reduce pain or opioid consumption after total knee arthroplasty: a systematic review and meta-analysis. JAMA Surg. 2017;152(10):1-13.

68. Thomas V. Pain: clinical manual Pain: clinical manual McCaffery Margo Pasero Chris Mosby 795pp. Nurs Stand. 2000;14(25):26.

69. Tkachuk GA, Harris CA. Psychometric properties of the Tampa Scale for Kinesiophobia-11 (TSK-11). J Pain. 2012;13(10):970-7.

70. Tripathi, KD. Essentials of medical pharmacology, 5th edition. New Delhi: Jaypee Brothers Medical Publishers (P) LTD; 2003.

71. Turk DC, Okifuji A. Evaluating the role of physical, operant, cognitive and affective factors in the pain behaviors of chronic pain patients. Behav Modif 1997;21:259-80.

72. Ucurum SG, Kaya DO, Kayali Y, et al. Comparison of different electrotherapy methods and exercise therapy in shoulder impingement syndrome: a prospective randomized controlled trial. Acta Orthop Traumatol Turc. 2018;52(4):249-55.

73. van Tulder MW, Koes BW, Bouter LM. Conservative treatment of acute and chronic nonspecific low back pain. A systematic review of randomized controlled trials of the most common interventions. Spine. 1997;22:2128-56.

74. Vardeh D, Yong RJ, et al (Eds). Pain Med. doi:10.1007/978-3-319-43133-8_4.

75. Vargas-Schaffer G. Is the WHO analgesic ladder still valid? Twenty-four years of experience. Can Fam Physician. 2010,56(6):514-7.

76. Von Korff M, Ormel J, Keefe F, et al. Grading the severity of chronic pain. Pain. 1992;50:133-49.

77. Wardenaar KJ, Wanders RBK, Jeronimus BF, et al. The psychometric properties of an internet-administered version of the Depression Anxiety and Stress Scales (DASS) in a sample of Dutch adults. J Psychopathol Behav Assess. 2018;40(2):318-33.

78. Ware J Jr, Sherbourne CD. The MOS 36-Item Short-Form Health Survey (SF-36): I. Conceptual framework and item selection. Med Care. 1992;30(6):473-83.

79. Wijma JA, van Wilgen CP, Meeus M, et al. Clinical biopsychosocial physiotherapy assessment of patients with chronic pain: the first step in pain neuroscience education. Physiother Theory Pract. 2016;32:(5):368-84. doi:10.1080/09593985.2016.1194651.

80. Willis W, Westlund K. Neuroanatomy of the pain system and of the pathways that modulate pain. J Clin Neurophysiol. 1997;14(1):2-31.

81. Woolf C, Mannion R. Neuropathic pain: aetiology, symptoms, mechanisms, and management. Lancet. 1999;353(9168):1959-64.

82. Woolf CJ. Central sensitization: implications for the diagnosis and treatment of pain. Pain. 2011;152(3 Suppl.):S2-15.

83. World Health Organization. (2019). WHO's cancer pain ladder for adults. Available from https://www.who.int/cancer/palliative/painladder/en/. [26 August 2019].

84. Zigmond AS, Snaith RP. The hospital anxiety and depression scale. Acta Psychiatr Scand. 1983;67(6):361-70.

Mobility Aids and Orthosis

Shyam Ganvir

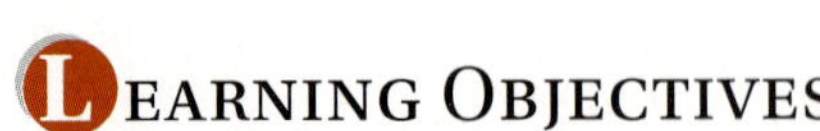 LEARNING OBJECTIVES

After reading this chapter, the readers should be able to:

- Discuss the concepts of walking, mobility, and disability
- Discuss the different mobility aids associated with the person with disabilities
- Describe the basic principles of mobility devices before providing appropriate mobility devices
- Contrast and compare the advantages and characteristic features of each mobility aid for gait training
- Discuss the characteristics of various mobility aids including assessment, measurement of each instrument
- Describe the guidelines for the selection and measurement of canes, crutches, and walkers
- Identify conditions to be considered in the selection of mobility aids
- Describe the preparation for gait training
- Identify the common gait patterns and techniques used with walking aids
- Discuss the mobility/walking aids for individuals with limb deficiency and spinal cord injury
- Describe the major parts of the upper extremity orthoses and the splints
- Describe the major parts of the shoe to the requirements of individuals fitted with lower extremity (LE) orthoses
- Describe the components of contemporary foot, ankle–foot, knee–ankle–foot, hip–knee–ankle–foot, trunk–hip–knee–ankle–foot, and trunk orthoses
- Identify the features of LE and trunk orthoses that are considered during the examination process
- Develop a plan of care when presented with a clinical case study

CHAPTER OUTLINE

- Mobility aids
  - Functions
  - Indications
  - Selection
- Preparation for walking/gait training
- Principles
- Types
  - Canes
  - Crutches
  - Walker
  - Wheelchairs
  - Area for wheelchair user training
- Mobility/walking aids for individuals with limb deficiency
  - Lower limb amputation
  - Spinal cord injury
- Orthotics in mobility
  - Objectives and functions
  - General principles
- Upper limb orthoses
  - Finger orthosis
  - Hand–finger orthosis
  - Wrist–hand–finger orthoses
  - Elbow orthosis
  - Shoulder orthoses
- Splints
  - Classification
  - General functions of splinting
  - Types of static splints
- Lower extremity orthoses
  - Shoes
  - Foot orthoses
  - Ankle–foot orthoses
  - Knee–ankle–foot orthoses
  - Hip–knee–ankle–foot orthoses
  - Trunk–knee–ankle–foot orthoses
- Trunk orthoses
  - Corsets
  - Rigid orthoses
  - Cervical orthoses
  - Scoliosis orthoses

INTRODUCTION

Mobility is defined as the ability to walk safely and independently. It is a critical requirement for performing activities of daily living (ADL) and instrumental activities of daily living (IADL). Mobility is also related to changes that are associated with aging in a person's body. Decline in muscle strength and mass, less mobile, and stiffer joints, along with gait changes affect an individual's balance and may significantly compromise their mobility. Mobility is crucial for maintaining independent living among the elderly population. If an individual's mobility is restricted, it may indirectly affect their activities of daily living.

Mobility aids are appliances that help people who experience walking difficulties.

- They enable some of the body weight to be distributed to the upper extremities and thus provide stability and indirectly the mobility of a patient.
- They enable persons with the disabilities to achieve mobility and independence, and access to these devices is a precondition for achieving equal opportunities, enjoying human rights, and living a dignified life.
- They are one of the most commonly used assistive technologies or devices.

> **Mobility assistive products** enable people to walk or move. They have specialized features to accommodate the individual needs. For example, in cerebral palsy, one may require a wheelchair with trunk or head supports to be able to maintain a good sitting position.

> **Assistive technology** can be defined as "An equipment or product which is available commercially or is modified or customized and is used to maintain, increase or improve the functional abilities of people with disability."

- Mobility devices are designed to maximize a user's personal mobility—this refers to their ability to change and maintain body position and walk and move from one place to another. Common examples include:
- Crutches
- Walking frames
- Wheeled walkers
- Wheelchairs
- Canes
- Mobility devices are appropriate for those who have difficulties in mobility as a result of various health conditions and impairments.
- When walking is not possible, or when the speed and range of ambulation are too low, the indicated mobility aid is the wheelchair or any one of the wheeled devices.

> **Positioning devices** are appliances that assist people with physical impairments who often have difficulty maintaining positions such as good lying, standing, or sitting positions for functional activities. They also assist those who are at risk of developing injuries because of improper positioning. The following devices can help overcome some of these difficulties: Wedges, chairs (e.g., corner chairs and special seats) and standing frames.

Individuals with physical and mobility impairments may experience difficulties in:

- Motor and/or fine motor functioning
- Locomotor and nonlocomotor functioning

Deficits and impairments may also occur in:
- Cognition
- Social skills
- Adaptive behavior skills
- Language ability
- Vision
- Hearing
- Other sensory areas

Individuals with physical and mobility impairments may experience:
- Stiffness and/or spasticity
- Loss of muscle strength

They may require assistance in learning, or activities of daily living. Individuals with physical and mobility impairments may need assistance in mobility, transfers, as well as ambulation. They may:
- Have a restricted range of motion
- Be reluctant to perform movement or
- Experience a perceptual or cognitive impairment.
- Experience pain, discomfort, depression or anxiety

Individuals with these impairments may need prolonged bed rest and may have medical comorbidities. They may also have musculoskeletal or neuromuscular impairments.

Physiotherapists support people with physical problems and movement. They see a physical movement as central to the health and wellbeing of an individual. They are trained to make the most of the potential available for active movement by promoting good health, treatment, and rehabilitation.

> **Physical impairment** is a disability that limits a person's physical capacity to move, coordinate actions, or perform physical activities.

Individuals with physical disabilities often utilize assistive devices or mobility aids such as crutches, canes, wheelchairs, and artificial limbs to obtain mobility.

> **Explanations of terms used: Abbreviations**
>
> **Impairment:** Any loss or abnormality of psychological, physiological, or anatomical structure or function in a human being.
>
> **Disability:** Any restriction or lack (resulting from an impairment) in the ability to perform an activity in the manner or within the range considered normal for a human being.
>
> **Full weight bearing (FWB):** Patient is allowed to bear full weight through the limb. They may require a walking aid for balance or to alleviate pain but not specifically to limit weight bearing.
>
> **Partial weight bearing (PWB):** Patient is NOT allowed to bear full weight through the limb and so will need aids such as a frame/wheeled frame or crutches to mobilize or a stand aid (such as an orbital seater or patient turner) to assist with transfer if patient is unable to limit weight bearing when stepping.

> **Nonweight bearing (NWB):** No weight bearing is allowed through the limb at all. The patient will require aids such as a frame/wheeled frame or crutches to mobilize or a stand aid (such as an orbital seater or patient turner) to assist with transfers if patient is unable to avoid weight bearing when stepping.
>
> **Ferrule:** A ferrule is a piece of metal or rubber enclosing the end of a stick to protect it and stop it from slipping. Most walking aids possess these.
>
> **Gait:** Walking pattern.

Disability is the difficulty encountered in any or all three areas of functioning: impairments (affecting body structure and functioning); activity limitations; and participation restrictions. According to the Equality Act, a person is considered disabled if the person has a physical or mental impairment that has a substantial or long-term adverse effect on the person's ability to carry out normal day-to-day activities. Locomotor disability can either be congenital or acquired and the nature of the built environment is very critical for persons with such disabilities. According to WHO statistics of 2008, 10% of 650 million persons with disabilities (PwDs) require a wheelchair, which reflects a huge need for wheelchair and resources needed by them.

- A built environment is defined as all buildings, spaces, and products that are created or modified by people. It consists of schools, workplaces, greenways, and transportation systems.
- The role of accessible, safe, well-designed built environments for health optimization and education is being recognized increasingly. This is due to surrounding social and physical environments that are likely to affect independence and individuals can experience a variety of conditions as they move in and out of different environments over their life course. Uneven or abrupt sidewalks, heavy human traffic, and inaccessible public transportation are some of the built environment characteristics that can hinder outdoor mobility and impact on a person's ability to function independently in a given community (e.g., shops, banks, lecture halls, and health services).

MOBILITY AIDS

Functions

Following are the functions of mobility aids:

- To improve balance
- To increase proprioception
- To decrease pain
- To reduce weight bearing on injured or inflamed structures
- To compensate for weak muscles
- To scan the immediate environment (for the visually impaired)

- To indicate to the bystanders of the disability of the individual (e.g., the white cane with a red tip indicates the user is visually impaired).

Indications

Indications for mobility aids include:

- Amputation
- Arthritis
- Cerebral palsy
- Poliomyelitis
- Muscular dystrophy
- Spinal cord injury
- Spina bifida
- Stroke
- Visual impairment
- Geriatric population
- Postoperative conditions

Selection

Selecting a walking aid relies upon:

- Diagnosis and prognosis of a given condition
- Upper and lower limb strength
- Type of gait
- Stability
- Extent of improvement or deterioration
  Other factors which affect the use of mobility aids are:
  - Motivation
  - Age
  - Acceptance
  - Relief from weight bearing
  - Coordination
  - Dynamic balance with body movement
  - Limb length discrepancy
  - Vision
  - Sensations

PREPARATION FOR WALKING/GAIT TRAINING

Walking/gait training preparation includes the below:

1. **Arms:** Good strength of shoulder extensors and adductors and elbow extensors will be needed. Before starting the gait training, the power of the muscles that are needed for walking must be assessed. The handgrip may also be tested to assess the power and mobility of hand muscles to grasp the hand piece.
2. **Legs:** Mobility and strength of lower limb (unaffected) muscles must be assessed for weight bearing.
   - NWB: Muscle and strength of the unaffected lower leg must be checked mainly hip abductors and extensors, ankle dorsiflexors, and plantar flexors. These muscles enable to bear strong weight.
   - PWB: Mobility and strength of both lower extremities must be assessed and strength training must be given as per the condition.
3. **Balance:** Static and dynamic balance must be checked in sitting as well as standing.

PRINCIPLES

Principles of providing appropriate mobility devices are as follows:

As per the convention on the rights of PwDs, the following key principles need to be considered:

- **Acceptability:** People with disabilities are actively involved in all stages of mobility device provision, making an active choice and control over the decisions that affect them. Factors such as efficiency, reliability, simplicity, safety, and esthetics should be taken into consideration to ensure that the devices and related services are acceptable to users.
- **Accessibility:** Mobility devices and related services are accessible to everyone with an identified need. Accessibility encompasses nondiscrimination, physical accessibility, and information accessibility. Provision of mobility devices should be equitable to avoid discrepancies between genders, age groups, impairment groups, socioeconomic groups, and geographical regions.
- **Adaptability:** Mobility devices and related services are adapted and modified to ensure they are appropriate as per the requirements of the individual. They consider all aspects of the individual's disability, i.e., impairments, activity limitations, participation restrictions, related health conditions, environmental factors (e.g., physical and social environment), and personal factors (e.g., gender, age, race, physical fitness, lifestyle, and habits).
- **Affordability** Mobility devices and related services must be affordable for persons with disabilities (PwDs) and their families, particularly in low-resource settings. Affordability refers to the extent to which an individual can pay for a device and/or its services.
- **Availability:** All relevant resources such as healthcare facilities, programs and services, human resources, materials, and products required for the provision of mobility devices should be available in sufficient quantity for the needs of the population. Also, they should be provided as close as possible to people's own communities.
- **Quality:** All relevant resources (health-care facilities, programs and services, human resources, and materials and products) should be of an appropriate quality. Product quality can be measured in terms of strength, durability, performance, safety, comfort, etc. Specific qualities of services can be measured in terms of compliance with staff training requirements and service guidelines. The overall quality of services can be measured in terms of outcomes, user satisfaction, and quality of life. Resource constraints or affordability should not necessarily compromise the quality.

TYPES

Mobility aids can be classified into the following types:

1. Stick (canes)
2. Crutches
3. Walkers (frames)
4. Wheelchair and its types
5. Tricycles

Canes

Canes or sticks are similar to crutches since they support the body's weight and help in load transmission. Walking sticks take away the body weight from the lower limb during walking and therefore can compensate for muscle weakness and reduce pain in the legs.

Features

Sticks can be wooden and metal, metal ones are adjustable and can be used easily for assessment purpose. Stick has handle, shaft, adjustable buttons, rubber ferrule, etc. **Figures 11.1A to C** show the types of sticks/canes.

A. **Standard cane:** It is also called a regular or conventional cane. It is made up of wood or aluminum or plastic and it has crook type of handle. The distal end has rubber ferrule which is almost 1 inch in diameter.

   Advantages: It is inexpensive and fits easily on any surface where space is limited.

   Disadvantages: It is not adjustable and its point of support is anterior to the hand.

B. **Standard aluminum cane:** This cane has the same design as the standard cane. It is made up of aluminum tubing, and it has a half-circle handle with molded plastic covering. They are adjustable within range of approximately 68–98 cm. The distal end has rubber ferrule of 1 inch in diameter. It also has a push button to adjust the height.

   Advantages: The height of cane is easily adjustable. It is lightweight and easily fits on stairs.

   Disadvantage: Its point of support is anterior to the hand. This cane is costlier than the standard cane.

C. **Adjustable aluminum offset cane:** The proximal component of the shaft of this cane has offset anteriorly

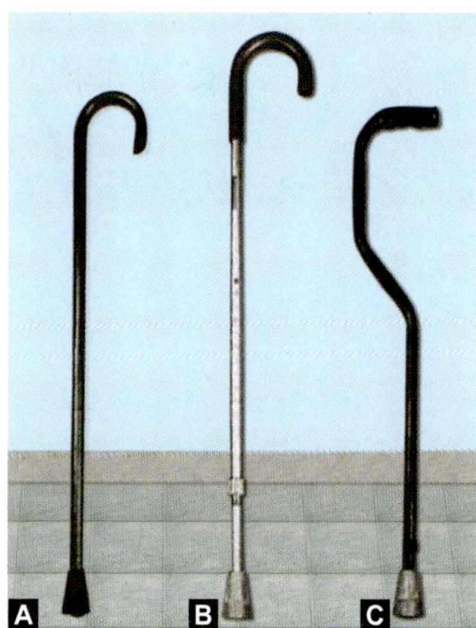

Figs. 11.1A to C: (A) Standard wooden cane; (B) Standard aluminum cane; (C) Adjustable offset cane.

creating a straight handle. It is made up of aluminum tubing with a plastic or rubber molded grip-shaped handle. The height can be adjusted approximately 65–98 cm by a push button mechanism. The diameter of the distal end rubber ferrule is 1 inch.

Advantages: The design of this cane allows bearing pressure over the center of the cane giving greater stability. This cane is also easily adjustable, lightweight, and fits easily on the stairs.

Disadvantages: This cane is costlier than standard or adjustable aluminum cane.

Measurement

Patient should be standing with elbow flexed and measurement is taken from the ulnar styloid process to the floor horizontally 15 cm from the heel.

Uses

The use of a walking stick or sticks can increase the stability and the confidence of a patient.

Types

Tripods and Quadripods

Tripods and quadripod stick are shown in **Figure 11.2**.

Features: Tripod and quadripod sticks are same as walking canes, but have three or four ferrules at the bottom, thereby providing more stability. A tripod or quadripod cane consists of a handle, a shaft and a base with three or four tips, in a manner that the cane can stand upright by itself. The tips give friction and prevent the cane from slipping over the ground.

Advantages: The cane is generally held in the hand on the side opposite to the injured or weak lower limb. It is brought forward and placed firmly on the ground before the legs, first the weak leg, followed by the strong leg.

Combination Cane and Seat

For patients who have difficulty in standing for more than a few minutes at a time, a cane can be provided combined

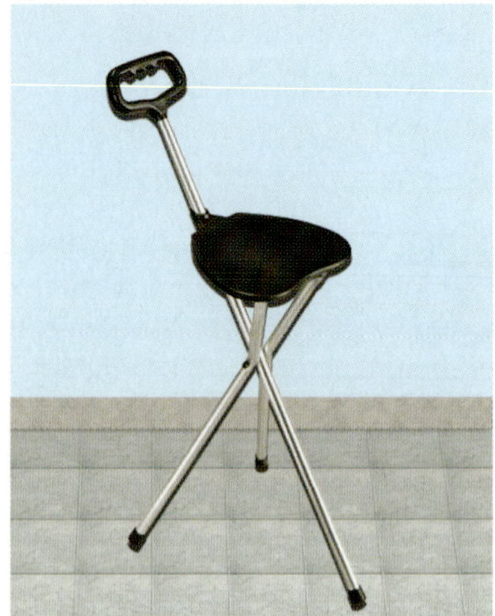
Fig. 11.3: Foldable cane with seat.

with a folding seat **(Fig. 11.3)**. They are lightweighted and have one or two legs when used as a cane for walking support. When folded out to a seat, they have three or four legs to support the weight of the individual when resting. They fold out easily into a chair having either a metal seat on three legs or a canvas seat on four legs. The height is usually adjustable.

White (Foldable) Cane

Description: People with visual disability use a white cane to detect objects in their path or to navigate through uneven terrains **(Fig. 11.4)**.

General features: It folds up easily when traveling and remains rigid while using.

Use: The cane is held such that the wrist is between the waist and the belly button, and swings left to right side as the user walks.

Gait Pattern: Cane

Gait pattern shows:
1. Starting position. The left lower extremity (LE) can be assumed to be the affected limb **(Figs. 11.5A to C)**.

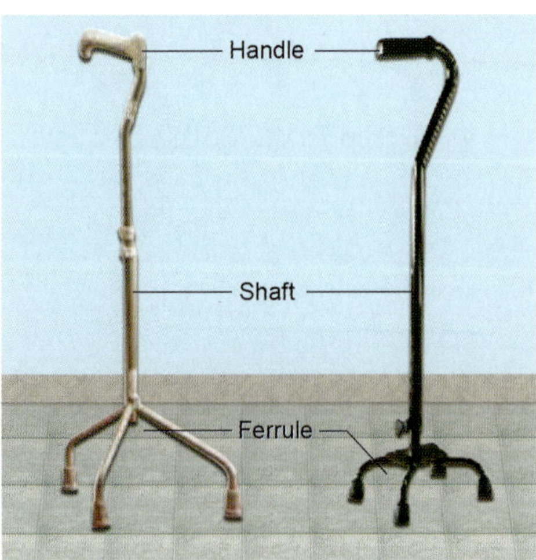

Fig. 11.2: Tripod and quadripod.

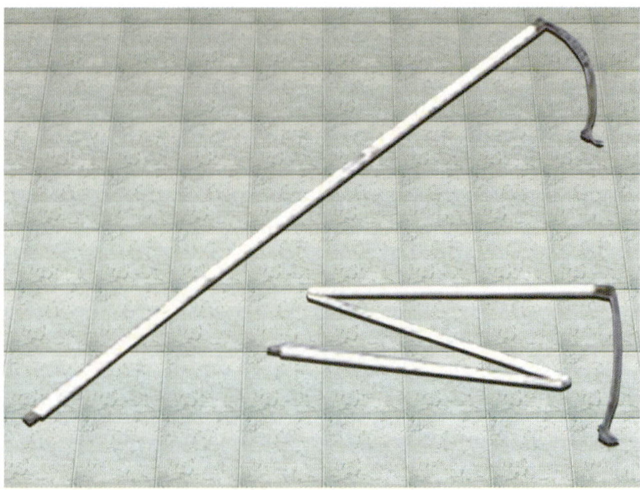
Fig. 11.4: Foldable cane.

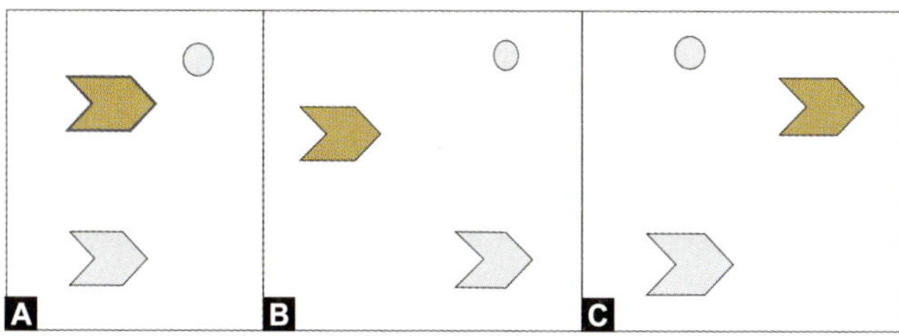

Figs. 11.5A to C: Gait pattern with cane.

2. The cane and the affected extremity are moved forward simultaneously.
3. The unaffected extremity is advanced.
4. The cycle is repeated.

Crutches

It helps in transferring the weight from the legs to the upper body.

Axillary Crutch

One part of an axillary crutch is placed against the rib cage under the axilla, while one holds onto the handgrip. It allows to transfer some or all of their weight from one lower limb to the upper body.

Features

Axillary crutches have an axillary bar, a hand piece, and double uprights which join distally with a single leg. They may be made of wood or a lightweight metal such as aluminum tubing. The axillary bar and often the hand piece have a coating or padding of soft plastic, rubber, or foam. The total height and the height of the hand piece can both be adjusted **(Fig. 11.6)**.

Measurement

The height of the crutches should be adjusted to achieve a space of two to three fingers between the top of the crutch and the armpit of the user (i.e., approximately 5 cm) in standing position. The hand piece should be adjusted so the elbow is slightly bent (15–30°) when standing straight.

Clinical Implication and Uses

The user should not rest their armpits on the axillary bar, to prevent axillary nerve passing under the arm being damaged, which can lead to "crutch palsy" (temporary or permanent loss of sensation or muscle control in some parts of the affected arm). It is used for short term only. Usually, two crutches are used together, one for each hand. When the injured, weak or disabled LE is NWB, the user begins by standing on the stronger leg. Both crutches are then progressed forward and placed on the ground, followed by the strong leg hopping to, or slightly past, the tips of the crutches.

When the injured weak or disabled lower limb is partially weight bearing, it is brought forward in line with the crutches. When climbing upstairs, each step is climbed by advancing the stronger leg first, followed by the impaired leg and crutches. When descending, the

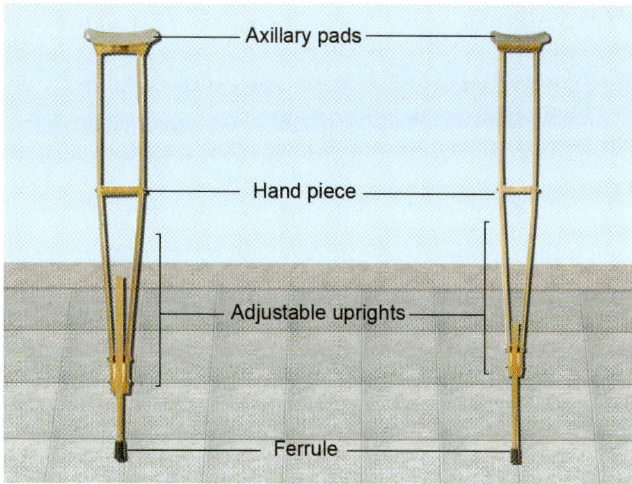

Fig. 11.6: Axillary crutch.

impaired leg is advanced first. If the crutches are used for balance, the right foot and left crutch are first moved forward followed by the other side.

Elbow Crutch

This crutch involves placing the arm into a metal or plastic curve and holding a handgrip. It has a perpendicular grip and vertical forearm support with a cuff that maintains the forearm in place. It allows the user to transfer part or all of their weight from one lower limb to the upper body.

General Features

Forearm crutches consist of a grip, cuff, shaft, and tip. The shaft and grip are made from a lightweight durable material/metal, usually aluminum **(Fig. 11.7)**. The grip is generally covered with a plastic material, which may be contoured.

The cuff is made of a plastic material that can either be open or closed. The tip is usually made of rubber available in different sizes and shapes. Most crutches can be adjusted in height between tip-to-grip and may also have adjustable grip-to-cuff height.

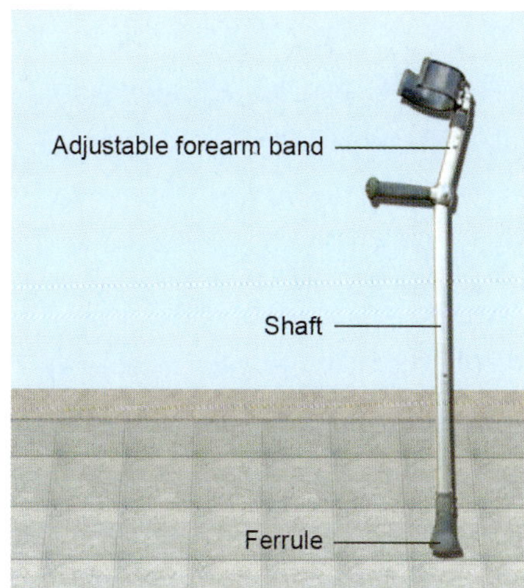

Fig. 11.7: Elbow crutch.

Measurement

The height of the crutches should be adjusted so the elbow is slightly bent (15–30°) when standing straight. While holding the grip, the cuff should lie 2.5–5 cm below the elbow.

Clinical Implication and Uses

Usually two crutches are used together, one for each side. When the injured, weak or disabled lower limb is NWB, the user starts by standing on the good leg. Both crutches are then advanced forward and placed on the ground, followed by the good leg hopping to, or slightly past, the tips of the crutches. Crutches should not be used in case of upper limb injuries which may be aggravated with their use.

If the injured, weak or disabled lower limb is partially weight bearing, it is brought forward in line with the crutches. When climbing upstairs, each step is climbed by advancing the good leg first, followed by the weak leg and crutches. When descending downstairs, the impaired leg is advanced first. When using the crutches for balance, the right foot and left crutch is first moved forward, followed by the left foot and right crutch.

Gutter Crutch

Also known as adjustable arthritic crutches or forearm support crutches **(Fig. 11.8)**.

General Features

These are additional types of crutches, composed of padded forearm support made up of metal, strap, adjustable hand piece, and rubber ferrule.

Measurement

If the patient is able to stand, measurements are from elbow to floor since it is the preferred position. It can be carried out with the patient lying with shoes on and is taken from the point of the flexed elbow to 20 cm lateral to the heel.

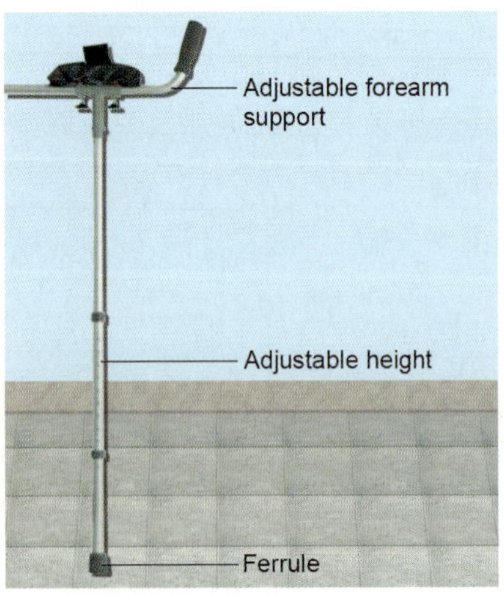

Fig. 11.8: Gutter crutch.

Uses

They are used for patients who are on PWB such as rheumatoid disease.

Walker

Walker is made up of a metal framework with four legs providing stability and support to the user. Some may have wheels (called rollators) or glides on the base of the legs, allowing the user to slide the walker rather than lifting it. A standard walker consists of a height-adjustable frame slightly wider than the user, has no wheels and no support devices other than handles. The user stands and walks behind and inside this frame, with the handles laterally and anterior to the hips. Walking frames or walkers are more stable than the others because their bases are quite large and the center of gravity falls within the base. They are prescribed for debilitated or elderly people who are usually confined to home, unable to climb stairs, and who have been advised not to venture outdoors.

Features

A walking frame consists of a frame having horizontal handgrips at the top, which attach to corresponding handles. The frame is generally made of lightweight metal tubing, such as aluminum tubing. All four legs have rubber tips/ferrules and are height-adjustable. They are often foldable and only rarely have a seat. It is often possible to have the tips exchanged to wheels (swivel or fixed, with or without push down breaks, cable breaks or castor breaks) or ski glides, converting the standard walking frame into a rollator.

Assessment

If the user needs to lean against the walker for balance, or if stability is a problem, a standard walking frame may be preferred compared to a rollator. However, the user should have the strength to pick it up and place it down. The height of the frame must be such that the handgrips lie with the crease of the user's wrist when he/she is standing straight with arms and shoulders relaxed. When holding the handgrips, the elbows should be slightly bent to about 15°.

Use

Walking cycle for the walker is as follows:
- Move the walker forward and place it on the ground
- Place one leg (affected lower extremity) first
- Then the other, inside the walker and repeat
  The user should keep their back upright at all times.

Types

There are three main types of walking frames:
1. The standard walking frame, including the pulpit frame
2. The reciprocal walking frame
3. The rollator

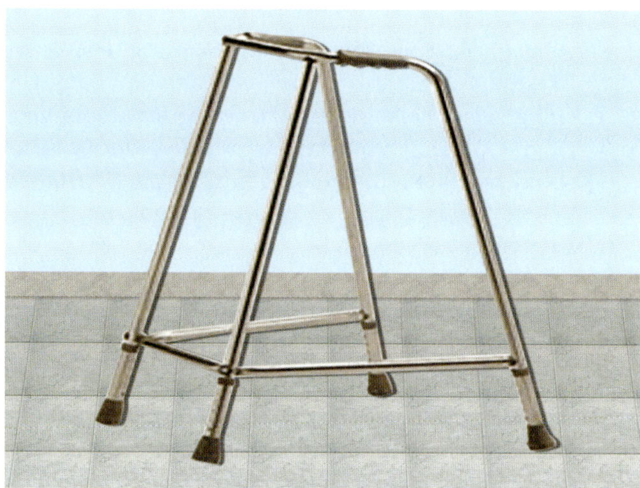

Fig. 11.9: Standard walker.

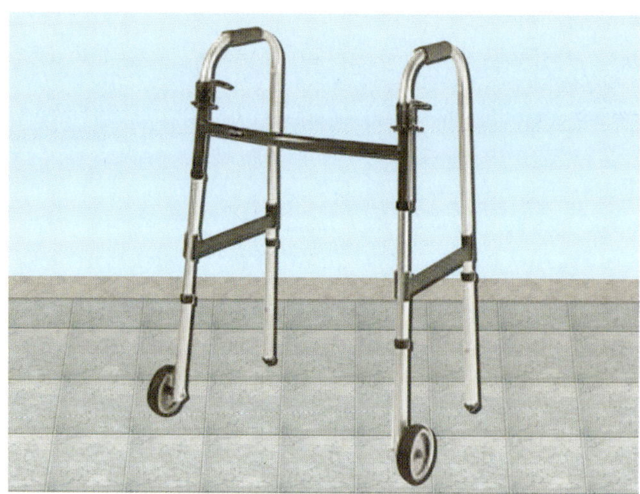

Fig. 11.11: Rollator walker.

Standard Walking Frame

The standard walking frame consists of four almost vertical aluminum alloy tubes arranged rectangular and joined on three sides by upper and lower horizontal tubes. One long side of the rectangle remains open. The vertical tubes, heights of which may be adjusted by means of spring-loaded catches have their lower ends fitted with rubber tips (ferrules) to prevent sliding and slipping. Handgrips on the upper horizontal tubes on each side help in grasping **(Fig. 11.9)**. Such a walker is light, rigid, stable, and easy to use. The user stands in the walking frame, lifts, and places the frame forward slightly away and then walks up to the frame while holding the handgrips.

Reciprocal Walking Frame

It is prescribed when the patient cannot lift the walker or need more stability. It is similar to the standard frame but with each side of the frame capable of being moved forward alternately. There are swivel joints between the front horizontal and vertical tubes **(Fig. 11.10)**. As the frame does not have to be lifted with each step, the patient's stability is increased. Stability is also more because the line of gravity always falls within the base (the parallelogram formed by the four uprights of the frame).

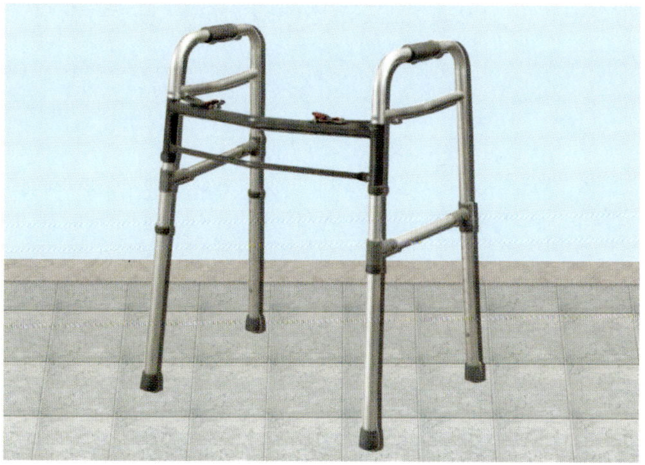

Fig. 11.10: Reciprocal walker.

Rollator Walkers

It is made up of a frame having four wheels, handle bars or seat so the user can rest as per their need. It also includes hand breaks for safety. It has built-in handgrips and three or more legs of which two or more have wheels which give support while walking. A rollator is a walker with two small casters at the front and two short legs at the back, protected by rubber ferrules **(Fig. 11.11)**. Care must be taken when recommending a rollator for elderly patients as it may roll too far forward and they may lose their balance. The rollator is best suited for children who may find it difficult to lift walkers. The patient:

- Holds the handgrips of the walker
- Lifts the rear legs just off the ground
- Wheels the rollator forward a short distance
- Lowers the rear legs on to the ground
- Then walks forward into the rollator holding the handgrips.

Assessment: A two wheeled walker is easy to use. The walker forward between steps, while allowing leaning against the walker when stepping forward. The legs with tips prevent the walker from rolling during the stepping phase. If the user does not require leaning onto the walker for balance, a four-wheeled walker is preferred.

Measurement: The height of the walker must be adjusted so the handgrips of the walker lie in level with the crease on the inside of the user's wrist, when they are standing straight with arms and shoulders relaxed. When holding the handgrips, the elbows should be slightly bent, at about 15°.

Uses: The walking cycle for the two-wheeled anterior walker is as follows: move the walker forward and place it on the ground. Place one leg (the affected limb) first, then the other, inside the walker, and repeat this cycle. The user should maintain their back upright at all times. If the walker is being used only for balance, the user can stand inside and walk normally, simply pushing along the walker.

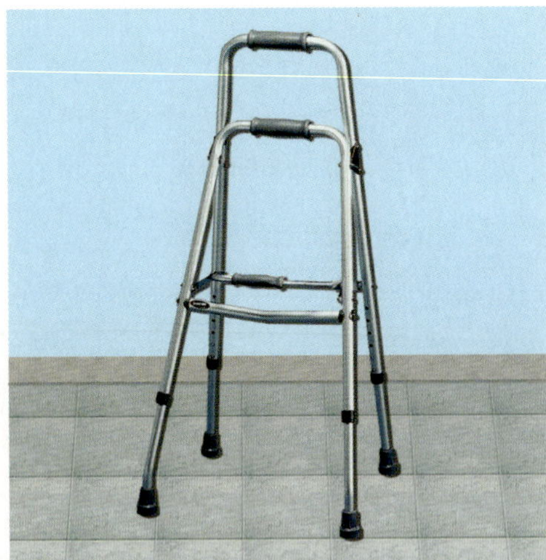

Fig. 11.12: Hemiwalker.

Hemiwalker

For those people who are having one-sided weakness from either a stroke or similar condition have the inability to use both their hands to grasp a standard walker but are able to grasp a walker with one hand. Hemiwalkers such as the adjustable aluminum side (hemi) folding walker are designed for such people. Hemiwalker is made up of two U-shaped pieces, which curve into two adjustable legs extending up to the floor; this provides four-legged support **(Fig. 11.12)**.

Hemiwalkers that have handles or handgrips at two levels are also available. Unlike the standard walker which is formed of a three-sided frame, hemiwalkers are made up of one-sided frame, but they also have reinforced frames with crossbars and sidebars.

The use of a hemiwalker to walk is done in a similar fashion as the cane. One should grasp the handle with hand, lift the walker forward to the side, just like how one tends to move a cane.

Gait Pattern: Standard Walker

Three types of gait patterns are there which can be used with a standard walker. These are full, partial, and NWB gaits.

1. **FWB gait:**
   - The walker is lifted forward about an arm's length.
   - Move the lower limb forward.
   - Move forward second LE past the first.
   - Repeat the cycle.
2. **Partial weight-bearing walking:**
   - The walker is lifted forward, about an arm's length.
   - The affected lower limb is taken forward. And body weight is moved partially onto this limb and partially via upper limb to the walker.
   - The unaffected lower limb is taken forward past the affected limb.
   - Repeat the cycle.

3. **NWB:**
   - Pick the walker and move it forward, about an arm's length.
   - Body weight is transferred through the upper limb to the walker. The affected LE is held anterior to the body but should not make contact with the ground.
   - The unaffected extremity is moved forward.
   - Repeat the cycle.

Crutch Walking Pattern

There are various kinds of gait patterns for individuals using crutches, such as:

Two-point gait pattern: This gait pattern is not very stable and a person requires very good balance to walk using a two-point crutch gait pattern **(Fig. 11.13)**.

For example:
1. Move the right-side lower limb and the left side crutch forward together.
2. Move the left side lower limb and right-side crutch forward together.
3. Repeat the cycle.

Three-point gait pattern: This type of walking pattern is useful when one affected lower limb has the inability to bear weight (which could be due to joint replacement, fracture, amputation, etc.). Just as the name suggests, this gait pattern involves three-point contact that includes the two crutch points and an unaffected lower limb on the floor **(Fig. 11.14)**.

For example:
1. Simultaneously move the affected (NWB) extremity and both crutches forward.
2. Followed by that take the unaffected (weight-bearing) lower limb forward.
3. Repeat the same.

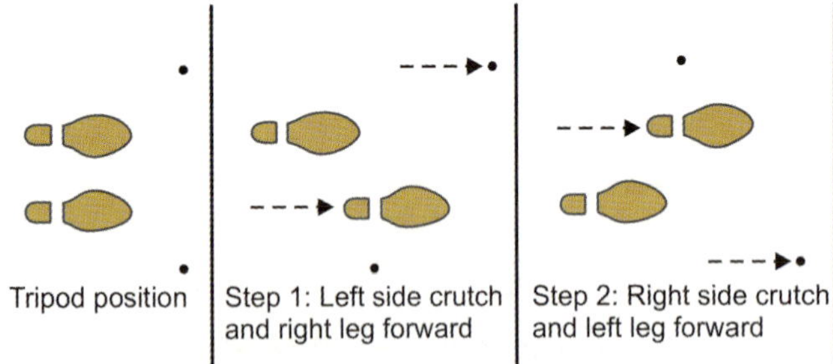

Fig. 11.13: Two-point gait pattern.

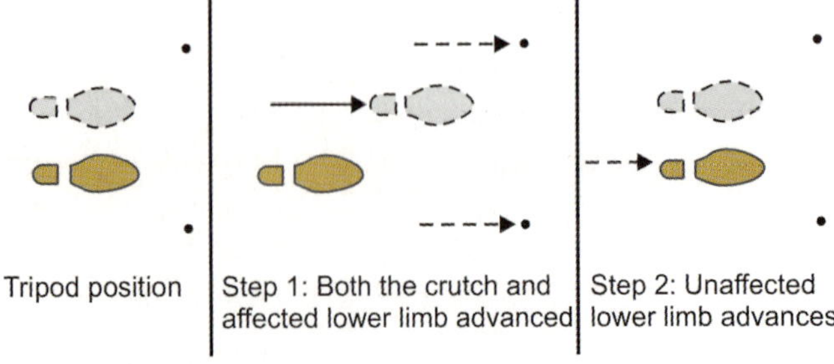

Fig. 11.14: Three-point gait pattern.

Fig. 11.15: Four-point gait pattern.

Four-point gait pattern: In people with problems of coordination, poor balance and muscle weakness in both LE, this type of gait pattern is very useful. It has the advantage of being a stable and slow gait pattern in comparison to the three-point gait pattern **(Fig. 11.15)**.

For example:

1. Move the right crutch forward
2. Move the left leg forward
3. Move the left crutch forward
4. Move the right leg forward
5. Repeat

Wheelchairs

The first wheelchair was produced by **Hebert Everest and Harry Jennings** in United States of America in 1993. The WHO has defined manual wheelchair as "Wheelchair propelled by the user or pushed by another person." Wheelchairs are helpful for people who are unable to take weight on their lower legs or those who are unable to walk. In other words, wheelchair is a chair that has wheels and is used by people who are unable to walk but have intact upper body function and strength.

Features

The basic manual wheelchair is composed of a seat and back rest (which provides the seating support system). It also consists of foot rest, one or two swivel castor wheels which are in front. There are two large wheels at the rear which have push rims. In some cases, there are levers that allow propulsion and steering manually by the user. The chair frame can be either rigid or foldable and is most commonly made up of aluminum or titanium **(Fig. 11.16)**.

Assessment

For providing maximum comfort and mobility to the user, a wheelchair should be fitted according to the individual, this also helps to prevent any sort of injury. A seat-to-back angle of 90–100° provides optimal sitting position for most of the users, along with it a knee angle of 90–120°. The feet as well as the thighs need to be properly supported by the footrest and seat/cushion respectively. The seat has to be narrow enough without touching the hip bones. Approximately half an inch of space on either side of the thighs should be provided. The correct seat depth is the one which permits with approximately an inch of space between the front sitting edge of seat or cushion to the posterior aspect of the knees. Usually, castors in front and the large wheels at rear have two to three positions of the wheel axle which allows the adjustment of the front and rear height of chair, respectively.

Uses

While using the wheelchair, the person should be as upright as possible, i.e., one should avoid leaning forward

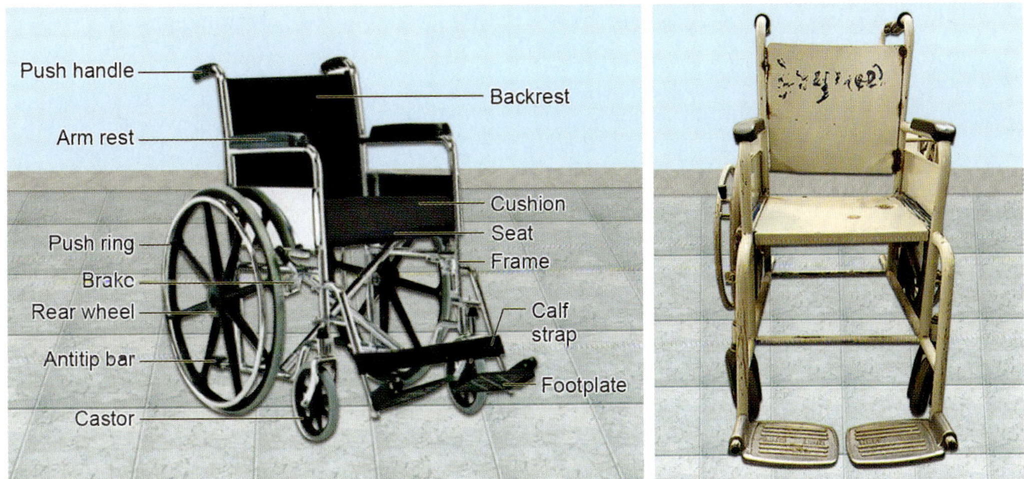

Fig. 11.16: Manual basic type of wheelchair.

or sliding backward in the seat. The importance of the wheelchair is as follows:

- To reduce immobility/being bed ridden
- To prevent secondary complications related to long-term recumbent position
- To increase involvement of the users in community activities
- To improve the opportunities for education, employment, and social interaction.

Instruction for Patients

Patients should always be instructed about the proper use and operation of a wheelchair. Make the patient sit in the chair with his feet on the footrest plates and then give him the instructions for the following maneuvers:

- Teach the patient locking and unlocking of wheel brakes.
- Demonstrate the hand placement for turning the rims and rolling the rims forward with even force to produce a straight-ahead movement.
- Teach the patient how to turn the wheelchair. Instruct the patient to make use of force on the left rim, to turn right, and application of force on the right turning rim to turn left.
- Ask the patient to show the wheelchair techniques, and provide necessary guidance.

Several precautions are required when orthopedic patients use a wheelchair, such as:

- Patient should not be using the chair as a racing vehicle.
- Patient should ask for assistance while entering elevators, passing through doorways, or while going through congested areas.
- Always instruct the patient that while getting in or out of the wheelchair, the braking devices must be set and the wheelchair should be braced against the wall or held. This would prevent the chair from tipping or rolling when he/she shifts weight or changes position.
- Instruct the patient to make use of safety belts.
- Educate the patient about ways of navigating through slopes and kerbs.

Common Problems

Some common problems with poor quality wheelchairs include:

- Poor quality seat and backrest upholstery tears or sags
- Castor wheels (axles, tires, bearings, castor forks) breakdown
- Rear wheels (wheel axle, push ring, spokes, bearings, tires) break or wear out
- Brakes tend to rust and become unusable with time
- Foot-rests also undergo wear and tear
- Cushions are either not provided or are of poor quality and quickly break down
- Removable parts can get lost

Types

Manual Push-Type Wheelchair

This wheelchair is like a manual basic wheelchair. It has push handles, which are designed so the wheelchair can be propelled by caregivers. The wheels at the rear do not have rims and are often smaller in size in comparison to the wheels of a manual basic wheelchair. Manual push-type wheelchairs are easy to maneuver (and often foldable) and light in weight. They are commonly used in places such as hospitals and airports for transport over very short distances.

General Features

Manual push-type or transport wheelchair comprises a frame, which is mostly foldable. It also has a seat and back rest. There are also arm rests (fixed or flip-up), foot rests, four wheels and push handles to move it. The front wheels are swivel castors. The rear wheels are fixed with wheel locks **(Fig. 11.17)**. Most of these wheelchairs have a flexible sling design, in which fabric of seat as well as backrest is stretched between the sides of the chair. Some transport wheelchairs have solid, one-piece bar footrests, but most provide separate, adjustable footrests.

Transport chairs are designed in a way that they are easy to transport and stow away. This factor is given priority over comfort. Some chairs are hybrids, that is they can be helpful to function of both as a rollator and a transport chair. Some of these chairs can tilt and recline, and some of these also provide the modification of adding accessories for extra support, such as head rests or calf supports.

Power-assisted Wheelchair

As the name suggests, power-assisted wheelchair is a wheelchair with add-on power assist feature. It is useful for users who have lesser upper body strength. The advantage of this wheelchair is the increased travel distance and propulsion efficiency along with the fact that it retains the functionality of a manual wheelchair **(Fig. 11.18)**.

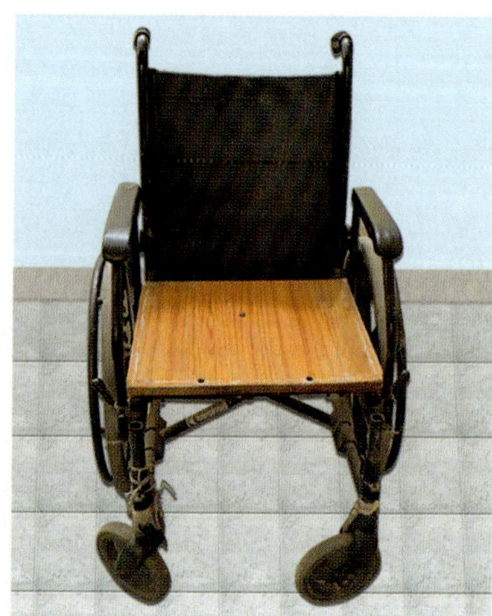

Fig. 11.17: Manual push-type wheelchair.

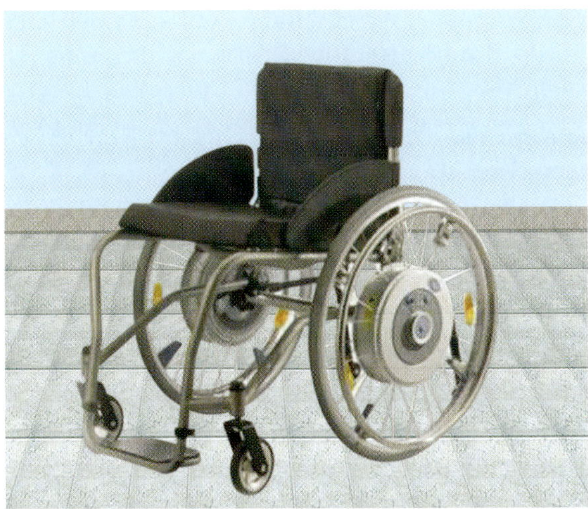

Fig. 11.18: Powered-assisted wheelchair.

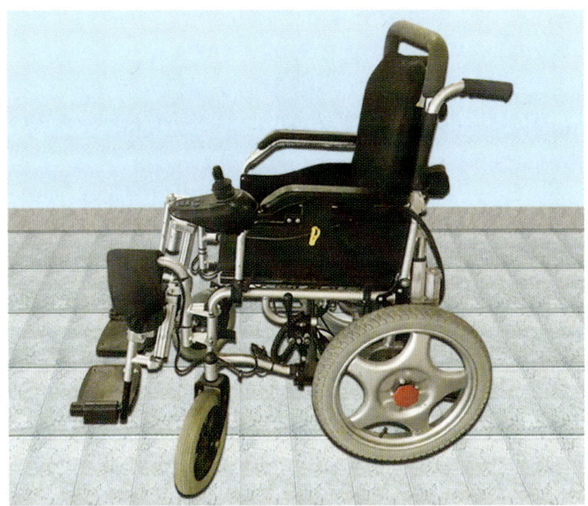

Fig. 11.19: Powered wheelchair.
Courtesy: Mission Health, Ahmedabad.

General Features

Manually driven wheelchair can be transformed to a power-assisted wheelchair by adding one of three types of accessories:

1. Replacement of regular wheel with power-assisted wheels, along with battery-powered motors in the hubs. The power sensor in the wheel will sense the pressure which is applied on push rims by the user and activate the motors proportionately. In some cases, the wheels come with a joystick, which makes it possible to alternate between manual and electrically powered configuration as per the necessity. In both cases, in order to prevent the wheelchair from tipping over backward, antitip wheels/bars are attached.

2. At the back of the wheelchair that is somewhere in between the rear wheels, an external motor with one or more wheels is attached. The power sensor in the wheel either senses the movement of the wheelchair, which helps to provide the assisting power, or it can be controlled by a joystick, and as per the need, it can be turned on and off.

3. At the back of the chair, a device with two small motor-powered wheels can be attached. This can be done in a way that the wheels are in close contact with the rims of the existing wheels. When the cylinders spin, so do the wheels. The device can sense movements of the wheelchair, and provide assisting power accordingly, or is controlled by a joystick and as per the need can be turned on or off.

Clinical Pearl

There are various types of the wheelchairs, and a single wheelchair will not suffice the needs of all patients when considering their physical and environmental needs. The most useful wheelchair for a user is the wheelchair that can give the benefit of safety and comfort. It also has to fulfill the user's physical and environmental needs and help the users to become more mobile and participate in the community.

Foldable wheelchairs are used for transportation. A wheelchair can have extra support padding or cushions to address postural needs.

Wheelchairs, Powered/Electrical

Description

A wheelchair that is powered by an electric motor is most commonly used by severely impaired people or those people who have reduced upper body strength and hence are unable to propel a manual wheelchair.

General Features

Electrically powered wheelchair comprises a seat and back rest (seating support system), along with armrests and footrests **(Fig. 11.19)**. This wheelchair is usually propelled by two large wheels. For this, the motor power is derived from some integral source of electric power. This wheelchair can either be front- or rear-wheel driven. It also has two smaller additional wheels/castors, which provide mid-wheel drive with four smaller wheels/castors. Scooters are a kind of electrically powered wheelchair having three or four wheels and a tiller for direct steering. The user directs the wheelchair to move at the desired speed and/or in the desired direction of travel by means of a control device. The standard control device is a small joystick which can be mounted on armrest. Some other control devices can be used depending on the severity of the user's disability (like allowing for steering by the chin).

Powered chairs provide four standard powered seating options: seat elevation, tilt in space, leg elevation, and recline. The manual adjustments that can be done are seat angle, seat depth, seat-surface height, footrest length and position, backrest height, armrest height, back angle, head support height, and forward/backward position.

Assessment and Fitting

Along with the physiotherapist (or other trained staff), the user should always assess if the electrically powered chair is essential especially in comparison to other

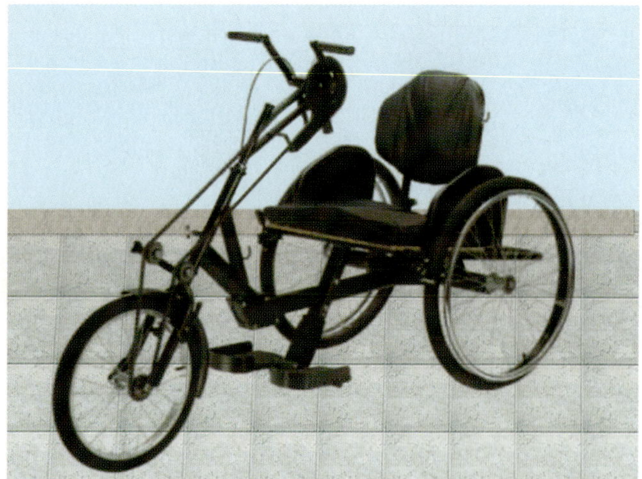

Fig. 11.20: Tricycle.

available alternatives. The chair should be fitted as per the requirements of the individual and as per the user's size and impairment.

Tricycles

Description
The tricycle functions like a bicycle. It has one wheel in front which is used for steering and has two rear wheels **(Fig. 11.20)**. A tricycle wheelchair is steered by the user by using his/her hands. In comparison to the basic wheelchair, a tricycle is more robust on uneven terrain.

Features
Tricycle wheelchairs comprise of frame with a seating system. Along with that, there are hand pedal(s) and three wheels. The wheels can be positioned either in a delta configuration, i.e., one front wheel and two rear wheels, or a tadpole configuration, i.e., two front wheels and one rear wheel. Delta configurations are most commonly used.

Different propulsion and steering configurations exist:
- **Propulsion and steering function are separate:** A turning handle/hand pedal is turned with one hand, and vehicle is steered with the other hand by turning the front wheel with a tiller. These can be one-hand drive, in which the hand pedal is positioned at one side only, or a two-hand drive, with hand pedals at both sides.
- **Propulsion and steering function are integrated:** Two pedals are positioned in front of the user, centrally. Both the pedals are useful for steering and propelling. The relative position of the pedals can coincide or be turned to 180° (similar to normal bicycles).
- **Propulsion and steering function are integrated:** The front wheel is attached with a tiller or steering wheel that helps the user propel and steer the chair. Propulsion is achieved either by pushing and pulling the tiller or by steering the wheel back and forth as if rowing.
- **Clip-ons:** The wheel in front is integrated with the function of propulsion and steering (configuration 2 or 3). It is clipped onto a normal wheelchair, converting it into a tricycle. It can be removed in situations where a basic push-rim wheelchair is needed, e.g., when the

user is indoors or accessing a toilet. As clip-ons are always front-wheel drive, it makes it difficult to climb steep hills.

Assessment and Fitting
A wheelchair should be fitted to the individual for the user to experience maximum comfort and mobility. It also helps to prevent injuries. A seat-to-back angle of 90–100° provides an optimal sitting position for wheelchair users and a knee angle of 90–120°. The feet as well as the thighs should be well supported by the footrest and a proper cushion/seat, respectively. The seat should be as narrow as possible without touching the hip bones. There should be approximately half an inch of space on either side of the thighs. The correct seat depth is the one that permits 1 inch of space between the front edge of the cushion to the posterior aspect of the knees.

Use
Training on how to transfer in and out of the tricycle and how to operate (propel and steer) are necessary.

Standing Frames (Adjustable)

Description
Used by persons relying on a wheelchair for mobility.
- Gives an alternative position other than sitting, by supporting the user in a standing position.
- Standing frames useful for the bones in the legs by preventing osteoporosis.
- They improve the circulation and digestion.
- Help to improve/maintain range of motion, reduce contractures.
- Manage pressure ulcers.
- Increase strength and endurance.

A standing frame can be static or mobile and is often equipped with a table.

General Features
There are five different types of standing frames that all include features for foot/heel fixation, knee fixation, and seat/back support:
1. **Upright/vertical standing frames:** These are the basic type of standing frames. They comprise a bottom plate with foot restraints and two vertical bars. Between these bars the person can stand with the help of suspended chest supports, pelvic supports, and knee supports. Another possibility of use is a foot plate/base and one vertical bar, to which knee, pelvic, and optionally chest supports are attached.
2. **Sit-to-stand frames,** which aid in transferring activity, consist of a planar seat, knee pads, foot plates, back support, a chest pad or chest strap, and a lifting system. The lifting system is capable of stopping at any angle between sitting and standing and is most often controlled by a gas spring lift, operated by a caregiver, or a hydraulic pump or battery-driven lift, which can also be managed by the user. These frames can either have tips or wheels/castors. Optional and additional components may include a tray, chest vest or straps, alternative options for seating and back rest, head

supports, hip or thigh supports, lateral supports, foot straps, pelvic belt, handgrips, push handles, and seat angle locators.

3. **Prone, supine, or multiposition standers** can be tilted to different degrees. Usually, the person in the frame cannot control their position. In multiposition standers, the person can be reversed, i.e., be placed in either prone or supine positions, depending on their abilities and requirements.
4. **Mobile standers** can either be sit-to-stand, prone or upright standers, with an incorporated system that allows the user to propel themselves while in a standing position. These are for users who have good head control and upper body strength.
5. **Active/dynamic standers** are less rigid standing frames that allow simultaneous movement of arms and legs in a reciprocal motion **(Fig. 11.21)**.

Assessments and Fitting
People with the following conditions often use standing frames:
- Muscular dystrophy
- Spina bifida
- Multiple sclerosis
- Cerebral palsy
- Stroke or
- Spinal cord injury (SCI) (paraplegics/quadriplegics)

Contraindications for using a standing frame include:
- Severe contractures
- Cardiac/circulatory issues
- Osteogenesis imperfecta
- Severe osteoporosis

Prior to commencement of standing program, a physiotherapist has to be consulted. All standing frames can be modified according to the need of the individual, i.e., kneepads, hip straps, and chest pad and in some cases foot plates/straps and headrest, are height-/width-/depth-adjustable.

Use
Proper instructions from the physiotherapist are essential. The suggested standing duration is either from 12 to 60 minutes/day, or multiple short durations of standing which could be more beneficial than one prolonged period.

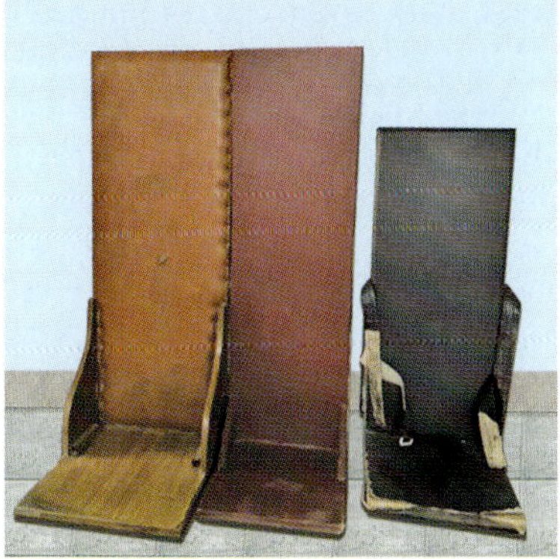
Fig. 11.21: Standing frames.

Area for Wheelchair User Training

A user training area is required for teaching:
- Transfers and health education
- Wheelchair handling, care, and maintenance
- Mobility skills and techniques to transfer **(Figs. 11.22A to E)**

MOBILITY/WALKING AIDS FOR INDIVIDUALS WITH LIMB DEFICIENCY

Individuals who have undergone amputation require a proper rehabilitation program as early as possible and are in need of compensatory aids to attain functional independence. The prescription of a proper assistive device or walking aid will require a multidisciplinary team assessing various factors.

Lower Limb Amputation

In order to restore the functional ambulation and independency, the person with an amputation can use a walking aid, which can be temporary or permanent. The selection of aid depends on the fitness level, strength, balance, and the risk of falls.
- The walking aid will allow weight bearing on the affected lower limb and compensate the risk of fall.
- Early mobilization following amputation is now an essential component in the rehabilitation program of all amputees.
- To mobilize the patient by allowing him to hop using a frame or crutches only allows the stump to hang down taking no active part in the exercise.
- The apparatus designed by Little (1971) comprised of a single compartment pneumatic sleeve long enough to extend from the groin to below the amputation stump. It was enclosed by a tubular frame, having at its lower end an extension tube to a solid ankle cushion heel (SACH) foot. The structure was changed so that it provides greater stability of the stump within the pneumatic sleeve and to give improved end support. The stability was improved by dividing the air space in the sleeve into anterior and posterior compartments which communicated with each other via a small transfer port. Improved end support was achieved by using a small subsidiary air bag placed in the lower part of the main pneumatic sleeve and invaginated on itself to support the end of the stump. Simple webbing slings supported the distal end of the pneumatic sleeve in the frame and allowed adjustments in length to be made. A simple support frame was designed with a padded safety ring at the upper end and a simple rocker in place of the SACH foot at the distal end.

Uses

The Roehampton pneumatic walking aid is suitable for patients of widely differing build. It may be used for

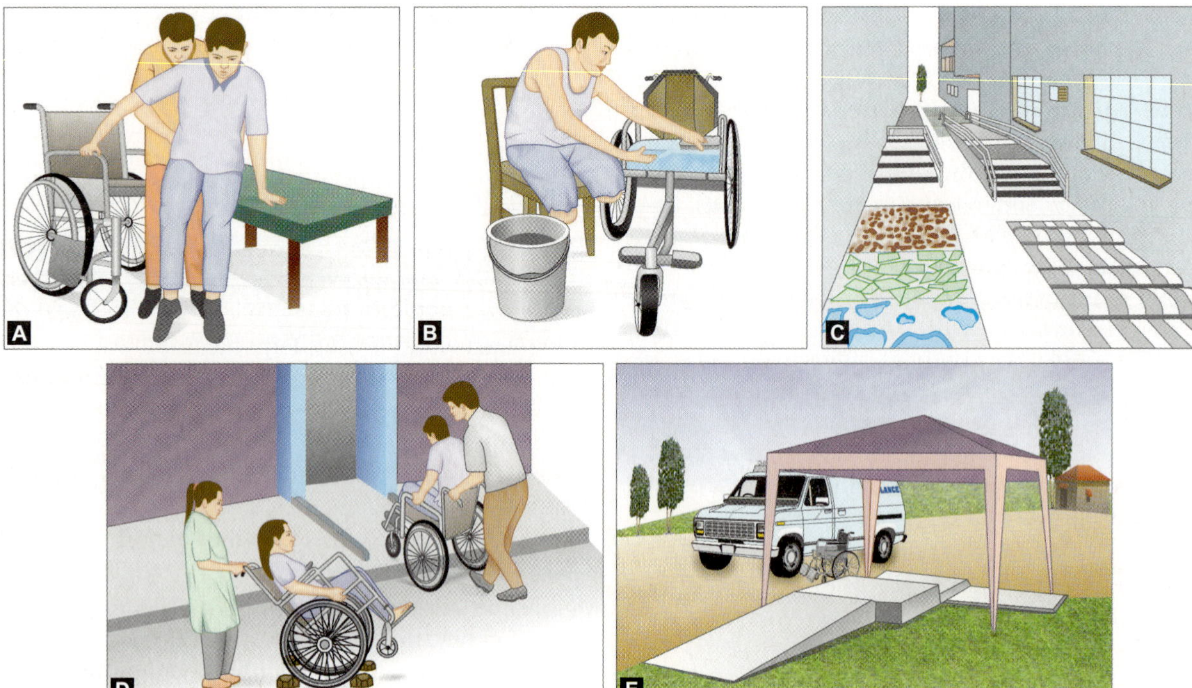

Figs. 11.22A to E: Area for wheelchair user training. (A) Transfers and health education can be taught in a clinical area, client's home, or outreach setting. Equipment: Basic equipment such as a bed to wheelchair practice transfers is helpful; (B) Wheelchair handing, care, and maintenance can be taught in the clean area of a workshop, or in any other suitable location. Equipment: Basic wheelchair is needed; (C) Mobility skills are commonly taught outside; however, indoors are also fine. A purpose-built outdoor mobility skills area can simulate the different surfaces that wheelchair users will need to be able to traverse in their daily life, such as rough ground, soft ground, drains, speed bumps, kerbs, steps, and stairs. In an integrated service, the mobility skills area may be used by people with other mobility impairments. For example, people learning to use a prosthetic limb, or regaining walking skills after an injury; (D) Where there is no space for a dedicated mobility skills area, identify existing spaces that can be safely used for mobility skills training. Avoid areas where there are a lot of people coming and going and aim to find a range of different obstacles; (E) Portable mobility skills training equipment can be fabricated and set up wherever a wheelchair service is being delivered. The illustration on the right shows portable mobility skills equipment set up under a shade shelter.

below- and through-knee amputations and with a slightly modified sleeve for above-knee cases.

Application

To apply the walking aid, the patient is seated between parallel bars with his stump extended in front of him. The small end-support air bag is positioned over the distal end of the stump and held in position as the long pneumatic sleeve is pulled over this and up to the groin. The frame of the prosthesis is then passed over the pneumatic sleeve and held in place until inflation is complete. The end-support bag is partially inflated, then the main air bag is inflated to a pressure of 40 mm Hg using a simple foot pump and pressure gauge. The gauge and pump are removed and the inflating tube is sealed off with a spigot. The patient can then stand so that minor adjustments can be made, and is then able to walk with a stiff knee gait. When the patient bears weight on the socket, the air pressure in both bags will rise to 60 mm Hg or more.

The apparatus can be worn continuously for a period of 2 hours and can be used as many times as is necessary in the course of a single day (two times a day is usual in the course of normal rehabilitation). However, when commencing exercise on the sixth postoperative day or at any time before complete wound healing, the air bag is inflated for 5–10 minutes only during the first day of use, and thereafter, the time is increased progressively. The appliance is a walking training aid.

Spinal Cord Injury

Spinal cord injury leads to deficits of movement, but more essentially, it may restrict a patient's ability to carry out self-directed, purposeful movements, which are required to perform all activities. SCI usually causes paralysis, which is permanent of some of the large and powerful skeletal muscles of the body. The location of the injury along the spine correlates roughly to the cumulative amount of paralysis that is seen. The less distal the site of injury, the greater the involvement. Trauma which occurs at the spinal column can affect the transmission of the nerve signals to all parts of the body served by the injury site and beyond.

Spinal cord injuries are usually incomplete in nature, meaning rarely there is complete function loss or bilateral symmetry of effects below the site of the injury (lesion). Let's consider two common kinds of paralysis: paraplegia and quadriplegia.

Spinal cord injury causes damage to the nerve cells which prevents signals from the brain to reach the muscles. SCI leads to weakness and spasticity in the limbs and trunk. The injury disrupts nerve signals for sensation that leads to parts of the body to be without sensation or cause abnormal sensations, such as burning or tingling. All these impairments cause difficulty in walking. Hence, in SCI, gait training with walking aids is essential to help the patient regain quality of life.

Walking is the most important goal for patients with SCI. There are currently various mechanical as well as electromechanical devices, orthotics and walking aids, which have been developed to help SCI patients to walk. As ambulation for routine activities (such as shopping) will require a person to walk distances more than 250 m, an average patient walking with aids will frequently need to walk for at least 10 minutes, which would probably mean arriving at the destination in exhaustion. SCI patients using assistive walking devices require extra energy. The amount of extra energy used will depend on the assistive device used, whereas some patients have only one possible mode and device to use.

Assistive devices may include:

- Special walkers that have safety straps at hips and trunk
- A standard walker with no wheels on the legs
- A rolling walker (walker with two wheels on front legs), if balance is a little better
- A rolling walker with forearm platforms, if arms are weak
- A rollator walker (walker with four wheels and a basket), if balance is good enough to walk in the community
- One or two forearm crutches, if better strength and balance is present, but with a weak grip
- One or two quad canes with four tips at the bottom, if patient has good strength and balance and fair grip.

All of these conditions must be kept at the forefront of planning for mobility and will be mentioned from time to time in the text that follows.

Transfer

The initial and simplest tasks of SCI mobility begin with rising from a reclining position, from which seated tasks, ambulation, or wheeled mobility can proceed. When starting from a bed, the person must first be able to sit up.

- A paraplegic or quadriplegic with good shoulder strength may be able to sit up without assistance.
- Some may prefer to use an overhead handle, often called a trapeze, or a looped strap, to pull up into a sitting position.
- Sometimes, a hospital-type bed, with a powered drive to the articulated back section, can raise the person to a sitting position from which he can turn and let his legs off the bed in preparation for standing.
- A standing transfer, even with an attendant assisting is desirable because the weight is borne on the legs, but not by the attendant or a transfer device.

If the legs are capable of supporting body weight, with or without bracing, the person may develop greater independence.

Standing Aids

Paraplegics and quadriplegics, although unable to stand unassisted, can derive both physiological and psychological benefits from standing. Being able to stand allows a wheelchair user to reach work surfaces and interact with standing people at their level. There are static devices, called standing frames that hold a person in a standing position by binding him to an upright, rigid structure.

Ambulation

Walking is the most common form of mobility for humans and the mode most desired by people who have limitations that diminish or eliminate their ambulation abilities. Where there is any possibility of a mechanism to regain the ability to walk or move about in a standing posture, even if it is slow and requires great expenditure of energy, a person often prefers to ambulate rather than use wheeled mobility. Even temporary standing, without walking, can be used to enable a person to get through narrow entryways, such as toilet compartments, bathrooms, and closets. The desire to remain upright has sustained the development and application of torso and leg braces, standing aids, and even artificial stimulation of paralyzed muscles by externally supplied electrical signals—functional electrical stimulation. At a lesion level around high thoracic, the instability of the torso suggests that ambulation may be less secure and more demanding of energy than wheeled mobility.

Stability

One of the more important considerations in assuring the fullest functional mobility of the SCI patient is stabilizing the proximal parts of the body in order to facilitate the most controlled movements of the distal portions. The person fitted with the finest of upper limb orthoses or supplied with the most elaborate vehicle control system will be substantially incapable of adequate performance if the body is not appropriately stabilized.

Wheeled Mobility

When walking is not an option, or when the upper limits of speed and range of ambulation are too low for the mobility needs of the person or the occasion, the indicated mobility aid is the wheelchair or any one of a variety of wheeled devices. The basic, most familiar form of the wheelchair is a shiny, tubular metal, open-framed structure that has four wheels, two small casters in front and two large drive wheels in the rear. For a chronic user, a wheelchair should be very carefully sized and the components and accessories selected should assure the efficiency of operation, postural support, and prevention of medical complications of disability.

Wheelchairs are one of the most commonly used assistive devices, providing wheeled mobility for people with a mobility disability. WHO estimates that 1% of any population needs a wheelchair. This means that globally more than 70 million people need a wheelchair.

ORTHOTICS IN MOBILITY

Introduction

Orthosis is an external appliance used over the body part. Several definitions have been given to the term orthosis.

- An orthosis is an external appliance worn to restrict or assist motion or to transfer load from one area of the body to another.
- An orthosis is defined as any medical device applied to, or around, a bodily segment in the case of physical impairment or disability.
- It is a device applied to the body to stabilize, immobilize, prevent or correct deformity, protect against injury promote healing or assist function.

An **orthotist** is the health-care professional who designs, fabricates, and fits orthoses for the limbs and trunk, and a **pedorthist** is the health-care professional who designs, fabricates, and fits only shoes and foot orthoses.

Objectives and Functions

The functions of orthosis and objectives of orthotic prescription are summarized as follows:

- To immobilize or support a body part for rest or stabilization, e.g., fracture bracing
- To increase range of motion (ROM)
- To help strengthening muscles, e.g., dynamic splint
- To correct a contracture deformity, e.g., Milwaukee brace
- To maintain alignment of body segment, e.g., shoe modification
- To reduce pain, e.g., spinal corset
- To stabilize a displaced or injured part, e.g., four post collar.

General Principles

- **Use of forces:** Orthoses utilize forces to limit or assist movements, for example:
  - Rigid material spanning a joint prevents motion, e.g., posterior tube splint.
  - A spring in a joint is stressed by one motion and then recoils to assist the opposite desired motion e.g., leaf spring orthosis.
- **Sensation:** An orthotic device often covers skin areas and decreases sensory feedback. Proprioception should be preserved where possible.
- **Correcting a mobile deformity:** A flexible deformity may be corrected by an orthosis, like the one given in genu recurvatum or mobile scoliosis. The corrective force must be balanced by proximal and distal counter forces (three-point force systems).

- **Fixed deformity:** If a fixed deformity is accommodated by an orthosis, it will prevent the progression of the deformity.
- **Adjustability:** Orthotic adjustability is indicated for children to accommodate their growth and for patients with progressive or resolving disorders.
- **Maintenance and cleaning:** The orthosis should be simple to maintain and clean.
- **Application:** The design should be simple for easy donning and doffing. The more complicated the gadget, the less likely it is to be accepted for permanent use.
- **Limitation of movement:** Limiting motion to reduce pain, e.g., knee brace.
- **Gravity:** Gravity plays an important role in upper limb orthosis, especially in those joints where the heaviest movement masses are present. For example, a Rolyan shoulder cuff can be used in hemiplegia to prevent subluxation of the shoulder, which is the largest joint prone for the deleterious effects of gravity.
- **Comfort:** The orthosis should be easy to wear and comfortable to use. This can happen only if the forces meant for correction are distributed over the largest area possible.
- **Utility:** The orthosis must be useful and serve a real purpose. If one hand is functional and normal, an upper extremity orthosis for the affected side may not be used as most activities of daily living can be performed with the good hand.
- **Cosmesis:** Cosmesis is important especially in the hand. A functional but unsightly orthosis is often rejected if the patient values appearance over function.
- **Duration:** Use only as indicated and for as long as necessary.
- **Appropriateness:** It should allow joint movement wherever appropriate.

UPPER LIMB ORTHOSES

Devices applied to hand and wrist are conventionally called hand splints. Hand splints are an important adjunct to the management of neuromusculoskeletal problems affecting hand or the whole upper limb.

Upper limb orthoses can be described by the joints or segments that they cross and any special design features incorporated. These should also be described as a:

- Static
- Dynamic or
- Hybrid system

A static orthosis remains fixed in one position with no movement across the joint. A dynamic orthosis increases or decreases the movements across the joint. In contrast to lower limb orthoses, many upper limb orthoses can be fabricated from a kit or purchased off the shelf from a catalog or medical supplier.

Finger Orthosis

There are three common types of finger orthoses used:
1. For fracture, ligamentous injury, inflammatory disease a static gutter splint, or circumferential splint is used to eliminate motion across interphalangeal (IP) joints **(Fig. 11.23)**.
2. For contracture across an IP joint, a dynamic finger orthosis with spring wire or rubber bands is used.
3. For progressive deformity from disease, such as rheumatoid arthritis, a specialized finger orthosis called a ring orthosis can be used. This is used to control swan neck deformity and Boutonniere's deformity.

Hand–Finger Orthosis

These are commonly used to control the digits or metacarpophalangeal (MCP) joints from a device positioned across the palmar or dorsal surface of the hand.
- For rheumatoid arthritis at the base of the thumb or de Quervain's tendonitis, the thumb can be controlled with a static hand-finger orthosis stabilizing the thumb commonly called a thumb spica.
- Median nerve injury at the distal forearm or wrist will cause loss of motor function of the thumb. A short opponens orthosis is fabricated from plastic to position the thumb opposite the fingers while maintaining the first web space.
- Ulnar nerve injury causes "intrinsic minus" hand positioning with hyperextension of the MCPs. This can be treated with a hand-finger orthosis with MCP block in slight flexion. This allows better functioning of the long finger flexors and extensors.
- Flexion–extension contracture across the MCP joints can be treated with a dynamic hand–finger orthosis commonly called a knuckle bender using spring wire or rubber bands.

Wrist–Hand–Finger Orthoses

These devices range from very simple, off-the-shelf products to complex, and custom-made devices.
- The simplest and most common device to cross the wrist is the cock-up splint for carpal tunnel syndrome. This device positions the wrist in its neutral or slightly extended position to minimize pressure within the carpal tunnel.
- Stroke patients with little or no function in the affected hand can be positioned properly with a static wrist–hand–finger orthosis, maintaining the wrist in neutral, MCPs in slight flexion, and IP joints in extension. The thumb must always be maintained in its position of opposition to the fingers.
- Low radial nerve injury causes wrist drop and inability to extend the fingers. A dynamic wrist–hand–finger orthosis with extension positioning of the wrist and fingers using outriggers and rubber bands should be used. The patient can still flex the fingers and wrist for grasp and functional activities. However, when the patient relaxes, the rubber bands extend the fingers to open the hand.
- With C6-level quadriplegia, active wrist extension is preserved but finger flexion and grasp are lost. A tenodesis or flexor hinge orthosis is commonly used to restore grasp or prehension. This is a dynamic wrist–hand–finger orthosis that uses active wrist extension to drive the second and third fingers against the thumb for grasp. There are several designs available both by kit and custom fabrication.

Elbow Orthosis

Flexion or extension contractures at the elbow are common after immobilization of the upper limb from fractures, burns, surgery, or other injuries. A dynamic elbow orthosis with adjustable tension in flexion or extension is commonly used to stretch the contractures. Elbow orthoses with adjustable ROM joints are also available postoperatively to slowly restore active movement at the joint as healing occurs **(Fig. 11.24)**.

Shoulder Orthoses

Generally, there are two types of devices applied across the shoulder joint **(Fig. 11.25)**:
1. In acute injury or surgery, the shoulder can be fixed in nearly any position using an airplane or gunslinger type of device. This provides unloading of the weight of the limb to prevent subluxation of the glenohumeral joint, and can allow limited or no movement for healing of soft or bony tissues.

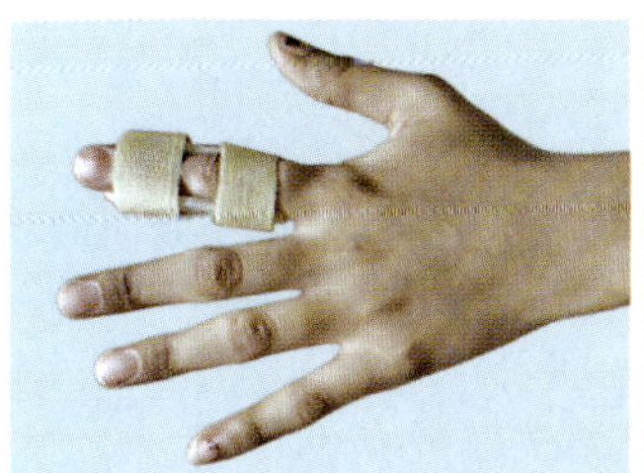
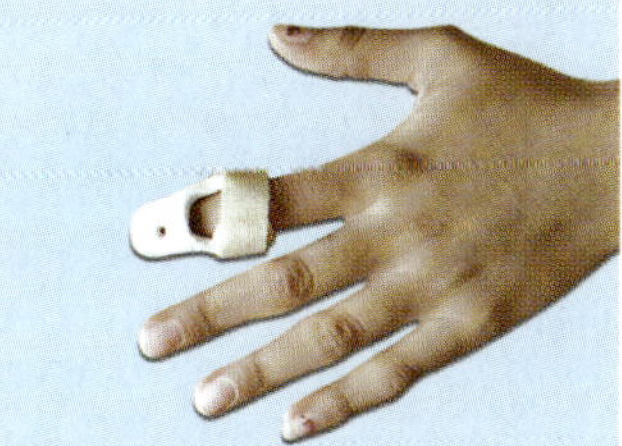

Fig. 11.23: Finger splint.

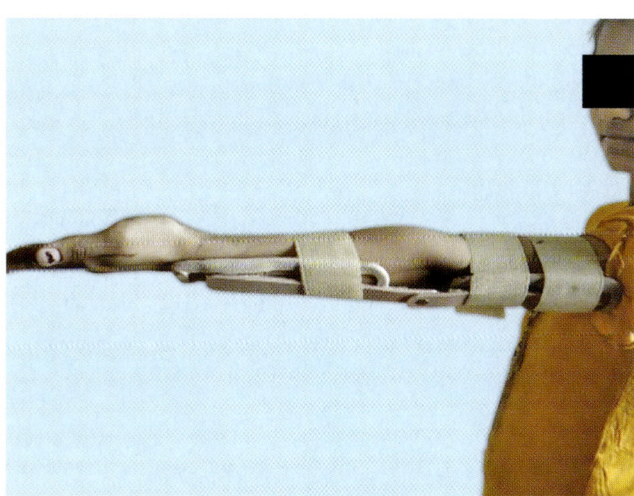

Fig. 11.24: Elbow orthosis.

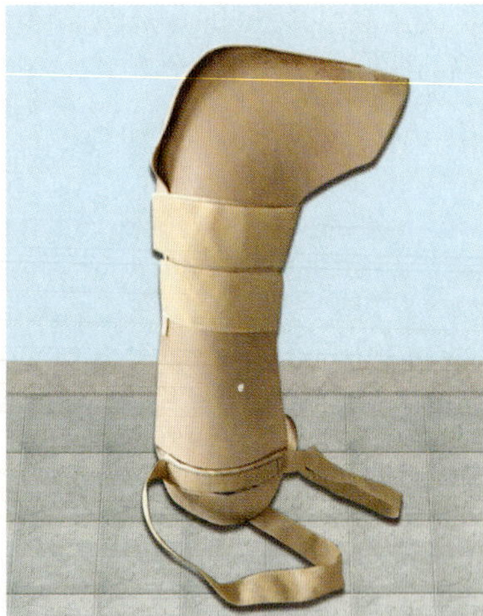

Fig. 11.25: Shoulder orthosis.

2. Following stroke or brachial plexus injury, the gleno-humeral joint may be at risk for subluxation and chronic pain. A nonelastic humeral cuff or sling can be applied to maintain glenohumeral positioning.

SPLINTS

Technically the term splint refers to a temporary device that is part of a treatment program.

Classification

Splints can be classified into the following:
- Static
- Dynamic

Static Splints

Static splints have the following characteristics:
- Static splints have no moving parts
- Prevent motion
- Are used to rest or rigidly support the splinted part.

Uses

These are used to stretch joint contractures progressively or align specified joints after a surgical procedure for optimal healing.

Disadvantages

Immobilization causes atrophy and stiffness.

Dynamic Splints

Dynamic splints are moving splints; their parts permit, control, or strengthen movement. The movement in a dynamic splint may be intrinsically powered by another body part or by electrical stimulation of the patient's muscles. Extrinsic power may be provided by elastic bands or pulleys.

Uses

It provides prehension and also static positioning of the hand in a functional position.

General Functions of Splinting

General functions of splinting are as follows:
- To prevent undesirable movements
- To provide a functional position for the hand
- To reduce pain
- To hold fractured bone ends in position until they are united
- To maintain the position after reduction of a dislocation until the joint capsule is healed
- To strengthen specific muscles
- To promote grip and pinch
- To diminish muscle spasm

Types of Static Splints

Airplane Splint

The airplane splint maintains the shoulder in abduction and external rotation. It immobilizes shoulder and elbow joint. It consists of chest, arm, forearm, and wrist pieces joined to one another almost at right angles **(Fig. 11.26)**.

Indications

Indications are as follows:
1. Erb's palsy
2. Supraspinatus tendon rupture
3. Avulsion of the greater tuberosity of the humerus
4. Tuberculous arthritis of the shoulder joint
5. Paralysis of the deltoid muscle
6. Abduction fracture of the neck of the humerus

Advantages and Disadvantages

Advantages and disadvantages are:
- The advantages of this splint are that it keeps the shoulder joint in its optimal position and does not confine the patient to the bed.
- The disadvantages are that it is inconvenient for the patient and that it tends to slide down the torso.

Cock-up splint

The cock-up splint immobilizes or stabilizes the wrist in dorsiflexion with volar or dorsal support. It may be static or

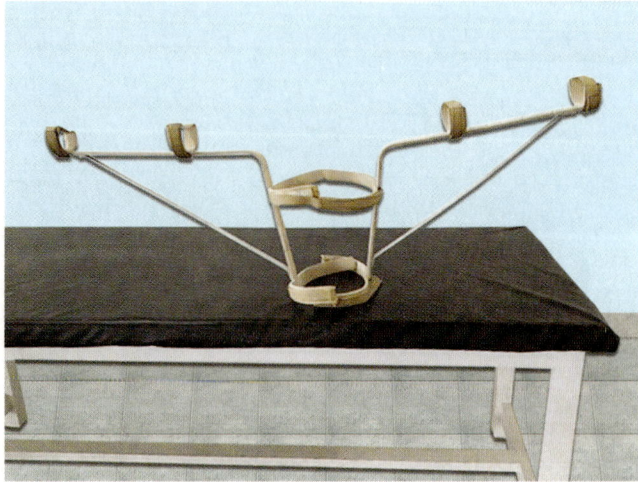

Fig. 11.26: Airplane splint.

dynamic. It allows full MCP flexion and carpometacarpal motion of the thumb. The splint should be worn all the time except during exercise and bath **(Figs. 11.27 and 11.28)**.

Indications

Wrist drop (radial nerve palsy), hemiplegia.

Knuckle Bender Splint

It maintains the MCP joint in 90° flexion and IP joint in extension.

Functions

Functions of knuckle bender splint:
- Immobilization of fingers.
- It provides support and stabilizes the wrist in extension.
- It maintains the transverse palmar arch.
- It assists in prehension.

Indications

Indications of knuckle bender splint are as follows:
- Total claw hand
- Ulnar claw hand

C-splint

This splint maintains the thumb in abduction and partial rotation and supports second metacarpal. It also stretches the first web space.

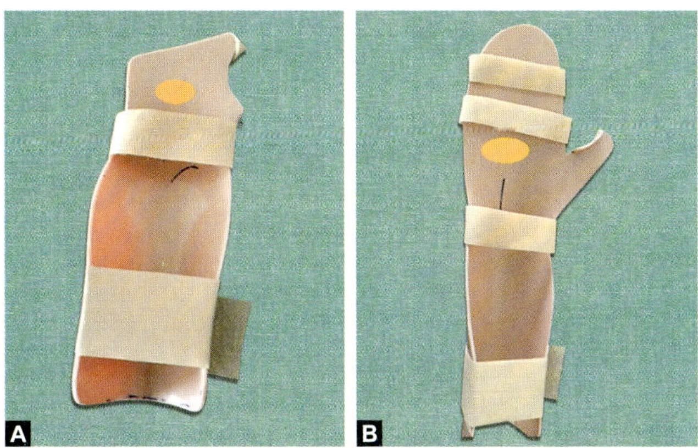

Figs. 11.27A and B: Static cock-up splint: (A) Half and (B) Full.

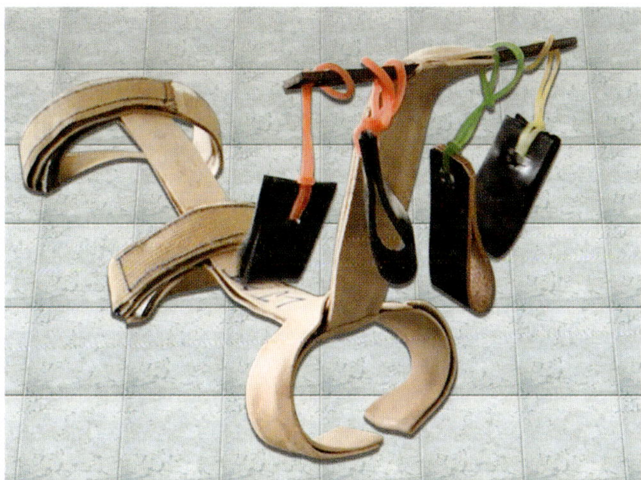

Fig. 11.28: Dynamic cock-up splint.

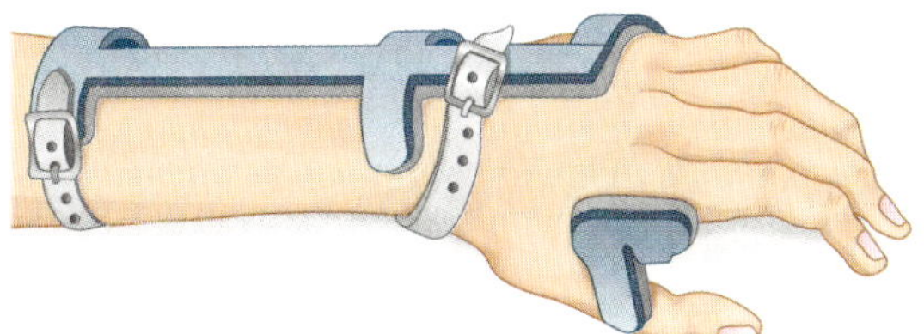

Fig. 11.29: Wrist hand orthosis (short opponens).

Indications

Indications for C-splint are as follows:
- Median nerve injury
- Contracture
- Burns

Opponens Splints

Short Opponens Splint

The short opponens splint maintains thumb in abduction and partial rotation under the second metacarpal. The wrist and other fingers are free **(Fig. 11.29)**.

Functions
- Immobilization of the thumb
- Improves prehension by providing a stable position against which the fingers can pinch
- Protects the joint from pain
- Stretches the web space.

Indications
- Low median nerve injury
- Opponens transfer (6 weeks after surgery postoperative splint).

Dorsal Long Opponens Splint

This splint holds the thumb in abduction and partial rotation under the second metacarpal and, in addition, supports the wrist dorsally in a functional position. The wrist is in 20–30° of dorsiflexion, and the thumb is abducted and rotated under the second metacarpal, with the MCP joint in 0–5° of flexion. The IP joint is free unless required to be held in extension. Other fingers are free.

Function

The function of dorsal long opponens splint is to immobilize and protect the thumb.

Indications
- Scaphoid fracture
- Bennett's fracture
- De Quervain's tenosynovitis

LOWER EXTREMITY ORTHOSES

Lower extremity orthoses range from shoes used for clinical purposes to trunk–hip–knee–ankle–foot orthoses (THKAFOs). Characteristics and functions of the principal FOs, ankle–foot orthoses (AFOs), knee–ankle–foot orthoses (KAFOs), hip–knee–ankle–foot orthoses (HKAFOs), and THKAFOs and trunk orthoses (TOs), together with the clinically important attributes of shoes, are given below.

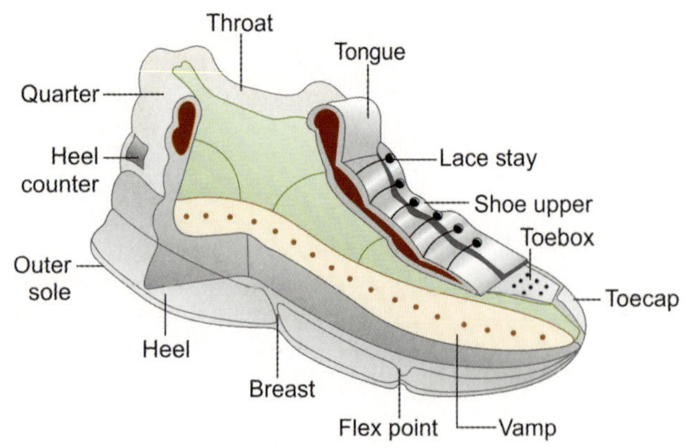
Fig. 11.30: Components of shoe.

Shoes

The shoe **(Fig. 11.30)** is the foundation for most LE orthoses. Each part of the shoe contributes to the efficacy of orthotic management and offers many options for selection. Shoes transfer body weight to the ground and protect the wearer from the terrain and the weather.

For the individual with an orthopedic disorder, footwear can serve two additional purposes:
1. It reduces pressure on sensitive deformed structures by redistributing force toward pain-free areas.
2. It serves as the foundation for AFOs and more extensive bracing.

Upper

The upper portion of the shoe has following features:
- The portion of the shoe over the dorsum of the foot is the upper.
- It consists of an anterior component called the vamp and the posterior part, the quarter. In a laced shoe, the vamp contains the lace stays, which have eyelets for shoelaces.
- For most orthotic purposes, a Blucher lace stay is preferable; it is distinguished by the separation between the anterior margins of the lace stays and the vamp **(Figs. 11.31A to C)**.
- The alternate design is the Bal, or Balmoral, lace stay, in which the lace stay is continuous with the vamp.
- *Quarter* height is another consideration in shoe prescription. The low-quarter terminates below the malleoli and is satisfactory for most clinical purposes. This style does not restrict foot or ankle motion. If the patient will be wearing a plastic orthosis molded about the ankle, it is not necessary to go to the additional expense of providing a high-quarter shoe for ankle support. A high-quarter shoe, covering the malleoli, is indicated to cover the foot having rigid pes equinus. It is also appropriate to augment foot stability in the absence of an AFO. The high-quarter shoe, however, is more difficult to don and more expensive than a comparable low-quarter one.

Sole

The *sole* is the bottom portion of the shoe. For use with a riveted metal attachment between shoe and orthosis, the sole should have an outer and an inner sole. Leather soles absorb little impact shock and provide minimal traction as compared to natural or synthetic rubber soles. To absorb shock, the shoe may have a resilient outer sole, inner sole, or insert.

Older people should wear shoes with firm, slip-resistant outsoles to reduce the risk of falling. The outer sole should not contact the floor at the distal end; the slight rise of the sole is known as *toe spring*, which allows a rocker effect at late stance.

Heel

The *heel* **(Fig. 11.32)** is the portion of the shoe adjacent to the outer sole, under the anatomical heel.
- A broad, low heel provides the greatest stability and distributes force between the back and front of the foot most evenly.
- Slight heel lifts increase the contraction of the medial gastrocnemius and the tibialis anterior.
- A higher heel places the ankle in greater plantar flexion range and forces the tibia forward. The high heel transmits more stress to the metatarsals and knee. The higher heel also reduces tension on the Achilles tendon and other posterior structures and accommodates rigid pes equinus.

Reinforcements

Reinforcements located at strategic points preserve the shape of the shoe. *Toe boxing* in the vamp protects the toes from stubbing and vertical trauma; it should be high enough to accommodate hammer toes or similar deformity. The *shank* piece is a longitudinal plate that reinforces the sole between the anterior border of the heel and the widest part of the sole at the metatarsal heads. A corrugated steel shank is necessary if an orthotic attachment is to be riveted to the shoe. The *counter* stiffens the quarter and generally terminates at the anterior border of the heel. The patient with pes valgus, however, should have a shoe with a long medial counter that provides

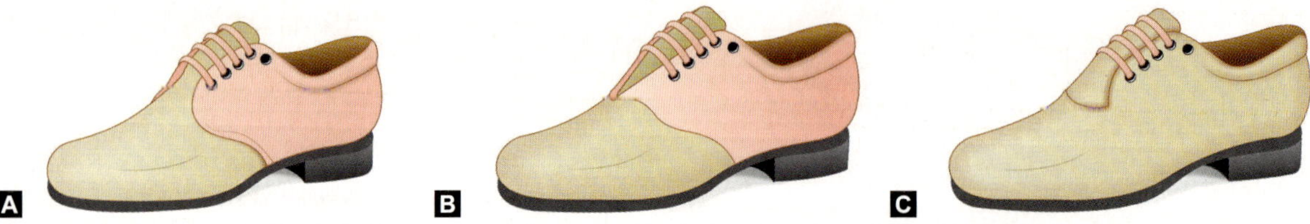
Figs. 11.31A to C: Types of shoe laces: (A) Blucher; (B) Balmoral; (C) Modified balmoral.

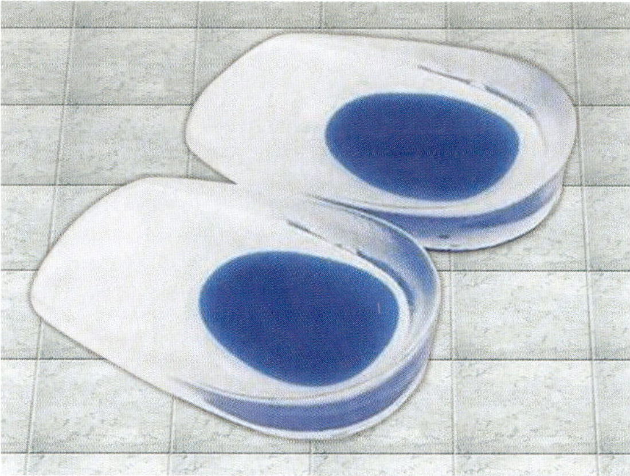

Fig. 11.32: Heel.

reinforcement along the medial border of the foot to the head of the first metatarsal, thus resisting the tendency of the foot to collapse medially **(Fig. 11.33)**.

Last

The *last* is the model over which the shoe is made. The last, whether of traditional wood, custom-made plaster, or computer-generated design, remains with the manufacturer; the shoe shape duplicates the last's contour. A given shoe size may be achieved with many lasts, each transmitting different forces to the foot. Consequently, the physical therapist should ascertain that the shoe shape fits the foot satisfactorily, rather than relying on a particular shoe size. The patient with a markedly deformed foot requires a shoe made over a special last, either a factory- or custom-made one **(Figs. 11.34A to C)**.

Foot Orthoses

Foot orthoses are appliances that apply forces to the foot. These may be an insert placed in the shoe, an internal modification affixed inside the shoe, or an external modification attached to the sole or heel of the shoe. They can enhance function by relieving pain. This may be accomplished by transferring weight-bearing stresses to pressure-tolerant sites, protecting painful areas from contact with the shoe, correcting alignment of a flexible segment, or accommodating a fixed deformity. Inserts can also improve the wearer's transition during stance phase, by altering the rollover point in late stance and by equalizing foot and leg lengths on both limbs. In many

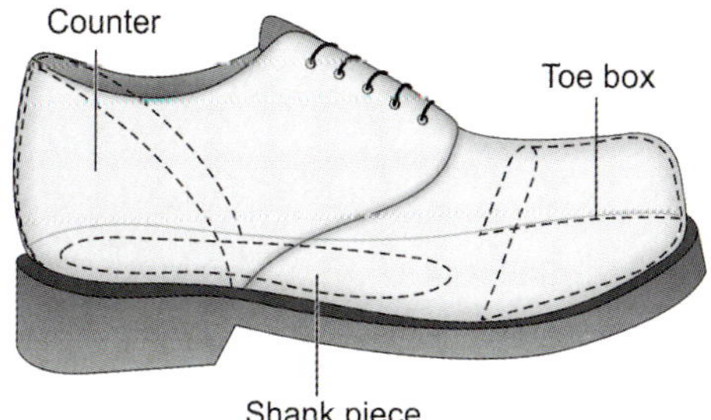

Fig. 11.33: Reinforcement.

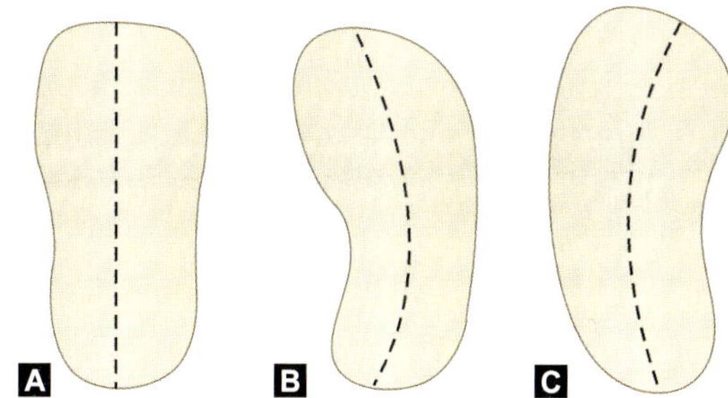

Figs. 11.34A to C: Types of last. (A) Straight; (B) Inflared; (C) Outflared.

instances, a particular therapeutic aim can be achieved by a variety of devices.

Internal Modifications

Both inserts and internal modifications **(Fig. 11.35)** reduce shoe volume, so proper shoe fit must be judged with these components in place. An insert permits the patient to transfer the orthosis from shoe to shoe.

Inserts made of resilient materials, such as the rubber, viscoelastic plastics (e.g., Sorbothane and Viscolas), or polyethylene foam, reduce impact shock and shear, thus protecting painful or insensitive feet. A full-length insert tends to reduce gait unsteadiness by improving proprioception from the increased foot contact area. Longitudinal arch supports are intended to prevent depression of the subtalar joint and flattening of the arch (pes planovalgus, pes planus). Insert orthoses are also used to relieve pain and activity limitation associated with pes cavus. The *metatarsal pad* is a convex component that may be incorporated in an insert or may be a resilient domed piece glued to the inner sole so that its apex is under the metatarsal shafts. The pad transfers stress from the metatarsal heads to the metatarsal shafts and is effective in reducing plantar pressure particularly in patients with diabetic neuropathy.

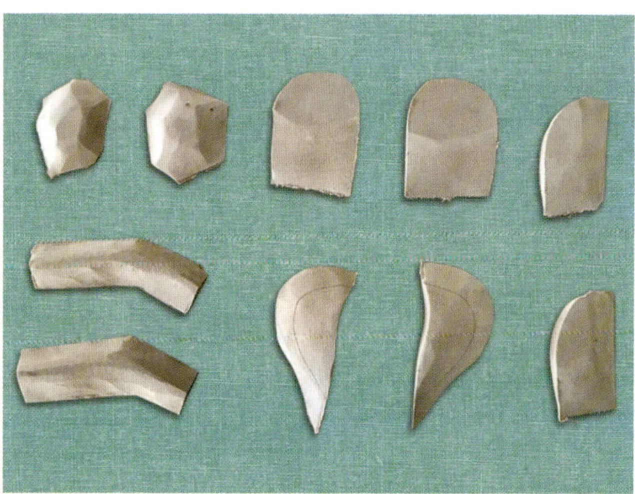

Fig. 11.35: Various internal modifications.

External Modifications

An external modification ensures that the patient wears the appropriate shoes and does not reduce shoe volume but will erode as the individual walks and is somewhat conspicuous. A *heel wedge* is a frequently prescribed external modification. It alters the alignment of the rearfoot. A medial heel wedge, by applying laterally directed force, can aid in realigning flexible pes valgus or can accommodate rigid pes varus by filling the void between the sole and the floor on the medial side. A cushion heel is made of resilient material to absorb shock at heel contact. Because it provides slight plantar flexion, the cushion heel is indicated when the patient wears an orthosis with a rigid ankle.

Sole wedges alter medial–lateral forefoot alignment. A lateral wedge shifts weight-bearing to the medial side of the front of the foot. It compensates for fixed forefoot valgus, allowing the entire distal foot to contact the floor.

Ankle–Foot Orthoses

The AFO **(Fig. 11.36)** is composed of a foundation, ankle control, foot control, and a superstructure.

Foundation

The foundation of the orthosis consists of the shoe and a plastic or metal component.

Insert

A plastic or metal insert or foot plate foundation has several advantages.

- Because internal modifications can be incorporated in it, the insert provides good control of the foot.
- It must be worn with a shoe that closes high on the dorsum of the foot to retain the orthosis.
- The insert facilitates donning the orthosis because the shoe can be separated from the rest of the brace.
- The insert also permits interchanging shoes, assuming that all shoes have been made on the same last.

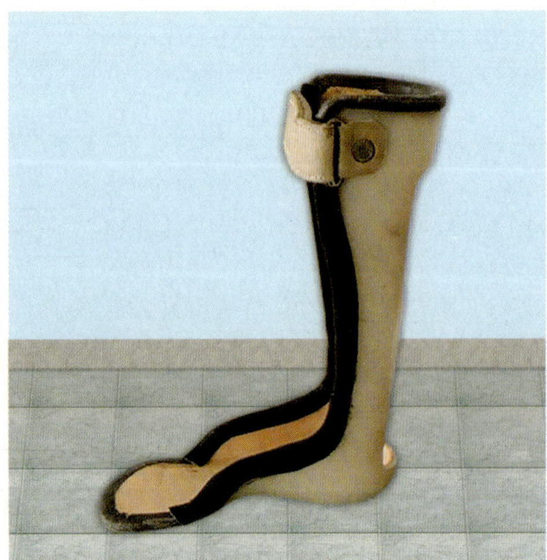

Fig. 11.36: Ankle–foot orthosis.

- Less expensive shoes, such as sneakers, can be worn because the foundation does not need to be riveted to the shoe.
- Because the insert is usually made of a thermoplastic material, such as polyethylene or polypropylene, the orthosis with an insert is relatively lightweight.

The orthotist creates a plaster model of the patient's leg, then modifies the model, removing plaster in areas where the orthosis is to apply substantial pressure, and adding plaster where pressure relief is required. Thermoplastic is then heated and molded over the modified plaster model.

Stirrup

The stirrup has the following features:
- An older foundation for the AFO is the steel stirrup, a U-shaped fixture, the center portion of which is riveted to the shoe through the shank.
- The arms of the stirrup join the brace uprights at the level of the anatomical ankle, providing congruency between orthotic and anatomical joints.
- The *solid stirrup* is a one-piece attachment that provides maximum stability of the orthosis on the shoe **(Fig. 11.37A)**.
- The split stirrup has three segments. The central portion has a transverse rectangular opening. Medial and lateral angled side pieces fit into the opening. The split stirrup simplifies donning the orthosis because the wearer can detach the uprights from the shoe. If a central piece is riveted to another shoe, the shoes can be interchanged. The extremely active client may dislodge a side piece from its receptacle unintentionally. The split stirrup is bulkier and heavier than a solid stirrup **(Fig. 11.37B)**.

Ankle Control

Ankle control specifies the following characteristics:
- Most AFOs are prescribed to control ankle motion by limiting plantar flexion and/or dorsiflexion, or by assisting motion.
- The patient with dorsiflexor weakness or paralysis risks dragging the toe during swing phase.
- Dorsiflexion assistance can be provided by a *posterior leaf spring* that arises from a plastic *insert*. During early stance, as the patient applies force to the braced foot, the upright bends backward slightly. When the patient progresses into swing phase, the plastic recoils forward to lift the foot. Thinner, narrower plastic permits relatively greater motion. Motion assistance can also be achieved with a steel dorsiflexion spring assist incorporated into each stirrup.
- An orthosis with a dorsiflexion spring assist is noticeably bulkier than the posterior leaf spring model.
- Both types of spring assist yield slightly into plantar flexion at heel contact, affording the wearer protection against inadvertent knee flexion. A joint placed in

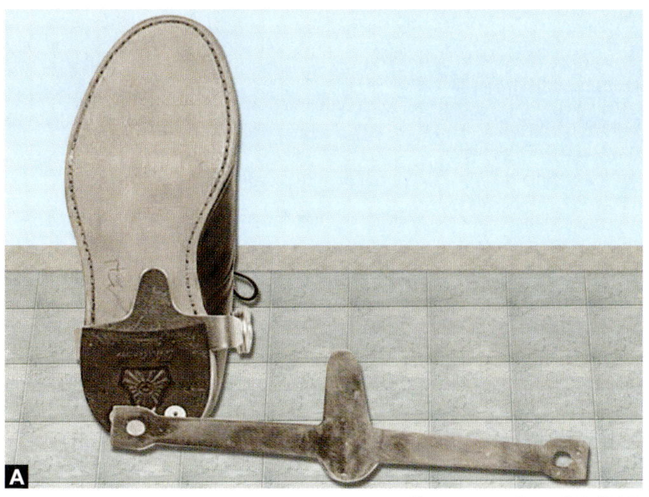

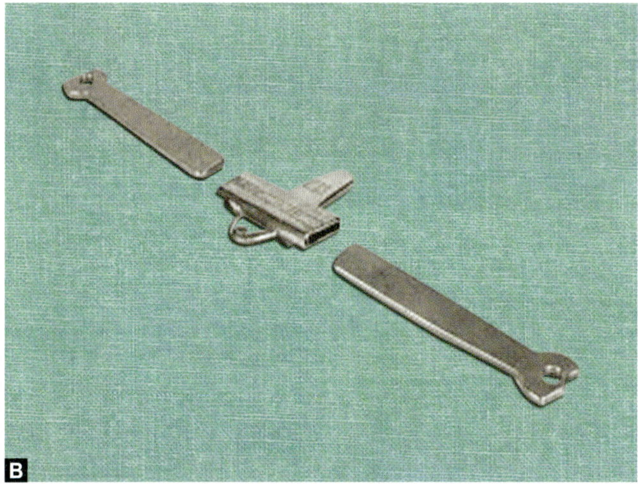

Figs. 11.37A and B: (A) Solid stirrup; (B) Split stirrup.

a plastic hinged AFO or a steel posterior stop can be incorporated in the stirrup **(Fig. 11.38)**. The posterior stop also imposes a flexion force at the knee during early stance, preventing the knee from hyperextending.

- Healthy adults walking with the ankle fixed in plantar flexion consumed more oxygen than when walking with AFOs which kept the foot in neutral position.
- Adults with hemiplegia who wore AFOs demonstrated increased cadence, walking speed, step length, and ankle dorsiflexion and the AFO enabled some patients to walk with increased stride length and cadence.
- A hinged AFO with full-length insert and posterior stop improves early stance stability for subjects with hemiplegia.
- The alignment of a solid AFO should be individualized to achieve optimal function. Adults with hemiplegia complicated by plantar flexor contracture walk with less plantar flexion and greater knee flexion when wearing either an AFO with posterior stop or a solid AFO.
- Functional electric stimulation is an alternative to an AFO for some adults with stroke and other central neuropathies. Various commercially available systems all incorporate a cuff on the proximal leg; the interior of the cuff contains a skin electrode over the peroneal nerve. The electrode is stimulated by a self-contained electrical unit. As compared to walking with an AFO, subjects report more positive results, particularly during swing phase.
- Children with hemiplegic cerebral palsy improved weight-bearing on the paretic limb while wearing either a posterior leaf spring AFO or a hinged AFO with plantar flexion.

Foot Control

Foot control can be described by the following:
- Medial–lateral motion can be controlled with a solid ankle AFO **(Fig. 11.39)**.
- The rigidity of the orthosis can be increased by:
  - Using thicker or stiffer plastic
  - Corrugating the plastic
  - Forming the edges with a rolled contour or
  - Embedding carbon fiber reinforcements
- A solid ankle AFO or a hinged solid ankle AFO also controls frontal and transverse plane foot motion of children with cerebral palsy to a limited extent.
- Less effective is a metal and leather orthosis to which a leather valgus (or varus) correction strap is attached. The valgus correction strap is sewn to the medial portion of the shoe upper near the sole, and buckles around the lateral upright, exerting a laterally directed force to restrain pronation. The varus correction strap has opposite attachments and force application. Either strap, although adjustable, complicates donning.

Superstructure

The proximal portion of the orthosis, the superstructure, consists of one or two uprights, and a shell, band, or brim **(Fig. 11.40)**. Plastic AFOs usually have a single upright or shell. Both the solid ankle and the hinged solid ankle AFOs

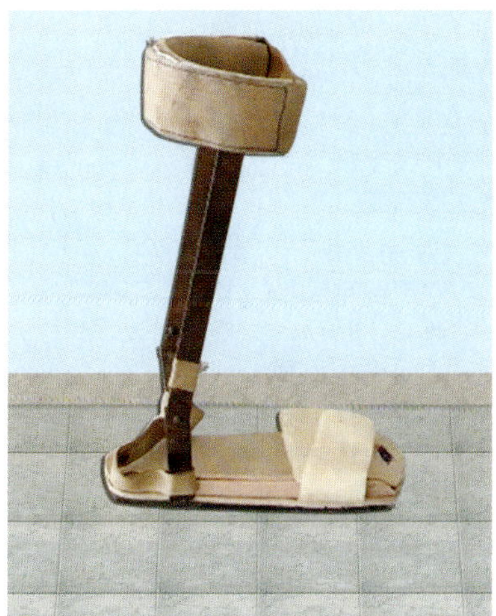

Fig. 11.38: Ankle–foot orthosis.

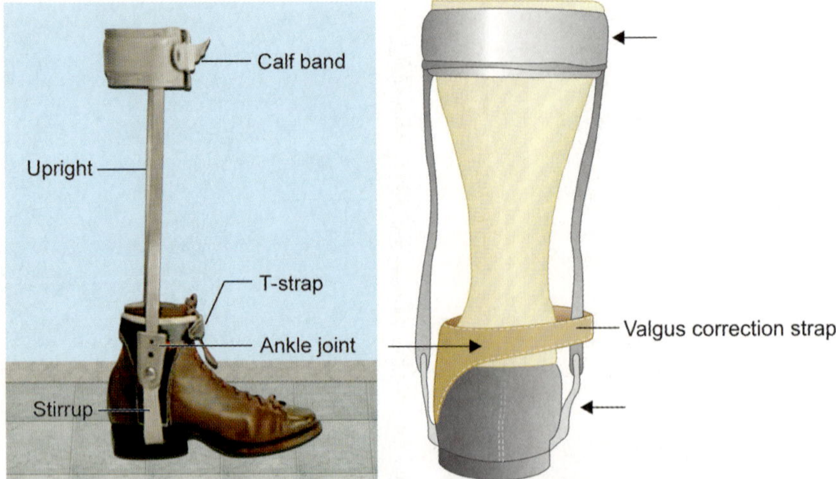

Fig. 11.39: Foot control.

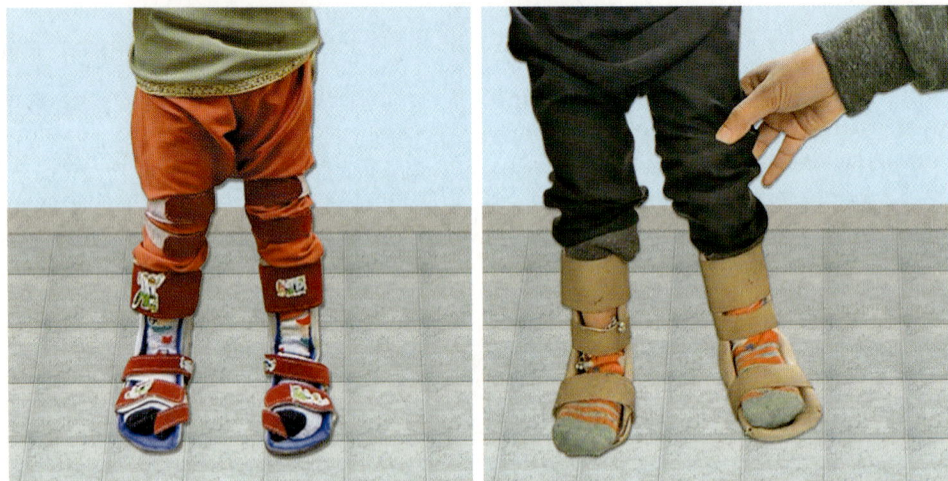

Fig. 11.40: Solid ankle–foot orthosis.

have a posterior shell extending from the medial to the lateral midline of the leg, thus providing excellent medial–lateral control and a broad surface to minimize pressure. The posterior leaf spring AFO has a single posterior upright that does not contribute to frontal or transverse plane control.

- The *spiral AFO* **(Fig. 11.41)** is a design in which single upright spirals from the foot plate around the leg, terminate in a proximal band.
- It may be made of polypropylene, nylon acrylic, or carbon fiber.
- The spiral orthosis controls, but does not eliminate, motion in all planes.
- Metal and leather orthoses usually have medial and lateral uprights to maximize structural stability. Occasionally, a single side upright will suffice when the patient insists on a less conspicuous orthosis and the person is not expected to exert undue force. Some AFOs have an anterior upright, thereby avoiding pressure and shear stress on the calf and Achilles tendon.

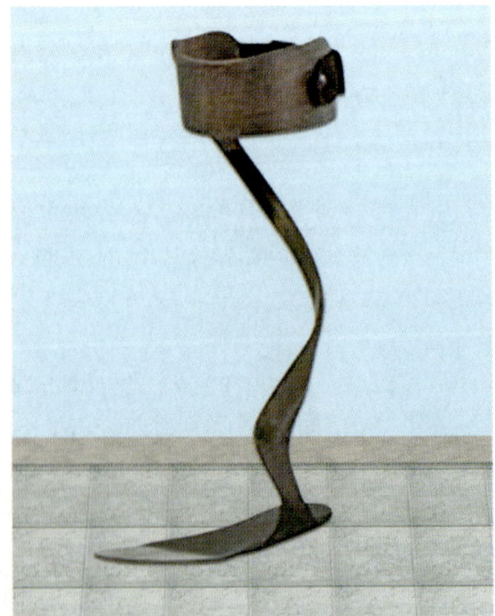

Fig. 11.41: Spiral ankle–foot orthosis.

Knee–Ankle–Foot Orthoses

Individuals with more extensive paralysis or limb deformity may benefit from KAFOs, which consist of:

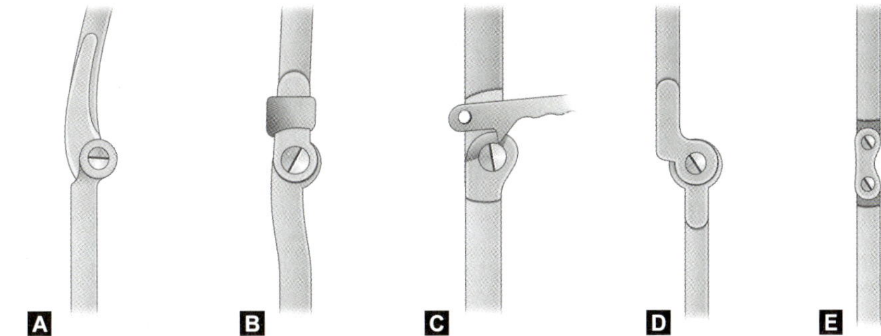

Figs. 11.42A to E: Types of knee joints. (A) Free motion; (B) Drop lock; (C) Swiss lock; (D) Off-set; (E) Dual axis.

- Shoe
- Foundation
- Ankle control
- Knee control
- Superstructure

Knee–ankle–foot orthoses often include foot control. The shoe, foundation, ankle control, and foot control of the KAFO may be selected from the components already described. Patients with poliomyelitis who wore carbon-composite KAFOs walked better than with leather/metal or plastic/metal KAFOs. Donning a plastic and metal KAFO is appreciably faster than putting on a metal and leather orthosis because the shoe can be separated from the rest of the orthosis.

Shoes

The shoe is the foundation for most LE orthoses. Each part of the shoe contributes to the efficacy of orthotic management and offers many options for selection. Shoes transfer body weight to the ground and protect the wearer from the terrain and the weather.

Foundation

The foundation of the orthosis consists of the shoe and a plastic or metal component.

Ankle Control

Ankle control specifies the following:
- Most AFOs are prescribed to control ankle motion by limiting plantar flexion and/or dorsiflexion, or by assisting motion.
- The patient with dorsiflexor weakness or paralysis risks dragging the toe during swing phase.
- Dorsiflexion assistance can be provided by a *posterior leaf spring* that arises from a plastic insert. During early stance, as the patient applies force to the braced foot, the upright bends backward slightly. When the patient progresses into swing phase, the plastic recoils forward to lift the foot. Thinner, narrower plastic permits relatively greater motion. Motion assistance can also be achieved with a steel dorsiflexion spring assist incorporated into each stirrup.

Knee Control

Knee control includes the following:
- The simplest knee joint is a hinge.
- Because most KAFOs include a pair of uprights, the orthosis has a pair of knee hinges **(Figs. 11.42A to E)** that provide medial–lateral and hyperextension restriction while permitting knee flexion.
- The *offset joint* **(Fig. 11.43A)** is a hinge placed posterior to the midline of the leg. When the wearer stands and walks on a level surface, the individual's weight line falls anterior to the offset joint, stabilizing the knee in extension during the early stance phase of gait. The offset joint does not hamper knee flexion during swing or sitting. The joint may, however, flex inadvertently when the wearer walks on ramps **(Figs. 11.42A to E)**.
- The most common knee control is the drop ring lock **(Fig. 11.43B)**. When the client stands with the knee fully extended, the ring drops, preventing the uprights from bending. Although both medial and lateral joints should be locked for maximum stability, manipulating a pair of drop ring locks is inconvenient, unless each upright is equipped with a spring-loaded *retention button*. The button permits the wearer to unlock one upright, then attend to the other one without having the first lock drop. The buttons also enable the physical

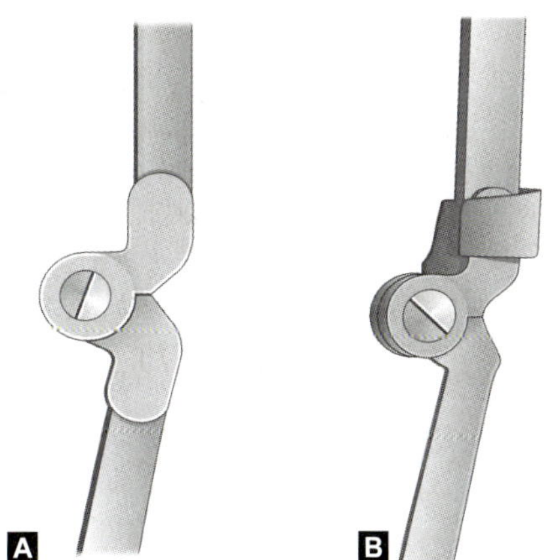

Figs. 11.43A and B: (A) Knee joint-offset hinge; (B) Hinge with drop ring rock.

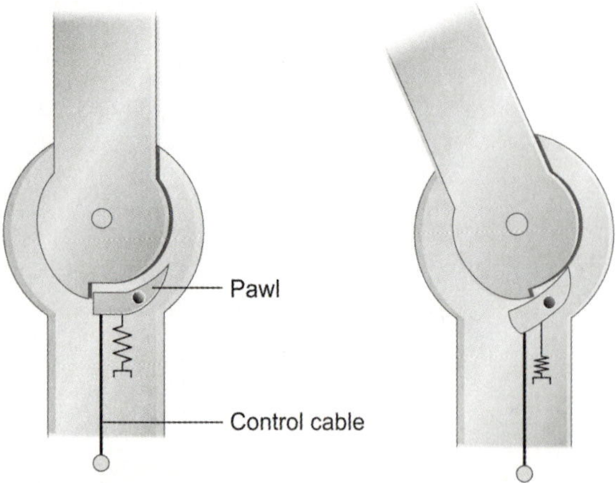

Fig. 11.44: Pawl lock.

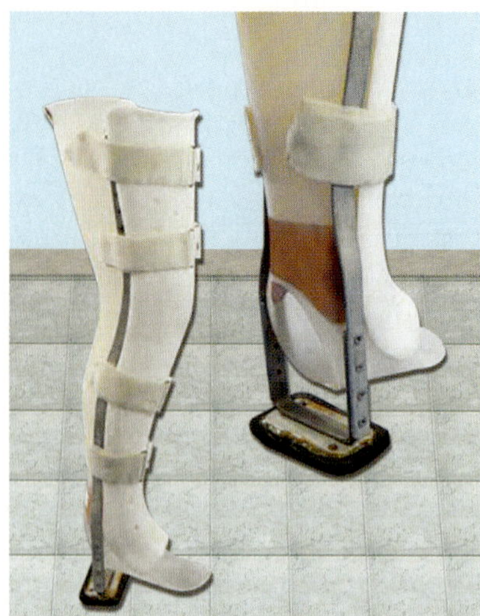

Fig. 11.45: Pattern bottom.

therapist to give the patient a trial period of walking with the knee joints unlocked.

- The *pawl lock with bail release* provides simultaneous locking of both uprights. The pawl is a spring-loaded projection that fits into a notched disk **(Fig. 11.44)**.
- The patient unlocks the brace by pulling upward on the posterior bail. Some people are agile enough to be able to nudge the bail by pressing it against a chair. The bail is bulky and may release the locks unexpectedly if the wearer is jostled against a rigid object.
- The offset joint and knee joints with basic drop ring or pawl locks are contraindicated in the presence of knee flexion contracture. If one cannot achieve full passive knee extension, an adjustable knee joint such as the fan lock, serrated lock or ratchet lock is required. Such joints usually have a drop ring lock for stability in the partially flexed attitude.

Superstructure

Following are specified for superstructure:

- Thigh bands provide structural stability to the orthosis. If the distal portion of the limb cannot tolerate FWB, then the proximal thigh band may be shaped to form a weight-bearing brim.
- To eliminate all weight-bearing through the LE, the orthosis must include a weight-bearing brim, a locked knee joint, and a pattern bottom **(Fig. 11.45)**.
- The pattern is a distal extension that keeps the foot on the braced side off the floor.
- To maintain a level pelvis, the patient must also wear a lift on the opposite shoe; the height of the lift should equal the height of the pattern.

Hip–Knee–Ankle–Foot Orthoses

Addition of a pelvic band and hip joints converts the KAFO to an HKAFO **(Fig. 11.46)**.

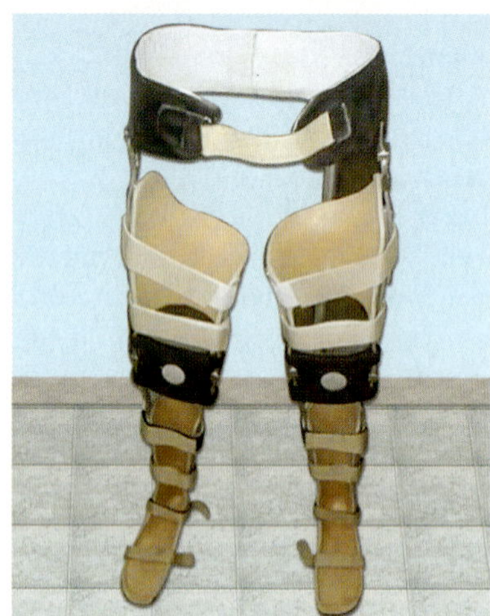

Fig. 11.46: Hip–knee–ankle–foot orthosis.

Hip Joint

Hip joint of an orthosis is described as follows:

- The usual hip joint is a metal hinge that connects the lateral upright of the KAFO to a pelvic band.
- The joint prevents abduction and adduction, as well as hip rotation.
- If the patient requires only control of hip rotation, a simpler alternative to the hip joint and pelvic band is a webbing strap. To reduce internal rotation, the strap resembles a Silesian belt on prosthesis. The center of the strap is riveted to the rear of a waist belt. Each end of the strap is attached to the proximal end of the lateral upright. To reduce external rotation, a strap joins the lateral uprights of the KAFOs, passing anteriorly at the level of the groin.
- If flexion control is required, a drop ring lock is added to the hip joint.
- A two-position lock stabilizes the patient in hip extension for standing and walking, and at 90° of hip flexion for sitting.

Pelvic Band

An upholstered metal band anchors the HKAFO to the trunk. The band is designed to lodge between the greater trochanter and the iliac crest on each side. HKAFOs are not used very often because they are much more awkward to don than KAFOs, and, if the hip joints are locked, they restrict gait to the swing-to or swing-through pattern. The pelvic band may be uncomfortable when the wearer sits **(Fig. 11.47)**.

Trunk–Hip–Knee–Ankle–Foot Orthoses

This orthoses has following features:
- Patients who require more stability than provided by HKAFOs may be fitted with THKAFOs **(Fig. 11.48)** which incorporate a lumbosacral orthosis attached to KAFOs. The pelvic band of the TO serves as the pelvic band used on HKAFOs.
- Because the THKAFO is very difficult to don and is heavy and cumbersome, it is seldom worn after the client is discharged from the rehabilitation program.
- Alternative orthoses providing standing stability, with or without provision for walking, are available for some individuals with paraplegia.

TRUNK ORTHOSES

Trunk orthoses (TO) may be used in association with LE orthoses or may be worn to reduce disabilities caused by low-back pain, cervical spine injuries, scoliosis, or other skeletal or neuromuscular disorders. By supporting the trunk, the orthosis assists in controlling spinal motion; however, forces that the orthosis exerts are modified by the skin, subcutaneous tissue, and musculature that surround the vertebral column, and, in the case of higher orthoses, by the thoracic cage. Patients with SCI benefit from TOs in two ways:

1. The orthoses control the motion of the lumbar region, with or without thoracic control.
2. They compress the abdomen to improve respiration.

Individuals with cervical lesions may need to wear an orthosis that restrains neck motion until stability is achieved by surgery or other means. A special group of TOs is intended for children and adolescents with scoliosis.

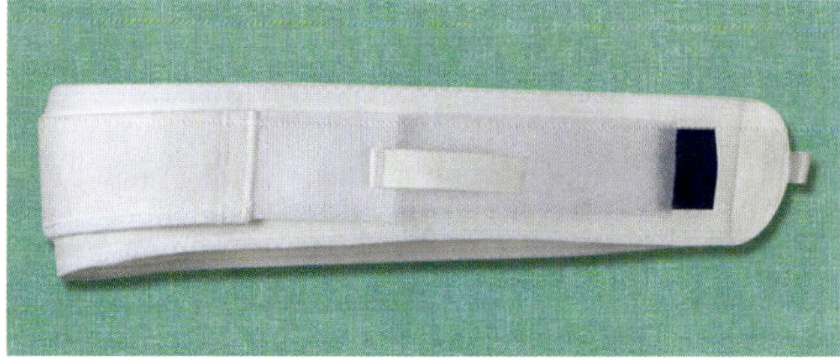

Fig. 11.47: Pelvic band.

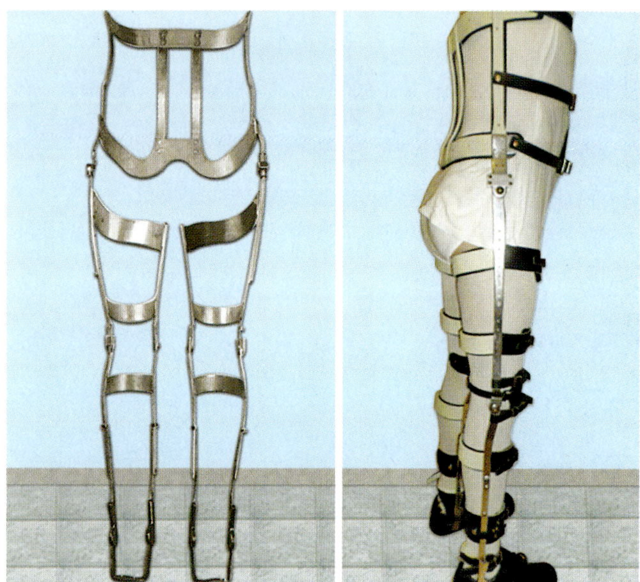

Fig. 11.48: Trunk–hip–knee–ankle orthosis.

Corsets

The corsets have following characteristics:
- If abdominal compression is the sole goal, a corset will suffice.
- It is a fabric orthosis that has no horizontal rigid structures, although many have vertical rigid reinforcements.
- The corset may cover only the lumbar and sacral regions or may extend superiorly as a thoracolumbosacral corset.
- The primary effect of a corset is to increase intra-abdominal pressure, although the orthosis does reduce frontal movement.
- Some individuals with low back disorders find that corsets relieve pain. The efficacy of orthotic intervention to reduce or prevent low back pain remains controversial. The increase in intra-abdominal pressure reduces stress on posterior spinal musculature, thus diminishing the load on the lumbar intervertebral disks.

Rigid Orthoses

These orthoses include:
- Most lumbosacral and thoracolumbosacral orthoses include a corset or a fabric abdominal front to compress the abdomen.
- Rigid orthoses are distinguished by the presence of horizontal, as well as vertical, rigid plastic or metal components.
- Motion limitation is accomplished by a series of three-point pressure systems, in which force in one direction is counteracted by two forces in the opposite direction.

Lumbosacral Flexion, Extension, Lateral, and Control Orthoses

A typical example of a rigid TO is the *lumbosacral flexion, extension, lateral control (LS FEL) orthosis* also known as a *Knight spinal orthosis* **(Fig. 11.49A)**.

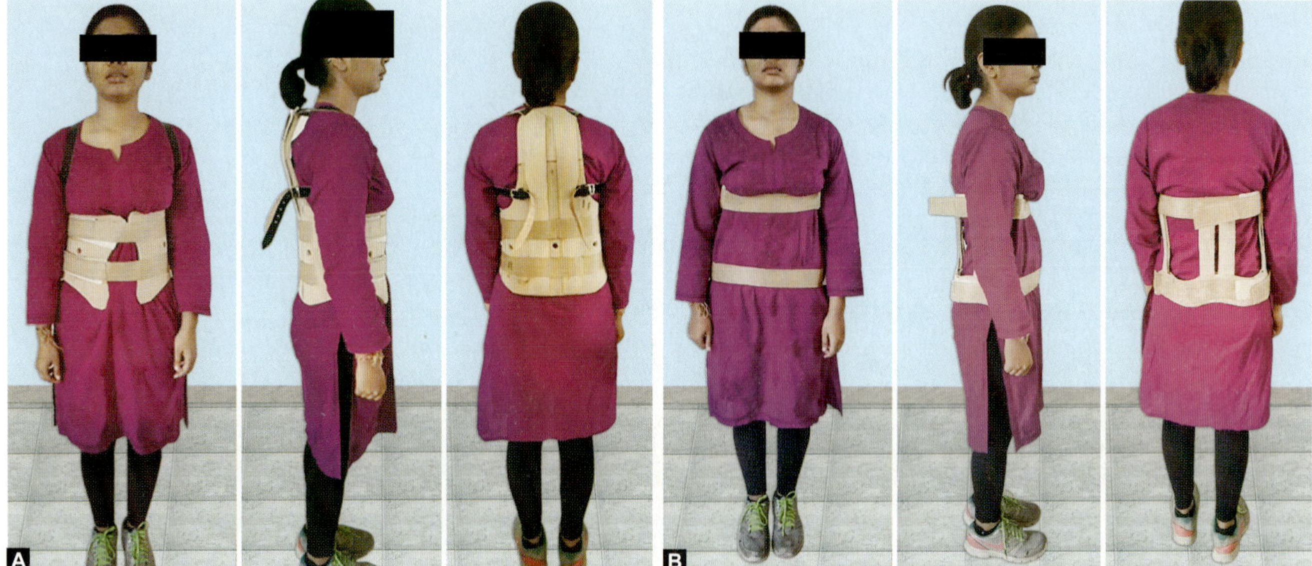

Figs. 11.49A and B: (A) Knight, (B) Taylor brace.

- This appliance includes a pelvic band, which should provide firm anchorage over the midsection of the buttocks, and a thoracic band, intended to lie horizontally over the lower thorax without impinging on the scapulae. The bands, which may be foam-lined rigid plastic or leather-upholstered metal, are joined by a pair of posterior uprights on either side of the vertebral spines, and a pair of lateral uprights placed at the right and left lateral midlines of the torso.
- A corset or abdominal front completes the LS FEL orthosis. The orthosis restrains flexion by a three-point system consisting of posteriorly directed force from the top and bottom of the abdominal front or corset and an anteriorly directed force from the posterior midportion of the orthosis.
- Extension is controlled by posteriorly directed force from the midsection of the abdominal front or corset and anteriorly directed force from the upper and lower posterior segments. The lateral aspects resist lateral flexion.
- Other rigid lumbosacral orthosis are made entirely of polyethylene with removable replaceable liners.

Thoracolumbosacral Flexion, Extension, and Control Orthoses

These orthoses include the following:
- Also called a *Taylor brace* **(Fig. 11.49B)**, the *thoracolumbosacral flexion, extension control (TLS FE) orthosis* consists of a pelvic band, posterior uprights terminating at midscapular level, an abdominal front or corset, and axillary straps attached to an interscapular band.
- This orthosis reduces flexion by a three-point system consisting of posteriorly directed force from the axillary straps and the bottom of the abdominal front or corset, and anteriorly directed force from the midportion of the posterior uprights.

- Extension resistance is provided by posteriorly directed force from the midsection of the abdominal front or corset and anteriorly directed force from the pelvic and interscapular bands.

Trunk movement restriction is evident when the wearer walks. A plastic *thoracolumbosacral jacket* limits trunk motion in the frontal, sagittal, and transverse planes providing maximum support.

Cervical Orthoses

Cervical orthoses are classified according to design characteristics. Minimal motion control is provided by collars that encircle the neck with fabric, resilient foam **(Fig. 11.50A)**, or rigid plastic. The therapeutic benefit of collars remains controversial.
- The *Philadelphia collar* has mandibular and occipital extensions and a rigid anterior strut; it is sometimes used for upper cervical injuries.
- For moderate control, a *four-post orthosis* is used **(Fig. 11.50B)**. Usually, it has two anterior adjustable posts joining a sternal plate to a mandibular plate and two posterior uprights connecting a thoracic plate to an occipital plate. The sternal plate is strapped to the thoracic plate, and the occipital plate is strapped to the mandibular plate. If the cervical orthosis does not fit properly, motion restriction is compromised.
- Maximum orthotic control of the neck may be achieved either with a *Minerva* or a *halo orthosis*. The Minerva orthosis is a noninvasive appliance that has a rigid plastic posterior section extending from the head to the midtrunk; the superior portion is held in place by a forehead band. The halo orthosis has a circular band of metal that is fixed to the skull by four tiny screws. Uprights connect the halo to a thoracic vest. Recent investigations confirm that the halo vest allowed cervical fractures to heal, particularly fractures of the second cervical vertebra.

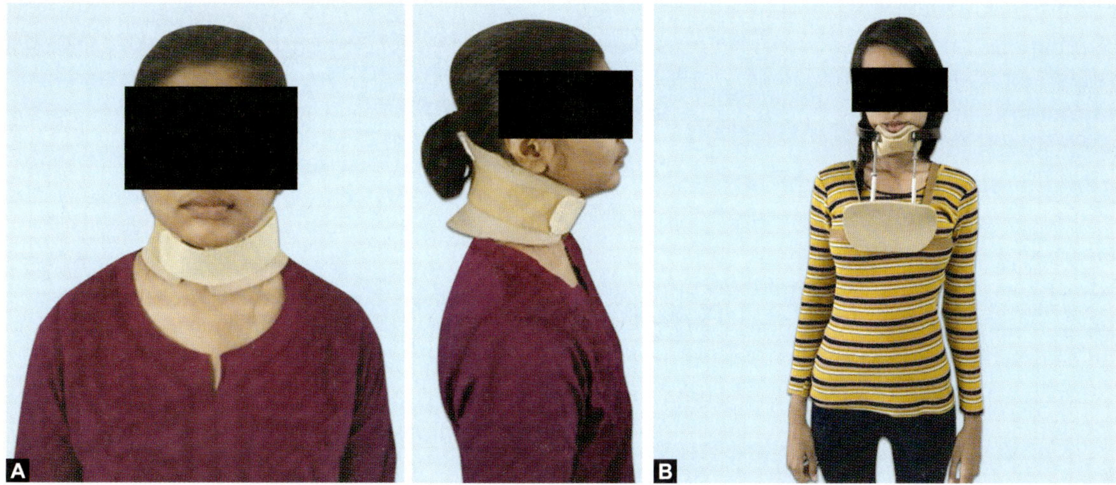

Figs. 11.50A and B: (A) Foam cervical collar; (B) Four-post orthosis.

By limiting upper trunk motion, this orthosis reduces stride length, and results in temporary atrophy of neck muscles.

Scoliosis Orthoses

Children and adolescents with kyphoses or thoracic, thoracolumbar, or lumbar scoliosis may be fitted with a thoracic lumbar sacral orthosis (TLSO) that applies:

- Distraction
- Derotation
- Bending forces to realign the vertebral column and thoracic cage.

Brace effectiveness depends on the flexibility of the patient's torso and snugness of contact with the wearer's trunk. Although substantial improvement is evident when the orthosis is worn, long-term follow-up indicates that the major achievement is that the orthosis prevents the curve from increasing beyond its original contour. Bracing diminishes the likelihood of surgical correction of scoliosis.

Clinical Pearl

Orthotic management is most effective for curves <35° Cobb angle. Orthosis for scoliosis are most effective on patients who have curves in the midthoracic or more inferior portions of the trunk.

Although wearing it for short time is better tolerated by adolescents, the classic protocol, which requires the youngster to wear the orthosis snugly 23 hours each day, is associated with more favorable results. Patients with larger curves achieve some curve reduction from bracing.

Braces do not impair standing balance. Psychological factors, rather than the type or duration of brace wear, appear to be more important in self-reported quality of life among those for whom scoliosis braces are prescribed. Adults with scoliosis do not benefit from orthoses.

- The Milwaukee orthosis, the oldest of contemporary orthosis for scoliosis, is still prescribed. It consists of a frame composed of a pelvic girdle, two posterior uprights, an anterior upright, and a superior ring that can be hidden by clothing. Various pads are strapped to the frame to apply corrective forces **(Fig. 11.51A)**.
- The Boston orthosis usually does not extend as high as the Milwaukee orthosis; its foundation is a mass-produced plastic module that the orthotist alters to fit the individual patient **(Fig. 11.51B)**. Effectiveness is enhanced by snugly strapping the interior pads to the torso. Long-term results are favorable, with patients preferring it to surgery.

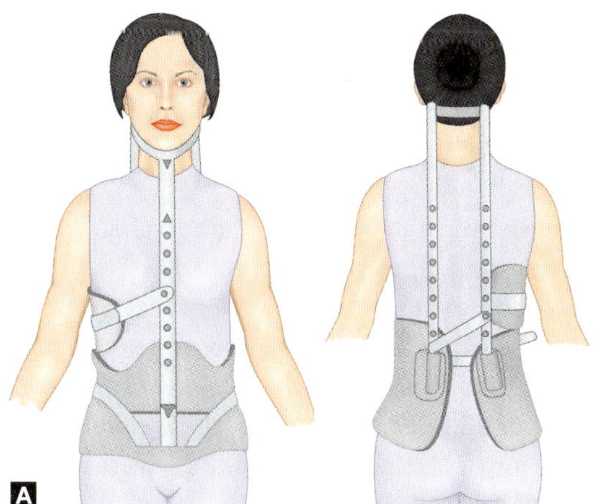

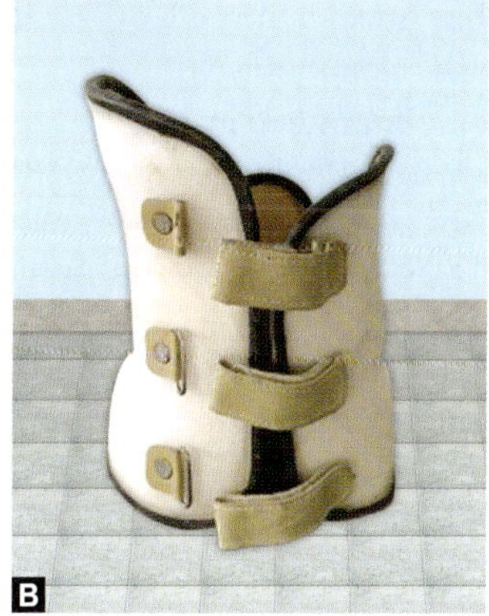

Figs. 11.51A and B: (A) Milwaukee orthosis; (B) Boston orthosis.

- The Wilmington orthosis is another option; it is a custom-made thoracolumbosacral jacket intended to guide the trunk to straighter alignment.

Night bracing is an alternate approach to scoliosis management. When the patient is in bed the effects of gravity are minimized allowing substantial corrective forces to be applied. Nevertheless, there is a higher risk of progression.

Both the Charleston bending brace and the providence brace provide overcorrection of the spinal curve on the recumbent patient. Scoliosis orthoses are also used for adolescents with hyperkyphosis.

SUMMARY

Mobility aids are appliances used to help people who have difficulty in walking. **Assistive technology** is used to increase, maintain, or improve the functional capabilities of individuals with disabilities. Assistive devices make it possible for individuals with disabilities to take part in life's activities, at home, school, work, and in the community. Persons with physical impairment disabilities often use assistive devices or mobility aids such as crutches, canes, wheelchairs and artificial limbs to obtain mobility. Wheelchair propulsion on a level surface requires a relatively low rate of energy expenditure, which is comparable to normal walking. Although wheelchair use has advantages in terms of energy expenditure, patients with SCI often cannot ambulate independently with a wheelchair because of environmental barriers. Therefore ambulation training of suitable SCI patients with orthotics and walking aids is a must.

This chapter has focused on the upper and LE and TOs. The most frequently prescribed orthoses and orthotic components have been presented. **Orthosis is** an orthopedic device designed to support, correct, compensate, accommodate, and prevent further deformity and aid movement to an injured or weakened limb or spine. Orthoses can be useful for chronic conditions, acute injury, and injury prevention. Orthoses are a nonsurgical, removable, and relatively cost-effective treatment for many joint and muscular conditions. Orthoses can be constructed of plaster, wood, leather, metal, cloth, or plastic. Most orthoses employ lightweight thermoplastic materials. The thermoplastic sheets are molded to fit body parts exactly, and some shall be reshaped repeatedly as the treated body part changes shape. Orthoses are classified into two: static and dynamic (functional) orthoses. **Orthoses** are devices applied externally to restore and/or improve functional and structural characteristics of the muscles, skeleton and nervous systems. In general, conditions include those resulting from trauma, sports, and work-related injuries.

Case Scenario

CASE STUDY 1
Patient History and Current Problem
The patient is a 63-year-old man who was diagnosed with poliomyelitis at 3 years of age. He sustained complete paralysis of the left LE and left foot and ankle. During childhood, he wore bilateral knee–ankle–foot (KAFO) orthoses and ambulated with a four-point gait using a pair of axillary crutches. When he was 21, he had a left ankle and subtalar fusion. He was fitted with a left KAFO, which included a stirrup foundation, posterior ankle stop, drop ring knee lock, knee pad, and leather-covered calf and thigh bands. For the next 40 years, he wore the same brace and had the leather and shoe replaced whenever needed. He used a cane in the left hand when he walked outdoors. He returned to the rehabilitation department today complaining of pain in the right knee and fatigue. He also said that his brace tears his stockings at the knee. He is curious about new orthotic developments.

Past Medical History
History of poliomyelitis.

Social History
The patient is a reference librarian. He enjoys visiting his grandchildren, attending the theater, and participating in political campaigns.

Physical Therapy Examination Findings
- Cognitive status: Alert, oriented, memory intact
- Endurance: Limited, primarily restricted by discomfort in his left knee
- Vision: Intact with corrective lens
- Blood pressure: 135/74
- Respiratory rate: Within functional limits (WFL)

Range of Motion Examination
- Right and left hip, knee ROM = WFL
- Left foot and ankle = no motion
- Right foot and ankle = reduced

Sensation
- All modalities within functional limits (WFL) bilaterally in both limbs
- Sensation in both upper limbs WFL

Strength: Manual Muscle Test Grades
- Left hip = grade 2
- Knee, ankle = grade 0
- Left and right UL = WFL
- Right hip = grade 4
- Knee = grade 3.

Orthotic Examination
Uprights malaligned permitting 20° knee hyperextension. Posterior ankle-stop worn, permitting 10° plantar flexion. Leather on calf and thigh bands is worn.

Balance
Standing
- Static: Good; able to maintain the static position for unlimited period
- Dynamic: Good on level surface
Sitting: Good.

Gait

Patient walks slowly with a left KAFO with considerable trunk bending to the left. Bending reduces when he uses a cane in the right hand. He reports that he has great difficulty ascending and descending ramps. Additional findings include the following:

- Overall decrease in speed of movement
- Broad walking base
- Circumducts right leg
- Right knee hyperextends within the orthosis
- Right ankle plantar flexion limited by orthosis
- Left foot and ankle immobile

Functional Status

- Independent in transfers: sit-to-stand; floor-to-stand transfer
- Independent in all basic activities of daily living (BADL)
- Independent in approximately 85% of IADL

Patient-desired Outcome and Goals

- Walk without knee pain
- Improve endurance
- Improve appearance
- Reduce the frequency of torn stockings in the vicinity of the knee

Guiding Questions:

1. Explain the modification in orthoses which can be helpful for patient.
2. Describe the physiotherapy management for this patient.
3. State any recent advances in assistive aids and devices which can help this patient.

CASE STUDY 2

The patient is a 60-year-old man with left hemiparesis. He was treated regularly in the inpatient physical therapy department for 5 months. He was discharged with a home program consisting of exercises to promote strength, joint mobility, endurance, gait training, and balance training.

Past Medical History

The patient was in fairly good health until 6 months ago, when he woke up in the early morning he felt sudden giddiness and faintness. He felt weakness in his left upper and LE and felt difficulty to stand independently. Then his relatives brought him to a nearby local hospital and admitted there for the further treatment. He was conscious. After stabilizing the vitals, the physiotherapy treatment was started regularly within 2 days. He was admitted for physiotherapy treatment for 5 months.

Social History

The patient is a retired driver.

Physical Therapy Examination Findings

- Cognitive status: Alert, oriented, memory intact
- Vision: Intact with corrective lens
- Cardiopulmonary system: Vital signs seated at rest—blood pressure 140/86, heart rate 84, respiration within normal limits (WNLs)
- Endurance: Fair, tolerance to activity is approximately 30 minutes
- Neuromuscular

- Sensation: Both upper and lower extremities—sharp/dull, light touch, temperature, and proprioception all WNL bilaterally.
- Reflexes: Superficial reflexes are normal but deep reflexes are diminished.

Range of Motion

- Goniometric examination
- Right upper and LE ROM: WNL
- Left upper and LE ROM: Reduced then normal limit

Observational Gait Analysis (General Findings)

- Overall decrease in speed of movement
- Diminished, awkward weight transfer hip/pelvis (bilateral)
- Decreased pelvic rotation
- Diminished hip flexion knee

Gait

The patient is a functional ambulator using a walker. Gait is slow, with longer steps on the left side; without the walker he leans to the left side. He can climb stairs slowly, using the handrail.

Strength

- Right upper extremity and LE = grade 4
- Left upper extremity and LE = grade 3+

Balance

Standing

- Static: poor
- Dynamic: poor

Sitting: WFL

Examination of Function

- Patient dependent on transfers: Bed, chair. Requires assistance in mobility.
- Patient is dependent on all BADL.
- Patient is dependent on approximately 60% of IADL.

Patient-desired Outcomes

- Walk without depending on walker when outdoors
- Improve endurance
- Improve balance
- Improve gait
- Improve coordination

Guiding Questions:

1. Formulate a problem list.
2. Design a plan of care to address the outcomes desired.
3. Discuss a long-term follow-up plan.

Review Questions

1. Describe the functions of mobility aids and factors to be considered while selecting a mobility aid.
2. What are the different types of sticks and canes used in rehabilitation?
3. Describe the types of walkers in detail.
4. Discuss a standard wheelchair along with its parts.
5. What are the functions and general principles of orthosis?
6. Discuss the parts of a shoe and various foot orthosis used in foot conditions.
7. What are the parts of ankle–foot orthosis? Discuss each in detail.
8. What is a pattern bottom?
9. Describe the orthosis used in scoliosis.
10. Discuss (a) Philadelphia collar and (b) Minerva orthosis.

SECTION 2: Intervention Strategies

BIBLIOGRAPHY

1. Arva J, Paleg G, Lange M, et al. RESNA Position on the Application of Wheelchair Standing Devices.Assistive Technology. 2009;21:161-8.
2. Braddom RL (Ed). Physical medicine and rehabilitation. Philadelphia, PA: W.B. Saunders; 2000. pp. 263-352.
3. Clarke P, Ailshire JA, Bader M, et al. Mobility disability and the urban built environment. Am J Epidemiol. 2008;168:506-13.
4. Cuccurullo SJ (Ed). Physical medicine and rehabilitation board review. New York, NY: Demos Medical Publishing; 2004. pp. 409-87.
5. Delisa JA (Ed). Physical medicine and rehabilitation: principles and practice. Philadelphia, PA: Lippincott, Williams, and Wilkins; 2005. pp. 1325-91.
6. Guide To walking aids: canes, crutches, and walkers. AbleData.
7. Hesse S, Herrmann C, Bardeleben A. A new orthosis for subluxed, flaccid shoulder after stroke facilitates gait. J Rehabil Med. 2013;45:623-9.
8. Joint position paper on the provision of mobility devices in less resourced settings. World Health Organization; 2011.
9. Mark W. Standing tall: the benefits of standing devices. 2012. Available from: https://scia.org.au/assistive-technology-equipment-modifications/
10. McFarland SR. Mobility and mobility devices for the spinal cord injured person. 1987;11(4): 215-24.
11. O'Sullivan SB, Schmitz HJ, Fulk GD. Physical rehabilitation, 6th edition. Jaypee Brothers Medical Publishers; New Delhi; 2004.
12. O'Sullivan SB. Physical rehabilitation, 5th edition, Jaypee Brothers Medical Publishers, New Delhi; 2006.
13. Redhead RG. The early rehabilitation of lower limb amputees using a pneumatic walking aid. Prosthet Orthot Int. 1987;7:88-90.
14. Scott H. An evaluation of the amputee mobility aid (AMA) early walking aid. Prosthet Orthot Int. 2000;24:39-46.
15. Sinha AG, Tripathy SK, Sharma R. Orthoses and prostheses and assistive devices for physiotherapists; 2012.
16. Spinal Cord Injuries Australia. Wheelchair selection: power chairs. Available from: https://www.who.int/disabilities/technology/wheelchairpackage/en/
17. Spinal cord injury and gait training; 2011.
18. Sunder S. Textbook of rehabilitation. 3rd edition. Jaypee Brothers Medical Publishers, New Delhi; 2020.
19. Ulkar B. Energy expenditure of the paraplegic gait: comparison between different walking aids and normal subjects. Int J Rehabil Res. 2003;26(3): 213-7.
20. Wheelchair service training package. World Health Organization. Available from: https://www.who.int/disabilities/publications/technology/wheelchairguidelines/en/
21. World Health Organization. Guidelines on the provision of manual wheelchairs in less resourced settings; 2008.

Yoga

Megha Jayswal, Megha S Sheth

LEARNING OBJECTIVES

After reading this chapter, the readers should be able to:
♦ Describe the history and philosophy of yoga
♦ Understand the basic concepts of yoga
♦ Gain knowledge regarding the different asanas and their implications
♦ Understand the technique of performing Suryanamaskar, Pranayama and Savasana
♦ Gain knowledge about the benefits of Suryanamaskar, Pranayama and Savasana
♦ Discuss the role of yoga in the rehabilitation process
♦ Understand the relationship between yoga and physiotherapy

CHAPTER OUTLINE

- Yoga as traditional medicine
- Reasons leading to modification of the mind
  - Pramana
  - Viparyaya
  - Vikalpa
  - Nidra
  - Smriti
  - Chitta vikshepa
- Limbs or stages of yoga
  - Yama
  - Niyama
  - Asana
  - Pranayama
  - Pratyahara
  - Dharana
  - Dhyana
  - Samadhi
- Yogasana
  - Hints and cautions
- Suryanamaskar
  - Basic features
  - Technique
- Savasana (the corpse pose)
  - Technique
  - Advantages
  - Indications
- Pranayama
  - Hints and cautions
  - Posture
  - Kumbhakas
  - Ujjayi pranayama
  - Surya bhedana pranayama
  - Nadi shodhana pranayama
  - Viloma pranayama
- Yoga and physiotherapy
- Benefits of yoga
  - Musculoskeletal improvements and posture control
  - Neuropsychological benefits of yoga
  - Physiological benefits of yoga
  - Benefits of yoga: psychological and spiritual wellness

INTRODUCTION

The word "yoga" is originated from an ancient Indian "Sanskrit" language root "Yuj." The literal meaning of Yuj is "to unite," "to harness," with the meaning also "to direct," "to concentrate" (the mind, thoughts, etc.). In Indian thought, everything is permeated by supreme universal spirit, Parmatma or God of which human individual spirit, Jeevatma is a part. Yoga teaches us the means by which jeevatma can be in communion with or united to parmatma and so secure liberation (Moksha). Another meaning of yoga is the union of the winds within our inner body.

Yoga is practice, not theory. Yoga relies on mutuality, integration, and, interconnection, not separation and isolation. Just as it is difficult to understand a swimming manual, unless one has seen some water, and it is even easier if one has tried to swim; similarly, an attempt to understand yoga intellectually without experience of its practice will only confuse the intellect or make it appear mystical or complicated. Self-experience abolishes all speculative doubts.

YOGA AS TRADITIONAL MEDICINE

World Health Organization (WHO) has classified yoga as a mind–body practice and considered it as an integrative and complementary health practice. Traditional medicine (TM) has been defined as "including diverse health practices, approaches, knowledge and beliefs incorporating plant, animal, and/or mineral based

medicines, spiritual therapies, manual techniques and exercises applied singularly or in combination to maintain well-being, as well as to treat, diagnose or prevent illness."
—WHO

Depending on the therapies involved, WHO has classified yoga as "nonmedication therapies," as it is executed primarily without using medication. TM is drawing more and more attention in terms of health care provision and health sector reform. It is based on the needs of individuals. TM relies on a belief that each individual has her or his own composition and social circumstances, which result in different responses to "causes of disease" and "treatment." Different individuals may require different treatments even if, according to modern medicine, they suffer from the same disease.

REASONS LEADING TO MODIFICATION OF THE MIND

Patanjali defines yoga as "chitta vritti nirodaha," which means that yoga has an ability to calm the fluctuations of the mind (chitta vritti). Patanjali has described five chitta vritti as follows **(Fig. 12.1)**:
1. Pramana (correct knowledge or valid cognition)
2. Viparyaya (misconception or wrong knowledge)
3. Vikalpa (imagination)
4. Nidra (sleep)
5. Smriti (memory)

Pramana

The experiences an individual has using the five senses of the human body determine the validity of the knowledge. However, it may sometimes happen that the individual may be misled by the five senses, e.g., a mirage. Hence, according to Patanjali, along with perception by the five senses to determine the validity of knowledge, it is important to have a practical application as well.

Acquiring knowledge requires the following:
1. **Pratayksha (direct experience):** Application of the five senses to acquire knowledge
2. **Anumana (inference):** Ability of the individual to analyze a situation and apply logical reasoning to determine the validity of the situation
3. **Agamah (trustworthy testimony):** Ability to trust someone else's knowledge and experience.
   The process of acquiring knowledge also requires anubhava or experience.

Viparyaya

False knowledge or misconception occurs due to the deceptive look of an object. Every individual perceives things in her/his own manner. For the same object, two individuals can have different thoughts regarding it. The goal of yoga is to make the mind calm, so that the person can see things for what they are, without appreciating them to be something else.

Vikalpa

Imagination works in a more subtle way than Pramana or Viparyaya. It makes an individual believe something that is nonexisting or not true. The mind cannot differentiate the real from the imagined. This has a strong impact on an individual's personality—if one thinks positive thoughts about his/herself, one believes them and develops a positive personality, whereas if one thinks negative thoughts about his/herself, one develops a negative personality. This leads to happiness or suffering in our lives. Yoga helps in developing a positive state of mind that creates a positive environment around us, helping us lead a good life.

Nidra

Nidra means "sleep." During sleep, the mind is diverted to oneself and it provides a state of relaxation and refreshment. Inadequate or loss of sleep reduces the ability to concentrate on things and negatively impacts mood, which leads to poor functioning. According to Patanjali, deep sleep occurs when heaviness overcomes the mind and there are no other activities taking place. Heaviness can occur due to exhaustion or boredom or any other reason. Its occurrence is not governed by the time of the day and can occur at any time of the day. Yoga involves various meditation techniques that help gain this state of Nidra or deep sleep.

Smriti

Memory is the mental retention of experiences gained through consciousness. Memory cannot be differentiated as being true or false. Memories affect the mood of an individual—recalling pleasant memories creates a pleasant mood, whereas recalling bad memories creates a bad mood.

Patanjali enumerates **five causes of chitta vritti** creating pain (klesha). These are:
1. *Avidya:* Ignorance or nescience
2. *Asmita:* Feeling of individuality which may be physical, mental, intellectual, or emotional, which limits the person and distinguishes them from the group
3. *Raga:* Attachment or passion
4. *Dvesha:* Aversion or revulsion
5. *Abhinivesha:* Love or thirst for life.

Chitta Vikshepa

The **distractions and obstacles** that hinder the aspirant's practice of yoga are:
- *Vyadhi:* Sickness that disturbs the physical equilibrium
- *Styana:* Lack of mental disposition of work
- *Samasya:* Doubt or indecision
- *Pramada:* Indifference or insensibility

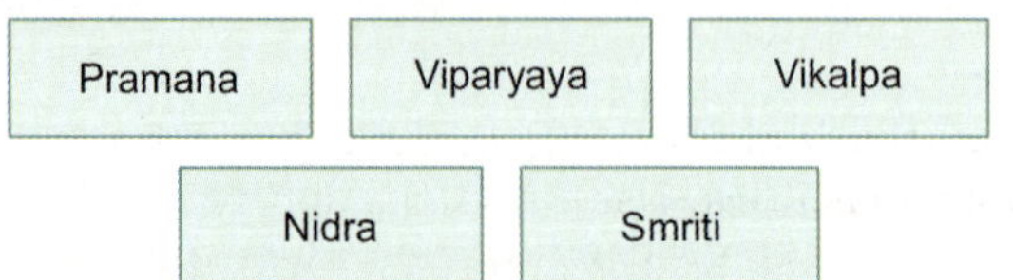

Fig. 12.1: Chitta vritti described by Patanjali.

- *Alasya:* Laziness
- *Avirati:* The rousing of the desires when the sensory objects possess the mind
- *Bhranti Darshana:* False or invalid knowledge or illusion
- *Alabdha Bhumikatva:* Failure to concentrate or attain continuity of thoughts so the reality cannot be seen
- *Anavashthitattva:* Instability in holding on to concentration.

LIMBS OR STAGES OF YOGA

Saint Patanjali has enumerated the eight limbs or stages of yoga for the quest of the soul **(Fig. 12.2)**. They are:
1. Yama (universal moral commandments)
2. Niyama (self-purification by discipline)
3. Asana (posture)
4. Pranayama (rhythmic control of the breath)
5. Pratyahara (withdrawal and emancipation of the mind from the domination of the senses and exterior objects)
6. Dharana (concentration)
7. Dhyana (meditation)
8. Samadhi [a state of superconsciousness brought about by profound meditation, in which the individual aspirant (sadhaka) becomes one with the object of his meditation—Paramatma or the universal spirit].

Yama

Yama means moral or ethical disciplines—the great commandments surpassing creed, country, age, and time. These commandments are the rules of morality for the individual and society, which if not followed bring untruth, chaos, violence, covetousness, dissipation, and stealing. The emotions of greed, desire, and attachment are the roots of these evils. They only bring ignorance and pain. Patanjali tries to eliminate the root of these evils by modifying one's ability of thinking along the five principles of yama. These commandments are:
1. *Ahimsa (nonviolence):* Not to inflict physical or mental pain to anybody.
2. *Satya (truth):* The simple meaning of satya is reality.
3. *Asatya (nonstealing):* The practitioner controls their desires and reduces their wants.

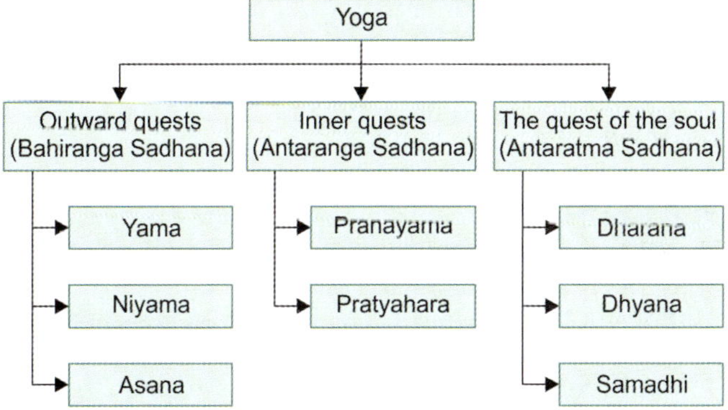

Fig. 12.2: Limbs of yoga.

4. *Brahmacharya (continence):* The simple meaning of brahmacharya is to lead a controlled sex life, even as a householder living in a society. Righteousness and virtue should guard the demand. Raw sense enjoyment must not be the motive.
5. *Aparigraha (noncoveting):* The meaning of aparigraha is not to collect. We should only have as much as is necessary.

Niyama

Niyama are the rules of conduct that need to be applied to individual discipline. Sage Patanjali has listed five niyama, which are: shaucha (purity), santosha (contentment), tap (austerity), swadhyaya (self-study), and Ishwar pranidhana (dedication to the Lord).
1. *Shaucha:* The word "shaucha" means cleanliness or purity. It involves both the physical cleansing as well as cleansing of the mind of its disturbing emotions such as passion (kama), anger (krodha), greed (lobha), pride (mada), lust (moha), delusion, and hatred. Good habits such as bathing purify the body externally, whereas asana and pranayama cleanse it internally.
2. *Santosha:* Santosha is a state of satisfaction, i.e., contentment. The mind that is not content, cannot concentrate. Differences arising among people because of race, creed, wealth, and learning distract the mind and it cannot become focused (ekagra). So simple meaning of santosha is that the yogi feels the lack of nothing and so he is naturally content.
3. *Tap:* Tap involves self-discipline and austerity. To be efficient, tolerant, and victorious over difficulties is the simplest meaning of tap. It is the conscious effort to achieve ultimate union with the divine and to lose all wishes and desires, which act as barriers in the way of this goal.
4. *Swadhyaya:* "Swa" means "self" and "adhyaya" means "study or education." Swadhyaya, therefore, is the education of the self. It brings knowledge and puts an end to ignorance. To make life healthy, happy and peaceful, it is essential to study divine literatures regularly. By swadhyaya, sadhaka (practitioner) understands the nature of their soul better and gains communication with the divine.
5. *Ishwara Pranidhana:* To surrender all of one's actions and will to God is Ishwara Pranidhana. When the priority of "I" and "mine" disappears, the individual soul reaches the full growth. Person who knows that all creations belong to the Lord will not be egotistic or drunk with power.

Asana

Asana is the third limb of yoga. Asanas are postures and not only gymnastic exercises. A steady and pleasant posture prevents instabilities of mind and produces mental equilibrium. Unlike other systems of physical training that need large playing field and costly equipment, Asanas can be done alone as the limbs of the body provide the necessary weights and counter weights. Asanas help maintain a fine physique, which is strong and elastic without being muscle bound and stiff. They keep the body free from the disease. A soul without the body can be likened to a bird which has been deprived of its power to fly. The yogi conquers the body through the practice of asanas, making it a fit vehicle for the spirit. To yogi, the body is an instrument of attainment, neither the impediment to his spiritual liberation nor is it the cause of its fall.

The names of the asanas are significant as they exemplify the principle of evolution. The names are based on:

1. Vegetations like padmasana (lotus)
2. Insects like salabhasana (locust)
3. Aquatic animals and amphibians like matsyasana (fish)
4. Birds like mayurasana (peacock)
5. Quadrupeds like ustrasana (camel)
6. Creatures that crawl like serpent bhujangasana (snake)
7. The human embryonic state called "garbhapinda"
8. Legendary heroes like Hanuman and sages such as Bharadvaj and Vashishtha.

Dualities such as body and mind, fame and shame, gain and loss, victory and defeat, mind and soul disappear through mastery of the asanas, and the sadhaka then passes on to pranayama.

Pranayama

Prana means breath, life, vitality, or energy. It also suggests the soul as opposed to the body. Ayama means length or expansion. Pranayama thus indicates extension of breath and the way to control it. This control is over all the functions of breathing, namely

- Inhalation or inspiration, which is termed "Puraka" (filling up)
- Exhalation or expiration, which is called "Rechaka" (emptying the lungs)
- Retention or holding the breath, a state where there is no inhalation or exhalation, which is termed "Kumbhaka."

  There are two states of Kumbhaka, namely
  1. When breathing is suspended after full inhalation, but before exhalation begins known as Antara Kumbhaka
  2. When breathing is suspended after full exhalation but before inhalation begins known as Bahya Kumbhaka.

"Antara" means "inner," while "bahya" means "outer." In both these types, breathing is suspended and restrained. Every living creature unconsciously breathes prayer "Soham" (Sah=He, Aham=I, the immortal spirit am I) with each inward breath. With each exhalation, each creature prays "Hamsah" (I am He). The yogi fully realizes the significance of this ajapa-mantra (unconscious repetitive prayer) and so is released from all the fetters of their soul.

Prana in the body of an individual (jeevatma) is part of the cosmic breath of the universal spirit (parmatma). Through practice of pranayama, an attempt is made to harmonize the individual breath with cosmic breath.

Pratyahara

"Pratyahara" means "gathering toward." The mind receives sensory impulses from the outside world and the body and also from extrasensory perception from the self. In pratyahara, the extrovert senses are filtered out, and they are turned inward. With the inward turned eyes and ears, one can experience optical and auditory extrasensory perceptions.

Dharana

When "chitta," the mind, consciousness, and intelligence is confined to and concentrated upon a certain place in the body, it is dharana. The mind should be made to think of one point in the heart or between the two eyebrows on the forehead.

Dhyana

When dharana continues for a long time, it becomes "Dhyana"—meditation. In dhyana, there is no movement in the body and the mind intelligence unit. Meditation is a subjective experience and cannot be taught. It is an incredible state that has to be experienced. It releases all tension. In meditation, the flow of energy is continuous and stable. The awareness of time and space lost.

Samadhi

The merging of the individual's consciousness in the object of meditation is a total consummation called "Samadhi." When an uninterrupted flow of the individual's awareness gets absorbed in the object of "meditation," their "consciousness" loses its identity and becomes one with the object.

YOGASANA

Hints and Cautions

1. *Cleanliness:* Before practicing asanas, the bladder should be emptied and bowel evacuated. If the practitioner is constipated or it is not possible to evacuate the bowel before the practice of asanas, start with Sirsasana or Sarvangasana and their variations.
2. *Food:* Asanas should preferably be performed on an empty stomach. If it is difficult, a cup of tea or coffee or milk may be taken before practicing. If the practitioner has had heavy meal before starting the practice, allow at least 4 hours to elapse after. Food may be taken an hour after completing the asanas after the meal.
3. *Bath:* A bath should be taken both before and after practicing asanas. It cleans the body and refreshes mind. Asanas become easier after taking a bath. After doing them, the body feels sticky due to perspiration and it is desirable to bathe around 15 minutes later.

4. *Time:* The best time to practice the asanas is either early morning or late in the evening. A regular practice in the morning is helpful in improving the performance at work. Practice after work can help in relieving the stress and fatigue of the day and making one fresh and calm.
5. *Sun:* After being out in the hot Sun for several hours, one should not practice asanas.
6. *Place:* They should be done in a clean, airy place, free from noise and insects. Do not perform asanas bare feet or on an uneven place but on a folded blanket laid on a level floor.
7. *Cautions:* No undue strain should be felt in the facial muscles, eyes, or ears and in breathing during the practice.
8. *Closing the eyes:* In the beginning, one can keep the eyes open. Then it will be known what is being done and where one can go wrong. When perfection is achieved in a particular asana, only then one can keep eyes closed.
9. *Mirror:* Using mirror while performing asanas can give a visual feedback to the practitioner about her/his assumed posture. If doing the asanas in front of a mirror, keep it perpendicular to the floor and let it come down to ground level. Use a mirror without a frame.
10. *Breathing:* In all the asanas, breathing should be done through the nostrils only and not through the mouth. The practitioner should focus on not holding the breath while performing the asana or holding the position. Follow the instructions regarding breathing given in the technique section.
11. *Savasana:* After completing the practice of asanas always lie down in Savasana for at least 10–15 minutes, as this will eliminate fatigue.
12. *Special provision for persons suffering from hyper-tension:* Do not start with Sirsasana and Sarvangasana. First practice Paschimottanasana, Uttanasana, and Adho Mukha Savasana before attempting topsy-turvy poses such as Sirsasana and Sarvangasana.
13. *Special warning for persons having ear infections or displaced retina:* Those suffering from these conditions should not attempt topsy-turvy poses.
14. *Special instructions for women*
    - *Menstruation:* Avoid practicing asanas during the menstrual period. Under any circumstances, do not stand on your head nor perform Sarvangasana, during the menstrual period. If the flow is in excess of normal, Upavishtha Konasana, Virasana, Baddha Konasana, Paschimottanasana, Janu Shirshasana, and Uttanasana will prove beneficial.
    - *Pregnancy:* During the first 3 months of pregnancy all the standing poses and forward bending asanas may be done with mild movements, but no pressure should be felt on abdomen. Upavistha Konasanacan and Baddha Konasana can be practiced throughout the pregnancy, as these two

Clinical Pearl

A complete assessment should be performed before prescribing any asanas. All contraindications must be ruled out. Under no circumstances, should performing the asanas aggravate the pain or any other symptom that may be present. Consult a specialist when in doubt.

asanas will strengthen the pelvic muscles and reduce the labor pain considerably. Pranayama without retention (kumbhaka) may be practiced throughout pregnancy, as regular deep breathing will help considerably during labor.

- *After delivery:* During the first month after delivery, no asanas should be performed. Thereafter, they may be practiced mildly and progressed gradually. After 3 months of delivery all the asanas can be performed with comfort.

SURYANAMASKAR

"Surya" and "Namaskar" are Sanskrit words meaning "Sun" and "salutation" or "worship," respectively. Hence, Suryanamaskar means **salutation of the Sun.** Surya Namaskar is a dynamic exercise. It is based on the concept of mobilizing and stretching the entire spine through the maximum range available for flexion and extension via a set of alternative forward and backward postures **(Fig. 12.3).**

Basic Features

Basic features are as follows:
- *Physical postures:* There are 12 physical postures, which correspond to the signs of zodiac.

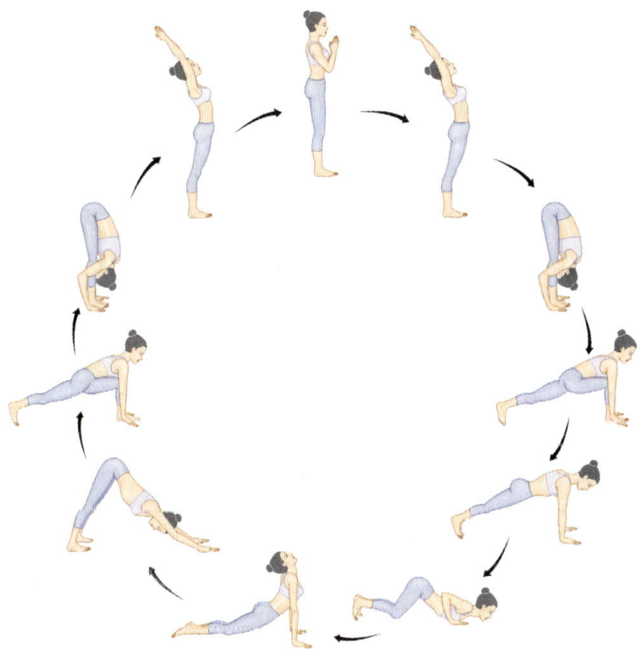

Fig. 12.3: Suryanamaskar poses.

- *Breathing:* Each position is associated with inhalation, exhalation, or retention of breath.
- *Mantras:* Mantras are associated with each of the 12 positions of Suryanamaskar. They are evocative sounds and through their power of vibration have subtle, but powerful and penetrating, effects on the mind and body.
- *Awareness:* The practitioner should be well aware of every movement and breathing pattern taking place.
- *Relaxation:* Any relaxation technique can be adopted, but best method is Savasana. During relaxation, allow the heart rate (HR) and respiratory rate (RR) to return to normal. It is also a must to feel the mental peace and awareness.

Technique

1. Pranamasana (prayer pose) **(Fig. 12.4)**
   - Stand erect with the feet together.
   - Place both the palms together in prayer position in front of the chest.
   - Close the eyes and try to relax the entire body.
   - Breathing: Breath normally
   - Mantra: Om Mitray Namah
2. Hasta Uttanasana (raised arm pose) **(Fig. 12.5)**
   - Raise both arms above the head keeping hands separated by a shoulder's width.
   - At the end of the movement extend the head, arms and upper trunk backward.
   - Breathing: Inhale while raising the arms.
   - Mantra: Om Ravaye Namah.
3. Padahastasana (forward bending pose) **(Fig. 12.6)**
   - Bend forward, place the palms on the ground either in front or side of the feet.
   - Keep knees straight.
   - Try to touch the knees with the forehead.
   - Do not apply any force to attain the final position or give any jerky movement.
   - Breathing: Exhale while bending forward.
   - Mantra: Om Suryaya Namah.

4. Ashwa Sanchalasana (equestrian pose) **(Fig. 12.7)**
   - Stretch the right leg backward as far as possible—sit on your bent left leg.
   - In the final position, the toes and knees of the extended right leg should be in contact with the ground.

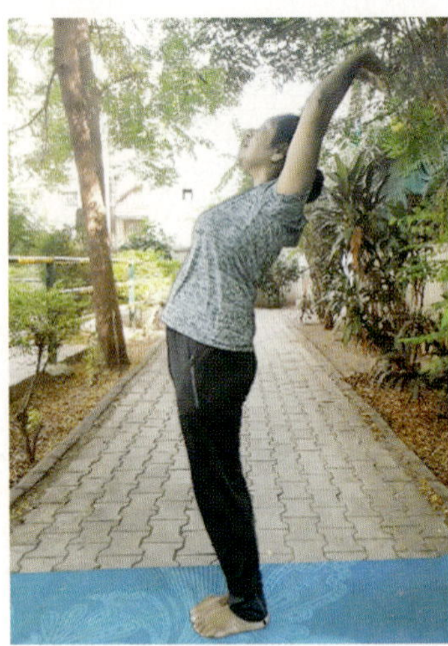

Fig. 12.5: Hasta Uttanasana (raised arm pose).

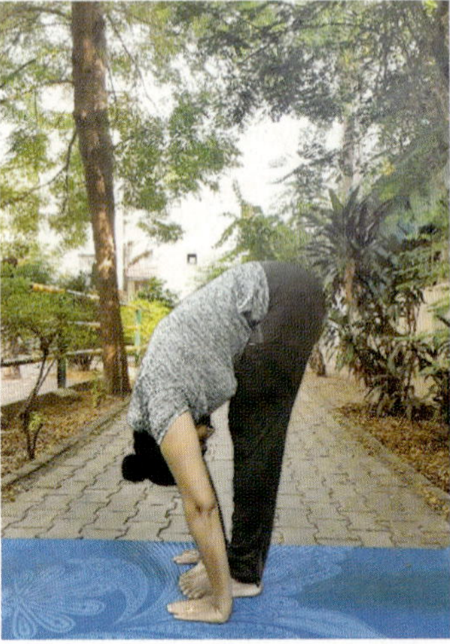

Fig. 12.6: Padahastasana (forward bending pose).

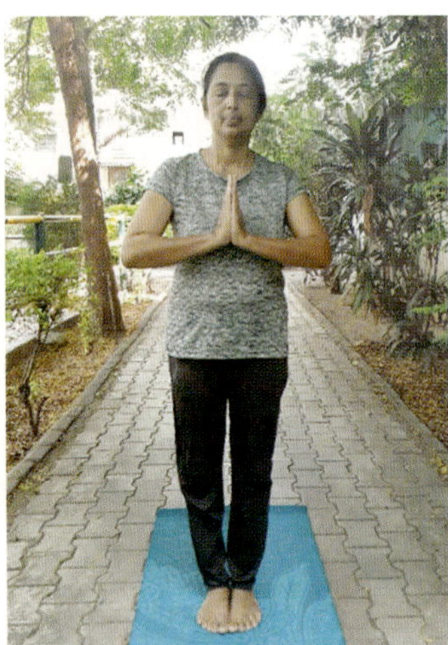

Fig. 12.4: Pranamasana (the prayer pose).

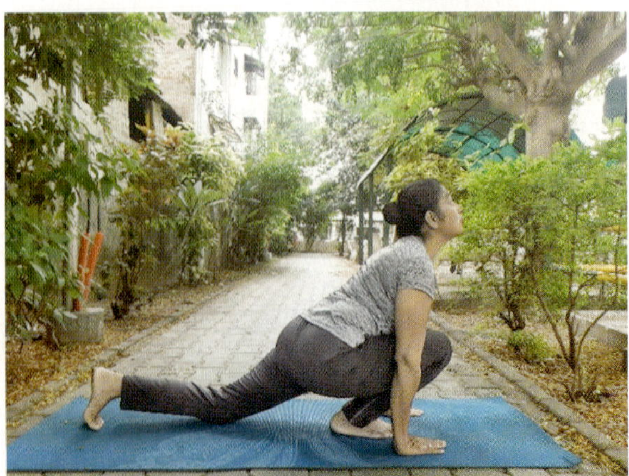

Fig. 12.7: Ashwa Sanchalasana (equestrian pose).

- Extend the neck and arch the spine as much as possible without straining.
- Breathing: Inhale deeply as the body moves forward.
- Mantra: Om Bhanave Namah.

5. Parvatasana (mountain pose) **(Fig. 12.8)**
   - Raise the right knee.
   - Simultaneously lower the head toward the floor.
   - Stretch the left leg backward and place it with right leg.
   - Raise the buttock as high as possible and lower the head between two hands, so that it makes a triangle.
   - Try pressing the heels of both feet toward the ground.
   - Breathing: Exhale while performing movement.
   - Mantra: Om Khagaya Namah.

6. Ashtanga Namashkara (worship with eight points) **(Fig. 12.9)**
   - This position is called so because in the final pose eight points of the body are in contact with the ground—two palms, two knees, two heels, chest, and chin/head.
   - Lower the body to the ground.

- Bend the legs and place the knees in contact with the ground.
- Bend the arms and lower the trunk toward the ground.
- Keep the chin or forehead on the floor.
- Keep the chest along with the floor.
- Finally raise the abdomen and hips slightly off the ground.
- Breathing: Exhale, hold the breath outside, do not inhale.
- Mantra: Om Pushne Namah.

7. Bhujangasana (cobra pose) **(Fig. 12.10)**
   - Lower the hips to the ground.
   - Straighten the arms.
   - Take the head and back upward and backward till the naval level.
   - Breathing: Inhale while performing the movement.
   - Mantra: Om Hiranyagarbhaya Namah.

8. Parvatasana (mountain pose) **(Fig. 12.11)**
   - Same as position five.
   - Lift buttock upward.
   - Keep the arms, legs straight.

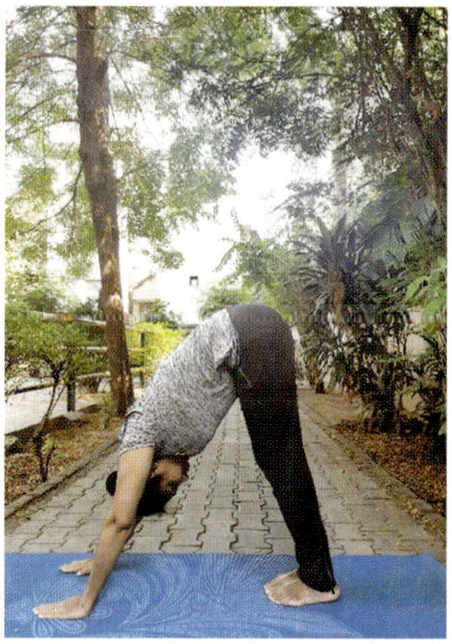

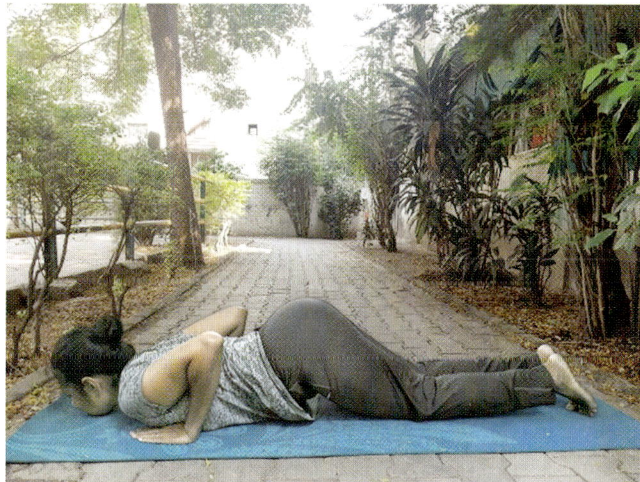

Fig. 12.8: Parvatasana (mountain pose).

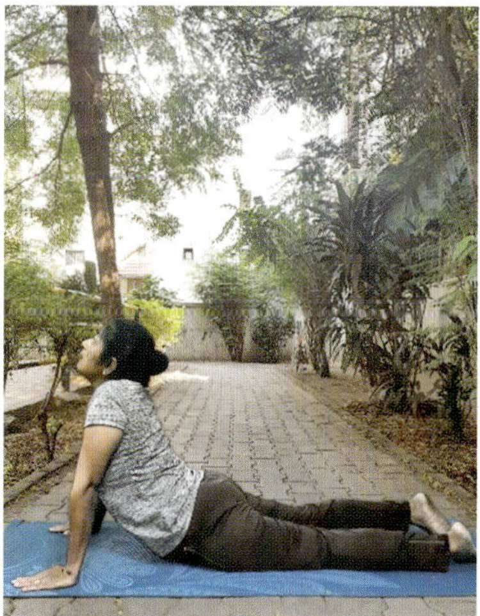

Fig. 12.10: Bhujangasana (cobra pose).

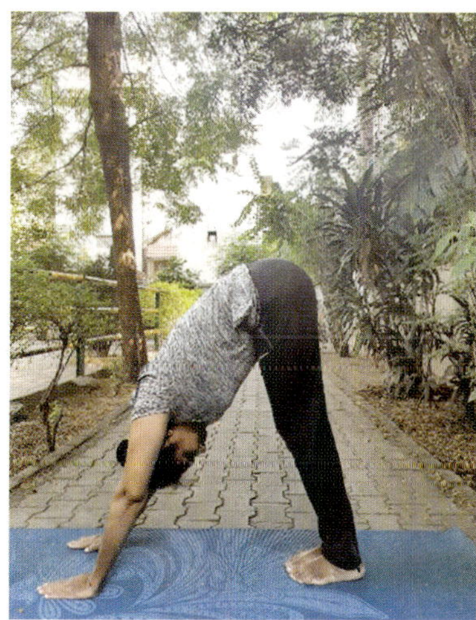

Fig. 12.9: Ashtanga Namashkara (worship with eight points).

Fig. 12.11: Parvatasana (mountain pose).

- Heels should be pressed toward the ground.
- Breathing: Exhale, while performing the movement.
- Mantra: Om Marichaye Namah.

9. Ashwa Sanchalasana (equestrian pose) **(Fig. 12.12)**
   - Same as position four.
   - Stretch the other leg backward.
   - Raise the head upward, arch the back downward.
   - Position of hands and foot must not be changed.
   - Breathing: Inhale.
   - Mantra: Om Adityay Namah.
10. Padhastasana (forward bending pose) **(Fig. 12.13)**
    - This position is same as position three.
    - Lower the head toward ground.
    - Raise the buttock.
    - Keep the right foot parallel to the left foot.
    - Straighten the legs and try to touch the forehead to the knees.
    - Breathing: Exhale as you move head toward the knees.
    - Mantra: Om Savitre Namah.
11. Hasta Uttanasana (raised arm pose) **(Fig. 12.14)**
    - This position is same as position two.
    - Straighten the whole body.

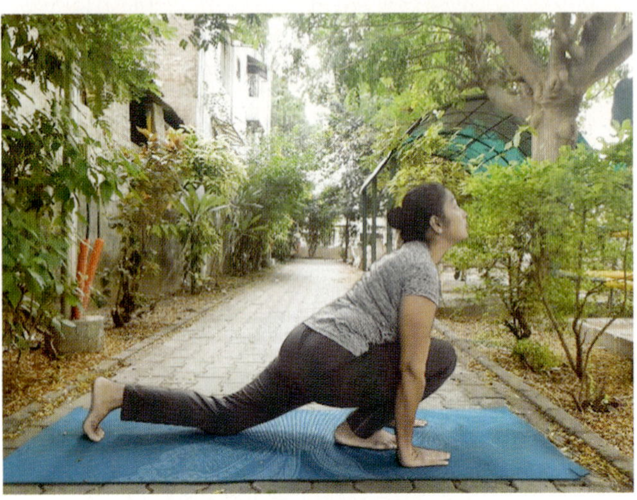

Fig. 12.12: Ashwa Sanchalasana (equestrian pose).

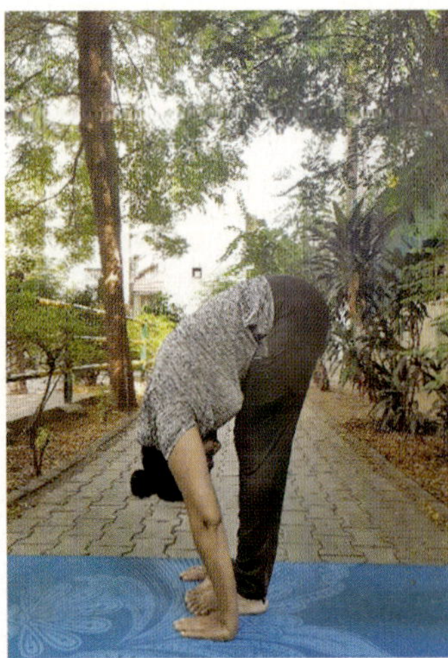

Fig. 12.13: Padhastasana (forward bending pose).

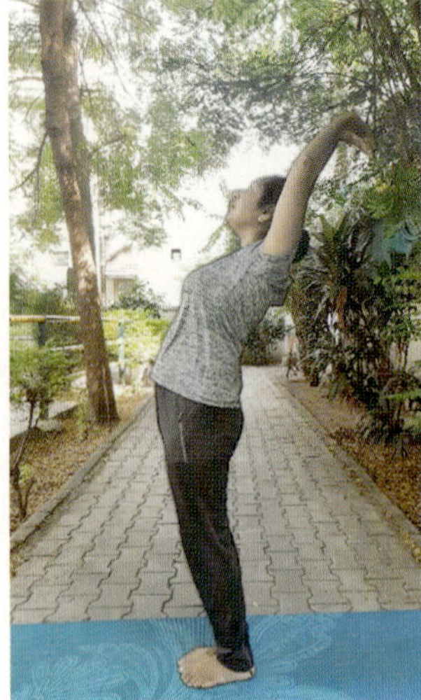

Fig. 12.14: Hasta Uttanasana (raised arm pose).

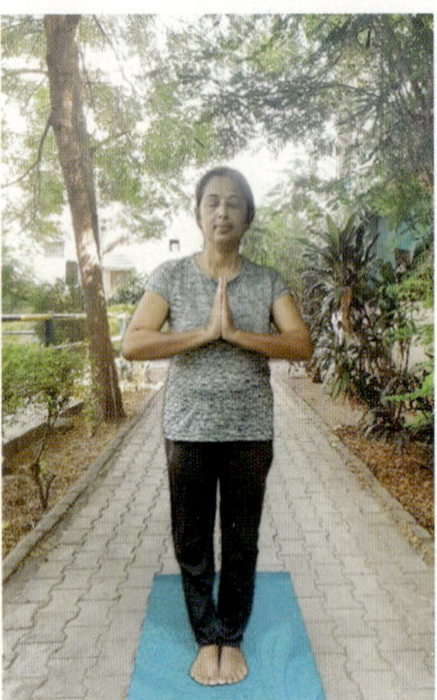

Fig. 12.15: Pranamasana (prayer pose).

- Raise the arms over the head.
- Bend (extend) back, neck, head, and arms backward.
- Breathing: Inhale
- Mantra: Om Arkay Namah.
12. Pranamasana (prayer pose) **(Fig. 12.15)**
    - This final pose is same as position one
    - Bring the palms together and hold them in front of the chest
    - Relax the whole body
    - Breathing: Exhale, breathe normally
    - Mantra: Om Bhaskaray Namah.

SAVASANA (THE CORPSE POSE)

It is also known as Mrtasana (dead man's pose).

Technique

The following instructions are to be followed:

- Lie flat on the back with center of forehead, chin, sternum, umbilicus, and pubis in a single line **(Fig. 12.16)**.

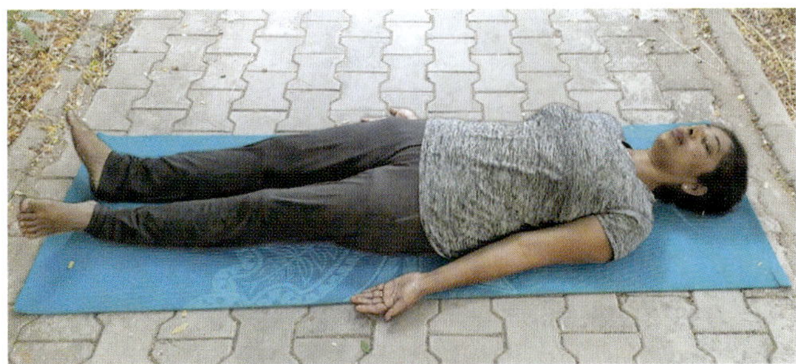

Fig. 12.16: Savasana.

- Keep arms slightly away from the side of the body, palms facing upward.
- Legs should be straight and slightly separated.
- Eyes should be closed.
- Breathe normally with full awareness.
- Try to feel different parts of the body in contact with the floor.
- If the muscles of the buttocks are tensed, then release them.
- Now try to feel the contact between the ground and the right heel for a few seconds.
- Repeat the same with the left heel.
- Now feel the contact between the floor and the right arm, right hand, left arm, left hand, the middle of the back, each shoulder blade, back of the head, and finally the whole body.
- Spend a few seconds at each point.
- Now try to release the tension from right hand, left hand, legs, each joint, and finally the whole body.
- Throughout the practice problems or worries may keep appearing. Do not suppress the thoughts if they occur, and merely continue to direct the attention to the relaxation of the different parts of the body and try to breathe relaxed and normally.
- One attains a relaxed state mentally and physically. When the practice is finished, gently move and clench the hands, move feet and slowly open the eyes.
- During the asana, do not go to sleep and be fully aware of the breath and the relaxed state of body and mind.

Advantages

- Reduces physical, mental and emotional stress, strain and fatigue of all kind
- Gives total relaxation to the body
- Soothes nerves and mind
- Reduces basal metabolic rate, pulse, and blood pressure

Indications

- Physical and mental fatigue and tension
- Insomnia, anxiety, neurosis, and phobia
- Stress-related disease, asthma, diabetes, peptic ulcer, colitis, and angina pectoris
- High blood pressure, tachycardia, and hyperthyroidism

PRANAYAMA

Hints and Cautions

Cleanliness and Food

- Before starting pranayama, the bowel should be evacuated and the bladder emptied. This leads to comfort in Bandhas.
- Preferably pranayama should be performed on empty stomach, but if this is difficult, a cup of milk, tea, or coffee may be taken. Allow at least 6 hours to elapse after a meal before practicing pranayama.
- Light food may be taken half an hour after pranayama practices.

Time and Place

The facts regarding time and place in pranayama are as follows:

- According to Hatha Yoga Pradipika, pranayama should be practiced four times a day, in the early morning, noon, evening, and midnight, with 80 cycles at a time. This is hardly possible in modern age. What is therefore recommended is to practice at least 15 minutes a day, but the 80 cycles are for intensely devoted practitioners, and not for the average house holder.
- The best season in which to start the practice are spring and autumn when the climate is equable.
- Pranayama should be practiced in a clean airy place, free from insects. Since noise creates restlessness, practice should be during quite hours.

Posture

The posture for pranayama can be described as follows:

- Breathing in pranayama practices is done through the nose only, except in Sitali and Sitkari.
- Pranayama is best done sitting on the floor on a folded blanket. The postures suitable are Siddhasana, Virasana, Padmasana **(Fig. 12.17)**, and Baddha Konasana.
- During practice, no strain should be felt in the facial muscles, eyes and ears, or in the neck muscles,

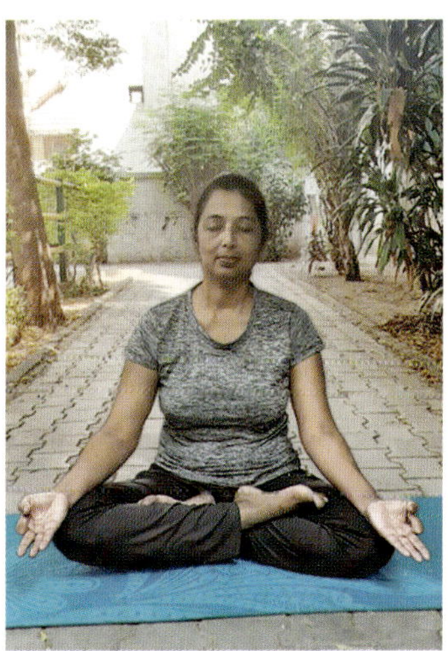

Fig. 12.17: Padmasana.

shoulders, arms, thighs, and feet. The thighs and arms should be relaxed deliberately since they are unconsciously tensed during pranayama.

- Keep the tongue passive or saliva will accumulate in the mouth. If it does, swallow it before exhalation (rechaka) not while holding the breath (kumbhaka).
- During inhalation and retention, the rib cage should expand both forward and sideways, but the area below the shoulder blades and armpits should only expand forward.
- To start with, there will be perspiration and trembling, which will disappear in course of time.
- In all the pranayama practices done in a sitting posture, the head should hang down from the nape of the neck, the chin resting in the notch between the collarbones on the top of the breastbone.
- Keep the eyes closed throughout as otherwise the mind will wander after outside objects and be distracted. The eyes, if kept open, will feel a burning sensation, and irritability.
- No pressure should be felt inside during the practice of pranayama.
- The left arm is kept straight, the back of the wrist resting on the left knee. The forefinger is bent toward the thumb, its tip touching the tip of the thumb. This is the Jnana Mudra **(Fig. 12.18)**.
- The right arm is bent at the elbow and the hand is kept on the nose to regulate the even flow of breath and to gauge its subtlety. The tips of the ring and little fingers control the left nostril and the tip of the thumb controls the right nostril when Nasika Mudra **(Fig. 12.19A)** or Nasagra Mudra **(Fig. 12.19B)** is assumed.
- Yogi observes details such as time, posture, and an even breath rhythm, and is alert and sensitive to the flow of prana within them.
- Asanas should never be practiced immediately after pranayama. Allow an hour to elapse before starting asanas.
- Pranayama, however, may be done not <15 minutes after mild practice of asanas.
- When deep, steady, and long breathing cannot be maintained rhythmically, stop. Do not proceed further.
- Try to achieve an even ratio in inhalation (Puraka) and exhalation (Rechaka).

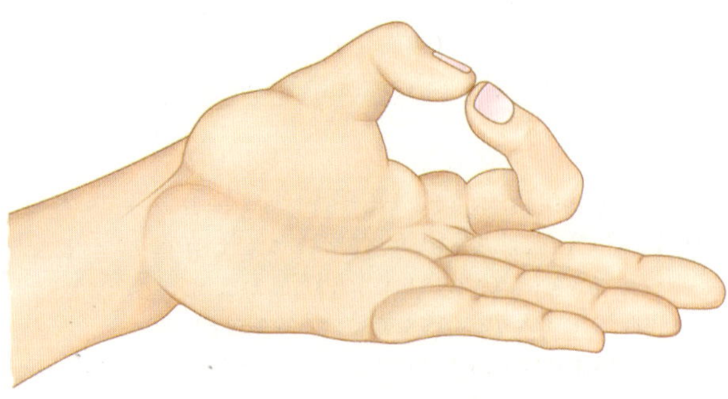

Fig. 12.18: Jnana Mudra.

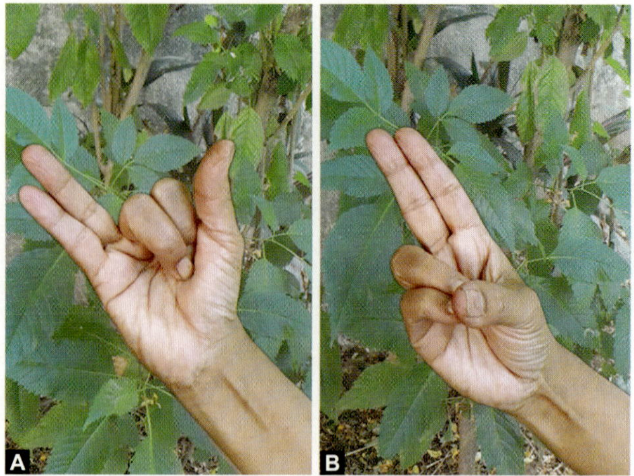

Figs. 12.19A and B: (A) Nasika Mudra; (B) Nasagra Mudra.

- After completing any pranayama, practice always lie down on the back like a corpse in Savasana for at least 5–10 minutes in silence.

Kumbhakas

"Kumbhakas" can be described as follows:

- Thorough mastery of inhalation and exhalation is essential before any attempt is made to learn antra kumbhaka.
- Bahya kumbhaka (restraint following exhalation) should not be tried until antra kumbhaka has become natural.
- Valsalva maneuver is a common unconscious and involuntary phenomenon that may occur during the practice of kumbhaka, which should be avoided.
- If it is found difficult to hold the breath (kumbhaka) after each inhalation or exhalation, do some cycles of deep breathing and then practice kumbhakas.
- If the rhythm of inhalation or exhalation is disturbed by holding the breath, lessen the duration of kumbhaka.
- Sometimes constipation occurs in the initial stages following the introduction of kumbhaka. This is temporary and is relieved in a few days.
- Since the eyes are closed throughout the practice of pranayama, the passage of time is noted by the mental repetition (japa) of a sacred word or name.

Ujjayi Pranayama

The prefix "ud" means upward or superiority in rank. It also means blowing or expanding. "Jaya" means "conquest," "victory," "triumph," or "success." If looked at from another point of view, it implies restraint or curbing. Like a proud conqueror, who puffs out his chest, Ujjayi involves maximal inhalation of air within the lungs where the chest inflates completely.

Technique

Following is the technique for Ujjayi Pranayam:

1. Any comfortable position such as Padmasana, Siddhasana, or Virasana can be chosen for sitting **(Fig. 12.20)**.

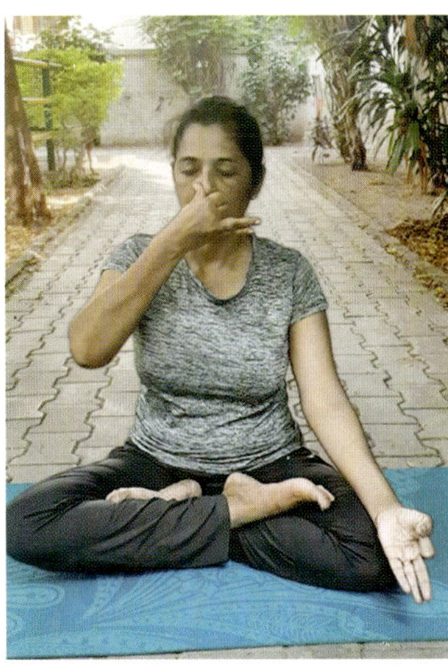

Fig. 12.20: Pranayama.

2. Keep the back erect and rigid. Lower the head to the trunk. Rest the chin in the notch between the collar-bones just above the breast-bone. (This is the Jalandhara Bandha)
3. Stretch the arms out straight and rest the back of the wrist on the knees. Assume the Jnana Mudra **(Fig. 12.18)**. (Join the tips of the thumbs to the tips of the index fingers, keeping the other fingers extended.)
4. Close the eyes.

Clinical Pearl

Persons suffering from pathological conditions of eyes and ears (such as glaucoma and ear infection) should not attempt to hold the breath.

5. Exhale completely.
6. Now the Ujjayi method of breathing begins.
7. Take a slow, deep, steady breath through both the nostrils.
8. Fill the lungs up to the brim. This filling up is called puraka (inhalation). Inflation of the abdomen during inspiration should be avoided.
9. The entire abdominal area from the pubis up to the breast-bone should be pulled back towards the spine.
10. Hold the breath for a second or a two.
11. Exhale slowly, deeply and steadily, until the lungs are completely empty. This exhalation is called Rechaka.
12. A pause should be taken before drawing a fresh breath. This waiting period is called Bahyakumbhaka.
13. The process described from points 2–12 completes one cycle of Ujjayi Pranayama.
14. The cycle should be repeated for 5–10 minutes and the eyes should remain closed for the entire process.
15. Lie on the floor for Savasana.
16. This is the only pranayama which can be done at all times of the day and night.

Effects

Ujjayi Pranayama helps in improving the vital capacity (VC), removal of secretions, improving endurance and gives a calm and refreshing feeling. Ujjayi without kumbhaka, done in reclining position, can be used for hypertension or coronary artery diseases patients.

Surya Bhedana Pranayama

Surya is the Sun. Bhedana means to pierce, to break or pass through. In this pranayama, the prana passes through the pingala or suryanadi, i.e., right nostril. After doing kumbhaka, the breath is exhaled through the left nostril, which is the path of Ida nadi.

Technique

The following steps are to be performed:
1. Any comfortable position such as Padmasana, Siddhasana, or Virasana can be chosen for sitting.
2. Keep the back erect and rigid. Lower the head to the trunk. Rest the chin in the notch between the collar-bones just above the breast-bone. (This is the Jalandhara Bandha)
3. Stretch the left arm. Rest the back of the left wrist on the left knee. Perform Jnana with the left hand.
4. Bend the right arm at the elbow. Bend the index and middle fingers towards the palm, keeping them passive. Bring the ring and little fingers towards the thumb.
5. The right thumb should be placed on the right aspect of the nose beneath the nasal bone and the ring and little fingers should be placed on the left aspect of the nose just beneath the nasal bone, slightly above the nostrils.
6. Press the ring and the little fingers to block the left side of the nose completely.
7. Press and close the right nostril with the right such that it makes the outer edge of the right nostril parallel to the lower edge of the cartilage of the septum.
8. The right thumb is bent at the top joint and the tip of the thumb is placed at a right angle to the septum.
9. With slow and deep inhalation, control the opening of the right nostril with the tip of the thumb. Fill the lungs to the brim (puraka).
10. Then block the right nostril so that both are now blocked.
11. Hold the breath for about 5 seconds (antra kumbhaka).
12. Keep the right nostril completely closed and open the left nostril partially exhaling the air out slowly and deeply (rechaka).
13. During the exhalation regulate the rhythmic flow of air from the left nostril by adjusting pressure with the ring and little fingers, so that the outer edge of the left nostril is kept parallel to the septum. The pressure should be exerted from inner sides of the tips of the fingers.
14. This completes the cycle of Surya Bhedan Pranayama. Continue with more cycles at a stretch from 5 to 10 minutes, according to capacity.

15. All the inhalations in Surya Bhedan are from the right nostril and all the exhalations from the left nostril.
16. Each inhalation and exhalation should last for the same length of time.
17. Lie down in Savasana after completing pranayama.

Effects

In Surya Bhedana Pranayama, the lungs have to work more and they are filled more slowly, steadily, and fuller than in Ujjayi Pranayama. It increases digestive power, soothes and invigorates the nerves, and cleans the sinuses.

Nadi Shodhana Pranayama

Nadi is a tubular organ of the body such as an artery or a vein for the passage of prana or energy. Shodhana meaning purifying or cleansing. So the objective of Nadi Shodhana Pranayama is the purification of the vessels.

Technique

The methods mentioned below are to be followed:
1. Follow step 1 to 8 of Surya Bhedana Pranayama.
2. Exhale out fully through the right nostril while controlling the opening of the right nostril with the inner aspect of the right thumb.
3. A slow deep inhalation should then be performed through the right nostril, controlling the opening with the tip of the right thumb. Fill the lungs to the brim (puraka), keeping the left nostril completely closed using the ring and little fingers.

Clinical Pearl

People suffering from low blood pressure will derive benefit but those with hypertension or other cardiac pathologies should not hold their breath after inhalation (antra kumbhaka) whilst practicing this pranayama.

4. After full inhalation, block the right nostril completely with the pressure of the ring and little fingers on the left nostril. Exhale slowly, steadily and deeply through left nostril. Empty the lungs completely (rechaka).
5. After full exhalation through the left nostril, change the pressure on it by adjusting the fingers. In the changed position, the tips of the ring and little fingers exert the pressure.
6. A slow deep inhalation is then performed through the left nostril, filling the lungs completely (puraka).
7. After the full inhalation through the left nostril, block it and exhale through the right nostril (rechaka).
8. This completes one cycle of NadiSodhana Pranayama. Here the rhythm of breathing is as follows:
   a. Exhale through the right nostril.
   b. Inhale through the right nostril.
   c. Exhale through the left nostril.
   d. Inhale through the left nostril.
   e. Exhale through the right nostril.
   f. Inhale through the right nostril and so on.

Stage (a) above is the preparatory one. The first real cycle starts at stage (b) and ends at stage (e).
9. Do 8–10 cycles at a stretch.
10. Inhalation and exhalation from each side should take the same time.
11. In a progression, attempt may be made to retain breath (antra kumbhaka) after inhaling.
12. Attempt to hold after the exhalation (bahyakumbhaka) should only be made once antra kumbhaka is mastered.
13. Always conclude by lying down in Savasana.

Effects

The blood receives a larger supply of oxygen by this pranayama than normal breathing. The mind becomes still and lucid.

Viloma Pranayama

Loma means "hair." "Vi" denotes negation or privation. Viloma thus means against the hair, against the natural order of the things. In Viloma Pranayama, inhalation or exhalation is not one uninterrupted continuous process but is interrupted by several phases.

Technique

Stage 1:
1. A sitting or supine lying posture may be used for Viloma Pranayama.
2. Inhale for 2 seconds, pause for 2 seconds holding the breath, again inhale for 2 seconds holding the breath, and continue like this until the lungs are completely full.
3. Now hold the breath for 5–10 seconds (antra kumbhaka) according to the capacity.

Clinical Pearl

People suffering from cardiovascular diseases must not attempt to hold their breath (kumbhaka).

4. Exhale slowly and deeply as in Ujjayi with an aspirate sound (huuum).
5. This completes one cycle of the first stage of Viloma Pranayama.
6. Repeat 10–15 cycles of this first stage at a stretch.

Stage 2:
7. Rest for a minute or two.
8. Then take a deep breath without any pauses as Ujjayi Pranayama with a sibilant sound (ssssssa). Fill the lungs completely.
9. Hold the breath from 5–10 seconds (antra kumbhaka), keeping the Mula Bandha grip.
10. Exhale for 2 seconds and pause for 2 seconds. Again exhale for 2 seconds, pause for 2 seconds and continue like this until the lungs are completely emptied.
11. This completes one cycle of the second stage of Viloma Pranayama.

Table 12.1: Asanas used in various pathologies/disorders.

Pathology/symptom	Asanas
Obesity	Garudasana, Gomukhasana, Pawanmuktasana, Ardhachandrasana, Ekapada Rajakapotasana
Diabetes	Supta Virasana, Halasana, Janu Sirsasana, Paschimottanasana, Nadi Sodhana Pranayama, Pawanmuktasana
Hypertension	Supta Baddha Konasana, Janu Sirsasana, Nadi Sodhana Pranayama, Dhyana, Adho Mukha Virasana, Savasana
Hypotension	Uttanasana, Salamba Sarvangasana, Adho Mukha Savasana, Salamba Sirsasana, Ustrasana, Dhanurasana, Parvottanasana
Arthritis, low back pain	Supta Baddha Konasana, Supta Virasana, Bhujangasana, Ustrasana, Garudasana, Salbhasana, Dhanurasana
Respiratory disorders such as COPD, chronic bronchitis, and asthma	Supta Baddha Konasana, Supta Virasana, Bhujangasana, Paschimottanasana, Ujjayi Pranayama, Nadi Sodhana Pranayama, Janu Sirsasana, Adho Mukha Savasana, Yoga Mudra
Cerebral disorders, e.g., migraine, insomnia, and memory impairments	Supta Baddha Konasana, Uttanasana, Salamba Sarvanagasana, Sirsasana, Savasana, Sanmukhi Mudra
GI disorders, e.g., constipation and peptic ulcers	Supta Virasana, Supta Baddha Konasana, Pawanmuktasana, Janu Sirsasana, Yoga Mudra, Ujjayi Pranayama, Nadi Sodhana Pranayama
Acidity	Supta Baddha Konasana, Paschimottanasana, Makarasana, Janu Sirsasana, Savasana, Nadi Sodhana Pranayama
Gynecological problems, e.g., menstrual disorders, PCOS, and dysmenorrhea	Virasana, Supta Virasana, Baddha Konasana, Supta Baddha Konasana, Paschimottanasana, Janu Sirsasana

(COPD: chronic obstructive pulmonary disorders; GI: gastrointestinal; PCOS: polycystic ovarian syndrome)

Effects

The first stage helps those suffering from hypotension. The second stage is beneficial for persons suffering from hypertension. The second stage of Viloma should only be done when lying down by persons suffering from hypertension.

YOGA AND PHYSIOTHERAPY

Yoga, as adjunctive therapy and a way of promoting and maintaining wellness, offers an excellent example of the mind–body connection. It has been suggested that yoga has diverse clinical and nonclinical applications in the physiotherapeutic process. This is mainly attributed to the degree of complexity and multidimensionality of influences that is apparent in both yoga exercises and physiotherapy as continuous processes.

On the conceptual level, the similarities between yoga and physiotherapy include physiological, psychological, social, educational, and spiritual dimensions of human health. When yoga exercises are combined with physiotherapeutic processes, both in clinical and nonclinical settings, they can affect various body systems and structures such as the musculoskeletal, nervous, endocrine, visceral, and immune system. This would be beneficial for patients with orthopedic, neurological, metabolic and psychosomatic disorders **(Table 12.1)**. Nevertheless, the main strength of this form of activity is that all the body's dimensions (i.e., cells, tissues, and organs) can be influenced simultaneously within one entire system.

BENEFITS OF YOGA

Musculoskeletal Improvements and Posture Control

Some researchers suggest that yoga exercises can influence the musculoskeletal and nervous systems via automobilization or mobilization of both joints and nerves respectively. For example, the "Cobra" pose (Bhujangasana) and one of McKenzie's static procedures are almost the equivalent and can directly lead to improvement of pain symptoms of cervical and low back pain. This suggests that there could be direct similarities between these two approaches and the compatibility of their essence. From the physiotherapeutic outlook, somatic dysfunction can be released and flexibility and range of movement improved. Yoga as a set of "static dynamic procedures" can be considered as a means to "self-mobilization" of the nervous system and the joints of spine and limbs, with regard to physiotherapeutic processes. This point of view has been supported by a research, having demonstrated that patient conditions improved considerably after 6 months of yoga practice, with some markers of incorrect posture completely disappearing such as poking chin, asymmetry of the shoulders, and shortening of the back extensors and pectorals. Findings from another exploratory study suggest that yoga practice may decrease anterior pelvic tilt, improve hip extension, and increase stride length, and that yoga programs especially designed according to individual needs may offer a cost-effective means of preventing or reducing age-related changes in these indices of gait function. Physiotherapists specialized in orthopedic manual therapy might be particularly interested in the beneficial effects of yoga exercises on the musculoskeletal system, scoliosis prevention, passive correction of multidimensional pelvic distortion, increased range of motion in spinal column, postural reeducation, and improved blood circulation in vertebral arteries as well as the prevention of soft tissue injury.

Neuropsychological Benefits of Yoga

Yoga techniques seem to stimulate the right hemisphere of the brain and increase alpha wave frequencies. Patients practicing yoga may also show a significant reduction in the number of mistakes during static motor performance as well as improvement in sensory-motor performance. It may also lead to enhanced processing ability of the central nervous system and eye-hand coordination. It can be suggested that physiotherapists could utilize yoga to promote the recovery processes among stroke patients and improve their function.

Physiological Benefits of Yoga

Practicing yoga exercises leads to stimulation of the autonomic nerve plexuses and the endocrine system by an increased pressure in the abdominal wall. Thus it is suggested that yoga asanas enhance lung function together with increased strength and endurance of respiratory muscles and improve the performance of the cardiorespiratory system, leading to increased VC. It also normalizes blood pressure; reduces HR, RR; and increases red blood cell volume and improves immunity. There has been significant reduction in the amount of oxygen consumed with decreased breath rate and increased breath volume found. Yoga can also significantly decrease fatigue. More precisely, yoga "intervention" increases regression of coronary lesions and coronary atherosclerosis in patients with severe coronary artery disease, whilst simultaneously improving myocardial perfusion. Yoga also improves risk factor profile, symptomatic status, and functional class. Patients who perform regular yoga exercises require revascularization procedures (coronary angioplasty or bypass surgery) less frequently.

From the physiotherapy perspective, yoga may be considered as an appropriate way of using body postures that offers enhanced cardiopulmonary function, i.e., improved breathing patterns or blood vessel contraction as well as various physiological benefits.

Benefits of Yoga: Psychological and Spiritual Wellness

Yogasanas have shown considerable reduction in the symptoms of depression and anxiety. They can also decrease oxidative stress and relieve tensions leading to better concentration and relaxation. This may be partially explained by the work of Shannahoff-Khalsa, who demonstrated that yogasanas increase serotonin and dopamine and decrease cortisol secretion. Studies on the effects of yoga on cognitive functions have shown improvements in memory and vigilance levels. Yoga techniques were found to be effective in treating obsessive–compulsive disorder, phobias, major depressive disorders, and grief. It has also been proven effective in insomnia and other sleep disorders as well as post-traumatic stress disorder. Yoga can also improve fear management through its assisting effects in coping mental challenges and soothing effects in controlling anger by helping patients to turn negative thoughts into positive ones as well as facilitating rehabilitation of patients prone to antisocial behaviors. Yoga offers a new path to positive mental health. It also helps to free individuals from drug dependency (substance abuse and addictive disorders) and its associated problems. Yoga techniques can enhance well-being, mood, stress tolerance, and mental focus. Yoga promotes personal development by encouraging individual initiative and self-belief and helps to bring about improvements in attitude and health behavior. Yoga asanas are observed as an open door to self-realization and creation of the union of the mind, body, and spirit. The results indicate an improvement in various parameters such as better sense of well-being, improved effectiveness, self-confidence, better interpersonal relationship, lowered irritability levels, increased attentiveness, and an optimistic outlook in life as some of the beneficial effects enjoyed by the yoga practitioners indicated by feedback score. Among yoga practitioners significant improvements in perceived self-efficacy may also improve coping and stress management. Improvements in quality of life scores are also observed.

It can be hypothesized that during yoga exercises the similar psychological and spiritual resources are employed by practitioners as used by physiotherapists in order to improve the patients' functional recovery. If verified, this hypothesis may be a useful adjunct both to patients intended to develop their spiritual or psychological features as well as to physiotherapists who might consider expanding their holistic approach as therapists using yoga's essence. Furthermore, physiotherapist, manual therapists, chiropractors, or osteopaths could consider yoga as a way of "mental mobilization" insofar as the individual performs postures that comprise elements of enhanced self-development, self-efficacy, or positive mind states such as optimism

Table 12.2 shows figures of common asanas used in physiotherapy.

SUMMARY

Yoga is an ancient science developed in India. Yoga works on all the aspects of the life of an individual—physical, physiological, psychological, and spiritual. It is based on the concept of governing our own selves by freeing our minds of all the fluctuations and bringing a sense of inner calm. Though the schools of yogic practice

Table 12.2: Common asanas used in physiotherapy.

Name of the asana	Pose
Pawanmuktasana	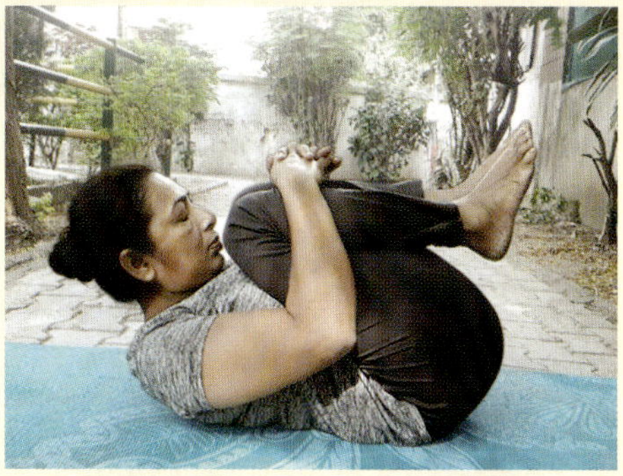
Virasana	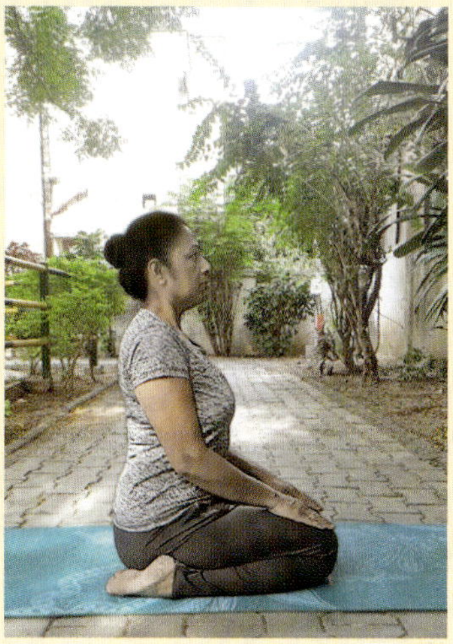
Adho Mukha Virasana	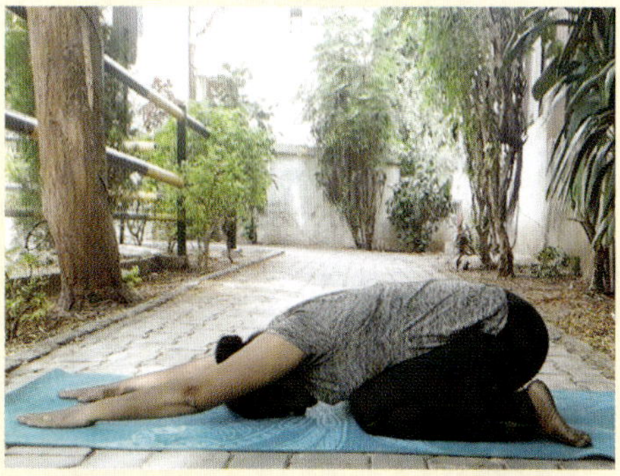
Halasana	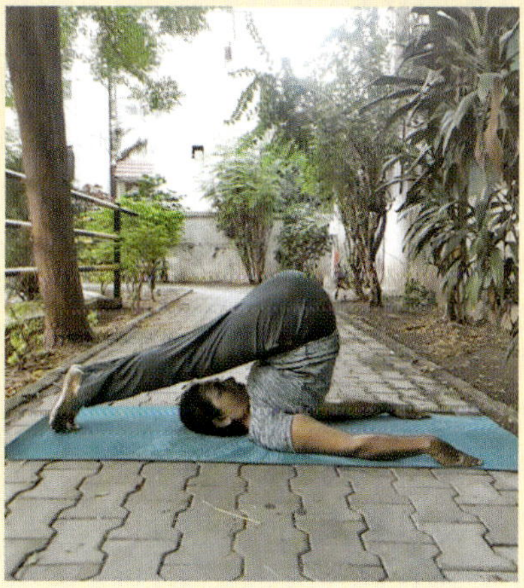

Contd...

Contd...

Name of the asana	Pose
Salabhasana	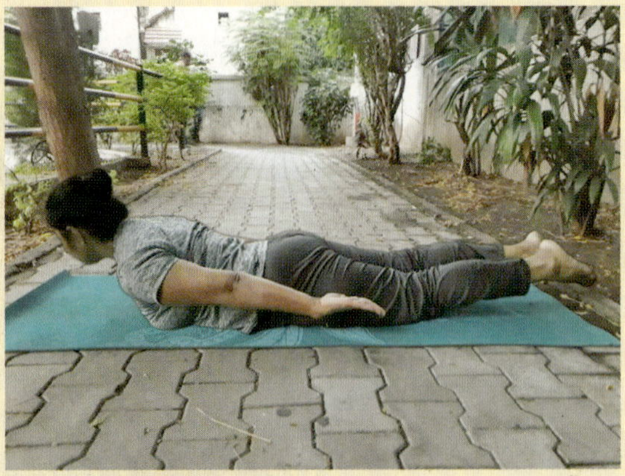
Makrasana	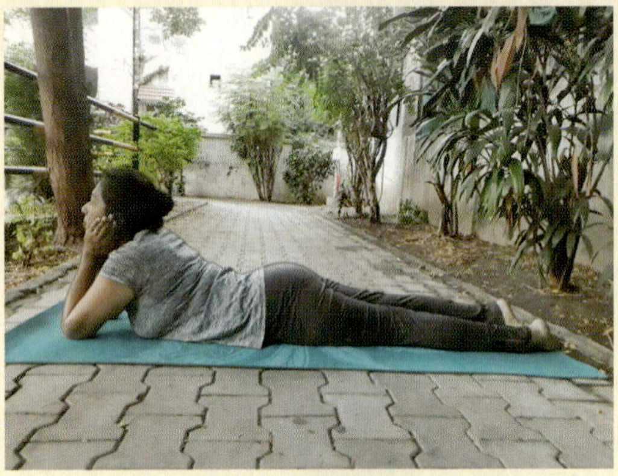 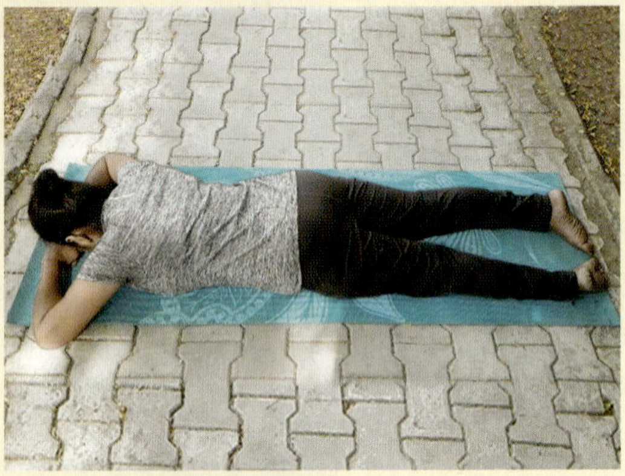
Paschimottanasana	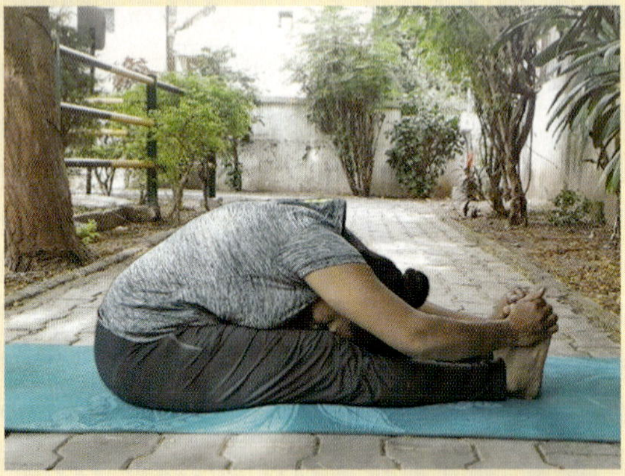
Ardha Paschimottanasana/ Janu Sirsasana	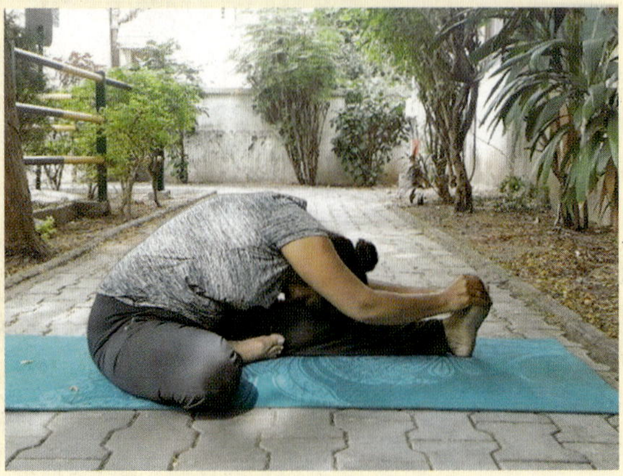

Contd...

Contd...

Name of the asana	Pose
Baddha Konasana	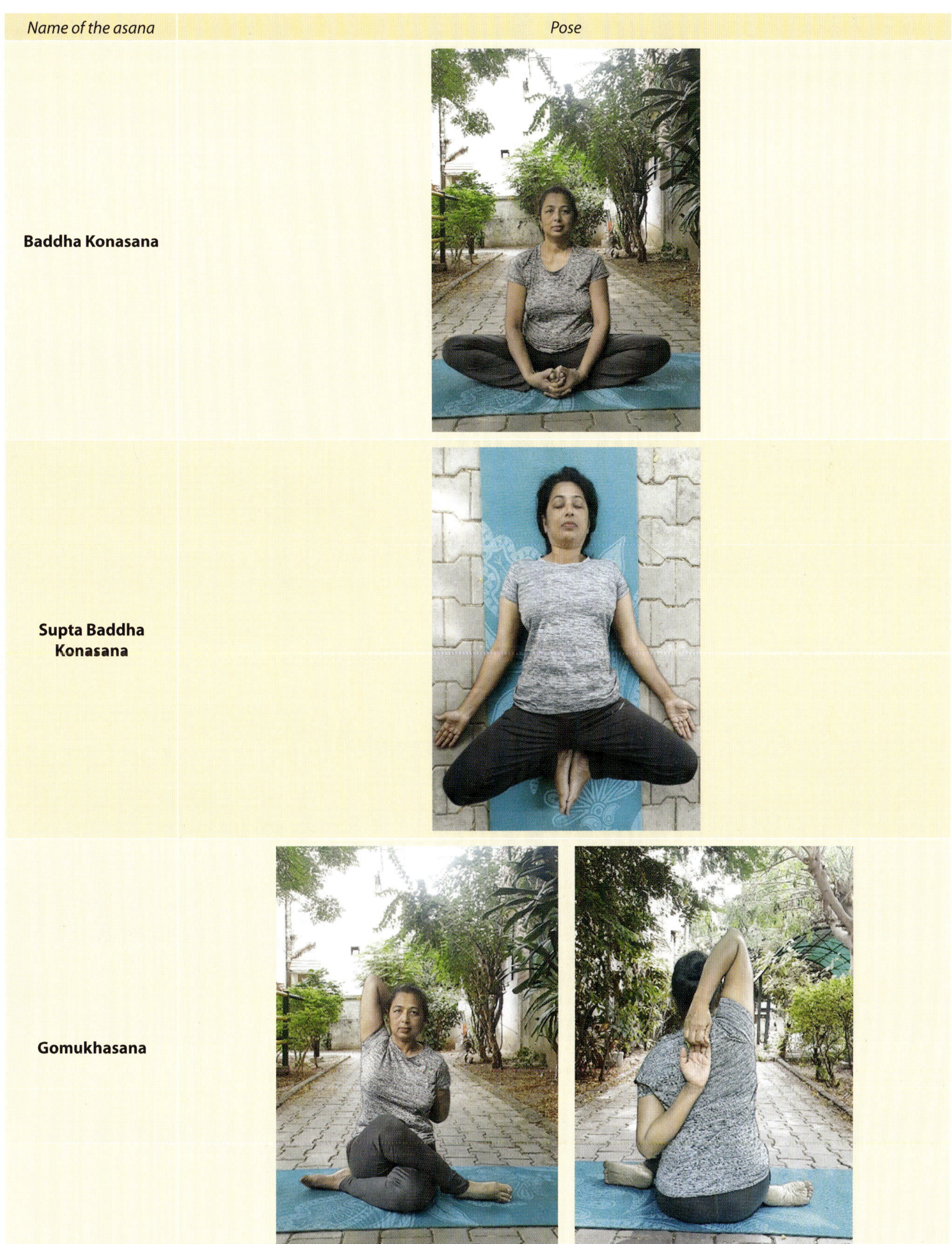
Supta Baddha Konasana	
Gomukhasana	

Contd...

Contd...

Name of the asana	Pose
Salamba Sarvangasana	
Sanmukhi Mudra	

differ in the execution, the nature of all yogic practices is psychophysiological. Regular yogic practice creates a sense of well-being, improves body mechanics and efficiency, improves concentration and memory, and elevates the mood of an individual. In the modern world, the practice of Yoga has gained popularity due to its therapeutic benefits. Yoga can be used by rehabilitation professionals as an adjunct therapy or allied therapy to aid the individual improve better. Yoga has proved to be beneficial in several musculoskeletal disorders such as back pain, arthritis, and spondylitis. It also helps improve cognitive and neurological symptoms, gastrointestinal disorders, gynecological disorders, etc. Yoga practices aid the individual to achieve a wholesome life.

Review Questions

1. How does yogasana help in physical and mental well-being?
2. What is Suryanamaskar? Describe how it is done.
3. Write a short note on the benefits of yogasana.
4. What are the benefits of Suryanamaskar?
5. Describe the five fluctuations of mind described by Patanjali.
6. Describe Savasana in detail.
7. Explain the procedure and benefits of pranayama.
8. Explain the stages of yoga.

BIBLIOGRAPHY

1. Bhagat S. Alternative therapies, 1st edition. New Delhi: Jaypee; 2004.
2. Bhavanani AB, Madanmohan, Udupa K. Acute effect of Mukhbhastrika (a yogic bellows type breathing) on reaction time. Indian J Physiol Pharmacol. 2003;47:297-300.
3. DiBenedetto M, Innes KE, Taylor AG, et al. Effect of a gentle Lyengar yoga program on gait in the elderly: an exploratory study. Arch Phys Med Rehabil. 2005;86:1830-7.
4. Iyengar BKS. The illustrated light on yoga, 10th edition. New Delhi: HarperCollins; 2005.
5. Luskin FM, Newell KA, Griffith M, et al. A review of mind/body therapies in the treatment of musculoskeletal disorders with implications for the elderly. Altern Ther Health Med. 2000;6:46-56.
6. Patel N. Yoga and rehabilitation, 1st edition. New Delhi: Jaypee; 2008.
7. Posadzki P, Parekh S. Yoga and physiotherapy: a speculative review and conceptual synthesis. Chin J Integr Med. 2009;15(1):66-72.
8. Posadzki P. Yoga in aspect of manual therapy. J Man Med. 2005;9:9-20.
9. Posadzki P. Yoga in aspect of neuromobilisations. J Man Med. 2006;10:15-26.
10. Raghuraj P, Telles S. Right uninostril yoga breathing influences ipsilateral components of middle latency auditory evoked potentials. Neurol Sci. 2004;25:274-80.
11. Roach GM, McNally C. The essential yoga sutra: Ancient Wisdom for Your Yoga. USA: Doubleday/ Random House; 2005.
12. Romanowski W. Theory and methodics of relaxation and concentration exercises. Warsaw: National Medical Publishing; 1973. p. 91.
13. Savic K, Pfau D, Skoric S, et al. The effect of Hatha yoga on poor posture in children and the psychophysiologic condition in adults. Med Pregl. 1990;43:268-72.
14. Shannahoff-Khalsa DS. An introduction to Kundalini yoga meditation techniques that are specific for the treatment of psychiatric disorders. J Altern Complement Med. 2004;10:91-101.
15. Sleboda R. Influence of integrated yoga system and kinesiology on motor system among children at the age of 8. Kraków: Academy of Physical Education in Kraków; 2002
16. Swami Vivekanand. Patanjali Yoga Sutras: Sanskrit text with transliteration, translation and commentary.
17. Telles S, Naveen KV. Yoga for rehabilitation: an overview. Indian J Med Sci. 1997;51:123-7.
18. Telles S, Praghuraj P, Ghosh A, et al. Effect of a one-month yoga training program on performance in a mirror-tracing task. Indian J Physiol Pharmacol. 2006;50:187-90.
19. The Yoga Sutras of Patanjali. Introduction, Commentaries, and Translation. http://www.rainbowbody.net/HeartMind/sutramud.htm
20. WHO Traditional Medicine Strategy 2002–2005. World Health Organization Geneva.
21. Wilczynski J. Scoliosis-diagnosis and treatment. Kielce: Wszechnica Świętokrzyska Publishing; 2000. pp. 33-4.
22. Williams KA, Petronis J, Smith D, et al. Effect of Lyengar yoga therapy for chronic low back pain. Pain. 2005;115:107-17.

Assistive Technology and Environment Modification

Anu Arora

For people without disability, technology makes things easier,
For people with disabilities, technology makes things possible

— Jeudy Heumann

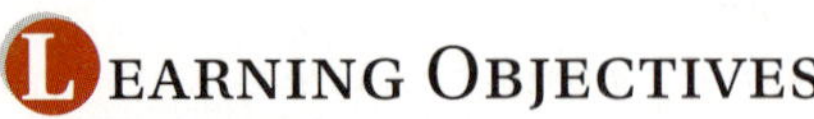# LEARNING OBJECTIVES

After reading this chapter, the readers should be able to:

♦ Comprehend the concept of assistive devices. Provide a brief overview of assistive technology (AT) devices and services through definitions (ICF and ISO)
♦ Understand the benefits of and barriers to assistive technology
♦ Gain knowledge about the use of AT in various domains, including subjects with neurological disorders, communication disorders, motor–sensory impairments, and cognitive/learning disabilities
♦ Discuss and apprise various environmental modifications, which may assist to overcome barriers to enhance level of function
♦ Make a shift towards the newer technologically driven approaches to rehabilitation in various communities

CHAPTER OUTLINE

- Empowering abilities through assistive technology
- Introduction to assistive technology: definition, purpose, and goals
- Human activity assistive technology model
- Assistive technology: areas of application
  - Self-maintenance
  - Self-advancement and self-enhancement
- Salient features and types of assistive technology
- Assistive technology for management of neurological conditions (stroke, Parkinson's disease, etc.)
- Assistive technology devices for students with special needs
  - Learners with disabilities
  - Augmentative and alternative communication
- Devices for daily life
- Assistive technology for mobility impairments
- Assistive technology and International Classification of Functioning, Disability and Health
- Benefits of assistive technology
- Barriers to assistive technology
- Assistive technology: future trends and applications
- Environmental modifications
  - Types of environmental modifications
  - Environmental modifications for elderly
  - Environmental modifications at workplace
- Assistive technology: the path ahead

EMPOWERING ABILITIES THROUGH ASSISTIVE TECHNOLOGY

Evidence in literature is suggestive of the use of technology in varying levels of sophistication to assist human functioning in day-to-day tasks.

The essence of a truly egalitarian society lies in its inclusivity and the recent advances in technology are not just making life easier for the able bodied but are also providing crucial assistance for person with varying level of disabilities to enhance their function at individual level and constructive participation at the community level.

The use of technology for rehabilitation of people with special needs, thereby empowering them to enhance their capabilities and quality of life is the latest challenge that the rehabilitation professionals of today's era face.

INTRODUCTION TO ASSISTIVE TECHNOLOGY: DEFINITION, PURPOSE, AND GOALS

Assistive technology (AT) has been referred to in literature as an umbrella term for both assistive products/devices and related services. AT refers to "any item, piece of equipment, or product system, whether acquired commercially off the

Goal of Assistive Technology

The goal of assistive technology is to compensate for absent or impaired abilities and enable occupational performance.

shelf, modified or customized, that is used to increase, maintain, or improve functional capabilities of individuals with disabilities."

The International Classification of Functioning, Disability and Health (ICF) defines assistive products and technology as any product, instrument, equipment, or technology adapted or especially designed for improving the functioning of a person with a disability. Drawing from the ICF, the International Organization for Standardization defines assistive products more broadly as any product, especially produced or generally available, that is used by or for persons with disability for any or all of the following purposes:

- To protect and support
- To measure or substitute for body functions/structures and activities
- To prevent impairments
- To decrease activity limitations or participation restrictions
- To train
- To enhance community participation.

This includes devices, equipment, instruments, and software system seen as an open system, which is dynamic and interacts with the environment. In this model, AT is seen as a means of enabling the person, who is unable to complete a task using existing resources.

The terms "assistive technology," "adaptive equipment," and "assistive devices" are generally used interchangeably. Adaptive equipment/devices refer to equipment designed to help persons with disabilities to compensate for functional limitations. These equipment range from simple, long-handled reacher for those unable to bend over to complex, computerized environmental control systems.

HUMAN ACTIVITY ASSISTIVE TECHNOLOGY MODEL

The Human Activity Assistive Technology (HAAT) Model depicts the relation between various components and AT system. It represents how AT devices can assist in improving the level of functioning. It constitutes of four main subsections:

1. **The human-technology interface** that represents the interaction between the subject and the technology device and is dependent upon on the physical abilities of the user. The success of a device can be determined by the ease with which it can be maneuvered by the subjects using it. For example, in people with severe disabilities, head movements are used to control the assistive equipment such as speech-generating devices, environmental control systems, assistive reading and writing tools, and powered wheelchairs. Further, adaptive interfaces include eye gaze, "sip and puff" systems, chin control devices, and switches configured to provide a specific output, eye gaze tracking technology that can be set to track the coordinated movements of two eyes. Single eye movement can also be utilized as a cue when a person does not have normal binocular movements. **Dragon Naturally Speaking** software is included in many popular operating systems for speech recognition.

2. The **processor** to which the information is relayed via a mechanical or electrical linkage that interprets it to create an activity output.

3. The **resultant activity output** that refers to the outcome of the AT activation, e.g., writing a text.

4. The **environmental** interface that modulates the response according to input from the environment.

ASSISTIVE TECHNOLOGY: AREAS OF APPLICATION

Assistive technology enables the subjects to accomplish not just their activities of daily living (ADLs) but also tasks of occupations and roles. AT can assist in:

- Self-maintenance
- Self-advancement
- Self-enhancement

Self-maintenance

Basic ADLs include activities such as independence in toilet activities, mobility, eating, bathing, dressing, grooming, and communication. These can be assisted by ATs such as electric toothbrushes and electric shavers, which can increase competency with personal care tasks.

Instrumental ADLs (IADLs) can also reap benefit from AT. Text telephones or the erstwhile telecommunication device for the deaf and hands-free or adapted telephones enable telephonic conversations as well as e-shopping.

Electronic Aids to Daily Living (EADLs) are devices used by individuals with mobility impairments to manipulate one or more electronic devices. Subjects with significant disabilities can manage their personal space (i.e., control lights, fans, or the volume on a TV or stereo and opening/locking of main doors) through the use of EADLs. The many benefits of EADLs include decreased physiological cost index of performing the activity, better vocational opportunities, positive psychosocial impact, increased independence, and thereby better quality of life. An example for EADL is Mini Relax by Ablenet, wherein the scanning switch access uses infrared for transmission and controls up to six functions of one appliance just like a remote control.

Self-advancement and Self-Enhancement

Self-advancement and self-enhancement through AT is achieved when subjects can perform roles and participate in activities that otherwise would not have been possible for them. Some examples could be the use of AT to promote education in visually impaired or using EADLs to remotely control entertainment systems to make living in home environment much more comfortable.

Some of the most desirable features in AT include:

- Availability
- Accessibility
- Affordability
- Adaptability
- Acceptability
- Quality

SALIENT FEATURES AND TYPES OF ASSISTIVE TECHNOLOGY

Table 13.1 describes the types and features of AT on the basis of complexity.

Table 13.1: Types of assistive technology (AT): On the basis of complexity.		
	Low-technology AT	*High-technology AT*
Characteristics	• Simple • Cheaper • Nonelectronic devices	• Sophisticated • Electronic devices • Usually fairly expensive • Often requires extensive training to ensure they are used to their fullest potential
Utilization	Improves a person's ability to carry out a work task for successful employment of people with disabilities	Invaluable in the successful employment of people with significant impairments
Examples	• Dressing aids • Pencil grips • Picture-based communication boards for persons who are nonspeaking • Magnifiers • Antifatigue standing mats to improve standing tolerance • Footrests • Wrist supports • Padded grips • Alternative keyboards	• Power wheelchairs **(Fig. 13.1)** • Computers • AAC devices • Remote controlled devices • Voice recognition • Screen reading technologies • Gaming • VR • Robotics

(AAC: augmentative and alternative communication; VR: virtual reality)

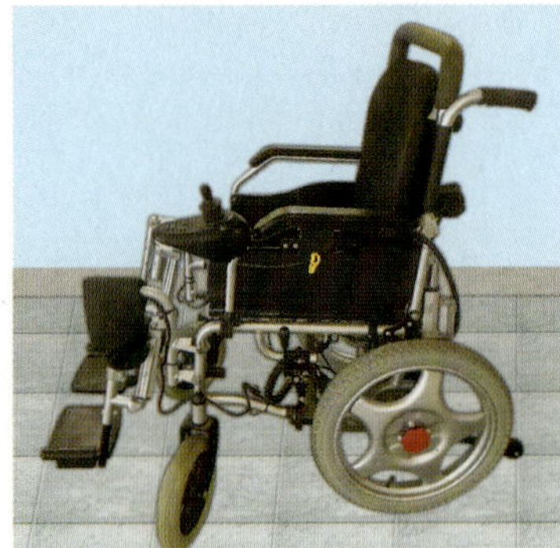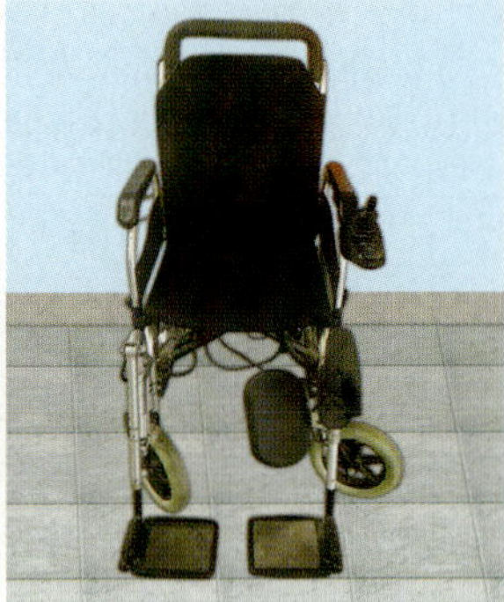

Fig. 13.1: Power wheelchair.
Source: Pic courtesy: Mission Health, Ahmedabad.

Table 13.2 describes the types and features of AT on the basis of utility.

Table 13.2: Types of assistive technology: On the basis of utility.	
Assistive technology types	*Assistive technology examples*
Mobility	• Walking stick, crutch, walker, wheelchair, splints, artificial limbs, and standing frame • Adapted furniture, cutlery, toilet seat, etc.
Cognition	• Reminders: Manual and automatic, adapted smart phones, task lists, and scheduler • Adapted games, picture-based instructions
Hearing aids and vision	Head phones, hearing aids, amplified listening devices such as telephones, sound-emitting balls, Braille-enabled board games, screen reader for computers, and Braille-transformed texts spectacles and magnifiers
Communication	Flash cards, electronic communication devices, recorders, amplifiers, etc.

ASSISTIVE TECHNOLOGY FOR MANAGEMENT OF NEUROLOGICAL CONDITIONS (STROKE, PARKINSON'S DISEASE, ETC.)

An emerging prospect to amend the therapeutic efficiency of stroke rehabilitation is through the use of AT. AT in the form of virtual reality (VR)/games can provide an enriched environment that can be modified in terms of its content and complexity. The multisensory feedback (visual, auditory as well as sensory) is utilized for attaining not just cognitive but also physical engagement. The computer aided visual feedback systems using VR and augmented reality such as Augmented Reflection Technology probably activate mirror neurons for rehabilitation of motor impairments especially to improve function.

Autonomous training with technology uses many principles of motor rehabilitation that have been proven to be effective modalities for stroke rehabilitation such as:

- Intensive and active execution of exercises
- Relevance of exercises to daily activities
- Varied and interactive exercise regimes
- Along with feedback from the therapist

There is now evidence to support the idea that subtle motor changes, which occur in very early, possibly preclinical stages of frank manifestation symptoms associated with Parkinson's disease can be detected through appropriate technology, where these impairments can be unmasked through activities of increased complexity (temporal or cognitive load).

All of us do not have equal talent, but all of us must have an equal opportunity to develop our talents.

—John F Kennedy

ASSISTIVE TECHNOLOGY DEVICES FOR STUDENTS WITH SPECIAL NEEDS

Learners with Disabilities

Children with disabilities, according to the Convention on the Rights of Persons with Disabilities, include children

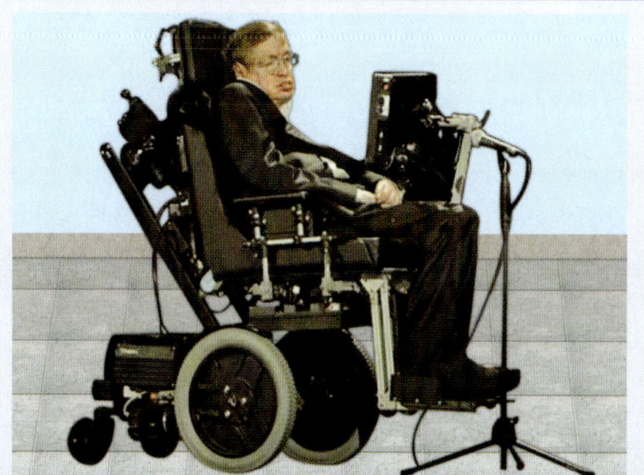

Stephen Hawking: Accidental ambassador for assistive technologies.

Despite suffering from the progressive neurodegenerative impact of amyotrophic lateral sclerosis, Stephen Hawking, the legendary physicist, could make significant contributions to scientific literature as assistive technology filled in for his functional limitations. Assisted by his recognizable wheelchair and computer-generated voice, he demonstrated the value of technological solutions to increase the quality of life, independence, and integration of people with physical and communication disabilities. Stephen Hawking's speech-generating devices system combined with relatively simple technology together in a unique and functional way wherein he managed a tablet computer with an infrared switch that he controlled with cheek movements. Stephen Hawking inadvertently became the spokesmodel for the use of assistive technologies who promoted the concept that physical limitation cannot hamper the human mind.

"who have long-term physical, mental, intellectual, or sensory impairments, which in interaction with various barriers may hinder their full and effective participation in society on an equal basis with others." Examples of some common impairments include:

- Autism
- Blindness
- Brain injury
- Cerebral palsy
- Congenital anomalies
- Down syndrome
- Hearing loss
- Intellectual and learning disabilities
- Muscular dystrophy
- Spina bifida
- Traumatic spinal cord injury
- Speech impairments
- Visual loss

These constitute the most stigmatized and excluded groups of children around the world. They are likely to have poorer health, less education, and less economic opportunity when they grow up leading to disparities between children with and without disabilities. Access and efficient utilization of assistive devices in this community promotes **inclusivity**. An educated child with a disability aided by appropriate AT will have:

- Better participation
- Greater opportunities for employment
- More self-reliance

This further assists them to utilize their potential to lead fulfilling lives, thus contributing to economic, social, and cultural vitality of their communities. AT supports children to access and enjoy their rights and participate in things they value thus bridging the disparities between children with and without disabilities.

The role of AT in support of students with disabilities is clearly seen in the use of software programing that compensates for reading or writing difficulties and enables the learner to more successfully master higher order learning tasks. Such tasks could be:

- Communication
- Mobility
- Self-care
- Household tasks
- Family relationships
- Education
- Engagement in play and recreation.

AT can enhance the quality life not only of affected children but of their families too.

Augmentative and Alternative Communication

The communication impairments may be a result of:

- Motor speech disorders (such as dysarthria or dyspraxia)
- A cognitive and language disorder (such as global developmental delay)

- A pervasive developmental disorder or autism spectrum disorder
- A chromosomal abnormality (including Down's syndrome)
- Mental retardation
- A brain injury
- Cerebral palsy
- A neuromuscular disorder [such as muscular dystrophy or spinal cord injury (SCI)]

Augmentative and alternative communication (AAC) includes devices that substitute or supplement communication skills and facilitate language learning. Augmentative communication options are appropriate for any subject whose natural speech and writing does not enable him or her to express himself or herself to all listeners in all environments and for all pragmatic communication purposes. The DynaVox/Tango and the Picture Exchange Communication System are some AAC systems, which use pictures to help people with significant delays in speech development, such as those with autism. Mayer–Johnson's Board Maker Plus! are software packages that use pictures, voice, sound, and animations as learning tools.

The most important features of AAC devices can be thought of as:

- Access options
- Vocabulary and syntax organization
- Pragmatic language function supports
- Language output.

Mouse, eye gaze tracking, and head tracking systems can be considered directed selection and rely on the mouse pointing options of AAC devices that are hosted by computer or tablet systems. A standard mouse or trackpad or with "mouse emulators" can accomplish this task.

DEVICES FOR DAILY LIFE

Assistive technology devices promote independent living and provide choices for decision-making across environmental demands and intrinsic barriers. It is vital to consider following before prescribing any type of AT device:

- The tasks at hand
- The strengths and limitations of the individual
- The features of devices

To manage eating, handles on utensils can be built up or handles can be angled to facilitate grasping and manipulation. Suction devices can be added to the bottom of plates to prevent them from moving and to provide stability, food preparation can be accomplished through a one-handed can opener, mechanical "reachers" to get items off shelves, jar openers, and bowls with suction devices to prevent spilling.

Speaking of liquid level indicators, Braille and talking scales and measures, and the use of Braille Dymo™ tape to label microwave ovens, stoves, and canned goods are some options to be considered for visually impaired individuals.

For subjects with intellectual disabilities and autism spectrum disorders (ASD), visual prompting systems such as pictorial cues using charts and video prompts using DVD players, computers, or handheld devices have been used to teach multistep tasks hook-and-loop tape instead of ties on shoes helps fasten shoes.

For bathing, handheld shower heads, shower chairs, wall grab bars, and scrub sponges with handles can be used by individuals with motor challenges. For individuals who have low vision, the bathroom should include high-contrast colors rather than the typical white found in many showers and bathtubs. Colored towels and mats and contrast on shower chairs help individuals discern items needed for grooming. Supportive frame can all provide options for individuals depending on their abilities to maneuver, position themselves, and sit upright while attending to their personal needs with dignity and independence.

Also, an alarm system can be installed near the toilet for the individual to call for assistance if needed. Finally, grab bars can provide support as an individual transfers on and off the toilet.

Examples of AT/environmental modifications to enhance function are as follows **(Figs. 13.2 A to C)**:

- A hearing aid or low-vision glasses to overcome functional impairments.
- Protective headgear can ensure the physical well-being of subjects with epilepsy and enable them to participate in activities important for social well-being.
- A pressure relief cushion in a wheelchair can protect a child or adult with paralysis from pressure sores and associated fatal infections.
- A communication board can support a subject with speech difficulties to express him/herself.
- A screen reader can make it possible for a subject who cannot see to access information on the web.
- A splint can enable a person to join the family at a cultural event.
- An alternative way of showing time can help a subject with an intellectual disability to keep his appointments.

ASSISTIVE TECHNOLOGY FOR MOBILITY IMPAIRMENTS

Subjects with mobility impairments are often seen with myriad needs and abilities.

AT solutions for some could be crutches, a scooter, or a wheelchair (Described in detail in Chapter 11). While for others, simple environmental modifications such as eliminating physical barriers by widening of doorway or building ramp instead of stairs may be all that is required.

While others might have a need for automobile hand controls, sit skis for downhill skiing, a van with an attached lift. Subjects who use wheelchairs might also need to be driving a wide range of motor vehicles as well as bicycles

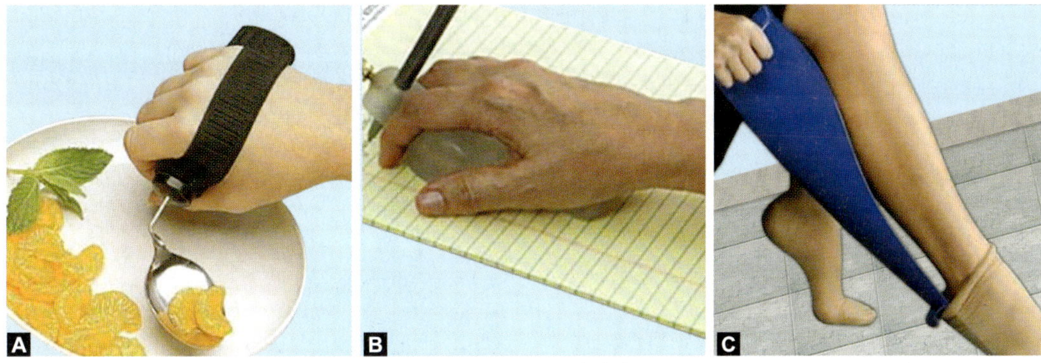

Figs. 13.2A to C: Assistive devices to aid basic activities of daily living. (A) Eating; (B) Writing; (C) Grooming.

using specially customized hand controls for turning and braking.

For someone with upper body mobility impairment, such as poor hand control or paralysis, assistive devices might include alternate keyboards or other input methods to access a computer.

Mobility devices, which are prescribed to augment the ambulatory function, may be effective through one/more of following functions:

- To broaden a patient's base of support
- To improve balance and stability
- To offload weight from the lower limbs to help alleviate joint pain
- To compensate for muscle weakness or injury

The achievables from such a mobility aid prescription include:

- Improved independent mobility
- Reduced disability
- Delayed functional decline
- Decrease in the burden of care.

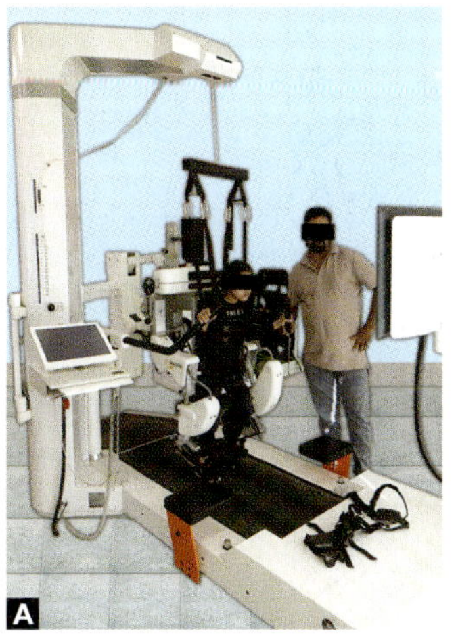
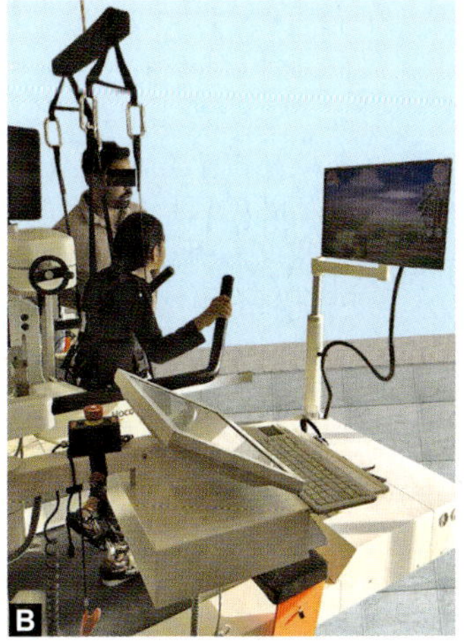
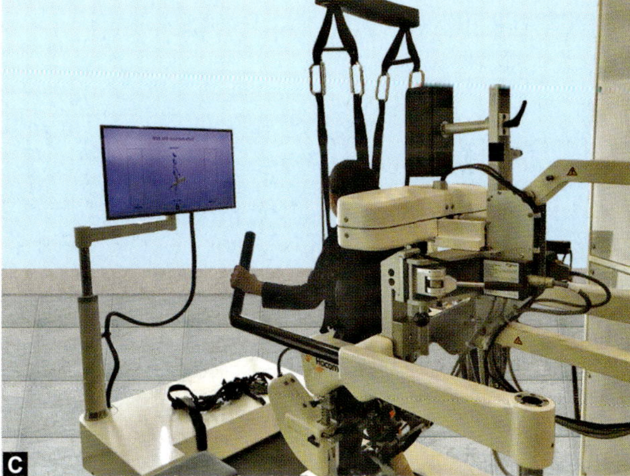
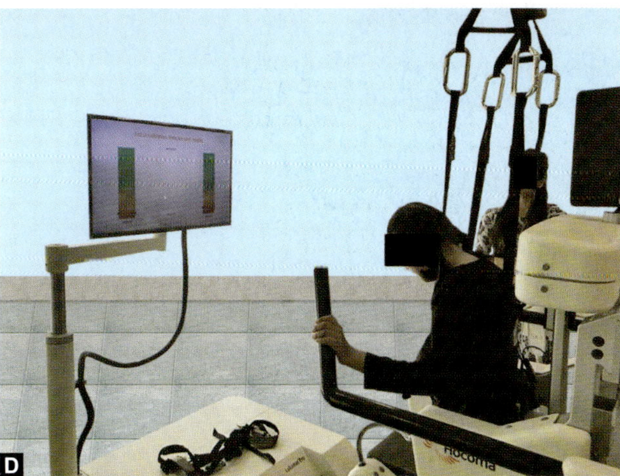
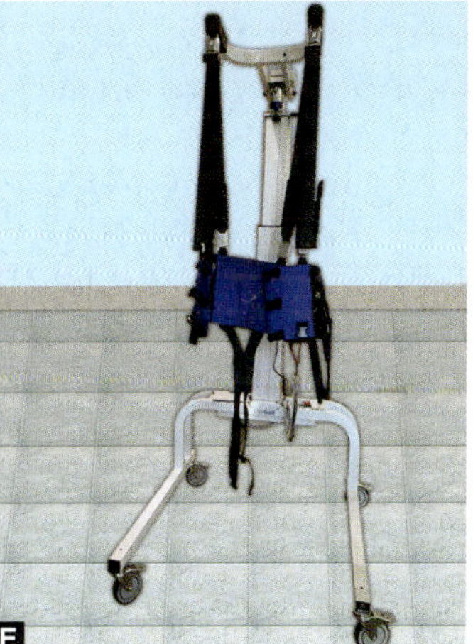
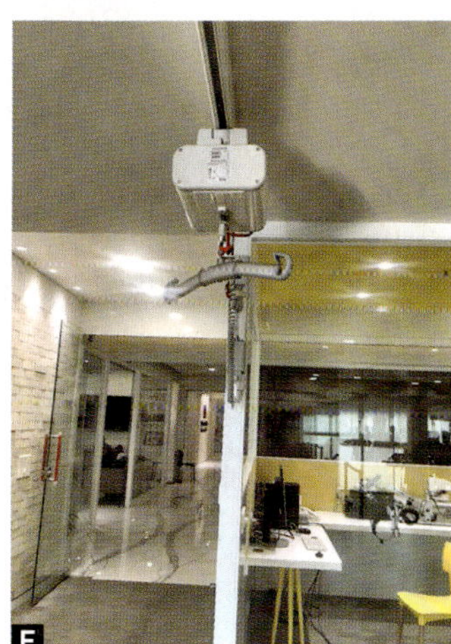

Figs. 13.3A to F

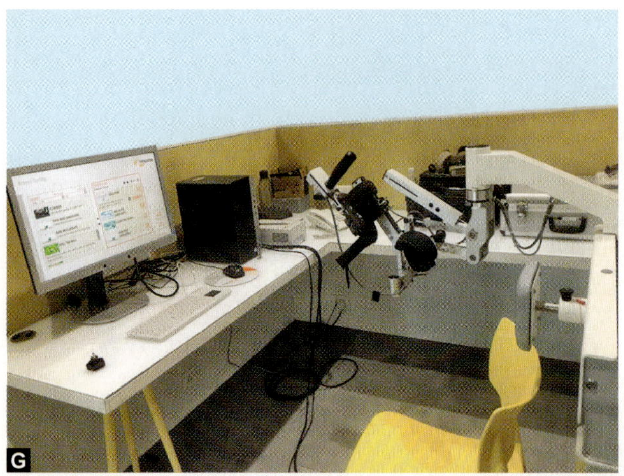
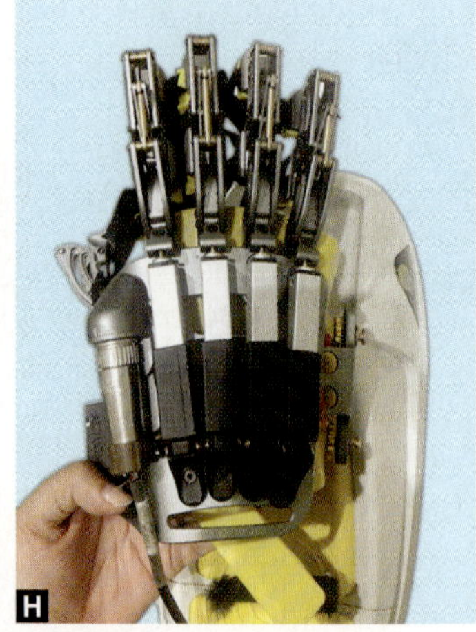
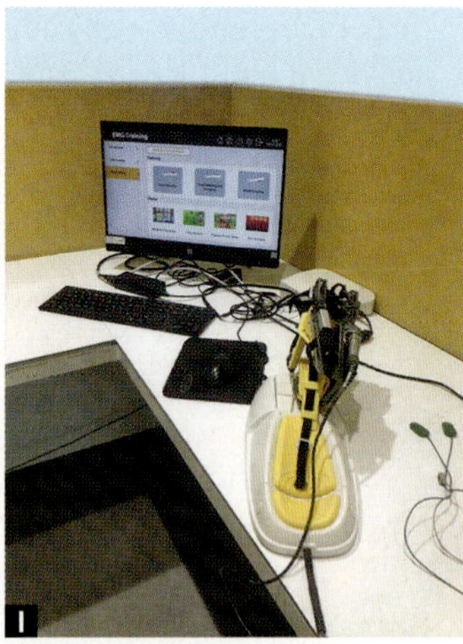

Figs. 13.3G to I

Figs. 13.3A to I: Devices and equipment used by physiotherapists to assist patients: (A) Use of robotics and assistive technology to improve locomotion; (B) Using task or goal-oriented training to improve locomotion; (C) Computer-guided training to improve locomotion; (D) Using feedback to improve locomotion; (E) Body weight-supported locomotor training device; (F) Hoists to assist in positioning; (G) Use of biofeedback and robotics to improve upper extremity function; (H) Robotic hand; and (I) Use of robotics and biofeedback to improve hand function.
Source: Pic courtesy: Mission Health, Ahmedabad.

ASSISTIVE TECHNOLOGY AND INTERNATIONAL CLASSIFICATION OF FUNCTIONING, DISABILITY, AND HEALTH

To facilitate agreement about the concept of disability, the World Health Organization (WHO) has developed a global common health language, the ICF, which moves away from a "consequences of diseases" classification (1980 version) to a "components of health" classification (2001). Using the common language of the ICF can help health-care professionals to communicate the need for health care and related services, such as the provision of AT for persons with disabilities.

In the ICF, function is understood as occurring at three levels:

1. At the level of the body part or system
2. At the level of the person (activities)
3. At the level of the person in society (participation)

Function is seen as a consequence of an interaction between an individual's health conditions and their environment and personal factors. Contextual environmental and personal factors mediate function at each level in positive and negative ways.

In ICF terminology, AT may be utilized to serve dual purpose of **enhancing function at an individual level and improving participation at community level (Table 13.3).**

Planning of AT for persons with disabilities is an engagement that has the possibility to decrease activity limitations and participation restrictions and, in turn, improve the quality of life of individuals with disabilities.

While a total knee replacement surgery not only directly impacts the patient's body structure and function, but hopefully also the surgery impacts ambulation and therefore his ability to participate in routine work. Prescribing a walker may directly impact ambulation,

Table 13.3: Role of assistive technology in various domains of International Classification of Functioning, Disability, and Health.

Body structure and function	AT in the form of force sensors helps detect muscle strength
Individual level activities	Gaming devices and virtual reality provide immersive environments to provoke motor responses to stimuli that are otherwise difficult to provide by therapist
Community participation and contextual factors	Activity monitors, accelerometers provide information on timing as well as quantity of physical activity

thus permitting improved work attendance, however, does not impact knee function. Recommending work site adaptations may improve participation but not the patient's body function or their ability to ambulate **(Box 13.1).**

BENEFITS OF ASSISTIVE TECHNOLOGY

Assistive technology is a powerful tool to increase independence and augment participation.

BOX 13.1: Simulation: Use of AT for various phases of rehabilitation of Mr A, a patient of early Parkinson's disease.

Assessment: Force sensors to detect subtle motor deficits in preclinical stage, activity monitors to record total duration of activity as well as diurnal variation in the activity.

Management: Use of virtual reality to create enriched simulated environment to modulate the patient response through gaming.

Strengthening evidence: The sharing of evidence regarding the impact of treatment approaches apprises the researcher for future research questions as well as solutions to them.

An environment with barriers restricts potential while an environment that facilitates enables the opportunities. The barriers could not just be social (e.g., negative attitudes) but also environmental where appropriate assistance is not provided. AT helps the subjects become mobile, communicate more effectively, see and hear better, and participate more fully in community. Moreover, AT helps the person with disability to access and enjoy their rights, do things they value, and bridge disparities between the persons with and without disabilities. AT furnishes the accession to and participation in educational, social, and recreational opportunities and empowers greater physical and mental function and improved self-esteem. These self-reliant, economically independent subjects are not a financial burden on the society anymore.

By facilitating the participation and inclusion of persons with disabilities in all aspects of life, AT boosts self-image, self-esteem, and sense of self-worth.

BARRIERS TO ASSISTIVE TECHNOLOGY

Disability has been recognized as the outcome of the interaction between person with an impairment and an environment with barriers, which in turn hinders his participation on an equal basis with others in the community. AT can play an important role in removing such barriers.

However, the following factors could become key barriers (**APPEAL**) in this process:

- Lack of **awareness**
- Lack of **product** and services
- Lack of trained **personnel** to assess needs and provide appropriate AT
- **Economic** barriers pertaining to cost
- **Access** to AT
- Lack of **legal support**, policies, and national programs.

The barriers to rehabilitation service provision can be overcome through a series of actions, including the following:

- Appropriate and accurate assessment prior to prescription of AT keeping in mind:
  - The tasks at hand
  - The strengths and limitations of the subject
  - The features of devices
- Strengthening human resources for rehabilitation
- Increasing the use and affordability of technology and assistive devices and putting in place funding mechanisms that address barriers related to financing of rehabilitation
- Promoting collaborative research with knowledge sharing between personnel
- Using technical expertise and clinicians along with inputs from stakeholders
- Bringing reforms in policies, laws, and delivery systems.

ASSISTIVE TECHNOLOGY: FUTURE TRENDS AND APPLICATIONS

Though we have been using Unified Parkinson's Disease Rating Scale to assess motor symptoms associated with Parkinson's disease, such scales are not sensitive enough to detect subtle changes early in the disease process. In such scenarios, AT is being used to develop a quantitative assessment tool to detect and document fine motor deficits based on the ability to control grip force output.

Robot-mediated neurorehabilitation is an emerging domain that incorporates progression in robotics with neurological science and rehabilitation requirements to devise novel, efficient, and accessible management regimes. The goal of robotic rehabilitation devices is to assist therapists in performing the types of activities and exercises they believe give their patients the best chance of a functional recovery.

Robotic technology provides consistent training for extended periods of time while collating data to evaluate progress. Robots can be used to assess performance before, after, and during an intervention, along with providing targeted intervention consistently and repetitively depending on the extent of impairment.

Robotic rehabilitation systems present evaluation methods that are based on the biomechanical data they acquire and process using specific software (e.g., INMOTION, IPAM, AMADEO, ARMEO, and T-WREX).

Robot-assisted system, INMOTION software (INMOTION EVAL), based on multiple regression models, calculates Fugl–Meyer Assessment (FMA), Motor Status Score (MSS), Motor Power (MP), and Modified Ashworth Scale (MAS) from the robot-based metrics.

Use of these functional outcome measures in collaboration with robotics provides the best metrics for assessing the effectiveness of rehabilitation.

From the first robotic device designed specifically for rehabilitation, the MIT-Manus, in 1992, an end-effector type of robot for treating the poststroke upper limb, we have come a long way toward greater automation with **robot-assisted telerehabilitation.** Telerehabilitation leverages telecommunications, computing technology, and remote sensing to enable both the delivery and assessment of rehabilitation services from a distance.

In contrast to traditional assessments that require one-on-one interaction with a therapist, objective assessment of motor function using data collected by rehabilitation robots can enable consistent, reliable, and automatic assessment of motor function without a subjective bias.

ENVIRONMENTAL MODIFICATIONS

The components of the environment can be evaluated in terms of following three domains:

1. Objective assessment using technology. For example, global positioning systems allow objective assessment of the structural layout of communities

and neighborhoods, including the transportation and infrastructure consisting of roads, crosswalks, and the location of buildings and houses.
2. Observational assessments.
3. Questionnaire-based self-report approaches asking about the impact the environment has on subject's level of participation.

Community environmental health assessment is another approach of environmental assessment that uses a systematic process to identify environmental health risks and create a practical action plan to address key environmental health issues within a target population (Details of assessment of environment can be found in Chapter 9).

Environmental modifications can be broadly defined to serve two purposes:
1. Physical adaptations to the home/workplace/community setup, required by the subject's plan of care indispensable for the health, welfare, and safety of the individual
2. Adaptations that enable the subject to function with greater independence in his native environment whether it is his place of residence or his workplace.

Environmental modifications made in home as well as external environment serve as an effective compensatory strategy to overcome environmental barriers and improve the ADL and IADL performance of subjects with functional limitations.

All environmental changes that are adopted must satisfy the following key concerns:
- Accessibility
- Independent functioning
- Enhanced safety
- Increased involvement in a life situation, i.e., participation.

A clear and systematic review of various kinds of environment modifications that can be undertaken is presented in the following sections.

Types of Environmental Modifications

The types of environmental modifications are as follows:
I. Alterations to the physical environment
   Examples:
   1. **Layout modification**, e.g., increasing the width of a door to make it easily accessible for wheelchair or crutch-aided ambulation
   2. **Use of adjustive/adaptive equipment**, e.g., wheelchairs, standing frames, gait trainers, lifts, augmentative communication devices, and recreational items such as swings or tricycles.
   3. **Architectural modifications**, e.g., provisions for ramps, rails, hand grabs, bathroom modifications.

II. Alterations to the way of using modalities
   1. Increase awareness amongst the subjects about using the environment in a modified way (always turn on lights before entering a room for an individual who has low vision).

2. Use everyday items to achieve goals (use of a portable phone for safety).

III. Enhancement of support from people:
   1. Educate the caregivers (proper transfer techniques, how to use a lift).
   2. Engage social services/NGO/vocational trainers/ ergonomists to assist in appropriate environmental modifications.

Guidelines for some generic environmental features that may be very effective in improving function

Ramps and Handrails

Following are the instructions in the usage of ramps and handrails:
- All pathways to patient areas should be level or have ramps to ensure patients have safe and independent access. These features are an important prerequisite for making our external environments friendly to persons with disability.
- Pathways to commonly accessed places should be flat or ramped where necessary.
- Ramps should be added (at a gradient of 1:20) if there is a rise to the door.
- Handrails should be included, wheresoever possible (about 85–95-cm high).

Doorways

The given instructions are to be followed regarding doorways:
- Door openings must be at least 90-cm wide to ensure easy entry for wheelchair.
- Sliding doors that open outwards promote ease of ambulation.
- All emergency exits should remain unobstructed.
- Operational devices on doors, such as levers or pull handles, should be easy to grip with one hand.

Showers and Washrooms

The guidelines for showers and washrooms are as follows:
- Showers should have a seat 45–50-cm high, positioned for easy access to the water source
- A grab bar at a height of 85–95 cm, next to the toilet, should be secured around the wall
- The wash basin and its taps should be placed low enough to be reached by someone in a wheelchair.

Environmental Modifications for Elderly

Functional independence in the elderly is dependent upon their capacity to function in their everyday environment. However, the sensory–motor changes associated with aging might compromise the elderly person's independence. While the sensory changes in vision, smell, hearing, and touch may deprive the aged of essential sensory cues, the decline in strength and endurance may negatively impact their adaptive capacities.

Consequently, older persons may misinterpret cues from the environment or may experience sensory deprivation. Therefore individuals may need higher thresholds of stimulation to continue to function in the environment.

Under these circumstances, the physiotherapists' role becomes very crucial toward accurate assessment of physiological changes and environmental interactions thereby suggesting appropriate modifications to assist independence at individual as well as community level. Strong evidence in literature exists to support the role of these in reducing fall risk and improving functional outcomes.

Various environmental factors may act as barriers to independent functioning in the elderly. Most important amongst them are the architectural barriers. Common examples of the same include staircases without bannisters, elevations without provision for slow rising ramps and curbs without appropriately placed cutouts. Addition of the above can easily enhance community ambulatory status of elderly. Following are some of the recommended Environmental Modifications to enhance independence in participation in elderly:

- Avoidance of highly polished floor in public areas
- Slow pedestrian crossing signals
- Installation of stall bars at intersections
- Benches for rest pauses in public places
- The height of curbs/step heights and public transportation medium like bus train height to be restricted (around 150 mm)

Modifying environmental challenges will prove as an effective and efficient strategy to promote independence in ADLs as well as participation. **Table 13.4** shows sensory changes, etiology and suggested modifications in the elderly for the vision.

Hearing loss that occurs with age can cause decreased awareness of environmental signals, poor communication skills and, eventually, social isolation. Age-related hearing loss can occur because of:

- Conductive loss
- Sensorineural loss
- Combination of both.

Sensory changes, etiology and suggested modifications in the elderly for auditory system are shown in **Table 13.5**.

Environmental Modifications at Workplace

Where mainstream technologies have proven to be quite effective into optimization of work performance at workplace, there is an ever expanding range of alternative and specialized technologies designed to address the needs of an employee with an injury or disability.

Assistive devices play an important role in workplace accommodations. Standard seating can be replaced with an alternative design such as a sit–stand stool or saddle seat. Computer access may be easier or more efficient using an ergonomic keyboard and trackball or voice recognition in place of a standard keyboard and mouse. Adaptations to standard technology (e.g., use a wrist support, back cushions on existing seating, padded handles on equipment, or a mount for a telephone handset) to position the equipment can all be utilized to enable employee functioning. In subjects with physical impairments, the use of integrated autocorrect feature in the keyboards is also an important assistive feature to help during typing.

Table 13.4: Sensory changes, etiology, and suggested modifications in elderly (vision).		
Sensory change **Vision**	*Probable causes*	*Suggested modification*
Field	Age-related changes in the structures of the eye and in external ocular structures	Lower height for signages such as traffic and street signs
Acuity	Increased thickness of the lens which affects amount of light allowed to reach the retina, loss of elasticity of the lens, decrease in changes in iris and pupil	Visual aids (glasses, contact lenses), handheld magnifier, large print signs and labels, etc.
Illumination	Age-related decrease in pupillary size, changes in the refractory media, and a reduction in retinal cones and rods, neural changes	UV-absorbing lenses, focused lights, gooseneck lamps, etc.
Glare	Increased opacity of lens, which diffuses light	Lamp shades, curtains to prevent direct glare, nonglare floors, flat paints, matt instead of shiny materials such as glass to prevent indirect glare
Dark adaptations	Smaller pupils that limit the amount of light reaching the periphery of the retina, metabolic changes in the retina. Decreased efficiency of the rods to respond to low levels of light	Night-lights with red bulbs; pocket flashlights, automatic light timers, and light switches at point of entry to a room
Colors and contrasts	Decreased efficiency of the rods to respond to low levels of light	White lettering on black background, warm colors to highlight handrails, steps, and mats that contrast with plates/floor, use of red light stimulates the cones and is suggested to function in dark
Depth perceptions	Related to loss of color discrimination	Avoid patterned floor surfaces

Table 13.5: Sensory changes, etiology, and suggested modifications in elderly (auditory).

Sensory change Auditory	Probable causes	Suggested modification
Conductive hearing loss	Impacted cerumen, perforation of the tympanic membrane, serum/pus in the middle ear, etc.	Hearing aids, pocket amplifiers, speak directly into the individual's ear, to increase the speaker's volume, increasing bass and turning down treble on radios, televisions; smoke alarms, telephones, and doorbells with visual cues such as flashing lights; insulating acoustic materials to minimize background noise
Sensorineural hearing loss (presbycusis)	Dysfunction in conversion of sound waves to electrical signals	Frequency-selective amplification by adjusting the treble and bass to compensate for loss of high frequency, cochlear implants
Taste and smell	Number of taste buds decreases with age	Use of spices, herbs, and flavorings to enhance foods; feel for bulges in canned goods to detect spoilage; check date of stored frozen foods. Smell adapt smoke detectors with loud buzzers; and place flowers in living areas

ASSISTIVE TECHNOLOGY: THE PATH AHEAD

Assistive technology devices promote independent living and provide choices for decision-making across environmental demands and intrinsic barriers.

The fundamental principle behind the success of any rehabilitation program lies in the identification of the most appropriate AT or orthosis or augmentative communication devices, which encourage social integration of the subject as a productive, effective, and appreciated member of the community.

This goal ultimately relies on the capability of the therapist in understanding the finer nuances of the anatomical, biomechanical aspects of the condition along with language and communication skills and sensitivity toward the subjects' individual preferences and desires.

Basic technical know-how utilized in collaborative efforts with engineers, architects, interior designers, etc. will help therapists to carve out creative, out-of-the-box effective solutions to barriers in their subjects' level of functioning.

The field of AT is in nascent stage but fast developing one of rapid change and growth. Newer frontiers of research and technology are being pushed to develop an understanding that persons with disabilities are persons with abilities who need assistance to unmask untapped potentials.

SUMMARY

Assistive technology can be referred to as *a tool/device* used to increase, maintain, or improve the functional capabilities of individuals with disabilities while performing everyday tasks such as getting dressed, moving around, or controlling his or her environment, learning, working, or engaging in recreational activities.

As such, AT has found its application in myriad conditions such as neurological conditions, students with special needs, and at workplace. From low-tech modified reachers to high-tech VR, immersive gaming to robotics,

AT has come a long way to promote independent living and provide options for decision-making across environmental demands and intrinsic barriers. This has brought in the need for physiotherapists to apprise themselves of the recent inventions in the field of AT to be able to provide holistic state-of-the-art management to their patients and clients.

Review Questions

1. Discuss the concept of assistive technology.
2. Discuss the purpose of prescribing AT as per ISO.
3. What are the goals that one aims to achieve with the prescription of AT?
4. Describe the Human Activity Assistive Technology (HAAT) Model in terms of its subsections.
5. What are the most important areas of application of assistive technology?
6. What do mean by Electronic Aids to Daily Living (EADL)? Explain giving suitable examples.
7. Discuss assistive technology in terms of its areas of application, salient features, and types (on the basis of complexity and utility).
8. What is the role of assistive technology for the management of neurological conditions?
9. What role can assistive technology devices play In the life of students with special needs and learners with disabilities?
10. Discuss AAC and its role in improving function in persons with speech impairments.
11. In what all ways, can AT be used for meeting the daily needs of persons with disability?
12. How can assistive technology address problems faced by subjects with mobility impairments?
13. How does assistive technology assist function in terms of ICF?
14. Discuss the common barriers to assistive technology. What actions can be taken to overcome them?
15. Discuss assistive technology in terms of future trends and applications.
16. What are environmental modifications? Discuss their characteristic features and types.

17. Discuss the guidelines for some generic environmental features for improving function.
18. Discuss environmental modifications to improve activity and participation in elderly population.
19. Discuss environmental modifications to improve functioning at workplace.

BIBLIOGRAPHY

1. Anon. (2019). [online] Available from https://www.researchgate.net/publication/327500822_Need_of_Technical_Educational_Integration_in_Disability_Sector_for_Differently-abled_Empowerment.
2. Cifu D, Kaelin D, Kowalske K, et al. Braddom's physical medicine & rehabilitation. 5th edition. Elsevier; 2016.
3. Craig A, Moses P, Tran Y, et al. The effectiveness of a hands-free environmental control system for the profoundly disabled. Arch Phys Med Rehabil. 2002;83(10):1455-8.
4. Frontera W and DeLisa J. Physical medicine and rehabilitation. 4th edition. Philadelphia: Lippincott Williams & Wilkins; 2005.
5. O'Sullivan S, Schmitz T, Fulk G. Physical rehabilitation, 6th edition. Philadelphia, PA: F.A. Davis Company; 2014.
6. Pradhan S, Brewer B, Carvell G, et al. Assessment of fine motor control in individuals with Parkinson's disease using force tracking with a secondary cognitive task. J Neurol Phys Ther. 2010;34(1):32-40.
7. Rigby P, Ryan S, Campbell K. Electronic Aids to Daily Living and quality of life for persons with tetraplegia. Disabil Rehabil: Assist Technol. 2010;6(3):260-7.
8. Un.org. Convention on the Rights of Persons with Disabilities (CRPD). United Nations Enable; 2019. [online] Available from https://www.un.org/development/desa/disabilities/convention-on-the-rights-of-persons-with-disabilities.html.
9. World Health Organization. (2019). International Classification of Functioning, Disability and Health (ICF). [online] Available from https://www.who.int/classifications/icf/en/. [Accessed December 30, 2019].

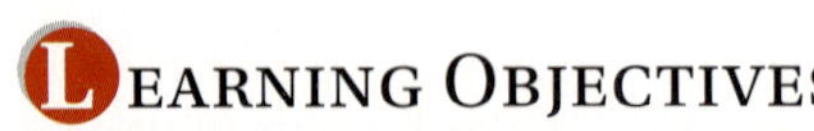

LEARNING OBJECTIVES

After reading this chapter, the readers should be able to:

- Understand the prerequisites for improvement in motor function across various neurological conditions
- Understand the concepts of motor control and motor learning
- Understand the stages and theories of motor learning
- Understand the constraints associated with the process of motor control and learning
- Understand the interventions which aim to improve motor function and motor-learning strategies
- Understand the interventions which aim to improve static and dynamic motor control
- Formulate strategies to improve postural control, balance, agility, coordination, gait with the use of impairment interventions, and compensatory or augmented interventions

CHAPTER OUTLINE

- Prerequisition for improvement in motor function
- Motor control
  - Hierarchical theory of motor control (old theory)
  - Systems theory of motor control (contemporary theory)
- Motor learning
  - Measures
  - Theories
- Stages of motor learning
- Constraints on motor control and learning

- Interventions to improve motor function and motor-learning strategies
- Interventions to improve motor control
  - Improvement in flexibility
  - Improvement of motor performance (strength, power, and endurance)
  - Improvement of muscle endurance and fatigue
- Interventions to improve postural control and balance
  - Interventions to improve reactive balance control
  - Interventions to improve sensory selection and utilization for balance

  - Interventions using augmented feedback
- Interventions to improve coordination and agility
- Interventions to improve gait and locomotion
- Interventions to induce relaxation
- Neurodevelopmental treatment
- Neuromuscular facilitation
- Sensory stimulation techniques
- Biofeedback
- Neuromuscular electrical stimulation
- Compensatory interventions

INTRODUCTION

Training motor function incorporates retraining the motor system with the use of strategies. In order to develop an appropriate strategy, it is important to understand the role of central nervous system (CNS) and how the disease processes may affect the neuronal network. Motor control and motor-learning theories enable to design an intervention which best suits to the impaired motor function along with targeted treatment to the various impairments, activity limitations, and participation restrictions.

PREREQUISITION FOR IMPROVEMENT IN MOTOR FUNCTION

Before one begins working on improvement of function, the following should be understood:

- Thorough understanding of CNS pathologies
- Resulting impairments (primary and secondary) and activity limitations
- Participation restrictions and contextual factors (personal and environmental)
- Clear understanding of neural processes for movement production and learning

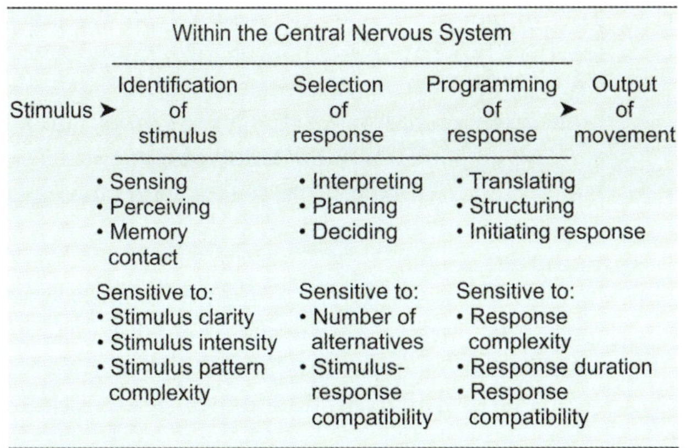

Fig. 14.1: Model of information-processing stages of movement control.

- Knowledge of recovery
- Neural plasticity post–CNS injury.

MOTOR CONTROL

Motor control is an area of study dealing with the understanding of the neural, physical, and behavioral aspects of biological movement **(Fig. 14.1)**.

Hierarchical Theory of Motor Control (Old Theory)

Hierarchical theory views motor control to proceed in only descending direction (top-down) from higher to lower centers, with the cortex dominating on the control.

Systems Theory of Motor Control (Contemporary Theory)

Systems theory describes the process by which various brain and spinal centers work cooperatively to accommodate the demands of intended movements. Systems theory assumes a shifting locus of neural control, referred to as a **distributed model of control**, so large areas of CNS may be engaged for complex motor tasks whereas relatively few centers are engaged for more discrete movements. This type of multilevel control allows for the control of a number of separate independent dimensions of movement, known as **degrees of freedom**.

MOTOR LEARNING

Motor learning is defined as a set of internal processes associated with practice or experience leading to relatively permanent change in the capability for motor skill.

Learning a motor skill is a complex process (e.g., learning to play piano by a subject without CNS injury/ learning to reach for a glass of water or learning to stand up from a chair by a subject with CNS injury) which requires spatial, temporal, and hierarchical organization of CNS.

Measures

1. Changes in CNS can be understood by changes in motor behavior of the task. Improvement in **performance** is used to measure the learning that results from clear understanding of the task and practice it.
2. It is possible to practice enough to temporarily improve performance but not to retain the learning of the task. **Retention** is viewed to be a better measure of learning which is measured by **retention test** [ability of the learner to demonstrate the skill over time and after a period of no practice **(retention interval)**]. Performance after retention interval may decrease slightly but should return to original level within relatively few practice trials called warm-up decrement in performance, e.g., learning to ride a bicycle in adulthood which was learned in childhood.
3. **Adaptability** is defined as the ability to adapt and refine a learned skill to changing task and environmental demands, e.g. subjects who have learned to transfer from wheel chair to mat can apply same learning principles to other types of transfers such as wheelchair to car or wheelchair to tub/subjects who have learned to stand from sitting on therapy stool can apply same learning principles to stand from a chair at home.
4. **Resistance to contextual change** is the adaptability required to perform a motor task in altered environmental situations, e.g., subjects who have learned a skill to walk with a cane on indoor level surface should be able to apply that learning to new and variable situations while walking outdoor or in a mall.

Theories

Adams' Theory of Motor Learning Based on Closed-Loop Control (Closed-Loop Theory)

It was postulated that sensory feedback from ongoing movement is compared with stored memory of the intended movement (perceptual trace) to provide the CNS with a reference of correctness and error detection. The stronger the perceptual trace developed through practice, the greater the capability of the learner to use closed-loop processes for learning movements. This theory helps to explain learning that occurs during slow, linear-positioning responses but failed to explain learning under conditions of rapid movements (open-loop control process) or learning that occurs in the absence of sensory feedback.

Schmidt's Schema Theory

Schema is defined as a rule, concept, or relationship formed on the basis of experience which can be viewed as a generalized motor program (GMP).

Schema allows storage into short-term memory of initial conditions such as body position and weight of object, relationships between movement elements, movement outcomes, and sensory consequences of movement. This information is abstracted into motor memory (procedural memory) that is defined as memory for movement or motor information.

Recall schemas are used to select and define relationship among past parameters, past initial conditions, and past movement outcomes produced by these combinations.

Recognition schemas are used to evaluate movement responses and are based on information of relationships among past initial conditions, past movement outcomes, and the sensory consequences produced by these combinations.

Practice of variety of movement tasks with different contexts and outcomes would improve learning through the development of expanded rules or schema.

STAGES OF MOTOR LEARNING

Stages of motor learning include the following:
1. **Cognitive stage:**
   - In this stage of learning, learner develops overall understanding of the skill **(cognitive map)**.
   - This stage is viewed as **"what to do"** phase of learning which requires high level of cognitive processing to explore the task discarding unsuccessful strategies and retaining successful strategies to execute the task (trial and error).
   - Progression is from the initial disorganized and clumsy pattern of movement to more organized movements so change in performance can be observed readily following intervention.
   - Learner is **dependent on vision** for early learning. **Close environment** without distractors (stable and predictable) facilitate learning in this stage.
2. **Associative stage:**
   - In this stage of learning, **refinement of motor pattern** is achieved through continued practice.
   - This stage is viewed as **"how to do"** phase of learning where there is well-organized speed, timing, accuracy, pattern and coordination of movement, greater consistency, less error, and less extraneous movement following practice.
   - Dependency of vision decreases with **increased reliance of proprioception.**
3. **Autonomous stage:**
   - In this stage of learning, **motor performance becomes largely automatic** following practice which needs minimal attention of the learner. The motor programs are so reined that they can almost **"run themselves."**
   - Movements are highly organized in terms of spatial and temporal aspects of movement, error free with little interference from environmental distractions.
   - The stage is viewed as **"how to succeed"** phase of learning where the learner is targeting the personal goals for the task. Learner is able to perform well in **open environment** (changing, unpredictable environment with distractors).

CONSTRAINTS ON MOTOR CONTROL AND LEARNING

Table 14.1 shows the difference in intact CNS and post CNS injury that may be the reason for the constraints on motor control and learning.

Table 14.1: Difference between intact central nervous system (CNS) and post CNS injury.

Characteristics of intact CNS	Characteristics post CNS injury
- Presence of functionally linked synergies - Presence of reciprocal actions of agonist–antagonists - Executed movements are similar to intended movements - Well-regulated balance and postural control	- **Impaired muscle tone** (hypertonia or hypotonia) spasticity and coactivation of agonist–antagonist muscles resulting in fixed abnormal resting postures with stiff and limited movements - **Hyperactive stretch reflexes** and inadequate recruitment of motor neurons challenges activation of muscle and greatly reduced movements in terms of speed, number and range - **Impaired voluntary movement** (difficulty initiating a movement, difficulty in controlling timing and force, difficulty in controlling speed and direction, disorganization of functionally linked synergies) - **Asynchronization in reciprocal actions** of agonist–antagonist muscles - Highly stereotyped and limited movements (presence of abnormal **obligatory synergies** poststroke) - Impaired activation of muscles needed to maintain the balance resulting in **impaired balance** which demands increased conscious control - Constraints due to **sensory impairments** (reception or perception) - Additional constraints due to **musculoskeletal impairments** (weakness, contracture, postural deformity) - **Impaired cognition** (attention, planning, problem solving, emotional stability) - **Cardiovascular impairment** (limited endurance) - **Fatigue** (mainly due to disease or secondary) - Delayed, disorganized, or absent motor learning - Inaccurate "reference of correctness" due to failed or inaccurate feedback

INTERVENTIONS TO IMPROVE MOTOR FUNCTION AND MOTOR-LEARNING STRATEGIES

One needs to determine patient's strengths and limitations and develop collaborative functional goal with plan of care **(Fig. 14.2 and Tables 14.2–14.4).**

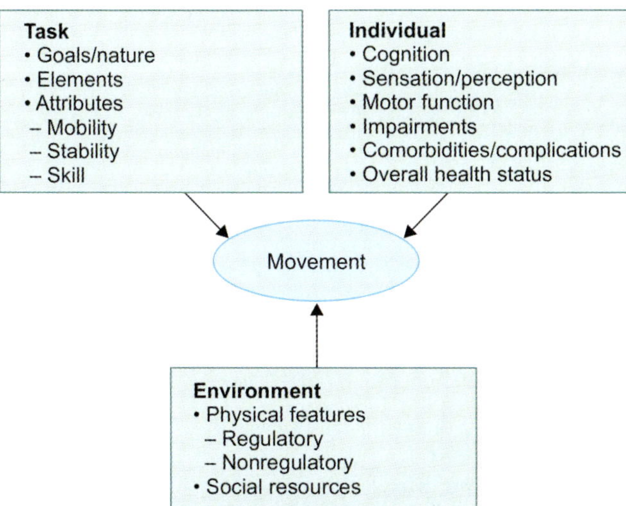

Fig. 14.2: Interaction between the task, the individual, and the environment.

Table 14.2: Interventions to improve motor function and functional independence.

Therapeutic outcome: Improved motor function and functional independence	
Restorative Interventions	
Functional Training	**Motor-learning Strategies**
Task-specific training:	Development of strategy
• Functional mobility skills	Feedback
• Activities of daily living	Practice
Environmental context	Transference
Behavioral shaping	Active decision-making
Safety-awareness training	
Impairment-Specific and Augmented Interventions	
Impairment Interventions	**Augmented Interventions**
Muscle strength, power, endurance	Neurodevelopmental treatment
Flexibility	Neuromuscular facilitation
Balance and Postural control	Sensory stimulation
Coordination and agility	Biofeedback
Locomotion and gait	Neuromuscular electrical stimulation
Aerobic capacity/endurance	
Relaxation	
Compensatory Interventions	
Substitution training	Assistive/supportive devices

Table 14.3: Types of augmented feedback.

Concurrent feedback	Feedback is presented during the movement, KP information is provided, e.g., information regarding joint position; importance of forward weight shift to move the COM over the BOS during sit-to-stand training; or biofeedback; best used for highlighting information that is not readily available from intrinsic feedback and if it is linked to active problem-solving
Terminal feedback	Feedback that is following the movement
Immediate feedback	Feedback is given immediately after the movement is completed
Delayed feedback	• Feedback that is provided after a brief time. The delay allows the learner some time for introspection and self-assessment, e.g., a delay of 5-second • Feedback given after prolonged delays is avoided, especially if some other movements that are not related to the task occurring in between. This leads to degrading of the learning
Summary feedback	Feedback presented after a set number of trials, e.g., after every 4th trial or every 6th or every 10th trial
Faded feedback	Feedback is given first following each trial, then less frequently after blocks of trials, e.g., after the 1st trial progressing to every 5th trial, then to every 7th trial
Bandwidth - KR feedback	Feedback given only when performance moves out of the boundaries of correct performance; error range allowed is predetermined (e.g., top and bottom range of errors is determined)
Blocked feedback	• One source of feedback is given; KS is presented about the same segment on consecutive trials, then the learner processes a limited information regarding the task, e.g., during gait training. KR is presented about knee segment only on successive trials • Blocked KR improves performance of the identified segment but may not lead to improvement in performance and learning of the whole task (multiple segments); performance deteriorates once KR is withdrawn
Variable (random) feedback	• Feedback is provided from multiple sources; KR about different segments is presented on successive trials; e.g., during gait training, KR about various body segments (trunk, hips, knees) is presented on subsequent trials • Random KR is better in improving both performance and learning of a task. It encourages the learner to process a wider range of information regarding the task

Table 14.4: Types of practice and practice parameters.

Types of Practice	
Massed practice	It is a sequence of practice with rest times in which the rest time is lesser than the time for which practice is done
Distributed practice	Practice and interval is spaced such that the practice lime is equal to or less than the rest time
Practice Sequence	
Blocked practice	A practice sequence that is organized around one task performed over and over again, and uninterrupted by practice of any other task
Random practice	A practice series in which variety of tasks are in an order being random across trials
Practice Order	
Blocked order	The repeated practice of a task or group of tasks is done in order; three trials of task 1, three trials of task 2., followed by three trials of task 3 (e.g., 111222333)
Serial order	A predictable and repeating order; where practice of multiple tasks is done in the following order (e.g., 123123123)
Random order	An order of multiple tasks that is non-repetitive and non-predictable (e.g., 123321311)
Practice Strategies	
Mental practice	A practice strategy in which performance of the motor task is imagined or visualized without overt physical practice
Part/whole practice	The whole task is broken into component parts which are practiced, before the whole task is practiced
Transfer training	The task performance is better as a result of experience or practice with some other task • Motor skills are acquired in one training experience that enhances acquisition of similar or related skills (positive learning) • Motor skills are acquired in one training experience that interferes acquisition of other skills (negative learning)
Practice of lead-up activities	The complex tasks are practiced as a combination of versions of simple tasks

INTERVENTIONS TO IMPROVE MOTOR CONTROL

Interventions that help to improve motor control can be targeted to:

Improvement in Flexibility

- Prolonged periods of disuse and immobility along with motor dysfunction following neurological injury will lead to muscle tightness, contracture, atrophy, joint stiffness, and postural deformity (secondary impairments).

- Need of proactive intervention in stroke, traumatic brain injury, spinal cord injury
- Targeted intervention in chronic and irreversible diseases, e.g., Parkinson disease, multiple sclerosis, amyotrophic lateral sclerosis to limit sequelae and degree of disability.

Benefits

- Maintain joint flexibility
- Maintain tissue extensibility
- Maintain physical ability and function
- Improve circulation and tissue nutrition to limb
- Pain inhibition

Therapeutic Approaches

- **Range of motion (ROM) exercises** (AROM, AAROM, PROM, ROM exercises in proprioceptive neuromuscular facilitation (PNF) patterns, ROM in functional training activities)
    - Caution—excessive force is contraindicated in patients at risk of osteoporosis and heterotopic ossifications.
- **Passive stretching:**
    - The end position (greatest tolerated length) is held for at least 20–30 seconds and stretch is repeated 4–5 times depending on patient's tolerance.
    - Slow prolonged muscle stretch at maximal end range → minimize muscle spindle activation and reflex contraction → firing of Golgi tendon organ (GTO) → inhibition of stretched muscle using the mechanism of autogenic inhibition.
- **Joint mobilization:**
    - **Therapeutic heat modality** (hot pack if no sensory impairment) premotor control exercises, warm-up period of exercises, e.g., calisthenics or low-resistance cycling, cold modalities to cool muscles and decrease muscle spasm and physiological splinting.
    - **Low load prolonged stretch** (15–30 minutes) using mechanical pulleys and weights or specialized orthotic devices, prolonged position on tilt table can be used for stretching.
- **Facilitated stretching:**
    - Use of neuromuscular inhibition techniques (hold-relax and contract relax) to inhibit and elongate muscles (superior to static stretching when active contractions are used)
    - Not effective with very weak or paralyzed muscles or chronic contractures.

Stretching and positioning for patient with spasticity:

- Use constant, firm manual contact over bony or nonspastic area.
- Avoid direct pressure on spastic muscles.
- Slow, repeated rotations of limb to gain elongation of shortened spastic muscles.
- Position the limb in newly gained range to provide prolonged stretching (optimal timing 10 minutes).

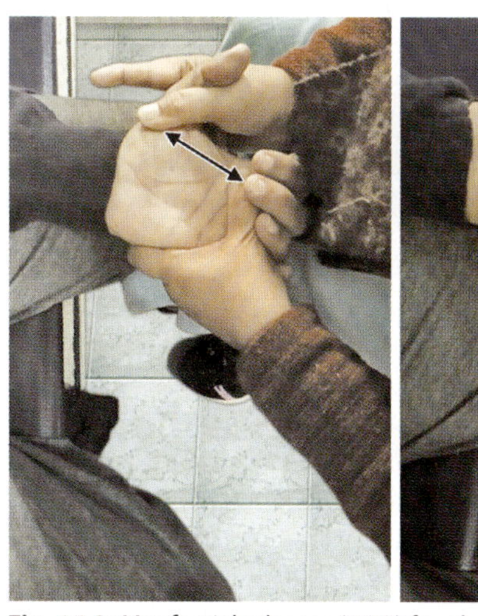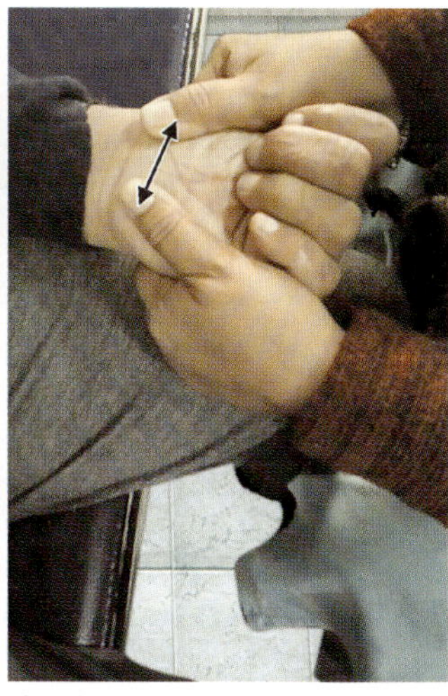

Fig. 14.3: Myofascial releases (MFR) for elongating the first web space in a hemiplegic patient (*Note:* Arrows indicate the direction of force applied at facial level of touch).

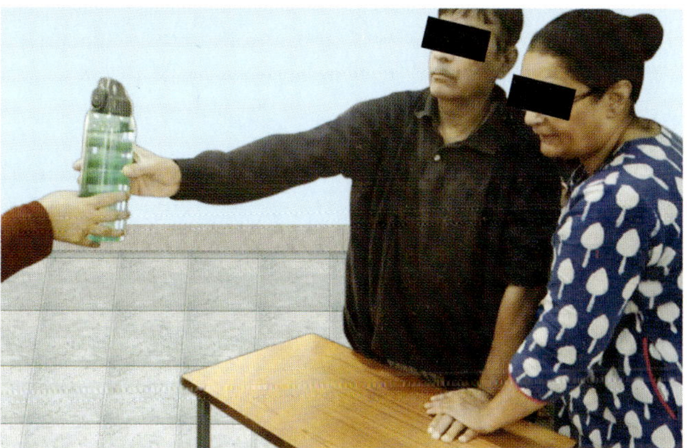

Fig. 14.4: Strategy to improve the flexibility of shortened structures of upper extremity in modified plantigrade position.

Figure 14.3 shows technique of myofascial release for elongating first web space. **Figure 14.4** shows strategies to improve flexibility in modified plantigrade position.

- Serial casts—serial application (7–10 days) of cast material for 1–6 weeks duration
- Adjustable orthosis

ROM for patients with hypotonia:

- Hypotonia (low tone) with weak or paralyzed muscles, joint instability, and deformity are reflected in patients with lower motor neuron (LMN) syndrome.
- Care should be taken of end-range joint instability and risk of hyperextension injury while giving PROM exercise in subjects with hypotonia. Use supportive and protective devices to prevent injury and postural asymmetry during functional training.

Improvement of Motor Performance (Strength, Power, and Endurance)

- Motor performance is the capacity of a muscle or group of muscles to generate forces.
- Neural factors influencing muscle performance are motor unit recruitment (number, type), motor neuron firing patterns, and efficiency of cooperative synergistic patterns.
- Biomechanical factors influencing muscle performance are initial muscle length and tension, muscle fiber composition, fuel storage and delivery, speed and type of contraction, and movement arm.
- Patients undergoing neurorehabilitation are commonly having disruption of motor neurons from central pathways and reduction in muscle force production. (This is a primary impairment)
- Prolonged periods of disuse and immobility result in decreased neural activity, atrophy, and weakness. (This is a secondary impairment)

Therapeutic Approaches

- PNF (functionally based synergistic movement in diagonal plane)
- Bobath approach
- Aquatic exercises
- Strength training progressive resisted exercises (PRE) (current research has shown that it is possible to increase strength without additional detrimental effects on tone and movement control) (**Table 14.5**)
- Task-specific training

Improvement of Muscle Endurance and Fatigue

- Fatigue is defined as the inability to contract a muscle repeatedly over time (decrement in force production). So, the exercise cannot be sustained and exercise tolerance is reduced.
- Following are the various sites of fatigue in neuromuscular disease such as multiple sclerosis, Guillian–Barre syndrome, postpolio syndrome, chronic fatigue syndrome:
  - The CNS (central fatigue)
  - The peripheral nerves or neuromuscular junction
  - The muscle itself

There is a risk of acute exercise overdose producing exhaustion and possibly injury.

Fatigue management can be done by the following techniques:

- Energy conservation techniques
- Activity pacing
- Lifestyle modifications
- Regular rest periods during the day
- Improved sleep using relaxation techniques and medications
- Use of activity logs
- Ergonomic changes
- Stress management

The patient should be trained to self-monitor fatigue using Borg rating of perceived exertion (RPE) and instructed to keep their activities at an RPE level of "somewhat hard" (14 or lower using the 6–20 RPE scale).

Table 14.5: Exercise guidelines for strength training.

Determinants	Parameters of exercise
Type of muscle contraction	Isometric, eccentric, concentric exercise
Mode of exercise training	• Open chain (isolating one segment): isotonic and isokinetic exercises • Closed chain: kinetic chain weight-bearing exercises (e.g., step-ups, modified squats) • Circuit training: combination of varied methods • Aquatic exercise • Synergistic patterns may be more efficient for improved function (based on specificity principle), e.g., PNF patterns with manual resistance
Type of resistance/equipment	Free weights, pulleys, elastic bands, mechanical resistance machine, isokinetic resistance (dynamometry), manual resistance, body weight, water resistance (aquatics)
Intensity: Exercise load that best challenges the pattern (based on overload principle)	Use submaximal loads • With weighs, load is typically 60–80% 1-RM with a goal • Very weak individuals can start at 50% 1-RM and less than 10 repetitions • Exercise progression: increase repetitions, number of sets, or load as tolerated; adjust the exercise load on the basis of exercise responses, strength measures, perceived exertion, and fatigue threshold
Number of repetitions and sets, number of exercises per set	Initial frequency is typically 3 sets of 10–15 repetitions or as tolerated
Duration	Total time of resistance training: typically 15–30 minutes per session or as tolerated
Frequency	Typically 2–3 days/week, depending on intensity and level of impairment disease
Warm-up and cool-down periods	Include 5–10 minutes of warm-ups (calisthenics, stretching, ROM exercises) and 5–10 minutes of cool-down (muscle relaxation, stretching)
Additional considerations	• Movements should be slow and controlled • Progression should occur in small increments • Intensity should be reduced with sudden onset of fatigue and exhaustion • Intensity should be reduced with prolonged and severe delayed onset muscle soreness • Maintenance of regular breathing pattern, while avoiding straining/Valsalva • The interactions of exercise and medications should be considered • Exercise is contraindicated in some patients (e.g., with severe atrophic polio and recent weakness or ALS with muscle grades <3/5)
Outcomes	• Strength training should be related to functional tasks • Focus the patient on improvements in functional performance in terms that are understandable and meaningful

(ALS: amyotrophic lateral sclerosis; PNF: proprioceptive neuromuscular facilitation; RM: repetition maximum)

Therapeutic Approaches

- Simple overground walking program
- Treadmill training **(Fig. 14.5)**
- Ergometry (two-limb, four limb)
- Recumbent stepper
- Therapeutic aquatics

Intensity: Moderate (40–70% of maximal oxygen consumption)

Contraindication: High-intensity aerobic exercises

Frequency: 3–5 days/week with 20–30-minute sessions/alternatively, multiple 10-minute sessions.

INTERVENTIONS TO IMPROVE POSTURAL CONTROL AND BALANCE

Interventions that help improve postural control and balance are:

- **Postural control** is the ability to control the body's position in space for stability and orientation.

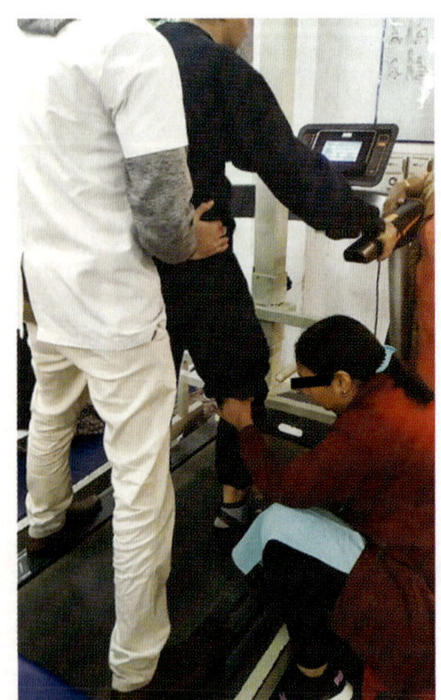

Fig. 14.5: Treadmill training in a patient with spastic quadriparesis following traumatic brain injury.

- **Postural orientation** is the ability to maintain normal alignment relationships between various body segments and between body and environment.
- **Static postural control (stability)** is the ability to maintain stability and orientation with center of mass (COM) over base of support (BOS) with body at rest.
- **Dynamic postural control (controlled mobility)** is the ability to maintain stability and orientation with COM over BOS while parts of body are in motion.
- **Factors contributing to impaired postural control:**
  - Tonal imbalances (hypotonia, hypertonia, dystonia)
  - Weakness
  - Impaired voluntary control
  - Hypermobility (ataxia, athetosis)
  - Impaired reciprocal actions of antagonists (cerebellar dysfunction)
  - Impaired proximal stabilization
  - Sensory hypersensitivity (tactile-avoidance reactions)
  - ROM restrictions
  - Increased anxiety or arousal (high sympathetic "fight-or-flight" state)
- **Characteristics of postural instability:**
  - Excessive postural sway
  - Wide BOS
  - Low- or high-guard position
  - Difficulty moving the limbs while maintaining posture
  - Holding onto an object in the environment
  - Loss of balance/fall
- **Techniques to improve static postural control:**
  - Quick stretch
  - Tapping
  - Resistance
  - Approximation
  - Manual contact
  - Rhythmic stabilization technique of PNF **(Fig. 14.6A)**
  - Demand more active and challenging postures **(Fig. 14.6B)**
  - Use of elastic resistance bands or aquatic loading (proprioceptive loading)
  - Stabilize static posture on moveable surface
  - Training for ankle strategy—small range, slow velocity shifts progressing to holding steady
  - Training for hip strategy—larger shifts in COM approaching LOS and/or faster body sway motions characterized by early activation of proximal hip and trunk muscles (AP displacement → activation of hip flexors and extensors; lateral displacement → hip abductors: standing with feet together, tandem standing, single-limb stance).
  - For patients with hyperkinetic disorders such as ataxia and athetosis—alternate isotonic contractions can be used allowing only very small range movements progressing to deceasing range, use aquatic therapy.

- Steady state, anticipatory (self-initiated), and reactive (external perturbation) balance control need to be practiced using activities focusing on static and dynamic postural control.
- **Techniques to improve dynamic postural control:**
  - PNF extremity patterns on static posture, e.g., chop/reverse chop pattern
  - Use of dynamic therapy tools (therapy ball, wobble board, balance mat)—limb movement on dynamic surface unilateral → bilateral → reciprocal **(Fig. 14.7)**
  - Use of resistance (elastic bands, weighted ball or weight cuffs) on ankles or wrists
  - Dual task training (catching and throwing a ball, batting a balloon or kicking a ball)
  - Cognitive task while doing motor task (spelling forward or backward, remembering a list, counting backward by 3s)
  - Training for stepping strategy—perturbations evoking COM displacements, variety of voluntary stepping movements, e.g., marching in place; anterior, posterior, lateral, or crossed side steps

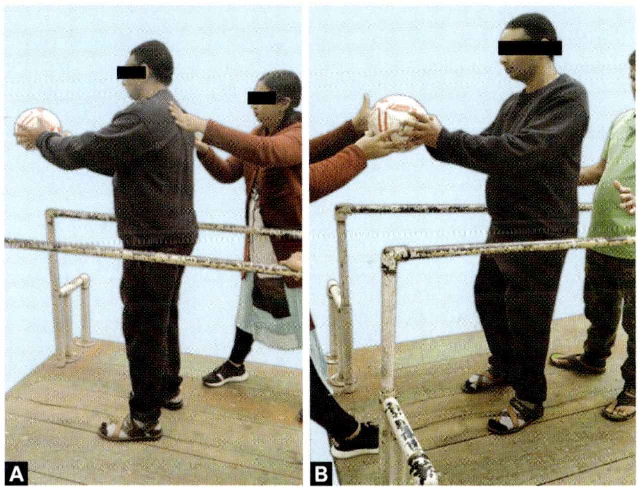

Figs. 14.6A and B: Strategies to improve static postural control in standing.

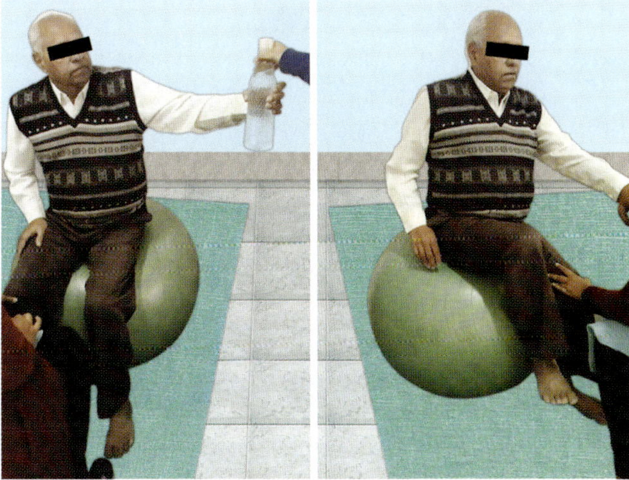

Fig. 14.7: Strategies to improve postural control on dynamic surface in sitting.

progressing from small to large step; tandem stepping to crossed stepping; elastic resistance band around pelvic to improve the strength of stepping responses.

Interventions to Improve Reactive Balance Control

Interventions that help to improve reactive balance control are:
- Use gentle manual pulls or pushes to shoulders or hips
- Use moving platforms to provide perturbations
- Tai Chi training

Interventions to Improve Sensory Selection and Utilization for Balance

Following are the tips to help in sensory selection and utilization for balance:
- Somatosensory inputs (proprioceptive and tactile)—challenged by changing the support surface (flat surfaces, e.g., floor to compliant surfaces such as low-to-high carpet pile to dense foam) **(Fig. 14.8)**.
- Visual inputs—challenged by closing the eyes or blindfolding; reduced visual cues (low light); inaccurate vision (petroleum-coated lenses in a pair of eyeglasses, flickering lights).
- Vestibular inputs—challenged by reducing both visual and somatosensory inputs through sensory conflict situations.
- Practicing the task in variable environments—challenged by walking on smooth terrain to uneven terrain to moving surfaces such as escalator or elevator.
- Patient with significant sensory loss will require assistance in shifting toward the intact systems to monitor and adjust balance using compensatory training strategies (use of assistive devices).
  For example,
  - Patients with diabetic neuropathy → LE proprioceptive loss → train visual system.

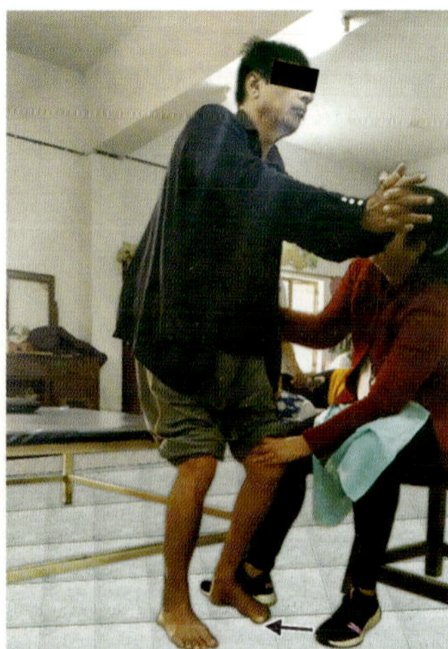

Fig. 14.8: Strategy to load paretic lower extremity by sit to stand with altered foot position.

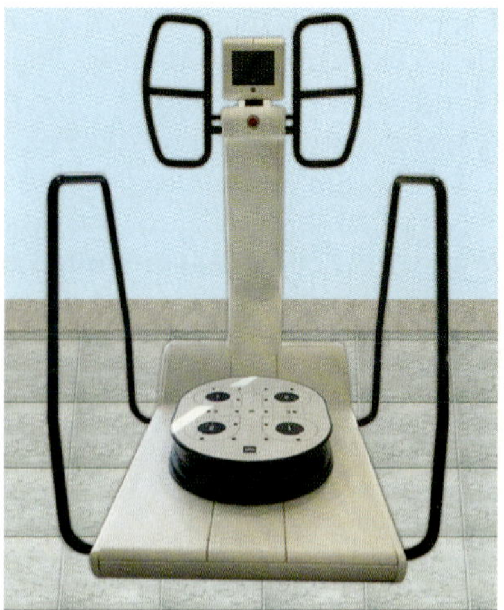

Fig. 14.9: Advanced balance training can be done using modern technologies.

- Patients with low vision → balance training with eyeglasses.

Interventions Using Augmented Feedback

Augmented feedback training can be given using biofeedback cane with auditory signals, limb load monitor, posturography **(Fig. 14.9)**, although symmetrical weight bearing can be gained by balance retraining using posturography, generalization of balance training to functional skills needs specific task-oriented training.

- **Strategies to improve safety and reduce fall risk:**
  - Patient education and lifestyle counseling regarding fall provoking activities
  - Avoid sedentary lifestyle and encourage active lifestyle incorporating regular exercises and walking
  - Review of medicines in consultation with physician
  - Education regarding compensatory training strategies in likelihood of fall—leaning forward to widen BOS, crouching down to lower COM, or proper shoes to increase friction
  - Use of assistive devices.
- **General tips for balance training:**
  - Selection of position required for activities of daily living (ADL)/work/participation/recreation
  - Assurance for safety (use of aids, e.g., human assistance/supervision, gait belt, or overhead harness) **(Fig. 14.10)** and building patient confidence
  - Postural re-education (tactile/verbal/visual cues)
  - Sensory selection and organization
  - Kinesthetic awareness of "True Vertical"
  - Manipulation of COM–BOS ($\uparrow$COM, $\downarrow$BOS)
  - Progress from closed environment to open (more variable) environment to real-life setting of home or community for better functional carryover
  - Repetition and practice

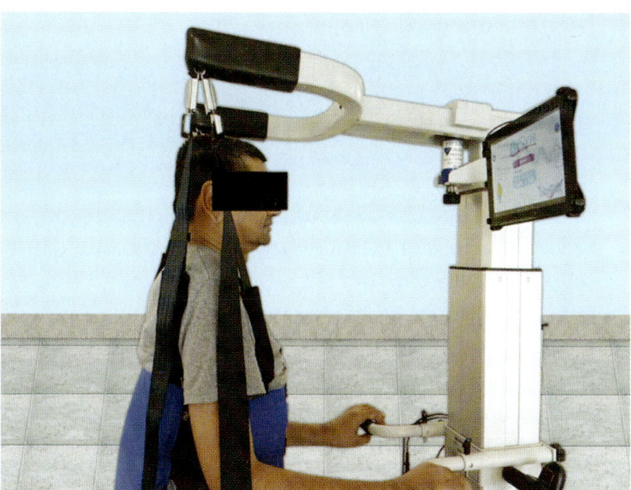

Fig. 14.10: Use of overhead harness for the safety of the patient.
Courtesy: Mission Health, Ahmedabad

INTERVENTIONS TO IMPROVE CO-ORDINATION AND AGILITY

- **Co-ordination** is the ability to execute smooth, accurate, and controlled movements.
- **Agility** is the ability to perform coordinated movements combined with upright standing balance.
- Ataxia is defined as uncoordinated movement that manifests when voluntary movements are attempted which influences gait, posture, and patterns of movement.

Causes

Cerebellar disease or lesions (e.g., cerebellar atrophy, tumor, multiple sclerosis, traumatic brain injury, stroke, hereditary ataxias, chronic alcoholism).

Characteristics

- Hypotonia (related to disruption of afferent input from stretch receptors and/or lack of CB's facilitatory efferent influence on fusimotor system)
- Generalized weakness (asthenia)
- Hypermobility
- Impaired synergistic actions with movement decomposition so movement is performed in a sequence of component parts rather than as a single, smooth activity (dyssynergia)
- Impaired ability to judge the distance or range of movement (dysmetria)
- Impaired ability to perform rapid alternating movements (dysdiadochokinesia)
- Intentional tremor (involuntary oscillatory movement resulting from alternate contractions of opposing muscle groups)
- Impaired posture (excessive lumbar lordosis, anterior pelvic tilt, hip flexion, knees hyperextension, more weight bearing on heels)
- Postural instability (excessive postural sway, wide BOS, high-guard position, handhold, frequent loss of balance)

- Impaired gait pattern (ataxic gait—broad BOS, poor upright stance stability), arms held away from the body to improve balance (high guard position), irregular stepping patterns in distance and direction
- Impaired motor learning (inability of cerebellum to timely and correctly utilize feedback to modulate movement)
- Nystagmus—rhythmic, quick, oscillatory, back-and-forth movement of eyes
- Titubation—rhythmic oscillations of head
- Dysarthria [scanning speech—one-word-at-a-time quality (slow, slurred, hesitant, prolonged syllables, inappropriate pauses; word use, selection and grammar intact but melodic quality of speech is altered)].

Techniques

- Use of light resistance, e.g., weight cuffs, elastic bands, weighted trunk vest, weighted walkers and canes, and water resistance (slow the limb and trunk movement, reduce dysmetria and tremors)
- PNF resistive technique of rhythmic stabilization, dynamic reversals, or dynamic-reversal-hold
- Augmented feedback (biofeedback, rhythmic auditory stimulation using metronome or music)
- Devices promoting reciprocal movements and timing (cycle ergometer, motorized treadmill with overhead harness).

INTERVENTIONS TO IMPROVE GAIT AND LOCOMOTION

Gait training and locomotion have been described in Chapter 11: Mobility Aids and Orthosis and Chapter 13: Assistive Technology and Environment Modification along with management of various conditions.

INTERVENTIONS TO INDUCE RELAXATION

Stress results from various factors such as:
- Loss of motor control which was previously present
- Pain
- Inability to execute functional tasks which were previously performed with ease
- Loss of control in life decisions
- Becoming passive

Sympathetic nervous system responses (fight or flight) are typically heightened. Therapies promoting engagement of parasympathetic responses along with an increase in alpha brain waves can thus be used.

NEURODEVELOPMENTAL TREATMENT

Neurodevelopmental treatment can be described as follows:
- Developed by Dr Karel (physician) and Berta Bobath (physiotherapist) in the late 1940–1960.
- Abnormal muscle tone, abnormal postural reflexes were identified as key problems in patients with CNS injury.

- Primary focus on specialized handling for inhibition of spastic muscle and abnormal reflex pattern and promotion of normal movements based on the hierarchical theory with top-down control (largely refuted by more recent studies on nervous system).
- Current neurodevelopmental treatment is based on newer theories of motor control (systems theory and distributed model of CNS control).
- Impaired tone and coordination, weakness, and limited ROM are found to be contributing factors for loss of motor control.
- Postural control is considered to be foundation for all skill learning and is challenged progressively.
- Handling techniques and key point of control (e.g., shoulder, pelvis, hands, feet) directed at supporting body segments and moving to more active control to functional use.
- Use of sensory stimulation (facilitation and inhibition via primarily proprioceptive and tactile inputs).
- Facilitation of postural alignment and stability and excessive tone and abnormal movements inhibited.

NEUROMUSCULAR FACILITATION

It refers to facilitation, activation, or inhibition of muscle contraction and motor responses **(Table 14.6)**.

- Facilitation is an enhanced capacity to initiate a movement response through increased neuronal activity and altered synaptic potential. An applied stimulus may lower the synaptic threshold of alpha motor neuron but may not be sufficient to produce an observable movement response.
- Activation refers to the actual production of movement response and implies reaching a critical threshold level for neuronal firing.
- Inhibition refers to the decreased capacity to initiate a movement response through altered synaptic potential. Increased synaptic threshold makes it more difficult for neuron to fire and produce movement.
- Combination of spinal and supraspinal inputs acting on alpha motor neuron will determine whether a muscle response is facilitated, activated or inhibited.
- Resistance, quick stretch, tapping/repeated quick stretch, prolonged stretch, joint approximation, and joint traction are examples of various neuromuscular facilitation techniques **(Fig. 14.11)**.

General guidelines for facilitative techniques:

- Additive—application of several inputs simultaneously, e.g., quick stretch, resistance and verbal cues (combined application has better motor response than single stimulation—property of spatial summation within CNS).

Table 14.6: Neuromuscular facilitation techniques.

Stimulus	*Response*	*Comments*
Resistance: Applied manually, using body position/gravity, or mechanically	Facilitates both intrafusal and extrafusal muscle contraction; hypertrophies extrafusal muscle fibers; enhances kinesthetic awareness (muscle spindle)	• With very weak muscle, use light resistance; isometric and eccentric contractions before concentric. Maximal resistance can produce overflow from strong to weak muscles within the same synergistic pattern or to contralateral extremities
Quick stretch to agonist	Facilitates both intrafusal and extrafusal agonist muscle contraction (stretch reflex)	• Optimally applied in the lengthened range • A low-threshold response, relatively short-lived: can add resistance to maintain contraction
Tapping/repeated quick stretch over tendon or muscle belly	Facilitates both intrafusal and extrafusal agonist muscle contraction (stretch reflex)	• Tapping over muscle belly produces a weaker response than over the tendon. Tapping over a muscle is used to enhance holding in a weight-bearing position
Prolonged stretch: Slow, maintained stretch, applied at maximum available lengthened range	Inhibits or dampens muscle contraction and tone due to peripheral reflex effects (stretch-protection reflex)	• Positioning; inhibitory splinting, casting; mechanical low-load weights using traction
Joint approximation: Compression of joint surfaces, using manual pressure or position/gravity: weighted vest or belt	Facilitates postural extensors and stabilizing responses (cocontraction); enhances joint awareness (joint receptors)	• Approximation applied to top of shoulders or pelvis in upright weight-bearing positions facilities postural extensors and stability (e.g., sitting, kneeling, or standing) • Used in PNF extensor extremity patterns, pushing actions
Joint traction: Manual distraction of joints; wrist and ankle cuffs	Facilitates joint motion, enhances joint awareness (joint receptors)	• Joint mobilization uses slow, sustained traction to improve mobility, relieve muscle spasm, and reduce pain • Used in PNF flexor extremity patterns, pulling actions

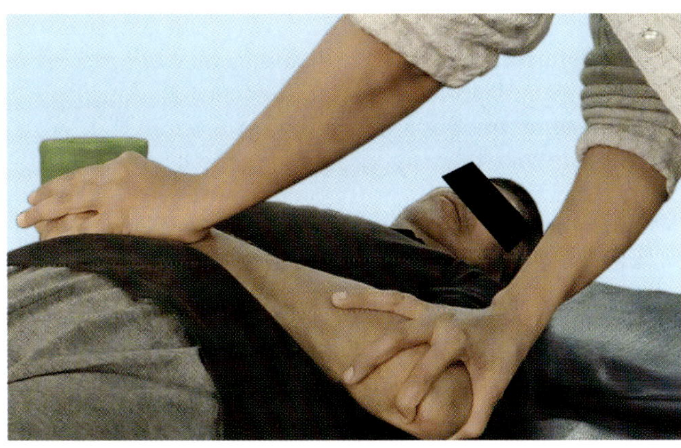

Fig. 14.11: Proprioceptive neuromuscular facilitation technique for upper extremity.

- Repeated stimulation—better motor response following temporal summation within CNS.
- Fast adapting, phasic receptors (touch) and phasic Ia muscle spindle endings → effective in initiating and shaping dynamic movements.

- Slow adapting tonic receptors (joint receptors, GTOs) and static II muscle spindle endings → effective in monitoring and regulating postural responses.
  - Factors affecting patient response: level of intactness of CNS, arousal, specific level of activity of motor neurons.
  - Stimulation is contraindicated for patients with hyperactivity and high arousal (use inhibition/ relaxation techniques).
  - Facilitation techniques are not appropriate for patients who have adequate voluntary control.

SENSORY STIMULATION TECHNIQUES

Following are the techniques for sensory stimulation:
- Sensory stimulation refers to the structured presentation of stimuli to improve attention and arousal levels and enhance sensory selection and discrimination **(Table 14.7)**
- Optimal stimulation for desired response
- Sensory receptors adapt overtime

Table 14.7: Sensory stimulation techniques.

Stimulus	Response	Comments
Maintained pressure: Firm manual pressure to midline back abdomen; mechanical pressure via cones, pads	Calming effect, generalized inhibition, decreased fight or flight responses; desensitizes skin	• Useful with patients with agitation and high arousal (e.g., the patient with TBI) • Can be combined with other relaxation techniques (deep breathing, imagery, quiet environment) • Also useful for patients with hypersensitivity (e.g., the patient with tactile defensiveness)
Slow, repetitive stroking: Applied to midline back	Calming effect, generalized inhibition, decreased fight or flight responses	• Performed while patient is prone or in supported sitting (head and arms resting on table top) • Can use massage lubricant; stroke on either side of the spine; applied for 3–5 minutes • May be contraindicated with very hairy surface
Light touch: Brisk, stroking	Facilitates muscle can elicit protection/flexor withdrawal response	• Low threshold response, accommodates rapidly • Can be used to initially mobilize patients with low response levels (e.g., the patient with TBI who is minimally responsive)
Neutral warmth: Retention of body heat through body wraps (Ace wraps, towel wraps, snug-fining clothing gloves, socks, tights); air splints, tepid bath	Calming effect, generalized inhibition, decreased fight or flight responses	• Useful for patients with high arousal or increased sympathetic activity • Overheating should be avoided, may produce rebound effects
Prolonged cooling: Immersion in cold water; ice wraps, ice massage; coding suit	• Decreases neural and muscle spindle firing • Provides inhibition of muscles and painful muscle spasm • Decreases metabolic rate of tissues	• Monitor effects carefully can produce sympathetic arousal, withdrawal or fight-or-flght responses • Contraindicated in patients with sensory deficits, generalized arousal, autonomic instability, and vascular problems
Slow vestibular stimulation: Constant, repetitive rocking manually assisted in side lying or sitting; mechanical (rocking chair): therapy ball: hammock	Calming effect, generalized inhibition, decreased fight or flight responses	Useful with patients who are hypertonic, hyperactive, or who demonstrate high arousal or tactile defensiveness (e.g., the patient with TBI who is agitated)
Rapid vestibular stimulation: Rapid movements, fast spinning in a chair, mesh net	Heightens postural responses, movements	Useful for patients with hypotonia (e.g., an individual with Down syndrome); patients with sensory integrative dysfunction (e.g., a child with hyperactivity); patients with bradykinesia (e.g., a patient with PD) can activate sympathetic arousal responses

Approaches:
- Sensory re-education
- Tactile kinesthetic guiding
- Repetitive sensory practice
- Desensitization

BIOFEEDBACK

Biofeedback can be described as:
- Electromyographic biofeedback (EMG-BFB) can be used to assist the patient with severe motor weakness (muscle grades trace, poor or fair or deficient sensory feedback systems) to regain neuromuscular control.
- BFB is also indicated to increase the contraction of a muscle, train voluntary inhibition, or muscle spasm and decrease muscle guarding.
- Cochrane Database of Systematic Review on effects of EMG-BFB for motor function recovery following stroke found evidence from a small number of individual studies to suggest that EMG-BFB along with standard physiotherapy produced improvements in motor power, functional recovery, and gait quality when compared to standard physiotherapy alone.

NEUROMUSCULAR ELECTRICAL STIMULATION

Neuromuscular electrical stimulation (NMES) can be described as follows:
- Neuromuscular electrical stimulation is used to stimulate contraction in very weak muscles to improve motor function with electrodes placed directly over the muscle to be stimulated.
- Contraction is elicited by depolarizing motor neurons with larger motor units and greater number of type II fibers firing first.
- Uses—to re-educate muscle, improve ROM, decrease edema, treat disuse atrophy, reduce spasticity with stimulation of weak antagonist, reduce flexor tone and posturing of hand and improve functional grasp in patients with stroke, reduce shoulder subluxation.

- In functional electrical stimulation (FES) **(Figs. 14.12A and B)**, microprocessor is used to recruit muscles in a programed synergistic sequence for the purpose of improving functional movements.
- In poststroke hemiparesis, peroneal nerve stimulation using FES is found to be effective in assisting dorsiflexion (drop foot) and improving walking.
- FES can be combined with body-weight support and treadmill.
- Patients with incomplete SCI have been stimulated to exercise on bicycle ergometers (FES ergometry) and walk.

COMPENSATORY INTERVENTIONS

Compensatory interventions can be described as follows:
- Compensatory training strategies permit the patient to perform a specific task using alternate limbs and/or alternate movement patterns so that he is able to perform an old task in a new manner.
- For example, patient with hemiplegia dresses using less affected upper limb and trunk movements; functional rolling or transfers done by paraplegic patient with a lot of intact muscles and tricks; or wheelchair locomotion using upper limbs.
- Adaptive compensation is a result of alternative or new movement patterns.
- Substitutive compensation is the result of using different parts of the body, effectors, to accomplish the task.
  - **Steps:** Cognitive awareness of movement deficiency; suggestion, simplification, and adoption of a new way to accomplish the functional task; practice and relearning of old task with a new pattern; practice of the functional task in real-life setting; energy conservation techniques.
  - **Criticism:** Focus on less-involved segments suppressing recovery of patients and contribution to learned nonuse of impaired segments, so need not be used in patients with potential

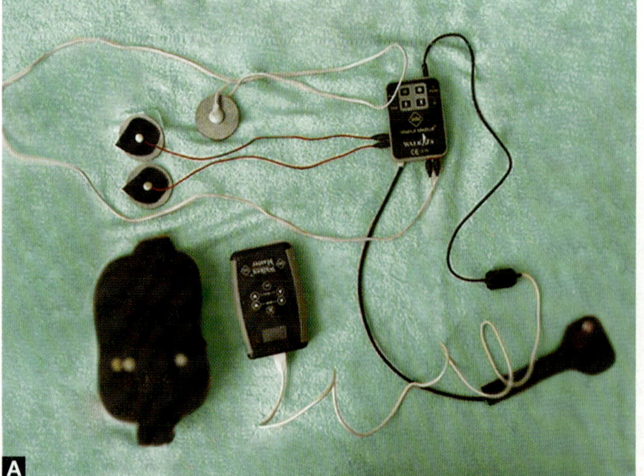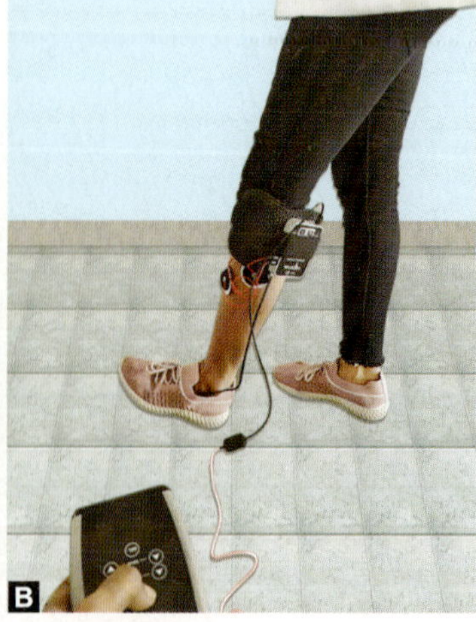

Figs. 14.12A and B: (A) Functional electrical stimulation apparatus; (B) Use of functional electrical stimulation for facilitation of walking.
Courtesy: Viral Shah (PT). Lakshya Neuro Rehab, Ahmedabad, India)

recovery. Compensatory training can lead to the development of splinter skills which are skills acquired in a manner inconsistent with skills the individual already possesses. Splinter skills cannot be easily generalized to other task variations or to other environments.

- It is the only realistic approach in patients with limited recovery or patients with significant impairments and functional limitations with little or no expectation for additional recovery.

Clinical Pearl

Elongate–align–activate–functional use—"use it or lose it"

SUMMARY

This chapter provides a detailed framework for strategies to improve motor function (motor control and motor learning) by taking into consideration various aspects of treatment interventions. Theories of motor learning to improve motor performance are explained to enable the process of clinical decision making and help therapists to focus on strategies that can be used to promote skilled performance. Interventions to promote adaptability of skills for function in day-to-day living in household, work, and community have been discussed. While selecting interventions, the therapist must consider those with the greatest chance of success and must also take into consideration other factors, such as ability to deliver care, cost-effectiveness, age of the patient, comorbidities, social support, and prognosis. Carefully planned and structured treatment protocols help the patient and their caregivers to develop meaningful skills over the long course of neurological condition.

Review Questions

1. Define motor control and motor learning.
2. What are the theories and stages of motor learning?
3. Describe strategies to improve motor learning. Explain the types of augmented feedback.
4. Discuss the various constraints on motor control and motor learning post–CNS injury.
5. Discuss the strategies used to improve postural control.
6. What is neurodevelopmental technique?
7. Write a short note on proprioceptive neuromuscular facilitation.
8. What is neuromuscular electrical stimulation (NMES)?
9. Describe the outline and management of cerebellar dysfunction.

BIBLIOGRAPHY

1. American College of Sports Medicine. ACSM's exercise management for persons with chronic diseases and disabilities, 4th edition. Philadelphia, PA: Lippincott Williams and Wilkins; 2016.
2. Bernstein N. The coordination and regulation of movement. London: Pergamon; 1967.
3. Bogataj U, Gros H, Kljajic M. The rehabilitation of gait in patients with hemiplegia: a comparison between conventional therapy and multichannel functional electrical stimulation therapy. Phys Ther. 1995;75:490.
4. Cauraugh J, Light K, Kim S, et al. Chronic motor dysfunction after stroke: Recovering wrist and finger extension by electromyography triggered neuromuscular stimulation. Stroke. 2000;31:1360.
5. Daly J, Ruff R, et al. Feasibility of combining multi-channel functional neuromuscular stimulation with weight-supported treadmill training. J Neurol Sci. 2004;255:105.
6. Embrey DG1, Haltz SL, Alon G, et al. Functional electrical stimulation to dorsiflexors and plantar flexors during gait to improve walking in adults with chronic hemiplegia. Arch Phys Med Rehabil. 2010;91:687.
7. Eng JJ. Strength training in individuals with stroke. Physiother Can. 2004;56:189-201.
8. Etnyre B, Lee E. Chronic and acute flexibility of men and women using three different stretching techniques. Res Q. 1988;59:222.
9. Fasen JM, O'connor AM, Schwartz SL, et al. A randomized controlled trial of hamstring stretching: comparison of four techniques. J Strength Cond Res. 2009;23(2):660.
10. Ferrante S1, Pedrocchi A, Ferrigno G, et al. Cycling induced by FES improves the muscular strength and motor control of individuals with post-acute stroke. Eur J Phys Rehabil Med. 2008;44:159.
11. Gatts SK, Woollazott MH, et al. Neural mechanisms underlying balance improvement with short term Tai Chi training. Aging Clin Exp Res. 2006;18:7-19.
12. Gritsenko Y, Ashworth N, et al. Upper-extremity functional electric stimulation-assisted exercises on a workstation in the subacute phase of stroke recovery. Arch Phys Med Rehabil. 2007;88(7):833-9.
13. Hale L, Fritz V, Goodman M. Prolonged static muscle stretch reduces spasticity—but for how long should it be held? J Physio. 1995;51:3.
14. Kamm K, Thelen E, Jensen J. A dynamical systems approach to motor development. In: Rothstein J (Ed). Movement science. Alexandria, VA: American Physical Therapy Association; 1991. pp. 11-23.
15. Levin M, Kleim J, Wolf S, et al. What do motor "recovery" and "compensation" mean in patients following stroke? Neurorehabil Neural Repair. 2009;23:313.
16. Li F1, Harmer P, Fisher KJ, McAuley E, et al. Tai Chi and fall reductions in older adults: a randomized controlled trial. J Gerontol A Biol Sci Med Sci. 2005;60:187-94.
17. Lindquist AR, Prado CL, Barros RM, et al. Gait training combining partial body-weight support, a treadmill, and functional electrical stimulation on poststroke gait. Phys Ther. 2007;87:1144.
18. Meilink A, Hemmen B, Han S, et al. Impact of EMG-triggered neuromuscular stimulation of the wrist and finger extensors of the paretic hand after stroke: a systematic review of the literature. Clin Rehabil. 2008;22:291.
19. Miller G, Light K. Strength training in spastic hemiparesis: should it be avoided? NeuroRehabilitation. 1997;9(1):17-28
20. Osternig LR1, Robertson RN, Troxel RK, et al. Differential response to proprioceptive neuromuscular facilitation (PNF) stretch technique. Med Sci Sports Exerc. 1990;22:106.
21. Powell J1, Pandyan AD, Granat M, et al. Electrical stimulation of wrist extensors in poststroke hemiplegia. Stroke. 1999;30(7):1384-9.

22. Prentice W. Therapeutic modalities in rehabilitation, 4th edition. New York, NY: McGraw Hill Medical; 2005.

23. Riolo L, Fisher K. Is there evidence that strength training could help improve muscle function and other outcomes without reinforcing abnormal movement patterns or increasing reflex activity in a man who has had a stroke? Phys Ther. 2003;83:844.

24. Roche A, Laighin G, Coote S. Surface-applied functional electrical stimulation for orthotic and therapeutic treatment of drop-foot after stroke—a systematic review. Phys Ther Rev. 2009;14:63.

25. Schimdt R, Lee T. Motor control and learning: a behavioral emphasis. 5th edition. Champaign, IL: Human Kinetics; 2011.

26. Sharp S, Brouwer B. Isokinetic strength training of the hemiparetic knee: effects on function and spasticity. Arch Phys Med Rehabil. 1997;70:1231.

27. Shumway-Cook A, Woollacott M. Motor control theory and practical applications, 5th edition. Baltimore, MD: Lippincott Williams and Wilkins; 2017.

28. Smith GV1, Silver KH, Goldberg AP, et al. Task-oriented exercise improves hamstring strength and spastic reflexes in chronic stroke patients. Stroke. 1999;30:2112.

29. Taggart H. Effects of Tai Chi exercise on balance, functional mobility, and fear of falling among older women. Appl Nurs Res. 2002;15:235.

30. Teixeira-Salmela LF1, Olney SJ, Nadeau S, et al. Muscle strengthening and physical conditioning to reduce impairment and disability in chronic stroke survivors. Arch Phys Med Rehabil. 1999;80:1211.

31. Triolo R, Bogir K, et al. Lower extremity applications of functional neuromuscular stimulation after spinal cord injury. Top Spinal Cord Inj Rehabil. 1999;5:44.

32. Wang R, Chan R, Tsai M. Functional electrical stimulation on chronic and acute hemiplegic shoulder subluxation. Am J Phys Med Rehabil. 2000;79:385.

33. Woodford HJ, Price CIM. EMG biofeedback for the recovery of motor function after stroke. Cochrane Database Syst Rev. 2007;(2):CD004585. doi: 10.1002/14651858.CD004585.pub2.

34. Yang YR1, Wang RY, Lin KH, et al. Task-oriented progressive resistance strength training improves muscle strength and functional performance in individuals with stroke. Clin Rehabil. 2006;20:860.

35. Yan T, Hui-Chan C, Li L. Functional electrical stimulation improves motor recovery of the lower extremity and walking ability of subjects with first acute stroke: a randomized placebo controlled trial. Stroke. 2005;36:80.

15
CHAPTER

Ischemic Heart Diseases

Neepa H Pandya

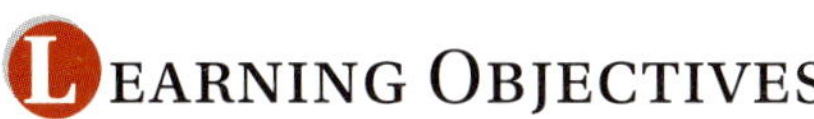

LEARNING OBJECTIVES

After reading this chapter, the readers should be able to:
- Recognize the risk factors of ischemic heart disease (IHD) and their modifications
- Describe the etiology, pathophysiology, clinical presentation, and sequelae of IHD
- Describe the process of IHD and its effect on exercise performance
- Identify side effects of common medications on exercise performance
- Understand specifics of exercise prescription and monitoring
- Understand outcomes of cardiac rehabilitation program
- Describe the role of physiotherapist in terms of intervention, patient-related instruction, coordination, and communication

CHAPTER OUTLINE

- Risk factors
- Pathophysiology
- Assessment
- Management of ischemic heart disease
  - Pharmacological management
  - Revascularization
- Exercise performance
- Exercise limitation
  - Exercise training
- Cardiac rehabilitation
  - Exercise prescription and monitoring
  - Aerobic training
  - Risks of exercise training
  - Boundaries of exercise session
  - Contraindications for exercise participation
  - Strength training
  - Monitoring
- Outcomes
- Psychosocial issues in ischemic heart disease

INTRODUCTION

At the dawn of the 20th century, India has witnessed an epidemiological transition and an abrupt rise in incidence of IHDs—progressive atherosclerotic disease involving coronary vasculature, crossing the global average. The prevalence of coronary heart disease has increased from 1 to 10% in urban population and <1 to 4–6% in rural population. A corresponding rise in the risk factors, such as physical inactivity and lack of inclusion of vegetarian diet, is also observed pan-India with increasing incidences of early age of onset, high fatality rate, and loss of productive midlife years.

The functional limitations associated with IHD depend on site and extent of atherosclerosis and the availability of normally perfused myocardium. The common signs and symptoms of IHD are:
- Chest pain
- Dyspnea

Definition of Ischemic Heart Disease.

Ischemic heart disease (IHD) is a reduction of myocardial blood supply in response to demand, associated with coronary artery disease resulting in an acute or chronic cardiac disability significantly affecting patient's exercise capacity to various degrees.

- Fatigue
- Syncope
- Palpitations
- Sudden death

This chapter intends to provide basic information on the mechanism of development of heart disease and its effects on physical activity, as physical inactivity is an independent predictor of development of IHD, and physiotherapists are primarily involved with exercise prescription and monitoring as a part of primary and secondary prevention programs. Along with viewing the different aspects of exercise prescription, here is an attempt to look into rationale of prescription and relative merits of exercise prescription indices. Modifications due to beneficial effects of coronary interventions on physical performance are mentioned wherever appropriate.

RISK FACTORS

Certain positive and negative risk factors are identified for the development of coronary vascular disease, which are enlisted in **Table 15.1**.

Certain risk factors have been reported for the development of coronary heart disease in India such as:

- Dyslipidemias
- Smoking
- Diabetes
- Hypertension
- Abdominal obesity
- Psychosocial stress
- Unhealthy diet
- Physical inactivity

This emphasizes the need of specific preventive measures to combat the epidemic.

PATHOPHYSIOLOGY

Coronary atherosclerosis is a chronic, progressive disease. Atherosclerotic changes in coronary arteries culminate into various degrees of myocardial damage, reflecting in corresponding electrocardiogram (ECG) leads, wall motion anomaly on 2D-echocardiogram, while clinically presenting mostly as angina, are the mainstay of IHD.

Sclerotic changes in coronary vessels and process of plaque formation secondary to smoking and other risk factors precede actual incidence of myocardial infarction (MI) and symptoms of angina by many years. These are associated with endothelial dysfunction, vascular inflammation, and accumulation of lipids, macrophages, platelets, thrombin, calcium, and fibrous connective tissue within the inner lining of coronary arteries. These changes are more commonly seen at proximal epicardial coronaries' bifurcation due to sheer stress generated by turbulent flow at the branching of the arteries.

Over a period of time, these atherosclerotic changes associated with vascular remodeling result in stenosis of coronary lumen and impairment of normal coronary blood flow. Blood flow through significantly narrowed lumen is inadequate to provide for increased demands on myocardium such as exercise, meals, emotional stress, and sexual activity. Reduction of 50% in the diameter of any major artery (left main, left anterior descending, left circumflex, right coronary artery) is considered clinically significant, is responsible for majority myocardial infarctions, and calls for possible medical and/or surgical intervention aiming at minimizing metabolic load and stabilizing blood supply. Lesions creating ~30% obstruction are unstable; can rupture, fissure, swell, or undergo combination of these processes; and lead to abrupt and complete obstruction and occurrence of acute MI. Lesions with 70% or greater stenosis are more commonly seen with myocardial ischemia and angina owing to collateral vessel development. Other factors affecting blood flow dynamics such as length and uniformity of the lesion also play a significant role in judging the critical value of stenosis.

Table 15.1: Risk factors for the development of coronary vascular disease.

Risk factor	Defining criteria	Modification
Age	Men ≥45 years, women ≥ 55 years	Nonmodifiable
Family history	Myocardial infarction, coronary revascularization or sudden death before 55 years in father or first-degree male relative or before 65 years in mother or first-degree female relative	Nonmodifiable
Cigarette smoking	Current smokers or who has quit before 6 months or exposure to environmental tobacco smoke	Modifiable
Sedentary lifestyle	Not participating in at least 30 minutes moderate-intensity physical activity 3 days/week for at least 3 months	Modifiable
Obesity	BMI ≥30 kg/m^2 or waist girth >102 cm (40 inches) in males and 88 cm (35 inches) in females	Modifiable
Hypertension	SBP ≥140 mm Hg or DBP ≥90 mm Hg or on antihypertensive	Modifiable
Dyslipidemia	• LDL ≥130 mg/dL • HDL <40 mg/dL • Total cholesterol ≥200 mg/dL • Lipid lowering drugs	Modifiable
Prediabetes	• Impaired fasting glucose between 100 and 125 mg/dL • Impaired glucose tolerance oral glucose value after 2 hours 140–199 mg/dL	Modifiable
Negative risk factor	Defining criteria	
HDL	≥60 mg/dL	Modifiable

(HDL: high-density lipoprotein; BMI: body mass index; SBP: systolic blood pressure; DBP: diastolic blood pressure; LDL: low-density lipoprotein)

Myocardial infarction is the necrosis of myocardial muscle cells and permanent loss of contractility following cessation of blood supply lasting more than a few seconds. The severity of MI depends on:

- The mass of myocardium rendered ischemic
- Duration of ischemia
- Metabolic requirement of myocardium during compromised blood flow
- Availability of collaterals to provide blood flow

Location of ischemia during MI corresponds to area supplied by the blocked artery, with areas of milder and reversible ischemia and injury surrounding focus of necrosis, leaving room for early intervention such as thrombolysis or emergency revascularization processes (primary angioplasty in MI) **(Box 15.1)**.

The site of MI takes almost 6 weeks to heal and after initial 24 hours and hemodynamic stability, instead of total rest, controlled increases in activity may lead to a reduced likelihood of myocardial remodeling as observed by Myers et al.

Figure 15.2 explains the sequence of events associated with the development of angina.

ASSESSMENT

Assessment of a patient having IHD includes history taking, examination, and exercise tolerance testing (ETT). Presenting symptoms of the patient include discomfort such as pain, tightness or squeezing feeling in the chest, neck, jaw, upper back, shoulder or arms; dizziness or faintness; shortness of breath; rapid or irregular heartbeats or palpitations. A classic presentation of angina is the Levine sign **(Fig. 15.3)** along with retrosternal chest discomfort **(Box 15.2)**. The discomfort may be precipitated by physical or emotional stress, exposure to cold, etc. It is generally relieved by nitroglycerin pills.

Medical history taking should include cardiovascular risk factors such as hypertension, dyslipidemia, obesity, and diabetes. Any previous occurrence of MI or any previous cardiac procedure viz. bypass graft or angioplasty should be asked about. Presence of any orthopedic problems such as arthritis should also be noted as they might affect the ambulation, hence affecting the ETT. Any

---

BOX 15.1: Progression of Ischemia in IHD.

Due to pattern of coronary blood flow, endocardium is the first one to be rendered ischemic. Subendocardial MI may progress to involvement of the entire thickness of the wall (transmural MI) **(Fig. 15.1)**.

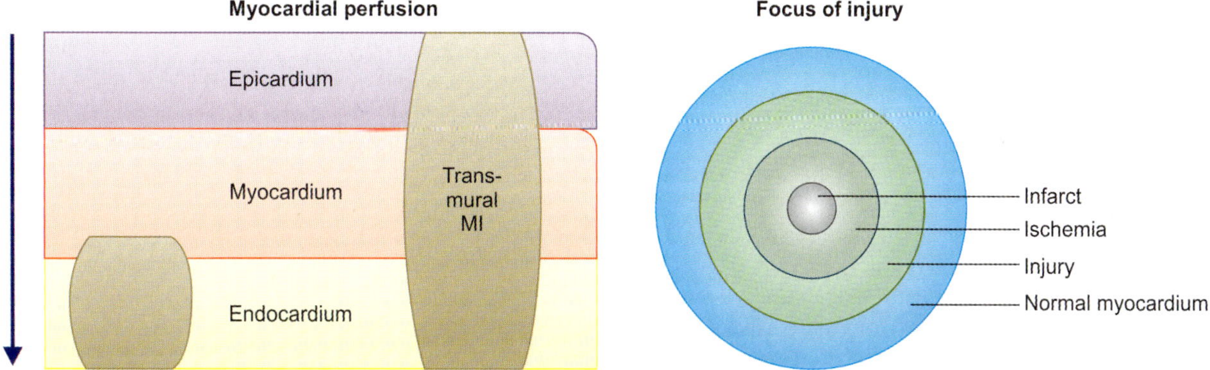

Fig. 15.1: Pathophysiology of myocardial infarction (MI).

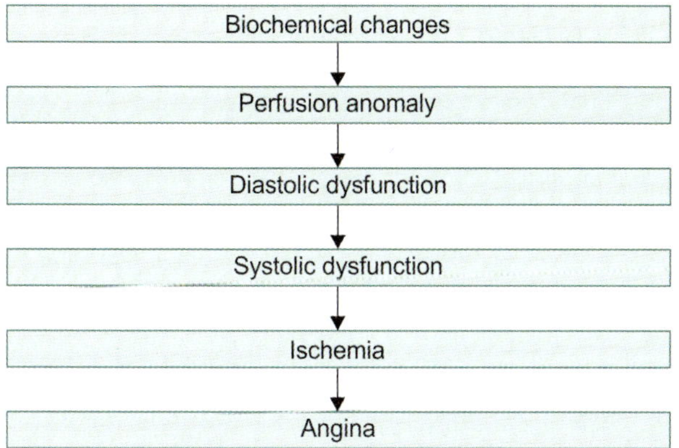

Fig. 15.2: The ischemic cascade.

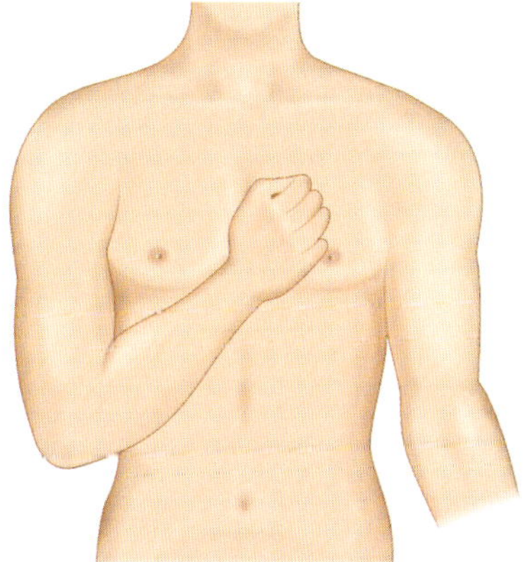

Fig. 15.3: The Levine sign.

BOX 15.2: Physical signs associated with angina.

The Levine sign is a clenched fist over the chest, used by the patient to describe ischemic chest pain or discomfort. Other signs such as the palm sign (palm to the chest), the arm sign (touching the left arm with the right hand), and pointing sign (pointing with one finger) are also used by patients.

respiratory illness should be asked for. Any personal habits such as smoking, tobacco consumption, and dietary habits should be reported. Previous physical examination findings such as murmurs, clicks, and presence of other abnormal heart sounds should be noted. Medications consumed by the patient should be documented along with their potential side effects, dosing intervals, and adherence to the drug regime. Documenting the patient's exercise history is essential as it gives the examiner an idea about the level of routine physical activity done by the patient and the possible lifestyle of the individual. Family history of any cardiac illness needs to be noted. Occupational history stressing a detailed evaluation of the physical and psychological demands of the work, is essential.

Physical examination of the individual should include the following components:

- Body mass index (BMI), waist–hip ratio (WHR), and waist circumference (WC)
- Vitals examination—blood pressure (BP), heart rate (HR) (rate and rhythm), pulse rate (PR) (rate and rhythm), body temperature, and SpO$_2$
- Auscultation of breath and heart sounds
- Measurement of the jugular venous pressure (JVP)
- Examination related to any orthopedic, neurological, pulmonary, or associated medical condition that may be present
- Examination of the chest and arm or leg wounds for signs of healing in case of postoperative cases
- Musculoskeletal examination including strength, flexibility, endurance, and balance
- In the case of patients operated via median sternotomy, sternal stability should be assessed by identifying any movement, pain or clicking in the sternum.

Diagnostic blood work exhibits increased levels of enzymes CPK MB and troponin I-markers of myocardial cell damage. An echocardiogram shows corresponding regional wall motion anomaly, reduction in left ventricular ejection fraction (LVEF), and changes in left ventricular cavity size and wall thickness. ECG shows ST segment elevation in leads corresponding to the ischemic area in subendocardial MI, whereas in transmural MI ST elevation, T wave inversion, presence of Q wave and some loss of R wave are seen. Other laboratory tests include electrolytes (potassium, calcium, and magnesium levels), complete blood count, renal and liver function tests, blood sugar and cholesterol levels, and arterial blood gases. Chest radiographs and cardiac catheterization also reveal important findings.

Stress testing or ETT should be performed to deduce the ability of the cardiovascular and pulmonary systems to accommodate the increasing metabolic demands. For individuals not able to perform the test, pharmacologic stress testing using persantine or adenosine may be performed. ETT may be performed with continuous monitoring of the patient using ECG, echocardiography or nuclear imaging. The test is concluded positive for ischemia when the myocardial oxygen supply fails to meet the myocardial oxygen demand at any given point during the test.

Assessment of the patient's aerobic capacity and endurance is crucial before starting any rehabilitation protocol. A simple and effective means to measure the aerobic capacity is the six-minute walk test (6 MWT). Other tests such as 12 MWT, bicycle tests, and step tests may also be used depending on the functional capacity of the subject.

MANAGEMENT OF ISCHEMIC HEART DISEASE

Pharmacological Management

Various combinations of pharmacological interventions are recruited in patients with myocardial ischemia with or without revascularization process largely aiming at reduction in risk factors, metabolic load on compromised myocardium and better central and peripheral hemodynamics.

Table 15.2 enlists common medications used in MI and their potential effects on exercise performance **within the therapeutic dose.**

Table 15.2: Effects of medications on exercise performance.

Sl. No.	Drugs	Side effects
1.	Diuretics	Precipitate ventricular ectopy False-positive test result in presence of hypokalemia/hypomagnesemia
2.	Beta-blockers	Decrease submaximal and maximal HR
3.	Vasodilators, ACE inhibitors, angiotensin receptor blockers	Hypotensive episodes post exercise
4.	Calcium channel blockers	Increase exercise tolerance
5.	CNS active drugs	Attenuating effects on HR and BP
6.	Antiarrhythmic drugs	False-negative or false-positive test results
7.	Digitalis	Causes ST depression
8.	α-receptor blockers	Reduce BP, exercise performance remains the same

(ACE: angiotensin-converting enzyme; CNS: central nervous system; HR: heart rate)

Revascularization

Atherosclerotic lesions resulting in 50% or greater stenosis in coronary artery are considered clinically significant and are an indication for revascularization procedure. Revascularization processes such as coronary artery bypass graft (CABG) and percutaneous transluminal coronary angioplasty (PTCA) are performed with the purpose of:

- Increasing blood flow and oxygen delivery to ischemic myocardium beyond the level of lesion
- Reducing or eliminating potential consequences/manifestations of ischemia
- Reducing cardiovascular morbidity and mortality

Coronary artery bypass graft involves a surgical procedure bypassing the sclerotic coronary artery with saphenous vein/internal mammary artery/radial artery through median sternotomy on a beating heart or using a heart–lung machine. Internal mammary artery has a 10-year patency of 93% compared to saphenous vein that has 60%. Recent advances of minimally invasive surgery on beating heart through intercostal incisions using fiber optical scope have been developed. Almost 50% patients are asymptomatic at 10 years after CABG.

On determination of coronary anatomy and ventricular function through cardiac catheter, CABG is indicated in cases of:

- Anginal symptoms refractory to pharmacological therapy
- PTCA is contraindicated
- Left main coronary artery disease (CAD)
- Triple vessel disease
- Double vessel disease
- Left ventricular dysfunction
- Proximal left anterior descending coronary artery lesions
- Diffuse/left main coronary lesion with significant myocardium at risk.

Coronary artery bypass graft patient is at risk because of one or more of the following complications in the postoperative phase:

- Thoracic pain
- Wound related issues
- Pleural pathology
- Retained secretion
- Reduced vital capacity
- Diaphragm dysfunction
- Embolism.

Percutaneous transluminal coronary angioplasty (PTCA) involves plaque compression and redistribution along with stretching of vessel wall using a balloon/double-lumen dilatation catheter.

Risks and possible complications associated with PTCA are:

- Bleeding at catheter insertion site
- Thrombosis/damage to the blood vessel at insertion site
- Thrombus within the lumen of artery treated by PTCA
- Infection at catheter insertion site
- Cardiac arrhythmias
- Myocardial infarction
- Chest pain
- Rupture of coronary artery, requires CABG.

EXERCISE PERFORMANCE

Exercise Limitation

Patients with history of MI exhibit reduction in cardiorespiratory fitness (50–70% age and gender predicted). Exercise limitation in IHD is due to inability to increase stroke volume, HR, or both diminishing cardiac output rather than impairments of peripheral extraction of oxygen. Loss of large mass of myocardium significantly compromises myocardial contractility and results in inability to increase stroke volume in response to exercise, clinically presenting as exertional hypotension. Restriction in rise of HR is largely due to beta-blockers, intrinsic disease of sinoatrial, or atrioventricular node or appearance of angina symptoms which may or may not be accompanied by ECG changes.

Maximal heart rate during exercise and heart rate recovery are two commonly used indices to evaluate the effects of rehabilitation and exercise training. It is important to optimally define and carefully monitor heart rate during training sessions to attain maximum benefit while preventing complications associated with unduly high intensity. While a normal heart responds to the increase in demand of exercise by the increase in HR, stroke volume, and myocardial contractility, heart with MI shows disproportionate reduction in diastole in response to increased HR resulting in reduced myocardial perfusion, leading to ischemia in presence of stenotic artery. Contraction and relaxation at high rates lead to ATP deficiency during exercise which results in ischemia and angina. Diastolic dysfunction increases filling pressure and pulmonary capillary wedge pressure resulting in dyspnea and increased pulmonary stiffness, increased work of breathing, diffusion distance, interstitial pulmonary edema, intrapulmonary shunt, and desaturation. In addition, diastolic deficit leads to systolic dysfunction and reduced ejection fraction accompanied by increased wall tension, coronary resistance and reduction in oxygen delivery to myocardium further compounding angina and dyspnea. A subnormal increase in HR (chronotropic incompetence) in response to exercise also contributes to an inadequate increase in contractility. Administration of calcium channel blockers and beta-blockers reduces the contractility and HR, respectively, thereby reducing the metabolic demands on compromised myocardium. Patients' medication prescription must be carefully noted during exercise testing as well as training sessions. The effects of common medications on exercise performance are discussed earlier in the chapter. **Figure 15.4** explains the exercise limitation and dyspnea in cardiac patients.

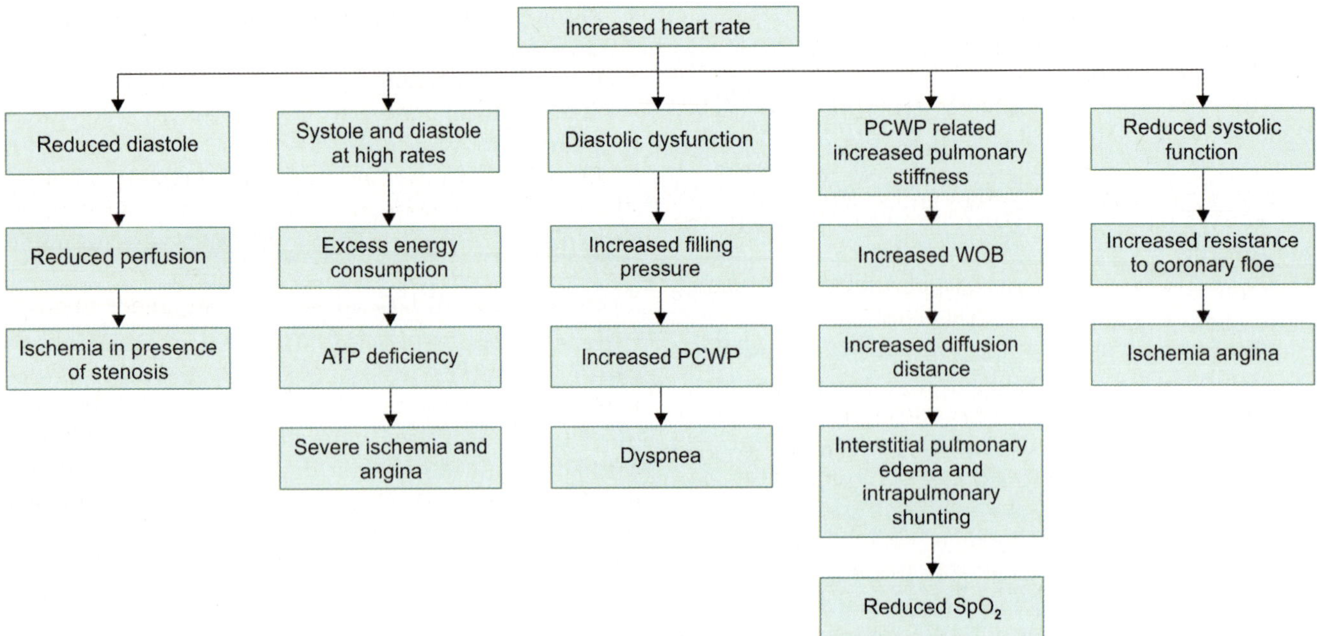

Fig. 15.4: Exercise limitation in myocardial infarction (MI).
(ATP: adenosine triphosphate; WOB: work of breathing; PCWP: pulmonary capillary wedge pressure)

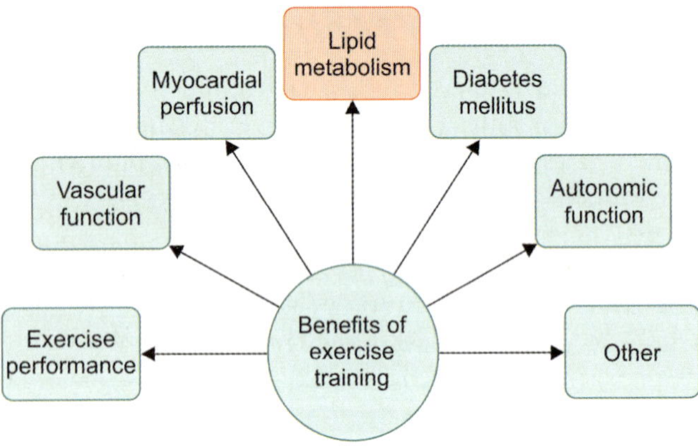

Fig. 15.5: Benefits of exercise training.

Exercise Training

Human physical exercise performance can improve multifold in response to gradually and systematically progressive external stimuli. **Figure 15.5** shows various areas of improvement following exercise training in IHD patients.

Vascular changes include regression of stenosis, collateral formation, and improved endothelial function along with increased sensitivity of resistance vessels to metabolic vasodilators and increased number of endothelial progenitor cells and angiogenic cells promoting angiogenesis. Reduction in blood viscosity, platelet activation, and thrombin generation also play a role in halting the progress of the disease. Other changes are:

- Increase in pretraining VO_{2max} ~20% (inversely proportionate to baseline fitness)
- Improvement in ventilatory response to exercise
- Improvement in ventilatory threshold
- Reduced rate-pressure product and anginal symptoms
- Increased heart rate variability
- Modest decrease in fat stores, blood pressure
- Decrease in total blood cholesterol, serum triglycerides, LDL
- Increased vagal tone and decreased adrenergic activity
- Decreased coronary inflammation marker C-reactive protein.

It is generally accepted that angina pectoris occurs at a certain myocardial oxygen demand which is clinically assessed as **rate-pressure product** [systolic blood pressure (SBP) × HR]. Patient should be closely monitored to maintain exercise training intensity below angina threshold known through exercise tolerance test. Exercise training of **adequate intensity** increases this angina threshold, attenuates the progress of atherosclerosis, and increases event-free survival as observed by Taylor and Anderson. A study done by Hambrecht et al. showed that over a training period of 12 months, patients with exercise training progressed better compared to coronary angioplasty in terms of exercise capacity, event-free survival, and cost effectiveness. Belardinelli et al. found that compared to sedentary counterparts, patients who underwent combination of PTCA and exercise training exhibited 26% more increase in peak O_2 uptake, 27% more improvement in health related quality of life (HRQOL) and 20% more reduction in cardiac events. These changes are largely attributed to restored autonomic balance, improved endothelial function, reduction in blood pressure, and afterload improving left ventricular function. Exercise-related myocardial hypertrophy as observed in athletes and chronic heart failure (CHF) patients is not observed in IHD patients.

Hofmann et al. found that successful revascularization favorably alters exercise response largely by increasing blood flow and oxygen supply, eliminating ECG changes of ischemia and exertional angina especially in patients who exhibit exertional angina at lower work rates. The potential mechanism behind augmented exercise responses are:

- Better ventricular contractility and wall motion
- Normalized chronotropic response and heart rate recovery
- Reduction in exertional hypotension and exercise-related arrhythmia.

According to American Heart Association, cardiac rehabilitation training is recommended to all CABG patients during in-patient phase and emphasizes walking as walk distance is a strong independent predictor and guide to prognosis than gains in VO_{2max} which improves by 20% post revascularization.

CARDIAC REHABILITATION

Cardiac rehabilitation is a process of optimizing cardiovascular health in patients with cardiac disease or surgery. It has three important components:

1. Exercise training
2. Risk factor modification
3. Stress reduction

Ornish et al., noted in "A Lifestyle Study" that a quintet of physical exercise, strict vegetarian diet, smoking cessation, stress management strategies, and group psychosocial support exhibited regression of stenosis that was sustained over a period of 5 years compared to progressive stenosis observed in a control group. This study reinforces the role of multidisciplinary approach to cardiac rehabilitation with emphasis on risk factor modification. The cardiac rehabilitation team comprises a cardiologist, cardiothoracic surgeon (in operated cases), nurse, physiotherapist and occupational therapists, nutritional expert, social worker, and a clinical psychologist.

Exercise Prescription and Monitoring

The purpose of the exercise prescription is to reduce the risk of progressing IHD and increase exercise tolerance while providing a safe and effective exercise program. American College of Sports Medicine (ACSM) recommends a combination of aerobic training, strength training, and flexibility exercises. Foster et al. note that patients with CABG are able to begin the exercise program sooner, progress at a faster rate but are at risk of deconditioning and contracture of shoulder musculature secondary to surgery-induced soft tissue injury. Flexibility exercises should be started in the in-patient phase, while exercise requiring heavy workload should be commenced after 12 weeks of surgery.

American Association of Cardiovascular and Pulmonary Rehabilitation marks the phases of cardiac rehabilitation from I to IV as:

- Phase I: In-patient phase
- Phase II: Immediate post-discharge phase lasting about 12 weeks
- Phase III: Intermediate phase lasting 4–6 months
- Phase IV: Maintenance phase lasting lifelong as patient maintains heart-healthy lifestyle.

Phase II requires intensive ECG and clinical monitoring and supervision and intensive risk factor modification. In Phase III, patient has stabilized and ECG monitoring is required only if indicated by signs and symptoms.

During phase of hospitalization and immediate post–hospital phase, the goal is to prevent deterioration, and hence, exercise frequency is more important than intensity. To avoid the risk of rerupture of the plaque, catecholamine release induced arrhythmias and myocardial rupture, mobility begins after 24 hours rest and hemodynamic stability where exercise intensity is targeted at 20 beats above resting HR (10 beats if patient is on beta-blockers) with subjective rating of perceived exertion (RPE) of easy to moderate [2–3 on New scale **(Table 15.3)**/10–12 on Old Borg Scale **(Table 15.4)**]. Exercises can begin as bed-side activity twice a day to progressive hall ambulation and stair climbing 3–4 times/day.

After about 6 weeks, while site of infarct has fairly stabilized the goal shifts to functional recovery and prevention of further events. Exercise prescription here is highly related to patient's functional ability that is ideally determined from symptom-limited exercise test. In the absence of an exercise test, training can be commenced and progressed at low work rates with supervision for symptoms **(Box 15.3)**.

The Coronary Revascularization Outcome Questionnaire (CROQ) is a reliable and valid tool that can be used for monitoring the prognosis of cardiac patients undergoing PTCA and CABG. It has two separate questionnaires for PTCA and CABG patients. It also provides separate questionnaires for pre and post-operative phase.

Table 15.3: The original Borg scale.	
Score	*Level of exertion*
6	
7	Very, very light
8	
9	Very light
10	
11	Fairly light
12	
13	Somewhat hard
14	
15	Hard
16	
17	Very hard
18	
19	Very, very hard
20	

Table 15.4: The modified Borg scale/RPE scale.

Score	Level of exertion
0	Nothing at all
0.3	
0.5	Extremely weak just noticeable
0.7	
1	Very weak
1.5	
2	Weak little
2.5	
3	Moderate
4	
5	Strong heavy
6	
7	Very strong
8	
9	
10	Extremely strong "maximal"
11	

(RPE: rating of perceived exertion).

BOX 15.3: The Borg scale.

The rating of perceived exertion (RPE) is a reliable and valid indicator of the exercise intensity. The individual rates their subjective level of exertion during exercise through means of a scale. The original scale was developed by Gunnar Borg, and hence, it is referred to as the Borg scale. The original Borg scale is a category scale ranging from a score of 6 to 20. The modified Borg scale or the RPE scale is a ratio scale ranging from 0 to 10.

Aerobic Training

Generalized exercises using large muscles of body three times a week for 12 weeks are beneficial for cardiac patients. Sattelmair et al. reinforce that the training effect is dose-dependent. The components of the dose are intensity, frequency, time, and type of exercises. The three primary components—intensity, frequency, and duration—are interrelated with each other where one impacts the other in the process of exercise prescription. For example, when intensity and duration are greater, frequency should be lower. As per a study by Schonhr et al., among primary components, intensity is the most important component as threshold for intensity is very well defined and provokes larger changes in performance ability than changes in either frequency or duration and is associated with the reduction in mortality. The side effects are also more likely with inappropriately high intensity of exercise than with frequency and/or duration. The mode of exercise can be chosen according to the patient's functional requirements and their convenience. Treadmill walking **(Fig. 15.6)** is usually more commonly used than cycling **(Fig. 15.7)** or

cross-trainer **(Fig. 15.8)**. Cross trainer and rowing require higher energy consumption and can be added to exercise program as progression from cycling and treadmill. Stepping can also be used for aerobic training, but care needs to be taken in individuals affected with osteoarthritis

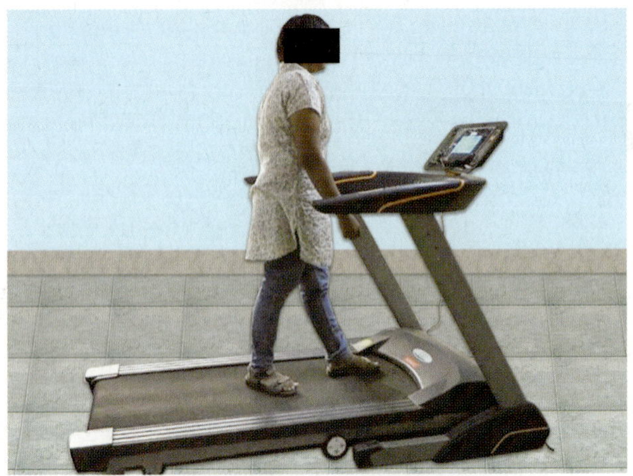

Fig. 15.6: Treadmill walking.

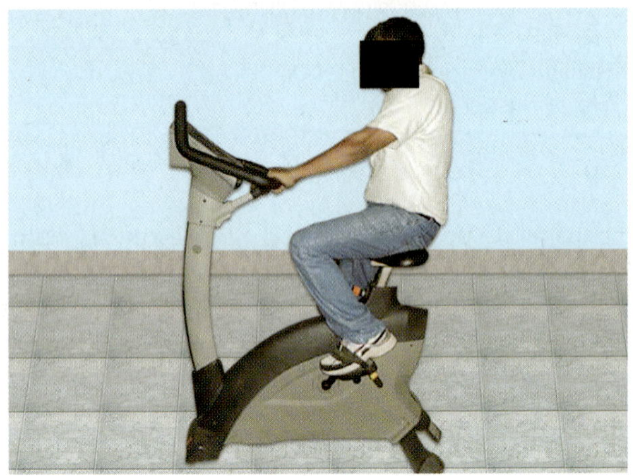

Fig. 15.7: Cycling.

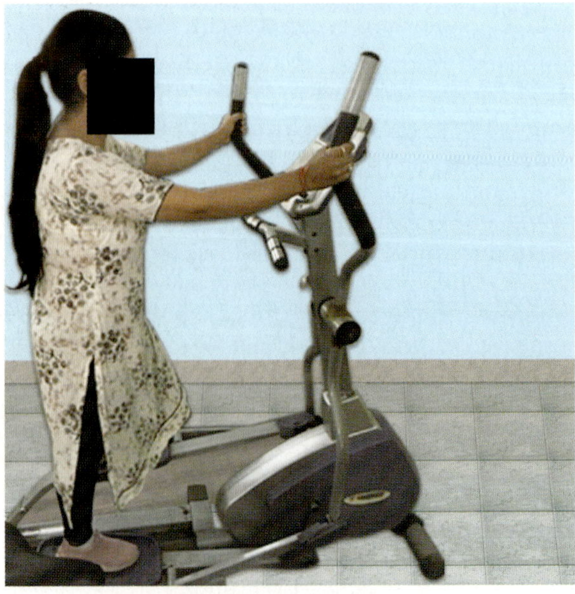

Fig. 15.8: Cross-trainer.

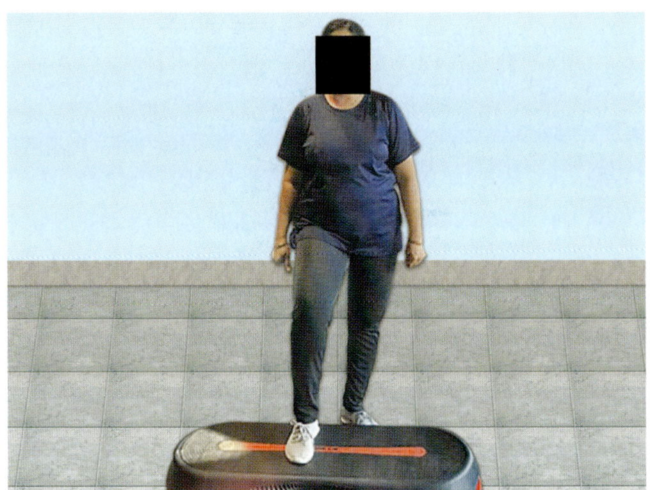

Fig. 15.9:. Stepping.
Courtesy: Mission Health, Ahmedabad

Table 15.5: Markers of exercise intensity.

Markers of exercise intensity	Reference value
VO_{2max}	• 60–80% of VO_{2max} • 40/50–80% of VO_2 reserve
Heart rate	• 55–65–90% MHR • 40/50–85% heart rate reserve
RPE	12–13 or 3–5 moderate to hard

(MHR: maximum heart rate; RPE: rating of perceived exertion)

(Fig. 15.9). **Table 15.5** enlists various markers of exercise intensity during this phase.

Meyer et al., observed that in patients with IHD, ventilatory threshold is reached earlier than ischemic threshold and whenever direct measures are available, 90% of ventilatory threshold should be considered more appropriate than age and gender-matched VO_2 reserve. The intensity associated with ventilatory threshold is linked more closely to RPE and elevation of catecholamines. Also, the inability to comfortably carry out a conversation (the talk test) is closely related to ventilatory threshold and is a simple method to ensure that appropriate intensity is not exceeded **(Box 15.4)**.

Objective markers of exercise prescription should be accompanied by subjective perception of effort reflected by RPE. Borg concluded that RPE relates well to metabolic rate and relative HR, and though less specific, it is possible to prescribe reasonably accurate intensity using RPE. As an

Being able to freely converse, or passing the so-called talk test assures that the ventilatory threshold has not been exceeded and ensures that the objective markers of exercise prescription are achieved. Asking the patient to recite any 30–50 words paragraph and then asking "Can you still talk comfortably?" serve as a convenient and practical evaluation strategy. If patient does not answer "Yes," then ventilatory threshold is exceeded and the patient is asked to step down the intensity by one stage. Investigators have used "the pledge of allegiance" for convenience but any paragraph of appropriate length can be used.

additional measure, observation of relationship between power output and HR, an HR performance curve should be noted to avoid hazards associated with disproportionate increases in HR as positive deflection point relates more closely to exercise intensity than maximum heart rate (MHR) and heart rate reserve. Foster et al. suggest that prescription through metabolic equivalent calculation overestimates energy expenditure as it is formulated using younger healthy individuals. ACSM recommendations for aerobic training in IHD are presented in **Table 15.6**.

Risks of Exercise Training

Though cardiac rehabilitation programs are safe for appropriately assessed patients, there is still some risk of morbidity and mortality associated with exercise training that largely results from inappropriately high intensity. Complication rates in adults are viewed in terms of person-hours and are observed to be 20 times less compared to exercise testing. The incidence of exertion related complications is lower in more active individuals. Battista et al. recommend preparticipation screening in older individuals; lower exercise intensity in the early weeks of exercise programs and inclusion of subjective performance evaluation and exercise prescription strategies such as RPE and the talk test are recommended as defending strategy.

Boundaries of Exercise Session

American College of Sports Medicine emphasizes exercise prescription at an intensity that avoids occurrence of signs and symptoms of exercise intolerance along with significant electrocardiographic changes. If ST depression

Table 15.6: Aerobic training in CAD.

Mode	Goal	Intensity	Frequency	Duration	Time
Large muscle activity	• Increase aerobic capacity • Decrease BP and HR response • Decrease submaximal myocardial O_2 demand • Decrease risk factors • Increase ADLs	• RPE 11–20 • 40–80% HR reserve	≥3 days/week	• 20–30 minutes session • 5–10 minutes warm-up and cool down	4–6 months

(CAD: coronary artery disease; ADL: activities of daily living; HR: heart rate; RPE: rating of perceived exertion)

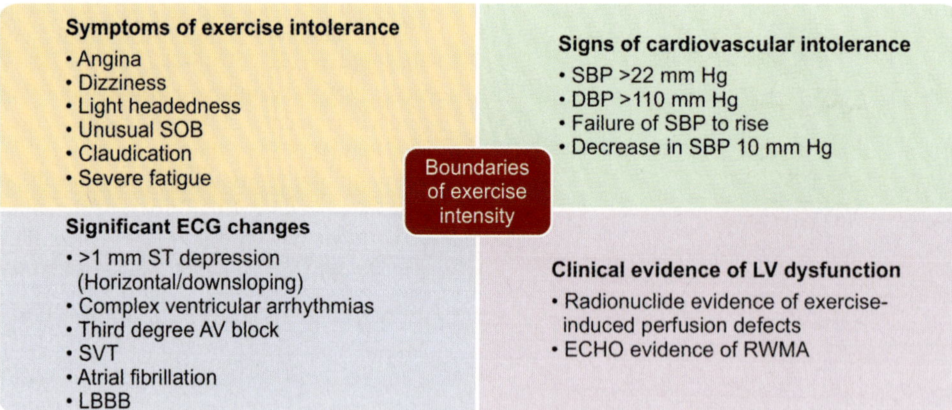

Fig. 15.10: Boundaries of exercise intensity for exercise prescription.
(SOB: shortness of breath; SBP: systolic blood pressure; DBP: diastolic blood pressure; SVT: supraventricular tachycardia; LBBB: left bundle branch block; AV: atrioventricular; LV: left ventricular; RWMA: regional wall motion abnormality)

is observed, exercise intensity may be revised to 10 beats below incidence intensity, recommend Foster et al. If any of the signs/symptoms presented in **Figure 15.10** is noticed during exercise training session, the session should be terminated and patient should be treated for the same.

Contraindications for Exercise Participation

In view of patient safety, patients with certain conditions are not permitted to participate in the exercise program. The contraindications are enlisted in **Figure 15.11**.

Strength Training

Strength training is an important component of exercise prescription aiming at better neuromuscular function and improving response to demands of activities of daily living (ADL), occupational and recreational activities. Resistance training **(Figs. 15.12A to F)** is recommended after a patient has stabilized during conventional training, though left ventricular function remains stable during resistance training in normal individuals, CAD, and CHF patients. ACSM indicates resistance training in:

- Four to six weeks after MI/CABG
- One/two weeks after PTCA without MI
- For four to six weeks in phase II
- Diastolic blood pressure (DBP) <105 mm Hg
- Peak exercise capacity >5 METs
- Not compromised by CHF, arrhythmias, or unstable symptoms.

Clinical Pearl

Exercise should be designed to recruit variety of muscle groups balancing agonist and antagonist function. While exercises are prescribed at some percentage of 1 RM, due to pressor response it is advisable to monitor exercises with RPE. Valsalva maneuver and end range hold should be avoided. Different muscle recruitment should be given priority over increase in number of repetitions for progressing the exercise.

Table 15.7 presents an example of strength training session.

Monitoring

It is essential to monitor the patient's exercise response to ensure optimum risk-benefit ratio of exercise training.

Heart Rate and Rhythm

There is a linear relationship between heart rate and workload. Workload is presented as Watts on a cycle ergometer and speed/grade on a treadmill. Beta-blockers due to their suppressive effect on sympathetic system limit the increase in heart rate.

Failure to increase the heart rate with the increase in workload is a concern, and patient must be evaluated for blood pressure, respiratory rate, skin color, and cognition.

Heart Rate Recovery

Cole's study on heart rate recovery noted that on cessation of exercise a rapid reactivation of vagal tone in the first 30 seconds to 1 minute is a major determinant of fall in heart rate along with oxygen deficit. As decreased vagal activity is associated with increased risk of death, decrease in heart rate recovery immediately after exercise is predictive of increased mortality. The impact of heart

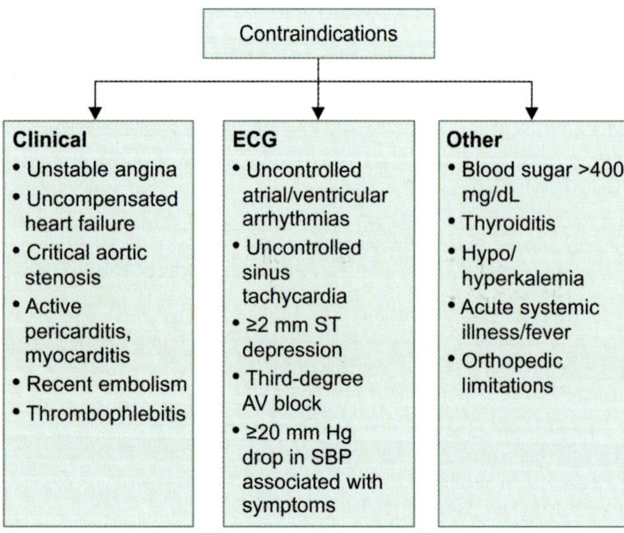

Fig. 15.11: Contraindications of exercise training.

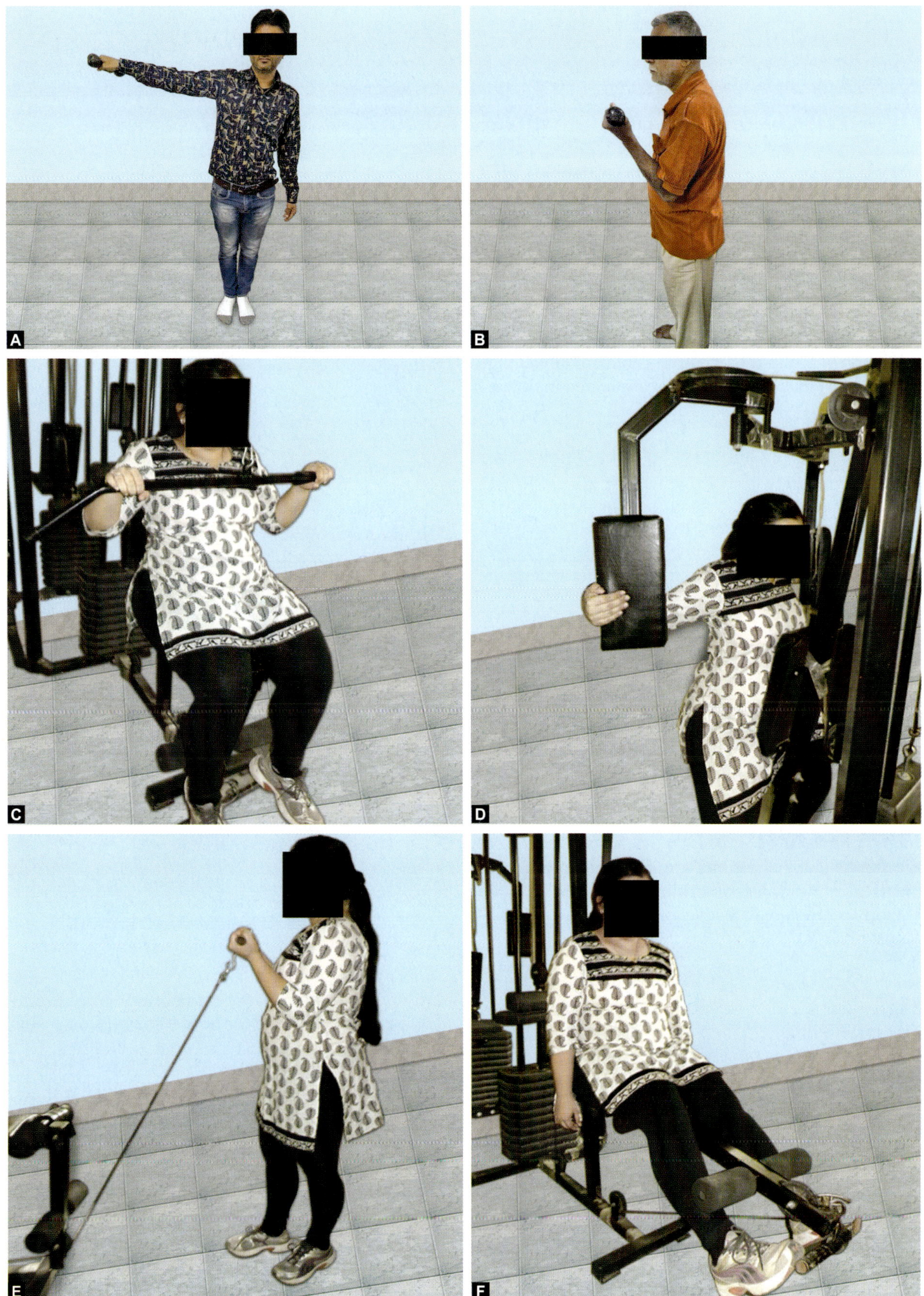

Figs. 15.12A to F: Strength training: (A) Strengthening of shoulder abductors; (B) Strengthening of elbow flexors; (C) Latissimus dorsi; (D) Scapula retractors; (E) Elbow flexors; (F) Knee extensors.

Table 15.7: Strength training for exercise training.

Mode	Goal	Intensity	Frequency	Duration	Time
Circuit training	• Leisure, occupational activities, and ADL • Increase muscle strength and endurance	• 30–40% of 1 repetition maximum (RM) for upper body • 50–60% of 1 RM for lower body	• 2–3 days/week • 2–4 sets of 12–15 repetitions • Gradually increase resistance	Variable	4–6 months

rate recovery varies with impaired left ventricular function and medications such as digoxin, beta-blockers, and chronotropic incompetence.

Respiratory Rate, Rhythm, and Dyspnea

Rate and depth of respiration increase with exercise. Dyspnea with or without exertion is a concern and can be accompanied by anxiety and must be evaluated in detail.

Blood Pressure

Blood pressure (BP) should be taken before and immediately after exercise with patient in the same position. BP should be taken during exercise to ensure a linear increase of blood pressure with the increase in workload. For each 10% increase of MHR, SBP is expected to increase 12–15 mm Hg. DBP changes are low in amplitude, and it remains the same or changes by 10 mm Hg.

ACSM considers abnormal responses to blood pressure indications to stop physical activity. These include:

- Failure of SBP to rise as exercise continues
- Hypertensive response to exercise with SBP≥200 mm Hg and/or DBP >110 mm Hg
- Progressive fall in SBP of 10–15 mm Hg (exertional hypotension).

Electrocardiography

Telemetric monitoring of ECG is an established method of monitoring heart rate, rhythm, and ST-T changes during exercise sessions. Subjective evaluation of RPE and talk test should accompany objective measures.

Symptoms

Patient should be monitored for symptoms enlisted below to observe signs of excessive effort:

- Persistent dyspnea
- Dizziness or confusion
- Pain
- Severe leg claudication
- Excessive fatigue
- Pallor, cold sweat
- Ataxia
- Pulmonary rales

Patients should be informed about late symptoms such as prolonged fatigue, insomnia, and sudden weight gain due to fluid retention.

OUTCOMES

Table 15.8 enlists the effects of cardiac rehabilitation on various risk factors. It is noteworthy that the impact of exercise alone has lesser evidence and found to be less effective as confirmed in a study by Wenger et al. **Table 15.9** lists the outcome measures commonly used in IHD population.

Table 15.8: Outcomes of cardiac rehabilitation program.

Risk factor	Outcome
Smoking	Significant benefit in smoking cessation
Lipids	Improved lipid profile
Body weight	Improvement in BMI and body composition
Hypertension	Modest impact on lowering BP
Psychosocial function	Improvement in various measurements of psychosocial status and function

Table 15.9: Outcome measures used for IHD patients.

Outcome measure	Description
Heart rate and rhythm	Must be assessed at rest and during activity. Both the absolute values and the relative changes in the rate and rhythm on a daily basis must be noted
Heart sound auscultation	Presence of normal heart sounds S1 and S2 should be noted. Murmurs, if any present, should be documented
Breath sound auscultation	Bronchial, bronchovesicular, and vesicular sounds should be auscultated. Presence of any abnormalities in the normal lung sounds and any adventitious sounds should be documented
JVP	JVP should be measured and recorded. It signifies increased filling pressures in the heart
Peripheral edema	Presence of edema should be noted with the type of edema—pitting or nonpitting and the stage of edema
Muscle strength	Muscle strength of all the muscles of the body should be measured, especially the major muscle groups of the lower and upper extremity and trunk. The classical manual muscle testing method may be employed or more functional tests may be used. Muscle strength of inspiratory muscles should also be measured

(IHD: ischemic heart disease; JVP: jugular venous pressure)

PSYCHOSOCIAL ISSUES IN ISCHEMIC HEART DISEASE

Cardiovascular diseases have a large proportion of mortality in India (255–525 per 100,000 population in men and 225–299 per 100,000 population in women). The mortality rate in India due to cardiovascular diseases is 30–42% higher compared to the global burden. There has been a rapid increase in the number of hospitalizations due to IHD. IHD affects not only the individual but also their family and friends. Absence from work, high cost of management, and increased morbidity following IHD impose a lot of pressure on the individual and the family. Patients undergoing surgery have to go through a lot of lifestyle modifications. Inability to cope up with these changes leads to failure of the surgery and increased risk of mortality. Majority of the patients are able to follow through these changes but around 25% of them have difficulties in long-term compliance. They develop negative emotions such as rage, anxiety, and depression and often fail to return to their premorbid state of work or pleasure in spite of being physically fit to do so. They feel as if they are different and are being coddled or overprotected by their family members, they may be stressed about recurrence or may not be open to making dietary changes due to cultural issues. Such emotional changes lead to anxiety and depression in the patients in the long-term.

Since the heart is one of the most vital organs of the human body, in matters dealing with the cardiac system, the treating health personnel are usually more concerned about the physical state of the body. But the psychological state of the patient should not be overlooked. Adequate attention should be given to the psychological, spiritual, and cultural problems of the patient, and consultation should be given accordingly. Psychological interventions to manage such issues have been discussed in detail elsewhere.

SUMMARY

Exercise training aims at improvements in exercise capacity, reductions in all-cause mortality, and improved HRQOL through physical exercises of adequate intensity, frequency, time, and type of exercises observing boundaries of risks associated with exercise training that is largely contributed through excessively high intensity. Cardiac rehabilitation, in addition to promote physical activity, includes smoking cessation, stress management, nutritional changes, and medication; improves exercise capacity as well as favorably modifies risk factors associated with CAD.

Case Scenario

CASE STUDY

A 69-year-old male presented with shortness of breath, chest pain, and difficulty in doing activities.

Past medical history: He has diabetes mellitus since 12 years (on glucose-lowering agents), hypertension since 15 years (on antihypertensives), and dyslipidemia (maintained by a controlled diet).

Personal history: He has been smoking around 20 cigarettes per day since childhood.

Family history: He has a positive family history with a brother and sister having acute MI episodes at age 64 and 72 years, respectively.

Socioeconomic history: The patient is a retired (since 6 years) office manager. He lives with his wife, son, daughter-in-law, and two granddaughters and comes from an upper-middle-class family.

Investigations: Chest radiograph revealed no significantly abnormal findings. CT angiography revealed 90% occlusion in right coronary and 85% occlusion in anterior descending and circumflex arteries. Echocardiogram reveals ventricular dysfunction and a LVEF of 50%. ECG reveals sinus rhythm with a normal heart rate and ST segment depression.

Physical examination: Heart rate and respiratory rate were found to be 106 beats/min and 24 breaths/min, respectively, blood pressure was 100/68 mm Hg, and SpO_2 was 99%. Pulmonary assessment and heart sound auscultation revealed normal findings.

Surgical details: The patient was treated with bypass grafting for all the three arteries with saphenous vein graft under general anesthesia. The patient is currently on day 2 post surgery.

Guiding Questions:
1. What would be the therapist's approach regarding the assessment of the patient?
2. List the possible complications that might occur at this stage.
3. Plan a rehabilitation protocol for this patient during his stay at the hospital and immediately after discharge.

Review Questions

1. How will you evaluate a 67-year-old male presenting with chest pain? What will be the course of management for the same?
2. Explain the risk factors and pathophysiology of coronary artery disease in detail.
3. Describe the diagnostic procedures used for IHD.
4. Explain the pharmacological management of IHD.
5. How does IHD impact the exercise performance of an individual?
6. Explain cardiac rehabilitation in detail.

BIBLIOGRAPHY

1. American College of Sports Medicine. ACSM's guidelines to exercise testing and prescription, 9th edition. LWW; 2014.
2. Anderson L, Oldridge N, Thompson DR, et al. Exercise-Based Cardiac Rehabilitation for Coronary Heart Disease: Cochrane Systematic Review and Meta-Analysis. J Am Coll Cardiol. 2016;67(1):1-12.
3. Belardinelli R, Paolini I, Cianci G, et al. Exercise training intervention after coronary angioplasty: the ETICA trial. J Am Coll Cardiol. 2001;37(7):1891-900.
4. Bohm M, Ukena C. Heart rate responses to exercise: Impact on myocardial ischemia and left ventricular function. Medicographia. 2012;34:395-9.
5. Borg G. Borg's perceived exertion and pain scales. Champaign, IL: Human Kinetics; 1998.
6. Cole CR, Foody JM, Blackstone EH, et al. Heart rate recovery after submaximal exercise testing as a predictor of mortality in a cardiovascularly healthy cohort. Ann Intern Med. 2000;132(7):552-5.
7. Foster C, Cadwell K, Crenshaw B, et al. Physical activity and exercise training prescriptions for patients. Cardiol Clin. 2001;19(3):447-57.
8. Foster C, Porcari JP, Battista RA, et al. The Risk in Exercise Training. Am J Lifestyle. Med. 2008;2(4): 279-84.
9. Foster C, Porcari JP, Cadwell K et al. Ischaemic cardiovascular disease, Clinical Exercise Physiology: Application and Physiological Principles, LWW; 2004. pp. 29-41.
10. Franklin B. ACSM's exercise management for persons with chronic diseases and disabilities. 3rd edition; 2009:pp.49-65.
11. Gupta R, Mohan I, Narula J. Trends in Coronary Heart Disease Epidemiology in India. Ann Glob Health. 2016;82(2):307-15.
12. Hambrecht R1, Walther C, Möbius-Winkler S, et al. Percutaneous coronary angioplasty compared with exercise training in patients with stable coronary artery disease: a randomized trial. Circulation. 2004;109(11):1371-8.
13. Hofmann P, Pokan R, Preidler K, et al. Relationship between heart rate threshold, lactate turn point and myocardial function. Int J Sports Med. 1994;15:232-37.
14. Karimi-Moonaghi H, Mojalli M, Khosravan S. Psychosocial complications of coronary artery disease. Iran Red Crescent Med J. 2014;16(6), e18162.
15. Kulik A, Ruel M, Jneid H, et al. Secondary prevention after coronary artery bypass graft surgery: a scientific statement from the American Heart Association. Circulation. 2015;131(10):927-64.
16. Leon AS, Franking BA, Costa F, et al. Guidelines for cardiac rehabilitation and secondary prevention programs, 3rd edition. Champaign, IL: Human Kinetics: 1999, p. 109.
17. Meyer K, Samek L, Pinchas A, et al. Relationship between ventilatory threshold and onset of ischemia in ECG during stress testing. Eur Heart J. 1995;16:623-30.
18. Myers J, Goebbels U, Dzeikan G, et al. Exercise training and myocardial remodeling in patients with reduced ventricular function: one year follow up with MRI. Am Heart J. 2000;139:252-61.
19. Ornish D, Scherwitz LW, Billings JH, et al. Intensive lifestyle changes for reversal of coronary heart disease. JAMA. 1998;280:2001-7.
20. Prabhakaran D, Jeemon P, Roy A. Cardiovascular diseases in India: current epidemiology and future directions. Circulation. 2016;133(16):1605-20.
21. Sattelmair J, Pertman J, Ding EL, et al. Dose response between physical activity and risk of CAD: a meta-analysis. Circulation. 2011;124:789-95.
22. Schonhr P, Marott JL, Jensen JS, et al. Intensity versus duration of cycling, impact on all cause and CHD mortality. Eur J Prevcardiol. 2012;19:73-80.
23. Taylor R, Brown A, Ebrahim S, et al. Exercise based rehabilitation for patients with CAD: systematic review and meta-analysis of RCTs. Am J Med. 2004;116:682-92.
24. Wenger NK, Froelicher ES, Smith LK, et al. Cardiac rehabilitation. Clinical practice guideline no 17, 1995.

Chronic Obstructive Pulmonary Disease

Neepa H Pandya

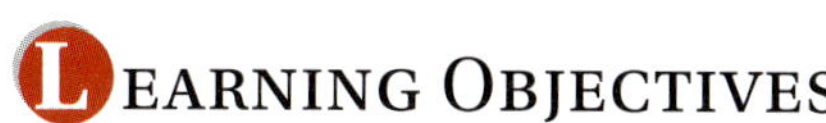LEARNING OBJECTIVES

After reading this chapter, the readers should be able to:

♦ Describe the etiology, classification, pathophysiology, and diagnosis of chronic obstructive pulmonary disease (COPD)
♦ Describe the medical and surgical management of COPD
♦ Describe the assessment of a patient having COPD
♦ Identify the goals and outcomes of pulmonary rehabilitation (PR)
♦ Learn to manage acute exacerbation episodes in COPD
♦ Determine the impact of COPD on exercise performance and learn about the benefits of exercise training in COPD
♦ Understand pulmonary rehabiliation of a patient with COPD
♦ Describe and manage the psychosocial issues associated with COPD.

CHAPTER OUTLINE

- Respiratory anatomy
- Respiratory physiology
- Risk factors
- Classification
- Pathophysiology
- Diagnosis
  - Clinical presentation
  - Spirometry
  - Other tests
- Impairments associated with chronic obstructive pulmonary disease
  - Impairments of ventilation
- Impairments of gas exchange
- Cardiovascular impairments
- Impairments of muscular function
- Pathophysiology of muscular dysfunction
- Other impairments
- Management
  - Medical management
  - Surgical management
- Pulmonary rehabilitation
  - Assessment
  - Management of acute exacerbations
- Management of dyspnea
- Secretion removal techniques
- Exercise training
- Outcomes of pulmonary rehabilitation
- Psychosocial issues in chronic obstructive pulmonary disease

OVERVIEW

Chronic obstructive pulmonary disease (COPD) is the fourth leading cause of death globally and results in poor health-related quality of life (HRQOL), loss of productivity and increased financial burden. COPD is marked by progressive airway obstruction in chronic bronchitis and alveolar destruction in emphysema presenting as debilitating dyspnea and various degrees of physical activity intolerance. Eventually, this proceeds to systemic involvement largely to compensate for respiratory changes culminating into multiorgan dysfunction. About 80% of COPD is caused by active and passive smoking along with occupational and indoor pollution. Owing to a large reserve of pulmonary system, patients remain asymptomatic for a considerable period, presenting with irreversible pulmonary changes later on.

RESPIRATORY ANATOMY

The skeleton of the pulmonary system comprises the thoracic cage which consists of 12 pairs of ribs, 12 thoracic vertebrae, sternum, and the costal cartilages. The respiratory pathway can be divided into an upper and a lower respiratory pathway. The upper respiratory pathway comprises the nose, pharynx, and larynx, whereas the lower respiratory pathway comprises the tracheobronchial tree. The tracheobronchial tree can be further divided

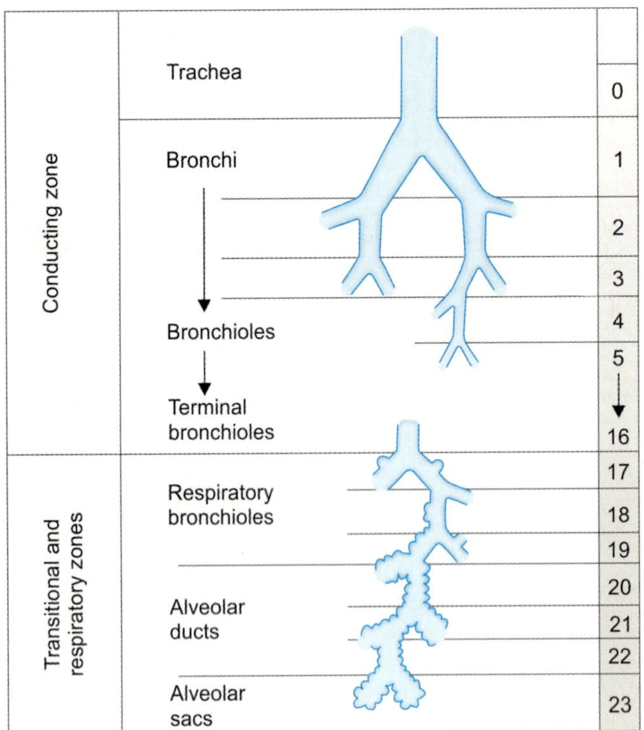

Fig. 16.1: Tracheobronchial tree.

into—a nonrespiratory conducting pathway (trachea, bronchi, and bronchioles) and the respiratory unit. There are approximately 23 generations (divisions) of bronchi in the human airway **(Fig. 16.1)**.

- First four generations: Main, lobar, and segmental bronchi
- Fifth to seventh generation: Subsegmental bronchi
- Eighth to twelfth generation: Bronchioles—conducting
- Twelfth to sixteenth generation: Terminal bronchioles—pathways
- Seventeenth to nineteenth generation: Respiratory bronchioles
- Twentieth to twenty-second generation: Alveolar ducts
- Twenty-third generation: Alveolar sacs.

The lungs are the organs where the respiration actually occurs. The lungs are divided into lobes—upper, middle, and lower for the right lung and upper, lower, and lingula for the left lung. Each lobe of the lung is divided into bronchopulmonary segments—10 for the right lung and 8 for the left lung. The acinus forms the functional unit of the lungs. The acinus is formed by the respiratory bronchioles, alveolar ducts, alveolar sacs, and the alveoli. Each lung is covered by a thin double-layered membrane called the pleura. Pleural fluid is present between the two layers of pleura (parietal and visceral layers) to allow frictionless movement of the lungs.

RESPIRATORY PHYSIOLOGY

During breathing, air moves from the nose or the mouth, through the conducting airways to reach the distal respiratory unit which comprises the respiratory

bronchiole, alveolar ducts, alveolar sacs, and alveoli. This movement of air from the nose or mouth through the conducting pathways is known as ventilation. The gas exchange that occurs within the body is termed as respiration. It can be internal or external. External respiration is the gaseous exchange that occurs through the alveolar capillary membrane between the atmospheric air in the alveoli and the pulmonary capillaries. Internal respiration refers to the gaseous exchange at the cellular level between the capillaries and the cells of various tissues in the body. The process of respiration is described in **Figure 16.2.**

RISK FACTORS

Incidence of COPD is proportional to long-term cumulative exposure to noxious gases and particles. Global Initiative for Chronic Obstructive Lung Disease (GOLD) describes the followings as the risk factors for COPD:

1. **Tobacco smoke**: Cigarette, pipe, cigar, water pine, *bidi*, and other types of tobacco smoking in various countries. Environmental tobacco smoking also increases incidence of COPD.

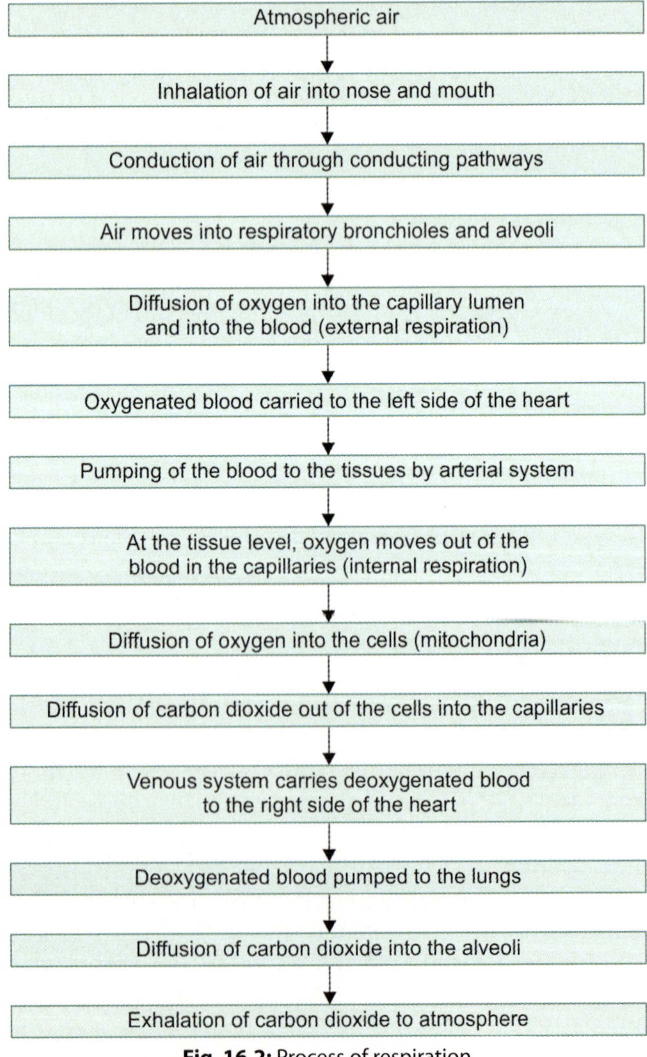

Fig. 16.2: Process of respiration.

2. **Indoor air pollution**: Biomass fuel used for cooking in poorly ventilated spaces.
3. **Occupational exposures**: Organic and inorganic dusts, chemical agents and fumes.
4. **Outdoor air pollution**: Though it appears to have a smaller effect on development of COPD, it increases the load on the lungs.
5. **Genetic factors**: Severe deficiency of alpha-1 antitrypsin.
6. **Age and sex**: Aging and female gender increase risk for COPD.
7. **Socioeconomic status**: Risk of developing COPD is more due to exposure to air pollutants, crowding, poor nutrition and infections.
8. **Asthma and airway hyperreactivity**: Airflow limitation induced by bronchoconstriction puts patients at a risk of COPD.
9. **Chronic bronchitis**: Increases frequency and intensity of exacerbations.
10. **Infections**: History of severe childhood respiratory infection is associated with reduced lung function and increased respiratory symptoms in adulthood.

CLASSIFICATION

The GOLD (Global Initiative for Obstructive Lung Disease) classification of severity of COPD is based on post bronchodilator spirometric values **(Table 16.1)**.

PATHOPHYSIOLOGY

Chronic bronchitis is a long-lasting inflammation of the bronchi caused by prolonged irritation of the bronchial mucosa. Diagnosis is based on the presence of cough and sputum production for more than 3 months for 2 consecutive years. This obstruction is confirmed by office spirometry reflecting as reduction in measures of maximal expiratory flow (FEV$_1$, FEF 25–75%). Enlarged mucous secreting glands and an increase in the number of mucous-secreting cells, the goblet cells lining the walls of the airway characterize the disease. These changes are associated with symptoms of chronic cough and increasing mucous expectoration as the disease progresses **(Fig. 16.3)**.

Emphysema is characterized by permanent destruction of gas conducting parts of the airway, the alveoli, and gas exchange units of the lungs. Due to loss of elastin, structure of the alveolar walls and bronchioles are not maintained, and the resultant destruction and collapse are permanent, making airflow difficult and leading to air trapping

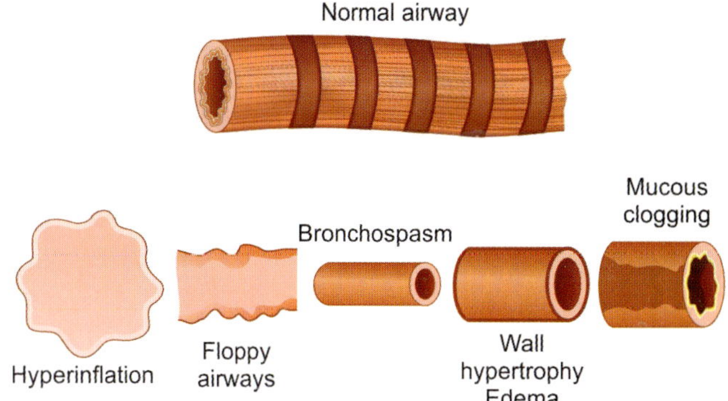

Fig. 16.3: Airway obstruction.

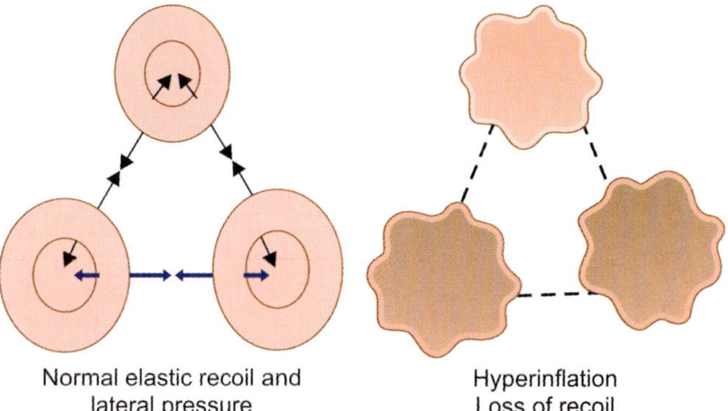

Fig. 16.4: Loss of lateral pressure and elastic recoil.

eventually resulting in hyperinflation. Hyperinflation is reflected in pulmonary function test (PFT) as reduction in forced vital capacity (FVC), increase in residual volume (RV) and functional residual capacity (FRC). This hyperinflation induces high energy cost of breathing and imposes limitations on the ability to increase tidal volume. Thoracic cage is held in inspiratory position at rest to accommodate hyperinflation putting inspiratory muscles at mechanical disadvantage further increasing work of breathing (WOB) **(Fig. 16.4)**.

Both chronic bronchitis and emphysema are progressive especially in the presence of irritants such as smoking. The airway irritation in chronic bronchitis leads to a chronic inflammatory process that can progress to emphysema. As emphysema progresses, increasing amount of lung tissue is destroyed and patient has to depend on external oxygen for exercise, activities of daily living (ADL), and eventually at rest. Smoking cessation halts the progress of the disease but existing lung destruction is irreversible. **Figure 16.5** explains the course of the disease and compensation by other systems.

BODE [**b**ody mass index (BMI), airflow **o**bstruction, **d**yspnea, **e**xercise capacity] index **(Table 16.2)** and its modification developed by Celli et al. effectively predict 5 years' survival in patients with airway obstruction. It derives prediction from amount of obstruction, MMRC (**M**odified **M**edical **R**esearch **C**ouncil) dyspnea scale, BMI, and degree of exercise tolerance on 6-minute walk test (6-MWT).

Table 16.1: GOLD severity staging system.		
Stage	Severity	Post bronchodilator FEV$_1$ % predicted
1.	Mild	≥80%
2.	Moderate	50% ≤FEV$_1$<80%
3.	Severe	30%≤FEV$_1$<50%
4.	Very severe	<30%

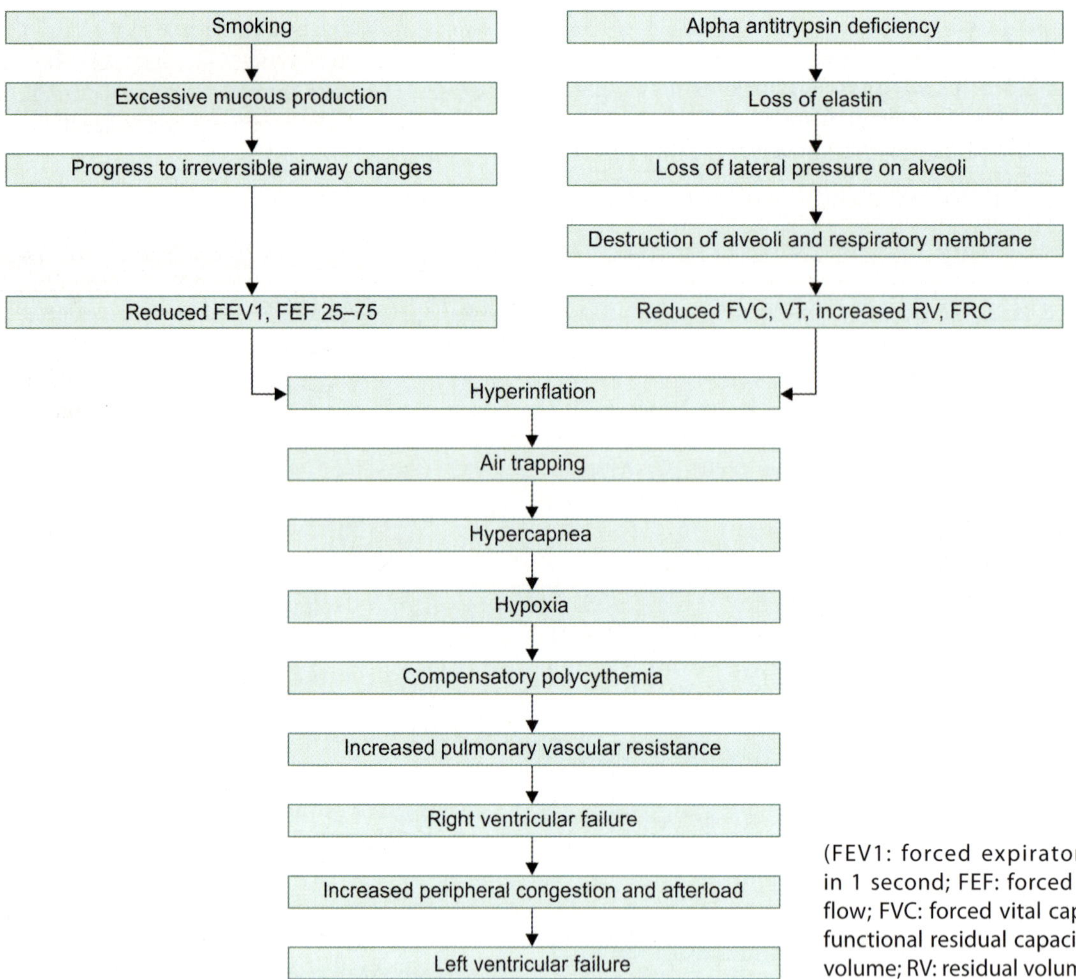

Fig. 16.5: Course of the disease.

Table 16.2: Body mass index (BMI), airflow obstruction, dyspnea, exercise capacity index.

Variable	Points			
	0	1	2	3
BMI (kg/m^2)	<21	≥ 21		
FEV1% predicted	≥65	50–64	36–49	≤35
Dyspnea MMRC scale	0–1	2	3	4
Walk distance (6-MWT) (m)	≥350	250–349	150–249	≤149

(6-MWT: 6-minute walk test; MMRC: Modified Medical Research Council)

Table 16.3: Distinguishing features between chronic obstructive pulmonary disease (COPD) and asthma.

	COPD	Asthma
Current smoker or ex-smoker	Almost always	May be possible
Age <35 years	Infrequent	Frequent
Chronic productive cough	Common	Uncommon
Dyspnea	Persistent and progressive	Variable
Paroxysmal nocturnal dyspnea	Common	Uncommon

DIAGNOSIS

The diagnosis of COPD is suspected based on the clinical presentation and examination findings and confirmed by means of spirometry. Asthma forms the principal differential diagnosis and can be ruled out based on the clinical examination findings **(Table 16.3)**.

Clinical Presentation

COPD is considered in patients around 40 years of age with complaints of chronic cough and/or persistent dyspnea that is progressive in nature and increases with physical exercise along with exposure to risk factors mentioned above. Other clinical findings such as wheeze, sputum production, and frequent exacerbations during winter and seasonal episodes might be present along with dyspnea and chronic cough. The patient may appear cachexic in severe cases.

Physical examination may occasionally reveal a barrel-shaped chest (increased anterior–posterior diameter) due to loss of lung elastic recoil and hyperinflation. There is reduced thoracic excursion and an increased WOB.

BOX 16.1: Cricosternal distance.

- It is the distance between the cricoid cartilage and suprasternal notch, measured by fingers.
- The normal distance is 3–4 fingers. If the distance is <3 fingers, it suggests lung hyperinflation. However, this measure is less reliable since the size of the fingers varies between individuals.

Hypertrophy of the muscles of ventilation is observed. The length–tension relationship of the ventilator muscles is altered as a result of chronic hyperinflation. Paradoxical movement of the lower ribs may be seen in severe cases due to flattening of the diaphragm and change in alignment of its fibers. Reduction of the cricosternal distance on examination and reduction of cardiac dullness on percussion will be present **(Box 16.1)**.

Auscultation will reveal the presence of wheeze due to obstructed bronchi and bronchioles. Crackles may be heard as well due to the presence of secretions. The patient may exhibit pursed lip breathing. In advanced stages of COPD, cyanosis and clubbing may also be seen.

Spirometry

Spirometry is fundamental to the diagnosis of COPD. Diagnosis is confirmed by office spirometry that indicates $FEV_1/FVC<70\%$ post bronchodilator administration suggesting persistent airflow limitation. FEV_1 is <80% of the predicted volume. RV and FRC are increased. Though the diagnosis is confirmed by spirometry, due to weak correlation between FEV_1 and patients' impairments, symptomatic assessment along with evaluation of comorbidities must be undertaken. In general, the PFT will conclude air trapping, increased midexpiratory time, and low work and normal or increased lung compliance.

Other Tests

Sputum culture may be done to exclude other infective pathologies or confirm the presence of infection. Serial home peak flow measurements can be done if diagnostic doubt related to asthma persists. In the case of a history of hypertension, cardiac disorder or hypoxia or if clinical signs such as tachycardia, edema, and cyanosis are present, electrocardiography or echocardiography can be done.

Chest X-ray findings in chronic bronchitis are nonspecific. Increased bronchovascular markings and cardiomegaly may be seen. An emphysema chest X-ray may show signs of lung hyperinflation such as flattened diaphragm, reduced size of the heart, and occasionally bullous changes. Increased anteroposterior diameter of the chest may be seen on the lateral view. Computed tomography (CT) scan is also done in COPD cases to exclude other differential diagnoses. CT scan in chronic bronchitis may show bronchial wall thickening and scarring with fibrosis and bronchovascular irregularity. CT scan in emphysema may show destruction of the alveolar

septum and subsequent enlargement of the airspace. Centrilobular emphysema is seen in the upper lobes, whereas panacinar emphysema is seen in the lower lobes.

Series of arterial blood gas analysis exhibits progressive hypercapnea and later on development of hypoxia as the disease progresses.

IMPAIRMENTS ASSOCIATED WITH CHRONIC OBSTRUCTIVE PULMONARY DISEASE

As the disease advances, there is an involvement of various systems, leading to progressive limitation of physical activity and development of dyspnea **(Figs. 16.6A and B)**.

Impairments of Ventilation

Impairments of ventilation include:

- Increased airway resistance, expiratory flow obstruction
- Reduced elastic recoil, air trapping, hyperinflation
- Increased WOB to overcome airway resistance
- Mechanical disadvantage of respiratory muscles
- Increased dead space and dead space ventilation (VD)/tidal ventilation ratio
- Ventilatory muscle fatigue

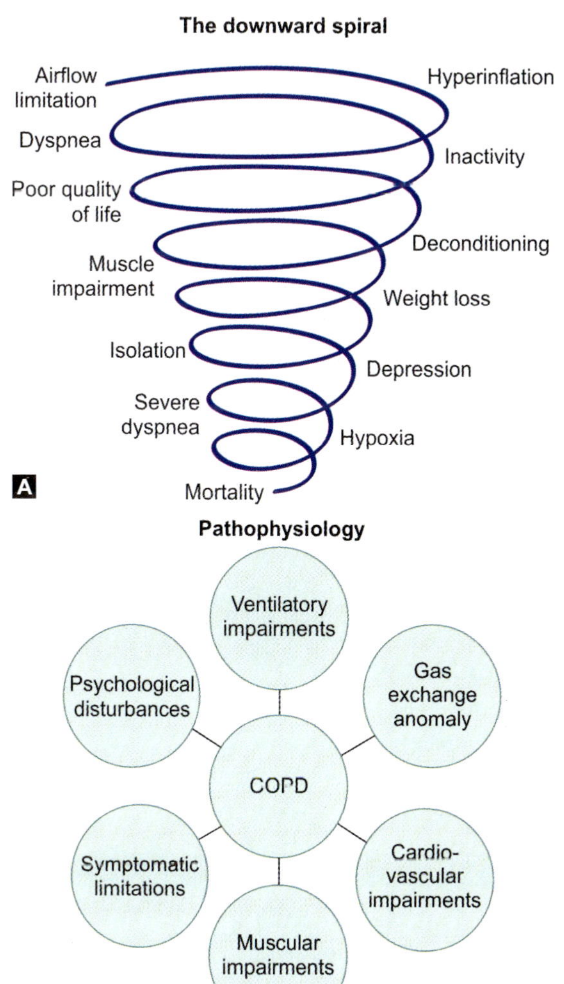

Figs. 16.6A and B: (A) Dyspnea spiral; (B) Impairments associated with COPD.

- Ventilatory failure with inadequate alveolar ventilation, hypoxia, and hypercapnia.

Impairments of Gas Exchange

Impairments of gas exchange are as follows:
- Chronic bronchitis causes ventilation perfusion inequality
- Emphysema destructs alveolar–capillary membrane, increases dead space and loss of diffusing capacity
- High V/Q (ventilation/perfusion) anomaly: Increased alveolar dead space, increased ventilator requirement, and WOB
- Low V/Q anomaly: Venous admixture causing hypoxia that worsens during exercise.

Cardiovascular Impairments

Cardiovascular impairments include:
- Hypoxia
- Destruction of capillary bed
- Reflex pulmonary vasoconstriction
- Increased pulmonary vascular resistance.

Impairments of Muscular Function

Causes of impairments of muscular function:
- Reduced physical activity
- Tobacco use
- Inflammation
- Chronic use of corticosteroids
- Low levels of anabolic hormones
- Nutritional depletion
- Reduced amino acid metabolism
- Hypoxia and hypercapnia.

Pathophysiology of Muscular Dysfunction

Pathophysiology of muscular dysfunction is as follows:
- Reduced aerobic capacity
- Shift from type I to type II fibers
- Reduced mitochondrial and capillary density
- Reduced oxidative enzymes
- Increased intramuscular fat content
- Disuse atrophy, reduced cross-sectional area
- Other—Malnutrition, age, hypoxia, medications
- Progressive deconditioning associated with dyspnea.

Other Impairments

Other impairments include:
- Chronic anxiety
- Depression
- Social isolation.

MANAGEMENT

Management of COPD is aimed at:
- Reduction in breathlessness
- Increase in exercise capacity
- Skeletal muscle strengthening
- Improvement in HRQOL.

Secondary aims are:
- Prevention and treatment of exacerbations
- Slow disease progression
- Prolong survival.

The management of COPD includes the following components:
- Assessment and monitoring the disease
- Reduction of risk factors
- Management of stable COPD
- Management of acute exacerbations.

COPD should be diagnosed as previously discussed in the chapter. The risk factors associated with the disease should be tried to be eliminated or the exposure should be reduced. Exposure of tobacco, occupational dusts, air pollutants, chemicals, etc. should be reduced as much as possible. Management of stable COPD can incorporate a step-wise incremental approach based on the severity of the condition. Health education can improve the patient's ability to cope with the illness and aid in accomplishing the goal of smoking cessation. Management of acute exacerbations usually requires medical interventions and mechanical ventilation.

Medical Management

Medical management in COPD comprises patient education, smoking cessation, pharmacological therapy, and supplemental oxygen administration.

Education

It is the responsibility of the primary care physician as well as the other medical professionals involved in the rehabilitation of the patient with COPD, to educate the patient and their family about the condition through written information at the time of diagnosis. They should be guided to a healthcare professional who may be specializing in the area and may have more experience. The information provided should cover an explanation about COPD and its symptoms, advice regarding smoking cessation, avoiding passive smoke exposure and other risk factors, management of dyspnea, and the benefits of physical activity and pulmonary rehabilitation (PR). The importance of adherence to medication regime and the complications of the disease should be explained to the patient and the caregivers. Pneumococcal and influenza vaccination should be offered to people with COPD to reduce the rate of infection. Self-management techniques for management of acute exacerbation episodes should be taught to the patient. Management strategies include adjustment of the short-acting bronchodilator used by the patient to treat their symptoms, short course of oral corticosteroids, addition of oral antibiotics in case of change in sputum color, volume or thickness, and consulting their health care professional. If the patient complains of anxiety and depression symptoms, a cognitive–behavioral component should be added to their self-management plan. For patients at risk of hospitalization, the family members should be explained about the need of hospitalization and what is to be expected then.

Smoking Cessation

As discussed earlier, smoking forms a major contributor in the development of COPD. Smoking cessation is the most therapeutic and cost-effective management strategy to reduce the risk of developing COPD and reducing the rate of progression. Tobacco-dependence treatments are an extremely effective means of smoking cessation. Studies have demonstrated that smoking cessation leads to better lung function and better survival rates in COPD patients. It improves QOL and symptoms and also reduces hospital stay and hospitalization. Practical counseling and the use of social support as part of treatment and outside treatment are effective forms of counseling. COPD patients exhibit a higher resistance to smoking cessation than smokers not having any associated pathologies due to higher dependence on smoking, higher number of pack years and older age. They are at a higher risk of developing depressive symptoms, and hence, chances of success are less and relapse rate may be higher.

Two types of smoking cessation strategies can be used: Pharmacological strategies and psychosocial interventions.

1. **Pharmacological strategies** include nicotine replacement therapy (NRT) and nonnicotine replacement drugs such as bupropion, nortriptyline, and varenicline. NRT can be prescribed in the form of nasal or oral spray, lozenge/tablet, patches, gum or inhaler. The pharmacological agents help in controlling the withdrawal symptoms and the craving and urge to have nicotine.

2. **Psychological interventions** include self-aid materials, brief interventions delivered by therapists, group therapy, individual counseling, or a combination of all approaches. Regular monitoring of cigarette use and affective states should be done. Long-term psychological interventions can promote abstinence for longer periods. Face-to-face counseling sessions are more beneficial than telephonic counseling sessions. Individual sessions or group therapy sessions can be continued once a week for at least 4 weeks after the quit attempt. A "make every contact count" approach (a large-scale behavioral change program) should be adopted as it reaches more number of people, creating a healthier population and improving health outcomes. The "Five A's" five-step program can be used to guide healthcare professionals working in the field of smoking cessation **(Table 16.4)** [Agency for Healthcare Research and Quality website. Five major steps to intervention (The "Five A's")].

The use of electronic cigarettes or E-cigarettes (EC) in the form of NRT and as an alternative to cigarette smoking has become increasingly popular in the recent years. Several researchers have studied and concluded the use of ECs to be

Table 16.4: The "Five A's."	
1. Ask	Identification of all tobacco users at each visit
2. Advise	Strong urge using a clear and personalized approach to all tobacco users to quit
3. Assess	Determination of the patient's willingness to quit
4. Assist	Aiding the patient by helping them form a quit plan and providing pharmacotherapy and counseling
5. Arrange	Scheduling a follow-up meeting

beneficial in ameliorating the effects of COPD and cigarette smoking. ECs have proven to be a beneficial smoking substitute as they are less harmful than tobacco smoke and they maintain a smoking experience without actually smoking, hence reducing withdrawal symptoms. However, more recent studies have concluded that EC smoke exposure can lead to inflammation, emphysema and increased vulnerability toward development of viral and bacterial infections. EC aerosols tend to increase interleukin-8 production in primary airway smooth muscle cells regardless of their nicotine concentration, leading to stimulation of lung neutrophilic inflammation, much similar to cigarette smoke. The decision to use ECs as an alternative to cigarettes should be made cautiously. Complete smoking cessation using other forms of NRT and behavior therapy is always a better choice than using EC. If however, the patient keeps relapsing, the use of ECs may be considered. Conclusively, the effectiveness and safety of EC are uncertain.

Pharmacological Management

It is generally the first line of management. Pharmacological management reduces symptoms and the frequency and severity of exacerbations; it improves the health status and exercise capacity. It usually involves the administration of bronchodilators, corticosteroids and other medications such as methylxanthines and phosphodiesterase type-4 inhibitors **(Table 16.5)**.

Acute exacerbations are treated with corticosteroids, short-acting bronchodilators, antibiotics, and supplemental oxygen. Use of inhalers is extremely common among COPD patients. However, the choice of inhaler device should be individually tailored. The importance of education and training in the use of the inhaler device should be stressed enough. Patient should be given appropriate instructions and demonstration of the use of the inhaler device. During acute exacerbations nebulizers are preferred over inhalers and oxygen is used with caution as a driving gas. Other pharmacologic treatments for COPD include alpha-1 antitrypsin augmentation therapy, antitussives, and vasodilators.

Supplemental Oxygen

Long-term administration of oxygen therapy (>15 h/day) in patients with chronic respiratory failure increases the survival in patients with severe hypoxemia at rest. It

Table 16.5: Commonly used drugs in management of chronic obstructive pulmonary disease.

Drug	Comments	Side effects
β-agonists	Short acting, serves as emergency medication	Peripheral vasodilatation, increased heart rate Skeletal muscle tremor Increased insulin, free fatty acid (FFA) Decreased PaO_2, myocardial necrosis
Theophylline	Long acting, sustained bronchodilatation over 24 h	Headache, seizures, cerebral vasoconstriction, gastrointestinal (GI) irritation, myocardial irritability
Anticholinergic	More sustained effect as an additive measure	Uncommon in therapeutic doses Dry mouth
Anti-inflammatory		Hypothalamic-pituitary-adrenal axis suppression Centripetal obesity Muscle atrophy Osteoporosis Hypertension
Cromolyn	Decreases airway reactivity Inhibits immunoglobulin E (IgE) dependent histamine release from lungs	GI irritation Increased cough Headache Dermatitis
Antibiotics	Used for acute exacerbations	Anaphylactic shock, urticaria, GI irritation
Expectorants	Breaks down polymeric structure of mucous	Severe bronchospasm if not accompanied by a bronchodilator

does not lengthen the time to death or the time to first hospitalization or provide any beneficial effects in the case of stable COPD or patients having resting or exercise-induced moderate arterial oxygen levels.

Ventilator support is provided during acute exacerbations or even in the case of stable COPD patients and in those having obstructive sleep apnea (OSA). Acute exacerbations and acute respiratory failure are managed with noninvasive ventilation (NIV) in the form of noninvasive positive pressure ventilation to reduce morbidity and mortality rates. Stable COPD and OSA are managed with continuous positive airway pressure.

Surgical Management

Surgical management is reserved for patients not responsive to pharmacological management. Surgical interventions include **(Table 16.6)**:

Table 16.6: Interventional therapy in chronic obstructive pulmonary disease (COPD).

Procedure	Details
Lung volume reduction surgery	Improves survival in severe upper lobe emphysema patients with low postrehabilitation exercise capacity
Bullectomy	Decreases dyspnea, improves lung function and exercise tolerance
Transplantation	In appropriately selected severe COPDs lung transplantation improves QOL and functional capacity
Bronchoscopic interventions	Reduce FRC, improve exercise tolerance, health status and lung function following 6–12 months of treatment

(FRC: functional residual capacity; QOL: quality of life)

- Bronchoscopic lung volume reduction (BLVR)
- Lung volume reduction surgery (LVRS)
- Bullectomy
- Total lung transplantation.

Bronchoscopic Lung Volume Reduction

Even though LVRS has been an established surgical approach in COPD, especially in upper lobe emphysema associated with significant air trapping and hyperinflation, it has a considerable rate of mortality and morbidity. Bronchoscopic techniques which are minimally invasive have provided a safer alternative with reduced surgical morbidity. They aim to close the airways to the hyperinflated regions so that no gas enters the region and the air already present there is reabsorbed over a period of days or weeks. Three approaches exist for BLVR:

1. Lung sealant
2. One-way endobronchial valve (EBV) or intrabronchial valve
3. Endobronchial coils.

EBVs and coils have better therapeutic outcomes and are considerably efficacious in patients remaining symptomatic with maximal medical therapy but not likely to tolerate or benefit from LVRS.

Lung sealant surgeries involve inserting biologically active reagents into peripheral airways. It acts as a tissue glue that seals the target area and causes permanent atelectasis. The procedure involves removal of dead emphysematous tissue and replacing it with an organized scar, thus making the procedure irreversible.

Similar to LVRS, EBVs aim to remove the less-functional and hyperinflated areas of the emphysematous lung. It is a one-way valve that allows expiration of air and expulsion of secretions from the treated area but does not allow reinflation. It reduces the lobar volume and eventually leads to full lobar collapse. This reduces the lung hyperinflation and improves dyspnea, exercise capacity and QOL. The intrabronchial valve also works on similar principles, but it is made of a nickel–titanium alloy wire frame, unlike the EBV which is made of a wire mesh and a lumen that has a one way valve.

Endobronchial coils are nitinol (nickel–titanium alloy) coils, approximately 10–15 cm in length. They are placed via bronchoscopy, and they are specially designed to regain their shape after deployment as they exhibit a shape memory effect. They compress the emphysematous tissue and improve the lung mechanics and elasticity of the adjacent lung tissue. The compression of the lung tissue by the coils results in reduced hyperinflation of the affected part and a reduction in the lung volume through better transmission of the elastic recoil pressure. Reduction in the airflow to the affected part of the lung causes a redistribution of the airflow to the healthier parts of the lung. It improves lung function and compliance, diaphragm function and leads to an increase in the expiratory pressure and flow.

Lung Volume Reduction Surgery

In the last two and a half decades, LVRS has emerged as an effective treatment option as it offers superior benefits than any medical treatment. It is a surgical procedure of removal of emphysematous lung tissue for the reduction of lung hyperinflation and expansion of the remaining functional lung. It can be done via staged thoracotomy, median sternotomy, or video-assisted thoracic surgery (VATS) either unilaterally or bilaterally. It produces long-term increments in exercise capacity, lung function, QOL, and survival rate. LVRS has the most beneficial outcome in patients with upper lobe emphysema.

Bullectomy

Similar to LVRS, bullectomy can also be done via thoracotomy/sternotomy or VATS. Bullae that usually form in COPD lungs are removed to allow expansion of surrounding healthy tissue. VATS is the more preferred option since it causes lesser pain and morbidity and allows earlier function. Bullectomy, however, would only benefit those having large bullae, as small multiple bullae scattered throughout the lung parenchyma cannot be removed using bullectomy.

Lung Transplantation

Lung transplantation is an effective therapeutic option but it cannot be considered for patients of advanced age and having multiple comorbidities. It is the removal of diseased lung(s) and replacement with new healthy functioning lung(s). But it is difficult to get an organ donor and even if an organ does become available, the patient many times cannot be saved till then. An ideal candidate for lung transplantation is the one who has no other associated major comorbidities and has advanced COPD.

Over 70% of the lung transplants in COPD are double lung transplants. Lung transplantation does improve functional capacity and health, but it does not prolong survival. It is also limited due to the high cost and lesser number of organ donors. Complications include rejection, bronchiolitis obliterans, and infections. Physiotherapy following transplant surgeries is described in Chapter 39.

PULMONARY REHABILITATION

Pulmonary rehabilitation (PR) has shown to be the most effective strategy to improve shortness of breath (SOB), health status, and exercise tolerance **(Box 16.2)**. It is a team approach to improve patients' HRQOL, reduce exacerbations, and effectively manage symptoms. The team comprises a physician, dietician, physiotherapist, occupational therapist, social worker, and psychologist **(Fig. 16.7)**.

PR should be included in the management of every COPD patient who has a dyspnea score of ≥3 on the MRC scale and who is functionally disabled due to the symptoms of COPD. Patients who are not able to walk or have had an episode of acute myocardial infarction or angina pectoris should not be put on PR regimes. PR programs should be individually tailored and should be multicomponent and multidisciplinary. They should include disease education, nutrition advice, physical training, and psychological and behavioral interventions.

A physiotherapist's focus is on:
- Managing dyspnea
- Effective removal of secretions
- Prevent further progression of the disease and acute exacerbations
- Increasing exercise capacity
- Social integration and prevention of isolation.

Assessment

Assessment of the patient having COPD is essential to form an individually tailored PR program. Assessment needs to be done during and at the time of termination as well and not just before commencing the PR program. The assessment, similar to the management, is led by the pulmonary physician. The assessment includes a general interview, past medical history, symptom assessment, physical examination, systems review (especially musculoskeletal and neurological), pain assessment, diagnostic tests,

---

BOX 16.2: Definition of pulmonary rehabilitation.

The American Thoracic Society and European Respiratory Society have defined PR as follows:

"Pulmonary rehabilitation is a comprehensive intervention based on a thorough patient assessment followed by patient tailored therapies that include, but are not limited to, exercise training, education, and behavior change, designed to improve the physical and psychological condition of people with chronic respiratory disease and to promote the long-term adherence to health-enhancing behaviors."

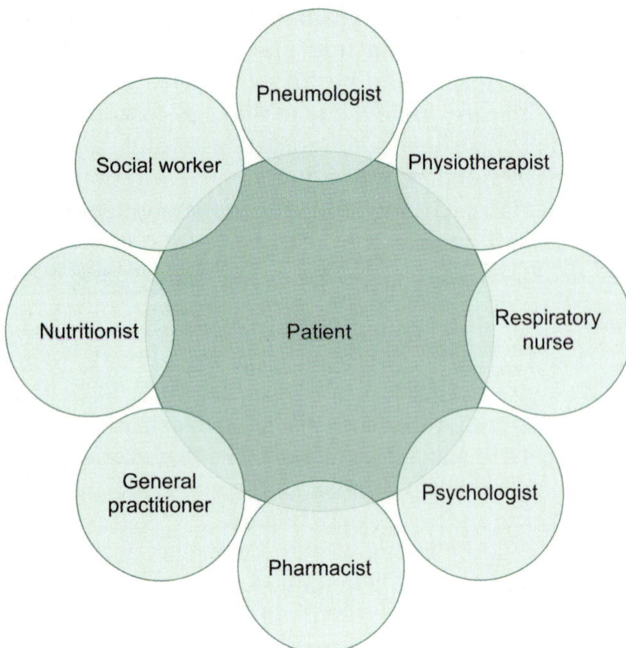

Fig. 16.7: Disciplines involved in pulmonary rehabilitation program.

exercise tolerance testing (ETT), pulmonary function testing, nutritional and psychological evaluations, ADL assessment, and disease-specific questionnaires.

Management of Acute Exacerbations

Exacerbations are acute episodes of worsening of the respiratory symptoms which require additional therapy for management. They negatively impact the health status of the individual, increase rates of hospitalization and disease progression. They are characterized by increased airway inflammation, mucus production, and gas trapping. Acute exacerbations can be classified based on the management required to treat them **(Table 16.7)**.

Exacerbations may be triggered by viral or bacterial infections, air pollutants, ambient temperature, etc. When treating an acute exacerbation, the goal is to minimize the consequences of the current exacerbation and reduce the possibility of subsequent effects. When the patient presents to the emergency room, a preliminary evaluation is performed by the healthcare professional and the decision to hospitalize the patient or not is made. Short-acting β-agonists are primarily given to the patient as bronchodilator. Systemic corticosteroids and antibiotics should also be used as indicated, but not for more than 5–7 days. NIV should be the first mode of ventilation to be used for COPD with acute respiratory failure.

Table 16.7: Classification of acute exacerbations.	
Mild	Treated with SABD alone
Moderate	Treated with SABDs and antibiotics; oral corticosteroids may or may not be administered
Severe	Patient requires hospitalization or visit to emergency room

(SABD: short-acting bronchodilators)

ATS defines dyspnea as *"a subjective experience of breathing discomfort that is comprised of qualitatively distinct sensation that varies in intensity. The experience derives from interactions among multiple psychological, physiological, social and environmental factors and may induce secondary physiological and behavioral changes".*

Management of Dyspnea

Debilitating dyspnea is a very common symptom amongst COPDs of various degrees of obstruction **(Box 16.3)**. The mechanism of development of dyspnea and its relation with deconditioning is discussed earlier in the chapter. While changes in FEV_1 mark the diagnosis of COPD, its poor correlation with physical impairments requires added evaluation of dyspnea—a signal of inadequate ventilation.

From rehabilitation perspective, it is important to evaluate dyspnea during exercise, ADL and 6-MWT as it relates to QOL and influences and predicts general health better than other parameters. **Figure 16.8** shows symptomatic management of dyspnea.

Metabolic load on muscles can be reduced by dose-dependent effect of exercise training, breathing retraining, pharmacological therapy and supplemental oxygen by decreasing central drive and impedance. Ventilatory muscle load can be optimized by:

- Minimizing the use of steroids
- Ventilatory muscle training
- Supplemental oxygen
- Nutrition
- Positioning
- Partial ventilatory support.

Most therapists are well versed with positions and relaxation techniques used to relieve dyspnea. Following

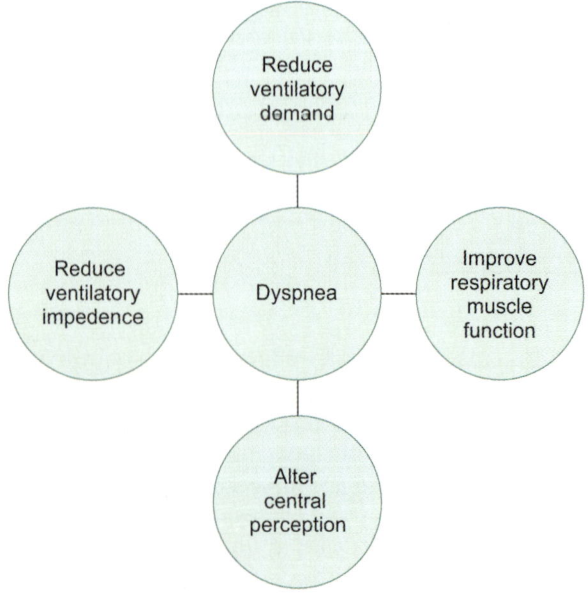

Fig. 16.8: Dyspnea management strategies.

strategies are known to reduce central perception of dyspnea:

- Cognitive–behavioral approaches
- Education
- Self-management of medication regimens
- Monitoring triggers
- Relaxation techniques
- Biofeedback
- Music
- Hypnosis
- Self-talk.

Secretion Removal Techniques

Excessive mucous production and obstruction due to plugging of airways result in increased risk of infection. It is a common modifiable feature in chronic bronchitis. Therefore airway clearance is an important target in management of COPD. External forces in manual or mechanical form loosen secretions, and in combination with gravity-assisted position and breathing methods aid in airway clearance. Most of these can be performed by patient themselves reducing dependence on health professional. Wang observes that efficient use of airway clearance techniques results in favorable outcomes in exacerbations, gas exchange, symptoms, sputum clearance, exercise tolerance and antibiotic use.

Specific techniques are:

- Postural drainage
- Autogenic drainage
- Forced expiratory technique
- Percussion
- Vibrations
- Coughing.

Mechanical aids include:

- Positive expiratory pressure (PEP) mask
- High-frequency chest oscillations
- Oscillatory positive expiratory pressure.

Exercise Training

As there is no cure for COPD, training aims at functional recovery in:

- Increased exercise capacity
- Improvement in muscle strength
- Independence in ADL
- Improved social interaction

- Prevention of progression of disease and episodes of acute exacerbations.

Training of 6–12 weeks at an appropriate intensity aims at increasing VO_2 peak, increase in ventilatory threshold and lactate threshold along with desensitization to dyspnea, efficient breathing pattern and improvement in ADL. Changes induced by aerobic training are sustainable up to 2 years. **Table 16.8** is an example of aerobic training session and **Table 16.9** is an example of strength training that aims at improving ADL, better lean body mass, and increasing the number of repetitions. Arm exercises are often associated with breathlessness in people with COPD. The available data analysis by McKeough suggests a small improvement in breathlessness observed in arm training group compared to the number of training that was not evident comparing arm leg exercise group with combined arm and leg exercise group or arm endurance training.

Exercise Performance in Chronic Obstructive Pulmonary Disease

Reduction in Exercise Capacity

A healthy individual utilizes around 80% of the lung capacity even during heavy exercise. Due to large reserve of respiratory system, limitations in exercise performance are not evident for a long time and patients remain asymptomatic till the entire reserve is exhausted.

Figure 16.9 explains various factors leading to limitations of physical activity. Lung destruction due to hyperinflation leads to air trapping and holds thoracic cage in inflated position. Along with malnutrition and chronic corticosteroid usage, respiratory muscles are at mechanical and metabolic disadvantage and fail to improve ventilation. In response to resultant hypoxia and hypercapnia there is increased respiratory rate with the increase in VD as well as intrapulmonary shunt, worsening chronic hypercapnia and hypoxia, symptomatically presenting as cyanosis. Compromised thoracic musculature cannot meet with this added demand for ventilation that is further compounded during exercise. An extra demand for exercise at this juncture leads to exercise intolerance and exertional dyspnea that leads to demotivation toward physical activity. Thus a compromised ventilatory mechanism and mechanism of gas exchange mentioned earlier in the chapter result in exertional dyspnea and reduction in physical activity. Even in the absence of true ventilatory limitation, exercise

Table 16.8: Aerobic training for chronic obstructive pulmonary disease.

Frequency	Intensity	Time	Type	Comment
1–2 sessions 3–5 days/week	RPE 11–13	30 min session Shorter initially	Walking, cycling, swimming	Monitor dyspnea, supplement O_2 if $SpO_2 < 80\%$

Table 16.9: Strength training in chronic obstructive pulmonary disease.

Frequency	Intensity	Time	Type	Comments
2–3 days/week	Low resistance, high repetition	–	Free weights, isokinetic machines	Incorporate in activities of daily living

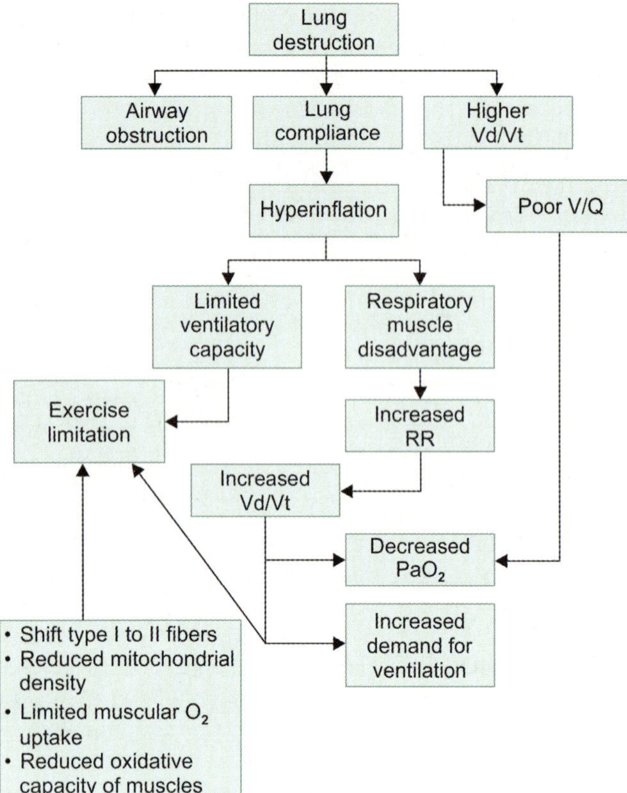

Fig. 16.9: Exercise limitation in chronic obstructive pulmonary disease.. (Vd: volume of dead space; Vt: tidal volume; V/Q: ventilation/perfusion ratio; RR: respiratory rate)

can be limited by physical deconditioning, cardiovascular impairments and reduced pulmonary blood flow in response to hypoxia. Deconditioned muscles accumulate lactic acid at relatively low work rates and increase CO_2 output due to bicarbonate buffering thereby increasing ventilatory demand. Peripheral muscle atrophy, reduced capillary density, increased intramuscular fat content and reduced oxidative capacity due to shift from type I to type II fibers, reduced mitochondrial density and reduced mitochondrial biogenesis proceed to reduced peripheral oxygen extraction and activity limitation. Prolonged rest and progressive reduction in activity lead to further deconditioning augmenting dyspnea at smaller workloads. This sets in a vicious cycle between physical inactivity and breathlessness.

This cycle leads to more rest, reduced social interaction, reduced ADL and recreational activities in a patient leading to social isolation and depression along with relevant anxiety about chronic disease.

Benefits of Exercise Training

Existing lung destruction and pulmonary dysfunction in COPD are irreversible, limiting the effect of exercise training, while the effect of exercise training is more attributed to peripheral changes than central. Peak O_2 delivery during training does not increase with endurance training, while there are significant improvements in O_2 extraction and cellular bioenergetics. However,

exercise-induced muscular changes are much smaller compared to age-matched controls as observed by Sala. A study by Rochester suggests that any level of physical activity results in favorable improvements in oxygen utilization, work capacity, and anxiety. While both low- and high-intensity exercises lead to increased exercise endurance; gains in aerobic fitness are observed only in high-intensity training (**Box 16.4**).

Exercise Prescription

Exercise prescription incorporates four variables—mode, frequency, intensity, and duration. During exercise, it is vital to monitor the heart rate, respiratory rate, rate of perceived exertion (RPE), oxygen saturation, and blood pressure. If the oxygen saturation falls below 90%, supplemental oxygen may be required.

Exercise Mode

Various modes of exercises are available for COPD patients, e.g., walking (walking on a treadmill, a track, supported walking using a walker, etc.), cycling, swimming, rowing, aerobic dance exercises, step exercise, strength training, and arm ergometry. Aerobic exercises involving the lower extremities, viz. walking, cycling, are used more often than others since they are more functional. A combination of upper and lower extremity training provides better outcomes than anyone alone. A combination of aerobic and strength training known as *circuit training* can also be utilized as it gives a wholesome improvement in function and endurance. In more severe, debilitated patients, interval training is a better choice. Interval training consists of several bouts of short high-intensity exercise periods alternated with low-to-moderate intensity exercise periods used for recovery. Whatever form of exercise is chosen, it is vital to include a warm-up and cool-down period to avoid musculoskeletal injuries and other complications that may arise, such as arrhythmias, orthostatic hypotension, and bronchospasm.

Exercise Frequency

The frequency of an exercise session in COPD patients may vary from three to five times a week to once or twice daily sessions. The frequency depends on the intensity that can be achieved by the patient and the duration for which it can be maintained. A lower frequency is used for patients who are more stable [patients who can exercise for 20–30 minutes within the target heart rate (THR)]. A higher frequency of exercise training (once or twice daily) is used for patients who have low and very low functional abilities. With a frequency of 2–3 sessions per week, a minimum of two sessions should be supervised. The whole rehabilitation program can be continued for 6–8 or 4–12 weeks depending on the severity of the condition.

Exercise Duration

Exercise duration carries more significance in COPDs than exercise intensity. The goal should be achieving 20–30 minutes of continuous exercise at the set intensity. However, if such durations cannot be obtained (like in the case of severe COPD), the patient should be allowed to pace himself or take intermittent rest period to achieve a total duration of 20–30 minutes.

Exercise Intensity

Exercise intensity can be prescribed using four parameters—oxygen consumption, heart rate reserve, rating of perceived exertion, and as a factor of the peak workload.

ETT gives the functional capacity of the individual as a measure of the maximal oxygen consumption. For patients with mild-to-moderate disease, a moderate or moderate-to-vigorous intensity can be prescribed **(Table 16.10)**. For patients with more severe disease, it is not advisable to reduce the exercise intensity as it proves to be of no benefit, but rather they should be advised interval training.

While treating a pulmonary population like COPD, it is not essential to use the THR as a factor determining the exercise intensity. But, the heart rate (HR) needs to be monitored throughout the exercise session, to be aware of the age-predicted maximum heart rate, the upper limit during the exercise test and other factors influencing the HR, such as medications.

With COPD patients, it is better to use rate of perceived exertion (RPE) or the rating of perceived dyspnea, to allow the patient to regulate the exercise intensity based on their own perception rather than the therapists. An RPE rating of 12–14 is sufficient to produce the desired effect.

Exercise intensity prescription in COPD patients can be done using a combination of physiological parameters as well. As mentioned earlier, cases of severe COPD cannot tolerate higher intensity training sessions for longer periods. Hence, interval training, where short bouts of high-intensity training are interspersed with rest periods of moderate-to-low intensity training, is used to attain beneficial effects of exercise.

Clinical Pearl

For patients with more severe disease, interval training can be considered over reduction in exercise intensity

Peak workload is another parameter that can be considered while deciding exercise intensity. An exercise intensity that is equivalent to a higher percentage of the peak workload or peak exercise capacity of an individual has better physiological and physical outcomes than an intensity corresponding to a lower percentage of peak workload. There is a direct relationship between the training outcome and the exercise intensity, meaning that a higher intensity produces a better outcome, whereas lower intensity produces insufficient outcome. However, a lower intensity training will have better adherence. The 6-MWT can be used to determine the peak VO_2, and hence, the results of 6-MWT can be used to determine the exercise capacity. The workload intensity in a 6-MWT is approximately 80% of the average speed attained during the test.

Exercise intensity needs to be carefully chosen as presence of dyspnea and desaturation associated with activity make estimation of work capacity difficult. Therefore, prescribing exercise at a standard percentage of peak is unrealistic in COPDs, suggest Simmons et al. Zacarias et al. observed that defining lactate threshold is difficult in COPDs rendering lactate threshold and associated tools less useful markers of exercise intensity. The presence of comorbidities also restricts patients from participation in the program or requires individual prescription. Under such circumstances, subjective definition of workload in terms of RPE is more appropriate.

Various Components of Exercise Training

Aerobic Training

Aerobic training conditions the ambulatory muscles, improves the cardiopulmonary fitness, increases the physical activity, and reduces the dyspnea and other related symptoms. The aerobic training program consists of a check-in period, warm-up, the aerobic exercise session, and the cool-down period. The check-in period involves the recording of baseline vital information. The warm-up period consists of exercises that increase the body vitals in a gradual manner to get the body systems prepared for the exercise session. For patients performing continuous training, the warm-up lasts for 5–10 minutes. It may last longer for severe patients as they will require rest periods during warm-up too. The aerobic session will comprise single or multiple modes of aerobic exercises up to the intensity decided by the therapist, for 20–30 minutes. Cycling **(Fig. 16.10)** is less energy consuming than treadmill walking **(Fig. 16.11)** but activity should be chosen

Table 16.10: Exercise intensity based on the percentage of maximal oxygen consumption (VO_{2max}).

Exercise intensity	Percentage of VO_{2max}
Low exercise intensity	<40
Moderate exercise intensity	40–60
Moderate-to-vigorous exercise intensity	>60

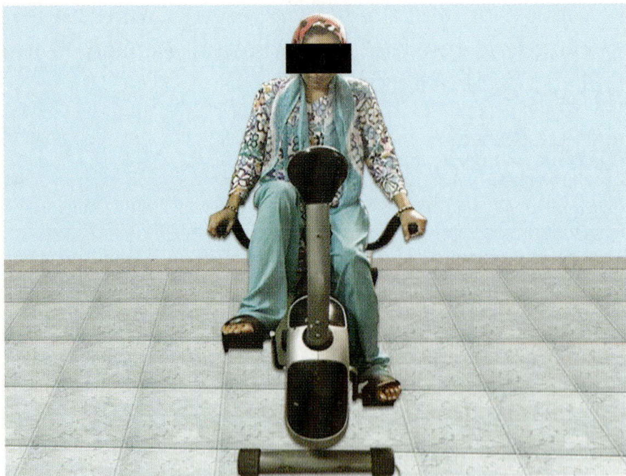

Fig. 16.10: Aerobic training using cycling.

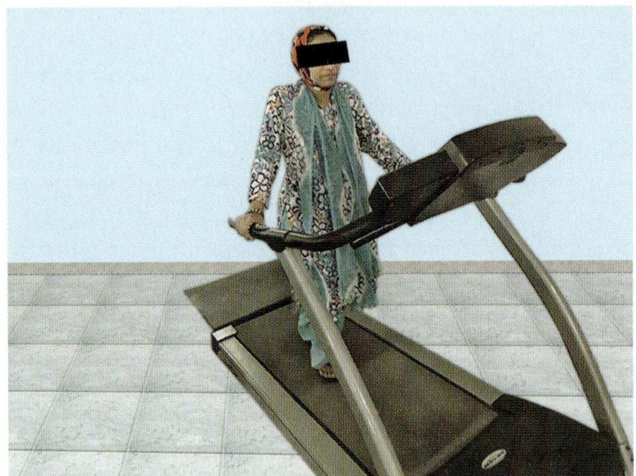

Fig. 16.11: Aerobic training on treadmill.

in accordance with ADL. The cross-trainer or elliptical can also be used for aerobic training **(Figs. 16.12A and B)**. The cool-down period follows immediately after the aerobic session. The purpose of cool-down period is to gradually slow the vitals to their original baseline. Stretching exercises can be performed in the cool-down period or after it to maintain muscle integrity and avoid soreness. Avoiding Valsalva maneuver should be emphasized to the patient during the whole training session.

Strength Training

Strength training is particularly indicated in patients having severe muscle atrophy and dyspnea. It improves muscle mass and strength. A combination of aerobic and strength training has several beneficial effects. It decreases the risk of falls and improves the bone mineral density in older individuals suffering from COPD. The resistance used (intensity and type), frequency, and mode of training should be decided by the therapist after a detailed evaluation of the cardiopulmonary and musculoskeletal systems of the patient. Strength training causes much less dyspnea and, therefore, is easier to tolerate compared to the aerobic training. American College of Sports Medicine (ACSM) recommends 1–3 sets of 8–12 repetitions 2–3 times/week with an initial load equivalent to 60–70% of 1 repetition maximum. The load should be gradually increased over time.

Upper Limb Training

The upper extremities are critical for several ADL, viz. bathing, grooming, and toileting. Upper extremity training is thus, crucial in an exercise program designed for patients with COPD. Upper extremity training includes aerobic (arm ergometry) as well as strength training (resistance exercises with free weights, elastic bands, etc.). Muscles of biceps, triceps, pectorals, latissimus dorsi, etc. are usually targeted. Upper limb training in patients with COPD improves upper extremity muscle strength and endurance, reduces metabolic demands during upper extremity activities and improves the general sense of well-being. People on long-term steroid therapy are at risk, as they have reduced bone mineral density as a side effect of steroid use. The osteoporosis is more pronounced in the thoracic vertebrae making them vulnerable to wear and tear and increasing the risk of sustaining compression fractures. Post-surgical patients should be refrained from arm ergometry for a period of 6 weeks to allow healing of incisions.

Flexibility Training

It is imperative to educate the patient about the importance of a good body posture and body mechanics and include appropriate exercises in the rehabilitation

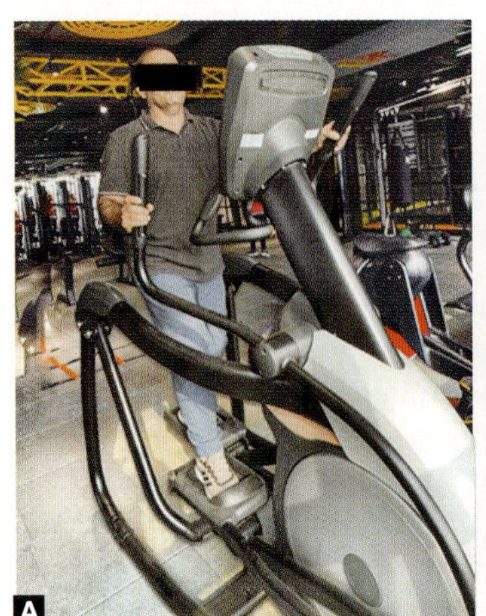

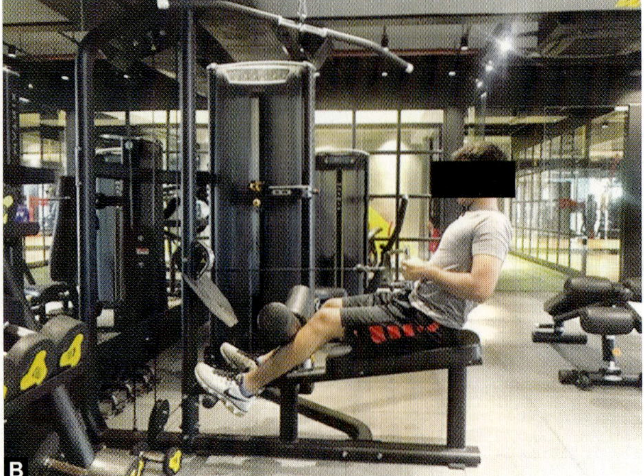

Figs. 16.12A and B: Aerobic training on (A) Cross-trainer; (B) Rowing machine.
Courtesy: Mission Health, Ahmedabad, India.

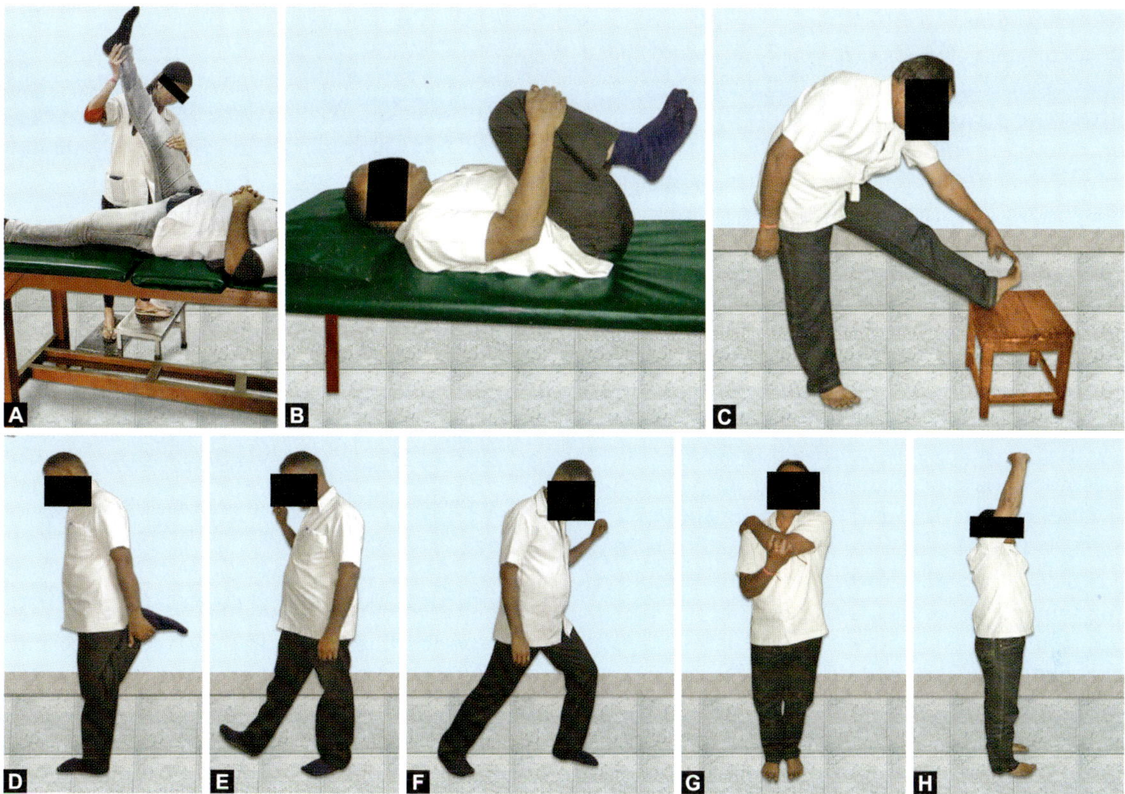

Figs. 16.13A to H: Flexibility training.

program. Reduced flexibility and muscular imbalance lead to a faulty posture. Postural deviations are associated with a reduced pulmonary function, QOL, bone mineral density, and increased WOB. Correction of posture using strengthening and flexibility training **(Figs. 16.13A to H)** improves the alignment of the muscles and body segments and eventually the respiratory mechanics.

Balance exercises should also be incorporated in the rehabilitation program, especially in older individuals. Flexibility and balancing exercises should be incorporated in the program 3–5 days/week and ADL aiming at better ROM, balance, and gait.

Inspiratory Muscle Training

American College of Clinical Pharmacy (ACCP)/ American Association of Cardiovascular and Pulmonary Rehabilitation (AACVPR) joint guidelines recommend that inspiratory muscle training (IMT) **(Fig. 16.14)** should be considered in stable COPD patients who exhibit respiratory muscle weakness despite optimum medical therapy. A large scale multicenter trial is required to foster the recommendation though. Vogitazis et al. noted that during intense exercise, reduced intercostal muscle perfusion, adequate blood flow to quadriceps and plateau in cardiac output limit the energy supply to working muscles. A study by Gosselink et al. and Ramirez et al. observed improvement in both strength (high intensity, low repetitions) and endurance (low intensity, high repetitions) of inspiratory muscles by enhancing pulmonary oxygen uptake and inducing ribcage remodeling partially addressing the issue

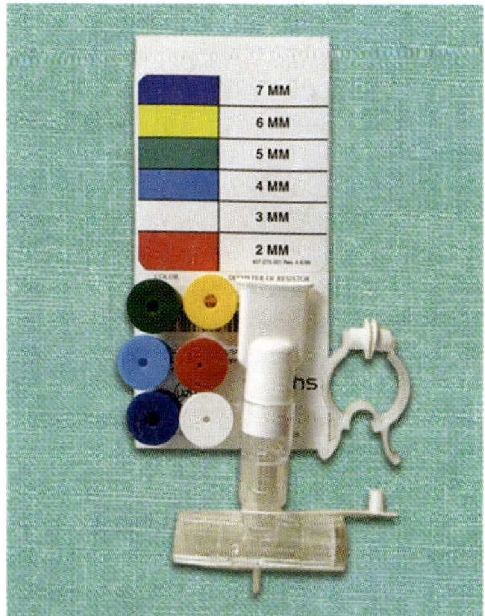

Fig. 16.14: Inspiratory muscle trainer.

of reduced energy supply. IMT using threshold devices has shown to improve inspiratory muscle strength, exercise capacity, and QOL but failed to exhibit an added effect on PR outcomes note Beaumont et al. Following the principles of specificity and overload, initial load is recommended at 30% P_iMax and supervision for oxygen desaturation and dyspnea. Training should be carried out 3 times/week for 8 weeks, progressively increasing load as symptoms permit. Outcomes measures should be P_iMax, dyspnea, HRQOL, and exercise capacity as studied by Hill et al. Weiner et al. recommend maintenance training as changes augmented through IMT decline over a period of a year if maintenance training is not continued.

Breathing Techniques

Breathing techniques **(Figs. 16.15 to 16.17)** are beneficial in improving dyspnea as a slow, relaxed and deep respiration reduces the dead space and carbon dioxide retention. Pursed lip breathing and diaphragmatic breathing are usually helpful in patients with COPD. Other devices such as acapella, flutter, and incentive spirometer can also be used for the strengthening of respiratory muscles and improving ventilatory capacity **(Figs. 16.18A to G)**.

Neuromuscular Electrical Stimulation

Neuromuscular electrical stimulation (NMES) can be used as an adjunctive therapy in individuals who are severely debilitated and are bed bound or suffer from extreme muscle weakness. A muscle contraction produced by NMES does not pose any cardiovascular demand, does not cause dyspnea and does not involve the cognitive or psychological aspects of movement. It is also relatively inexpensive and can be administered at home. It improves the walking capacity in severe COPD cases.

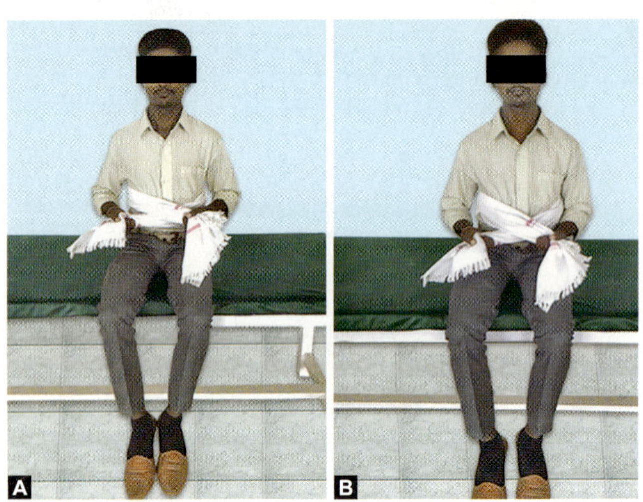

Figs. 16.15A and B: Segmental breathing exercises using towel: (A) Inhalation; (B) Exhalation.

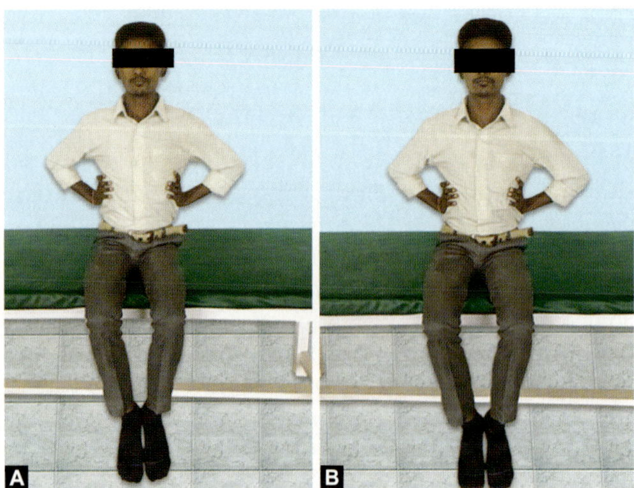

Figs. 16.16A and B: Segmental breathing exercises: (A) Inhalation; (B) Exhalation.

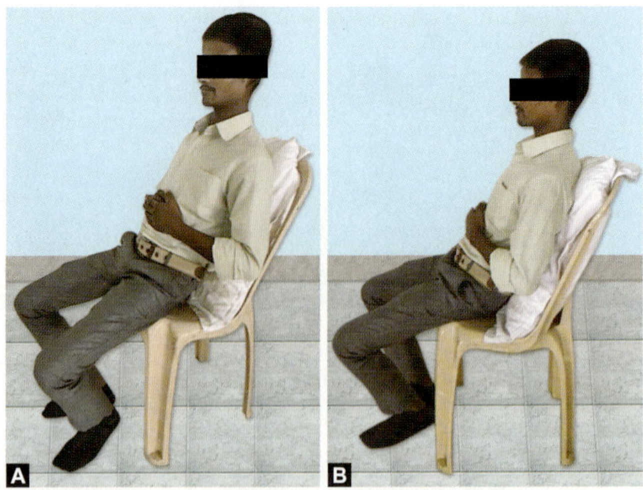

Figs. 16.17A and B: Diaphragmatic breathing exercises in sitting: (A) Inspiration; (B) Expiration.

Outcomes of Pulmonary Rehabilitation

PR improves BMI, 6-minute walk distance, and dyspnea suggesting better survival in patients with airflow obstruction in reference to BODE Index. HRQOL questionnaires suggest improvement in functional limitation and ADL. **Table 16.11** enlists AACVPR recommendations for outcome measures in PR.

The St George's Respiratory Questionnaire can be used to evaluate the effect of PR. It is a respiratory disease–specific questionnaire designed to evaluate the effect of the disease on overall health and perceived well-being. It consists of 50 items that are divided into two parts—symptoms and activity and impacts. There are three components—symptoms, activities, and impact. The score ranges from 0 to 100 with a higher score representing more limitations **(Appendix)**.

PSYCHOSOCIAL ISSUES IN CHRONIC OBSTRUCTIVE PULMONARY DISEASE

Similar to any other major conditions, COPD too affects the psychological well-being of the patients with COPD. Patients with COPD have a higher prevalence of anxiety and depression than any other psychological disorder. The pathophysiology of depression and anxiety in COPD is not clearly understood.

Smoking forms one of the major risk factors of COPD. Smoking and depression have a direct impact on each other. Depressed individuals are at higher risk of commencing smoking, and it is more difficult for them to quit smoking. On the other hand, smoking activates the nicotinic acetylcholine receptors, which sequentially leads to depression. A possible mechanism for the presence of depression in patients with COPD may be the inflammation of the lung that "overspills" into a systemic inflammation. Another possible mechanism may be the hypoxia caused by COPD that can cause the arterial saturation levels to be lowered, ultimately causing periventricular white matter lesions that are indicative of depression. Other factors such

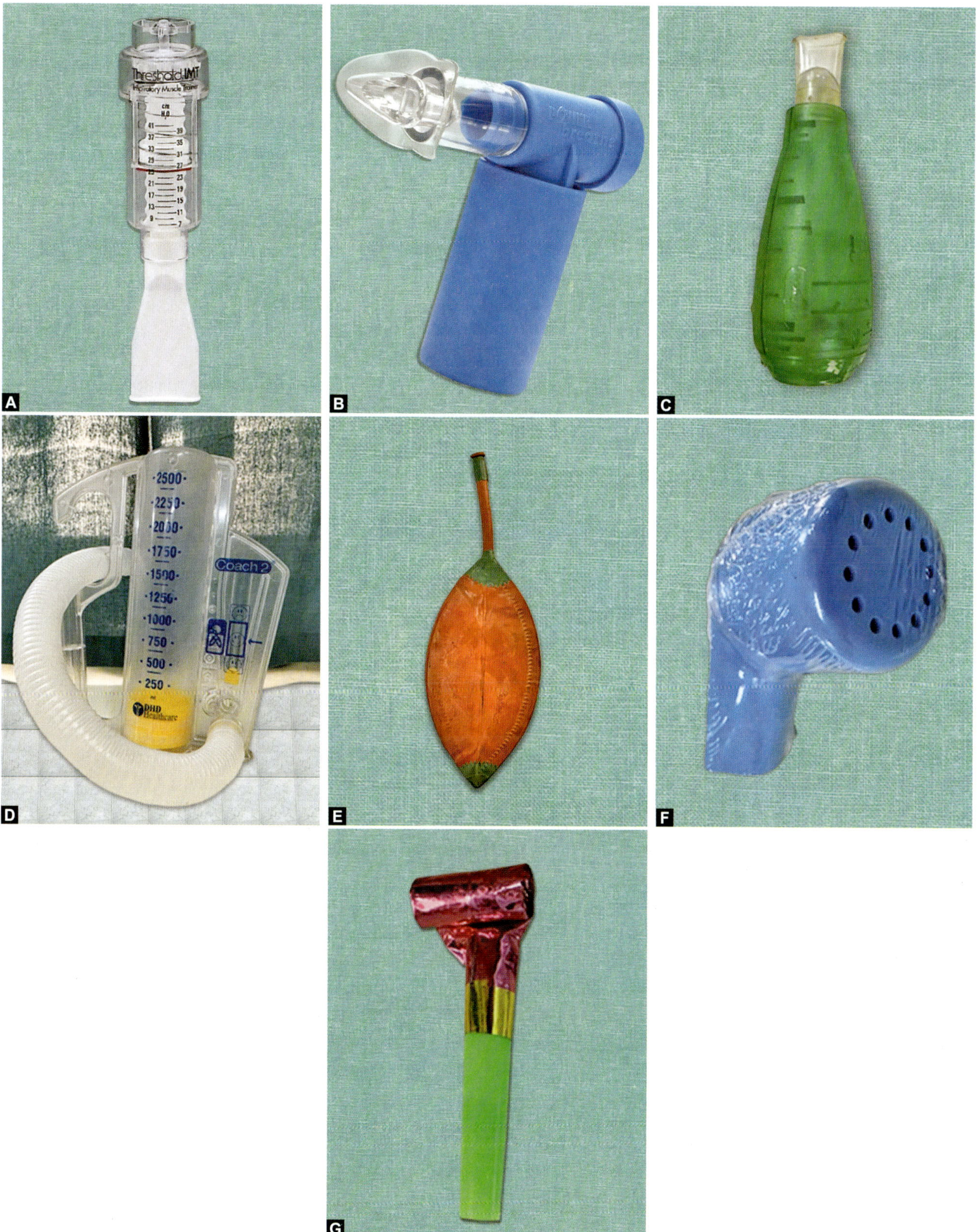

Figs. 16.18A to G: Devices for breathing exercises: (A and B) Pressure threshold device; (C) Acapella; (D) Volume spirometer; (E) Red rubber balloon; (F) Flutter; (G) Whistle.

Table 16.11: Outcome measures of pulmonary rehabilitation.

Core components	Clinical	Behavioral	Health	Service
Management	BODE ADL	Self efficacy	• Morbidity • Mortality	Performane measures
Exercise testing and training	Max/submaximal monitoring	Compliance energy expenditure		
Strength flexibilty	1 RM grip flexibility			
Breathing retraining		PLB inhaler mucous clearance		
Bronchial hygiene				
Nutrition and weight	BMI skinfold abdominal circumference	Diet		
Psychosocial	Mood cognition	Coping strategies social network sexual dysfunction		
Smoking cessation	Pack-years			

(BODE: **B**MI, airflow **o**bstruction, **d**yspnea, **e**xercise capacity; BMI: body mass index; ADL: activities of daily living; PLB: pursed-lip breathing)

as reduced functional capacity, reduced QOL, severity of the symptoms, and amount of assistance required during ADL are also associated with depression in COPD cases.

Hyperventilation is one of the features frequently seen in COPD. Hyperventilation lowers the CO_2 levels, causing respiratory alkalosis. This may cause dyspnea in COPD, building up to a panic attack.

Depression and anxiety are related to an increased rate of mortality and nonadherence to the drug regime. They increase the risk of hospitalization and the frequency of exacerbations. They are associated with persistent smoking, poor QOL, reduced physical and social functioning, worsening of dyspnea and fatigue.

Anxiety inventory for respiratory disease and brief assessment schedule depression cards can be respectively used for evaluation of anxiety and depression in COPD. Other than these scores, geriatric depression scale and 15-item short form can be used for depression and hospital anxiety and depression scale and the geriatric anxiety inventory can be used for anxiety.

Management of psychological issues in COPD is similar to other populations. The treatment can be divided into psychological and pharmacological. Psychological treatment consists of cognitive–behavior therapy, self-management, and relaxation.

SUMMARY

COPD comprises largely of chronic bronchitis and emphysema predisposed by continuous exposure to various risk factors. The diagnosis is confirmed by office spirometry and clinical symptoms. It is associated with central and peripheral changes in exercise performance partially reversible with pharmacological treatment, physical activity, and exercise of appropriate intensity, frequency, and duration. Physical exercises involving upper limbs, lower limbs, and ventilatory muscles in adequate intensity exhibit favorable changes in exercise capacity, symptoms and HRQOL that are sustained through maintenance exercise sessions.

Case Scenario

CASE STUDY

A 63-year-old man presents to the emergency department with a complaint of shortness of breath (SOB).

History of present illness: The patient has had sudden and severe SOB since the past 2–3 years. The SOB has gradually worsened over the years and has now debilitated him so much that he cannot perform his ADL without feeling out of breath. Since the past 1 week, the SOB has become worst and he has developed a productive cough with yellow-colored sputum. The coughing has been present since 3–4 years (longer than the SOB). He does not complain of any chest pains, fever or chills. He complains of reduced sleep and sleep disturbances due to breathing difficulties at night.

He is a current smoker for the past 40 years and has smoked around 20 cigarettes every day.

No significant medical or surgical history. No family history related to cardiopulmonary disorders or SOB.

Social and environmental history: He lives with his wife who is 59-years-old. He has two sons, both of whom are settled abroad. He lives on the second floor of the building but uses a lift and usually drives a four wheeler to commute at all places he visits.

Occupational history: He is a retired building contractor (retired since 4 years). He retired as per his wish and not on being compelled by his condition.

Examination: The patient is conscious and well aware of his surroundings. Vitals are normal. Dyspnea is grade 4 on the New York Heart Association (NYHA) scale. Posture examination reveals a forward head posture, leaning forward, and greater use of accessory muscles of respiration. He has grade II clubbing in his nails. There are no signs of cyanosis. Lower extremities or upper extremities show no signs of edema.

Chest examination: Reveals paradoxical movement of ribs in the lower segments. Chest shape is altered, it is barrel shaped. Auscultation of heart sounds is unremarkable. Breath sounds are reduced overall the zones bilaterally. Wheeze and crackles are heard in the lower and middle zones post anteriorly and posteriorly on both sides.

Musculoskeletal examination: The patient has a generalized reduced muscle strength in all the muscles of the body.

Medical tests and investigations: Chest X-ray shows flattened diaphragm with increased anteroposterior diameter and opacities in the middle and lower lobes bilaterally. Routine blood tests are normal with slightly reduced hemoglobin. Exercise tolerance test could not be conducted at this stage. Spirometry revealed FEV_1 <50% of age predicted, and FEV_1/FVC as <0.70 postbronchodilator administration.

Guiding Questions:
1. What is the possible diagnosis of the patient?
2. Calculate the number of pack years for this patient.
3. How will you perform an exercise tolerance test for this patient?
4. Describe a plan of care for this patient.

Review Questions

1. How will you assess and manage a 59-year-old female with COPD?
2. Describe pulmonary rehabilitation in detail.
3. Describe the effect of COPD on exercise performance and the benefits of exercise training.
4. Explain the risk factors, pathophysiology, and diagnosis of COPD.
5. Write short notes on:
   a. BODE index
   b. Classification of COPD
   c. Medical and surgical management of COPD
   d. Impairments associated with COPD
   e. Management of acute exacerbations in COPD

BIBLIOGRAPHY

1. Agency for Healthcare Research and Quality. Five major steps to intervention (the "5 A's"). [website] Available from www.ahrq.gov/professionals/clinicians-providers/guidelines-recommendations/tobacco/5steps.html.
2. American College of Sports Medicine. ACSM's exercise management for persons with chronic diseases and disabilities, 3rd edition. Champaign, IL: Human Kinetics; 2009.
3. Anthonisen N, Skeans MA, Wise RA, et al. The effects of a smoking cessation intervention on 14.5-year mortality: a randomized clinical trial. Ann Intern Med. 2005;142:233-9.
4. Beaumont M, Couturaud F, Reychler G, et al. Effects of inspiratory muscle training in COPD patients: a systematic review and meta-analysis. Clin Respir J. 2018;12(7):2178-88.
5. Bozier J, et al. Heightened response to e-cigarettes in COPD. ERJ Open Res. 2019;5(1):00192-2018.
6. Bronstad E, Rutting S, Xenaki D, et al. High-intensity knee extensor training restores skeletal muscle function in COPD patients. Eur Resp J. 2012;40:1130-36.
7. Celli BR, Cote CG, Marin JM, et al. The body-mass index, airflow obstruction, dyspnea, and exercise capacity index in chronic obstructive pulmonary disease. N Engl J Med. 2004;350:1005-12.
8. Global Initiative for Chronic Obstructive Lung Disease. Global update on the diagnosis, management and prevention of chronic obstructive pulmonary disease. 2018 report.
9. Gosselink R, De Vos J, Heuvel SP, et al. Impact of inspiratory muscle training in patients with COPD. What is the evidence? Eur Resp J. 2011;37:416-25.
10. Hartman JE, Vanfleteren L, Rikxoort E, et al. Endobronchial valves for severe emphysema. Eur Respir Rev. 2019;28:180121.
11. Hill K, Cecins N, Eastwood P, et al. Inspiratory muscle training for patients with chronic obstructive pulmonary disease: a practical guide for clinicians. Arch Phys Med Rehabil. 2010;91(9):1466-70.
12. LeMura L. Clinical exercise physiology-application and physiological principals, 1st edition. Pennsylvania, PA: Lippincott Williams and Wilkins; 2004.
13. McKeough, Velloso M, Lima V, et al. Upper limb exercise training for COPD. Cochrane Database Syst Rev. 2016;(11):CD011434.
14. Morjaria JB, Mondati E, Polosa R. E-cigarettes in patients with COPD: current perspectives. Int J Chron Obstruct Pulmon Dis. 2017;12:3203-10.
15. Polosa R, Jaymin B, Umberto P, et al. Health effects in COPD smokers who switch to electronic cigarettes: a retrospective-prospective 3-year follow-up. Int J Chron Obstruct Pulmon Dis. 2018;13:2533-42.
16. Pumar MI, Gray C, Walsh J, et al. Anxiety and depression—important psychological comorbidities of COPD. J Thorac Disease. 2014;6(11):1615-31.
17. Ramirez-Sarmiento A, Orozco L, Guell R, et al. Inspiratory muscle training in patients with chronic obstructive pulmonary disease: structural adaptation and physiologic outcomes. Am J Respir Crit Care Med. 2002;166:1491-97.
18. Rise AL, Bauldoff GS, Carlin BW, et al. Pulmonary rehabilitation: ACCP/AACVPR evidence based clinical practice guidelines. Chest. 2007;131:4S-42S.
19. Rochester CL. Exercise training in chronic obstructive pulmonary disease. J Rehabil Res Dev. 2003;40:59-80.
20. Sala E, Roca J, Marrades R, et al. Effects of endurance training on skeletal muscle bioenergetics in chronic obstructive pulmonary disease. Am J Respir Crit Care Med. 1999;159(6):1726-34.
21. Simmons DN, Berry MJ, Hayes SI, et al. The relationship between %HR Peak and %VO2 peak in patients with COPD. Med Sci Sports Exerc. 2000;32:881-6.
22. Spruit MA, Singh SJ, Garvey C, et al. ATS/ERS task force on pulmonary rehabilitation. An official American Thoracic Society/European Respiratory Society statement: key concepts and advances in pulmonary rehabilitation. Am J Respir Crit Care Med. 2013;188:e13-64.
23. Temitayo OI, Ojo O. Evaluating the effectiveness of smoking cessation in the management of COPD. Br J Nurs. 2016;25(14):786-91.
24. Vogitazis I, Athanasopoulos D, Habazettl H, et al. Intercostal blood flow limitation during exercise in COPD. Am J Respir Crit Care Med. 2010;182:1105-13.
25. Wang M. Airway clearance techniques for patients with stable COPD: a rapid review. Toronto: Health Quality Ontario; 2015.
26. Welling J, Slebos DJ. Lung volume reduction with endobronchial coils for patients with emphysema. J Thorac Dis. 2018;10(Suppl. 23):S2797-805.
27. Weiner P, Magadle R, BeckermanM, et al. Maintenance of inspiratory muscle training in COPD patients: one year follow-up. Eur Resp J. 2004;23:61-5.
28. Zacarias EC, Neder J, Cendom S, et al. Heart rate at the estimated lactate threshold in patients with COPD: effects on target exercise intensity for dynamic exercise training. JCRP. 2000;20:369-76.
29. Zafeiris L, Stavroula S, Eleni A, et al. 12 weeks of interval training induces clinically meangiful effects in amount and intensity of daily activities in COPD. Available from : http// ow.ly/Rzx13002awp
30. Vogiatzis I, Nanas S, Rouss C. Interval training as an alternative modality to continous exercise in patients with COPD. European Respiratory Journal. 2002 20:12-19.
31. Marla K, Mika N, Roger S et al. Interval versus continous training in Individuals with chronic obstructive pulomary disease—A systematic review. Thorax. 2010;65;157-64.

APPENDIX: ST GEORGE'S RESPIRATORY QUESTIONNAIRE (SGRQ)

This questionnaire is designed to help us learn much more about how your breathing is troubling you and how it affects your life. We are using it to find out which aspects of your illness cause you most problems, rather than what the doctors and nurses think your problems are.

Please read the instructions carefully and ask if you do not understand anything. Do not spend too long deciding about your answers.

Before completing the rest of the questionnaire:

Please tick in one box to show how you describe your current health:

Very good	Good	Fair	Poor	Very poor
☐	☐	☐	☐	☐

St George's Respiratory Questionnaire
Part 1

Questions about how much chest trouble you have had over the past 3 months.

Please tick (✓) one box for each question.

	Most days a week	Several days a week	A few days a month	Only with chest infections	Not at all
1. Over the past 3 months, I have coughed:	☐	☐	☐	☐	☐
2. Over the past 3 months, I have brought up phlegm (sputum):	☐	☐	☐	☐	☐
3. Over the past 3 months, I have had shortness of breath:	☐	☐	☐	☐	☐
4. Over the past 3 months, I have had attacks of wheezing:	☐	☐	☐	☐	☐

5. During the past 3 months how many severe or very unpleasant attacks of chest trouble have you had?

Please tick (✓) one:

More than 3 attacks	☐
3 attacks	☐
2 attacks	☐
1 attack	☐
no attacks	☐

6. How long did the worst attack of chest trouble last?
(Go to question 7 if you had no severe attacks)

Please tick (✓) one:

A week or more	☐
3 or more days	☐
1 or 2 days	☐
Less than a day	☐

7. Over the past 3 months, in an average week, how many good days (with little chest trouble) have you had?

Please tick (✓) one:

No good days	☐
1 or 2 good days	☐
3 or 4 good days	☐
Nearly every day is good	☐
Every day is good	☐

8. If you have a wheeze, is it worse in the morning?

Please tick (✓) one:

No	☐
Yes	☐

St George's Respiratory Questionnaire

Part 2

Section 1

How would you describe your chest condition?

Please tick (✓) one:

The most important problem I have ☐

Causes me quite a lot of problems ☐

Causes me a few problems ☐

Causes no problems ☐

If you have ever had paid employment

Please tick (✓) one:

My chest trouble made me stop work altogether ☐

My chest trouble interferes with my work or made me change my work ☐

My chest trouble does not affect my work ☐

Section 2

Questions about what activities usually make you feel breathless these days.

Please tick (✓) in **each box** that
applies to you **these days**

	True	False
Sitting or lying still	☐	☐
Getting washed or dressed	☐	☐
Walking around the home	☐	☐
Walking outside on the level	☐	☐
Walking up a flight of stairs	☐	☐
Walking up hills	☐	☐
Playing sports or games	☐	☐

Section 3

Some more questions about your cough and breathlessness these days.

Please tick (✓) in **each box** that
applies to you **these days**

	True	False
My cough hurts	☐	☐
My cough makes me tired	☐	☐
I am breathless when I talk	☐	☐
I am breathless when I bend over	☐	☐
My cough or breathing disturbs my sleep	☐	☐
I get exhausted easily	☐	☐

Section 4

Questions about other effects that your chest trouble may have on you these days.

Please tick (✓) in *each box* that
applies to you *these days*

	True	False
My cough or breathing is embarrassing in public	☐	☐
My chest trouble is a nuisance to my family, friends or neighbors	☐	☐
I get afraid or panic when I cannot get my breath	☐	☐
I feel that I am not in control of my chest problem	☐	☐
I do not expect my chest to get any better	☐	☐
I have become frail or an invalid because of my chest	☐	☐
Exercise is not safe for me	☐	☐
Everything seems too much of an effort	☐	☐

Section 5

Questions about your medication, if you are receiving no medication go straight to section 6.

Please tick (✓) in *each box* that
applies to you *these days*

	True	False
My medication does not help me very much	☐	☐
I get embarrassed using my medication in public	☐	☐
I have unpleasant side effects from my medication	☐	☐
My medication interferes with my life a lot	☐	☐

Section 6

These are questions about how your activities might be affected by your breathing.

Please tick (✓) in *each box* that applies to you
because of your breathing

	True	False
I take a long time to get washed or dressed	☐	☐
I cannot take a bath or shower, or I take a long time	☐	☐
I walk slower than other people, or I stop for rests	☐	☐
Jobs such as housework take a long time, or I have to stop for rests	☐	☐
If I walk up one flight of stairs, I have to go slowly or stop	☐	☐
If I hurry or walk fast, I have to stop or slow down	☐	☐
My breathing makes it difficult to do things such as walk up hills, carrying things up stairs, light gardening such as weeding, dance, play bowls or play golf	☐	☐
My breathing makes it difficult to do things such as carry heavy loads, dig the garden or shovel snow, jog or walk at 5 miles per hour, play tennis or swim	☐	☐
My breathing makes it difficult to do things such as very heavy manual work, run, cycle, swim fast or play competitive sports	☐	☐

Section 7

We would like to know how your chest usually affects your daily life.

Please tick (✓) in *each box* that applies to
you *because of your chest trouble*

	True	False
I cannot play sports or games	☐	☐
I cannot go out for entertainment or recreation	☐	☐
I cannot go out of the house to do the shopping	☐	☐
I cannot do housework	☐	☐
I cannot move far from my bed or chair	☐	☐

St George's Respiratory Questionnaire
Part 3

Here is a list of other activities that your chest trouble may prevent you doing (You do not have to tick these, they are just to remind you of ways in which your breathlessness may affect you):

Going for walks or walking the dog

Doing things at home or in the garden

Sexual intercourse

Going out to church, pub, club or place of entertainment

Going out in bad weather or into smoky rooms

Visiting family or friends or playing with children

Please write in any other important activities that your chest trouble may stop you doing:

....

....

....

....

Now would you tick in the box (one only) which you think best describes how your chest affects you:

It does not stop me doing anything I would like to do ☐

It stops me doing one or two things I would like to do ☐

It stops me doing most of the things I would like to do ☐

It stops me doing everything I would like to do ☐

Thank you for filling in this questionnaire. Before you finish would you please check to see that you have answered all the questions.

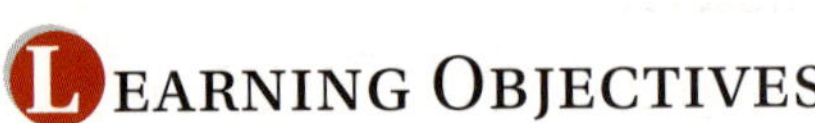

CHAPTER 17

Peripheral Vascular Diseases

Mariya Jiandani

LEARNING OBJECTIVES

At the end of this chapter, the readers will be able to:
- Understand basic concepts of anatomy, physiology, and pathophysiology of arterial, venous, and lymphatic system
- Understand the differences between the three peripheral vascular systems
- Identify the risk factors and common disorders pertaining to them
- Identify the components of comprehensive assessment of peripheral vascular system
- Design an appropriate physiotherapeutic plan of care for peripheral vascular diseases
- Understand the cause of arterial and venous ulcers, their assessment, and management.

CHAPTER OUTLINE

- Anatomy and physiology of peripheral vascular systems
  - Arterial system
  - Venous system
  - Lymphatic system
- Diseases of peripheral vascular system
  - Arterial diseases
  - Venous diseases
  - Lymphatic disorders
- Assessment of peripheral vascular disease
  - Clinical evaluation
  - Test for arterial dysfunction
- Tests for venous dysfunction
- Functional evaluation
- Management of vascular disorders
  - Management of arterial disorders
  - Rehabilitation for venous and lymphatic insufficiency
- Vascular ulcers and healing
  - Wound healing
  - Factors delaying wound healing
  - Assessment of wound
  - Wound management
  - Objectives of management
- Electrotherapy in vascular disorders
  - Burst transcutaneous electrical nerve stimulation
  - Electrical stimulation
  - High-voltage electrical stimulation
  - Laser
  - Hydrotherapy
  - Ultrasound
  - Ultraviolet rays
  - Radiant heat
  - Hyperbaric oxygen therapy for non-healing wounds

INTRODUCTION

The human circulatory system is designed uniquely to provide nutrients, oxygen, and clear waste. The central pumping mechanism of the heart is continued into intricately designed tubular system of the peripheral vessels. Peripheral vascular system is an extension of cardiovascular system, made up of three systems, i.e., arteries, veins, and lymphatics. The arterial and venous systems are connected through a dense capillary network. The structure of arterial and venous system is based on the function they perform. Peripheral vascular disease (PVD) is often associated with underlying cause such as cerebrovascular accident, coronary artery disease, aneurysm, and amputations. Physiotherapist is an integral part of the team. Diseases of peripheral vascular system often lead to major functional impairments and impaired quality of life. Physiotherapists identify impairment and functional limitation and plan physiotherapy intervention appropriately.

ANATOMY AND PHYSIOLOGY OF PERIPHERAL VASCULAR SYSTEMS

The peripheral vascular system is divided into two basic systems—the arterial and venous. The third system the lymphatics is coordinated with venous to take up the excess extracellular fluids and tissue products. It is also a defense system to protect against the pathogens. The basic design of vascular framework is of three layers:

1. **Tunica intima:** Innermost layer composed of endothelium, connective tissue, and basement membrane.

2. **Tunica media:** Middle layer composed of smooth muscles
3. **Tunica adventitia:** Outermost layer composed of elastic and collagenous fibers.

Arterial System

Arteries are the muscular and elastic vessels, which perform the function of carrying oxygen-rich blood at high pressures to the entire body. Pressure within the artery varies with the distance from the heart. Major vessels closer to the heart have higher pressures than distal smaller arteries. They are more elastic in nature, e.g., aorta and its branches and pulmonary arteries, whereas distal vessels are more muscular, e.g., radial, popliteal, temporal, and occipital. Smallest arteries are muscular type and are called arterioles, which have 1–2 layers of smooth muscles in their walls. They generate peripheral resistance and regulate diastolic blood pressure. The contractile nature allows the vessel to constrict and dilate under the control of autonomic nervous system. Arteries are accompanied by veins and nerves, and together they form the neurovascular bundle.

The exchange of nutrients for waste products takes place in microscopic vessels called capillaries. These structures allow diffusion or passage of oxygen and nutrients into organs and tissues. It is governed by hydrostatic pressure, osmotic pressure, and properties of capillary wall. The capillaries terminate in venules, which in turn channel blood into larger veins and back to the heart through the largest veins; the superior and inferior vena cava. The walls of arteries are much thicker compared to veins as it has to sustain higher pressure of the blood that flows through them.

Venous System

Veins are capacitance vessels. They have a capacity to distend (expand) readily to store a high volume of blood, even at a low pressure. Their function is to receive deoxygenated blood and take it to the heart. Veins are made of three coats like arteries but are not well defined and have poor muscle and elastic tissue content. Tunica intima is made up of one thin layer of endothelial cells and has the smallest amount of connective tissue. The amount of collagen in tunica media is greater than that of elastic and smooth muscle fibers. This leads to inability to contract. Hence, the vein is dependent on system of valves to assist the return of blood to the heart. The valves in veins maintain unidirectional flow of blood against gravity. The valves are formed from the tunica intima layer. As blood moves toward the heart, the valves are open; however, when the blood attempts to flow back, the flaps fill with blood, closing the valves and preventing the reflux of blood. They are more common in lower extremity where the gravitational force is maximum. As blood moves from arteries through capillaries, venules, and veins, the pressure reduces. Vascular competency and skeletal

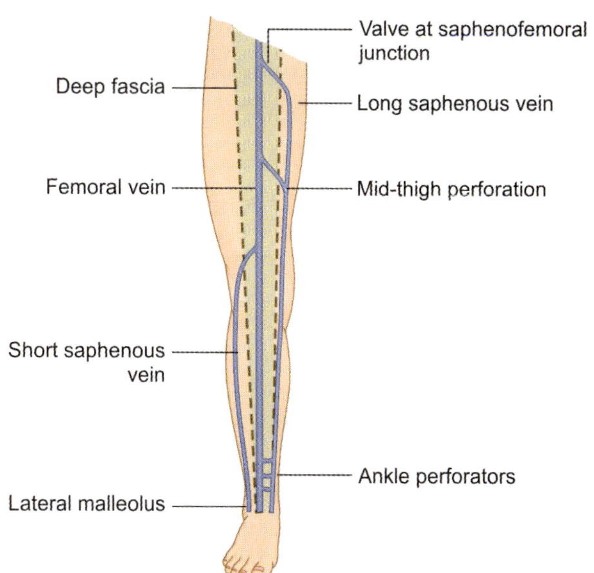

Fig. 17.1: Venous system.

muscle contraction are driving forces for the blood to flow. Contraction of skeletal muscle surrounding the vein causes milking effect on the vessel, propelling the blood to flow forward through the vein towards the heart. The calf muscle is therefore also called the second heart.

The venous system is divided into superficial veins, perforators or communicators, and deep veins **(Fig. 17.1)**. **Superficial veins:** The long saphenous veins pass up the medial malleolus behind the knee and through a defect of the fascia to join the femoral vein in the groin. The short saphenous vein passes up the lateral side of the back of the calf and through the fascia to join the popliteal vein behind the knee. These superficial veins drain from the skin. Their walls have smooth muscles, which are under control of autonomic nervous system.

Deep veins: There are three groups of veins accompanying the artery in the calf and large venous sinuses in the calf muscle. These drain into popliteal then femoral and finally into iliac and join to form inferior venae cava. The two systems communicate at the saphenofemoral junction in the groin, saphenopopliteal in the knee, at mid-thigh level through the hunterian perforator, and at the ankle through Cockett's perforators.

Table 17.1 shows the differences between the arteries and veins.

Lymphatic System

The lymphatic system is an extensive network of collecting vessels, lymph nodes, and lymph organs. It serves as a transport channel for fluid and proteins from the interstitium to return back to bloodstream. The lymph vessels from the lower extremity drain into the lymph nodes in the groin, which is further taken by lymphatics into iliac and para-aortic nodes. Lymphatics draining the gut join those from the legs at cisterna chyli from which

Table 17.1: Differences between arteries and veins.

		Arteries	Veins
1.	Direction of blood flow	Conducts away from heart	Conducts toward the heart
2.	General appearance	• Rounded • More muscular	Irregular often collapsible with position. Ability to dilate can accommodate 80% of total volume
3.	Pressure	High	Low. Pressure is affected by gravity and posture
4.	Wall thickness	Thick	Thin
5.	Relative oxygen concentration	Higher in systemic arteries and lower in pulmonary arteries	Lower in systemic veins and higher in pulmonary veins
6.	Valves	Not present	Present most commonly in limbs and veins inferior to the heart

the lymphatic duct travels up through the chest along the vertebral column. Lymphatics from the arm then join the system, which ultimately drains into the left subclavian vein. The negative intrathoracic pressure aids lymph flow, lymph formation, and transport **(Fig. 17.2)**.

Lymphatic capillaries take up lymph, a protein-rich exudate from blood vessels. Tissue fluid enters these lymphatic vessels in between discontinuous button-like cell junctions via larger collecting lymphatic vessels and ultimately the thoracic duct, it is returned to the blood vasculature through the lymphaticovenous connections at the junction of the jugular and subclavian veins. In the intestine, specialized lymphatic vessels, so-called lacteals, take up dietary fat and fat-soluble vitamins to transport them to the venous circulation.

The flow of lymph toward the heart is maintained due to various factors such as contraction of valve, skeletal muscle pump, peristalsis of gastrointestinal tract (GIT), rhythmic contraction of walls of large lymphatics and interstitial fluid pressure, negative intrathoracic pressure during inspiration, and suction effect in veins. Lymph finally drains into the right lymphatic duct, which opens into right subclavian vein, and the thoracic duct, which opens into left subclavian vein.

Lymphatic glands are the first line of defense of immune system and functions closely with the cardiovascular system to maintain the homeostasis and the fluid volumes in the body. It absorbs and transports fatty acids and fats as chyle from the digestive system and removes interstitial fluid from tissues. The lymph node filters water and electrolytes but retains proteins and lipids. Bacteria and other toxic substances are destroyed by macrophages.

DISEASES OF PERIPHERAL VASCULAR SYSTEM

Peripheral vascular disease (PVD) is an important cause of morbidity and mortality. Detailed history and clinical evaluation are important to determine the type of disease, its extent, prognosis, and treatment intervention strategies.

Arterial Diseases

Arterial insufficiency is generally as a result of atherosclerosis **(Fig. 17.3)**. **Atherosclerosis** is a chronic, complex inflammatory condition of elastic and muscular arteries affecting both large and small vessels. The major risk factors associated with it are smoking, diabetes mellitus, altered triglycerides, and hypertension. They are divided into acute and chronic. The spectrum of disease

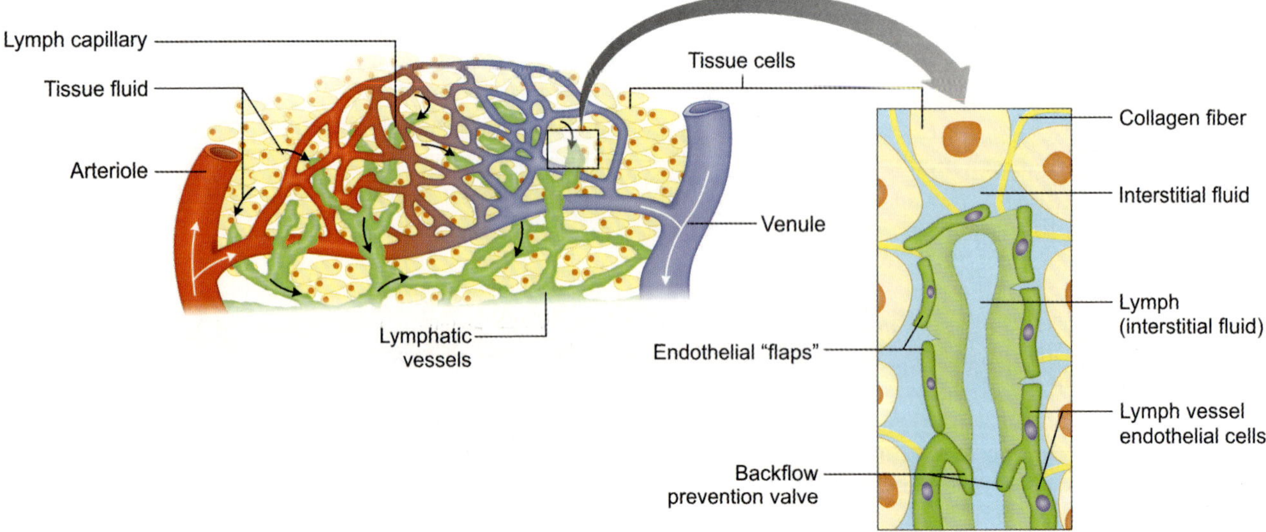

Fig. 17.2: Lymphatic system.

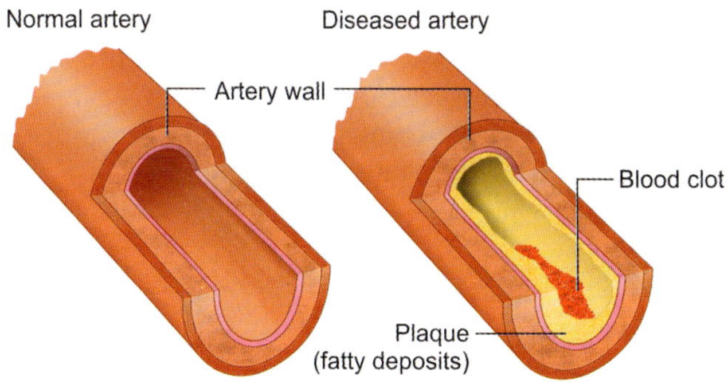

Fig. 17.3: Diseased artery.

seen with atherosclerosis is coronary artery disease, cerebrovascular disease, and peripheral arterial disease. Patients with one manifestation often have coexisting other underlying vascular disease. Atherosclerotic arterial disease does not manifest itself clinically till the critical threshold of 75% stenosis is reached. The severity of a lesion and symptomatic presentation depends on absolute vessel diameter, length of lesion, presence of other multiple lesions, and presence of collateral blood flow. Collaterals are seen in chronic lesions, whereas in acute there is no collateral circulation to combat ischemia. Blood flow through diseased vessel also depends on viscosity, hematocrit, and aggregability of red blood cells.

Acute arterial diseases are a result of **thrombosis and embolism**. A sudden cessation of blood flow associated with acute pain and cold limb, usually requiring surgical intervention in emergency is the most common presentation. The thrombus when it blocks the atherosclerotic vessel causes turbulent flow within the lumen, which activates platelets causing a partial or complete obstruction of the lumen **(Fig. 17.4)**. A fragment of arterial thrombus may break away and lodge in smaller diameter artery distally, resulting in ischemic condition of another portion of the artery.

The patient presents with **(Fig. 17.5)**:

- Pain
- Pallor
- Paresthesia
- Pulselessness
- Paralysis and gangrene.

Arterial emboli most commonly originates from the heart, as in the left atrial fibrillation commonly seen in mitral valve disease or mural thrombus after infarction or from atheroma from aorta.

A large embolus can lodge in distal aorta blocking both common iliac arteries affecting both limbs or in the femoral or popliteal artery where the affected limb will be painful, pulseless, pale, and paralyzed.

Chronic Arterial Insufficiency

Arteriosclerosis is thickening, hardening, and loss of elasticity of arterial walls. Atherosclerosis is the most common form of arteriosclerosis, associated with endothelial damage and the formation of fat deposits within the vessel wall lining, eventually leading to plaque formation. Atherosclerosis affects the vascular structure and vascular reactivity. Normal endothelium-dependent mechanism of vascular relaxation is impaired, which predisposes the vessel to excessive vasoconstriction.

Arteriosclerosis Obliterans

The vessel walls of the arterial system undergo degeneration losing their elasticity and becoming sclerotic. Development of atherosclerotic plaque in systemic arteries reduces the lumen due to significant stenosis, hence reducing the blood flow to regions distal to area of occlusion. This reduction in blood flow creates an imbalance between oxygen supply and demand, causing ischemia especially during effort to develop in affected areas, typically calf, thigh, or buttock. As there is an

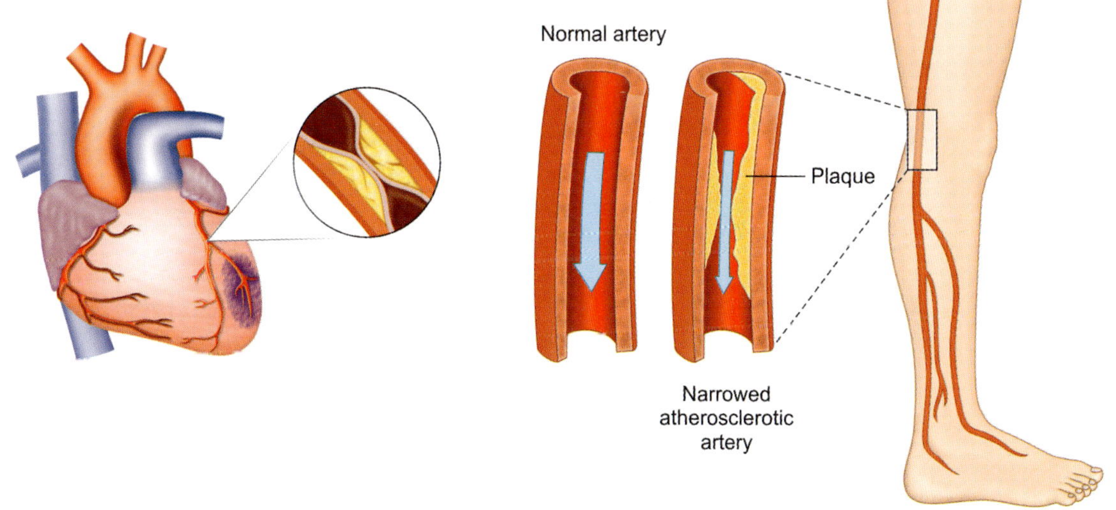

Fig. 17.4: Arterial disease.

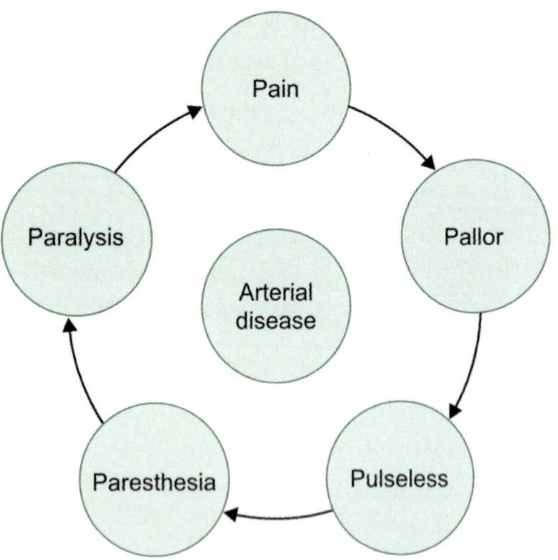

Fig. 17.5: Five Ps of arterial disease.

accumulation of lactate and metabolites, local sensory receptors are stimulated that causes the pain of intermittent claudication. Clinically patient presents with pain in the affected muscle on exertion, which occurs at a fixed distance or threshold and relieved on rest. This is known as **intermittent claudication**. Claudication is defined as a reproducible discomfort or fatigue in the muscles of the lower extremity that occurs with exertion and is relieved within 10 minutes of rest. The calf musculature is most commonly affected. If the lesion is higher as in femoral the whole extremity or if in common iliac, bilateral extremity may be affected. The threshold of intermittent claudication is associated with approximate 50% occlusion.

A proportion of patients with widespread disease reach a stage where the arterial perfusion is not sufficient at rest. In supine position the benefit of gravity to improve circulation due to increased hydrostatic pressure which improves flow in high resistance vessels is lost and rest pain ensues. The pain is severe and disturbs sleep. The patient may sit with legs hanging in order to aid gravity for circulation. It may be associated with trophic changes, absent pulses, and cold extremities. It may mark the development of gangrene where the cell death (necrosis) occurs due to insufficient blood supply. The digits mummify and turn black. Severe stenosis results in necrosis in the ischemic tissues and leg amputation is indicated.

Various factors limit blood flow to the limb:
- Those that limit flow such as plaque, stenosed vessels, inadequate collaterals, increased fibrinogen, platelet aggregation, which can ensue due prolonged immobility.
- Endothelial dysfunction, which impairs vasodilation response to decreased nitric oxide in skeletal muscle.
- Factors such as thromboxane, serotonin, endothelin, which increase vasoconstriction.

Peripheral arterial disease is also associated with distortion and impaired function of mitochondria in calf muscle.

The cycles of ischemia/reperfusion lead to the generation of reactive oxygen species with oxidative stress and inflammation, endothelial activation, mitochondrial dysfunction, muscle fiber-type switching, activation of apoptosis, and myofiber degeneration. Arterial insufficiency may be associated with distal motor neuropathy, which may independently affect muscle performance (**Fig. 17.6**).

Aortoiliac Disease

The aorta because of its wide lumen does not generally get affected. It may be blocked by thrombosis extending up from iliac vessels up to the level of renal arteries.

Leriche Syndrome

Leriche syndrome consists of buttock claudication and impotence. It results from occlusion of distal aorta and the common, external and internal iliac arteries. Femoropopliteal disease is very common; superficial

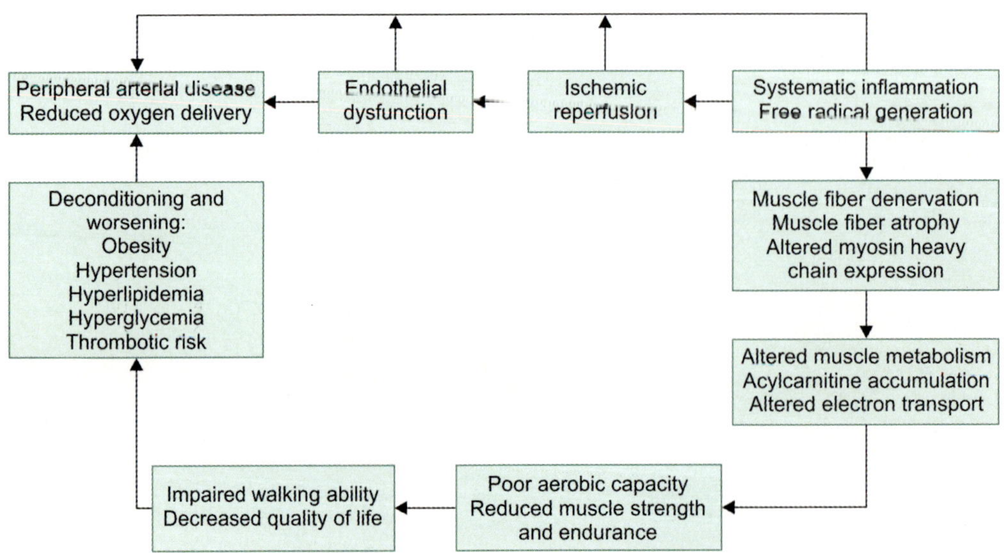

Fig. 17.6: The cycle of disability in intermittent claudication.

femoral artery is commonly affected as it passes beneath the adductor muscles with diffuse plaques in the distal vessels.

Thromboangiitis Obliterans

Also known as **Buerger's disease** occurs primarily in young males who are smokers and tobacco users. It is nonatherosclerotic inflammatory disorder affecting medium and small vessels of the extremity beginning distally and moving proximally. There seems to be a direct correlation between the disease manifestation and cigarette smoking. The inflammatory reaction appears to be due to nicotine sensitivity, which allows invasion of lymphocytes. The rest pain is usually the initial symptom followed by intermittent claudication. It results in sequential necrosis of digits.

Diabetic Vascular Disease

Diabetics suffer major problems with their metabolism of lipids and carbohydrates eventually leading to early atherosclerosis. Diabetes affects the smaller vessels (microangiopathy), affecting the microcirculation producing ischemic ulcers and isolated necrosis of digits. These are further worsened due to nonhealing, infection, and peripheral neuropathy.

Spasmodic Arterial Disorders

Raynaud's syndrome, acrocyanosis, and erythromelalgia form a spectrum of disorders caused by vasospasm or excessive dilatation of affected vessels. Raynaud's phenomenon refers to spasm of arterioles affecting the digits, along with intermittent pallor of the skin. Etiology may be idiopathic or secondary to condition such as scleroderma. Clinical manifestation of **Raynaud's syndrome** is intermittent attacks of cyanosis of the digits when exposed to cold or emotional trauma. It is usually bilateral and more commonly seen in women. Warming the extremity may restore back the color. The thumb is rarely involved. Pain may not be present but paresthesia could be present. Small ulcerations are generally seen at the tip of the finger. The distal pulses are generally palpable. There may not be any symptoms of intermittent claudication. The digits experience cycles of cyanosis followed by redness and reflex vasodilation. **Acrocyanosis** is cyanosis of distal extremities. It typically affects hands and fingers or the feet and toes. **Erythromelalgia** is bilateral vasodilatation affecting the extremities, especially the feet. It is marked by redness, burning and throbbing sensations, and increased skin temperature.

Thoracic Outlet Syndrome

An abnormal rib developed over the seventh cervical vertebra or a tough fibrous band attached on the first rib may compress subclavian artery stenosing it. An aneurysm commonly forms distal to the narrowing and together with pressure on plexus may cause tingling and weakness in the forearm and Raynaud's syndrome in hand.

Hand Arm Vibration Syndrome

This is vasospastic arterial dysfunction similar to Raynaud's. Frequently develops spasm with or without tingling, sensory losses along both median and ulnar distribution, and weakness of hand.

Aneurysm

It is localized dilatation of an artery. Atheromatous aneurysm most commonly occurs in abdominal aorta but may also occur in iliac, femoral, and popliteal arteries. Clinical diagnosis is based on finding of pulsatile swelling. It is a result of weakening of vessel wall.

False aneurysm: A hematoma may occur secondary to injury to artery, needle puncture, or an arterial surgical anastomosis and organize to form a false aneurysm, the lumen of which is in communication with arterial system and wall of which is composed of clot.

Complications

Complications include:
- Arterial ulcers are formed due to long-standing nonhealing wounds and ischemia **(Fig. 17.7A to C).**
- Gangrene and amputation of the extremity at higher levels.
- Peripheral sensory and motor neuropathy due to ischemia to nerves.

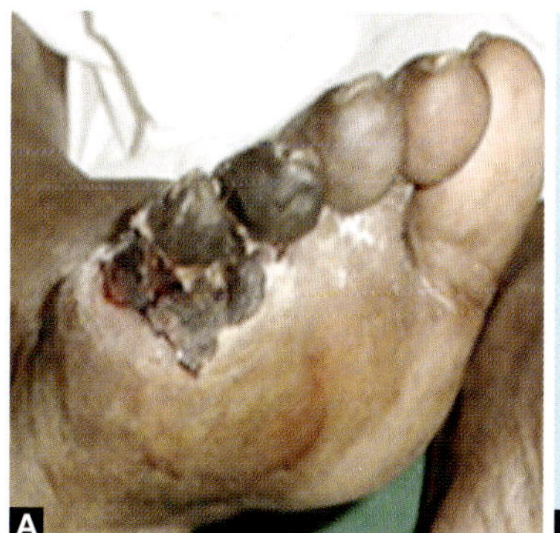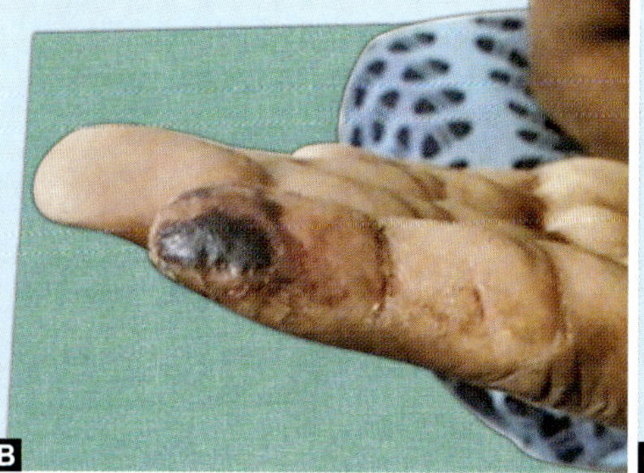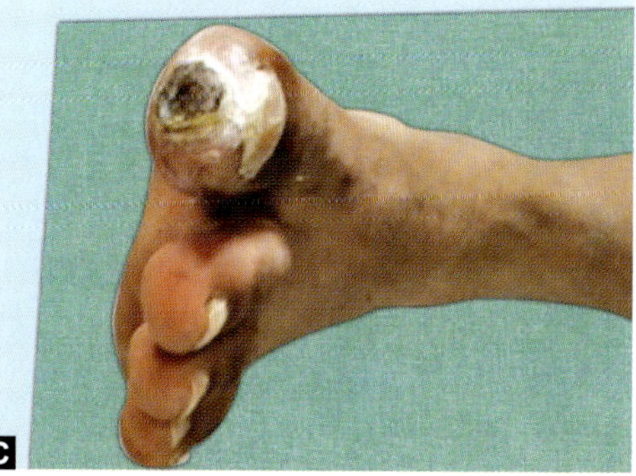

Figs. 17.7A to C: (A) Gangrenous mummified digits; (B) Discoloration tip of finger; (C) Nonhealing wound.

Venous Diseases

Venous disorders are more common than the arterial disorders. The veins of the leg consist of superficial and deep system separated by fascia and joined by perforators or communicators. Phlebitis of superficial and deep veins is common and related to injury and inflammation, whereas valve incompetency is related to gravitational stresses and other factors and as sequel to deep vein thrombosis (DVT).

Acute Venous Disease

Venous thrombosis or phlebothrombosis is generally considered as a contraindication for physical therapy. It is defined as occlusion of blood flow in the vein secondary to coagulation. It is generally associated with inflammation of tissues surrounding the veins called periphlebitis. It is usually caused by infection or injury, e.g., indwelling catheters, formation of a blood clot in the presence of venous inflammation or injury. The pain is generally described as deep ache in the muscle such as "Charlie Horse," which is relieved by rest. Superficial venous thrombosis can be identified as a cord-like structure palpated along the affected vein. It may be associated with redness and swelling.

Venous stasis is a major risk factor for **DVT (Fig. 17.8)**. DVT is manifested as:

- Increased painful palpation of calf
- Edema of the affected limb
- Painful passive stretch of the vein (Homans signs)
- Warm extremity

It is associated with reduced blood flow as a result of:

- Bed rest
- Immobility due to lower extremity fractures, spinal cord injury
- Postoperative
- During long journeys where the blood flow is stagnant
- In autoimmune disorders

In supine position during immobility along with sluggish blood flow due to lack of active pumping, there is also a constant pressure on the calf muscle by the contact of bed. Changes in vessel wall, platelet aggregation, and altered coagulation profile contribute to formation of thrombus. Thromboembolism can occur wherein a fragment of thrombus detaches and dislodges in smaller vessel obstructing blood flow, most commonly brain and lungs (**pulmonary embolism**) wherein the mortality is very high. When pulmonary embolism occurs, patient complains of chest pain, breathlessness, and hemoptysis.

Varicose Veins

Primary varicosities: Cause is generally linked to family or occupation where prolonged standing is required. Obesity, pregnancy, and constipation can contribute to the problem. It affects women more than men. It is due to malfunction of the valves in superficial veins. Most commonly, there is an incompetent valve at saphenofemoral junction, causing backflow down the long saphenous vein. This leads to dilatation and tortuousness of long saphenous veins and its tributaries. It can occur in short saphenous veins and both can be incompetent together. The common problem is cosmetic appearance and aching legs **(Fig. 17.9)**.

Secondary varicose veins: This generally follows DVT, which destroys the valves in deep veins causing gross reflux through the perforators into superficial venous system. This leads to chronic venous insufficiency (CVI).

Chronic Venous Insufficiency

It is a syndrome resulting from chronic venous hypertension in the erect posture either on standing or exercise. Venous valves when begin to fail and lose their ability to close properly lead to venous reflux. The calf muscle pump can also be affected. In addition, people with poor mobility loose the functioning of venous plexus of the foot. This plexus located in the arch of the foot is responsible for shunting of the blood through the venous system with each step.

The venous pressure which is around 90 mm Hg at rest reaches around 200 mm Hg in the deep venous system during calf muscle contraction. After contraction, it drops down to 10 mm Hg in deep and 30 mm Hg in superficial system, allowing a gradient of flow from superficial

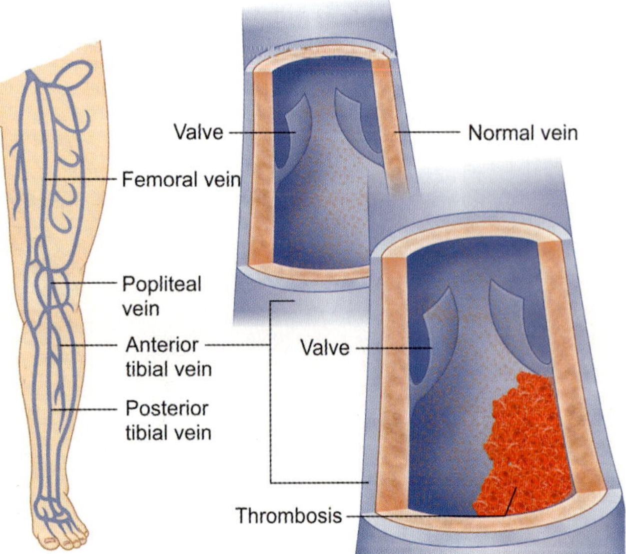

Fig. 17.8: Deep vein thrombosis.

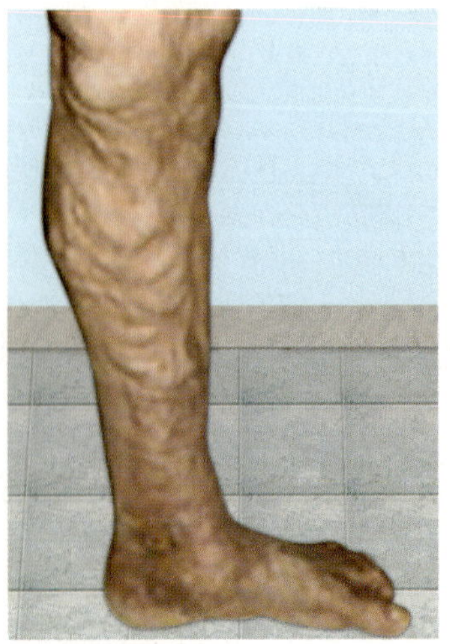

Fig. 17.9: Varicose veins.

venous system to deep venous system. With pathology, the pressure in deep venous system does not lower but may remain higher than the superficial system reversing the gradient. There is increased venous hypertension and congestion leading to edematous lower extremity, erythema, and dermatitis. It causes stasis pigmentation **(Fig. 17.10)** due to hemosiderin, a dark staining pigment, which is a by-product of lysed red blood cells that causes internal stain of affected limb. Macrocirculatory and microcirculatory dysfunction which results in increased venous hypertension can become chronic and debilitating leading to the formation of ulcerations **(Figs. 17.11 and 17.12)**.

There are various theories to the microcirculatory components of this disease, which leads to subsequent ulcerations.

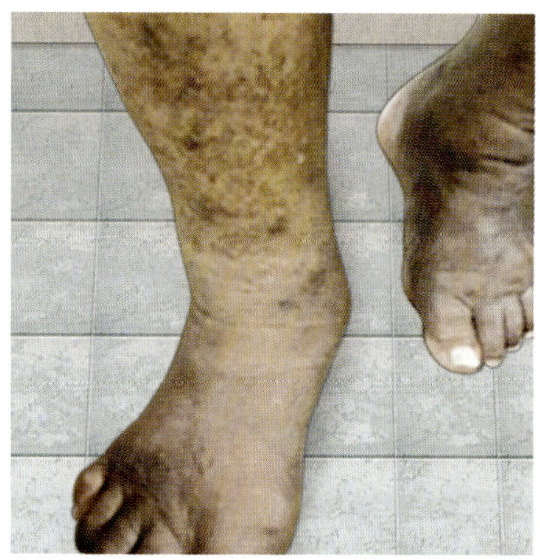

Fig. 17.10: Edema and pigmentation due to stasis.

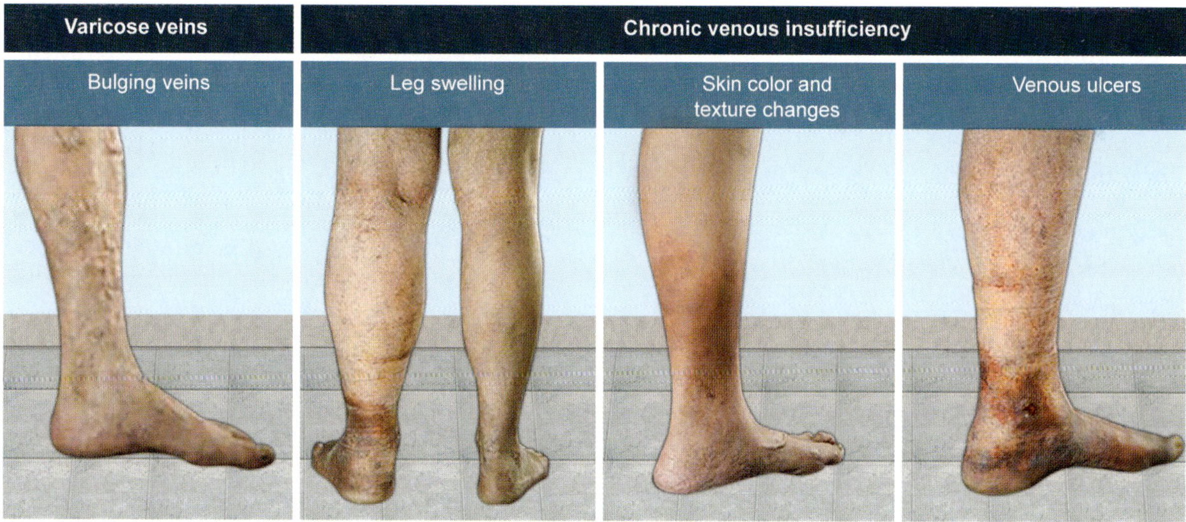

Fig. 17.11: Chronic venous insufficiency.

The fibrin cuff theory: First described by Browse and Burnand, it states that the elevated venous pressure allows leakage of fibrinogen through the pores of distended veins. This fibrinogen forms a cuff around the vessel. This reduces tissue fibrinolysis through a cascade of events, leading to a decreased tissue oxygenation and repair. The skin begins to develop lipodermatosclerosis.

The leukocyte trapping theory: The neutrophils trapped in the endothelial lining become activated and release cytokines that damages vessel wall (Coleridge Smith et al.). Fibrin deposition, tissue death, and scarring occur together called lipodermatosclerosis.

Ischemia-reperfusion injury (Greenwood et al.): Damage and death of tissues occur due to release of free radicals, which are released due to reperfusion of ischemic tissues.

Complications

Hemorrhage: Occurring from minor trauma to dilated vein. The bleeding can be profuse.

Ulcers: The dysfunction of communicating and perforating veins leads to the formation of ulcers along the medial aspect of lower extremity. If vascular incompetence

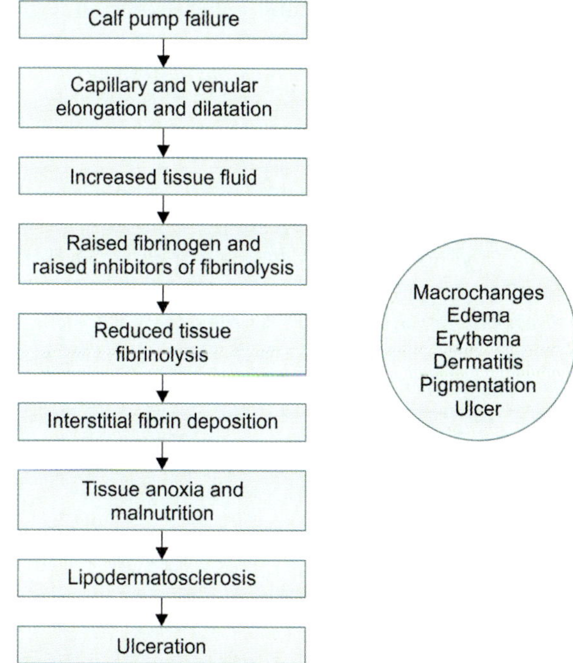

Fig. 17.12: The cascade of events in chronic venous insufficiency.

develops in the perforators and reflux is significant, high pressures can develop at the junction of the superficial veins and perforating veins. This leads to tissue ischemia and ultimately to skin ulcer. Long-standing ulcers can be malignant (Marjolin's ulcer), can lead to periostitis if on tibia, and an equinus deformity.

Lymphatic Disorders

The principal physiological function of the lymphatic vasculature is to take up fluid, leaking out of blood capillaries into interstitial spaces in the tissue, and to return it to the blood circulation. Any failure to effectively do so results in lymphedema, a chronic, disabling and disfiguring condition. Limb edema occurs because of osmotic forces created by these molecules, which retain fluid. Chronic fibrosis tends to occur with skin changes. Although some contractility may occur in lymphatics, most fluid movement is passive due to squeezing of lymph vessels by adjacent muscle contractions. Lymphedema is generally hard and is nonpittable. Kinmonth et al., classified lymphedema into primary and secondary.

Primary lymphedemas are those in which no other disease process or intrinsic abnormalities can be identified. They are sometimes hereditary. Most cases without an apparent hereditary factor are classified as per age.

- Congenital lymphedema usually presents at birth or at an early age and can be unilateral or bilateral.
- Lymphedema praecox occurs around puberty before the age of 35 due to inability of lymphatic system to cope up with the tissue protein handling due to hormonal changes.
- Lymphedema tarda develops after the age of 35 due to a result of deterioration of barely adequate lymph vessels.

Secondary lymphedema are those which are caused due to an extrinsic disease process. They result from obstruction, obliteration, or functional insufficiency of the lymphatics secondary to a pathological cause. Here, the previously normal lymphatics have been damaged.

- Filariasis **(Fig. 17.13)** is caused by infection through mosquito bites with filarial worms. These parasites move up the lymphatics blocking them and causing massive edema and appearance commonly known as elephantiasis. Scrotal edema is also common.
- The other common cause is surgical resection of lymph nodes as in radical mastectomy or irradiation in treatment of malignancy.

  Lymphedema is also classified based on clinical and lymphographic finding (Browse and Stewart).

- **Distal obliteration** where in total absence or reduction in number of distal lymphatics; mild edema of both ankles and lower legs. It constitutes 80% of primary lymphedemas.
- **Proximal obliteration** usually involves the entire limb and is unilateral.

  Prof Kinmonth on the basis of lymphangiography classified lymphedema into:

- **Aplasia** wherein no lymphatics are formed as in Milroy's disease

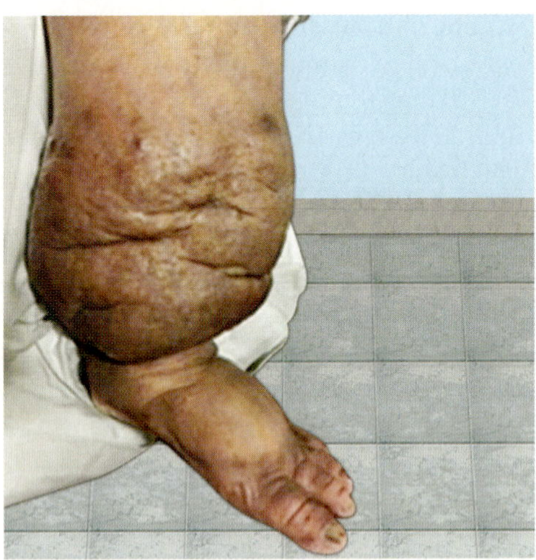

Fig. 17.13: Secondary lymphedema.

- **Hypoplasia** where lymphatics are present but less than normal
- **Hyperplastic** with incompetent valves allowing backflow of lymph, causing leakage from skin, sometimes in chest producing pleural effusion and in abdomen causing ascites. A concise summary of disease, pathogenesis and functional consequence is presented in **Table 17.2.**

ASSESSMENT OF PERIPHERAL VASCULAR DISEASE

A detailed **history** and evaluation can differentiate arterial from venous dysfunction. It is important to identify a coexisting arterial and venous dysfunction as venous disorders need elevation whereas arterial disorders obtain relief in dependent position.

Age is an important factor in consideration of diagnosis—atherosclerosis is more common in old age, whereas Buerger's and Raynaud's are diseases of young. Varicose veins are commonly seen in middle-aged. Primary lymphedema is seen at young age, whereas secondary lymphedema occurs in middle and old age.

Associated risk factors are an equally important consideration.

- Diabetes, dyslipidemia, hypertension
- Addictions (tobacco, cigarette) in suspected arterial disease
- Occupational history (prolonged standing)
- Dietary habits
- Bowel habits (constipation)
- Physical activity
- History of malignancy, surgical removal of lymph nodes or irradiation, mosquito bite goes in favor of lymphatic disorders.

Pain at rest, on activity, or at the end of the day guides toward the nature of vessel involved.

- **Intermittent claudication** is characterized by pain in the calf, foot, thigh, or buttock which increases with walking; typically disappears quickly at rest or stopping the

Table 17.2: Functional consequence of peripheral vascular disease.

Disease	Pathology	Functional consequence
Acute arterial occlusion	Thrombosis and embolism	• Reduced blood flow
Peripheral atherosclerotic disease	Atherosclerosis	• Decreased vasodilator function
Thromboangiitis obliterans	Inflammatory and thrombotic	• Increased arterial stiffness
Raynaud's	Vasospastic	• Impaired hyperemic response
		• Impaired arterial remodeling
		• Increased inflammatory activation
		• Impaired energy production
		• Impaired oxygen utilization
		• Increased reactive oxygen species
		• Reduced skeletal muscle content
		• Adverse skeletal muscle remodeling
		• Increased atherosclerotic progression
Thrombophlebitis	Inflammatory and thrombotic	• Increased activation of inflammatory markers
Deep vein thrombosis	Embolic and thrombosis	• Increased free oxygen radicals
Varicose veins	Structural defect of walls	• Impaired venous valve function
		• Impaired venous pressure
Chronic venous insufficiency	Valve dysfunction and increased venous pressure	• Reduced skeletal muscle content
		• Adverse skeletal muscle remodeling
Primary lymphedema	Lymphatics absent or not formed	• Increased protein in tissues
Secondary lymphedema	Removal or destruction of lymph channels or lymph nodes	• Increased fluid retention
		• Impaired inflammatory response

activity. It refers to the pain that occurs in a muscle with inadequate blood supply causing ischemia on demand. The pain does not occur with sitting or standing (unless in critical ischemia), is reproducible and more severe when walking upstairs or uphill, and is described as a cramp that disappears within 2 minutes after stopping the exercise. It has to be differentiated from neurogenic claudication due to lumbar canal stenosis, where the pain is relieved only by stooping or bending forward.

- Rest pain that develops at night, awakens the patient, or requires analgesics for relief is considered more severe than claudication.
- **Critical limb ischemia** is persistently recurring ischemic rest pain for 2 weeks which requires regular analgesics for more than 2 weeks or ulceration or gangrene of the foot or toes. The ankle systolic blood pressure is generally <50 mm Hg.
- Prominence of veins in the leg, swelling in the extremity toward the evening, and aching legs that is relieved with elevation are more complaints of venous disorders. Occupation that demands prolonged standing has common sufferers.
- Swelling of the leg around ankle and a little higher which may be painful is an important feature commonly seen in patients with on prolonged bed rest, post-surgical, fractures of long bones.

Clinical Evaluation

Observation

Observation includes:
- Observation of skin for (pigmentation, ulceration, trophic changes), attitude of limb and gait pattern forms a crucial part of evaluation.
- Look at the resting position of the limb. Is it dependent to relieve ischemic pain or is it kept in elevated position to relieve engorgement of veins?
- Observe affected limb for wasting or trophic changes such as abnormal nail growth, decreased leg and foot hair, and dry skin as in arterial disorders.
- Skin color for cyanosis or pallor or blackish discoloration with mummified digits in arterial dysfunction.
- Prominence of tortuous veins, edema, discoloration as hemosiderin staining, loss of skin creases; fibrotic skin is seen in venous disorders. Weeping skin is seen in CVI.
- If the patient has itching, redness it may be due to eczema.
- Wet wound or oozing ulcers with irregular margins seen near the medial malleolus or gaiter areas are indicative of venous disease.
- Scar may be seen as a result of healed ulcers or previous operation of varicose veins.
- Redness and associated swelling with peeling of skin are seen in inflammatory reactions (cellulitis).
- Swelling or edema: Look for increase in size of the limb and shape of the limb. Palpate and check for pitting. If the edema is nonpittable, it generally indicates chronicity as may be seen in CVI. Pitting edema may be caused by DVT, venous insufficiency, and early stages of lymphedema. Nonpitting edema (no skin indent) that remains unchanged overnight is rare, and a disturbance in the lymph flow should be considered as a possible cause.
- Inspection of the skin will reveal deepened natural creases, thickened cutaneous folds, pronounced soft

local swelling, and fibrosis. The skin cannot be easily lifted up. Legs appear like huge columns.

- DVT and reflex sympathetic dystrophy are painful conditions with edema. CVI may cause some aching. Lymphedema is usually painless. Skin ulcerations are not seen in lymphatic disorders.
- Check if the edema disappears with elevation. The swelling of the extremity due to the accumulation of protein-rich fluid in the tissues is usually not relieved by elevation and is in most patients also associated with inflammatory reactions, fibrosis, and overgrowth of adipose and connective tissue in the affected areas. In later stages of non-pitting edema, fibrosis with abnormalities such as cysts, fistulas, papillomas, hyperkeratosis is seen. There is an increased susceptibility to infections.
- A subjective feeling of fatigue, heaviness, pressure, or tightness is present in the affected region. This may be associated with numbness and tingling.

Edema is measured using girth measurement with reference to bony points to allow consistency of tracking changes. Measurement of calf circumference should be obtained in all patients with suspected lower extremity thrombophlebitis. This should be done with the patient standing and the feet 30 cm apart. The maximum circumference is recorded and a significant difference exists if the two sides differ by 1.5 cm in males and 1.2 cm in females. Figure of 8 measurements around the ankle can be done. Volumetrics is a quantitative system to measure edema. It is alternative method of measuring limb size by immersing the limb in a tank of water to a predetermined anatomical landmark and measuring

Table 17.3:	Grades of lymphedema by the International Society of Lymphology.
Grade 1	No pitting, larger fibrotic limb, skin, and nail changes
Grade 2	No pitting, larger fibrotic limb, skin, and nail changes
Grade 3	Elephantiasis, thick skin with huge folds, marked skin deterioration

the volume displaced. Depending on the appearance of skin and edema, lymphedema can be graded. **Table 17.3** describes the grades of lymphedema by the International Society of Lymphology.

Mobility and gait are affected in all the vascular dysfunctions due to pain, loss of range, strength, and presence of ulcers. Gross motor examination to assess the range of motion and strength is important. It is important to test the strength of calf and foot muscles. Sensory testing is done using light touch and pressure. Monofilament testing can be done if available to rule out neuropathy. Temperature of the skin can be assessed using thermistor, test tube, or palpating. Altered temperature compared to unaffected limb or proximal part can provide important insight into vascular dysfunction. Skin is cold to touch in arterial, whereas it is warm in venous dysfunction.

Test for Arterial Dysfunction

Pulse

Palpation of distal arteries such as brachial, radial, femoral, popliteal, dorsalis pedis, and posterior tibial is very important **(Fig. 17.14)**. Palpation should be done using the fingertips and intensity of the pulse graded on a scale

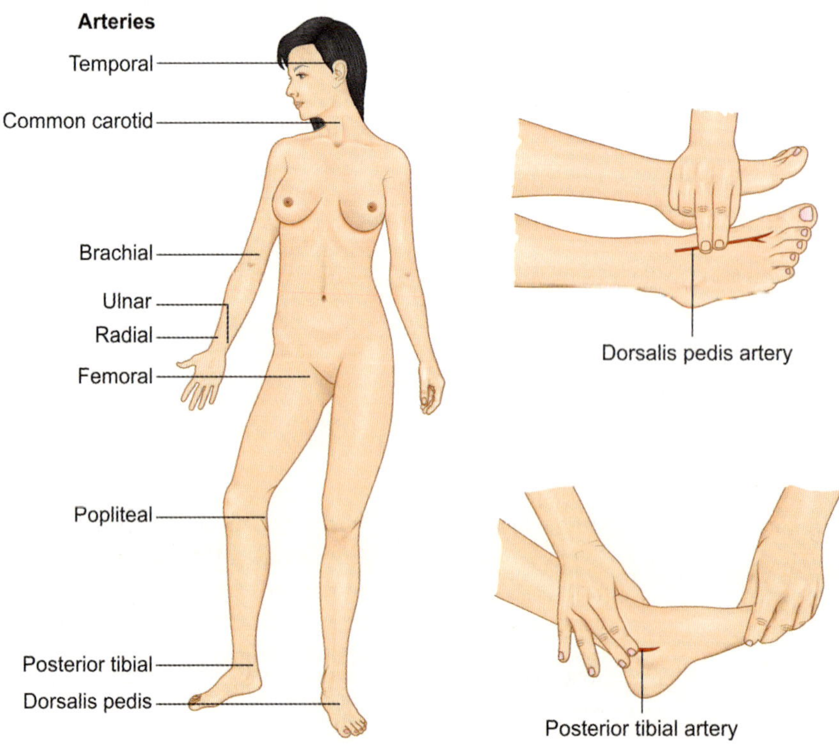

Fig. 17.14: Palpation of arteries.

<table>
<tr><td>BOX 17.1: Grades of pulses.</td></tr>
</table>

0 – – indicating no palpable pulse
1+ – indicating a faint, but detectable pulse
2+ – suggesting a slightly more diminished pulse than normal
3+ – is a normal pulse
4+ – indicating a bounding pulse

of 0 to 4+ where **(Box 17.1)**. It may not be possible to feel the pulses, Doppler should be used. Pulses are compared with normal extremity. Auscultation on the vessel with stethoscope may help identify turbulent blood flow (Bruit) that indicates the possibility of partial blockage.

Ankle–Brachial Index

It is a simple noninvasive test performed with Doppler ultrasound for diagnosing peripheral–arterial disease. The dorsalis pedis artery or posterior tibial artery is located with the Doppler. A blood pressure cuff is then placed around the calf and inflated until cessation of audible signals. The cuff is then slowly released until the signal is heard. At this point, the pressure readings are recorded as ankle pressure. The procedure is repeated for the upper extremity with the cuff around the arm over the brachial artery and Doppler on radial artery. The upper extremity pressure obtained is called brachial pressure. The ratio of ankle-to-brachial pressure is called ankle–brachial index (ABI). The 2007 Inter-Society Consensus for the Management of Peripheral Arterial Disease (TASC II) defines the cutoff value of ABI 0.90 or less for diagnosing peripheral artery disease (PAD) by using the higher of the two ankle pressures in calculating ABI. A normal ABI at rest but decreases by 15–20% on exertion is also considered as diagnostic of PAD **(Fig. 17.15 and Table 17.4)**.

Severe ischemia is assumed with ABI of 0.5 at rest and 0.15 after exercise. It indicates multilevel disease. Indices of 0.4 or less are generally considered indications for amputations.

Segmental pressures can also be assessed to determine different pressures and levels of vascular flow. Falsely elevated ABI of more than 1.2 with a history of claudication and/or rest pain can be indicative of arterial disease. It is generally seen in diabetics and calcified vessels which have low compressibility. If pressure readings during cuff inflation exceed 200 mm Hg or the sound does not disappear, arteriosclerosis or calcified vessels are suspected. ABI is recorded as unattainable in view of noncompressible artery.

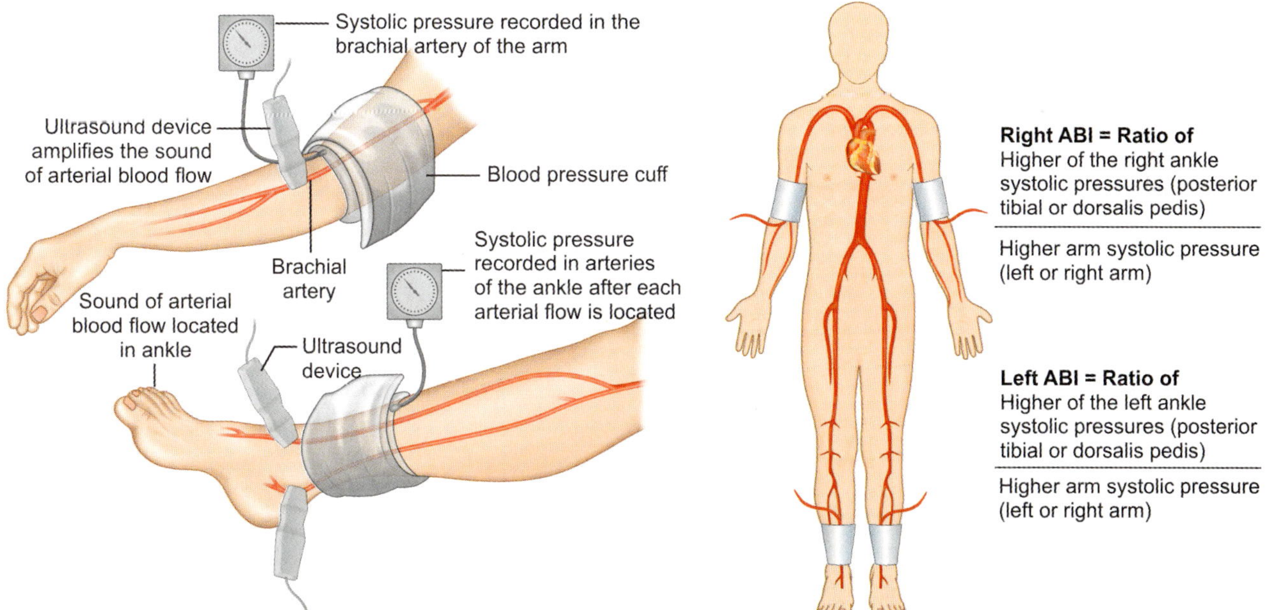

Fig. 17.15: Measurement of ankle–brachial index.

Table 17.4: Ankle–brachial index.		
Ankle–brachial index	Possible indication	Associated symptoms
>1.2	Falsely elevated	Intermittent claudication/rest pain
0.95–1.2	Normal	–
0.8–0.9	Mild disease	Intermittent claudication
0.5–0.8	Moderate disease	Rest pain
<0.5	Severe disease	Rest pain/gangrenous changes

Pole Test (for Falsely Elevated Ankle–Brachial Index)

In patients with leg ischemia the level of elevation at which the foot takes on significant pallor correlates to the level of disappearance of Doppler signal disappears over the distal artery. In a calcified artery, this level represents the systolic blood pressure. Using a calibrated pole that converts the height of ankle elevation into mm Hg, the systolic blood pressure can be assessed based on disappearance of Doppler sound on dorsalis pedis on elevation of the leg. Calibrations on the pole are marked at 13 cm intervals that correspond to 10 mm Hg. The upper extremity value is determined as usual. In absence of a pole, the vertical distance in centimeters between the bed and height of the ankle at which sound disappears is noted. This value can be multiplied by 0.735 to give systolic pressure.

Cold Provocation Test

Hand or foot to be tested is put in cold water (10–15°C) for 1–10 minutes. Visible cyanosis and blanching indicate vasospasm. Skin temperature can be measured over time to note the rate of digital rewarming. Clinical categories of various level of acute limb ischemia is described in **Table 17.5**.

Tests for Venous Dysfunction

Venous Filling Time

This test is used to assess both arterial and venous systems. The patient is positioned supine and affected extremity is elevated to empty blood from superficial veins of the limb. Next, the patient hangs the limb over the edge of the bed into a dependent position. Time is recorded when veins of top of foot have filled. Normal filling time is approximately 15 seconds. A time greater than 15 seconds is indicative of arterial disease and less than 15 seconds suggests venous insufficiency.

Rubor of Dependency

It is performed similar to venous filling test. The patient is positioned supine and the color of both the feet is examined. The affected limb is then elevated for several seconds and lowered back to the original position. The time is recorded for testing the color of affected foot with stationary foot. In arterial disease, it may take more than 20–30 seconds for color to return and it will be bright red. If the color returns immediately, then it may indicate venous insufficiency.

Schwartz Test

In standing position, when a lower part of the long saphenous vein in the leg is tapped, impulse is felt at the saphenous junction or at the upper end of the visible part of the vein. It signifies continuous column of blood due to valvular incompetence.

Brodie–Trendelenburg Test

The purpose is to assess incompetency of saphenofemoral valve and functioning of valves within the communication system.

- The lower extremity is elevated to approximately 75° with the patient supine to empty the veins. This may be hastened by milking the veins proximally.
- A tourniquet is placed around the thigh to prevent superficial venous backflow.
- The patient is asked to stand up quickly so that extremity is in dependent position.

If the superficial veins start filling up without release of the tourniquet on standing, it indicates incompetent communicating system or perforators that allow the flow of blood from deep to superficial veins. On release of tourniquet, if the varices fill rapidly from above, it indicates incompetent saphenofemoral valve. In both the cases test is considered positive and is an indication for surgery. To test short saphenous vein, the same test is done with tourniquet at saphenopopliteal junction.

Tourniquet Test

The purpose is to identify the position of incompetent communicating vein. Test is performed as Trendelenburg test. Tourniquet is tied around the thigh or leg at different levels. By moving the tourniquet down the leg in steps, one can determine if mid-thigh, lower thigh, or low leg perforators are incompetent. If the vein above the tourniquet fills up but those below remain collapsed, it indicates incompetent veins above tourniquet. Similarly, if veins below the tourniquet fill up but above remain empty, it indicates an incompetent system below tourniquet.

Table 17.5: Clinical categories of acute limb ischemia.

Category	Description/prognosis	Findings		Doppler finding	
		Sensory loss	Muscle weakness	Arterial	Venous
I. Viable	Not immediately threatened	None	None	Audible	Audible
II. Threatened					
a. Marginally	Salvageable if promptly	Minimal (toes) or none	None	Inaudible	Audible
b. Immediately	Salvageable with immediate revascularizaton	More than toes associated with rest pain	Mild-moderate	Inaudible	Audible
III. Irreversible	Major tissue loss or permanent nerve damage inevitables	Profound anesthetic	Profound paralysis (rigor)	Inaudible	Inaudible

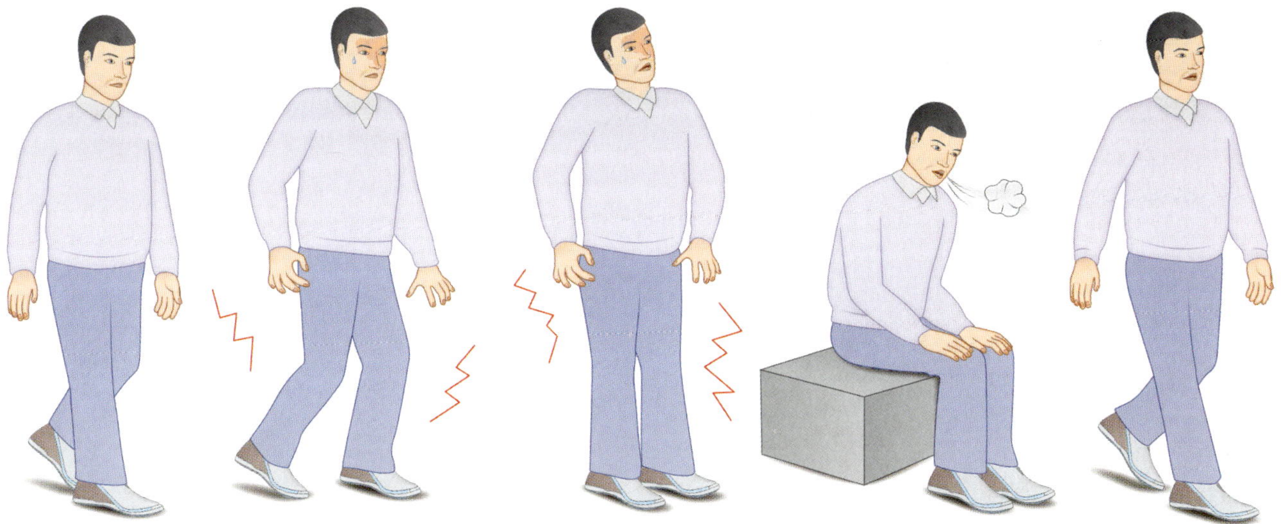

The first noticeable symptom of PAD may be intermittent claudication. This is leg discomfort, pain or cramping that develops with activity is relieved with rest, and recurs upon resuming activity. The pain is most often noticed in the calf, but may also be felt in the buttocks or thighs.

Fig. 17.16: Claudication.

Cuff Test

It is used to assess the presence of DVT. It is performed by placing a blood pressure cuff around the lower leg and inflating the cuff. If the patient is unable to tolerate a cuff pressure higher than 40 mm Hg, there is a high probability of DVT. The test can be augmented by forcefully squeezing the calf muscle or passive dorsiflexion of the calf. A positive result is severe pain by the patient (+ **Homans Sign**).

Stemmers Test

The purpose is to assess for lymphedema. Inability to pick up a fold of skin at the base of the second toe of the affected extremity indicates a positive test for lymphedema or lymphostasis.

Air Plethysmography

It is noninvasive vascular examination for both arterial and venous systems. It is used to detect minute changes in leg volume and can be performed during static or postural changes or during exercise. It provides a quantitative measure of venous reflux, calf pump, and residual venous volume after exercise.

Reflux Test

The Doppler is used to listen for reflux over major veins in the lower extremity. Easiest to assess is great saphenous vein. The probe is placed over the saphenous vein to detect an audible signal of venous blood flow. The vessel sound can be augmented by squeezing the extremity distal to the probe to detect for obstructions as well as determine proper placement of probe. To listen for reflux, the extremity should be squeezed proximal to the probe. No audible signal should occur unless there is valvular incompetence.

Invasive Test for Vascular Insufficiency

Venography and arteriography are contrast dye studies to examine patients' vascular system. Lymphangiography and lymphoscintigraphy are studies done to know about lymphatic system.

Functional Evaluation

Grading Claudication

A classical symptom of peripheral arterial disease is pain on walking fixed distance which is relieved on stopping or rest. The pain recurs upon resuming activity. This is referred to as claudication. The distribution of pain is generally calf but can be in buttock also. It depends on site of disease **(Fig. 17.16).** Claudication pain can be based on the perception as no pain, moderate, intense and maximal pain **(Box 17.2)**.

The time at which the patient first begins to feel claudication symptoms is defined as the **initial claudication time** (also called pain-free walking time). The workload which brings on claudication is considered the initial training workload. Furthest distance patient is able to walk is termed as **absolute claudication distance**. Clinical staging of arterial disease is done on the basis of symptoms and distance walked. There are two classifications Fontaine's and Rutherford's **(Table 17.6)**.

BOX 17.2: Claudication pain perception scale.

Claudication pain perception scale:
0 – No pain
1 – Onset of pain
2 – Moderate pain
3 – Intense pain
4 – Maximal pain

Table 17.6: Clinical staging based on claudication.

Fontaine's classification		Rutherford's classification			
Stage	Symptoms	Grade	Category	Symptoms	
1	Asymptomatic	0	0	Asymptomatic	
2	Intermittent claudication	I	1	Mild claudication	
2A	Distance to pain onset >200 m	I	2	Moderate claudication	
2B	Distance to pain onset <200 m	I	3	Severe claudication	
3	Pain at rest	II	4	Ischemic rest pain	
4	Gangrene, tissue loss	III	5	Minor tissue loss	
–	–	III	6	Major tissue loss	

Claudication remains stable in 80% of patients. Risk of limb loss (amputation) at 5 years is 4–7% and at 10 years is 12%.

Assessment of functional impairment and health-related qauality of life **(HRQOL)** in patients with claudication should be incorporated into the evaluation of all treatments for symptomatic PAD. Functional ability is an individual's ability to perform normal daily activities required to meet basic needs, to fulfill usual roles, and to maintain health and well-being. For people with PAD, this includes the ability to walk distances without pain. HRQOL is a multidimensional concept that includes domains related to physical, mental, emotional, and social functioning and focuses on the impact that health status has on quality of life.

Patients with PAD have a significant **functional impairment**. Overall, patients with claudication have an ≈50% reduction in peak oxygen consumption (VO_2) compared with an age-matched healthy cohort. Tests to measure functional capacity and claudication are:
- Six-minute walk test
- Short physical performance battery includes:
  1. Four-meter walking velocity
  2. Repeated chair rise
  3. Standing balance.

Impairment according to ambulatory distance on 6-minute walk test:
- Greater than 150 m is mild
- 50–150 m is moderate
- Less than 50 m is considered severe

Treadmill Testing Protocols

Treadmill exercise performance has been the most common outcome measurement used to measure changes in walking endurance and peak exercise capacity in response to exercise interventions in patients with PAD. A graded treadmill exercise test modifies the load during treadmill testing, has better test–retest reliability than constant-load treadmill testing, and is the preferred method of treadmill testing in randomized trials of PAD.

Gardner–Skinner protocol (1991): Treadmill speed is held constant at 2 mph. Treadmill grade begins at 0% and increases 2% every 2 minutes.

Modified Gardner protocol: The speed begins at 0.5 mph and a grade of 0 and speed is increased by 0.5 mph every 2 minutes until 2.0 mph is achieved. When a speed of 2.0 mph is reached, the treadmill grade is increased by 2% every 2 minutes.

Hiatt protocol (1990): Treadmill speed held constant at 2 mph. Treadmill grade begins at 0% and increases by 3.5% every 3 minutes.

Bronas/Treat–Jacobson protocol (2009): Treadmill speed begins at 2 mph. Treadmill grade begins at 0% and increases by 3.5% every 3 minutes through 10.5% grade (12 minutes, stage beginning with stage 5), the treadmill grade is kept constant at 10.5% and the speed increases by 0.5 mph every 3 minutes.

- The walking impairment questionnaire (WIQ)
- Vascular quality of life questionnaire (VascuQoL)
- Peripheral artery questionnaire (PAQ)
- Impact of PAD on quality of life questionnaire

The above questionnaires have been used to measure patient-reported perceptions of their walking ability or HRQOL after exercise interventions. The WIQ, PAQ, VascuQoL, and Impact of PAD on quality of life questionnaire are PAD-specific measures; in that, they were developed specifically to measure limitations in walking or HRQOL in people with PAD.

The WIQ is a disease-specific questionnaire widely used to assess the ability of patients with claudication to walk defined distances and speeds and to climb stairs. In addition, the questionnaire evaluates claudication severity and the presence of other (nonclaudication) symptoms that could potentially limit walking. The WIQ was validated against treadmill walking in patients with claudication and has been used extensively in these patients to evaluate changes in community-based walking ability resulting from an exercise training program, stenting, and pharmacological agents.

It has also been shown to improve mortality risk prediction models. Scores range from 0 to 100, with higher scores indicating better community-based walking ability.

MANAGEMENT OF VASCULAR DISORDERS

Clinical Pearl

Acute arterial and venous disorders may not need immediate physical therapy intervention rather need immediate medical and surgical intervention.

Management of Arterial Disorders

Pharmacotherapy

Pharmacotherapy includes:
- In acute arterial occlusion heparinization is indicated.
- Pentoxifylline increases the flexibility of RBCs and helps them to reach microcirculation in a better way so as to increase the oxygenation.
- Low-dose aspirin for antithrombin activity.
- Dipyridamole and warfarin may improve time to claudication.

Table 17.7: Target therapy for peripheral arterial disease.	
Lipid-lowering therapy	• Treatment with statin for all PAD patients to target LDL cholesterol <100 mg/dL • Target LDL cholesterol <70 mg/dL for high-risk patients
Hypertension treatment	• Treat to target blood pressure <140/90 mm Hg (<130/80 mmHg for patients with diabetes or chronic kidney disease) • Consider ACE inhibitor in hypertensive patients • Use of beta-blockers is not contraindicated in PAD
Smoking cessation	• Provide comprehensive smoking intervention program • Consider pharmacotherapy to support smoking cessation
Antiplatelet therapy	• Treat with asprin 75–325 mg or clopidogrel 77 mg • Treat with aspirin + thienopyridine in patients with acute coronary syndrome or coronary or peripheral stent

(PAD: peripheral arterial disease; LDL: low-density lipoprotein; ACE: angiotensin-converting enzyme)

- Beta-blockers may decrease time to claudication. Target therapy involves treatment of risk factors and maintaining health targets **(Table 17.7)**.

Surgical Intervention

Surgical procedures may include thrombectomy, embolectomy, endarterectomy for removal of thrombus or revascularization through bypass such as:
- Femoropopliteal bypass
- Aortoiliac or aortobifemoral
- Axillofemoral bypass
- Percutaneous transluminal balloon angioplasty is also carried out for larger vessels.

Postoperative care, pain relief, and wound care are important. Remobilize the patient and maximize function. Work on maintaining venous return with active muscle pumping. Progress quickly to weight-bearing ambulation to tolerance. Avoid hip and knee flexion to reduce the risk of graft occlusion. Care should be taken to avoid movements that would kink the graft and cause turbulent flow.

Vascular rehabilitation program includes patient education and exercise. It improves walking distance and claudication.

Patient Education

It is important that the patient is explained the disease process its prognosis, reversibility, and importance of behavior modification for lifestyle to control risk factors.

Smoking Cessation

Patients should be assisted with counseling and developing a plan for quitting that may include pharmacotherapy (varenicline, bupropion, nicotine replacement therapy), behavioral therapy, and/or referral to a smoking cessation program.

Weight Reduction

Obesity is associated with increased relative risks for total mortality and cardiovascular diseases. Moreover, body mass index has also been shown to be directly associated with total cholesterol, blood pressure, and blood glucose levels. Abdominal fat distribution, but not total body fatness, is associated with peripheral arterial occlusive disease, independently of concurrent cardiovascular risk factors. Weight loss can improve insulin sensitivity and increase high-density lipoprotein cholesterol (HDL-C). It may also improve claudication distance.

Diet and Physical Activity

The risk of PAD is inversely related to previous levels of physical activity suggesting a protective effect of exercise. Trials have also clearly demonstrated that walking capacity is increased by exercise training in patients with claudication and regular exercise coupled with risk factor modification, especially smoking cessation, is the cornerstone of conservative therapy for intermittent claudication. There is also evidence for the benefit of diet rich in fruit, nuts, vegetables, fish, and mono-unsaturated vegetable oils.

Foot and Skincare

Exposure of feet to more warm and cold temperature should be avoided. Trauma even minor such as nail paring or pressure points in the feet should be avoided. Dryness on feet and legs should be avoided. Plantar aspect of feet should be inspected daily. Footwear should be appropriate. Use of ankle–foot orthosis and microcellular rubber insoles are also found to be beneficial.

Exercise

It is the mainstay of rehabilitation program. A program of supervised exercise training is recommended as an initial treatment modality for patients with intermittent claudication. Potential mechanism underlying benefits of exercise are shown in **Figure 17.17**. Exercise improves perfusion, inducts angioneogenesis, increases collaterals, improves muscle metabolism and hence increses walking efficiency. Supervised program should be performed for a minimum of 30–45 minutes, in sessions performed at least 3 times per week for a minimum of 12 weeks. The patient should be made to walk until he/she reaches a claudication pain score of 3 (intense pain) on the four-point scale. Time should be allowed for ischemic pain to subside before resuming exercise. Initially, patients may need to start with a minimum of 10 minutes of exercise and gradually progress intermittently to accumulate a total of 30–60 min/day. Gradually, the time is increased by 5 min/day biweekly. As individuals can walk beyond 10

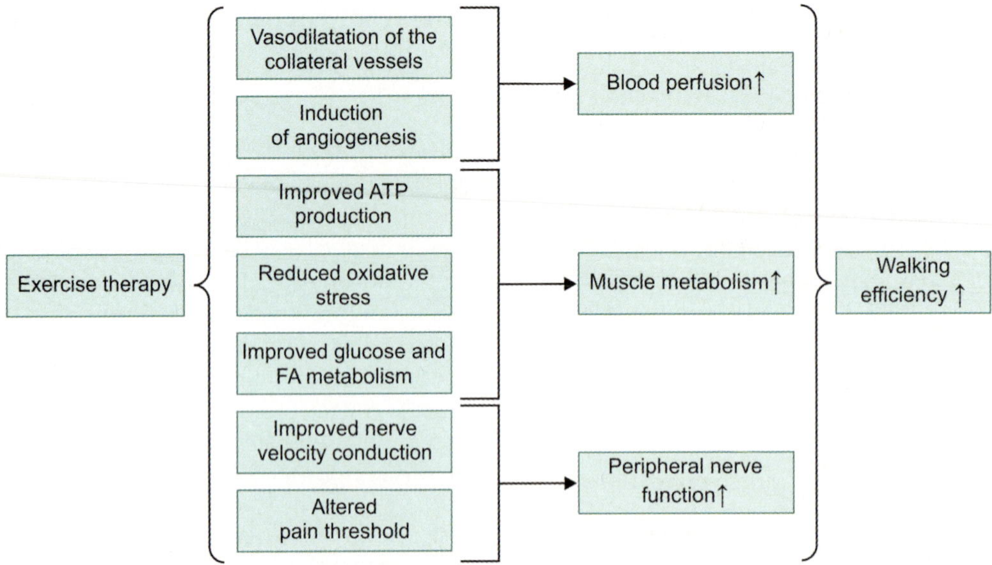

Fig. 17.17: Potential mechanisms underlying benefits of exercises (to add from the end). (ATP: adenosine triphosphate; FA: fatty acid)

minutes without reaching prescribed claudication level, grade or speed of exercise prescription should be changed such as to induce claudication within 5–10 minutes of walking session.

Training using an interval training approach leads to an increase in the initial and maximum absolute distance that can be walked without pain. The exercise program should be designed to target the cardiovascular disease risk factors that are often associated with PAD.

Clinical Pearl

Based on a meta-analysis of exercise rehabilitation programs, Gardner and Poehlman concluded that the optimal exercise program for improving claudication distances uses intermittent walking to near maximal pain during a program of at least 6 months duration. Gardener et al., suggested that stair climbing might offer an advantage over treadmill walking for patients with claudication.

Weight-bearing aerobic exercise such as walking, treadmill, and nonweight bearing exercise such as arm ergometry can be prescribed. Warm-up and cooldown for 5–10 minutes before and after each session (longer in cold weather) is a must.

The Oxford Radeliffe Hospital program suggests four basic exercises:
1. Alternate heel raising in standing
2. Simultaneous heel raising in standing
3. Step-ups on to a low bench
4. Toe walking

Table 17.8 shows the recommendations for exercise prescription AHA 2016 and **Table 17.9** shows evidence-based 2016 AHA guidelines.

Buerger Exercise

Buerger exercise intended to improve feet and legs circulation was first described by Buerger in 1926 and

Table 17.8: Recommendations for exercise prescription AHA 2016.

Intensity	40–60% maximal workload based on baseline treadmill test or workload that brings on claudication within 3–5 min during a 6-MWT
Claudication intensity	Moderate-to-moderate/severe claudication as tolerated
Session duration	30–50 min of intermittent exercise; goal is to accumulate at least 30 min of walking exercise
Work:rest ratio	Walking duration should be within 5–10 min to reach moderate to moderately severe claudication followed by rest until pain has dissipated (2–5 min)
Frequency	3 times per week supervised. Aerobic exercises 3–5 days/week
Progression	Every 1–2 week increase duration of training session to achieve 50 min
Mode	Nonweight-bearing exercises in case of ulcer on plantar aspect. Weight-bearing exercise such as walking, treadmill, ergometry, circuit training
Resistance exercise	At least 2 days/week
Program duration	At least 12 weeks
Maintenance	Lifelong maintenance program at least 2 times per week

then modified by Allen in 1930. To relieve the symptoms in patients with lower limbs arterial insufficiency, Buerger exercises drained engorged vessels by using postural changes and stimulated peripheral circulation by modulating gravity and applying muscle contractions. The duration of each position varies in accordance with patient's tolerance or the velocity of color changes.

Table 17.9: Evidence-based guidelines AHA 2016.

COR	LOE	Recommendations
I	A	In patients with claudication, a supervised exercise program is recommended to improve functional status and QoL and to reduce leg symptoms
I	B-R	A supervised exercise program should be discussed as a treatment option for claudication before possible revascularization
IIa	A	In patients with PAD, a structured community- or home-based exercise program with behavioral change techniques can be beneficial to improve walking ability and functional status
IIa	A	In patients with claudication, alternative strategies of exercise therapy, including upper-body ergometry, cycling, and pain-free or low-intensity walking that avoids moderate-to-maximum claudication while walking, can be beneficial to improve walking ability and functional status

(COR: class of recommendation; LOE: level of evidence;
B-R: B-randomized)

- The first position should last as long as it is necessary to blanch the extremity. This varies considerably, but 2 minutes of elevation at 45° is usually sufficient **(Fig. 17.18A)**.
- The second position is carried out by the patient sitting on the side of the bed with the feet hanging down. During this phase, which should also last 2 minutes, the patient should systematically move the ankle and toe through all its ranges. The dorsal–plantar foot flexion can also help the patients to exercise their Achilles tendon to avoid contracture or joint stiffness that leads to further foot deformity **(Fig. 17.18B)**.
- The third position is carried out with the patient lying flat in bed with the feet either under the electric cradle or, better still, with the feet covered with a light warm blanket, and should last 5 minutes. It improves leg reperfusion when the gravity effects are withdrawn **(Fig. 17.18C)**.

The three positions consist of a cycle and there should be from three to six cycles in a sequence, with two to four sequences a day. The exercises should be carried out with accuracy, a timepiece at the bedside or in the patient's hand being essential.

Vasotrain

Vacuum compression therapy provides alternating cycles of positive and negative pressure in which the affected extremity rests inside the airtight cylinder. In the negative pressure cycle, the vessels are dilated and blood flows in the extremity. During positive pressure cycle, the vessel is compressed gently to push the blood out of the extremity. This device improves wound condition.

Rehabilitation for Venous and Lymphatic Insufficiency

The rehabilitation is tailored to the specific needs of each patient. It depends not only on the severity of cardiovascular

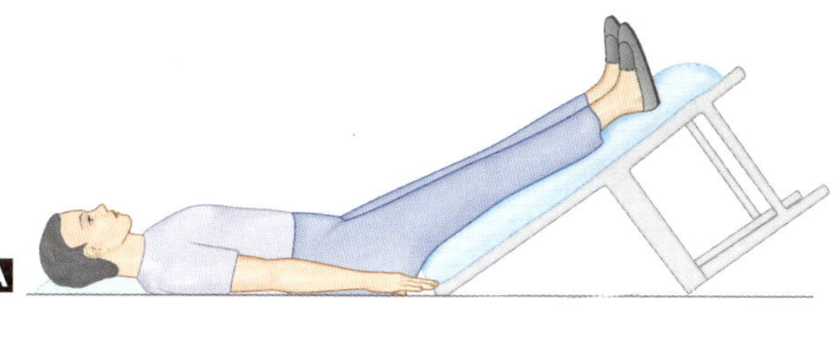
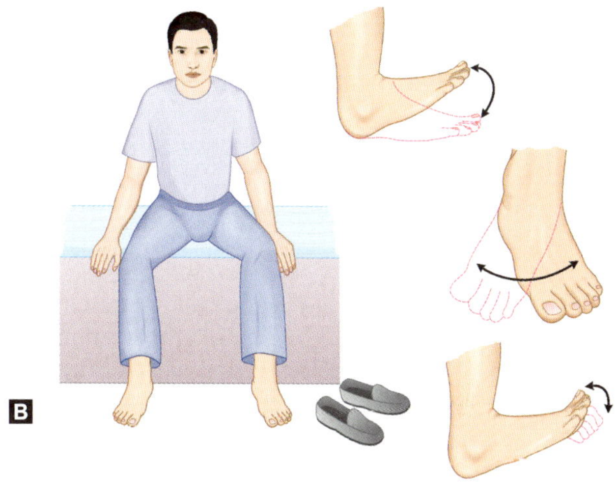
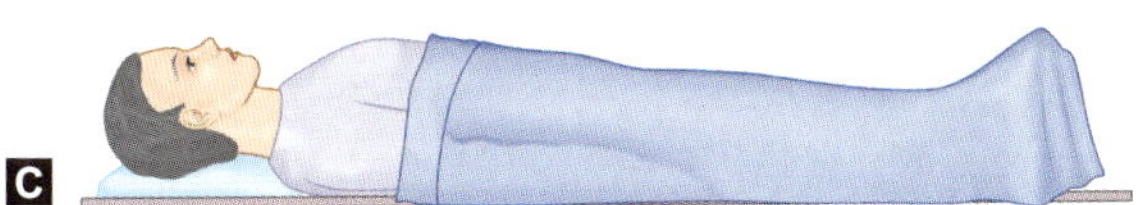

Figs. 17.18A to C: Buerger exercise.

disease (CVD) and location and pattern of venous lesions but also on age, motor deficits, comorbidities, and psychosocial conditions. The objectives of management for both lymphatic and venous disorders are the same, hence they are discussed together. For further details on lymphedema assessment and management, readers are requested to refer to Chapter 37: Cancer.

Pharmacotherapy and Surgical Interventions

Deep Vein Thrombosis

As the risk of distal DVT (calf-vein DVT) propagation to proximal DVT is 20%, recurrence is 30% and post-thrombotic syndrome is 20% along with associated risk of fatal embolism immediate treatment is recommended.

- Anticoagulation is recommended for 6–12 weeks with initiation of low molecular weight heparin and then to oral warfarin.
- Fibrinolytic agent such as streptokinase is given for free thrombus.
- Thrombectomy and intracaval filters are used to prevent the emboli from reaching the heart.

Prophylactic Prevention of Deep Vein Thrombosis

The prophylactic prevention of DVT is as follows:
- Proper positioning of the legs is required with no pressure on the calf.

- During major surgeries, pressure bandage is tied on the legs.

  Various measures like the following are used to prevent sluggish flow of blood:
- Graduated static compression
- Elastic stockings
- Electrical compression of calf muscles
- Pneumatic compression

  As smoking increases the blood viscosity, it should be discontinued prior to surgery.

  Patients on oral contraceptives or estrogens should stop drug 6–8 weeks prior to elective surgery.

Postdetection of DVT: To reduce risk of postphlebitic syndrome
- Minimize activity for the first few days
- Elevate affected limb
- Advise graded elastic compression stockings
- In calf-vein thrombosis, bed rest is recommended for 72 hours which is followed by graded mobilization.
- In the case of proximal vein thrombosis, bed rest is advised for 4–7 days followed by graded mobilization.
- Gradient elastic stocking should be worn during mobilization.
- It is safe to mobilize patients with DVT when managed with low molecular weight heparin (LMWH) and compression dressings.

Management of Varicose Veins

Pharmacotherapy

Pharmacotherapy includes:
- Calcium dobesilate improves lymph flow; macrophage mediated proteolysis and reduces edema.
- Diosmin, which is micronized purified flavonoid fraction, protects venous wall and valve. It is anti-inflammatory, profibrinolytic, antiedema, and lymphotropic.

Surgery

Surgery includes:
- Injection sclerotherapy—where complete sclerosis of venous walls is achieved by injecting sclerosants in the vein.
- Surgeries such as Trendelenburg operation which is juxtafemoral flush ligation of long saphenous vein
- Vein stripping
- Ligation of perforators and short saphenous vein.
- Endovenous LASER ablation.

Patient Education

Patient education is as follows:
- Elevation and compression are of paramount importance in management of venous and lymphatic disorders.
- The patient should be educated in lifestyle changes and self-care.
- They should be advised to walk frequently, especially during working hours, preferably in the middle of the day or before/after work while always wearing compression stockings.
- Legs should be elevated during breaks and whenever possible.
- Preferably use specially designed seats at work.
- The foot end of the bed should be raised by 10–20 cm with blocks to obtain an angle of approximately 10° while sleeping. This is not recommended for patients with cardiac or pulmonary failure, peripheral arterial disease, and hiatal hernia.
- Skin should be maintained moist and prevent drying out and cracking of the skin.
- Constrictive clothing and jewelry in the case of females should be avoided. Wear loose clothes favoring respiratory movements.
- Footwear should be comfortable shoes with low heels (<3 cm), supplied by insoles in case of foot dysmorphisms.
- Sunbathing, sauna, hot thermal baths, and mud baths should be avoided.

Elevation

It is important that the patients elevate the affected limb and sleep with the arm or leg elevated. The reduced swelling should be maintained by application of low-stretch elastic garments Elevation is advised at least for 20–30 minutes for minimum twice daily.

Exercises in Venous Disorders

The blood return from the lower limbs is a result of three kinds of forces:
1. Propulsion by residual capillary pressure
2. Blood acceleration by muscular pumping
3. Thoracoabdominal blood aspiration

Rehabilitative measures aim to increase the efficacy of all mechanisms involved in blood acceleration and aspiration.

Exercising enhances microvascular endothelial function, resulting in increased venous flow, even if exercises are performed with other parts of the body. Accordingly, in order to increase the blood propulsion at the venular level, any kind of physical activity should be intensified and sedentary habits completely discouraged. Muscular contractions squeeze intermuscular veins and intramuscular venous networks (muscular pumps) acceleration blood flow. A coordinated chain of muscular pumps is sequentially activated during walking, respectively, the plantar, calf, thigh, and gluteal pumps.

In patients with severe CVI, plantar loading, joint flexibility, and muscular efficiency are more impaired than in age-matched subjects. Hence, it may be necessary to correct plantar abnormalities, to increase muscular efficiency, joint mobility, as well as to optimize function and coordination of the different pumps.

The plantar pump plays a very important role. The hemodynamic effects of the plantar pump are similar to those of the calf and that correction of plantar loading by insoles improves venous return and quality of life in an equally efficient manner as provided by compression stockings. Plantar loading hence must be routinely evaluated and corrected as needed in all patients with CVI. Rehabilitation of the calf pump mainly consists of exercises of dorsal and plantar foot flexion with increasing load. These can be performed according to different protocols. Individually tailored physiotherapeutic exercises may include a mix of stretching the muscles and repeated contractions and relaxations, calf muscle and intrinsic strengthening to improve the plantar and calf pump, mobility of all joints including the ankle, tarsals and intertarsals, and tarsometatarsal and phalangeal joints.

Gait reeducation helps to increase the efficacy of the plantar and leg pumps by promoting heel-to-toe gait pattern and discouraging the shuffling gait. The correct sequence of weight bearing on the calcaneus (emptying of the veins of the lower leg and of the anterior muscular compartment), weight bearing on the mid-foot (emptying the plantar reservoir), and weight bearing on the anterior foot (emptying the veins of the calf) helps in activating the calf and plantar pump.

Compression

Clinical application of compression is for the control of peripheral edema due to vascular and lymphatic dysfunction. It can also be used to prevent DVT, facilitate healing of venous ulcer, and shape amputation stump. Both static and intermittent pneumatic compression (IPC) can increase circulation since both can increase the hydrostatic pressure in the interstitial pace outside the blood and lymphatic vessels. Grades of compression stockings are shown in **Table 17.10**.

Class	Support	Pressure mm Hg	Condition
I	Light	18.4–21.1	• Mild varices • Venous hypertension in pregnancy
II	Medium	25.2–32.3	• Pronounced varices • Moderate oedema • Inflammation of superior veins
III	Strong	36.5–46.6	• Severe varices • Post resolution of ulcer post thrombotic syndrome • Mode oedema
IV	Heavy	>59	• Lymphedema • Elephantiasis

Table 17.10: Grades of compression stockings.

Intermittent pneumatic compression (IPC) devices are designed for automatic decongestion by exposing the limbs to compression via pneumatic cuffs similar to a boot or a sleeve. The apparatus consists of pneumatic pump with a series of controls that regulate sequence of inflation and deflation, amount of pressure applied and ratio of inflation and deflation. It mimics calf pump action and has shown to facilitate wound healing. Inflation pressures should never exceed patient's diastolic pressure.

An ABI assessment should be performed to rule out arterial disease. If ABI range from 0.95 to 0.75, one has to be cautious. After limb girth has stabilized appropriate vascular compression garments are advocated.

There can be a continuous single compartment or sequential where the sleeve will consist of multiple compartments that are inflated and deflated in sequence. Sequential apparatus generally has 10–12 cells. With multiple gradients, sequential chambers apply differentiated compression in order to move the edema from the periphery to the center of the limb. The patient is supported comfortably with the limb in elevation. The limb is placed in a double-skinned plastic tube which is alternately inflated and emptied. Inflation–deflation ratio would be around 3:1. Pressure should start low and increase to about 60–100 mm Hg. Low-pressure pneumatic compression (30–60 mm Hg) can be quite effective and is less risky compared to high-pressure compression that has complications.

Contraindications include cellulitis, thrombophlebitis, atrial congestion, abdominal and thoracic venous occlusion, ischemia of the extremities, and cardiac failure. The use of any kind of compression therapy requires an adequate arterial blood supply to the limb. This treatment is **contraindicated in ischemic limbs** because it can prevent arterial blood flow and promote severe ischemia or even necrosis. It must be ensured that there is no edema in the corresponding quadrant of the trunk, and it is emptied by manual lymphatic treatment before and after the compression treatment.

Complete Decongestive Therapy

This is the best global treatment of lymphedema as per the international guidelines of the International Society of Lymphology. It includes elevation, manual lymph drainage, compressive bandages, hygiene measures, and decongestive exercises. The majority of studies emphasize that IPC should be used as a supplement to complete decongestive therapy (CDT) and its components.

The therapy comprises two phases:
1. **The intensive phase**: It consists of the mobilization of fluid and the initiation of a decrease in the proliferated connective tissue.
2. **The maintenance phase**: It maintains the swelling reduction and aims for the optimization of connective tissue reduction.

Intensive phase includes:
- Manual lymph drainage
- Lymphological compression bandages
- Exercises adapted to the age and general health of the patient
- Self-treatment measures and skincare.

Maintenance phase includes:
- Self manual lymphatic drainage by the patient
- Compression therapy (compression garments during the day and multiple layer compression bandages in the night)

- Exercises
- Skin care

In early lymphedema, CDT measures are applied daily of short duration. In late lymphedema, the necessity and duration of therapy increase for both phases. Generally, the patient needs at least 2–4 weeks of intensive treatment and maintenance for months or for years. Elevation of the limb is maintained as discussed earlier.

Manual Lymphatic Drainage

Manual lymphatic drainage (MLD) begins with non-edematous quadrants adjacent to the trunk of affected extremity. Proximal congestion in trunk, groin, buttock, axilla are cleared first to make space for fluid from distal areas. Central regions are emptied first to increase the collateral lymphatics and form alternative drainage pathway to carry more lymph over to normally draining areas or lymphotomes and deeper collectors of normal region. Lymph is gently forced across lymphatic watersheds. Massage also moves tissue fluid into the initial and collecting lymphatics and through its lymph nodes. Often, the optimum drainage pathways in the palliative care patient are blocked by hard fibrous regions, ulcers, pressure sores, radiation burns, metastases, scar tissue, etc. The interstitial fluid of the obstructed quadrant is drained into neighboring edema-free quadrant after drainage of trunk. All strokes are applied from the center to the periphery, so as to drain the proximal regions and prepare them to receive stagnated lymph from the distal regions. It is proximal to distal, performed once or twice daily for approximately 45 minutes duration for 4–6 weeks. MLD is intended to stimulate lymph nodes, prevent further swelling, improve muscle pump function, and increase rhythmic contractions of the lymphatics to enhance their activity so that stagnant lymphatic fluid can be rerouted.

There are four main strokes: stationary circles, scoop technique, pump technique, and rotary technique with a phase of "pressure," or working phase, and a relaxation phase, or resting phase. In the **working phase**, stretch on the lymphatic structures increases its activity, and this, in combination with the slight pressure of the hands, achieves drainage of the lymph fluid in the desired direction. In **resting phase**, the lymphatics are refilled with lymph from the periphery. Pressure is of lower intensity and just adequate so as not to damage or alter the superficial lymphatics.

Compression Therapy

Compression therapy is a very important tool in the treatment of lymphedema and preserves the gains of lymphatic drainage. Short stretch bandages are most beneficial. Bandaging is essential, and with satisfactory compression, a reduction of edema can be observed in the absence of MLD. Compression bandages should remain on the extremities until the next session of MLD. They are either applied to exert a specified pressure on the tissues or serve as a resistive layer against pressure of the muscles. Bandages increase tissue pressure, inhibit outflow from capillaries, prevent tissue fluid transfer associated with gravity, and improve venous return. The distal part of the affected limb is bandaged at the highest pressure that is reduced proximally. Additionally, when the limb is in motion, short-stretch bandages maintain their integrity as the muscles contract against them, provide a semirigid support structure when the muscles reach working pressure, and reduce capillary filtration resulting in further edema reduction.

Lymphedema Rehabilitation Exercises

Exercise enhances protein absorption and increases lymphatic transport due to increases in inspiration and expiration and the cyclic decrease in intrathoracic pressure. Exercise should be designed with the objective of reducing lymphedema volume, improving muscle strength, maintaining mobility, and improving quality of life. Exercises applied are stretching, aerobic, and resistance. Exercises with light weight have been proved not to affect the volume of lymphedema adversely.

Any exercise program should consider the safety and limits of each patient's abilities. The movements should be pain free and nonexhausting. Breathing exercises should be encouraged in rest periods. Exercises should be done with elastic garments to exert pressure on the capillaries and improve the lymphatic return. The exercises follow a specific sequence to move lymph away from congested areas. Exercise first the proximal areas of the body to clear central collecting vessels and then involve distal muscle groups to mobilize peripheral edema to central lymph vessels. Exercises are generally done in elevated position. Static dependent positions are avoided. Avoid overstretching and high-intensity exercise. Gradually increase repetitions to avoid fatique. Exercises are to be done twice daily for 20–30 minutes.

Skincare

The skin of patients is susceptible to inflammation and infection and is usually very sensitive, dry, and itchy due to disturbances of skin metabolism as a result of the macro- and microcirculation alterations. Water, moisturizing factors, and lipids should be restored using medical skin products. Vaseline and paraffin decrease the effectiveness of the compressive garments.

Skin should be dried completely after a bath or shower, especially deep skin folds, to minimize the risk of liquid "chambers" leading to cutaneous fungal infection. Products for skin care should be used sparingly and applied with gentle massaging movements. Compression garments should not be applied if the products have not been fully absorbed.

VASCULAR ULCERS AND HEALING

Physical therapist is frequently involved with the management of wound on the affected extremity. Wound progresses through three phases of healing. Pressure sores

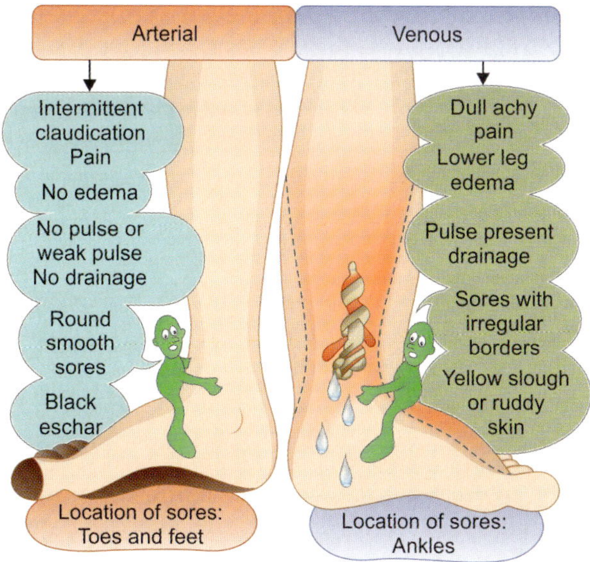

Fig. 17.19: Differences in arterial and venous wounds.

and leg ulcers are the most common types of chronic wounds. Venous insufficiency, arterial insufficiency, and diabetes are responsible for 80–90% of leg ulcers. Venous ulcers are recurrent, larger and involve the gaiter area, whereas arterial ulcers have punched out appearance, are dry, and smaller with or without gangrenous changes. **Figure 17.19** highlights the difference between the arterial and venous ulcers.

Wound Healing

The different phases of wound healing include the following:

1. *Inflammatory phase:* Day 0–10. A phagocytic phase characterized by vasodilatation, migration of leukocytes, release of histamine, and stimulation of nociceptive receptors. It is the reaction of immune system to injury. Migration of granulocytes and macrophages are facilitated due to release of platelet-derived growth factor and epidermal growth factors. Oxygen is the primary nutrient. The neutrophils, mast cells, and macrophages facilitate healing. Macrophages bridge the gap between the inflammatory phase and proliferative phase of healing.

2. *Proliferative phase:* Day 3–20. It is characterized by formation of granulation tissue, wound contraction and reepithelialization. A collagen matrix is formed due to accumulation of fibroblast in the wound. This along with vascular network is known as granulation tissue. The presence of myofibroblasts assists with wound contraction to decrease the size of the wound and facilitate epidermal cell migration from wound edges. Contact inhibition occurs when migration of epidermal cells meets at the center of the wound. At this time, epidermal cell migration ends and stratification of these cells occurs leading into the third and final phase of healing.

3. *Maturation phase:* Day 9–2 years. Remodeling occurs during this phase. There is an organization of collagen structure with the increase in tensile strength of scar tissue.

Factors Delaying Wound Healing

Multiple factors delay wound healing:
- Age
- Poor blood supply
- Cytotoxic topical agents
- Poor wound management
- Presence of infection

Assessment of Wound

Identify if the lesion is primary or secondary and which stage of healing.

Type and amount of drainage: What is the kind of drainage? Clear shiny exudate (serous) with yellow appearance or red bloody drainage (sanguinous) or pinkish-red color (serosanguinous) or indicates healthy wound.

Bright yellow, thick, slightly (seropurulent), thick cloudy, or opaque exudate (purulent) malodorous indicates contamination and infection. Culture for growth and antibiotic sensitivity needs to be done to identify organism. Look for the presence or absence of edema and surrounding periwound area for pain, inflammatory reaction. Visual assessment of lesion noting the floor of ulcer, surrounding skin, edges whether spreading or indolent.

Measurement of wound area: It can be measured using tape measure or ulcer tracing. Ulcer tracing is a method wherein a piece of cellophane paper is sterilized with normal cleansing agent and placed over the wound **(Fig. 17.20)**. A second cellophane paper is placed over it and tracing is done. This is then put over the graph paper to assess the surface area. Photographic or computer digitalization of wounds can be done. Volume measurement can be carried out by filling a large syringe with saline to a known volume

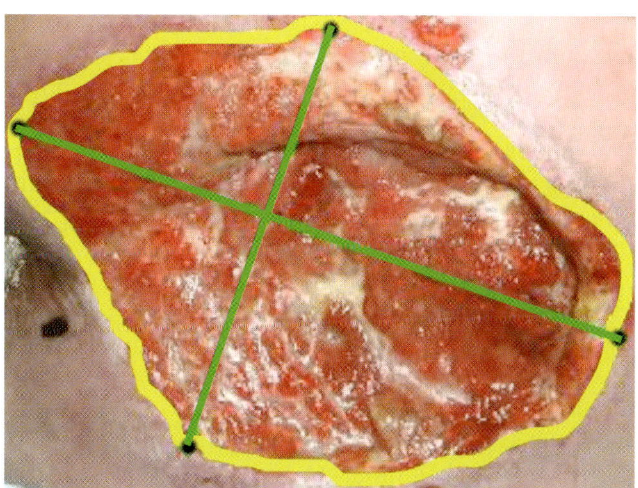

Fig. 17.20: Measurement of wound.

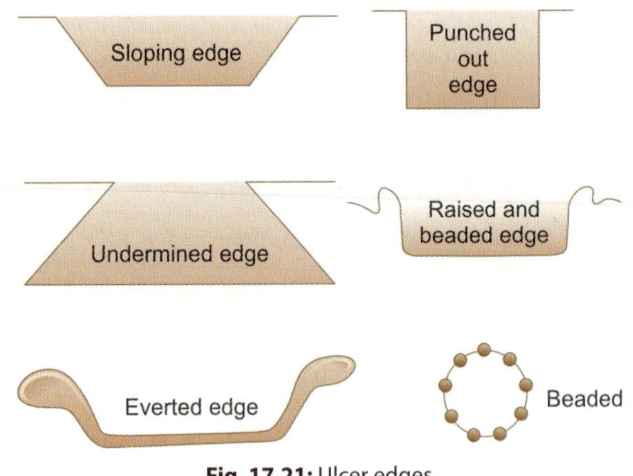

Fig. 17.21: Ulcer edges.

and slowly injecting the fluid till it levels with surrounding skin **(Fig. 17.21)**.

Marking and measuring are important to understand the response of ulcer to intervention and progress of healing.

Wound Management

Providing a moist environment optimizes wound healing by enabling collagen synthesis, autolytic debridement, angiogenesis, and better granulation tissue. It also enhances epidermal cell migration and optimizes immune system function. It also increases patient comfort and compliance with dressing changes. Moisture retentive dressings meet the ideal criteria for healing and protect against secondary infection.

Debridement

Slough or dead necrotic tissue needs to be debrided. A nonselective method of debridement such as hydro-therapy, wet–dry dressing, and radical surgical debridement would remove all tissues and harm the delicate healing tissue as well. Selective debridement protects the healing tissue and eliminates necrotic tissue. Sharp debridement by using scalpel, scissors, or tweezers to remove necrotic tissue can be done. Autolytic is using a moist environment where patients own body cleanse the wound. Enzymatic debridement involves using topical ointments impregnated with enzymes placed directly on the wound to assist the debridement. Maggot debridement therapy or biosurgery involves sterile newly hatched larvae placed on chronic wounds and held in place with dressings or biobag for 2–5 days before removal.

Wound Dressings

Topical agents: Antiseptics, disinfectants and/or antimicrobials, antibiotics and analgesics can be directly applied on the wounds.

Gauze dressings: The type of dressing selected for a wound has profound effect on healing time. The choice of dressing depends on presence or absence of infection, drainage whether dry or excessive, presence of

granulation tissue, cavities and tunnelling and periwound area are used when less than 50% granulation tissue is present. It can be used to successively support a cavity wound but should not be used to aggressively pack any shape of the wound. It is an effective secondary dressing if used for heavy exudate.

Absorbent dressings: Used for moderate to highly exudating wounds or venous ulcers. They include semipermeable foams, calcium alginate dressings, hydrophilic fiber dressing, absorbent antimicrobial dressing, and collagen dressings. Semipermeable foams are developed from absorbent polyurethane material, hydrophilic in nature and allow for rapid uptake of fluid to control heavily exudating wounds.

Calcium alginate dressing: Manufactured from seaweed derivative indicated for highly exudating wounds. As wound exudate reacts with dressing a gel matrix is formed which controls exudate and provides moist healing environment. When exudate is less, the dressing can be moistened with saline to provide moisture to wound.

Hydrophilic fiber dressing: They are synthetic highly absorbent similar to calcium alginate.

Absorbent antimicrobial dressings: These are ready dressings with antibiotics.

Collagen dressings: Developed from bovine hide acts as hemostatic agent. With continuous use they accelerate healing.

Hydrocolloid dressing: They are developed from gel-forming polymer material combined with impermeable backing to create an occlusive environment over the wound. Low-to-moderate exudates colloid material reacts with exudate to form a gel matrix but has minimal absorbent capacity. The benefits of occlusive environment include development of a moist healing environment, promotion of autolytic debridement, and the creation of new capillaries in the wound called angiogenesis.

Hydrogel dressing: Composed of amorphous gels or incorporated into sheets or island dressing. Intended to hydrate a dry desiccated wound bed. They are indicated for wounds with eschar and have no absorbing capacity.

Semipermeable film dressing: Have a high moisture permeability vapor rate. Allow the transfer and exchange of important gases through dressing while providing a fluid-proof barrier **(Fig. 17.22)**.

Vacuum-assisted closure: Includes special surgical foam and an occlusive drape connected to programmable pump to create controlled subatmospheric pressure. It

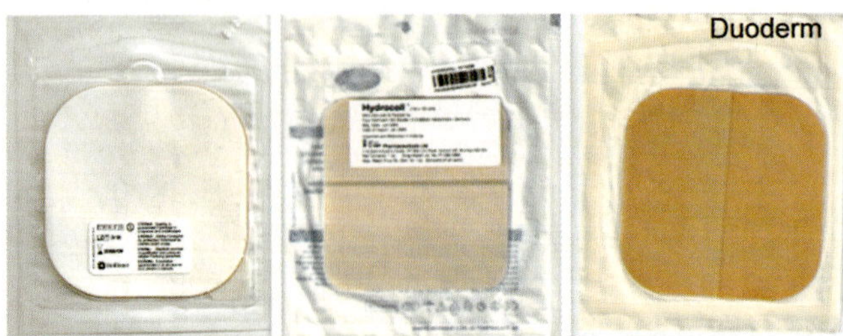

Fig. 17.22: Dressings.

is recommended to start with a continuous pressure of 50–125 mm Hg and continue to intermittent pressure, applying a constant negative pressure value from second change of dressing which is done every 3 days. It has been shown to promote rapid wound edge approximation, formation of granulation tissue, and reepithelialization. All necrotic tissue must be debrided. The wound is dressed with antibiotic-impregnated gauze. Sterile foam is trimmed to match the appropriate size of the wound. Hastens wound contraction. Increases success rates of split skin grafts. Untreated osteomyelitis and fistulas are contraindications.

Unna boot: In absence of inflammation or cellulitis. Further covered with a layer of dry gauze/stockinet/elastic bandage 30 mm Hg means pressure below malleolus reduces to 6 mm Hg below knee. Wound care and external compression are contained in one unit. Changed twice weekly prevents the patient from scratching and further damage. It provides physical support to improve calf muscle pump.

Four-layered high-compression bandage: Sequential application of orthopedic wool, cotton crepe, elastic wrap bandage, cohesive bandage with weekly dressing. System creates 40 mm Hg of mean pressure at ankle which decreases to 17 mm Hg below knee.

Objectives of Management

Edema reduction as it inhibits circulation and hence local metabolism and repair. As it may thrombose minute vessels in the skin and subcutaneous tissues causing further degradation. Edema may limit movement especially if organized and adhesive. There may be pain, and it may be culture medium for bacteria to spread infection.

- Elevation frequently for 20–30 minutes at least twice daily.
- Lie on the floor with legs vertical, supported by wall.
- Massage slow deep kneading, squeeze kneading to soften edema. Effleurage to drain fluid proximally. Careful around ulcer area and surrounding skin to soften edema and mobilize the skin.
- Bandaging to reduce edema and support veins: Local pressure by well-shaped pads to the malleolar hollows and over varicose veins. Held by crepe or confirming bandage. It should be retained during treatment sessions and night. Self-bandaging to be taught with correct tension and patterns. To be removed and retied to avoid pressure imprint on the skin. At least three bandages, one on one spare and one wash bandage are applied over stockinet. From toes to tibial tubercle over foot ankle.

Mobilization of the tissues in the floor and edges of ulcer: To soften and increase vascularity of tissues and hasten more rapid, nonadherent healing of ulcer.

Mobilize stiff joints: Attempt to mobilize any joint that may be limited with movement and then maintain range of movement. Patient may have a limited range of movement due to edema or because of supporting bandage to maintain dressings and control edema. Joints may be stiff with adaptive shortening and possible contraction of periarticular structures.

Exercise program for intrinsics of foot, leg, and thigh and therapeutic techniques such as hold relax, slow reversal, rhythmic stabilization should be considered due to disuse and reduced blood supply.

Gait reeducation and posture: Patients adopt faulty gait and posture; they should be advised to improve progressively as a part of restoration to normal function. Foot pressures can be evaluated during various phases of gait to guide toward correct gait pattern.

Weight bearing and walking: In the case of plantar wound, pressure reduction through strict bed rest or use of non-weight-bearing gait is recommended to hasten healing. Total contact walking cast for midfoot and forefoot neuropathic ulcers, molded double rocker plantar shoes, ankle–foot orthosis, and posterior walking splint is recommended.

ELECTROTHERAPY IN VASCULAR DISORDERS

Burst Transcutaneous Electrical Nerve Stimulation

Transcutaneous electrical nerve stimulation (TENS) caused reductions in wound sizes of up to 60%, increases of 35% in blood flow in ulcers, and 15% in the intact skin surrounding the ulcer. In addition, TENS provided faster healing following foot amputation, decreased the number of reamputation cases in individuals with diabetes, and relieved pain during stimulation. Increased perfusion associated with electrical stimulation (ES) may be associated with increased vascular endothelial growth factor (VEGF). The full benefits of ES on perfusion may not be realized after a single treatment since gene expression reverts to basal levels after a short duration. ES may have a bimodal effect on perfusion through an initial release of stored VEGF followed by a later increase in gene expression of VEGF. Daily ES might allow secretion of VEGF to remain above basal levels throughout the healing process.

Electrical Stimulation

Electrical stimulation (ES) can be used in both acute and chronic wounds. In the 17th century, gold leaf was used to prevent scarring from smallpox. Later on, gold leaves were applied directly to wounds to improve wound healing. John Wesley, an 18th-century electrotherapist, listed cases of pain relief following ES for suspected cases of angina, headaches, and pains in the feet. Currently, there is a substantial body of work that supports the effectiveness of ES for wound healing. Treatment is safe, effective, and well tolerated. ES has been suggested to reduce infection, improve cellular immunity, increase perfusion, and accelerate wound healing. It has a galvanotaxis effect on cells.

Faradic-type current: Faradism under pressure is used to drain pitting kind of edema with electrodes over anterior tibial and dorsal aspect of foot and calf and plantar aspect of foot for a period of 10–15 minutes, each with an intensity of current sufficiently strong to produce a firm contraction. Assistance from contracting calf muscles with faradic current and elastic recoil of the bandage during relaxation phase helps in draining edema. Capillary pressure on the digits should be tested before and frequently during the treatment to ensure bandage is not too tight to obstruct the circulation. It is important to keep ulcer area dry throughout treatment and not to disturb the ulcer dressing. Increasing discomfort requires immediate removal of bandage.

High-voltage Electrical Stimulation

Electrical Stimulation produces muscle contraction and relaxation; it increases the venous and lymphatic flow. Among different electrical current forms, high-voltage stimulation is clinically indicated for acute and chronic pain, to increase the speed of tissue regeneration, neuromuscular reeducation, to increase the venous blood flow and absorb the edema. HVPC directly on the wound does the following: attraction of neutrophils, macrophages, and epidermal cells which facilitate debridement and reepithelialization of wound that is advanced using anodal pole. Cathodal pole increases fibroblastic activity.

LASER

The exact mechanism by which low-level LASER therapy (LLLT) facilitates wound healing is largely unknown. However, several theories may help explain the enhanced wound contraction observed here. In vitro studies have shown an increase in fibroblast proliferation after irradiation, suggesting that LLLT therapy may facilitate fibroplasia during the repair phase of tissue healing. LASER irradiation transforms fibroblasts into myofibroblasts. Myofibroblasts are directly involved in granulation tissue contraction, and increased numbers could lead to facilitated wound contraction.

Hydrotherapy

The use of whirlpools, pulsed lavage, and syringe irrigation causes mechanical debridement of nonviable tissue and promotes granulation tissue. It is contraindicated in venous insufficiency as whirlpool can increase venous pressure and congestion. In arterial insufficiency, heat dissipation may be compromised.

Ultrasound

Ultrasound is directly applied to the wound by use of coupling media. It is more effective in inflammatory phase. Both thermal and nonthermal effects promote healing—nonthermal for acute wounds and arterial insufficiency and thermal for chronic wounds.

Ultraviolet Rays

Ultraviolet C (UVC) (200–280 nm) is highly antimicrobial and can be directly applied to acute wound infections to kill pathogens without unacceptable damage to host tissue. Ultraviolet B (UVB) (280–315 nm) has been applied to the wounded tissue to stimulate wound healing, UVA (315–400 nm) has distinct effects on cell signaling but has not yet been widely applied to wound care. For chronic wounds to decrease bacterial load and initiate an inflammatory response secondary to erythema created. Ultraviolet C (UVC) rays are more used.

Radiant Heat

Infrared increases local wound and skin temperatures facilitating higher metabolic rates and improves circulatory activity to the wound. Extreme heat or cold is contraindicated in peripheral arterial diseases as sensations may be affected.

Hyperbaric Oxygen Therapy for Nonhealing Wounds

"Hyper" means increased and "baric" relates to pressure. Hyperbaric oxygen therapy (HBOT) refers to intermittent treatment of the entire body with 100% oxygen at greater than normal atmospheric pressures. While undergoing HBOT, the pressure is increased up to two times in 100% oxygen. This increased pressure, combined with an increase in oxygen to 100%, dissolves oxygen into the blood and in all body tissues and fluids at up to 20 times normal concentration greatly increasing oxygen concentration in all body tissues, even with reduced or blocked blood flow; stimulates the growth of new blood vessels to locations with reduced circulation, improving blood flow to areas with arterial blockage; causes a rebound arterial dilation after HBOT, resulting in an increased blood vessel diameter greater than when therapy began, improving blood flow to compromised organs.

This elevation in oxygen tension induces significant positive changes in wound repair process by directly enhancing fibroblast replication, collagen synthesis, crosslinking, and rapid capillary growth. At the cellular level, HBOT increases leukocyte bactericidal activity and has a direct effect on anaerobic organism. It also stimulates platelet-derived growth factor (PDGF) receptor sites in wound. It is found to be an effective adjunct therapy for diabetic foot, compromised amputation sites, nonhealing and vascular insufficiency ulcers.

Ozone: It is an allotrophic form of oxygen. It is panvirucidal and panbacterial agent. Ozone improves epithelialization and granulation tissue and promotes healing.

SUMMARY

Physical therapist is an integral part of the team for patients with vascular and lymphatic disorders for prevention and rehabilitation. Very often physiotherapy is a neglected part of management. In recent years, the therapeutic options have expanded significantly, providing a challenging and rewarding therapeutic intervention. Though interrelated, each vascular system is unique in its structure and function. The movement impairments associated with all three systems are profound. This chapter is an attempt to sensitize the reader to various problems associated with vascular dysfunction and its management approach.

Case Scenario

CASE STUDY 1

Mr Sabnis, 46 years old, resident of Jalna, farmer by occupation (left nearly 2 years back), bidi smoker since 15 years, complains of tingling numbness in forefoot and pain in calf on walking 100 m. His CT angiography reveals complete occlusion of left common iliac artery up to bifurcation and right external iliac artery up to bifurcation of common femoral artery. He is operated 5 days ago for common femoral bypass.

Guiding Question:

1. Discuss his impairments and management.

CASE STUDY 2

Mrs Sharma, 54 years old, supervisor by occupation, is a chronic uncontrolled diabetic with ischemic heart disease. She complains of pain in lower extremity on walking and sometimes at rest. She gives history of little finger amputation 1 month back, now is referred for nonhealing wound of right great toe.

Guiding Question:

1. Plan her management. What are the outcome measures you would consider?

CASE STUDY 3

Mrs Tambe, 46 years old, homemaker, complains of fatigue and edema (pittable) around both malleoli since 2 years. She cannot wear dresses as her legs have veins standing out. Her skin around the ankle and foot is pigmented and itchy. She is scared that it may just break.

Guiding Question:

1. Discuss her impairments, highlighting the assessment, management, and outcome.

Review Questions

1. Discuss the differences in structure and function of arterial and venous systems.
2. Discuss the functional assessment for people with arterial and venous dysfunction.
3. Discuss the rationale for therapy with arterial, venous, and lymphatic dysfunction.
4. Give the characteristic of arterial and venous ulcers.
5. Discuss the factors affecting healing of wounds.
6. What is the role of electrotherapy in peripheral venous disease?
7. What are the different kinds of dressing used for healing of wounds?

BIBLIOGRAPHY

1. Abergel RP, Meeker CA, Lam TS, et al. Control of connective tissue metabolism by lasers: recent developments and future prospects. J Am Acad Dermatol. 1984;11(6):1142-50.
2. Allen AW. Recent advanced in the treatment of circulatory disturbance of the extremities: results contained in the peripheral circulatory clinic of the Massachusetts general hospital. Ann Surg. 1930;92:931-46.
3. Allen AW. Recent advances in the treatment of circulatory disturbances of extremities. Annals of Surgery. 1930;92 (5):931-46.
4. Anderson JL, Halperin JL, Albert NM, et al. Management of patients with peripheral arterial disease—compilation of 2005 and 2011 AHA guideline recommendations. Circulation. 2013;127:1425-43.
5. Badimon L, Padró T, Vilahur G. Atherosclerosis, platelets and thrombosis in acute ischaemic heart disease. Eur Heart J Acute Cardiovasc Care. 2012;1(1):60-74.
6. Baker LL, Chambers R, DeMuth SK, et al. Effects of electrical stimulation on wound healing in patients with diabetic ulcers. Diabetes Care. 1997;20(3):405-12.
7. Bottomley JM. The insensitive foot in U.K. Geriatric rehabilitation manual. 2nd edition. Chapter 42. Edinburgh; New York: Churchill Livingstone Elsevier; 2007.
8. Buerger L. The circulatory disturbances of the extremities. Ann Surg. 1926;83:157.
9. Caggiati A, de Maeseneer M, Cavezzi A, et al. Rehabilitation of patients with venous diseases of the lower limbs: state of the art. Phlebology. 2018;33(10):663-71.
10. Caldwell K, Prior SJ, Kampmann M, et al. Upper body exercise increase lower extremity venous blood flow in deep venous thrombosis. J Vasc Surg Venous Lymphat Disord. 2013;1:126-33.
11. Chang C-C, Chen M-Y, Shen J-H, et al. ACSM guidelines for exercise testing and prescription. A quantitative real-time assessment of Buerger exercise on dorsal foot peripheral skin circulation in patients with diabetes foot. Medicine (Baltimore). 2016;95(46): e5334.
12. Cosmo P, Svensson H, Bornmyr S, et al. Effects of transcutaneous nerve stimulation on the microcirculation in chronic leg ulcers. Scand J Plast Reconstr Surg Hand Surg. 2000;34(1):61-4.
13. Cueni LN, Detmar M. The lymphatic system in health and disease. Lymphat Res Biol. 2008;6(3-4):109-22.
14. Das S. Chapter 7. Examination of varicose veins. In: A manual on clinical surgery, 13th edition. Kolkata: 2018. pp. 100-8.
15. Das S. Chapter 8. Examination of lymphatic system. In: A manual on clinical surgery, 13th edition. Kolkata; 2018. pp. 109-21.
16. de Moura RM, Gomes Hde A, da Silva SL, et al. Analysis of the physical and functional parameters of older adults with chronic venous disease. Arch Gerontol Geriatr. 2012;55:696-701.
17. Finsen V, Persen L, Løvlien M, et al. Transcutaneous electrical nerve stimulation after major amputation. J Bone Joint Surg Br. 1988;70(1):109-12.
18. Grey J, Harding K, Enoch S. ABC of wound healing. Venous and arterial leg ulcers. Br Med J. 2006;332:7537.
19. Gupta A, Avci P, Dai T, et al. Ultraviolet radiation in wound care: sterilization and stimulation. Adv Wound Care (New Rochelle). 2013;2(8):422-37.
20. Hamburg NM, Balady GJ. Exercise rehabilitation in peripheral arterial disease: functional impact and mechanisms of benefit. Circulation. 2012;123(1):87-97.
21. Hamner JB, Fleming MD. Lymphedema therapy reduces the volume of edema and pain in patients with breast cancer. Ann Surg Oncol. 2007;14(6):1904-8.
22. Hopkins JT, McLoda TA, Seegmiller JG, et al. Low-level laser therapy facilitates superficial wound healing in humans: a triple-blind, sham-controlled study. J Athl Train. 2004;39(3):223-229.

23. Jackson BS. Chronic peripheral arterial disease. Am J Nurs. 1972;72:928-934.

24. Karadibak D, Yavuzsen T, Saydam S. Prospective trial of intensive decongestive physiotherapy for upper extremity lymphedema. J Surg Oncol. 2008;97(7):572-7.

25. Khan S, Cleanthis M, Smout J, et al. Life-style modification in peripheral arterial disease. Eur J Vasc Endovasc Surg. 2005;29:2-9.

26. Klonizakis M, Tew G, Michaels J, et al. Exercise training improves cutaneous microvascular endothelial function in post-surgical varicose vein patients. Microvasc Res. 2009;78:67-70.

27. Koul R, Dufan T, Russell C, et al. Efficacy of complete decongestive therapy and manual lymphatic drainage on treatment-related lymphedema in breast cancer. Int J Radiat Oncol Biol Phys. 2007;67(3):841-6.

28. Kumar D, Savarna, Pritam K, et al. Role of physiotherapy in prevention and management of lymphedema in post-operative breast cancer patients. OncoExpert. 2016;2(2):11-5.

29. Milani RV, Lavie CJ. The role of exercise training in peripheral arterial disease. Vasc Med. 2007;12:351-8.

30. Morgan MB. Vascular quality of life questionnaire (VascuQol). J Vasc Surg. 2001;33(4):679-87.

31. Murphy T, Cutlip DE, Regensteiner JG, et al. Supervised Exercise versus Primary stenting for claudication resulting from aortoiliac peripheral arterial disease. Circulation. 2012;125:130-9.

32. Nicolaï SP, Kruidenier LM, Rouwet EV, et al. The walking impairment questionnaire: an effective tool to assess the effect of treatment in patients with intermittent claudication. J Vasc Surg. 2009;50(1):89-94.

33. Norgren L, Hiatt WR, Dormandy JA, et al. Inter-society consensus for the management of peripheral arterial disease (TASC II). Eur J Vasc Endovasc Surg. 2007;33:1-S75.

34. Parmenter BJ, Dieberg G, Smart NA. Exercise training for management of peripheral arterial disease: a systematic review and meta-analysis. Sports Medicine. 2015;45(2)231-44.

35. Pourreau-Schneider N, Ahmed A, Soudry M, et al. Helium-neon laser treatment transforms fibroblasts into myofibroblasts. Am J Pathol. 1990;137(1):171-8.

36. Regensteiner JG, Hiatt WR. Walking impairment questionnaire (WIQ). J Vasc Surg. 1996:23;104-15.

37. Regensteiner JG, Steiner JF, Hiatt WR. Low level physical activity recall questionnaire. J Vasc Surg. 1996; 23:104-15.

38. Saggini R, Bellomo RG, Iodice P, et al. Venous insufficiency and foot dysmorphism: effectiveness of viscoelastic rehabilitation systems on veno-muscle system of the foot and of the calf. Int J Immunopathol Pharmacol. 2009;22(3 Suppl.):1-8.

39. Spertus J, Jones P, Poler S, et al. Peripheral artery questionnaire (PAQ). Am Heart J. 2004;147(2):301-8.

40. Sriram Bhat M. Manual of surgery, 6th edition. New Delhi: Jaypee Publishers; 2016. pp. 169-221.

41. O'Sullivan SB, Schmitz TJ, Fulk GD, et al. Physical rehabilitation, 6th edition. FA Davis Company, Philadelphia; 2014.

42. Thakral G, Lafontaine J, Najafi B, et al. Electrical stimulation to accelerate wound healing. Diabet Foot Ankle. 2013;4:1-9.

43. Treat-Jacobson D, McDermott MM, Bronas UG, et al. Optimal exercise programs for patients with peripheral artery disease: A scientific statement from the American Heart Association. Circulation. 2019;139:e10-33.

44. Tzani I, Tsichlaki M, Zerva E, et al. Physiotherapeutic rehabilitation of lymphedema: state-of-the-art. Lymphology. 2018;51(1): 1-12.

45. Uhl JF, Gillot C. Anatomy of the veno-muscular pumps of the lower limb. Phlebology 2015;30:180-93.

46. Vignes S, Porcher R, Arrault M, et al. Long-term management of breast cancer-related lymphedema after intensive decongestive physiotherapy. Breast Cancer Res Treat. 2007;101(3):285-90.

Spinal Disorders

Sheshna Rathod, Dinesh Sorani

Ⓛ EARNING OBJECTIVES

At the end of this chapter, the readers will be able to:

- Understand the basic anatomy of the spinal column
- Learn the classification models of neck pain
- Describe the detailed evaluation of cervical spine
- Understand the clinical presentation of models of neck pain based on International Classification of Functioning, Disability, and Health (ICF)
- Understand the physiotherapy management of different models of neck pain
- Perform a detailed evaluation of lumbar spine
- Understand the clinical presentation of models of low back pain based on ICF
- Understand physiotherapy treatment for back pain
- Gain knowledge of T4 syndrome
- Understand the pathomechanics, clinical presentation and physiotherapy management of sacroiliac (SI) dysfunction
- Gain knowledge of the pathomechanics, clinical presentation, evaluation and physiotherapy management of ankylosing spondylitis (AS)
- Describe the pathophysiology, clinical presentation and physiotherapy management of scoliosis

CHAPTER OUTLINE

- Cervical spine
- Classification models of neck pain
  - Neurological or nonspecific
  - Clinical condition
  - Pathoanatomical
  - Response to movement
  - Treatment based
- Evaluation
  - History
  - Observation
  - Palpation
  - Examination
- Clinical presentation
  - Neck pain with mobility deficits
  - Neck pain with movement co-ordination Impairments
  - Neck pain with headache
  - Neck pain with radiating pain
- Physiotherapy management
  - Neck pain with mobility deficits
  - Neck pain with movement coordination impairments
  - Neck pain with headache
  - Neck pain with radiating pain

- Lumbar spine
- Classification of back pain
- Evaluation
  - Observation
  - Palpation
  - Examination
- Clinical presentation
  - Acute/subacute low back pain with mobility deficits
  - Acute low back pain with movement co-ordination impairments
  - Subacute/chronic low back pain with movement co-ordination impairments
  - Acute low back pain with related (referred) lower extremity pain
  - Acute/subacute/chronic low back pain with radiating pain
  - Acute and subacute low back pain with related cognitive and affective tendencies
  - Chronic low back pain with generalized pain

- Physiotherapy management
  - Acute/subacute low back pain with mobility deficits
  - Acute low back pain with movement coordination impairments
  - Subacute/chronic low back pain with movement co-ordination impairments
  - Acute low back pain with related (referred) lower extremity pain
  - Acute/subacute/chronic low back pain with radiating pain
  - Acute/subacute low back pain with related cognitive or affective tendencies
  - Chronic low back pain with related generalized pain
- Miscellaneous conditions
  - T4 syndrome
  - Sacroiliac joint dysfunction
  - Ankylosing spondylitis
  - Scoliosis

INTRODUCTION

The spinal column consists of 33 vertebrae and their respective intervertebral disks. The spinal column can be divided into 7 cervical, 12 thoracic, 5 lumbar, 5 fused sacral, and 3 or 4 coccygeal vertebrae. The cranium attaches at the top of the spine at atlanto-occipital joint, the pelvis connects at the bottom of the spine via sacroiliac (SI) joint. The ribs attach to the spine in the thoracic region.

The chapter explains the various pathologies that involve the spine, their etiology, epidemiology, clinical features, examination, and physiotherapy management. Medical management of the pathologies usually involves pain management that is described in the Chapter 10: Pain Assessment and Management. Surgical management is beyond the scope of this chapter.

CERVICAL SPINE

The cervical spine is particularly susceptible to degenerative changes because normal day-to-day activities require frequent movements of the head and cervical spine. The inevitable degeneration process leads to injury, altering the precision of movement that negatively impacts the rate and type of degeneration **(Box 18.1)**.

CLASSIFICATION MODELS OF NECK PAIN

Introduction

Literature of neck pain depicts various classification models of neck pain **(Box 18.1)**.

Neurological or Nonspecific

As the diagnosis is completed and individual is ruled out of red and yellow flags for spinal pathology, the condition is stamped as being nonspecific (mechanical) or having neurological involvement. However, most of the individuals have mixed pain, probably due to the fact that radicular (neurological) pain is usually caused by degenerative conditions that predispose a person to nociceptive (nonspecific) pain, which makes for an unclear classification system.

Red flags include:
- Fracture around cervical spine
- Neoplasm
- Infection
- Cervical myelopathy
- Upper cervical ligamentous instability

BOX 18.1: Classification models of neck pain.

Traditionally neck pain can be classified by the pathoanatomical model. However, recently there has been a shift from the pathoanatomical model of diagnosis toward the development of prognostic tests that can separate a heterogeneous population into treatment-oriented subgroups that will inform patient management and be cost effective.

- Vertebral artery insufficiency
- Inflammatory disease

Yellow flags for neck pain include:
- Fear of movement
- Fear of increasing pain with work
- Believing that pain is harmful and uncontrollable
- Expecting the worse and passive attitude to rehabilitation

Clinical Condition

This is a sign- and symptom-based medical model and utilizes terms such as cervical spondylosis, cervicogenic headache, etc.

Pathoanatomical

This is a structurally based medical model that focuses on the structure involved or dysfunction, e.g., facet joint, intervertebral disk, and myofascial. However, the pathoanatomical model has proven limited to the correlation between diagnosis and clinical decisions regarding treatment management plans because different diagnoses often exhibit similar symptoms.

Response to Movement (Centralization)

Based on McKenzie model of centralization and peripheralization, the patient can be classified as centralized (those who respond through centralization phenomenon) and non-centralized (those who do not respond through centralization phenomenon).

Treatment Based

This classification is proposed by Childs (2004) and is adapted in clinical practice guidelines linked to International Classification of Functioning, Disability, and Health (ICF). The classification is as follows:
- Neck pain with mobility deficits
- Neck pain with movement co-ordination impairments [WAD (Whiplash-associated disorder)]
- Neck pain with headache (cervicogenic)
- Neck pain with radiating pain (radicular)

EVALUATION

History

Evaluation of a patient with cervicogenic symptoms consists of a detailed history and examination procedure.

Rule out red flags such as:
- Fracture around cervical spine
- Neoplasm
- Infection
- Systemic disease
- Vertebral artery insufficiency (presence of drop attacks, dizziness, dysphasia, dysarthria, diplopia)
- Cervical myelopathy (presence of sensory disturbance of hands, muscle wasting of intrinsic muscles of hand, unsteady gait, positive Hoffman's reflex, hyperreflexia)

- Upper cervical ligamentous instability
- Neurological injury (bowel and bladder dysfunction, progressive neurological deficit in upper and lower extremities).

Observation

Postural alignment should be observed along with observation of anatomical movements of neck into flexion-extension, side flexion, and rotation to both sides. Nodding movements of head should be observed to find any restriction/deviation from normal and patient's willingness to do the movement.

Palpation

Following are the benefits of palpation:
- Palpation of bony landmarks **(Figs. 18.1 and 18.2)** in static posture and during movements may help therapist to find any motion restrictions or deviations in cervical and thoracic column.
- Palpation of muscles may help identify spasm, tenderness, trigger points, and swelling in cervical region.

  Myofascial trigger points (MTrPs) are hypersensitive, painful areas over a taut band of muscle. They produce localized and referred pain to other structures with mechanical stimulation.

Examination

Range of Motion

The motion can be classified as per the following:
- Active and passive movements of the cervical spine should be assessed. End feel is felt at the end of passive movement.

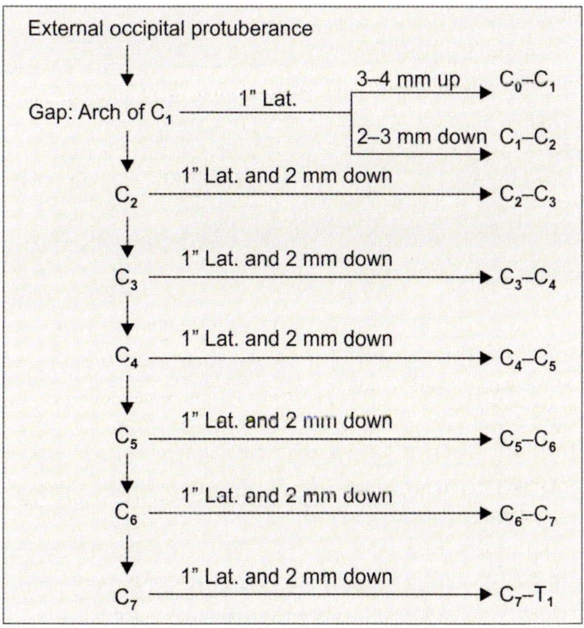

Fig. 18.1: Surface landmarks of cervical spine.

- Tightness of muscles such as pectorals, scalene, upper trapezius, and sternocleidomastoid should be assessed.
- Accessory movements (intersegmental mobility testing): Pain response and segmental mobility are assessed through accessory movements including joint play **(Figs. 18.3A and B)** at all vertebral levels. Intersegmental mobility testing reveals characteristic restriction.

Strength

Following are the methods for measuring strength:
- Muscle strength should be objectively measured for muscles of cervical region including superficial and deep muscles, scapular, and thoracic region.
- Deep muscles can be assessed using a pressure biofeedback unit clinically through craniocervical flexion test.
- Endurance is also one of the important components of assessment. It is assessed by measuring for how long a patient is able to hold the position of the neck in flexion, extension, side flexion, rotation and tucked in chin.

Sensations and Reflexes

Sensations should be checked in respective dermatomes corresponding to cervical nerve roots. Reflexes should be checked for differences on both sides including biceps, brachioradialis, triceps, and jaw jerk.

Functional Assessment

Neck disability index and similar tests can be used to assess patient's day-to-day activities and to detect change in daily functions over time.

Special Tests

Most common special tests performed on cervical spine according to suspected pathology are craniocervical flexion test and deep neck flexor endurance test (for deep neck flexors), foraminal compression test, distraction test, and upper limb neurodynamic tests (for neurological symptoms).
- *Craniocervical flexion test:* Craniocervical test is performed with patient in crook lying position with head and neck in neutral position. A pressure biofeedback unit is placed between the cervical lordotic curve and the surface of table and inflated up to 20 mm Hg **(Figs. 18.4A and B)**. While keeping the occiput steady, the patient performs chin tucks at five graded increments (22, 24, 26, 28, and 30 mm Hg) holding each position for 10 seconds. 10 seconds rest is allowed between each stage. Trick movements such as unwanted activation of superficial muscles of cervical region should be avoided. A normal response is considered when pressure is increased between

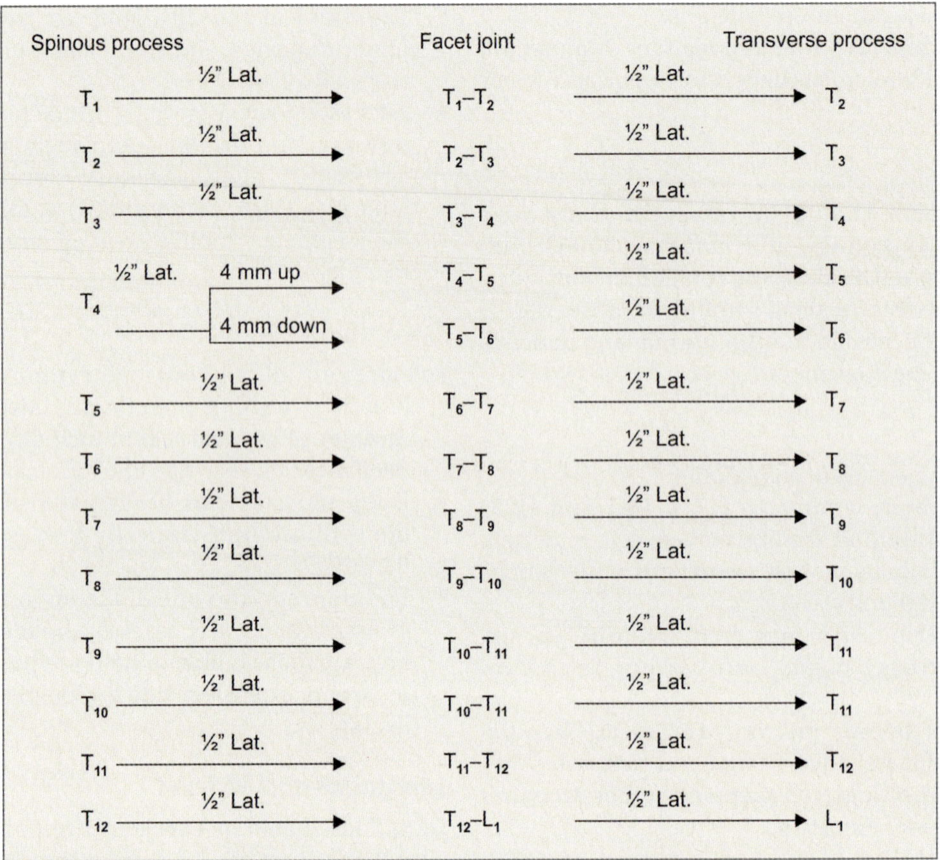

Fig. 18.2: Surface landmarks for thoracic spine.

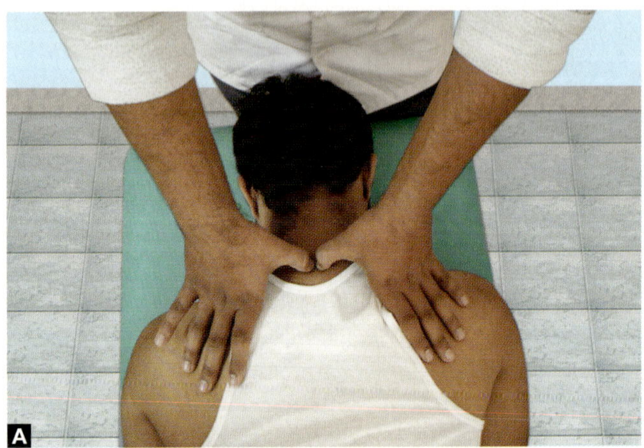

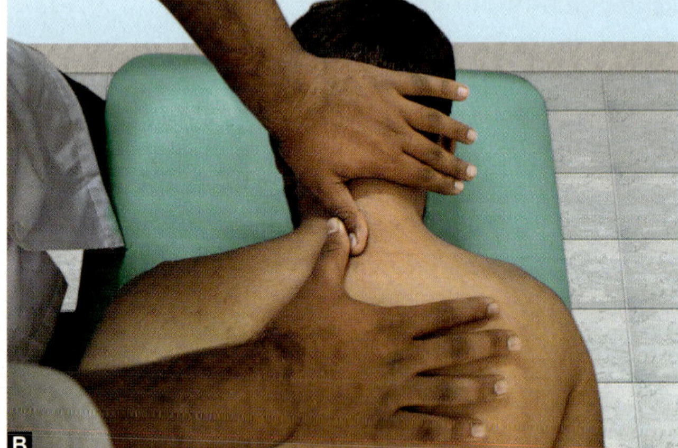

Figs. 18.3A and B: Joint play techniques for cervical spine.

26 and 30 mm Hg and maintained for 10 seconds without any trick movements. Scoring is based on activation score (pressure achieved and held for 10 seconds) and performance index (increase in pressure × number of repetitions).

- *Deep neck flexor endurance test:* Patient is in crook lying position and patient is asked to lift the head with chin in retracted position **(Figs. 18.5A and B)**. Patient is asked to maintain the position for as long as possible.
- *Foraminal compression test:* Patient is in sitting position and therapist stands behind the patient. Test is performed in three stages:

1. First stage includes compression in neutral.
2. Second stage includes compression with head in extension.
3. Third stage includes compression with head in extension and rotation to the unaffected side and then rotation to affected side with compression **(Figs. 18.6A to D)**.

If symptoms are present with one stage, therapist does not proceed to next stage. Test is termed as positive if pain radiates into affected upper limb.

- *Distraction test:* Test is performed if patient complains of radicular symptoms. Patient is in sitting position and

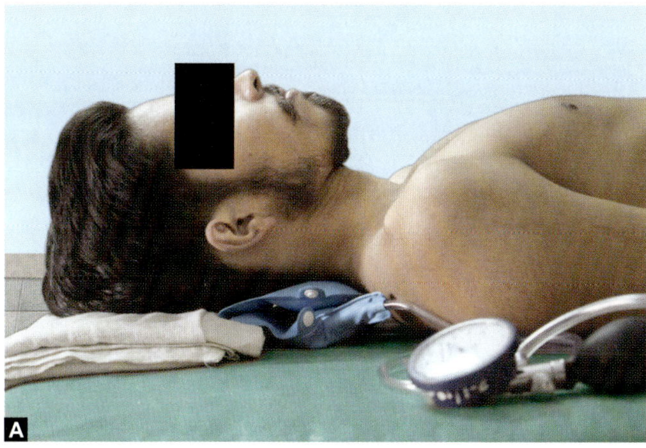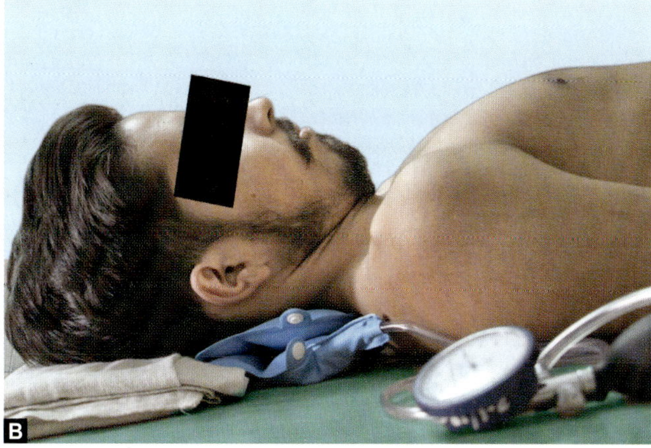

Figs. 18.4A and B: Craniocervical flexion test: (A) Starting position and (B) End position.

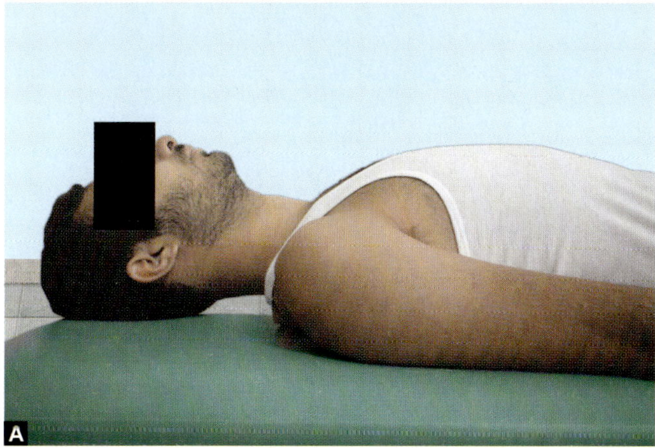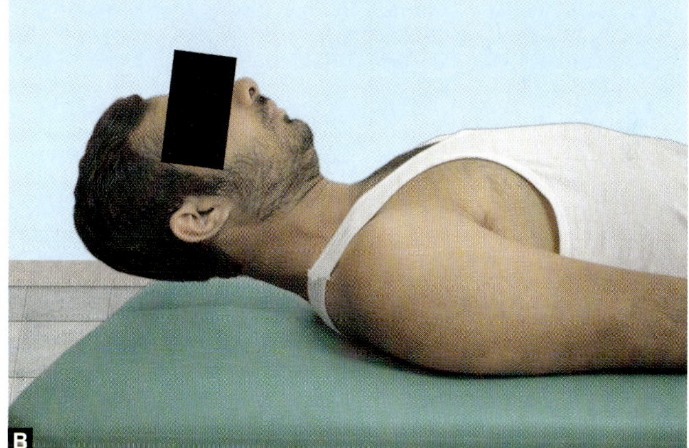

Figs. 18.5A and B: Deep neck flexor endurance test: (A) Starting position and (B) End position.

therapist stands beside the patient. Therapist's one hand is placed under patient's chin and other around occiput and the therapist gently lifts the head of the subject. Test is considered positive if pain is decreased or relieved while lifting head.

- *Upper limb neurodynamic tests:* Tests are performed with patient in supine lying position and therapist in walk standing position on the side of the plinth. Test starts with performing on unaffected side first, moving on to the affected side. Position of shoulder is followed by forearm, wrist, fingers, and elbow **(Table 18.1)**. Each phase is added one by one till the symptoms are produced. Test is considered positive on reproduction of radicular symptoms.

Fibromyalgia

Differential diagnosis of neck pain is to be considered with fibromyalgia, as the latter is a clinical presentation along with:

- Widespread pain
- Chronic fatigue
- Paresthesia
- Anxiety
- Sleep disturbances along with psychosomatic complaints.

Modified fibromyalgia criteria are:

- Widespread pain index (WPI) ≥7 and symptom severity scale (SSS) score ≥5 OR WPI of 4–6 and SSS score ≥9.
- Generalized pain, defined as pain in at least four of five regions, must be present.
- Jaw, chest, and abdominal pain are not included in generalized pain definition.
- Symptoms have been generally present for at least 3 months.
- A diagnosis of fibromyalgia is valid irrespective of other diagnoses. A diagnosis of fibromyalgia does not exclude the presence of other clinically important illnesses. If the above three conditions are met, patient is confirmed of having fibromyalgia.

CLINICAL PRESENTATION

Neck Pain with Mobility Deficits

Common Symptoms

The general symptoms of neck pain with mobility deficits are:

- Central and/or unilateral neck pain.
- Limitation in neck motion that consistently reproduces symptoms.

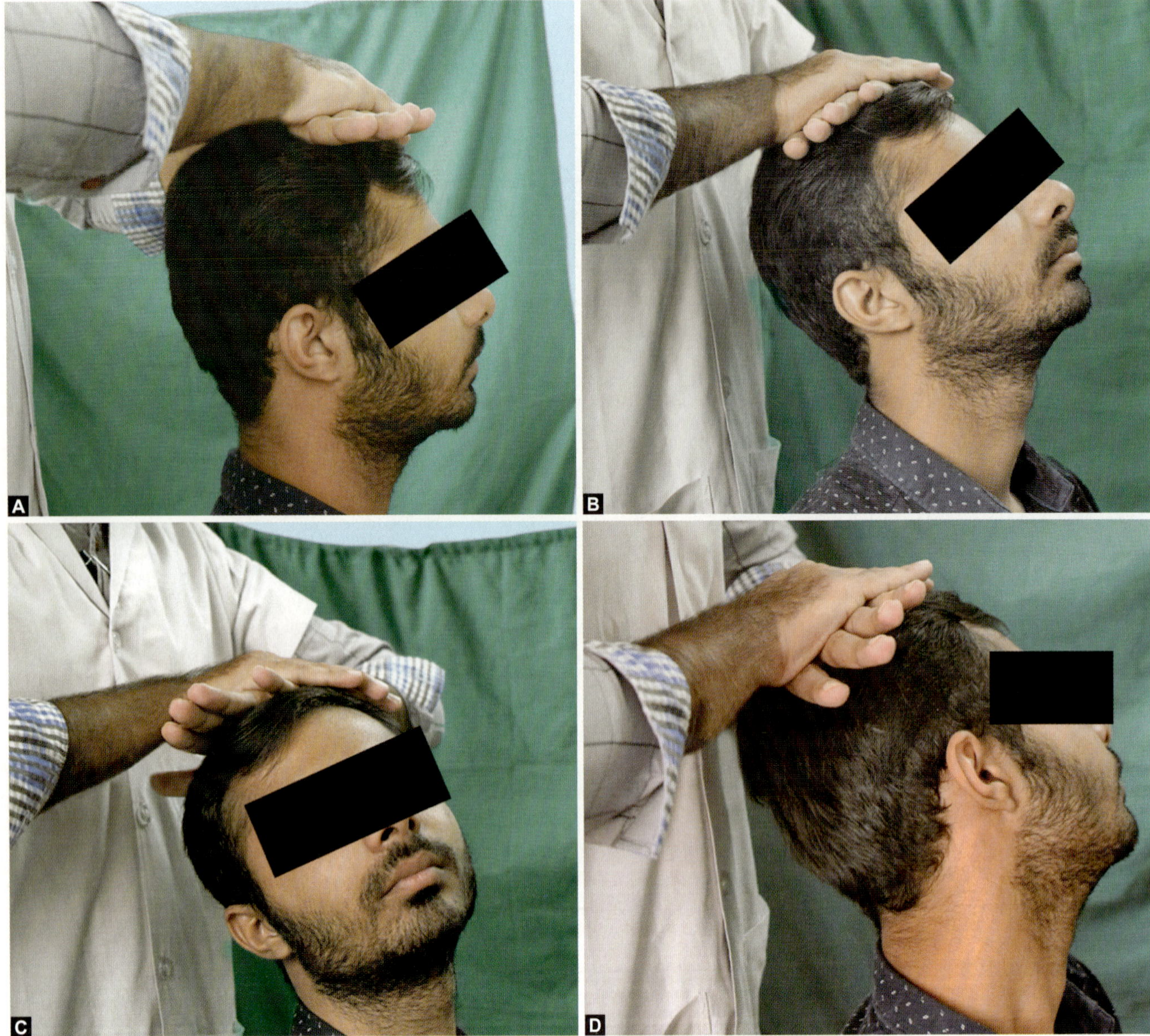

Figs. 18.6A to D: Foraminal compression test: (A) In neutral; (B) In extension; (C and D) In extension and rotation.

Table 18.1: Upper limb neurodynamic tests.

Joint	Median, anterior interosseous nerve and nerve roots (C5, C6, C7)	Median, musculocutaneous, and axillary nerve	Radial nerve	Ulnar nerve and nerve roots (C8 and T1)
Shoulder	Depression and 110° abduction	Depression, 10° abduction and lateral rotation	Depression, 110° abduction and medial rotation	Depression, 10–90° abduction and lateral rotation
Elbow	Extension	Extension	Extension	Flexion
Forearm	Supination	Supination	Pronation	Supination or pronation
Wrist	Extension	Extension	Flexion and ulnar deviation	Extension and radial deviation
Fingers and thumb	Extension	Extension	Flexion	Extension
Cervical spine	Opposite side flexion	Opposite side flexion	Opposite side flexion	Opposite side flexion

- Onset of pain associated with recent awkward movement or position.
- Associated (referred) shoulder girdle or upper extremity pain may be present.

Expected Examination Findings

Expected findings of the examination are:
- Limited cervical range of motion (ROM).
- Neck pain reproduced at end ranges of active and passive motions.
- Restricted cervical and thoracic segmental mobility.
- Neck pain and referred pain reproduced with provocation of the involved cervical or upper thoracic segments or cervical musculature.
- Deficits in strength of cervical, thoracic, and scapular muscles and deficits in motor control may be present in individuals with subacute or chronic neck pain.

Neck Pain with Movement Co-ordination Impairments (Whiplash-Associated Disorder)

Common Symptoms

The general symptoms of WAD are:
- Mechanism of onset linked to trauma or whiplash
- Associated (referred) shoulder girdle or upper extremity pain
- Associated varied nonspecific concussive signs and symptoms
- Dizziness/nausea
- Headache, concentration, or memory difficulties; confusion; hypersensitivity to mechanical, thermal, acoustic, odor, or light stimuli; heightened affective distress.

Expected Examination Findings

Examination findings expected are:
- Positive craniocervical flexion test.
- Positive neck flexor muscle endurance test.
- Positive pressure algometry **(Fig. 18.7)**.
- Strength and endurance deficits of the neck muscles.

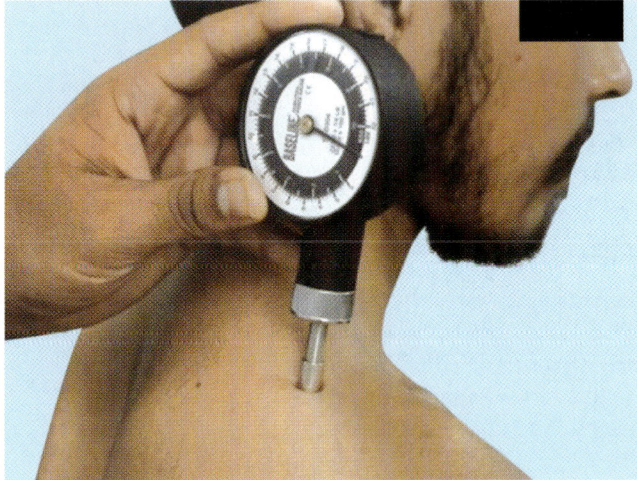

Fig. 18.7: Technique for pressure algometry.

- Neck pain with midrange motion that worsens with end range positions.
- Point tenderness may include MTrPs.
- Sensorimotor impairment may include altered muscle activation patterns, proprioceptive deficit, postural balance or control.
- Neck and referred pain reproduced by provocation of the involved cervical segments.

Neck Pain with Headache (Cervicogenic)

Common Symptoms

The common symptoms of cervicogenic headache are:
- Noncontinuous, unilateral neck pain, and associated (referred) headache.
- Headache is precipitated or aggravated by neck movements or sustained positions/postures.

Expected Examination Findings

Expected examination findings are:
- Positive craniocervical flexion test
- Headache reproduced with provocation of the involved upper cervical segments
- Limited cervical ROM
- Restricted upper cervical segmental mobility
- Strength, endurance, and co-ordination deficits of the neck muscles.

Neck Pain with Radiating Pain (Radicular)

Common Symptoms

Following are the general symptoms of neck pain with radiating pain:
- Neck pain with radiating (narrow band of lancinating) pain in the involved extremity
- Upper extremity dermatomal paresthesia or numbness, and myotomal muscle weakness.

Expected Examination Findings

Expected examination findings of neck pain with radiating pain are:
- Neck and neck-related radiating pain reproduced or relieved with radiculopathy testing: positive test cluster includes upper-limb nerve mobility, foraminal compression test, cervical distraction, cervical ROM.
- May have upper extremity sensory, strength, or reflex deficits associated with the involved nerve roots.

PHYSIOTHERAPY MANAGEMENT

Neck Pain with Mobility Deficits

Acute

Physiotherapy management to deal with acute neck pain with mobility deficits:
- *Cervical mobilization or manipulation along with thoracic manipulation:* Both are equally valuable in

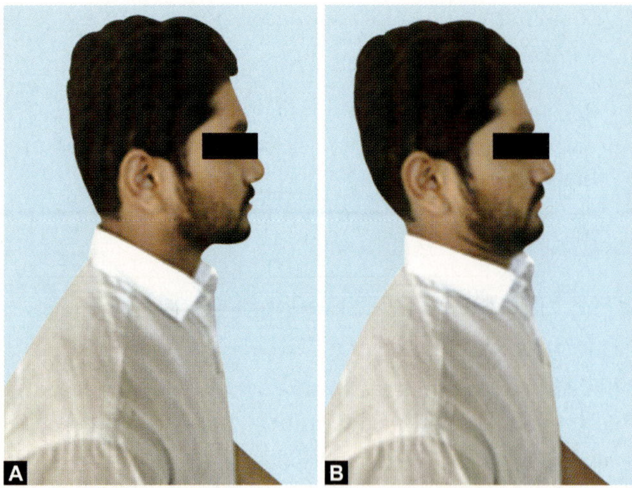

Figs. 18.8A and B: Chin tuck exercises.

relieving pain and disability in the short term. Central posteroanterior glide and transverse glide at respective spinous processes, lateral posteroanterior glide at respective facet joints are found to be beneficial. Detailed techniques of mobilization and manipulation are beyond the scope of this chapter.

- *ROM:* Active movements of cervical region including movements such as flexion, extension, side flexion, rotation, and chin tucks **(Figs. 18.8A and B)** can be done. Patient is positioned either in sitting or standing. Full movements within pain-free range are allowed.
- *Stretching of tight muscles:* Stretching can be applied passively by the therapist or self-stretching can be taught to the patient **(Table 18.2)**.

Traction can be used as a part of stretching exercises. Traction includes mechanical or manual traction. Manual traction for cervical spine given with patient in supine lying and therapist standing at the head end of the table. The therapist may place fingers of both hands under the occiput or one hand on frontal region and the other under occiput or using a belt to reinforce hands. Patients head position may be flexion, extension, or side flexion. If the head is moved in flexion more traction force is directed over lower cervical spine. Apply the traction force by leaning backward **(Figs. 18.10A to C)**.

- *Strengthening exercises*
  - Strengthening exercises include isometric exercises **(Table 18.3)** and dynamic exercises (concentric and eccentric contraction).
  - Isometric exercise for cervical region:
    - Manual resistance by therapist: Position of patient is in sitting. Therapist is standing behind the patient and places the hand on the patient's forehead for flexion, places the hand against the side of the head for side flexion, places the hand on the back of the head for extension and for rotation places the hand superior and lateral to the eye. Then the patient is asked to press against therapist's hand without allowing the movement to occur **(Figs. 18.11 A to D)**.
    - Self-resistance: Position of patient is in sitting. Patient places both hands on the forehead for flexion, places one hand against the side of the head for side flexion, places both hands on the back of the head for extension and for rotation places one hand superior and lateral to the eye. Then the patient is asked to press against the hand without allowing the movement to occur.
  - Isometric exercise for scapular muscles can be performed as described in **Table 18.3.**
  - Dynamic Strengthening can be performed in the same positions as mentioned in **Figures 18.11 A to D**.
  - Strengthening of deep muscles of cervical region also plays a crucial role. It involves core stability exercises for cervical spine. Deep neck flexors of cervical spine can be activated through craniocervical flexion (chin tuck) exercises. Lower cervical and upper thoracic extensors can be activated with patient in prone lying with forehead on the plinth, arms by the sides and performing

Table 18.2: Stretching techniques.		
Muscle	*Passive stretching*	*Self-stretching*
Pectoralis major	• Position of therapist: Behind the patient • Position of patient: Sitting with hands behind the head • Procedure: Ask the patient to breathe in and bring elbows out to the side and hold it as patient breathes out **(Fig. 18.9)**	• Position of patient: Standing facing the corner • Procedure: Arms in reverse T or V against wall. Ask the patient to lean forward from ankle
Suboccipital muscles	• Position of therapist: Behind the patient • Position of patient: Sitting • Procedure: Palpate C2 spinous process and stabilize it. Ask the patient to do gentle chin tucks	• Position of patient: Sitting • Procedure: Instruct to perform chin tucks and then bring the chin toward larynx. Gentle pressure can be applied over the occiput region with palm of the patient's hand to reinforce the movement
Upper trapezius	• Position of therapist: Behind the patient • Position of patient: Sitting with ipsilateral hand behind the back • Procedure: Therapist hand over patient's head. Perform cervical flexion, rotation to tight side and side flexion on opposite side	• Position of patient: Sitting with ipsilateral hand behind the back • Procedure: Patient uses contralateral hand to provide stretch with neck flexion, rotation to tight side, side flexion on the opposite side

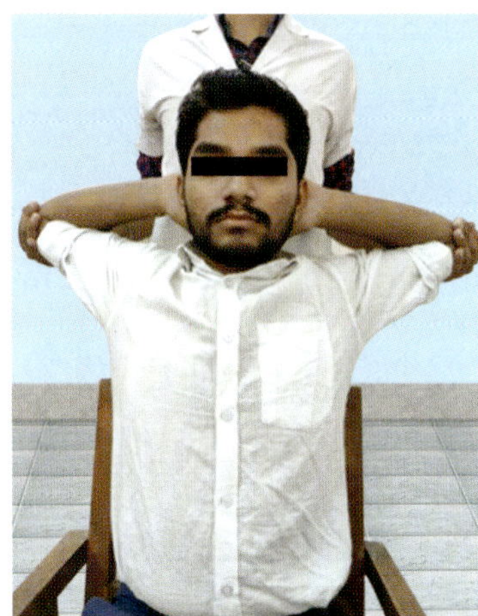

Fig. 18.9: Stretching of pectoral muscles.

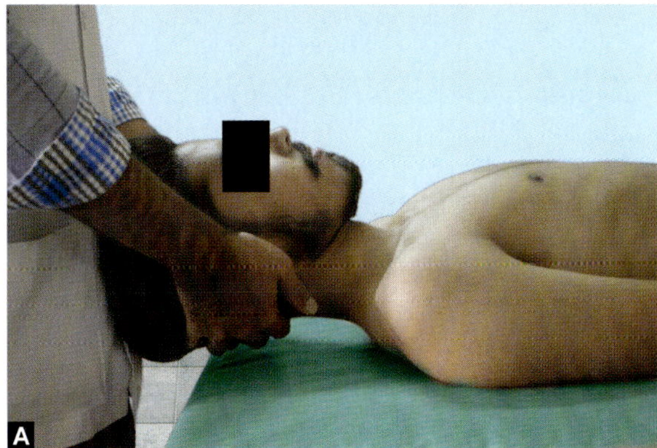

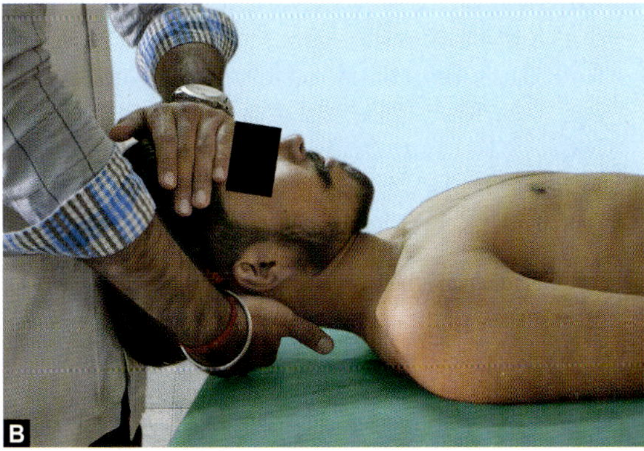

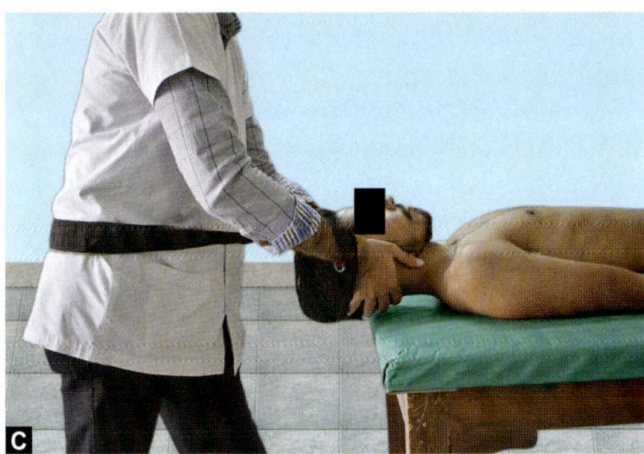

Figs. 18.10A to C: Techniques for manual traction with various hand placement: (A) Over occiput; (B) One over forehead and one occiput; and (C) With belt.

Table 18.3: Scapular isometrics.

Muscle	Patient position	Therapist resistance
Depressors	Side lying	Inferior angle of scapula
Elevators	Side lying	Spine of scapula
Protractors	Sitting	Lateral border of scapula
Retractors	Sitting	Medial border of scapula

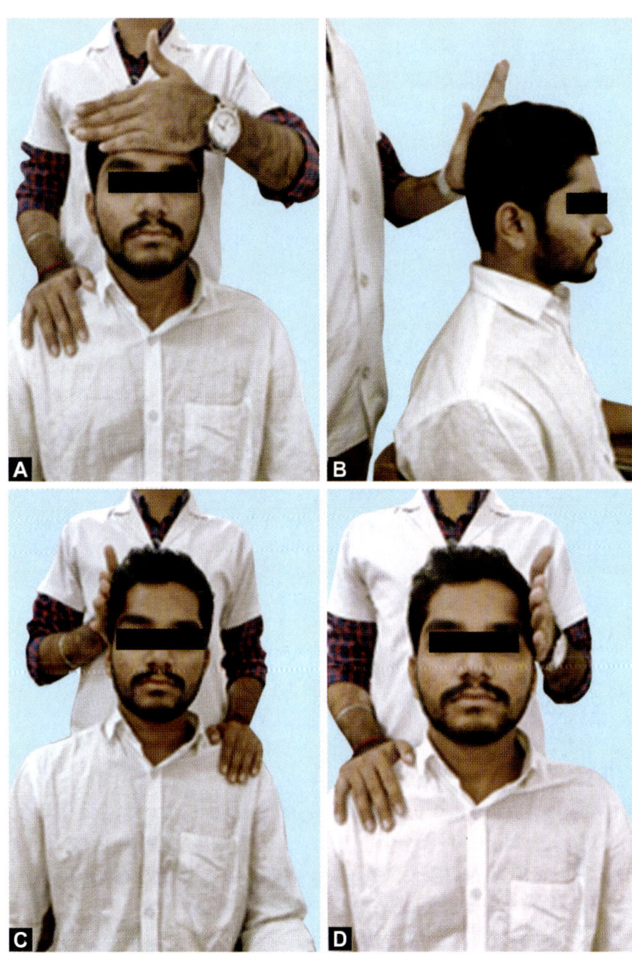

Figs. 18.11A to D: Hand placement for manual isometrics: (A) Flexors; (B) Extensors; and (C and D) Side flexors.

chin tucks. Gradually, progressive limb loading can be added to the treatment.

- Core stability exercises are performed in progression from one starting position to another in sequence (**Table 18. 4**). Chin tucks are maintained throughout all the repetitions. Limb loading can be done as a progression, once the patient has mastered the skill of maintaining chin tucks throughout one limb loading then progress to other limb loading position.
- Endurance training involves holding exercises mentioned in **Table 18.4** for prolonged period of time
- General fitness training (stay active)
- Advice to stay active plus home cervical ROM and isometric exercise

Table 18.4: Core stability exercises for cervical spine.	
Muscles / **Cervical flexors**	**Cervical and thoracic extensors**
Position • Supine lying • Sitting • Sitting on physio-ball • Standing with support • Standing without support/standing on unstable surface	• Prone with forehead on the plinth • Quadruped • Standing with support • Standing without support/standing on unstable surface
Limb loading • 90° shoulder flexion • 90° shoulder abduction • External rotation of the shoulder with arms at the sides • Full range shoulder flexion diagonal patterns of bilateral upper limbs simultaneously • Functional activities such as pushing/pulling/lifting	• Prone with arms by the side and externally rotating shoulder and retract scapulae • Prone with arms at 90° shoulder abduction, external rotation of the shoulder and horizontally abduct shoulder and retract scapulae. Prone lying with full bilateral flexion of shoulder • Prone lying with arms at 90° shoulder abduction, external rotation of the shoulder with elbow extension and horizontally abduct and retract scapulae • Diagonal patterns of upper limbs and lastly functional activities such as pushing/pulling/lifting

Subacute

Physiotherapy management to deal with subacute neck pain with mobility deficits:

- Cervical mobilization or manipulation along with thoracic manipulation.

   Central posteroanterior glide and transverse glide at respective spinous processes, lateral posteroanterior glide at respective facet joints are found to be beneficial. Detailed techniques of mobilization and manipulation are beyond the scope of this chapter.

- Endurance exercise for cervical, scapular, and thoracic muscles.

Chronic

Physiotherapy management to deal with chronic pain with mobility deficits:

- Cervical mobilization or manipulation along with thoracic manipulation.
- Cervical, scapular, and thoracic muscles' exercises that involve active ROM exercises, stretching, and strengthening and endurance exercises.
- Postural correction exercises
- Aerobic conditioning by walking, running, cycling, aerobic dancing, or swimming. The mode of aerobic exercises should be suggested based on access and convenience of the patient. Precautions are to be considered before starting with aerobic exercises. Painful movement/position should be avoided during exercises. Exercises should be performed with proper warm-up and cooldown and within the tolerance of patient.
- Co-ordination exercises include eye, head, and neck co-ordination exercises, proprioception exercises include head relocation practices.
- Cognitive–behavioral therapy may be helpful in chronic neck pain patients. It includes mental imagery,

relaxation techniques, and behavioral modifications such as pacing and graded exposures. Detailed techniques of cognitive–behavioral therapy are beyond the scope of this chapter.

- "Stay active" lifestyle approaches.
- Physical agents:
  - Dry needling can be beneficial in relieving pain in immediate and short term.
  - Low-level laser (GaAlAs with 830 or 904 nm) is found to be beneficial in relieving pain and improving function immediately and after 6 months follow-up also. Intermittent mechanical traction is beneficial for short-term period. There are a variety of physical agents used in clinical practice but statistical evidence does not support it.

Neck Pain with Movement Co-ordination Impairments (Whiplash-Associated Disorder)

Acute if Prognosis is for a Quick and Early Recovery

Ways to deal with acute WAD:

- Education: advice to remain active performing day-to-day activities.
- Pain-free cervical ROM and postural balance exercises at home.
- Monitor for any acceptable progress.
- Minimize cervical collar use.

Subacute if Prognosis is for a Prolonged Recovery Trajectory

Following are the ways of dealing with subacute WAD:

- Patient counseling
- Physical agents such as cryotherapy, thermal modalities, or transcutaneous electrical nerve stimulation (TENS)
- Active cervical ROM exercises

- Stretching, strengthening, and endurance exercises of cervical, scapular, and thoracic muscles
- Cervical mobilization grade I and II
- Core stability for cervical spine.

Chronic

Following are the ways of dealing with chronic WAD:
- Patient education for prognosis and pain management.
- TENS is found to be beneficial for reducing pain immediately following treatment.
- Cervical mobilization.
- Cervical, scapular, and thoracic muscles strengthening, endurance, stretching exercises.
- Cognitive–behavioral therapy.
- Vestibular rehabilitation (detailed techniques of vestibular rehabilitation are mentioned in Chapter 27: Vestibular Rehabilitation)
- Core stability for cervical spine.

Neck Pain with Headache (Cervicogenic)

Acute

Physiotherapy management to deal with acute neck pain with headache:

C1-2 self-SNAG (sustained natural apophyseal glide): It is sustained glide to facet joint throughout the movement. Patient is in sitting/standing with horizontal pressure continuously applied through thin rubber strap at C1 and simultaneously patient rotates the head on one side.

Subacute

Physiotherapy management to deal with subacute neck pain with headache:
- Cervical manipulation and mobilization
- C1-2 self-SNAG.

Chronic

Physiotherapy management to deal with chronic neck pain with headache:
- Cervical and thoracic mobilization/manipulation
- Exercise for cervical and scapulothoracic region: Strengthening and endurance exercise
- Core stability exercises for cervical muscles.

Neck Pain with Radiating Pain (Radicular)

Acute

Ways to deal with acute neck pain with radiating pain:
- Cervical ROM exercises in pain-free ranges, core stability exercises, cervical and scapular isometric exercises.
- Low-level LASER: 905 nm LASER is found to be beneficial in reducing pain and improving function. There are a variety of modalities used but research evidence does not support the use of it in acute conditions.
- Cervical collar

Chronic

Ways to deal with acute chronic pain with radiating pain:
- Stretching and strengthening exercises for cervical, scapular, and thoracic muscles
- Cervical and thoracic mobilization/manipulation
- Intermittent cervical traction.

LUMBAR SPINE

Lumbar spine is the most mobile region of vertebral column next to cervical spine. Thus it is more prone to be associated with pain and disability. Abnormal postures during day-to-day activities and degeneration of spine with aging lead to a disabling condition such a low back pain (LBP).

CLASSIFICATION OF BACK PAIN

In the field of physical therapy, there are four primary LBP classification systems:
1. The mechanical diagnosis and therapy classification model described by McKenzie
2. The movement system impairment syndromes model described by Sahrmann
3. The mechanism-based classification system described by O'Sullivan
4. The treatment-based classification system described by Delitto et al.

Classification based on ICF:
- Acute LBP with mobility deficits
- Subacute LBP with mobility deficits
- Acute LBP with movement co-ordination impairments
- Subacute and chronic LBP with movement co-ordination impairments
- Acute LBP with related (referred) lower extremity pain
- Acute LBP with radiating pain
- Subacute and chronic LBP with radiating pain
- Acute and subacute LBP with related cognitive and affective tendencies
- Chronic LBP with generalized pain.

EVALUATION

Evaluation of a patient with LBP symptoms consists of a detailed history and examination procedure. Certain red flags should be ruled out before proceeding any further in the evaluation **(Box. 18.2).**

Observation

Postural alignment should be observed along with observation of anatomical movements of lumbar spine into flexion-extension, side flexion, and rotation to both sides. Movements should be observed to find any restriction/deviation from normal and patient's willingness to do the movement.

BOX 18.2: Red flags for low back pain.

Rule out red flags such as:
- Tumors (constant pain not affected by position or activity, worse at night, unexpected weight loss)
- Cauda equina syndrome (urine retention, fecal incontinence, saddle anesthesia, sensory, or motor deficits in L4, L5, and S1 areas)
- Infections
- Spinal compression fracture
- Abdominal aneurysm (back, abdominal, or groin pain; presence of peripheral vascular disease or coronary artery disease and associated risk factors; palpable abdominal aortic pulse)

Palpation

Following are the benefits of palpation:

- Palpation of bony landmarks **(Fig. 18.12)** in static posture and during movements may help therapists to find any motion restrictions or deviations in lumbar region.
- Palpation of muscles may help identify spasm, tenderness, trigger points, and swelling in lumbar region.

MTrPs are hypersensitive, painful areas over a taut band of muscle. They produce localized and referred pain to other structures with mechanical stimulation.

Examination

Range of Motion

Active and passive movements of the lumbar spine and hip should be assessed. End feel is felt at the end of passive movement. Lumbar active range of movement can be assessed with bubble goniometer.

For flexion, patient is in standing position. At starting position, one bubble goniometer is placed over the sacrum, and the second one is placed over the T12–L1 vertebral junction. The two different angles are noted and the difference between them is calculated. The resultant angle will be the starting angle. At the end position, both the bubble goniometer in position the person bends forward and downward. In this newly achieved position, measure the angles of both bubble goniometer and calculate the difference between them. This resultant angle will be the ending angle. Now measure the difference between this starting angle and ending angle. This difference will be the angle of lumbar spine flexion. Stabilize the pelvis during the movement.

For extension, patient is in standing position. At starting position, one bubble goniometer is placed over the sacrum, and the second one is placed over the T12–L1 vertebral junction. The two different angles are noted and the difference between them is calculated. The resultant angle will be the starting angle. At the end position with both the bubble goniometer in position, the person bends backward. In this newly achieved position, measure the angles of both bubble goniometer and calculate the difference between them. This resultant angle will be the ending angle. Now measure the difference between this starting and ending angle. This difference will be the angle of lumbar spine extension. Stabilize the pelvis during the movement.

For lateral flexion, universal goniometer can be used in standing position. Alignment of stable arm is over the sacrum aligned vertically downward at the midline, alignment of fulcrum is at the junction of L5 and S1 vertebra, and alignment of movable arm is from the L5–S1 junction to T12–L1 junction. As the person bends laterally movable arm moves along with the trunk movement. The angle between the stable and movable arm is measured. Stabilize the pelvis during the movements.

Alternative method of measuring ROM is with a measure tape. The person is in the standing position for

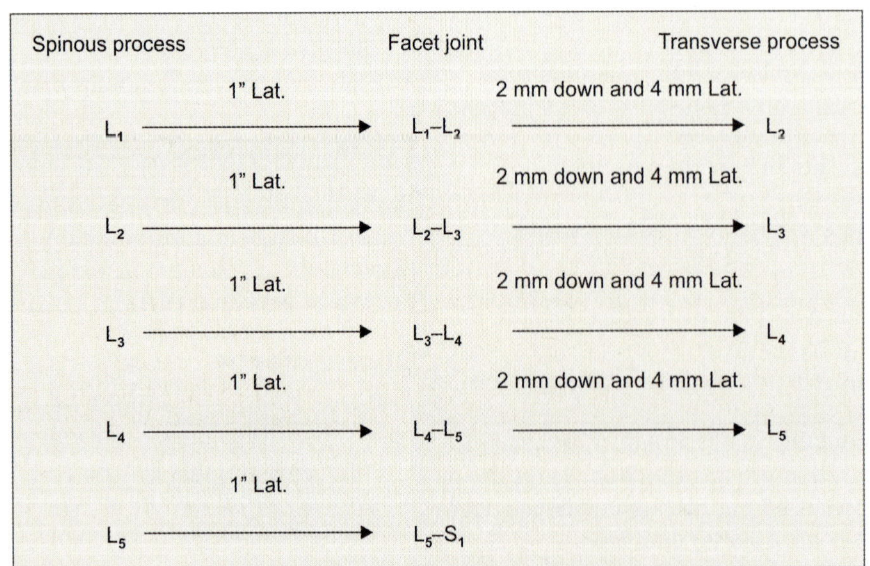

Fig. 18.12: Surface landmarks of lumbar spine.

BOX 18.3: Centralization versus peripheralization.

When symptoms ascend upward to back from leg and are localized to back on repeated spinal movements, it is termed as centralization. When symptoms descend down to the leg on repeated spinal movements, it is termed as peripheralization.

lumbar flexion (**Modified Schober's Test**)—mark the first point at lumbosacral junction, second point 10 cm above the first mark and third point 5 cm below the first mark. Measure the distance between the second and third mark then ask the person to perform the movement and again measure the distance at the end of ROM. The difference in the distance is the range of flexion. For lumbar extension (Modified Schober's Test)—mark the first point at lumbosacral junction, second point 10 cm above the first mark and third point 5 cm below the first mark. Measure the distance between the second and third mark then ask the person to perform the movement and again measure the distance at the end of ROM. The difference in the distance is the range of flexion.

Repeated movements of lumbar spine in flexion, extension, side flexion in standing, supine and prone lying should be performed to assess centralization and peripheralization (**Box 18.3**).

Painful arc with flexion or return from flexion is positive if the patient complains of pain during movement but not at the end ranges of movements. **Reversal of lumbopelvic rhythm** is present if the patient while returning from a forward bent position bends knees and extends hips first followed by anterior tilting of the pelvis. **Gower sign** is positive if the patient uses hands to push against the anterior thighs in a sequential distal to proximal manner to diminish the load on the low back when returning to the upright position from a forward bent position.

Accessory Movements (Intersegmental Mobility Testing)

Pain response and segmental mobility are assessed through accessory movements including joint play at all vertebral levels. Intersegmental mobility testing reveals characteristic restriction.

Strength and Endurance

Muscle strength should be objectively measured for muscles of lumbar region including superficial and deep muscles, hip region. Deep muscles can be assessed using pressure biofeedback unit clinically through abdominal drawing in maneuver. Endurance is also one of the important components of assessment. It is assessed by measuring for how long a patient is able to hold the position of the trunk in flexion, extension, side flexion, and rotation (**Table 18.5**).

Strength of transversus abdominis is assessed by positioning patient in prone over a pressure biofeedback unit that is inflated to 70 mm Hg (**Fig. 18.13**). The patient is instructed to draw in the abdominal wall for 10 seconds

Table 18.5: Isometric and dynamic test for lumbar spine.

Tests	Position	Procedure	Grades
Dynamic abdominal endurance test **(Fig. 18.14A)**	Crook lying	Patient tucks in chin and curls trunk up till scapula is cleared off the plinth	Number of repetitions patient is able to perform task in 1 minutes is recorded
Isometric abdominal test	Crook lying	Holding the above position	• Normal (5): Hands behind the back and holding for 20–30 seconds • Good (4): Arms crossing the chest and holding for 15–20 seconds • Fair (3): Arms straight and holding for 10–15 seconds • Poor (2): Arms straight and clearing top of scapula and holding for 1–10 seconds • Trace (1): Unable to raise more than head off
Dynamic extensor endurance test **(Fig. 18.14B)**	Prone lying with hips and pelvis stabilized with straps and upper body outside the plinth with support on table	With arms crossed around chest patient extends trunk	Number of repetitions patient is able to perform task in 1 minutes is recorded
Isometric extensor test	Prone lying on plinth	Same as above	• Normal (5): Hands behind the head, lifting head and chest and holding for 20–30 seconds • Good (4): Hands at the sides, lifting head and chest and holding for 15–20 seconds • Fair (3): Hands at the sides, lifting sternum and holding for 10–15 seconds • Poor (2): Hands at the sides, lifting head and holding for 1–10 seconds • Trace (1): Slight contraction of muscle with no movement

Contd...

Contd...

Tests	Position	Procedure	Grades
Dynamic side bridge test **(Fig. 18.14C)**	Side-lying position with upper body resting on elbow with knees 90° flexed	Patient lifts pelvis off the plinth and straighten the spine	Number of repetitions patient is able to perform task in 1 minute is recorded
Isometric side bridge test	Same as above	Same as above	• Normal (5): Able to lift pelvis and holding for 10–20 seconds • Good (4): Able to lift pelvis holding for 5–10 seconds • Fair (3): Able to lift pelvis and holding for less than 5 seconds • Poor (2): Unable to lift the pelvis of the plinth

without inducing pelvic motion while breathing normally. The maximal decrease in pressure is recorded. Muscle endurance of transversus abdominis is measured by number of 10 seconds hold up to 10 repetitions.

Tightness of Muscles

Muscles such as iliopsoas, hamstring, and rectus femoris should be assessed.

- Tightness of the iliopsoas is checked by patient in supine lying position, then therapist flexes one knee of the patient and brings it towards the chest. If tightness of iliopsoas is present, then the straight leg rises off the plinth.
- Tightness of rectus femoris is assessed with patient in prone lying position and therapist passively flexes the patient's knee. It tightness of rectus femoris is present, then hip on same side will spontaneously flex.
- Tightness of hamstring is assessed in supine lying with hips flexed at 90° and knees bent. Patient actively extends knee as much as possible while grasping the thighs to maintain hip at 90° flexion. If tightness of hamstring is present, then tested leg will not be able to extend the knee beyond 20° of knee flexion.

Sensations and Reflexes

Sensations should be checked in respective dermatomes corresponding to lumbar nerve roots. Reflexes should be checked for differences on both sides including knee and ankle.

Functional Assessment

Oswestry disability index, Roland–Morris disability questionnaire, and Quebec back pain disability scale can be used to assess patient's day-to-day activities and to detect change in daily functions over time.

Special Test

Common special tests performed for lumbar spine include slump test, straight leg raise (SLR) test, and prone instability test.

- *Prone instability test:* Patient position is prone lying and therapist applies posterior to anterior pressure over spinous processes of lumbar spine. Pain is noted on application of pressure. In second position, patient lifts both legs off the plinth and again therapist applies posterior to anterior pressure over spinous processes of lumbar spine. Test is positive if pain is present in first position and subsides in second position.

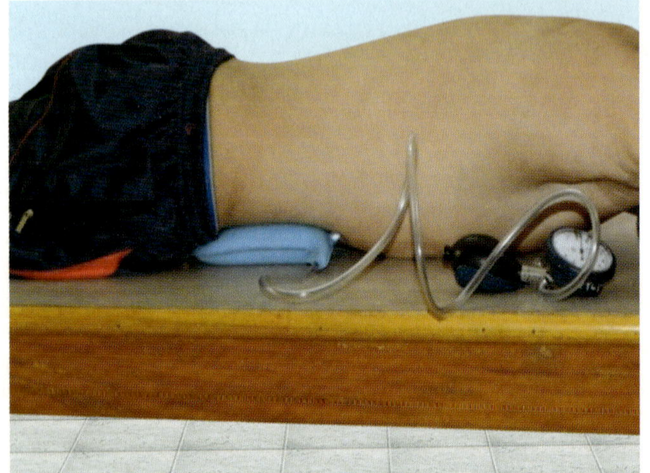

Fig. 18.13: Transversus abdominis assessment.

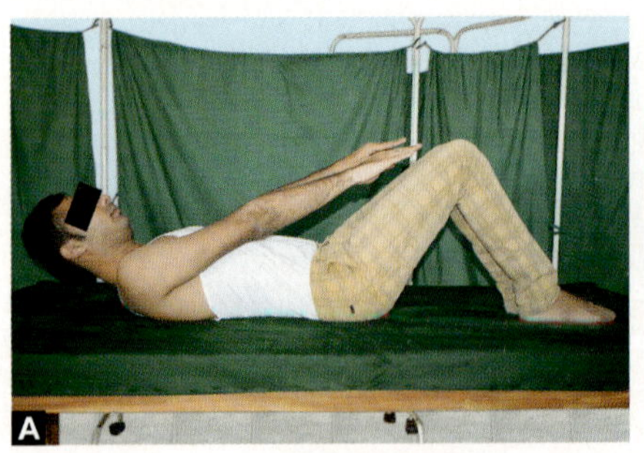
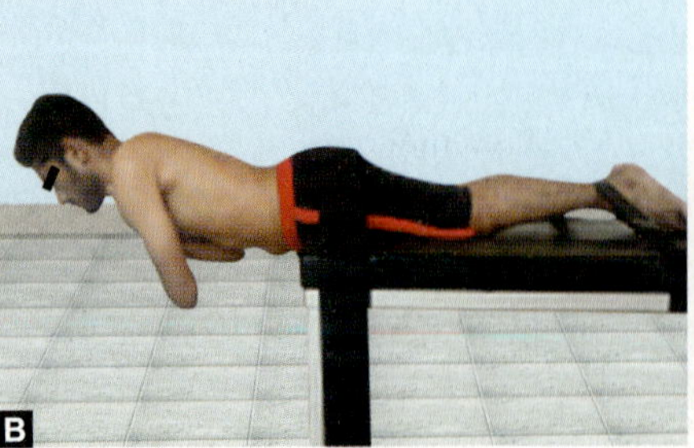
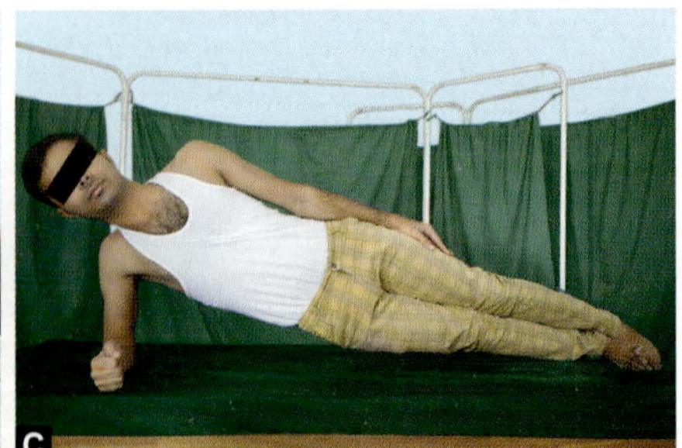

Figs. 18.14A to C: (A) Abdominal endurance test, (B) Extensor endurance test, and (C) Side bridge test.

Table 18.6: Straight leg raising and its modifications.

Joint	Sciatic and tibial nerve	Tibial nerve	Sural nerve	Common peroneal nerve
Hip	Flexion and adduction	Flexion	Flexion	Flexion and medial rotation
Knee	Extension	Extension	Extension	Extension
Ankle	Dorsiflexion	Dorsiflexion	Dorsiflexion	Plantarflexion
Foot	–	Eversion	Inversion	Inversion
Toes	–	Extension	–	–

- *Straight leg raise:* Tests are performed with patient in supine lying position and therapist in walk standing position on the side of the plinth. Tests start with performing on unaffected side first moving to affected side (**Table 18.6** and **Figs. 18.15A to D**). Position of hip is followed by ankle. Test is positive on reproduction of radicular symptoms. Test positive between 35° and 70° of hip flexion is suggestive of sciatic nerve root involvement and test positive beyond 70° of hip flexion is suggestive of joint pain.
- *Slump Test:* Patient is in sitting position with hands behind the back and therapist in walk standing position on the side of the patient. Sequential steps are to be followed while performing the test (**Figs. 18.16A and B**). Slumped position is adapted that places thoracic and lumbar spine in flexion and hip is at 90° flexion. Further, therapist passively flexes cervical spine, extends knee and dorsiflexes ankle. Test is positive on reproduction of radicular symptoms. Test assesses structures such as spinal cord, cervical and lumbar nerve roots and sciatic nerve.

Clinical Pearl

Mental impairment measures such as fear-avoidance beliefs questionnaire, pain catastrophizing scale, Örebro musculoskeletal pain screening questionnaire should be used when necessary (Chapter 10: Pain Assessment and Management).

CLINICAL PRESENTATION

Acute/Subacute Low Back Pain with Mobility Deficits

Common symptom: Low back, buttock, or thigh pain. In acute condition duration of symptoms is 1 month or less.

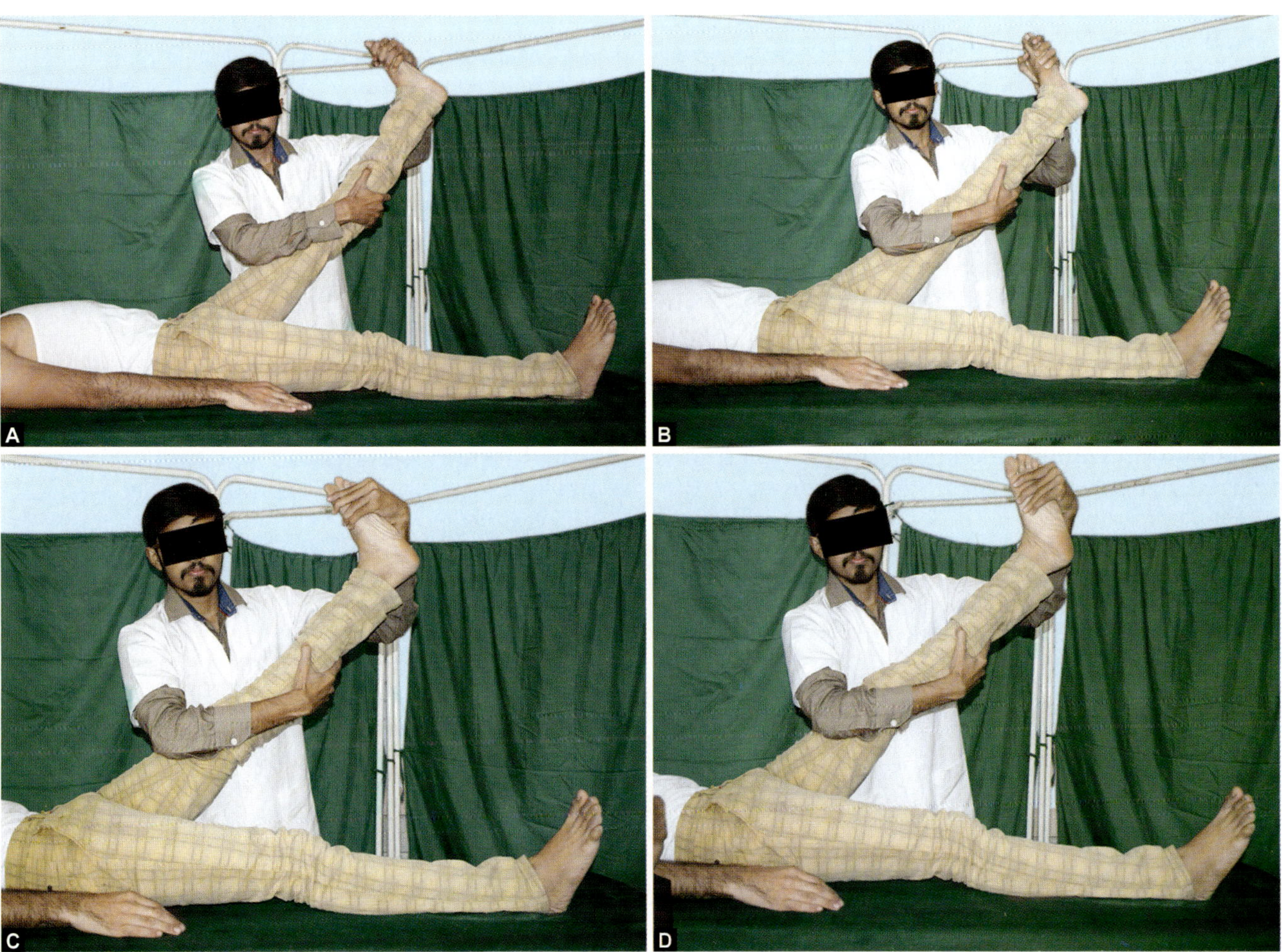

Figs. 18.15A to D: Straight leg raising test and its modifications.

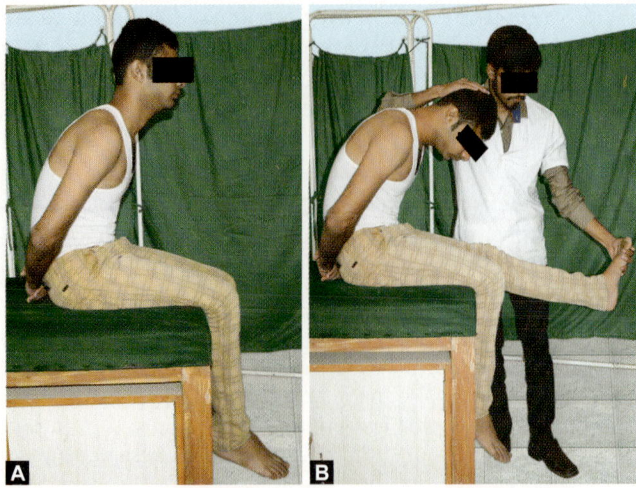

Figs. 18.16A and B: Slump test: (A) Starting position and (B) End position.

Expected Examination Findings

Following are the expected findings:
- Restricted spinal ROM
- Restricted segmental mobility
- Symptoms reproduced with end range movements of spine in subacute conditions.
- LBP and related lower extremity pain are reproduced with provocation of involved vertebral segments.

Acute Low Back Pain with Movement Co-ordination Impairments

Common symptom: Acute exacerbation of recurring LBP with associated lower extremity pain.

Expected Examination Findings

Following are the expected findings:
- Symptoms reproduced with initial- and midrange of spinal movement.
- LBP and related lower extremity pain are reproduced with provocation of involved vertebral segments.
- Movement co-ordination impairments with flexion and extension movements of lumbar region.

Subacute/Chronic Low Back Pain with Movement Co-ordination Impairments

Common symptom: Exacerbation of recurring LBP with associated lower extremity pain.

Expected Examination Findings

Following are the findings:
- Symptoms reproduced with midrange of spinal movement and worsens with end range in subacute condition. Symptoms reproduced with sustained end range in chronic conditions.
- LBP and related lower extremity pain are reproduced with provocation of involved vertebral segments.
- Segmental hypermobility is present.

- Mobility, strength, and endurance deficits in thoracic, lumbar, and pelvic region.

Acute Low Back Pain with Related (Referred) Lower Extremity Pain

Common symptom: LBP with associated lower extremity pain that worsens with flexion activities and sitting.

Expected Examination Findings

Following are the findings:
- Centralization with repeated movements or position is present
- Lateral trunk shift
- Reduced lumbar lordosis
- Symptoms reproduced worsening with end range
- Mobility, strength, and endurance deficits in thoracic, lumbar, and pelvic region.

Acute/Subacute/Chronic Low Back Pain with Radiating Pain

Common symptom: LBP with associated lower extremity pain—paresthesia, numbness, and weakness in lower extremity.

Expected Examination Findings

Following are the expected examination findings:
- Symptoms reproduced with initial- to midrange of spinal movement in acute conditions. Symptoms reproduced with midrange and worsen with end range of spinal movement in subacute conditions. Symptoms reproduced with sustained end range of spinal movement in chronic conditions.
- LBP and related lower extremity pain are reproduced with provocation of involved vertebral segments by lower limb tension tests, straight leg raising test, and slump tests.
- Strength, sensory, and reflex deficits may be present.

Acute and Subacute Low Back Pain with Related Cognitive and Affective Tendencies

Common symptom: Acute or subacute LBP with associated lower extremity pain.

Expected Examination Findings

Following are the expected examination findings:
- Positive responses for depressive symptoms
- High scores on Fear Avoidance Belief Questionnaire and Pain Catastrophizing Scale.

Chronic Low Back Pain with Generalized Pain

Low back pain or related lower extremity pain with duration more than 3 months. Presence of depression, fear-avoidance belief, and pain catastrophizing. Generalized pain that is not consistent with other impairments mentioned above.

PHYSIOTHERAPY MANAGEMENT

Introduction

Goals of treatment based on classification of low back pain are mentioned in **Table 18.7**.

Acute/Subacute Low Back Pain with Mobility Deficits

Following are the ways to deal with acute/subacute low back pain with mobility deficits:

- **Manual therapy procedures** (manipulation/mobilization) to diminish pain and improve segmental spinal or lumbopelvic motion. Central posteroanterior glide and transverse glide at respective spinous processes, lateral posteroanterior glide at respective facet joints are found to be beneficial. Detailed techniques of mobilization and manipulation are beyond the scope of this chapter.

- **Therapeutic exercises** to improve or maintain spinal mobility that focuses on co-ordination, strength, and endurance of lumbar muscles. Stretching exercises to stretch tight muscles such as rectus femoris and iliopsoas and hamstrings **(Table 18.8)**.

Abdominal bracing is performed in crook lying position. Ask the patient to breathe in and out and then gently and slowly push out waist without drawing abdomen inward or moving back or pelvis.

Isometric abdominals are traditionally performed with patient in crook lying position and therapist places hand below the lumbar spine. Ask the patient to isometrically contract the abdominals such that pressure is exerted on the therapist hand placed below. Trick movements such as pressing down from feet or head, breathe holding should be avoided. **Isometric back extensors** are traditionally performed with patient in supine lying and asking the patient to press down from head and heels simultaneously on the plinth.

Table 18.7: Goals of treatment based on the classification of low back pain.

Back pain	Goals of treatment
• Acute low back pain with mobility deficits • Acute low back pain with movement co-ordination impairments • Acute low back pain with radiating pain	• Reducing pain • Improve mobility of the involved spinal segments
• Acute low back pain with related (referred) lower extremity pain	Focused on centralizing the patient's symptoms
• Subacute low back pain with mobility deficits • Subacute low back pain with movement coordination impairments • Subacute low back pain with radiating pain	Focused on movements that increase movement tolerances in the mid to end ranges of spinal movements
• Chronic low back pain with movement co-ordination impairments • Chronic low back pain with radiating pain	Focused on movements that increase movement tolerances in the end ranges of spinal movements
• Acute and subacute low back pain with related cognitive and affective tendencies • Chronic low back pain with generalized pain	Addresses the cognitive and affective tendencies and pain behaviors with patient education and counseling

Table 18.8: Stretching techniques for lumbar spine.

Muscle	Passive stretching	Self-stretching
Rectus femoris	• Position of patient: Prone • Position of therapist: Walk standing beside the patient • Procedure: After stabilizing pelvis grasp over distal leg and flex the knee. Further stretch can be applied by extending the hip simultaneously	• Position of patient: Standing • Procedure: Grasp the ankle of leg and flex the knee of one lower limb with hip extension
Iliopsoas	• Position of patient: Supine at the edge of the plinth and opposite limb is flexed at the knee and hip • Position of therapist: Walk standing beside the patient stabilizing opposite leg • Procedure: Downward pressure is applied over anterior aspect of distal thigh	• Position of patient: Prone • Procedure: Raise the trunk on hands with pelvis on the plinth
Hamstrings	• Position of patient: Supine • Position of therapist: Walk standing beside the patient stabilizing opposite leg and supporting lower leg on arms • Procedure: With knees in extension take hip into flexion as far as possible	• Position of patient: Supine with towel behind the thigh • Procedure: Perform straight leg raise and pull with towel to move hip on more flexion

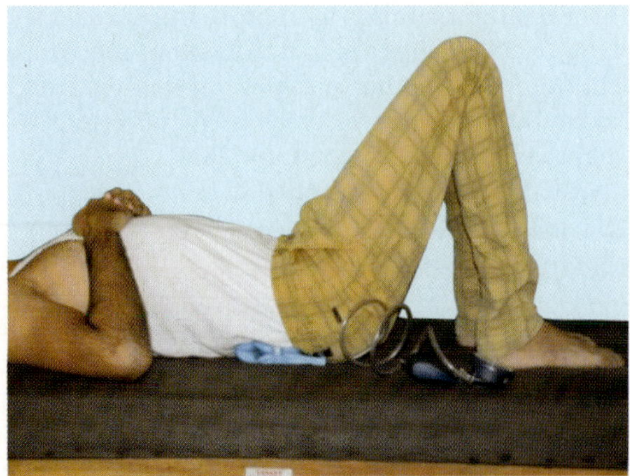

Fig. 18.17: Abdominal drawing in maneuver with pressure biofeedback unit.

Abdominal drawing in maneuver is performed in crook lying or quadruped position. Ask patient to gently draw in or hollow the abdomen while maintaining normal breathing **(Fig. 18.17)**. The instructions were given to breathe in and out and then, without breathing in, to slowly draw in the abdomen, keeping the spinal position steady. Avoid trick movements such as movements of the pelvis and spine, breath holding, rib elevation, and bulging of the abdomen. If patient is facing difficult in performing, the exercise feedback can be provided by pressure biofeedback unit. Once mastered, the same maneuver can be performed in sitting, standing, and other functional positions.

Dynamic and endurance exercises—before proceeding with any of the dynamic and endurance exercises, spinal bias should be assessed. Spinal bias is the movement of relief of symptoms, e.g., if patient is having relief in flexion movement then use flexion as exercises **(Table 18.9 and Figs. 18.18A to G)**. Bias is not the opposite of the painful movement, relief of pain should be checked.

Endurance training involves holding exercises mentioned in **Table 18.9** for prolonged period of time.

Core stability exercises are being performed in progression from one starting position to another in sequence. Abdominal drawing in maneuver is maintained throughout the whole repetition **(Table 18.10 and Figs. 18.19A to C)**. Limb loading can be progressed once the patient has mastered the skill of maintaining abdominal drawing in maneuver throughout one limb loading then progress to other limb loading position.

Patient education that encourages the patient to return to an active lifestyle should not overdo exercises, patient should be actively participating in treatment, instructions of prevention such as ways to do exercises, do activities that minimize stress, modification in home and work environment.

Acute Low Back Pain with Movement Co-ordination Impairments (Spinal Instabilities)

Following are the ways to deal with acute low back pain with movement coordination impairments:

Table 18.9: Exercises for lumbar spine.

Exercise	Position	Procedure
Curl up	Crook lying	Lift shoulders until scapulae clear the plinth. Arms are horizontal. Alteration in arm position to folding around chest and then behind the head
Diagonal curls up	Crook lying	While performing curls up reach opposite knee with one hand and then alternate
Knee to chest	Supine lying	Single: Bring one knee by flexing toward the chest Double: Bring both the knees toward the chest
Single straight leg raising	Supine lying with one knee flexed	Lift extended lower limb with knee straight and then alternate with other lower limb
Back extension	Prone lying with lower limb stabilized	Lift head and trunk up till clearing of sternum. Arms are by the side of the trunk. Alteration in arm position to folding around chest and then reaching overhead
Leg extension	Prone lying with thorax stabilized	Lift both lower limbs alternately

- Core stability with its progression to maintain the involved segment.
- Use of temporary external devices such as lumbar corsets to provide stability.
- Home advice includes maintaining positions/movements in symptom relief positions and maintains an active lifestyle, should not overdo exercises, instructions of prevention such as ways to do exercises, do activities that minimize stress, modification in home and work environment.

Subacute/Chronic Low Back Pain with Movement Co-ordination Impairments (Spinal Instabilities)

Following are the ways to deal with spinal instabilities:

- Core stability with its progression to maintain the involved segment.
- Isometric abdominals and back extensors, dynamic and endurance training for lumbopelvic region should be advised as described above. Exercises such as isometric, dynamic, and endurance training for hip muscles should be incorporated.
- Home advice includes maintaining positions/movements in symptom relief positions and maintaining an active lifestyle, should not overdo exercises, instructions of prevention such as ways to do exercises, do activities that minimize stress, modification in home and work environment.

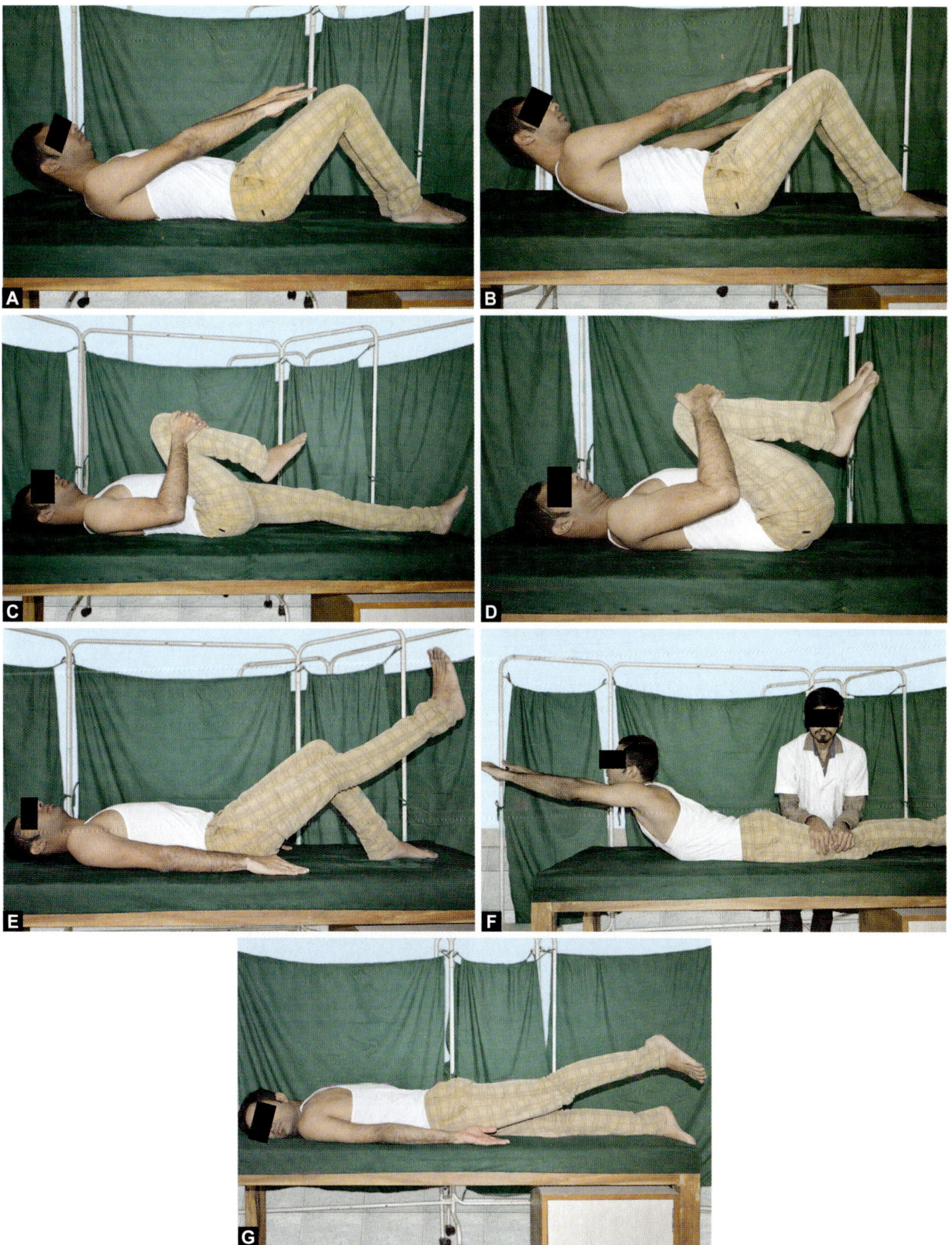

Figs. 18.18A to G: (A) Curls up; (B) Diagonal curls up to the left; (C) Single knee to chest; (D) Double knee to chest; (E) Straight leg raising; (F) Back extension; and (G) Leg extension.

Acute Low Back Pain with Related (Referred) Lower Extremity Pain (Flat Back Syndrome, Lumbago due to Displacement of Intervertebral Disk)

Following are the ways to deal with acute low back pain with related lower extremity pain:

- **Therapeutic exercises based on spinal bias**: Extension approach that includes exercises focusing on spinal extension such a prone lying with or without pillows below the chest, prone on elbows, prone on hands, sustained back extension in prone, sustained extension in standing. Following this, certain joint mobilizations can be used.
- **Core stability** with its progression to maintain the involved segment.

Traction can be manual or mechanical. Manual traction is difficult on the part of the therapist to apply for lumbar spine **(Figs. 18.20A and B)**. Position of patient for manual

Table 18.10: Core stability for lumbar spine.

Muscles	Abdominals		Trunk extensors
Position	Crook lying	Quadruped	Prone
Limb Loading	• Heel sliding to extend knee • Bend leg to 90° hip flexion • Lift straight leg to 45° hip flexion • Bent leg fall out	• Flex one upper limb • Extend one lower limb by sliding on mat • Extend one lower limb by lifting off mat • Flex one upper limb and extend contralateral lower limb	• Extend one lower limb • Extend both lower limb • Lift head, arms, and both lower limbs

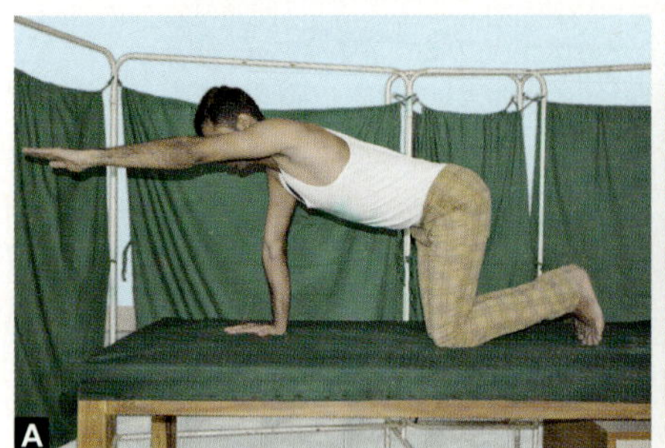
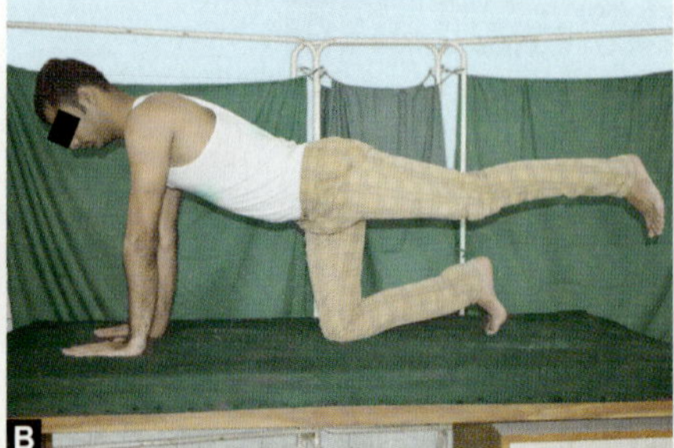
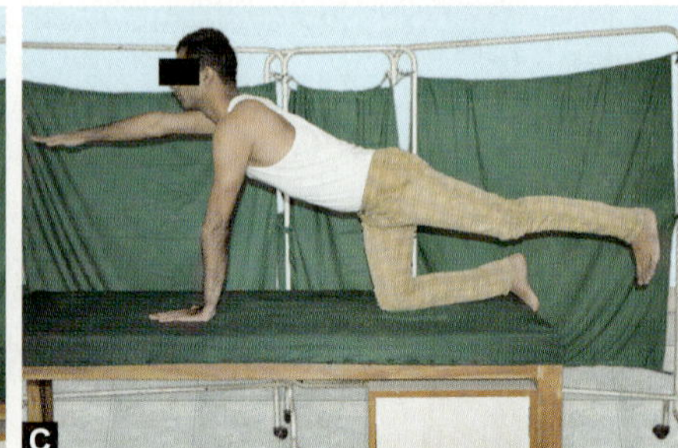

Figs. 18.19A to C: Core stability exercises in quadruped position.

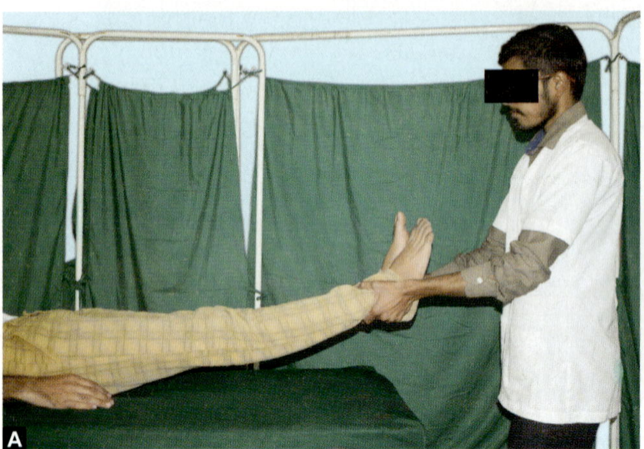
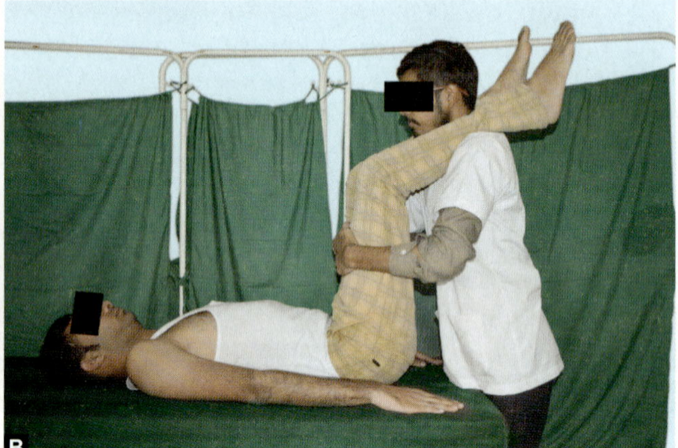

Figs. 18.20A and B: Manual traction: (A) in extension; (B) in flexion.

traction is supine lying with thorax stabilized by harness. Assistant stands at the head end of the plinth and holds the patient's arms. Therapist position is at the leg end and in walk standing position facing the patient. To apply traction in extension, patient's legs are extended and therapist pulls at the ankles, and to provide traction in flexion, patient's legs are flexed at the hips and lower leg rests over therapist's shoulder and traction pull is given by therapist's hands wrapped around the patient's thigh. Mechanical traction can be applied with appropriate traction force, i.e., half of patient's body weight. Duration of mechanical traction should be less than 15 minutes for intermittent traction.

■ With changing times, modern technology has grown. Spinal decompression has become immensely popular in recent times for the management of symptoms of low back and cervical region. It causes decompression of the spine, leading to reduced pressures over the nerves **(Fig. 18.21)**.

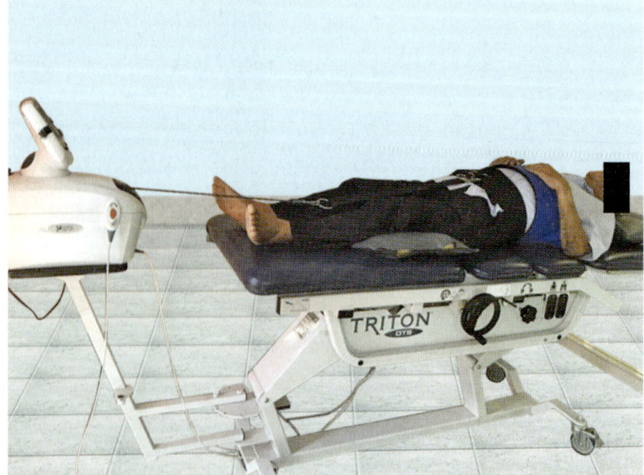

Fig. 18.21: Spinal decompression being applied to the patient for low back.
Courtesy: Mission health, Ahmedabad.

- Patient education for positions of centralization that should be assumed and maintain an active lifestyle.

Acute/Subacute/Chronic Low Back Pain with Radiating Pain (Lumbago with Sciatica)

Following are the ways to deal with lumbago with sciatica:

- Patient education to maintain position that decreases compression on involved nerve roots.
- Manual or mechanical traction as described earlier.
- Nerve mobility exercises to improve the mobility of neural elements. Assume a position of straight leg raising test that puts tension on involved neural tissues, maintain the stretched position, and then release it by moving one of the joints such that it glides the nerve.

Acute/Subacute Low Back Pain with Related Cognitive or Affective Tendencies (Low Back Pain, Disorder of Central Nervous System, Specified as Central Nervous System Sensitivity to Pain)

Following are the ways to deal with acute or subacute low back pain with related cognitive or affective tendencies:

- Patient education and counseling to address specific classification exhibited by the patient (i.e., depression, fear-avoidance, pain catastrophizing).
- Cognitive–behavioral therapy may be helpful in patients. It includes imagery, relaxation techniques, and behavioral modifications such as pacing and graded exposures. Detailed techniques of cognitive–behavioral therapy are beyond the scope of this chapter.

Chronic Low Back Pain with Related Generalized Pain (Low Back Pain, Disorder of Central Nervous System, Persistent Somatoform Pain Disorder)

Following are the ways to deal with chronic low back pain with related generalized pain:

- Patient education and counseling to address specific classification exhibited by the patient (i.e., depression, fear avoidance, and pain catastrophizing). Cognitive–behavioral therapy may be helpful in chronic back pain patients. It includes imagery, relaxation techniques, and behavioral modifications such as pacing and graded exposures.
- Low-intensity, prolonged (aerobic) exercise activities. Aerobic conditioning by walking, running, cycling, aerobic dancing, or swimming. Type of aerobic exercises should be suggested based on access and convenience of the patient. Precautions are to be considered before starting with aerobic exercises. Painful movement/position should be avoided during exercises. Exercises should be performed with proper warm-up and cooldown and within the tolerance of patient.

T4 Syndrome

T4 syndrome is a collection of symptoms resulting from autonomic dysfunction of upper thoracic spine leading to pathologic condition at affected level and extending up to occiput proximally and either ipsilateral or contralateral upper limbs distally. The name is a little misleading since it is used to describe such symptoms at any thoracic level from which sympathetic nerves originate. Evans suggested it be named "Upper thoracic syndrome" to make it more specific and descriptive, but the name has not been used that often. T4 syndrome is more common in females than males and usually occurs after the age of 35 years.

Pathophysiology

Evans described the pathophysiology behind the T4 syndrome. Vasomotor fibers (preganglionic fibers) descend down the spinal cord, emerging as the ventral roots and horns, pass through the dorsal root ganglion and later emerge as a part of the spinal segmental nerve. From here, the sympathetic fibers join the sympathetic chain after leaving the segmental nerve. The sympathetic chain then passes down the neck of the ribs with varying areas of the ganglia. Branching of the sympathetic chain at the costovertebral joints provides sympathetic supply to the heart, esophagus, and the abdominal viscera. The other fibers either ascend or descend along the length of the vertebral column synapsing with postganglionic neurons (above T1 or below L2–L3) and finally leave the sympathetic chain and join a peripheral nerve. The sympathetic fibers are vulnerable to damage via stretching or compression following any degenerative changes (presence of osteophytes) in the vertebral column, particularly the thoracic spine. Along their course in the peripheral nerve, the sympathetic fibers leave the nerve and join an artery in a neurovascular bundle, taking control of the blood pressure regulation via vasoconstriction **(Fig. 18.22)**.

The head and neck receive their sympathetic supply through fibers from T1–T4, while the upper extremities receive it through T2–T5. Due to such kind of arrangement of sympathetic supply, symptoms are more commonly seen in the cervical region and the upper extremities **(Box 18.4)**.

Examination

- Patient may present with pain, sensory symptoms, and occipital headache.
- Pain is present in upper back, scapular, interscapular region, neck, arms, forearms, and chest.
- Nocturnal pain may disturb sleep.
- Prolonged sitting or bending activities aggravate symptoms.
- Sensory symptoms are vague and ill-defined and include paresthesia in hands (unilateral/bilateral).
- Abnormal postures such as increased thoracic kyphosis or flat back posture.

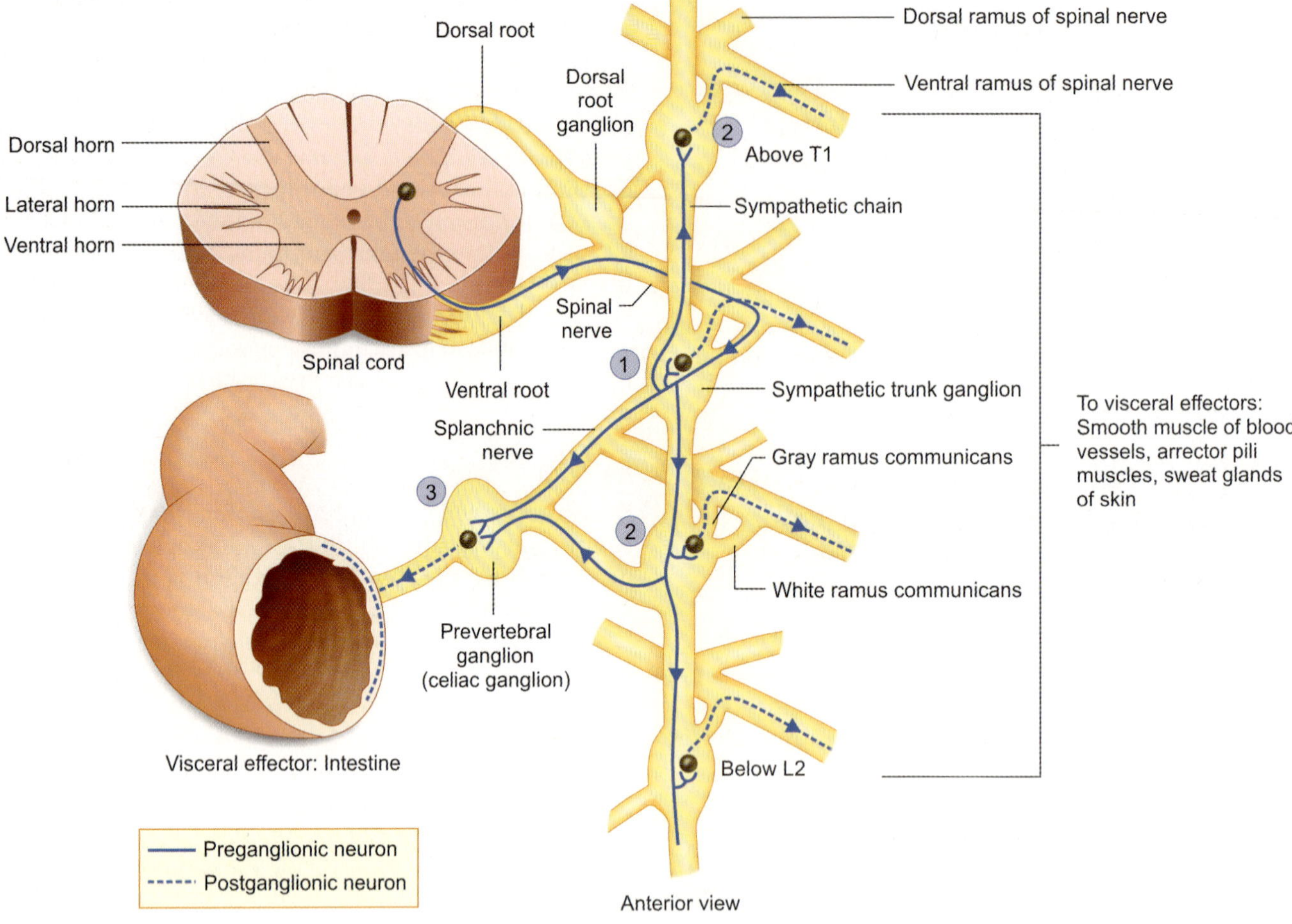

Fig. 18.22: Sympathetic chain.

- Tenderness present over T4 vertebral level.
- Allodynia and hyperalgesia are found over hypomobile segment.
- Trigger points are found around shoulder and upper trapezius.
- Tightness is present in pectorals and scalene.
- Accessory movement examination reveals pain and hypomobility of the affected segment of thoracic spine (palpated as shown in **Fig. 18.2**).
- Sensory examination reveals decreased light touch and pinprick occipital region, cervical region, and shoulders.
- Proprioception and vibration are affected in involved extremity.
- Grip strength is also decreased with affected extremity.
- Cervical ranges are painful and limited.

T4 syndrome is an exclusion diagnosis based on present clinical findings or radiological findings. There are no valid clinical criteria for the diagnosis of T4 syndrome. Investigations—both pathological and radiographic—do not aid in the diagnosis but can be used for ruling out other pathologies. Electrodiagnostic tests are found to be negative. Upper limb neural tissue tension test (ULTT) may be positive **(Table 18.1)** but do not correlate with the involved hypomobile segment. Differential diagnoses should include cardiac problems, thoracic outlet syndrome, lower cervical roots involvement, and carpal tunnel syndrome.

Physiotherapy Management

Techniques to deal with T4 syndrome are:
- **Mobilization and manipulation of thoracic spine**: Central posteroanterior glide and Transverse glide at respective spinous processes, lateral posteroanterior glide at respective facet joints are found to be beneficial. Detailed techniques of mobilization and manipulation are beyond the scope of this chapter.
- **Stretching and strengthening exercises:** Stretching of pectorals as mentioned in **Table 18.2**, stretching of scalene, scapular isometrics as mentioned in **Table 18.3** and thoracic muscle strengthening exercises.
- **Myofascial techniques** can be used to relieve trigger points and improve fascial mobility. They also help in improving physical function and postural stability.
- **Postural correction exercises:** Scapular retraction, chin tucks, and thoracic extension exercises.

There is a lack of high-quality evidence for diagnosis and treatment of T4 syndrome; it can be used as diagnosis of exclusion.

> **BOX 18.4:** Clinical features of T4 syndrome.
>
> Evans gave a symptom complex of a typical patient with T4 syndrome.
> - **Age:** Usually above 35 years
> - **Posture:** Forward head posture with increased angulation or kyphosis at the cervicothoracic junction, reduced kyphosis at the thoracic spine
> - **Occupation:** Requiring frequent and prolonged bending or stooping, e.g. surgeons, electricians, and hand-work skilled workers
> - **Onset:** Usually associated with a change in working habits, e.g. job change and taking up new recreational activity
> - **Symptoms frequently present (may be unilateral or bilateral):**
>   - Glove type of paresthesia covering all the digits, hand or forearm
>   - Hot or cold hands
>   - Heaviness in the arm
>   - Feeling of or actual swelling in the hand
>   - Nondermatomal aching or pain in the arm and/or forearm
>   - Crushing or bursting type of pain
> - **Symptoms occasionally present:**
>   - Pain and stiffness around the chest wall or in focal areas anteriorly or posteriorly
>   - Pain or stiffness in the interscapular area
>   - Nocturnal pain or night disturbances
>   - Sensation of water gushing or ants creeping in the affected area
>   - Tension tests may be positive with typical symptoms.
>   - Cervical spine symptoms may be present
> - **Objective signs:**
>   - Bluish discoloration of the hands along with warmth or cold
>   - Stooped posture
> - **Examination findings:**
>   - Symptoms not affected by active spinal movements
>   - Reduced joint play at thoracic segments (may elicit pain)
>   - Palpation of rib angles elicits symptoms
> - **Physiotherapy may include:**
>   - Mobilization of upper thoracic spine or lower cervical spine or rib angles
>   - Ultrasound application
>   - Exercises, correction of posture, self-mobilization of thoracic spine, ergonomic advices

Sacroiliac Joint Dysfunction

SI dysfunction is termed as altered movement and position of SI joint associated with or without pain. Pain may be localized to SI joint or referred to lumbar region, buttocks, lower limb, hip, or groin.

Common Presentations of Sacroiliac Joint Dysfunction

Rotational malalignment

Rotational malalignments are as follows:
- It is a fixation of ilium in excessive anterior or posterior rotation in relation to sacrum in sagittal plane.
- If it is in anterior direction, it is termed as anterior rotational malalignment, and if it is in posterior direction, it is termed as posterior rotational malalignment.

- Causes can be fall or combination of bending, lifting, and twisting incident. Females are more prone to develop this pathology during pregnancy due to anatomical and physiological changes occurring in the body. Asymmetrical forces exerted by spine (scoliosis), pelvis (tension in pelvic floor muscles) and lower extremity (true/apparent limb length discrepancy, Trendelenburg gait, change in weight bearing due to painful areas in lower limbs) can be the reason for the malalignment.
- Spasm in iliacus, gluteus maximus, and piriformis muscles can be present in patients with rotational malalignment.

Upslip and downslip

Upslip and downslip and their causes:
- Upward fixation of ilium in relation to sacrum results in upslip, whereas downward fixation of ilium in relation to sacrum results in downslip in frontal plane.
- Causes for upslip may be traumatic upward force or injury to muscle that pulls ilium upward.
- Typical findings of upslip include upward position of anterior superior iliac spine (ASIS), iliac crest and posterior superior iliac spine (PSIS) in relation to sacrum and opposite ilium, leg will be shorter equally in sitting–lying test.
- Causes for downslip include history of excessive traction through lower limbs.

Outflare and inflare

Outflare and inflare and their association:
- Movement of ilium outward in relation to sacrum is outflare and movement of ilium inward in relation to sacrum relates to inflare in transverse plane.
- Outflare is associated with posterior rotational malalignment, while other causes are tight posterior SI joint ligaments, tight adductors, and gracilis muscles. On palpation, ASIS will be away from umbilicus and PSIS near gluteal cleft.
- Inflare is often associated with anterior rotational malalignment. Other causes include tight anterior SI joint ligaments, strong contraction of transverses abdominis, tight abductors, and piriformis muscles. On palpation, ASIS will be near umbilicus and PSIS away from gluteal cleft.

Evaluation

Evaluation of a patient with SI dysfunction consists of a detailed history and examination procedure. Type of pain may range from dull aching to sharp stabbing. Pain is aggravated with changes in positions such as supine to side lying, supine to sitting, sit to stand, walking, one leg standing, climbing, or bending forward.

Observation

Postural alignment of spine, pelvis, and lower extremity should be observed. Abnormal alignment of lower extremity may also predispose to SI joint pain such as excessive foot pronation which can lead to genu valgum and internal rotation at hip which in turn alters the position of SI joint. Determine limb length discrepancy.

Palpation

Palpation of bony landmarks in static posture and during movements may help therapist to find any motion restrictions or deviations of spine. Palpation of muscles may help identify spasm and tenderness.

Examination

In the following ways, the patient can be examined:

- *Range of movement:* Assess for hip and lumbar ROM (as previously mentioned under the heading "Lumbar Spine").
- Asymmetric lumbar-pelvic rhythm may be present. Symmetric lumbar pelvic rhythm is combined movement of lumbar spine and pelvis during maximum forward flexion of trunk as if bending forward to touch the floor in standing position. Initial movement is lumbar flexion followed by anterior pelvic tilt while bending forward, whereas return to upright position is initiated with posterior pelvic tilt followed by lumbar extension.
- Tightness should be assessed in quadriceps, hamstrings, iliopsoas (as mentioned under the heading "Lumbar Spine"), hip abductors, hip adductors, and piriformis **(Table 18.11)**.
- Muscle strength of hip and lumbar muscles (as mentioned under the heading "Lumbar Spine") should be assessed.
- Special tests for diagnosis SI dysfunction include **(Table 18.12)**:
  - Flexion, abduction, and external rotation (FABER) test
  - Gaenslen's test
  - Pelvic compression test
  - Sitting–lying test

Differential diagnosis for SI dysfunction includes:

- Piriformis syndrome
- Hip pathology
- Lumbar disk pathology
- Facet joint pain
- Rheumatoid arthritis (RA)
- Ankylosing spondylitis (AS)
- Myofascial pain
- Trochanteric bursitis
- Visceral referred pain
- Malignancy

Physiotherapy Management

- Patient education regarding proper ergonomics in activities of daily living and work environment.
- Modalities such as:
  - Ultrasound with or without phonophoresis
  - Short wave diathermy
  - Moist heat
  - Cryotherapy
  - Transcutaneous electrical nerve stimulation is found to be beneficial in addition to therapeutic exercises.

  Pulsed ultrasound with mark space ratio 1:4, frequency of 1 MHz, and output of 1 W/cm^2 for 5 minutes is found to be beneficial in reducing pain and improving function.
- Activity modification by rest and avoiding movements that cause aggravation in pain.
- SI joint belts provide stabilization and proprioceptive feedback. Patients are advised to use belts specifically during standing and walking activities.
- Pregnant patients have hypermobile and lax SI joints; thus stretching and mobilization techniques should be avoided.
- SI joint and lumbar manipulations are found to be helpful in decreasing pain and functional disability. Mobilization with movement along with taping is found to be beneficial in reducing pain and improving function. Detailed techniques of mobilization and manipulation are beyond the scope of this chapter.
- Stretching exercises for iliopsoas, rectus femoris, hamstrings (as mentioned in **Table 18.8** under the heading "Lumbar Spine").
- Strengthening exercises for gluteus medius and gluteus maximus.
- Core stability exercises of lumbar spine (as mentioned under the heading "Lumbar Spine").

Table 18.11: Tests for tightness in various muscles of hip.

Test	Position	Procedure	Interpretation
Abduction contracture test	Supine with both ASIS in level	Perform hip adduction. Normal hip adduction is 30° before ASIS moves	If ASIS moves before 30° of hip adduction and muscle stretch is felt then test is positive for hip abductors tightness
Adduction contracture test	Supine with both ASIS in level	Perform hip abduction. Normal hip abduction is 30–50° before ASIS moves	If ASIS moves before 30–50° of hip abduction and muscle stretch is felt then test is positive for hip adductors tightness
Piriformis	Side lying with tested leg up with hip 60° flexion and knee flexion	Therapist stabilizes hip with one hand and presses downward from the knee	If pain is present in piriformis muscle then test is positive for tightness

(ASIS: anterior superior iliac spine)

Table 18.12: Special tests for sacroiliac (SI) joint.

Test	Position	Procedure	Interpretation
FABER test **(Fig. 18.23A)**	Supine lying with foot of tested leg on knee of unaffected leg	Therapist slowly lowers knee of test leg toward the plinth	Positive test—test leg's knee remains above opposite straight leg along with pain on SI joint of tested side
Gaenslen's test **(Fig. 18.23B)**	Side lying with tested side up. Lower leg is flexed against the chest	Therapist stabilizes the pelvis while extending the hip of uppermost leg	Pain over SI joint of uppermost side indicates positive test
Pelvic compression test **(Fig. 18.23C)**	Side lying	Therapist places hands over upper iliac crest and applies vertically downward force toward plinth compressing pelvis	Pain over SI joint indicates positive test
Sitting–lying test **(Figs. 18.24A and B)**	Supine lying	Note for the level of medial malleoli and then ask patient to sit up in long sitting and note for level of medial malleoli	If one malleolus moves up proximally than the other one, it suggests function leg length discrepancy due to SI dysfunction

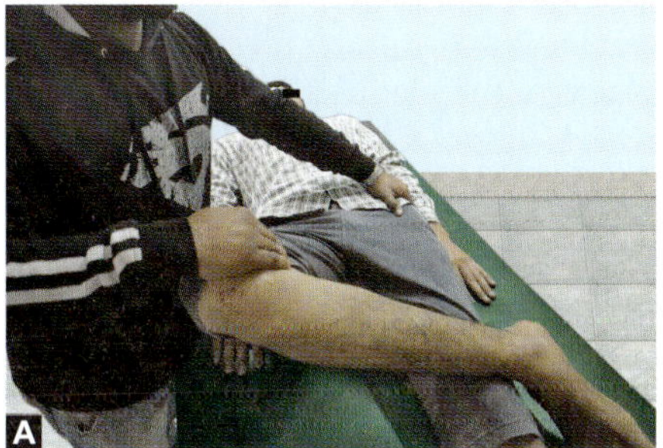
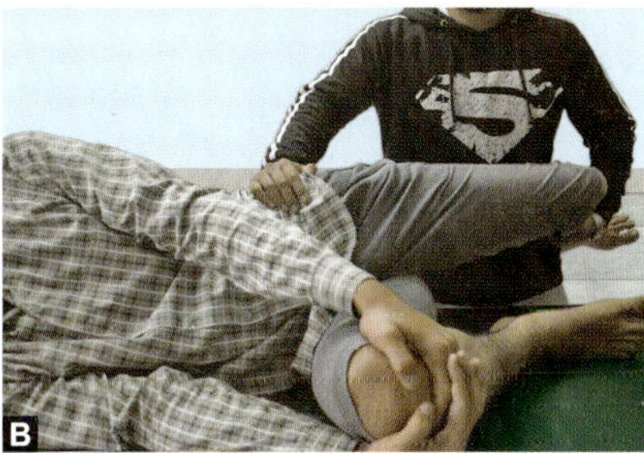
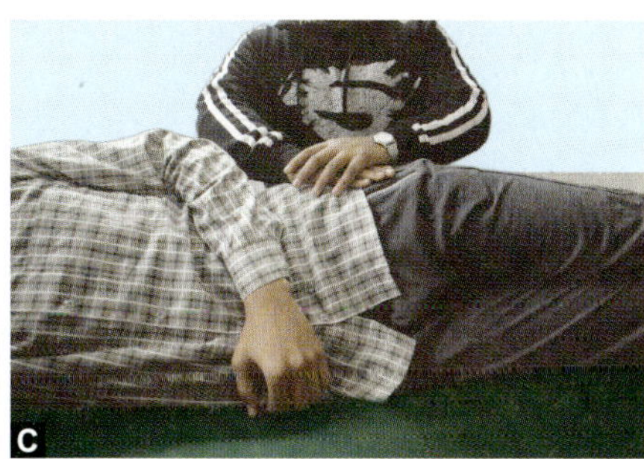

Figs. 18.23A to C: (A) FABER test, (B) Gaenslen's test; and (C) Pelvic compression test.

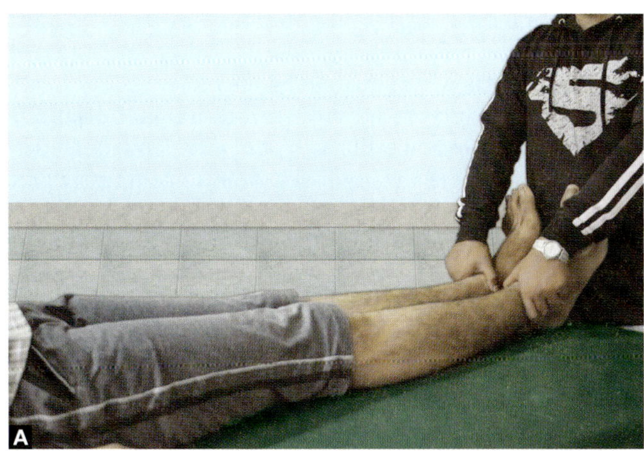
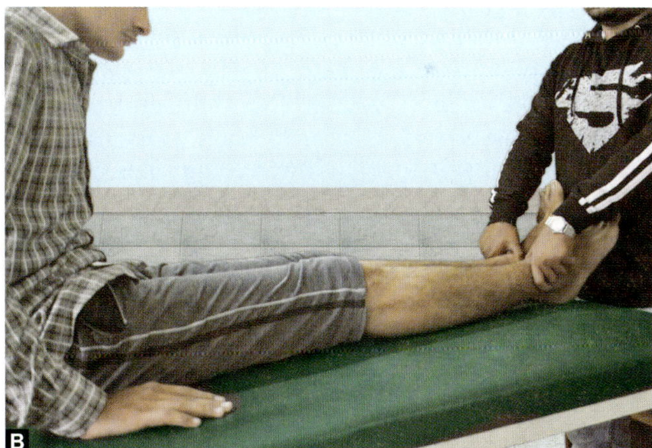

Figs. 18.24A and B: Sitting–lying test: (A) Supine lying; and (B) Long sitting.

- Orthotics and shoe modifications can be used to correct lower limb deformities and limb length discrepancy.

Ankylosing Spondylitis

Ankylosing spondylitis (AS) is a chronic inflammatory disease affecting SI joints and spine. It is a type of seronegative spondyloarthropathy having HLA B27 (Genetic marker) positive. Pathognomonic feature of AS is bilateral SI pain. Patient has insidious onset of pain and tenderness over SI joint, morning stiffness in spine, fatigue, and decreased chest expansion. Primary pathology includes enthesitis (inflammation occurring at site of muscle insertion). Other extraskeletal manifestations include weight loss, acute iritis, apical pulmonary fibrosis, conduction defects due to aortitis, and C1–C2 subluxation. X-ray findings reveal symmetric SI joint narrowing, bamboo spine (fusion of vertebrae leading to obliteration of spinal curves), syndesmophyte formation (bridging osteophytes) and squaring of vertebrae.

AS should be differentiated from RA, which is also an inflammatory disease affecting synovial joints. In RA, there is simultaneous symmetrical involvement three or smaller distal small joints initially along with subcutaneous nodules. Later joints get deformed leading to swan neck deformity, boutonniere deformity, and mallet finger. It even affects spinal column in the later stage of the disease.

Evaluation

Evaluation of a patient with AS symptoms consists of a detailed history and examination procedure. Bath Ankylosing Spondylitis Disease Activity Index (BASDAI) is a valid and reliable tool to assess levels of back pain, fatigue, peripheral joint pain and swelling, localized tenderness and duration, and severity of morning stiffness in patient with AS.

Observation

Postural alignment should be observed along with observation of anatomical movements of spine including cervical and thoracolumbar movements. Movements should be observed to find any restriction/deviation from normal and patient's willingness to do the movement.

Palpation

Palpation of bony landmarks as mentioned earlier in the chapter in static posture and during movements may help therapist to find any motion restrictions or deviations of spine. Palpation of muscles may help identify spasm and tenderness.

Examination

In the following ways, the problem can be examined:

- *Range of motion:* Active and passive movements of spine should be assessed. End feel is felt at the end of passive movement. Bath Ankylosing Spondylitis Metrology Index (BASMI) is a valid and reliable measure to assess cervical rotation, tragus to wall distance, lumbar flexion, lumbar side flexion, and intermalleolar distance. Modified Schober's test is helpful to assess lumbar flexion and extension as described earlier in the chapter.
- *Accessory movements (intersegmental mobility testing):* Pain response and segmental mobility are assessed through accessory movements including joint play at all vertebral levels. Intersegmental mobility testing reveals characteristic restriction.
- Strength and endurance of spinal muscles should be assessed as mentioned earlier in the chapter.
- Tightness of muscles such as pectorals, scalene, upper trapezius, iliopsoas, hamstrings, and rectus femoris should be assessed.
- Balance assessment and cardiorespiratory function should be checked (including chest expansion, 6-minute walk test).
- *Functional assessment:* Bath Ankylosing Spondylitis Functional Index (BASFI) is a reliable and measure for assessing physical functions such as bending, reaching, changing positions, standing, turning and climbing stairs using visual analog scale. Bath Ankylosing Spondylitis Global Score (BAS-G) is an indicator of patient's well-being over the last week and last 6 months.

Sufficient monitoring and evaluation at regular intervals are important in patient with AS to modify exercises according to the need, build up patient confidence, and competence to the exercise.

Physiotherapy Management

Physiotherapy management is mainly emphasized on **mobility exercises** of spine and peripheral joints. Goals for mobility exercises vary in early stage to later stage of disease. In the early stage, the goal is to restore full ROM and normal posture, whereas in the later stage, it is the maintenance of the existing ROM. Exercise intensity, frequency, duration, and type of exercise are customized to individual need of the patient. Exercises can be modified according to pain, fatigue, cardiorespiratory involvement, ankylosis, osteoporosis, and impairment in balance. Progression in exercises can be made according to patient response to exercise.

- In early stages, sleeping in prone position and using towel roll behind lumbar spine in sitting helps to maintain lumbar lordosis. Joint mobilizations (grade I and II) to uninvolved segments for decreasing pain.
- Core stability and scapular stabilization exercises as mentioned earlier in the chapter.
- Stretching and strengthening exercises for the involved segments.
- Balance exercise, cardiopulmonary fitness (including incentive spirometry, chest mobility, and aerobic exercises), and fatigue management.
- Regular physical activity should be encouraged to promote physical well-being and functional outcomes. No one activity is better than other so general physical activity should be advised.
- Group therapy and regular follow-up assessment help patient to adhere to exercise programs.

Scoliosis

Scoliosis and its classification and causes:

- Scoliosis is termed as lateral curvature of spine with rotatory component. Rotation of vertebrae is on the convex side of spine.
- It can be classified into structural and nonstructural (functional) scoliosis.
- Structural scoliosis is an irreversible lateral curvature with fixed rotation of vertebrae. Posterior rib hump is visible in thoracic spine on forward bending.
- Causes for structural scoliosis encompass neuromuscular diseases, rickets, hemivertebrae, osteomalacia, and lastly it can be idiopathic.
- Idiopathic scoliosis has been defined as a torsional deformity of the spine, with several torsional regions joined by a junctional zone, every region including a variable number of morphologically lordotic vertebrae translated and rotated to the same side.

Table 18.13: Classifications of idiopathic scoliosis.		
Chronological (years)	*Angular (degrees)*	*Topographical*
• Infantile (0–2) • Juvenile (3–9) • Adolescent (10–17) • Adult (18+)	• Low (up to 20) • Moderate (21–35) • Moderate to severe (36–40) • Severe (41–50) • Severe to very severe (51–55) • Very severe (56+)	• Cervical (up to C6, C7) • Cervicothoracic (C7–T1) • Thoracic (T1–T12) • Thoracolumbar (T12–L1) • Lumbar (L1 to down)

- Functional scoliosis is reversible and changes with forward bending, realigning pelvis, and correcting limb length discrepancy. Functional scoliosis can be due to limb length discrepancy, muscular spasm following pain, and habitual postures.
- Idiopathic scoliosis commonly appears during the phase of growth spurts and progresses during these phases. Progression of idiopathic scoliosis ends once puberty is achieved or spinal osseous growth ends. Screening of idiopathic scoliosis is important at school for early detection of deformity and commencing early treatment.

Classifications of Idiopathic Scoliosis by International Scientific Society on Scoliosis Orthopaedic and Rehabilitation Treatment

Based on the report by the International Scientific Society on Scoliosis Orthopaedic and Rehabilitation Treatment, idiopathic scoliosis can be classified as follows **(Table 18.13)**:

- Chronological—based on the age of the child at which deformity was diagnosed.
- Angular—based on Cobb's angle. Cobb's angle is measured on standing anterior–posterior X-ray of spine. It is the angle between intersecting lines drawn perpendicular to the top of the first tilted vertebrae and the bottom of the last tilted vertebrae of the curve.
- Topographic—based on anatomical site of spinal deformity in frontal plane **(Table 18.13)**.
- Rigo—based on specific principles of correction required by brace design and fabrication.

Evaluation

Evaluation of a patient with scoliosis symptoms consists of a detailed history and examination procedure. It is mandatory to collect family and personal clinical history and perform medical and neurological evaluation.

Observation

Postural alignment should be observed. Any deviation from normal should be observed. Ask patient to perform Adam forward bending test. Esthetics is a major concern for patient. It can be evaluated using many scales such as:

- Trunk Esthetic Clinical Evaluation
- Posterior Trunk Symmetry Index
- Anterior Trunk Symmetry Index
- Photographic evaluations

Palpation

Palpation of bony landmarks as mentioned earlier in the chapter in static posture and during movements may help therapist to find any deviations of spine. Palpation of muscles may help identify spasm and tenderness.

Examination

In the following ways, the problem can be examined:

- *Range of motion:* Active and passive movements of spine should be assessed. Scoliometer to measure rib hump appears on forward bending. It is a measure angle of trunk rotation. A novel tool scoligauge app (smartphone aided measurement) is also helpful in measurement of angle of trunk rotation.
- *Accessory movements (intersegmental mobility testing):* Pain response and segmental mobility are assessed through accessory movements including joint play at all vertebral levels. Intersegmental mobility testing reveals characteristic joint laxity/hypermobility.
- Strength and endurance of spinal muscles should be assessed as mentioned earlier in the chapter.
- Tightness of muscles such as pectorals, scalene, upper trapezius, iliopsoas, hamstrings, and rectus femoris should be assessed.
- Cardiorespiratory function should be checked including chest expansion.
- *Functional assessment:* SRS-7 (Scoliosis Research Society-7) is a seven-item questionnaire to measure functional outcome in patients.

Physiotherapy Management

Goals of management for idiopathic scoliosis include:
- Improving esthetics
- Improving the quality of life
- Decreasing disability and back pain
- Promoting psychological well being
- Limiting progression in adulthood
- Improving breathing function
  Bracing is recommended to treat idiopathic scoliosis. It is used in patients with Cobb's angle above 20±5°. Brace should be designed according to the curve of the deformity taking consideration to correct deformity in all planes. It should not restrict breathing pattern. It is worn full time and not less than 18 hours a day at the beginning of the treatment. Wearing a brace is proportionate to severity of deformity, age of patient, and goals of treatment. Wearing time for brace is gradually decreased with end of vertebral bone growth and while performing stabilization exercises. Brace should be changed according to the growth/development of the curve.

Table 18.14: Examples of stretching exercises for correcting right thoracic scoliosis.

Position of patient	Position of therapist	Stabilization	Procedure
Prone with left upper limb in flexion and right upper limb besides the trunk **(Fig. 18.25)**	Walk standing on the side of the patient	Over the pelvis	Ask the patient to touch right knee with right hand and hold the position
Kneel sitting with abdomen resting on thighs and arms flexed bilaterally with hands resting on plinth **(Figs. 18.26A and B)**	Walk standing on the side of the patient	Over the pelvis	Ask the patient to walk the hands on the right side and hold the position
Quadruped position **(Figs. 18.27A and B)**	Walk standing on the side of the patient	Over the pelvis	Ask the patient to walk the hands on the right side and hold the position
Right side lying with towel roll at apex of the curve (on the plinth or at the edge of the plinth)	Walk standing on the side of the patient	Over the pelvis	Ask the patient to take top upper limb into full abduction and hold the position

Physiotherapeutic scoliosis specific exercises (PSSE): PSSE consists of autocorrection in 3D, training in activities of daily living, stabilizing corrected posture and patient education. They are used to prevent or limit progression of deformity in idiopathic scoliosis. These exercises are customized according to the curve pattern, patient's need and treatment phase. Various approaches are given by different schools of scoliosis as follows:

- The Lyon approach: It combines PSSE with bracing. The goals motivate patient with bracing, patient education (awareness of postural defects), increase ROM, neuromuscular control of the spine, respiration, and ergonomics. This protocol considers patient's age, postural imbalance, and Cobb's angle. Awareness of deformity is implied with visual biofeedback from mirrors and videotape recording. It enhances thoracic kyphosis with lumbar lordosis and side bending correction, core stability, breathing exercises, proprioception, and balance exercises. It avoids spinal extension exercises and exercises that cause shortness of breath.

- The Schroth method: The goals are spinal corrections, postural training, teach home-exercise program, support help for self-help, and pain prevention and coping strategies.
  - *The Schroth "50×Pezziball" exercise:* Patient sits on a Swiss-ball in front of a mirror and performs active auto self-correction using the wall bar.
  - *The Schroth prone exercise:* Corrects lumbar curve with the activation of the iliopsoas muscle (right hip flexion) and corrects the thoracic curve using shoulder traction and shoulder counter.
  - *The Schroth "Sail" exercise:* Patient stands with two poles and performs active stabilization. It is a type of stretching exercises.
  - *The side-lying exercise:* It corrects lumbar scoliosis. Patient lies on the convex side with roll below the curve to align the spine horizontally. Patient upper limb is supported on chair and leg on low stool. The method also includes rotational breathing exercise, mobilization, and flexibility in the spine and between ribs. Activation of iliopsoas, the quadratus lumborum, and erector spinae muscles help to correct curve.

- Scientific exercise approach to scoliosis (SEAS): It focuses on regaining postural control and improving spinal stability through exercises. Self-correction can be achieved through patient education and awareness of the deformity. Various spinal stability exercises can be used and incorporated in activities of daily living. It believes in a team approach involving patient's family.
  - SEAS exercises in brace includes prone lying and lift thorax away from sternal part of brace, standing and pulling abdomen inward away from brace.
  - Breathing exercises and stretching exercises **(Table 18.14)** are also integral part of the method.
  - Endurance and strengthening exercises of abdominals, trunk extensors, lower limb, and scapula-humeral muscles are focused.

- Barcelona Scoliosis Physical Therapy School: Based on the principles of Schroth method to improve scoliosis by muscle activation and rotational angular breathing. It includes exercises in supine, side lying, prone, and muscle cylinder exercises.

- Dobomed: Emphasize thoracic kyphosis and lumbar lordosis with correction of curve in frontal plane in closed kinetic chain. It includes exercises in cat and camel exercises in quadruped position with stabilization of pelvis and shoulder girdle.

- Side shift: Based on the theory that repetitive side bending movement of spine will correct the deformity

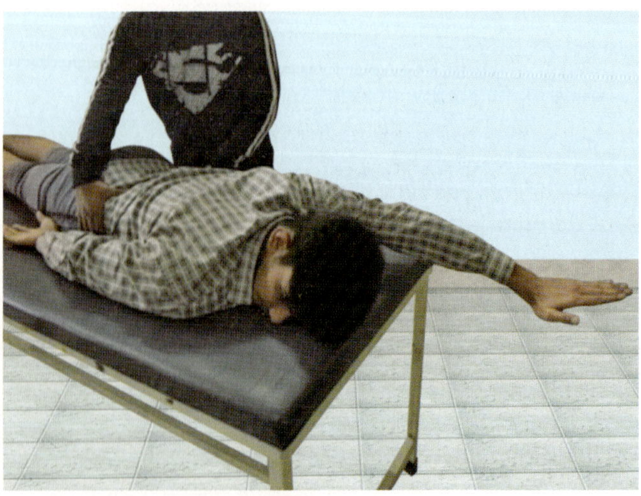

Fig. 18.25: Stretching exercises for scoliosis in prone lying.

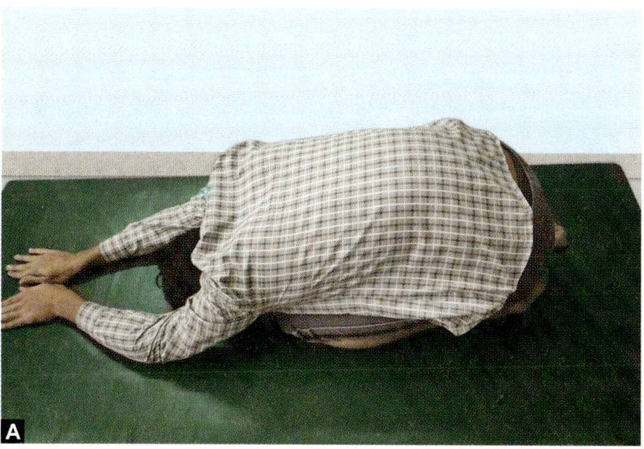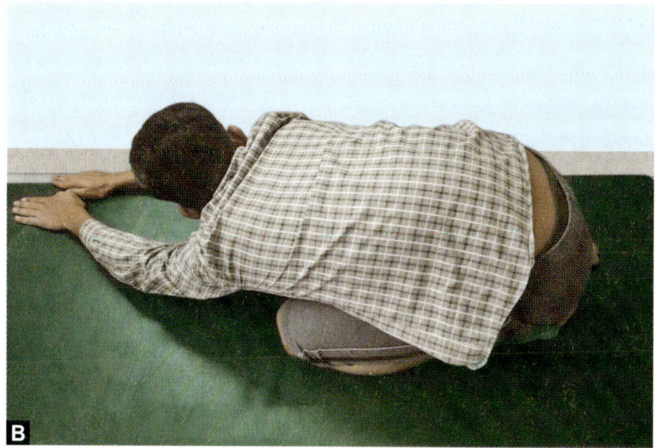

Figs. 18.26A and B: Stretching exercises for scoliosis in kneel sitting: (A) Starting position and (B) End position.

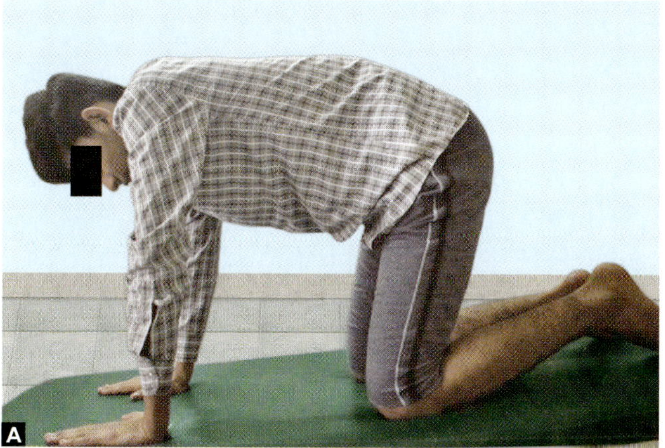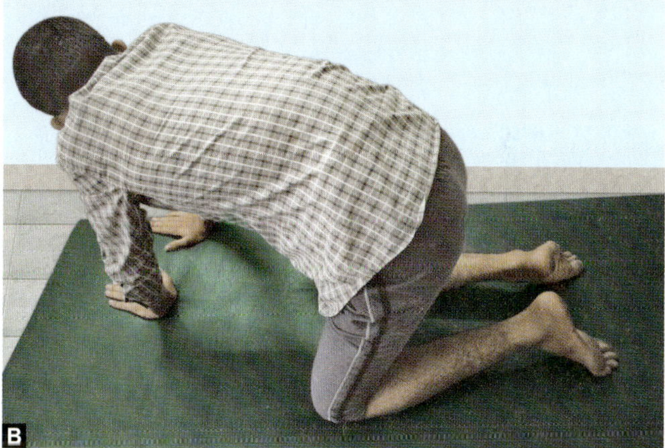

Figs. 18.27A and B: Stretching exercises for scoliosis in quadruped: (A) Starting position and (B) End position.

in frontal plane. It includes hitching exercise in standing where heel on the side of convexity is lifted with hip and knees straight. Hitch shift exercises for double scoliosis (e.g., left lumbar and right thoracic scoliosis) include standing where heel on the side of convexity in lumbar is lifted with hip and knees straight and the stabilize lumbar region with one hand and shift trunk on concavity side of thoracic region. Bird-dog and plank exercises are performed maintaining the side shift position. Side-shifting exercises incorporated with balance exercises in standing are also included.

- Functional individual therapy for scoliosis: Variety of physiotherapy exercises interventions are selected for correction of deformity. Main goals are:
  - Awareness of existing deformity of spine and direction of scoliosis
  - Sensory-motor balance training
  - Myofascial release
  - Lumbo-pelvic stabilization
  - Correction of shift
  - Facilitation of corrective breathing in functional positions and while wearing brace
  - Postural re-education
  - Autocorrection in activities of daily living
  - Decrease or stabilization of the scoliosis curvatures.

For double curves, stabilization is provided on one curve and then the exercises are performed. For double curves, exercise in high sitting position with resisted hip flexion and reaching diagonally with upper limb may be helpful. For example, if patient has left thoracic and right lumbar scoliosis, resisted left hip flexion and right upper limb should be diagonally raised overhead.

Gentle mobilizations, soft tissue release techniques, respiratory exercises, and correction of limb length discrepancy are being traditionally used for treatment of idiopathic scoliosis, but there is a lack of high-quality research evidence supporting them.

SUMMARY

The chapter on spinal disorders comprises various conditions that affect spinal column, its evaluation based on physiotherapy, and respective physiotherapy treatment. It includes ICF-based classification for neck pain and LBP along with its detailed clinical presentations. The chapter discusses about signs and symptoms, evaluation and physiotherapy management for T4 syndrome, SI dysfunction, AS, and scoliosis in detail. Proper physical evaluation of condition is of paramount importance for effective physiotherapy treatment.

Case Scenario

CASE STUDY 1

Cervical Neck Pain with Radiating Pain

Suratben is a 52-year-old housewife with a complaint of gradual onset of neck pain, heaviness in left upper limb and tingling over index, and middle and ring finger of left hand. X-ray shows degenerative changes in cervical spine.

On observation patient has forward head posture.

Grade 1 tenderness is palpated over nape of neck and spasm over bilateral upper trapezius.

Cervical ranges of movements are full but painful. On examination, weakness of rhomboids and deep cervical flexors is present. Hypoesthesia is found over index, middle, and ring finger of the left hand. Grip assessment reveals weakness in grip on the left side.

Compression, distraction, Upper limb tension tests 1 and 2, and Phalen's and reverse Phalen's test are found to be positive.

Neck disability index reveals moderate disability (22/44).

Clinical diagnosis is cervical spondylosis with Carpal tunnel syndrome.

Guiding Questions:

1. Discuss the possible impairments, activity limitations, and participation restrictions for the above case.
2. How would you differentiate this condition from other conditions according to treatment-based classification of neck pain?
3. Plan the short-term goals for management for the abovementioned patient.
4. Explain the procedure to assess strength of neck and scapular muscles.

CASE STUDY 2

Neck Pain with Cervicogenic Headache

Mr. Shah is a 35-year-old computer operator.

He has a gradual onset of pain over left side of nape of neck and occipital region.

Pain aggravated by prolonged work on computer.

On observation, he has forward head posture and increased kyphosis.

Grade 2 tenderness is present below nuchal line. Craniocervical flexion test is found to be positive. Hypomobility is present in upper cervical region.

Clinical diagnosis is mechanical neck pain with cervicogenic headache.

Guiding Questions:

1. Describe how do you differentiate between upper and lower cervical spine involvement.
2. Describe craniocervical flexion test.
3. Explain accessory movements at cervical spine.
4. Plan a physiotherapy management for the above case.

CASE STUDY 3

Acute Low Back Pain with Referred Lower Extremity Pain

Ritesh Bhai is a 40-year-old salesman with a complaint of sudden onset of LBP with associated right lower extremity pain. Pain aggravates with prolonged sitting, bending down forward, and while activities of sneezing or coughing.

On observation, lateral trunk shift and decreased lumbar lordosis are visible.

On examination, centralization is found with repeated extension movements and peripheralization with flexion movements. Strength and endurance deficits are present in muscles of lumbar region. Tightness in bilateral hamstrings and calf is present. Right side SLR (basic) test exacerbates the symptoms at 40°.

Oswestry disability score is 50/100.

Clinical diagnosis is posterolateral disc prolapse in lumbar region.

Guiding Questions:

1. Explain centralization and peripheralization.
2. Explain SLR test and its modifications.
3. How would you differentiate this condition from other conditions according to the classification of low back pain based on ICF?
4. Discuss possible impairments, activity limitations, and participation restrictions for the above case.

CASE STUDY 4

Chronic Low Back Pain with Generalized Pain

Mrs Desai is a 45-year-old housewife complaining of LBP since last 1 year.

She shows positive responses for depressive symptoms. She depicted high scores on Fear Avoidance Belief Questionnaire and Pain Catastrophizing Scale.

She has a generalized pain over back that is not specific to any vertebral segment. Provocation tests do not reproduce symptoms. No restriction in spinal ROM or segmental hypomobility is found.

Clinical diagnosis is LBP with generalized pain.

Guiding Questions:

1. How would you differentiate this condition from other conditions according to the classification of low back pain based on ICF?
2. Plan management for relieving pain in the above case.
3. Describe the scales of mental impairment measure.

CASE STUDY 5

Ankylosing Spondylitis

Mr Patel is a 55-year-old shopkeeper complaining of difficulty in sleeping in supine lying, difficulty in turning around at work and fatigue.

X-ray reveals squaring of cervical and lumbar vertebrae and syndesmophytes.

Past history of LBP since 9 years. Patient has a medical history of hypertension.

On observation, patient has forward head, kyphotic, and flat back posture. Gait shows decreased swing phase.

Pain is present over nape of neck, lumbar and SI joint, hip joints, and shoulder joints. Pain is aggravated in morning with stiffness.

ROM of cervical, thoracic, lumbar, hip, and shoulder are restricted. Muscle strength is good in available ROM. Tightness is present in pectoralis major (B/L), hamstrings (B/L), iliopsoas (B/L), and calf (B/L). On 6-minute walk test, patient covered less distance due to fatigue, short step length, and less endurance. Chest expansion is reduced.

Functional assessment shows severe disability.

Clinical diagnosis is AS.

Guiding Questions:

1. Discuss possible impairments, activity limitations, and participation restrictions for the above case.
2. How would you differentiate this condition from other conditions?
3. Plan physiotherapy management for the abovementioned patient.
4. Explain Bath Ankylosing Spondylitis Metrology Index (BASMI), Bath Ankylosing Spondylitis Functional Index (BASFI), and Bath Ankylosing Spondylitis Global Score (BAS-G).

Review Questions

1. Explain the classification model of neck pain based on treatment.
2. Write a short note on various abnormal postures of spine.
3. Depict surface landmarking for cervical spine.
4. Explain craniocervical flexion test and deep neck flexor endurance test.
5. Describe upper limb tension tests.
6. Demonstrate stretching exercises for pectorals, upper trapezius, and suboccipital muscles.
7. Demonstrate the core stability for cervical spine.
8. Demonstrate scapular isometrics and manual traction techniques for cervical spine.
9. Explain the classification model of low back pain based on ICF.
10. List down red flags for low back pain.
11. Depict surface landmarking for lumbar spine.
12. Explain the isometric and dynamic test of strength and endurance for muscles of lumbar spine.
13. Define centralization and peripheralization.
14. Describe tightness assessment of hamstrings, rectus femoris, and iliopsoas.
15. Explain the various therapeutic exercises for low back pain specific to spinal bias.
16. Demonstrate core stability exercises for lumbar spine.
17. Explain various traction techniques for lumbar spine.
18. Explain neural mobility for upper limb and lower limb.
19. Discuss T4 syndrome.
20. Explain common presentations of SI joint dysfunction.
21. Demonstrate tests to check tightness of hip muscles.
22. Demonstrate various special tests to rule out SI dysfunction.
23. Describe ankylosing spondylitis and its clinical presentations.
24. Discuss the evaluation of ankylosing spondylitis.
25. Discuss scoliosis and its classification.
26. Explain Adam's forward bending, Cobb's angle, and rib hump.
27. Demonstrate the various exercises for correcting scoliosis.
28. Explain physiotherapeutic-specific scoliosis exercises.

BIBLIOGRAPHY

1. Berdishevsky H, Lebel VA, Bettany-Saltikov J, et al. Physiotherapy scoliosis-specific exercises–a comprehensive review of seven major schools. Scoliosis Spinal Disord. 2016;11(1):20.
2. Blanpied PR, Gross AR, Elliott JM, et al. Neck pain: revision 2017: clinical practice guidelines linked to the international classification of functioning, disability and health from the orthopaedic section of the American Physical Therapy Association. J Orthop Sports Phys Ther. 2017;47(7):A1-83.
3. Brown K, Luszeck T, Nerdin S, et al. The effectiveness of cervical versus thoracic thrust manipulation for the improvement of pain, disability, and range of motion in patients with mechanical neck pain. Phys Ther Rev. 2014;19(6):381-91.
4. Childs MJ, Fritz JM, Piva SR, et al. Proposal of a classification system for patients with neck pain. J Orthop Sports Phys Ther. 2004;34(11):686-700.
5. Delitto A, Erhard RE, Bowling RW. A treatment-based classification approach to low back syndrome: identifying and staging patients for conservative treatment. Phys Ther. 1995;75(6):470-85.
6. Dellito A, George SZ, Whitman JM, et al. Low back pain clinical practice guidelines linked to the international classification of functioning, disability, and health from the orthopaedic section of the American physical therapy association. J Orthop Sports Phys Ther. 2012;42(2):A1-57.
7. Evans P. The T4 syndrome: some basic science aspects. Physiotherapy. 1997;83(4):186-9.
8. Fernandes S. Comparative effectiveness of mulligan mobilisation and mulligan taping technique in sacroiliac joint dysfunction-randomized clinical trial (doctoral dissertation); 2010.
9. Foley BS, Buschbacher RM. Sacroiliac joint pain: anatomy, biomechanics, diagnosis, and treatment. Am J Phys Med Rehabil. 2006;85(12):997-1006.
10. Graham N, Gross AR, Carlesso LC, et al. An ICON overview on physical modalities for neck pain and associated disorders. Open Orthop J. 2013;7(Suppl. 4):440.
11. Hall CM, Brody LT. Therapeutic exercise: moving toward function, 4th edition. Philadelphia: Lippincott Williams & Wilkins; 2018. p. 734.
12. Hall T, Chan HT, Christensen L, et al. Efficacy of a C1-C2 self-sustained natural apophyseal glide (SNAG) in the management of cervicogenic headache. J Orthop Sports Phys Ther. 2007;37(3):100-7.
13. Hamidi-Ravari B, Tafazoli S, Chen H, et al. Diagnosis and current treatments for sacroiliac joint dysfunction: a review. Curr Phys Med Rehabil Rep. 2014;2(1):48-54.
14. Hefford C. McKenzie classification of mechanical spinal pain: profile of syndromes and directions of preference. Man Ther. 2008;13(1):75-81.
15. Kamali F, Shokri E. The effect of two manipulative therapy techniques and their outcome in patients with sacroiliac joint syndrome. J Bodyw Mov Ther. 2012;16(1):29-35.
16. Karas S, Pannone A. T4 syndrome: a scoping review of the literature. J Manipulative Physiol Ther. 2017;40(2):118-25.
17. Kisner C, Colby A, Borstad J. Stretching for improved mobility. In: Therapeutic exercise; foundations and techniques, 7th edition. New Delhi, India: Jaypee Publishers; pp. 117-21.
18. Kisner C, Colby A, Borstad J. The shoulder and shoulder girdle. In: Therapeutic exercise; foundations and techniques, 7th edition. New Delhi, India: Jaypee Publishers; 2018. pp. 599-601.
19. Kisner C, Colby A, Borstad J. The spine: exercise and manipulation interventions. In: Therapeutic exercise; foundations and techniques, 7th edition. New Delhi, India: Jaypee Publishers; 2018. pp. 473, 499, 505, 516-25, 529, 531-5.
20. Koh HW, Cho SH, Kim CY. Comparison of the effects of hollowing and bracing exercises on cross-sectional areas of abdominal muscles in middle-aged women. J Phys Ther Sci. 2014;26(2):295-9.
21. Liu L, Huang QM, Liu QG, et al. Effectiveness of dry needling for myofascial trigger points associated with neck and shoulder pain: a systematic review and meta-analysis. Arch Phys Med Rehabil. 2015;96(5):944-55.
22. Magee D. Cervical spine. In: Orthopedic physical assessment, 6th edition. Amsterdam, Netherlands; Elsevier publication: 2014. p. 156.
23. Magee D. Orthopedic physical assessment, 6th edition. Amsterdam, Netherlands; Elsevier publication: 2014. pp. 578-81, 598-602, 670-1, 721-9, 180-87.
24. Millner JR, Barron JS, Beinke KM, et al. Exercise for ankylosing spondylitis: an evidence-based consensus statement. In: Seminars in arthritis and rheumatism, vol. 45, no. 4. WB Saunders; 2016. pp. 411-27.
25. Negrini S, Donzelli S, Aulisa AG, et al. 2016 SOSORT guidelines: orthopaedic and rehabilitation treatment of idiopathic scoliosis during growth. Scoliosis Spinal Disord. 2018;13(1):3.
26. O'Sullivan P. Diagnosis and classification of chronic low back pain disorders: maladaptive movement and motor control impairments as underlying mechanism. Man Ther. 2005;10(4):242-55.
27. Prather H. Sacroiliac joint pain: practical management. Clin J Sport Med. 2003;13(4):252-5.
28. Racicki S, Gerwin S, DiClaudio S, et al. Conservative physical therapy management for the treatment of cervicogenic headache: a systematic review. J Man Manip Ther. 2013;21(2):113-24.
29. Ribeiro DC, Belgrave A, Naden A, et al. The prevalence of myofascial trigger points in neck and shoulder-related disorders: a systematic review of the literature. BMC Musculoskelet Disord. 2018;19(1):252.
30. Ribeiro S, Heggannavar A, Metgud S. Effect of mulligans mobilization versus manipulation, along with mulligans taping in anterior innominate dysfunction—A randomized clinical trial. Indian J Phys Ther Res. 2019;1(1):17.
31. Sahrmann S, Azevedo DC, Van Dillen L. Diagnosis and treatment of movement system impairment syndromes. Braz J Phys Ther. 2017;21(6):391-9.
32. Sahrmann S. Diagnosis and treatment of movement impairment syndromes. Missori: Elsevier Health Sciences; 2001.
33. Schamberger W. Common presentations and diagnostic techniques. In: The malalignment syndrome. London: Churchill Livingstone: 2002. pp. 5-86.
34. Wang WT, Olson SL, Campbell AH, et al. Effectiveness of physical therapy for patients with neck pain: an individualized approach using a clinical decision-making algorithm. Am J Phys Med Rehabil. 2003;82(3):203-18.
35. Wolfe F, Clauw DJ, Fitzcharles MA, Goldenberg DL, Hauser W, Katz RL, et al. 2016 revisions to the 2010/2011 fibromyalgia diagnostic criteria. Seminars in Arthritis and Rheumatism 2016;46(3):319–29. [PUBMED: 27916278].
36. Zochling J. Measures of symptoms and disease status in ankylosing spondylitis: Ankylosing Spondylitis Disease Activity Score (ASDAS), Ankylosing Spondylitis Quality of Life Scale (ASQoL), Bath Ankylosing Spondylitis Disease Activity Index (BASDAI), Bath Ankylosing Spondylitis Functional Index (BASFI), Bath Ankylosing Spondylitis Global Score (BAS-G), Bath Ankylosing Spondylitis Metrology Index (BASMI), Dougados Functional Index (DFI), and Health Assessment Questionnaire for the Spondylarthropathies (HAQ-S). Arthritis Care Res. 2011;63(S11):S47-58.

Shoulder Conditions

Deepak B Anap

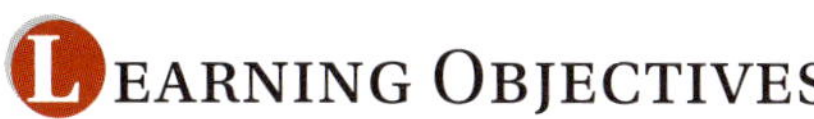 LEARNING OBJECTIVES

After reading this chapter, the readers should be able to:
- Describe the etiology, pathophysiology, and clinical presentation of various pathologies related to the shoulder joint
- Describe the evaluation process to be followed for shoulder joint assessment
- Describe the medical and surgical management for various pathologies related to the shoulder joint
- Describe the physical therapy management for various pathologies related to the shoulder joint
- Describe the various operative procedures performed on the shoulder joint and their postoperative physiotherapy management

CHAPTER OUTLINE

- Frozen shoulder
  - Related pathophysiology and etiology
  - Clinical signs and symptoms
  - Stages of frozen shoulder
  - Assessment
  - Management
- Rotator cuff pathology
  - Epidemiology
  - Etiology
  - Pathology
  - Supraspinatus tendinitis
  - Infraspinatus tendinitis
  - Physical examination
  - Diagnosis
  - Management
- Shoulder instability
  - Classification
  - Factors affecting instability
  - Assessment
  - Management
- Supraspinatus tendinopathy
  - Etiology
  - Pathomechanics
  - Clinical features
  - Investigations
  - Assessment
  - Management

- Subscapular tendinopathy
  - Causes
  - Clinical features
  - Investigations
  - Assessment
  - Management
- Bicipital tendinopathy
  - Causes
  - Biomechanical causes
  - Clinical features
  - Assessment
  - Investigations
  - Management
- Subacromial bursitis
  - Etiology
  - Pathology
  - Assessment
  - Management
- Osteoarthritis of the shoulder joint
  - Epidemiology
  - Risk factors
  - Pathophysiology
  - Clinical features
  - Examination
  - Management
- Acromioclavicular and sternoclavicular joints
  - Clinical features
  - Management

- Scapular dyskinesis
  - Clinical features
  - Assessment
  - Management
- Labral tear
  - Etiology
  - Clinical features
  - Diagnostic procedures
  - Special tests
  - Management
- Thoracic outlet syndrome
  - Etiology
  - Types
  - Clinical signs and symptoms
  - Investigations
  - Assessment
  - Management
- Shoulder rehabilitation
  - Electrotherapy modalities
  - Shoulder range of motion/mobility exercises
  - Active assisted range of motion exercises
  - Stretching exercises
  - Strengthening exercises
  - Proprioceptive exercises

INTRODUCTION

The shoulder complex is formed by the combination of three joints:

1. The glenohumeral (GH) joint formed by the humerus and glenoid cavity of scapula.
2. The acromioclavicular (AC) joint formed by the acromion process of the scapula and the sternum.
3. The sternoclavicular (SC) joint formed by the sternum and clavicle **(Fig. 19.1)**.

The scapulothoracic (ST) joint, though not being a true joint, allows a lot of movement of the scapula on the thoracic cavity, is also considered to be a part of the shoulder complex. The shoulder joint is a rather unstable and incongruent joint since it has to provide a lot of mobility and the need is more dynamic than static. The stability is provided by the muscular forces generated surrounding the joint or the so-called dynamic stabilization, which is mainly factored by the rotator cuff (RC). The contradictory and competing demands of mobility and stability that are placed on the shoulder girdle, make it greatly susceptible to dysfunction and disability.

This chapter discusses the common pathologies occurring at the shoulder complex and the strategies used to manage them. It should be mentioned however that each individual is different in their own way, and there can be no standardized approach to manage any specific condition. Hence, the competent professional should always note the impairments and limitations faced by the patient and treat accordingly.

FROZEN SHOULDER

Introduction

It is also called adhesive capsulitis. It is a painful condition in which the movements of shoulder become limited. Frozen shoulder **(Fig. 19.2)** is a specific condition that has a natural resolution and needs to be treated in a different manner than other pathologies.

The history of frozen shoulder dates back to 1872, when Duplay had named the same condition as periarthritis. Later in 1934, Codman named it as frozen shoulder, and in 1945, Naviesar coined the term "Adhesive Capsulitis" (even though there are no actual adhesions formed in the capsule).

Related Pathophysiology and Etiology

Frozen shoulder is commonly associated with the following conditions:

- Rheumatoid arthritis (RA) and osteoarthritis (OA)
- Traumatic arthritis
- Postimmobilization arthritis or stiff shoulder
- Diabetes
- Idiopathic frozen shoulder **(Box 19.1)**.

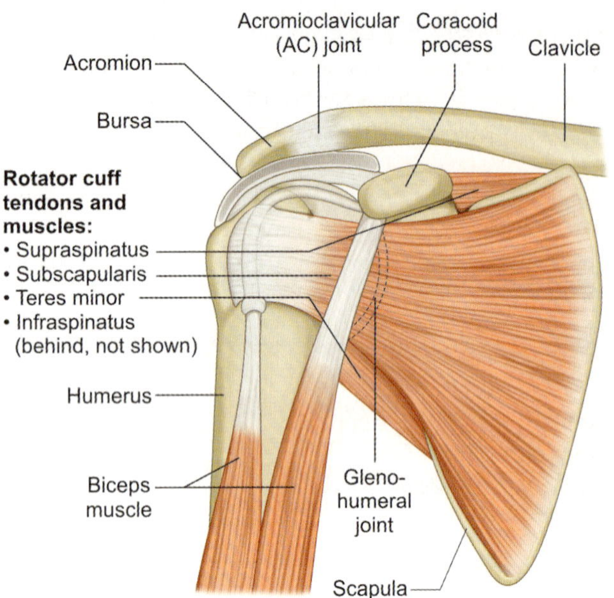

Fig. 19.1: The shoulder complex.

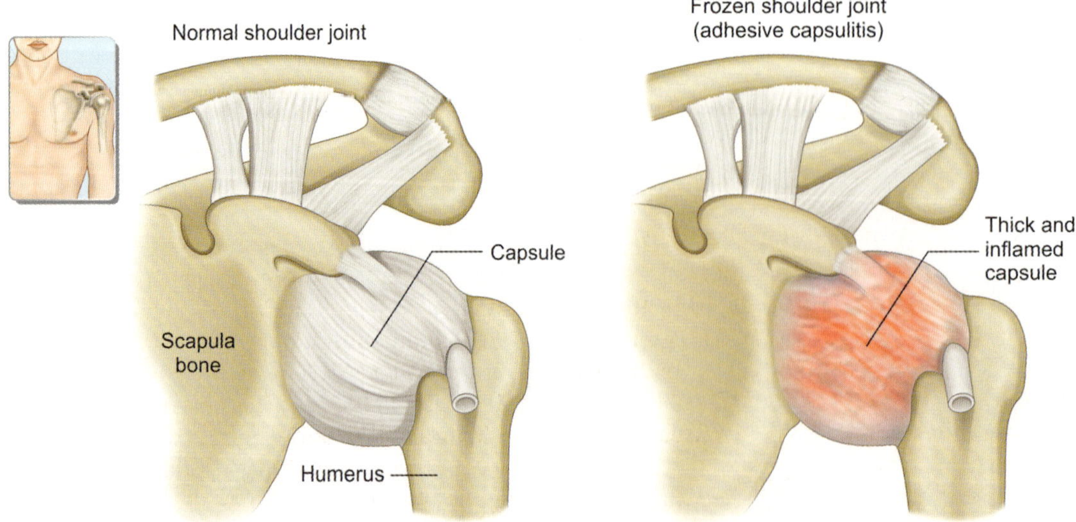

Fig. 19.2: Frozen shoulder.

> **BOX 19.1:** Classification of frozen shoulder.
>
> Frozen shoulder may be primary (idiopathic) or secondary. Secondary frozen shoulder is most commonly associated with diabetes mellitus. Other associated pathologies are Dupuytren's disease, hyperthyroidism, hypothyroidism, hypoadrenalism, stroke, cardiac disease, Parkinson's disease, etc.

> **BOX 19.2:** Hallmarks for the diagnosis of frozen shoulder.
>
> • Insidious shoulder stiffness
> • Severe pain, even at night
> • Loss of active and passive external rotation range of motion.

Clinical Signs and Symptoms

History

Details of the patients include:

- Age—40-60 years
- Women more affected than men
- Nondominant shoulder more affected than dominant **(Box 19.2)**.

There are three phases in adhesive capsulitis:

1. *Acute phase:*
   - Pain and muscle guarding limit the motion, usually external rotation and abduction.
   - Pain may radiate below elbow and disturb sleep.
   - Tenderness immediate below acromion process.
2. *Subacute phase:*
   - Capsular tightness
   - Motions affected in capsular patterns
3. *Chronic phase:*
   - Progressive restriction of GH joint capsule
   - Limited motion
   - Decreased joint play
   - Significant loss of function with inability to reach overhead, outward, or behind the back.
   - Aching is usually at the deltoid region.

Stages of Frozen Shoulder

The stages of frozen shoulder are discussed below:

Stage 1:

- Characterized by a gradual onset of pain that increases with movement and is present at night.
- Loss of external rotation motion with intact RC strength is common.
- The duration of this stage is usually less than 3 months.

Stage 2 (often referred to as the "freezing" stage):

- Characterized by persistent and more intense pain even at rest.
- Motion is limited in all directions and cannot be fully restored with an intra-articular injection.
- This stage is typically between 3 and 9 months.

Stage 3 ("frozen" stage):

- Characterized by pain only with movement, significant adhesions, and limited GH motions, with substitute motions in the scapula.
- Atrophy of the deltoid, RC, biceps, and triceps brachii muscles may be noted.
- This stage is between 9 and 15 months.

Stage 4 ("thawing" stage):

- Characterized by minimal pain and no synovitis but significant capsular restrictions from adhesions.
- Motion may gradually improve during this stage.
- This stage lasts from 15 to 24 months or longer.
- Some patients never regain normal range of motion (ROM).

Assessment

Observation

Following are the observations made:

- Posture: Soft tissue adaptation can occur with habitual poor posture (adduction and internal rotation with arm by the side); disuse atrophy may be seen.
- Muscle tightness as a result of overactivity, rather than adaptive shortening, can also result in perceived contracture.
- Commonly tightness or overactivity of pectoralis minor leads to protracted shoulder.

Examination

Examination includes:

- Tenderness on palpation
- Temperature changes
- Presence of edema or effusion
- Mobility and feel of superficial tissues and muscles
- Active range of motion (AROM)—range and quality of movement
  - Behavior of pain and resistance throughout the ROM
  - Provocation of any muscle spasm.
- Passive range of motion (PROM)—to check for available ROM
  - End feel
  - Capsular pattern
- Accessory joint movement
- Muscle testing

Management

Treatment in the initial phase is directed at pain relief. Pain-free activities should be allowed to maintain ROM. Nonsteroidal anti-inflammatory drugs (NSAIDs) or other forms of analgesics may be administered. Later, the goal is to increase the ROM and strength.

Manipulation under anesthesia or surgical release may be used for long-standing chronic stages not responding to conservative management.

ROTATOR CUFF PATHOLOGY

Introduction

The RC comprises the supraspinatus, infraspinatus, teres minor, and the subscapularis. The RC is responsible for the dynamic stability and the rotation of the humerus on the glenoid. The term RC pathology includes:

- Tear
- Inflammation
- Degeneration
- Tendonitis

  Rotator cuff tears (RCT) are usually associated with pain, weakness, and reduced ROM.

Epidemiology

Rotator cuff injuries (RCI) form almost 50% of the shoulder injuries. RCI are more prevalent beyond 40 years of age. The prevalence rate is 25% in those above 50 years of age. It occurs more often in athletes participating in sports involving repetitive overhead activities such as swimming, basketball, badminton, tennis, and volleyball. There is no gender predilection. Most of the RCT do not cause pain or the patients are not bothered by the pain.

Etiology

Following are the etiologies of RC pathology:

- Repetitive overhead activities
- Fall while catching or throwing objects
- Microtrauma caused due to impingement of the RC
- Degenerative changes

Pathology

Rotator cuff injury can extend from inflammation to full-thickness tears. Supraspinatus is the most commonly torn muscle. It undergoes atrophy, has reduced fatigue resistance (due to reduction in slow muscle fibers), reduction in vascularity, and fibrosis postinjury. Degenerative tears show an increased number of fibroblasts, neovascularity, and loss or reduction in the amount of collagen and fatty infiltration.

Tendinitis is commoner in supraspinatus and infraspinatus tendons. This occurs due to repetitive motions, restricted space to function (subacromial space restricted by coracoacromial arch) and poor vascularity of these tendons, leading to inability to heal following microtrauma. Calcium deposition occurs in chronic cases, complicating the healing further. Bursitis is also commonly associated with tears and tendinitis of the RC **(Box 19.3)**.

Supraspinatus Tendinitis

Following are the clinical signs of supraspinatus tendinitis:

- Inflammation in the supraspinatus tendon
- Tenderness present over the tendon (inferior to anterior aspect of acromion with hand behind the back).
- Painful arc with overhead activities
- Positive impingement clinical signs

Infraspinatus Tendinitis

Following are the clinical signs of infraspinatus tendinitis:

- Inflammation in the infraspinatus tendon
- Occurs as deceleration injury due to overload during repetitive or forceful throwing activities.
- Tenderness present over the tendon (inferior to posterior corner of acromion with horizontal adduction and external rotation of humerus).
- Painful arc with overhead, forward and cross-body activities.
- Positive impingement clinical signs

Physical Examination

Physical examination may reveal the following findings:

- Tenderness on palpation in the subacromial region.
- Atrophy of the RC muscles (seen over the infraspinatus fossa).
- In severe cases, scapula may be protracted and abducted.
- Altered scapulohumeral rhythm
- Positive painful arc (pain during 60–120° of active arm elevation)
- Positive impingement sign: Neer and Hawkins–Kennedy (pain during passive elevation of the arm); indicates subacromial impingement.
- Positive empty can test (inability to hold against resistance at 90° scaption and internal rotation of the shoulder)—indicates weakness of supraspinatus due to tear.
- Positive full can test (inability to hold against resistance at 90° scaption and external rotation of the shoulder)—indicates weakness of supraspinatus due to tear.
- Presence of dropping sign or external rotation lag sign (inability to hold arm in external rotation by the side and subsequent dropping of forearm to neutral position)—indicates infraspinatus tear.
- Positive liftoff sign (inability to raise the hand off the back when the hand is placed at the back)—indicates subscapularis tear **(Box 19.4)**.

BOX 19.3: Neer's classification of rotator cuff pathology.

- Stage I: Edema, hemorrhage (patient is usually under 25 years of age)
- Stage II: Tendonitis/bursitis and fibrosis (patient is usually 25–40 years of age)
- Stage III: Presence of bone spurs and tendon rupture (patient is usually >40 years of age).

BOX 19.4: Palpation of a rotator cuff defect.

Codman described a technique to palpate the rotator cuff defect. The examiner needs to palpate using a finger placed anterior to the acromion process. A defect can be palpated just anterior to the acromion in shoulder extension and under the acromion during shoulder in flexion.

Diagnosis

Radiographic investigations show narrowing of subacromial space or degenerative changes (e.g., bone spur). Magnetic resonance imaging (MRI) may reveal inflammatory or degenerative changes or tear in the substance of the tendon. MRI and ultrasonography (USG) are more reliable techniques to be used.

Management

Medical management involves administration of oral NSAIDs, steroids and hyaluronic injections into the site of pain or tear.

Surgical Management

Surgical management is required in RCT. RC repair is the most commonly used technique for RCI. Partial tears may be treated with debridement procedures but full-thickness tears would require RC repair. Surgery is indicated in cases of severe pain or weakness, severe debility, chronic tears, full-thickness tears, or recent acute injuries. The repair may be a traditional open approach or a mini open approach. Nowadays, arthroscopic repairs are used more often. However, there are chances of reinjury or repair failure. Biologic repair is a novel technique that has been developed to reduce these risks. It involves the application of growth factors and/or cells to promote healing of the RC tendons. It has shown potential to restore the normal histologic structure of RC postinjury. Acromioplasty or subacromial decompression may be performed in cases of acromial degeneration and presence of bony spurs that may restrict the subacromial space.

Physiotherapy Management

Physiotherapy is the first line of management for RC pathologies.

Aims

Physiotherapy management aims at:
- Reduction of pain
- Promotion of healing
- Maintaining and improving integrity and mobility of soft tissues
- Improvement of biomechanics
- Improvement of movement patterns
- Reduction of disability.

The physiotherapy management usually includes heat therapy and occasionally transcutaneous electrical nerve stimulation (TENS) or interferential therapy (IFT) for relief of pain, ultrasound (US) therapy for reducing inflammation, passive and active ROM exercises, strengthening of the RC and other scapular muscles, and correction of any scapular dyskinesia (taping may be used in the acute phase).

SHOULDER INSTABILITY

Introduction

Shoulder joint has a relatively unconstrained bony architecture, leading to greater mobility and lesser stability. The structures mainly responsible for the stability of the glenohumeral (GH) articulation are the capsule, surrounding ligaments and muscles, the RC, and the labrum. This kind of arrangement provides for a greater freedom of movement but leaves the joint vulnerable to instability after dislocation, particularly in the case of a traumatic event.

Shoulder instability **(Figs. 19.3A to C)** is termed as the inability to maintain the humeral head in the glenoid fossa. Under nonpathological states, the static and dynamic stabilizers of the shoulder joint create a balanced net joint reaction force. If the integrity of any of these structures is disrupted, instability ensues.

Classification

Various classification systems exist to classify the instability—etiology, direction, severity, frequency, hyperlaxity, voluntary, static versus dynamic, radiography, treatment, surgical pathology, treatment, bilaterality, and muscle patterning **(Fig. 19.4)**. Etiology, severity, direction, and frequency are the most commonly used in the clinical practice.

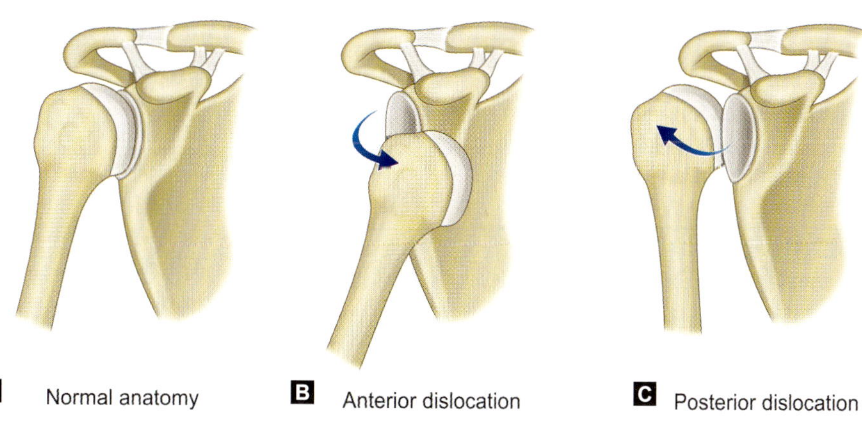

Figs. 19.3A to C: Types of shoulder instability.

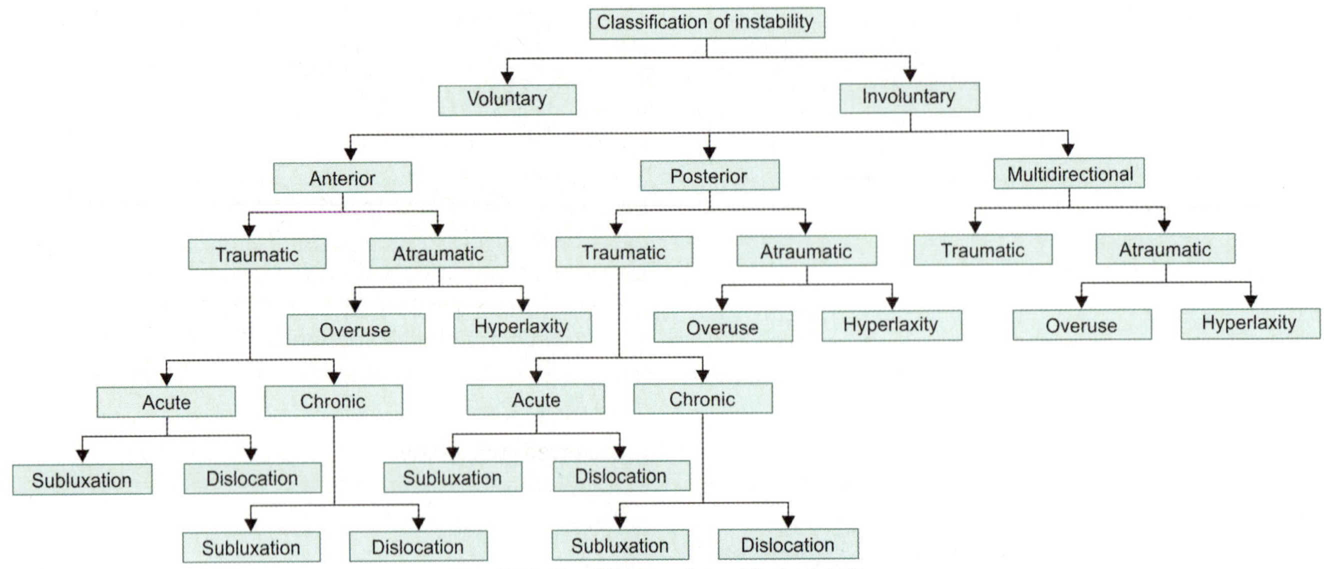

Fig. 19.4: Classification of shoulder instability.

Combinations of the abovementioned features are also used to develop new classification systems, e.g., the FEDS (frequency, etiology, direction, severity) classification system.

Acronyms such as **TUBS** (traumatic instability, unidirectional, with Bankart lesion and typically responding to surgery) and **AMBRI** (atraumatic, multidirectional, with bilateral shoulder findings, responding to rehabilitation, with inferior capsular shift) have also been developed historically to classify majority of the instabilities. However, these do not provide adequate information to differentiate instability from soft tissue hyperlaxity.

Factors Affecting Instability

Volition or Position

Instability can be voluntary (nonpositional) or involuntary (positional). Voluntary instability can be seen in individuals having personality disorders. Such individuals can dislocate their shoulders on a voluntary basis by muscular contractions. Individuals with involuntary instability may also be able to demonstrate dislocation with elevation of the arm, but they tend to avoid these positions even during functional tasks.

Direction

Instability can be unidirectional or multidirectional. Among unidirectional instabilities, anterior instability is the most common. With athletes, multidirectional instability is also often seen.

Unidirectional instability usually occurs following a single acute traumatic event or multiple or single low energy instability events. Low energy instability events may or may not be associated with soft tissue hyperlaxity. In the presence of soft tissue hyperlaxity, capsulolabral lesions are less likely, and the cause may be an open or patulous capsular tissue leading to recurrent shoulder dislocations.

> **BOX 19.5:** Humeral and glenoid sided defects.
>
> - Humeral-sided defects—Hill–Sachs lesion:
>   - An impaction injury to the posterosuperolateral humeral head occurring in association with anterior instability events
>   - Occurs with an anteroinferior dislocation of the humeral head causing the humeral head to abut the anterior glenoid rim and compression fracture of the humeral head
>   - A line of condensation seen on internal rotation radiographs is diagnostic
> - Glenoid-sided defects—Bankart lesion:
>   - Lesion of the anterior part of the glenoid labrum caused by recurrent anterior dislocations and subluxations
>   - Associated with absent or poorly developed medial glenohumeral ligament
>   - Appears as a true fracture fragment containing a portion of the anterior glenoid rim
> - Glenoid-sided defects—chronic attritional glenoid erosive changes:
>   - More chronic erosive changes occurring over time secondary to recurrent instability or a low energy compression fracture
>   - Appears rounded off with blunt edges

However, in the absence of soft tissue hyperlaxity, capsulolabral lesions are highly common. With traumatic cases, associated chondral and osteochondral lesions are often seen **(Box 19.5)**.

Multidirectional instability is the instability in at least two or three directions. Most commonly seen are anterior and posterior instability associated with an inferior subluxation or dislocation.

Cause

Glenohumeral instability can be atraumatic or traumatic. Traumatic instability can be diagnosed based on the history of the patient. A stress applied to the shoulder when it is externally rotated and abducted or a blow to the posterolateral aspect of the shoulder in the anterior direction may be few of the causes. Atraumatic instability is seen with individuals having a generalized hyperlaxity of all joints or in individuals not having hyperlaxity but instability due to overuse.

Frequency or Chronology

Based on the frequency or chronology, instability can be acute or chronic. Chronic instability can be subdivided into recurrent episodes of instability or a locked dislocation since a long time.

Assessment

History

A comprehensive detailed history should include:
- The occupation of the patient (if they are athletes—then the type of sports should be enquired about)
- Mechanism of injury (nature of injury and direction and amount of force sustained)
- Number of episodes
- If any treatment has been taken previously

Examination

Examination should include the following:
- Visual inspection of the entire anterior and posterior aspect of the shoulder girdle noting any asymmetry between affected and unaffected sides (position of the shoulder, winging of scapula, atrophy of muscles and AC position) during both static and dynamic states.
- Skin should be inspected for any previous scarring to assess the state of patient's collagenous tissues.
- Posture examination: Patient may hold the shoulder in a protected position—adduction and internal rotation with the elbow supported by the other limb or in a sling; "sulcus sign" **(Fig. 19.5)** may be present in case of inferior dislocation or subluxation; posterior dislocation may show a prominent coracoid.
- Spasm of the trapezius and other scapular muscles may be present.
- Diffuse tenderness may be found at the AC joint, SC joint, medial border of scapula, biceps tendon, acromion, and greater tuberosity.
- Warmth and swelling may be rarely present, but if present indicate an active inflammatory process.
- ROM may be limited due to pain and inflammation; active ROM testing may be associated with crepitus and clicking or popping sounds.
- ROM testing of the other areas such as thumb, knee, and elbows should be done to assess generalized laxity.
- Integrity of the RC needs to be examined.
- Strength of the RC and other surrounding muscles needs to be assessed.
- Assessment of joint play may reveal hypermobility at the GH joint.

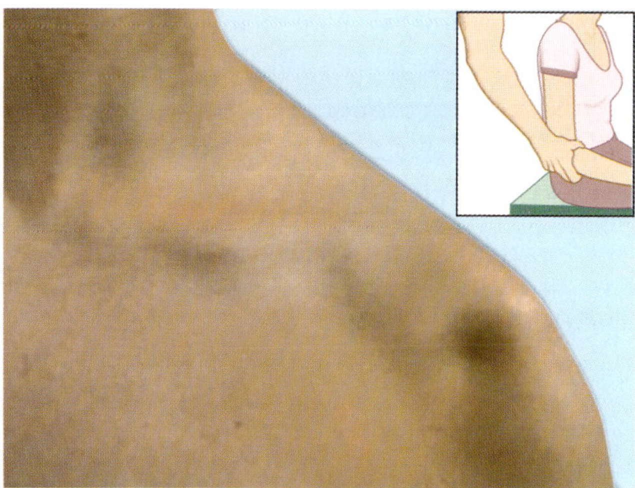

Fig. 19.5: Sulcus sign.

- A thorough neurologic examination should be included in the assessment considering motor, sensory and reflex changes; joints proximal and distal to the shoulder should be assessed (cervical spine, AC and SC joints and elbow and hand); dysesthesias and paresthesias should be noted.
- Shoulder should be evaluated for a possible injury to biceps/labral complex and the posterior labrum—O'Brien's active compression test, biceps load test, crank test, and dynamic labral shear test **(Box 19.6)**.
- Provocative tests may help to confirm the direction of instability **(Box 19.7)**.
- Psychological assessment of the patient should also be done to differentiate between positional and nonpositional instability; the DSM-5 Self-Rated Level 1 Cross-Cutting Symptom Measure can be used for this purpose.

Management

Conservative Management

Physiotherapy forms the mainstay of conservative management. It should be impairment-based and response-driven.

BOX 19.6: Assessment of biceps/labral complex.

"3-pack examination" including O'Brien sign active compression test, throwing test, and palpation of bicipital tunnel has excellent sensitivity and reliability and can be used as an ideal screening tool.

BOX 19.7: Provocative tests to confirm instability.

- Apprehension test for anterior and posterior instability
- Anterior and posterior drawer test for anterior and posterior instability, respectively
- Hyperabduction test for inferior instability
- Jobe's relocation test
- Load and shift test
- Anterior jerk test

Goals of Physiotherapy Management

Goals of physiotherapy management are as follows:
- Patient education to prevent recurrence
- Postural correction
- Improving motor control of shoulder and scapular muscles
- Strengthening of dynamic stabilizers of the shoulder
- Stretching of tight structures

Surgical Management

The most common procedures performed are:
- Open capsular shift
- Arthroscopic thermal capsulorrhaphy

Open procedures exhibit the advantage of better results with minimal risk of redislocation in cases of primarily soft tissue injuries and minimal osseous involvement. Arthroscopic procedures have the benefit of decreased loss of motion in the acute postoperative phase, decreased morbidity, faster recovery, and ability to assess concomitant injuries.

Postoperative rehabilitation begins in the immobilization phase (4–6 weeks) with active and passive ROM exercises in the protected range. Full ROM can be achieved by 8 weeks. Progressive resisted exercises can be started after 10–12 weeks. Return to sports is usually after 3 months for noncontact and low impact sports and 6 months for contact and high impact sports.

SUPRASPINATUS TENDINOPATHY

Tendinopathy of the supraspinatus muscle **(Fig. 19.6)** is a frequent cause of shoulder pain. The tendon of the supraspinatus commonly impinges under the acromion as it passes between the acromion and the humeral head. This mechanism is multifactorial.

Etiology

Extrinsic and intrinsic factors predisposing to supraspinatus tendinopathy are described in **Table 19.1**

Table 19.1: Etiological factors related to supraspinatus tendinopathy.

Extrinsic factors	Intrinsic factors
Primary impingement:	Acromial morphology (i.e., hooked acromion, presence of an os acromiale or osteophyte, calcific deposits in the subacromial space, all of which predispose to primary impingement)
Increased subacromial loading	Acromioclavicular atrhrosis (inferior osteophytes)
Trauma (direct macrotrauma or repetitive microtrauma)	Coracoacromial ligament hypertrophy
Overhead activity (athletic and nonathletic)	Coracoid impingement
Secondary impingement:	Subacromial bursal thickening and fibrosis
Rotator cuff overload/soft tissue imbalance	Prominent humeral greater tuberosity
Eccentric muscle overload	Impaired cuff vascularity
Glenohumeral laxity/instability	Aging (primary)
Long head of the biceps tendon laxity/weakness	Impingement (secondary)
Glenoid labral lesions	Primary tendinopathy
Muscle imbalance	Intratendinous
Scapular dyskinesia	Articular side partial-thickness tears
Posterior capsular tightness	Calcific tendinopathy
Trapezius paralysis	

Pathomechanics

Pathomechanics related to impingement leading to a painful arc is shown in **Figure 19.7**.

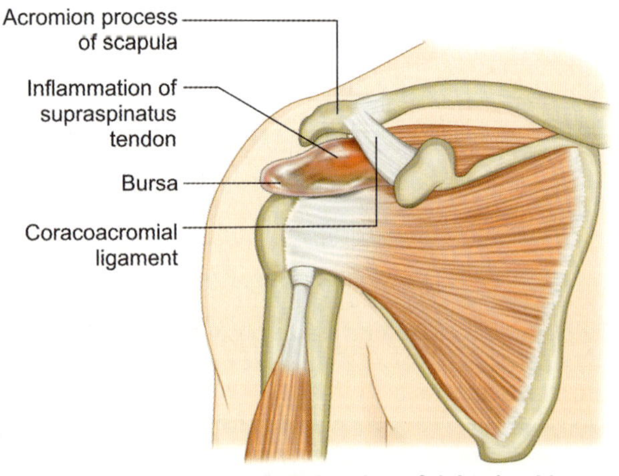

Fig. 19.6: Supraspinatus tendinopathy.

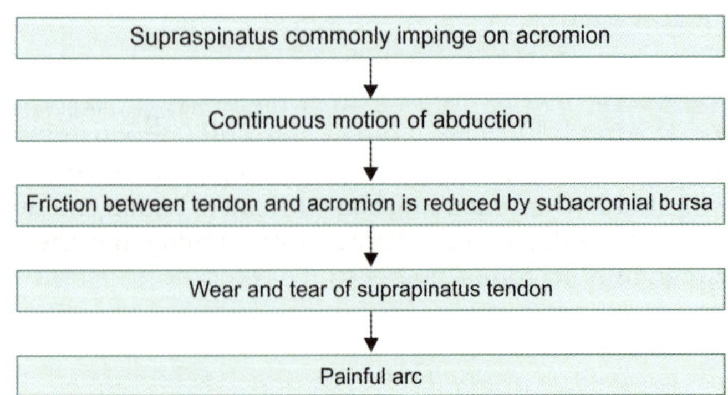

Fig 19.7: Pathomechanics in supraspinatus tendinopathy.

Clinical Features

Following are the clinical features:

- Subdeltoid aching
- Pain increases with reaching
- Pain is felt after frequent repetitive activity at, or above shoulder.
- Patient feels weakness of resisted abduction and forward flexion, especially with pushing and overhead movements.
- Patient has difficulty sleeping at night due to pain, especially when lying on the affected shoulder, and with an inability to sleep.
- Patient has difficulties with simple movements, such as brushing hair, putting on a shirt, or jacket, or reaching the arm above shoulder height.
- Patient has a limited ROM in the shoulder.
- Patient had a former shoulder trauma.

Investigations

Investigations include blood investigations, e.g., white cell counts, search for abnormal blood biochemistry and inflammatory markers, as well as radionuclide imaging and MRI and USG.

Assessment

The following special tests can be performed for confirming the diagnosis:

- Painful arc
- Special tests
  - Neer's test
  - Hawkins–Kennedy test
  - Supraspinatus challenge test or "the empty can" sign or Jobe's test
  - Drop arm test
  - Impingement test

Management

Conservative management includes ice, rest, anti-inflammatory and analgesic drugs and physical therapy. If conservative management fails, surgical management may be opted.

Goals of physical therapy management:

- Reduce pain and inflammation
- Reduce muscle atrophy
- Improve motor control of the muscles
- Normalize arthrokinematics of the girdle

SUBSCAPULAR TENDINOPATHY

It is usually caused by an inflamed subscapularis tendon or degeneration of the tendon. This can lead to impingement syndrome with the head of humerus becoming impinged under the roof of the shoulder structure.

Causes

The causes of subscapular tendinopathy are as follows:

- Overloading
- Incorrect use or degeneration of tendon

Clinical Features

Following are the clinical features:

- Pain on anterior aspect of shoulder or in axilla
- Difficulty in lifting heavy objects
- Difficulty in rotational movements

Investigations

Below tests can be performed:

- MRI
- USG

Assessment

The following special tests can be done assessed:

- Liftoff test: Sensitivity 25%; specificity 92%
- Bear hug test: Sensitivity 75%; specificity 56%
- Belly press test: Sensitivity 45%; specificity 92%
- Napoleon test: Sensitivity 41%; specificity 80%

Management

Mild symptoms usually relieve with 1–2 weeks of rest. Most of the cases go into recurrence resulting in scar formation. To eliminate this scar tissue, techniques such as massage, friction, and exercise therapy can be used. Resisted and proprioceptive exercises may be used for further rehabilitation.

BICIPITAL TENDINOPATHY

Bicipital tendinopathy is the inflammation of the tendon of long head of biceps **(Fig. 19.8)**. The long head of biceps lies in close approximation with the glenoid labrum and the RC, and hence becomes usually involved in any pathology of those structures.

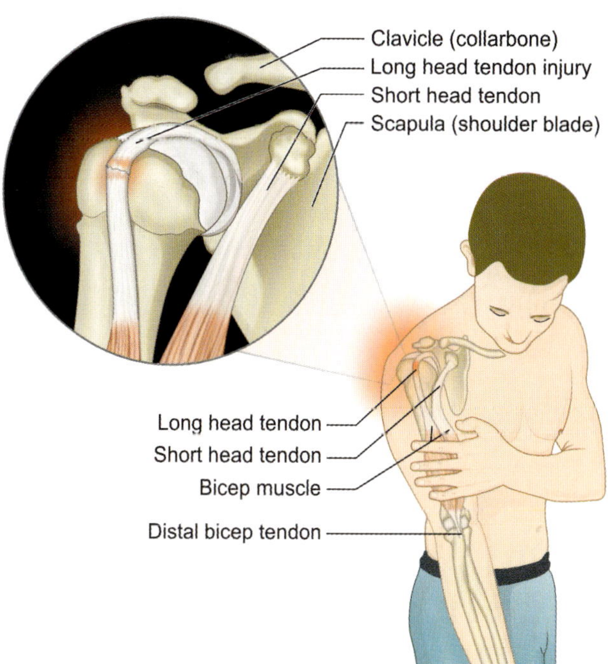

Fig. 19.8: Bicipital tendinitis.

Causes

The causes of bicipital tendinopathy are as follows:
- Age—because of degeneration
- Repeated trauma—overhead throwing, racquet players
- Improper biomechanical circumstances and movement patterns.

Biomechanical Causes

Biomechanical causes are:
- Coracoacromial ligament thickening
- Impingement in the subacromial space
- Acromial apophysis fusion
- Rotator cuff tear (RCT), particularly those that involve the subscapularis tendon
- Persistent RCT (>3 months)

Clinical Features

Following are the clinical features:
- Insidious onset
- Deep, throbbing pain in anterior shoulder
- Pain increases on lifting objects
- Pain localized in bicipital groove and might radiate toward insertion of deltoid muscle.
- Pain worsens at night, especially if patient sleeps on the affected shoulder.
- Pain aggravated by overhead reaching, pulling, lifting, and repetitive activities
- Active elbow flexion painful
- Biceps instability: anterior shoulder clicking or popping sensation.

Assessment

The following special tests can be done:
- Tenderness in bicipital groove
- Special tests:
  - Yergason test
  - Neer's test
  - Hawkins test
  - Speed test.

Investigations

Below tests can performed:
- Arthrography
- Bicipital groove view radiography **(Table 19.2)**
- MRI
- USG
- Tendon sheath swelling

Table 19.2: Dimensions of bicipital groove.

	Transverse view (mm)	Longitudinal view (mm)
Women	≥4.6	≥2.5
Men	≥5.5	≥2.8

Management

Conservative management includes pain management using NSAIDs and acetaminophen. For pain unmanageable by these drugs, corticosteroids may be used. In cases where conservative management fails, surgical management may be tried using biceps tenotomy or tenodesis through an arthroscopic or open procedure.

Goals of Physiotherapy Management

- Relief of pain and inflammation
- Education of patient regarding correct technique for use of upper limb
- Improving ROM and flexibility
- Improving joint stability and muscle strength
- Correction of abnormal posture
- Improving speed of movement, endurance and proprioception

Physiotherapy Management

- Avoidance of the pain causing movement or activity is advised in the early phase. The patient should be educated about the correct technique of movement. Cryotherapy or Transcutaneous Electrical Nerve Stimulation (TENS) may be used for pain relief. Phonophoresis with an anti-inflammatory agent may also be used for relief of pain and inflammation. Stretching of the scapular muscles, rotator cuff and posterior capsule may be used for improving and maintaining the ROM. Stretching of low back muscles and hamstrings must also be incorporated in the program as tightness of these muscles also causes an imbalance of the scapula and shoulder ligaments.
- A slow progressive resisted exercises program should be started to optimize the collagen tissue formation during the healing of the tendon. Strengthening of the scapular muscles, rotator cuff and biceps should be included. Emphasis should be made on the correction of scapulohumeral rhythm. High speed activities and proprioceptive training should be included in the physiotherapy regime.

SUBACROMIAL BURSITIS

Bursitis is a common cause of shoulder pain that occurs due to inflammatory changes in the shoulder bursa. The most prevalent bursal pathology is the subacromial bursitis. The subacromial space is lined by the acromion, coracoid, proximal fibers of the deltoid, and the coracoacromial ligament superiorly and the supraspinatus muscle inferiorly.

Etiology

Following are the etiologies of subacromial bursitis:
- Repetitive overhead activities
- Subacromial impingement
- Subacromial hemorrhage

- Crystal deposition
- Direct trauma
- Infection
- Autoimmune or inflammatory pathologies such as RA

Pathology

The changes shown in **Figure 19.9** are common for all stages of bursitis.

Bursitis has three **stages or phases**:

1. Phase I (acute phase)—local inflammation with thickened synovial fluid; painful overhead movements
2. Phase II (chronic phase)—chronic inflammatory process in the bursa; constant pain which may lead to weakness and subsequent rupture of surrounding tendons and ligaments
3. Phase III (recurrent bursitis)—in patients exposed to repetitive trauma or overhead movements.

Normally, the bursa is not impinged during any overhead activities or at rest. At rest, it protrudes laterally, saving itself from the impingement. When overhead activities are performed, the bursa rolls under the acromion, reducing the space. But the reduction in space is not that great to produce an impingement. However, due to repetitive movements or trauma, the bursa gets inflamed and hence gets impinged during overhead activities and gradually during rest as well.

If the bursitis goes unattended, it may result in deposition of calcium within the substance of the bursa causing calcific bursitis of the shoulder, which is very difficult to manage.

Assessment

History

Details of the patients include:

- Age usually over 30 years
- Female predominance seen
- Pain on the anterolateral aspect of shoulder.
- May have a history of trauma, e.g., fall on the shoulder or repetitive overhead activities.
- Duration of symptoms may vary from 1 month to 1 year.

Physical Examination

Physical examination includes following:

- Clinical signs of impingement may be present.
- Patient will complain of localized pain on overhead movements (both active and passive).

- Tenderness present over anterolateral aspect of the shoulder below the acromion.
- Warmth and mild swelling may be present in the area.
- Painful resisted abduction of the shoulder beyond 75–80°.
- Crepitus may be palpated in some individuals.

The disability in arm, shoulder, and hand (DASH) questionnaire may be used to quantify the disability of the patient. It is a 30-item questionnaire rated on a 5-point Likert scale. The Shoulder Pain and Disability Index (SPADI) may also be used to measure shoulder pain and disability. It consists of 13 items–5 for pain and 8 for disability.

The Constant–Murley score is a more comprehensive score comprising of a variety of parameters rated on a 100-point scale. The parameters can be categorized into four subscales–pain (15 points), activities of daily living (20 points), strength (25 points), and ROM (forward elevation, abduction, internal, and external rotation of the shoulder) (40 points). A higher score indicates a higher quality of function and vice versa **(Box 19.8)**.

Management

Medical management includes ingestion of oral NSAIDs and corticosteroids and injections using corticosteroids or other analgesics with or without US guidance.

Surgical management includes bursectomy primarily which can be an open or arthroscopic procedure. Surgery is usually indicated for recalcitrant cases that are not responsive to conservative management. Other surgeries include subacromial decompression or acromioplasty and RC repair in case of associated RCT.

Physiotherapy Management

Goals of Physiotherapy Management

Physiotherapy management should have the following goals:

- Prevent further injury
- Improve mobility
- Restore scapular control and scapulohumeral rhythm
- Improve the strength of RC muscles
- Improve endurance, power, and agility of the shoulder muscles.

Most often, the physiotherapy management comprises the application of cold, US, active, resisted, and proprioceptive exercises. Though US is conventionally used for the majority of the cases of bursitis, its effectiveness has not been proven in the literature. Phonophoresis may

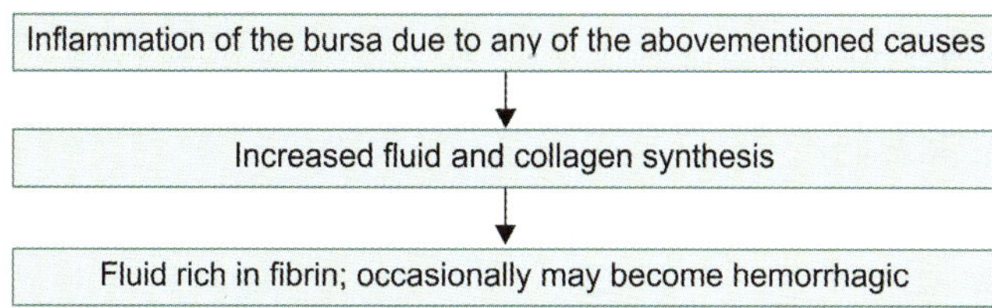

Fig. 19.9: Pathological changes in bursitis.

BOX 19.8: Differential diagnoses for subacromial bursitis.

- AC joint OA
- Biceps tendinitis
- Impingement syndrome
- Adhesive capsulitis
- Rotator cuff tendinitis/tear

(AC: acromioclavicular; OA: osteoarthritis)

also be applied using any anti-inflammatory agents. For calcific bursitis of the shoulder, iontophoresis using acetic acid can also be used.

In the acute phase, the bursa should be protected by avoiding all activities that may cause pain. A shoulder sling may be advised or taping may be applied for the protection and correction of any postural abnormalities. Scapular stabilization exercises may be given for improving scapular control. Codman's pendulum exercises can be used for improving or maintaining mobility and reducing stiffness.

For athletes, endurance and agility training form an important part of the rehabilitation and should be more focused on. Sports-specific training should be given to improve agility and endurance.

OSTEOARTHRITIS OF THE SHOULDER JOINT

Degeneration of the shoulder or the GH joint involves degeneration of the articular cartilage lining the bones and the subchondral bone underneath, leading to a reduction in joint space **(Fig. 19.10)**.

Epidemiology

Osteoarthritis (OA) is the most common rheumatic pathology. Studies have reported a prevalence of 3% in China in the year 2016 and 5% in Korea in 2015 for shoulder OA. In Korea, the prevalence has reduced from 16.1% primary OA to 1.3% prevalence of secondary OA. Japan has a prevalence of 17.4%. The rate is higher among former athletes (33%). Shoulder joint is the third most common joint to be affected with OA, following knee and hip.

Risk Factors

Following risk factors are involved:
- Age
- Female gender
- Athletic activities
- Occupations involving repetitive activities of the shoulder, e.g., window cleaner and school teacher.

Pathophysiology

The pathology behind the degeneration is similar to that seen in knee OA. The degenerative process causes a progressive and gradual breakdown of the mechanical and biochemical components of the articular cartilage, joint capsule, and the bone. This increases the friction between the surfaces during any movement causing further wear and tear of the structures, leading to a vicious cycle of pain and disability.

There are two types of OA—primary and secondary **(Table 19.3)**. Primary OA is diagnosed when there is a presence of no predisposing factors leading to OA. Secondary OA occurs as a result of joint trauma, dislocation or instability, previous surgeries, inflammatory arthropathies, avascular necrosis, infection, congenital malformations, or major joint injuries such as RCT.

Shoulder OA, even though less common than knee or hip OA, can be equally debilitating. Limitation of shoulder can cause depression, anxiety, and performance limitations at the workplace.

Clinical Features

Following are the clinical features:
- Old age
- History of trauma, dislocation, or previous surgery
- Deep aching type of pain in the posterior aspect of the shoulder, aggravated by movement.
- Occasional nocturnal pain
- Stiffness of the shoulder joint (not lasting more than 30 minutes)
- Crepitus during movement
- Occasionally in severe cases, joint effusion may be seen **(Box 19.9)**.

Examination

Examination of a shoulder having mild OA changes may not reveal any significant findings other than pain, mild hypomobility and crepitus during movement **(Table 19.4)**. Examination of advanced arthritic joints may reveal severe pain during movement and, also at rest, reduced ROM of the shoulder and surrounding joints, hypomobility, reduced muscle strength, and severe functional restriction. Inflammation of the surrounding tendons and bursae are also quite common, secondary to the degeneration of the joint.

Western Ontario Osteoarthritis of the Shoulder index is a shoulder and OA-specific measurement tool. It is reliable,

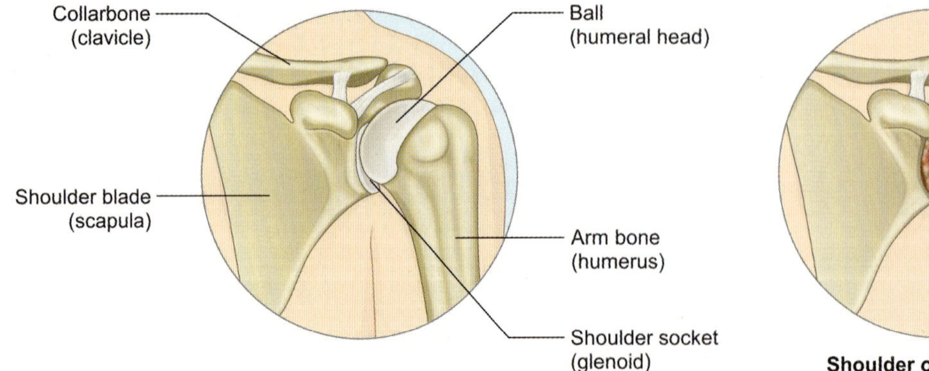

Fig. 19.10: Osteoarthritis of the shoulder.

Table 19.3: Classification of glenohumeral osteoarthritis.

Classification	Etiology
Primary	Unknown
Secondary	
Atraumatic osteonecrosis	• Corticosteroid therapy • Cytotoxic drugs • Obesity • Gaucher's disease • Lipid metabolism disorders • Sickle cell disease • Radiation • Alcohol induced
Postinflammation	• Postinfection arthritis • Crystal arthropathies • Rheumatoid arthritis • Rotator cuff arthropathy
Postsurgical	• Capsulorrhaphy arthropathy • Intra-articular implants (screws, etc.) • Overtight anterior capsule repair
Post-traumatic	• Dislocation • Proximal humerus malunion • Post-traumatic avascular necrosis • Subluxation

BOX 19.9: Red flags in differential diagnosis of shoulder osteoarthritis.

• Infection
• Tumor or malignancy
• Unreduced dislocation
• Inflammatory oligo- or polyarthritis
• Systemic inflammation

Table 19.4: Differential diagnosis of shoulder osteoarthritis (OA).

Clinical feature	Possible diagnosis
History	
Joint effusion	• OA • RA • Septic arthritis
Morning stiffness that improves on activity	RA
Nocturnal pain	• RC pathologies • Impingement syndrome
Pain or "clunking" sound with overhead activity	Labral disorders
Pain radiating along the arm	Cervical spine disorders
Stiffness aggravated by activity, relieved with rest	OA
Physical examination	
Decreased cervical ROM	Cervical spine disorders
Crepitus during movement	• OA • RA

Contd...

Contd...

Clinical feature	Possible diagnosis
Reduced ROM in capsular pattern	• OA • Adhesive capsulitis or soft tissue injury
Erythema along with warmth	• Septic arthritis • RA
Tenderness along shoulder joint line	OA
Radiography	
Joint space narrowing	• Arthropathy following RC tear • OA • RA
Marginal joint erosions	RA
Normal joint	Adhesive capsulitis
Osteophytes, subchondral sclerosis	OA

(RA: rheumatoid arthritis; RC: rotator cuff; ROM: range of motion)

valid, and highly responsive. The instrument has 19 items describing 4 domains—pain and physical symptoms (6 items); sports, recreation, and work function (5 items); lifestyle function (5 items); and emotional function (3 items).

Radiographic changes can also not be appreciated in the initial phases. However, advanced pathologies may show degenerative changes such as bony erosion, osteoporosis, osteophytes, cysts, and joint space narrowing. MRI is of great importance in detecting early clinical signs of degeneration in the articular cartilage. Computed tomography (CT) scanning may help identify any articular defects.

Management

Medical Management

Medical management of shoulder OA is similar to OA of the hip and knee and can be referred from Chapter 21: Hip Conditions and Chapter 21: Knee Conditions.

Surgical Management

Various surgical options **(Table 19.5)** exist for the management of shoulder OA but the decision depends

Table 19.5: Surgical procedures performed for shoulder osteoarthritis (OA).

Surgical procedure	Description
Debridement	Removal of mechanical irritants, loose bodies, or cartilage flaps
Synovectomy	Removal of synovial membrane of the joint
Capsular release	Release of inflamed and stiff contracted capsule
Arthrodesis	For patients not suitable for arthroplasty; joint is fused to limit pain and mobility
Arthroplasty	Replacement of the surfaces of the joint by metal implants; treatment of choice for severe OA

on the age, extent of damage, and the disability faced by the patient. Joint preservative surgeries (capsular release, arthroscopic debridement, interposition arthroplasty, corrective osteotomies, etc.) are more commonly preferred for the younger patient. Arthroscopic debridement with capsular release forms the most common procedure performed.

Physiotherapy Management

Goals of physiotherapy management:
- Reduce pain
- Improve ROM
- Improve muscle strength and endurance
- Improve stability of the joint
- Improve function
- Patient education regarding the nature and the prognosis of the pathology.

ACROMIOCLAVICULAR AND STERNOCLAVICULAR JOINTS

It is imperative for the examiner to evaluate the AC and the SC joints in a shoulder case. Commonly presented pathologies of the AC and the SC joints include overuse syndrome, hypomobility, and dislocation or subluxation.

Overuse of the AC and the SC joints leads to the development of arthritic changes in them. They are commoner in post-traumatic conditions. AC joint arthritis of the nontraumatic variety occurs in individuals having repeated movements at the waist level, e.g., grinding, packaging, and construction work or those involved in diagonal extension, adduction, and internal rotation motions, e.g., tennis or volleyball.

Hypomobility of the SC and AC joints is often associated with faulty postures, e.g., depression or retraction. Hypomobility may lead to thoracic outlet syndrome (TOS) in the long run. Instability at the AC and SC joints occurs following trauma such as fall on the outstretched arm or on the shoulder. Hypermobility following trauma is usually of the permanent nature.

Clinical Features

Following are the clinical features:
- Local pain over involved joint or ligament
- Painful arc with shoulder elevation
- Pain with *horizontal* movements
- Hypermobility or hypomobility on joint play assessment.
- If TOS is present, neurological and vascular symptoms may be present.
- Reduced ROM
- Reduced endurance and strength

Management

For hypermobile joints, rest in a sling is provided. Gentle ROM exercises may be initiated to maintain the mobility

of the GH joint. For hypomobile joints, mobilization may be added to the rehabilitation program.

SCAPULAR DYSKINESIS

Scapular dyskinesis, also known as the **SICK** (**s**capular malpositioning, **i**nferior medial border prominence, **c**oracoid pain and malposition and dys**k**inesis of scapular movement) scapula, is an overuse syndrome where alteration in normal scapular kinematics is seen **(Fig. 19.11)**.
- Bony causes—thoracic kyphosis, clavicle fracture, nonunion or shortened malunion.
- Joint causes—high-grade AC instability, AC arthrosis and instability, GH joint internal arrangement.
- Neurological causes—cervical radiculopathy, long thoracic or spinal accessory nerve palsy.
- Soft tissue cause—tightness of pectoralis minor and biceps short head

↓

Anterior tilt and protraction due to their pull on coracoid
- Posterior muscle tightness

↓

Glenohumeral internal rotation deficit

↓

Winging of the scapula on the thorax with reduced humeral internal rotation and horizontal abduction
- Alteration in periscapular muscles

↓

Shoulder impingement

↓

Serratus anterior strength and activation decreases

↓

Shoulder pain

↓

Loss of posterior tilt and upward rotation

↓

Dyskinesis
- Alteration of upper trapezius and lower trapezius force couple

↓

Delayed onset of lower trapezius

↓

Alter scapular upward rotation and posterior tilt

↓

Decrease linear measures of subacromial space
- Increase impingement symptoms
- Decrease RC strength
- Increase strain on anterior GH ligaments
- Increase risk of internal impingement.

Clinical Features

Following are the clinical features:
- Symptoms of isolated SICK scapula: Anterior shoulder pain (most common), posterior superior scapular

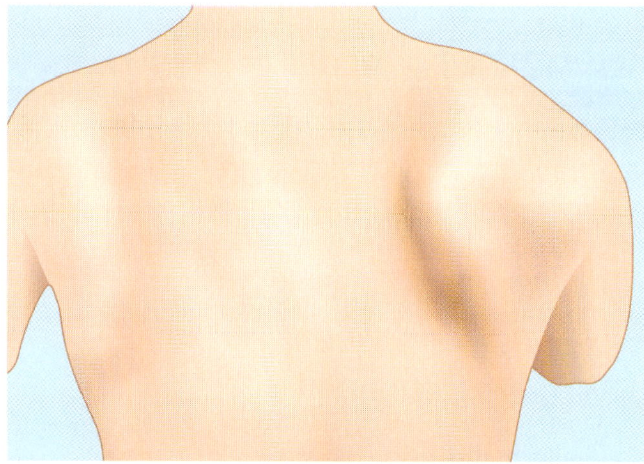

Fig. 19.11: Scapula dyskinesis.

pain, superior shoulder pain, proximal lateral arm pain or any combination of above.

- Posterosuperior scapular pain may radiate into the ipsilateral paraspinous cervical region or patient may complain of radicular/TOS type symptoms.
- The onset is almost always insidious.
- Pain and/or tenderness around the scapula when using the arm overhead or carrying heavy objects with the arm at the side.
- Snapping or popping sensation around the scapula with shoulder movement.
- Loss of strength with shoulder and arm use.
- Asymmetrical posture (affected side usually sits lower).
- Winging of the scapula
- Instability of the shoulder

Assessment

Assessment includes the following:

- **Clinical observation of scapular dyskinesis**
  Kibler classification of scapular dysfunction (Fig. 19.12):
  - **Type 1 or inferior dysfunction:** The primary external visual feature is the prominence of the inferior angle as a result of anterior tilting of the scapula in the sagittal plane. Inferior pattern

presentation is better visualized while in the hands-on-hips position or during eccentric lowering from overhead elevation. According to Kibler, type 1 pattern is most commonly found in patients with RC dysfunction.

- **Type 2 or medial dysfunction:** The primary external visual feature is the prominence of the entire medial scapular border due to internal rotation of the scapula in the transverse plane. As with type 1, the type 2 presentation becomes more evident in the hands-on-hips position and during active eccentric lowering from overhead. Medial pattern dysfunction most often occurs in patients with GH joint instability.
- **Type 3 or superior dysfunction:** Characterized by excessive and early elevation of the scapula during upper extremity elevation. This pattern has been referred to as compensatory shoulder hiking or shrug and is most often seen in patients with RC dysfunction and deltoid-RC force couple imbalances.
- **Symptom altering tests:**
  - **Scapular retraction test:** Baseline active ROM and pain are evaluated. This test is positive if pain is reduced as the therapist assists active elevation by applying a posterior tilt and external rotation motion to the scapula. This application may be used in conjunction with other tests such as Neer's, Hawkins–Kennedy, and Jobe's relocation.
  - **Scapular assistance test:** Baseline AROM and pain are evaluated. The therapist then applies an assist to scapular dynamics. This test is positive if ROM is increased or pain is reduced as the therapist manually assists scapular upward rotation during active UE elevation.
  - **Lateral scapular slide test (LSST):** Measurements are taken from spine of scapulae to T2/T3, inferior angle of scapulae to T7/T9 and superior angle of scapulae to T2. The measurements are taken in three positions, sitting/standing with arms resting on the side, hands on the waist, thumbs posteriorly

Dyskinetic patterns fall into three categories characterized by:

Type 1: Prominence of the inferomedial border of the scapula

Type 2: Prominence of the entire medial border

Type 3: Prominence of the superomedial border

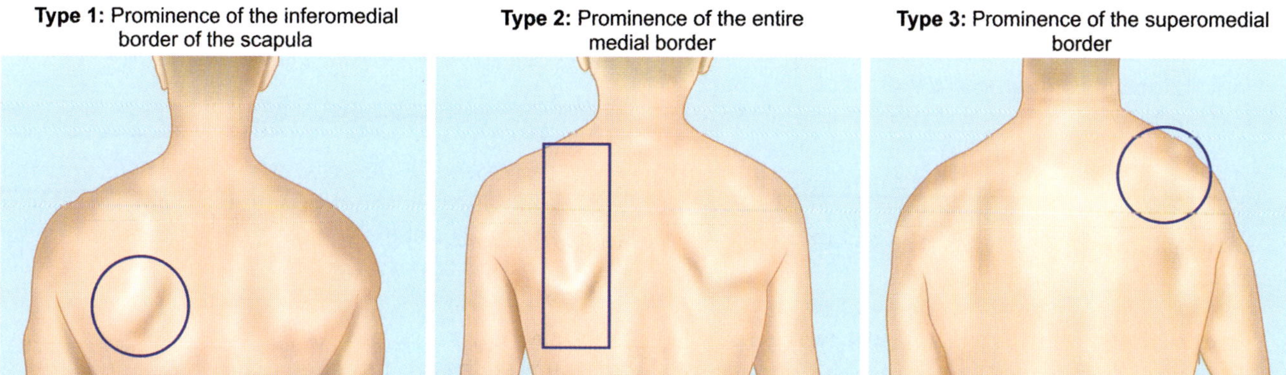

Fig. 19.12: Types of scapular dysfunction.

(45° abduction), and 90° abduction and maximal internal rotation. Measurement should not vary more than 1–1.5 cm, more the 1.5 cm difference significant.

- **Isometric scapular pinch test:** Patient in standing position and is asked to actively squeeze or retract the scapulae together as hard as possible.
  - *Normal response:* An individual able to hold the squeeze or 15–20 seconds without any burning pain or noticeable weakness.
  - *Positive:* Burning pain present.
  - *Watch for:* Patient relaxing the contraction.
- **Scapular load test:** As in position for LSST, manual load is applied in anterior, posterior, inferior, or superior direction to the arm, and scapula should not move more than 1.5 cm.
- **Wall pushup test:** Patient performs wall pushups for 15–20 times. Weakness of scapular muscles (mainly serratus anterior) or winging usually shows up with 5–10 pushups. For stronger or younger population, perform the test on floor.

Management

Physiotherapy Management

Physiotherapy management should involve the following goals:

- Reducing pain and inflammation
- Improving mobility of posterior capsule and pectoralis minor.
- Improving scapular control
- Improving the strength of scapular muscles
- Postural correction

LABRAL TEAR

It is an injury to the glenoid labrum which is attached to the margin of glenoid cavity.

Superior labrum anterior-posterior (**SLAP**) tear is classified into seven types:

1. Type I concerns degenerative fraying with no detachment of the biceps insertion.
2. Type II is the most common type and represents a detachment of the superior labrum and biceps from the glenoid rim.
3. Type III represents a bucket-handle tear of the labrum with an intact biceps tendon insertion to the bone.
4. Type IV lesions, the least common type represents an intrasubstance tear of the biceps tendon with a bucket-handle tear of the superior aspect of the labrum.
5. Type V: A Bankart lesion that extends superiorly to include a Type II SLAP lesion.
6. Type VI: An unstable flap tears of the labrum in conjunction with a biceps tendon separation.
7. Type VII: A superior labrum and biceps tendon separation that extends anteriorly, inferior to the middle GH ligament.

Etiology

Following are the etiologies:

- Age
- Acute trauma
- Repetitive throwing
- Hyperextension
- A fall on an outstretched arm
- Heavy lifting
- Direct trauma

Clinical Features

Following are the clinical features:

- Sensations of painful clicking and/or popping with shoulder movement
- Loss of GH internal rotation ROM
- Pain with overhead motions
- Loss of RC muscular strength and endurance
- Loss of scapular stabilizer muscle strength and endurance
- Inability to lie on the affected shoulder.

Diagnostic Procedures

Tenderness to palpation at the rotator interval, i.e., space between supraspinatus tendon, subscapularis tendon, and coracoid process, is considered diagnostic.

Special Tests

Following special tests should be conducted:

- Positive anterior drawer
- Anterior slide test: specificity 91.5%; sensitivity 78.4%
- Biceps load test: I and II specificity 96.9%; sensitivity 90.9%
- O'Brien test: specificity 98.5%; sensitivity 100%
- Anterior apprehension test
- Positive relocation test
- Clunk test
- Crank test: specificity 67–88%; sensitivity 13–81%
- Speeds test
- Yergason's test
- Compression rotation test
- Dynamic labral shear test

Management

Management has been discussed along with instability.

THORACIC OUTLET SYNDROME

It is a term used to describe a group of disorders that occur when there is compression, injury, or irritation of the nerves and/or blood vessels (arteries and veins) in the lower neck and upper chest area (**Fig. 19.13**).

Etiology

Anatomical defects: Inherited defects that are present at birth (congenital) may include an extra rib located above

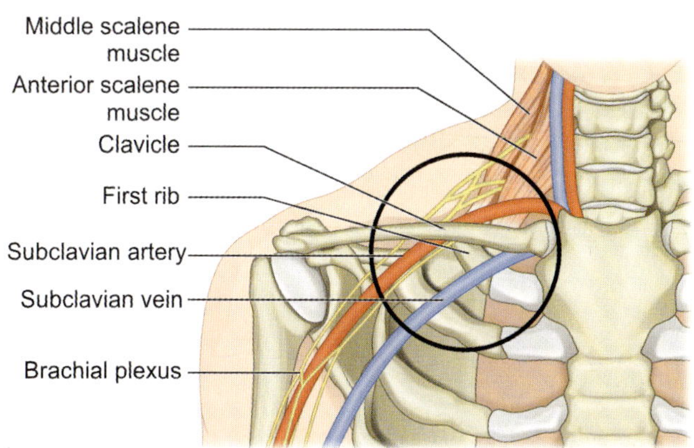

Fig. 19.13: Thoracic outlet.

the first rib (cervical rib) or an abnormally tight fibrous band connecting spine to your rib.

Poor posture: Drooping of shoulders or holding the head in a forward position can cause compression in the thoracic outlet area.

Trauma: A traumatic event, such as a car accident, can cause internal changes that then compress the nerves in the thoracic outlet. The onset of symptoms related to a traumatic accident often is delayed.

Repetitive activity: Doing the same thing repeatedly can, over time, wear the body's tissue. One may notice symptoms of TOS if the job requires repetition of the movement continuously, such as typing on a computer, working on an assembly line or lifting things above the head, as when were stocking shelves. Athletes, such as baseball pitchers and swimmers, also can develop TOS from years of repetitive movements.

Pressure on joints: Obesity can put an undue amount of stress on the joints, as can carrying around an oversized bag or backpack.

Pregnancy: Because joints loosen during pregnancy, clinical signs of TOS may first appear during pregnancy.

Types

Neurogenic (neurological) TOS: This most common type of TOS is characterized by compression of the brachial plexus.

Vascular TOS: This type of TOS occurs when one or more of the veins (venous TOS) or arteries (arterial TOS) under the clavicle are compressed.

Nonspecific-type TOS: This type is also called disputed TOS. Some doctors do not believe it exists, while others say it's a common disorder. People with nonspecific-type TOS have chronic pain in the area of the thoracic outlet that worsens with activity, but a specific cause of the pain can not be determined.

Clinical Signs and Symptoms

According to types of TOS:
Neurological TOS:
- Muscle wasting in the thenar or hypothenar eminence (Gilliatt–Sumner hand)

- Numbness or tingling in the arm or fingers
- Pain or aches in neck, shoulder, or hand especially on medial side
- Weakening grip

Vascular TOS:
- Discoloration of the hand (bluish color)
- Arm pain and swelling, possibly due to blood clots
- Blood clot in veins or arteries in the upper area of body
- Lack of color (pallor) in one or more of the fingers or entire hand
- Weak or no pulse in the affected arm
- Cold fingers, hands, or arms
- Arm fatigue with activity
- Numbness or tingling in fingers
- Weakness of arm or neck
- Throbbing lump near clavicle

Investigations

Electromyography (EMG), CT-scan, MRI, X-ray, US, angiography, arteriography and venography, and nerve conduction velocity (NCV) tests can be performed.

Assessment

Physical Examination

Physical examination includes:
- Posture: Forward head or rounded shoulders may lead to muscle tightness of levator scapula, scalenes, suboccipitals, and pectoralis minor.
- Palpation of the scalenes, cervical musculature, upper trapezius, pectoralis minor, and periclavicular region should reveal any musculature or tissue that is tender, tight, or in spasm.
- Cervical ROM, shoulder ROM, pectoralis minor flexibility, scalene flexibility, and upper trapezius flexibility.
- Muscle testing for strength
- Sensation
- Reflexes
- Respiratory pattern

Special Tests

1. **Roos test:** The patient stands and abducts shoulders to 90°, externally rotates the shoulders, and flexes the elbows to 90°. The patient then opens and closes the hand slowly for 3 minutes. The test is positive if the patient is unable to complete the test or experiences heaviness, numbness, tingling, or pain.
2. **Adson's test:** The examiner locates the radial pulse while arm is held in extension, external rotation, and slight abduction. The patient is instructed to take a deep breath and turn head toward the test arm while extending the neck. If there is compression, the radial pulse will be diminished or absent. The goal of this test is to tense the anterior and middle scalenes.

3. **Costoclavicular test:** The examiner palpates the radial pulse and then draws the patient's shoulder down and back. If the pulse disappears, the test is positive. The goal of this test is to provide compression of the costoclavicular space.
4. **Halstead maneuver:** The examiner palpates the radial pulse and applies downward traction on the test extremity while the patient's neck is hyperextended and rotated to the opposite side. Absence of the pulse indicates a positive test.
5. **Wright test (hyperabduction test):** The examiner palpates the radial pulse and hyperabducts the arm so the hand is brought overhead with the elbow and arm in the coronal plane. The patient takes a deep breath and may rotate or extend the neck for additional effect.
6. **Allen maneuver:** The examiner palpates the radial pulse while positioning the shoulder in external rotation and horizontal abduction. The patient then rotates the head away from the test side.

Management

Management of neurogenic TOS consists of gentle rehabilitative exercises, behavior modification, posture correction, manual therapy, stretching exercises, trigger point release, etc. Surgical management includes first rib excision, scalenectomy, and fibrotic band lysis.

For venous TOS, physical therapy carries a little less role. Conservative management comprises rest, elevation of the limb, and anticoagulant therapy. Stent placement and surgical decompression of axillo-subclavian venous system are possible surgical options.

SHOULDER REHABILITATION

When designing a rehabilitation program for patients with an unstable shoulder (GH joint instability), it is important that the following key factors should be considered:

- Onset of pathology
- Degree of instability and the effect of their functions
- Frequency of dislocation (chronic vs. acute)
- Direction of instability (posterior, anterior, or multidirectional)
- Concomitant pathologies (Bankart lesion, Hill–Sachs lesion, a reverse Hill–Sachs lesion, etc.)
- End range neuromuscular control
- Activity level

When considering all of these seven key factors, each patient will have a different rehabilitation program.

The **common problems** faced by each patient are:

- Pain and inflammation
- Reduced ROM
- Reduced flexibility
- Reduced strength

Electrotherapy Modalities

Transcutaneous electrical nerve stimulation (TENS), IFT, and US are the most frequently used modalities **(Figs. 19.14**

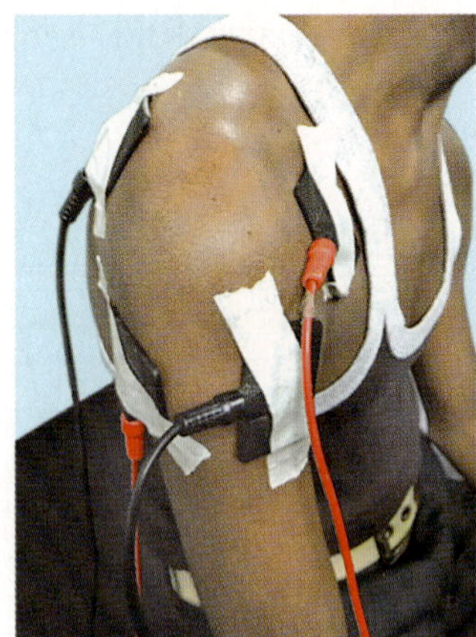

Fig. 19.14: Application of interferential therapy (IFT) to the shoulder joint.

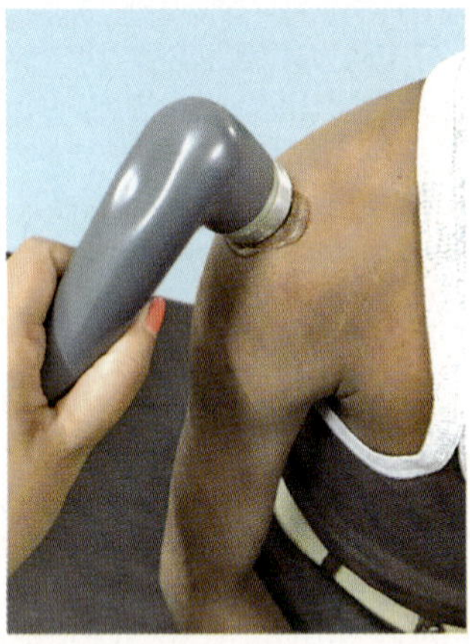

Fig. 19.15: Application of ultrasound for shoulder.

and 19.15). Ice packs are of huge benefit for acute injuries. In addition to these, heat therapy, shortwave diathermy, and LASER can also be applied.

Shoulder Range of Motion/Mobility Exercises

Shoulder Pendulum Exercises

They facilitate range of motion (ROM) of the joint and do not require a muscle contraction.

This exercise is most recommended for many shoulder conditions, including:

- RCT
- Adhesive capsulitis (frozen shoulder)
- Labral tears
- Clavicle fractures
- Shoulder dislocations

When performed correctly, these exercises help decrease joint stiffness and prevent adhesions and contractures as well as increase circulation and improve healing. They induce relaxation of the surrounding muscles.

These exercises mimic the movement of a clock pendulum and are excellent rehabilitation tools after shoulder injury. They use gravity and momentum to create motion rather than muscle strength. It is important to do these exercises correctly since active ROM exercises, those that use muscle strength, are often contraindicated in early recovery stages.

Standing Pendulum Exercises (Fig. 19.16)

This exercise uses the weight and momentum of the arm to encourage movement at the shoulder joint, while maintaining inactivity of the injured or repaired muscles.

Lying Pendulum Exercises (Fig. 19.17)

- This exercise helps relax the muscles of the shoulder and neck and allows for passive ROM of the shoulder joint.
- It is best for people who have a difficult time with the standing exercise due to balance or back pain.

Weighted Pendulum Exercises

Following are the uses of weighted pendulum exercises:

- This advanced pendulum exercise uses a dumbbell or wrist weight for an added pull on the shoulder joint **(Fig. 19.18)**.
- A 2006 study compared weighted and unweighted pendulum exercises. They concluded that adding 3.3 lb (1.5 kg) to standing pendulum exercises does not cause an increase in muscle activation when performed correctly, and they can be used during the initial rehabilitation period.

Shoulder Pulley Exercises

Pulleys have been used in postoperative shoulder rehabilitation with the intention of improving ROM and developing strength.

- The pulling should be with the good arm.
- The exercises should be done slowly and with control.

1. **Shoulder flexion (Fig. 19.19):**
   - The patient sits on a chair.
   - The pulley handles are grasped with both hands.
   - The pulley is pulled down on with the good arm. This will lift the injured arm up over the head. It is pulled as high as the patient can and held for some time.
   - Relax and repeat.

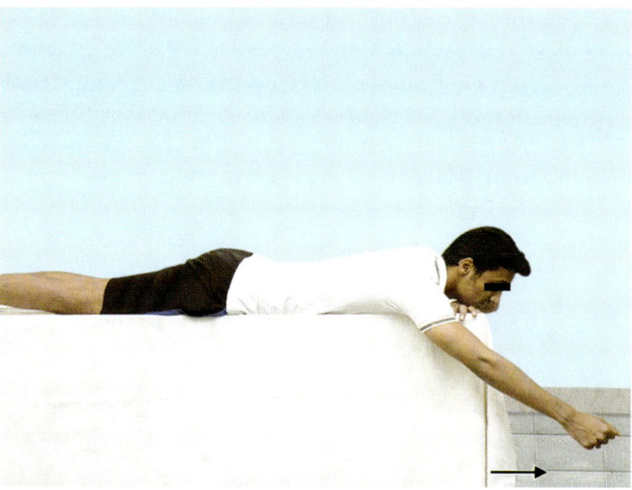

Fig. 19.17: Pendulum exercises without weight performed in prone position to neuromodulate pain and provide range of motion to gelnohumeral joint.

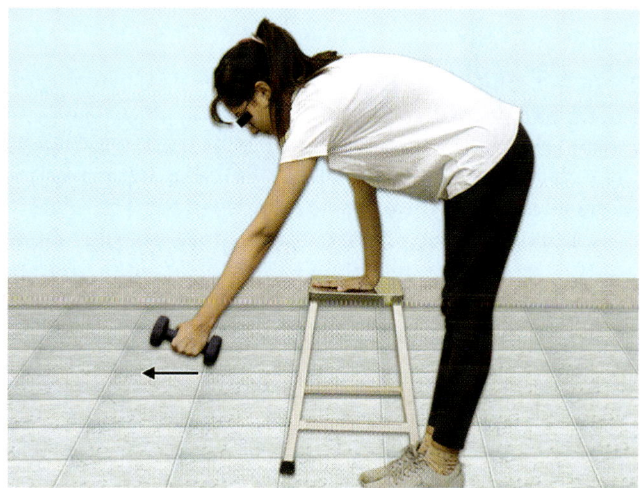

Fig. 19.18: Weighted pendulum exercises.

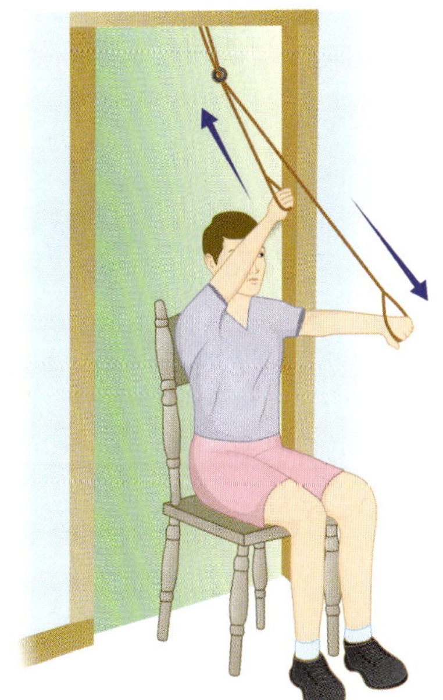

Fig. 19.19: Pulley exercises for shoulder flexion.

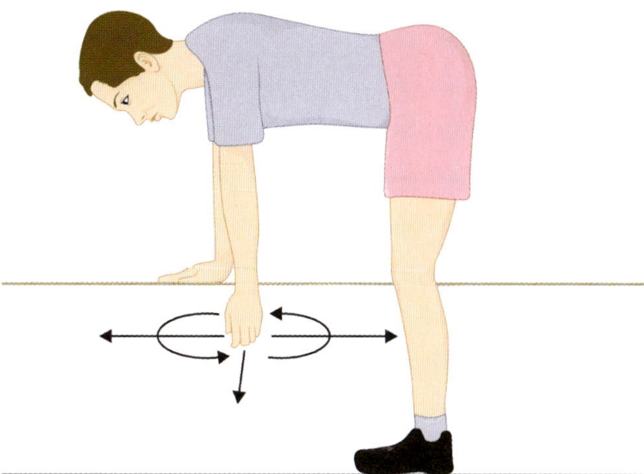

Fig. 19.16: Pendulum exercises in standing.

2. **Shoulder abduction (Fig. 19.20):**
   - The patient sits sideways.
   - The pulley handles are grasped and the patient pulls the injured arm up to the side as high as possible. The patient is instructed to pull down with the good arm. This will help to raise the injured arm.
   - Hold, relax and repeat.
3. **Shoulder internal rotation (Fig. 19.21):**
   - The patient stands with the back toward the pulleys.
   - The patient tries to reach over the head with the good arm and tries to grasp the handle.
   - The patient tries to reach behind the back with the injured arm (as if trying to touch the spine with the thumb) and grasps the other handle.
- The patient is then asked to pull down with the good arm and hold. This should pull the injured arm further up the back.
- Relax and repeat.

Active Assisted Range of Motion Exercises

Shoulder Wand Exercises

- **Wand exercise, flexion:** The patient stands upright and holds a stick in both hands, palms down. He/she is asked to stretch the arms by lifting them over the head, keeping the arms straight. Hold for 5 seconds in that position and return to the starting position. Repeat 10 times seperately for flexion to internal rotation **(Figs. 19.22A to D)**.
- **Wand exercise, extension:** The patient stands upright and holds a stick in both hands behind the back. The patient is instructed to move the stick away from the back. Hold this position for 5 seconds. Relax and return to the starting position. Repeat 10 times.
- **Wand exercise, external rotation:** The patient stands upright and holds a stick in both hands, shoulder by the side of the trunk and elbow at 90° flexion. He is asked to use the uninjured arm to push the injured arm out away from your body. The elbow of the injured arm is kept at the side while it is being pushed. Hold the stretch for 5 seconds. Repeat 10 times.
- **Wand exercise, internal rotation:** The patient stands upright and holds a stick in both hands, shoulder by the side of the trunk and elbow at 90° flexion. The patient is asked to pull the stick with the uninjured arm and the injured arm is pulled toward the body. Hold this position for 5 seconds and then go back to the starting position. Repeat 10 times.
- **Wand exercise, shoulder abduction, and adduction:** The patient stands and holds a stick with both hands, palms facing away from the body. The stick is rested against the front of the thighs. The uninjured arm is used to push the injured arm out to the side and up as high as possible. Keep the arms straight. Hold for 5 seconds. Repeat 10 times.

Self-glide Exercises to Improve Mobility

Various positions can be assumed as shown in **Figures 19.23 A to C** to improve the gliding of the shoulder joint (GH joint).

Stretching Exercises

Posterior Shoulder Capsule Stretch

The following steps need to be followed for posterior shoulder capsule stretch:
- The involved arm is brought across in front of body as shown **(Fig. 19.24)**.
- The elbow is held with the other arm.
- The patient is asked to gently pull the arm across the chest until a stretch is felt in the back of shoulder.

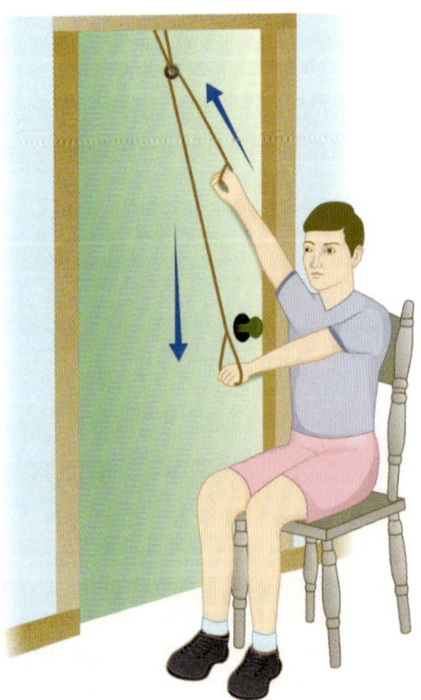

Fig. 19.20: Pulley exercises for shoulder abduction.

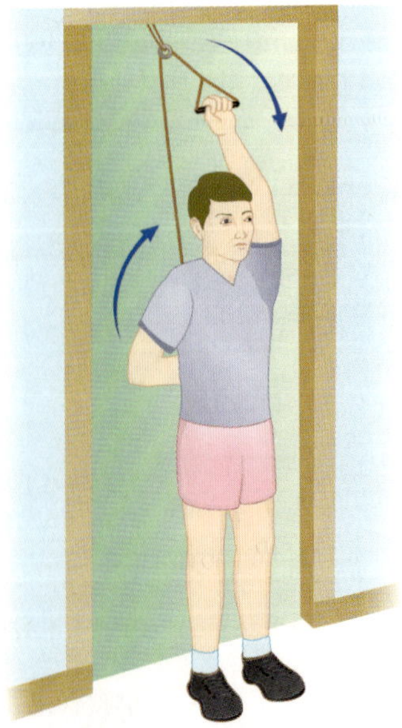

Fig. 19.21: Pulley exercises for rotation.

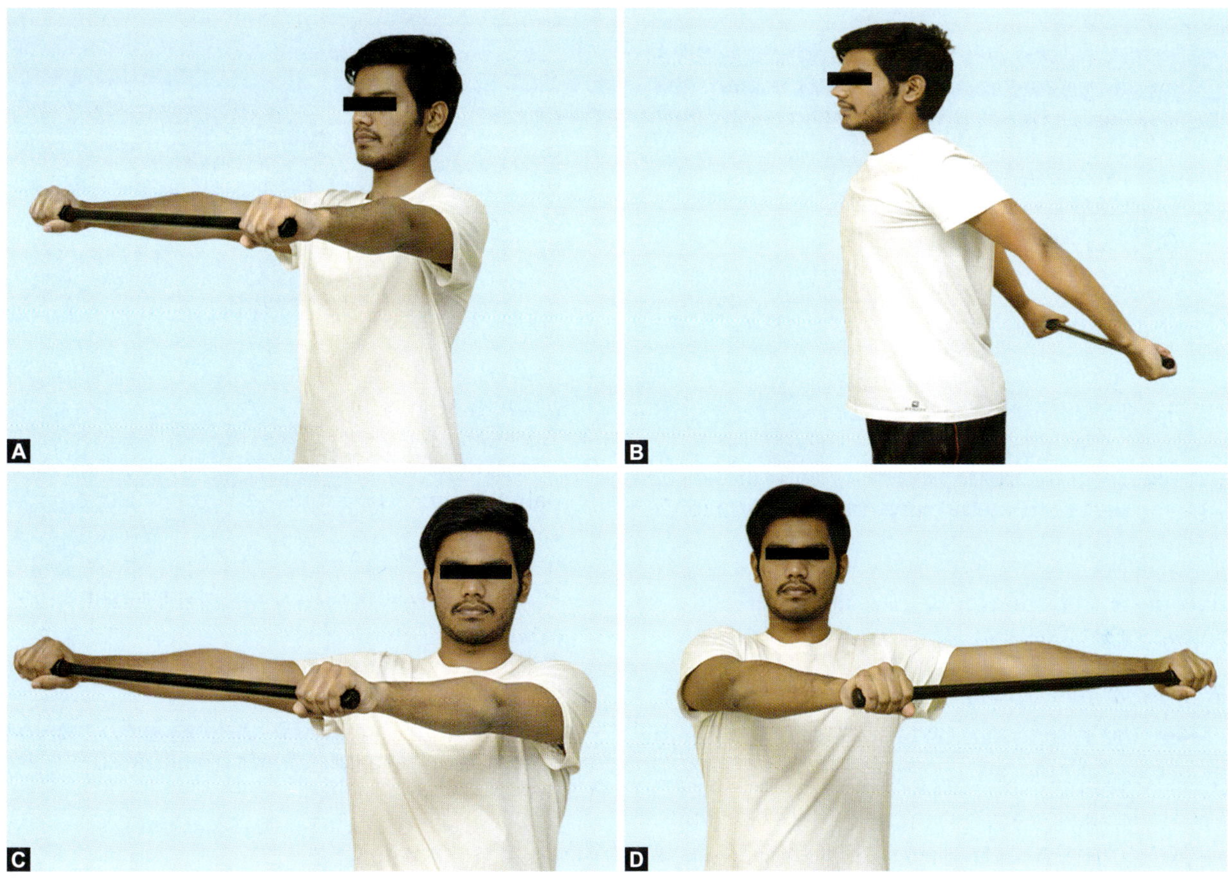

Figs. 19.22A to D: Wand exercises: (A) Flexion; (B) Extension; (C) Adduction; (D) Abduction.

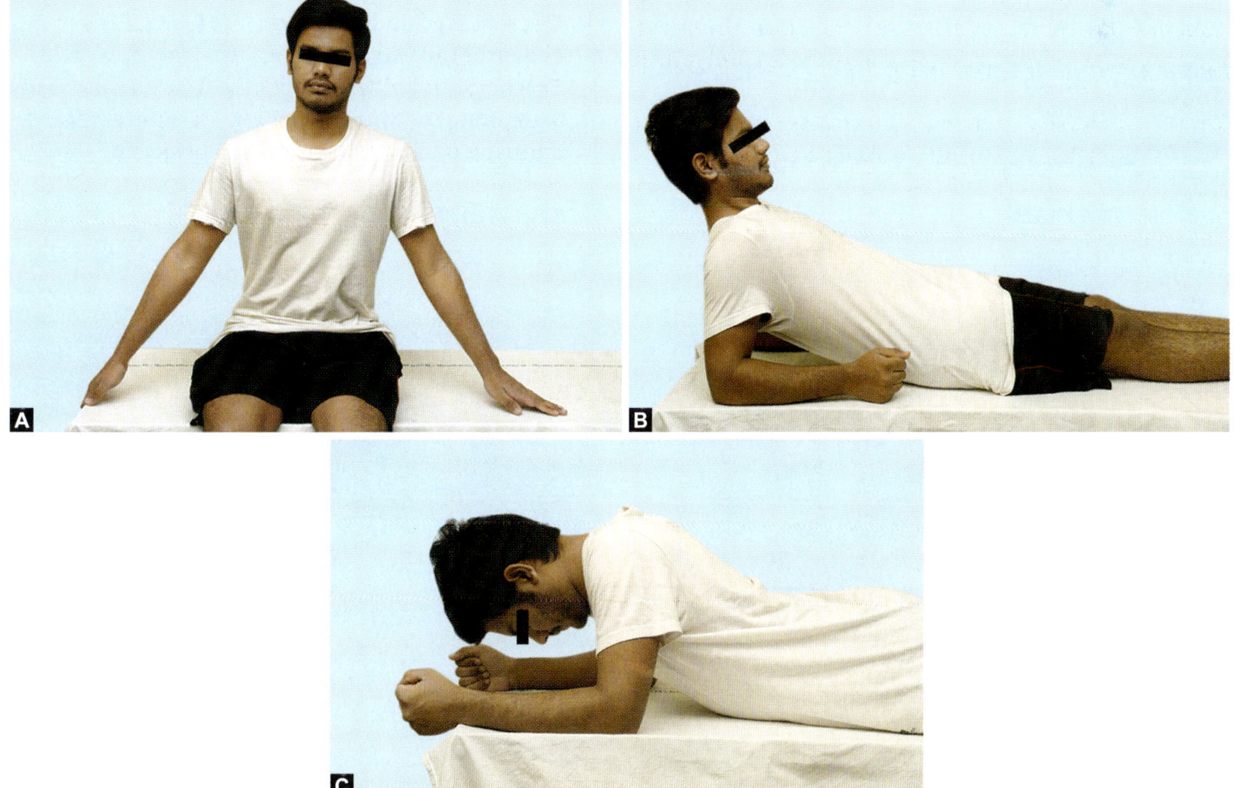

Figs. 19.23A to C: Self-glide exercises. (A) Inferior; (B) Anterior glide; (C) Posterior glide.

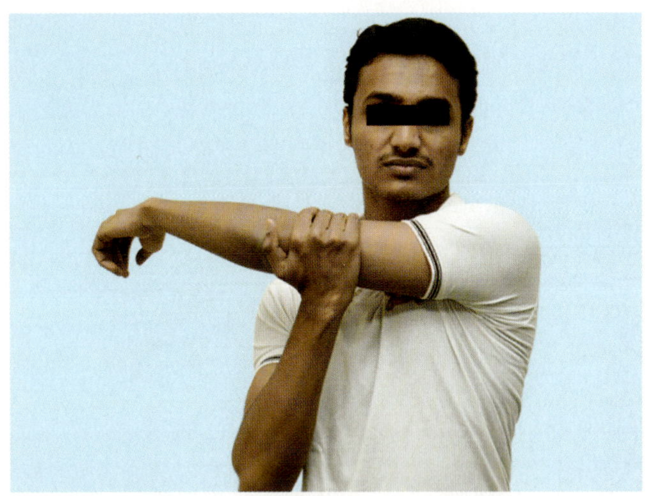

Fig. 19.24: Posterior capsule stretching.

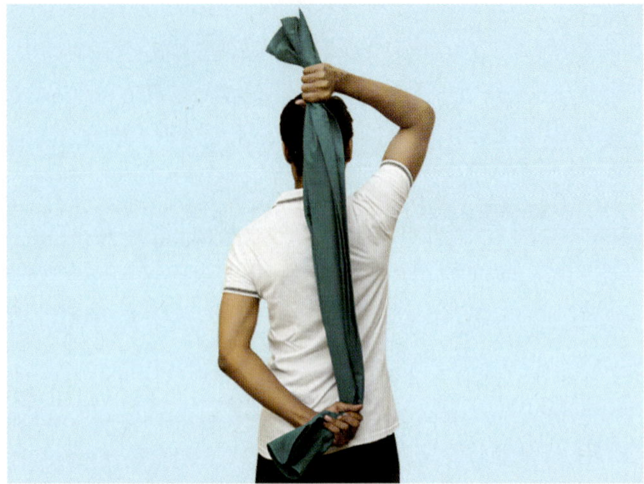

Fig. 19.26: Towel stretch.

- Hold the end position for 10–15 seconds.
- Repeat for 5–6 times.

Inferior Shoulder Capsule Stretches

The following steps need to be followed for inferior shoulder capsule stretches:
- The involved arm is raised over and behind the head with the elbow bent **(Fig. 19.25)**.
- The elbow or wrist of involved arm is grasped with the uninvolved arm.
- The patient is asked to pull gently until a stretch is felt.
- Hold the end position for 10–15 seconds.
- Repeat for 5–6 times.

Shoulder Internal Rotation with Towel Stretch—Behind Backstretch

The following steps need to be followed:
- The involved arm is placed behind back as far as possible **(Fig. 19.26)**.

- The other arm is held over the shoulder with the towel as shown.
- The patient is asked to grasp the towel with the involved arm.
- The patient is then asked to slowly pull upward with uninvolved arm until a gentle stretch is felt.
- Hold, relax, and repeat.
- Hold the end position for 20–30 seconds.
- Repeat for 5–6 times.

Pectorals Stretch—Standing at the Corner

The following steps need to be followed:
- The patient stands in a corner **(Fig. 19.27)**.
- The arms are placed at chest level on the wall.
- The patient is asked to gently step forward, keeping back straight.
- Then the patient returns to start position.
- Hold the end position for 20–30 seconds.
- Repeat for 5–6 times.

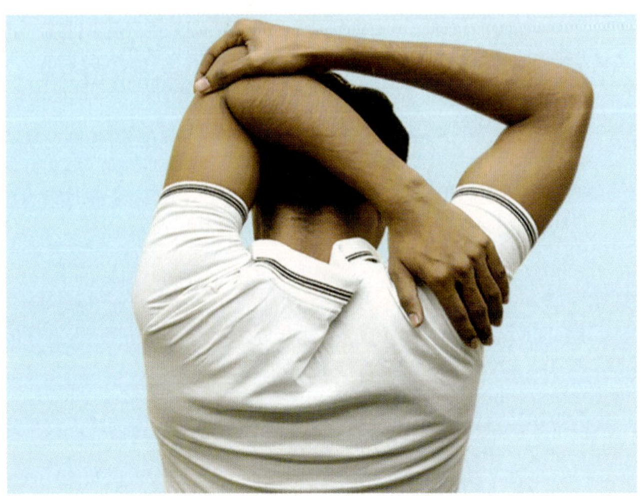

Fig. 19.25: Inferior capsule stretching.

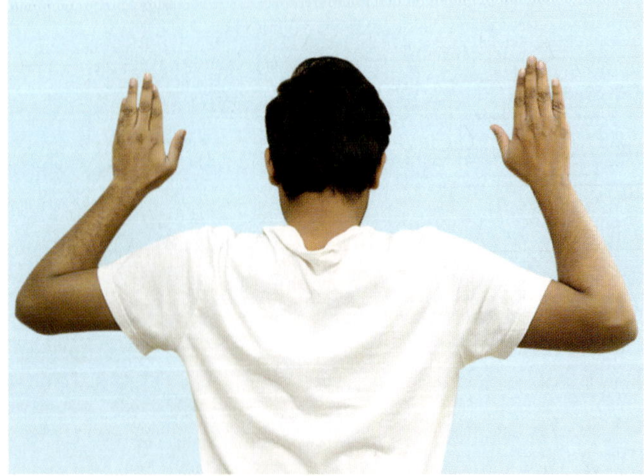

Fig. 19.27: Pectoral stretching.

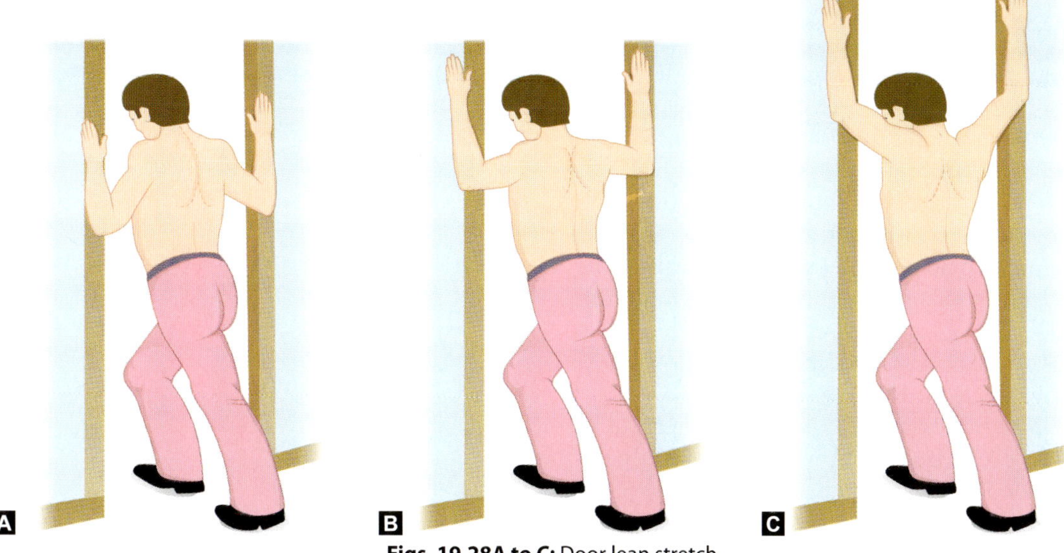

Figs. 19.28A to C: Door lean stretch.

Door Lean

Follow the below steps:

- The patient stands in front of a doorway placing both arms on the wall slightly above the head **(Figs. 19.28A to C)**.
- The patient is asked to slowly press the body in the forward direction until one feels a stretch in the front shoulder.
- Hold for 15–30 seconds.
- Repeat this three times.

Shoulder External Rotation Stretch at Doorway

Follow the below steps:

- The patient stands at the edge of the doorway **(Figs. 19.29A and B)**.
- The arms are kept at the side with the elbow bent to 90°.

- The hand of the involved arm is placed on the door frame.
- The patient is asked to slowly turn away from the doorway until a gentle stretch is felt.
- Hold end position for 10–15 seconds.
- Repeat for 5–6 times.

Shoulder Stretch

Follow the below steps:

- The patient is asked to squeeze the shoulder blades back and together **(Fig. 19.30)**.
- Hold for 5 seconds.
- Then the patient is asked to pull the shoulder blades downward.
- Hold for 5 seconds.
- Relax and repeat 10 times.

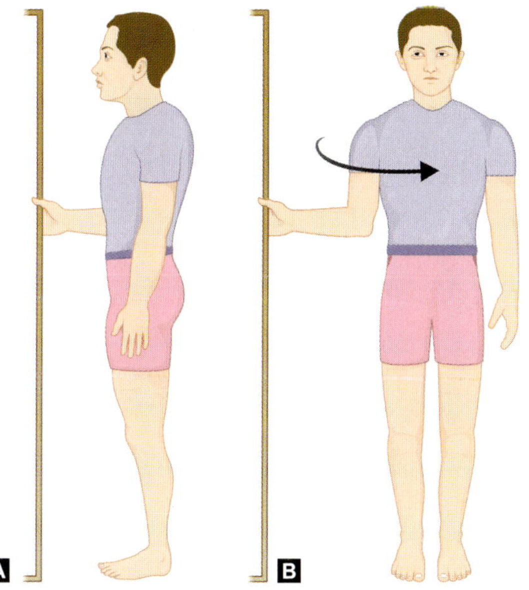

Figs. 19.29A and B: Shoulder external rotation stretching.

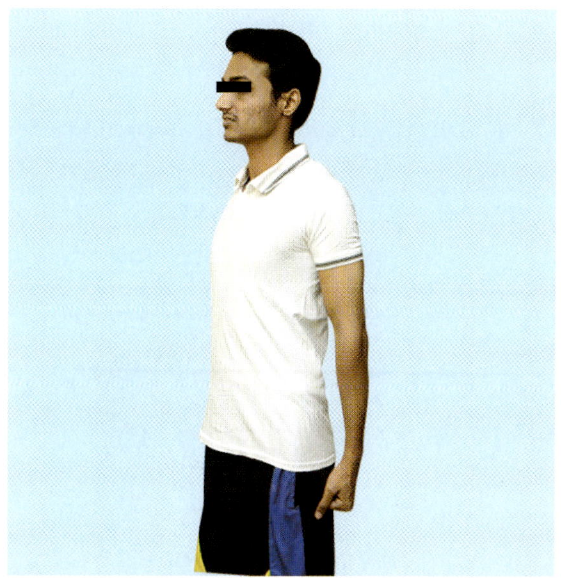

Fig. 19.30: Shoulder stretch.

Strengthening Exercises

Shoulder Isometric Exercises

Isometric Shoulder Flexion

One should follow the below steps:
- To start with shoulder flexion, the patient stands facing a wall **(Fig. 19.31)**.
- He/she is asked to bend the elbow of the shoulder that is to be exercised and make a fist.
- A folded towel is placed between the fist and the wall, and the patient is asked to gently press the hand into the wall.
- Hold for 5 seconds, and then slowly release.
- Repeat the exercise for 10–15 times.

It should be kept in mind that there is no need to try to push the wall over. The patient just presses gently into the wall to activate the shoulder muscles. This is especially important if one is just starting isometric exercise after shoulder surgery. If the exercise causes pain, then the exercise should be stopped.

Shoulder Abduction Isometric Exercise

One should follow the below steps:
- The patient stands about 6 inches from a wall, turning the body so it is perpendicular to the wall **(Fig. 19.32)**.
- The shoulder to be exercised should be close to the wall.
- The patient makes a fist and presses it into the wall.
- One may wish to use a folded up towel for a little extra comfort. The patient gently presses into the wall as if you are trying to lift the arm out to the side.
- Hold it there for 5 seconds.
- Slowly release pressure on the wall. Again, no need to push the wall over; gentle pressure will do.
- Repeat the exercise 10–15 times.

Isometric Shoulder External Rotation

Follow the below-mentioned steps:
- Isometric shoulder external rotation is an exercise that can help strengthen the RC muscles, specifically teres minor and infraspinatus **(Fig. 19.33)**.

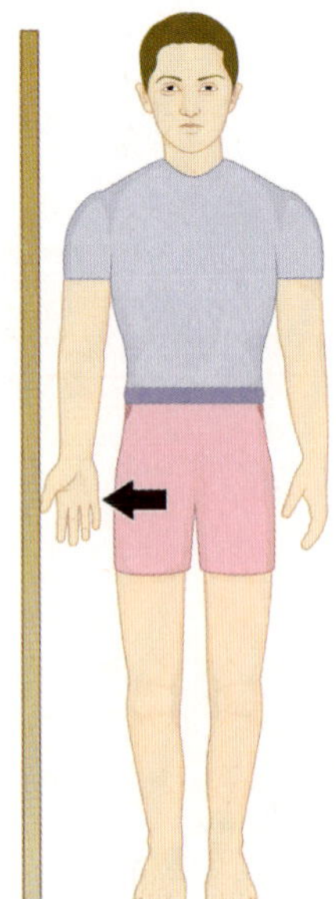

Fig. 19.32: Isometric shoulder abduction exercise.

- The patient stands perpendicular to a wall about 6 inches from it. The shoulder to be exercised should be closest to the wall.
- The elbow is bent to 90°, the patient makes a fist and is asked to press the back of the hand into the wall as if rotating the arm outward. A small towel can be used for a little padding, if needed.
- The patient is asked to gently press into the wall for about 5 seconds.
- Slowly release pressure on the wall.
- The exercise is stopped if any increased pain is felt.
- Repeat the exercise 10–15 times.

Isometric Shoulder Internal Rotation

Follow the below-mentioned steps:
- To perform isometric shoulder internal rotation, the body is positioned so that the patient is facing an outside corner of a wall or facing a door frame **(Fig. 19.34)**.

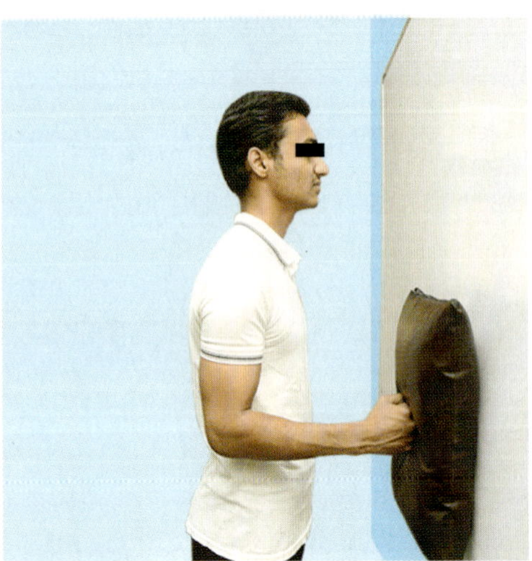

Fig. 19.31: Isometric shoulder flexion exercise.

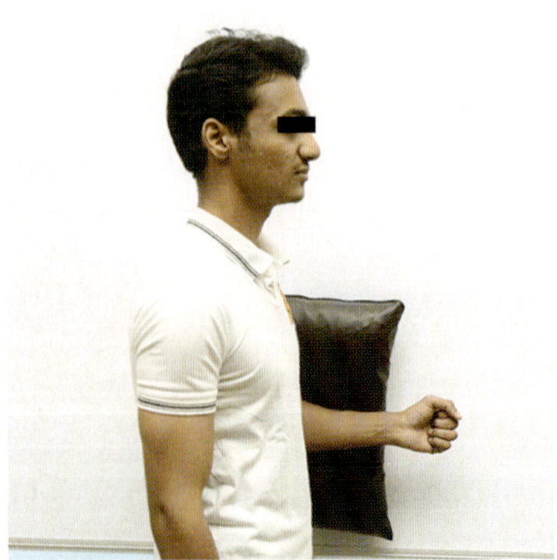

Fig. 19.33: Isometric shoulder external rotation.

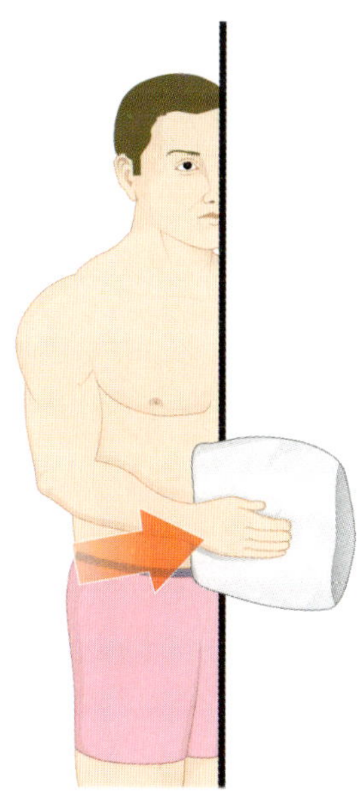

Fig. 19.34: Isometric shoulder internal rotation.

- The patient should be facing the wall, and the shoulder that is being exercised should be near the door opening or corner of the wall.
- The patient is asked to bend the elbow 90°, make a fist, and gently press into the corner wall or door jamb as if trying to rotate the hand inward toward the belly button.
- It is important to remember that no motion should occur in the shoulder during the exercise. A small folded towel can be used for padding.
- Press and hold for 5 seconds, and then slowly release.
- Repeat 10–15 repetitions.

Isometric Shoulder Extension

Follow the below-mentioned steps:

- To perform isometric shoulder extension, the patient stands about 6 inches away from a wall with the back facing it **(Fig. 19.35)**.
- The patient keeps the elbow straight so the hand is down near the hip.

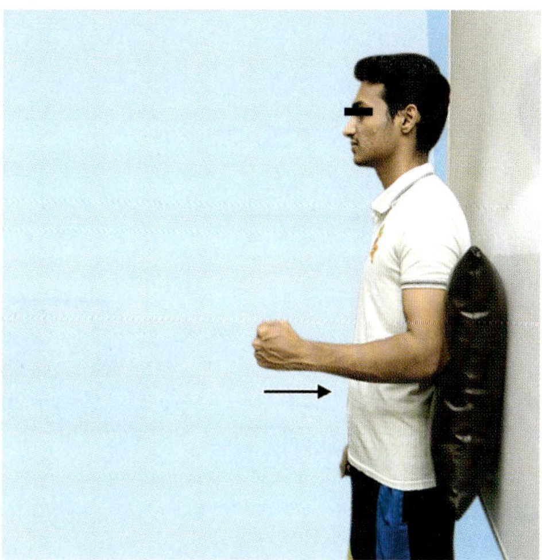

Fig. 19.35: Isometric shoulder extension exercise.

- The patient is asked to make a fist and gently press it into the wall behind him/her.
- One should remember that very little motion should occur at the shoulder.
- Hold the pressure against the wall for 5 seconds and then release slowly.
- Repeat the exercise 10–15 times.
  - Shoulder isometrics can be performed up to three times per day, but the physical therapist should decide the frequency based on the specific condition and the duration of the problem.
  - Once the patient starts regaining shoulder muscle activation, one can progress to shoulder isometrics with dynamic resistance.

Shoulder Strengthening with Mechanical Resistance

Shoulder Rotator Cuff and Scapular Strengthening Program

External rotation:

- The Theraband is attached at waist level to a doorknob or post **(Figs. 19.36A and B)**.
- The patient is asked to stand sideways to the door and facing straight ahead.
- Feet should be kept shoulder width apart and the knees are kept slightly flexed.
- The elbow is placed next to the side with the hand as close to the chest as possible (the patient can think of the elbow as being a hinge on a gate).
- The patient grasps one end of the band and is asked to pull the band all the way through until it is taut.
- The patient is asked to take the cord in the hand, "set" the shoulder blade and move the hand away from the body as far as it feels comfortable.
- Return to the start position.

Internal rotation (Figs. 19.37A and B):

- The Theraband is attached at waist level in a doorknob or post.

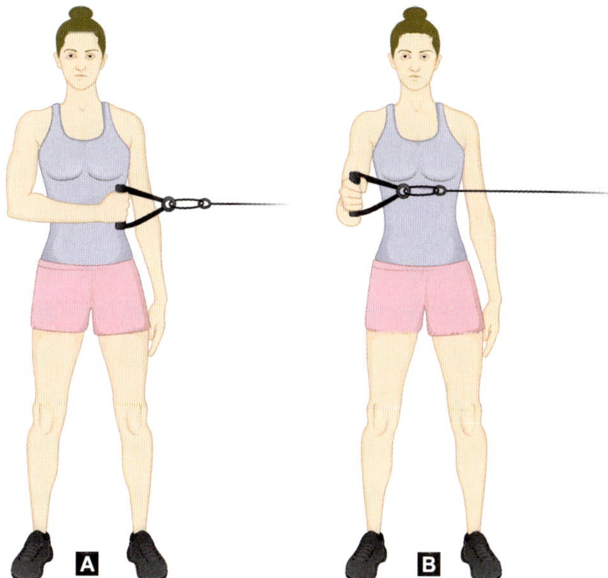

Figs. 19.36A and B: Strengthening of external rotators using Theraband.

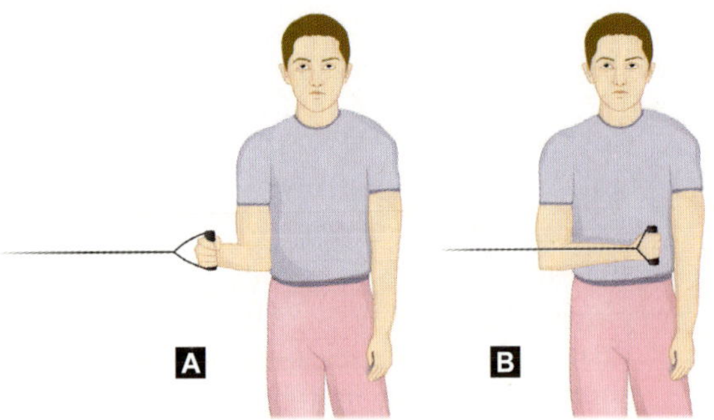

Figs. 19.37A and B: Strengthening using internal rotators using Theraband.

- The patient stands sideways to the door and looks straight ahead.
- Feet are kept shoulder width apart and the knees are slightly flexed.
- The elbow is placed next to the side and is flexed at 90° (think of this elbow as being a hinge on a gate).
- The patient grasps one end of the handle and pulls the cord all the way through until it is taut.
- Taking the cord in the hand, "set" the shoulder blade and move the hand toward the belly as far as it feels comfortable, or to where the endpoint of pain limits you.
- Return to the start position.

Lateral raises (Figs. 19.38A and B):
- The patient stands with the arm at the side with the elbow straight and the hands rotated so that the thumbs face forward.
- The patient is asked to raise the arm straight out to the side, palm down, until the hands reach shoulder level.
- One should remember not to raise the hands higher than the shoulder.
- A pause is given and the patient is asked to slowly lower the arm.

Standing forward flexion ("full-can") exercise (Fig. 19.39):
- The patient stands facing a mirror with the hands rotated so that the thumbs face forward.

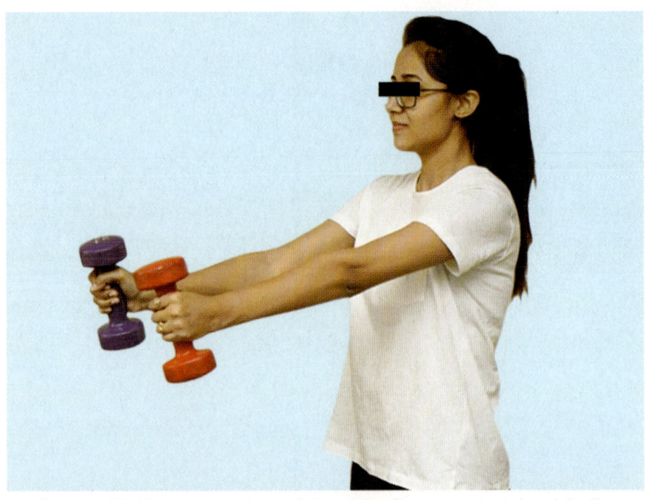

Fig. 19.39: Strengthening of shoulder flexors using dumbbells.

- While keeping the shoulder blade "set" and keeping the elbows straight, the patient is asked to raise the arms forward and upward to shoulder level with a slight outward angle (30°).
- The patient is asked to pause for 1 second and slowly lower and repeat.

Side-lying external rotation (Fig. 19.40):
- Lying on the nonoperated or unaffected side, the patient is asked to bend the elbow to a 90° angle and keep the operated or affected arm firmly against the side with the hand resting on the abdomen.
- By rotation at the shoulder, the patient raises the hand upward, toward the ceiling through a comfortable ROM.
- Hold this position for 1–2 seconds.
- Slowly lower the hand.

Prone extension (Fig. 19.41):
- The starting position for this exercise is that the patient bends over at the waist so that the affected arm is hanging freely straight down.
- Alternatively, the patient is asked to lie face down on the bed with the operated/affected arm hanging freely off of the side.

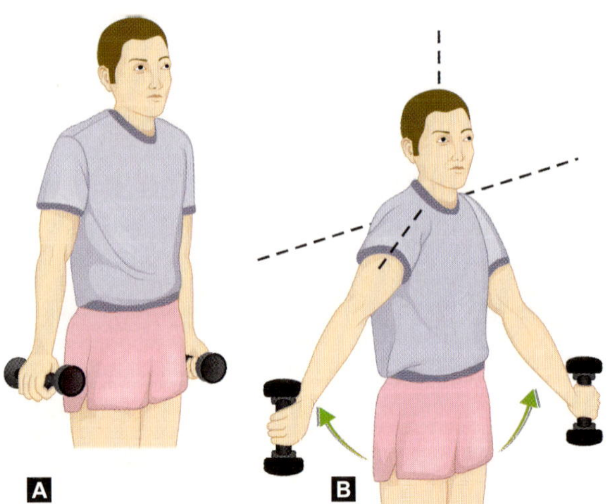

Figs. 19.38A and B: Lateral raises.

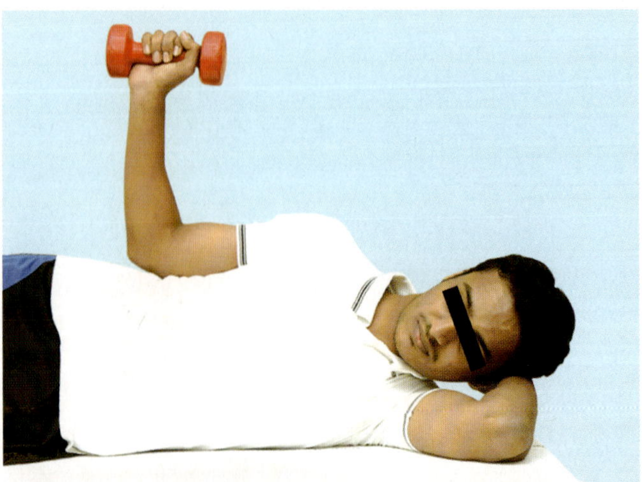

Fig. 19.40: Strengthening of external rotators in side-lying position.

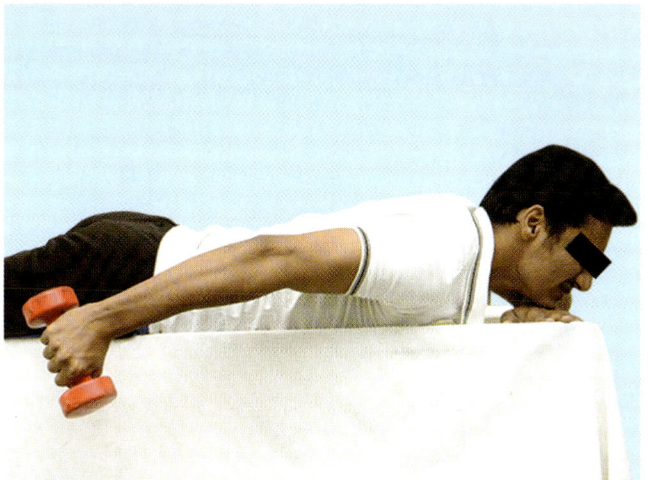

Fig. 19.41: Strengthening of shoulder extensors in prone lying.

- While keeping the shoulder blade "set" and keeping the elbow straight, the patient is asked to raise the arm backward toward the hip with the thumb pointing outward.
- The patient is asked not to lift the hand past the level of the hip.

Prone rowing exercise (Fig. 19.42):
- The starting position for this exercise is the patient is asked to bend over at the waist so that the affected arm is hanging freely straight down.
- Alternatively, patient is asked to lie face down on the bed with the operated/affected arm hanging freely off the side of the plinth.
- While keeping the shoulder blade "set," the patient is asked to raise the arm toward the ceiling while bending at the elbow. The patient is asked to draw the elbow along the side of the body until the hands touch the lower ribs.
- The patient is instructed to always return slowly to the start position.

Prone horizontal abduction ("Ts") (Fig. 19.43):
- The starting position for this exercise is to ask the patient to bend over at the waist so that the affected arm is hanging freely straight down.

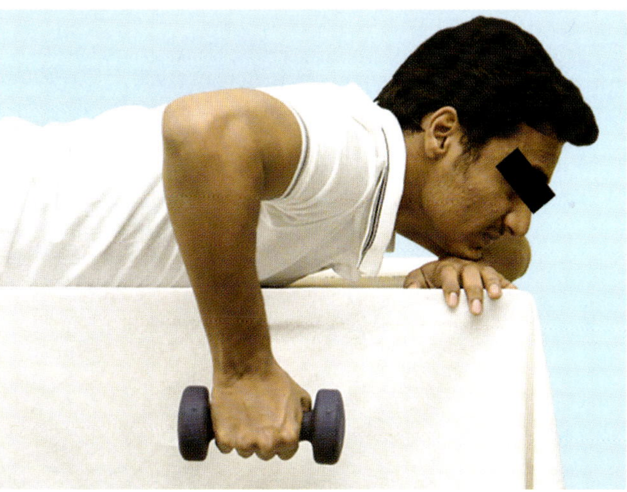

Fig. 19.43: Horizontal abductors strengthening in prone lying.

- Alternatively, the patient is asked to lie face down on the bed with the operated/affected arm hanging freely off the side.
- The hand is rotated so that the thumb faces forward.
- The patient is asked to keep the shoulder blade "set" and the elbows straight.
- The patient is then instructed to slowly raise the arm away from the body to shoulder height, through a pain-free ROM (so that the hand now has the thumb facing forward and aligned with the cheek).
- Hold that position for 1–2 seconds and slowly lower.
- The height of the raise of the arm is limited to 90°, or in other words, horizontal to the floor.

Prone scaption ("Ys") (Fig. 19.44):
- The starting position for this exercise is to ask the patient to bend over at the waist so that the affected arm is hanging freely straight down.
- Alternatively, the patient is asked to lie face down on the plinth with the operated/affected arm hanging freely off the side.
- The patient is instructed to keep the shoulder blade "set" and the elbows straight.
- The patient is asked to slowly raise the arm away from the body and slightly forward through a pain-free ROM

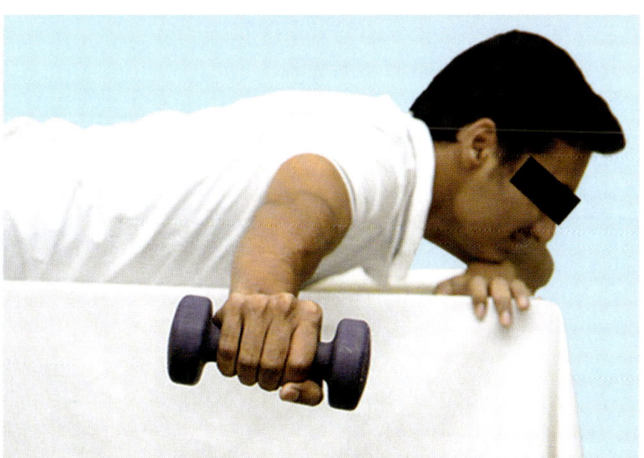

Fig. 19.42: Prone rowing exercises.

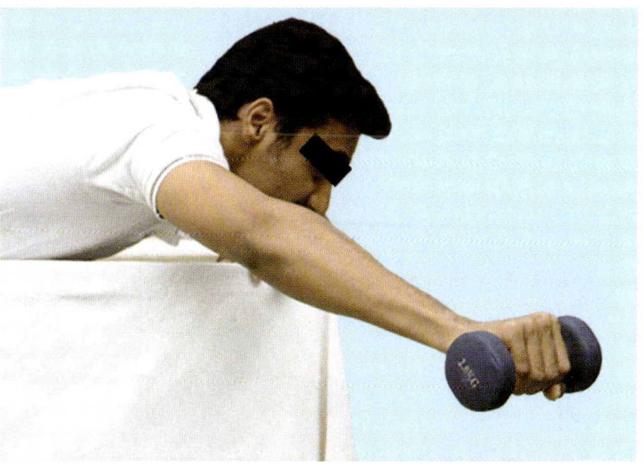

Fig. 19.44: Prone scaption exercise.

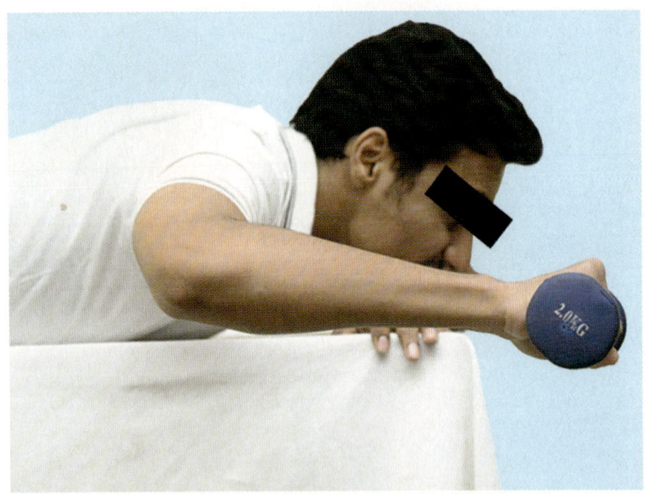

Fig. 19.45: Prone external rotation at 90° abduction.

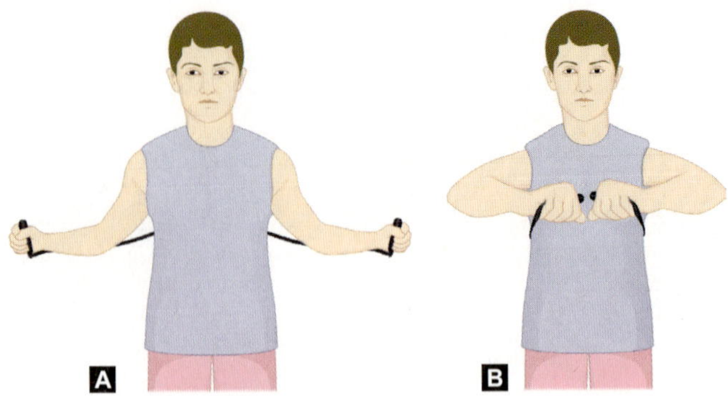

Figs. 19.47A and B: Dynamic hug exercises.

(so that the hand now has the thumb facing up, and is aligned with the forehead).

- Hold that position for 1–2 seconds and slowly lower.
- The height to raise the arm is limited to 90°, or in other words, horizontal to the floor and not more.

Prone external rotation at 90° abduction ("Us") (Fig. 19.45):

- The patient is asked to lie face down on a table with the arm hanging over the side of the table.
- He/she is then asked to raise the arm to shoulder height at a 90° angle to the body.
- While holding the arm in this position, the patient is asked to rotate the hand upward, until the hand is even with the elbow.
- Hold 1 second and then ask the patient to slowly let the hand rotate to the starting position and repeat.

"Ws" (Fig. 19.46):

- With the tubing attached in front, the patient stands with the tubing in both hands with the elbows bent at 90° and fixed at the side.

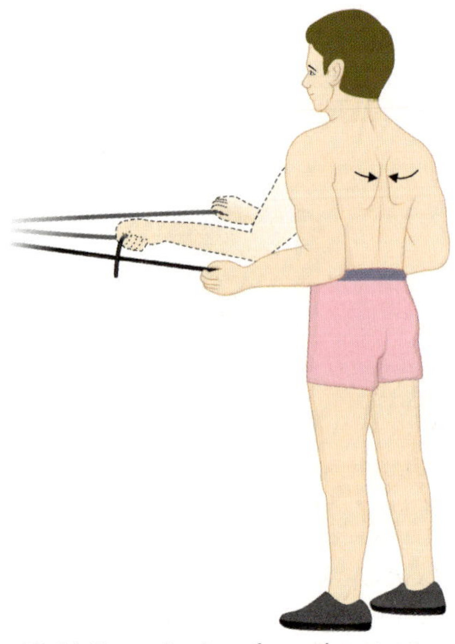

Fig. 19.46: Strengthening of scapular retractors.

- The patient is asked to pull the band outward, keeping the elbow at the side.
- The arms of the patient rotate outward making the shape of a "W."

Dynamic hug (Figs. 19.47A and B):

- The tubing is attached behind the patient at shoulder height.
- The patient is asked to grip both ends of the tubing in the hands with the tubing on the outside of the patient's shoulders.
- The patient is instructed to pull the band forward and slightly downward in a "hugging" motion or as if wrapping both arms around a small tree.
- Pause and return slowly to the starting position.

Scapular Stabilization Exercises

Scapular dysfunction might occur in response to inappropriate or deficient training habits, traumatic injury; microtrauma-induced muscle strains that affect normal scapulohumeral rhythm, or inhibition caused by shoulder pathology. Stability of the ST joint depends on coordinated activity of the surrounding musculature. The scapular muscles must dynamically position the glenoid so that efficient GH movement can occur. When weakness or dysfunction of the scapular musculature is present, normal scapular positioning and mechanics may become altered. When the scapula fails to perform its stabilization role, shoulder complex function is inefficient, which can result not only in decreased neuromuscular performance but also may predispose the individual to injury of the GH joint. As the patient's scapular neuromuscular control improves, open-chain scapular stabilization exercises may be initiated. Adding open-chain exercises can increase the endurance capacity of selected muscles, and they can be performed incorporating the entire kinetic chain.

Exercise 1: Blackburn prone horizontal scaption Ts (Fig. 19.48A).

- Neutral: The patient is asked to lie face down on the table, with a towel under the forehead for support.
- The patient starts with arms hanging straight down with palms facing in.

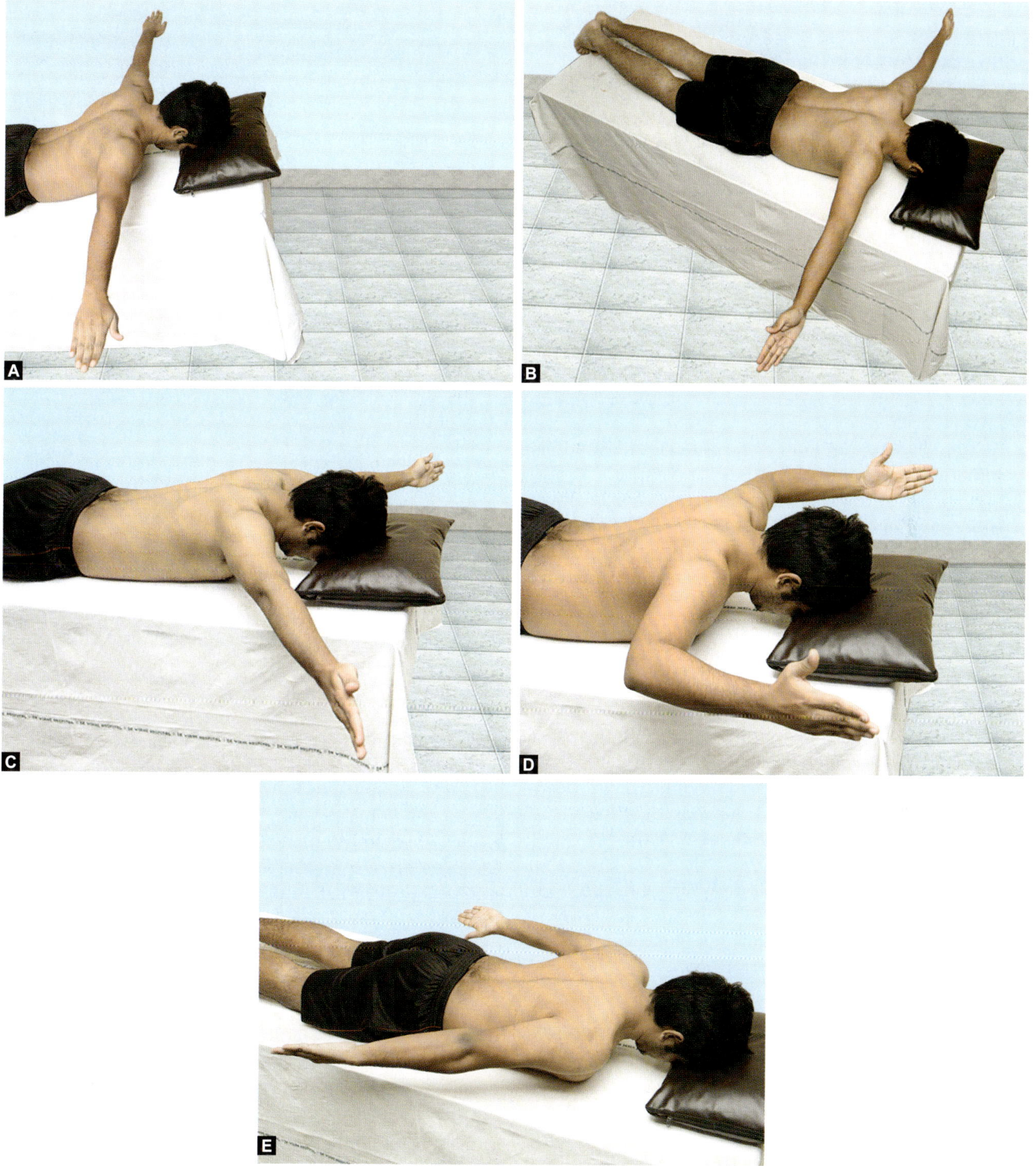

Figs. 19.48A to E: Scapular stabilization exercises (Blackburn exercises 1-5).

- The patient is asked to raise arms straight up to the side and return back slowly.
- The patient is instructed not to extend beyond the level of the shoulder/back and not to swing arms.
- 2–3 sets of 10–15 reps are performed.

Exercise 2: Blackburn prone horizontal scaption Ts **(Fig. 19.48B)**.

- Thumb up: The patient is asked to lie face down on table, with towel under the forehead for support.
- The patient starts with arms hanging straight down with palms facing toward head.
- The patient is asked to raise arms straight up to the side with thumb toward the ceiling and not move beyond the shoulder level.

- The patient is instructed to return slowly and not swing arms.
- 2–3 sets of 10–15 reps are performed.

Exercise 3: Blackburn prone horizontal scaption Ys **(Fig. 19.48C).**

- Neutral: The patient is asked to lie face down on the table, with the towel under the forehead for support.
- The patient starts with arms hanging straight down with palms facing in.
- The patient is asked to raise arms up at a 45° angle making a "Y" with palms facing the ground and not to move beyond the shoulder level.
- The patient is asked to return slowly and not swing arms.
- 2–3 sets of 10–15 reps are performed.

Exercise 4: Blackburn prone horizontal scaption Ws **(Fig. 19.48D).**

- Thumb up: The patient lies face down on the table, with the towel under the forehead for support.
- The patient starts with arms hanging straight down with palms facing toward head.
- The patient is asked to raise arms straight up to the side with the thumb toward the ceiling and not move beyond the shoulder level.
- He/she is asked to return slowly and not swing arms.
- 2–3 sets of 10–15 reps are performed.

Exercise 5: Blackburn prone horizontal extension **(Fig. 19.48E).**

- The patient lies face down on a table, with the towel under the forehead for support.
- The patient starts with arms hanging straight down with palms facing away from the body.
- The patient is asked to raise arms behind into extension, with thumbs facing the ground.
- The patient is instructed not to move beyond body level.
- He/she is asked to return slowly and not swing arms.
- 2–3 sets of 10–15 reps are performed.

Wall Ball Circles

This is a very effective close chain exercise for improving the stability of scapular muscles and proprioception **(Fig. 19.49).**

- The patient is asked to stand facing a flat wall.
- With feet–shoulder width apart, he/she is then instructed to extend one hand forward and press a medicine ball up against the wall with a flat palm about shoulder height off the ground.
- The patient is also instructed to not let the ball drop.
- Using palm only, the patient then rolls the ball around in small circles both clockwise and counter-clockwise.

Proprioceptive Exercises

Conditions that may Require Weight-bearing Shoulder Exercises

People with certain conditions may benefit from shoulder weight-bearing and balance exercises in quadruped or in

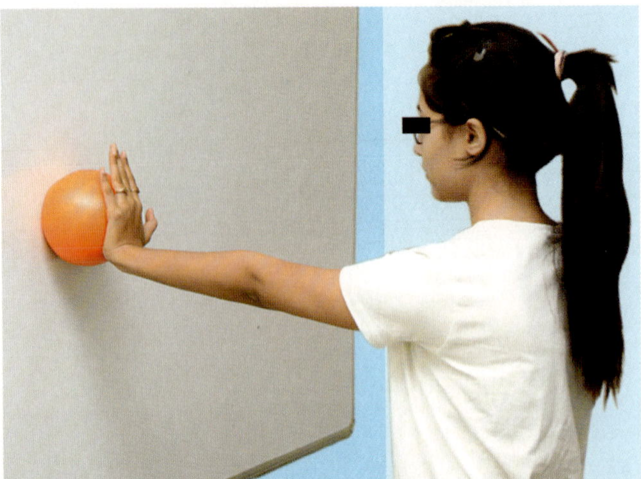

Fig. 19.49: Wall ball circles.

the plank position. Any upper extremity injury or condition may cause limitation of balance and proprioception in the shoulder or arm. The physiotherapist may recommend the patient exercises to improve the overall balance through the arms during rehab. Working on specific exercises to improve upper extremity proprioception can help the patient regain normal use of the arm. The physical therapist may choose to use various exercises and exercise progression to help recovery after a shoulder or arm injury or surgery.

Exercising the shoulders in a quadruped or weight-bearing position, such as a plank, activates muscles around the RC and shoulder blade. These muscles work when a person lifts the arms overhead or during activities that require one to push or pull something. They may become impaired after an injury or surgery around the shoulder that requires a period of immobilization. During this immobilization time, the shoulder or arm may be healing, but it may also be losing strength, the ROM, and proprioception.

Shoulder Exercise Progression in a Weight-bearing Position

If a physical therapist chooses to prescribe weight-bearing shoulder and arm exercises, he or she will likely follow a progressive program. The progress is from simple to more advanced exercises.

Before starting with weight-bearing shoulder exercises, the therapist should ensure that the shoulder strength and stability are adequate enough for the patient to bear weight through the arm. The patient should be performing RC strengthening exercises with a resistance band and supine dynamic shoulder stabilization exercises before starting weight-bearing exercises as part of rehabilitation.

A typical progression of weight-bearing shoulder proprioception exercises may include **(Figs. 19.50A to D):**

1. **Quadruped weight shifts:** The patient is asked to get in a position of crawling. Then, they are instructed to rock slowly left and right and forward and backward for 30–60 seconds.

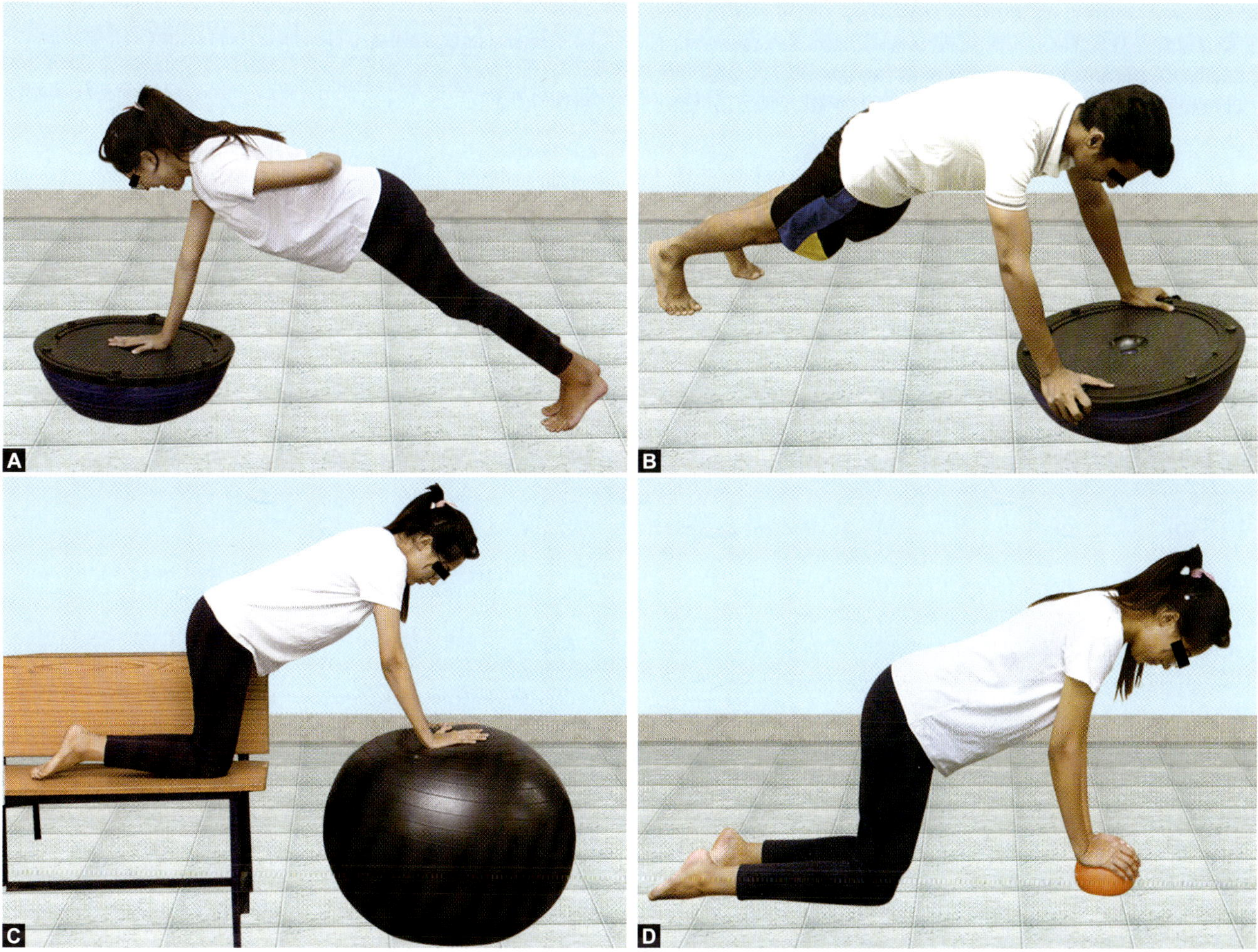

Figs. 19.50A to D: Various exercises to improve proprioception.

2. **Quadruped weight shifts on an unsteady surface:** The above exercise is repeated with a small pillow underneath the hand of the injured shoulder. Using a rubber ball under that hand can also increase the challenge of this exercise.

3. **Quadruped position with opposite arm motions:** The patient is in the quadruped position and is asked to lift the noninjured arm up until it is parallel to the floor. The patient has to hold this position for a few seconds and then return to the start position. About 10–15 repetitions can be done. The therapist and patient should make sure to keep the shoulder right over the hand while performing the exercise. One also needs to remember that the noninjured hand moves, so the shoulder that needs to be worked is bearing the body weight.

4. **Quadruped position with arm motion on an unsteady surface:** Exercise 3 above is performed with the hand on a pillow or small ball.

5. **Quadruped position on a biomechanical ankle platform system (BAPS) board:** A BAPS board for ankle proprioception can be used for upper extremity balance as well. The patient is asked to position the hands on the BAPS board and keep it steady while performing weight shifts in the quadruped position. This exercise can only be done in a physiotherapy clinic and not as a part of a home exercise program.

6. **Plank position weight shift:** Once the patient has gained adequate strength and stability, the patient can move away from the quadruped position and repeat the sequence in the plank position. Getting into the plank pose, the patient can then shift weight from side to side and forward and backward.

7. **Plank position on an unsteady surface:** The plank with weight shifts in Exercise 6 can be repeated while keeping the hand on an unsteady surface.

8. **Plank position on a BAPS board:** While keeping hands steady on a BAPS board, the patient can be asked to perform the plank position weights shifts.

9. **Bionic osscillatory stabilization unit (BOSU) Walkovers:** A BOSU can also be used for shoulder balance and proprioception training. The patient is asked to get in the plank position with hands on the BOSU, and then "step" sideways with one hand and then the other. The patient can also "walk" side to side over the BOSU with both hands. The therapist must make sure that the patient maintains a steady plank with abs engaged. About 10 repetitions of the lateral walkovers with the BOSU can be performed.

10. **Lateral upper extremity walking with resistance bands:** A resistance band is looped around the wrists, and the patient is asked to get in the plank position. The patient is then instructed to walk the hands sideways, keeping tension on the band as one goes. The therapist should ensure that the patient maintains a stable core by keeping the abs engaged, while he/she walks the hands sideways about 10 steps to the left and 10 to the right. The patient's feet are going to have to walk along sideways too.

Clinical Pearl

If any exercise causes pain, the PT should ensure that the patient is performing the exercise correctly and be sure that it is right for that patient.

The progression starts with a basic crawling position and progresses to advanced dynamic motions for the shoulders with resistance and on unsteady surfaces. The physical therapist should be able to decide when it is time to progress through each stage of the exercise progression.

Each patient may or may not be able to or need to make it through the entire progression. For some people, simple quadruped weight bearing is enough to improve shoulder balance and function. For other people, especially those who participate in high-level athletics, there may be a need to progress through to the advanced upper extremity exercises to fully recover.

SUMMARY

The shoulder is a complex structure comprising of three bones—humerus, clavicle, and scapula and three structural and one functional joint. It has greater mobility but less stability; as a result, it becomes vulnerable to greater trauma and injury and subsequent pathologies. Also, the greater mobility leads to a higher prevalence of overuse injuries. Assessment of each pathological condition is unique, and there can be no general outlook toward it. Provocative tests exist for each condition to confirm the diagnosis. Management in most cases is conservative, unless there is greater trauma and recurrence of the pathology. Surgical management is rarely required. Conservative management mainly focuses on pain relief and physical therapy. In addition to rehabilitation of the GH joint, it is essential to pay attention to the AC and SC joints as well. A comprehensive rehabilitation program focusing on pain relief, correction of any muscle imbalances, strengthening of the RC and other shoulder and scapular muscles, retraining of neuromuscular control, and proprioceptive exercises is of utmost importance to manage shoulder pathologies and reduce the chances of recurrence to a minimum.

Case Scenario

CASE STUDY

A 56-year-old male presents with a complaint of shoulder pain and inability to elevate the shoulder. The pain has been gradual in onset, increasing since the past 1 month. The limitation of movement has also become worse throughout the same period. The doctor consulted an orthopedician 2 days back, who advised him rest and analgesics. The pain has reduced after taking the medicines but the restriction persists.

- Past history—none
- Personal history—sleep disturbances due to pain
- Family history—none
- Medical history—diabetes mellitus since 5 years; on medications (metformin 500 mg/day) but currently under control
- Occupational history—bank clerk; desk job requiring him to work on the computer for 8–9 hours.

Examination

The following was examined:

- Pain—at the anterior and posterior aspect of shoulder, dull aching in character, aggravated by any shoulder movement and sleeping on affected side and relieved by rest and hot water fomentation, Visual Analog Scale score 7/10
- Posture—guarded posture with arm in adduction and internal rotation
- Tenderness—along the GH joint border (Grade II)
- Warmth and swelling—absent
- Tightness—pectoralis major and minor
- ROM testing—active and passive ROM both reduced for all the motions of shoulder
- Joint play of shoulder—hypomobility present at the GH joint in all directions
- End feel—capsular end feel for all movements
- Strength testing—reduced muscle strength of RC muscles and scapular muscles because of pain
- Functional assessment—patient having difficulty with overhead activities, dressing upper body, grooming, etc.

Guiding Questions:

1. What can be the possible diagnosis of the patient?
2. List out the impairments of the above-mentioned patient.
3. Write down the management plan for this patient.

Review Questions

1. Describe the assessment and management of a 64-year-old male presenting with frozen shoulder.
2. Explain the classification of shoulder instability.
3. Describe the assessment of osteoarthritis of the shoulder.
4. Write short notes on the following:
   a. Stages of frozen shoulder.
   b. Subacromial bursitis.
   c. Proprioceptive exercises for the shoulder.
   d. Kibler classification of scapular dysfunction.
   e. Neer's classification of rotator cuff pathology.

BIBLIOGRAPHY

1. Agarwal S, Raza S, Moiz JA, et al. Effects of two different mobilization techniques on pain, range of motion and functional disability in patients with adhesive capsulitis: a comparative study. J Phys Ther Sci. 2016;28(12):3342-49.
2. Arrigo G, Cesare AD, Safran MR, et al. Short-term effectiveness of hyperthermia for supraspinatus tendinopathy in athletes, a short-term randomized controlled study. Am J Sports Med. 2006;34(8): 1247-53. (Evidence level: 1B).
3. Aydin N, Sirin E, Arya A. Superior labrum anterior to posterior lesions of the shoulder: diagnosis and arthroscopic management. World J Orthop. 2014;5(3):344-50.
4. Brewster C, Schwab DR. Rehabilitation of the shoulder following rotator cuff injury or surgery. J Orthop Sports Phys Ther. 1993;18(2):422-6.
5. Cho HJ, Morey V, Kang JY, et al. Prevalence and risk factors of spine, shoulder, hand, hip, and knee osteoarthritis in community-dwelling Koreans older than age 65 years. Clin Orthop Relat Res. 2015;473(10):3307-14.
6. Cricchio M, Frazer C. Scapulothoracic and scapulohumeral exercises: a narrative review of electromyographic studies. J Hand Ther. 2011;24:322-34.
7. Davies GJ, Dickoff-Hoffman S. Neuromuscular testing and rehabilitation of the shoulder complex. J Orthop Sports Phys Ther. 1993;18:449-58.
8. Faruqi T, Rizvi TJ. Subacromial bursitis. In: StatPearls. Treasure Island, FL: StatPearls Publishing; 2019. [Internet] Available from https://www.ncbi.nlm.nih.gov/books/NBK541096/).
9. Fu FH, Harner CD, Klein AH. Shoulder impingement syndrome: a critical review. Clin. Orthop. 1991;269:162-73.
10. Gigliotti D, Xu MC, Davidson MJ, et al. Fibrosis, low vascularity, and fewer slow fibers after rotator-cuff injury. Muscle Nerve. 2017;55(5):715-26.
11. Gouttebarge V1, Inklaar H, Backx F, et al. Prevalence of osteoarthritis in former elite athletes: a systematic overview of the recent literature. Rheumatol Int. 2015;35(3):405-18.
12. Heiderscheit BC, McLean KP, Davies GJ. The effects of isokinetic vs. plyometric training on the shoulder internal rotators. J Orthop Sports Phys Ther. 1996;23:125-33.
13. Itoi E. Rotator cuff tear: physical examination and conservative treatment. J Orthop Sci. 2013;18(2):197-204. doi:10.1007/s00776-012-0345-2.
14. Kibler WB. Shoulder rehabilitation: principles and practice. Med Sci Sports Exerc. 1998;30(4 Suppl.):S40-50.
15. Kobayashi T, et al. Prevalence of and risk factors for shoulder osteoarthritis in Japanese middle-aged and elderly populations. J Shoulder Elbow Surg. 2014;23(5):613-9.
16. Kuhn JE, Lebus V GF, Bible JE. Thoracic outlet syndrome. J Am Acad Orthop Surg. 2015;23(4):222-32.
17. Lephart SM, Pincivero DM, Giraldo JL, et al. The role of proprioception in the management and rehabilitation of athletic injuries. Am J Sports Med. 1997;25(1):130-7.
18. Martin JK, Phillip WM, Brian GL. Frozen shoulder: evidence and a proposed model guiding rehabilitation. J Orthop Sports Phys Ther. 2009;39(2):135-48.
19. Milgrom C, Schaffler M, Gilbert S, et al. Rotator-cuff changes in asymptomatic adults. The effect of age, hand dominance and gender. J Bone Joint Surg Br. 1995;77:296-8.
20. Millett PJ, Gobezie R, Boykin RE. Shoulder osteoarthritis: diagnosis and management. Am Fam Physician. 2008;78(5):605-11.
21. Oh JH, Chung SW, Oh CH, et al. The prevalence of shoulder osteoarthritis in the elderly Korean population: association with risk factors and function. J Shoulder Elbow Surg. 2011;20(5):756-63.
22. Peterson M, Butler S, Eriksson M, et al. A randomized controlled trial of eccentric vs. concentric graded exercise in chronic tennis elbow (lateral elbow tendinopathy). Clin Rehabil. 2014;28(9):862-72. (Evidence Level: 1A).
23. Roche SJ, Funk L, Sciascia A, et al. Scapular dyskinesis: the surgeon's perspective. Shoulder Elbow. 2015;7(4):289-97.
24. Silliman JF, Hawkins RJ. Classification and physical diagnosis of instability of the shoulder. Clin Orthop Relat Res. 1993;291:7-19.
25. Taylor SA, Newman AM, Dawson C, et al. The "3-pack" examination is critical for comprehensive evaluation of the biceps-labrum complex and the bicipital tunnel: a prospective study. Arthroscopy. 2017;33(1):28-38.
26. Varacallo M, Musto MA, Mair SD. Anterior shoulder instability. In: StatPearls. Treasure Island, FL: StatPearls Publishing; 2019. [Internet] Available from https://www.ncbi.nlm.nih.gov/books/NBK538234.
27. Wang ZL, et al. Research progress on biologic repair of rotator cuff injury. Tianjin Med J. 2018;46(2):211-5.
28. Zhang JF, Song LH, Wei JN, et al. Prevalence of and risk factors for the occurrence of symptomatic osteoarthritis in rural regions of Shanxi Province, China. Int J Rheum Dis. 2016;19(8):781-9.

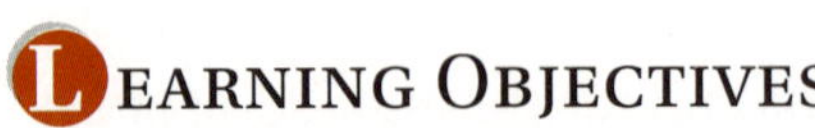

20
CHAPTER

Elbow, Wrist, and Hand Conditions

Ajit Dabholkar, Tejashree Dabholkar

LEARNING OBJECTIVES

At the end of this chapter, the readers will be able to:

- Describe pathophysiology and clinical presentation, disease course, and common clinical manifestations in common elbow, wrist, and hand disorders
- Identify the common medical diagnostic procedures and describe the common clinical assessment skills in common elbow, wrist, and hand disorders
- Develop the technical and clinical skills and knowledge of up-to-date information, which includes evidence-based view in physiotherapy for the treatment of common musculoskeletal conditions affecting the elbow, wrist, and hand
- Analyze and interpret patient data, formulate realistic goals with clear treatment guidelines for better patient outcomes
- Explain in brief common therapeutic goals along with their purpose and rationale with relevant clinical pearls and clinical case studies

CHAPTER OUTLINE

INTRODUCTION

Musculoskeletal disorders of the elbow, forearm, wrist, and hand result in pain, loss of function, and decreased productivity in the general population. They usually affect limb function, social activities, and the ability to work and difficulty in activities of daily living.

Fortunately, most such episodes last for a brief period of time and do not affect over long term. However, in a significant proportion of the population, such problems are sufficiently severe, disabling, and persistent leading to loss of employment, long-term pain, and dependence. Often, if unresolved, these disorders may become recurrent or may keep relapsing. The World Health Organization's International Classification of Functioning, Disability, and Health (ICF) provides a framework for rehabilitation practitioners to address physical and psychological impairments, along with subsequent activity limitations and participation restrictions resulting from problems affecting the upper limb that affect an individual's ability to perform daily life activities.

The ICF model combines medical diagnosis and levels of functioning and disability, to predict needs of an individual. The goal of ICF is to shift the focus from cause, or diagnosis, to impact, or function. The model integrates the diagnosis and subsequent impairments of overall function within the context of environmental and personal factor constraints.

The key to musculoskeletal rehabilitation is to understand the timelines of healing and to follow treatment guidelines with sound clinical reasoning and promote interventions that are safe and appropriate with competence in differential diagnosis targeting the right tissue from the toolbox of techniques to a given diagnosis.

Overview

A complete understanding of unique anatomy and biomechanics of elbow, wrist and hand forms the basis for clinical evaluation and formulation of thorough and comprehensive treatment program

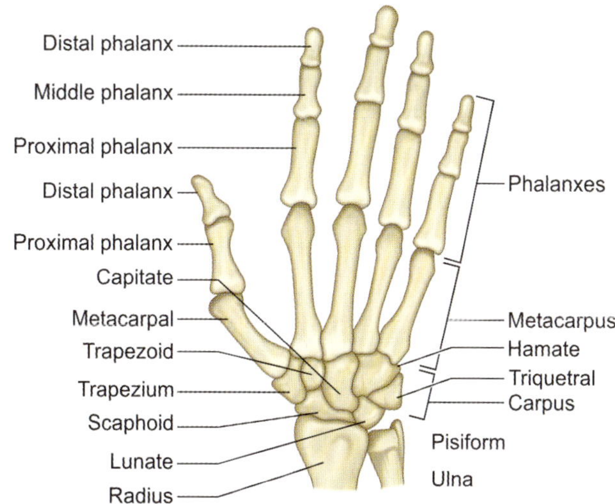

Fig. 20.2: Anatomy of wrist and hand.

for patients with elbow, wrist, and hand dysfunction **(Figs. 20.1 and 20.2)**.

Normal elbow function is vital to the participation in most simple daily activities, as well as for higher level actions such as sports. Prehensile function of the hand is interdependent on the shoulder complex, joint stability of the wrist and upper arm, efficient tendon gliding, and precise feedback from nerve. The principles of stability, mobility, rhythm, and balance apply to the interlink of the complex interplay between joints of upper extremity. The restoration of function requires knowledge of the complex anatomic relationships and applications of skilled rehabilitation efforts. The examination of the entire upper extremity and trunk in clinical evaluation is imperative, since it hugely relies on the kinetic chain. The primary role of the entire upper limb—shoulder, arm, elbow, and forearm—is to place the hand in its proper position of function. Thus it is relevant to understand the common conditions of the same.

REHABILITATION OF POST-TRAUMATIC STIFF ELBOW

Clinical Presentation and Pathophysiology

Post-traumatic stiff elbow is a frequent and disabling complication and poses serious challenges for its management. Stiffness of elbow is defined as flexion <120° and loss of extension >30°. Stiffness of elbow causes difficulty in placement of hand in space and hence limits the functional capacity. The exact incidence of post-traumatic elbow stiffness is difficult to estimate because of its multifactorial pathogenesis and variable time of manifestation.

Regan and Reilly postulated three potential factors for an elbow to be so prone for stiffness:
1. Complex articular congruity
2. Brachialis muscle covering the elbow and predisposing it to myositis ossificans
3. Prolonged immobilization in the presence of unstable fixation.

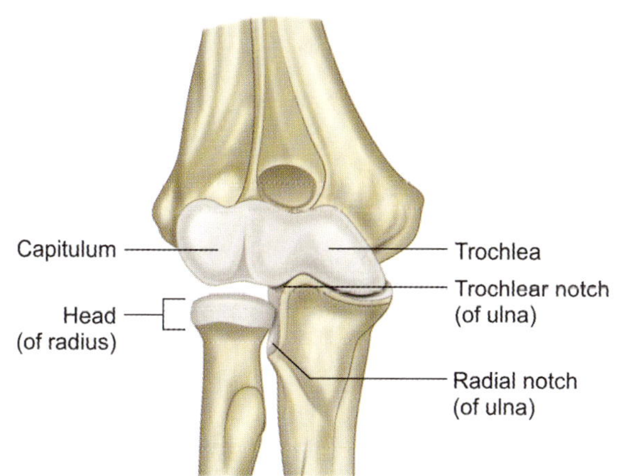

Fig. 20.1: Anatomy of elbow joint.

The stiffness of elbow is multifactorial.

- Intrinsic contractures are due to intra-articular pathology. The intrinsic causes that limit from deep to superficial to joint motion are joint surface incongruity, osteophytes, synovitis and joint capsule and ligaments contracture.
- Extrinsic contractures are extra-articular pathology: The extrinsic causes of joint limitation are contractures of muscle–tendon units, fascial/fibrous supporting tissue that are not tendons or ligaments and skin.

There are two classification systems of stiff elbow:

1. Kay's classification is based on the offending structure:
   Type 1—Soft tissue contracture
   Type 2—Soft tissue contracture with ossification
   Type 3—Nondisplaced articular fracture with soft tissue contracture
   Type 4—Displaced articular fracture with soft tissue contracture
   Type 5—Post-traumatic bony bars
2. Morrey's classification is based on etiology and its location and is classified as:
   - Intrinsic
   - Extrinsic
   - Mixed

An elbow capsule, which is contracted, is much thicker than normal and has collagen disorganization and fibroblast infiltration.

Evaluation

The nature of an individual's pain, its quality and behavior in different scenarios and over a 24-hour period is important to assess:

- The presence of neuropathic pain, weakness, clumsiness, paresthesia, or anesthesia.
- Locking or mechanical symptoms.
- Any deformity, muscle wastage, previous scars, metal implant, along with edema, color changes and trophic changes in the elbow, forearm and hand, should be noted.
- A hard end feel suggests a bony block to motion, whereas a softer end feel may be indicative of soft tissue contracture.
- Crepitus appreciated during movement may signify degenerative changes or a nonunited fracture, whereas restriction of forearm motion with a positive grip and grind test, where the forearm is axially loaded and rotated, may be a result of radiocapitellar joint pathology.
- Passive motion also allows the therapist to try and differentiate between joint and muscle length contributions to elbow range. A difference in elbow extension range with the forearm in pronation and then in supination may signify a decrease in biceps length. Physiological motion restriction may be as a result of limitation of accessory range of motion (ROM).

Therefore, positive findings can be used to plan a treatment protocol. Upper limb neural dynamic testing should be performed where neural involvement is suspected.

Intervention Strategies

The intervention strategies are as follows:

1. **Orthoses**
   - Static progressive splints (turnbuckle splints) **(Fig. 20.3)** place the tissues at maximally tolerable load and then as the tissues stretch, the load decreases. This uses the viscoelastic properties of the tissues as per which the tissue tension decreases over time when placed at a constant length.
   - The dynamic splints use springs or rubber bands. They use the principles of creep; changing length under constant load.
   - Both methods aim to produce plastic deformation of tissues leading to permanent lengthening. Both the types of splints are effective for managing elbow contractures.
   - Static progressive stretching three times 30 min/day in each direction should be the first line of treatment in patients with post-traumatic and postsurgical elbow stiffness. If this fails or is not applicable due to osseous reasons of stiffness, surgical intervention should be considered.

   Review of literature has shown a paucity of reports concerning stretching exercises, local heat application, and joint mobilization even though these are widely used modalities. The benefit of all the modalities is highest in the first 3 months. However, it continues till 1 year. Physiotherapists should emphasize on pain control measures while employing conservative methods of treatment, and due care should be taken as to prevent exacerbation of the existing condition.

2. **Heat on stretch application in the desired motion:** Moist heat before an exercise session will influence tissue extensibility.

3. **Combination of gentle passive, active, and active assisted exercises:** The focus should be on duration of stretch, end range stretch should be gentle, prolonged, and to the point of resistance or mild discomfort.

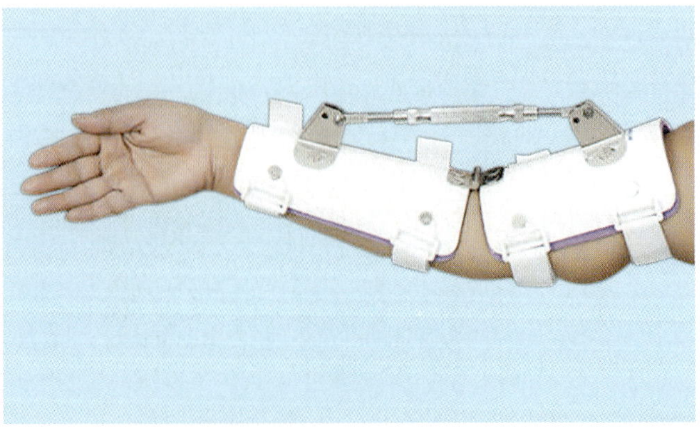

Fig. 20.3: Turnbuckle splint.

Clinical Pearl

Use of dumbbell (2 or 3 lb to hold on stretch) may increase muscle cocontraction, spasm, or microtearing.

4. **Capsule or ligamentous tightness:** Continuous ultrasound at 3 MHz, 1.0 W/cm^2 for 5 minutes.
5. **ROM exercise:** Early mobilization (active mobilization), continuous passive motion, and active assisted techniques **(Figs. 20.4 to 20.6)** may be used.
6. Home exercise program need to be shown to adhere to the exercise regime.
7. **Strength:** PRE using free weights, wall pulleys, theraband (isometric, concentric, and eccentric), manual resistance, etc.
8. Proprioceptive neuromuscular facilitation (PNF) patterns can be encouraged and later performed with resistance, e.g., proprioceptive exercise (close kinetic chain) and neuromuscular control exercise.
9. Prolonged stretching (contraction–relaxation exercise, joint mobilization techniques **(Fig. 20.7)**.
10. Mobilization with movement techniques.

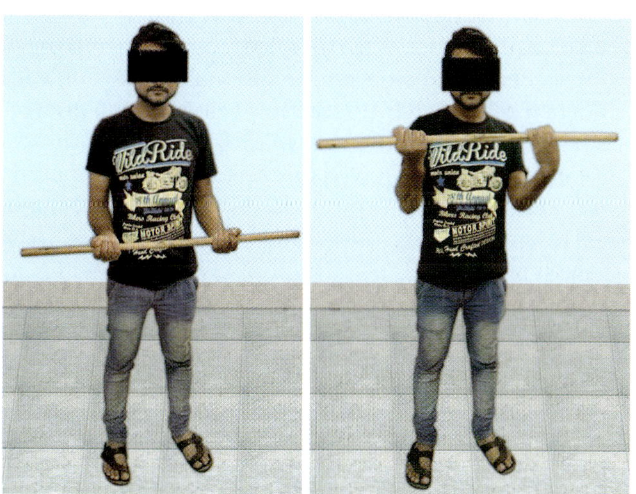

Fig. 20.4: Active assisted exercises using stick.

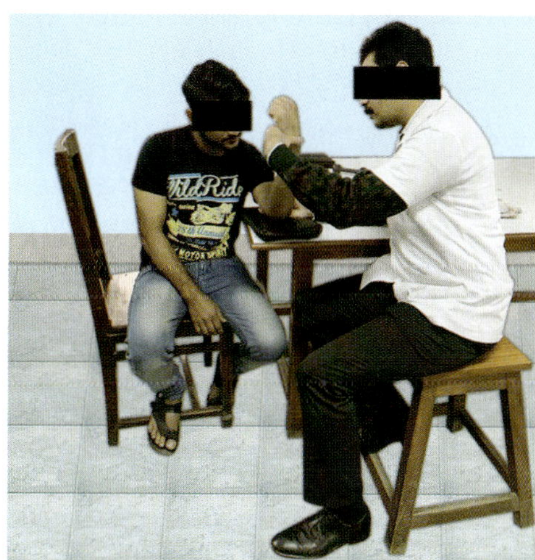

Fig. 20.5: Active assisted exercises using manual assistance by therapist.

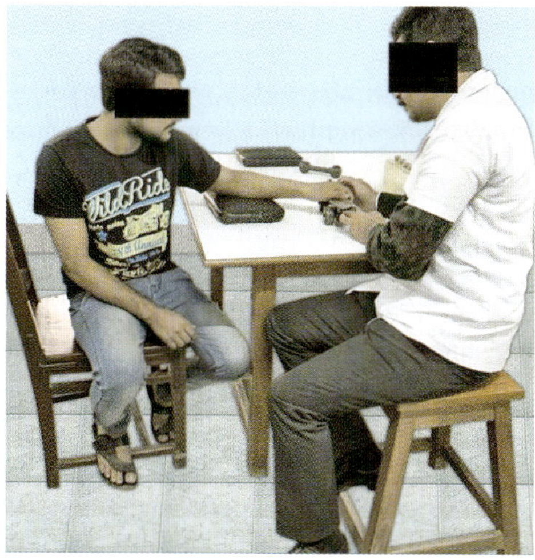

Fig. 20.6: Active assisted exercises using skate.

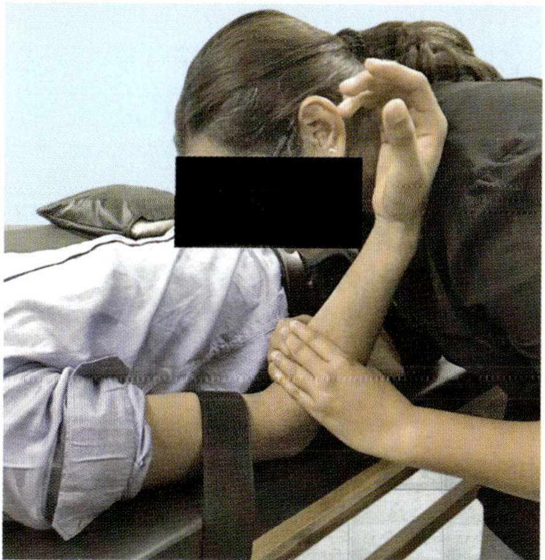

Fig. 20.7: Passive mobilization of the elbow.

Other techniques: Manipulation under anesthesia, surgical release and, recently, botulinum toxin A have been considered for treatment due to its pronounced results in children. Those undergoing internal fixations after fracture showed improvement in ROM and function following intraoperative injection into the elbow flexors.

BOX 20.1: Key points.

According to Wilk et al. (2004), rehabilitation is important to prevent the ill effects of immobilization and helps against placing excessive stress on healing tissues. While progressing a patient from one rehabilitation stage to the other, careful consideration should be made. Therapists should tend to evidence-based protocols and individualize them as per needs of the patients.

Chinchalkar and Szekeres (2004) propose that a five-step rehabilitation process should be used. This involves the appropriate diagnosis, pain and inflammation control, early protected motion, neuromuscular control, and integrating motion into the whole kinetic chain.

LATERAL ELBOW TENDINOPATHY

Clinical Presentation and Pathophysiology

Lateral elbow tendinopathy (LET) is the most appropriate clinical diagnostic term. Lateral epicondylalgia, lateral epicondylosis, and tennis elbow and/or lateral epicondylitis are considered as inappropriate terms to use, due to pathophysiological, anatomical, and etiological factors involved.

LET is related to sports or arm work pain disorder and is defined as a cause of pain in the lateral epicondyle **(Fig. 20.8)** that failed healing tendon response rather than inflammatory or may be degenerative. It is characterized by the absence of inflammatory cells, glycosaminoglycans, and proteoglycans; disorganized and immature collagen vascular hyperplasia; and the increased presence of fibroblasts. The most commonly involved structure is the origin of the extensor carpi radialis brevis (ECRB).

LET occurs commonly between 30 and 60 years of age. It tends to be more severe and of longer duration in females. The most commonly affected arm is the dominant arm.

Diagnosis and Assessment

The commonly presenting complaints of patients with LET are pain and decreased function, both of which affect activities of daily living. Pain can be reproduced with one of the following ways:

1. Palpation on the facet of the lateral epicondyle.
2. With the elbow in extension, resisted wrist extension **(Cozen's test)** and/or resisted middle finger extension.
3. Gripping activities.

Mill's test: While flexing the wrist stretches the common extensor tendon and gives pain.

The Patient-Rated Tennis Elbow Evaluation (PRTEE) questionnaire is a standardized, quantitative, and quick measure to describe pain and functional disability in LET patients. Evaluating the cervical and thoracic spine and testing neurodynamics of the radial nerve are also helpful to determine the contribution of spinal component to pain.

Management Strategies

Patient Education

Patients with LET can be reassured that the condition will resolve gradually with adequate rest and time. Instructions can be given to avoid pain-provoking activities. Ergonomic advice should focus on minimizing work tasks that require deviated wrist postures, forceful exertions, and highly repetitive movements.

Exercise Therapy

The following exercise therapy is to be done:

- Applying gradually increasing resistance on wrist extensor muscles is useful. Some studies suggest using eccentric over concentric exercise while others recommend equal effects with both.
- For patients with reactive tendinopathy or irritable symptoms, gentle, pain-free isometric contractions 30–60 seconds in duration, performed daily, with wrist extended up to 20–30° and elbow flexed at 90°, may be more appropriate than eccentric exercise, which may aggravate pain. Progression can be made by either increasing the duration of contraction (up to 90 seconds) or by increasing the load (through free weight or resistance tubing).
- Motor control impairments, such as dissociation of wrist from finger extension and retraining of wrist alignment during gripping should also be added with exercises.
- Concentric **(Figs. 20.9A and B)** and/or eccentric exercise of wrist extensors is preferable for patients with degenerative-stage tendinopathy, starting with flexed elbow and progressing to restricting end-of-range wrist flexion, when the ECRB tendon experiences greater compression and more pain. Eccentric training induces hypertrophy and increases tensile strength, thereby reducing the strain on the tendon during movement.
- **Stretching:** Passive wrist flexion exercises with variable angles of elbow extension and forearm pronated maintain the length of musculotendinous unit and provide stretching effect.
- **Orthosis:** Forearm counter strap and a customized wrist extension orthosis (positioning the wrist in 30–40° of extension) provide adequate pain control by unloading of the wrist extensors **(Figs. 20.10A to C)**.

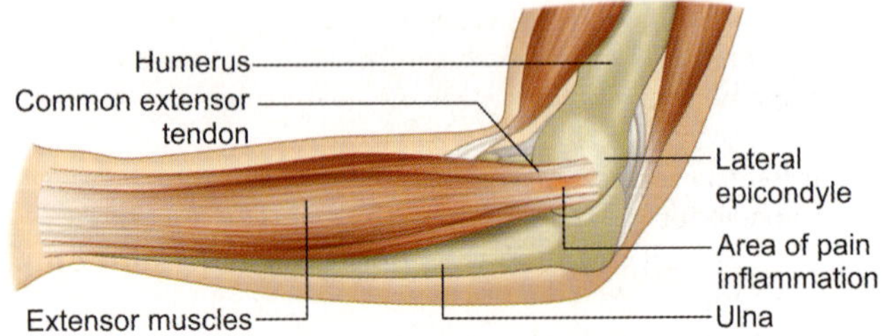

Fig. 20.8: Inflammation site in tennis elbow.

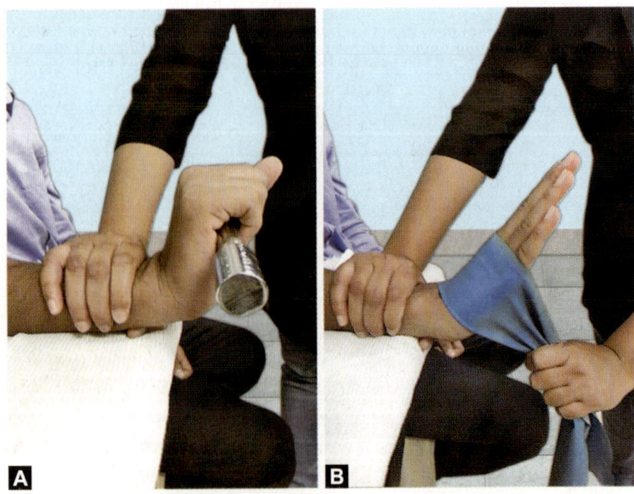

Figs. 20.9A and B: Concentric strengthening of wrist extensors: (A) Using dumbbell; (B) Using Theraband.

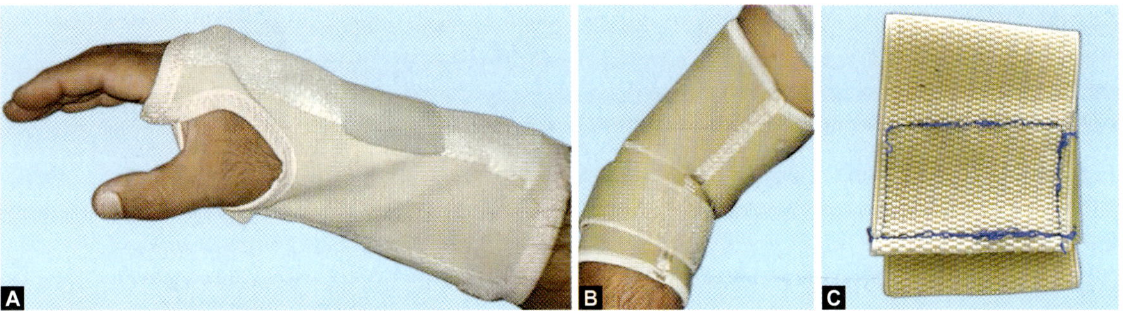

Figs. 20.10A to C: (A) Wrist extension orthosis; (B) Elbow sleeve; (C) Elbow band.

- **Electrotherapy:** Ultrasound can be applied along with other therapeutic interventions. Iontophoresis with dexamethasone sodium phosphate causes short-term pain relief during acute phase. Other modalities, such as low-level LASER therapy (LLLT) and extracorporeal shock wave therapy (ESWT), also reduce pain. 904 nm LASER is known to be beneficial in the short term as compared to placebo, but LASER and other active interventions do not differ much in the short term or long term. ESWT may reduce pain but results are inconclusive.

- **Acupuncture:** Acupuncture is proven to be better than placebo and more effective than US for pain relief and provides short-term treatment benefit.

- **Manual therapy:** Manual therapy techniques to the elbow, wrist, and cervicothoracic spine provide immediate pain relief and improvement in function in people with LE. Evidence for the immediate effects of manual therapy techniques on pain and grip strength and for short-term clinical benefits when used along with graduated exercise hold moderate strength.
  - Ulnar–humeral lateral glide and radial head posteroanterior glide can be used following Mulligan's mobilization with movement, where the patient performs the pain-producing movement in conjunction with sustained mobilization.
  - Cyriax: Deep friction massage and Mill's manipulation. Deep transverse friction (DTF) combined with Mill's manipulation is performed immediately after DTF. These two components must be used together in the order mentioned to account as Cyriax intervention. Patients must follow the protocol three times a week for 4 weeks.

- **Multimodal program:** A multimodal program of Mulligan's mobilization-with-movement and exercise are better than wait and see. Placebo injection in the short term, and in the long term, is superior to corticosteroid injection.

- **Other treatments:** In the presence of tendinopathy, counseling should be offered to the patient for second-line interventions, such as prolotherapy injections or nitric oxide patches. In the case of severe pain with lateral collateral ligament (LCL) or tendon tears on imaging, early referral to an orthopedic surgeon may be made.

Clinical Pearl

One plausible reason for persistent pain in lateral elbow tendinopathy (LET) is the sensitization of the nervous system given the reduced thresholds to nociceptive withdrawal and greater temporal summation.

Previously, it has been shown that people with LET have widespread hyperalgesia (i.e., enhanced pain response to various stimuli), which is associated with high pain levels, decreased function, and longer symptom duration.

Some tips for equipment: Use racquet with midsize frame with medium flexibility to lower the string tension; large handle, submaximal grip; new tennis balls; grip bands to handle; learn correct stroke mechanics from coach.

GOLFER'S ELBOW

Clinical Presentation and Pathophysiology

Medial epicondylitis, often called "golfer's elbow," is a common pathology. Repetitive forced wrist extension and forearm supination during activities involving wrist flexion and forearm pronation results into flexor–pronator tendon degeneration **(Fig. 20.11)**. This can result in structural breakdown and irreparable fibrosis or calcification gradually.

Medial epicondylitis is tendinopathy of the medial common flexor tendon of the elbow due to overload or

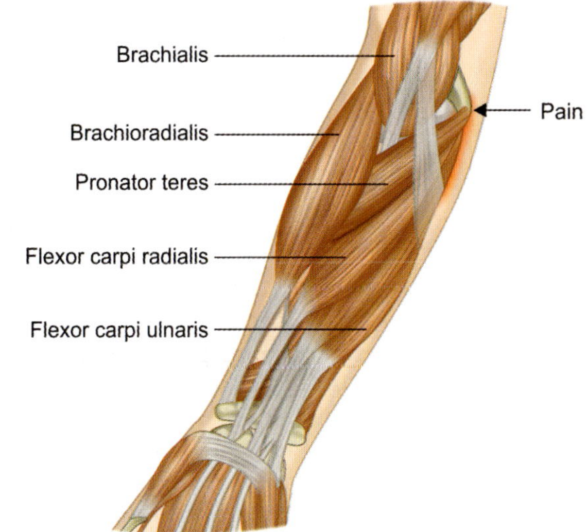

Fig. 20.11: Inflammation site in golfer's elbow.

overuse. During the late cocking and acceleration phase, pitchers and overhead throwing athletes often develop this condition due to high energy valgus forces. In golfers, it is thought to occur from the top of the backswing to just before ball impact. However, more than 90% of cases are not sports related. Labor-intensive occupations with forceful, repetitive activities, including professions in carpentry, plumbing, and construction, are also implicated.

Risk factors for developing medial epicondylitis in athletes include:

- Training errors
- Improper technique

Equipment, or functional risk factors, include:

- Lack of strength, endurance, or flexibility.

Occupation-related risk factors include:

- Heavy physical work
- Excessive repetition
- High body mass index
- Smoking
- Presence of comorbidities
- High psychosocial work demands

Medial epicondylitis is an overuse tendinopathy because of chronic repetitive concentric or eccentric loading of the wrist flexors and pronator teres (PT), which leads to angiofibroblastic changes. Repetitive activity leads to recurrent microtears within the tendon and subsequent tendinosis.

Physical Examination

In physical examination, the following factors are monitored:

- Physical examination may reveal tenderness up to 5–10 mm distal and anterior to the medial epicondyle, accompanied by soft tissue swelling.
- Resisted wrist flexion, forearm pronation, or forceful grip may be weakened as compared to the contralateral side and may worsen the elbow pain.
- Elbow flexion contracture secondary to pain and guarding can develop; however, most patients present with normal passive and active ROM of the elbow and wrist.
- Peripheral neurovascular status is usually normal. Patients should be examined for the presence of other pathologies such as ipsilateral signs of cervical radiculopathy, particularly of the C6 and C7 roots, since these patients may be at increased risk of developing medial epicondylitis secondary to an imbalance of forearm muscles.

Management

Initial management should include cessation of aggravating activities, including decreasing their volume, frequency, or intensity.

Once acute symptoms are relieved, flexor–pronator mass stretching and strengthening should be addressed. During each phase of rehabilitation, the patient should perform targeted exercises with increasing repetition and speed. The initial goal is to return to full and pain-free ROM.

- Wrist and elbow movements are emphasized, with open chain exercises (non-weight-bearing) and self-directed passive stretching techniques.
- In overhead throwers and nonathletes with concomitant shoulder pathology, shoulder ROM is emphasized. The goal is full, pain-free ROM at the wrist and elbow. If a baseline flexion contracture exists, elbow extension may require support with extension block bracing. Passive ROM and eccentric contractions are avoided initially to inhibit excessive stress on the tendon. Once pain-free functional motion arc is achieved, strengthening of the tendon begins. Concentric open and closed chain exercises, with progressing weight and repetitions to increase flexor–pronator mass power, are then initiated.
- Strength exercises should focus on eccentric activity. But concentric strengthening should also be incorporated in the program (**Figs. 20.12A and B**).
- Various modalities that may provide relief include dry needling, ESWT, LLLT, electrical stimulation, iontophoresis, and ultrasound/phonophoresis.
- Soft tissue and manipulation techniques appear to allow more vigorous stretching, resulting in better and faster recovery from the symptoms of medial epicondylitis. Night splint with a cock-up wrist splint may be helpful. A counterforce brace can unload the tendon, decreasing pain. Elbow taping with kinesiology taping may also be useful.

All patients, particularly throwers, achieve benefit with strengthening exercises of the shoulder girdle and scapular stabilization exercises. Core and lower body strengthening helps in throwing mechanics and activities involving moderate to heavy resistance. Reconditioning of the upper limb to maintain tendon excursion and strength during rigorous tendon stress is vital in preventing undue stresses around the elbow and to prevent recurrence of symptoms.

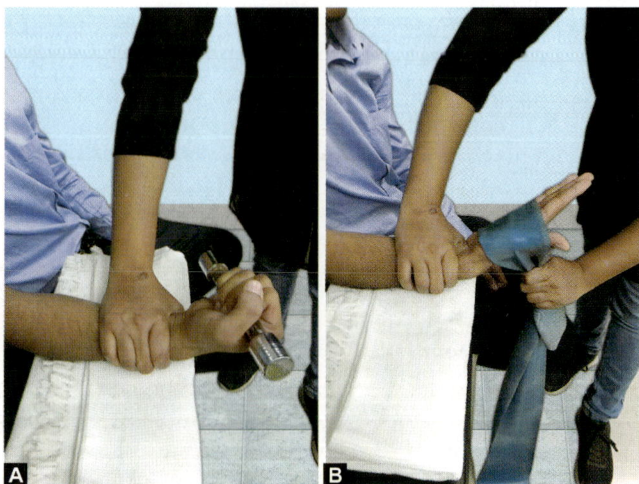

Figs. 20.12A and B: Concentric strengthening of wrist flexors: (A) Using dumbbell; (B) Using Theraband.

- **Sports-related strategies:** While selecting golf clubs, the length, shaft weight, club head weight, and club head strike zone should be considered. Proper technique is particularly important, especially in the case of amateur athlete. Medial epicondylitis is common in the trail arm of the swing, than that in the lead arm. This is due to secondary to greater valgus stress and is more likely in amateur golfers than in professionals, who use the lead arm in a protective manner to obtain optimum swing speed and power without excessive stress. In tennis, racquet size, weight, head weight, strike zone, and string tension can influence stress at the elbow. Vibration dampeners directly attached to the strings can be useful in amateurs. Poor forehand stroke mechanics is a cause of medial elbow stress. Late ball strike, with the racquet head behind the elbow at contact, may be a significant contributor to medial epicondylitis. It can worsen with an open stance technique, particularly with a topspin stroke, which works on rapid angular acceleration to the disadvantageous strike point.
- **Surgical options:** Surgical debridement is mainly used in those with persistent symptoms despite an aggressive regimen of conservative therapy for 4–6 months. Elite athletes with definitive tendon disruption appreciable on MRI are an exception to this guideline.

Surgical management includes release of the common flexor tendon at the epicondyle and debriding the pathologic tissue. In mini-open muscle resection, removal of degenerative tissue of the flexor carpi radialis is done. Fascial elevation and tendon origin resection is another useful technique.

Clinical Pearl

The differential diagnosis of medial epicondylitis is broad and includes neuropathy (such as C6 or C7 radiculopathy, cubital tunnel syndrome, ulnar or median neuropathy, ulnar neuritis, anterior interosseous nerve entrapment, or tardy ulnar nerve palsy) and ligamentous injury (such as ulnar or medial collateral ligament instability, sprain, or tear). It also includes intra-articular issues such as adhesive capsulitis, arthrofibrosis, or loose bodies; osseous concerns such as medial epicondyle avulsion fracture, or osteophytes; myofascial difficulties, including flexor or pronator strain; tendinopathy (lateral epicondylitis, triceps tendonitis); synovitis; valgus extension overload; or dermatologic concerns (e.g., herpes zoster).

ELBOW INJURY IN THROWING ATHLETES

Introduction

Athletes of all ages and skill levels participate increasingly in sports involving overhead arm motions, thus making elbow injuries common. Among these injuries, lateral epicondylitis occurs in over 50% of athletes using overhead arm motions. Soft tissue and bony injuries around the elbow are very common and usually linked to overuse.

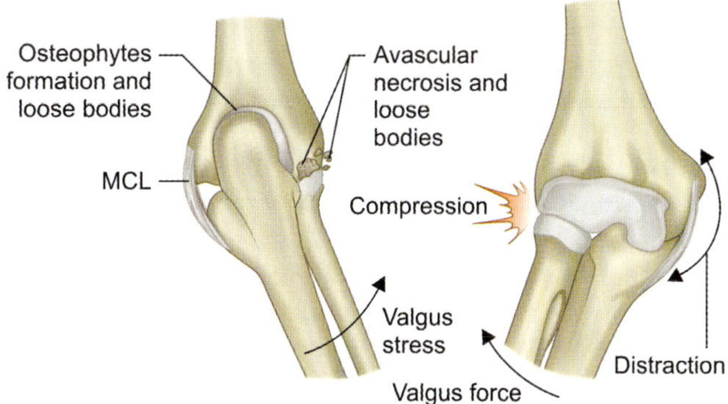

Fig. 20.13: Valgus extension overload in the elbow. (MCL: medial collateral ligament)

Valgus extension overload syndrome: Valgus extension overload **(Fig. 20.13)** is a syndrome of symptoms and physical findings commonly seen in overhead athletes because of altered throwing biomechanics. High valgus loads with rapid elbow extension cause a combination of forces.

- Tensile stress along the medial compartment [ulnar collateral ligament (UCL), flexor–pronator mass] causes tears.
- Shear stress in the posterior compartment (posteromedial tip of the olecranon and trochlea/olecranon fossa) leads to spurring and osteoarthritis.
- Compression laterally on the radial head and capitulum leads to osteochondral lesions especially in young patients.

Table 20.1 shows the description of medial tension injury types at the elbow.

Ulnar collateral ligament injuries: Repetitive near-failure tensile stresses cause microtrauma of the anterior bundle leading to ligament attenuation or failure, either partial or complete. High-demand throwers respond to conservative treatment in rare conditions.

Ulnar neuritis: Osteophyte irritation, muscle hypertrophy compression, or nerve subluxation occur due to traction

Table 20.1: Description of medial tension injury types.	
Medial tension injury type	**Description**
I	MCL injury, MCL subacute injury with inflammation, MCL partial tear, MCL complete tear
II	Posteromedial impingement, chondromalacia, osteophyte formation, olecranon stress fractures, and loose bodies
III	Flexor–pronator injury, medial epicondylitis, partial rupture of flexor–pronator muscle type
IV	Ulnar nerve entrapment, cubital tunnel syndrome, ulnar nerve subluxation, and lateral compression injury
V	Radiocapitellar overload syndrome, lateral elbow pain, capitellum and radial head chondromalacia, capitellum and radial head osteochondritis dissecans

(MCL: medial collateral ligament)

resulting from valgus stress. This presents with paresthesias in the fourth and fifth digits while throwing and dull pain in the elbow or forearm.

Olecranon osteophytes: Osteophytes can cause pain due to impingement during the deceleration phase and recurrent impingement may fracture the osteophytes, giving rise to loose bodies.

Olecranon stress fractures: Maybe due to posterior impingement or excessive force of the triceps on olecranon. Pain occurs over the olecranon during deceleration and follow-through phases. Early lesions without sclerosis may be managed conservatively.

Osteochondritis dissecans of the capitellum: Lesions of the capitellum are common due to compressive stress on the lateral elbow. This may compromise the subchondral blood supply, particularly in adolescents, leading to osteochondral degeneration and possible loose body formation.

Medial humeral epicondyle apophysitis (Little Leaguer's elbow): Caused by direct traction of the common flexor–pronator tendon on the epiphysis. Pain occurs during the late cocking and early acceleration phases of throwing. On the other hand, medial epicondyle avulsion generally affects more skeletally mature adolescents and occurs due to either repeated microtrauma or acute elbow dislocation.

Injury Prevention and Rehabilitation

Wilk et al. in 1995 described the following phases of rehabilitation after elbow injuries:
a. Immediate controlled motion
b. Immediate strengthening
c. Dynamic stabilization
d. Functional progression

Various risk factors exist for elbow injuries in young athletes such as elevated single game and total season pitch counts, playing the position of pitcher or catcher, poor throwing biomechanics, and pitching while fatigued account for an increased risk for elbow injury. Identification of the risk factors for elbow injury has helped in the prevention of elbow injuries by limiting the number of throws for young athletes round the year.

Fleisig and Andrews in 2012 made certain recommendations for injury prevention. These include proper throwing mechanics and utilization of the core and lower extremities throughout the throwing motion, identifying and addressing in-game fatigue, limiting total game and total season pitches, avoiding pitching on multiple teams in multiple leagues, and complete cessation of throwing for at least 2–3 months per year.

Throwing rehabilitation helps in prevention of injury, treatment for minor pathology, and during recovery after surgical intervention. While training is individually tailored, most programs follow a similar regimen. First, major deficits are addressed, including core stabilization, leg strengthening, and global flexibility; and finally players complete a graduated throwing program and return to sport. This allows for progressive focus on the upper extremity kinetic chain, including scapular stabilizers, rotator cuff, and distal arm musculature. The entire process concludes over a 3–12-month period based on severity of initial injury.

Clinical Pearl

Principles of treatment—PEACE and LOVE

P: Protection	Refrain activities and movements that aggravate pain during the first few days after injury
E: Elevation	Elevate the injured limb higher than the heart as often as possible
A: Avoid anti-inflammatories	Avoid taking anti-inflammatory medications since they impede tissue healing
C: Compression	Use elastic bandage or taping to reduce swelling
E: Education	Avoid unnecessary passive treatments and medical investigations and let nature play its role
L: Load	Let pain guide gradual return to normal activities. Body usually signals when it's safe to increase load
O: Optimism	Condition the brain for optimal recovery by being confident and positive
V: Vascularization	Choose pain-free cardiovascular activities to increase blood flow for repair of the tissues
E: Exercise	Restore mobility, strength, and proprioception by using an active approach to recovery

COMPLEX REGIONAL PAIN SYNDROME

Introduction

The International Association for the Study of Pain (IASP) proposed the term "complex regional pain syndrome (CRPS)" in 1993. There are synonyms used for CRPS, e.g., reflex sympathetic dystrophy, neurodystrophy, pain dysfunction syndrome, and minor or major causalgia. The IASP definition of the syndrome states, "CRPS Type I is a syndrome that usually develops after an initiating noxious event, is not limited to the distribution of a single peripheral nerve, and is apparently disproportioned to the inciting event. It is associated at some point with evidence of edema, changes in skin blood flow, abnormal sudomotor activity in the region of the pain, or allodynia or hyperalgesia (Merskey et al 1994)."

There are two types of CRPS, I and II. In type I, nerve lesion is not identified but in type II nerve lesion is evident. Type II CRPS generally develops after an injury of peripheral nerve, branches or trunk.

Etiology and Demographic Features

Individual of any age can develop CRPS but it is common around the age of 35 years old. Women are frequently involved. Mostly, CRPS occurs secondary to trauma. It is common in 20% of fracture cases. Wrist and hand are common areas to get involved. Trauma leads to initiation of process of tissue healing. Inflammatory phase initiated but in CRPS it lasts abnormally leading to vicious cycle. Physiological changes such as vasoconstriction, edema, and hyperalgesia continue. This is labeled sympathetic over activity. Nociceptive impulses going to brain spreads over wider areas sensitizing more nociceptors.

Clinical Signs

The following clinical signs are observed:
- Pain: Severe, constant, burning associated with hyperpathia and allodynia
- Shiny, dry, scaly skin, brittle nail, and thick hair on involved extremity **(Fig. 20.14)**.
- Skin temperature changes such as cold or excessive sweating
- Change in skin color such as redness
- Edema of hand
- Limitation of movement, tremors or dystonia.

Stages of Complex Regional Pain Syndrome

Stage I (acute phase): Duration lasts approximately 1–3 months **(Fig. 20.15)**.
- Spontaneous onset of pain is common in CRPS. Pain is disproportionate to extent of trauma hyperesthesia, i.e., abnormal pain sensitivity to minor cutaneous pressure is a significant finding.
- Redness, warmth, and shiny skin are common features.
- Functional discomfort and restriction is common.
- Significant edema is seen. Post-traumatic plaster of Paris removal sometimes gives similar findings which make it difficult for clinician to identify and diagnose CRPS at an earlier stage.

Stage II (dystrophic phase): Duration lasts approximately 3–6 months.

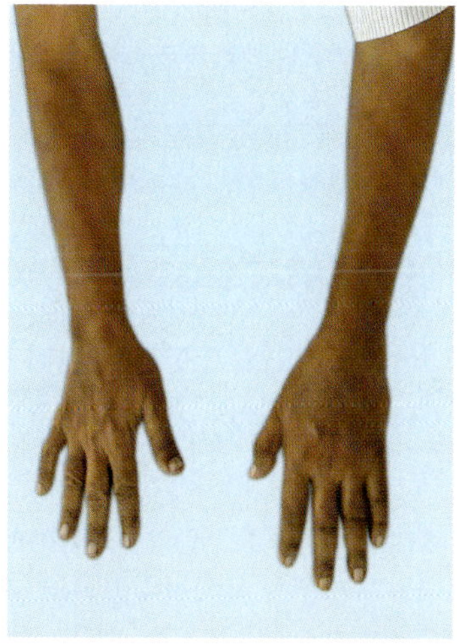

Fig. 20.14: Reflex sympathetic dystrophy (RSD) in the left hand.

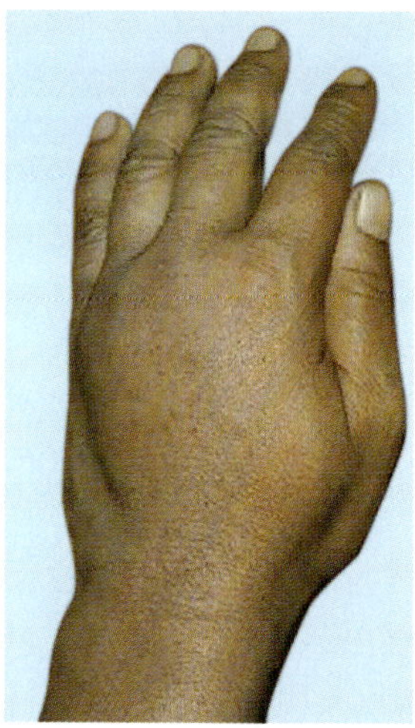

Fig. 20.15: Stage 1 complex regional pain syndrome (CRPS).

- Bluish discoloration with cold skin is a common feature. In Indian population, this discoloration may be seen as blackish discoloration.
- Brittle and sharp nails are common features.
- Spontaneous pain progressively decreases.
- Edema may decrease but gets organized which can affect finger mobility significantly.
- Atrophy of muscles and fibrosis is common
- Deformity of the hand is seen.
- Demineralization and loss of bone matrix is a characteristic radiographic feature of this stage.
- Patient may either recover or move ahead toward sequel.

Stage III (atrophic phase): This phase may last from 12 to 24 months.

The third stage involves irreversible trophic changes, intractable pain involving the entire limb, flexor tendon contractures, marked muscle atrophy, severe joint limitations and limb immobility, and marked bone deossification. Articular stiffness and tendon adhesions are common.

Management

When "physiotherapy" is used as adjuvant treatment along with medical treatment, it gives very good functional outcomes especially for type I CRPS.

Goals of physiotherapy in CRPS are:
1. Quick reduction of pain.
2. Abnormal skin temperature reduction.
3. Treatment of reduced mobility and edema.
- **Edema control**
  - The excessive fibrosis also impedes the flow of lymphatic fluid, which enhances edema. It is important to start early controlled motion. Active repeated finger flexion and dynamic splinting redistributes this fluid to lower tissue pressure areas. This loosens the skin in proximity to the joint axis, which decreases the effort needed for finger flexion.
  - Active ROM exercise should be encouraged to increase venous and lymphatic outflow.

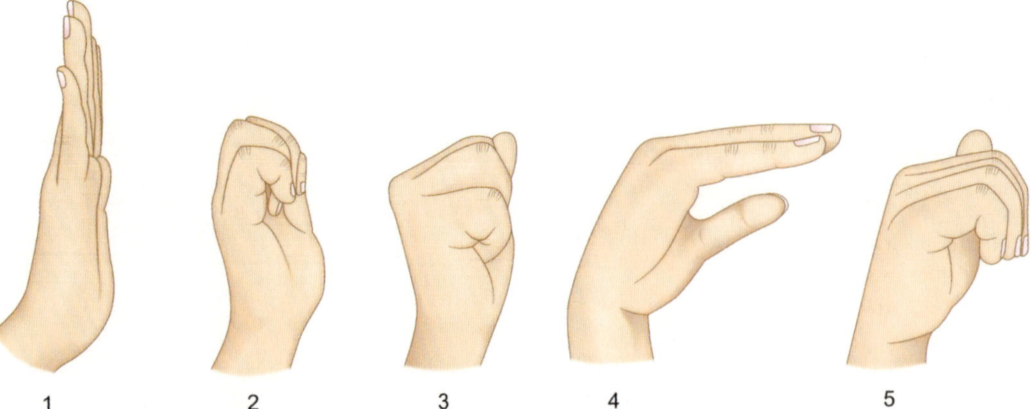

Fig. 20.16: Tendon gliding exercise.

- Encourage active wrist extension exercise (gentle fist), tenodesis. Resume functional activities and activities of daily living (ADL) (self-care tasks).
- **Tendon gliding exercises:** Differential tendon gliding and active finger flexion help restore ROM **(Fig. 20.16)**.
- **Desensitization program:** Touch and massage the area providing non-noxious stimuli.

Other Strategies

Physiotherapy should begin at an early stage, or soon after diagnosing the condition, since this enhances rapid improvement.

- TENS can be used in the treatment of CRPS-I but lacks sufficient evidence.
- Mirror therapy works on pain management in CRPS. Activation of mirror neurons helps to create an illusion of functional limb.

Increased mobility is essential for the reduction of edema and pain management. Multidisciplinary approach helps to build up trust from patient and increase patient compliance.

- Maintaining active or passive movement of subjects is essential throughout management but it needs to be done within pain threshold.
- Other adjunct therapies such as hypnosis are vital in some of the cases.

Physiotherapy in the stage II aims to gain a good functional outcome.

- Treatment measures such as fluid therapy, ultrasound, electrical stimulation, manual mobilization techniques; progressive muscular rehabilitation helps to gain mobility.
- Use of dynamic flexion or extension orthosis helps to sustain achieved range. But utmost concern is about edema control and pain management.

Guideline for the management of CRPS suggests early diagnosis and treatment in order to avoid secondary physical complications associated with disuse of the affected limb. Psychological consequences associated with secondary complications are reduced due to early detection.

Four pillars of management of CRPS are recommended:
1. Patient education
2. Pain management
3. Physical and vocational rehabilitation
4. Psychological intervention.

Physiotherapist following these four aspects related to management would be able to manage cases of CRPS effectively.

Clinical Pearl

Early and immediate treatment of CRPS leads to better outcome than delay in treatment. Early gentle AROM without increase in pain monitors swelling because this can lead to permanent joint stiffness.

CRUSH INJURIES OF HAND

Introduction

Fractures and crush injuries are common traumatic conditions of wrist and hand involvement. Crush injuries are the injury where more than one structure is involved. Crush injuries of upper quadrant are common as upper extremity is frequently used at work, e.g., for protection or at home for operation of various appliances. Due to significant industrialization, human and machine interface has increased, which becomes common cause of industrial hand injuries. High impact compressive force can damage multiple structures of hand along with inflammatory reaction to injury which can damage soft structures of hand significantly.

Common Causes of Crush Injuries

There can be multiple mechanisms leading to hand injuries such as machine press, ringer injury, degloving injury, saw or injury due to sharp edges, blast or bullet injuries **(Box 20.2)**.

- Industrial hand injury
- Fall from height
- Road traffic accidents
- Blast or bomb injuries
- Bullet/gunshot/chopper

Multiple structures can be involved in crush injuries but extent of involvement may vary as described below:

- Superficial skin abrasion to complete skin damage—As there is no evidence that early coverage has more advantages; hence, surgery can be done within 4–6 days after injury to avoid possible infection. Options for surgery can be skin grafts, local or rotational flaps, free or pedicle flaps, etc. Expertise of surgeon is essential for successful recovery.
- Tendons can get lacerated or may have partial to complete tear—both flexor and extensor tendons can get involved but requirements for healing and rehabilitation is different for flexor and extensor tendons. Tendons heal by both intrinsic as well as extrinsic healing mechanism. Intrinsic healing does not allow adhesion formation. Early mobilization is encouraged to avoid postoperative adhesion formation.
- Bone fractures involved could be stable or unstable.
- Joint injury or dislocation could be present.
- Nerve damage can be just compression to complete cut of major nerves of upper quadrant. Preoperative and intraoperative assessment and decision-making is important to decide timing of nerve repair. In the case of avulsion and crush injuries, the extent of damage is not apparent and time is needed to decide the exact picture of nerve damage.
- Vascular damage may extend from capillary involvement to major arterial cut—simple test to assess perfusion is to pierce the pulp with needle and observe bleeding which should be bright red in color. Dark blue blood or absent bleeding can be due to venous obstruction or perfusion inadequacy. Use of pulse oximeter, ultrasound, or arteriography can give a clear picture. Arterial repair is essential with injuries.

Zones of the hand (**Fig. 20.17**) give significant insight into type of structures involved and extent of prognosis (**Table 20.2**). Though the zone of injury can be smaller, further damage caused by inflammation and swelling can broaden the zone of injury. Hence, it is essential to do early diagnosis and intervention. Patient anxiety, pain, alcohol intoxication as well as willingness to cooperate affect the accuracy of diagnosis.

Diagnosis and Assessment

Clinical examination of the patient is an essential key to diagnose subclinical injuries (**Table 20.3**). Key points present in **Table 20.4** should be considered while taking history.

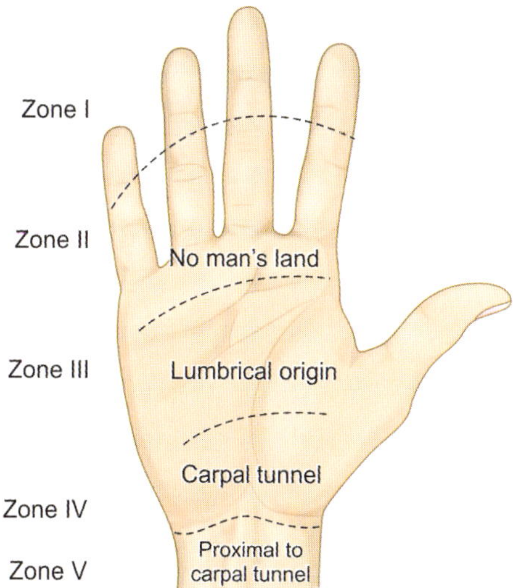

Fig. 20.17: Zones of hand.

Table 20.2: Zones of the hand.

Zones of the hand (Fig. 20.17)	Description
Zone I	Region between PIP joint and the point where the FDP tendon inserts into base of distal phalanx
Zone II	Region between distal palmar crease to PIP joint
Zone III	Distal to carpal tunnel up to level of fibro osseous tunnel
Zone IV	Area of carpal tunnel from where nine flexor tendons and the median nerve pass
Zone V	Area proximal to carpal tunnel in the distal third of the forearm

(FDP: flexor digitorum profundus; PIP: proximal interphalangeal).

Table 20.3: Hand assessment.

1	Mobility of hand joints: Mobility of joints can be assessed using linear or angular measurement system. Modified Buck–Gramcko evaluation system can be a good measure of assessment
2	Sensation
3	Functional evaluation: Essentially there is lot of difference of opinion about exact time of functional evaluation. Jebsen hand function test and Purdue Peg Board can be helpful to assess functional outcome
4	Swelling that can be assessed with volumetric analysis or by figure-of-eight method (described in detail in Chapter 37)

Physiotherapeutic Management

Edema Control

Edema affects the natural healing process; hence, control of edema is necessary. Elevation, compression, and active exercises are the main lines of treatment. In the case of hand edema, it settles on the dorsum of hand since the skin is loose and pulls metacarpophalangeal joints toward

Table 20.4: Key points to be considered while taking history.
1. Dominance: Involvement of dominant hand leads to higher disability level
2. Occupation: Demand put up by occupation gives guideline about type and extent of rehabilitation required
3. Informant gives significant information related to mechanism of injury
4. Type of injury
5. Date of surgery
6. Number of structures involved
7. Associated injuries

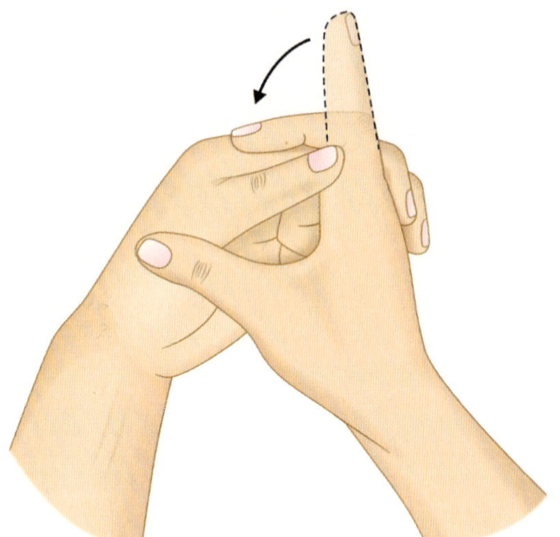

Fig. 20.18: Bunnel block exercise.

extension and interphalangeal (IP) joints toward flexion. Excessive elevation of the hand is avoided in some cases such as free flaps or revascularization. Compressive wrapping, gloves, retrograde massage, or intermittent pneumatic compression devices are essential for edema control. Active simple exercises or use of neuromuscular electrical stimulation as an adjunct to active exercises can be used. Simple Bunnel block exercises can benefit patients to reduce edema **(Fig. 20.18)**.

Desensitization and Sensory Re-education

Neuroma and hypersensitive scars are common in complex crush injuries. Hence, desensitization plays a significant role. Sensory re-education is essential for such hand as only functional recovery without good sensory reeducation is of no use.

Initially, patients are asked to rank the discomfort felt with different textures when the sensitive skin area is massaged. Different texture pieces can be used, ranging from soft cotton to Velcro hooks approximately 10×10 cm. Arm is placed comfortably, supported by the body or a table. Patients are instructed to perform the massage in the same direction, with the same speed and pressure every time until numbness occurred, for between 2 and 5 minutes.

Exercises/Mobilization

Experimental studies by Gelberman et al. reported that mobilization of the tendon increases the strength of the tendon repair, whereas complete immobilization during the healing phase of flexor tendon injuries frequently results in rapid formation of peritendinous scarring and adhesions. Due to early mobilization, the formation of adhesions is reduced by stimulating the intrinsic healing mechanism. Various protocols for managing flexor as well as extensor tendon injuries do exist. Various mobilization protocols are available for the management of flexor as well as extensor tendon injuries:

- Controlled active mobilization by Kleinert
- Controlled passive mobilization by Duran
- Indianapolis: Early active motion protocol (recent)
- Washington regimen (Kleinert's+Duran's): Recent protocols are available. All of these protocols are based on basic principle of wound healing.

Prevention of Complications

Stiffness of wrist and hand, Volkmann ischemic contracture, CRPS, and rupture of repaired structures are some of the frequently seen complications. Preventive measures and close supervision with examination is essential throughout rehabilitation to avoid any of the above mentioned complications.

Clinical Pearl

Role of finger flexors and wrist extensors are important in hand function. The importance of maintenance of first web space and opposition is critical in thumb injuries. Wrist stability, functional sensibility is utmost important for functional use of hand.

RHEUMATOID HAND

Introduction and Pathophysiology

Rheumatoid arthritis (RA) is a systemic inflammatory condition of the synovial tissue **(Fig. 20.19)**.

- Joint destruction in RA is due to interaction of diseased synovial tissue and normal joint tissue. Inflamed synovium attracts neutrophils into the synovial fluid.

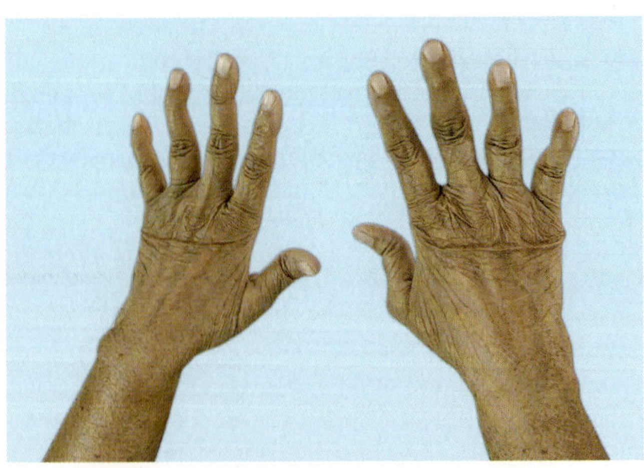

Fig. 20.19: Rheumatoid arthritis (RA) of the hand.

- Matrix degrading enzymes, produced by multiple cell types, destroy cartilage and bone as the disease progresses and the hyperplastic synovium surfaces over the articular cartilage and gradually over underlying subchondral bone.
- The diseased synovium forms "pannus" of RA by adhering to the cartilage and bone. Diseased synovium secretes fluid that causes distention of joint capsule and eventually leads to ligament injury along with joint instability.
- Loss of normal architecture of tendons and its function is common as perivascular inflammation can affect muscles especially intrinsic hand muscles that are more susceptible to the disease.
- Tendon rupture either due to attrition or ischemia is a common feature. Extensor pollicis longus (EPL) and flexor pollicis longus are commonly ruptured.

Stages of Rheumatoid Arthritis

Clinically there are four stages of RA **(Box 20.3)**.

Table 20.5 shows the 2010 RA classification criteria by ACR.

BOX 20.3: Stages of rheumatoid arthritis.

Stage I: Redness, warmth, swelling, severe pain.
Stage II: The pannus formed by inflamed synovium starts invading soft tissues leading to tenosynovitis, decreased mobility, pain is reduced.
Stage III: Joint deformity and soft tissue involvement occurs commonly.
Stage IV: Significant joint deformity, instability, bony or fibrous ankyloses.

Table 20.5: Rheumatoid arthritis classification criteria: Domains, categories, and point scores as per 2010 criteria.

Domain	Category	Point score
A	Joint involvement (0–5 points)	
	1 large joint	0
	2–10 large joints	1
	1–3 small joints (large joints not counted)	2
	4–10 small joints (large joints not counted)	3
	>10 joints including at least one small joint	5
B	Serology (at least one text needed for classification; 0–3 points)	
	Negative RF and negative ACPA	0
	Low positive RF or low positive ACPA	2
	High positive RF or high positive ACPA	3
C	Acute-phase reactants (at least one test needed for classification; 0–1 points)	
	Normal CRP and normal ESR	0
	Abnormal CRP or abnormal ESR	1
D	Duration of symptoms	
	<6 weeks	0
	>6 weeks	1

(ACPA: anti-citrullinated protein antibodies; CRP: C-reactive protein; ESR: erythrocyte sedimentation rate)

Clinical Features

Clinical features include the following:

- Affection of synovial lining of joints such as radiocarpal joint, scapholunate joint, midcarpal joint, subluxation of carpus, and distal radioulnar joint.
- Bilateral symmetrical involvement is commonly seen.
- **Deformities:** Following deformities in the joints are commonly seen as given in **Table 20.6** and **Figure 20.20**. Clinical differentiation of osteoarthritis of hand and RA of hand is possible through examination as shown in **Table 20.7**.

Management of Rheumatoid Hand

Management is essentially dependent upon assessing strength, mobility, and neurological and functional evaluation of wrist and hand.

1. **Joint protection** principles consist of techniques that can be applied to all activities. Improper use of joints can cause deformity, whereas joint protection techniques help performing activities in order to reduce risk of deformity.
2. Respect for **pain** is essential. It is advisable to cease doing activities before one reaches the point of discomfort or pain. Limit activities that cause pain that lasts more than 1 hour after the activity has been stopped. Patient should be advised to balance activity and rest. Planning rest periods during longer or more difficult activities is helpful. Resting for 10 minutes during an activity can help a patient restore energy for further task. Gentle passive mobilization techniques can be used for pain relief and maintaining joint mobility **(Figs. 20.21A to E)**.
3. **Activity pacing**: Patient is asked to stop the activity in between, which he or she cannot avoid. This eliminates excessive pain and fatigue later. Prioritizing activities helps to perform better in demanding tasks. Patient should consider factors such as the type of activity, length of time, and difficulty before beginning and then plan difficult activities for "peak" energy times. Take frequent breaks in between long tasks.
4. **Ergonomic advice:**
   - Use larger and stronger joints for activities when possible and distribute the weight over noninvolved or stronger joints. For example, patient can use the hip to push open doors, and the feet to shut lower drawers.
   - Avoid being in one position for prolonged periods of time. Plan adequate rest. Change the joints position. Stretch and relax the joints. Avoid positions of deformity.
   - Maintain or use the joints in optimal alignment and proper posture.
   - Maintain proper weight, since additional weight can stress weight-bearing joints (hip, knees, feet, and back).
   - Use adaptive equipment such as jar openers and button hooks.

Table 20.6: Common deformities seen in rheumatoid arthritis.

Joint	Factor affecting deformities
Metacarpophalangeal joint—Volar subluxation or ulnar deviation	1. Proliferative synovitis of joint leading to stretching and fragmentation of collateral ligaments 2. Decreased stability of joint can lead to progressive deformity. Intrinsic muscle weakness creates imbalance 3. Extrinsic extensor tendons affects MP joint ulnar drift along with flexor tendons
Swan neck deformity of fingers	A zigzag collapse of the IP joints with proximal IP joint hyperextension and distal IP joint flexion, as a result of muscle–tendon imbalance and /or joint laxity
Boutonniere deformity of fingers	This deformity has three components: 1. Flexion of the PIP joint 2. Hyperextension of DIP joint 3. Hyperextension of MCP joint Alteration in muscle tendon balance can lead to this deformity
Swan neck deformity of thumb	Characterized by MP joint hyperextension and IP joint flexion along with adduction of metacarpal. Synovitis and capsular distension of CMC joint causes this deformity
Boutonniere deformity of thumb	Characterized by MP joint flexion and IP joint hyperextension along with adduction of metacarpal. Synovitis and capsular distension of MP joint causes this deformity
Radial deviation deformity of thumb	Characterized by radial deviation deformity of MP joint with secondary adduction of thumb metacarpal

(DIP: distal interphalangeal; IP: interphalangeal; MCP: metacarpophalangeal; CMC: carpometacarpal)

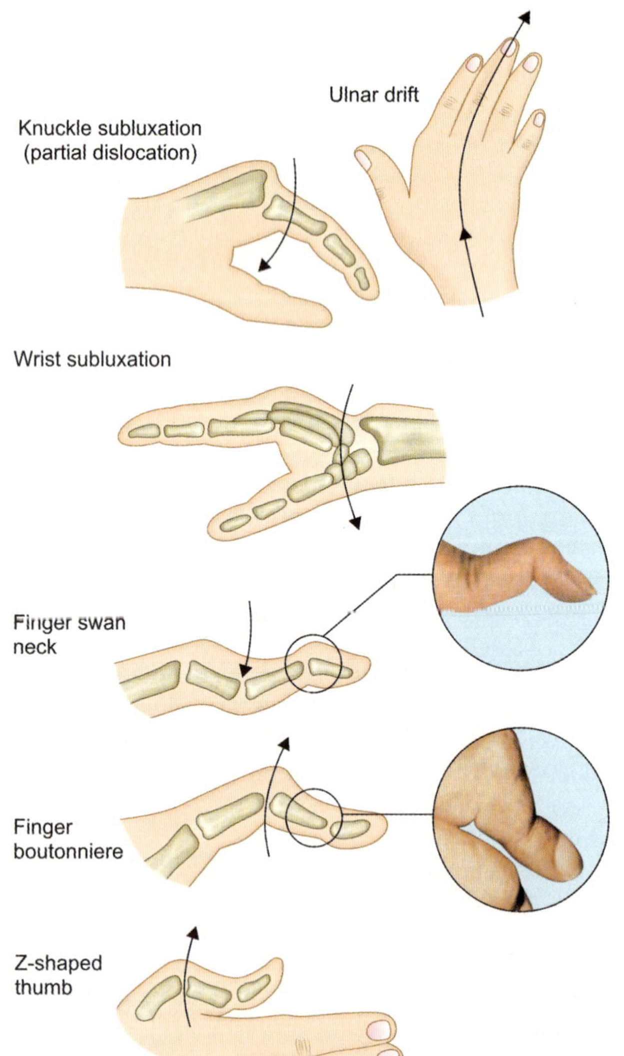

Fig. 20.20: Common deformities of rheumatoid arthritis (RA) hand.

Table 20.7: Difference between rheumatoid arthritis and osteo-arthritis.

Rheumatoid arthritis	Osteoarthritis
It is a chronic inflammatory condition and is an autoimmune disease	Degenerative joint disease, which occurs due to deterioration of cartilage
It can occur even in childhood and is more common in females. Typical age of occurrence of rheumatoid arthritis is between 30 and 60 years	It generally occurs at the age of 45 years in males, and 55 years in females
Usually, it is symmetrical, the same joints on both sides are affected, particularly in hands, elbows, wrists, feet, knees, ankles, and neck	Usually single joint involvement and asymmetrical involvement seen
	Heberden's nodes are common manifestation. Commonly seen at distal interphalangeal (DIP) joint

Special Exercise Considerations for the Hands

There are some special exercises considered for hands:

- Avoid tight grasp, and use a relaxed grip and enlarged handles.
- Avoid pressure on the back of knuckles [metacarpophalangeal (MCP) joints].
- Whenever possible, make use of both hands.
- Avoid repetitive hand activities such as using a screwdriver.
- Avoid pressure over the thumb tip, e.g., pushing snaps together, opening car doors, and ringing doorbells.

A study done by Hoenig et al., described the significance of home exercise protocol and insisted that

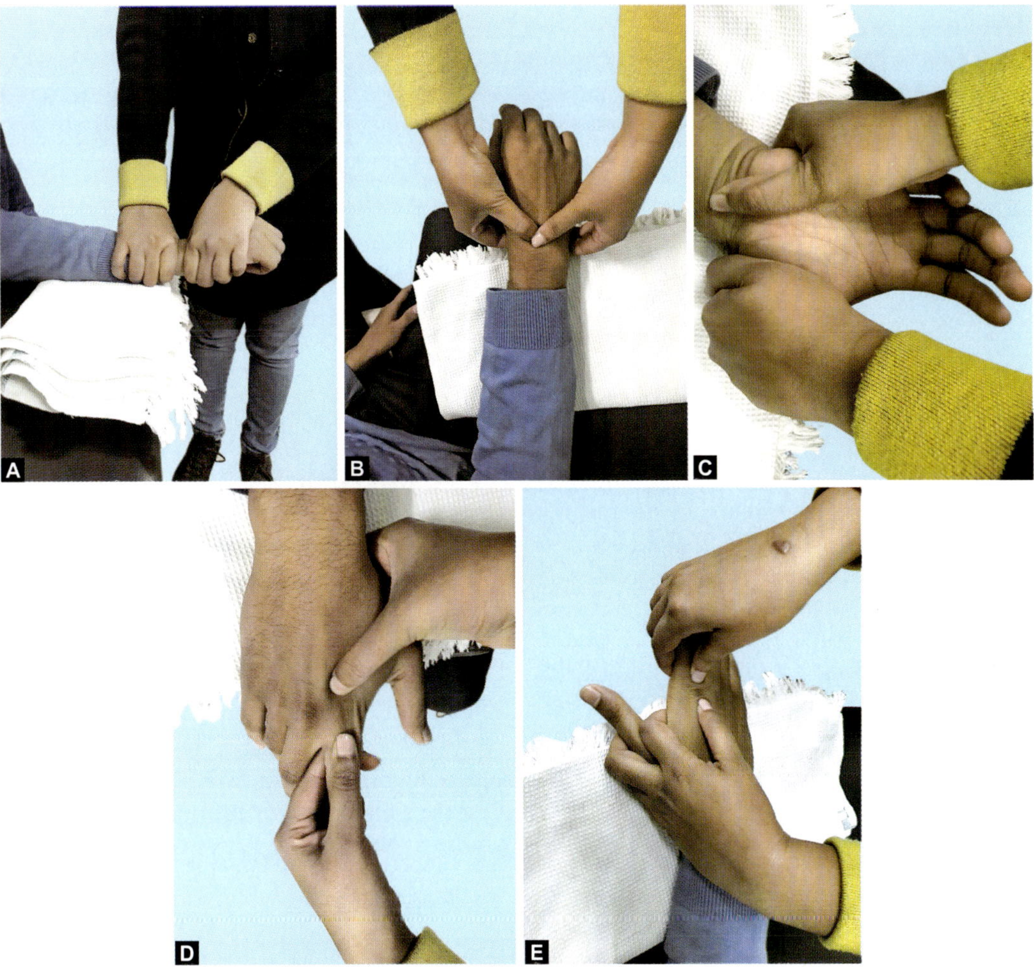

Figs. 20.21A to E: Joint mobilization techniques for wrist and hand.

temporary use of home hand exercises has acceptable side effects and is an effective means of increasing grip strength. Physiotherapy and particularly exercise therapy improves the functional status of the rheumatoid hand in short term favorably. Different opinions exist about benefit of exercises in RA but recent studies suggest that the benefits of exercise outweigh its possible detriments. A single standard treatment never applies to all those with RA. Instead, treatment program should be individualized to each person's needs, considering the severity; presence of other medical problems, and their individual lifestyle and preferences. Dynamic individually tailored strength training is safe to include as a part of an overall rehabilitation program for patients with RA.

The aim of **electrotherapy** is pain relief and improving muscle strength. One of the greatest benefits of physiotherapy modalities is facilitation of exercise performance.

- Heat therapy reduces stiffness and pain and causes muscle relaxation. It increases collagen extension in tendons, reduces joint stiffness, relieves pain, increases pain threshold, alleviates muscle spasm, and improves intra-articular circulation in RA. Paraffin wax bath is particularly useful for treating the rheumatoid hand. When followed by active hand exercise, it results in significant improvement in the ROM and grip function. Apply heat for 20 minutes every 2–3 hours. Heat should not be applied in the presence of discoloration or swelling.

- Cold therapy reduces swelling and inflammation. Cryobaths are very effective for pain control, reduction of joint swelling, and improving hand grip. Ice can be applied for 15 minutes but no longer than 20 minutes. Suitable modes of application could be used in the form of crushed ice, cold gel, frozen bag of peas, chemical cold packs, ice blocks, and ice water. The ice should not be held in any one spot for more than 3 minutes. Always use cloth or towel to hold the ice. Consistent check of circulation is essential to avoid any adverse effect of cryotherapy. Contrast bath can be considered in some of the patients.

Exercise therapy plays a great role in fighting against rheumatic disability.

Counseling plays an essential role in RA. Acceptance of the disease is of utmost importance so as to make the patient physically independent and be proactive in managing symptoms.

Provision and education of use of **assistive devices** such as splints, orthoses, helps to enhance performance

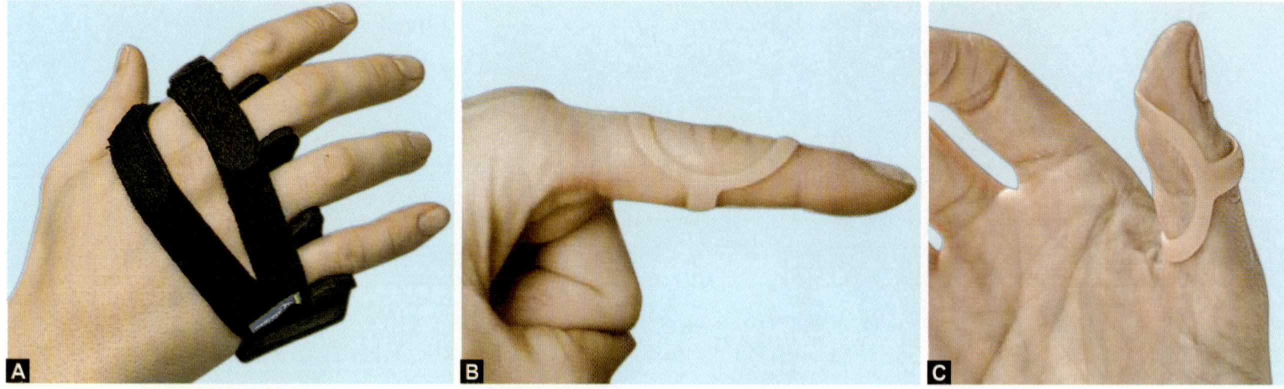

Figs. 20.22A to C: (A) Ulnar drift splint; and (B and C) oval-8 for boutonniere of index and thumb.

of RA patients. Stage I patient of RA can be benefited by resting splints at night. This splint helps for decreasing pain, inflammation, and spasm. In stage II, night splint is useful for rest and to decrease pain. In stage III, splints are applied with the intention to slow down the progression of deformity.

Metacarpophalangeal ulnar drift (MUD) splint **(Fig. 20.22A)** is helpful for passive correction of ulnar drift and patient acceptance is also good. The oval-8 splint **(Figs. 20.22B and C)** is available in a variety of sizes and is made of metal. These splints are well tolerated by patients as they do not interfere with ADLs. Boutonniere deformity splint gives good passive extension, proximal interphalangeal (PIP) extension with a distal interphalangeal extension block. Due to less acceptance of this splint, patient is advised to wear it at night. Splinting also prevents volar subluxation of the carpus on radius, distal ulnar dorsal subluxation, and is useful in carpometacarpal (CMC) joint stabilization for RA thumb.

Clinical Pearl

There are various clinical practice guidelines for managing rheumatoid arthritis and favorable recommendations are proposed. Readers are advised to go through NICE guidelines, Ottawa panel evidence-based guidelines, and Strengthening and Stretching for RA of Hand (SARAH) trial.

PERIPHERAL NERVE INJURIES AND ENTRAPMENT NEUROPATHY

Introduction

Ulnar, median, and radial are the three common nerves supplying the upper quadrant. Involvement of these nerves can be in the form of radiculopathy, mononeuropathy, or entire nerve trunk involvement as in brachial plexus injury. Radiculopathy is a process that affects the nerve root, most commonly due to a herniated disk. Dysfunction of a single peripheral nerve is called mononeuropathy. Brachial plexopathy involves the entire plexus, or parts of the plexus like trunk lesions. In a cord level lesion, pattern of weakness and numbness depends upon the part of the

---

BOX 20.4: Causes of entrapment with examples.

Cause of entrapment	Example
Nerve opposing bone	Ulnar nerve at the level of elbow
Closed spaces	Area of carpal tunnel
Adjacent structures	Median nerve at the level of elbow, adjacent to the brachial artery

plexus involved. Entrapment neuropathy is also common. Certain sites are likely for nerve entrapments/injuries as shown in **Box 20.4**.

Assessment

Assessment should be as follows:

- Both passive and active ROM should be measured and recorded with the help of a suitably sized goniometer.
- Composite grip strength and pinch strength of various types of grips **(Figs. 20.23 and 20.24)**, as measured by a commercially available dynamometer and pinchometer **(Figs. 20.25 and 20.26)**, are also helpful in understanding the effects of a peripheral nerve injury.
- Sensory assessment is divided into five levels:
  1. Sympathetic response (ninhydrin, wrinkle test)
  2. Detection (Semmes–Weinstein monofilament)
  3. Discrimination [two-point discrimination (2PD)]
  4. Quantification
  5. Recognition

Combined, these five categories create a continuum of sensibility function, which ranges from simple, non-subjective responses to the highly complex identification process.

Standardized hand function tests that measure a wide range of hand coordination and dexterity levels are currently available for assessing the functional repercussions of peripheral nerve injury. The instruments are:

- The Valpar work samples measure total extremity strength and coordination related to work skills
- Jebsen hand function test for hand co-ordination
- The minnesota rate of manipulation tests measure relatively gross hand coordination

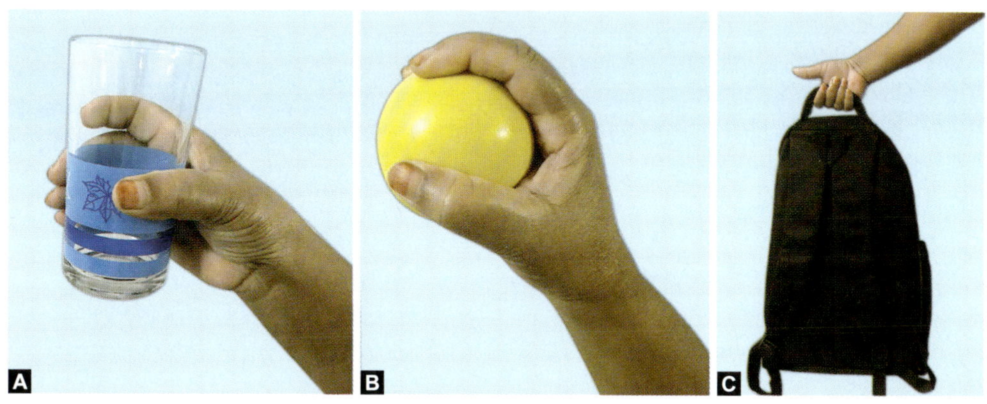

Figs. 20.23A to C: Types of power grips: (A) Cylindrical grip; (B) Spherical grip; (C) Hook grasp.

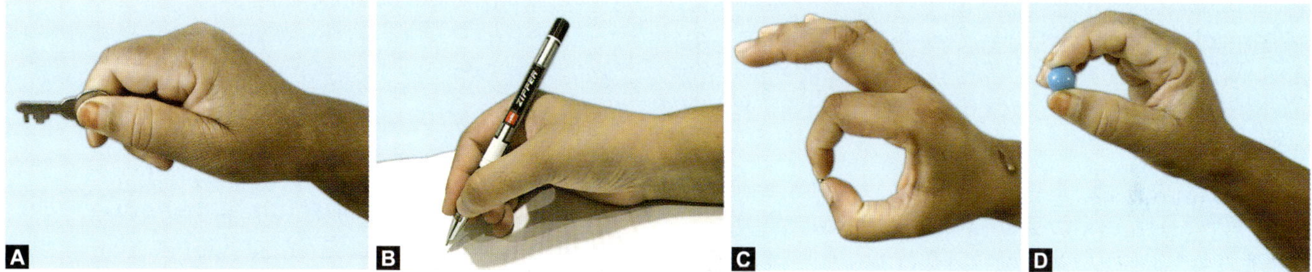

Figs. 20.24A to D: Types of prehension grips: (A) Lateral prehension grip; (B) Three jaw chuck grasp;
(C) Tip-to-tip prehension; (D) Pad-to-pad prehension.

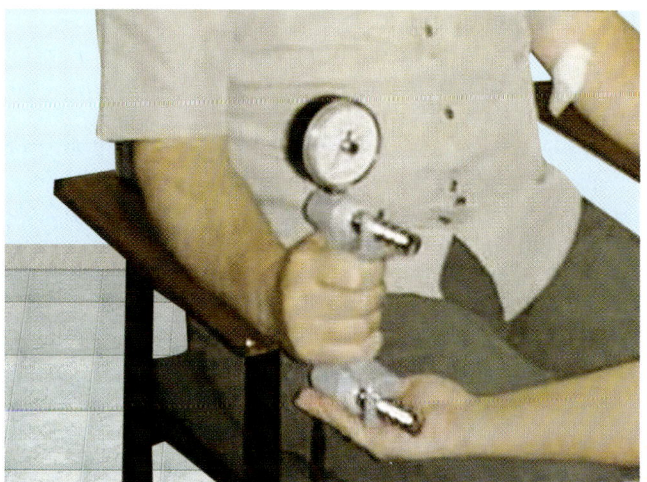

Fig. 20.25: Measurement of grip strength using JAMAR
dynamometer.

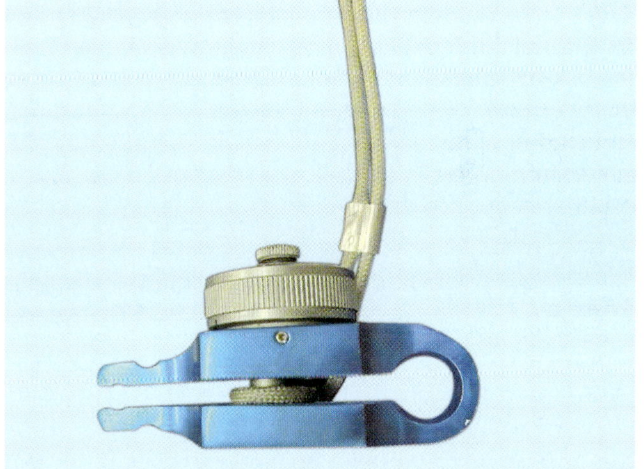

Fig. 20.26: Pinch gauge to measure strength
of pinch.

- For the finer dexterity requirements the Purdue Peg Board (PPB)
- The Crawford Small Parts Dexterity Test

Standardized assessment tests should be chosen according to the general capacities of the patient population to be studied and the type of data required.

Rehabilitation of Peripheral Nerve Injuries

Sensory Re-education

Rehabilitation in the case of anesthesia aims at protecting patients from traumas to which he/she is exposed. Patient may be unprotected from hot or cold burns or sharp objects, etc. due to anesthesia. They need to perform and memorize simple actions several times a day to preserve body mapping.

In the case of hyposensitivity, rehabilitation relies on the brain's neuroplasticity. Patient is encouraged to react to tactile stimulation and reorganizing the pathways. Global exercises are incorporated when patient has recovered sufficiently. Familiar objects of different shapes and textures are used. Furthermore, memory is used to recognize a stimulus; hence, it is likely that familiar shapes, textures, and objects will be more easily recognized than specific treatment objects, and therefore functional sensibility may improve more rapidly and, possibly, to a larger extent.

Motor Strengthening

Denervated muscles can undergo atrophy hence therapists have to strive to prevent fibrosis. Early contraction of muscles is facilitated; massage kneading techniques help to prevent fibrosis. Facilitation techniques based on percussions and stretching are encouraged as signs of regrowth are observed. Muscle trophicity can be maintained using electrical stimulation for denervated or partially innervated muscles.

Range of Motion

Maintaining ROM is essential throughout recovery phase as stiffness or contractures make it difficult to have good dexterity of hand. Static splinting of hand in functional position helps to sustain optimum hand function.

Median Nerve

Anatomy

It is a mixed nerve arising from C6 to T1 roots and passes through posterior cord (C6–C7) and medial cord (C8–T1) **(Fig. 20.27)**. At the level of forearm, it passes through the two heads of PT where it gives an anterior interosseous branch, which innervates the flexor digitorum profundus (index finger), the flexor pollicis longus, and pronator quadratus. Palmar cutaneous branch of median nerve arises from

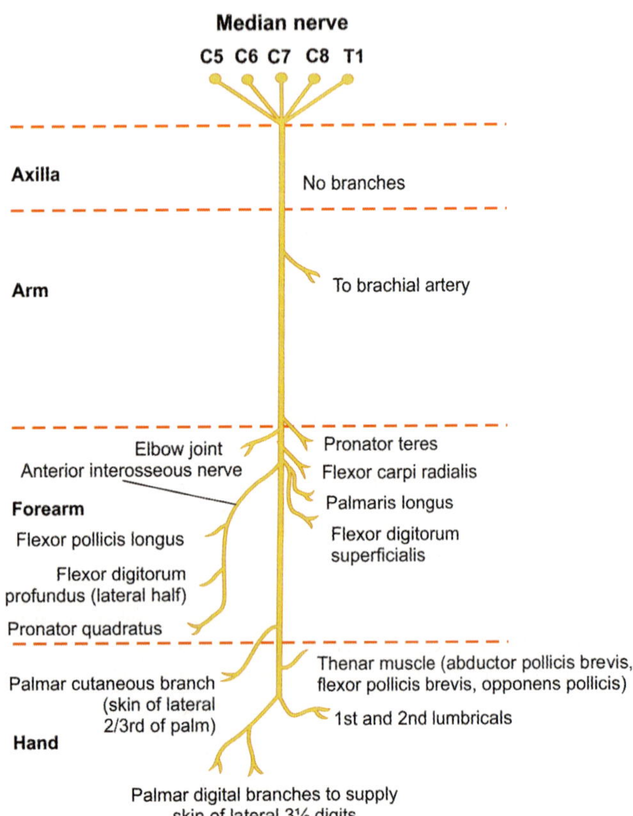

Fig. 20.27: Median nerve course.

BOX 20.5: Causes of Median nerve involvement.

- Axillary level-root involvement
- Trauma
- At the level of arm, median nerve commonly does not get injured or entrapped
- Forearm-pronator teres syndrome
- Anterior interosseous nerve involvement
- Vascular reasons—brachial artery involvement
- Glass cut injuries at the wrist level
- Carpal tunnel syndrome
- Carpal fractures
- Volkmann's ischemic contracture

lateral side 6 cm above the wrist palmar flexion crease. At carpal tunnel area, median nerve enters wrist. The causes of median nerve involvement are given in **Box 20.5**.

Clinical Presentation of Median Nerve Involvement

Clinical presentation of median nerve involvement includes the following:

1. **Sensory loss:** Median nerve innervates.
   - Palmar side of the first three digits and the radial half of the fourth digit.
   - Dorsal side of two distal phalanges of the index and third finger and the radial side of the distal two phalanges of the fourth finger.

   Sensory loss in these areas can be a common presentation as shown in **Figure 20.28**.

2. **Motor weakness:** At motor level, it innervates the muscles of anterior compartment of forearm, **except** flexor carpi ulnaris and the two medial heads of the flexor digitorum profundus. It also innervates two radial side lumbrical muscles and intrinsic muscles of the thenar eminence such as abductor pollicis and superficial fascicle of the flexor pollicis brevis. The

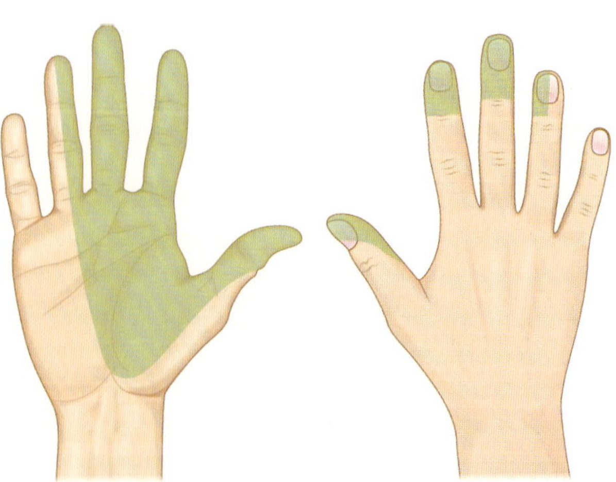

Fig. 20.28: Sensory loss in median nerve.

anterior interosseous branch innervates the flexor digitorum profundus (index finger); the flexor pollicis longus and pronator quadratus. Weakness of these muscles is common.

3. Functional loss in terms of inability to hold objects as there is thumb involvement leading to pointing index and ape thumb deformity.

4. Trick movements are seen in many patients where muscles supplied by intact nerves like ulnar try and compensate the action. Observation of functional tasks is helpful to report these trick movements.

Rehabilitation of Peripheral Nerve Involvement

Splints like C-bar **(Fig. 20.29)** help to avoid first web space contracture and enhance good thumb positioning and function. Dynamic splints like knuckle bender helps to achieve lumbrical positioning and prevent claw hand position.

Surgical options: In long-standing case options such as Riordan Opponensplasty where ring flexor digitorum superficialis (FDS) is transferred for abductor pollicis brevis (APB) or extensor indicis proprius transfer to APB is preferred. In any of these tendon transfer procedures, aim is to achieve thumb opposition. Muscle reeducation after transfer procedure and strengthening of donor muscles before transfer is aimed at.

Clinical Pearl

Splinting to prevent adduction contracture of the thumb is addressed by proactive splinting.

Ulnar Nerve

Anatomy

Ulnar nerve is a mixed nerve that originates from C8 and T1 nerve roots and extends along the internal head of triceps **(Fig. 20.30)**. It passes between the two heads of the flexor carpi ulnaris. In the mid-forearm, it gets ventral and passes along the FDS toward the Guyon's canal in the wrist. It then gives of four branches: motor branch supplies muscles of hypothenar eminence, interossei, third and fourth lumbricals, adductor pollicis, deep bundle of flexor pollicis brevis. Sensory branch supplies fifth and half of the fourth finger. The most radial branch supplies flexor

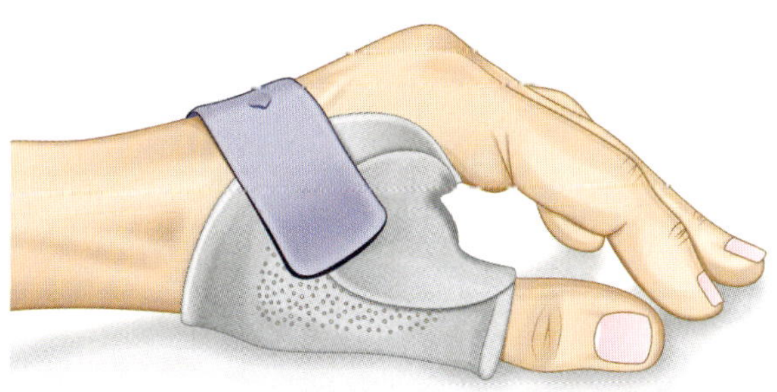

Fig. 20.29: Thumb splint to prevent adductor contracture.

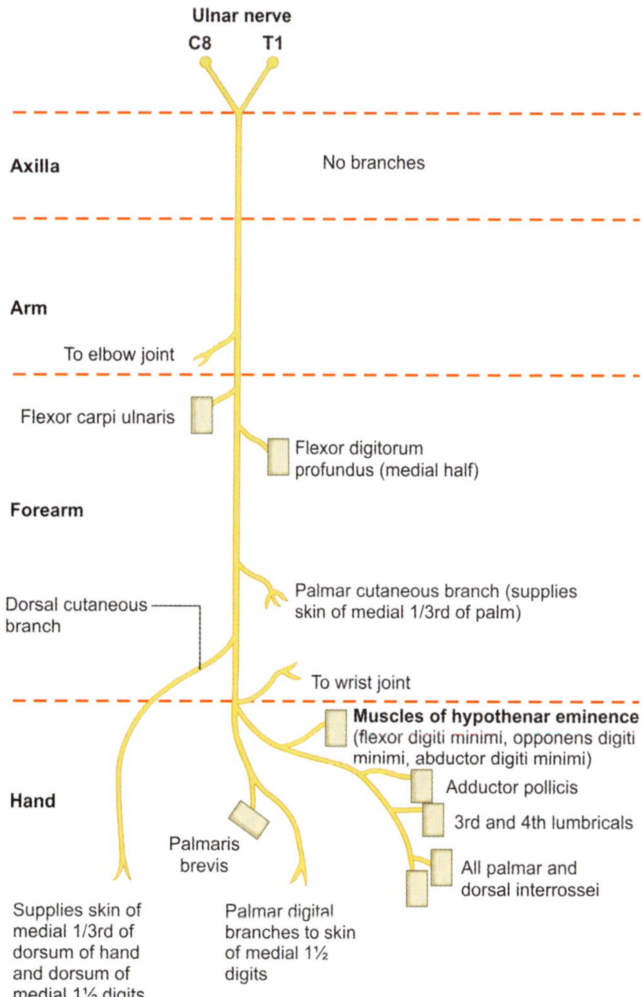

Fig. 20.30: Ulnar nerve course.

carpi ulnaris and two medial heads of the flexor digitorum profundus. In the forearm and hand, it innervates all the intrinsic hand muscles except for the two radial lumbricals, the opponens pollicis, the APB and superficial bundle of flexor pollicis brevis. Causes of ulnar nerve involvement are shown in **Box 20.6**.

Clinical Features

Following are the clinical features:

- Injury at the elbow is characterized by paresthesia and numbness over the fourth and fifth digits. It is usually characterized by tingling or numbness along the little finger.
- Pain over the medial forearm
- Lumbricals and flexor digitorum profundus muscle weakness and weakness of abduction and/or adduction of the fingers
- Examining the hand reveals ulnar claw characterized by hyperextension of the metacarpophalyngeal joints and flexion at the distal and proximal IP joints of the ring and the little finger.
- **Froment's sign or Book test:** In **Figure 20.31**, the thumb IP joint on the left side is seen to have flexed because of weakness of adductor pollicis.

BOX 20.6: Causes of ulnar nerve involvement.	
1. Overuse injuries of elbow	Overuse of forearm muscles such as flexor carpi ulnaris can entrap the ulnar nerve at the level of elbow
2. Larger carrying angle	When arms are held out at sides with palms facing forward, forearm and hands should normally be about 5–15° away from the body. This is called carrying angle. Females have a larger carrying angle than males. Due to fractures at the elbow carrying angle may become excessive leading to stretch on ulnar nerve
3. Tardy ulnar nerve palsy	Nonunion of lateral condyle fracture leads to cubitus valgus deformity, which could affect ulnar nerve
4. Fracture of ulnar	A fall over the elbow or a direct blow to the medial aspect of the elbow causes ulnar nerve palsy associated with pisiform fracture
5. Leprosy	Ulnar nerve is common to get involved in leprosy patients at the level of elbow
6. Glass cut injuries at wrist or forearm can directly affect ulnar nerve	

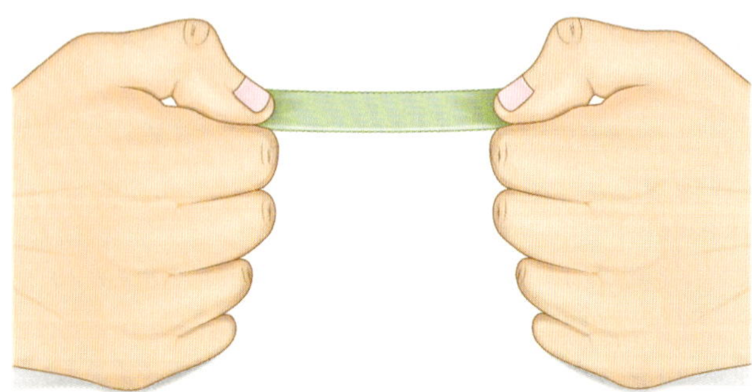

Fig. 20.31: Froment's sign.

- When asked to adduct the thumb (such as holding a pencil in the web space), patient will instead hyperflex the IP joint to compensate for loss of the adductor and MP joint instability. Adductor pollicis weakness causes instability of the MP joint; unopposed action of the thumb extensors causes MCP hyperextension deformity and unopposed activity of the thumb flexors causes IP joint hyper flexion deformity.
- **Wartenberg's sign** (little finger abduction)

The little finger remains abducted. Due to unopposed ulnar insertion of extensor digiti quinti, little finger shows more severe claw deformity, as opposed to ring finger, because of the inherently more laxity in little finger MP joint volar plate.

Rehabilitation Following Ulnar Involvement

Rehabilitation of ulnar nerve is done with same techniques as for median nerve.

- **Strengthening protocol:** The muscles involved in compression at the level of the elbow are flexor carpi ulnaris and fourth and fifth fingers' deep flexors. But symptoms depend on extent of fiber compression.
- Reinforcement techniques are encouraged. It is always better to train muscles for functional task through strengthening. Training intrinsic muscles and hypothenar muscles is essential for gaining strong grip.
- Special attention given for proprioception, coordination, and dexterity training.

Orthotic Management

In initial stage of injury, the role of orthosis is to give rest to the nerve. Static splints are used. If compression is at the level of elbow, splint with elbow flexed at 30° is preferred. This avoids undue pressure on nerve at elbow. Compression at the level of Guyon's canal will be helped by a splint which maintains wrist in neutral **(Fig. 20.32)**.

Surgical Management

Surgical management can be done by the following ways:

- **Adductor pollicis deficit:** Substitution of the adductor pollicis by FDS of long finger passed through interosseous membrane, over and under extensor carpi ulnaris (ECU) as a distal pulley; crossing beneath extensor digitorum communis (EDC), and into adductor insertion, anchoring tendon into bone.
- **Boyle's procedure:** Transfer of brachioradialis (rerouting around third MC to adductor pollicis)
- **Metacarpophalangeal arthrodesis:** Tendon transfer may not be possible at times, due to lack of muscles, so MP arthrodesis of hypermobile thumb MP joint will provide stability and some strength gain.

Intrinsic muscles deficit (**Burkhalter transfer**): Transfer of APL to first dorsal interossei.

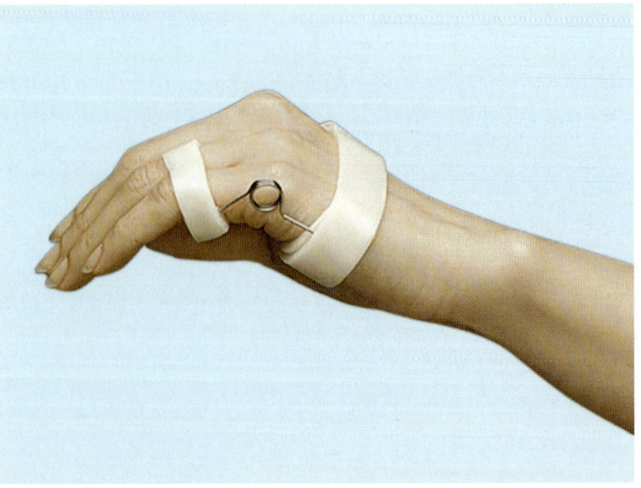

Fig. 20.32: Knuckle bender splint for ulnar nerve involvement.

Clinical Pearl

An elbow pad can be provided to protect the vulnerable cubital tunnel area, which patients' may continue wearing if there is persistent hypersensitivity.

Radial Nerve

Anatomy

The radial nerve is a mixed nerve arising from the posterior branches of spinal nerves, C5 to C8, and T1 **(Fig. 20.33)**. Near radial head, it splits into two branches, namely posterior interosseous nerve and superficial branch of radial nerve. Posterior branch of radial nerve supplies ECU, extensor digitorum, and extensor digiti minimi. Anterior branch innervates abductor pollicis longus (APL), EPL, extensor pollicis brevis (EPB), and extensor indicis. The causes of radial nerve involvement are mentioned in **Box 20.7**.

Clinical Features

Wrist drop **(Fig. 20.34)** is a common clinical feature where patient is not able to extend at the level of wrist or fingers. Sensory loss on dorsum of hand is significant especially first web space. For strong gripping force, extension of wrist is essential, which maintains a good length tension relationship but due to inability of wrist extension grip becomes weak.

Rehabilitation

The features of rehabilitation can be described as follows:

- Inflammation surrounding nerve can be managed in initial stages through cryotherapy, massage that could decrease perineural inflammation.

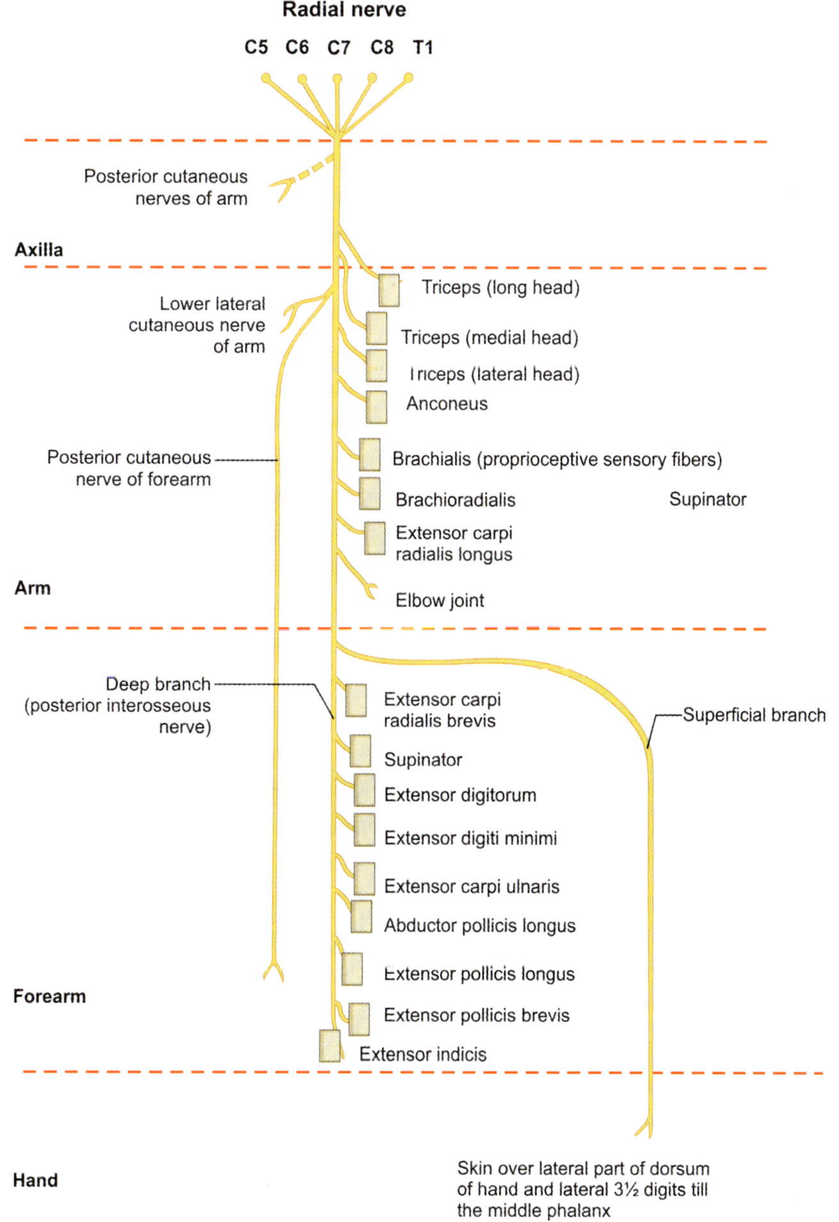

Fig. 20.33: Radial nerve course.

- Pressure in the axilla of inappropriate crutch height can affect radial nerve.
- Vascular cause affecting radial artery supplying radial nerve.
- Arm-fracture of the distal humeral one-third can affect radial nerve near humeral spiral groove. Compression due to prolonged pressure or an overinflated tourniquet kept for a long time can affect nerve.
- Saturday night palsy: Excessive prolonged pressure in the proximal part of arm.
- Posterior interosseous nerve syndrome: Nerve compression at the level of supinator arch, which can be secondary to repetitive movement in patients who have an anatomical predisposition like thick Arcade of Frohse or tumor.

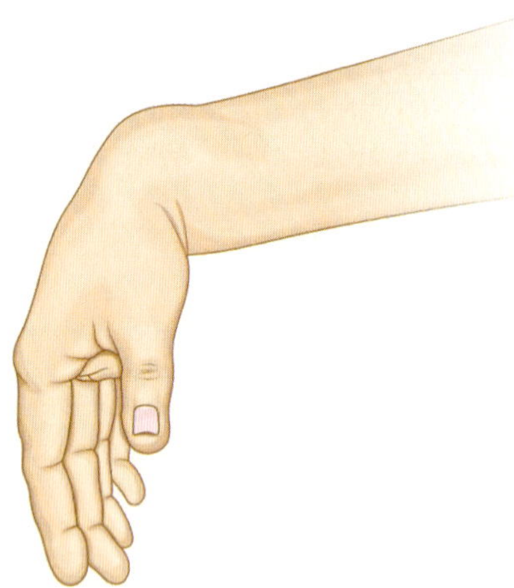

Fig. 20.34: Wrist drop (radial nerve injury).

- **Strengthening:** Muscles affected by radial nerve compression in posterior interosseous nerve syndrome are the ECRB, supinator, extensor carpi ulnaris, extensor digitorum, extensor digiti minimi, APB, and extensor indicis.
- Reinforcement of these muscles is essential where gradual progression from static to intensive strengthening protocol can be encouraged.
- Proprioception, dexterity, and coordination are given utmost importance.
- Sensory involvement is seen mainly with superficial branch of radial nerve damage. Sensory re-education protocol is followed similar as for median and ulnar nerve.

Orthotic Management

Static splint that allows the wrist to rest in 20° of extension is helpful for the prevention of wrist contractures.

Dynamic cock-up splint can be suggested for further recovery **(Fig. 20.35)**.

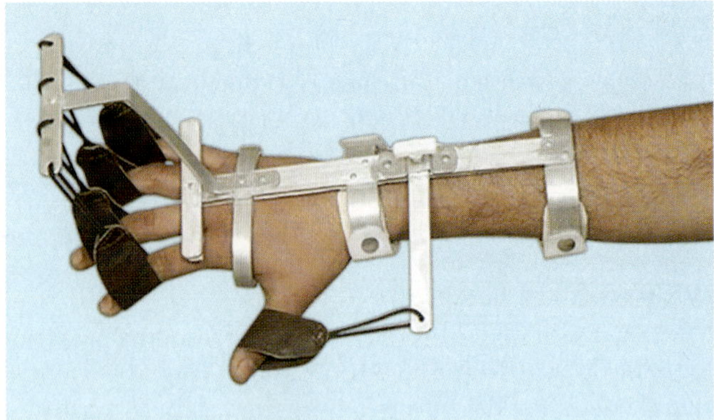

Fig. 20.35: Dynamic cock-up splint.

Surgical Management

The procedures of surgical management are as follows:

- Tendon transfer for high radial nerve palsy. Pronator teres is inserted onto the ECRB. Palmaris longus is inserted onto the EPL and EPB. Flexor carpi radialis is inserted onto the EDC. Tenodesis of the APL around the brachioradialis prevents a flexion adduction contracture of the thumb.
- Low radial nerve palsy. ECRB tenodesis to the extensor carpi radialis longus for compensating radial deviation. APL, EDC, and EPL are the commonly affected muscles.

Clinical Pearl

Avoid forceful wrist extension and supination in radial nerve palsy. Behavioral modification should be considered in long term for better patient outcome.

CUMULATIVE TRAUMA DISORDERS OF HAND AND WRIST

Musculoskeletal disorders related to the hand and wrist can take a variety of forms, such as cumulative trauma disorder (CTD), repetitive strain injury, occupational repetitive microtrauma, repetitive motion injury, overuse syndrome, carpal tunnel syndrome (CTS), and repetitive stress disorder. Predominantly repetitive motion hand disorders are caused due to constant flexion and extension motions of wrist and fingers. Chronic, repetitive hand and wrist movements, especially with the hand in "pinch" position, are the most stressful for small joints. Wrist joint in an abnormal or awkward position; or working for too long a period without rest or altering of hand and forearm muscles; mechanical stresses to digital nerves from sustained grasping of sharp edges on instrument handles; forceful work; long use of vibratory instruments and also due to proximal joint involvement are common contributory factors.

Risk of developing musculoskeletal disorder (MSD) increases when the same or similar parts of the body is continuously used, with few breaks or rest. Highly repetitive

> **BOX 20.8:** Common types of cumulative trauma disorders of hand.
>
> - Carpal tunnel syndrome
> - Guyon's canal syndrome
> - Pronator teres syndrome
> - Tenosynovitis and tendinitis, e.g., DeQuervain's, trigger digits

tasks can cause fatigue, tissue damage, discomfort, and eventually injury. This can also occur if the level of force is low and the work postures are not awkward.

The common types of CTDs are mentioned in **Box 20.8**.

Carpal Tunnel Syndrome

Pathoanatomical Factors

Typical CTS symptoms include numbness and tingling along the median nerve distribution of the hand and in more severe cases, loss of muscle strength. Median nerve pathology affects all nerve functions distal to the site of lesion and, sometimes, pain extends proximally up to the shoulder. Pathoanatomical factors include high carpal tunnel pressure, ischemic changes within the nerve, and adjacent structures compressing on the nerve.

Clinical Course

Symptom duration and severity of nighttime symptoms should be assessed. The presence of a positive Phalen's test, thenar muscle wasting, and prior nonsurgical interventions should also be assessed, since they have been shown to influence results with nonsurgical management.

As per some evidences, frequency of symptoms (mild demonstrating more intermittent symptoms and moderate demonstrating more constant symptoms) seems to be a factor that distinguishes mild from moderate CTS, and thenar muscle atrophy is the clinical sign that distinguishes patients with severe CTS from those with mild or moderate disease.

Risk Factors

The intrinsic risk factors such as obesity, age, and female sex play a significant role. The occupational risk factor of forceful hand exertions has strongest association with CTS. In a patient with suspected CTS, clinicians should use SWMT (Semmes-Weinstein monofilament test) using the 2.83 or 3.22 monofilament as the threshold for normal light touch sensation **(Figs. 20.36A and B)** and static 2-point discrimination (2PD) on the middle finger to aid in determining the extent of nerve damage. Those with suspected moderate to severe CTS should be assessed for any radial finger using the 3.22 filament as the threshold for normal. In those with suspected CTS, Katz hand diagram, Phalen's test, Tinel's sign, and carpal compression test should be used to determine the likelihood of CTS and interpret test findings.

Outcome Measures for Assessment

Activity limitations—self-report measures:
- Boston carpal tunnel questionnaire
- Carpal Tunnel Questionnaire-Symptom Severity Scale (CTQ-SSS)
- CTQ-FS (Functional Scale)
- The DASH.

Activity limitations—physical performance measures:
- Purdue Peg Board (PPB)
- DMPUT (Dellon-modified Moberg pick-up test) to assess dexterity (compare with established normative values for age and sex).

Physical impairment measures:
- SWMT
- Static 2PD on the middle finger
- Phalen's test
- Tinel's sign
- Carpal compression test
- Grip strength and tip or three-point pinch strength to assess strength.

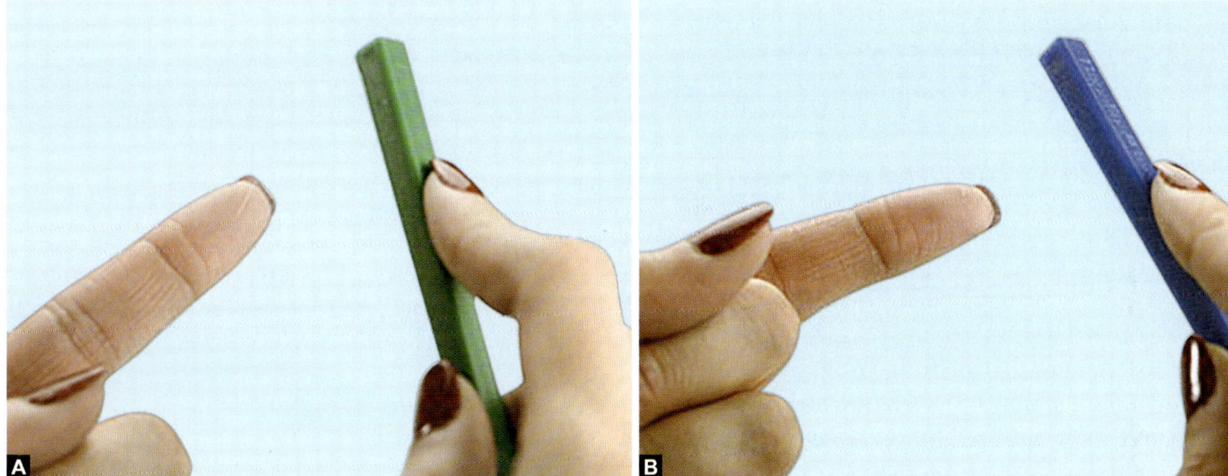

Figs. 20.36A and B: Semmes–Weinstein monofilament test.

Electrodiagnosis

Electrodiagnosis can be explained as follows:

- Nerve conduction study is more useful than needle electromyography (EMG) because of the underlying pathophysiology of focal demyelination in CTS.
- The key finding for CTS is conduction slowing localized to the segment of the median nerve passing through the carpal tunnel.
- In early and mild CTS, mild sensory nerve conduction slowing across the carpal tunnel may be the only abnormal finding.
- The peak latency of the median sensory nerve action potential is typically delayed or prolonged.
- Median motor nerve conduction is usually recorded over the APB muscle.
- Delay in distal motor latency suggests CTS.
- Needle EMG can reveal denervation by the presence of membrane instability, such as fibrillation potentials and positive sharp waves, and altered motor unit morphology.

Intervention Strategies

Intervention strategies include the following:

- Educating the patients regarding the effects of mouse use on carpal tunnel pressure and assisting them in developing alternate strategies for the use of arrow keys, touch screens, or alternating the mouse hand.
- Keyboards with reduced strike force are recommended for patients with CTS who report pain with keyboard use. A neutral-positioned wrist orthosis worn at night provides short-term symptom relief and functional improvement for those seeking nonsurgical management.
- Superficial heat for short-term symptom relief is helpful, application of microwave or long-wave diathermy for short-term pain and symptom relief in mild-to-moderate idiopathic CTS is useful. A trial of IFC (interferential current) for short-term pain symptom relief in adults with idiopathic, mild-to-moderate CTS may also be preferred.
Contraindications should be taken into consideration before choosing any intervention.
- Phonophoresis for mild-to-moderate CTS may be used.
- Manual therapy, directed at the cervical spine and upper extremity, for individuals with mild to moderate CTS may help in the short term.
- A combined orthotic/stretching program may be used in mild to moderate CTS who do not have thenar atrophy and have normal 2-point discrimination. Those undergoing treatment for clinically significant improvement should be monitored carefully.

Tendonitis and Tenosynovitis

Tendons of wrist and hand are covered by membranous tendon sheath. Excessive repetitive stress without rest can lead to inflammation of tendon sheath and resultant painful limitation of motion. Swelling and crepitation while performing movement of wrist are felt. Commonly involved tendon of wrist complex is dorsal extensor of wrist and the long abductor and short extensor of thumb. This anatomic site is termed "snuffbox." Tendonitis in this area is called **DeQuervain's disease**. Tenderness over tendon is common.

Finkelstein test: Flexion of thumb and cupping it under the thumb can reproduce the symptoms. Pinching and holding by thumb becomes difficult. As any profession of patient demands holding of small instrument and maneuvering, this pain can restrict lot of activities. Essential activities of daily living can also become difficult due to pinching force.

Guyon's Canal Syndrome

Ulnar nerve passes across the narrow Guyon's canal (**Fig. 20.37**) formed between pisiform bone and hook of the hamate. Volar carpal ligament forms roof of the canal. Pressure on this area while performing procedures can lead to sensory involvement of volar and dorsal aspect of ring and little finger. Weakness of intrinsic hand muscles, flexor digitorum profundus of ring and little finger, and flexor carpi ulnaris is common.

Pronator Teres Syndrome

Median nerve pierces the forearm between two heads of PT muscles near antecubital area. Tenderness in the area of forearm and paresthesia on excessive pronation leads to confirmation of entrapment of median nerve.

Management of Cumulative Trauma Disorders

Therapists play unique role in gaining information related to symptoms and their relation with injury. Through

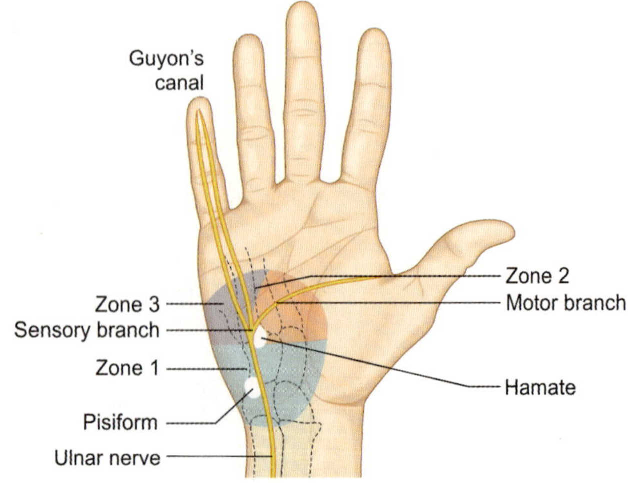

Fig. 20.37: Guyon's canal.

exercises, activity, and work simulation therapist can try and replicate the symptoms. This helps to establish relation between CTD, stages, and patient response. Rehabilitation of CTDs goes through three phases.

Symptom Control

To control the symptoms, the following are to be taken care of:
- Therapist needs to re-evaluate appropriate rest period and time off work period.
- Modification of work schedule
- Splinting
- Ergonomic aids
- Task analysis and modification

All abovementioned points can help to achieve appropriateness of rest period.

Use of various modalities such as the following help to take care of pain associated with activity and helps to sustain through this phase.
- Icing
- TENS
- Ultrasound
- Biofeedback
- Therapeutic massage
- Relaxation taping
- Manual edema mobilization

Strengthening Phase

Strengthening needs to be progressed carefully as people with CTDs experience no symptoms immediately but experience symptoms 12–24 hours later. Exercise protocol for tenosynovitis needs to be little vigorous as dynamic exercises given repetitively may cause gliding of tendon within sheath and irritation of tendon. In CTDs where nerves get entrapped in hypertrophied muscles, strengthening of specific muscle needs to be delayed.

Conditioning Phase

People with CTDs should be progressed to conditioning exercises when sufficient amount of strength is gained. Conditioning involves gradual increase of both intensity and duration. Stretching to gradually increase flexibility of tendon, muscle, and nerve is essential but a therapist needs to keep close supervision of symptom aggravation.

Return to Work

Therapist needs to do a detailed job analysis and task analysis before taking decision of return to work. Ergonomic tools, such as Rapid Upper Limb Assessment, Rapid Entire Body Assessment, and Occupational Repetitive Actions, help to analyze biomechanical risk exposure in workers.

THE SPASTIC HAND

Introduction

Spasticity occurs from a variety of common central nervous system insults, including stroke, traumatic brain

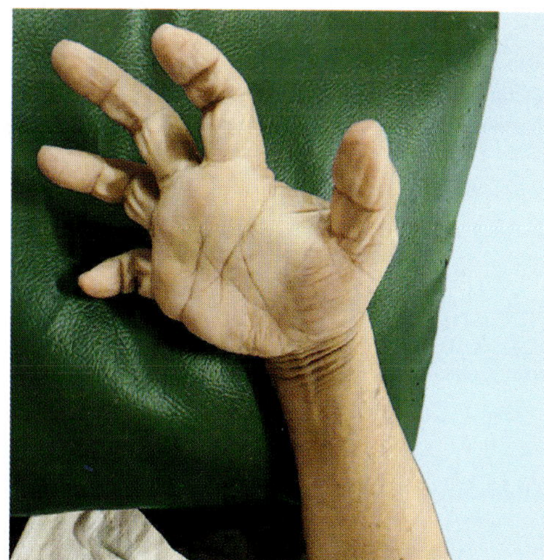

Fig. 20.38: The spastic hand.

injury, cerebral palsy, multiple sclerosis, and spinal cord injury. It is commonly defined as a motor disorder (**Fig. 20.38**) characterized by a velocity-dependent increase in tonic stretch reflexes, exaggerated tendon jerks, and often abnormal cutaneous and autonomic reflexes, muscle weakness, lack of dexterity, fatigability, and cocontraction of agonist and antagonist muscles.

Spasticity is a velocity-dependent increase in tonic stretch reflexes that results from a variety of disorders affecting the brain and spinal cord. Treatment of spasticity is considered when the increase in tone interferes with function, such as positioning, mobility, or daily cares, or is painful, or when it leads to complications such as contractures or skin breakdown.

Active finger extension and shoulder abduction are potential predictors of upper extremity recovery.

Evidences for Rehabilitation Management Poststroke

Hand Edema

In general, upper extremity elevation with the hand above the heart helps in edema management. When sitting or lying down, pillows assist with positioning the hand. Light retrograde massage can be used in stroke patients with varying evidences about many techniques of the treatment method. Compression gloves, sleeves, and wrapping for finger edema (e.g., Coban) can also be used but should be monitored frequently.

Active ROM should be gradually increased along with restoring alignment and strengthening weak muscles of the shoulder girdle. Stretching of the spastic muscles can be done to improve ROM and reduce spasticity (**Figs. 20.39A to C**). Self-ROM exercises can be used after a stroke when one arm or hand is unable to perform exercises on its own. During self-ROM, the less affected arm assists the affected arm or hand through the desired movement. Most importantly, self-ROM exercises make daily activities (e.g., dressing, grooming) easier.

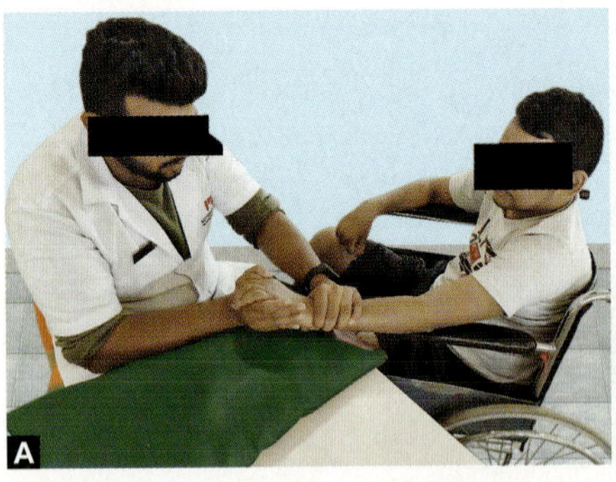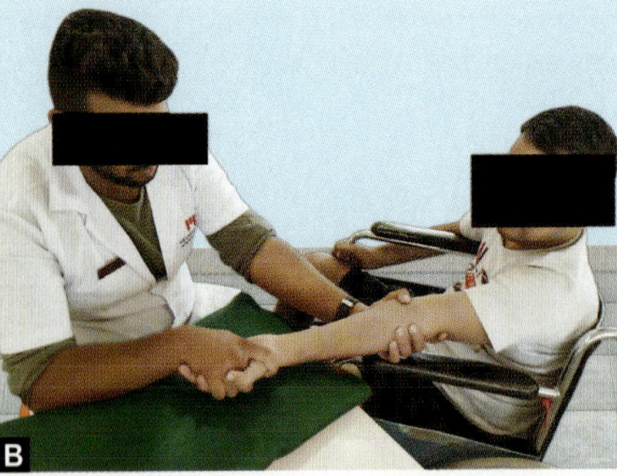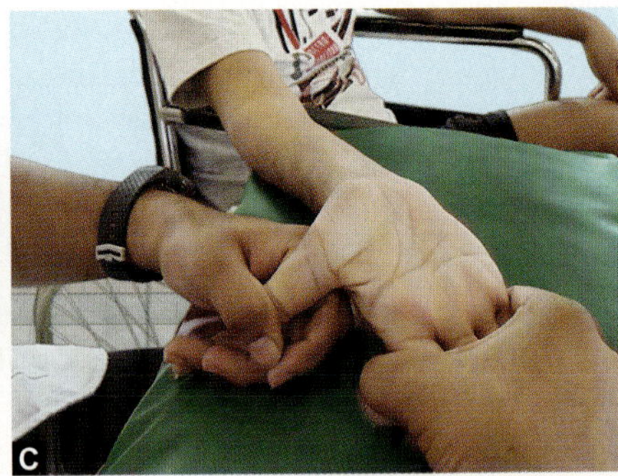

Figs. 20.39A to C: Stretching various muscles of the hand and wrist: (A) For wrist flexors; (B) For pronators; (C) For intrinsic muscles of the hand.

Role of Intensity of Therapy

Rehabilitation following stroke increases motor reorganization, while lack of it reduces reorganization; more intensive motor training in animals further increases reorganization.

Task-specific Training

Task-specific practice helps motor learning to occur. The best way to relearn a given task is retraining that task. Repetitive task practice may be superior to conventional training at improving upper extremity motor function following a stroke.

Sensory Motor Training

Whether or not sensorimotor training improves U/E function, compared to traditional techniques is controversial. However, bilateral arm training is equal to unilateral training or conventional therapy for improving upper extremity motor function.

Constrained-induced Movement Therapy (CIMT)

CIMT for acute and chronic stage of stroke:
- **CIMT for acute stage of stroke:** Modified constraint-induced movement therapy (mCIMT) holds strong evidence in comparison to traditional therapies in the acute stage of stroke.
- **CIMT for chronic stage of stroke:** Constraint-induced movement therapy and mCIMT also hold strong evidence in comparison to traditional therapies in the chronic stage of stroke.

Strength training: Strength training increases grip strength following stroke, which is also proven with strong evidence **(Fig. 20.40)**.

Mirror therapy: Mirror therapy in combination with other therapies or delivered alone improves motor function following stroke.

Mental practice: Mental practice improves upper extremity motor function when compared to standard care.

Upper extremity orthosis: Commonly used orthosis in hemiplegic upper extremity is the wrist–hand orthosis/splints, which can be either static/passive (volar, dorsal splints) or dynamic/active (e.g., SaeboFlex® **Fig. 20.41**).

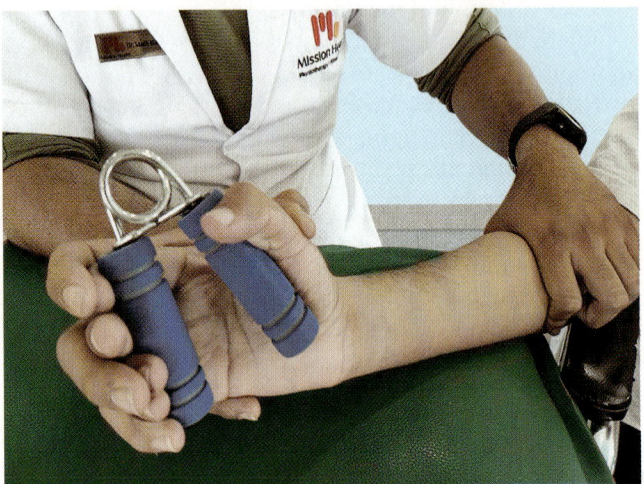

Fig. 20.40: Strength training using mechanical resistance.

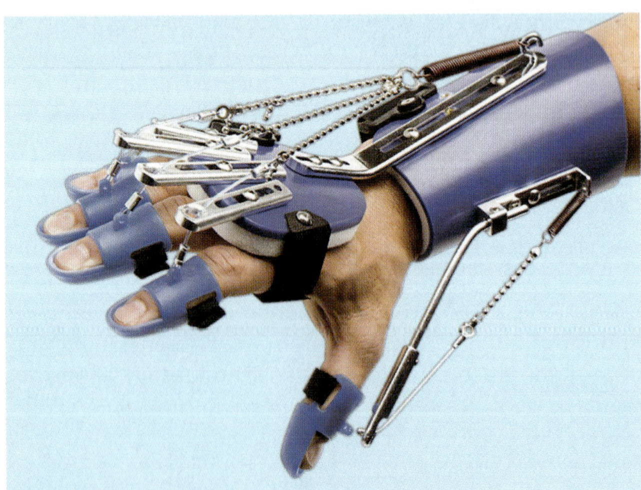

Fig. 20.41: SaeboFlex for stroke recovery.

Static hand splinting, however, does not improve motor function or reduce contracture formation.

EMG biofeedback: EMG biofeedback therapy is not superior to other forms of treatment and may not improve upper extremity motor function or spasticity.

Functional electrical stimulation: It improves upper extremity function in acute stroke (<6 months postonset) and chronic stroke (>6 months postonset) when combined with conventional therapy or delivered alone

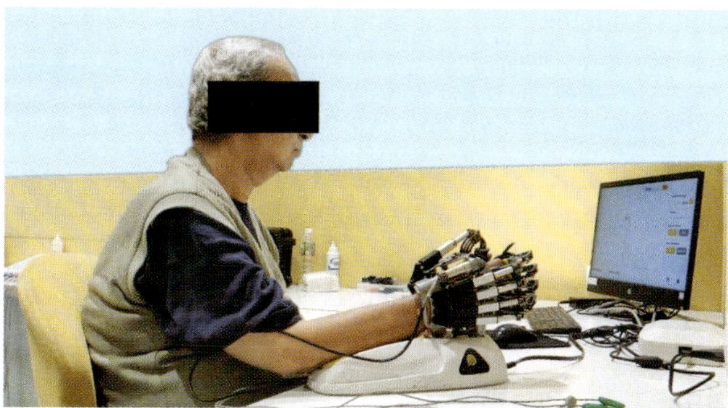

Fig. 20.42: Robotic training for the hand.
Courtesy: Mission Health, Ahmedabad

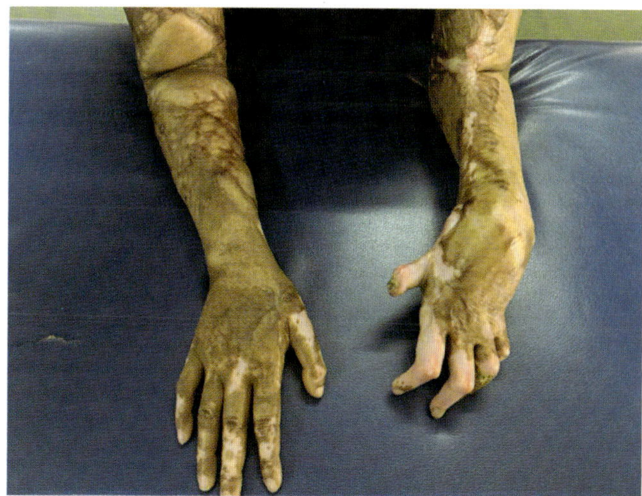

Fig. 20.43: The burnt hand.

Robotic training: Sensorimotor training with robotic devices improves upper extremity functional outcomes, and motor outcomes of the shoulder and elbow. However, robotic devices **(Fig. 20.42)** do not improve motor outcomes of the wrist and hand.

Virtual reality: It improves general functioning but may not aid functional independence.

Repetitive Transcranial Magnetic Stimulation and Transcranial Direct Current Stimulation

Impaired arm and hand motor function in addition to grasp and pinch may improve but wrist ROM may not improve. Anodal transcranial direct current stimulation (tDCS) and cathodal tDCS improve general upper extremity function but may not aid in dynamometric measures such as pinch, grasp, and grip strength. Dual repetitive transcranial magnetic stimulation (cathodal and anodal) stimulation improves dexterity and grip function.

Botulinum toxin: Treatment with botulinum toxin either alone or combined with therapy significantly decreases spasticity in upper extremity of stroke survivors. Most recent meta-analysis suggests moderate treatment effect for botulinum toxin A on function

Acupuncture/complimentary: Traditional acupuncture and electroacupuncture may not improve upper extremity function.

THE BURNT HAND

Rehabilitation following burn injuries starts from the day of injury, lasts for several years, and requires multidisciplinary efforts. A comprehensive rehabilitation program is vital to decrease patient's post-traumatic effects and improve functional independence **(Fig. 20.43)**.

Early rehabilitation is the key for maximizing long-term outcome, and improving patient compliance. When the various aspects of rehabilitation are introduced as an integral part of care from day one, irrespective of patient being inpatient or outpatient, they are easier for the patient to accept and follow rather than as an additional element to their care at a later date when contractures start developing.

Phases of Recovery

The phases of recovery are explained as follows:

1. **Emergent phase:** Generally considered the first 24–72 hours after injury. The goal is to evaluate the patient and help edema control and initiate and maintain active motion.

2. **Acute phase:** It generally extends from the emergent phase until wound closure. Wound closure may be either surgical closure or involves application of skin graft or by secondary intention healing. The goal of the therapist in this phase is to maintain ROM, tendon gliding, and muscle activity, to inhibit contraction, and maximize function. Early intervention is imperative for aligning collagen fibers that are deposited so that deformity caused by scar formation is reduced or prevented.

3. **Skin grafting phase:** Full-thickness burns require skin grafting to heal. Although deep partial-thickness burns will heal without grafting because of the prolonged healing time (>2 weeks) and resulting hypertrophic scarring and contraction, such wounds often are grafted when possible. It is important to obtain full ROM before grafting since the patient will need to be immobilized for up to 4–5 days after surgery. A splint that maintains the wrist in extension, MP in flexion, IP in extension, and the thumb between radial and palmar abduction, should be applied immediately after grafting for 4–5 days.

4. **Rehabilitation phase:** It is generally considered to extend from the time of graft adherence or wound closure to scar maturation. The primary goals during this are to protect the new spontaneous healed wound or the fragile graft, maintain joint mobility, increase function and strength, and inhibit scar contraction and hypertrophy.

Table 20.8: Anticontracture positioning for areas involved.

Area burnt	Contracture/difficulty experienced	Anticontracture position
Axillas or anterior and posterior axillary fold	Posterior axillary fold limited abduction, protraction when burns also to chest	Lying and sitting—arms abducted to 90° supported by pillows or foam blocks between chest and arms. Figure-of-eight bandaging or strapping to provide stretch across chest
Front of elbows	Elbow flexion	Elbow extension
Back of hands	MCP hyperextension, IP flexion adduction of thumb, wrist flexed	Wrist: 30–40° extended, MCPs: 60–70° flexion, IP joints in extension, thumb mid-palmar radial abduction
Palm of hand	Fingers adducted and flexed, palm pulled inwards	Wrist extended, minimal MCP flexion, fingers extended and abducted

(IP: interphalangeal; MCP: metacarpophalangeal)

5. **Anticontracture positioning**: Positioning is essential to influence tissue length by limiting or inhibiting loss of ROM secondary to formation of scar tissue as shown in **Table 20.8**.

Patients should adhere to a positioning regime in the early stages of healing and this requires teamwork and dedication. They also need encouragement to maintain anticontracture positioning most of the time (except for when carrying out exercise programs and functional activities), and not just during the therapy; family support is crucial at this stage to assist maintaining the correct position.

Treatment for Scar

Use of pressure: The purpose of pressure is to achieve a flat, soft, smooth, and pliable scar. Pressure after graft adherence or wound closure: Goal is not only to inhibit scar contraction and hypertrophy but also to inhibit vascular and lymphatic pooling and to avert hypersensitive, fragile skin. Although there is no scientific evidence, it has been shown that massage therapy not only reduces scar-related pain and itching but also increases ROM, reveals patients' anxiety, and improves their mood and mental status. Scar can be mobilized by kneading and lanolin massage and maintaining hydration with topical moisturizer. Commercially available custom-fit pressure gloves and inserts, interim pressure bandages or gloves may be used until patient can tolerate custom gloves. Closed fingertip gloves may be worn at night, while open fingertip gloves are recommended for day use.

Skin care: Application of total sunblock lotion. If the graft is exposed to the sun prematurely, it may tend to tan darker because of increase in melanin.

Splinting: Maintain ROM by opposing the force of contracting scar, usually during periods of patient inactivity. Traction may be used to correct scar contractures. Both static and dynamic splits can be used.

Clinical Pearl

Various complications occur after hand burn injury, which can result in limitations in everyday movements and in functional disorders. Edema occurs even in the early stage of burn injury; alters the fibrosis of muscle, tendon and skin; and impairs the joint structures, thus, inducing the occurrence of complications that are exacerbated in time. Thus early edema formation reduction would prevent these complications. Most effective method being a combination of compression wrap with continuous retrograde massage.

SPORTS-RELATED WRIST AND HAND INJURIES

Approximately 25% of all sports-related injuries involve the hand or wrist, and incidence is growing not only due to the competitive level of high school and collegiate athletes but also due to the activity level of the general population.

Appreciation of the anatomy and mechanism of injury is extremely helpful in diagnosing the pathology as depicted in **Table 20.9**. Early and accurate diagnosis minimizes the delayed problems of pain and dysfunction in hand injuries. As with any other sports injury the primary goal is to return the athlete to full participation as soon as possible without risking further injury or permanent disability.

Table 20.9: Overview of injuries, mechanism, and treatment.

Types of injuries	Mechanism of injury	Treatment
Radial-sided wrist injuries		
Scaphoid fracture	This hyperextension wrist injury tends to occur in a pronated, radially deviated hand	Immobilization in scaphoid cast for 8 weeks following by postimmobilization rehabilitation
Scapholunate ligament tears	Athlete in a position of impact with hyperextension, ulnar deviation, and supination of the wrist that can lead to these injuries	Minor: Conservative Major: Open reduction and repair with internal fixation

Contd...

Contd...

Types of injuries	Mechanism of injury	Treatment
Radial-sided tendinopathies		
DeQuervain's tenosynovitis	Repetitive thumb extension and abduction can lead to a thickening of the abductor pollicis longus and extensor pollicis brevis tendons as they pass under the first extensor compartment retinaculum	Conservative treatment for these tendinopathies begins by avoiding inciting events. Immobilization, stretching techniques, ice, and nonsteroidal anti-inflammatory medications can effectively diminish symptoms. Should symptoms persist, anesthetic/corticosteroid injections into the responsible tendon sheaths at the point of maximal tenderness can be of diagnostic and of therapeutic benefit
Intersection syndrome	Friction at the crossing of the tendons of the first extensor compartment as they pass over the tendons of the second extensor compartment (extensor carpi radialis longus and brevis) or a stenosing tenosynovitis within the second extensor compartment itself	
Tendonitis of the flexor carpi radialis	Repetitive wrist flexion or acute overstretching of the wrist	
Ulnar-sided wrist injuries		
Extensor carpi ulnaris injury	Injury may present as acute or chronic encompassing tendinosis, subluxation, dislocation, or rupture causing pain with or without mechanical symptoms on the ulnar side of the wrist. The pathophysiology involves repetitive microtrauma or a sudden traumatic episode during wrist flexion, supination, and ulnar deviation	Acute or chronic ECU tendinopathy can be managed with immobilization in wrist extension and ulnar deviation with progression to isometric and eccentric exercises
Ulnar abutment	As the wrist becomes more ulnar positive, the ulnocarpal joint experiences increased forces leading to ulnar-sided wrist pain. Ulnar positivity can be a normal anatomic variant, the result of distal radius physeal arrest (so-called "gymnast's wrist"), or as a dynamic condition with grip and pronation	• Conservative measures to decrease symptoms and avoid provocative activities can allow continued participation • Arthroscopic debridement and ulnar shortening are the mainstays of treatment
TFCC	In acute, tears of the TFCC can occur with hyperextension and pronation of the axially loaded, ulnar deviated wrist, micro- or repetitive trauma can cause peripheral tears to the TFCC with rapid supination-pronation of the ulnar deviated wrist	Immobilization, with or without physical therapy if ECU irritation is involved, for a period of 3 months can be helpful in alleviating symptoms. Symptomatic peripheral TFCC tears should be repaired either open or with arthroscopic assistance and typically require 3 months before return to play
Hook of the hamate fractures	Direct blows from a golf club with the ground or from a baseball bat while "checking" a swing can result in hook of the hamate fractures. Infrequently, repeated lesser impacts from the same can result in stress fracture	Immobilization, excision of the hook of the hamate fragment is currently the standard of care and has produced successful results with return to play in 6 weeks
Hand/finger injuries		
Thumb ulnar collateral ligament tears	Injury occurs from an abduction moment at the thumb MCPJ such as a fall onto an outstretched hand with the thumb abducted	Immobilization with a hand-based thumb spica splint or a cast with the IP joint free is appropriate for treating UCL partial tears with a firm endpoint to valgus stress testing at the MCPJ. For complete tears without an endpoint, surgery is recommended
Metacarpal/phalangeal fractures	Injuries occur from falls, direct blows, or crush during sporting activity, although stress fractures have rarely been noted in racquet sports	Many fractures can be treated nonoperatively if acceptable alignment can be maintained with immobilization. When conservative treatment is inadequate, operative fixation is indicated
Metacarpal fractures	Metacarpal base fractures occur from an axial load with the wrist in flexion	Closed or open reduction of the fracture stabilized with K-wires or screws is frequently needed
Phalangeal fractures	Shaft fractures of the proximal and middle phalanges can occur in a variety of patterns	Buddy taping and/or protective splint wear in acceptable alignment can allow fast return to play. Operative fixation with open versus closed reduction using either K-wires, screws, or plate and screws as fixation is sometimes required

Contd...

Contd...

Types of injuries	Mechanism of injury	Treatment
Central slip ruptures	Volar dislocation or forced flexion at the PIP joint can lead to acute rupture or chronic attenuation of the triangular ligament at the distal end of the central slip. Injury leads to the lateral bands migrating volarly with resultant PIP joint flexion and hyperextension at the DIP joint known as a boutonniere deformity	Splinting of the affected digit with the PIP joint in extension and PIP free is appropriate in order to allow the central slip tendon to heal in as closed to an anatomic position as possible
Sagittal band rupture	A boxer's knuckle refers to an injury of the sagittal band, which is the structure that normally keeps the EDC tendon centralized over the metacarpal head at the level of the MCPJ. The sagittal bands are composed of transverse, sagittal, and oblique fibers that can be injured by blunt trauma over the MCPJ with a clenched fist impact	Sagittal band injury without subluxation or dislocation can be treated with MCPJ extension splinting with the PIP joint free
Pulley ruptures	Closed annular pulley ruptures occur most commonly in rock climbers due to the high demand placed on the flexor tendon system in the hanging and crimping positions. Pulley ruptures typically involve the A2 or A4 pulleys and occur most often in the middle and ring fingers. Previous work has evaluated the force required to produce an A2 pulley tear and loads experienced during these vulnerable maneuvers finding they are at particular risk for climbers	Isolated pulley ruptures can be effectively treated nonoperatively with taping or pulley rings that externally provide support for the flexor tendon. However, in the case of multiple pulley ruptures, or failed nonoperative treatment, reconstruction is indicated
Jersey finger	Forceful hyperextension of the DIP joint leading to FDP avulsion, as seen with a jersey tearing away from a finger	Needs medical evaluation within 24–48 hours. Requires surgery within 10 days
Mallet finger	Mallet finger injuries refer to the disruption of the terminal extensor tendon from the distal phalanx, with or without an avulsed bony fragment	Conservative treatment with extension splinting of the DIP joint is appropriate for almost all mallet fingers, including those with bony fragments as long as there is no significant joint subluxation

(DIP: distal interphalangeal; EDC: extensor digitorum communis; IP: interphalangeal; K-wires: Kirschner wires; MCPJ: metacarpophalangeal joint; TFCC: triangular fibrocartilage complex tears; UCL: ulnar collateral ligament)

WRIST GANGLION

Ganglions of the wrist occur around articular capsules and tendons in the form of nodules. These changes are cavities with thin walls made of connective tissue filled with liquid or gel-like substance. Ganglions occur in 50–70% of all soft tissue tumors of the hand.

Pathophysiology

Ganglia are benign soft tissue tumors most commonly encountered in the wrist, but which may occur in any joint.
- Sixty to seventy percent of ganglion cysts are found in the dorsal aspect of the wrist and communicate with the joint via a pedicle. This pedicle not only usually originates at the scapholunate ligament, but also may arise from a number of other sites over the dorsal aspect of the wrist capsule.
- Thirteen to twenty percent of ganglia are found on the volar aspect of the wrist, arising via a pedicle from the radio scaphoid/scapholunate interval, scaphotrapezial joint, or the metacarpotrapezial joint, in that order of frequency.
- Ganglia arising from a flexor tendon sheath in the hand account for approximately 10% of ganglia.
- Occurrence in other joints as well as intraosseous and intratendinous ganglia is much less common. Microscopically, the *pedicle* contains a tortuous lumen, connecting the cyst to the underlying joint.

Clinical Picture

Clinical picture can be described as follows:
- On examination, wrist ganglia are usually 1–2-cm cystic structures, feeling much like a firm rubber ball that is well tethered in place by its attachment to the underlying joint capsule or tendon sheath.
- There is no associated warmth or erythema and the cyst readily transilluminates.
- The clinical presentation is usually adequate for diagnosis, and X-ray evaluation is rarely indicated (except in the case of "occult wrist ganglion" where MRI is needed to make a diagnosis).
- Symptoms include aching in the wrist that may also radiate up the patient's arm, pain with activity or palpation of the mass, decreased ROM and decrease grip strength. Volar ganglia may also cause paresthesias from compression of the ulnar or median nerves or their branches.

Management

Reassurance: The *spontaneous resolution* rate of untreated ganglion ranged 40–58% Therefore reassurance can be the option if the patients do not want any intervention.

Conservative treatment of choice is *aspiration*. Aspiration alone is one of the simplest ways to treat ganglion. However, it has high recurrence rates.

Becker suggested the use of *steroid injection* in treating ganglion, with 87% resolution rate, based on the initial theory that chronic inflammation may take part in the pathogenesis of ganglion. *Sclerotherapy* has been proposed to treat ganglion. Sclerosant can be injected into ganglion sac to damage the intimal lining and cause fibrosis to reduce the recurrence rate. Some advocated the use of hyaluronidase, which depolymerizes the hyaluronic acid present in ganglion content.

Surgical management: Techniques of *excising* the whole ganglion, including the cyst, its attachments to the scapholunate ligament, and the involved segment of joint capsule, to reduce the recurrence rate. It is now considered to be the most effective technique. *Arthroscopic resection* has the potential advantages of minimizing the surgical scar and permits evaluation of any intraarticular pathologic condition of either midcarpal or radiocarpal joints.

The goal of **physical therapy** is to restore the normal use of the hand. Therefore we need to regain full mobility of all the joints of the hand.

- ROM exercise
- Tendon gliding exercises
- Bunnel blocking exercises can be performed
- It's also important to reduce scar tissue to restore functional mobility, to improve ROM and to decrease pain. Scar tissue remodeling occurs as one starts to stretch and pull on it.
- Stretching of, in this case, the hand helps to align the collagen fibers to allow them to return to normal. This realignment of the collagen fibers makes the tissue better able to tolerate the forces that are placed on it during the day.
- Another way to help remodel scar tissue in the skin is massage. This can also help loosen any adhesions between the scar and the underlying tissue and fascia.

Stretching, scar massage along with flexibility, and strengthening exercises can help loosen the scar tissue and ensure that proper remodeling takes place. With specialized hand therapy, there is a lower recurrence rate and a faster recovery. Patients with a ganglion cyst are able to use their hand back, 2 week after the surgical excision.

SUMMARY

The primary role of the entire upper limb—shoulder, arm, elbow, and forearm is to place the hand in its proper position of function. The burden of these conditions may become exponentially high in the absence of rehabilitation.

Accurate evaluation of the patient's condition is a critical element in the rehabilitative process. The evaluative results provide information for establishing a diagnosis, setting realistic goals, planning a program of treatment and management, and determining a baseline for measuring progress.

The aim of physical therapy diagnosis or functional diagnosis is to diagnose movement system impairments to guide intervention for health optimization such that the disability can be minimized. The objective is clearly focused in the expertise of identifying clusters of movement system dysfunction and classifying them rather than diseases. Treatment effectiveness and prognosis are further mapped for a particular classification of movement system impairment using function as an outcome. This not only increases effectiveness of practice but also contributes to health care and research.

Case Scenario

CASE STUDY 1

A 49-year-old lady presented with the following symptoms.

Subjective findings: Pain on the outside of the right elbow with referral to top of shoulder and into the forearm. It aches most of the time and then becomes sharp with use. No tingling or numbness. No heat/cold/mottling of skin. No neck/thoracic pain.

Aggravating factors: Gripping (handbag), elbow flexion, or wrist extension. It increases on static positions for long, e.g., 30 minutes plus.

Relieving factors: Rest, but not for too long or it stiffens, Heat.

24 hours pattern: Very stiff for 1 hour in the morning. Aches in evening but depends on activity.

History: Gradual onset over 2 years, worse in the last 3 months, difficulty in doing household chores like cooking, no obvious trauma.

Observation: Poor posture, slouched flexed thoracic (mid spine), extended cervical spine (neck). Right forearm/elbow looks wasted in comparison to left (right handed). No swelling. Neck rotation to right is restricted other ranges are normal. No referred pain from neck. Shoulder ranges are normal.

Right elbow assessment: Tenderness present on lateral aspect of elbow. ROM and MMT is as follows:

- **Active movements** (patient performed): Moving the elbow itself was just a little stiff. Wrist extension (pullback) caused pain at the end of the range. Flexion (wrist down) produced a pull in the forearm muscles. Grip was weak and painful.
- **Passive movements** (physiotherapist performed): Elbow movements were full and normal. Bending the wrist with the elbow straight pulled in the spot.

- **Muscles:** Elbow flexion/extension no pain in all ranges. Wrist grip, hand, and thumb/finger extension all are immediately painful at the outside forearm muscles and tendon and into the lateral epicondyle.
- **Additional tests:** Nerve tension test produces restriction and pain in the forearm.

Guiding Questions:
1. What special tests can be done?
2. How will you manage this case?

CASE STUDY 2
Ulnar Neuropathy
A 49-year-old right-handed woman presents with a 3-week history of wrist pain and numbness and tingling in her right hand. There is no history of trauma or injury to the neck, elbow, or wrist. She works mostly at a desk job but has not had any changes in her work schedule. Physical examination of the wrist reveals no soft tissue swelling, muscle atrophy, or skin changes. She has painful wrist extension, as well as reproduction of the tingling in her fifth finger with tapping over the pisiform. Grip strength is normal and no other bony tenderness is appreciated

Guiding Questions:
1. What is the differential diagnosis? How will you confirm the diagnosis?
2. What is the physiotherapy management?

CASE STUDY 3
De Quervain's Tenosynovitis
A 31-year-old woman presents with several months of worsening radial left wrist pain that started insidiously. She denies any specific trauma. She has no numbness or tingling in the wrist, hand, or fingers. Her pain worsens with gripping and grasping, and with picking up her 9-month-old daughter. Physical examination reveals no discoloration and minimal soft tissue swelling along the radial styloid and anatomic snuffbox. There is soft tissue tenderness about the anatomic snuffbox and radial styloid. She has limited motion of the thumb, with pain mostly in extension and abduction. Her sensory and vascular examinations are unremarkable.

Guiding Questions:
1. What is the diagnosis and what tests can be done to confirm the same?
2. What are the physiotherapy options for management?

CASE STUDY 4
Carpal Tunnel Syndrome
A 55-year-old female presents with a complaints of "tingling" affecting the thumb, index, and middle fingers of the right hand. This symptom began spontaneously about 4 months previously and was not associated with any injury or change in her activities. She first noted this symptom at night when it disrupted her sleep, sporadically at the outset but in recent weeks on almost a nightly basis. She is employed as a computer operator. Her right hand is dominant. The physical examination of the right hand does not reveal abnormalities on inspection; in particular, the bulk of the intrinsic musculature of the hand, including the thenar eminence, is normal. There is no tenderness to palpation in the hand. The neurologic examination shows that the strength of the APB muscle is normal and is rated as grade 5. 2PD in the distribution of the median nerve is normal. The Phalen's test is positive. The Tinel's sign is positive—light tapping over the median nerve at the level of the carpal tunnel causes paraesthesiae radiating into the index and middle fingers.

Guiding Questions:
1. What special investigation can confirm the diagnosis? What will be the findings?
2. What are the possible causes for the condition?
3. What advice can be given to prevent symptoms?

CASE STUDY 5
Rheumatoid Arthritis
A 43-year-old female presented with a 4-month history of swelling and pain involving both of her hands, wrists, and feet. She complained of morning stiffness lasting 3 hours and was exhausted throughout the day. On two occasions, she had a low-grade fever and, for the prior few weeks, was unable to go to work. Her past medical history was unremarkable and there was no family history of generalized arthritis disorder. On physical examination, there was swelling, redness, and warmth involving the small joints of both hands and both wrists. Her grip strength was poor. There was a small joint effusion in the right knee. Both feet were very tender around the metatarsal-phalangeal joints. The rest of the examination proved routine.

Guiding Questions:
1. What are the deformities that can possibly occur? Describe each in detail.
2. What is the physiotherapy management in this case?

Review Questions

1. Mention modalities for the treatment of stiff elbow.
2. Mention the importance of eccentric muscle training in lateral elbow tendinopathy.
3. What is the role of manual therapy in lateral elbow tendinopathy?
4. What is the differential diagnosis of golfer's elbow?
5. Describe medial tension injury types in elbow.
6. What are the phases of rehabilitation after elbow injuries?

7. Which are the common injuries of elbow and what are the mechanisms of injuries?
8. Describe the stages of CRPS.
9. Describe the desensitization program in management of CRPS.
10. What are the common causes of crush injuries of hand?
11. What is the importance of edema management in hand injuries?
12. Which are the common deformities in rheumatoid hand and what are the splints for them?
13. Mention the joint protection program in RA hand.
14. What are the causes of median nerve injury?
15. What are the causes of ulnar nerve injury?
16. Describe splinting in peripheral nerve injury.
17. What are the types of cumulative trauma disorders?
18. What are the electrodiagnostic findings in carpal tunnel syndrome?
19. Describe the evidence-based view in management of spastic hand.
20. Which are the anticontracture positions in burnt hand?
21. Describe the common ulnar-sided wrist injuries.
22. What is the conservative management for ganglion cyst?

BIBLIOGRAPHY

1. Alfredson H, Pietilä T, Jonsson P, et al. Heavy-load eccentric calf muscle training for the treatment of chronic Achilles tendinosis. Am J Sports Med. 1998;26:360-6.
2. Amadio PC. Epidemiology of hand and wrist injuries in sports. Hand Clin. 1990;6:379-81.
3. Angelides AC, Wallace PF. The dorsal ganglion of the wrist: its pathogenesis, gross and microscopic anatomy, and surgical treatment. J Hand Surg. 19761(3):228-35.
4. Araghi A, Celli A, Adams R, et al. The outcome of examination (manipulation) under anesthesia on the stiff elbow after surgical contracture release. J Shoulder Elbow Surg. 2010;19:202-8.
5. Avery DM, Rodner C, Edgar C. Sports-related wrist and hand injuries: a review. J Orthop Surg Res. 2016;11:99.
6. Birkenmeier RL, Prager EM, Lang CE. Translating animal doses of task-specific training to people with chronic stroke in 1-hour therapy sessions: a proof-of-concept study. Neurorehabil Neural Repair. 2010;24(7):620-35.
7. Bisset LM, Vicenzino B. Physiotherapy management of lateral epicondylalgia. J Physiother. 2015;61:174-81.
8. Buljina AI, Taljanovic MS, Avdic DM, et al. Physical and exercise therapy for treatment of the rheumatoid hand. Arthritis Care Res. 2001;45(4):392-7.
9. Bunnell S. Surgery of the hand, 3rd edition. Philadelphia, PA: JB Lippincott; 1956.
10. Cailliet R. Soft tissue pain and disability, 2nd edition. New Delhi: Jaypee Publishers; 2005.
11. Casaubon LK, Boulanger JM, Glasser E, et al. Canadian stroke best practice recommendations: acute inpatient stroke care guidelines, update 2015. Int J Stroke. 2016;11(2):239-52.
12. Chin D, Jones N. Repetitive motion hand disorders. J Calif Dent Assoc. 2002;30(2):149-60.
13. Chinchalkar SJ, Szekeres M. Rehabilitation of elbow trauma. Hand Clin. 2004;20:363-74.
14. Clay NR, Clement DA. The treatment of dorsal wrist ganglia by radical excision. J Hand Surg. 1988;13(2):187-91.
15. Coombes BK, Bisset L, Vicenzino B. Management of lateral elbow tendinopathy: one size does not fit all. J Orthop Sports Phys Ther. 2015;45:938-49.
16. Dabholkar TA, Shroff R, Dabholkar A, et al. Effect of fatigue on hand function in dental profession. In: Ergonomics in caring for people. Singapore: Springer; 2018.
17. Dawson AS, Knox J, McClure A, et al. Stroke rehabilitation. In: Lindsay MP, Gubitz G, Bayley M, Phillips S (Eds). Canadian best practice recommendations for stroke care, 4th edition. Ottawa, ON: Heart and Stroke Foundation and the Canadian Stroke Network; 2013. pp. 1-97.
18. Dubois B, Esculier J. Soft-tissue injuries simply need PEACE and LOVE. Br J Sports Med. 2019. doi:10.1136/bjsports-2019-101253. Published online first: 03 August 19.
19. Ellenbecker TS, Reinold M, Nelson CO. Clinical concepts for treatment of the elbow in the adolescent overhead athlete. Clin Sports Med. 2010;29:705-24.
20. Erickson M, Lawrence M, Stegink Jansen CW, et al. Hand pain and sensory deficits: carpal tunnel syndrome—clinical practice guidelines linked to the International Classification of Functioning, Disability and Health from the Academy of Hand and Upper Extremity Physical Therapy and the Academy of Orthopaedic Physical Therapy of the American Physical Therapy Association. J Orthop Sports Phys Ther. 2019;49(5):CPG1-85.
21. Evans PJ, Nandi S, Maschke S, et al. Prevention and treatment of elbow stiffness. J Hand Surg Am. 2009;34:769-78.
22. Firestein G. Rheumatoid arthritis. In: Kelly's textbook of rheumatology, 9th edition. Philadelphia, PA: WB Saunders; 1997.
23. Fleisig GS, Andrews JR. Prevention of elbow injuries in youth baseball pitchers. Sports Health. 2012;4:419-24.
24. Geissler WB, Burkett JL. Ligamentous sports injuries of the hand and wrist. Sports Med Arthrosc Rev. 2014;22(1):39-44.
25. Gelberman RH, Botte MJ, Spiegelman JJ, et al. The excursion and deformation of repaired flexor tendons treated with protected early motion. J Hand Surg. 1986;11A:106-10.
26. Gelberman RH, Manske PR. Factors influencing flexor tendon adhesions. Hand Clin. 1985;1:35-42.
27. Gelberman RH, Woo SLY, Amiel D, et al. Influences of flexor sheath continuity and early motion on tendon healing in dogs. J Hand Surg. 1990;15A:69-77.
28. Gelberman RH, Woo SLY, Lothringer K, et al. Effects of intermittent passive mobilization on healing canine flexor tendons. J Hand Surg. 1982;7:170-5.
29. Gelberman RH, Woo SLY. The physiological basis for application of controlled stress in the rehabilitation of flexor tendon injuries. J Hand Ther. 1989;2:66-70.
30. Greendyke SD, Wilson M, Shepler TR. Anterior wrist ganglia from the scaphotrapezial joint. J Hand Surg. 1992;17(3):487-90.

31. Gustafsson L, Walter A, Bower K, et al. Single-case design evaluation of compression therapy for edema of the stroke-affected hand. Am J Occup Ther. 2014;68:203-11.

32. Haak M. Musculoskeletal disorders (lecture). Chicago, IL: Dental Ergonomics Summit American Dental Association; 2000.

33. Harden RN, Swan M, King A, et al. Treatment of complex regional pain syndrome: functional restoration. Clin J Pain. 2006;22:420-4.

34. Hoenig H, Groff G, Pratt K, et al. A randomized controlled trial of home exercise on the rheumatoid hand. J Rheumatol. 1993;20(5):785-9.

35. Hoogvliet P, Randsdorp MS, Dingemanse R, et al. Does effectiveness of exercise therapy and mobilisation techniques offer guidance for the treatment of lateral and medial epicondylitis? A systematic review. Br J Sports Med. 2013;47(17):1112-19.

36. Joyce ME, Jelsma RD, Andrews JR. Throwing injuries to the elbow. J Sports Med Arthrosc Rev. 1995;3:224-36.

37. Kibler WB, Press J, Sciascia A. The role of core stability in athletic function. Sports Med. 2006;36:189-98.

38. Kraushaar BS, Nirschl RP. Tendinosis of the elbow (tennis elbow). Clinical features and findings of histological, immunohistochemical and electron microscopy studies. J Bone Joint Surg Am. 1999;81:259-78.

39. Kwan M, Kennis W. Splinting programme for patients with burnt hand. Hand Surg. 2002;7:231-41.

40. Leslie BM. Rheumatoid extensor tendon ruptures. Hand Clin. 1989;5(2):191-202.

41. Limpisvasti O, ElAttrache NS, Jobe FW. Understanding shoulder and elbow injuries in baseball. J Am Acad Orthop Surg. 2007;15:139-47.

42. Magyar E, Talerman A, Mohacsy J, et al. Muscle changes in rheumatoid arthritis: a review of literature with study of 100 cases. Virchows Arch A Pathol Anat Histol. 1997;373(3):267-78.

43. Mannerfelt LG, Norman O. Attrition ruptures of flexor tendons in rheumatoid arthritis caused by bony spurs in the carpal tunnel: a clinical and radiological study. J Bone Joint Surg. 1969;51(2):270-7.

44. Merskey H, Bogduk K. Classification of chronic pain: definitions of chronic pain syndromes and definition of pain terms, 2nd edition. Seattle, WA: IASP Press; 1994.

45. Müller AM, Sadoghi P, Lucas R, et al. Effectiveness of bracing in the treatment of nonosseous restriction of elbow mobility: a systematic review and meta analysis of 13 studies. J Shoulder Elbow Surg. 2013;22:1146-52.

46. Nalebuff EA. Diagnosis, classification and management of rheumatoid thumb deformities. Bull Hosp Joint Dis. 1968;29(2):119-37.

47. Nassab R, Kok K, Constantinides J, et al. The diagnostic accuracy of clinical examination in hand lacerations. Int J Surg. 2007;5(2):105-8.

48. Neviaser RJ, Wilson JN, Gardner MM. Abductor pollicis longus transfer for replacement of first dorsal interosseous. J. Hand Surg Am. 1980;5(1):53-7.

49. Oerlemans HM, Oostendorp RA, de Boo T, et al. Adjuvant physical therapy versus occupational therapy in patients with reflex sympathetic dystrophy/complex regional pain syndrome type I. Arch Phys Med Rehabil. 2000;81:49-56.

50. Oerlemans HM, Oostendorp RA, de Boo T, et al. Pain and reduced mobility in complex regional pain syndrome I: Outcome of a prospective randomized controlled clinical trial of adjuvant physical therapy versus occupational therapy. Pain. 1999;83:77-83.

51. Paul R, Chan R. Nonsurgical treatment of elbow stiffness. J Hand Surg Am. 2013;38:2002-4.

52. Polkinghorn BS. A novel method for assessing elbow pain resulting from epicondylitis. J Chiropr Med. 2002;1(3):117-21.

53. Regan WD, Reilly CD. Distraction arthroplasty of the elbow. Hand Clin. 1993;9:719-28.

54. Rennie HJ. Evaluation of effectiveness of a metacarpophalangeal ulnar deviation orthosis. J Hand Therap. 1996;9(4):371-7.

55. Rettig AC. Athletic injuries of the wrist and hand. Part 1. Traumatic injuries of the wrist. Am J Sports Med. 2003;31(6):1038-48.

56. Richard R, Baryza MJ, Carr JA, et al. Burn rehabilitation and research: proceedings of a consensus summit. J Burn Care Res. 2009;30(4):543-73.

57. Shiri R, Viikari-Juntura E, Varonen H, et al. Prevalence and determinants of lateral and medial epicondylitis: a population study. Am J Epidemiol. 2006;164(11):1065-74.

58. Sims SE, Miller K, Elfar JC, et al. Non-surgical treatment of lateral epicondylitis: a systematic review of randomized controlled trials. Hand (NY). 2014;9(4):419-46.

59. Smith EM, Juvinall RC, Bender LF, et al. Flexor forces and rheumatoid metacarpophalangeal deformities: clinical implications. JAMA. 1966;198(2):130-4.

60. Stanton-Hicks M, Janig W, Hassenbusch S, et al. Reflex sympathetic dystrophy: changing concepts and taxonomy. Pain. 1995;63:127-33.

61. Stasinopoulos D, Johnson MI. 'Lateral elbow tendinopathy' is the most appropriate diagnostic term for the condition commonly referred-to as lateral epicondylitis. Med Hypotheses. 2006;67:1400-2.

62. Steinbrocker O, Traeger CH, Batterman RC. Therapeutic criteria in rheumatoid arthritis. JAMA. 1949;140(8):659-62.

63. Suen M, Fung B, Lung CP. Treatment of ganglion cysts. ISRN Orthop. 2013;1-7.

64. Taleisnik J. The wrist, 1st edition. New York, NY: Churchill Livingstone; 1985.

65. Tejashree K, Chhaya V. Compare outcome measures in flexor tendon repair of different zones following supervised controlled active mobilization. Indian J Physiother Occup Ther. 2014;8:256-60.

66. Thornburg LE. Ganglions of the hand and wrist. J Am Acad Orthop Surg. 1999;7(4):231-38.

67. Tophoj K, Henriques U. Ganglion of the wrist—a structure developed from the joint. Acta Orthop Scand. 1971;42(3):244-50.

68. Turner-Stokes L, Goebel A. On Behalf of the Guideline Development Group. Complex regional pain syndrome in adults: Concise guidance. Clin Med. 2011;11(6):596-600.

69. Vaughan-Jackson OJ. Attrition rupture of tendons in rheumatoid hand. J Bone Joint Surg. 1958;40A:1431.

70. Vinod AV, Ross G. An effective approach to diagnosis and surgical repair of refractory medial epicondylitis. J Shoulder Elbow Surg. 2015;24(8):1172-7.

71. Waugh EJ, Jaglal SB, Davis AM, et al. Factors associated with prognosis of lateral epicondylitis after 8 weeks of physical therapy. Arch Phys Med Rehabil. 2004;85:308-18.

72. Wilk KE, Azar FM, Andrews JR. Conservative and operative rehabilitation of the elbow in sports. Sports Med Arthrosc Rev. 1995;3:237-58.

73. Wilk KE, Reinold MM, Andrews JR. Rehabilitation of the thrower's elbow. Clin Sports Med. 2004;23:765-801.

Hip Conditions

Surendra Wani

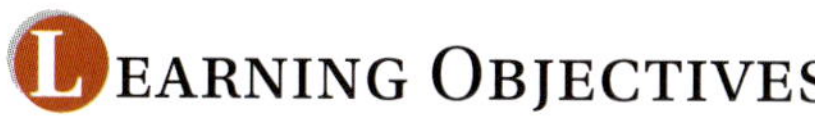LEARNING OBJECTIVES

After reading this chapter, the readers should be able to:

- Understand the basic anatomy of the hip joint
- Describe the evaluation process to be followed for hip joint assessment
- Describe the etiology, pathophysiology, and clinical presentation of various pathologies related to the hip joint
- Describe the medical management used for various pathologies related to the hip joint
- Describe the physical therapy management used for conditions related to the hip joint
- Describe the surgical management used for various pathologies related to the hip joint
- Describe the various operative procedures performed on the hip joint and their postoperative physiotherapy management

CHAPTER OUTLINE

- Evaluation of the hip joint
- Osteoarthritis
  - Etiology
  - Epidemiology
  - Pathophysiology
  - Classification
  - Clinical features
  - Diagnostic criteria
  - Investigations
  - Nonsurgical management
  - Physiotherapy management
  - Surgical management
- Legg–Calvé–Perthes disease
  - Etiology
  - Pathological features
  - Clinical features
  - Investigations
  - Prognosis
  - Management
  - Complications

- Developmental dysplasia of hip
  - Etiology
  - Pathological features
  - Clinical features
  - Investigations
  - Medical management
  - Surgical management
  - Physiotherapy management
- Slipped capital femoral epiphysis/slipped upper femoral epiphysis
  - Etiology and pathological features
  - Clinical features
  - Investigations
  - Morphological classification based on amount of deformity
  - Medical treatment
  - Physiotherapy
- Trochanteric bursitis
  - Etiology

- Pathological features
  - Clinical findings
  - Investigations
  - Medical treatment
  - Physiotherapy management
- Meralgia paresthetica
  - Introduction, etiology, and pathological features
  - Clinical features
  - Physiotherapy interventions
- Piriformis syndrome
  - Etiology
  - Clinical features
  - Physical examination
  - Investigations
  - Medical management
  - Surgical management
  - Physiotherapy management

INTRODUCTION

The hip joint is also known as the coxofemoral joint. It is a type of synovial joint of the ball and socket variety. Articulation between the acetabulum of pelvic bones and the head of the femur forms this joint. The acetabulum cavity is deepened by the acetabular labrum in which the hemispherical head of femur is accommodated. The hip joint is designed primarily for weight-bearing function and stability. It supports the weight of the trunk, arms, and head in static as well as dynamic postures. It provides three degrees of freedom as it allows flexion/extension in the sagittal plane, abduction/adduction in the frontal plane, and medial/lateral rotation in the transverse plane. The capsule of the hip joint has two sets of fibers, namely longitudinal and circular, which provides stability in all directions. However, the ligaments increase the anterior and posterior stability to hip joint. The intracapsular ligament is the ligament of the head of femur/ligamentum teres, which provides blood supply to the head through the branch of obturator artery. Extracapsular ligaments include iliofemoral (inverted Y-shaped ligament of Bigelow) anteriorly and pubofemoral and ischiofemoral ligaments posteriorly. Muscles of hip provide dynamic stability, which is contributed by hip flexors, extensors, abductors, adductors, and rotators. Hip is mainly innervated by the sciatic, femoral, and obturator nerves.

EVALUATION OF THE HIP JOINT

Meticulous and accurate assessment of the hip pain and related impairments will lead to correct diagnosis and its successful management.

Subjective examination includes getting history/information of symptoms from the patients; information about onset of symptoms, the mechanism of injury, details of pain and other symptoms, aggravating and easing factors, history of developmental disorders, etc.

While assessing the hip joint, the entire lower limb that includes lumbar spine, pelvis and the sacroiliac (SI) joint also should be focused. Mobility of hip with range of motion and joint play assessment should be done. The muscles should be assessed for their control, strength, and function. The muscle length of iliopsoas, quadriceps, hamstrings, adductors, and iliotibial band (ITB) must be tested. The nerves of the lower limb such as the sciatic, femoral, and obturator, must be checked for their neural tissue extensibility.

Lastly, the hip joint biomechanics is of utmost importance as a part of assessment as hip pain may be related to the whole lower limb biomechanics and function.

OSTEOARTHRITIS

Introduction

Osteoarthritis (OA) is a common form of arthritic condition that adults encounter during their middle age or later. OA is the most frequently reported joint condition with a prevalence of 22–39% in older people in India. Most commonly, it affects weight-bearing joints such as hip or knee. Progressive wear and tear (degeneration) of hip joint structures **(Fig. 21.1)** due to aging causes pain and stiffness in hip joint leading to difficulty in performing some activities of daily living such as full squats and walking. As OA progresses gradually over period of time, it requires the

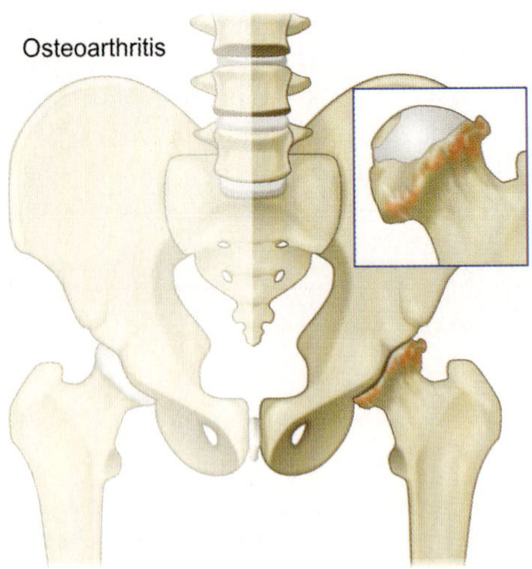

Fig. 21.1: Normal and arthritic hip joint.

early management to prevent further disability associated with it. Although there is no permanent cure for OA, there are various treatment strategies available to reduce pain and disability.

Etiology

Modifiable and nonmodifiable factors that may contribute to the development of the disease are:

- Advancing age
- Reduced physical activity
- Family history of OA
- Previous trauma/fracture to hip joint
- Increased body mass index (BMI)—obesity
- Deformities at hip—coxa vara/valga

Epidemiology

Osteoarthritis is one of the common rheumatic diseases with a prevalence of around 20–40% in India with females more affected than males. However, a systematic review conducted in the United States for the prevalence of radiographic hip OA reported 9.2% among people with age 45 years or more. OA has detrimental effect on activities of daily living (ADLs), including walking, stair climbing, and getting up from chair, leading to profound disability.

Pathophysiology

Osteoarthritis is a degenerative condition affecting mostly older people above 50 years of age and may occur in younger age-groups. Degeneration and fraying of articular cartilage of hip joint due to aging and increased stress over the joint and capsulo-ligamentous structures may further reduce joint space and form extra bony outgrowth/proliferation called osteophytes. This contributes to reduction in hip joint mobility causing functional impairments.

- Cartilage (connective tissue that has viscoelastic and compressive properties, which consist of type II collagen and proteoglycans) is mainly involved in OA.

- Degradative and synthetic enzyme actions arc balanced (dynamic remodeling) in extracellular matrix of cartilage to maintain good volume. In OA, degradative enzyme activity is increased causing reduction in collagen and proteoglycans from the extracellular matrix.
- Due to this loss, chondrocytes proliferate and later produce proteoglycans and collagen.
- Disease progresses with the progressive cartilage degradation in the form of fibrillation and erosion starting in superficial layers of cartilage and then involving whole cartilage.

Although OA is a disease of aging of cartilage, some differences are observed between the aging and osteoarthritic cartilage. Denatured type II collagen in more amounts is found in OA cartilage due to increased degradative enzyme activity than in aging cartilage along the differences in water content and ratio of chondroitin sulfate to keratin sulfate in both. The synthesis of matrix metallo-proteinase is increased in OA and presence of pro-inflammatory cytokines (e.g., IL-1) aggravates cartilage degradation causing further disability.

Classification

Primary OA: OA developed with no known cause or idiopathic in nature. It is generally due to physiological aging process, which leads to degeneration of joint.

Secondary OA: OA of hip developed secondary to trauma/injury, congenital acetabular dysplasia of hip and developmental disorders, infection, metabolic conditions, and neuropathic conditions.

Clinical Features

The symptoms of hip OA start with gradual onset of pain in and around the hip joint, which worsens with time. Morning pain and stiffness lasts for only a few minutes and subsides in 30 minutes or less, pain aggravates after prolonged sitting or physical inactivity, and movements and exercises of involved joint generally improve symptoms of OA. Extra features may include:

- Pain in the groin may or may not radiate to thigh or buttocks region (L2–L3 dermatome).
- Stiffness that may reduce after some steps of walking.
- Pain increases on exertion or prolonged standing or walking.
- Reduced hip joint movements/motion due to increased stiffness affect ability to transit from sitting to standing in chair, deep squats, and prolonged walking.
- Painful gait/limping gait on the side of involvement.
- Sometimes limb length discrepancy in unilateral involvement may be observed.

Diagnostic Criteria

Presently, there are no standard or specific criteria to measure and report the radiographic hip OA. The Kellgren and Lawrence grading method is commonly preferred

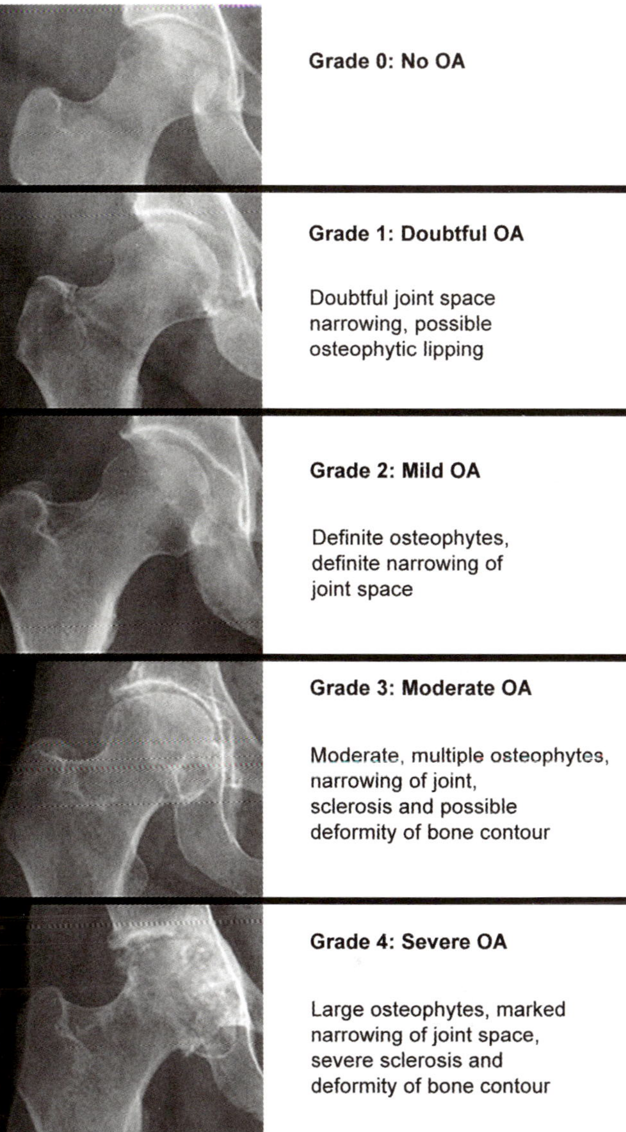

Fig. 21.2: The Kellgren and Lawrence grading of hip joint OA.
Soruce: Radiology, LTHT, Leeds general infirmary—Leeds/UK. (OA: osteoarthritis)

Table 21.1: Kellgren and Lawrence grading system for osteoarthritis (OA).

Grade	Radiologic findings
0	No radiologic findings of OA
1	Doubtful narrowing of joint space and possible osteophytic lipping
2	Definite osteophytes and possible narrowing of joint space
3	Moderate multiple osteophytes, definite narrowing of joint space, small pseudocystic areas with sclerotic walls and possible deformity of bone contour
4	Large osteophytes, marked narrowing of joint space, severe sclerosis, and definite deformity of bone contour

for the diagnosis of radiographic OA and its severity **(Fig. 21.2 and Table 21.1)**. However, this method relies on the presence of osteophytes around the joint, which was found to be weakly correlated with hip joint pain.

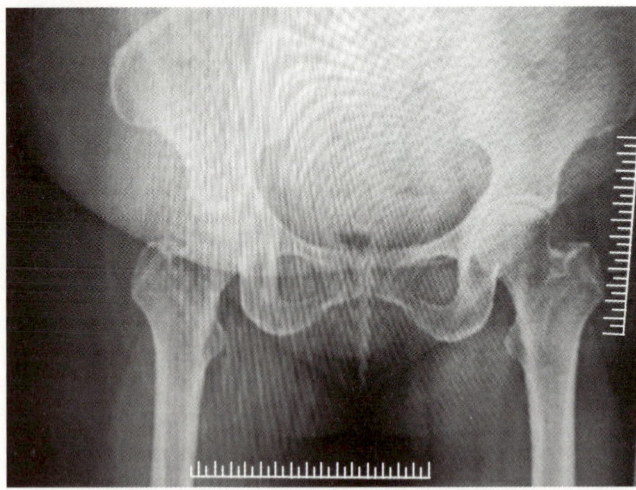

Fig. 21.3: Anteroposterior (AP) view X-ray of hip.

Investigations

Anteroposterior (AP)/lateral views of radiograph may show joint space reduction, mild-to-moderate sclerosis of articular surfaces, and presence of osteophytes at edges **(Fig. 21.3)**. Magnetic resonance imaging (MRI) scan or computed tomography (CT) may be advised for better visualization of bone and soft tissues around the hip.

Nonsurgical Management

Management depends upon the stage of the disease and the amount of disability.

Drugs

Paracetamol, nonsteroidal anti-inflammatory drugs (NSAIDs), acetaminophen, viscosupplementation (hyaluronan) or glucosamine sulfate, chondroitin sulfate, cyclooxygenase 2 inhibitors, or opioids sometimes oral or intra-articular corticosteroids/hyaluronic acids/platelet-rich plasma injections can be prescribed by an orthopedician for severe painful conditions.

Lifestyle Modifications

Lifestyle modifications such as avoiding deep squats, frequent stair climbing, prolonged standing or walking, use of western toilets, proper use of assistive devices such as a cane, crutches, or a walker to improve independence and also to protect the hip joint may reduce the progression of the disease. Patients are advised to reduce body weight by implementing weight reduction strategies (using low-impact activities—static cycling, aqua aerobics, swimming, etc.).

Physiotherapy Management

Aims of Management

In early stages of the disease, the aim should be focused on:

- Relieving pain
- Maintaining the joint mobility
- Improving strength of the lower extremity musculature
- Correction of any biomechanical malalignments
- Avoiding further progression of the disease
- Maximizing function and exercise capacity

Physiotherapy Interventions

- Superficial heat is preferred over cold, or contrast therapy although all reduce inflammation, improve metabolism and may block pain transmission in patients with OA. Transcutaneous electrical nerve stimulation (TENS) has beneficial effect on hip joint pain and can provide considerable symptomatic relief.
- Grade 1 or 2 Maitland or Kaltenborn mobilization, active and active assisted range of motion (ROM) exercises can be used to restore normal mobility and joint capsule flexibility. In moderate and advanced stages of OA, mobilization should be avoided due to high irritability of joint.
- Muscle strengthening program based on the principles of progressive resisted exercises with special focus to strengthen hip abductors should be advised **(Figs. 21.4 to 21.6)**. Hip muscle flexibility (hip flexors, adductors) should also be maintained to improve joint mobility.

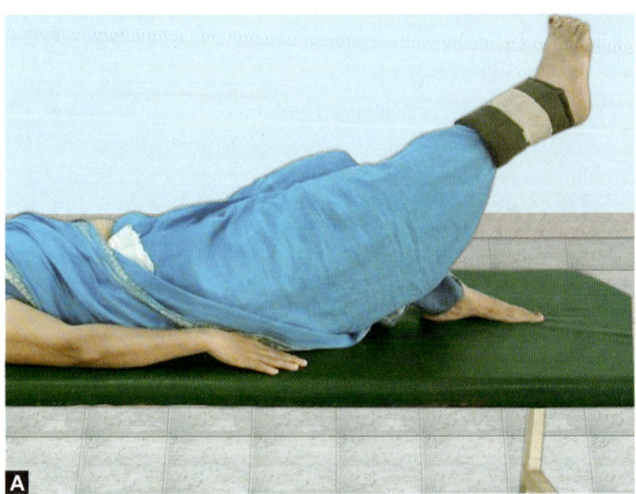
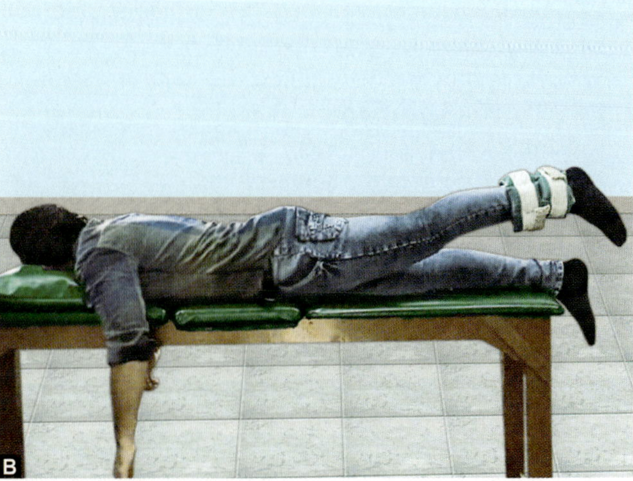

Figs. 21.4A and B: Strengthening of (A) hip flexors; (B) hip extensors.

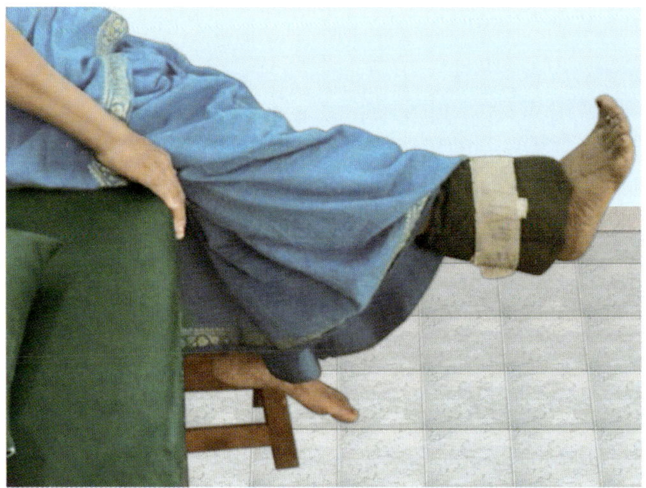

Fig. 21.5: Strengthening of quadriceps in high sitting.

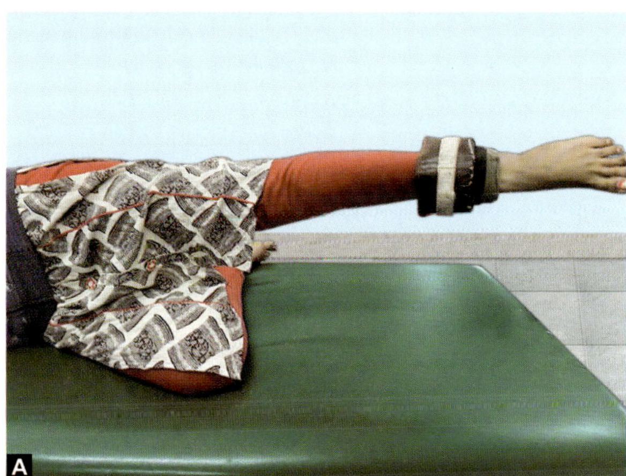

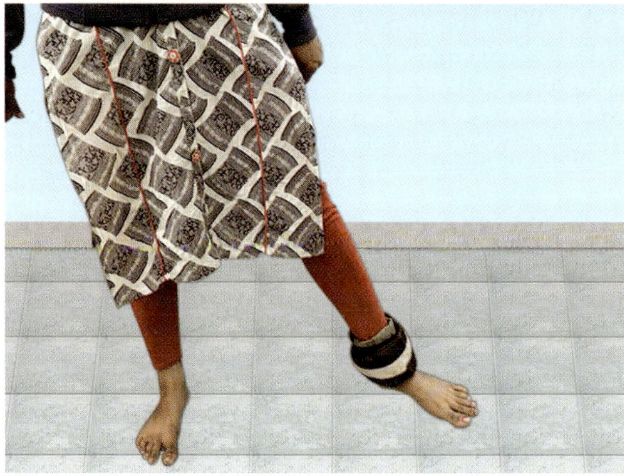

Figs. 21.6A and B: Strengthening of hip abductors in (A) Side lying; (B) Standing.

- Hydrotherapy or aquatic therapy may help to improve the joint mobility and improve strength of hip muscles without loading the joint.

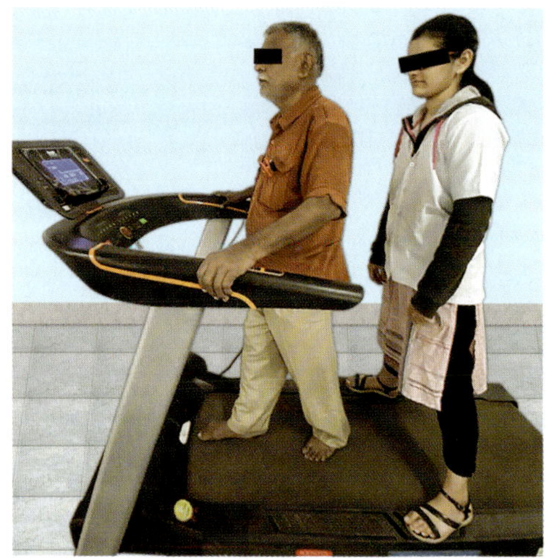

Fig. 21.7: Treadmill walking.

- Obesity reduction program [using aerobic exercises, e.g., treadmill walking **(Fig. 21.7)** or strengthening exercises] aids to reduce body weight, which relieves stress over the hip joint during weight-bearing activities.
- Limb length discrepancy can be treated with proper insole to equalize length.

Surgical Management

When disease has progressed to moderate or advanced stages or if patient does not get relief from conservative treatments, then the following surgical options are recommended:

- *Total hip arthroplasty:* To restore the normal hip joint function.
- *Partial hip replacement:* Replacement of the head of the femur with artificial prosthesis to restore normal hip joint function.
- *Femoral/pelvic osteotomy:* Osteotomy of femur/pelvis is done to reduce the pressure on hip joint by realigning, although this procedure is not used frequently.
- *Arthroscopic hip articular resurfacing procedure (chondroplasty):* The damaged articular surfaces of hip joint are smoothened by resurfacing and could be replaced with metal covering to allow frictionless movement at hip.
- Advanced techniques such as mesenchymal stem cell therapy, chondrocyte transplantation marrow stimulation techniques, osteochondral transplantation, autologous matrix-induced chondrogenesis, and autologous chondrocyte implantation are still under research and may have good outcomes.

Postoperative Physiotherapy

Postoperatively, physiotherapy is highly recommended in a prescribed protocol to restore and improve range of motion and subsequently strength, which is beyond the scope of this chapter. This is described in detail in Chapter 24: Arthroplasties.

LEGG–CALVÉ–PERTHES DISEASE

It is also known as Legg's stress fracture of femoral head/pseudocoxalgia/coxa plana/osteochondrosis of hip **(Fig. 21.8)**.

Introduction

Legg–Calvé–Perthes disease is a hip joint pathology having unknown cause, in which the femoral head undergoes ischemic necrosis. First explained by Waldenström in 1902, Perthes, Legg, and Calvé described the disease process in detail in 1910. Further, by 1922 Waldenström classified the disease into different stages as per the level of involvement or damage.

Etiology

The exact cause for avascular necrosis (AVN) in children is not known, but some assumptions have been reported previously.

- *Trueta's assumption:* In younger children, less than 3 years of age, arterial insufficiency of lateral epiphyseal artery and metaphyseal artery leads to AVN. At growing age between 4 and 8 years, AVN can be due to compression of single retinacular artery due to force of strong lateral rotators, positioning the hip in the extreme ranges, limiting the blood supply.
- According to Caffey, the blood supply to ossification centers at epiphysis is compromised leading to necrotic bone formation.

Predisposing factors include:
- Low birth weight babies
- Abnormal growth and development as per the child's chronological age.
- Dietary or environmental influences due to low socioeconomic status
- Any significant injury to the hip, e.g., during closed reduction of congenital hip dislocation.

Pathological Features

Perthes disease of hip is commonly confined to early age-group and has a male predisposition. It is due to ischemic changes in capitis femoral epiphysis because of loss of

Table 21.2: Classification of stage of Perthes disease.	
Waldenström pathological classification	*Modified Elizabethtown radiological classification*
Stage I: Initial stage of synovitis (1–3 weeks)	Stage Ia: Sclerosis of the epiphysis with no loss of height
	Stage Ib: Sclerosis of the epiphysis with loss of height but no fragmentation
Stage II: Stage of AVN (6–12 months)	Stage IIa: Early fragmentation with just one or two vertical fissures in the epiphysis on the AP or frog-leg lateral view
	Stage IIb: Advanced fragmentation with no new bone lateral to the fragmented epiphysis
Stage III: Fragmentation and resorptive stage (2–3 years)	Stage IIIa: Early "porotic" new bone formation at the periphery of the epiphysis covering less than a third of the epiphysis
	Stage IIIb: New bone formation of "normal" texture and covers more than a third of the epiphysis
Stage IV: Residual stage	Stage IV: Complete healing with no radiographically identifiable avascular bone

blood supply to femoral head or a part of the femoral head (AVN) affecting primary and secondary ossification centers. Also, imbalance of osteogenesis and resorption contributes to the femoral head deformity. And due to added blood supply from foveolar artery of ligamentum teres, the incidence of this disease is rare after the age of 8 years. Waldenström pathological classification and modified Elizabethtown radiological classification are shown in **Table 21.2**.

Clinical Features

- Insidious onset of symptoms.
- Generally seen in males between the age group of 3 and 10 years.
- Unilateral or bilateral involvement.
- Pain in hip joint which may radiate to groin region to medial aspect of thigh up to the knee joint.
- Pain is aggravated by hip movements, standing or walking, and relieved by rest.
- Antalgic gait followed by Trendelenburg gait.
- In initial stage of the disease child may hold the limb in hip flexion and slight abduction followed by gradual limitation in range of motion due to pain and stiffness—with maximal restriction in abduction and internal rotation.
- Positive Thomas test due to tight hip flexors.
- Atrophy in thigh muscles and limb shortening may be observed in later stages of the disease.

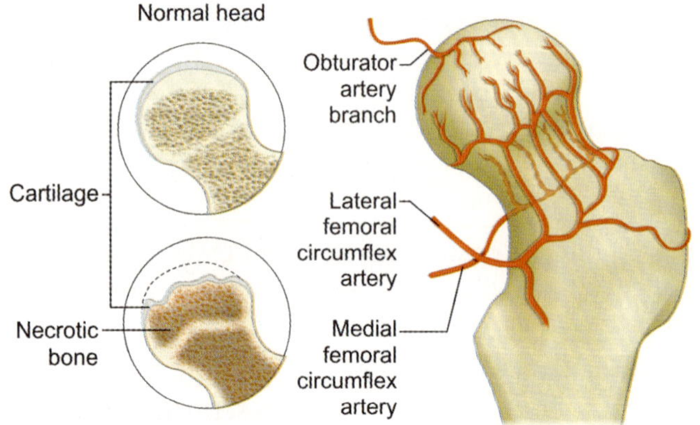

Fig. 21.8: Perthes disease.

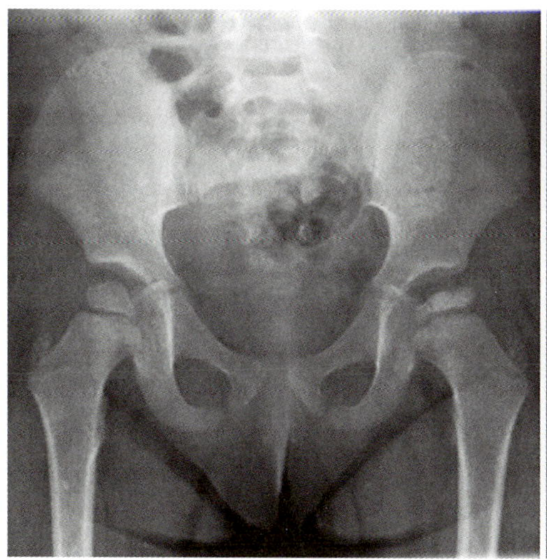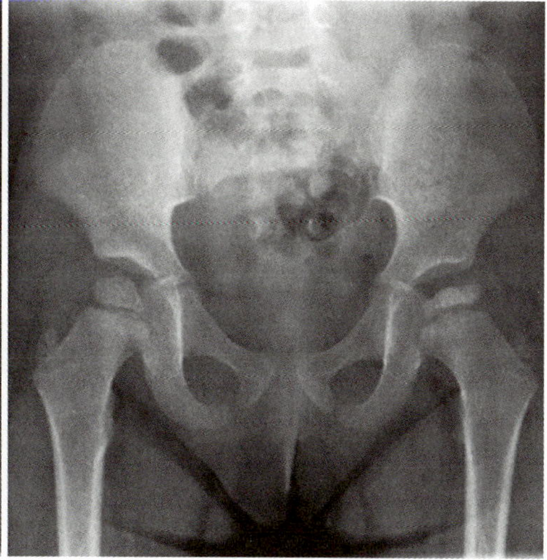

Fig. 21.9: Anteroposterior view radiograph of pelvis showing left side Perthes disease.

Investigations

Arthrography or MRI scan of hip joint is advised to visualize the actual shape of head and joint congruity, epiphyseal infarction, presence of deformity, etc.

Radiological findings may include **(Fig. 21.9)**:

- *Early stages:* Gage's sign (convex rounding of lateral margin of epiphysis) involving epiphyseal ossification center (EOC); small EOC and lateral shifting of femoral head (Waldenström's sign) best seen in frog-leg view; the distance between the medial pole of head and acetabular socket is increased; Salter's extrusion angle less than 50° (angle between the horizontal line from the bottom of acetabulum and perpendicular line drawn at the lateral ossified margin of acetabulum); sclerosis of femoral epiphysis.
- *Late stages:* Major findings in this stage include size of femoral head and neck is reduced, gap between the head and socket is increased, increase in bone mineral density, and mushroom-like appearance of femoral head.

Prognosis

Poor prognostic factors include severe involvement of EOC and femoral head, head-at-risk signs, and early closure of epiphyseal plate. **Tables 21.3 and 21.4** describe the classifications for outcomes of Perthes disease.

Management

Treatment is generally focused on reducing the femoral head in the acetabulum, reducing hip irritability, restoring almost full range of motion, achieving normal shape of femoral head, etc.

Medical Management

Patients aged less than 5 years at onset of disease are commonly managed conservatively by NSAIDs, resting the hip with skin traction in abduction frame, applying Petrie cast or Scottish Rite braces in abduction. However,

Table 21.3: The Stulberg classification for outcomes of Perthes disease.

Stulberg class	Description	Outcome
I	Normal, congruent hip	Arthritis does not develop
II	Spherical head, concentric in acetabulum on AP and frog-leg lateral; shortened femoral neck or abnormally steep acetabulum	
III	Ovoid, mushroom, or umbrella-shaped femoral head; not flat	Mild-to-moderate arthritis in adulthood
IV	Flat head and acetabulum (congruent joint)	
V	Flat femoral head, normal femoral neck, and acetabulum (incongruent joint)	Severe arthritis before 50 years of age

(AP: anteroposterior)

Table 21.4: Modified Herring lateral pillar classification.

Group	Description	Outcome
A	No loss of lateral pillar height	Excellent outcome
B	Lateral pillar with <50% loss of height	Good outcome
B/C	Thin pillar, loss of lateral pillar height at 50%	Intermediate outcome
C	>50% collapse of lateral pillar	Poor prognosis

older children require some surgical management—intertrochanteric femoral osteotomy or pelvic osteotomy having better outcomes.

Physiotherapy Management

Conservatively, exercises to maintain the available range at hip joint without aggravating pain are advised.

Postoperatively, after the immobilization of around 8–10 weeks in hip spica—initially, static contractions of hip and knee muscles, ankle toe movements, gentle passive range of motion exercises for flexion, extension, abduction with rotations as tolerated with precautions are advised. Active assisted exercises progressed to active hip movements particularly, to improve abduction and internal rotation. Strengthening of glutei, hamstrings, and quadriceps muscles is important followed by gait training in front of mirror in parallel bars.

Complications

Limb length measurement should be done. If there is a difference, a shoe raise can be given to prevent further complication of scoliosis. The conservatively managed hip may be more prone to OA of hip.

DEVELOPMENTAL DYSPLASIA OF HIP

Introduction

Developmental dysplasia of hip (DDH) is developmental disorder involving hip in which the hip joint has not formed normally and usually occurs before, during, or shortly after birth due to structural abnormalities, including dislocation, subluxation and instability, and dysplasia of the femoral head and acetabulum. It is more in first born babies, predominantly seen on left hip. This condition could be confused with coxa vara, posterior hip dislocation or paralytic hip dislocation, etc. The presence of hip dysplasia in growing children will result in abnormal gait pattern, reduced muscle strength, limb length discrepancy, hip deformity, and increased chances of OA hip and knee.

Etiology

- Hereditary predisposition to joint laxity
- Breech malposition
- Commonly seen in females as maternal relaxin, which is a ligament relaxing hormone in the mother during pregnancy, acts on the fetus's joints if the hormonal environment of the fetus is female
- Shallow acetabulum
- Oligohydramnios (low levels of amniotic fluid)

Pathological Features

Types of deformities in DDH are as follows:
- *Dislocated hip:* There is no articular contact between the femoral head and the acetabulum; may or may not be reducible.
- *Subluxated hip/dislocatable:* Femoral head is partially displaced from its original position having some contact with the acetabulum.
- *Subluxable hip:* Only excessive movement of femoral head is present.

- Acetebular dysplasia: Abnormal development of acetabulum with respect to its size, shape, or position.

Clinical Features

Most of the newborns presenting with mild dysplasia during initial few weeks after birth may resolve by eighth week of age. Progressive dysplasia needs intervention after 6 months of age. Screening is important because the prognosis is better with early diagnosis than when detected late, which may result in prolonged disability. Therefore physical examination is important for detection of DDH.
- Asymmetry of groin or gluteal skin creases (thigh folds) along with unequal knee heights.
- Observed by placing the child in a supine position with the hips and knees flexed.
- Limitation of movements of affected hip mainly hip abduction **(Fig. 21.10)**.
- Soft tissue clicking sound during hip movement.
- Sometimes not noticed until the child starts walking; child walks with a "peculiar gait"—Trendelenburg gait/waddling gait if bilateral involvement, though there might be no pain.
- Special tests that are positive: Barlow's test, Ortolani's test, Galeazzi's sign, and Trendelenburg's test.

Investigations

Real-time ultrasonography is an accurate method for observing hip during the first few months of life as plain radiograph may not be able to detect dysplasia for initial few months.

AP radiograph of pelvis would be reliable after 4–6 months with abnormal findings—no ossification of epiphysis of the femoral head (in child below age of 1 year), break in Shenton's line, sloping acetabulum, and lateral and upward displacement of femoral head **(Fig. 21.11)**.

Medical Management

The goal of management in early diagnosed infants is to attain stable, accurately reduced hip joint at an earliest

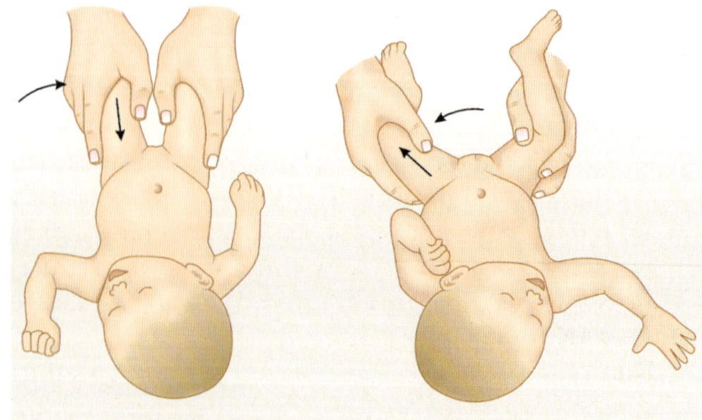

Fig. 21.10: Checking of hip movement and stability.

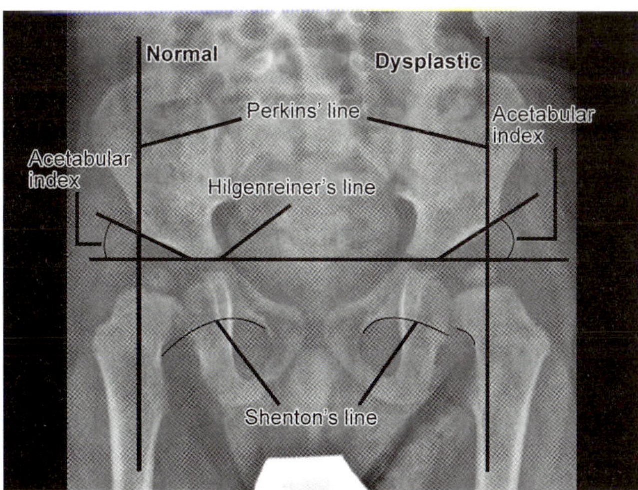

Fig. 21.11: Anteroposterior radiograph of pelvis.

possible age. The goals of treatment in children with persistent dysplasia are to prevent the complications such as early OA and may require hip arthroplasty at younger age.

- *To provide stability to hip joint:*
  - Orthoses allow better capacity to adapt the hip in normal position, and a better chance of good prognosis. Although some authors suggested that the Craig and the Von Rosen splints are superior to the Pavlik harness for maintaining stability and proper position while allowing free movement of the legs and easy care, the Pavlik harness is ideal treatment as it is safe and highly effective with good success rate for most of the children with less than 6 months of age and not recommended after 6 months. Safety measures for day care tasks, such as diapering, bathing, feeding, and dressing should be taught to the parent.
  - The use of an abduction brace orthosis (Plastazote and Ilfeld abduction orthoses) for some time is recommended for the children between the ages of 6–12 months for persistent acetabular dysplasia.
  - Closed reduction is achieved by applying weight traction to the limbs with the child either on a frame or in gallows suspension. Traction is maintained gradually to abduct the hips, a little more each day, until 80° of abduction is reached. Once reduced, it is maintained using hip spica or a frog-leg cast.
  - Closed reduction and fixation with hip spica: This is preferred when orthosis fails to maintain the stability at hip joint and performed under general anesthesia. Followed by splinting in the reduced position, moderate abduction is recommended for a minimum of 6 weeks.
- Diet modification is often done. Oral glucosamine comes from shellfish (although vegetarian options exist) and may help rebuild cartilage. An anti-inflammatory diet may help reduce inflammation. Ginger, garlic, green tea, and omega-3 fatty acids may have anti-inflammatory effects and can be found in fish and fish oil supplements, as well as in flaxseed, squash, collard greens, nuts, broccoli, cauliflower, and spinach. Inflammatory foods such as tomato, potato, eggplant, and red pepper should be avoided.

Surgical Management

- Open reduction and hip reconstruction through modified Smith–Petersen anterolateral approach: Recommended in children more than 18 months
- Salter's osteotomy
- Chiari's pelvic displacement osteotomy
- Pemberton's pericapsular osteotomy
- Pelvic osteotomy for persistent acetabular dysplasia

  After open reduction, a hip spica cast is given for 6 weeks for immobilization in 30° of abduction, flexion, and internal rotation. After immobilization period, supervised physiotherapy is recommended. However, Gather et al. in 2018 recommended early mobilization after hip reconstruction surgery in DDH for better outcomes.

Physiotherapy Management

- *Postoperatively, to reduce associated pain:* The application of ice on the painful regions helps to numb pain and reduce the inflammation.
- *To improve strength, range of motion, and functional activities:* Regular and low or nonimpact range of motion exercises and mild stretching can be given to improve range and to prevent contractures and stiffness in hip joint. Resistance exercises with manual resistance along with functional task training are recommended.
- Weight bearing and gait training are an integral part of rehabilitation, which has to be started after consultation with surgeon for better outcomes.

SLIPPED CAPITAL FEMORAL EPIPHYSIS/ SLIPPED UPPER FEMORAL EPIPHYSIS

Introduction

It is a common hip pathology presented in preadolescent and adolescents leading to short- and long-term morbidity. The head of the femur shifts off at the growth plate of the neck of the femur in a posteroinferior direction (migration of the epiphysis in metaphysis). Pain on hip movement, stiffness, and feeling of instability are the usual complaints in the affected hip. The condition usually builds up gradually over several weeks or months and is more common in males than females between the ages of 12 and 16; in girls, between the ages of 10 and 14 years.

Etiology and Pathological Features

- Idiopathic
- Individuals with endocrine disorders (such as hypothyroidism, hyperthyroidism, kidney failure,

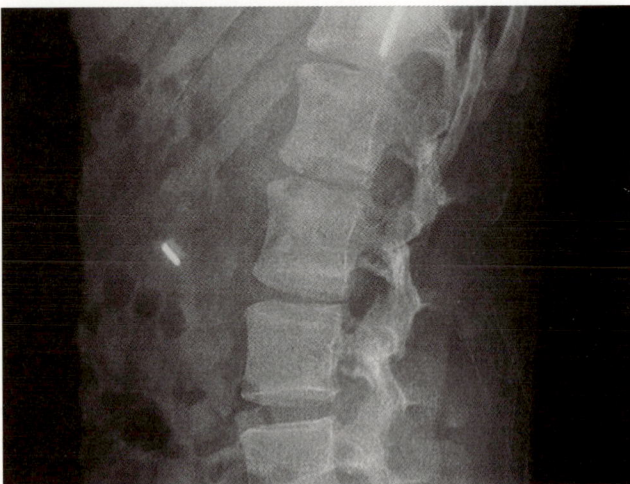

Fig. 21.12: Pelvic incidence.

hypopituitarism, and growth hormone deficiency) may have an association.
- Family history of slipped capital femoral epiphysis (SCFE).

Gebhart et al., in 2015 reported the variations in two common anatomic measurements using AP radiograph of pelvis:
1. Pelvic incidence (PI) **(Fig. 21.12)**
2. Acetabular retroversion in patients with SCFE.

They found that in patients with small PI, the pelvis is tilted anteriorly to maintain lumbar lordosis of the spine. This excessive anterior pelvic tilt would increase the stress on anterior aspect of hip joint and physis of the proximal femur. Because of increased stress on the hip along with other factors such as obesity, physeal sloping angle, femoral retroversion, and size of the epiphyseal tubercle, it could contribute to the development of SCFE.

Mechanical abnormalities such as
- Physeal instability
- Deformity at the neck/metaphysis level
- Pre-existing deformity of proximal femur and/or acetabulum may also be associated with SCFE.

Clinical Features

Types of SCFE (American Association of Orthopedic Surgeons):
- **Stable SCFE:** Patient can bear weight on the affected hip and walk independently with or without using crutches.
- **Unstable SCFE:** Patient cannot walk or bear weight, even with crutches. Unstable SCFE requires immediate management.

Symptoms:
- Patient with mild SCFE complains of intermittent pain in the groin, hip, knee, and/or thigh region since several weeks or months.
- Pain aggravates on hip activity and may present with limp during walk or run.

In severe or unstable SCFE cases:
- Sudden onset of pain, usually secondary to fall or injury
- Unable to bear body weight on affected extremity
- Externally rotated hip joint
- Limb length discrepancy, i.e., the affected limb may be shorter than the nonaffected limb.

Clinical examination findings of affected hip demonstrate:
- Severe pain at the end range of movement
- Restricted hip mobility—mainly medial rotation
- Severe muscle spasm around hip joint
- Limping or Trendelenburg or antalgic gait
- Sometimes atrophy of thigh muscles

Investigations

X-ray radiograph with AP and frog-leg lateral view of bilateral hip joint is usually done for diagnosis. The line of Klein (a *line* along the superior edge of the neck of the femur, i.e., from the lateral part of the superior femoral epiphysis) is an important finding on AP view X-ray, which detects SCFE. When the line of Klein does not intersect the outermost part of the femoral head epiphysis, then SCFE is usually present (also known as Trethowan's sign). Additionally, S sign in the frog-leg lateral view has more diagnostic accuracy for diagnosing *SCFE*. S sign is a curvilinear line drawn on the inferior margin of the proximal femoral head–neck junction along the proximal femoral physis. Discontinuity in the line is abnormal and may confirm SCFE **(Figs. 21.13 and 21.14)**.

Morphological Classification Based on Amount of Deformity

Using AP and lateral X-ray views, the linear displacement of the head on the neck or slip angle (angle between shaft and perpendicular to physis) is considered for grading:
1. Preslip (widening of the physis; no displacement)
2. Mild slip (up to 1/3 displacement, or up to 30° of head tilt)
3. Moderate slip (1/3–1/2 displacement; or 30–60° slip angle)
4. Severe slip (>1/2 displacement; >60° of slip angle).

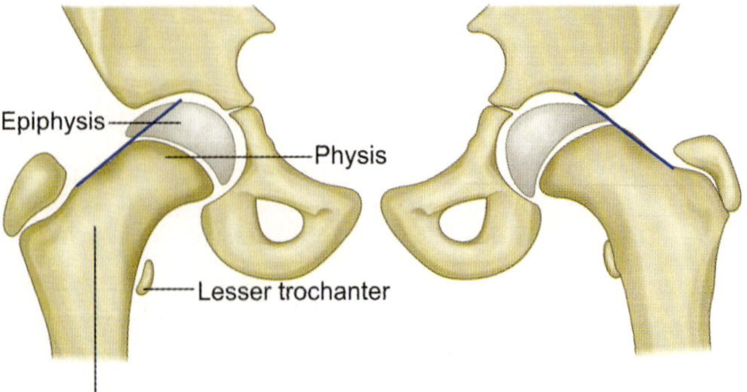

Fig. 21.13: Anteroposterior view bilateral hip and pelvis (line of Klein).

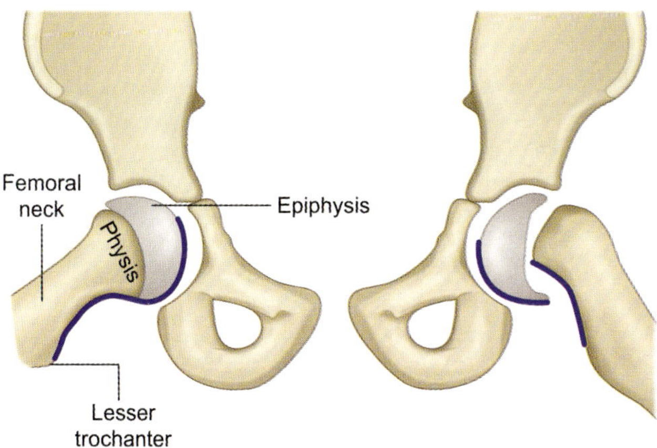

Fig. 21.14: Frog-leg view bilateral hip (S sign).

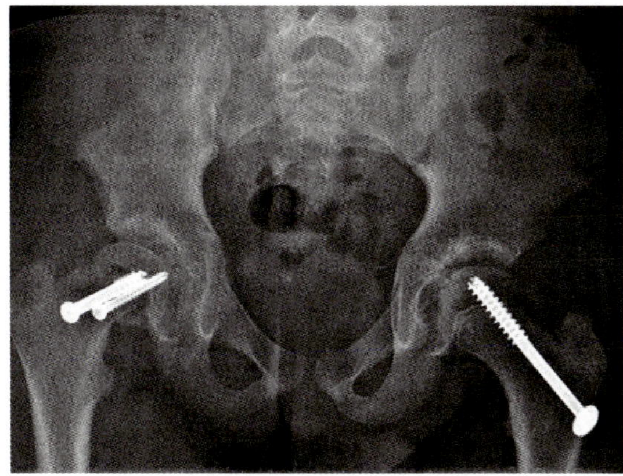

Fig. 21.16: Surgical intervention for developmental dysplasia of hip (DDH).

Medical Treatment

The goal of treatment is to prevent the further displacement of femoral head from slipping by surgical procedure. Early treated cases of SCFE have good prognosis with hip function. Suspected case of SCFE is initially treated with strict nonweight bearing walking/ambulation and wheel chair is advised.

Surgical stabilization (percutaneous fixation of the epiphysis) with in situ screw or Kirschner wires **(Figs. 21.15 and 21.16)** fixation of head on neck of femur is done by open reduction and internal fixation.

In situ fixation in the opposite hip, which is at high risk for SCFE, is done as a part prophylactic pinning.

Weight Bearing after Surgery

After surgery, strict nonweight bearing (NWB) walking using crutches or walker is advised for several weeks. And the weight-bearing decision is often taken by the surgeon based upon the current status of stability of head on neck of femur.

Physiotherapy

Gradual range of motion exercises can be started as early as tolerated (generally after 3–4 weeks or may be delayed further) with proper precautions to avoid dislocations in consultation with the surgeon. Early isometric exercises for hip muscles can be started to prevent atrophy and progressed gradually to improve strength isotonically. Gait training is also essential.

Participation in vigorous sport activities should be avoided for some period after starting weight bearing.

TROCHANTERIC BURSITIS

Introduction

Trochanteric bursitis is inflammation of the bursa superficial to the greater trochanter (GT) **(Fig. 21.17)** of the femur. When this bursa becomes irritated or inflamed, it causes pain in the hip. In chronic conditions, it may be called greater trochanteric pain syndrome. A bursa is a double-membrane sac filled with fluid located near a joint. It forms a sort of cushion to minimize friction between the soft tissue/bone interfaces and acts as a shock absorber during the movement of muscles and joints.

Commonly involved bursae are:

- Subgluteus medius bursa—located above the GT and underneath the insertion of the glutcus medius.
- Subgluteus maximus bursa—located between the GT and the insertion of the gluteus medius and gluteus maximus muscles.

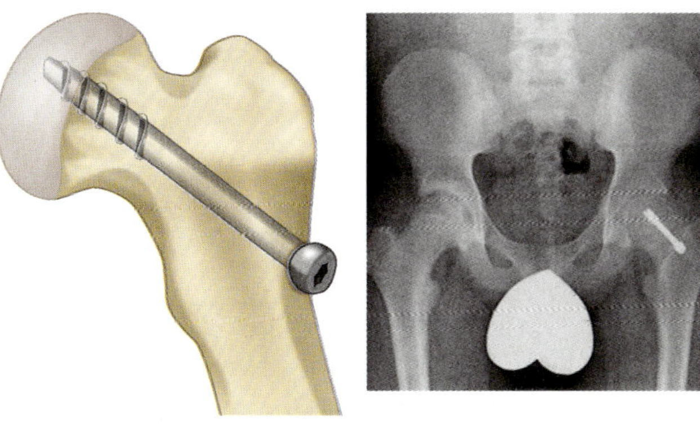

Figs. 21.15A and B: Surgical intervention in the form of screws for developmental dysplasia of hip.

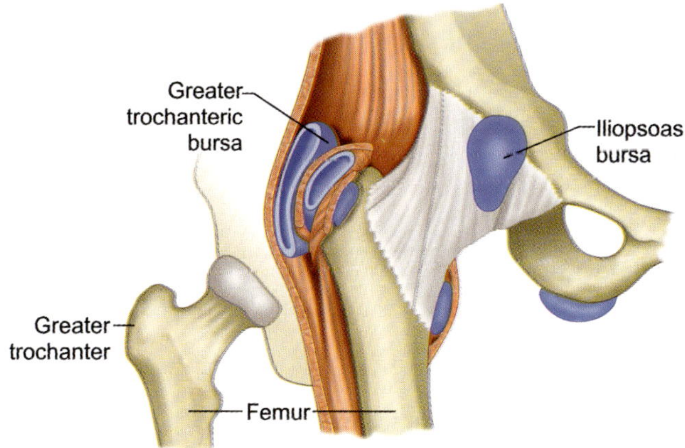

Fig. 21.17: Trochanteric bursa.

Etiology

- Standing asymmetrically for long periods of time with affected hip elevated and adducted and drooping of pelvis on nonaffected side
- Excessive walking or running—overuse injury
- Fall on GT/external trauma to GT
- Leg length discrepancy
- Dysfunction of gluteus medius muscle
- Overweight/obesity and especially in females than in males.

Pathological Features

Increased repetitive friction of the bursa against the GT causes irritation and inflammation, which in turn causes pain.

Clinical Findings

- Acute/chronic pain around the lateral region of hip.
- Swelling, increased local temperature, and tenderness on the lateral aspect of GT.
- Pain that may radiate down the lateral aspect of thigh.
- A snap felt in the lateral aspect of the hip.
- Pain is more during ascending stairs than descending stairs.
- Patient is unable to lie down on the affected side.
- Development of pain-related sleep disturbances.
- Decreased muscle flexibility and endurance of hip muscles.
- Sometimes antalgic gait.

Investigations

SOAP diagnostic approach, including subjective, objective assessment, and then planning treatment, should be followed:

- History of onset and about symptoms
- Palpation of bursa—for tenderness, temperature, etc.
- For provocative test—Ober's test
- X-ray to rule out GT fracture or ultrasonography to confirm the diagnosis
- MRI only if required.

Medical Treatment

- Analgesics/anti-inflammatory drugs—NSAIDs are given for pain and inflammation.
- Use of a cane or crutches during treatment to relieve pressure on bursa is advised for a week or more.
- If conservative management fails, then corticosteroid injections **(Fig. 21.18)** into the bursa will reduce the symptoms, but recurrence is often possible within the period of 3–6 months.
- When the bursa is suspected for infection, the examination of bursa fluid is advised and antibiotic therapy is started and fluid aspiration is done if required.
- Bursectomy of affected bursa is rarely needed.

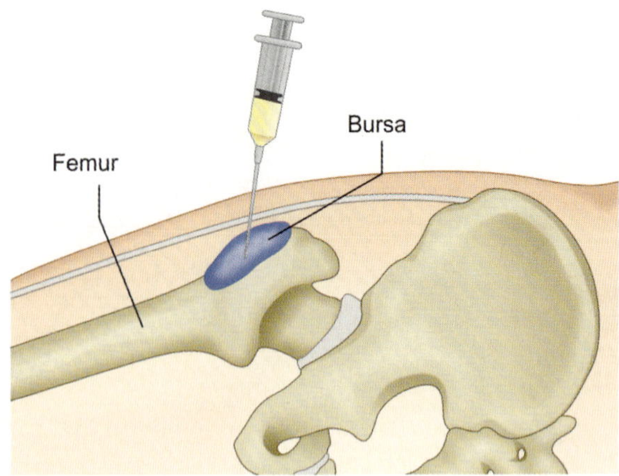

Fig. 21.18: Corticosteroid injection into trochanteric bursa.

Physiotherapy Management

- *To manage the pain and the inflammation:* Rest is given and aggravating activities are restricted, cryotherapy for at least 20 minutes three to four times in a day **(Fig. 21.19)**. Ultrasound therapy with accurate dosimetry should be chosen according to stage of condition to acquire desired effect.
  - Hip spica taping **(Fig. 21.20)** to provide additional support—Place a 1–2-inch object under the heel to slightly flex the hip. Using a 6-inch, double-length elastic bandage, wrap lateral to medial on the involved side at a slight downward angle. Wrap the bandage around the involved side and cross the anterior hip. Wrap the bandage around the back of the patient and around the anterior aspect of the involved side. Continue across the anterior aspect of the hip.
- *To improve strength and to restore the normal ROM:* Strengthening of gluteus medius, gluteus minimus along with stretching or myofascial release (MFR)

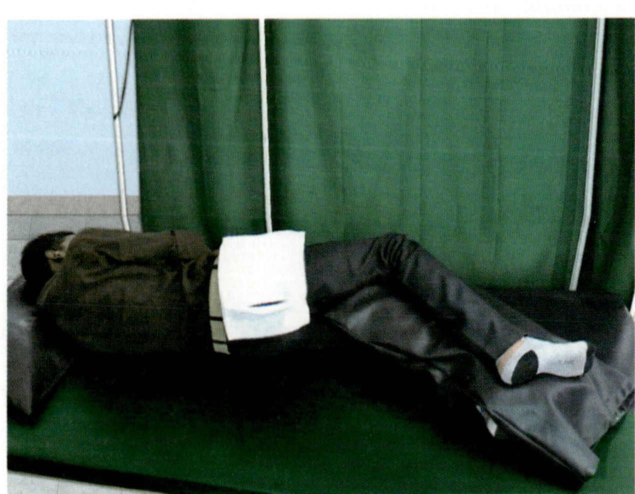

Fig. 21.19: Cold pack application for trochanteric bursitis.

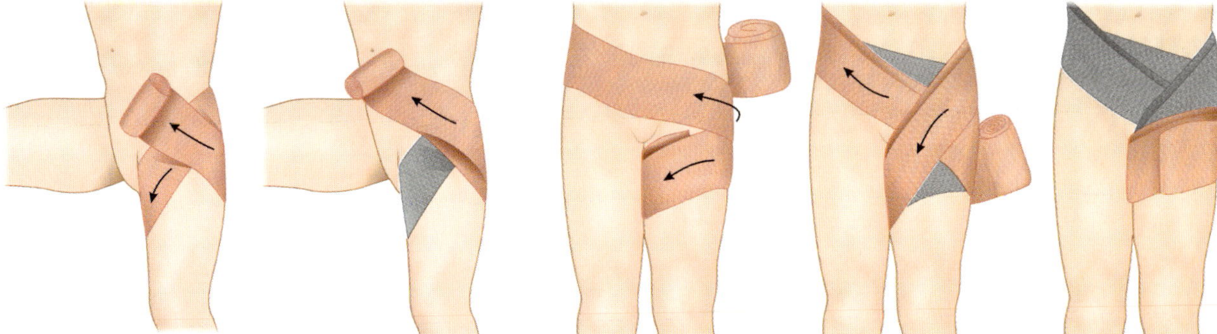

Fig. 21.20: Hip spica taping.

of ITB if ITB tightness is present is recommended as tolerated by the patient.

MERALGIA PARESTHETICA

Introduction, Etiology, and Pathological Features

Meralgia paresthetica (MP) or lateral cutaneous nerve (LCN) neuralgia or Bernhardt-Roth syndrome is associated with tingling, numbness, and burning pain in the lateral aspect of thigh. It is due to compression of lateral femoral cutaneous nerve (LFCN). It occurs mainly due to impingement or compression or irritation of LFCN when it exits pelvis. The common site of compression is entrapment of the nerve under inguinal ligament due to obesity (BMI ≥30), pregnancy, tight garments such as jeans, direct trauma, muscle spasm, scoliosis, iliacus hematoma, and limb length discrepancy or injury to the ligament during anterior approach for total hip arthroplasty or due to severe tightness of iliopsoas muscle. The other factors include obesity, diabetes mellitus, and aging process leading to symptoms resembling neuropathy.

Clinical Features

- Pain at lateral or anterolateral aspect of thigh region, which extends up to the knee and can extend in groin or buttocks (within the distribution of LFCN).
- May have associated burning sensation, tingling, and numbness.
- Sometimes sensory loss or hypersensitivity to heat and itching.

The differential diagnosis for MP could be lumbar canal stenosis, disk herniation, and nerve root radiculopathy. Neurodynamic testing suggested by Butler or Tinel's sign may confirm the diagnosis. For confirming the diagnosis, neurophysiological studies such as sensory nerve conduction, somatosensory evoked potentials, and nerve conduction block tests are recommended.

The medical management includes NSAIDs, rest, and injection vitamin B_{12}. Other factors include protection of that area if it is associated with sensory loss, avoiding tight clothing, etc. The other interventions include pulsed radiofrequency/ultrasound-guided LCN of the thigh (LCNT) nerve block using lignocaine/corticosteroids. The surgical intervention options include LCNT neurolysis and resection when conservative management fails which has good prognosis.

Physiotherapy Interventions

- TENS therapy for atleast 20 minutes over dermatomal distribution of LFCN.
- Manual therapy techniques mainly soft tissue release or manipulative techniques may release the nerve.
- MFR techniques/active release techniques for rectus femoris and iliopsoas.
- Transverse friction massage of inguinal ligament.
- Stretching for TFL, ITB along with hip muscles.
- Kinesiotaping may reduce the symptoms associated with MP.
- Acupuncture is also very helpful in managing pain and numbness.

PIRIFORMIS SYNDROME

Introduction

Piriformis is a flat muscle, which originates at the anterior surface of the sacrum, usually at the levels of vertebrae S2 through S4 and attaches to the superior medial aspect of the GT. It is a hip lateral rotator and hip abductor when hip is flexed. The sciatic nerve passes through the greater sciatic foramen below the piriformis muscle.

Piriformis syndrome is a condition caused by a shortened piriformis muscle, causing compression and irritation of sciatic nerve (sciatic nerve entrapment) and hence producing sciatica-like symptoms **(Fig. 21.21)**. Its clinical picture is similar to that of lumbar radiculopathy, primary sacral dysfunction, or innominate dysfunction; hence, it sometimes can be confusing.

Etiology

- Tightness of piriformis muscle causes sciatic nerve to get compressed in the greater sciatic foramen and causes symptoms radiating from the lower back downward to lateral aspect of thigh.

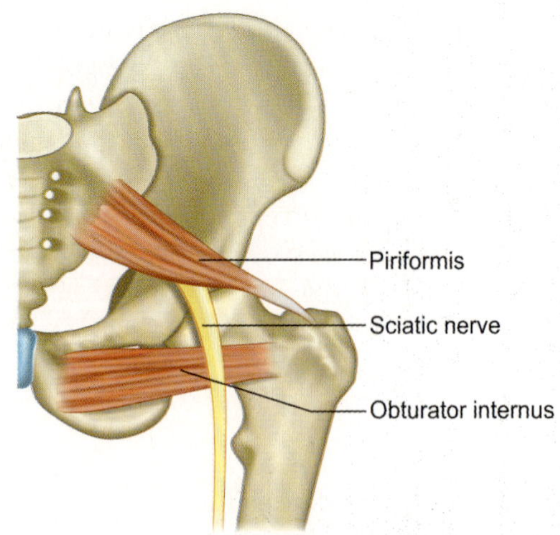

Fig. 21.21: Piriformis syndrome.
Source: Beckie Palmer, Stat Pearls Publishing LLC; 2019.

- Trauma over hip or buttocks region.
- Sitting for prolonged periods (taxi drivers, office desk workers, and bicycle riders).
- Anatomical anomalies such as bipartite piriformis muscle.

Clinical Features

- Patient complains of pain with sitting, standing, when rising from seated or squatting position or lying longer than 15–20 minutes, when getting out of bed.
- Pain in the buttock region, which aggravates on hip movements.
- Pain improves with ambulation and worsens with no movement.
- There is pain or paresthesia radiating from sacrum through gluteal area and down the posterior aspect of thigh, usually stopping above the knee.
- Difficulty in walking (e.g., antalgic gait, foot drop) is also seen along with numbness in foot and weakness in ipsilateral lower extremity.
- Inability to sit for a prolonged time.

Physical Examination

Positive findings would generally be piriformis muscle spasm, weak hip abduction and lateral rotation, pain, tingling, and numbness radiating from lower back region to the lower leg. There is tenderness seen in region of sacroiliac joint, greater sciatic notch, and piriformis muscle. Special tests, such as straight leg raising test, Pace's sign (contraction of the piriformis muscle with resistance to active hip external rotation and abduction may reproduce pain or asymmetrical weakness), Beatty maneuver (patient lies on the unaffected side and abducts the affected extremity, which elicits pain), Freiberg sign (pain with internal rotation of the extended hip), FAIR test (positive when the hip is passively flexed, adducted, and internally rotated by the examiner reproducing buttock pain radiating down the leg), and piriformis muscle tightness, may be positive. In chronic cases, gluteal muscle atrophy or shortening of ipsilateral limb may be observed.

Investigations

Electromyography could differentiate piriformis syndrome from intervertebral disk herniation. Radiographic studies have limited application to the diagnosis of piriformis syndrome. Although MRI and CT may reveal enlargement of the piriformis muscle. It is most useful when ruling out disk and vertebral pathologic conditions.

Medical Management

- Short-term rest
- NSAIDs (analgesics) and acetaminophen
- Muscle relaxants such as tramadol
- Although evidence for the efficacy of steroids in chronic cases is inconclusive, local corticosteroid injections may produce an anti-inflammatory effect
- Recently, botulinum toxin type B is used to relieve sciatic nerve compression and inherent muscle pain from a tight piriformis
- Regular doses of mannitol and vitamin B may reduce the symptoms of neuropathy.

Surgical Management

Endoscopic release (lateral release) of piriformis tendon and sciatic nerve exploration and decompression or removal of the scars around the nerve can be performed to relieve the recurring and chronic symptoms.

Physiotherapy Management

- *To reduce pain or paresthesia radiating downward from lower back:* TENS for a minimum of 20 minutes, ultrasound therapy for localized pain or if the presence of associated trigger points is seen in gluteal muscles.

  Hashemirad et al., in 2016 concluded that the use of K-taping for releasing trigger points in the piriformis muscle in a stretched position is effective in reducing pain and improving medial rotation (**Figs. 21.22A and B**).
- *To reduce muscle spasm:* Moist heat pack for 10–15 minutes.
- *To release the tightened muscle:* MFR or static piriformis muscle stretch for 30-second duration, Muscle energy technique for piriformis muscle preferably with reciprocal inhibition technique. A clinical case study done by Choi and Yoon in 2010 suggested MET technique to women complaining of piriformis syndrome helps to reduce pain significantly and improve passive flexion angle of the coxal articulation.
- Keskula and Tamburello in 1992 suggested that the treatment of piriformis syndrome should focus on the exercises for improving its strength, flexibility, and functional activities (**Fig. 21.23**).

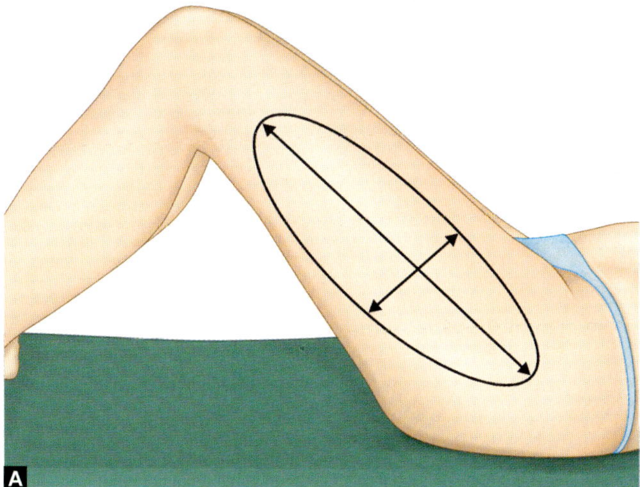

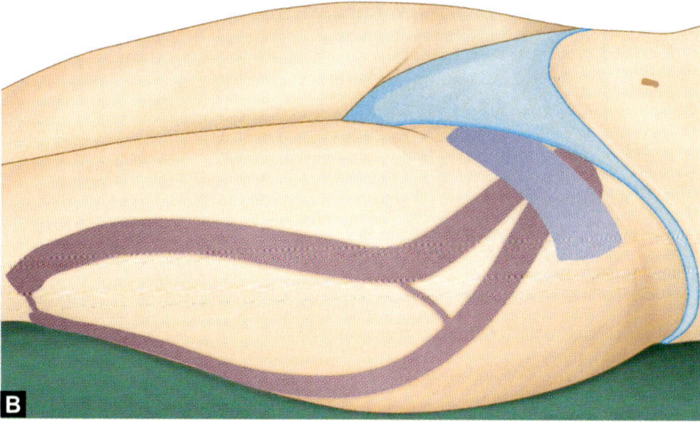

Figs. 21.22A and B: K-taping technique for piriformis syndrome.

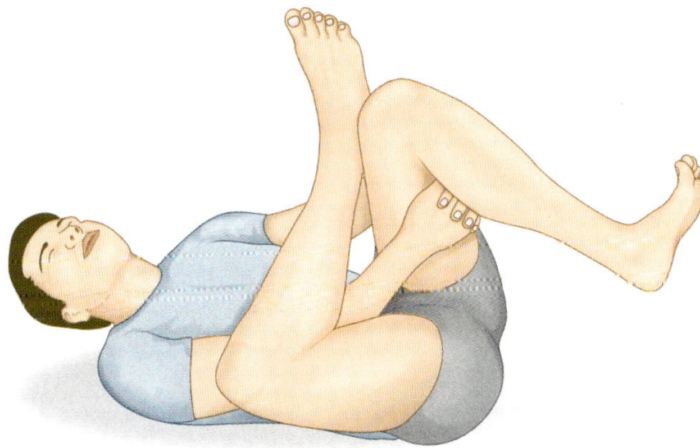

Fig. 21.23: Piriformis auto stretching.

Ergonomics for patients with piriformis syndrome:
- Avoid prolonged sitting.
- Stretching exercises as a routine warm up program before participating in sport activities.
- Recurrent pain can be treated and prevented by stretching exercises for at least 5–10 minutes before engaging in sitting or recreational activities.

SUMMARY

The hip joint is a synovial joint of the ball and socket variety. Due to the shallow acetabulum and the great

stresses borne by the hip, it becomes easily susceptible to degeneration and dislocation. The vasculature of the head of the femur is poorly developed, making it vulnerable to AVN in both adult and pediatric conditions. Evaluation of the hip joint is simple and does not require much effort. However, the management of any hip pathology is difficult since it requires immobilization and nonweight bearing for prolonged periods, increasing the chances of degeneration even further. Also, as it forms a connection between the lumbar spine and the lower extremity, it plays a vital role in locomotion and loading. Hip pathologies, if not treated well, may culminate into knee or lumbar spine pathologies. Medical management usually involves use of analgesics and anti-inflammatory agents. Surgical options differ based on the kind of pathology and the impairments caused by it. Physiotherapy management is crucial, since it allows the individual to get back to weight bearing and improves the function and quality of life. Strength and gait training form an important part of the physiotherapy management.

Case Scenario

CASE STUDY

A 51-year-old woman working as a clerk in government office presented with a diagnosis of early hip joint OA. The patient reported injury to her right leg when she fell down from her bike 3 months back. The patient continued her routine with mild pain over the hip region. Subsequently, the pain got worsened and later she had difficulty in hip movements during ADLs. The patient consulted with orthopedician. X-rays revealed the features of early OA in her right hip. And the patient was given some medications and referred to physiotherapy.

Pain Assessment

The patient described the area of pain as the right groin region and the pain referred to the anterior aspect of thigh. She also has low back pain occasionally on right side. The pain was of a subacute, intermittent, and dull aching type, which was aggravated by standing, walking, and relieved by rest in nonweight-bearing position. In morning, the patient felt mild pain and stiffness for nearly 45 minutes to 1 hour. As the day progressed, the patient's complaints get worsened.

Physical Examination

Mild tenderness was present over the medial joint line of hip and right sacroiliac joint, gluteal muscles were in spasm, and there was mild swelling in the inguinal region. Posture assessment was normal with the pelvis level and the GT and the gluteal folds in standing well aligned. The patient walked with an evident antalgic gait with reduced weight bearing on her right limb with a slight shift of upper body towards the same side during walking. Patient could walk independently with short step length and stride length on the right and decreased heel strike time to avoid weight bearing. Stance time on the right side was reduced significantly, whereas the base of support was increased with the absence of heel strike bilaterally.

ROM evaluation showed that active and passive ranges of motion were restricted and painful with abnormal capsular end-feel at all end ranges. Accessory motions of the hip were restricted and graded according to Kaltenborn and Stoddard as considerably hypomobile. The lumbar spine and knees appeared normal.

Manual muscle testing of pelvic, hip, and knee muscles revealed the strength to be grade 4. Tightness of hamstrings, piriformis, TFL was not tested due to hip pain at extreme ranges.

There was a 2-cm true limb length discrepancy on right compared to unaffected side.

Special tests for sacroiliac joints such as iliac compression and distraction, FABER's test, Gaenslen's maneuver were false positive.

Functional outcomes can be evaluated using following scales:
- Hip Disability and Osteoarthritis Outcome Score (HOOS)
- Intermittent and Constant Osteoarthritis Pain Index (ICOAP)
- Dutch Hip Disability and Osteoarthritis Outcome Score questionnaire
- Lower Extremity Functional Scale
- Harris Hip Score

Guiding Questions:
1. List out the impairments of the patient.
2. What can be the possible differential diagnoses for this patient?
3. What ergonomic advices should the therapist instruct the patient to follow?
4. Describe a physiotherapy management program for this patient.

Review Questions

1. Describe osteoarthritis under the following headings: (a) definition, (b) clinical features, (c) medical/surgical management, and (d) conservative physiotherapy management.
2. Explain the etiological factors, classification, clinical signs and symptoms, and medical management of Perthes disease.
3. Write down the causes, types of deformities, clinical features, diagnosis, and medical and surgical options of management of developmental dysplasia of hip.
4. Describe etiology, pathological features, clinical features, diagnosis, and medical and surgical options of management for slipped capital femoral epiphysis.
5. Describe etiology, clinical features, and medical and physiotherapy options for the management of trochanteric bursitis.
6. What are the clinical features and physiotherapy management for piriformis syndrome?
7. Add a note on clinical features and physiotherapy management for meralgia paresthetica.

BIBLIOGRAPHY

1. Beers A, Ryan M, Kasubuchi Z, et al. Effects of multi-modal physiotherapy, including hip abductor strengthening, in patients with iliotibial band friction syndrome. Physiother Can. 2008;60(2):180-8.
2. Bewyer DC. Iowa rationale for treatment of hip abductor pain syndrome. Orthop J. 2003;23:57-60.
3. Cashman JP, Round J, Taylor G, et al. The natural history of developmental dysplasia of the hip after early supervised treatment in the Pavlik harness. A prospective, longitudinal follow-up. J Bone Joint Surg Br. 2002;84(3):418-25.
4. Catterall A. The natural history of Perthes' disease. J Bone Joint Surg Br. 1971;53(1):37-53.
5. Chaitow L. Muscle energy techniques, 2nd edition. Edinburgh: Churchill Livingstone; 2001.
6. Choi HC, Yoon IJ. A clinical case study on piriformis syndrome with oriental medical treatment and muscle energy techniques. J Orient Rehab Med. 2010;20:209-17.
7. Dagenais S, Garbedian S, Wai EK. Systematic review of the prevalence of radiographic primary hip osteoarthritis. Clin Orthop Relat Res. 2009;467(3):623-37.
8. De Groot IB, Reijman M, Terwee CB, et al. Validation of the Dutch version of the hip disability and osteoarthritis outcome score. Osteoarthritis Cartilage. 2007;15(1):104-9. Level of quality C.
9. Denegar CR, Dougherty DR, Friedman JE, et al. Preferences for heat, cold, or contrast in patients with knee osteoarthritis affect treatment response. Clin Interv Aging. 2010;5:199-206.
10. Fredericson M, Cookingham CL, Chaudhari AM, et al. Hip abductor weakness in distance runners with iliotibial band syndrome. Clin J Sport Med. 2000;10(3):169-75.
11. Gather KS, von Stillfried E, Hagmann S, et al. Outcome after early mobilization following hip reconstruction in children with developmental hip dysplasia and luxation. World J Pediatr. 2018;14(2):176-83.
12. Gebhart JJ, Bohl MS, Weinberg DS, et al. Pelvic incidence and acetabular version in slipped capital femoral epiphysis. J Pediatr Orthop. 2015;35(6):565-70.
13. Gillingham BL, Sanchez AA, Wenger DR. Pelvic osteotomies for the treatment of hip dysplasia in children and young adults. J Am Acad Orthop Surg. 1999;7(5):325-37.
14. Grossman MG, Ducey SA, Nadler SS, et al. Meralgiaparesthetica: diagnosis and treatment. J Am Acad Orthop Surg. 2001;9(5):336-44.
15. Grossman MG, Ducey SA, Nadler SS, et al. Meralgiaparesthetica: diagnosis and treatment. J Am Acad Orthop Surg. 2001;9(5):336-44.
16. Hashemirad F, Karimi N, Keshavarz R. The effect of Kinesio taping technique on trigger points of the piriformis muscle. J Bodyw Mov Ther. 2016;20(4):807-14.
17. Iowa Orthop J. 2002;22; published by the Residents and Faculty of the Department of Orthopaedics, The University of Iowa.
18. Joseph B, Varghese G, Mulpuri K, et al. Natural evolution of Perthes disease: a study of 610 children under 12 years of age at disease onset. J Pediatr Orthop. 2003;23:590-600.
19. Kalichman L, Vered E, Volchek L. Relieving symptoms of meralgiaparesthetica using Kinesio taping: a pilot study. Arch Phys Med Rehabil. 2010;91(7):1137-9.
20. Keskula DR, Tamburello M. Conservative management of piriformis syndrome. J Athl Train. 1992;27(2):102, 104, 106-7, 110.
21. KNGF-guidelines for physical therapy in patients with osteoarthritis of the hip and knee. Supplement to the Dutch Journal of Physical Therapy. 2010;120(1).
22. Kollitz KM, Gee AO. Classifications in brief: the herring lateral pillar classification for Legg-Calvé-Perthes disease. Clin Orthop Relat Res. 2013;471(7):2068–72.

23. Kotlarsky P, Haber R, Bialik V, et al. Developmental dysplasia of the hip: what has changed in the last 20 years?. World J Orthop. 2015;6(11):886-901.

24. Leunig M, Casillas MM, Hamlet M, et al. Slipped capital femoral epiphysis: early mechanical damage to the acetabular cartilage by a prominent femoral metaphysis. Acta Orthop Scand. 2000;71(4):370-5.

25. Loder RT, Dietz FR. What is the best evidence for the treatment of slipped capital femoral epiphysis?. J Pediatr Orthop. 2012;32 Suppl 2():S158-65

26. Lustenberger DP, Ng VY, Best TM, et al. Efficacy of treatment of trochanteric bursitis: a systematic review. Clin J Sport Med. 2011;21(5):447-53.

27. Millis MB. SCFE: clinical aspects, diagnosis, and classification. J Child Orthop. 2017;11(2):93-8.

28. Millis MB. SCFE: clinical aspects, diagnosis, and classification. J Child Orthop. 2017;11(2):93-8. doi:10.1302/1863-2548-11-170025.

29. Nilsdotter AK, Lohmander LS, Klässbo M, et al. Hip disability and osteoarthritis outcome score (HOOS)--validity and responsiveness in total hip replacement. BMC Musculoskelet Disord. 2003;4:10. Epub 2003 May 30.

30. Ogura Y, Miyahara Y, Naito H, et al. Duration of static stretching influences muscle force production in hamstring muscles. J Strength Cond Res. 2007;21(3):788-92.

31. Orchard JW, Fricker PA, Abud AT, et al. Biomechanics of iliotibial band friction syndrome in runners. Am J Sports Med. 1996;24(3):375-9.

32. Pal CP, Singh P, Chaturvedi S, et al. Epidemiology of knee osteoarthritis in India and related factors. Indian J Orthop. 2016;50(5):518-22.

33. Parisi TJ, Mandrekar J, Dyck PJ, et al. Meralgiaparesthetica: relation to obesity, advanced age, and diabetes mellitus. Neurology. 2011;77(16):1538-42.

34. Rebich EJ, Lee SS, Schlechter JA. The S sign: a new radiographic tool to aid in the diagnosis of slipped capital femoral epiphysis. J Emerg Med. 2018;54(6):835-43.

35. Rutjes AWS, Nüesch E, Sterchi R, et al. Transcutaneous electrostimulation for osteoarthritis of the knee. Cochrane Database Syst Rev. 2009; (4) 88 :CD002823.

36. Sankar WN, Nduaguba A, Flynn JM. Ilfeld abduction orthosis is an effective second-line treatment after failure of Pavlik harness for infants with developmental dysplasia of the hip. J Bone Joint Surg Am. 2015;97(4):292-7.

37. Schwellnus MP, Mackintosh L, Mee J. Deep transverse frictions in the treatment of iliotibial band friction syndrome in athletes: a clinical trial. Physiotherapy. 1992;78(8):564-8.

38. Shamus J, Shamus E. The management of iliotibial band syndrome with a multifaceted approach: a double case report. Int J Sports Phys Ther. 2015;10(3):378-90.

39. Shipman SA, Helfand M, Moyer VA, et al. Screening for developmental dysplasia of the hip: a systematic literature review for the US Preventive Services Task Force. Pediatrics. 2006;117(3):e557-76.

40. Thomas SR. A review of long-term outcomes for late presenting developmental hip dysplasia. Bone Joint J. 2015;97-B(6):729-33.

41. Trummer M, Flaschka G, Unger F, et al. Lumbar disc herniation mimicking meralgiaparesthetica: case report. Surg Neurol. 2000;54(1):80-1.

42. Vassalou EE, Katonis P, Karantanas AH. Piriformis muscle syndrome: a cross-sectional imaging study in 116 patients and evaluation of therapeutic outcome. Eur Radiol. 2018;28(2):447-58.

43. Vedantam R, Bell MJ. Dynamic ultrasound assessment for monitoring of treatment of congenital dislocation of the hip. J Pediatr Orthop. 1995;15(6):725-8.

44. Vitale MG, Skaggs DL. Developmental dysplasia of the hip from six months to four years of age. J Am AcadOrthop Surg. 2001;9(6):401-11.

45. Wells D, King JD, Roe TF, et al. Review of slipped capital femoral epiphysis associated with endocrine disease. J Pediatr Orthop. 1993;13(5):610-4.

46. Wilkinson AG, Sherlock DA, Murray GD. The efficacy of the Pavlik harness, the Craig splint and the von Rosen splint in the management of neonatal dysplasia of the hip. A comparative study. J Bone Joint Surg Br. 2002;84(5):716-9.

Knee Conditions

Priyasingh Rangey

LEARNING OBJECTIVES

After reading this chapter, the readers should be able to:
- Understand the evaluation process to be followed for knee joint assessment
- Understand the etiology, pathophysiology, and clinical presentation of various pathologies related to the knee joint
- Understand the medical and surgical management used for the various pathologies related to the knee joint
- Formulate the physical therapy management used for the various pathologies related to the knee joint
- Understand the various operative procedures performed on the knee joint and their postoperative physiotherapy management.

CHAPTER OUTLINE

- Evaluation of the knee joint
  - Subjective assessment
  - Objective examination
  - Knee instruments and rating scales
- Pathologies related to the knee
  - Ligament injuries
  - Meniscus injuries
- Rheumatoid arthritis
  - Clinical presentation
  - Management
- Osteoarthritis
  - Pathophysiology
  - Classification of osteoarthritis
  - Diagnosis
  - Management
- Bursitis
  - Pathophysiology
  - Physical examination
  - Management
- Anterior knee pain syndrome
  - Patellofemoral pain syndrome
  - Chondromalacia patellae
  - Osteochondritis dissecans
  - Synovial plica syndrome
  - Fat pad irritation (Hoffa's syndrome)
  - Patellar tendinopathy
  - Osgood–Schlatter disease
- Iliotibial band syndrome
  - Etiology
  - Pathological features
  - Clinical features
- Investigations
  - Medical management
  - Physiotherapy interventions
- Iliotibial band syndrome
  - Etiology
  - Pathological features
  - Clinical features
  - Investigations
  - Medical management
  - Physiotherapy interventions
- Operative procedures of the knee
  - Anterior cruciate ligament reconstruction
  - Synovectomy
  - Arthroscopic procedures

INTRODUCTION

The knee joint is a complex structure that is made up of three bones—femur, tibia, and patella. It can be divided into three compartments—patellofemoral, medial, and lateral. Each of these compartments consists of a joint—patellofemoral and medial and lateral tibiofemoral. Since it is present at the end of two long bones, it is more susceptible to injury. In addition to that, the bony ends do not completely conform to each other. The stability is enhanced by surrounding ligaments and menisci. There are also several other structures, e.g., fat pad, plicae, and bursae that play an important role in the functioning of the knee **(Figs. 22.1A and B)**.

This chapter will try to uncover a few of the several pathologies related to the knee joint and also try to explain the techniques to assess and manage them.

EVALUATION OF THE KNEE JOINT

Evaluation of the knee joint consists of history taking and physical examination along with functional evaluation.

During the examination of any knee injury, the following points need to be considered:
- Mechanism of injury (MOI)
- Intensity of pain, instability, and disability
- Swelling—whether present or absent, and if present then the time of onset; type of swelling
- Past history.

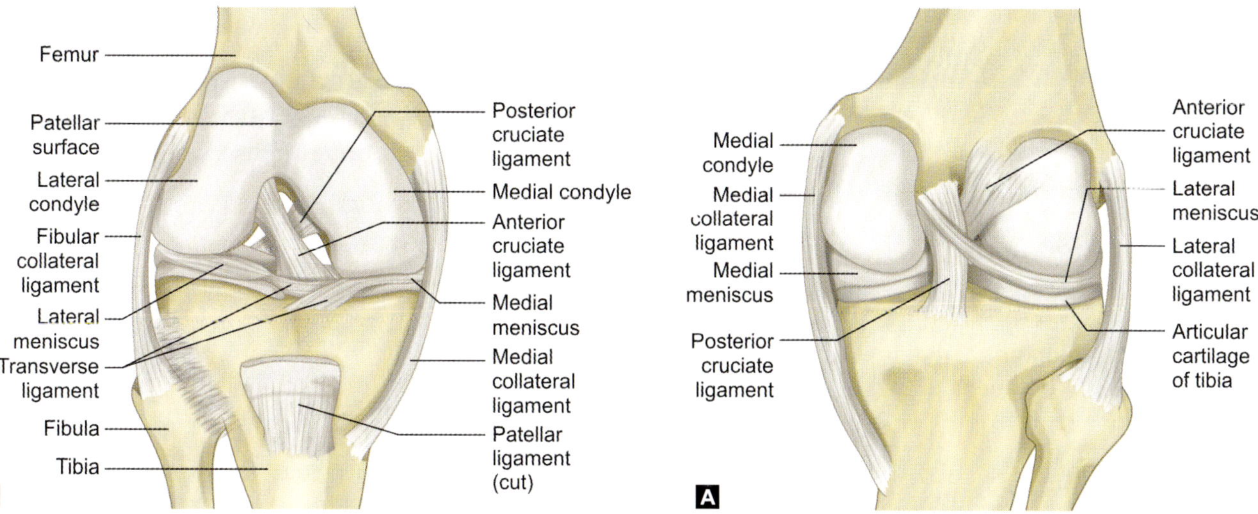

Figs. 22.1A and B: Structure of the knee joint: (A) Anterior view (B) Posterior view.

Subjective Assessment

History taking should focus on the precise MOI, since the MOI is many times indicative of several possible differential diagnoses. The amount of force that caused the injury, the direction of force, the position of the knee, the weight-bearing status of the leg, etc., should be noted. Speed of the movement of knee and the speed with which the patient is moving during injury can also be indicative of the structure involved, e.g., anterior cruciate ligament (ACL) injuries are common with deceleration. Hearing of any "pop," "snap," or "click" at the time of injury indicates ligament or meniscal injuries. Often, crepitation can be heard inside the joint during movement which may suggest degenerative changes.

The pain caused by any injury is an important indicator of the structure that may be injured and the extent of the injury. Location of the pain gives a reasonable indication of the location of the injured structure as shown in **Table 22.1**. Intensity of the pain is an indicator of the extent of tissue damage, except with Grade III sprains. Positions and movements that alter the pain can also provide guidance regarding the cause.

The amount of swelling and the time of onset of swelling can reflect whether the injury is intra-articular or extra-articular. Intra-articular swelling (hemarthrosis) is usually large (voluminous) and occurs rapidly (1–2 hours) following injury.

Presence of similar incidents in the past suggests recurrent injuries and it should be noted, as recurrent injuries are usually a sign of some weak or lax structure. Any functional disabilities should also be noted as they may be due to ligament or meniscal injuries. "Giving way" or locking of the knee is a noteworthy finding in meniscal injuries. Locking can also be seen in osteoarthritis (OA) due to the presence of loose bodies. Inability to bear weight on the affected limb is reported by individuals having severe pain.

Knee injuries in the past may lead to early degeneration of the joint. Meniscal injuries, ACL injuries, intra-articular fractures, and meniscectomy increase the incidence of the secondary degenerative changes.

In addition to the above-mentioned factors, the age of the patient is also an important variable. Degenerative changes of the knee occur around the age of 40 years. Ligament and meniscal injuries are more prevalent in the younger athletic population.

History taking is an integral part of the assessment procedure since it can streamline the process and avoid unnecessary questions and tests.

Table 22.1: Location of pain and related possible disorders.

Anterior knee pain	Posterior knee pain	Medial knee pain	Lateral knee pain
• Patellofemoral problems	• Popliteal tendonitis	• PFPS	• IT band syndrome
• Bursa (infra- and prepatellar)	• Popliteal cyst	• MCL injury	• Popliteal tendonitis
• Fat pad	• PCL injury	• Medial meniscus injury	• LCL injury
• Tendinosis		• Medial plica syndrome	• Lateral meniscus injury
• Osgood–Schlatter disease		• Pes anserine bursitis	• Lateral compartment OA
• Patellar fracture, subluxation or dislocation		• Medial compartment OA	• Biceps femoris tendonitis
		• Tibial plateau fractures	

(PCL: posterior cruciate ligament; PFPS: patellofemoral pain syndrome; MCL: medial collateral ligament; OA: osteoarthritis; IT band: Iliotibial band; LCL: lateral collateral ligament)

Clinical Pearl

The examiner should be cautious while assessing the knee joint as the knee is susceptible to infective conditions such as osteomyelitis and tuberculosis and also many benign tumors such as giant cell tumor. Symptoms such as fever and weight loss should be looked for as these are red flags.

Objective Examination

While evaluating any joint, it is important to evaluate the other joints associated with the kinetic chain as well. For knee joint, evaluation of the ankle and foot and hip and lumbar spine too needs to be performed. Physical examination should involve:

- Pain examination
- Swelling/effusion
- Any integumentary changes, evaluation of the wound or scar if present
- Local temperature
- Palpation of the joint to evaluate tenderness
- Range of motion (ROM) determination
- Contracture, tightness, or deformities if present
- Evaluation of end feels and joint play
- Evaluation of muscle tone, strength, endurance, and power
- Resisted isometrics
- Sensory system evaluation
- Limb length assessment
- Proximal and distal pulses to check circulation
- Assessment of knee reflexes
- Assessment of posture, gait, balance, and proprioception: Local posture examination of knee may show genu varum, valgum, tibia vara, and valgum. Gait assessment reveals reduced stance phase of the affected extremity, reduced swing phase of the unaffected extremity and reduced cadence. Antalgic or waddling type of gait is seen.
- Special tests **(Table 22.2)**

Table 22.2: Special tests commonly used for the knee joint.

Pathology	Special test
Medial instability	Valgus stress test
Lateral instability	Varus stress test
Anterior instability	Anterior drawer test, Lachman test
Posterior instability	Posterior drawer test, Lachman test, posterior sag sign
Meniscal lesions	Apley's test, Mcmurray's test, Thessaly test
Plica lesions	Hughston's plica test, Stutter test
Swelling/effusion	Brush test, patellar tap test, fluctuation test
Anterior knee pain syndrome	Clarke's test, McConnell test, Zohler's sign
Patellar instability	Apprehension test

- Functional evaluation
- Evaluation of physical function and quality of life

Knee Instruments and Rating Scales

1. **Western Ontario and McMaster Universities Osteoarthritis Index (WOMAC):** The WOMAC is a self-administered questionnaire comprising 24 questions. It has three distinct components—pain (5 questions), stiffness (7 questions), and physical function (17 questions). Each item is scored on a four-point Likert scale—none (0), mild (1), moderate (2), severe (3), and extreme (4). It has been used to evaluate patients having OA and rheumatoid arthritis (RA) of the knee joint and also following total knee arthroplasty (TKA). The minimal clinically important difference for TKA is around 15 points. WOMAC is a reliable and valid measure with intraclass correlation coefficient (ICC) ranging from 0.83 to 0.90 and Cronbach's alpha ranging from 0.70 to 0.93.

2. **International Knee Documentation Committee (IKDC) Subjective Knee Evaluation Form:** IKDC evaluation form was developed first in 1987 and several subsequent revisions have been made. It is used to evaluate subjects with sports injuries such as patellofemoral pain, articular cartilage lesions, and ligament and meniscus lesions. It has three domains: (1) symptoms which include pain, stiffness, swelling, locking/catching, and giving way; (2) sports and daily activities; and (3) current and preinjury knee function. Preinjury score is not included in the total score. There are 18 items—symptoms (7 items), sports participation (1 item), daily activities (9 items), and current knee function (1 item). Possible score range is 0–100 where 100 represents normal function with no limitation and symptoms. Minimal detectable change (MDC) has been reported as 8.8 and 15.6. Test–retest reliability is reported to be adequate for knee injury population.

3. **Knee Injury and Osteoarthritis Outcome Score (KOOS):** KOOS was developed for people with injuries that may lead to post-traumatic OA or subjects having post-traumatic OA. It consists of five domains: (1) frequency and severity of pain during functional activities; (2) symptoms such as intensity of knee stiffness, presence of swelling, catching, grinding, clicking and restriction of ROM; (3) difficulty during activities of daily living (ADL); (4) difficulty during sports and other recreational activities; and (5) knee-related quality of life (QOL). There are 42 items in total, which are scored on a five-point Likert scale of 0–4. Total scores are not used. The sum of individual domains is obtained and converted into a 0–100 score where 0 represents extreme problems and 100 represents no problems at all. All the five domains are reported to have adequate internal consistency and test–retest reliability. MDC ranges from 6 to 12 and 13.4 to 21.1 for knee injuries and knee OA, respectively.

4. **Lysholm Knee Scoring Scale:** The Lysholm scale is primarily used for ligament surgeries and cases of instability such as meniscal tears, OA, and cartilage lesions. It was first developed in 1982 and has eight items—limp, support, stair climbing, squatting, walking, running, and jumping and thigh atrophy. Individual items are scored differently. Lysholm scale has inadequate internal consistency for various knee pathologies and adequate reliability for knee injuries.

5. **Index of severity for OA of the knee:** The index of severity for osteoarthritis of the knee was developed by Lequesne et al. in the 1980s. Modifications were made to the original index in 1991 and later in 1997 when it was termed "algofunctional index." The modified index or the algofunctional index consists of three sections—pain or discomfort (five items), maximum distance walked (two items), and activities of daily living (four items). The minimum score for each section is 0 point and the maximum score is 8 points. The minimum and maximum scores for the index are 0 and 24 points, respectively. Based on the index score, the handicap of the subjects can be classified as none (0 points), mild (1–4 points), moderate (5–7 points), severe (8–10), very severe (11–13), and extremely severe (≥14 points). Cronbach's alpha for the knee Lequesne algofunctional index has been reported as 0.82.

PATHOLOGIES RELATED TO THE KNEE

Ligament Injuries

Anterior Cruciate Ligament Injuries

Anterior cruciate ligament (ACL) is completely stretched during extension and hyperextension of the knee and thus aids in checking hyperextension of the knee. ACL injuries are the most common ligament injuries seen in athletes. These injuries may occur in isolation or in association with other soft tissues such as other ligaments, menisci, and articular cartilage. They are equally prevalent in contact as well as non-contact sports. Male athletes are less likely to suffer from ACL injuries than female athletes. ACL injuries in females are 2–8 times more prevalent than males. One of the probable causes of this might be a greater hamstrings-to-quadriceps peak torque ratio in males than females. This means that males have a better recruitment of the hamstrings, whereas females have a more quadriceps dominant neuromuscular recruitment pattern. Hormonal effects of estrogen on ACL extensibility are also considered responsible for the greater incidence in females.

ACL injuries usually occur when excessive tensile force is applied on the ACL. These tensile forces may be generated by the athlete themselves, e.g., in non-contact sports, or may, be applied from external sources, e.g., contact sports. Running, jumping, and cutting during sports are very common phenomena that cause ACL injuries. Road traffic accidents (RTA) are also a common cause of ACL injuries when a significant amount of force strikes the knee. The incidence is much higher in young athletes of 14–19 years of age.

ACL injuries seldom occur in isolation. Medial or lateral collateral ligament (LCL) injuries occur in 1–5% of ACL injury cases. Meniscus injuries are commoner (38%) in association with ACL injuries. Articular cartilage lesions are also found in few (26%) patients.

Mechanism of Injury

Almost 70% of all sports-related ACL injuries are due to non-contact mechanisms. Various mechanisms may be responsible for ACL injuries **(Box 22.1)**. The weight-bearing status of the limb, position of the knee, speed of movement, and presence of external forces are considerable factors.

- Usually non-contact, deceleration injury
  - Foot planted on the ground; cutting or changing directions with the knee flexed
  - Valgus force with external rotation of the tibia or internal rotation of the femur **(Fig. 22.2)**.
  - Hyperextension of the knee while landing after a jump
- Contact injury—blow from the side of the knee on a planted foot.

Clinical Examination

History generally reveals the following findings:

- The patient reports an audible "pop," "snap," or "crack" at the time of injury.
- The patient may report the feeling of something coming out and going back inside at the time of injury.
- Severe, intense pain immediately after injury
- Immediate, profound disability
- Immediate swelling (in most cases hemarthrosis).

Examination immediately following injury is difficult due to the presence of hemarthrosis. Initial examination, even if possible, will not be able to reveal any significant

---

BOX 22.1: Causes of anterior cruciate ligament injuries.

- Anterior cruciate ligament (ACL) injuries occur due to large amounts of anterior shear forces being applied at the knee.
- Anterior tibial translation in combination with a valgus stress is the most common cause of ACL injuries.
- The existing literature demonstrates that a large posterior ground reaction force (GRF) might lead to generation of a large quadriceps muscle force, which may subsequently draw the knee anteriorly quite substantially.
- The presence of even a small knee flexion angle may cause an increase in the angle formed between the patellar tendon and the tibial shaft and the ACL elevation angle, rendering the ACL susceptible to greater loads.
- The addition of varus-valgus and rotation moments to the flexion moment might lead to injury to other surrounding structures along with the ACL.
- Higher amount of friction between the surface of the field and the shoes can also lead to ACL injuries.

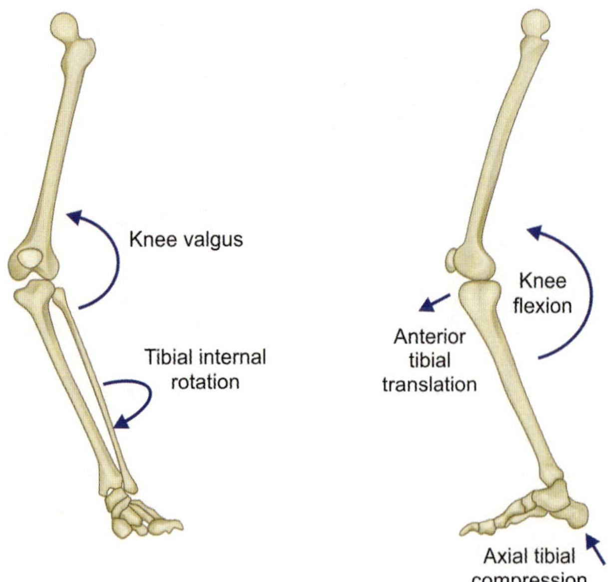

Fig. 22.2: Mechanism of injury of anterior cruciate ligament.

Table 22.3: Phases of anterior cruciate ligament rehabilitation and the symptoms associated with them.

Acute phase	Subacute phase	Return to activity phase
• Pain • Hemarthrosis • Diminished ROM • Weakness of the lower extremity • Inhibition of the quadriceps	• Full ROM • Resolution of effusion • Lower extremity strength sufficient enough to participate in dynamic weight-bearing exercises • No increment in instability episodes	• No instability • Isokinetic strength symmetry of >90%

(ROM: range of motion)

findings. Examination under anesthesia may be used or examination after aspiration of the hemarthrosis may be tried.

Examination reveals:

- Restricted ROM
- Not-so-localized tenderness—lateral joint line may be tender which reveals bone impaction at the time of injury; medial joint line tenderness may indicate injury to the medial meniscus along with the ACL.
- Reduced quadriceps strength (if swelling persists for long periods, chances of quadriceps weakness increase).
- Increased anterior tibial translation
- Positive Lachman's and anterior drawer test
- Pivot shift test positive if rotational injury present
- Feeling of knee "giving way"

Management

Fitzgerald GK et al., proposed a dynamic screening tool to identify subjects who could return back to function without ACL reconstruction (ACLR). These subjects were called "potential copers." The screening tool included four tests (single-leg hop test for distance, single-leg triple hop test, single-leg triple cross-over hop test, and 6-minute timed hop test), incidence of "giving way" episodes, knee outcome survey–activity of daily living scale—KOS-ADLS, and a self-reported global knee function rating score. Patients without any other associated injuries were identified as copers if they achieved:

1. ≥80% limb symmetry on all single-hop tests
2. >80% on KOOS-ADLs
3. >60% on the global knee function rating score
4. ≤1 episode of giving way

If a subject fails to achieve all of the above factors, they are identified as "non-copers" and are a likely candidate for ACLR.

The rehabilitation of ACL injuries is divided into three phases—acute, subacute, or neuromuscular training phase and return to activity phase. The phases are not only dependent on the time elapsed since injury but also on the presentation of the patient **(Table 22.3)**.

A few general precautions need to be taken by the patient and the therapist during the rehabilitation process:

- Weight bearing as tolerated (WBAT) with crutches or any other form of external aid during the acute phase.
- Report to the physician if the patient has any giving way episodes.
- Use of functional brace for enhanced stability
- Gradual return to function without being too eager and overstressing the ligament.

Surgical management of ACL injury is usually by ACLR. With the improvement in surgical techniques and expertise of the surgeons, the patients now prefer ACLR to non-operative management. ACLR is mentioned later in the chapter. Extensor lag can be one of the features in ACL injury managed conservatively or surgically **(Box 22.2)**.

Posterior Cruciate Ligament Injury

Posterior cruciate ligament (PCL) acts as a primary restraint to posterior tibial translation and as a secondary restraint to rotation, particularly between 90° and 120° of knee flexion. PCL injuries occur concurrently with ACL, medial collateral ligament (MCL), or posterolateral corner (PLC) injuries. They are almost always a part of multi-ligamentous injuries rather than isolated injuries. PCL injuries occur as a result of high-impact forces which commonly are seen in RTA or during sports.

Mechanism of Injury

Mechanism of injury is as follows:

- Posteriorly directed force to the anterior tibia while the knee is in flexion, e.g., dashboard injury or falling on a flexed knee.
- Hyperflexion of the knee joint
- Hyperextension of the knee joint.

BOX 22.2: Extensor lag.

Extensor lag or quadriceps lag is the inability to complete the full range of knee extension especially the last 15–20°. The passive limit of knee extension should be achieved without causing significant pain or discomfort and applying only mild force. Extensor lag may be physiological or pathological. Physiological lag is normal as it can be seen in healthy adult knees due to active insufficiency of rectus femoris. Pathological lag occurs due to factors such as:

1. Abnormal lengthening of quadriceps muscle, e.g. due to muscle rupture or fracture leading to bone shortening
2. Quadriceps muscle inhibition
3. Disuse atrophy.

Pathological extensor lag is usually seen after ACLR, TKA, or quadriceps tendon rupture and surgeries around the knee.

Extensor lag can be assessed by various methods. The most commonly used method is the active lag test. The subject is asked to sit erectly and extend the uninvolved knee fully with maximal dorsiflexion. They are then asked to extend the involved knee to the same level with maximal dorsiflexion. Inability to do so shows the presence of extensor lag. It is crucial for the examiner to differentiate between lag and lack. Extension lack is the inability to extend the knee passively as well as actively in contrast to the inability to extend the knee just actively in extensor lag mostly due to hamstring muscle tightness. It is also different from pure muscle weakness which is neurological. Lag is more of a biomechanical problem with much more strength needed to complete the last range of knee extension.

Extensor lag can be managed by strengthening the quadriceps. Isometric exercises of the quadriceps can be used in the initial program. Eccentric control of quadriceps muscle helps to recruit more fibers than concentric contractions. This can be progressed to progressive-resisted exercises for the quadriceps and closed chain exercises. Electrical stimulation to the quadriceps also helps in improving the strength and thereby reducing the extensor lag. If the lag is due to causes other than neuromuscular weakness or inhibition, other forms of management can be tried.

BOX 22.3: Grades of posterior cruciate ligament tear.

- Depending on the position of tibia relative to the femoral condyles:
- Normally, the tibia lies 1 cm anterior to the femoral condyles:
  - Grade A: Tibia lies anterior to the femoral condyles but the distance is reduced
  - Grade B: Tibia is level with the femoral condyles
  - Grade C: Tibia lies posterior to the femoral condyles
- Depending on the amount of laxity:
  - Grade I—0–5 mm laxity
  - Grade II—6–10 mm laxity
  - Grade III—>10 mm laxity

- Positive posterior drawer test or Lachman's test.

Chronic PCL injury patients exhibit anterior knee pain, instability, and difficulty in ascending stairs.

Management of Posterior Cruciate Ligament Injuries

Most of the PCL injuries can be managed nonoperatively. Severe injuries are generally immobilized in extension for 2 weeks. PCL has an inherent ability to heal, and hence, the prognosis is often good. In spite of this, while deciding the course of management, factors such as quadriceps strength and inherent joint laxity should be considered.

General precautions to be taken into consideration during PCL rehabilitation:

- Hyperextension of the knee and posterior tibial translation to be avoided in the initial stages of rehabilitation.
- Use of Jack or rebound PCL brace for the protection of a healing PCL.
- Progress from smaller to larger knee angles to avoid overstressing the PCL.

In the cases of severe grade III or C injuries, multi-ligamentous injuries or chronic PCL injury with severe instability, operative management may be considered. PCL reconstruction (PCLR) is not as common as ACLR. With recent arthroscopic advancements, there has been improvement in the outcome of PCLR. However, there is still paucity of studies dealing with long-term outcomes of these new procedures.

PCLR is done by replacing the injured PCL with a graft. This graft may be autograft (commonly patellar tendon) or allograft. Weight bearing and ROM are limited during the initial postoperative period. Activities involving the hamstrings are also avoided as these can cause posterior tibial translation. Weight bearing is gradually increased as the PCL heals and pain reduces. Returning to function is frequently after 8–12 weeks.

Medial Collateral Ligament Injury

Medial collateral ligament (MCL) is amongst the most commonly injured structures of the knee. MCL injuries are often found concomitant with ACL injuries. MCL is the primary stabilizer of the medial compartment at 20° knee flexion. Both medial and lateral collateral ligaments (LCLs) are taut during extension and lax during flexion.

- In cases of multiligamentous injuries, there may be some rotational component as well.

History

History includes:

- No distinct "pop" or "snap"
- Stiffness
- Posterior instability
- Inability to bear weight
- Pain over the posterior region of knee
- Pain during deceleration activities, e.g., descending stairs and during sprinting
- Pain during extreme flexion, e.g., kneeling

Clinical Examination

Clinical examination includes:

- Mild-to-moderate effusion
- Restricted ROM
- Increased posterior tibial translation **(Box 22.3)**

Mechanism of Injury

Like ACL injuries, MCL injuries too are sustained by a strong valgus force at the knee when the foot is planted on the ground.

History

History includes:

- Pain over medial aspect of the knee joint
- Patient may have felt or heard a "pop"
- Instability in grade III injuries or injuries concomitant with ACL injuries
- Most of the individuals with isolated tears are able to walk after the injury.

Clinical Examination

Clinical examination includes:

- Tenderness over medial aspect of the knee joint
- Swelling over medial aspect of the knee joint
- Increased lateral translation of tibia over femur
- Positive valgus stress test—increased laxity at 30° of flexion suggests MCL tear, increased laxity at 0° of flexion suggests concurrent injury to other postero-medial structures
- Antero-medial rotatory instability might also be present **(Box 22.4)**.

BOX 22.4: Grades of medial collateral ligament tear.

- Hughston in 1976 standardized the grades of MCL tear and further clarified them in 1994. He has given two related systems for classification—the severity system and the laxity system.
- Severity system **(Fig. 22.3)**:
    - Grade I: Tearing of a few fibers resulting in localized tenderness without instability
    - Grade II: Tearing of more fibers with generalized tenderness without instability
    - Grade III: Complete tear, with instability
- Laxity system (amount of laxity on applying valgus stress with knee at 30° of flexion):
    - Grade 1+—medial pain with 3–5 mm laxity
    - Grade 2+—medial pain with 6–10 mm laxity
    - Grade 3+—medial pain with >10 mm laxity

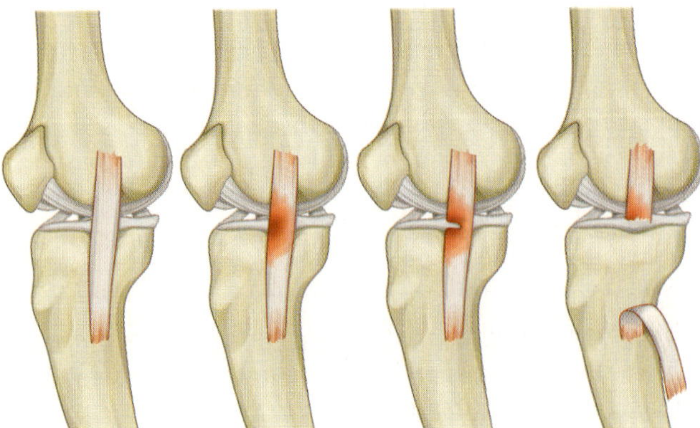

Fig. 22.3: Grades of MCL injury.
(MCL: medial collateral ligament)

Management

The management of MCL injuries is not only dependent on the grade of MCL tear but also on the presence of an ACL tear, meniscus tear, bone bruising, and capsular injury. In concomitant lesions of MCL and ACL, ACL injury takes priority and is managed surgically, whereas MCL is left to heal on its own. For isolated MCL injuries, non-operative management has been recommended as the mainstay treatment. According to a study by Logan CA et al., there was no significant difference between the athletic performances of football players having previous history of MCL injury who were treated surgically or nonsurgically. They also concluded that around 96% athletes had been treated nonsurgically.

A hinged knee brace should be advised for 4–6 weeks to the patient for support and protection of the joint. WBAT with crutches should be advised for initial painful period. With grade I injuries, return to function can be expected within 3–6 weeks. For grade II–III injuries, it may take 8–12 weeks.

When the injury is managed surgically, acute injuries are often repaired in contrast to chronic injuries that are reconstructed using autografts or allografts. Postoperatively, the use of hinged knee brace in 30° of knee flexion should be continued for 3 weeks, during which period the patient is allowed to walk only with toe-touch weight bearing. Knee flexion ROM should be limited to 90°, and strengthening exercises should be started while the brace is on. After 3 weeks, the use of brace may be discontinued and weight bearing can gradually be increased to full. Full ROM exercises can be advised after 3 weeks postoperative period.

Lateral Collateral Ligament Injury

Lateral collateral ligament (LCL) injuries are much less common than their medial counterpart. LCL injuries require a significant amount of force, and hence, they usually are associated with injuries to the surrounding structures [(posterolateral corner (PLC) injuries]. Isolated LCL injuries would require forces of lower intensity, which would disrupt only a few fibers. Consequently, isolated high-grade injuries are uncommon.

PLC injuries are now becoming increasingly prevalent. They are often associated with PCL or ACL injuries. PLC injuries usually involve injury to the LCL, arcuate ligament, popliteofibular ligament, posterolateral capsule, lateral meniscus, lateral head of gastrocnemius, and the iliotibial band. PLC structures act as the primary restraint to varus forces and posterolateral rotation of the tibia on the femur. They also act as secondary restraint to anterior and posteriorly directed forces. LCL is most taut in 0–30° of knee flexion range.

Mechanism of Injury

PLC injuries occur following varus, extension, and external rotatory forces at the knee in weight-bearing position. Knee hyperextension or adduction may cause PLC damage. A common cause can be direct trauma to the anteromedial knee.

History

History includes:

- Pain over lateral aspect of knee
- Lateral instability
- Difficulty in walking or climbing stairs

Clinical Examination

Clinical examination includes:

- Swelling over lateral aspect of knee
- Positive varus stress test—increased translation in 30° flexion is suggestive of LCL or PLC injury; later, when translation is tested in full extension, absence of laxity is suggestive of LCL alone.
- Increased medial translation of tibia on femur
- Tenderness over lateral aspect of knee
- Hyperextension or lateral thrust gait
- Occasionally, there might be an associated injury to the common peroneal nerve (CPN). In these rare cases, there might be diminished sensations over the CPN supplied area along with weakness in CPN supplied muscles. The patient may present with foot drop.

Management

Grade I and II injuries are commonly managed conservatively. Surgical management may be needed for grade III injuries.

Rehabilitation of Ligament Injuries

A number of distinct variables affect the rehabilitation of ligament injuries. Some of these variables may be:

- Degree of ligament injury
- Presence of any concomitant injuries
- Expectations of the patient regarding return to function.
- Presence of any other comorbidities such as diabetes and osteoporosis.
- Cooperation of the patient in avoiding activities that may further injure the structure.

Rehabilitation of ligament injury varies between individuals. There can be no standard guidelines to follow as each case and individual is unique in their own way. However, based on the general recommendations made by different studies and routine programs that are being followed, a general rehabilitation program has been documented below **(Table 22.4)**.

General impairments of the patient following ligament injury are as follows:

- Pain
- Swelling or hemarthrosis
- Diffuse or localized tenderness
- Instability
- Restricted ROM

Table 22.4: Rehabilitation of ligament injuries.

Phase of rehabilitation	Goals	Treatment protocol
Acute phase	Reduction of pain and hemarthrosis	• Cryotherapy and compression • Electrotherapy—ultrasound, TENS, LASER
	Facilitation of normal quadriceps activation and strengthening of quadriceps	• NMES • OKC: Simultaneous contraction of the quadriceps and hamstrings at 30, 60, and 90° and isometric quadriceps contraction at 60 and 90° for minimum ligament strain • CKC to incorporate quadriceps into a dynamic movement involving the lower extremity: cycling
	Restoration of pain-free ROM	• OKC knee extension limited within 30–100° of knee flexion • Grade I and II patellar mobilization
	Improve gait pattern	• Hip muscles and core muscles strengthening • Gait training with visual and auditory biofeedback (WBAT)
	Protection of healing tissues	Protective bracing
Subacute phase or neuromuscular training phase	Maximizing lower extremity and core muscle strength	• OKC muscle strengthening in full knee ROM • PRE for lower extremity muscles • CKC exercises to develop both lower extremity and core strength (planks, side-planks, step-ups, squats, etc.)
	Improve proprioception, balance and neuromuscular coordination **(Figs. 22.4 and 22.5)**	• Perturbation training from static to dynamic surface • Skill-specific training
	Improve cardiovascular conditioning	Cycling—increase in speed and duration
Return to activity phase	Improve and maintain proprioception, balance and neuromuscular coordination	• Agility and advanced skill-specific training • Plyometrics
	Improve cardiovascular conditioning	Running, cycling, swimming, etc.
	Improve flexibility	Stretching exercises

(CKC: closed-chain exercises; NMES: neuromuscular electrical stimulation; OKC: open-chain exercises; PRE: progressive resisted exercises; ROM: range of motion; TENS: transcutaneous electrical nerve stimulation; WBAT: weight bearing as tolerated)

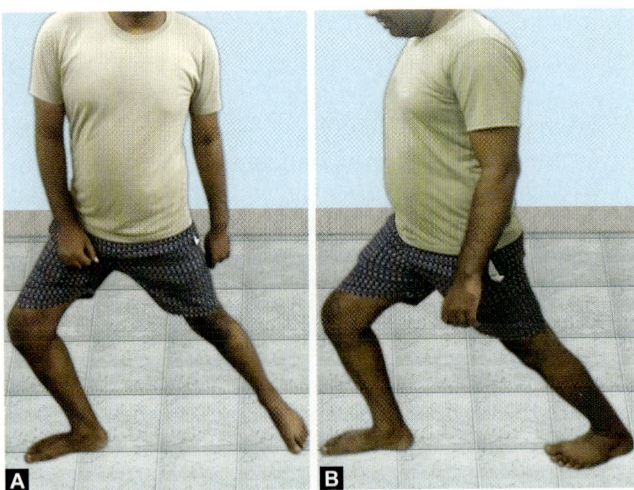

Figs. 22.4A and B: Patient performing lunges.

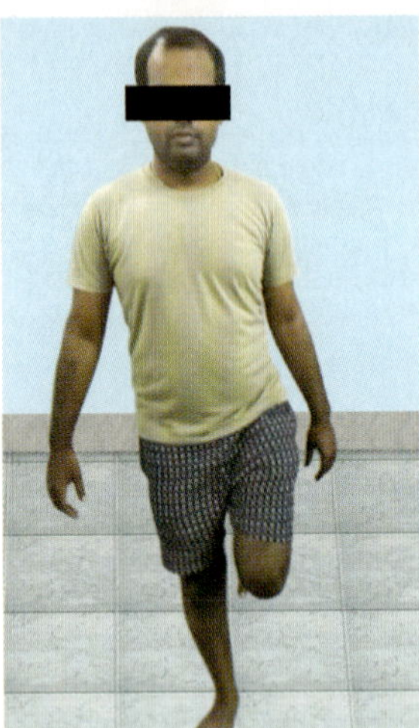

Fig. 22.5: One-leg standing.

- Inability to bear weight on the involved extremity
- "Giving way" or buckling
- Quadriceps inhibition
- Poor proprioception and neuromuscular control

Meniscus Injuries

Meniscal injuries may occur during sporting events or even during routine activities. The spectrum of meniscal injuries is vast; just like the structure and biomechanics of the menisci. The continuum of meniscal injuries has two ends—one that involves the younger age group and the other that involves the >40 years old age group. Meniscal injuries may occur in isolation or in association with other structures such as the ACL and MCL (O'Donoghue's or unhappy triad). Sports or other accidental injuries are commonly seen in conjunction with ACL or MCL or both. Meniscal tears seen in the older adult age group are often due to degenerative changes.

The menisci function to distribute stress across the knee joint in load-bearing positions, to stabilize the knee joint, act as shock absorbers, provide joint lubrication, provide nutrition to the articular cartilage, act as a restraint to hyperextension, and promote joint gliding. Only 10–30% of the peripheral medial meniscus border and 10–25% of the peripheral lateral meniscus border receive a direct blood supply. Rest of the meniscus receives nutrition through diffusion from the synovial fluid. Because of such poor vascularity, healing of tears in the central portion of the meniscus is poor and such injuries would usually require surgical interventions.

The medial meniscus is attached to the tibia anteriorly through the anterior horn at the intercondylar eminence, posteriorly through the posterior horn between the intercondylar eminence and PCL and peripherally by the coronary ligament. Since the medial meniscus is so firmly attached to the tibia, it moves with the tibia in certain directions. The posterior horn of medial meniscus is also attached to the almost half of the ACL. Medial meniscus is also attached to the MCL. Due to this attachment, most of medial meniscus injuries are associated with ACL and MCL injuries. The lateral meniscus is attached to the tibia only anteriorly through the anterior horn at the intercondylar eminence. Also, it has no attachments to the LCL or PCL. Due to this, the lateral meniscus is rather free to move. And because of this mobility, lateral meniscus injuries are rather infrequent than medial meniscus injuries. Medial meniscal injuries account for 10.8% and lateral meniscal injuries account for 3.7% of all sports-related knee injuries reported. Males are more frequently injured than females (4:1). Meniscal injuries due to nonsporting activities are more prevalent (account for around two thirds of total injuries) in the general population.

Meniscal cysts are found in about 10% of meniscus related pathologies. Meniscal cysts are pockets filled with fluid presumably extruded from a torn meniscus. These are mostly seen in lateral meniscus tears. The patient presents with localized pain and swelling over the joint line. A mass can sometimes, be palpated in the painful area.

Risk Factors

- For traumatic meniscal tears:
  - Soccer or rugby players
  - Waiting period of >12 months between ACL injury and reconstruction
- For degenerative meniscal tears:
  - Age >60 years
  - Male gender
  - Repetitive kneeling, squatting, or climbing stairs.

Mechanism of Injury

Mechanism of injury is as follows:
- External force causing hyperextension or hyperflexion
- Tibial rotation when the knee is flexed and the foot is weight bearing, e.g., sudden squatting or getting out of a car.

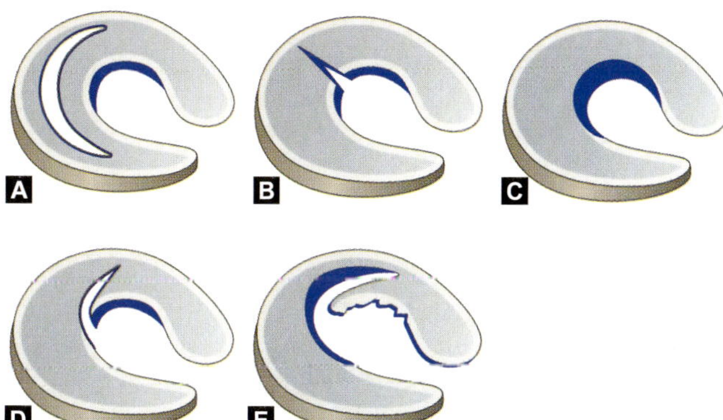

Fig. 22.6: Types of meniscal tears based on the patterns seen during arthroscopy.

Classification of Meniscal Tears

Meniscal tears can occur due to application of a large amount of force to a normal meniscus or due to application of a normal amount of force to a degenerated meniscus. Based on arthroscopic findings, meniscal tears can be classified as shown in **Figures 22.6 and 22.7**.

Around 81% of the meniscal tears are vertical longitudinal or oblique. Vertical longitudinal tears may be complete or incomplete. Complete vertical tears are called bucket handle tears since their shape resembles that of a bucket handle. Vertical tears are the most common reason for locking of the knee. The torn fragment comes to lie within the joint space between the two moving bones and prevents further movement, locking the knee into that particular range of movement. These tears are commonly found in conjunction with ACL tears. Oblique (flap) tears can also cause locking if the flap comes to lie between the bones. Complex tears are mostly degenerative in nature. Transverse or radial tears are commonly seen in isolation. Horizontal tears are found in the center of the meniscus, extending toward the periphery.

The International Society of Arthroscopy, Knee Surgery and Orthopaedic Sports Medicine gives the most detailed and reliable classification of meniscal tears. The classification is based on various parameters: tear depth, rim width, radial location, tear pattern, location of the tear relative to the popliteal hiatus, quality and length of the tear, and the amount and percentage of meniscus excised.

The prognosis of a tear can be decided based on the location of the tear as well. According to the location, a tear can be in (1) the red-red zone—which has good vascularity and hence excellent prognosis; (2) the red-white zone—which is vascular only at the periphery and has good

prognosis; and (3) the white-white zone—which has poor vascular supply and, hence, poor prognosis.

History

History includes:
- Pain over the medial or lateral aspect of knee
- "Locking" of the knee—inability of the knee to extend further than a point in the range.
- Inability to bear weight on the affected leg while walking.

Clinical Examination

Clinical examination includes:
- Pain at terminal ranges of flexion and extension
- Tenderness over the medial or lateral tibiofemoral joint line
- Swelling around the knee joint
- Restricted ROM
- Springy block end feel on extension
- Positive McMurray's and Apley's compression test

Management

The management of meniscal tear depends on the portion of the meniscus that is torn, the type of tear, tissue quality, and the presence of any other concomitant injuries. Tears that are present in the central nonvascular region are difficult to heal. Repeated locking episodes also warrant surgical management. Patient factors such as age, expectations after recovery, activity level, lifestyle, and general health should also be taken into consideration. The ultimate decision should be made by the consulting orthopedic surgeon after careful and meticulous consideration of the abovementioned factors.

Non-surgical Management

Non-operative management of the meniscal tear is the choice in younger individuals and when the tear lies in the vascular zone.

The goals of non-operative management are to:
- Relieve pain and inflammation
- Improve strength of muscles
- Improve flexibility
- Improve neuromuscular coordination and balance
- Improve proprioception
- Improve muscular and cardiovascular endurance

Acute phase: During the acute phase, the goal is relief of pain and swelling. Physiotherapy intervention consists of POLICE (Protection, Optimal Loading, Ice, Compression, and Elevation). POLICE is helpful during the initial 24–48 hours.

Figs. 22.7A to E: Classification of meniscal tears based on the patterns seen during arthroscopy: (A) Vertical longitudinal; (B) Transverse radial; (C) Horizontal; (D) Oblique; (E) Complex/degenerative.

Rehabilitative phase: The main goals during the rehabilitative phase include improvement of ROM, strength, proprioception, balance, and functional independence. During the rehabilitative phase, the progression of the exercises depends on the clinical presentation of the patient rather than the number of days lapsed. Weight bearing is gradually progressed as the pain declines and strength improves.

Interventions include:
- Electrotherapy, cold, and compression
- Full ROM active exercises
- Progressive resisted exercises (PRE) for lower extremity muscles especially quadriceps and hamstrings
- Closed kinetic chain (CKC) exercises—squatting, running, cycling, etc.
- Proprioceptive exercises

Surgical Management

The goal of surgical interventions for meniscal injury is to relieve pain, rehabilitate the patient to their preinjury level of functioning, and prevent early degeneration of the knee joint. Surgical management of meniscal tears can be done by three techniques: meniscal repair, meniscectomy, and meniscal reconstruction. A meta-analysis concluded that there is a lack of Level-I evidence to guide surgical management of meniscal tears. The choice of the surgical intervention is based on the patient's age, willingness to undergo major surgery, their general health, lifestyle, and their expectations regarding the outcome along with the location and type of tear.

Meniscectomy

Meniscectomy is removal of the meniscal tissue. It can be total or partial; open or arthroscopic. In the past, meniscus was considered to be vestigial structure which did not provide any substantial function. Hence, open total meniscectomy was the standard operation for meniscal tears in the 20th century. However, it was later established that total meniscectomy leads to an increased risk of developing OA and meniscus is an essential structure for joint lubrication and protection. Thus partial meniscectomy was accepted in lieu of total removal.

Even though partial meniscectomy preserves more meniscus tissue and produces better results than total meniscectomy, the benefit of using this procedure lies in the preservation of the peripheral rim that is vital to the shock absorption and joint protection function of the meniscus. An arthroscopic procedure is always a better option than an open procedure as it promotes early rehabilitation and leads to earlier recovery.

With increased understanding of the biomechanical structure and function of the menisci and advances seen in technology, new surgical interventions have been developed that can preserve almost all of the meniscus tissue. In spite of this, there can be cases that may warrant meniscectomy, but it is preferable to look for other options.

Rehabilitation after meniscectomy is shown in **Table 22.5**.

Meniscal Repairs

Similar to meniscectomy, meniscal repair can also be done either arthroscopically or by an open procedure. Arthroscopic procedures are preferred due to lesser tissue trauma, lesser chances of neurovascular injury, earlier recovery, and resultant better outcomes. Meniscal repair is the preferred choice for younger patients with no degenerative changes of the menisci, tears in the vascular outer one-third region and occasionally for tears in the inner two-third avascular region along with healing enhancement techniques. For older patients and most of the central tears, partial meniscectomy is performed.

Table 22.5: Rehabilitation post-meniscectomy.

	Maximum protection phase (0–1 week)	Moderate protection phase (1–3 weeks)	Minimum protection phase and return to function (3–8 weeks)
Goals	• Relieve inflammation • Relieve pain • Maintain active and passive ROM • Restore isolated muscle function	• Regain ROM • Improve weight bearing • Improve proprioception and balance	• Gain normal gait pattern • Improve lower extremity muscle strength • Maximize function
Interventions	• Electrotherapy • Cold and compression • WBAT with crutches • Active ROM exercises • Isometric exercises for quadriceps	• Stretching of lower extremity muscles • CKC exercises—squatting to 90° knee flexion, cycling • PRE for lower extremity muscles • FWB walking • Proprioceptive exercises on static and dynamic surfaces	• CKC exercises—gradually increasing the amount of knee flexion to full range • Gradual progression to plyometrics • Endurance activities such as running and jumping

(ROM: range of motion; PRE: progressive resisted exercises; WBAT: weight bearing as tolerated; CKC: closed kinetic chain; FWB: full weight bearing)

Biologic augmentation techniques are being developed to enhance the healing of meniscal tears. Some of these techniques are:

- **Synovial abrasion**: Surgical rasping instruments are used for abrasion of the synovial lining on both femoral and tibial surfaces of the meniscus, which stimulates a reparative response. It increases the production of several growth-promoting factors such as interleukin-I-alpha (IL-I-alpha), proliferating cell nuclear antigen (PCNA), platelet-derived growth factor (PDGF), and transforming growth factor-beta 1 (TGF-beta1). These growth factors promote healing of the meniscus. However, excessive synovectomy may hamper healing.
- **Vascular access channels (trephination)**: It is the application of a small incision in the vascularized meniscus to produce channels that can direct the blood flow from the vascular zone (red–red zone) to the avascular zone (white–white zone). It may help enable the proliferation of fibrovascular scar tissue in the damaged meniscus. Success rate of trephination has been found to be high (90%).
- **Fibrin clot**: Injection or topical application of fibrin clot into the damaged meniscal tissue may promote healing. It induces the proliferation of fibrous connective tissue which stimulates the formation of fibrocartilaginous tissue required for the repair of damaged meniscus. It can be used in conjunction with abrasion or trephination.
- **Growth factors**: Treatment with anabolic or catabolic growth factors is also growing in popularity. Growth factors stimulate the regeneration of damaged tissue by inducing the formation and inhibiting the degradation of extracellular matrix (ECM) essential for meniscal repair.

Rehabilitation After Meniscal Repair

After meniscal repair, the knee is immobilized at 0° of flexion and only toe-touch weight bearing is allowed for 2 weeks. Accelerated rehabilitation protocols allow early weight bearing and return to function by 10 weeks **(Table 22.6)**.

Meniscal Reconstruction

A meniscal deficiency can be reconstructed and/or transplanted using autografts, allografts, or substitutive materials.

Autologous tissues such as fat pad, periosteum, perichondrium, or tendon may be used to reconstruct the deficient meniscus. However, the results have not been satisfactory as the mechanical properties of the tissue are changed.

Meniscal allograft transplantations (MAT) are the most commonly performed meniscal reconstruction procedures. In 2015, the International Meniscus Reconstruction Experts Forum gave recommendations regarding the indications for MAT. These include unicompartmental pain following total or partial meniscectomy, along with revised ACLR when the deficient meniscus may be responsible for the failure of the previous procedure or along with articular cartilage repair. MAT has led to significant improvements in pain and function.

Varied materials have been developed and used as meniscal substitutes or scaffolds, but the efficacy of two materials has been proven satisfactory for clinical use—collagen meniscus implant (CMI®) and polyurethane polymeric implant (Actifit®). These are non-cellular biodegradable scaffolds having high porosity. Meniscal scaffolds are deemed fit only for individuals having an intact peripheral rim of the meniscus and not having significant damage to the articular cartilage post-meniscectomy. Both these implants have shown significant improvements in pain and function. However, few studies have reported negative outcomes such as immaturity of the scaffold and re-appearance of bone bruises on follow-up magnetic resonance imaging (MRI). Meniscal scaffolds give outcomes comparable to meniscal repair; however, when compared to MAT, their outcomes are unfavorable.

Table 22.6: Rehabilitation following meniscal repair.

	Maximum protection phase (0–2 weeks)	Moderate protection phase (2–4 weeks)	Minimum protection phase and return to function (4–8 weeks)
Goals	• Relieve inflammation • Relieve pain • Maintain muscle function	• Regain ROM • Improve weight bearing • Improve lower extremity muscle strength	• Gain normal gait pattern • Improve lower extremity muscle strength • Improve proprioception, coordination, and balance • Maximize function
Interventions	• Electrotherapy • Cold and compression • Isometric exercises for lower extremity muscles • Toe touch weight-bearing gait training with crutches	• Active ROM exercises up to 30–70° of flexion • PRE for lower extremity muscles • WBAT walking with crutches	• Active full ROM exercises • CKC exercises—gradually increasing the amount of knee flexion to full range • Gradual progression to plyometrics • Proprioceptive exercises on static and dynamic surfaces • Endurance activities such as running and jumping

(PRE: progressive resisted exercises; ROM: range of motion; WBAT: weight bearing as tolerated; CKC: closed kinetic chain)

Newer Trends for Meniscal Regeneration

Novel therapeutic techniques are being developed and made possible by tissue engineering. Tissue engineering is the application of biological and engineering principles to manufacture substituting material for damaged tissues. These substituting materials are a combination of biological scaffolds, cells, and various growth factors. Meniscal cells, chondrocytes, fat tissue, mesenchymal stem cells (MSC), or synovial cells may be used. 3D bioprinting meniscal regeneration is also an upcoming area of research. Animal studies have been performed and have shown short-term benefits. Tissue engineering and 3D bioprinting are next-gen technologies that will prove promising in the areas of implants and transplants.

RHEUMATOID ARTHRITIS

Rheumatoid arthritis (RA) has already been discussed in much detail in Chapter 20: Elbow, Wrist, and Hand Conditions. This chapter describes the details about RA of the knee. Among the population affected by RA, the prevalence of knee joint involvement is 14% at the age of 79.

Clinical Presentation

Systemic features:
- Weight loss
- Fever
- Easy fatigability
- Morning stiffness of the knee lasting >1 hour before maximal improvement (duration of morning stiffness is related to disease activity).

Features of the knee joint:
- Acute or subacute onset of pain and tenderness at and around the knee joint.
- Synovitis leading to increased girth of the knee **(Box 22.5, and Figs. 22.8A and B).**
- Instability due to destruction of surrounding ligaments and joint surfaces.

> **BOX 22.5:** Features of acute synovitis.
>
> Patients with acute synovitis of the knee may rarely present with *pseudo-thrombophlebitis*. The patient may present with swelling, warmth, and tenderness in the calf, which are findings consistent with thrombophlebitis. The presence of such symptoms is due to a draining popliteal cyst secondary to the RA fluid build-up in the posterior aspect of knee.

- Atrophy of quadriceps musculature
- Extension lag
- Inflammation of patellar and hamstrings tendons
- Reduced function
- Deformities—genu varum, genu valgum, and flexion deformity **(Fig. 22.9).**

Diagnosis of RA of the knee joint is made similar to the other joints, based on the revised criteria for classification of RA given by the American College of Rheumatology (ACR).

Management

Medical Management

Active RA in adults should be managed with a target of remission or low disease activity (for patients in whom remission is not possible) in mind. For people who may be vulnerable to radiological progression, i.e., anticyclic citrullinated peptide (anti-CCP) antibodies or bony erosions on X-ray during baseline evaluation, the target should be remission rather than low disease activity. Drug prescriptions should be meticulous since many drugs used for RA have teratogenic effects. The medical management of knee RA is similar to RA of the wrist and hand.

Physiotherapy Management

Goals of physiotherapy management are to:
- Relieve pain
- Improve joint flexibility
- Improve muscle strength

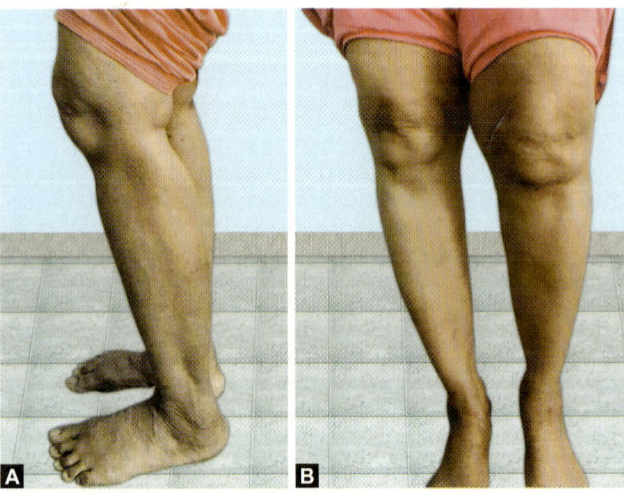

Figs. 22.8A and B: Swelling seen in rheumatoid arthritis of the knee joint.

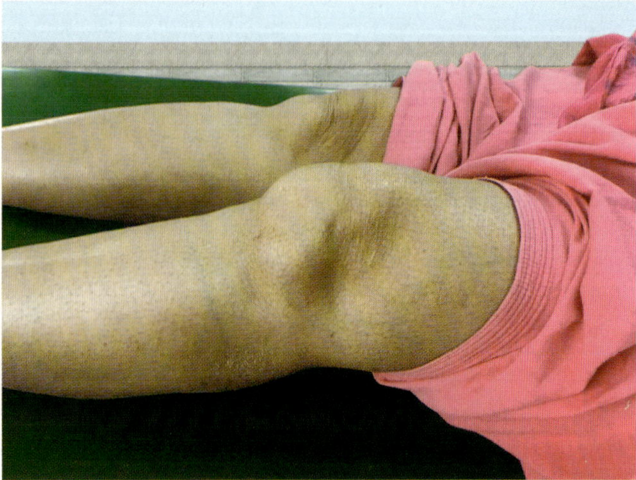

Fig. 22.9: Fixed flexion deformity of the knee joint in rheumatoid arthritis.

- Improve general fitness
- Encourage regular exercise
- Improve function

There is a strong recommendation for the use of physiotherapy interventions in RA, but there is a lack of consensus regarding the mode of delivery and the various parameters of treatment such as intensity, frequency, and duration. Exercises in various forms, e.g., aerobics, muscle strengthening exercises, high-intensity dynamic exercises, and low-intensity exercises have been recommended.

- **Electrotherapy:** Transcutaneous electrical nerve stimulation (TENS) and paraffin wax bath are recommended therapies for pain relief in RA. Low-level LASER therapy (LLLT), thermotherapy, ultrasound therapy, and electrical stimulation have also been recommended. Patient education and information also form a key component of the rehabilitation program.

- **Joint protection strategies:** During states of acute exacerbation, it is important to protect the joint from any additional damage. Variety of joint protection strategies exist. But, the one that the patient feels most comfortable and confident with should be used. Rest, knee braces, compression stockings, etc., may be used. Use of a cane while walking reduces the load on the knee by several folds. Knee is a joint that has a natural tendency to swell significantly because of its anatomical structure and biomechanical importance. A swollen knee attains a knee flexion attitude. During acute periods, the knee should be rested in about 25–30° of flexion. As the swelling subsides, the knees should be gradually extended. Splints made up of soft or firm material should be used to maintain the ROM and prevent deformities along with reducing the pain.

- **Therapeutic exercises:** Therapeutic exercises are useful for maintaining ROM rather than relieving pain or inflammation. The knee joint should be moved multiple times through full ROM to fulfill the purpose of maintaining ROM. During acute stages, the movement may be painful, but the benefits of exercises should be reinforced to the patient. Isometric contractions should be advised during acute stages to maintain the strength of the muscles. Progression to low-intensity isotonic contractions should be made gradually once the pain reduces. Activities such as walking, stair climbing, and squatting should be avoided in acute periods as they increase the intra-articular pressures in an inflamed knee joint. Stretching activities or exercises should be deterred from. During chronic stages, conditioning exercises such as swimming, cycling, and walking should be advised to improve the cardiovascular function and QOL. Even a minimal involvement of the knee joint in RA leads to weakness in the quadriceps, creating a muscular imbalance between quadriceps and hamstrings. This muscular imbalance is the cause of future deformities. Strengthening of the quadriceps in the initial period and, later on, strengthening of all the lower extremity muscles helps reduce the chances of developing deformities.

- **Aquatic exercises:** Aquatic therapy is as beneficial as land-based exercises in improving physical function and mobility in patients having RA. Aquatic therapy is believed to be of benefit because of the properties of water. It reduces pain and swelling, strengthens muscles using the hydrostatic pressure property of water, and the buoyancy helps to improve ROM and reduce joint loading. Temperature regulators in the pool can be used to warm water that can provide additional effects of thermotherapy. Thus aquatic therapy is a convenient alternative for individuals who face difficulties in exercising on land or are limited so much that they cannot perform exercises on land.

Surgical Management

For advanced late stage RA where the patient suffers from debilitating pain and ROM restriction, TKA has been shown to be a well-proven choice. Of the patients suffering from RA, 20–50% develop advanced destruction of the joints, so much so that they need to undergo arthroplasty, knee joint being one of the most affected joints. Since RA patients are administered immunosuppressant drugs, they are at a higher risk of developing postsurgical infections, irrespective of the joint involved. They also have a lower rate of healing, since many have a history of long-term corticosteroid use. The risk of deep vein thrombosis is lower in RA patients than any other condition. The reason for the same is, however, unknown.

OSTEOARTHRITIS

Osteoarthritis (OA) is a complex degenerative joint disease that is characterized by the destruction of the articular cartilage of the joint, osteophyte formation, subchondral bone thickening, inflammation of the synovial membrane, and pathological changes in the joint capsule **(Fig. 22.10 and Box 22.6)**.

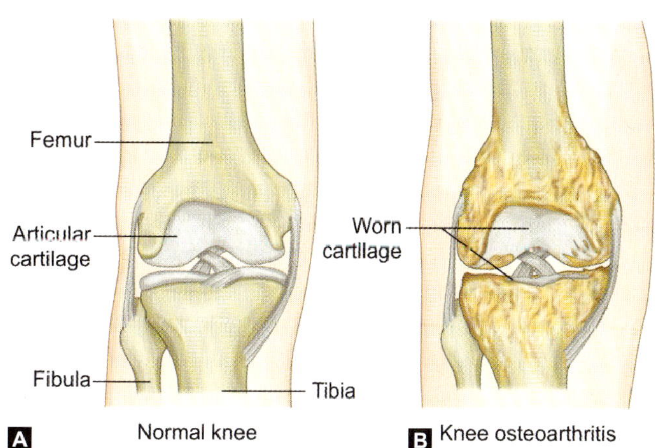

Figs. 22.10A and B: Cartilage destruction in osteoarthritis.

BOX 22.6: Definition of Osteoarthritis.

Osteoarthritis (OA) is defined by the Subcommittee on OA of the American College of Rheumatology Diagnostic and Therapeutic Criteria Committee as *"A heterogeneous group of conditions that lead to joint symptoms and signs which are associated with defective integrity of articular cartilage, in addition to related changes in the underlying bone at the joint margins."*

Osteoarthritis Research Society International (OARSI) defines OA as *"A disorder involving movable joints characterized by cell stress and extracellular matrix degradation initiated by micro- and macro-injury that activates maladaptive repair responses including pro-inflammatory pathways of innate immunity. The disease manifests first as a molecular derangement (abnormal joint tissue metabolism) followed by anatomic, and/or physiologic derangements (characterized by cartilage degradation, bone remodeling, osteophyte formation, joint inflammation and loss of normal joint function), that can culminate in illness."*

BOX 22.7: Risk factors for the development of osteoarthritis.

Multiple risk factors have been cited for the occurrence of OA:

- Old age
- Obesity
- Genetic factors
- Post-menopausal hormonal imbalance
- Low bone mineral density (osteoporosis and osteopenia)
- Vigorous physical activity
- Physical inactivity
- Knee joint injuries and deformities
- Meniscectomy
- Increased stress on the articular cartilage
- Muscular imbalance

Osteoarthritis is commoner among women than men, but the prevalence changes with increasing age. It is the commonest cause of locomotor disability among the elderly. The prevalence of OA of the knee joint is the highest. It is about 3.9% among the rural population and 5.5% among the urban population in India **(Box 22.7)**.

Pathophysiology

Initially, it was believed that the articular cartilage is the only structure that is involved in OA. But with passing years, new researches have provided the information regarding other structures such as the synovium and subchondral bone being concomitantly damaged and affected. Over the years, OA was believed to be a consequence of the constant wear and tear that takes place with age. The beginning of the 21st century brought about a change in the existing ideology with the discovery of inflammatory mediators in the synovium and other surrounding tissues.

OA was previously presumed to be a noninflammatory local degenerative disease. With the recent literature proving otherwise, OA has been accepted as a systemic, biomechanical, and inflammatory disease. A multitude of factors influences the development and progression of OA—joint shape and dysplasia, synovitis, obesity, complementary proteins, innate immunity, inflammaging, systemic inflammatory mediators, and metabolic diseases.

The articular cartilage can withstand tremendous amounts of forces but does not possess the property of healing even a minor injury. Due to this, it becomes highly vulnerable to undergo degenerative changes, progressively leading to OA. The primary cause leading to the cascade of pathological changes is not known. It is hypothesized that genetic factors, systemic factors, and biomechanical factors (abnormal forces on joints, biomechanical abnormalities or injuries) can contribute to the pathogenesis of OA.

The progression of OA can be divided into three stages:

1. Stage I: Proteolytic breakdown of ECM.
2. Stage II: Fibrillation and erosion of cartilage surface, followed by release of the breakdown products into the synovial fluid.
3. Stage III: Ingestion of the breakdown material by the synovial cells leading to synovitis and production of proteases and proinflammatory cytokines.

ECM breakdown is a sequential phenomenon that is triggered by some specific enzymes. The family of matrix metalloproteinases (MMP) has an important contribution to this initial ECM breakdown. Three groups from the MMP family have been found at elevated levels in the human osteoarthritic cartilage—the collagenases, the stromelysins, and the gelatinases. These MMPs cause the degradation of native collagen, proteoglycans, and denatured collagen, respectively. The activity of MMP is counter-balanced by tissue inhibitors of MMP (TIMP). A smooth regulated activity of MMP and TIMP retains the normal composition of ECM. However, in OA, the synthesis of MMP is increased beyond that of TIMP, leading to ECM breakdown.

The activity of MMP and TIMP is controlled by cytokines and growth factors. Cytokines can be grouped into three categories:

1. Catabolic (IL-1α, IL-1β, and TNF-α)
2. Regulatory and enzyme inhibitory (IL-6, IL-8, IL-4, IL-10)
3. Anabolic (growth factors, IGF, etc.)

IL-1β and TNF-α are the cytokines primarily responsible for the cartilage damage. They both enhance ECM degradation either by:

- Reducing the synthesis of macromolecules of ECM such as aggrecan, proteoglycans, and collagen.
- Stimulation of secretion of proteolytic enzymes from the chondrocytes.
- Inhibition of the secretion of inhibitors of the proteolytic enzymes.

A combination of the activity of the cytokines, proteolytic enzymes, and a reduced synthesis of the ECM results in the cartilage damage seen in OA.

There are physiological inhibitors that inhibit the activity of these catabolic cytokines. These cytokines need to bind to receptor sites over cell membranes in order to be efficient. There are receptor antagonists such as IL-1 receptor antagonist (IL-1Ra) which bind over the same site and compete with the catabolic cytokines. Also, there are soluble receptors that can bind to the cytokines and reduce their ability to bind to the receptor sites and anti-inflammatory cytokines that decrease the secretion of IL-1 and TNFα. A balance between the catabolic and anabolic activity of the cytokines retains the integrity of the cartilage.

Cytokines are not the only factors responsible for cartilage degradation. The activity of IL-1 and activated macrophages and neutrophils also leads to the generation of reactive oxygen species (ROS) such as superoxide (O_2^-), nitric oxide (NO), and nitrogen dioxide (NO_2). These ROS, mainly NO, can cause breakdown of collagen and aggrecan. They reduce the synthesis of hyaluronic acid that is an important component of ECM.

The homeostasis of an articular cartilage is maintained by a reciprocal interaction between the chondrocytes and the ECM. The chondrocytes produce the proteins and proteoglycans present in the ECM, which in turn are responsible for the metabolism of chondrocytes. This balance between the two components of cartilage is maintained by chondrocyte-ECM signaling which occurs by virtue of some specific adhesion molecules—β integrins. Within the family of β integrins, β_1 integrins are the most abundant, and they interact with several molecules, e.g., collagen. This interaction is critical for the prevention of the programmed cell death (apoptosis) of the chondrocytes. In OA, the chondrocytes are unable to discern the ECM signals and send reciprocating signals to the ECM, and this hampers the production of the ECM components.

The cascade that brings about the change in the chondrocyte function can be caused by various stresses such as mechanical, oxidative, or inflammatory.

Role of Synovial Inflammation

The cartilage has no vascular supply and is nourished through diffusion by the synovial fluid present in the joint cavity. The synovium provides nutrition to the chondrocytes and also removes the mechanical debris from the ECM. Synovitis can be detected clinically by the presence of effusion and signs of inflammation—redness, local hyperthermia, and pain. It can be detected on the MRI, sonogram, arthroscopy, or in histopathological reports. Synovitis, as seen in OA, can lead to cartilage destruction through the release of above-mentioned cytokines and reduced synthesis of TIMPs. Synovial macrophages are crucial for the synthesis of MMPs from the synovial cells. These synovial macrophages may also be involved in the development of osteophytes induced by transforming growth factor-β (TGF-β) through secretion of bone morphogenetic proteins (BMPs)—BMP-2 and BMP-4 or through the transmission and transduction of signals that may influence the MSC.

It has not yet been proven that the synovitis is a primary process that eventually leads to or is a secondary process that occurs in response to cartilage destruction. Based on these findings, novel strategies are being developed targeting the synovium to prevent progression of OA.

Role of the Subchondral Bone in Pathogenesis of Osteoarthritis

The subchondral bone has two distinct layers—the subchondral bone plate that is the compact layer adjacent to the calcified cartilage and the trabecular bone that lies adjacent to the medullary cavity. The thickness of the layers is variable depending on the location and the joint. The subchondral bone plate serves to provide support and the trabecular bone serves as a shock absorber since it is more elastic in nature. The subchondral bone follows the Wolff's law which states that the bone adapts in response to the amount of load placed over it. This adaptation of the bone is through osteoblastic and osteoclastic activities.

Bone remodeling is the process of removal of degraded or damaged bone cells by osteoblast and replacing them with new osteoblast precursors which later differentiate into mature cells. There is a time gap between these activities since osteoclastic activity takes weeks to remove the degraded bone and osteoblastic activity takes months to fill the new bone. This time gap leads to a transient state of osteoporosis. If during this period, unwanted stresses are being placed on the subchondral bone, then it may start to undergo damage. Initially, sclerosis of the subchondral bone may be seen, leading to reduced elasticity of the bone. The subchondral bone eventually undergoes thickening, which causes a reduction in the cartilage's ability to withstand mechanical loads, creating minor clefts and fissures in the deep zone of the cartilage. With time, these fissures may progress to the superficial zone of the cartilage and trigger the cascade of events leading to characteristic OA features.

Osteophytes in the Pathophysiology of Osteoarthritis

Osteophytes are bony outgrowths or projections. Osteophyte formation is one of the characteristic features of OA. There are three types of osteophytes:
1. Traction spurs—a physiological response located at the insertion of ligaments and tendons.
2. Inflammatory spur—syndesmophyte at the insertion of ligaments and tendons to the bone, e.g., ankylosing spondylitis.
3. Osteochondrophyte—the real osteophyte, which arises at the junction of the synovium and the bone.

Osteophytes may be symptomatic or asymptomatic based on their location. Osteophytes around the knee joint almost always cause pain and loss of function. They cause limitation of ROM and compression of surrounding structures like nerves.

Osteophytes are formed due to the differentiation of MSC in the periosteum into chondrocytes, followed by further differentiation and hypertrophy and, later on, calcium deposition in the matrix and bone-marrow formation. The osteophyte is covered by a layer of fibroblast-like cells that differentiate into chondrocytes. Hence, the osteophyte always remains covered by the cartilage. TGF-β and insulin-like growth factor-I (IGF-I) seem to have a role in the formation of osteophytes.

Classification of Osteoarthritis

The classification of OA was given by the sub-committee on the classification criteria of OA in 1986. They classified OA into two main categories:

1. Idiopathic OA—OA that was not related to any other known prior event or pathology
   a. Localized—involves a single joint.
      For the knee joint, the involvement can further be classified based on the compartment involved:
      - Medial tibiofemoral
      - Lateral tibiofemoral
      - Patellofemoral.
   b. Generalized—involves three or more areas.
2. Secondary OA—OA that was related to any other known prior event or pathology in the past
   a. Post-traumatic
   b. Congenital or developmental diseases
   c. Calcium deposition disease
   d. Other bone or joint disorders, e.g., RA and gout
   e. Other diseases such as endocrine disorders.

Knee OA can also be classified based on the number of compartments involved:

- Unicompartmental OA—when only one compartment of the knee joint is involved
- Bicompartmental OA—when two compartments of the knee joint are involved
- Tricompartmental OA—when all the three compartments are involved

Kellgren and Lawrence gave the radiological classification of the severity of OA in 1957, which divided OA into five grades based on X-ray findings **(Table 22.7)**.

Diagnosis

The diagnosis of OA is not as simple as it appears to the amateur therapist. OA may be masked behind several other related pathologies. Several pathologies such as chondromalacia patellae (CMP) and RA may give the appearance of OA. The patient with osteoarthritic changes in the knee will, in most cases, present with:

- History of mechanical dull aching knee pain aggravated by activity and relieved by rest
- Occasionally, calf pain or posterior thigh pain may also be present
- Swelling around the knee
- Stiffness in the morning and after prolonged inactivity.
- Crepitus
- Pain during stair climbing and walking on uneven terrain

Table 22.7: Kellgren Lawrence radiological classification of osteoarthritis.

Grade	Description	Radiological findings
Grade 0	None	Definite absence of X-ray changes (normal)
Grade 1	Doubtful	Doubtful joint space narrowing with possible osteophyte formation
Grade 2	Minimal	Possible joint space narrowing with definite osteophyte formation
Grade 3	Moderate	Definite joint space narrowing with moderate osteophyte formation, some sclerosis and possible deformity of bony ends **(Figs. 22.11A and B)**
Grade 4	Severe	Large osteophyte formation, severe joint space narrowing with marked sclerosis and definite deformity of bone ends

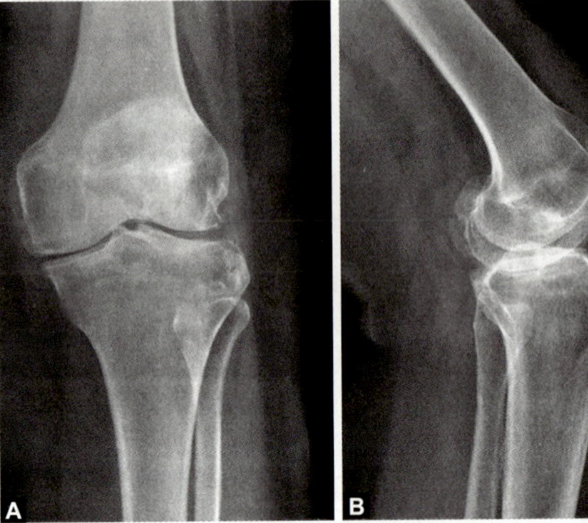

Figs. 22.11A and B: Radiograph suggesting Grade 3 osteoarthritis: (A) Anteroposterior; (B) Lateral view.

- Giving way or locking of the knee if ligaments or menisci are involved
- Deformities—flexion deformity of the knee, genu varum or valgum, genu recurvatum, patellar malalignment.
- Antalgic or waddling gait may be seen

ACR criteria for classification of idiopathic OA of the knee is a helpful aid in the diagnosis based on clinical, radiological, and laboratory findings **(Table 22.8)**.

Nowadays, with degeneration beginning at an earlier phase in life due to poor dietary and lifestyle choices, it has become difficult to evaluate patients with early OA. Hence, the therapist should always be cautious when using the ACR criteria since it considers the age to be an important factor. There might be several patients with advanced symptoms at early ages too and care should be taken to evaluate such patients thoroughly.

Table 22.8: American College of Rheumatology criteria for the diagnosis of osteoarthritis (OA).

Clinical	Clinical and radiological	Clinical and laboratory
Knee pain along with at least three out of the six following criteria:	Knee pain along with at least one out of the three following criteria:	Knee pain along with at least five out of the nine following criteria:
1. Age >50 years	1. Age >50 years	Age >50 years
2. Stiffness lasting <30 min	2. Stiffness lasting <30 min	Stiffness lasting <30 min
3. Crepitus	3. Crepitus	Crepitus
4. Bony tenderness	Along with osteophytes in the radiograph	Bony tenderness
5. Bony enlargement		Bony enlargement
6. No palpable warmth		No palpable warmth
		Erythrocyte sedimentation rate <40 mm/h
		Rheumatoid factor <1:40
		Synovial fluid shows signs of OA—clear, viscous or with WBC <2,000/mm^3

Management

Pharmacological Management

Pharmacological management of OA can be undertaken orally, topically, or in the form of intra-articular injections. The goals of pharmacological management are relief of pain, reduction of inflammation, and improvement of QOL and physical activity. **Table 22.9** gives a description of the common drugs used for OA.

With the better understanding of the pathophysiology of OA, newer techniques are being developed to limit or slow the progression of the degenerative changes seen in OA. Platelet-rich plasma (PRP) injections into the arthritic knee reduce pain more effectively compared to hyaluronic acid injections. PRP is a concentrated autologous blood product that possesses higher amounts of platelets. PDGFs contained within these platelets regulate certain biological processes in the tissues and cause a relief in the pain. It is a safe and minimally invasive procedure. A greater use of hyaluronic acid (HA) is also associated with a delay in total knee replacement (TKR). The role of MSC in the management of OA is also being explored. MSC injections may be effective in reducing pain and improving physical function. MSCs are the progenitors of any form of connective tissue, and hence, it could be hypothesized that the injection of MSCs in the joint cavity may trigger the differentiation into new tissue cells.

Non-pharmacological Management

Several guidelines have been put forward to explain the management of OA through non-pharmacological techniques. The goals of any non-pharmacological management are as follows:

- Reducing joint pain and stiffness
- Maintaining and improving joint mobility
- Reducing physical disability and handicap
- Improving health-related QOL
- Limiting the progression of joint damage

Table 22.9: Pharmacological management of osteoarthritis.

Route of administration	Drug	Adverse effects
Oral	Acetaminophen	Gastrointestinal and renal adverse effects such as stomach cramps, diarrhea, nausea, vomiting, decreased urine output
	NSAIDs (oral and topical)	Allergic reactions, peptic ulcers, diarrhea, constipation, dizziness
	Opioids	Drug tolerance and dependence, nausea, vomiting, respiratory depression
	Duloxetine	Constipation, dry mouth, diarrhea, excessive sweating, reduced appetite, hypertension
	Corticosteroids (oral and intra-articular injections)	Obesity, hypertension, osteoporosis, glaucoma, cataract, dermatological changes such as thinning of skin, acne, and purpura
	Glucosamine	Nausea, acidity, headache, skin reactions
Topical	Capsaicin	Burning, itching, and drying of skin, hyperalgesia
Intraarticular injections	Hyaluronic acid	Myalgia, arthralgia, muscle and joint stiffness, swelling of the joint

(NSAIDs: nonsteroidal anti-inflammatory drugs)

- Educating patients about the nature of the disorder and its management.

Physiotherapy Management

Based on the clinical practice guidelines, a physiotherapy regime can be developed. As mentioned earlier, obesity is a risk factor predisposing the individuals to OA. There is strong evidence for encouraging obese patients to lose weight, engaging in any form of physical activity, and strengthening and aerobic exercises either on land or in water. There is moderate evidence for self-management programs, use of walking aids, and the installation of lateral wedge insoles in the shoes for those suffering from medial compartment OA. There is weak evidence for the use of TENS, patellar taping, LLLT, massage therapy, use of knee braces, and use of medial insoles for lateral compartment OA. There is insufficient evidence for the use of manual therapy, physical agents or electrotherapeutic modalities, or valgus-directed force brace **(Table 22.10)**.

Table 22.10: Physiotherapy interventions that can be used for osteoarthritis knee.	
Physiotherapy intervention	*Description*
TENS or LLLT	Dosage parameters set according to individual patient and condition characteristics
Flexibility training	• Exercises to improve flexibility should be given. Rectus femoris, hamstrings, tendo-Achilles, and iliopsoas are prone to tightness • Frequency—6 times a week • Duration—30–60 s
Strengthening of all lower extremity muscles (particularly quadriceps including vastus medialis obliquus, hip abductors, gluteus maximus, hamstrings, and ankle plantarflexors)	• Frequency—3 times a week • Intensity—60–70% of 10 RM • Closed chain exercises are preferable to open chain, however, in the initial acute phase, open chain exercises would be preferred by the patient **(Figs. 22.12A to E)**
Aerobic exercises	• Frequency—3 times a week • Intensity—based on the symptoms of the patient and rate of RPE (Note: It should not aggravate the pain) • Type—walking is most preferred. Although, cycling and swimming will be preferred by the patient in the acute phase **(Fig. 22.13)** • Time—30–40 min with rest periods incorporated
Manual therapy	Mulligan or Maitland mobilization and different forms of PNF techniques can be used to improve strength and ROM and for pain relief
Proprioceptive and balance training	Begin with static surface and progress to dynamic surface
Physical agents (e.g., hot packs) **(Fig. 22.14)**	May be used to relieve pain and soreness due to the exercise

(LLLT: low-level laser therapy; RM: repetition maximum; ROM: range of motion; RPE: rate of perceived exertion; TENS: transcutaneous electrical nerve stimulation; PNF: proprioceptive neuromuscular facilitation)

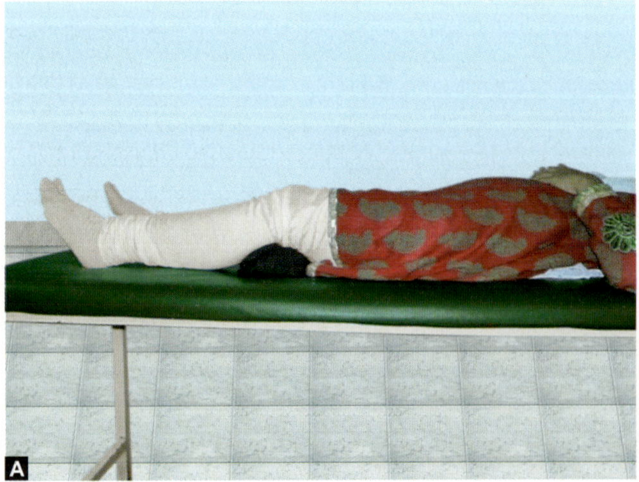
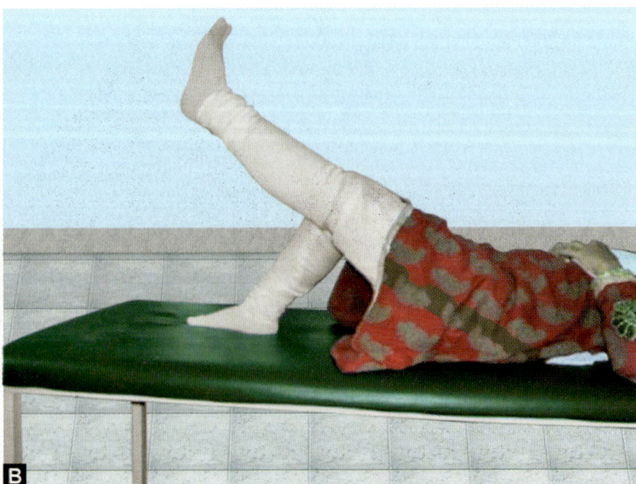

Figs. 22.12A and B

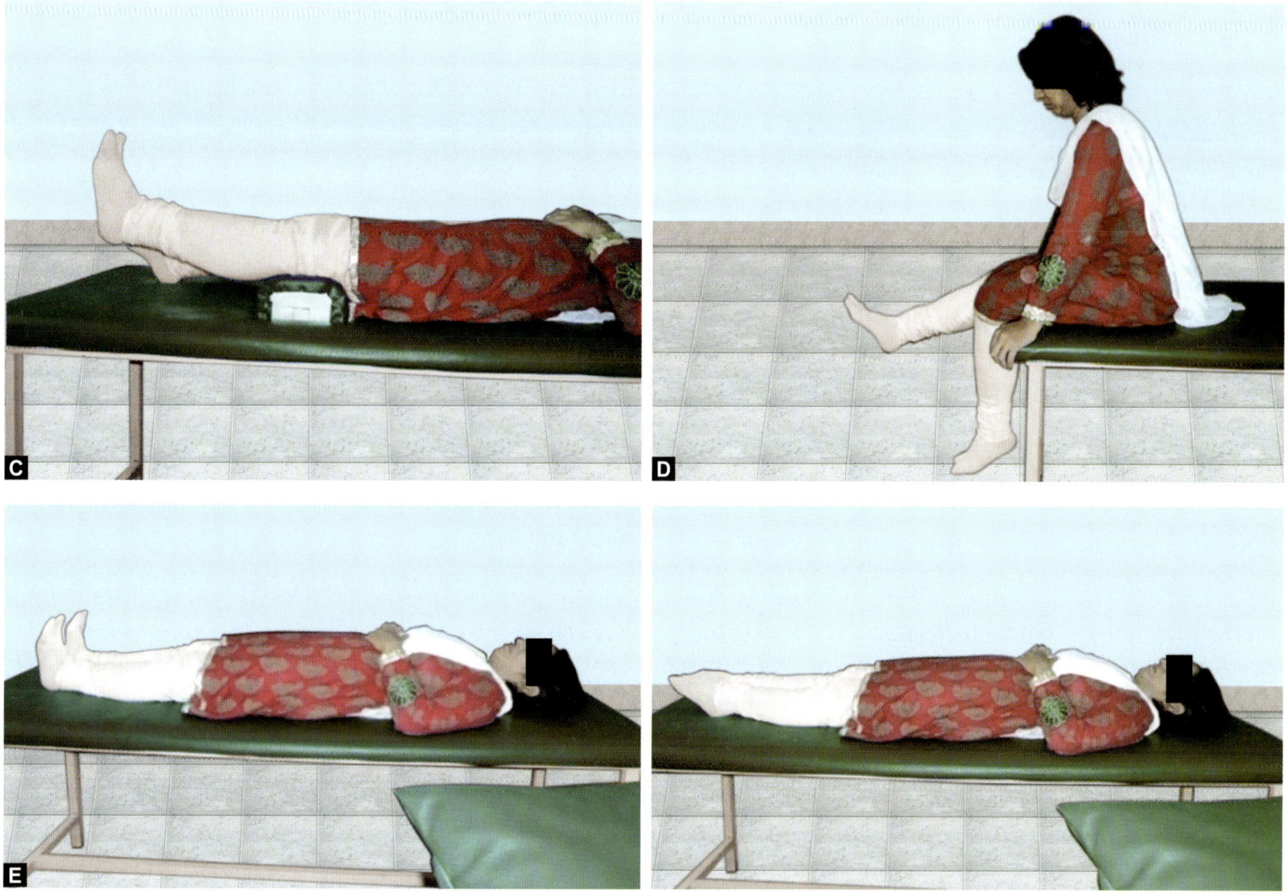

Figs. 22.12C to E

Figs. 22.12A to E: Active exercises for osteoarthritis of the knee: (A) Static quadriceps exercises; (B) Straight leg raise (SLR); (C) Short arc terminal extension; (D) High sitting knee extension; (E) Ankle toe movements.

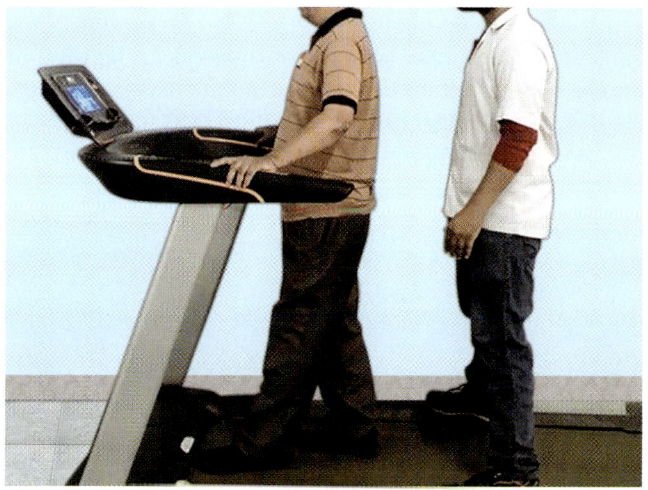

Fig. 22.13: Treadmill walking for osteoarthritis of the knee joint.

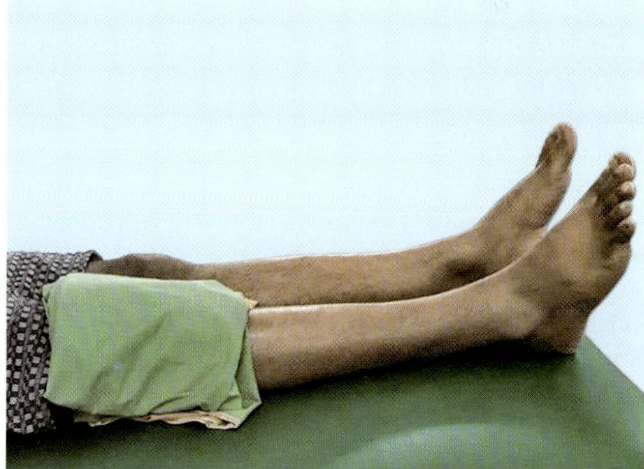

Fig. 22.14: Hot packs applied to the knee.

Often, the patient may suffer from severe pain and may not be able to perform aerobic or proprioceptive exercises in standing. In such cases, target matching foot stepping exercises have been found to be beneficial. Foot stepping exercises eliminate knee joint overloading by having the patient sit on a chair; enhance the endurance and proprioception by having the patient perform a high number of repetitions of stepping onto various pedals at high speeds and in multiple directions.

Virtual reality training (VRT): Both immersive and non-immersive type provide an interactive engaging motor-learning task that piques the patient and motivates them.

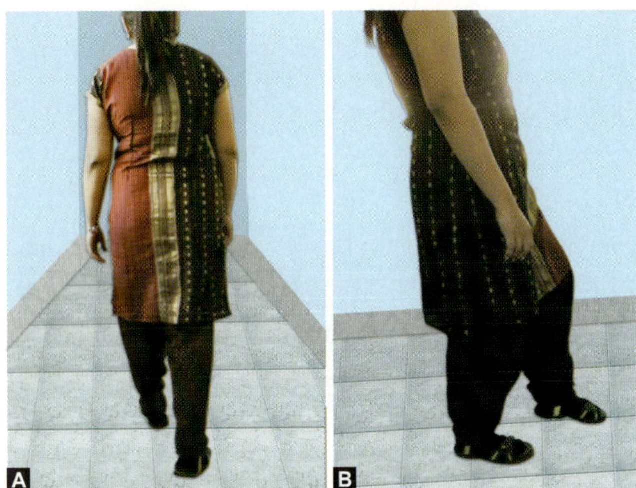

Figs. 22.15A and B: Retro or backward walking.

It relieves pain and enhances physical function and proprioception. The advantage of VRT over conventional methods of training is that the patient gets a new experience every time which keeps the activity new and the patient also gets a continuing biofeedback from the experience. However, the equipment required for such training is quite expensive and elderly patients might not be able to get a grasp of it easily.

Retro-walking or backward walking **(Figs. 22.15A and B)** is another exercise that has gained interest over the years. Retro-walking improves the muscle activation pattern, reduces the knee adductor moment during stance phase of the gait cycle, provides an augmented stretch to the hamstrings, and reduces patellofemoral joint reaction forces and eccentric loading of the patellar tendon. It, thereby, reduces pain and improves muscle strength, physical function, and the QOL in patients with OA knee.

Once the patient has a significant amount of symptom relief, they should be forwarded to a home care program. Patient education and home care are of utmost importance when dealing with OA patients since OA is not a curable pathology. Regular exercises reduce the chances of exacerbation of the symptoms and maintain or slow the progression of the pathology. Home-exercise programs with or without supervised exercise programs are capable of relieving pain and improving function and are more cost-effective and community friendly.

Lifestyle modification too forms an integral component of the rehabilitation of the patient with OA. Strengthening and neuromuscular training improve the stability provided to the joint, but in spite of this, there is a need to protect the joint from undue stress. Measures need to be taken to avoid loading of the joint excessively to reduce the degeneration. Avoiding squatting, prolonged standing and walking, repetitive stair climbing, cross-legged sitting, use of western type of toilets, etc., are some of the several joint protection strategies that may be used.

Alternative Therapies

Yoga and Tai chi are becoming increasingly popular in the management of OA. Yoga is an amalgamation of physical, psychological, and spiritual disciplines that originated in ancient India. The practice of yoga incorporates taking the body into various postures and holding them for a specific period of time. It reduces pain, improves function and mobility, and increases knee flexor and extensor strength in patients suffering from OA knee. Due to global trend of practicing yoga nowadays, it has gained immense popularity. Tai chi is an ancient art form of Chinese origin. It is a gentle form of exercise where the body flows into various postures without any retention of posture. It helps in relieving stress and also improves flexibility and strength. It also produces beneficial effects similar to physical therapy in improving physical function and QOL in OA patients.

Crenobalneotherapy or balneotherapy or spa therapy is a common practice for OA in some European and Middle Eastern countries. It is undertaken by various methods—using mineral water, regular hydrotherapy techniques, or even using mud sometimes. Although various clinical practice guidelines have either not recommended or proved it to be inappropriate, several reviews have cited the positive and long-term effects of spa therapy in reducing pain and stiffness and improving mobility and physical function.

Surgical Management

Cases with severe disability and debilitating pain that cannot be managed conservatively are managed surgically with arthroscopy, cartilage repair, osteotomy, or knee arthroplasty. Knee arthroplasty is the technique most commonly used nowadays. Arthroplasty can be total or partial depending on the compartments managed **(Figs. 22.16A and B)**. Detailed description and management following arthroplasty are described in Chapter 24: "Arthroplasties."

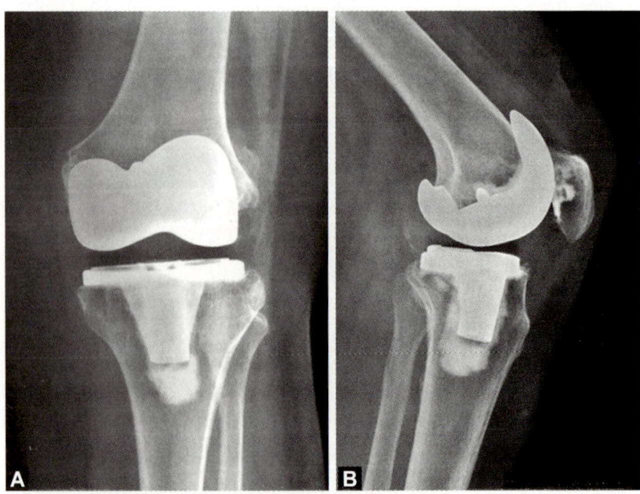

Figs. 22.16A and B: Radiograph showing bicompartmental knee arthroplasty: (A) Anteroposterior view; (B) Lateral view.

BURSITIS

Bursitis is the swelling or inflammation of bursa. A bursa is fluid-filled sac-like structure surrounding areas that are more prone to friction. Bursae act like a cushion and reduce the amount of pressure and friction that is generated between moving structures. The knee joint possesses around 11 bursae in all. The most commonly affected are the prepatellar, infrapatellar, suprapatellar, and pes anserine bursae **(Fig. 22.17)**.

As the name suggests, the prepatellar bursa is located anterior to the patella, between the patella and the overlying skin and superficial tissues. Prepatellar bursitis is more commonly known as Housemaid's knee, as it is commonly seen in people whose jobs necessitate repeated and prolonged kneeling positions, e.g., laborers and gardeners.

The infrapatellar bursa comprises two bursae—superficial and deep infrapatellar bursa. The superficial bursa lies between the skin and patellar tendon, whereas the deep infrapatellar bursa lies between the patellar tendon and tibia. Infrapatellar bursitis is also known as Clergyman's knee. Pes anserine bursitis involves the pes anserine bursa that lies deep to the pes anserine tendon (conjoined tendon of semitendinosus, sartorius, and gracilis muscles). It usually occurs in middle-aged females.

Suprapatellar bursa lies superior to the patella and extends from beneath the patella to posterior aspect of the quadriceps tendon. Suprapatellar bursitis occurs often in athletes due to direct trauma to the anterior aspect of the knee or due to microtrauma related to overuse.

Pathophysiology

The name bursitis is a misnomer, since all bursitis do not involve an active inflammatory process. Often, there might be swelling alone in the bursa. The bursa possesses the tendency to collapse upon itself under external pressure. Sometimes, the bursa may get irritated and synovial fluid may start building up inside it following some trigger. Secondary to this, the bursa fails to collapse when external pressure is applied and may get compressed between the external pressure and bone, muscles, ligaments, or tendons.

Physical Examination

Bursitis may be acute or chronic. Acute bursitis occurs secondary to trauma or infection, whereas chronic bursitis is associated with arthritis and other inflammatory arthropathies, overuse, and microtrauma.

Physical examination of a patient with acute bursitis will reveal:

- Pain
- Tenderness
- Warmth and erythema, if superficial bursae are involved
- Restricted ROM
- Painful knee movements
- Empty or late onset muscle spasm end feel

Physical examination in chronic bursitis does not reveal much since the inflammation subsides and the bursa undergoes thickening. Warmth and erythema may be absent. Movements may be pain free and pain may not be present at all in few cases.

Management

Bursitis, usually, is self-limiting. Conservative treatment helps in relieving the symptoms of pain and inflammation. It comprises protection and cryotherapy. Protection and prevention measures such as knee pads, taking frequent breaks, and avoiding pain aggravating movements such as squatting and kneeling for prolonged time can be advised. Nonsteroidal anti-inflammatory drugs (NSAIDs) and acetaminophen are the first-line drugs. For involvement of deep bursae, corticosteroid injections may be tried but the results remain unpredictable. Septic bursitis is treated with systemic antibiotic drugs. Complications such as septic arthritis may arise if not treated adequately. For recalcitrant cases, endoscopic or arthroscopic resection of the bursa can be done.

Physiotherapy Management

Physiotherapy management includes:

- Reducing pain and inflammation using patient education regarding avoidance of exacerbating activities, cryotherapy, ultrasound, or LASER.
- Maintain and improve ROM through active ROM exercises.
- Maintain and improve muscle strength especially quadriceps and hamstrings through PRE.
- Improve muscle flexibility through stretching.
- Improve proprioception through static and dynamic balance exercises **(Figs. 22.18A and B)**.
- Sport-specific skill and agility training.

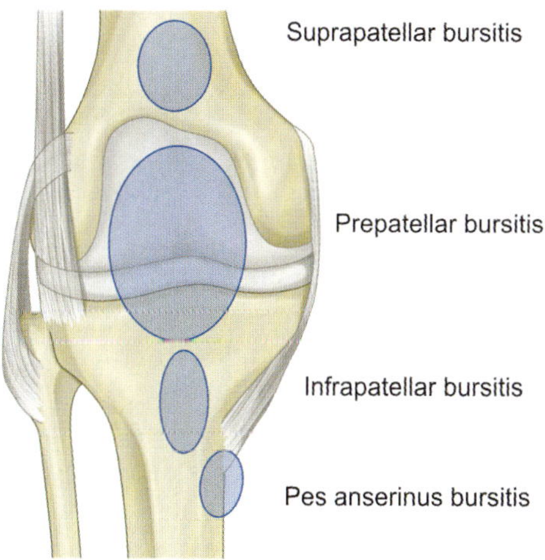

Fig. 22.17: Common knee bursitis.

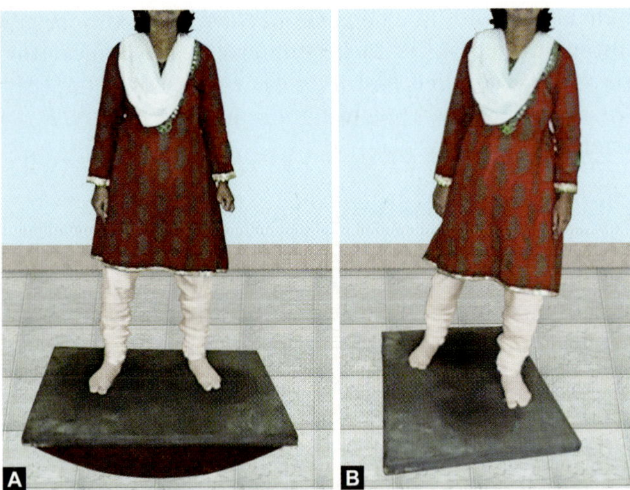

Figs. 22.18A and B: Proprioceptive exercises on dynamic surface (balance board).

ANTERIOR KNEE PAIN SYNDROME

Anterior knee pain syndrome is characterized by pain at the anterior aspect of the knee. It encompasses several pathologies such as patellofemoral pain syndrome (PFPS), CMP, and prepatellar bursitis. A few of the many pathologies that may give rise to anterior knee pain are discussed below.

Patellofemoral Pain Syndrome

The definition of PFPS is rather difficult. The diagnosis too is a rather tricky affair. PFPS belongs to the group of pathologies that are encompassed under the umbrella terminology of "anterior knee pain." PFPS is an exclusion diagnosis. The patient presents with the complaint of anterior knee pain but the diagnoses of plica syndrome, Sinding Larsen's disease, CMP, intra-articular pathology, peripatellar bursitis, or tendinitis are ruled out. It usually involves the patella and patellar retinaculum. The prevalence is higher in the adolescent and young adult population. Females are more affected than males.

Risk Factors

Risk factors for the development of PFPS include:
- Anatomic abnormalities (patella alta, hypoplastic medial patellar facet, etc.)
- Biomechanical abnormalities of the lower extremity (pes planus, foot pronation, increased Q angle, etc.)
- Hypermobile patella
- Tightness of the quadriceps, lateral patellar retinaculum, iliotibial (IT) band, or hamstrings.
- Overuse and trauma
- Past history of surgery

Etiology

The etiology behind the development of PFPS is uncertain. Three major contributing factors have been identified: muscular imbalance, biomechanical malalignment of the lower extremity (specifically the patella), and overactivity. These factors create abnormal stresses over the patella, which affects the normal tracking mechanism of the patella during flexion and extension movements. Pain occurs as a response to this abnormal tracking of the patella.

History

History includes:
- Gradual onset of symptoms
- Anterior and retropatellar knee pain ("Circle sign"—when asked about the location of pain, the patient draws a circle around the patella or places the hand over the anterior aspect of knee).
- Pain while descending stairs, kneeling, squatting, and cross-legged sitting (positive "Theatre sign"—pain following prolonged knee flexion).

Physical Examination

Physical examination includes:
- Patellar maltracking (positive "J sign")
- Tenderness over medial and lateral retinaculum
- Crepitus
- Normal ROM
- Occasional popping or clicking of patella during patient reported outcome measure (PROM).
- Decreased patellar mobility in medial direction or increased patellar mobility in lateral direction.
- Patellar tilt might be present
- Other related biomechanical abnormalities may also be present such as increased Q angle or pes planus.
- Positive patellar grind test
- Tightness of quadriceps, hamstrings, and lateral structures—lateral retinaculum, vastus lateralis (VL), IT band.
- Muscular imbalance between flexor and extensor groups.

Management

The management of PFPS should focus on a comprehensive rehabilitation plan that can help the patient get back to their daily activities and premorbid state. Medical management consists of rest, analgesics, and anti-inflammatory drugs. Bracing can be advised to protect the joint from any further stresses. A brace may not be helpful in relieving the symptoms but will definitely prevent further injury.

Physical therapy should consist of techniques to improve the tracking of the patella and reduce the muscular imbalance. Strengthening of the knee musculature, particularly the quadriceps helps in relief of symptoms. Improving flexibility of the tight structures by stretching or other similar means also helps. Patellar taping can be used to improve the tracking of the patella. In the cases of biomechanical abnormalities, orthoses should be advised to correct the malalignment. Use of excessively worn out or inappropriate footwear should be discouraged. Physical agents such as hot pack and cold pack can be used for pain relief. Ultrasound therapy relieves pain by reducing inflammation and also helps in healing of the tissues that might be damaged due to the maltracking.

A discrepancy between the activities of vastus medialis obliquus (VMO) and VL is a common finding in patients with PFPS. There is a delay in the onset of VMO activity compared to VL activity. This delay renders the VMO ineffectual to maintain the position of patella, leading to maltracking. Physical therapy treatment that incorporates biofeedback training is efficacious in correcting this delay.

Surgical management involves the release of the tight lateral retinaculum and proximal and distal realignment procedures to correct the malalignment of patella or other anatomic anomalies. Extremely rarely, when the patient is in severe pain that cannot be managed by any medical or surgical means, patellectomy is opted.

Chondromalacia Patellae

Chondromalacia patellae (CMP) or commonly known as the *runner's knee* is anterior knee pain that occurs due to softening of the articular cartilage on the posterior surface of the patella **(Fig. 22.19)**. The word literally means softening of the cartilage ("chondros" meaning cartilage and "malakia" meaning softening) in Greek language. Females seem to be more affected than males, probably due to an increased Q angle.

Etiology

The etiology in CMP is clearly understood. Repetitive trauma occurring due to overuse during athletic activity or routine daily activities, intra-articular injections using chondrotoxic drugs, or post-traumatic injuries can lead to CMP. Normally, the articular cartilage appears bluish-white in color and has a glistening appearance. In CMP, the cartilage at the center of the medial patellar facet becomes soft and swollen and appears dull and yellowish-white in color. With progression of the pathology gradually, there is a development of deep irregular fissures and the appearance becomes like that of a bunch of villous-like peelings of the cartilage that remain attached to the

subchondral bone. The surrounding area too becomes affected later, while the central area continues to erode to subsequently expose the bone. With passing time, the lateral facet too gets involved.

Outerbridge classification based on the arthroscopic appearance:
- Grade I—softening and swelling of cartilage
- Grade II—fragmentation and fissuring in ≤0.5 inches area
- Grade III—fragmentation and fissuring in >0.5 inches area
- Grade IV—erosion down to the bone.

History and Physical Examination

History and physical examination include:
- Anterior knee pain that is exaggerated by stair climbing, squatting, etc.
- Occasional history of trauma and subsequent immobilization.
- Effusion surrounding the knee
- Positive Clarke's sign
- Sometimes quadriceps weakness may be present
- Crepitus

Although Clarke's sign has been traditionally used for the assessment of CMP, it has been found to be of poor diagnostic value. The sensitivity (0.39) and specificity (0.67) are quite low, and hence, the use is not appropriate.

Management

There is no standardized plan of management for CMP. The management is individualized and symptom and need based. Medical management consists of advising the use of a dynamic brace, analgesics, and anti-inflammatory drugs. Physical therapy consists of cold pack for pain relief, ultrasound therapy for healing and reducing inflammation, quadriceps strengthening exercises (static and isokinetic), patellar taping, and mobilization.

Surgical management is carried out using both invasive and minimally invasive techniques. Arthroscopic procedures involve chondro-abrasion and release of the lateral retinaculum or plica. More extensive surgeries involve patellar resurfacing, patellectomy, or patellofemoral arthroplasty.

Osteochondritis Dissecans

Osteochondritis dissecans (OCD) is a subchondral bone lesion characterized by osseous resorption, delamination, and sequestration of the bone. Articular cartilage may or may not be involved. It is an idiopathic pathology. The lesion is located over the lateral aspect of the medial femoral condyle, possibly as a result of contact with a hypertrophic tibial spine. The etiology is unknown, but it is theorized that the pathology may be an outcome of repetitive microtrauma along with vascular impairment. If the OCD is not managed in the initial phase, it may progress to secondary OA.

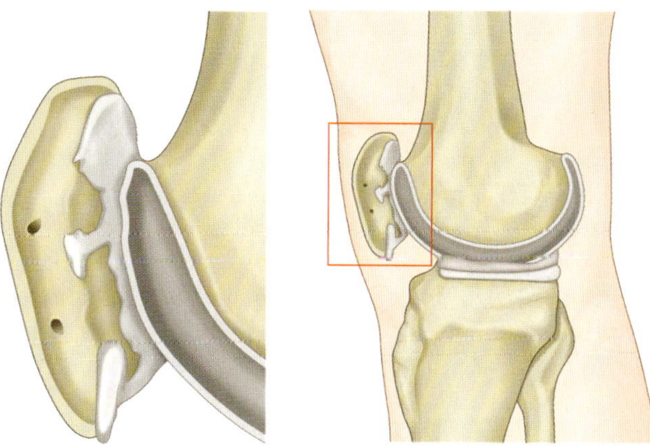

Fig. 22.19: Cartilage softening and damage in chondromalacia patellae.

Epidemiology

Epidemiology includes:
- More commonly seen in 10–20 years of age.
- Children in the 12–19 years age group are at three times higher risk than children in 6–11 years age group.
- Males almost four times more commonly affected than females.

Classification

Based on skeletal maturity:
- Juvenile—having an immature distal femoral physis; have the tendency to heal.
- Adult—having a mature distal femoral physis; follow a progressive-remitting course.

International Cartilage Repair Society classification of OCD:
- **Type I:** Stable lesion with a continuous but softened area covered by intact articular cartilage.
- **Type II:** Lesion with partial articular cartilage discontinuity, stable when probed.
- **Type III:** Lesion with complete articular cartilage discontinuity, but no dislocation ("dead in situ").
- **Type IV:** Empty defect, or defect with a dislocated fragment or loose fragment within the bed.

Clinical Presentation

Osteochondritis dissecans can clinically present as follows:
- Anterior knee pain that may be poorly localized and variable in intensity.
- Occasional episodes of locking and giving way; episodes may become frequent with increasing severity of pathology.
- Loose bodies may get detached from the bone end and cause locking and severe pain.

Management

Conservative management is successful in the cases of stable juvenile lesions. The healing takes around 6–18 months. Immobilization is given for a period of 1–2 weeks, followed by activity modification till 6 months or until complete symptomatic relief. High-impact activities may be resumed after complete symptomatic relief, a normal physical examination, and signs of healing on the X-ray.

For most of the adult cases and unstable juvenile cases or in cases where there is failure of conservative management, operative approach needs to be used. Subchondral drilling with K-wire placement is the most commonly used technique. Microfracture surgeries, osteochondral allografts or autografts, and periosteal patching techniques may also be considered.

Physical therapy treatment is usually delayed to allow for healing of the bone. Strengthening of the quadriceps, stretching to correct postimmobilization tightness, and electrotherapeutic modalities for pain relief play an essential role in the management of OCD.

Synovial Plica Syndrome

Normal synovial plicae are thin and pliable. Plica syndrome is characterized by the abnormal thickening of synovial plica, which is associated with edema and fibrosis. Chronic inflammatory changes in the knee joint lead to thickening and fibrosis of the plica, which causes pain and other impairments. The plica may, in rare cases, get impinged between the patella and femur during knee flexion. **Figure 22.20** shows the various plicae in the knee joint.

Clinical Presentation

Clinical presentation includes:
- Anterior, anteromedial, or anterosuperior knee pain
- Dull aching type of pain
- Pain aggravated by repeated movement of the knee or sustained flexion of the knee.
- Clicking, popping, and snapping sensation in the knee.

Physical Examination

Physical examination includes:
- Tenderness around the anterior or medial aspect.

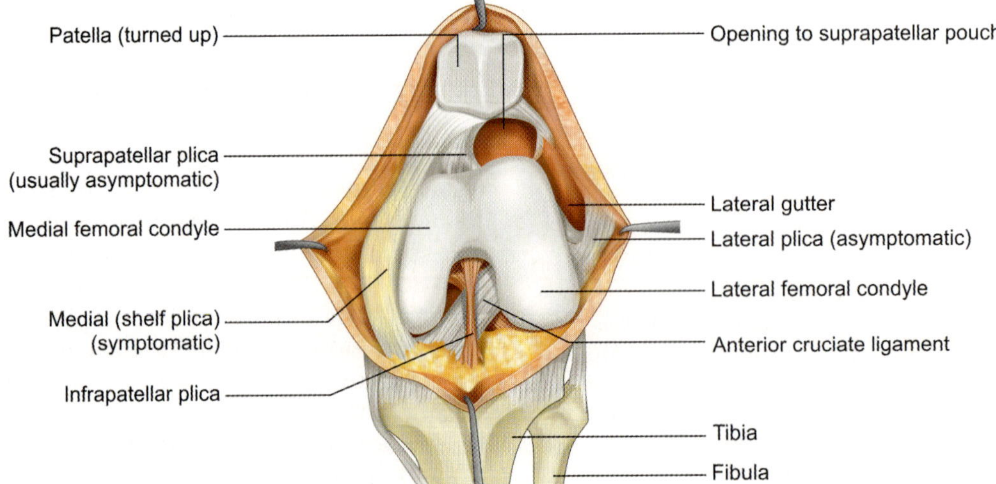

Fig. 22.20: Synovial plicae in the knee joint.

- Plica can be palpated on the medial patellofemoral joint line or suprapatellar aspect as a ribbon-like fold.
- Positive Hughston's and Stutter test.

Management

Activity modification to avoid high impact activities, e.g., jumping and squatting should be advised. NSAIDs and paracetamol can be prescribed for pain relief. Rest and ice application can be advised for milder intensities of pain. Strengthening of the quadriceps (specifically the VMO), patellar taping, and use of knee braces form the main physical therapy techniques. If conservative management fails, synovial resection through arthroscopy can be considered.

Fat Pad Irritation (Hoffa's Syndrome)

Fat pad irritation was first described by Albert Hoffa in the year 1904. It is often mistaken as PFPS or patellar tendinitis due to the close proximity of the structures. Hoffa's syndrome occurs due to acute or chronic inflammation of the infrapatellar fat pad **(Fig. 22.21)**.

Etiology

The infrapatellar fat pad is a richly innervated structure. Irritation or inflammation of the fat pad can be due to any of the following causes:

- Direct blow to the anterior aspect of the knee
- Genu recurvatum
- Posterior tilting of the patella
- Repetitive trauma to the knee which causes scarring of the fat pad
- Tight quadriceps.

Clinical Presentation

Clinical presentation includes:

- Anterior knee pain, may be localized over infrapatellar or retropatellar region.
- Patellofemoral crepitus
- Pain with activities causing stress over the PF joint, e.g., squatting, jumping, and climbing stairs.

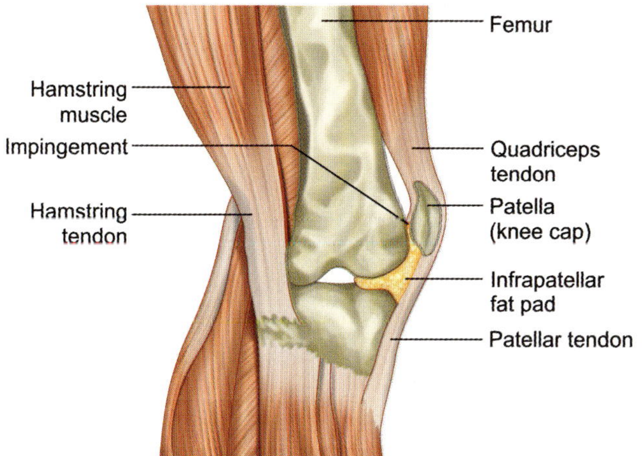

Fig. 22.21: Impingement of infrapatellar fat pad.

- Localized swelling
- Pain while walking in high-heeled shoes.

Physical Examination

Physical examination includes:

- Patellar tilt or genu recurvatum may be present
- Positive Hoffa's test
- Pain during hyperextension of the knee

Management

Medical management involves anti-inflammatory and analgesic agents. Anesthetics and steroids may be injected into the painful area for immediate relief. Physical therapy management includes application of ice to relieve pain and inflammation, quadriceps strengthening exercises, flexibility training, patellar taping, and correction of lower extremity biomechanics.

Patellar Tendinopathy

This pathology has been known by several terms—patellar tendonitis, patellar tendinopathy, patellar tendinosis or jumper's knee. The basic symptomatology remains the same irrespective of the name. The patient presents with anterior knee pain which is localized over the inferior pole of the patella. The incidence is higher among athletes, particularly sports that involve jumping. The incidence is >50% among basketball and volleyball players as opposed to 20% among soccer players.

Risk Factors

Risk factors for patellar tendinopathy include:

- Extrinsic risk factors including shoes, environmental conditions, types of conditioning activities, hard training surfaces, and higher training volumes.
- Intrinsic risk factors including tightness of the quadriceps and hamstrings, altered biomechanics of the knee joint, weight, BMI, strength of the quadriceps and hamstrings, waist-to-hip ratio, height of the arch of the foot, and limb length discrepancy.

Pathology

Cook and Purdam have proposed a continuum of tendon pathology that comprises three different stages, which are distinct but occur in succession.

1. **Reactive tendinopathy:** This stage involves a noninflammatory proliferative phenomenon in the cell and ECM that occurs in response to acute tensile and compressive loads, e.g., overload due to unaccustomed physical activity or falling directly onto the patellar tendon. Normally, as a response to tension or compression, the tendon stiffens but does not alter the thickness of the tendon significantly. But reactive tendinopathy leads to a short-term adaptive thickening of a portion of the tendon. This thickening reduces the stress by increasing the cross-sectional area. This quick short-term adaptation occurs as a temporary measure

till the long-term changes in the mechanical and structural properties of the tendon occur. The tendon returns to its normal structure if the overload is reduced or the overloading occurs at sufficient time gaps.

2. **Tendon disrepair:** This stage too attempts to heal the tendon during overloading but necessitates a larger breakdown of the ECM. This concludes with a significant increase in the number of chondrocytes and protein molecules, mainly proteoglycans in the matrix. Increased number of proteoglycans results in the segregation of the collagen and a disorganized ECM. These changes are more focal in nature and also lead to an increased vascularity. This stage is more difficult to revert since the tendons are less adaptive and stiffer. However, the reversal can be achieved by appropriate exercises that organize the ECM and with proper load management. This stage is seen in tendons that have been chronically overloaded or along a spectrum of ages.

3. **Degenerative tendinopathy:** There are large areas that are acellular due to cell death occurring as a result of apoptosis or trauma. These areas are filled with large volumes of ECM which is disorganized and highly vascular. There are huge amounts of matrix breakdown products. There is little to none capacity of reversal. This stage is commonly seen in older people.

Classification

Two systems of classification exist—Blazina classification system and the Victorian Institute of Sports Assessment (VISA) score.

Blazina classification system:
- Phase 1—pain only after exercise or activity.
- Phase 2—pain at the beginning and at the end of activity but absent after warm up.
- Phase 3—pain during and after activity.
- Phase 4—complete tendon rupture (added later on by Roels and colleagues in 1978).

VISA score: The VISA scale was developed in 1998. It is a questionnaire consisting of eight items that assess (1) symptoms, (2) simple tests of function, and (3) ability to play sport. The maximum score is 100, whereas the minimum score is 0. Six of the eight questions are scored on a visual analog scale from 0 to 10. A higher score indicates fewer symptoms. It has excellent short-term test–retest and interrater reliability (>0.95). It can be used as a measure to assess the efficacy of a treatment intervention.

Clinical Presentation

Clinical presentation includes:
- Anterior knee pain, localized over inferior pole of patella.
- Pain aggravated during activities causing overload or strong activity of quadriceps, e.g., squatting and jumping.

Physical Examination

Physical examination includes:
- Tenderness over patellar tendon
- Swelling over inferior aspect of patella
- Biomechanical abnormalities of the lower extremity
- Limb length discrepancy
- Tightness of quadriceps and hamstrings
- Positive resisted isometrics for quadriceps
- Positive Bassett's sign—tenderness on palpation of patellar tendon in knee extension when the tendon is relaxed, nontender patellar tendon in knee flexion when the tendon is taut.

Management

Conservative Management

Conservative management includes:
- Relative rest, avoiding of jumping activities, proper warm up and cool down prior to or after any activity.
- Use of NSAIDs and corticosteroids
- Cryotherapy—to relieve pain and inflammation
- Extracorporeal shockwave therapy for mechanical disintegration of calcium deposits and stimulation of tissue repair and regeneration.
- Application of a patellar counterforce strap or patellar taping.
- Plasma-rich protein injections
- Eccentric exercise program for strengthening of quadriceps and hamstrings.
- Transverse friction massage to breakdown the adhesions and stimulate normal alignment of fibers.
- Appropriate lower limb orthoses to correct biomechanical abnormalities.

Surgical Management

Surgical management includes:
- Arthroscopic debridement of affected tissue
- Arthroscopic resection of inferior pole of patella
- Arthroscopic removal of hypertrophic synovium and fat pad, sparing the patellar tendon.

Osgood–Schlatter Disease

Osgood–Schlatter Disease (OSD), also known as Lannelongue's disease, is the traction apophysitis of the tibial tuberosity. It was first separately described by two physicians Osgood and Schlatter in 1903, hence the name OSD. It is seen in growing children, in late childhood, usually the second decade of life. It has a waxing and waning character, resolving with the end of skeletal growth. It is commoner in boys than girls. The common age of presentation is 10–15 years in boys and 8–12 years in girls. It frequently occurs bilaterally. Activities involving running, jumping and kneeling, e.g., playing volleyball, and basketball tend to cause repeated stresses over the tibial tuberosity leading to OSD.

Risk Factors

Risk factors include:

- Age—boys 10–15 years; girls 8–12 years
- Gender—boys more affected than females
- Physical activity—children involved in any form of running, jumping, and kneeling
- Tightness and increased strength of quadriceps femoris
- Tightness of the hamstring muscles

Pathophysiology

Various theories have been proposed to explain the pathogenesis of OSD. However, the most commonly accepted theory suggests that OSD occurs due to repetitive strong forceful contractions of the quadriceps muscle over a weak apophysis of the tibial tuberosity. This results in an avulsion of the anterior segment, i.e., the secondary ossification center of the tibial tuberosity. Since OSD occurs in growing children, the avulsed segment continues to grow, ossify, and enlarge. The space between the avulsed fragment and the tibial tuberosity is then filled with fibrous tissue, in which case the avulsed fragment remains as a separate ossicle or it may undergo bony union, leading to a large tibial tuberosity. Mechanical factors may play a role in the weakening of the secondary ossification center. The length of the moment arm from the patellar tendon to the rotational axis of the knee joint plays a crucial biomechanical role. The length of the moment arm may vary depending on the position of patella (patella alta and baja), tibial tuberosity, the length of the patellar tendon, and its attachment.

Classification

Ehrenborg and Lagergren divided the bony maturation of the tibial apophysis into four stages based on radiologic appearances **(Table 22.11)**.

Hirano et al., studied the progress of OSD through MRI and classified it into five stages:

1. Normal: No abnormal signs.
2. Early: Signs of edema surrounding the tibial tuberosity.
3. Progressive: Partial avulsion and proximal pulling of the secondary ossification center.
4. Terminal: Complete separation of the avulsed part(s) of the secondary ossification center.
5. Healing: Intervening gap is filled with fibrocartilage that may ossify.

Clinical Presentation

Clinical presentation includes:

- Age—8–14 years
- Dull aching pain over anterior aspect of knee, particularly the tibial tuberosity.
- Pain with forceful contraction of quadriceps femoris.
- Pain exaggerates with jumping, running, climbing stairs, and kneeling.
- Swelling over anteroinferior aspect of knee

Physical Examination

Physical examination includes:

- Tenderness over tibial tuberosity
- Positive resisted isometrics of the knee extensors
- Tight quadriceps femoris and hamstrings
- Biomechanical abnormalities of the patella, e.g., patella alta or patella baja or tibial tuberosity leading to an abnormal Q angle.

Management

OSD is a self-limiting pathology. The primary goal of management is the relief of pain and swelling. The management of OSD is often conservative.

Conservative management

Conservative management includes:

- Rest
- Reduction of physical activity
- Oral anti-inflammatory drug administration
- Application of ice-packs
- Knee pads for patients involved in sports
- Knee immobilizer for patients with severe pain

Surgical Management

In chronic cases that remain unresolved with conservative treatment, surgical management provides beneficial results. Surgery serves most benefits after the individual has attained skeletal maturity. It can be done using open, bursoscopic, or arthroscopic procedures. Arthroscopic procedures are usually preferred as they lead to early rehabilitation and thus early recovery and are cosmetically more appealing to the patient. Surgical options include drilling or excision of the tibial tuberosity, tibial sequestrectomy, and insertion of bone pegs. Cases that show radiographic evidence of ossicles can be managed

Table 22.11: Ehrenborg and Lagergren classification of radiological maturity of tibial apophysis.

Stages	Description	Age (years)	Characteristics
Stage C	Cartilaginous stage	0–11	• Large amount of apophyseal cartilage • Absence of secondary ossification center
Stage A	Apophyseal stage	11–14	• Patellar tendon attaches to apophyseal cartilage • Secondary ossification center seen in apophysis
Stage E	Epiphyseal stage	14–18	• Patellar tendon attaching to bone • Presence of thin layer of insertional cartilage
Stage B	Bony stage	>18	• Patellar tendon attaches to tibial tubercle • Absence of apophyseal cartilage

with simple excision, whereas those showing evidence of associated apophysis bed deformity can be managed with trimming of the apophysis along with excision.

Any alteration in the position of the patella or the tibial tuberosity can be structurally corrected if that is found to be the cause of the OSD.

Physiotherapy Management

Physical therapy management forms a foundational basis for the management of OSD. The goals of physical therapy management are:

- Relief of pain
- Improving length of quadriceps and hamstrings
- Improving strength of quadriceps and maintaining balance between quadriceps and hamstrings strength.

Physiotherapy interventions include:

- Electrotherapeutic modalities for pain relief—ultrasound and ice pack give beneficial effects.
- Stretching of quadriceps, hamstrings, and IT band
- PRE for quadriceps and hamstrings
- Plyometric training

ILIOTIBIAL BAND SYNDROME

Introduction

The iliotibial band (ITB) syndrome (ITBS) is also known as ITB friction syndrome. It is one of the most common injuries around the knee and usually occurs due to overuse or repeated activities involving knee flexion and extension such as running, cycling, hiking, and walking long distances or full marathon athletes.

Etiology

- Incorrect training techniques such as inadequate warm-up, cool-down, and stretching
- Inadequate rest in between training sessions
- Improper/old footwear
- Excessive uphill and downhill running
- Anatomical abnormalities such as bowlegs, leg length discrepancy, supination of the foot, high or low arches, OA of knee, or excessive foot-strike force
- Weakness of hip abductor muscles in runners.

Pathological Features

It is a type of a nontraumatic overuse injury (repetitive stress disorder) of the connective tissues on the lateral part of the knee and thigh. ITB extends, abducts, and laterally rotates the hip and also stabilizes the knee joint during flexion and extension. During full knee extension, ITB lies anterior to the lateral femoral epicondyle; however, as the knee joint flexes to around 30°, the band moves posteriorly to the lateral femoral epicondyle. Therefore repeated flexion and extension of the knee cause friction between the band and the underlying lateral femoral condyle. Due to prolonged repeated irritation and friction, it leads to inflammation of the ITB leading to pain.

Clinical Features

- Pain on the lateral side of the knee usually 2 cm superior to the lateral joint line, which may radiate along the entire band up to the lateral aspect of thigh and hip.
- Usually starts with pricking sensation over the lateral aspect of knee joint may progress to sharp pain particularly during heel strikes.
- Occasionally, severe pain while walking or climbing upstairs and downstairs.
- Mild swelling along with the other signs of inflammation may appear at its insertion on tibia.
- Sometimes a snap may be heard when the band moves anterior and posterior.
- Subjective history of the patients, including questions about their pain, onset, occupation, exercising habits, overtraining, and foot wear, should be focused on.
- Some provocative tests such as Renne's test, Nobel's test, and Ober's test may be positive.

Investigations

MRI confirms the diagnosis showing thickening of distal portion of the ITB and has to be differentiated from biceps femoris tendinopathy, degenerative joint disease, lateral collateral ligament strain, myofascial pain, patellofemoral pain syndrome, stress fractures, meniscal injuries, etc.

Medical Management

Analgesics and anti-inflammatory medications—NSAIDs can be safely used. Sometimes corticosteroids such as dexamethasone, methylprednisolone, and hydrocortisone can be injected at the site of inflammation.

Orthopedic surgical interventions such as excision or release of the inflamed distal portion of the ITB or bursectomy are needed if conservative treatment fails.

Physiotherapy Interventions

- In acute pain, RICE therapy (absolute rest from running, ice, compression, and elevation) is used to decrease pain and inflammation followed by mild stretching techniques.
- To reduce inflammation, ultrasound therapy with phonophoresis to transport 10% hydrocortisone into subcutaneous tissues or iontophoresis shows beneficial effects.
- Radial shockwave therapy has proven to be effective in runners with ITBS by promoting healing and inhibiting nociceptors.
- Static stretching exercises to lengthen the ITB and tensor fascia lata (**Fig. 22.22**).
- MFR techniques using foam roller or instrument-assisted soft tissue release techniques can be used to release trigger points in band.
- Deep friction massage over ITB.
- Muscle energy technique for posterior innominate and counterstrain technique for psoas muscle would help in ITBS.

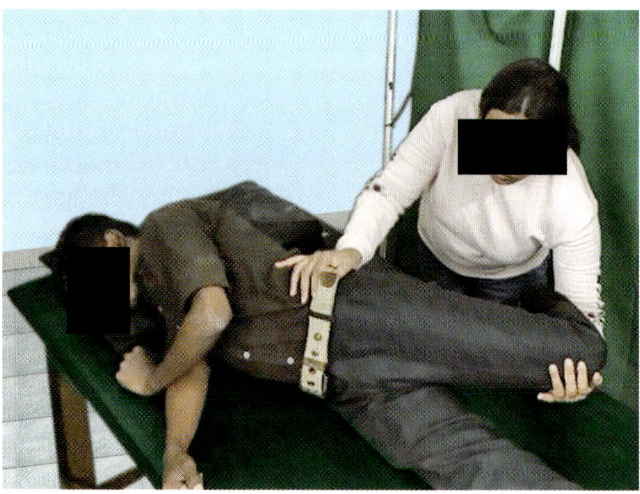

Fig. 22.22: Static stretching for iliotibial band.

- Exercise program for strengthening hip abductor muscles and the glutei.
- Exercises to improve neuromuscular control and reeducation of lower limb, including double leg squats **(Fig. 22.23)** progressing to single leg wall squats and single leg dead lifts.
- Activity modifications are important to prevent the further aggravation of patient's symptoms by decreasing the intensity of training, promoting adequate rest, modification of running habits, and engaging the athlete in some physical activities such as swimming to maintain the body conditioning rather than in running activities.
- Retraining with proper advice on surface, shoes and schedule is important to return to running.

OPERATIVE PROCEDURES OF THE KNEE

Anterior Cruciate Ligament Reconstruction

ACL injuries are highly prevalent and most of the injuries require reconstruction these days. ACLR has become a rather common procedure nowadays, since the healing of ACL is poor and an ACL deficient knee is likely to become

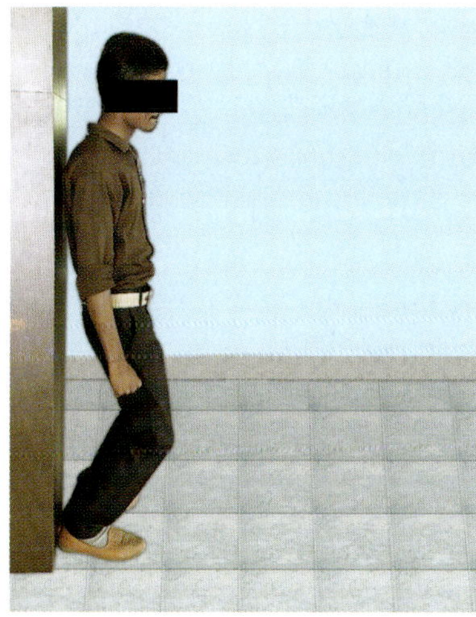

Fig. 22.23: Double leg squatting.

injured again and undergo arthritic changes earlier and at a much faster pace.

Indications

Indications are as follows:
- Severe instability of the joint due to a partial or complete ACL tear.
- Chronic ACL injury that has not healed and has led to severe pain and debility.
- Concomitant injuries to other structures, e.g., meniscus or MCL
- Increased risk of re-injury
- Frequent episodes of "giving way."

Procedure

ACLR is an arthroscopic procedure. As a common procedure, autografts are used. The surgeon is presented with two choices in such a case—bone-patellar tendon-bone graft or hamstring tendon graft that incorporates semitendinosus and gracilis tendons. The graft is harvested anteriorly or posteriorly depending on the choice of graft. It is prepared for implantation. The sites of tibia and femur are prepared for insertion of the graft by drilling bone tunnels. The graft is implanted at the appropriate position and bone plugs are used to secure the position. The knee is moved through full ROM to check the integrity of the graft. The incisions are closed and wound is wrapped.

Complications

Complications include:
- Pain
- Loss of ROM
- Instability
- Loss of muscle strength especially quadriceps
- Improper positioning of the graft
- Inadequate length of the graft tendon

Postoperative Rehabilitation

With newer techniques being developed, the accelerated approach of rehabilitation is commonly practiced now **(Table 22.12)**.

Synovectomy

Synovectomy is the surgical removal of the synovial lining of the knee joint. It can be done as an open procedure or arthroscopically. Concomitant tissue biopsy can be performed to confirm the diagnosis. Synovectomy is usually considered when the symptoms have not responded to conservative treatment even after 6–12 months.

Indications

Indications are as follows:
- Chronic inflammatory arthritides (e.g., RA and psoriatic arthritis)

Table 22.12: Rehabilitation post anterior cruciate ligament reconstruction.

	Clinical presentation	Goals	Management
Phase I (day 0 to 4 weeks)	• Pain and hemarthrosis • Poor quadriceps activation • Reduced ROM • Impaired gait and posture	• Protection of the healing structures • Control pain and swelling • Prevention of quadriceps inhibition • Maintain and improve ROM • Improve gait pattern	• Cryotherapy • Electrical stimulation using faradic current • Active ROM exercises within 0–90° • Protective bracing • WBAT with crutches • Quadriceps and hamstrings isometric contraction exercises • Patellar mobilization • Active ROM exercises of the hip and ankle • Cycling
Phase 2 (4–10 weeks)	• Reduced pain and swelling • Terminally restricted ROM • Reduced muscle strength • Improved weight bearing during gait	• Reduce pain and swelling • Strengthening of quadriceps • Progress to FWB • Normalize function	• Active full ROM exercises • Neuromuscular training • Close chain exercises—partial squats • PRE for strengthening of muscles • Proprioceptive training • Cycling
Phase 3 (10–16 weeks)	• Full ROM • Fairly normal gait pattern • Improved functioning of ADL	• Increase muscle strength and endurance • Improve proprioception and balance • Improve cardiopulmonary endurance • Prevention of reinjury	• Plyometrics • CKC exercises—squatting, jumping, etc. • Proprioception and agility training • Sport-specific skill training

(PRE: progressive resisted exercises; ROM: range of motion; WBAT: weight bearing as tolerated; CKC: closed kinetic chain)

- Hemophilia
- Benign neoplastic pathologies (e.g., osteochondromatosis)
- Septic arthritis of the knee
- Popliteal cyst

Contraindications

Contraindications include:

- End-stage disease with bony destruction, deformity, and instability
- Stiff joint
- Flexion deformity >25°

Physical Therapy Management

Goals:

- Relief of pain
- Wound care in case of open procedure
- Maintenance and improvement of quadriceps muscle strength
- Improving knee ROM
- Gait training

Plan of Care

Acute phase:

- Application of TENS or ice for relief of pain
- Static quadriceps exercises
- Calf pumping exercises
- Active knee ROM exercises in pain-free range for arthroscopic procedures
- Full weight bearing (FWB) walking (use of crutches or cane if required) for arthroscopic procedures, WBAT for open procedures.

Subacute phase:

- Active full ROM exercises of the knee and hip
- PRE for quadriceps and hamstrings
- FWB walking with emphasis on proper gait pattern
- Proprioceptive training on static surface

Return to activity phase:

- Continued strengthening of all lower extremity muscles
- Progression of proprioceptive training to dynamic surface.
- Aerobic activities, e.g., cycling, jogging, and running.

Arthroscopic Procedures

Knee arthroscopy is a minimally invasive procedure performed under general anesthesia. Two or three small incisions are made in the anterior aspect of knee that act as portals to insert the equipment inside the cavity.

Indications

Indications include:

- Meniscal repair and reconstruction
- Articular cartilage repairs
- Debridement
- Extraction of loose bodies
- Synovectomy
- Ligament reconstruction
- Fractures
- Biopsy

Postsurgical Physical Therapy Management

Acute phase (0–2 weeks): Usually, the patient can start FWB walking on the same day, unless unadvised by the medical professional or the surgeon. Wound care is important as there are chances of infection. Use of analgesics and cryotherapy can be made for pain relief. Active knee ROM exercises should be started on the first day.

Return to work phase (after 2 weeks): Since arthroscopic procedures are minimally invasive, routine activities can be resumed in the subacute phase. Strength training for the lower extremity should be started along with proprioceptive training and balance training. Closed chain exercises should be advised.

SUMMARY

Knee joint is a very complex joint comprising three different joints—medial and lateral tibiofemoral and patellofemoral joints. There are several structures viz. ligaments, menisci, and cartilage which can be damaged and lead to knee pain and other symptoms such as instability and inability to bear weight on the affected limb. ROM is easily lost and quadriceps atrophy or weakness is seen in majority of the patients. Medical and surgical management form important components of the rehabilitation but physiotherapy forms the mainstay of the treatment since knee pathologies usually make the joint vulnerable to degeneration. The key to complete recovery in case of any knee pathology is early rehabilitation specially focusing on strengthening the hip and knee musculature along with proprioceptive and neuromuscular training. Multiple or chronic injuries are treated surgically, but physiotherapy is required after surgery as well to regain complete function. Thus an early and multidisciplinary approach is required to manage knee pathologies.

Case Scenario

CASE STUDY 1

A 22-year-old male sustained an injury to the right knee while playing Kabaddi. He was tackled by an opponent and he sustained a fall with the foot planted on the ground, his femur in internal rotation and the leg in valgum. He heard a pop sound from his knee and could not stand from the ground. Later examination at the orthopedician revealed an increased anterior tibial translation and gross swelling. The patient was advised surgery but he declined and hence was advised analgesics, brace, and rest. The patient consulted a physiotherapist after 10 days of the injury on referral from the orthopedician.

Assessment

Pain examination: Pain is sharp in character and grossly spread over the entire knee. The patient reports a score of 9 on the numerical pain rating scale and states that the pain is aggravated with knee movements and weight bearing.

Local examination: Severe swelling and ecchymosis on the whole of right knee. Moderate warmth present in the same area.

Posture examination: Knee remains in flexion and weight cannot be borne on the extremity.

ROM: All hip, knee, and ankle ranges are restricted.

Muscle strength: The pain is so severe that the patient cannot bear any resistance, active movements are also painful, and hence, it cannot be measured accurately at this stage.

Joint play: Increased anterior translation of tibia on femur, painful.

Gait examination: Patient could not bear weight on the right extremity.

Guiding Questions:

1. What special test did the orthopedician perform?
2. What can be the possible diagnosis of the patient?
3. What can be the possible management plan for the patient?

CASE STUDY 2

A 56-year-old male presents left with knee pain since 6 months that has been gradually increasing in intensity. The pain is situated on the anterior aspect of the knee, dull aching in character and aggravated by squatting, stair climbing and prolonged sitting and standing. Morning stiffness is present and lasts for 10–15 minutes. Currently, he has been not taking any drugs.

Assessment

Local examination: Mild swelling over the superior and anterior aspect of the patella with mild warmth in the same area.

Posture examination: Genu valgum.

ROM: Active knee flexion is restricted on the left side with extension lag of 5°. Ankle dorsiflexion is reduced by 10° on the left side and 5° on the right. Hip flexion (SLR) ROM is 65° and extension ROM is 20°. Rest of the ranges are full.

Joint play: Reduced patellar mobility in all directions, reduced tibiofemoral gliding in anterior direction.

Muscle strength examination: Reduced strength of quadriceps, hamstrings, glutei, and calf muscles.

Tightness: Present in calf, hamstrings, and rectus femoris muscles.

Gait examination: Antalgic gait with reduced cadence and reduced stance phase on the left side and reduces swing phase on the right side. Knee flexion on the left side during swing phase is reduced.

Guiding Questions:

a. State the differential diagnoses for the patient.
b. What treatment plan will you formulate for the patient?
c. What functional scale can be used in this case?

Review Questions

1. Define osteoarthritis. Describe pathophysiology, classification, clinical features, and the physiotherapy management of osteoarthritis of the knee.
2. Discuss the rehabilitation of a 32-year-old male who has undergone right ACL reconstruction.
3. Describe the management of a 44-year-old female with RA of the knee.
4. Write short notes on:
   a. Physiotherapy following conservatively managed meniscal tear
   b. Physiotherapy management following meniscectomy
   c. Bursitis
   d. Assessment of PCL injury
   e. Chondromalacia patellae
   f. Diagnostic criteria of OA
   g. Classification of meniscal tears
   h. Grades of MCL tear
   i. WOMAC

BIBLIOGRAPHY

1. Altman R, Asch E, Bloch D, et al. Development of criteria for the classification and reporting of osteoarthritis. Classification of osteoarthritis of the knee. Diagnostic and Therapeutic Criteria Committee of the American Rheumatism Association. Arthritis Rheum. 1986;29(8): 39-1049.
2. Altman R, Lim S, Steen RG, et al. Hyaluronic acid injections are associated with delay of total knee replacement surgery in patients with knee osteoarthritis: evidence from a Large US Health Claims Database. PLoS One. 2015;10(12): e0145776.
3. Anderson AF, Irrgang JJ, Dunn W, et al. Interobserver reliability of the International Society of Arthroscopy, Knee Surgery and Orthopaedic Sports Medicine (ISAKOS) classification of meniscal tears. Am J Sports Med. 2011;39:926-32.
4. Antonelli M, Donelli D, Fioravanti A. Effects of balneotherapy and spa therapy on quality of life of patients with knee osteoarthritis: a systematic review and meta-analysis. Rheumatol Int. 2018;38:1807.
5. Anwar S, Alghadir A, Brismee J. Effect of home exercise program in patients with knee osteoarthritis: a systematic review and meta-analysis. J Geriatr Phys Ther. 2016;39(1):38-48.
6. Batterham SI, Heywood S, Keating JL. Systematic review and meta-analysis comparing land and aquatic exercise for people with hip or knee arthritis on function, mobility and other health outcomes. BMC Musculoskelet Disord. 2011;12:123.
7. Bergström G, Bjelle A, Sorensen LB, et al. Prevalence of rheumatoid arthritis, osteoarthritis, chondrocalcinosis and gouty arthritis at age 79. J Rheumatol. 1986;13(3):527-34.
8. Blazina ME, Kerlan RK, Jobe FW, et al. Jumper's knee. Orthop Clin North Am. 1973;4(3):665-78.
9. Boling M, Padua D, Marshall S, et al. Gender differences in the incidence and prevalence of patellofemoral pain syndrome. Scand J Med Sci Sports. 2010;20(5):725-30.
10. Brenneman EC, Kuntz AB, Wiebenga EG, et al. A yoga strengthening program designed to minimize the knee adduction moment for women with knee osteoarthritis: a proof-of-principle cohort study. PLoS One. 2015;10(9):e0136854.
11. Brindle T, Nyland J, Johnson DL. The meniscus: review of basic principles with application to surgery and rehabilitation. J Athl Train. 2001;36(2):160-9.
12. Brooks PM. Rheumatology. Med J Aust (Practice Essentials). 1998:8-45.
13. Brukner P, Clarsen B, Cook J, et al. Brukner and Khan's clinical sports medicine, 5th edition. Chennai, India: McGraw Hill Education (India) private limited; 2018.
14. Chen H. Diagnosis and treatment of a lateral meniscal cyst with musculoskeletal ultrasound: a case report. Case Rep Orthop 2015;432187. doi:10.1155/2015/432187.
15. Chopra A, Patil J, Billempelly V, et al. Prevalence of rheumatic diseases in a rural population in western India: a WHO-ILAR COPCORD Study. J Assoc Physicians India. 2001;49:240-6.
16. Chopra A, Saluja M, Patil J, et al. Pain and disability, perceptions and beliefs of a rural Indian population: a WHO-ILAR COPCORD study. WHO International League of Associations for Rheumatology. Community Oriented Program for Control of Rheumatic Diseases. J Rheumatol. 2002;29:614-21.
17. Collins NJ, Misra D, Felson DT, et al. Measures of knee function. Arthritis Care Res (Hoboken). 2011;63(11):S208-28.
18. Combe B, Landewe R, Lukas C, et al. EULAR recommendations for the management of early arthritis: report of a task force of the European Standing Committee for International Clinical Studies Including Therapeutics (ESCISIT). Ann Rheum Dis. 2007;66(1)34-45.
19. Cook JL. Purdam CR. Is tendon pathology a continuum? A pathology model to explain the clinical presentation of load-induced tendinopathy. Br J Sports Med. 2008;43(6):409-16.
20. Cowan SM, Bennell KL, Crossley KM, et al. Physical therapy alters recruitment of the vasti in patellofemoral pain syndrome. Med Sci Sports Exerc. 2002;34(12):1879-85.
21. Cowan SM, Bennell KL, Hodges PW, et al. Delayed onset of electromyographic activity of vastus medialis obliquus relative to vastus lateralis in subjects with patellofemoral pain syndrome. Arch Phys Med Rehabil. 2001;82(2):183-9.
22. Dan M, Philips A, Harris IA. Surgical interventions for patellar tendinopathy. Cochrane Database Syst Rev. 2018;(5):CD013034.
23. Danoff JR, Moss G, Liabaud B, et al. Total knee arthroplasty considerations in rheumatoid arthritis. Autoimmune Dis. 2013;185340.
24. Dhollander A, Verdonk P, Verdonk R. Treatment of painful, irreparable partial meniscal defects with a polyurethane scaffold. Midterm clinical outcomes and survivor analysis. Am J Sports Med. 2016;44:2615-21.
25. Dixit S, Difiori JP, Burton M, et al. Management of patellofemoral pain syndrome. Am Fam Physician. 2007;75(2):194-202.
26. Doberstein ST, Romeyn RL, Reineke DM. The diagnostic value of the Clarke sign in assessing chondromalacia patella. J Athl Train. 2008;43(2):190-6.
27. Drosos GI, Pozo JL. The causes and mechanisms of meniscal injuries in the sporting and non-sporting environment in an unselected population. Knee. 2004;11(2):143-9.
28. Ehrenborg G, Lagergren C. Roentgenologic changes in the Osgood-Schlatter lesion. Acta Chir Scand. 1961;121:315-27.
29. Escobar, AI, Quintana JM, Bilbao A, et al. Responsiveness and clinically important differences for the WOMAC and

SF-36 after total knee replacement. Osteoarthritis Cartilage. 2007;15(3):273-80.

30. Fernandes L, Hagen KB, Bijlsma JW, et al. EULAR recommendations for the non-pharmacological core management of hip and knee osteoarthritis. Ann Rheum Dis. 2013;72:1125-35.

31. Fitzgerald GK, Axe MJ, Snyder-Mackler L. A decision-making scheme for returning patients to high-level activity with nonoperative treatment after anterior cruciate ligament rupture. Knee Surg Sports Traumatol Arthrosc. 2000;8:76-82.

32. Forestier R, Forestier FBE, Francon A. Spa therapy and knee osteoarthritis: a systematic review. Ann Phys Rehabil Med. 2016;59(3):216-26.

33. Fox JM, Rintz KG, Ferkel RD. Trephination of incomplete meniscal tears. Arthroscopy. 1993;9:451-5.

34. Franchignoni F, Salaffi F, Giordano A, et al. Psychometric properties of self-administered Lequesne Algofunctional Indexes in patients with hip and knee osteoarthritis: an evaluation using classical test theory and Rasch analysis. Clin Rheumatol. 2012;31(1):113-21.

35. Frobell RB, Lohmander LS, Roos HP. Acute rotational trauma to the knee: poor agreement between clinical assessment and magnetic resonance imaging findings. Scand J Med Sci Sports. 2007;17:109-48.

36. Gholve PA, Scher DM, Khakharia S, et al. Osgood Schlatter syndrome. Curr Opin Pediatr. 2007;19:44-50.

37. Granan LP, Bahr R, Steindal K, et al. Development of a national cruciate ligament surgery registry: the Norwegian National Knee Ligament Registry. Am J Sports Med. 2008;36:308-15.

38. Grassi W, De Angelis R, Lamanna G, et al. The clinical features of rheumatoid arthritis. Eur J Radiol. 1998;27(Suppl. 1):S18-24.

39. Hirano A, Fukubayashi T, Ishii T, et al. Magnetic resonance imaging of Osgood-Schlatter disease: the course of the disease. Skeletal Radiol. 2002;31(6):334-42.

40. Hochberg MC, Altman RD, April KT, et al. American College of Rheumatology 2012 recommendations for the use of nonpharmacologic and pharmacologic therapies in osteoarthritis of the hand, hip, and knee. Arthritis Care Res. 2012;64(4):465-74.

41. Hsieh LF, Didenko B, Schumacher HR Jr, et al. Isokinetic and isometric testing of knee musculature in patients with rheumatoid arthritis with mild knee involvement. Arch Phys Med Rehabil. 1987;68(5 Pt. 1):294-7.

42. Hughston JC. The importance of the posterior oblique ligament in repairs of acute tears of the medial ligaments in knees with and without an associated rupture of the anterior cruciate ligament. Results of long-term follow-up. J Bone Joint Surg Am. 1994;76(9):1328-44.

43. Hurkmans EJ, Jones A, Li LC, et al. Quality appraisal of clinical practice guidelines on the use of physiotherapy in rheumatoid arthritis: a systematic review. Rheumatology. 2011;50(10):1879-88.

44. Jackson JP. Degenerative changes in the knee after meniscectomy. Brit Med J. 1968;2:525-7.

45. Jeong HJ, Lee SH, Ko CK. Meniscectomy. Knee Surg Relat Res. 2012;24(3):129-36.

46. Joshi VL, Chopra A. Is there an urban-rural divide? Population surveys of rheumatic musculoskeletal disorders in the Pune region of India using the COPCORD Bhigwan model. J Rheumatol. 2009;36:614-22.

47. Kaneuchi Y, Otoshi K, Hakozaki M, et al. Bony maturity of the tibial tuberosity with regard to age and sex and its relationship to pathogenesis of Osgood–Schlatter disease: an ultrasonographic study. Orthop J Sports Med. 2018;6(1).

48. Kavanaugh A, Cush JJ, Polisson RP. Educational Review Manual in Rheumatology. Rheumatoid arthritis: patho-genesis, clinical features, and treatment; 2007.

49. Kavuncu V, Evcik, D. Physiotherapy in rheumatoid arthritis. MedGenMed. 2004;6(2):3.

50. Kellgren JH, Lawrence JS. Radiological assessment of osteo-arthrosis. Ann Rheum Dis. 1957;16:494-502.

51. Kessler JI, Nikizad H, Shea KG, et al. The demographics and epidemiology of osteochondritis dissecans of the knee in children and adolescents. Am J Sports Med. 2014;42(2):320-6.

52. Kisner C, Colby LA, Borstad J. Therapeutic exercise: foundations and techniques, 7th edition. Philadelphia, PA: F.A. Davis Company; 2018.

53. Kohn MD, Sassoon AA, Fernando ND. Classifications in Brief: Kellgren-Lawrence classification of osteoarthritis. Clin Orthop Relat Res. 2016;474(8):1886-9.

54. Kraus VB, Blanco FJ, Englund M, et al. Call for standardized definitions of osteoarthritis and risk stratification for clinical trials and clinical use. Osteoarthritis Cartilage (2015) Apr 9. pii: S1063-4584(15)00899-7. doi:10.1016/j.joca.2015.03.036.

55. LaPrade CM, Civitarese DM, Rasmussen MT, et al. Emerging updates on the posterior cruciate ligament: a review of the current literature. Am J Sports Med. 2015;43(12):3077-92.

56. Laudy ABM, Bakker EWP, Rekers M, et al. Efficacy of platelet-rich plasma injections in osteoarthritis of the knee: a systematic review and meta-analysis. Br J Sports Med. 2015;49:657-72.

57. Lee PYF, Nixion A, Chandratreya A, et al. Synovial plica syndrome of the knee: a commonly overlooked cause of anterior knee pain. Surg J. 2017;3(1):9-16.

58. Lequesne MG. The algofunctional indices for hip and knee osteoarthritis. J Rheumatol. 1997;24:779-81.

59. Leroy A, Beaufils P, Faivre B, et al. Actifit(R) polyurethane meniscal scaffold: MRI and functional outcomes after a minimum follow-up of 5 years. Orthop Traumatol Surg Res: OTSR. 2017;103(4):609-14.

60. Lian OB, Engebresten L, Bahr R. Prevalence of jumper's knee among elite athletes from different sports: a cross-sectional study. Am J Sports Med. 2005;33(4):561-7.

61. Logan CA, Murphy CP, Sanchez A, et al. Medial collateral ligament injuries identified at the National Football League Scouting Combine: assessment of epidemiological characteristics, imaging findings, and initial career performance. Orthop J Sports Med. 2018;6(7): 2325967118787182. doi: 10.1177/2325967118787182.

62. Majewski M, Susanne H, Klaus S. Epidemiology of athletic knee injuries: a 10-year study. Knee. 2066;13:184-8.

63. Matsumoto H, Hagino H, Hayashi K, et al. The effect of balneotherapy on pain relief, stiffness, and physical function in patients with osteoarthritis of the knee: a meta-analysis. Clin Rheumatol. 2017;36(8):1839-47.

64. McAlindon TE, Bannuru RR, Sullivan MC, et al. OARSI guidelines for the non-surgical management of knee osteoarthritis. Osteoarthritis Cartilage. 2014;22:363-88.

65. Menkes CJ, Lane NE. Are osteophytes good or bad? Osteoarthritis Cartilage. 2004;12(Suppl. A):S53-4.

66. Mobasheri A, Batt M. An update on the pathophysiology of OA. Ann Phys Rehabil Med. 2016;59:333-9.

67. Mutsaerts ELAR, van Eck CF, van de Graaf VA, et al. Surgical interventions for meniscal tears: a closer look at the evidence. Arch Orthop Trauma Surg. 2016;136:361-70.

68. Naqvi U, Sherman Al. Medial collateral ligament (MCL) knee injuries. In: StatPearls [Internet]. Treasure Island, FL: StatPearls Publishing; 2019. Available from https://www.ncbi.nlm.nih.gov/books/NBK431095/. [Updated 2019 Jun 4].

69. National Institute for Health and Care Excellence (NICE) (2018). Rheumatoid arthritis in adults: management (NICE guideline NG100). Available from https://www.nice.org.uk/guidance/ng100/chapter/Recommendations.

70. Ottawa P. Ottawa Panel evidence-based clinical practice guidelines for electrotherapy and thermotherapy interventions in the management of rheumatoid arthritis in adults. Phys Ther. 2004;84(11):1016-43.

71. Outerbridge RE. The etiology of chondromalacia patellae. J Bone Joint Surg. 1961;43B(4):752-7.

72. Papoutsidakis A. Predisposing factors for anterior cruciate ligament injury. Br J Sports Med. 2011;45(2):e2.

73. Paterno MV. Non-operative care of the patient with an ACL-deficient knee. Curr Rev Musculoskelet Med. 2017;10(3):322-7.

74. Pelletier JP, Martel-Pelletier J, Howell DS. Etiopathogenesis of osteoarthritis. In: Koopman WJ (Ed). Arthritis & allied conditions. A textbook of rheumatology, 14th edition. Baltimore, MD: Williams & Wilkins; 2000. pp. 2195-2245.

75. Phisitkul P, James SL, Wolf BR, et al. MCL injuries of the knee: current concepts review. Iowa Orthop J. 2006;26:77-90.

76. Rangey PS, Sheth MS, Vyas NJ. Comparison of effectiveness of forward and backward walking on pain, physical function, and quality of life in subjects with osteoarthritis of knee. Int J Health Allied Sci. 2016;5(4);220-6.

77. Reinking MF. Current concepts in the treatment of Patellar tendinopathy. Int J Sports Phys Ther. 2016;11(6):854-66.

78. Renstrom P, Ljungqvist A, Arendt E, et al. Non-contact ACL injuries in female athletes: an International Olympic Committee current concepts statement. Br J Sports Med. 2008;42(6):394-412.

79. Roels J, Martens M, Mulier JC, et al. Patellar tendinitis (jumper's knee). Am J Sports Med. 1978;6(6):362-8.

80. Roos EM. Joint injury causes knee osteoarthritis in young adults. Curr Opin Rheumatol. 2005;17(2):195-200.

81. Roos H, Adalberth T, Dahlberg L, et al. Osteoarthritis of the knee after injury to the anterior cruciate ligament or meniscus: the influence of time and age. Osteoarthritis Cartilage. 1995;3:261-7.

82. Royal National Orthopedic Hospital. (2014). Rehabilitation guidelines for patients undergoing knee arthroscopy. Available from https://www.rnoh.nhs.uk/sites/default/files/downloads/knee_arthroscopy_rehabilitation_guidelines.docx.

83. Rush J. Open surgical synovectomy of the knee in rheumatoid arthritis. Orthop Traumatol. 1993;2(4):244-50.

84. Schuttler KF, Haberhauer F, Gesslein M. Midterm follow-up after implantation of a polyurethane meniscal scaffold for segmental medial meniscus loss: maintenance of good clinical and MRI outcome. Knee Surg Sports Traumatol Arthrosc. 2016;24(5):1478-84.

85. Schwartz A, Watson JN, Hutchinson MR. Patellar tendinopathy. Sports Health. 2015;7(5):415-20.

86. Shimomura K, Hamamoto S, Hart DA, et al. Meniscal repair and regeneration: current strategies and future perspectives. J Clin Orthop Trauma. 2018;9(3):247-53.

87. Smida M, Kandara H, Jlalia Z, et al. Pathophysiology of Osgood-Schlatter disease: does vitamin d have a role? Vitam Miner. 2018;7:2.

88. Snoeker BAM, Bakker EWP, Kegel CAT, et al. Risk factors for meniscal tears: a systematic review including meta-analysis. J Orthop Sports Phys Ther. 2013;43:352-67.

89. Stillman BC. Physiological quadriceps lag: its nature and clinical significance. Aust J Physiother. 2004;50(4):237-41.

90. Thomeé R, Augustsson J, Karlsson J. Patellofemoral pain syndrome: a review of current issues. Sports Med. 1999;28(4):245-62.

91. Thumboo J, Chew LH, Soh CH. Validation of the Western Ontario and McMaster University osteoarthritis index in Asians with osteoarthritis in Singapore. Osteoarthritis Cartilage. 2001;9(5):440-6.

92. Vaishya R, Azizi AT, Agarwal AK, et al. Apophysitis of the tibial tuberosity (Osgood-Schlatter disease): a review. Cureus. 2016;8(9):e780.

93. van der Kraan PM, van der Berg WB. Osteophytes: relevance and biology. Osteoarthritis Cartilage. 2007;15(3):237-44.

94. Visentini P, Khan K, Cook J, et al. The VISA score: an index of severity of symptoms in patients with jumper's knee (patellar tendinosis). J Sci Med Sport. 1998;1(1):22-8.

95. Volpin G, Dowd GSE, Stein H, et al. Degenerative arthritis after intra-articular fractures of the knee: long-term results. J Bone Joint Surg Br. 1990;72-B:634-8.

96. Wang C, Schmid CH, Iversen MD, et al. Comparative effectiveness of Tai Chi versus physical therapy for knee osteoarthritis: a randomized trial. Ann Intern Med. 2016;165:77-86.

97. Wang D, Graziano J, Williams RJ, et al. Nonoperative treatment of PCL injuries: goals of rehabilitation and the natural history of conservative care. Curr Rev Musculoskelet Med. 2018;11(2):290-7.

98. Xia P, Wang X, Lin Q, et al. Efficacy of mesenchymal stem cells injection for the management of knee osteoarthritis: a systematic review and meta-analysis. Int Orthop (SICOT). 2015;39:2363.

99. Zanon G, di Vico G, Marullo M. Osteochondritis dissecans of the knee. Joints. 2014;2(1):29-36.

100. Zhang W, Moskowitz RW, Nuki G, et al. OARSI recommendations for the management of hip and knee osteoarthritis, Part II: OARSI evidence-based, expert consensus guidelines. Osteoarthritis Cartilage. 2008;16:137-62.

Ankle and Foot Conditions

Surendra Wani

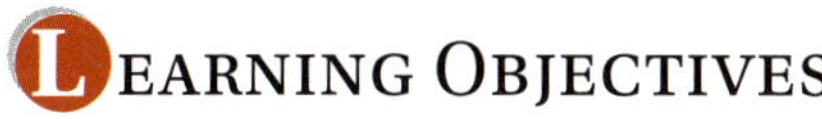EARNING OBJECTIVES

After reading this chapter, the readers should be able to:

- Understand the basic anatomy of the ankle and foot complex
- Describe the evaluation process to be followed for ankle and foot complex assessment
- Describe the etiology, pathophysiology, and clinical presentation of various pathologies related to the ankle and foot complex
- Describe the medical management used for the various pathologies related to the ankle and foot complex
- Describe the physical therapy management used for the various pathologies related to the ankle and foot complex
- Describe the surgical management and postoperative physiotherapy management used for the various pathologies related to the ankle and foot complex

CHAPTER OUTLINE

- Assessment
  - Evaluation of Functional Outcomes
- Congenital Talipes Equinovarus/Clubfoot
  - Etiology
  - Pathological Features
  - Clinical Features
  - Investigations
  - Management
- Pes Planus/Flat Foot
  - Etiology
  - Pathological Features
  - Clinical Features
  - Diagnosis
  - Management
- Plantar Fasciitis
  - Etiology
  - Pathological Features
  - Clinical Features
  - Investigations
  - Management
- Metatarsalgia
  - Etiology and Pathological Features
  - Morton's Metatarsalgia
  - Clinical Features

- Investigations
- Management
- Ankle Sprain
  - Etiology and Pathological Features
  - Clinical Features
  - Radiographic Evaluation
  - Management
  - Prevention
- Chronic Ankle Instability
  - Etiology
  - Clinical Features
  - Investigations/Diagnosis
  - Management
- Achilles Tendinitis
  - Etiology and Pathological Features
  - Clinical Features
  - Investigations
  - Management
- Rheumatoid Arthritis in Ankle Joint
  - Predisposing Factors
  - Pathological Features
  - Clinical Features
  - Investigations
  - Management

- Gouty Arthritis in Ankle Joint
  - Risk Factors and Etiology
  - Pathological Features
  - Clinical Features
  - Investigations
  - Assessment
  - Management
- Foot Drop
  - Etiology
  - Clinical Features
  - Investigations
  - Management
- Tarsal Tunnel Syndrome
  - Etiology
  - Pathological Features
  - Clinical Features
  - Investigations
  - Management

INTRODUCTION

The ankle joint is also known as the talocrural joint. It is a type of a synovial joint of hinge variety which is formed by the articulations between the tibia and fibula (the mortise) proximally and talus distally **(Fig. 23.1)**. It has only one degree of freedom, which permits the action of dorsiflexion and plantarflexion. The movement of inversion and eversion is produced at the subtalar joint. An articular capsule provides stability which surrounds the joint. The ligaments of the ankle joint are divided into medial and lateral ligaments. The medial ligament or the deltoid ligament consists of four ligaments that fan out from the malleolus. The lateral ligaments consist of three ligaments namely anterior talofibular, posterior talofibular, and calcaneofibular. The deltoid ligament resists the over-eversion of the foot and prevents the subluxation of the ankle joint, while the lateral ligaments resist the inversion and internal rotation stress. The movement of plantarflexion is produced by the gastrocnemius, soleus, plantaris, and posterior tibialis muscles [together called as tendoachilles (TA) or calf], and dorsiflexion is done by tibialis anterior, extensor hallucis longus, and extensor digitorum longus. The arterial supply to the ankle joint is from the malleolar branches of the anterior tibial, posterior tibial, and fibular arteries. It is innervated by the common peroneal nerve (CPN), tibial nerve, and superficial and deep fibular nerves.

The foot is a flexible structure that helps to maintain and stand upright on ground and allows activities, such as ambulation, running, and jumping. It is divided as forefoot, midfoot, and hindfoot. The forefoot consists of the tarsometatarsal, intermetatarsal, metatarsophalangeal, and interphalangeal joints. The midfoot consists of the talocalcaneonavicular, cuneonavicular joint, cuboideonavicular joint, intercuneiform joints, cuneocuboid joint, calcaneocuboid joint, and it also forms the arches of the foot. The hindfoot consists of the tibiofibular joint, ankle joint, and the subtalar joint.

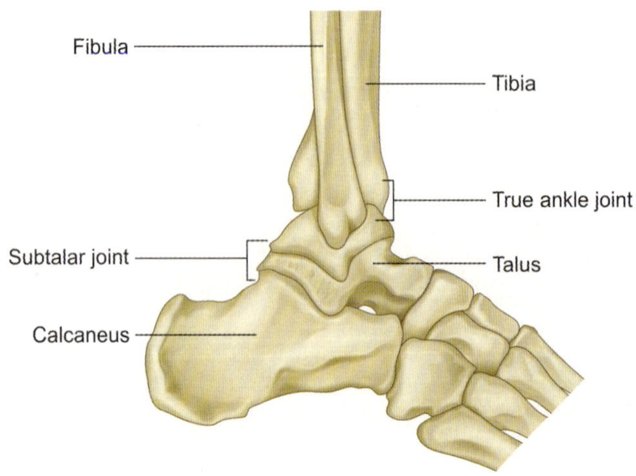

Fig. 23.1: The ankle complex.

ASSESSMENT

Assessment of the lower leg, ankle, and foot are essential to plan an efficient and successful treatment.

- The history taking must include questions about the onset, mechanism of injury, occupation, swelling, bruising, pain, abnormal sensations if any, type of footwear used, history of previous injury or surgery, and so on.
- The posture, movement patterns, and gait should be observed. Any deformities, such as hammer toes, claw toes, and hallux valgus should be properly inspected. Muscle wasting or signs of effusion must be duly noted.
- The joint lines, medial and lateral ligaments, Achilles tendon, and the muscles must be palpated. Palpation of the dorsalis pedis artery may indicate any compromise in the blood circulation.
- In the case of a referred pain or other neurological deficits, a complete neurological assessment must be performed.
- Active range of motion (AROM), passive range of motion (PROM), joint mobility, and muscle length and strength must also be tested.
- Various special tests may also be performed, e.g., squeeze test, windlass test, impingement sign of the ankle, navicular drop test, talar tilt test, and anterior of the drawer test of the ankle.
- A detailed kinesiological evaluation of ankle and foot in the gait laboratory can also be performed if indicated.

Evaluation of Functional Outcomes

Functional outcomes can be evaluated using the following scales:

- Foot and ankle ability measure (FAAM): It is a reliable scale for assessing ankle sprain of patients playing sports with r = 0.848.
- Foot and ankle outcome score: It is a reliable outcome measure for evaluating functional outcomes in patients with ankle sprain (r = 0.9).

CONGENITAL TALIPES EQUINOVARUS/CLUBFOOT

Introduction

Congenital talipes equinovarus (CTEV) is an idiopathic congenital deformity of the foot with following components: Talipes—related to talus bone; equinovarus—equinus related to plantar flexion; and varus—foot is supinated (inverted and adducted). Overall, incidence is 1 in 1,000 childbirths with male:female ratio of 2:1; may be presented unilaterally or bilaterally **(Fig. 23.2)**.

Etiology

Etiology includes:

- Idiopathic—it could develop in utero
- Increased intrauterine pressure leading to ischemia of calf muscles

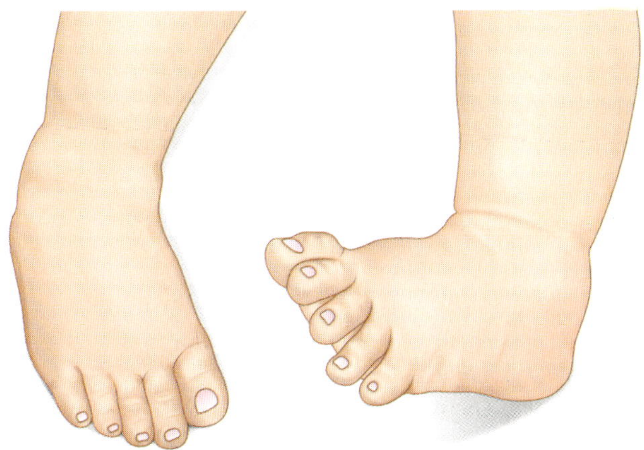

Fig. 23.2: Congenital talipes equinovarus.

- Genetic cause
- Can be associated with some congenital diseases—arthrogryposis multiplex congenital (AMC), myelodysplasia, tibial hemimelia, amniotic band syndrome (Streeter dysplasia), upper extremity and hand anomalies (common in this population), Pierre Robin syndrome, Opitz syndrome, etc.

Pathological Features

Contractures of following structures of ankle and foot contribute to this deformity:

- Tightness of muscles—flexor hallucis longus, flexor digitorum longus muscles—cavus of foot (C)
- Tightness of tibialis posterior—adduction of foot (A)
- Tightness of TA, tibialis posterior, tibialis anterior—varus (V)
- Tightness of TA—equinus deformity (E).

In addition, following structural bone malalignments contribute to the deformity:

- Medial twisting of midfoot and forefoot comparative to the hindfoot
- Talus is deviated medially and downwardly tilted
- Calcaneal varus
- Navicular and cuboid bones are shifted medially.

Clinical Features

Clinical features are as follows:

- Presence of deformity at foot with hindfoot in equinus and varus, midfoot in cavus, forefoot in adduction
- Small size of foot/underdeveloped calf muscles
- Deep creases on the back side of the heel
- Bony prominence may be felt on lateral side.

Investigations

CTEV is usually diagnosed in utero in the first trimester on ultrasonography (USG) scan. After birth, X-ray [anteroposterior (AP) and lateral views] reveals—kite's angle (angle between talus and calcaneus) <35°.

Management

Conservative Treatment

It is aimed at:

- To correct and maintain overcorrected deformity
- To prevent recurrence
- At proper gait training.

Meta-analysis carried out by Jin-Peng He et al., in 2017 indicates that **Ponseti procedure** of **serial casting (Fig. 23.3) with manipulation** (every week for 6–8 weeks followed by once in 2 weeks for next 6 months) is considered

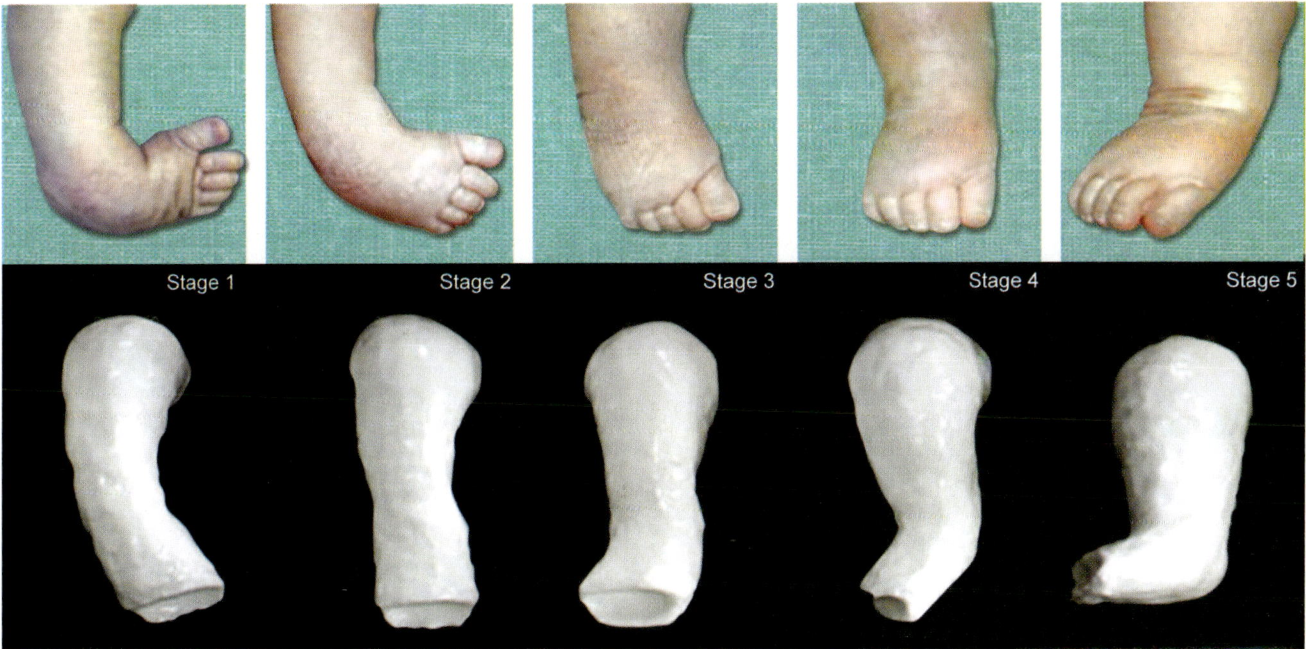

Fig. 23.3: Ponseti procedure of serial casting for congenital talipes equinovarus (CTEV).

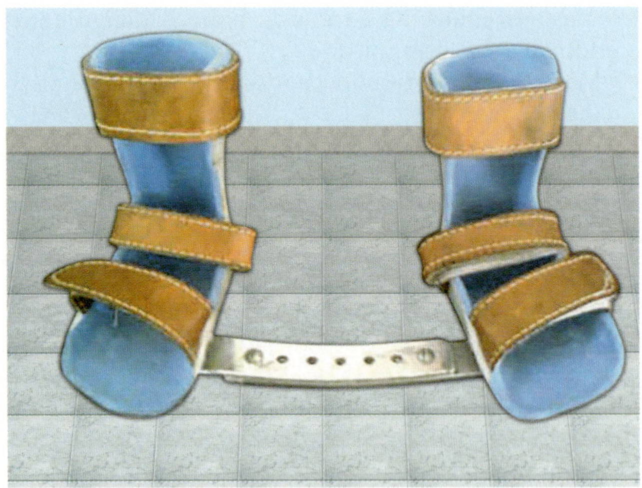

Fig. 23.4: Denis Browne splint.

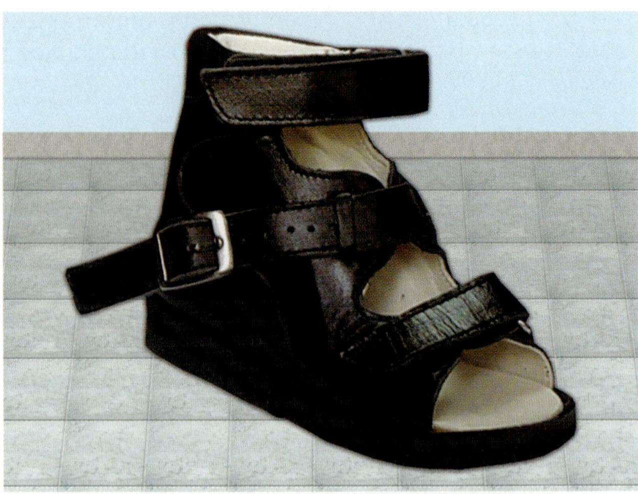

Fig. 23.5: Congenital talipes equinovarus (CTEV) shoe.

as safe, efficient, and standard method with around 90% success rate to avoid surgery. The **French method** of daily physical therapy, manipulation, and splinting is also known to be an option for conservative treatment. Once the correction is achieved, it is maintained in **Denis Browne splint (Fig. 23.4)/Phelps brace** up to 18–24 months of age. **CTEV shoes (Fig. 23.5)** are prescribed while walking till the skeletal maturity is attained.

For mild CTEV cases—physiotherapy treatment involves **manipulation by mother** (in correct order or sequence of forefoot adduction > inversion > followed by equinus correction to avoid midfoot break or rocker bottom foot) and stretching of calf muscles **(Figs. 23.6A to F)**. Maintenance of correction is done by **elastic adhesive strapping or kinesio taping** method. In moderate

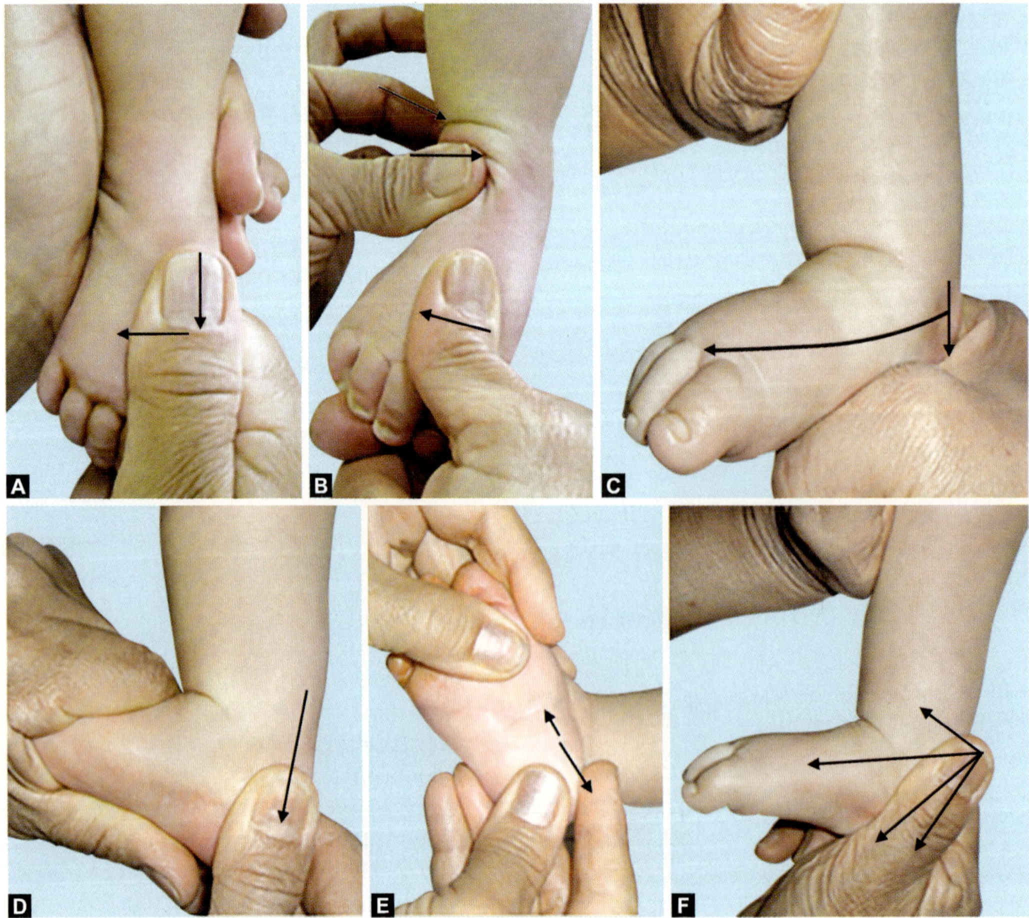

Figs. 23.6A to F: Functional manipulation by therapist/mother.

cases, manipulation should be done by therapist and maintained in position by above knee plaster cast with knee flexed in 90°.

Surgical Management

When conservative treatment fails or in infants with severe deformities of:

- Less than 3 years, soft tissue release forms the key management.
- For children of more than 3 years of age, bony corrections are required.

Surgical procedures, such as posteromedial soft tissue release and tendon lengthening, Dwyer's osteotomy, tendon transfers, medial column lengthening or lateral column shortening osteotomy, or cuboid decancelation, multiplanar supramalleolar osteotomy, talectomy, or rarely triple arthrodesis if required are used.

Physiotherapy Management

Physiotherapy management after surgery can be divided into two aspects: Postsurgical management and CTEV correction maintenance.

Active physiotherapy starts in moderate protection phase and is aimed at reducing pain if present, stiffness at ankle joint, maintaining corrected position of deformity, improving strength of foot and ankle muscles, proprioception, balance, and improving gait pattern.

Physiotherapy interventions include:

- Cryotherapy for pain relief
- Gentle-active or active-assisted movements of ankle and subtalar joint in sequence of correction/ manipulation
- Night splints
- Continuous passive motion to the ankle joint
- Stretching exercises of TA and posterior capsule of ankle joint
- Strengthening of ankle dorsiflexors, foot evertors, extensor hallucis longus, extensor digitorum longus, and intrinsic foot muscles
- Proprioception training in standing on stable surfaces, balance board, walking on inclined re-education board, etc.
- Gait training in all phases of gait with the help of proper assistive devices (walker, below-knee orthosis) or CTEV shoes if required.

CTEV correction maintenance is the same as described above.

PES PLANUS/FLAT FOOT

Introduction

Pes planus or flat foot is a postural deformity in which medial longitudinal arch is flattened or lost **(Fig. 23.7)**. It is called hyperpronation or overpronation of midfoot. In adults, congenital nonpathologic foot is present since

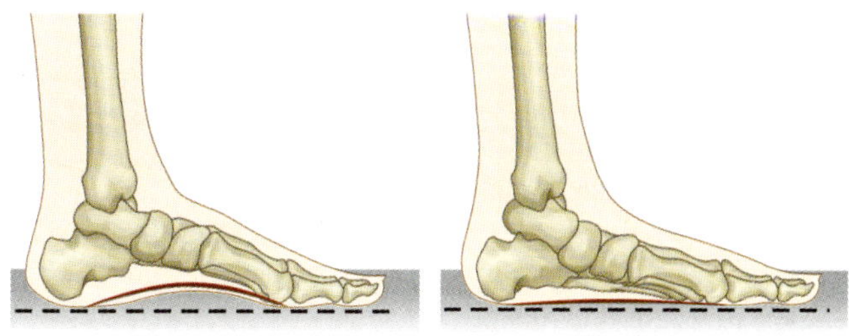

Fig. 23.7: Flat foot.

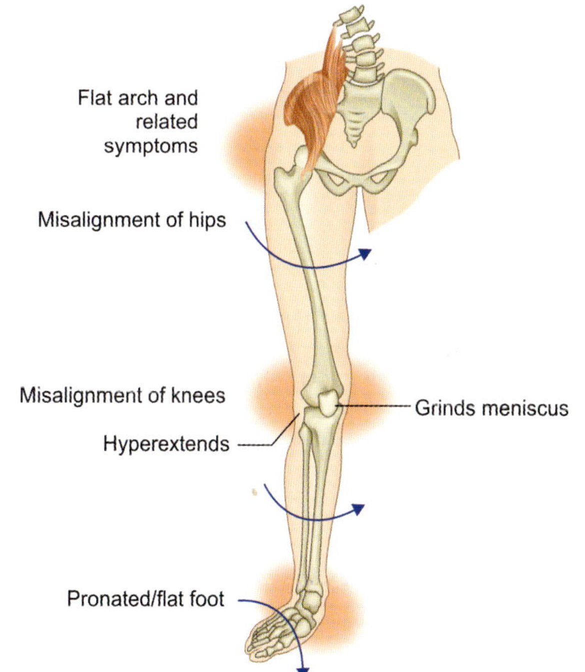

Fig. 23.8: Biomechanical alterations due to flat foot.

birth and pes planus (flat foot) deformity is acquired, which develops after skeletal maturity and called adult-acquired flatfoot deformity (AAFD).

It is a condition in which the apex of longitudinal arch of foot is flattened and the medial border of foot is nearly in contact with the ground leading to pronation of midfoot at subtalar and midtarsal joints and calcaneal valgus **(Fig. 23.8)**.

Etiology

Idiopathic Causes

Idiopathic causes are as follows:

- Congenital hypermobile foot/infantile/physiological flat foot: Due to excessive mobility at subtalar and midtarsal joints, laxity of ligaments may cause excessive foot pronation.
- Congenital rigid flat foot: Due to fibrous fusion of talus with calcaneus or navicular bone or congenitally vertical talus. Because of limited range at hindfoot, the forefoot and midfoot go into pronation.

Acquired Causes

Acquired causes include:

- Prolonged standing job
- Overweight body
- Inappropriate footwear
- Secondary to genu valgum, foot varus, and internal tibial torsion deformity for compensation may lead to flat foot and vice versa
- Osseous causes may include secondary to malunion of Pott's fracture, calcaneus/talus fracture, flaccid flat feet, peroneal muscle spasm or spasticity, rheumatoid arthritis (RA), and ligamental instability (deltoid, spring, calcaneonavicular, and calcaneocuboid ligaments)
- Flat feet may be associated with plantar fasciitis, shin splints, Achilles tendinitis, etc.

Pathological Features

Pathological features include:

- In flat feet, talus along with navicular bone shifts medially and downward to increase the weight of head, arms, and trunk on talar head leading to deformity.
- Flat foot consists of the following components: Abduction, eversion of foot with or without tibial and femoral internal rotation, severe tightness of TA, and hypermobility at subtalar and midtarsal joints.
- Physiological pes planus observed in infants generally disappears as age progresses after complete arch development.

Clinical Features

Pain over the foot after prolonged standing may be due to overstretching of medial structures and increased pressure on arch, stretch weakness of medial sided muscles, and ligaments. In chronic cases, sometimes heel pain due to plantar fasciitis, pain at first or second metatarsal region due to metatarsalgia during walking may be seen. Heel–toe movements are lost.

Diagnosis

Foot posture index is an observational measurement method to observe the foot in three planes in standing posture, which can help to diagnose flat feet **(Figs. 23.9A to F)**.

If required, then radiographs of foot (AP/lateral view) in weight-bearing position can confirm the joints under stress. Footprints on paper can be used for diagnosis and documentation purpose. Gait analysis or biomechanical analysis can be helpful in athletes to find out the relationships with adjacent joints causing problems.

Management

Conservative physiotherapy management is found to be effective and may vary as per the etiology of flat foot. Goals should be focused to:

- Reduce pain
- Improve active stability at ankle and foot
- Correct the flat feet biomechanically.

For pain reduction, the following can be used:

- Proper foot support/insole for medial arch **(Fig. 23.10)**
- Contrast bath
- Faradic foot bath
- Ultrasound therapy
- Soft tissue release technique
- Myofascial trigger point therapy
- Instrument assisted soft tissue manipulation (IASTM)
- Kinesio or rigid taping to correct and support medial arch **(Fig. 23.11)**
- Dry needling and acupuncture

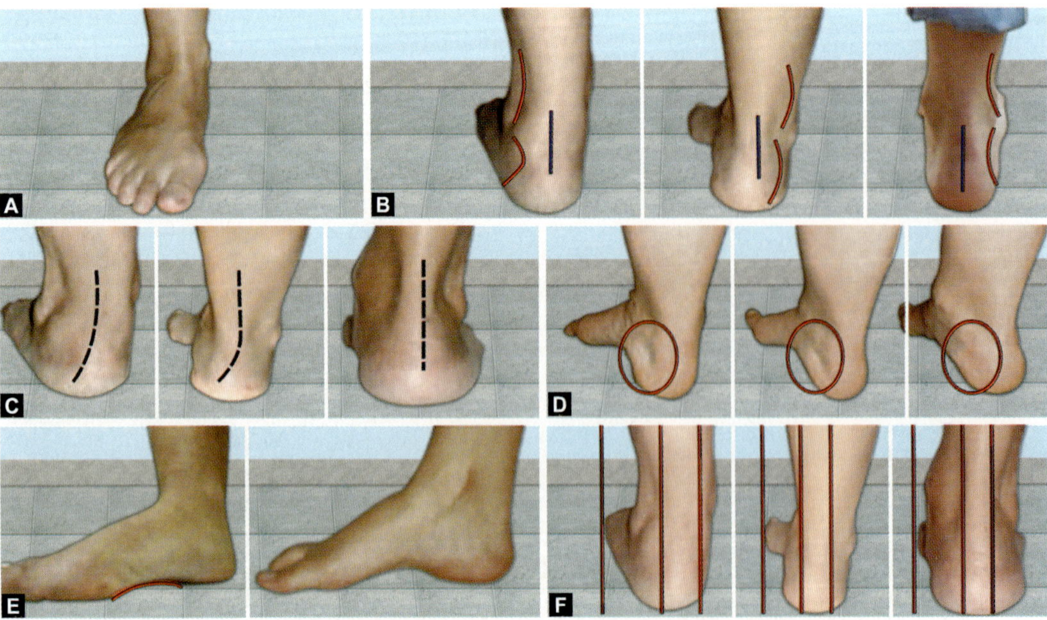

Figs. 23.9A to F: Foot posture index. (A) Talar head palpation; (B) Supra and infralateral malleolar curvature; (C) Calcaneal inversion/eversion; (D) Prominence of the talonavicular joint; (E) Congruence of the internal longitudinal arch; (F) Abduction/adduction of the forefoot with respect to the rearfoot.

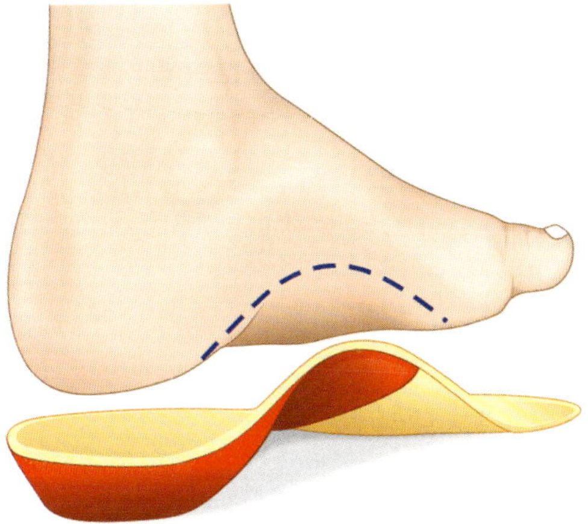

Fig. 23.10: Insoles for flat foot.

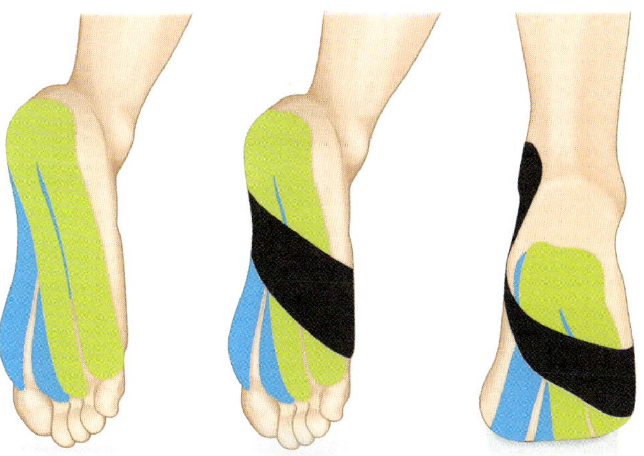

Fig. 23.11: Taping techniques for flat foot.

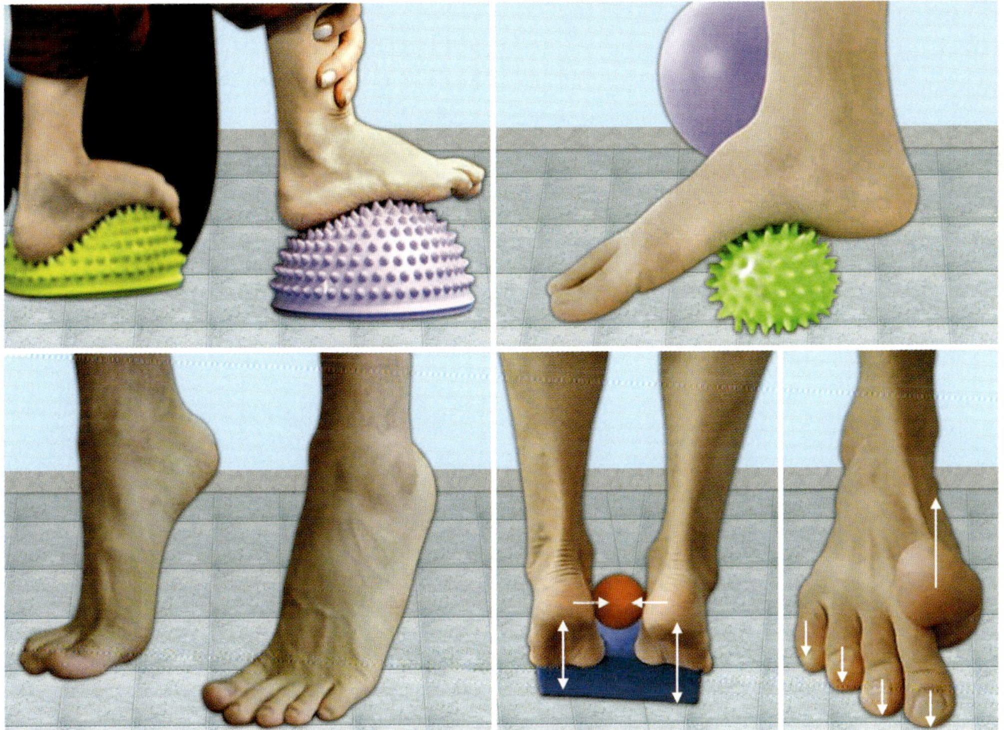

Fig. 23.12: Posture corrective exercises for the feet.

For biomechanical correction:

- Appropriate footwear with insole
- Foot posture corrective exercises actively and dynamic foot control exercises can be advised **(Fig. 23.12)**. Ergonomic advice may be given as required.
- If the cause is obesity, weight management advice can be given.

Self-management can include:

- Stretching of TA, peronei, and plantar fascia to maintain flexibility of foot
- Strengthening of intrinsic muscles of foot—toe curls, picking up objects from the ground
- Exercises to correct any ankle, knee, or hip joint malalignment leading to flat foot

- Proprioceptive and balance exercises—closed kinematic chain exercises, walking on slope and uneven surfaces such as sand and standing on wobble board **(Fig. 23.13)**. Agility and sport-specific training exercises for athletes have been found helpful. For athletes, physiotherapist should assess and improvise the landing technique during running or walking which can correct or prevent flat feet.

PLANTAR FASCIITIS

Introduction

It is among the most common foot disorders reported by patients. It is a chronic inflammation of plantar fascia and perifascial structures. The plantar fascia arises from

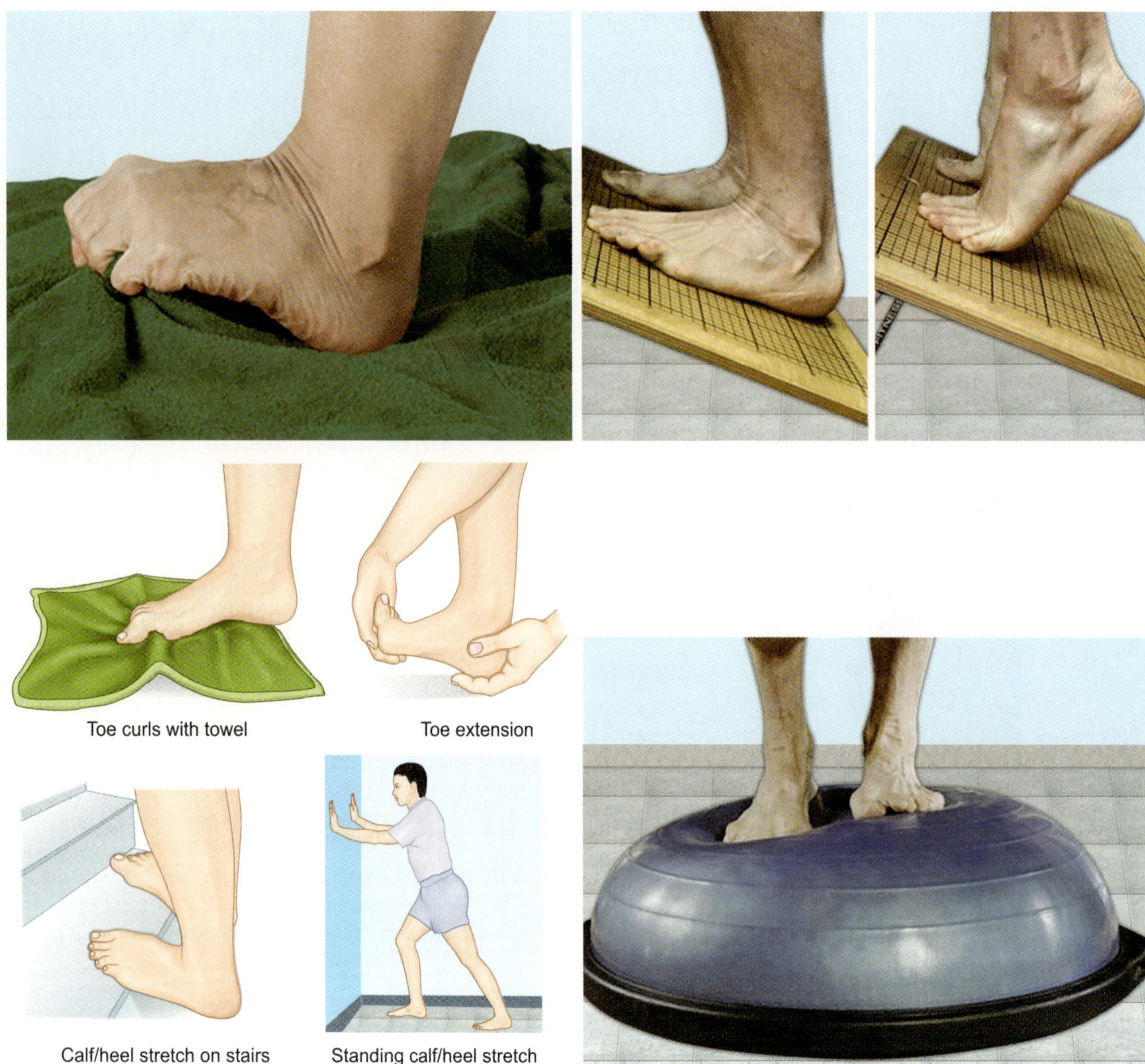

Toe curls with towel

Toe extension

Calf/heel stretch on stairs

Standing calf/heel stretch

Fig. 23.13: Active, stretching and proprioceptive exercises for foot.

calcaneus and inserts over the base of metatarsal heads. It is more common in females than men with active lifestyle between the age group of 40 and 60 years.

Etiology

Acute trauma to heel or fall on the heel, increase in BMI, excessive loading of sole during walking on uneven surfaces, microtrauma to fascia in athletes involved in running or jumping activities, and prolonged weight-bearing demands, such as standing at workplace, inappropriate footwear, and secondary to pes cavus or metatarsalgia can cause plantar fasciitis.

Pathological Features

Due to prolonged loading or microtrauma to plantar fascia during walking, running, or standing, there is repeated stress that leads to inflammation and irritation of plantar fascia. Prolonged stress may lead to microtears in fascia at the attachment to calcaneus that heals with extra fibrous tissues causing adhesions in fascia restricting the mobility and flexibility, leading to pain in heel. It may be associated with calcaneal spur, tightness of TA, plantar fascia, and reduced metatarsophalangeal mobility.

Clinical Features

Clinical features include:
- **Heel pain:** Gradual onset of pain at the inferomedial aspect of calcaneus or complete foot sole pain, initially only on weight bearing and relieved on rest and later even on rest. Inability to keep foot on ground especially in morning where the first few steps are painful, and then pain subsides and at the end of the day due to increased pain. Pain aggravation on climbing stairs, prolonged standing, or walking is also a complaint by patients.

- **Stiffness in foot:** Increases in morning or prolonged walking.
- **Tenderness:** Over the medial tuberosity of calcaneus/metatarsal heads, sometimes over the heel posteriorly.
- Reduced step length, stride length, decrease in stance time on affected side due to presence of pain and altered weight-bearing pattern of foot while walking.

Investigations

X-ray may be normal or show the presence of calcaneal spur, which can be the cause. USG can report the presence of inflammation of plantar fascia.

Management

Medical Management

Usually, pain killers and anti-inflammatory drugs are advised in acute stages. In chronic cases and cases unresponsive to conservative treatment, corticosteroid injections can be used. Surgical treatment, such as percutaneous plantar fascia release or endoscopic plantar fasciotomy is rarely needed.

Physiotherapy Management

Physiotherapy is an effective conservative treatment for plantar fasciitis and is aimed to reduce the inflammation, pain and to increase flexibility of fascia along with footwear modification and ergonomic advice.

- Pain—cryotherapy, paraffin wax bath, ultrasound with/without phonophoresis, cathodal galvanism, contrast bath, LASER, or more recent extracorporeal shock wave therapy can reduce inflammation of plantar fascia effectively. Manual therapy techniques, such as myofascial release, Maitland/Mulligan mobilization of ankle, or subtalar joint are found to be effective.
- To provide rest, relieve stress on plantar fascia—Kinesio taping **(Fig. 23.14)**, silicon or rubber custom-made foot orthosis/heel cushion, and regular use of soft sole footwear can be beneficial.
- Therapeutic exercises include plantar fascia and calf/TA stretching, intrinsic foot muscle strengthening, plantar fascia mobility using frozen bottle roll, etc.
- Ergonomic advice includes avoiding prolonged standing, use of optimal/shock-absorbing footwear, stretching of plantar fascia immediately after waking up, autostretching of plantar fascia, massage using tennis ball, etc.

METATARSALGIA

Introduction

Metatarsalgia (metatarsal pain) is a painful condition of plantar aspect of foot under the metatarsal heads. Frequently, it is associated with deformities of the first to fifth toes. However, when there is a sudden onset of pain with burning sensation over the outer aspect of forefoot while walking, then it is known as Morton's metatarsalgia.

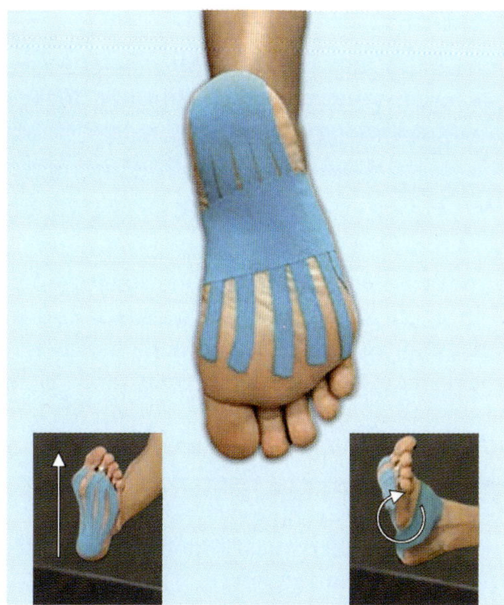

Fig. 23.14: Kinesio taping.

Etiology and Pathological Features

Increased metatarsal head loading due to presence of the following conditions increases abnormal stress on metatarsal heads leading to inflammation. During the push-off phase of gait cycle, great toe is designed to push the foot off the ground, but due to reduced great toe mobility, the extra load is placed on the remaining MTP joints resulting in pain and inflammation (MTP synovitis). Due to excessive repetitive loading of metatarsal heads, the degeneration and thickening of fatty cushion also contribute to local inflammation. The weakness of intrinsic foot muscles, tightness of plantar aponeurosis and plantar keratosis may be present.

- Pes cavus deformity
- Tightness of calf muscle
- Congenital Charcot–Marie–Tooth disease
- Prolonged use of high heel footwear
- Abnormal foot mechanics due to direct trauma, arthritis, infection
- Continuous use of poor quality shoes.

Morton's Metatarsalgia

Morton's metatarsalgia or Morton's neuroma is caused due to the entrapment of the common plantar digital nerves under the deep transverse metatarsal ligament. It commonly affects the intermetatarsal plantar nerves of second and third metatarsal spaces. There may be sudden onset of pain with burning sensation over the outer aspect of forefoot while walking.

Clinical Features

Clinical features include:

- Pain and swelling under the metatarsal heads
- Pain may radiate proximally to whole foot
- Pain may increase while walking or weight shifting
- Tenderness over the MTP joints.

Investigations

Plain radiograph may show the presence of foot deformities and occasionally show the presence of sesamoid bone under the metatarsal head.

Management

Medical Management

Usually, pain killers and anti-inflammatory drugs are advised in acute stages. In chronic cases and in cases unresponsive to conservative treatment, steroid injections can be used and surgical treatment may rarely be needed.

Physiotherapy Management

Physiotherapy is focused to:
- Reduce pain and swelling
- Correct any biomechanical abnormalities if present
- Strengthen weak musculature
- Improve function

Electrotherapeutic modalities, such as contrast bath, ultrasound therapy and acetic acid and dexamethasone iontophoresis may show short-term beneficial effect. Swelling can be treated with cryotherapy, contrast bath, faradic foot bath, etc.

Therapeutic exercises include plantar fascia, calf/TA stretching, intrinsic foot muscle strengthening, etc.

Ergonomic advices include avoiding prolonged standing, use of optimal/shock-absorbing footwear with flat heel, use of supportive shoes with extra padding under the heads (prefabricated orthotics) to relieve stress and semirigid prefabricated orthotics to support midfoot, control foot pronation, and distribute weight and pressure.

ANKLE SPRAIN

Introduction

The most common injury affecting the ankle is a sprain when ligaments get stretched beyond their capacity **(Fig. 23.15)**. It is common among all age groups ranging from mild to severe sprain.

Mild ankle sprains heal with rest and cryotherapy. However, mild-to-moderate sprains not treated with

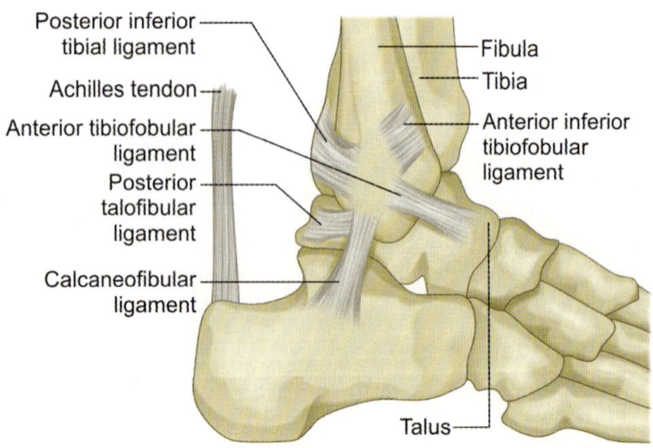

Fig. 23.15: Ligaments around ankle complex.

Table 23.1: Ligaments involved with type of injury.

Inversion injury (lateral ligaments)	Eversion injury (medial ligaments)
Sequentially anterior talofibular, calcaneocuboid, posterior calcaneofibular, and posterior tibiofibular ligaments	Deltoid and tibiofibular ligaments

appropriate treatment and rehabilitation may lead to recurrent ankle sprains, ankle instability, chronic ankle pain, etc.

Etiology and Pathological Features

Ankle/talocrural sprain is either possible on lateral or medial side, which may or may not be with rotational or twisting movement. Most common ligament injured is anterior talofibular ligament (ATFL), and involvement of other ligaments predicts the severity of ankle injury. The ligaments involved with type of injury are shown in **Table 23.1**.

Common mechanisms: Unexpected twisting at ankle during various functional activities, such as walking, running on uneven surfaces, missed step of stair or fall from height on ankle, wearing high heel shoe, sport-specific activities while playing badminton, tennis, football, etc.

ATFL sprain occurs when ankle undergoes plantar flexion–inversion stress. Additionally, calcaneocuboid ligament may be injured if the forefoot is stressed into supination or adduction, calcaneofibular ligament (CFL) may be injured due to increased inversion when the foot is in dorsiflexed position. Injury to deltoid ligament happens when the foot is stressed into external rotation and eversion in relation to lower leg.

Clinical Features

Acute ankle sprain cases usually present with:
- **Pain** of varying intensity that corresponds to the approximate area of injury which may or may not refer proximally to lower leg or distally to foot
- **Difficulty in weight bearing** on ankle while standing/walking
- Reduced movement because of muscle spasm and pain
- Intermittent giving away at ankle, and
- Joint effusion

In more severe sprains:
- Localized remarkable swelling lasts for several hours of injury
- Painful active movements at ankle
- Raised local temperature at local site of lesion
- Tenderness usually dictates the site of lesion.

Patients with chronic ankle sprain complain of:
- Dull aching pain which aggravates on stressing that ligament
- Organized swelling
- Reduced ROM at ankle
- Reduced proprioception
- Occasional instability

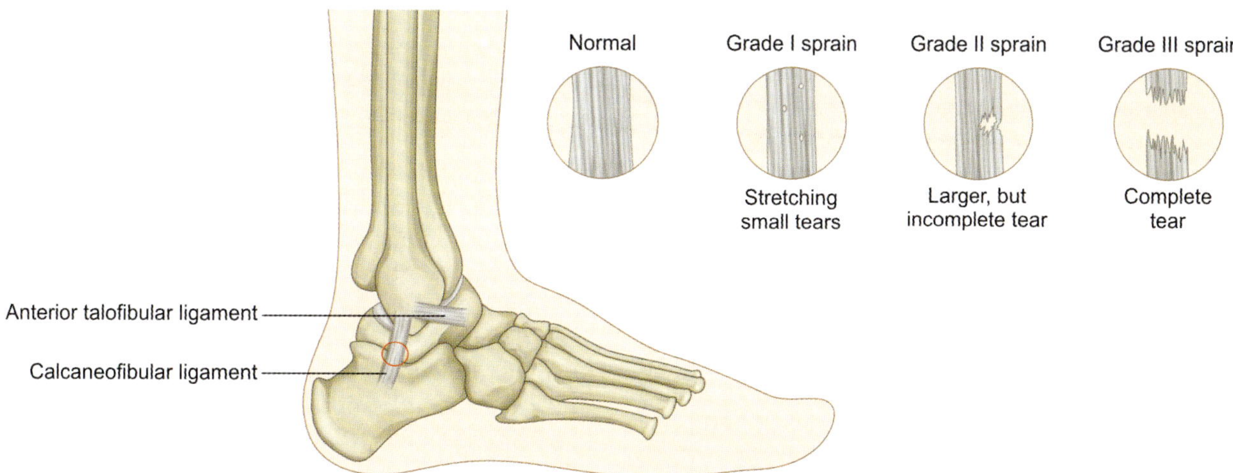

Fig. 23.16: Grades of ligament injury.

Intensity of pain and amount of disability following an injury may not compulsorily correlate with the severity. **Figure 23.16 and Box 23.1** shows the grades of ligament injury.

Radiographic Evaluation

X-rays are usually prescribed to rule out the presence of any fracture around the ankle joint.

- When the injury is due to forceful plantar flexion of foot, then lateral view of ankle joint is prescribed to confirm the anterior displacement of talus in relation to ankle, which confirms the injury to talofibular and CFLs.
- When the injury occurs with the foot in inversion and plantar flexion, the anteroposterior view is prescribed to confirm tilting of talus for confirming a tear of talofibular and calcaneofibular ligaments.
- During eversion sprain, an oblique view may confirm the injury to tibiofibular ligament due to separation of both malleoli.

Stress X-rays: X-rays can be taken in various positions of ankle to confirm the abnormal movement of ankle due to injury to ligaments.

Magnetic resonance imaging (MRI) scans: MRI scan may be prescribed following severe injury to ligaments to visualize the damage to adjacent cartilage or bone and also for better visualization of extent of ligament injury.

Management

Medical Management

Anti-inflammatory, analgesic drugs in acute stages with proper immobilization with elastic crepe bandage and plaster cast immobilization for 3–6 weeks following severe injury form the key management. Ankle corset is usually advised for chronic ankle sprain conditions.

Physiotherapy Management

All grades of ankle sprains can be treated in a three-phase program (mild sprain—up to 2 weeks and severe sprains may take up to 6–12 weeks):

1. **Maximum protection phase:** Rest, support the ankle, and reduce the swelling **(Box 23.2)**
2. **Moderate protection phase:** Restoring ROM, strength, and flexibility at ankle
3. **Minimum protection phase:** Maintenance phase with exercises and slowly return to functional activities followed by the activities requiring turning or twisting at ankle.

BOX 23.1: Grades of ankle sprains depending upon the amount of injury to ligaments, which may guide the designing of treatment plan.

Grade 1 sprain (mild): Slight overstretching causing microtears of the ligament fibers (<25% fibers torn) with mild tenderness (grade 1) and swelling around the ankle

Grade 2 sprain (moderate): Partial tear in the ligament fibers (25–50% fibers torn) with moderate tenderness (grade 2) and swelling around the ankle may be associated with slight instability

Special tests: Anterior drawer test, talar tilt test, and prone anterior drawer test may be positive

Grade 3 sprain (severe): Complete tear of the ligament (>75% fibers torn), severe throbbing pain, maximum tenderness, and severe swelling around the ankle along with significant instability with weak and painful resisted isometrics and increased joint play

---

BOX 23.2: POLICE principle.

Start POLICE protocol as early as possible after the injury. Earlier, the PRICE and RICE protocols were used. But studies have concluded based on Wolff's law that optimal loading stimulates the healing process since bones, tendons, ligaments, etc. require some loading to heal, and it also maintains nutrition of the structure. Optimal loading can be achieved through mechanical or manual interventions. At the ankle, contraction of the calf muscles may also help in relieving swelling by moving the fluid up the leg. Hence, weight bearing as tolerated should be advised rather than nonweight bearing.

The POLICE principle includes the following:

- Protection of ankle: Avoid full weight bearing, use of crutches for at least 2–3 days, avoid sudden forceful movements and support with the help of ankle binder or corset or air stirrup-type ankle brace. Unloading and stress shielding are required for shorter periods. Prolonged nonweight bearing leads to adverse effects.
- Optimal loading: Wolff's law states that an appropriate amount of loading is required to increase healing and maintain the nutrition of the injured structure. It also prevents atrophy and excessive scarring and maintains joint ROM.
- Ice (cryotherapy) can be applied immediately to reduce swelling by ice towels/ice packs for 20–30 minutes, 3–4 times in a day. Ice cold immersion method for 20 minutes (foot and lower leg immersed directly into ice-cold water tub) is effective for reducing pain, swelling, and inflammation.
- Compression of ankle to support and reduce swelling using elastic crepe bandage in minor sprains and plaster cast immobilization in severe sprains (grade 2 or 3).
- Elevation of ankle above the level of heart to reduce swelling by draining fluid proximally toward lymph nodes due to effect of gravity.

Physiotherapy exercises incorporated in the treatment regime are aimed to:

- Promote healing of ligament
- Prevent adhesions
- Improve ankle strength and proprioception
- Prevent recurrent or chronic ankle sprains

Maximum Protection Phase of Ankle Sprain

Intervention in the maximum protection phase of ankle sprain is as follows:

- Electrotherapeutic modalities, such as ultrasound therapy or LASER therapy are found to be effective after 2–3 days of injury to promote healing and repair of collagen found in ligaments. Icing can be continued.
- Elevation is maintained above the heart level in supine. Kneading/effleurage can be given from distal to proximal direction to clear the edema.
- Gentle free active movements in midrange without resistance or weight bearing in supine lying or preferably in whirlpool bath 3–4 times a day to reduce chances of ankle stiffness.
- Manual therapy should not be preferred in acute stages. However, current literature favors the combination of manual therapy along with supervised exercise program at both 4 weeks and 6 months as there might be presence of proximal tibiofibular, distal tibiofibular,

talocrural, or subtalar joint dysfunction following ankle sprain. Cleland et al. provided evidence for the effective use of manual therapy in grades 1 and 2 irrespective of stage of injury.

Techniques, such as high velocity, anterior glide to the head of the fibula on the tibia, low velocity, mid-to-end-range anterior-to-posterior oscillatory glides to the distal fibula, end-range longitudinal distraction to talocrural joint, mid-to-end-range anterior-to-posterior oscillatory glides to the talus on the distal tibiofibular joint, mid-to-end-range medial-to-lateral oscillatory glides to the medial side of the talus (or calcaneus), end-range anterior-to-posterior sustained glide to the talus in a weight-bearing position along with home exercise program twice a week for 4 weeks can be advised.

- Mild isometric strengthening exercises for ankle musculature.

Moderate and Minimum Protection Stage of Ankle Sprain

Moderate and minimum protection stage of ankle sprain includes the following:

- Active ROM exercises for foot and ankle, Kaltenborn mobilization techniques to improve joint play if required.
- Strengthening exercises: Progressive resistance training exercises using manual resistance **(Fig. 23.17)** or therabands/weights or bodyweight to improve strength. Intrinsic foot muscles strengthening should be included as well.
- Proprioception (balance) training: To reduce recurrent ankle sprain, proprioceptive training is important by a variety of modes—walking on sand, grass, uneven surface, single-leg stance on level ground followed by single-leg stance on wobble or balance board **(Figs. 23.18 to 23.21)** or Bosu ball with and without eyes open **(Fig. 23.22)**.
- Training of functional weight-bearing activities.

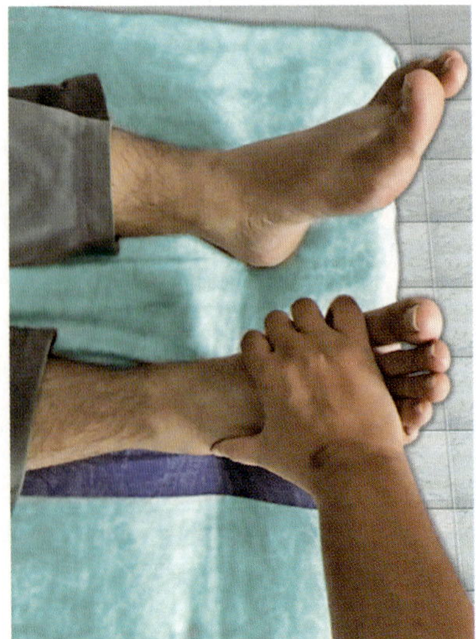

Fig. 23.17: Manual strengthening of ankle dorsiflexors.

Clinical Pearl

It is important to have a proper knowledge of dosimetry of electrotherapeutic modalities for acute conditions, or one ends up increasing the pain and inflammation.

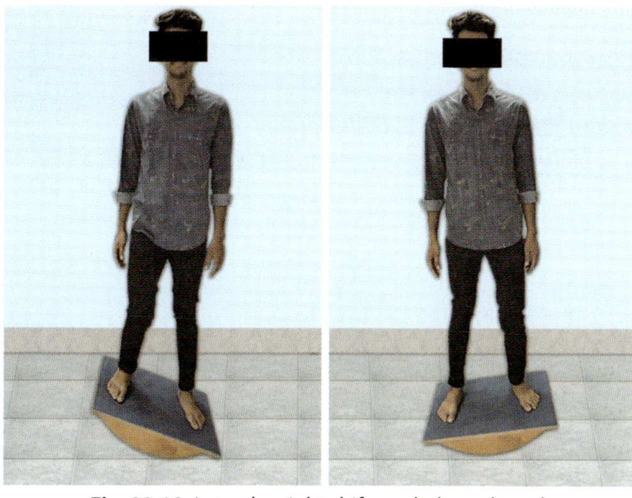

Fig. 23.18: Lateral weight shifts on balance board.

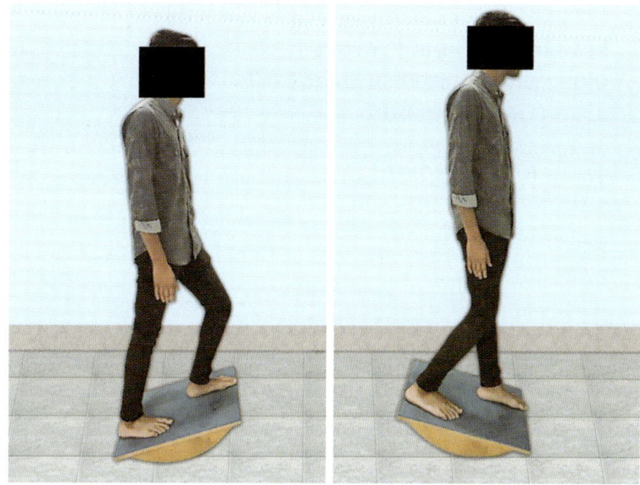

Fig. 23.19: Anteroposterior weight shifts on balance board.

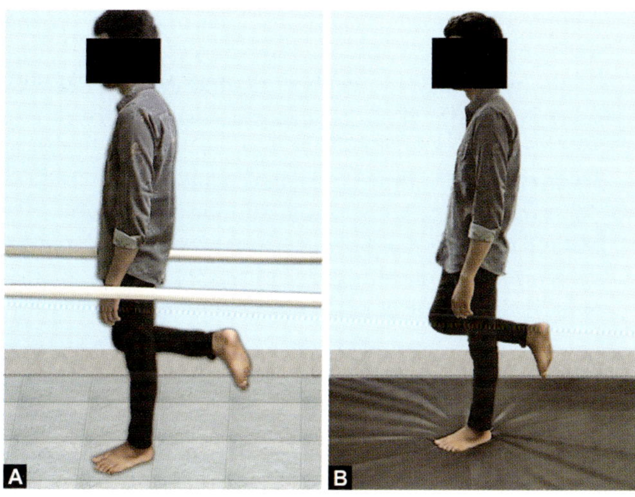

Figs. 23.20A and B: One leg standing on (A) floor (hard surface) and (B) mat (soft surface).

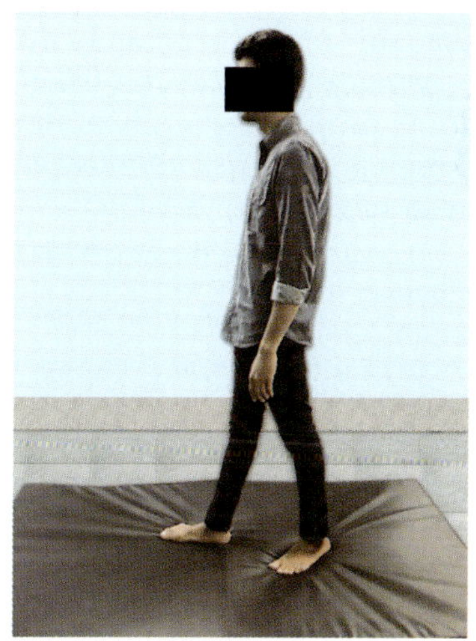

Fig. 23.21: Walking on mat (soft surface).

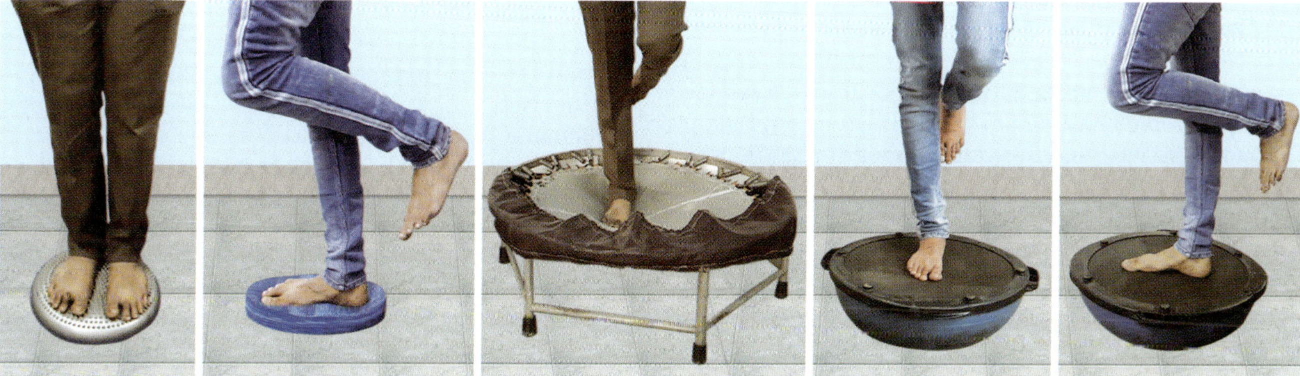

Fig. 23.22: Balance training.

- Endurance and agility exercises: After the pain reduces significantly, patient can be trained for improving agility and endurance as per the individual's functional requirement and age.

Surgical Management

For ankle sprains surgery is generally rare and is only required when conservative treatment fails and prolonged persistent ankle instability is present.

Surgical options may include: Watson–Jones modified operation/Chrisman and Snooks operation/Brostrom operation to repair lateral ligaments, and deltoid ligament repair for medial ankle instability are often suggested. Postoperative physiotherapy and rehabilitation follow the similar guidelines as discussed during the postoperative management of chronic ankle instability (CAI).

Prevention

Prevention of ankle sprains is possible by maintaining good muscle strength, balance, and flexibility at ankle joint. In addition, proper warm up before exercise and sports aids in reducing the risk of injury; elderly people should be careful when walking, running, or working on uneven surfaces; reduction of bodyweight, etc. also have been found effective.

CHRONIC ANKLE INSTABILITY

Introduction

Ankle sprain is reported to be among the most common recurrent injuries. Ankle sprain is a common athletic injury and about 20% of acute ankle sprain patients develop chronic ankle instability (CAI). Lateral ankle sprain affects the ATFL, the CFL, and/or the posterior talofibular ligament. Medial ankle sprain is not that common as the deltoid ligament is the strongest ligament in ankle and the assessment and management are the same as that of lateral ankle sprain. Following an acute ankle sprain deficits in postural control, proprioception, muscle reaction time, and strength typically occur which can lead to **CAI**. Chronic ankle sprain/instability is a continuation from the original impairments developed during the initial stages of acute ankle sprain.

CAI can be functional or mechanical in nature.
1. Functional instability depends on the patient-generated reports or complaints that could be accompanied by clinical laxity.
2. Mechanical instability can be identified by physical examination.

Etiology

Etiology includes:
- Chronic ankle sprain that did not heal completely.
- Recurrent ankle sprain within 6 months.
- The main cause of CAI is no accurate management of acute ankle sprain that may lead to CAI.

Clinical Features

Clinical features include:
- Sensation of instability at ankle due to medial, lateral, or multidirectional instability.
- Decreased proprioceptive abilities because of a loss of mechanoreceptors.
- Decreased strength of ankle invertor and evertor muscles.
- Postural control deficits
- Gait disturbances
- Balance deficits

Investigations/Diagnosis

Investigations/diagnosis includes:
- A complete clinical and physical assessment of the ankle is of utmost importance
- History of recurrent ankle sprain after an acute ankle sprain, of which grade and how it was managed, conservatively or surgically
- Patient self-reported functional ankle instability during his/her activities of daily livings (ADLs)
- Is the instability caused by postural control deficits, neuromuscular deficits, muscle weakness of ankle, and proprioceptive deficits?
- Positive anterior drawer test and talar tilt test
- Star excursion balance test in athletic individuals
- MRI is most useful for CAI. Ligament injury can be seen on MRI as swelling, discontinuity of fiber, a lax or wavy ligament, or nonvisualization.

Management

Physiotherapy Management

If management of acute ankle sprain is not done properly or not enough time is given for the ligament to heal, it may lead to CAI.

After assessing the individual, the presence of functional impairments are determined and treated:
- Strengthening of ankle musculature, i.e., invertors, evertors, plantarflexors, and dorsiflexors with resistance or therabands in long sitting open-chain exercises.
- Balance squat, lunges, and dorsiflexion and plantar flexion performed by weight bearing while standing on the Bosu ball. Time is maintained at 30 seconds per set, during which isometric training is done.
- 5-minute set of sensory-targeted ankle rehabilitation strategies (STARS) treatments consisting of calf stretching, plantar massage, ankle-joint mobilizations, and ankle-joint traction before each home balance-training protocol session—3 days/week, 20 min/session.
- Lace up ankle brace, aircast ankle brace
- Gait training

Four-week rehabilitation physiotherapy protocol followed by Donovan L et al. for 4 weeks is described below:
- **Range of motion exercises:** If joint play at talocrural, distal tibiofibular, proximal tibiofibular, or calcaneocuboid joints is a cause of restricted ROM

then, grade 2–3 Maitland's joint mobilization for 2 minutes can be given to improve range, dynamic balance, and self-reported function at ankle joint in patients with CAI as suggested by Hoch et al.

Active ankle and toe ROM exercises along with seated towel stretches and standing stretches to stretch calf, with the knee straight and bent.

- **Strengthening exercises:** Double-legged heel raises **(Fig. 23.23)**, double-legged forefoot raises, four-way manual ankle resistance, and D1 and D2 proprioceptive neuromuscular facilitation patterns for lower limbs may be helpful, four-way walks [walk on heels, toes **(Fig. 23.24)**, medial aspect, and lateral aspect of the foot at least for 10 minutes], single-leg heel raises **(Fig. 23.25)** and toe raises, and short foot exercises (SFEs), i.e., patients can pull the head of the first metatarsal to the calcaneus; theraband exercises to improve isometric and isotonic strength, etc., initially with less repetitions and later may increase repetitions.

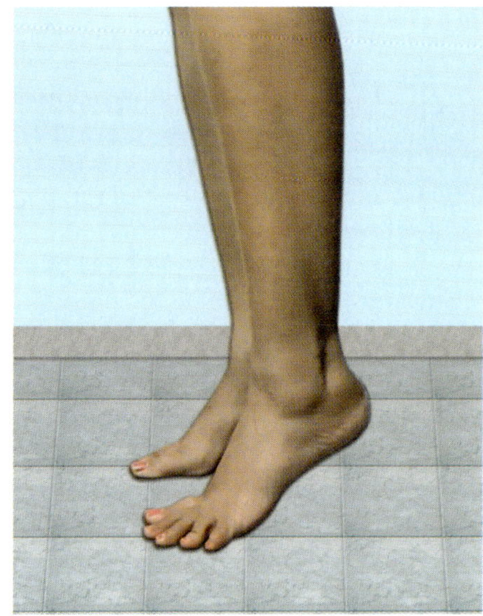

Fig. 23.23: Double-legged heel raise.

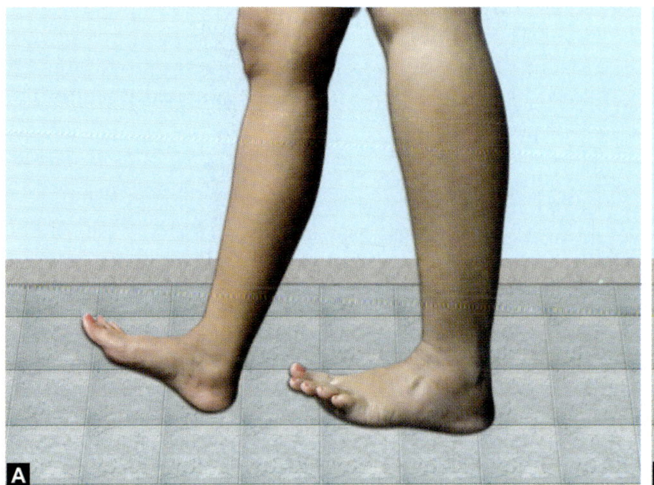

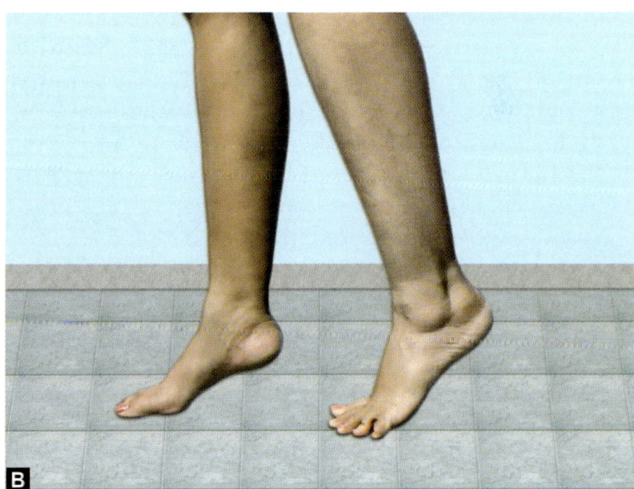

Figs. 23.24A and B: Walking on: (A) Heels; (B) Toes.

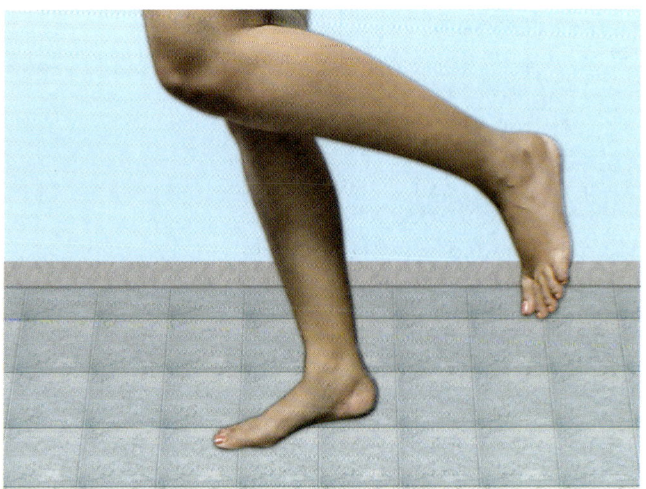

Fig. 23.25: One-legged heel raise.

- **Balance exercises:** As suggested by McKeon et al., balance exercises can be performed with eyes-open static, eyes-closed static, approaching tasks, hop to stabilization with and without foam, or unstable surface, etc.
- **Neuromuscular control:**
  - Single-limb stance with eyes open progress to closed, increasing time, and adding perturbations
  - Both single-limb stance once at a time—ball toss with increasing number of repetitions time, from stable to unstable surface
  - Single-limb stance kicking the medicine ball with increasing weight, resistance, and reps
  - Step-downs with single limb with proper support (railing) in all four directions.

- **Functional exercises:** Lunges, step-ups and step-downs, forward and backward running, zigzag walking, figure of 8 walking, jumps at place, jumping jacks followed by gait-training exercises.
- **Treadmill walking:** Treadmill walking as a part of functional training exercises advised for at least 15–30 minutes at self-selected speed.

Surgical Management

When patients with CAI fail to improve through a conservative management course and physical therapy, surgery is indicated.

- Anatomic direct repair, anatomic reconstruction with an autograft or allograft, and arthroscopic repair
- Primary repair: (1) identification and suturing of the torn ligament and (2) end-to-end repair on tension
- Ahlgren–Larsson technique: (1) augmentation by nearby fascia and (2) interosseous suture
- Augmentation by peroneal brevis flap: (1) Watson-Jones, (2) Evans, (3) Chrisman–Snook, and (4) Colville.

Postsurgically, rehabilitation stage is focused on improving ROM, strength, neuromuscular and proprioceptive balance, altered gait pattern. The physiotherapist can follow the guidelines as described above with proper precautions. The progression to next level of exercises should be based upon the level of stability achieved. Weight-bearing exercises should be started after the recommendation of the surgeon only.

ACHILLES TENDINITIS

Introduction

Achilles tendinitis (**Fig. 23.26**) is a soft tissue injury condition in which chronic irritation and inflammation of TA occur in athletes or nonathletes. TA is a continuation of calf muscles mainly active in basic functional activities, such as walking, stair climbing, running, and jumping. As it is involved in various functional tasks, it is more prone to develop inflammation or degeneration due to overuse. Achilles tendinitis can be an inflammation of TA at its insertion (insertional Achilles tendinitis) that occurs at any age; or inflammation of more proximal middle fibers (noninsertional Achilles tendinitis) that occurs in young active adult athletes, such as long-distance runners, football, volleyball, and tennis players.

Etiology and Pathological Features

Achilles tendinitis is specifically due to repetitive stress on tendon that may be related to sudden increase in intensity of exercise by an athlete or sudden increase in distance of running, overtraining; poor supportive footwear, sudden change of running surface or may be because of overuse of tight tendon without prior stretching or due to increase in friction between the bony spur at the insertion or degeneration of tendon due to aging, etc.

People with diabetes, tight and/or weak calf muscles, low endurance and strength of the calf muscles, poor core muscle strength, reduced ankle mobility, etc., are at risk of developing Achilles tendinitis. Tendinitis is often associated with the microtears in the tendon proximally or at its insertion due to overuse leading to swelling, fibrosis, marked thickening, calcification of tendon at insertion which leads to the formation of heel bony spurs causing chronic inflammation.

Clinical Features

Common clinical symptoms include:

- Pain and stiffness over TA usually more in morning
- Pain at the tendon or backside of heel that aggravates on stressing during various activities
- Swelling may be present throughout the day which worsens with activity
- Difficulty in walking and increased pain over the tendon during toe-off phase of gait cycle
- Tenderness over the site of inflammation along with reduced and painful plantar flexion range.

Investigations

X-ray can reveal the calcification at insertion or proximally in tendon or the presence of bony spur at its insertion.

Management

Medical Treatment

Medical treatment usually involves nonsteroidal anti-inflammatory drugs (NSAIDs) for reducing pain and swelling. Rarely, hydrocortisone injections in tendon are given.

Physiotherapy Management

Achilles tendinitis can be treated effectively with conservative treatment, may require a long duration of up to 3–6 months for complete relief.

- **Rest and support:** Reduce the activities that provoke pain, shift from high impact activities to low impact activities. The use of shoe having soft edge at the heel

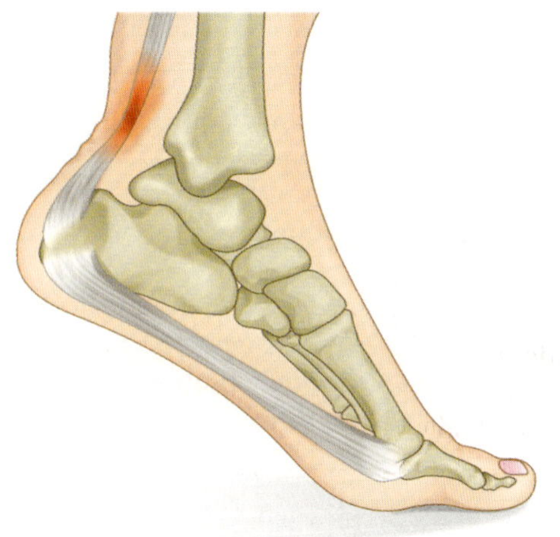

Fig. 23.26: Achilles tendinitis.

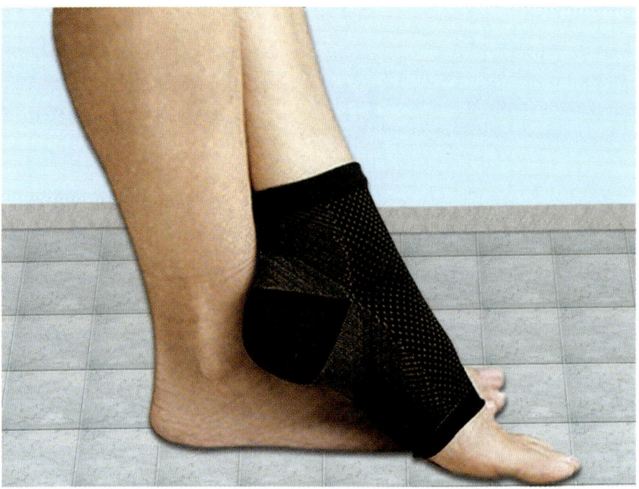

Fig. 23.27: Achilles heel sleeve.

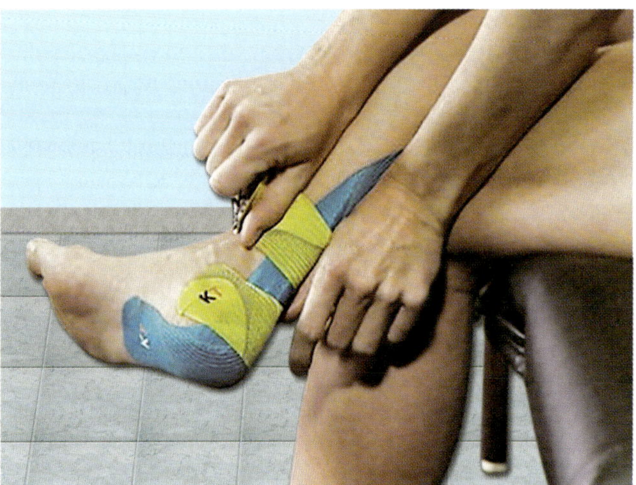

Fig. 23.28: Kinesio taping for Achilles tendinitis.

or soft heel cups or Achilles heel sleeve **(Fig. 23.27)** or Kinesio taping **(Fig. 23.28)** would reduce the irritation of TA tendon with shoe.

- **Cryotherapy:** 20 minutes of icing with ice packs over the painful area 4–5 times in a day to reduce swelling and pain.
- **Electrotherapy modality:** Ultrasound/LASER would help to reduce inflammation and promote healing. Extracorporeal shock wave therapy has satisfactory effects in Achilles tendinitis.
- **Exercise:** Active exercises of ankle followed by mild stretching of calf and soleus muscle. Foam rolling to stretch the calf muscles may be tried.
- Eccentric strengthening exercise for calf muscles may include bilateral or unilateral heel drop from higher step initially with knees extended; progressed to knees slightly flexed. Isometrics to calf muscles can be preferred before eccentric exercises. Eccentric exercises increase stress on tendon gradually to reduce swelling and pain. Eccentric exercise program may aggravate pain but it should not be intolerable for patient. The pain subsides as rehabilitation continues.

RHEUMATOID ARTHRITIS IN ANKLE JOINT

Introduction

Rheumatoid arthritis (RA) is an autoimmune, chronic inflammatory systemic disease of an unknown etiology affecting the synovial lining of joints as well as other connective tissues and joints becomes inflamed. This gradually destructs the joint. Commonly, it starts involving smaller joints of the hands and feet bilaterally and large joints may get involved later. In most of the patients with RA, ankle and foot get involved as the disease progresses.

Predisposing Factors

Predisposing factors include:
- Genetic predisposition (HLA-DR4 present in 70% of the patients)
- Infection
- Autoimmune response

Pathological Features

Rheumatoid arthritis causes an overactivity of the synovium. Therefore the synovium which results in the production of extrasynovial joint fluid. Also, there is swelling and inflammation of the joint. The excess fluid along with the inflammatory chemicals released by the immune system leads to joint destruction as well as destruction of the supportive ligaments and tissues of the joints and therefore deformities, such as claw toe or hammer toe are developed. It may also affect the blood vessels, nerves, and tendons.

Clinical Features

Clinical features include:
- Fever, weight loss, anemia
- Symmetrical joint involvement
- Pain
- Swelling
- Tenderness
- Decreased ROM
- Morning stiffness
- Dislocated toe joints
- Hammer toes, bunions
- Heel pain, TA pain
- Flatfoot
- Ankle pain
- Rheumatoid nodules

As the ankle and foot get involved, patients have:
- Difficulty in walking
- Stair climbing up and down
- Walking on uneven surface becomes painful.

Surgical Option

When conservative management up to 6 months is ineffective, then surgical options, such as gastrocnemius recession or debridement and tendon repair or transfer may be used.

In later stages:

- Flat foot deformity develops due to collapse of medial longitudinal arch due to weakened ligaments in midfoot.
- Deformities, such as hallux valgus (bunions), claw toes, hammer toe, and metatarsalgia are usually associated with RA.

Investigations

Investigations include:

- X-rays: Show marked joint destruction due to sclerosis, reduced joint space or deformity, etc.
- Computerized tomography (CT) scan or MRI scan: May be required to observe the status of ligaments and soft tissues around joint
- Ultrasonography (USG)

Management

Medical Management

Medical management includes:

- Analgesics/antiinflammatory drugs—NSAIDs
- Disease modifying antirheumatic drugs, e.g., sulfasalazine, methotrexate, and d-penicillamine
- Immunosuppressants (they have serious side effects), e.g., cyclophosphamide, azathioprine
- Corticosteroids, e.g., prednisolone.

Surgical Management

The most common surgery done in RA is "fusion"/arthrodesis.

Physiotherapy Management

Physiotherapy management is as follows:

- Rest: Stopping activities that aggravate pain.
- Swimming, static cycling, and other exercises that minimize the load placed on the foot may be done to maintain physical conditioning.
- Ice: For 20 minutes to reduce the acute pain and inflammation.
- Orthotics: They help to reduce the pain and prevent deformities and callous formation, e.g., shoe inserts and braces, such as lace-up ankle braces to provide stability.
- Transcutaneous electrical nerve stimulation can be used to reduce pain (**Fig. 23.29**).
- To minimize joint stiffness and maintain available ROM, AROM, PROM, or active-assisted ROM exercises as tolerated are given.
- Gentle joint mobilization techniques using grade I and grade II oscillations may be used to reduce pain and maintain the joint play.
- Joint protection and energy conservation techniques must be taught to the patient, e.g., alternate activities to avoid fatigue, increase rest during flare period of the disease, avoid deforming positions for prolonged time, frequently change of positions, every 20–30 minutes.

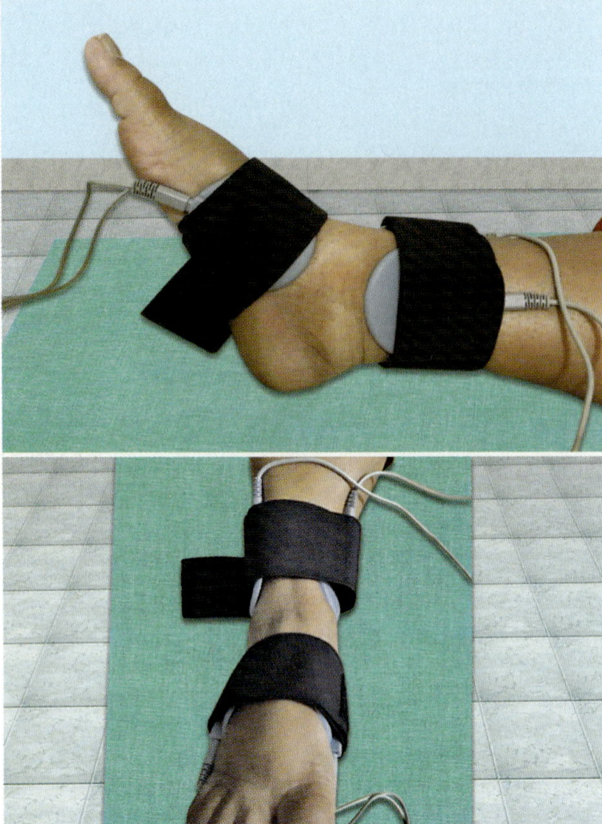

Fig. 23.29: Transcutaneous electrical nerve stimulation for ankle joint rheumatoid arthritis.

- Balneotherapy (mineral bath) is a therapy in which Spa bath with mineral water or thermal waters containing substances, such as sulfur, radon, and carbon dioxide are used. Systematic review carried out by Verhagen AP et al., concluded that balneotherapy is not more beneficial than no treatment in patients with RA.

GOUTY ARTHRITIS IN ANKLE JOINT

Introduction

Gout is a form of an inflammatory arthritis caused by the build-up of uric acid crystals in the joints or its surrounding tissues. The joint of the great toe is the most commonly affected joint. However, the disease also affects the joints, such as foot, ankle, knee, hand, and elbow joints.

Risk Factors and Etiology

Risk factors and etiology include:

- Age and gender—males in the age range from 30 to 45 years
- Obesity
- High alcohol intake
- Positive family history

- High intake of foods rich in purines (e.g., some seafoods and meats)
- Use of diuretics in kidney or heart diseases
- Long-standing kidney disease
- Metabolic syndromes, such as diabetes and heart diseases.

Pathological Features

The monosodium urate crystals are formed as a result of metabolic changes, such as increase or decrease in the sodium urate level or as a result of mechanical trauma. These crystals are then deposited into the joint space or the tissues that lead to an inflammatory response which causes an acute attack of gouty arthritis. After the acute attack, the symptoms of gouty arthritis may disappear, but the crystals (microtophi in the synovium) still persist in the joint along with low-grade inflammation. Hence, the disease may progress or may appear as acute exacerbation.

Persistent inflammation and crystals in the joint may lead to joint destruction. Clinically, the disease may start with asymptomatic hyperuricemia, acute flares of arthritis, intercritical gout, and if hyperuricemia is untreated, it may lead to advanced gout leading to chronic gouty arthritis, tophi formation, and joint destruction.

Clinical Features

Clinical features include:
- Severe night pain in big toe along with the signs of inflammation—calor (heat), dolor (pain), rubor (redness), tumor (swelling) at the ankle joint
- Stiffness at ankle joint may lead to reduced ROM
- Sometimes subcutaneous nodules dorsal aspect of foot.

Investigations

Investigations include:
- X-rays may show joint destruction along with tophi formation **(Fig. 23.30)**
- Joint fluid test—presence of white blood cells may contain uric acid crystals

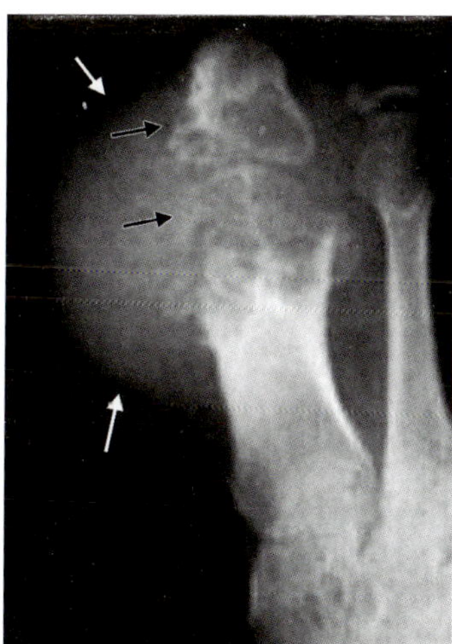
Fig. 23.30: Radiographic changes in gout.

- Blood test—high uric acid levels
- Dual-energy CT scan

Assessment

Subjective history should include the family history, dietary habits and history of alcohol consumption, onset, pain assessment, area of current symptoms, diurnal variations, aggravating and relieving factors, etc. Physical examination includes observation of redness, swelling, deformities, and gait; joint examination include site of tenderness, AROM, PROM, end feels, accessory movements if it is chronic case, muscle strength and endurance, gait assessment, etc.

Management

Medical Management

Medical management includes:
- NSAIDs, such as indomethacin, naproxen, and fenoprofen are the preferred choice of drugs.
- Colchicine is the second choice of drug.
- Oral prednisolone
- Intra-articular corticosteroids may be given when medium or large joints are involved.
- Probenecid or febuxostat are often used to reduce uric acid levels

Surgical Management

In case of severe deformity and pain in joint require surgical removal of tophi, Joint arthrodesis or even Joint arthroplasty.

Lifestyle Modifications

Following changes may prevent frequent gout attacks:
- Exercise regularly to maintain joint mobility and bodyweight.
- Drink plenty of water
- Avoid alcoholic drinks
- Avoiding meat and seafoods

Physiotherapy Management

Physiotherapy management guidelines of RA can be followed for treatment of gouty arthritis also.

FOOT DROP

Introduction

Foot drop refers to a flaccid, paralytic condition involving the dorsiflexor muscles of ankle which may result in difficulty while walking due to involvement CPN. CPN divides into deep and superficial peroneal nerves that provide sensory and motor innervation to the lower limb. Therefore both sensory and motor symptoms are generally present after the CPN palsy. Usually, paralysis of tibialis anterior, extensor hallucis longus, extensor digitorum longus, extensor digitorum brevis and peroneus longus, brevis, and tertius muscles are present.

Etiology

Etiology includes:

- Direct traumatic injury to CPN secondary to fracture of neck of fibula
- Compression of the nerve by tight bandaging or plaster or a splint in lower leg
- Involvement of CPN in leprosy or Hansen's disease
- Various neurological conditions involving muscular deficiency, such as poliomyelitis, cerebral palsy, stroke, multiple sclerosis, amyotrophic lateral sclerosis, Charcot–Marie-Tooth disease
- Tibialis anterior muscle strain; TA rupture
- Lower motor lesion (severe cases of prolapsed intervertebral disk (PIVD)/lumbar canal stenosis) affecting CPN
- Lumbar myelopathy

Clinical Features

Clinical features include:

- Loss or reduced sensation over lateral aspect of knee in proximal third of the calf, posterolateral aspect of the calf and over the lateral malleolus, lateral aspect of foot, and fourth and fifth toes (hypoesthesia)
- Abnormal sensations (paresthesia), such as tingling and numbness on the dorsal aspect of foot and ankle or lower leg
- Inability to dorsiflex in nonweight bearing (NWB) position and during heel strike phase
- Dragging of foot while walking, i.e., reduced ability or inability to produce toe clearance in the swing phase due to reduced strength of ankle and foot dorsiflexor muscles (high steppage gait for compensating dorsiflexion).

Investigations

Electrophysiological studies are required for accurate diagnosis. Electromyographic findings of dorsiflexors show spontaneous activity and represent neurogenic picture. CPN conduction velocity findings may show reduced conduction velocity or conduction block in CPN.

Management

Medical and Surgical Management

- If drop foot is caused by myotomal weakness in lumbar radiculopathy, treatment may involve lumbar nerve root decompression especially L4 nerve root.
- Secondary to neurotmesis injury, the following surgical options can be considered:
  - Internal/external neurolysis
  - Nerve repair, end-to-end repair: Epineural/fascicular, neurotization using intercostal nerve/accessory nerve/cervical plexus within 1 year
  - Partial neurorrhaphy
  - Complete neurorrhaphy with suture, or
  - Autogenous nerve grafting (often with the sural nerve)

- Tendon transfer surgery using tibialis posterior muscle tendon as a substitute to dorsiflexors.
- Sometimes, TA lengthening is required for gaining dorsiflexion in the ankle joint.

Physiotherapy Management

Physiotherapy management is as follows:

- To achieve the functional position, to support the foot and to prevent equinovarus deformity of the ankle: Ankle foot orthosis with dorsiflexion stop at ankle neutral position.
- To maintain the properties of the denervated muscles: Stimulation of the paralyzed muscles using interrupted galvanic current to ensure a good blood supply and for maintaining muscle properties followed by faradic stimulation or functional electrical stimulation (FES) once the regeneration and muscle activity starts.
- To maintain ROM of joints: Passive ROM exercises with end range stretch to maintain muscle length and flexibility of dorsiflexor and plantar-flexion motion followed by active assisted and active exercises as per the recovery.
- To maintain the skin texture: The skin should be kept moisturized to prevent skin tropic skin changes.
- To prevent external infection and wounds: Soft shoes with preferably toe windows should be worn to avoid wounds. Skin of the foot should be kept dry. Proper hygienic measures should be taken for infection prevention.
- Total period of immobilization after surgical management is around 6 weeks in splint and after immobilization—gradually ROM exercises along with muscle strengthening exercises and FES would be beneficial.
- Re-education of transferred tendons after the period of nonweight bearing, faradic stimulation is preferred in initial stages to train the transferred muscle for its new action. Electromyography (EMG) biofeedback technique is found to be a facilitator for faster re-education. During nonweight-bearing phase, strengthening can be started in open-chain positions using manual resistance, weights, and therabands. Weight-bearing training can be done on a weighing scale as a visual cue and patient is trained from partial to full weight bearing as indicated by surgeon. Later, gait training can be started in parallel bars, on even ground, uneven ground, and stairs.
- Proprioceptive training can be started on wobble board or Swiss ball.

TARSAL TUNNEL SYNDROME

Introduction

Tarsal tunnel syndrome (TTS) is a condition of compression or entrapment neuropathy in which the tibial nerve gets compressed under the flexor retinaculum when it passes through the tarsal tunnel. The tarsal tunnel is a narrow fibro-osseous space that is present behind and inferior to the medial malleolus. The medial wall of the tarsal tunnel is formed by flexor retinaculum and forms the lower and upper margin of the tunnel. The medial surface of talus and calcaneus along with distal medial surface of tibia forms the bottom of tunnel. The medial malleolus lies in front of the tunnel. Tendons of the posterior tibialis, flexor digitorum longus, and flexor hallucis longus, posterior tibial artery and vein, as well as posterior tibial nerve (L4-S3), pass through tarsal tunnel.

Etiology

Tarsal tunnel syndrome is divided into intrinsic and extrinsic etiologies:

- Extrinsic factors include poorly fitted shoes, trauma to ankle, biomechanical abnormalities valgus/varus foot deformity, postoperative hypertrophied scarring, and generalized lower limb edema.
- Intrinsic causes include tendinopathy, tenosynovitis, perineural fibrosis, osteophytes formation in ankle, tightened retinaculum, and space-occupying lesion, and nerve ischemia due to arterial insufficiency.

Pathological Features

Compression of the posterior tibial nerve or one of its two branches, the lateral or medial plantar nerve (neuropraxia) within the tarsal tunnel leads to TTS. It is common in patients having previous history of trauma or ankle sprains.

Clinical Features

Clinical features include:

- Tingling/paresthesia sensations (hyperesthesia or dysesthesia) sometimes associated with numbness in ankle and foot region
- Plantar heel pain—shooting pain that worsens as the day progresses
- Aggravated by weight-bearing activities, such as standing or walking.

Investigations

Investigations include:

- The Valleix phenomenon (symptoms may radiate proximally up to lower leg) when tapping the entrapped nerve.
- Positive Tinel sign, triple compression stress test.
- Plain radiographs of the ankle and foot—osteophytes, hindfoot varus and valgus, tarsal coalition, or evidence of fracture.
- EMG and nerve conduction velocity findings may include distal motor latencies of 7.0 ms or more, prolonged sensory latencies of more than 2.3 ms, sensory action potential more likely to be abnormal than motor, decreased amplitude of motor action potentials of abductor hallucis or abductor digiti minimi.

Management

Medical Management

Medical management includes:

- Antiinflammatory drugs, vitamin B-complex supplements
- Corticosteroid injections if required.

Surgical Management

Surgery is indicated when conservative management fails or when the exact cause of entrapment is confirmed.

- Removal of space-occupying lesion
- Surgical release of the flexor retinaculum from its proximal attachment near the medial malleolus for surgical decompression tibial nerve and its branches or release of the deep fascia of the abductor hallucis muscle.

Physiotherapy Management

Goals are to reduce pain, swelling, and increase flexibility of soft tissue structures.

- Treatment generally involves cryotherapy or contrast bath in acute stage, ultrasound therapy to reduce inflammation, plantar arch taping to maintain medial longitudinal arch, University of California Berkeley Laboratory (UCBL) orthosis, calf stretching, soft tissue release of plantar fascia; neural tissue mobilization using SLUMP test or tibial nerve glide progression (foot everted and dorsiflexed) to improve nerve mobility, tibialis posterior strengthening in subacute stage—weight-bearing exercises balance/proprioceptive training in late stages of TTS.
- The therapist should educate the importance of appropriate footwear to avoid tight-fitting shoes.

SUMMARY

The ankle joint forms one of the most important joints of the body since it bears the stress of the whole body along with bearing stresses related to ambulation, running, uneven terrains, etc. The ankle and foot form a complex amalgamation of various joints that allow locomotion possible. Due to its complexity and the amount of load it bears, the ankle is vulnerable to various injuries. Improper biomechanics, improper footwear, muscle imbalances, and poor ergonomics lead to recurrent injuries in the ankle and foot complex. Pain and swelling are the most common and important clinical features. Swelling surrounding the ankle joint is a difficult challenge for the treating professional. Management is essentially conservative, including pharmacological and physiotherapy management. Pharmacological management is based on the use of NSAIDs and analgesics along with supplements. Physiotherapy management includes ultrasound therapy, cryotherapy, iontophoresis, strengthening exercises, and proprioceptive training. Static and dynamic balance training are vital to the physiotherapy regime to avoid recurrent injuries. Lifestyle modification, use of orthoses, and appropriate footwear should be advised to the patient to avail long-term benefits and reduce chronic instability.

Case Scenario

CASE STUDY

A 16-year-old athlete at a local sports club ground sustained a massive inversion twist at his left ankle (landed foot) while kicking a football with his right limb. Pain and swelling occurred immediately after injury over anterolateral aspect of ankle. The pain was sharp shooting in nature and aggravated with ankle–toe movements. He was having difficulty in weight bearing on his left ankle. He followed rest for 2 days. On the third day as the pain (VAS-8) did not subside, he went to an orthopedician and got a radiograph. No fracture was detected. He is presently on anti-inflammatory drugs and referred for physiotherapy.

Physical Assessment

Physical assessment is as follows:

Local examination: Mild swelling and redness along with Grade 2 tenderness was elicited at lateral joint line over the anterior edge of the fibula.

Posture examination: Standing with partial weight bearing on left side with foot slightly inverted and plantar flexed. No other significant deviations were observed.

Range of motion: All motions at ankle and subtalar joint are restricted due to pain.

Joint play: Slight hypermobile (Grade 4) anteroposterior glide at ankle.

Muscle strength: Reduced strength of ankle muscles and resisted isometrics were weak and painful.

For swelling: Figure-of-eight measurements was done at ankle and a difference of 4.5 cm was recorded.

Gait pattern: Altered gait parameters such as slower gait speed, reduced cadence, reduced step length, reduced swing phase on right side with reduced base of support.

Special tests: Anterior drawer test, talar tilt, external rotation stress test, fibular translation test.

Guiding Questions:

1. State the differential diagnosis for the patient.
2. State the confirmatory diagnosis for the patient.
3. What treatment plan will you formulate for the patient?

Review Questions

1. Describe etiology, pathological features, clinical features, medical treatment of CTEV. Explain the role of physiotherapist in management.
2. Describe physiotherapy management in pes planus deformity.
3. Write a short note on metatarsalgia.
4. Describe the short- and long-term management of ankle sprain.
5. Explain the causes, clinical features, and management of chronic ankle instability.
6. Explain the physiotherapy management for the 20-year-old runner who is recently diagnosed with Achilles tendinitis.
7. Describe the physiotherapy management of a case of foot drop secondary to fracture fibular head.
8. Write a short note on clinical features and etiology of tarsal tunnel syndrome.

BIBLIOGRAPHY

1. Akbari M, Karimi H, Farahini H, et al. Balance problems after unilateral lateral ankle sprains. J Rehabil Res Dev. 2006;43(7):819-24.
2. Al-Mohrej OA, Al-Kenani NS. Chronic ankle instability: current perspectives. Avicenna J Med. 2016;6(4):103-8.
3. Burcal CJ, Trier AY, Wikstrom EA. Balance training versus balance training with STARS in patients with chronic ankle instability: a randomized controlled trial. J Sport Rehabil. 2017; 26(5):347-57.
4. Cleland JA, Mintken P, McDeviit A, et al. Manual physical therapy and exercise versus supervised home exercise in the management of patients with inversion ankle sprain: a multicenter randomized clinical trial. J Orthop Sports Phys Ther. 2013;43(7):443-55.
5. De Ridder R, Willems TM, Vanrenterghem J, et al. Effect of a home-based balance training protocol on dynamic postural control in subjects with chronic ankle instability. Int J Sports Med. 2015;36:596-602.
6. Dimeglio A, Canavese F. The French functional physical therapy method for the treatment of congenital clubfoot. J Pediatr Orthop B. 2012;21(1):28-39.
7. Donovan L, Hart JM, Saliba SA, et al. Rehabilitation for chronic ankle instability with or without destabilization devices: a randomized controlled trial. J Athl Train. 2016;51(3):233-51.
8. Díaz López AM, Guzmán Carrasco P. Effectiveness of different physical therapy in conservative treatment of plantar fasciitis: systematic review. Rev Esp Salud Publica. 2014;88(1):157-78.
9. Feger M, Donovan L, Hart JM, et al. Effect of ankle braces on lower extremity muscle activation during functional exercises in participants with chronic ankle instability. Int J Sports Phys Ther. 2014;9(4):476-87.
10. Grieve R, Palmer S. Physiotherapy for plantar fasciitis: a UK-wide survey of current practice. Physiotherapy. 2017;103(2):193-200.
11. He J-P, Shao JF, Hao Y. Comparison of different conservative treatments for idiopathic clubfoot: Ponseti's versus non-Ponseti's methods. J Int Med Res. 2017;45(3):1190-99.
12. Hertel J. Functional instability following lateral ankle sprain. Sports Med. 2000;29(5):361-71.
13. Hoch MC, Andreatta RD, Mullineaux DR, et al. Two-week joint mobilization intervention improves self-reported function, range of motion, and dynamic balance in those with chronic ankle instability. J Orthop Res. 2012;30(11):1798-804.
14. Hong CH, Lee YK, Won SH, et al. Tarsal tunnel syndrome caused by an uncommon ossicle of the talus: a case report. Medicine (Baltimore). 2018;97(25):e11008.
15. Ju S-B, Park GD, Effects of the application of ankle functional rehabilitation exercise on the ankle joint functional movement screen and isokinetic muscular function in patients with chronic ankle sprain. J Phys Ther Sci. 2017;29(2):278-81.
16. Komagamine J. Bilateral Tarsal tunnel syndrome. Am J Med. 2018;131(7):e319.
17. McKeon PO, Ingersoll CD, Kerrigan DC, et al. Balance training improves function and postural control in those with chronic ankle instability. Med Sci Sports Exerc. 2008;40(10):1810-19.
18. Towiwat P, Chhana A, Dalbeth N. The anatomical pathology of gout: a systematic literature review. BMC Musculoskelet Disord. 2019;20:140.

19. Uematsu D, Suzuki H, Sasaki S, et al. Evidence of validity for Japanese version of foot and ankle ability measure. J Athl Train. 2015;50(1):65-70.

20. van den Akker-Scheek I, Seldentuis A, Reininga IH, et al. Reliability and validity of the Dutch version of the foot and ankle outcome score (FAOS). BMC Musculoskelet Disord. 2013;14:183.

21. Verhagen AP, Bierma-Zeinstra SM, Boers M, et al. Balneotherapy (or spa therapy) for rheumatoid arthritis. Cochrane Database Syst Rev. 2015;(4):CD000518.

22. Vulpiani MC, Trischitta D, Trovato P, et al. Extracorporeal shockwave therapy (ESWT) in Achilles tendinopathy. A long-term follow-up observational study. J Sports Med Phys Fitness. 2009;49(2):171-6.

23. Yates B. Merriman's assessment of the lower limb, 3rd edition. New York: Churchill Livingstone; 2009. ISBN 978-0-08-045107-7.

24. Zuckerman SL, Kerr ZY, Pierpoint L, et al. An 11-year analysis of peripheral nerve injuries in high school sports. Phys Sportsmed. 2019;47(2):167-73.

Arthroplasties

Nipa Shah

LEARNING OBJECTIVES

After reading this chapter, the readers should be able to:

♦ Understand what arthroplasty is
♦ Describe hip arthroplasty and its types
♦ Describe indications, contraindications, and related complications of total hip arthroplasty
♦ Gain knowledge about various surgical approaches with its precautions for hip arthroplasty
♦ Compare advantages and disadvantages of cemented and uncemented prosthesis
♦ Describe the preoperative role of physical therapist and postoperative physiotherapy according to its phases and explain how to progress to next phase of rehabilitation
♦ Describe the guidelines for participation in sport, recreational, and fitness activities following THA
♦ Understand basics of knee arthroplasty, its types, indications and contraindications
♦ Explain in detail about surgical approaches, various implant design, and types of implant fixation of knee arthroplasty
♦ Enlist intraoperative and postoperative complications of knee arthroplasty
♦ Understand exercise precautions following knee arthroplasty
♦ Describe preoperative role of physical therapist and postoperative physiotherapy according to its phases and explain about criteria to progress
♦ Write about recommendations of physical activities for fitness and recreation after knee arthroplasty
♦ Describe shoulder arthroplasty with its types
♦ Give details about indication, surgical procedures, and implant designs of shoulder arthroplasty
♦ Describe detailed rehabilitation following shoulder arthroplasty with precaution to consider in different phases of rehabilitation.

CHAPTER OUTLINE

- Hip arthroplasty
  - Indications for total hip arthroplasty
  - Complications
  - Surgical techniques
  - Physiotherapy management
- Total knee arthroplasty
  - Indications
  - Contraindication
  - Surgical techniques
  - Implant designs
  - Implant fixations
  - Surgical approach
  - Complications
  - Physiotherapy management
- Shoulder arthroplasty
  - Indications for total shoulder arthroplasty
  - Designs of prosthetic implants
  - Operative procedure
  - Postoperative positioning and immobilization

INTRODUCTION

Arthroplasty can be defined as an orthopedic surgical procedure in which a joint's articular surface is realigned or replaced or remodeled. Arthroplasty is usually done to relieve pain and restore function to the joint.

In the last 45 years, the most common form of arthroplasty which is till date used successfully is the surgical replacement of joint surface with prosthesis. Joint replacement surgery is performed most commonly in large joints, such as shoulder, knees, and hip.

The goal of the procedure is pain relief and restoration of normal function and mobility in the damaged joint.

HIP ARTHROPLASTY

Introduction

Hip arthroplasty (or **hip replacement** surgery) involves replacement of the hip joint with prosthetic implant to reduce pain and improve mobility. Total replacement and a hemi (half) replacement are the two ways in which hip replacement surgery **(Fig. 24.1)** can be performed. A total hip replacement (THR) or a total hip arthroplasty (THA) involves replacement of both the acetabulum and the femoral head, whereas in hemiarthroplasty usually only the femoral head is replaced. Hip replacement is currently one of the most common musculoskeletal surgical procedures but satisfaction of the patient, both short- and long-term varies widely.

Indications for Total Hip Arthroplasty

Indications for THA are as follows:
- Osteoarthritis—THA is most commonly performed in joint failure caused by osteoarthritis.
- Other indications include rheumatoid arthritis (RA),
- Traumatic arthritis, protrusio acetabuli, avascular necrosis (AVN),
- Fractures of hip joint
- Bone tumors.
- Arthritis associated with ankylosing spondylitis, Paget's disease, and juvenile RA
- Failure of conservative management or previous joint reconstruction procedure

Contraindications of THA are shown in **Box 24.1**.

Complications

Recent research suggests that 2–10% of patients during and after a THR surgical procedure, tend to develop some sort of complications. The following are the most commonly occurring complications that are observed in the clinical setting:
- **Dislocation:** Though there are lesser chances of dislocation in anterior approach
- **Abductor insufficiency:** Mostly occurs in direct lateral approach
- Prosthetic loosening and implant wear or intraoperative fracture
- Nerve injury (associated with specific surgical approaches):
  - Direct lateral approach—femoral nerve, superior gluteal nerve
  - Direct anterior approach—femoral cutaneous nerve
  - Posterior approach—sciatic nerve
- Infection and/or sepsis of the wound
- Deep-vein thrombosis (DVT) or pulmonary emboli
- Atelectasis and lower respiratory tract infection
- Leg length discrepancy.

> **BOX 24.1:** Contraindications of total hip arthroplasty (THA).
>
> **Relative contraindications:**
> - Absent or relative insufficiency of the abductor musculature
> - Localized infection, especially bladder, skin, chest, or other local regions
> - Any kind of neurological deficit which is progressive in nature
> - Any process causing rapid bone destruction
> - Patients requiring extensive dental or urologic procedures, such as transurethral resection of the prostate, should have performed this before total joint replacement
>
> **Absolute contraindications:**
> - Active infection in the joint
> - Infection or sepsis that is systemic in nature
> - Neuropathic hip joint
> - Malignant tumors that may not allow adequate fixation of the components
> - Severe paralysis of the muscle surrounding the joint

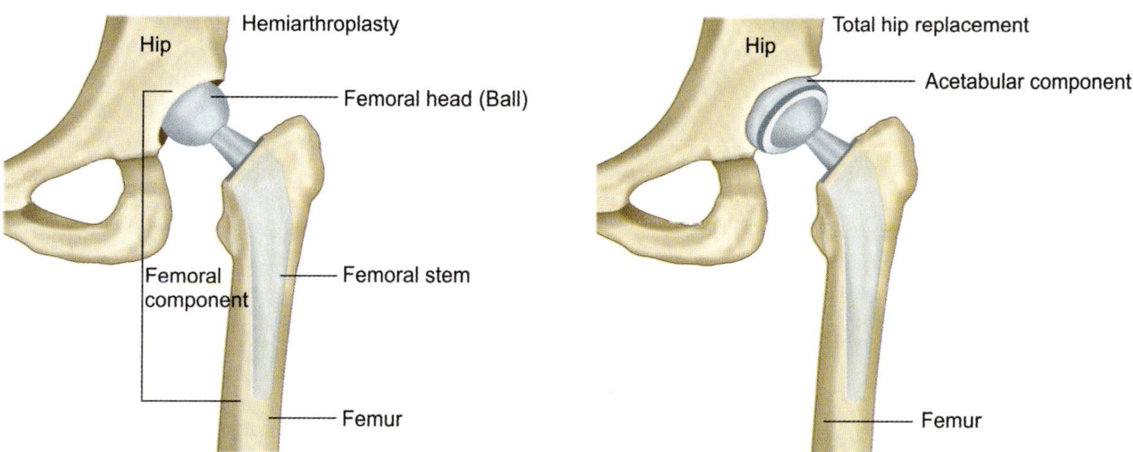

Fig. 24.1: Hemiarthroplasty and total arthroplasty.

Surgical Techniques

Surgical Approaches

There are several surgical approaches for THR **(Fig. 24.2)**, but commonly used approaches—anterior, lateral, and posterior—are described with the major precautions following THA **(Box 24.2)**.

Posterior approach surgery is the most common approach used for THR surgery. This method has the major advantage that it spares the abductor muscle group and it also provides good visualization of the femur and acetabulum.

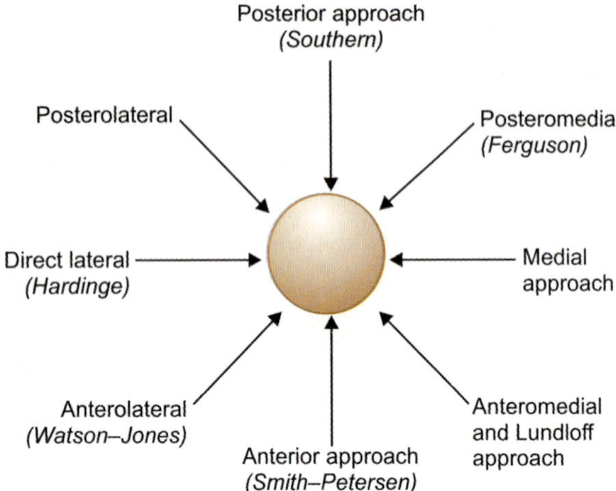

Fig. 24.2: Various approaches for hip arthroplasty.

<table>
<tr><td colspan="1" style="background:#2b7bb9;color:white;text-align:center">BOX 24.2: Precautions following THA.</td></tr>
</table>

Posterior/posterolateral approaches:

Range of motion (ROM): Avoid hip flexion >90°, adduction, internal rotation

Activities of daily living (ADLs):
- Do not cross legs or feet
- Transfer to the unaffected side from bed to chair or chair to bed
- Avoid sleeping and resting in side lying position, and in supine position an abduction pillow must be used
- In standing, do not twist the upper body
- Sleep in supine lying only for the first 6 weeks
- Avoid sitting in low, soft chairs or stools
- Use a raised toilet seat
- Use some forms of aids while putting on socks/shoes ,underwear for first 6 weeks to avoid excessive hip flexion.

Anterior approach

ROM:
- Avoid flexion at the hip >90°.
- Avoid hip extension, external rotation, and adduction.
- Do not perform active, antigravity hip abduction for at least 6–8 weeks if the gluteal medius was incised and repaired, or trochanteric osteotomy was done

ADL
- Do not cross legs
- Never step back to avoid hyperextension
- Use a pillow between legs when rolling
- Sleep on surgical side when side lying

Direct anterior approach surgery has the benefit of being less invasive and damaging for muscles, capsules, ligaments, and nerves. Recent research shows that this approach has a better rehabilitation time and functional outcome. As the direct anterior approach has lowered risk of dislocation in comparison to a posterior approach, the direct anterior approach is indicated in patients with muscle imbalance, such as cerebral palsy or stroke.

Direct lateral approach involves division of tensor fascia lata, vastus lateralis, and gluteus medius. Disruption of the abductor mechanism that is commonly associated with this approach often leads to postoperative weakness and gait abnormalities.

The use of minimally invasive surgery is becoming popular, as it causes:
- Less soft tissue trauma
- Quicker recovery rates
- Reduced postoperative pain.

In minimally invasive procedures, length of incision is defined as ≤10 cm. Long-term follow-up and comparison studies are needed to verify these facts.

> A 2018 survey of the Canadian Arthroplasty Society and American Association of Hip and Knee Surgeons, using an electronic questionnaire format to determine how commonly they prescribed precautions and equipment, reported 44% of surgeons universally prescribing precautions while about one-third never prescribed precautions. The utilization of a posterior approach for the THA was a significant risk factor for implementing postoperative hip precautions.

Materials Used

The articulating prostheses (femoral and acetabular components) are made of any of the following materials:
- Metal-on-polyethylene (PE)
- Metal-on-metal and
- Ceramic-on-ceramic
- Ceramic-on-PE.

Important properties of these prostheses are stability against dislocation and fixation in bone tissue and friction coefficient. In some rare cases, there can be a complication of osteonecrosis which tends to occur due to erosion of the two components rubbing against each other.

- Recent studies have concluded that there is 95% less wear and tear with **vitamin E–infused PE** when compared to other liners.
- One of the most recent advances in hip replacement implants has been the development of **newer PE (plastic)** that lasts much longer and has very low wear rates than conventional PE.
- The newly developed highly **cross-linked PE** plays a significant role. Cross-linked PE created by radiating and reheating the PE implants, allows the plastic to strengthen its molecular structure through a cross-linking process.

Cemented—Uncemented Prosthesis

A **cemented** prosthesis is designed in a way that there is a layer of bone cement which is typically an acrylic polymer called **polymethylmethacrylate (PMMA)**. It lies in between the patient's natural bone and the prosthetic joint component.

A **cementless** prosthesis, which is known as press-**fit prosthesis**, has a rough surface or a porous coating, which encourages the natural bone to grow on it. Some prosthetic components have screws or pegs that help to hold the bone and prostheses in place till the time a new bone growth can create a secure attachment.

Cement fixation is routinely used for patients with osteoporosis and poor bone stock and typically with elderly patients. In contrast to that, cementless fixations are more often the choice for the patients under 60 years of age and those who are physically active and have good bone quality.

Cemented implants are cheaper than the uncemented implants. Better short-term clinical outcomes mainly improved pain and early pain-free full weight-bearing, are obtained from cemented fixation **(Box 24.3)**.

Physiotherapy Management

Preoperative Management

Preoperative management includes the following:

- Assessment of pain, ROM, muscle strength, balance, leg length, ambulatory status, gait, and functional ability.
- Documentation of patient's status as well as patient education about the procedure and postoperative precautions with their rationale including positioning and weight-bearing.

- Exercises and functional training for early postoperative days including bed mobility, transfers, and gait training with assistive devices.

Li Wang, Jessica Moodie, et al. conducted a systematic review and meta-analysis titled—"Does preoperative rehabilitation for patients planning to undergo joint replacement surgery improve outcomes?" They concluded that rehabilitation can help improve the early postoperative pain and function among patients undergoing joint replacement. Though the effects of it remain too small and short-term to be considered clinically important and did not cause any change in the key outcomes of interest (i.e., costs, length of stay, and quality of life).

Postoperative Management

Immobilization

After THA, there is no need for immobilization, but operated limb should remain in position of slight abduction and neutral rotation. Abduction pillow or wedge is sufficient to maintain **(Fig. 24.3)** the position in supine lying.

Weight-Bearing Consideration

After cemented THA—patients are allowed weight-bearing as per tolerance immediately after surgery.

After cementless THA—recommendation varies from partial weight-bearing (toe touch) for almost 6–8 weeks to early weight-bearing.

Factors affecting weight bearing: Weight-bearing will be restricted in following conditions:

- Trochanteric osteotomy
- Use of bone graft
- Poor quality of patient's bone.

BOX 24.3: Advantages and disadvantages of cemented-uncemented prosthesis.	
Cemented	**Cementless**
Advantages	*Advantages*
• Bone cement allows prosthetic joint components fixation to a bone that is porous from osteoporosis	• It is believed that cementless components provide a better long-term bond between the prostheses and bones
• Antibiotic material can be added to the bone cement, which helps reduce the risk of postsurgical infection	• No chance of potential breakdown of cement with cementless components
• It allows early postoperative weight-bearing and reduces the duration of rehabilitation	
Disadvantages	*Disadvantages*
• A breakdown of the cement can cause the artificial joint to become loose, which leads to the requirement for another joint replacement surgery (revision surgery)	• Press-fit prosthesis are useful only in healthy bones. Patients with low bone density due to osteoporosis or other conditions are not eligible for these components
• There can be inflammation due to irritation of the surrounding soft tissue by the cement debris	• It may take 3 or more months for bone material to grow into a new joint component
• Though very rare, but the cement can enter the bloodstream and end up being lodged in the lungs, which can be a life-threatening condition. This risk is greatest for people who undergo spinal surgeries	• Patients need to postpone putting their full weight on new joints as it takes time for the natural bone to fully adhere to the new joint components

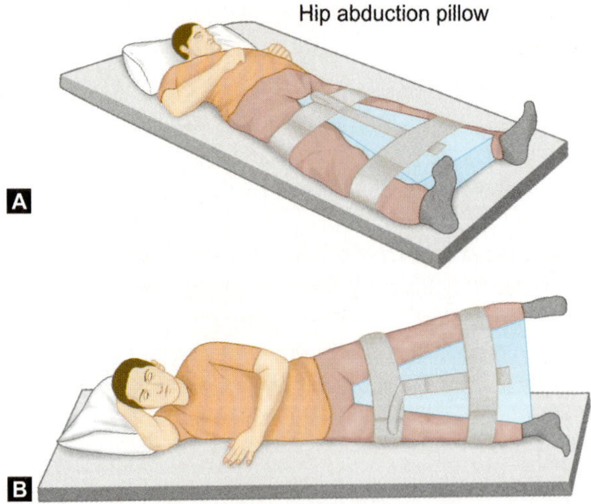

Figs. 24.3A and B: Abduction pillow.

A metaanalysis by Peng Tian, Zhi-jun Li et al. showed that early postoperative full weight-bearing in patients with uncemented THA proves to be safe and did not increase the risk of any complications postoperatively.

Maximum protection phase after traditional THA:
Goals and intervention: After a THR surgery, the early postoperative rehabilitation is done with the aim to restore mobility, strength, flexibility, and reduce pain.

Prevent vascular and pulmonary complication:
- Ankle pumping exercises prevent venous stasis, thrombosis, or pulmonary embolism
- Deep breathing exercise prevent respiratory complication.

Prevent postoperative dislocation of operated hip and achieve functional mobility (**Box 24.2**):
- Educate patient regarding dislocation and weight-bearing.
- Education and proper training to patient for positioning and joint protection strategies.
- Training for bed mobility and transfers including sit–stand.
- Immediately after surgery, ambulation with an assistive device (initially a walker or two crutches) has to be done by adhering to the weight-bearing restrictions and gait-related precautions. Progress to one crutch or a cane depending on pain, strength of hip abductors, and gait symmetry.
- Ascending and descending stairs with an assistive device, initially one step at a time (while ascending stairs, initiate with the sound leg, whereas while descending, lead with the operated leg).

Maintain strength and muscular endurance of upper limbs as well as nonoperated lower limb: Active-resistive exercises in functional movement patterns which target the muscle groups that are used during transfers and ambulation with assistive devices.

Prevent reflex inhibition and atrophy of muscles in the operated extremity: Submaximal muscle-setting exercises for the quadriceps, hip abductor muscles, and hip extensors—just enough to elicit a muscle contraction.

Regain active mobility and control of the extremity that has been operated on (**Figs. 24.4A to F**):
- While in bed:
  - Active-assisted (progressing to active) heel slides
  - Hip abduction/adduction within protected ranges (with a pillow between the thighs to prevent hip adduction past neutral)

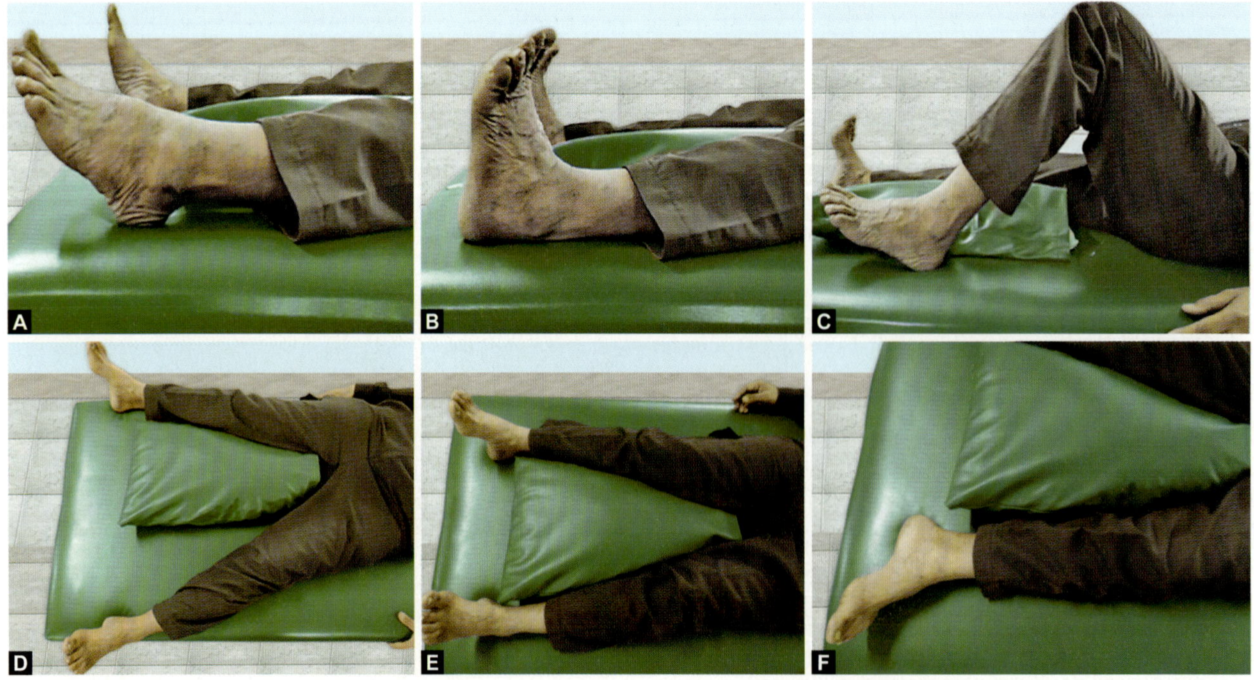

Figs. 24.4A to F: Exercises in bed: (A) Ankle ROM—plantar flexion; (B) Ankle ROM—dorsiflexion; (C) Heel slides; (D) Hip abduction; (E) Hip adduction; (F) Hip external rotation.

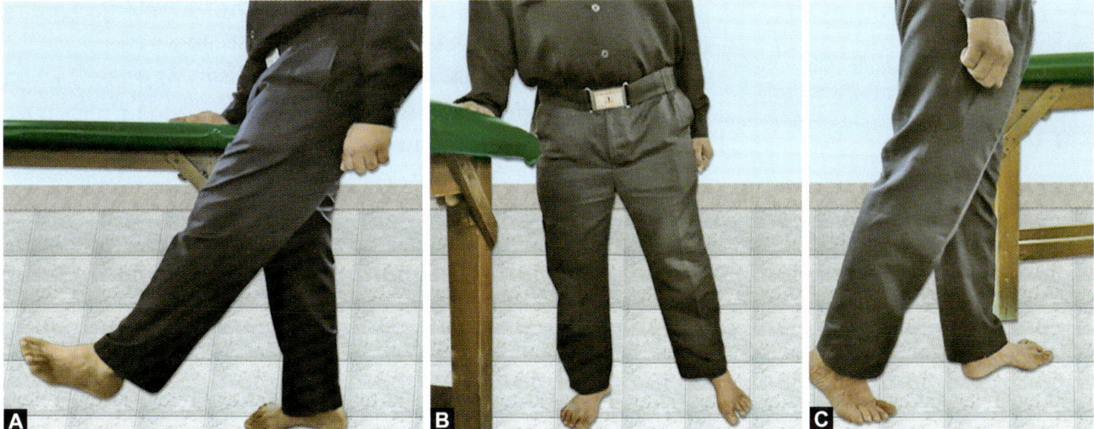

Figs. 24.5A to C: Hip pendular motion.

- Active hip rotation between external rotation (ER) and internal rotation (IR) to neutral depending on the surgical approach.

■ While seated in a chair: Active knee flexion and extension exercises, emphasizing terminal knee extension.

■ In the standing position **(Figs. 24.5A to C)**
  - Active hip ROM (forward and backward pendulum motions) with the knee flexed and extended and hands on a stable surface to maintain balance.
  - Bilateral, closed-chain, weight-shifting balance activities, heel raises, and mini-squats while maintaining symmetrical alignment but placing only the allowable amount of weight on the operated extremity.
  - Hip hiking while bearing the allowable amount of weight on the operated extremity.

Prevent flexion contracture of the operated part: Avoid using a pillow below the knee of the operated side.

Criteria to progress: The criteria to advance to the next phase of rehabilitation are highly dependent on weight-bearing and ROM restrictions; however, the following criteria typically must be met:

■ Well-healed incision with no signs of wound drainage or infection
■ Independent level-ground ambulation with one crutch or a cane or no assistive device if weight-bearing restrictions permit
■ Ability to bear full weight on the operated extremity without pain and with the knee fully extended, i.e., functional ROM of the hip
■ Muscle strength of operated hip: At least 3/5.

Moderate protection phase after traditional THA:

Goals and interventions: Regain muscular endurance and strength, with emphasizes on strengthening of hip abductors and extensors.

Clinical Pearl

Precaution: The initiation and progression of resistance training to strengthen hip abductor muscles are contingent on the integrity of the abductor mechanism.

■ Open-chain exercises of the operated leg while standing on the sound limb against light resistance, within the permissible ROM. To improve muscular endurance, emphasize on increasing the number of repetitions rather than the resistance.

■ Bilateral, closed-chain exercises help strengthen hip and knee extensors. For example, mini-squats against light-grade elastic resistance or holding light weights in both hands when unsupported standing is permitted **(Fig. 24.6)**.

■ Unilateral, closed-chain exercises, such as **(Fig. 24.7)**:
  - Forward as well as lateral step-ups (to a low step).
  - Partial lunges with the operated side foot forward (when full weight-bearing is allowed).
  - During step-ups and lunges, apply elastic resistance around the lateral thigh of the operated extremity to simultaneously strengthen the hip abductors and hip extensors.

■ *Resisted exercises* of other involved areas, as it helps to improve function.

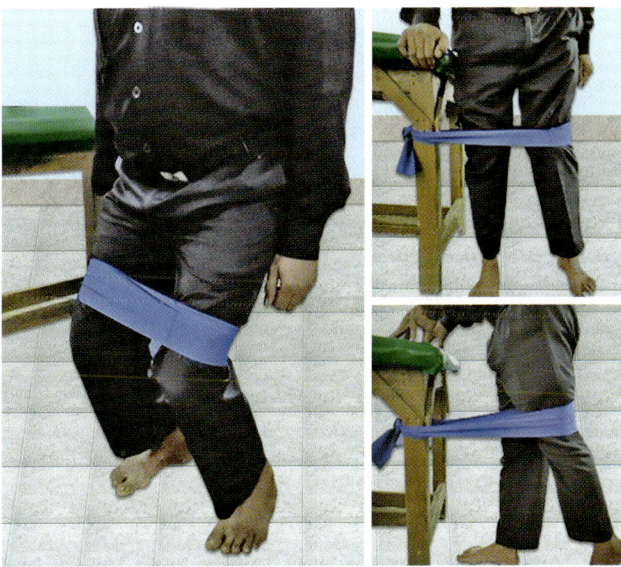

Fig. 24.6: Bilateral, closed-chain, and open-chain resisted exercises.

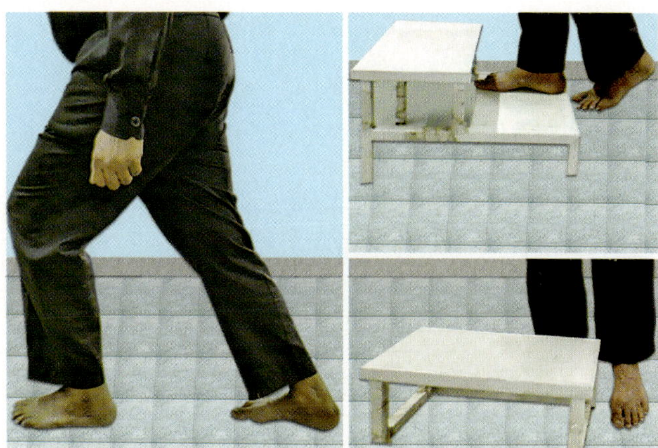

Fig. 24.7: Unilateral closed-chain exercises.

Improve cardiopulmonary endurance: Nonimpact aerobic conditioning program that involve progressive stationary cycling, swimming, or water aerobics can be advised.

Restoration of ROM while adhering to precautions:
- Gravity-assisted supine stretch to neutral in the Thomas test position. The patient is asked to pull the unaffected side knee to the chest while relaxing the operated hip. (at least 10° of hip extension beyond neutral is needed for a normal gait pattern.)
  Precaution: Check with the surgeon particularly if an anterior or anterolateral approach.
- Resting in prone position provides a prolonged passive stretch of the hip flexor muscles.
- Integrate gained ROM into functional activities.

Improve postural stability, balance, and gait:
- Progressive balance training: Activities in standing (weight shifting, lunges). Practice walking on uneven and soft surfaces to challenge the balance system.
- Gait: Continue cane use until weight-bearing restrictions are discontinued or if the patient has a positive Trendelenburg sign, indicating hip abductor weakness. Cane use is also recommended during extended period of ambulation to reduce muscle fatigue. Gait training should be done with proper emphasizes on an erect trunk with proper vertical alignment along with equal step lengths and a neutral symmetrical alignment of the pelvis and extremities.
- For selected patients, consider treadmill walking to practice a symmetrical gait pattern when full weight-bearing is permitted.

Criteria to progress: The criteria to progress to the advanced phase include the following:
- Pain-free ambulation with or without a cane and previous exercises
- Functional ROM and strength of the operated hip
- Independence in ADL.

Minimum protection phase and resumption of full activity after traditional THA: The final phase of rehabilitation begins usually around 12 weeks postoperatively. Returning to full-fledged functional activities may take at least a year.

Extended rehabilitation and modification of activities: Patients, especially those wishing to return to an active lifestyle, may benefit from an extended strength training program that targets the hip musculature that include the following:
- Incorporate strength, endurance, and balance training into simulated functional activities to prepare for independent activities.
- To improve muscular and cardiopulmonary endurance, progressively increase the duration and distance of a low-intensity walking program, 2–4 days a week.
- Through patient education, explain the significance of selecting or modifying activities to reduce the forces and demands that are placed on the prosthetic hip. If a patient's occupation involves heavy labor, vocational retraining, or a modification in work-related activities should also be suggested.

Clinical Pearl

While walking, patient should hold heavy objects on the same side of the operated hip. EMG studies have shown that the forces imposed on the abductor muscles of the operated hip are significantly lower than when the load is carried on the contralateral arm with and without cane usage. Theoretically, this attenuates the stress created on the hip replacement over time.

Leisure and Sport after Total Hip Replacement
Patient can gradually and safely return to low- and moderate-impact sports and fitness activities following THA. Recommendations regarding leisure and sport-related activities after hip replacement surgery are shown in **Table 24.1**. *Note*: These are only guidelines and one should check with a surgeon or other healthcare professional for specific case-related advice.

Accelerated Rehabilitation
Recently, accelerated rehabilitation has become more common particularly for patients under 60–65 years of age who have undergone minimally invasive THA and wish to resume an active lifestyle as quickly as possible following surgery. Although "accelerated rehabilitation" following minimally invasive THA has not been clearly defined, two characteristics stand out
- Exercises start on the day of surgery and discharge of patient day 2 postsurgery.
- A rapid progression to full weight-bearing during ambulation and discontinuing crutch and cane use as soon as possible in the rehabilitation program.

Before discontinuing use of an ambulation aid, it is important to regain sufficient strength of the hip abductors and extensors to maintain stability and symmetry during ambulation. With this in mind, it is clear that an individualized program of strengthening exercises must be an integral component of accelerated rehabilitation.

Table 24.1: Guidelines for participation in sport, recreational, and fitness activities following total hip arthroplasty.

Permitted	Permitted with experience	No consensus	Not recommended
• Road cycling • Brisk walking, swimming • Golf • Hiking • Ballroom dancing, canoeing/kayaking, square dancing • Sailing • Bowling • Water aerobics • Low-impact aerobics • Weight training	• Ice skating • Downhill skiing, cross-country skiing, stationary skiing • (Cross-country ski machine) • Doubles tennis • Pilates • Horseback and riding rowing • Inline skating	• Tai chi • Singles tennis • Volleyball • Handball • Rock climbing	• Jogging • Martial arts • Basketball • Baseball • Football • High-impact aerobics • Squash • Hockey

Source: Consensus guidelines based on a Survey of the Hip Society and American Association of Hip and Knee Surgeons.

TOTAL KNEE ARTHROPLASTY

Introduction

Total knee arthroplasty (TKA) or total knee replacement (TKR) is a widely performed orthopedic surgical procedure **(Fig. 24.8)**. In this, as the name suggests the articular surfaces of the knee joint (the femoral condyles and tibial plateau) are replaced. In about 50% of the cases, the patellar replacement also occurs. Patella replacement may be due to osteolysis, malt racking of the patella, or failure of the implant. Patella replacement is usually performed with the aim to restore the extensor mechanism.

Indications for Surgery

Indications for surgery are as follows:
- Severe knee pain causing functional impairment
- Radiographic evidence of severe arthritis
- A knee condition that has a severe impact on patient's quality of life (QOL) for at least 3–6 months
- Failure of conservative management or a previous surgical procedure.

Contraindications (Box 24.4)

BOX 24.4: Contraindication of total knee arthroplasty.

Absolute
- Joint infection
- Systemic infection or sepsis
- Painful solid knee fusion (usually due to repetitive stress disorders)
- Neuropathic arthropathy

Relative
- Very severe osteoporosis
- Debilitated poor health
- Extensor mechanism that is nonfunctioning
- Significant peripheral vascular disease

Surgical Techniques

Implant Components

Implants are usually composed of ceramic material, metal alloys, or strong plastic parts. Three bone surfaces are replaced in a TKR:

1. **The lower end of the femur**—around the end of femur (thighbone), the metal femoral component is used which curves around the distal surface of femur.
2. **The top surface of the tibia**—the tibial component is a flat metal platform with a cushion of durable and strong plastic, called PE.
3. **The back surface of the patella**—in some cases, the patella does not have to be replaced. The patellar component is a dome-shaped piece of PE, which duplicates the shape of the patella.

Components are designed in a way that metal borders with plastic which gives smoother movement and results in less wear and tear of the implant.

Types of Arthroplasty

The following are the types of arthroplasty according to number of compartment replaced:
- Unicompartmental implant—if only one side of the knee joint is damaged, then only medial or lateral joint surfaces are replaced **(Fig. 24.9B)**.

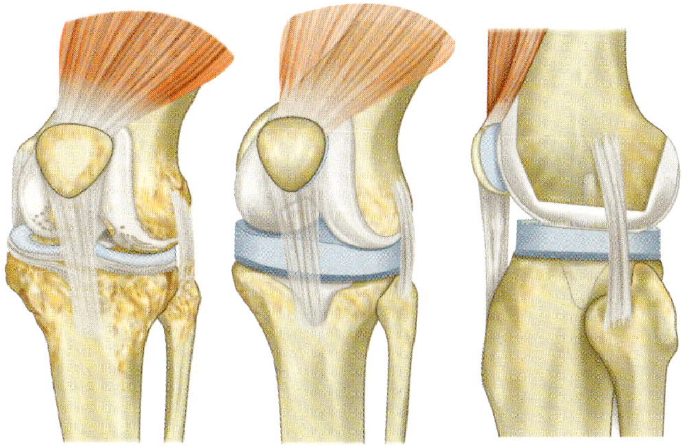

Fig. 24.8: Arthritic knee joint, AP, and lateral view of replaced knee joint.

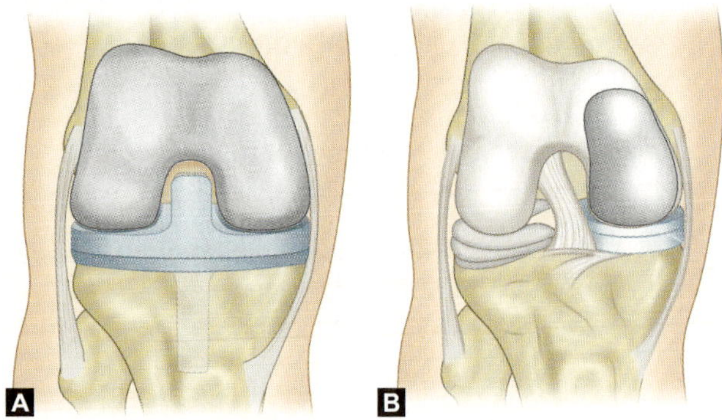

Figs. 24.9A and B: Types of knee arthroplasty:
(A) Total; (B) Unicompartmental.

- Bicompartmental implant—entire tibial and femoral surfaces are replaced.
- Tricompartmental implant—femoral, tibial, and patellar surfaces are replaced **(Fig. 24.9A)**.

Implant Designs

Posterior-stabilized Designs

One of the most commonly used types of implant is a posterior-stabilized component **(Fig. 24.10A)**. In this design, parts of the implant substitute for the posterior cruciate ligament (PCL) because the cruciate ligaments are removed. The tibial component has a raised surface along with an internal post which fits into a special bar (called a cam) in the femoral component. These components work together to perform the function of PCL: Preventing the thighbone from sliding forward too far on the tibia during knee flexion.

Cruciate-retaining Design

As the name suggests, the PCL is kept intact with this implant design (the anterior cruciate ligament is removed) **(Fig. 24.10B)**. For patients whose PCL is strong enough to continue stabilizing the knee joint, this implant proves to be appropriate.

Bicruciate-retaining Designs

Bicruciate-retaining components are relatively new in the market. The anterior cruciate ligament and PCL remain intact in this design. In this type of design, by saving both ligaments, the knee will function and feel like a nonreplaced knee. There still isn't enough evidence that demonstrates the pros and cons of this design.

Fixed- versus Mobile-Bearing Implant Designs

- Mobile-bearing implants **(Fig. 24.10C)**—a mobile-bearing knee has a rotating platform which is made up of PE. It is inserted between the femoral and tibial components. The top surface is congruent with the femoral implant (round-on-round articulation). The undersurface is flat that allows rotation and sliding of the tibial component (flat-on-flat articulation).

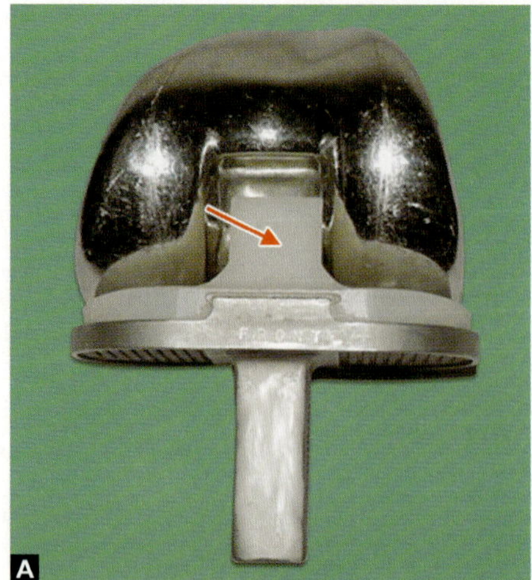

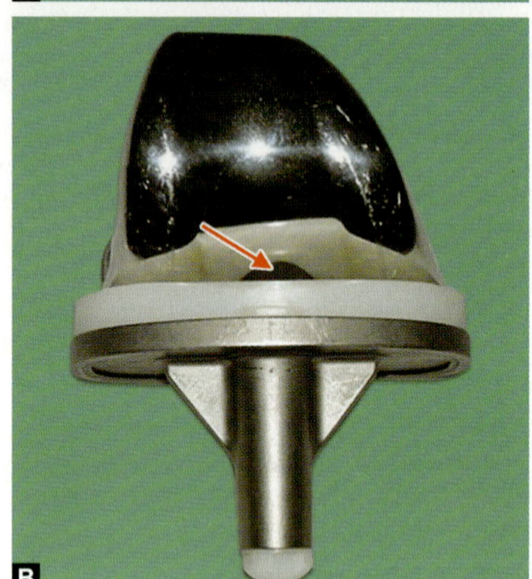

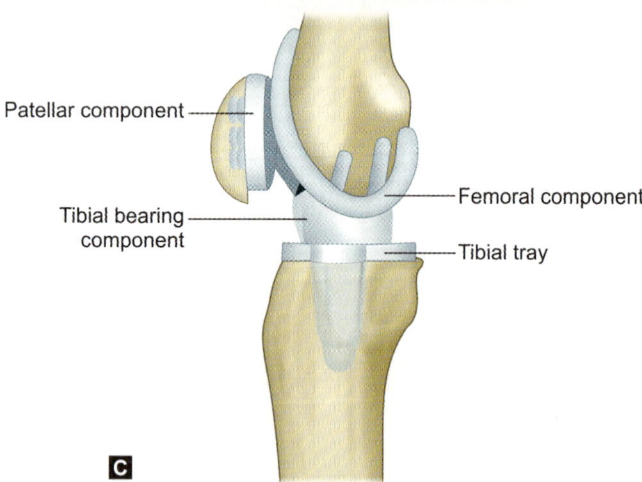

Figs. 24.10A to C: Implant designs for knee replacement: (A) posterior-stabilized design; (B) Cruciate-retaining design with implant (arrow) replace groove to accommodate PCL; (C) Mobile bearing design. (PCL: posterior cruciate ligament)

- Fixed-bearing implants—these implants do not have such insert.

  Mobile-bearing insert is designed in a way that permits patients with a few degrees of rotation to the medial and lateral sides of their knee. The purpose of this design is to decrease the long-term wear of the tibial component. A mobile-bearing knee design is recommended most often for the active patients who are younger than 55–65 years of age.

Implant Fixation

There are various kinds of fixations that can be used to connect knee implants to the bones.
- Cemented fixation—as the name implies, these implants are commonly held in place with a bone cement (PMMA).
- Cementless fixation—these implants are "press-fit" onto the bones. This type of fixation has to rely on new bone growing into the surface of the implant.
- Hybrid fixation—in hybrid fixation that is used for TKR, the femoral component is attached without cement, but the tibial and patellar components are attached with cement.

Currently, cemented fixation is used most often and cementless used least often. A surgeon's decision whether to employ hybrid fixation depends on the patient's age, bone quality, and expected activity level and the tightness of fit of the femoral component achieved during surgery.

Surgical Approach

Following are the surgical approaches:
- **Standard or minimally invasive** approaches with an incision (13–15 cm and 6–9 cm, respectively) along the midline or anteromedial aspect of the knee can be used. However, minimally invasive TKA involves a smaller incision and less soft tissue disruption, which decreases postoperative pain and increases the rate of postoperative recovery.
- **A quadriceps-splitting or a quadriceps-sparing approach** used to reach the capsule for an arthrotomy.

A series of surgical techniques are performed prior to inserting the implants. Contemporary TKA employs computer-assisted, image-guided surgery to ensure precise placement and alignment of the components.

Complications

Intraoperative complications during knee arthroplasty, such as the following are uncommon:
- Damage to a peripheral nerve (e.g., the peroneal nerve)
- An intercondylar fracture

Postoperative complications include:
- Joint instability
- Infection
- Wound-healing problems
- PE wear and prosthesis loosening
- DVT

Precautions following TKA are shown in **Box 24.5**.

Physiotherapy Management

Preoperative Management

The physical therapist should teach the patient some of the exercises before surgery that will help the patients understand the procedures. Also this will help the patients

BOX 24.5: Exercise precautions following TKA.
- Postpone side lying straight leg raises for 2 weeks after cemented and 4–6 weeks after cementless arthroplasty to avoid varus and valgus stresses
- Postpone-independent weight-bearing until strength of quadriceps and hamstrings is sufficient to stabilize the knee joint
- Any mobilization or manipulation techniques may not be appropriate, so take prior surgeon's opinion

after surgery, to be ready to practice a proper version of the relevant exercises. It is also necessary that the functional status of the patient before surgery is optimized, because it will later assist recovery.

The focus of a preoperative training program should be on:
- Functional lower extremity exercises
- Postural control
- Strengthening exercises for both of lower extremities.

Unfortunately, there is very limited evidence that supports the fact that preoperative physiotherapy leads to significant improvements in patient's lower limb strength, range of movement, pain or length of hospital stay following TKA.

Postoperative Management

Immobilization and Early Motion

After a primary TKA, the knee is immobilized in extension with a compression dressing for a day only, but after complicated revision arthroplasty, an immobilization of longer duration may be necessary.

During the initial postoperative period, until quadriceps control is re-established, it is recommended to have the patient wear a posterior extension splint during ambulation and also at night for a patient, especially for the patients who have difficulty achieving full knee extension after surgery or who had a significant preoperative knee flexion contracture.

In the past, continuous passive movement (CPM) was used routinely during a patient's hospital stay after TKA. At that time, a number of studies described the benefits of CPM, but the current evidence states that this intervention is insufficient to be used routinely in clinical practice. They concluded neither the ROM of knee joint nor the functional outcomes can be improved by CPM therapy. To add to it, the risk of incidence of adverse events and length of stay cannot be decreased by use of CPM.

Weight-bearing Consideration

After primary TKA, weight-bearing relies on the:
- Patient's age
- Type of fixation used
- Bone quality
- Type of prosthesis implanted
- Size

With cemented fixation, weight-bearing is allowed as per the tolerance immediately after surgery with the use

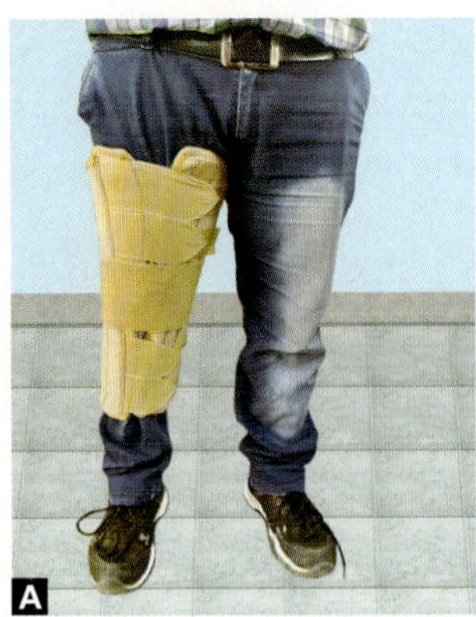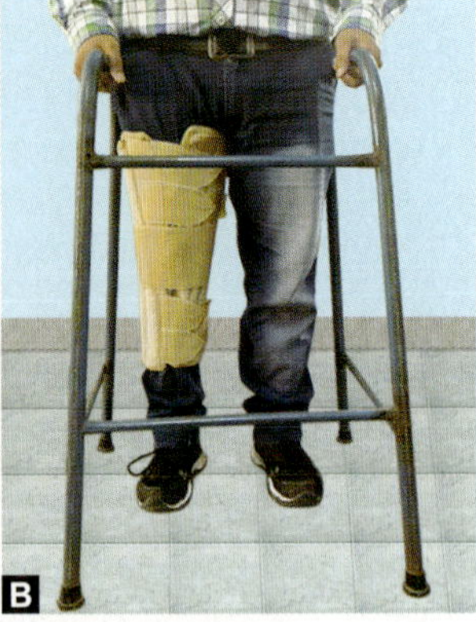

Figs. 24.11A and B: Knee immobilizer.

of crutches or a walker. Though during the first few postoperative days, use of a knee immobilizer **(Figs. 24.11A and B)** may be required.

With biological/cementless fixation, recommendations for weight-bearing vary from permitting only touch-down weight-bearing for 4–8 weeks while using crutches or a walker to weight-bearing as tolerated within a few days after surgery while using crutches or a walker.

Until the patient has achieved full or nearly full, active range of knee extension and optimal strength of the quadriceps and hip musculature to control the operated lower limb, ambulation without an assistive device, particularly outdoor walking is not advisable.

Rehabilitation is key to successful recovery from TKA and to optimizing joint function; however, the rising demand for TKA is stressing outpatient and in-home rehabilitation services.

A study of 41 patients who had total knee arthroplasty (TKA) suggested telerehabilitation as a possible solution. The experimental group received in-home telerehabilitation services via online videoconferencing. Investigators compared that group with a conventional home care/outpatient rehabilitation group. The authors recorded measures of range of motion, balance, strength, knee function, walking, and autonomy at three points over about 6 months. The study results showed that home telerehabilitation for TKA is a practical and effective alternative to conventional therapy.

Maximum protection phase: It extends about 4 weeks. The goal is to attain 90° of flexion of knee and full extension of knee by the end of this phase.

Goals and interventions: The following goals and exercise interventions are included in the initial phase of rehabilitation after TKA.

To prevent vascular and pulmonary complications:
- Ankle pumping exercises with the lower limb in elevation, immediately after surgery helps prevent venous stasis and decrease the risk of a DVT or pulmonary embolism
- Deep breathing exercises.

To control pain and swelling: Cold, compression, and elevation.

To minimize reflex inhibition or loss of strength of knee and hip muscles:
- Muscle-setting exercises of the quadriceps, hamstrings, hip abductor, and hip extensors
- Active-assisted and active straight leg raise (SLR) exercises.

To maintain ROM of hip and knee:
- Heel slides in a supine position and gravity-assisted knee flexion in high sitting position.
- To prevent knee flexion deformity—gravity-assisted or self-assisted knee extension in the supine or long sitting position by periodically placing a rolled towel under the heel and leaving the knee unsupported and pressing downward just above the knee with both hands. Avoid placing a pillow under the knee while lying supine to reduce the risk of developing a knee flexion contracture.
- Gentle inferior and superior patellar gliding techniques to prevent restricted mobility.
- Neuromuscular facilitation and inhibition technique, such as the agonist-contraction technique to decrease muscle guarding particularly in the quadriceps which will increase knee flexion.

To develop control of the knee extensors and to prevent an extensor lag:
- Active-assisted ROM progressing to active ROM (AROM) of the knee while seated and standing for antigravity knee extension and flexion, respectively. As weight-bearing on the operated lower extremity permits
- Terminal knee extension in standing
- Wall slides in a standing position
- Mini-squats and partial lunges
- Neuromuscular electrical stimulation or biofeedback is also recommended as an adjunct.

To maintain or improve strength of the contralateral lower extremity: Progressive resisted exercises (PRE) of nonoperated lower extremity particularly the quadriceps and hip extensors and abductors.

To improve trunk stability and balance:
- Trunk stabilization exercises
- Balance activities in sitting and weight shifting in bilateral stance while adhering to weight-bearing restrictions
- Gait training adhering to weight-bearing restrictions with use of appropriate assistive device
- Functional training (bed mobility, sit-to-stand transfers, and basic ADL).

Criteria to progress: Criteria to proceed to the next phase of rehabilitation include the following:
- Minimal swelling and pain
- Well-healed incision
- No signs of infection
- Independent basic ADL
- Ambulation with appropriate assistive device

- AROM approaching full or nearly full, active knee extension and 90° knee flexion.

Moderate protection/controlled motion phase: It begins around fourth week and extends to 8–12 weeks postoperatively. The goal is to gain approximately 110° of knee flexion and active knee extension to complete 0° along with gradual increase in lower limb strength and muscular endurance, balance, cardiopulmonary endurance, and additional functional mobility.

The goals and exercise interventions:

To increase endurance and strength of hip and knee musculature:

- Multiple-angle isometrics and low-intensity dynamic resistance exercises of the quadriceps, hamstrings, and hip musculature (extensors, abductors, and external rotators) against a light grade of elastic resistance or a cuff weight around the ankle.
- Resisted SLRs in various positions to increase the strength of hip and knee musculature.
- As weight-bearing allows, continue or begin closed-chain exercises including resisted terminal knee extension in standing **(Fig. 24.12C)**, standing wall slides, mini-squats **(Figs. 24.12A and B)**, partial lunges, and the sit-to-stand task emphasizing proper lower extremity alignment. Include scooting forward and backward on a wheeled stool to improve functional control of the knee.
- Step-ups and step-downs (initially using a low step and increasing the height of the step) forward and then lateral. To progress, perform step-ups against elastic resistance **(Figs. 24.13A and B)**.
- Stationary cycling with the seat positioned as high as possible helps to increase knee extension.
- Continue strengthening exercises for the nonoperated lower extremity.

Continue to increase knee ROM:

- Low-intensity stretching of hip flexors hamstrings, and calf muscles or hold–relax technique to increase knee flexion and extension if limitation persists.
- Stationary cycling with seat lowered, to emphasize flexion of knee.
- Grade III inferior or superior patellar mobilization techniques to increase knee flexion or extension,

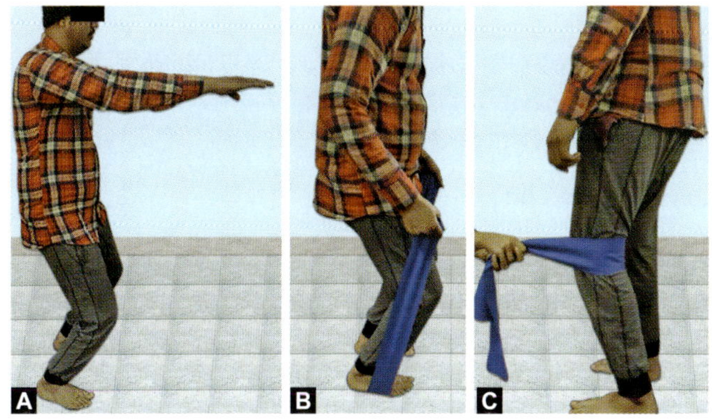

Figs. 24.12A to C: (A) Mini-squat; (B) Mini-squat with resistance; (C) Closed-chain resisted last degree extension.

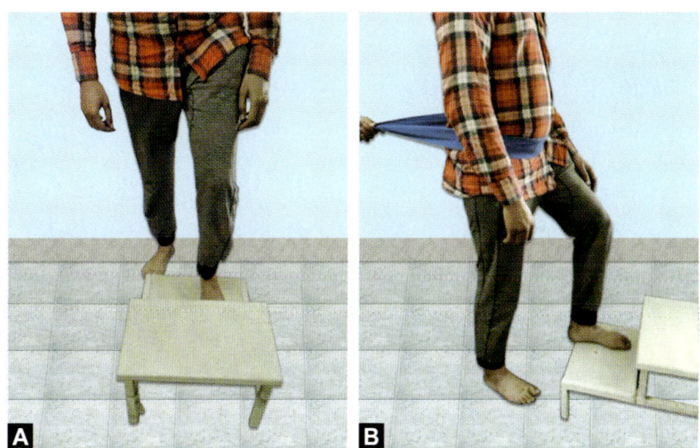

Figs. 24.13A and B: (A) Step up and step down; (B) Step up and down with resistance.

respectively, if insufficient patellar mobility is restricting ROM.

To improve standing balance and trunk stability:

- Trunk stabilization exercises
- Proprioceptive and balance training progressing from bilateral to unilateral stance on stable surface, then to balance activities on an unstable surface **(Figs. 24.14 to 24.16)**
- Functional reaching activities while standing or stooping
- Tandem walking, grapevine walking initially in parallel bars for safety.

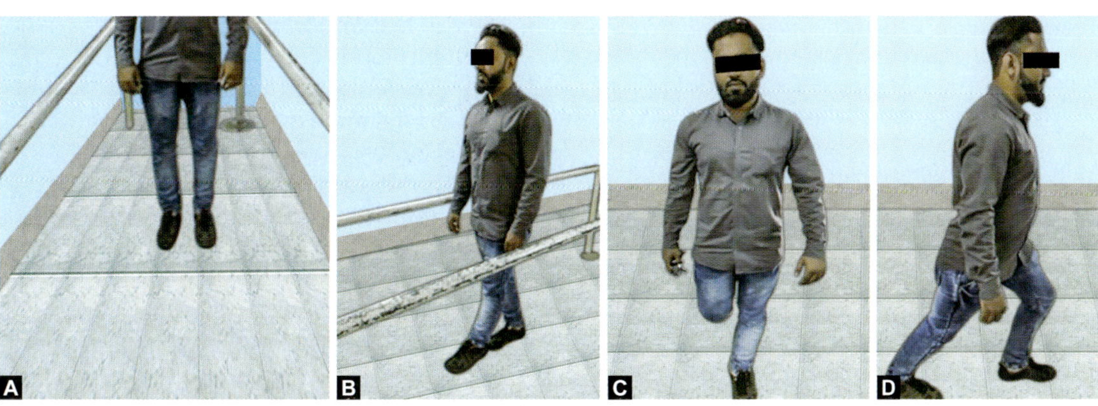

Figs. 24.14A to D: Proprioceptive training on stable surface.

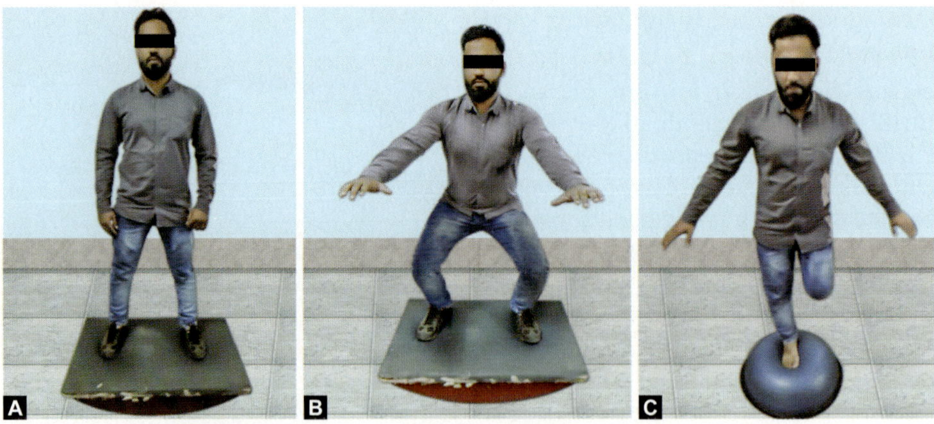

Figs. 24.15A to C: Proprioception training on unstable surface.

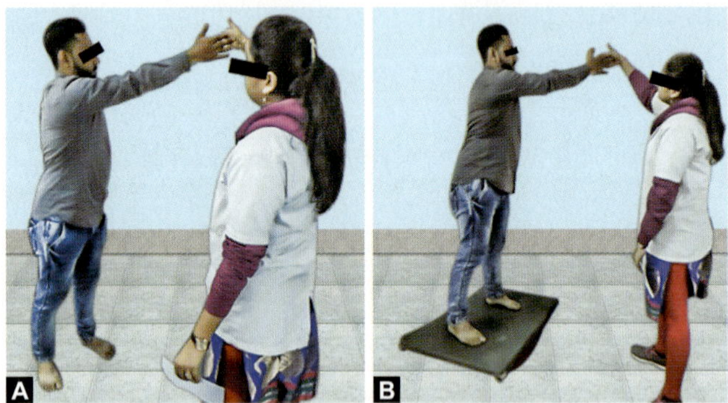

Figs. 24.16A and B: Reach out activities on stable and unstable surface.

Precaution: A progression of balance activities for patients with TKA is typically safe to begin about 8 weeks postoperatively but must be based on the ability to control the knee during stance, weight-bearing restrictions, and the absence of pain.

Continue to improve functional mobility:
- Symmetrical heel–toe walking, ambulation on a variety of surfaces and inclines, kneeling and getting up to a standing position, and ascending and descending stairs.
- Functional exercises: Backward walking, side-stepping, marching, and stepping over small objects.

Following total knee arthroplasty (TKA) or UKA, patients often report difficulty kneeling or the inability to kneel even a year after surgery. Although many functional activities, such as housework and gardening involve kneeling, patient education about this skill often is not included in postoperative rehabilitation. Jenkins et al. conducted a single-blind, prospective, randomized, and controlled study and suggested that kneeling advice and instruction should be included in postoperative rehabilitation after partial knee replacement. The findings of this study may have implications for patients who have undergone TKA.

Improve cardiopulmonary endurance: Aerobic conditioning on a stationary cycle or upper body ergometer, emphasizing increased duration.

Criteria to progress: Criteria to proceed to the final phase of rehabilitation are following:
- Full knee extension (no extensor lag)
- 110° knee flexion
- Quadriceps/hamstring and hip muscle strength: 4/5 muscle compared to uninvolved leg
- Minimal to no pain during exercises and ambulation with or without a cane.

Minimum protection/return to function phase: It begins at about 8 weeks and extends approximately to 12 weeks postoperatively.

Exercises:
- Task-specific strengthening exercises.
- Continue proprioceptive and balance training.
- Advanced functional training and continued cardiopulmonary conditioning (pool activities, walking, and stationary cycle), so that the patient regains the endurance, power, strength, and balance needed to return to a full level of functional activities in the community.

Advanced activity phase (*Weeks 12 and beyond*).
Goals:
- Maintain and/or improve the strength and endurance of lower limb musculature.
- Allow patients to return to advanced level of function, such as recreational sports.
- Return to normal life and routine.

Current trends favor a higher level of athletic activity among people post-TKR surgery. However, this return to high-impact sports should be properly assessed for any potential negative impact on the implant.

For recreational sports, patients are advised to participate in low-impact physical activities after TKA to reduce the risk of component wear and mechanical loosening over time and the premature need for revision arthroplasty.

For the patient who wishes to participate in athletic activities after TKA, there are a number of considerations.

Table 24.2: Recommendations of physical activities for fitness and recreation.

Highly recommended	Recommended if experienced before TKA	Not recommended
• Stationary cycling • Water aerobics • Swimming • Table tennis • Walking • Golf (preferably with golf cart) Ballroom or square dancing	• Road cycling • Rowing • Low-impact aerobics • Doubles tennis • Speed/power walking • Cross-country skiing (machine or outdoor • Bowling, canoeing	• High-impact aerobics • Jogging, running • Basketball, volleyball • Singles tennis • Baseball, softball • Handball, racquetball, squash • Water skiing • Football, soccer • Tumbling, gymnastics

(TKA: total knee arthroplasty)

Factors that impact participation include:
- The level of demand (intensity and load) of an athletic activity
- A patient's body weight, overall level of fitness
- Preoperative experience with the activity and the technical quality of the knee replacement and related soft tissue balancing or reconstruction.

Physical activities for fitness and recreation that are highly recommended, recommended with caution, or not recommended after TKA are noted in **Table 24.2**.

SHOULDER ARTHROPLASTY

Total shoulder replacement or **total shoulder arthroplasty** (TSA) is a surgical procedure in which the diseased or damaged ball and socket joint of the shoulder is replaced with prosthesis **(Figs. 24.17A to C)**. These prostheses are composed of high-density PE glenoid component and metal humeral components.

A reverse TSA (RTSA) refers to a similar procedure. In this the prosthetic socket and metal ball are switched. This means that the metal ball is attached to the shoulder blade and a plastic socket is attached to the top of upper arm bone. This procedure is useful when the rotator cuff function is permanently and severely lost. By reversing the joint the deltoid has a greater influence on the improvement of the active shoulder ROM and function.

Hemiarthroplasty refers to only one surface, humeral head is replaced.

Indications for Total Shoulder Arthroplasty

Underlying pathologies causing severe deterioration of one or both surfaces of glenohumeral (GH) joint, causing significant pain and loss of upper extremity function includes:
- Osteoarthritis
- Rheumatoid arthritis (RA)
- Rotator cuff tear or arthropathy
- AVN (caused by fractures or long-term steroid use)
- Post-traumatic degenerative joint disease
- Severe proximal humerus fractures (hemiarthroplasty).

Designs of Prosthetic Implants

They range from unconstrained (gives more mobility than stability, used more when rotator cuff is intact) to semiconstrained to constrained provide varying amount of mobility and stability.

Operative Procedure

This involves anterior approach using deltopectoral incision—release of subscapularis—anterior capsulotomy—exposure of bony components.

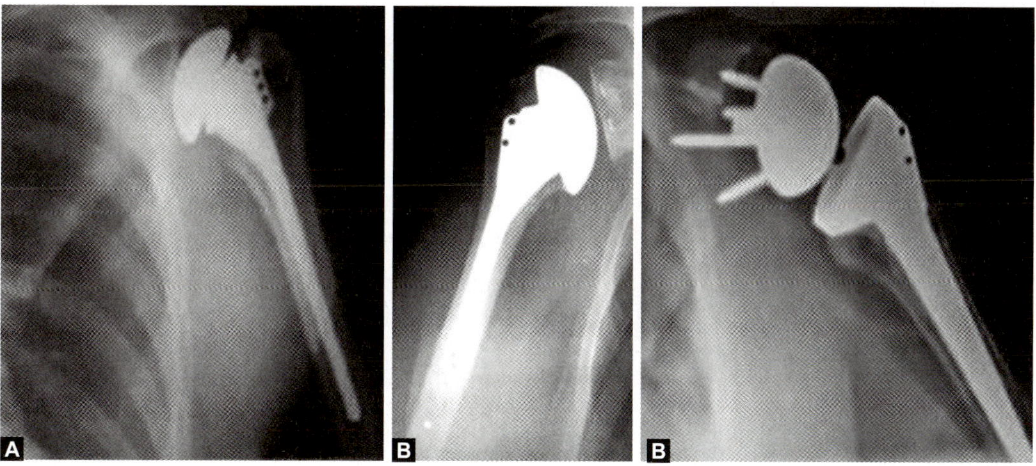

Figs. 24.17A to C: Types of shoulder arthroplasty: (A) Hemiarthroplasty; (B) Total shoulder; (C) Reverse total shoulder.

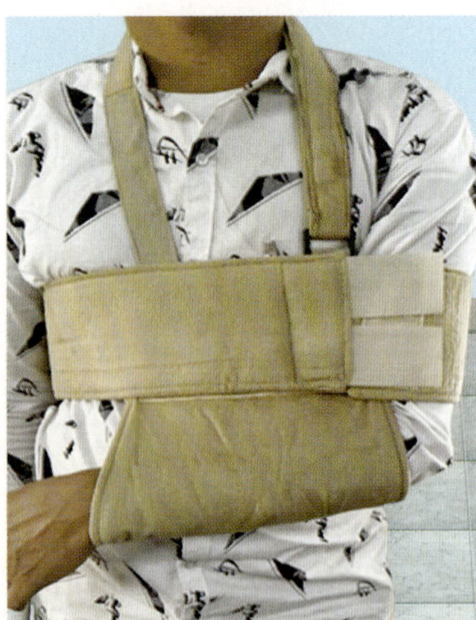

Fig. 24.18: Shoulder immobilizer.

Postoperative Positioning and Immobilization

Patients will be in a shoulder immobilizer **(Fig. 24.18)**, a sling during day and night for the first week and in crowded areas for the first month. A patient who underwent a cuff repair or other soft tissue reconstruction may need to wear sling until sufficient healing has occurred. A patient who has undergone RTSA wears a shoulder immobilizer (sling and swathe) continuously for at least 3–4 weeks following surgery except for daily personal hygiene and periodic PROM (pendulum exercises) during the day.

Guidelines for Progression of Exercises

The guidelines during each phase of rehabilitation after TSA, RTSA, or hemiarthroplasty described here are drawn from recent published protocols available. It is important to note that these criteria and suggested timelines for progression of exercises and functional activities must be adapted to each patient based on periodic evaluations of the patient's status and ongoing communication between the therapist and the surgeon.

Maximum Protection Phase of Rehabilitation

Begins on the first postoperative day and extends for 4–6 weeks. The emphasis of this first phase is patient education, pain control, and initiation of ROM exercises to prevent adhesions and restore shoulder mobility as early as possible.

Precautions:

- Avoid shoulder AROM
- No excessive shoulder motion behind back, especially IR
- In supine lying, a small pillow or towel roll can be placed behind the elbow to avoid shoulder hyperextension/anterior capsule stretch/subscapularis stretch
- No lifting of objects
- No driving for 3 weeks
- No stretching or jerky movements (particularly ER)
- No giving support to body weight by hand on involved side.

Goals and treatment:

Control pain and inflammation:
- Use of a sling or splint for comfort
- Use of cryotherapy especially after exercise.

Maintain mobility of adjacent joints:
- Active movements of the spine and scapula (while wearing the shoulder sling and after it can be removed for exercise)
- AROM of the hand, wrist, and elbow when the arm can be removed from the sling.

Restore shoulder mobility:
- Passive forward flexion in supine to tolerance
- Gentle ER in scapular plane to available PROM, usually around 30° (attention: particularly with shoulder in extension, do not produce undue stress on the anterior joint capsule)
- IR until the forearm rests on the chest
- Pendulum (Codman's) exercises. Encourage the patient to periodically remove the sling and gently swing the arm during ambulation at home
- Later during this phase, progress to supine self-assisted shoulder ROM (elevation and rotation) by assisting with the sound hand and later using a wand or dowel rod
- Then progress to self-assisted shoulder ROM with a wand in sitting or standing by performing "gear shift" exercises
- Resting the arm on a table and sliding it forward
- Self-assisted reaching movements (to the nose, forehead, or over the head as comfort allows) to simulate functional movements
- For some patients, transition to active (unassisted) shoulder ROM is often possible by 4 weeks
- Functional activities with the elbow at waist level, such as hand to face and writing, are permissible.

Minimize muscle inhibition, guarding, and atrophy:
- Gentle muscle setting of shoulder musculature (excluding the internal rotators) with the elbow flexed and the shoulder in the plane of the scapula or neutral.
- Scapular stabilization exercises in nonweight-bearing positions. Target the serratus anterior and trapezius muscles **(Figs. 24.19A and B)**.

Criteria to progress to next phase:
- At least 90° of PROM of flexion and abduction elevation
- At least 45° of ER and 70° of IR in the plane of the scapula with minimal pain.
- No pain during resisted, isometric IR of the subscapularis.

Moderate Protection/Controlled Motion Phase

It begins at about 4–6 weeks postoperatively and extends to at least 12–16 weeks and focuses on gradually establishing active (unassisted) control, dynamic stability, and strength of the shoulder while continuing to increase ROM.

Precautions: Although it is safe to place increasing stresses (stretching or resistance) on periarticular soft

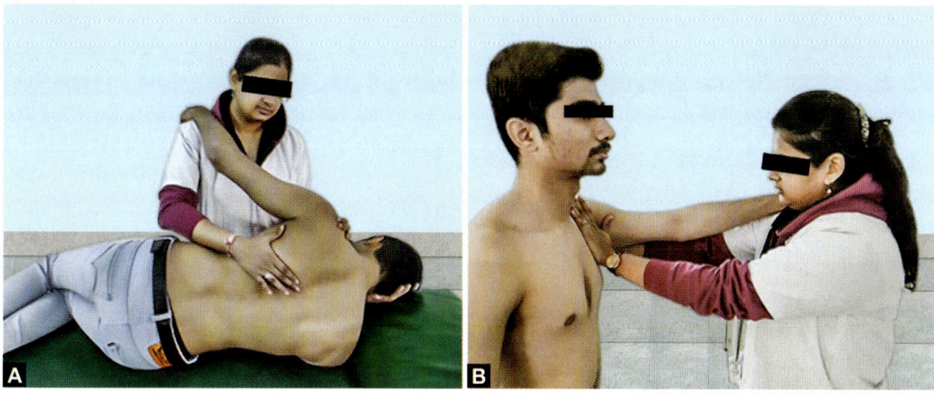

Figs. 24.19A and B: Nonweight-bearing scapular stabilization exercise.

tissues, it should be performed gradually not to irritate healing tissues. Therefore continue with short but frequent exercise sessions (preceded by application of heat and followed by cold). Avoid heavy weight lifting and weight-bearing on affected hand.

Goals and Treatment

Continue to increase ROM of the shoulder:

- Transition from passive or assisted ROM to low-intensity, pain-free stretching in all anatomical and diagonal planes of motion to achieve intraoperative ROM
- Gentle joint mobilization techniques for specific capsular restrictions
- Gentle self-stretching exercises to increase elevation, IR/ER, extension, and horizontal adduction/abduction.

Develop active control and dynamic stability and improve muscle performance (strength and endurance) of the shoulder:

- Continue or gradual transition to active shoulder ROM exercises, initiating antigravity abduction with correct GH rhythm
- Scapular and GH joint stabilization exercises progress from nonweight-bearing to light weight-bearing positions **(Figs. 24.20A and B)**. (For patients who have had an RTSA, maintain nonweight-bearing precautions for up to 12 weeks postoperatively.)

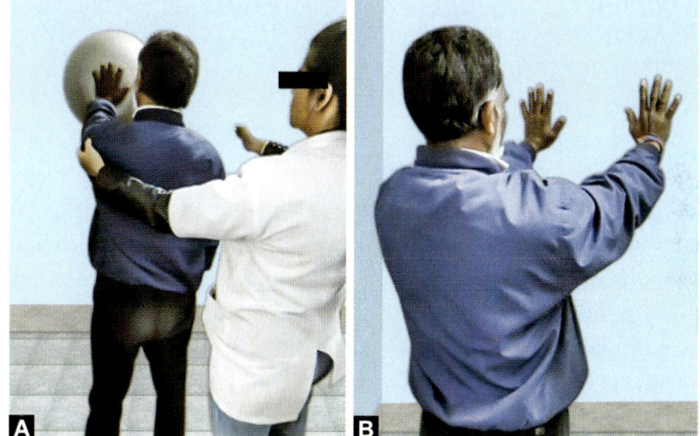

Figs. 24.20A and B: Closed-chain scapular stabilization exercises.

- Pain-free, low-intensity (submaximal) resisted isometrics of shoulder muscles, particularly the rotator cuff, including the subscapularis or any other repaired muscle–tendon units.
- Scapular strengthening exercises **(Figs. 24.21A to C)**.

Increase muscular and cardiopulmonary endurance: Upper extremity endurance training with stationary ergometer or a portable reciprocal exerciser on a table.

Criteria to progress:

- Full or at least 130–140° PROM of the shoulder flexion or abduction.

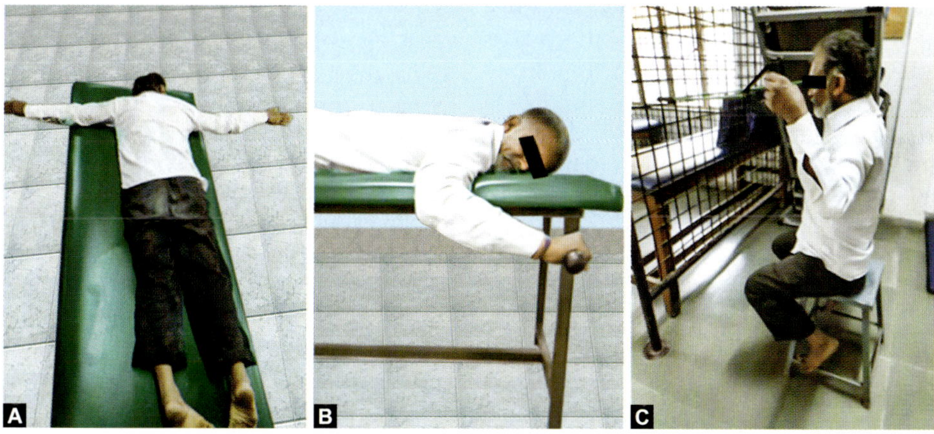

Figs. 24.21A to C: Strengthening of scapular muscles.

- In the plane of the scapula, at least 60° pain-free, passive ER and 70° IR.
- Active (unassisted), antigravity elevation of the arm to at least 100–120° in the plane of the scapula.

Minimum Protection/Return to Function Phase

It usually begins around 12–16 weeks postoperatively and typically extends for several more months. Focus is on pain-free strengthening of the shoulder girdle for dynamic stability and functional use of the upper extremity for progressively more demanding tasks. For optimal results, the home exercise program has to be continued for at least 6 months or longer, and functional and recreational activities may need to be modified.

Goals and Treatment

Continue to improve or maintain shoulder mobility:
- End-range self-stretching
- Grade III joint mobilization and self-mobilization, if appropriate.

Continue to improve neuromuscular control and muscle performance of the shoulder:
- Pain-free, low-load, high-repetition progressive resisted exercise (PRE) of shoulder musculature. Position the patient in a variety of gravity-resisted positions.
- Closed-chain, resisted shoulder exercises, gradually increasing the amount of weight-bearing through the upper extremity.

Return to most functional activities (typically 4–6 months postoperatively):
- Use of the operated upper extremity for progressively more advanced functional activities.
- Use of the operated upper limb for lifting, carrying, pushing, or pulling activities against increasing loads.
- Recreational activities, such as swimming and golf are possible.
- Modification of high-demand, high-impact work-related or recreational activities to avoid imposing excessive forces on the GH joint that could lead to loosening or premature wear of prosthetic implants.

SUMMARY

This chapter provides an understanding about total joint replacement surgery. Detailed information about specific types of joint replacement—such as for the hip, knee, and shoulder—are given. Postoperative rehabilitation is important following total joint replacement in order to ensure pain-free function of the joint and improve the QOL of the patient. Hence, this chapter addresses arthroplasty management across the continuum from assessment to surgery to rehabilitation and recovery to everyday living. For that complete knowledge regarding recent advances in implant design, different surgical approaches and related precaution are explained. It is recommended that a proper pre- and postoperative rehabilitation program plays a significant role in decreasing the length of hospitalization and the incidence of early complications. The time-based guidelines provided for progression of exercises during each phase of rehabilitation after arthroplasty along with proper precautions are given. Few criteria are also reported for progress of the patient from one phase of rehabilitation to next. Recommendations for participation in physical activities or recreation following arthroplasty are also given.

Case Scenario

CASE STUDY 1

A 56-year-old man working in a courier company since 30 years has to do cycling, walking, and climbing/descending stairs to deliver couriers. 1 week ago he has undergone THR with minimally invasive posterolateral approach for severe degenerative arthritis of hip, having severe pain and gait abnormality. He is walking in tolerated weight-bearing with walker. He is the only earning person in his family and wants to return to his job as early as possible.

Guiding Questions
1. Can you start accelerated rehabilitation program for this patient? Outline a plan for rehabilitation.
2. Make a list of suggestions and home modifications to follow the related precautions.
3. Can he return to his job? To help him meet his goals, design a sequence of progression according to his occupation demanding activities.

CASE STUDY 2

Patient was a 62-year-old obese female presenting to outpatient PT 5 days post left TKA. She is having knee pain and AROM is lacking in 10° of extension with 80° of flexion possible. Her long-term goals are to be able to perform all household work, reduce weight, and enjoy traveling with her family in vacation.

Guiding Questions
1. Explain the evaluation procedure; determine criteria to advance to next phase of rehabilitation.
2. Design exercise protocol to meet those criteria and to meet her desired goals.
3. Can you start aerobic training for her? How will you train her to return to full level of functional activities?

CASE STUDY 3

A 74-year-old left-handed female with chronic shoulder pain, resistant to conservative treatment underwent a left TSA for the treatment of significant osteoarthritis 10 days ago. Both she and her husband are retired, in good health and independent in all ADLs, and have proper financial and moral support of all family members. The patient reported that prior to surgery she enjoyed playing with her grandchildren, socializing with neighbors and going to nearby temples. She is wearing a sling to protect the operated shoulder.

Guiding Questions
1. Which precautions will you take into consideration while designing your exercise protocol in current status?
2. Which information is necessary to ask the surgeon regarding status of soft tissues?
3. Describe the series of graded exercise to develop the control and dynamic stability of the shoulder to return to her function goal and healthy and happy life.

Review Questions

1. Explain in detail about pre- and postoperative physiotherapy for THR.
2. Describe types of TKR based on component design, surgical approach, and fixation.
3. Describe each phase of rehabilitation after TKA with goals and interventions.
4. Describe indications and contraindications of total hip and knee arthroplasty.
5. Explain in detail about exercise guidelines and precautions during intervention after shoulder arthroplasty.

BIBLIOGRPAHY

1. Affatato S. Perspectives in total hip arthroplasty: advances in biomaterials and their tribological interactions. London: Woodhead Publishing; 2014.
2. Alecci V, Valente M, Crucil M, et al. Comparison of primary total hip replacements performed with a direct anterior approach versus the standard lateral approach: perioperative findings. J Orthopaed Traumatol. 2011;12:123-9.
3. Aumiller WD, Dollahite HA. Advances in total knee arthroplasty. JAAPA. 2016;29(3):27-31.
4. Bader R, Steinhauser E, Zimmermann S, et al. Differences between the wear couples metal-on-polyethylene and ceramic-on-ceramic in the stability against dislocation of total hip replacement. J Mater Sci Mater Med. 2004;15(6):711-18.
5. Bonutti PM. Minimally Invasive Total Knee Arthroplasty — Midvastus Approach. In: Hozack WJ et al. (Eds). Minimally Invasive Total Joint Arthroplasty. Springer, Berlin, Heidelberg; 2004. pp. 139-45.
6. Boudreau S, Boudreau E, Higgins L, et al. Rehabilitation following reverse total shoulder arthroplasty. J Orthop Sports Phys Ther. 2007;37(12):734-43. [Serial online].
7. Brent Brotzman S, Wilk KE. Clinical orthopedic rehabilitation. 2003.
8. Brotzman SB, Wilk KE. Clinical orthopedic rehabilitation, 2nd edition. Philadelphia, PA: Mosby; 2003. pp. 125-250.
9. Cameron H, Brotzman SB. The arthritic lower extremity. In: Brotzman SB, Wilk KE (Eds). Clinical orthopedic rehabilitation, 2nd edition. Philadelphia, PA: Mosby; 2003. pp. 441-74.
10. Carli AV, Poitras S, Clohisy JC, et al. Variation in use of postoperative precautions and equipment following total hip arthroplasty: a survey of the AAHKS and CAS membership. J Arthroplasty. 2018;33(10):3201-5.
11. Chechik O, Khashan M, Lador R, et al. Surgical approach and prosthesis fixation in hip arthroplasty world wide. Arch Orthop Trauma Surg. 2013;133(11):1595-600.
12. Colby LA, Kisner C. Therapeutic exercise. Foundations and techniques, 6th edition. F.A. Davis; 2012. 778-88.
13. Colby LA, Kisner C. Therapeutic exercise. Foundations and techniques, 6th edition. FA Davis; 2012. pp. 553-61.
14. Colby LA, Kisner C. Therapeutic exercise. Foundations and techniques. FA Davis; 2012. pp. 721-25.
15. Dargel J, Oppermann J, Brüggemann G, et al. Dislocation following total hip replacement. Dtsch Arztebl Int. 2014;111:51-2.
16. Donatelli RA (Ed). Physical therapy of the shoulder, 4th edition. St. Louis, MO: Churchill Livingstone; 2004. pp. 529-45.
17. Dooley P. Total knee replacement: understanding patient-related factors. BCMJ. 2016;58(9):514-19.
18. D'Antonio JA. Complications of total hip and knee arthroplasty: lessons learned. In: Hozack WJ, Krismer M, Nogler M, et al. (Eds). Minimally invasive total joint arthroplasty. Heidelberg: Springer; 2004. pp. 304-8.
19. Garcia-Rey E, Cruz-Pardos A, Garcia-Cimbrelo E. Alumina-on-alumina total hip arthroplasty in young patients: diagnosis is more important than age. Clin Orthop Relat Res. 2009;467(9):2281-9.
20. Goyal D, Bansal M, Lamoria R. Comparative study of functional outcome of cemented and uncemented total hip replacement. J Orthop Traumatol Rehabil. 2018;10:23-8.
21. Gregory T, Hansen U, Emery R, et al. Developments in shoulder arthroplasty. Proc Inst Mech Eng. H. 2007;221(1):87-96. [Serial online].
22. Gustke K, et al. Quadriceps sparing minimally invasive total knee replacement: initial experience and comparison to a matched set of non-MIS total knee replacements. Orthopaedic Proceedings 2006 88-B:SUPP_I, 90-90.
23. Hoppenfeld S, DeBoer P, Buckley R. Surgical exposures in orthopaedics: the anatomic approach. Philadelphia, PA: Lippincott Williams and Wilkins; 2009.
24. Huber EO, de Bie RA, Roos EM, et al. Effect of pre-operative neuromuscular training on functional outcome after total knee replacement: a randomized-controlled trial. BMC Musculoskelet Disord. 2013;14:157.
25. Jenkins C, Barker KL, Pandit H, et al. After partial knee replacement patients can kneel, but they need to be taught to do so: a single-blind. Randomized controlled trial. Phys Ther. 2008;88(9):1012-21.
26. Kline PW, Melanson EL, Sullivan WJ, et al. Improving physical activity through adjunct telerehabilitation following total knee arthroplasty: randomized controlled trial protocol. Phys Ther. 2019;99(1):37.
27. Kloiber J, Goldenitsch E, Ritschl P. Patellar bone deficiency in revision total knee arthroplasty. 24. Orthopade. 2016; 45(5):433-8.
28. Kuster MS. Exercise recommendations after total joint replacement: a review of the current literature and proposal of scientifically based guidelines. Sports Med. 2002;32(7):433-45.
29. Kwok IH, Paton B, Haddad FS. Does pre-operative physiotherapy improve outcomes in primary total knee arthroplasty?—a systematic review. J Arthroplasty. 2015;30(9):1657-63.
30. Lindalen L, Nordsletten L, Høvik Ø, et al. E-vitamin infused highly cross-linked polyethylene: RSA results from a randomised controlled trial using 32 mm and 36 mm ceramic heads. Hip Int. 2015;25(1):50-5.
31. Mahendra G, Pandit H, Kliskey K, et al. Necrotic and inflammatory changes in metal-on-metal resurfacing hip arthroplasties: relation to implant failure and pseudotumor formation. Acta Orthop. 2009;80(6):653-9.
32. Manner PW, et al. Knee replacement implants American Academy of Orthopaedic Surgeon in orthoinformation; April 2016.
33. Matsen Iii F, Boileau P, Walch G, et al. The reverse total shoulder arthroplasty. Instr Course Lect. 2008;57:167-74. [Serial online].
34. Mulvey TJ, et al. Complications associated with total knee arthroplasty. In: Pellicci PM, Tria AJ, Garvin KL (Eds). Orthopedic knowledge update 2. Hip and knee

reconstruction. Rosemont, IL: American Academy of Orthopedic Surgeons; 2000. p. 323.

35. Neumann DA. An electromyographic study of the hip abductor muscles as subjects with hip prostheses walked with different methods of using a cane and carrying a load. Phys Ther. 1999;79(12):1163-73.

36. Pagnano MW, Papagelopoulas PJ, Rand JA. Uncemented total knee arthroplasty. In: Morrey BF (Ed). Joint replacement arthroplasty, 3rd edition. Philadelphia, PA: Churchill Livingstone; 2003. pp. 993-1001.

37. Pagnano MW, Papagelopoulas PJ, Rand JA. Uncemented total knee arthroplasty. In: Morrey BF (Ed). Joint replacement arthroplasty, 3rd edition. Philadelphia, PA: Churchill Livingstone; 2003. pp. 993-1001.

38. Peak EL, Parvizi J, Ciminiello M, et al. The role of patient restrictions in reducing the prevalence of early dislocation following total hip arthroplasty. J Bone Joint Surg Am. 2005;87(2):247-53.

39. Petis S, Howard JL, Lanting BL, et al. Surgical approach in primary total hip arthroplasty: anatomy, technique and clinical outcomes. Can J Surg. 2015;58(2):128-39.

40. Proposed rehab protocol for total knee replacement. https://www.losangelessportssurgeon.com/pdf/total-knee-replacement-po.pdf.

41. Ranawat CS, Rasquinna VJ, Rodriguez JA. Results of cemented total hip replacement. In: Pellicci PM, Tria AJ, Garvin KL (Eds). Orthopedic knowledge update. 2. Hip and knee reconstruction. Rosemont, IL: American Academy of Orthopedic Surgeons; 2000. p. 181.

42. Rand JA. Cemented total knee arthroplasty: techniques. In: Morrey BF (Ed). Reconstructive surgery of the joints, 2nd edition. New York, NY: Churchill Livingstone; 1996. p. 1389.

43. Robertson NB, Warganich T, Ghazarossian J, et al. Implementation of an accelerated rehabilitation protocol for total joint arthroplasty in the managed care setting: the experience of one institution. Adv Orthop Surg. 2015; Article ID 387197|7.

44. Röttinger H. Minimally invasive anterolateral surgical approach for total hip arthroplasty: early clinical results. Hip Int. 2006;16(4):42-7.

45. Schmitt J, Lange T, Günther KP, et al. Indication criteria for total knee arthroplasty in patients with osteoarthritis—a multi-perspective consensus study. Z Orthop Unfall. 2017;155(5):539-48.

46. Stockton KA, Mengersen KA. Effect of multiple physiotherapy sessions on functional outcomes in the initial postoperative period after primary total hip replacement: a randomized controlled trial. Arch Phys Med Rehabil. 2009;90(10):1652-7.

47. Tian P, Li ZJ, Xu GJ, et al. Partial versus early full weight bearing after uncemented total hip arthroplasty: a meta-analysis. J Orthop Surg Res. 2017;12(1):31.

48. Tsur A, Volpin G. What are the recommendations for sport activity following total hip or total knee arthroplasty?. Harefuah. 2013;152(11):647-8, 688.

49. Vaishya R, Vijay V, Demesugh DM, et al. Surgical approaches for total knee arthroplasty [retracted in: J Clin Orthop Trauma. 2019 Jul-Aug;10(4):835]. J Clin Orthop Trauma. 2016;7(2):71–79.

50. Verywell Health. Orthopedics—hip and knee—replacements implants. http://orthopedics.about.com/od/hipkneereplacement/a/implants.htm. (Accessed July 23, 2018).

51. Vogel LA, Carotenuto G, Basti JJ, et al. Physical activity after total joint arthroplasty. Sports Health. 2011;3:441-50.

52. Volpe S, Craig JA. Postoperative physical therapy management of a reverse total shoulder arthroplasty. Orthop Phys Ther Pract. 2009;21(2):11-17.

53. Wang L, Lee M, Zhang Z, et al. Systematic review and metaanalysis—does preoperative rehabilitation for patients planning to undergo joint replacement surgery improve outcomes. BMJ Open. 2016;6(2):e009857.

54. Whiteside LA. Fixation in total knee replacement: bone ingrowth. In: Pellicci PM, Tria AJ, Garvin KL (Eds). Orthopedic knowledge update, 2. Hip and knee reconstruction. Rosemont, IL: American Academy of Orthopedic Surgeons; 2000. p. 275.

55. Wilcox R, Arslanian L, Millett P. Rehabilitation following total shoulder arthroplasty. J Orthop Sports Phys Ther. 2005;35(12):821-36. [Serial online].

56. Yang X, Li GH, Wang HJ, et al. Continuous passive motion after total knee arthroplasty: a systematic review and meta-analysis of associated effects on clinical outcomes. Arch Phys Med Rehabil. 2019;100(9):1763-78.

Amputation and Prosthesis

Rutvik Purani, Srishti S Sharma

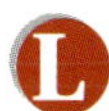 **LEARNING OBJECTIVES**

After reading this chapter, the readers should be able to:
- Understand the major concepts involved in amputation surgery, along with etiological factors responsible for amputation
- Understand tissue healing in each amputation
- Gain knowledge on the evaluation and management of an amputee while designing an effective plan of care with better understanding of the prosthesis
- Understand various prosthetic designs for upper limb and lower limb amputation
- Gain knowledge about the parts of each prosthetic design in detail, along with importance of static and dynamic prosthetic checkout
- Understand common gait deviations in lower limb prosthesis
- Understand the role of physiotherapist in management of individuals with upper and lower limb amputation.

CHAPTER OUTLINE

- Levels of amputation
- The surgery
- Healing process
- The postsurgical dressings
- Physical therapy examination and intervention
  - Postsurgical phase
  - Preprosthetic phase
- Upper extremity prostheses
  - Terminal devices for upper limb prosthesis
  - Prosthetic replacements for the wrist and forearm
  - Donning and doffing of prosthesis
  - Controls training
  - Functional use and vocational training
- Lower limb prostheses
  - Lower limb prostheses: prescription and factors affecting prescription
  - Prosthetic types and parts
  - Prostheses for partial foot amputation: toe fillers, spring shanks, shoe inserts
  - Terminal devices
  - Syme's prosthesis
  - Transtibial prostheses
  - Transfemoral prosthesis
  - Prosthesis for disarticulation
  - Bilateral lower limb amputation prosthesis
- Prosthetic examination
  - Prosthetic evaluation for transtibial prosthesis
  - Gait deviations in a transtibial prosthesis
  - Prosthetic evaluation for transfemoral prosthesis
  - Gait deviations in a transfemoral prosthesis
- Determining prosthetic potential
  - Functional outcome measures

INTRODUCTION

India is a vast nation with considerable number of individuals in the community with various disabilities. Amputation is one of the major health burdens on the families, society, and on medical services as well. Traumatic limb amputation is a catastrophic event that devastates the victim's life not only physically but also psychologically.

Acquired amputation is commoner than congenital causes. Peripheral vascular disease along with associated comorbidities, such as diabetes, atherosclerosis, and immunologic and cardiac disease, continues to be the major cause of lower limb amputation. In upper extremity (UE), trauma is the leading cause of limb loss, accounting for 80% of amputations with the vast majority limited to digital amputations. Hence, the inclusion of patient education regarding diabetes and diabetic foot care should be emphasized in the plan of care (POC) by the physical therapists. Early patient education and proper foot care have significant positive impact on the reduction of amputation. Trauma, resulting from motor vehicle accidents, gunshots, or war, is the second leading cause of amputation. Other causes of acquired amputations consist of infections, such as gangrene, nerve injuries, benign, or malignant tumors. The absence of part or complete extremity is mostly included in congenital skeletal deficiency; however, sometimes, it is discussed along with congenital amputations.

Individuals with such amputations are often young adults, more frequently men, and have often been involved in an active lifestyle before amputation. The incidence of salvage procedures following osteogenic sarcoma has been significantly reduced owing to advancement in the better procedures, effective chemotherapy, and quality imaging techniques. Deciding between amputation and limb salvage following trauma is complex and relies on various factors. Factors influencing the limb salvage procedures include the age of the patient, the size of the tumor, and the potential for future growth if the patient is young. When the injuries are not immediately life-threatening, the decision to amputate versus attempting limb salvage must be based on an assessment of the approach that will most effectively restore function and return the individual to their preinjury activities. Limb salvage of the lower extremity (LE) requires more surgeries involves longer hospital stays, delays weight-bearing, and slows the return to preinjury activities compared to amputation. Functional demands of upper extremity (UE) make it a requirement for salvage procedures. Irrespective

of the cause of amputation, physical therapist has a great role in rehabilitation.

Amputation is defined as the "removal of part or all of a body part enclosed by skin." The word "amputation" has been derived from the Latin word "Amputare" (to excise, to cut out).

LEVELS OF AMPUTATION

An international classification system to define the amputation levels was formulated by the Task Force on Standardization of Prosthetic–Orthotic Terminology in 1974. **Figures 25.1 and 25.2** show the anatomical levels of amputation of upper and lower extremity. **Tables 25.1 and 25.2** describe the levels of amputation and some salient features of each amputation in brief.

THE SURGERY

Various surgical procedures may be performed, as the surgeon tries to maintain the greatest bone length and preserve all possible joints. Broad anterior and posterior skin flaps are used for transfemoral amputation and transtibial amputation without vascular impairments, while with jeopardized circulation, long posterior flaps are used in transtibial amputation as they have better blood supply than anterior skin. An angular medial–lateral incision referred to as the *skew flap* places the scar away

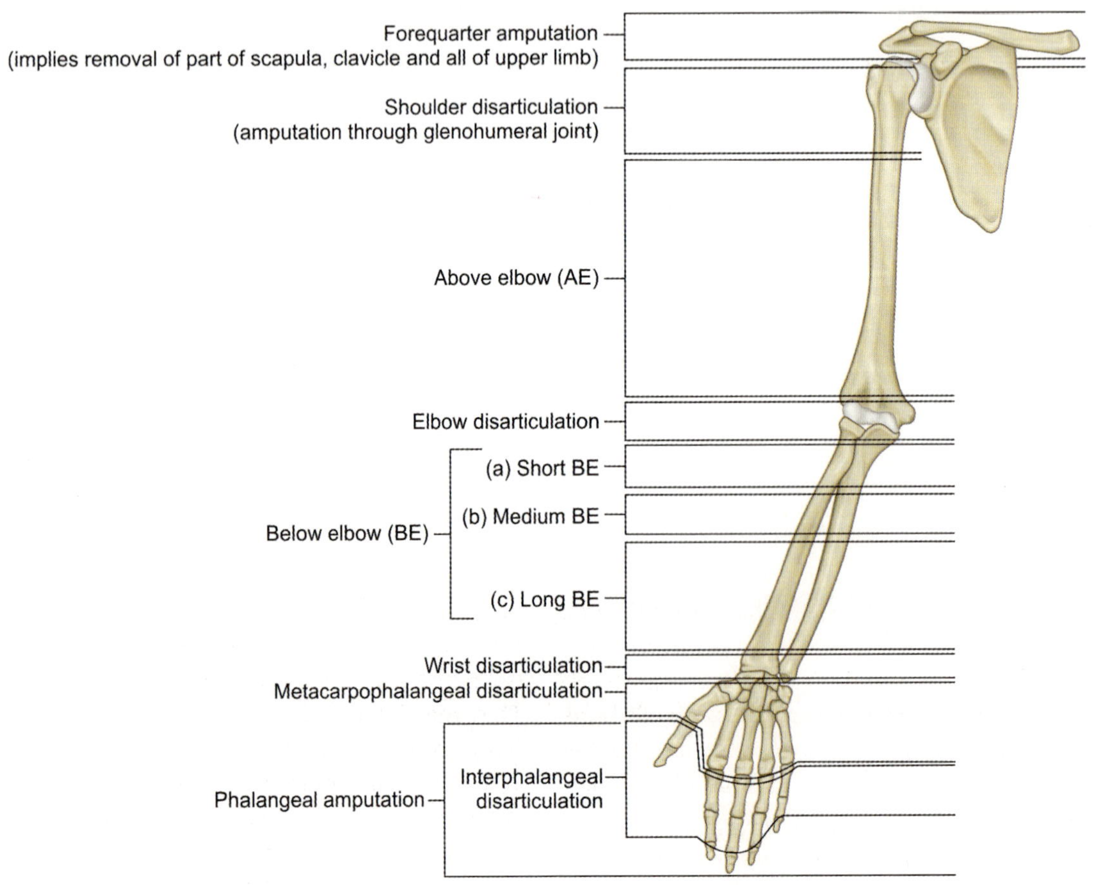

Fig. 25.1: Levels of upper extremity amputation.

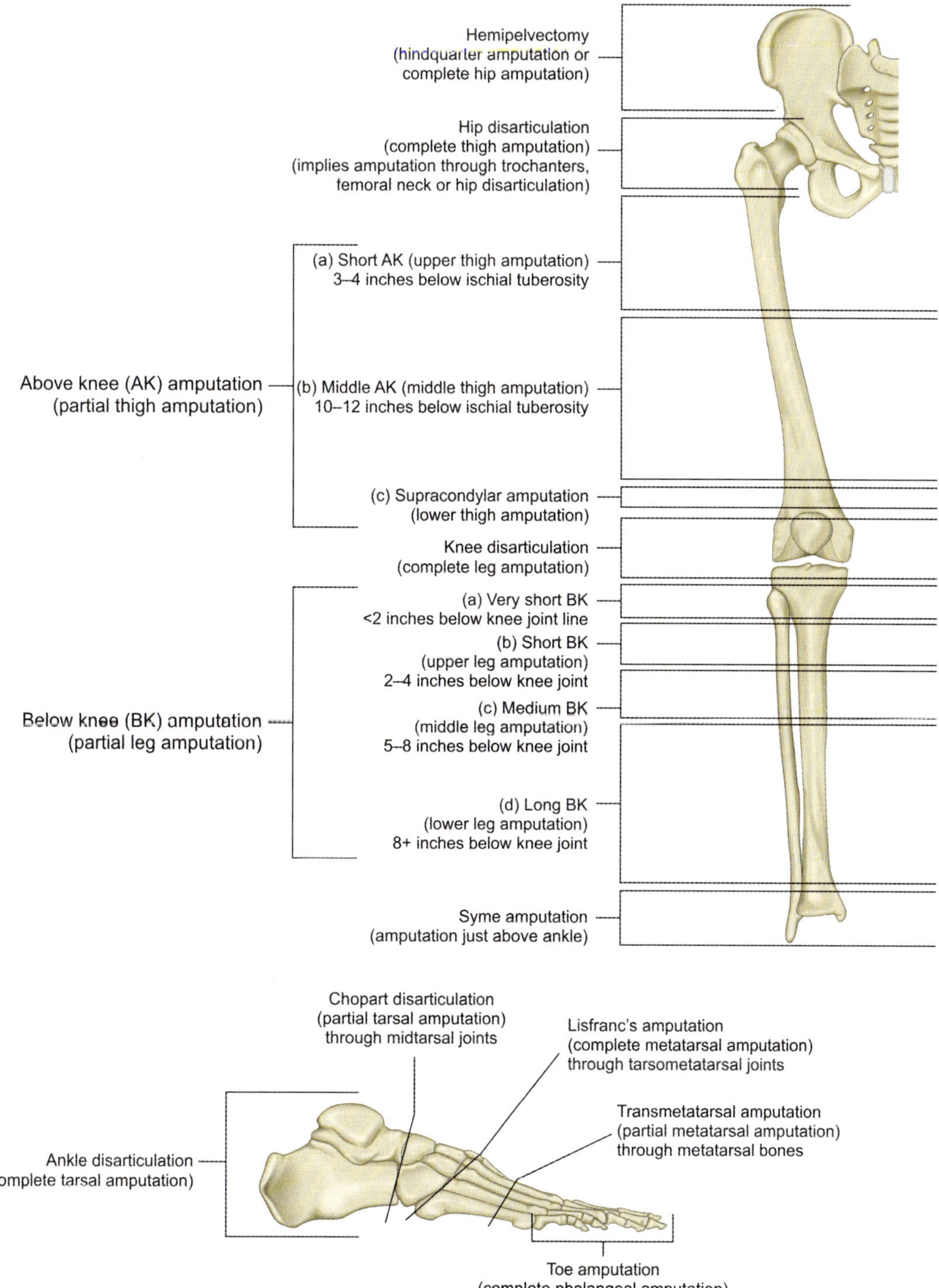

Fig. 25.2: Levels of lower extremity amputation.

from bony prominences, which is a problem with the long posterior flap. *Myoplasty* refers to the procedure in which the cut ends of the anterior and posterior compartment muscles are attached to each other, over the end of a bone, whereas in *Myodesis,* the ends of the muscles are attached to the end of the bone and is rare as it involves longer surgical hours, and more trauma to bone.

To overcome the complication of *neuromas* (a collection of nerve cell ends), surgeons pull down major nerves under some tension and then cut them sharply allowing them to retract into the soft tissue of the residual limb (RL). *Neuromas* are usually the source of pain, interfering with the prosthetic wear, as they are formed close to the scar. They may later require revision or resection. The sharp bony ends are smoothened and rounded; in transtibial amputation, the anterior segment of distal tibia is beveled to reduce the pressure between prosthetic socket and end of the bone. Under normal physiological tension, tissue layers are approximated as the incision is closed with sutures. A drainage tube may be inserted as necessary.

Table 25.1: Upper extremity amputations.

Partial hand	• Fingertip injuries have been divided into several zones to facilitate the choice of techniques for microsurgical procedures • Zones DP-I, DP-IIA, DP-IIB, and DP-III have been proposed for this purpose considering the feasibility of arterial and nerve anastomosis • Varying levels of grip impairment
Transcarpal	• Intact forearm pronation and supination as well as wrist flexion and extension as the tendons from forearm wrist flexors and extensors can be attached to the carpal bones
Wrist disarticulation	• Radius is separated from the carpal bones • Retained supination and pronation • Long lever arm for lifting, but cosmetically disfiguring
Transradial	• Level at least 2 cm above the wrist • Difficulty in supporting a myoelectric prosthesis due to the weight if forearm residual limb is too short • With a minimum of 4–5 cm of ulna resection, active elbow flexion is possible (biceps is reinserted into ulna in proximal level amputation)
Elbow disarticulation	• Enhanced suspension and rotational control as lever arm is greater due to the length and presence of the humeral epicondyles
Transhumeral	• Distance from the tip of the olecranon to the distal end of the resected humerus should be at least 10 cm to get a good stump for better prosthetic fitting • Arthrodesis should be done to prevent abduction contractures for transections through the humeral neck. Too short transhumeral amputations may be considered a modified shoulder disarticulation
Shoulder disarticulation	• Coverage/padding is done by deltoid, and acromion (usually the distal third) and coracoid process may have to be amputated
Scapulothoracic amputation	• Indicated for malignancy, necrotizing fasciitis, or trauma • The entire arm, the scapula, and generally most of the clavicle • Cosmetically unappealing

(DP: distal phalanx)

Table 25.2: Lower extremity amputation.

Metatarsal ray resection	• Metatarsal bone(s) and toe(s) are removed resulting in a narrow foot • Diminished push-off—if the first or second rays are removed Fourth and fifth ray resections are better tolerated
Transmetatarsal	• Done through the metatarsals, just proximal to the metatarsal heads Potentially provides lower morbidity and mortality and better functional results
Lisfranc	• Done at tarsometatarsal junction where all phalanges and metatarsals are removed Unopposed pull from the ankle plantar flexors can result in a fixed ankle plantar flexion contracture
Chopart	• Navicular, cuboid, cuneiforms, metatarsals, and phalanges are resected as it is done through midtarsal joint • Equinovarus contracture due to the action of gastrocnemius/soleus Callus formation over the foot at its anterior and inferior portion
Pirogoff	• Done between tibia and calcaneus by removal of phalanges, metatarsals, cuneiforms, navicular, cuboid, talus, and part of the calcaneus followed by calcaneotibial arthrodesis • A longer limb with lesser limp than the Syme's amputation • Instability resulting from failure of fusion of the calcaneus to the tibia Greater vulnerability to bursitis and ulcerations as the skin overlying the Achilles tendon insertion does not tolerate weightbearing well
Boyd	• Amputation is done between the ankle mortise and calcaneus where phalanges, metatarsals, cuneiforms, navicular, and cuboid, part of the sustentaculum tali, talus, and cartilage are removed A little longer than the Syme's amputation, and end-bearing on weight-tolerant skin
Syme's (ankle disarticulation)	• Talus, calcaneus, cuneiforms, cuboid, navicular, metatarsals, and phalanges and parts of the malleoli are removed More suitable weight-bearing for short distances as compared to partial foot amputation
Transtibial or BKA	• Distal tibia and fibula and those of the foot and ankle are amputated • Generally, 5–7 inches below the joint line through the tibia and fibula • Usually the fibula is sectioned 1 cm (3/8 inches) proximal to the distal tibia • >50% of tibial length is resected in long BKA, while in short BKA, <20% of tibial length is amputated

(Contd...)

(Contd...)

Knee disarticulation (through the knee joint)	• Done when there is insufficient skin coverage for a BKA or when there is <4 cm or 1.5 inches of viable tibia remaining • Reduced chances of osteomyelitis if the bone is left intact • Long lever arm for ambulation is provided by long femur • Better for children as growth of femur can occur since femoral epiphysis remains intact • Fitting of prosthesis is difficult
Transfemoral amputation or AKA **(Fig. 25.3)**	• About 25% success rate of prosthesis usage • Prosthetic ambulation is less successful as compared to other lower levels • >60% of femoral length is resected in long AKA, while in short AKA, <35% of femoral length is amputated
Hip disarticulation	• Higher mortality rate and infrequently performed • Entire lower limb from hip joint is resected • Substantial challenges for rehabilitation
Hemipelvectomy	• Performed for malignancies of the upper thigh, hip joint, or pelvis and osteomyelitis of the pelvis or proximal femur • Pelvis is separated at either the sacroiliac joint or just laterally through the ala of the ilium • The pubic bone can be sectioned 1 cm lateral to the symphysis
Hemicorporectomy	• Performed for extensive bladder cancer, rectal malignancies that involve the entire pelvis, and intractable decubiti • Amputation of both lower limbs and pelvis below L4 and L5 vertebrae

(AKA: above-knee amputation; BKA: below-knee amputation)

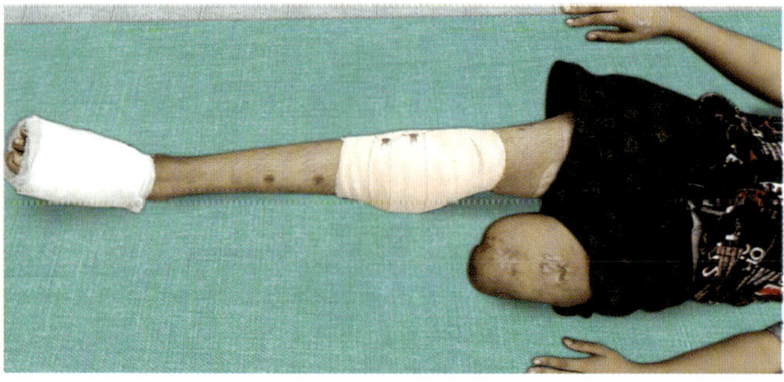

Fig. 25.3: Transfemoral amputation with healed incision.

HEALING PROCESS

Several factors affect the course of healing in each patient. Postoperative infection is the major concern for patients with contaminated wounds from injury, infected foot ulcers, etc. Other factors affecting the healing include the severity of the vascular problems, diabetes, renal disorders, or cardiac diseases. Smokers have a higher rate of infection as compared to nonsmokers as reported by one study.

THE POSTSURGICAL DRESSINGS

Variable options regarding the postoperative dressing to control the edema are available for the surgeons. Excessive edema can compromise the healing and can cause pain. Commonly used dressings are outlined in **Table 25.3.**

Soft dressings: Oldest method of postsurgical management, *soft dressings* are of two forms: the elastic wrap and the elastic shrinker **(Fig. 25.4)**. Commercial shrinkers are preferred in some places over traditional ace wrapping. They require little skill in donning and can

Table 25.3: Types of postsurgical dressings.

Type of dressing	Advantage	Disadvantage
Soft dressing	Easy application	Little edema control
	Inexpensive	Minimal RL protection
	Easy access for incision	Requires frequent rewrapping
Shrinkers	Easy application	Used only when sutures are removed
	Inexpensive	Requires frequent change as shrinks
Semirigid dressing	Better edema control than soft dressing	Needs frequent changing
	Protects RL	No access to incision
Rigid dressing	Excellent edema control	No access to incision
	Excellent RL protection	More expensive than other dressings
	Control of pain	Requires proper training for use

(RL: residual limb)

be pulled over the RL. Elastic wraps are usually applied postsurgically with moderate compression in figure-of-eight pattern.

Rigid dressings: They are also known as immediate postoperative prosthesis (IPOP) and may be handmade from plaster of Paris by the surgeon or a prosthetist and they usually follow the general configuration of the prosthetic socket. They are not adjustable or removable.

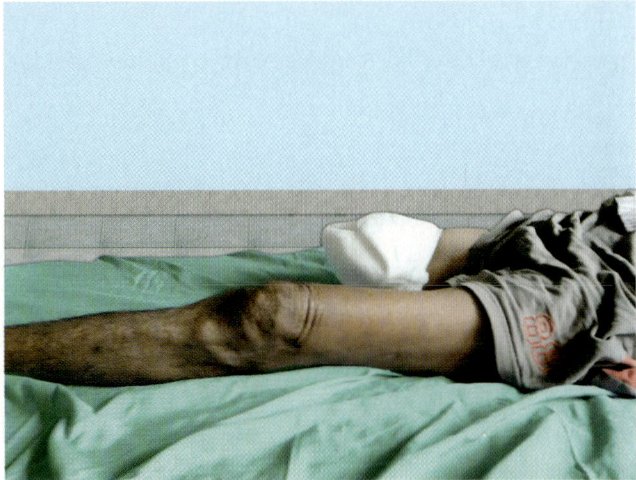

Fig. 25.4: Transfemoral amputation under dressing.

Removable rigid dressings (RRDs) are also available, which may be handmade from plaster or prefabricated from plastic materials and come in different sizes. Prefabricated RRDs are adjustable as the limb changes and may be removed for wound inspection as and when required.

Semirigid dressings: Semirigid dressings, such as Unna's dressing gauze impregnated with a compound of zinc oxide, gelatin, glycerin, and calamine may be applied sometimes. Earlier, the use of an *air splint* to control postoperative edema was made to aid in early ambulation. The air splint is a plastic double-wall bag that is pumped to the desired level of rigidity. The RL is covered with an appropriate postoperative dressing and inserted into the bag which allows wound inspection, but the constant pressure does not intimately conform to the shape of the RL, and the plastic is hot and humid requiring frequent cleaning.

PHYSICAL THERAPY EXAMINATION AND INTERVENTION

The major steps essential for the management of any individual include mainly five steps. They are examination, evaluation, diagnosis, prognosis, and intervention. Early rehabilitation has a greater potential for successful prognosis. A delay might result in the development of complications, such as joint contractures, general debilitation, and depression. Rehabilitation team comprising of physiatrist, prosthetist, physiotherapist, occupational therapist, social worker, and vocational counselor is essential **(Box 25.1)**. In scenarios where large number of amputees are dealt with especially regional centers, a less formal coordination of efforts between surgeons, physiatrists, prosthetists, and therapists in the community can provide effective care to most individuals with an amputation who lack access to specialized centers.

Box 25.2 describes the data necessary to develop a plan of care (POC) for the patient following amputation. The information obtained on initial examination and

BOX 25.1: Rehabilitation team for management of amputees.	
Team member	*Role*
Surgeon	Performs the surgical process of amputation
Physiatrist	Evaluation of patient, prescription of physiotherapy, occupational therapy, prosthesis, vocational rehabilitation, coordination between team members
Rehabilitation nurse	In-patient care of the patient, nursing, dressing, and hygiene needs of the amputee
Physiotherapist	Evaluation and treatment through postsurgical and prosthetic phase, long-term rehabilitation
Occupational therapist	Evaluation and treatment through postsurgical and prosthetic phase, training in activities of daily living
Psychologist	Counseling of the patient, motivating and coping through impact of amputation
Prosthetist	Prescription, measurement, fabrication and fitting of prosthesis
Social worker	Counseling and coordinating with NGOs, GOs, agencies, and community for welfare of amputees
Vocational counselor	Identifying the capacity, educating, and training with vocational skills, placement in the appropriate vocation

subsequent evaluation will influence discharge planning and future care. Depending on the critical findings, the therapist designs the POC that, of course, aims at the goals. The phases of rehabilitation are divided into two: (1) the duration between surgery and discharge from the hospital—the postsurgical phase and (2) the duration from hospital discharge to prosthetic fitting—the preprosthetic phase. A third phase, although less popular but equally important, is that of preoperative care where patients' expectations are discussed, questions answered, goals discussed, and the POC outlined. Limited time is available for the therapist to treat a patient in the hospital, to achieve the desired goals. The intervention must be aimed at preparing for discharge from acute care and to some form of follow-up care, be it in an acute rehabilitation facility, through a home health service or agency, or an outpatient facility.

Postsurgical Phase

The major goals of management during postsurgical phase include (1) patient education, (2) positioning, (3) balance and transfers, (4) mobility, (5) RL care, and (6) care of remaining extremity.

<table>
<tr><td>

BOX 25.2: Postsurgical assessment.

History

- Demographics, family history, and socioeconomic status
- Preamputation status, work, and leisure activities

Systems review

- Cause of amputation, coexisting medical conditions
- Vital signs, pain review, review of medications
- Looking for complications (deep vein thrombosis, pulmonary embolism, congestive heart failure)

Skin

- Scar (healed/adherent/invaginated/flat), lesions
- Moisture (moist, dry, scaly), sensation (absent, diminished, hyperesthesia)
- Grafts (location, type, healing), dermatological lesions (psoriasis, eczema, cysts)

Residual limb length

- Bone length (transtibial limbs measured from medial tibial plateau; transfemoral limbs measured from ischial tuberosity or greater trochanter)
- Soft tissue length (note redundant tissue)

Residual limb shape

- Cylindrical, conical, bulbous end, etc.
- Abnormalities ("dog ears," adductor roll), specific circumferential measurements

Cardiovascular

- Pulses (femoral, popliteal, dorsalis pedis, posterior tibial)
- Color (red, cyanotic), temperature, edema (circumference measurement. water displacement measurement, caliper measurements)
- Pain (type, location, duration), trophic changes
- Aerobic capacity, dyspnea, perceived exertion

Motor examination

- Range of motion of all possible joints (residual limb, unaffected side)
- Strength of major muscle groups (residual limb, unaffected side)

Neurological

- Pain [phantom (differentiate sensation or pain), neuroma, incisional, from other causes]
- Neuropathy
- Cognitive status (alert, oriented, confused)
- Emotional status (acceptance, body image)

Functional status (current and prior abilities)

- Transfers (bed to chair to toilet, to car)
- Balance (sitting, standing, reaching, moving)
- Mobility (ancillary support, supervision, closed and open environments, steps, curbs)
- Home/family situation (caregiver, architectural barriers, hazards)
- Activities of daily living (ADLs) (bathing, dressing)
- Instrumental ADLs (cooking, cleaning)

Quality of life, psychological status, motivation

- Vocational evaluation (analysis of role and environment, functional capacity for task)

</td></tr>
</table>

Patient Education

Throughout the rehabilitation program, the physical therapist continuously answers the questions and provides the information to the patient and caregivers. Emphasis is given to the development of a home program and the patient should be motivated to be as mobile as possible. Early involvement of a peer visitor might provide the patient insight and understanding of the healing and rehab process, coping strategies, and assurance that there is support available throughout the entire process. Supportive counseling may be required to validate patients' anxieties, assist with involving their support system, and provide coping strategies through the entire process especially in dealing with the immediate loss of limb. Good nutrition is essential for all wound healing. A multivitamin with minerals is suggested for wound healing, and advices regarding maintenance of good hydration should be given since any wound drainage in excess as loss of fluid from the wound/incision site would put the patient at risk for dehydration.

Positioning

Prevention of hip flexion contractures and encouraging the patient to spend some time in the prone position if at all possible is very essential in above-knee amputation as well as below-knee amputation. A pillow beneath the RL while the patient is supine is never recommended, nor is prolonged sitting. The RL should be placed with both hip and knee in extension **(Figs. 25.5A to D)**. In the initial days, the patient will want to avoid side-lying on the amputated side.

Balance and Transfers

Individuals with bilateral amputations require the intervention to improve sitting balance which is usually not a problem with a unilateral amputation. Standing balance exercises on the remaining extremity can be very effective in helping the individual regain their proprioceptive sense that might help them to use crutches during the period before prosthetic fitting. In the early postsurgical phase, the person should learn to transfer the weights on the normal extremity to protect the RL from possible injury against the chair or bed.

Mobility

Most of the therapists fit patients with a walker, although independent mobility with crutches is preferable as it is much more beneficial. The flexibility is greater in accomplishing activities of daily living (ADL) on crutches, whereas there is more stability in a walker. Partial weight-bearing gait is initiated with addition of pylon and foot if the patient has good control of weight-bearing with IPOP. It is critical that the patients with compromised vascularity or diabetes protect their RL by wearing a shoe on the remaining foot.

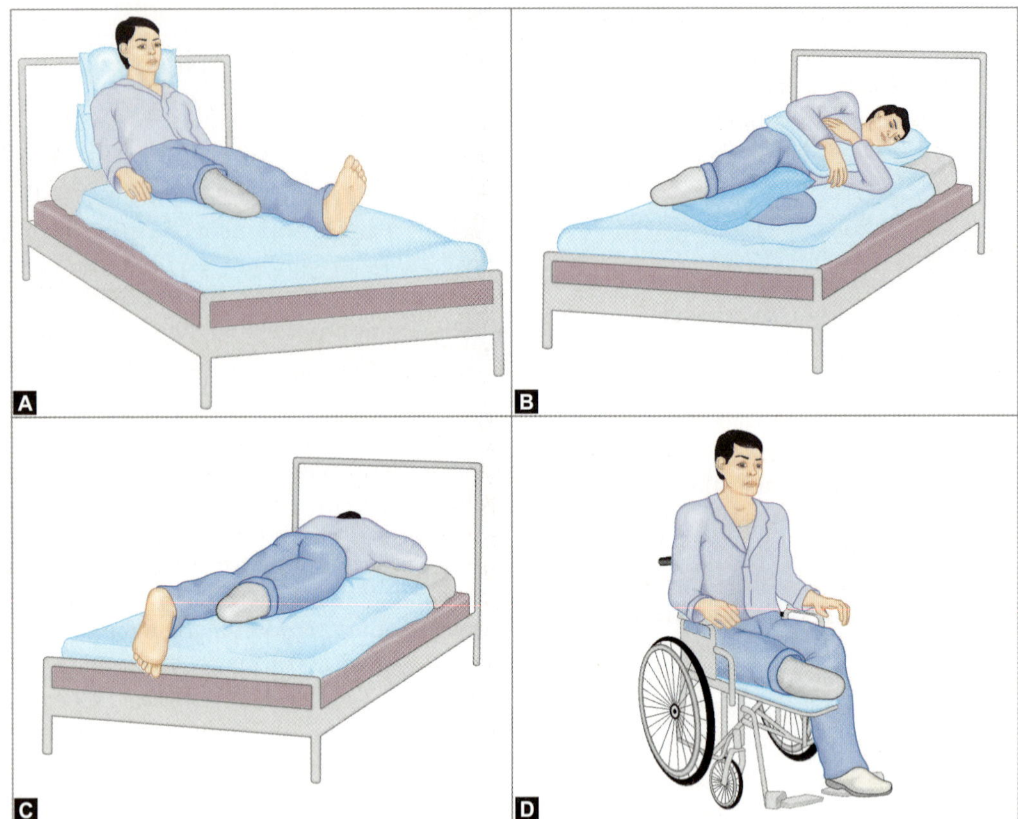

Figs. 25.5A to D: Positions for a transtibial amputation: (A) Avoidance of use of pillow beneath the residual limb; (B) Sleeping on the unamputated side to avoid discomfort to the residual limb; (C) Placing the residual limb in hip and knee extension; (D) Use of amputee board to prevent knee flexion contractures.

Residual Limb Care and Residual Limb Pain

Teaching the patient and family about how to wrap the limb, how to protect the RL while moving in bed or any other transfer activities must be emphasized by the physical therapist. Physical therapist needs to carefully monitor the excessive bleeding or draining through the cast. The patient can be encouraged to move the limb gently within a pain-free range. Gentle hip extension with the knee straight, while lying on normal limb side, is an excellent exercise for patients with transtibial amputations. Any resistive exercises for the RL are contraindicated during this period.

Pain assessment should begin preoperatively with treatment through all phases of rehabilitation. Residual limb pain can occur due to a neuroma, improper wrap, entrapped scar, alteration in blood flow, insufficient nutrition, or disrupted sleep pattern. Preferably, the patient's pain should be managed prior to any physical activity, wound care, or management of the residual limb, and rated by the visual analog pain scale. Pain should be minimized since controlled pain will allow maximal mobility and rehabilitation during inpatient and outpatient phases. Treatment may include pharmacological treatment including anticonvulsants, antidepressants, nonsteroidal anti-inflammatory drugs (NSAIDs), opioids, lidoderm patches, and topical analgesics, such as capsaicin cream allowing active rehab participation. Medication should be provided prior to dressing changes and rehab sessions. It is relevant for the therapist to be aware of the side effects of medications as side effects might include orthostatic hypotension, lethargy, disinterest, and cognitive impairment. Nonpharmacological measures will include desensitizing by tapping, stimulation with varied textured fabrics, transcutaneous electrical nerve stimulation (TENS), acupuncture, and biofeedback.

Care of the Remaining Lower Extremity

It is necessary to evaluate the status of the remaining extremity and teach the patient and family proper care, as the majority of individuals need to undergo amputation because of poor circulation. Often sutures and staples are left in place in the dysvascular amputee up to 1 month postoperatively. If staples are removed, Steri-Strips are applied and allowed to remain in place until they separate and fall off. It is important to mobilize the scar once wound healing is complete. The prime time to attempt to mobilize the incision line and prevent adhesions to the underlying tissue is when the scar is not yet mature. Pressure is applied above and below the incision line mobilizing the incision. Olive oil, cocoa butter, and vitamin E cream are some of the agents used to facilitate massage and prevent dryness.

Once the prosthetic wearing is initiated, an adherence along the suture line could result in skin breakdown, delaying ambulation. One approach to wound healing might be electrical stimulation which facilitates healing by increasing capillary density, improving tissue oxygenation, and aiding granulation tissue formation and fibroblastic activity. Bioelectrical activity is normally present in skin, but during tissue injury, the electrical field is diminished and cells have difficulty in migrating for tissue repair. The synthesized electrical activity generates a signal to the cells, which is essential to the cascade reaction to achieve wound healing. Electrical stimulation has bacteriostatic properties that help to reduce the number of bacteria by generating galvanotaxis in the wound.

Preprosthetic Phase

A careful monitoring and preprosthetic assessment is required, once the patient has been discharged from the hospital, till he has been fitted with a definitive prosthesis. Circumferential measurements of the RL at regular intervals are taken once the postoperative edema has subsided and then continued regularly throughout the period. Exact anatomical landmarks are carefully noted to avoid errors during repeat measurements. Other necessary information to be gathered about the RL includes the condition of the skin, sensation, and joint proprioception and, most importantly its shape, whether it is conical, bulbous, or cylindrical. **Table 25.4** enlists the landmarks for measurements of transtibial and transfemoral RL.

Range of motion (ROM) is necessary for the both amputated side as well as normal lower extremity. Hip flexion contractures are very crucial to note as without hip extension, the patient can neither stand nor bear the weight. **Manual muscle testing (MMT)** is also performed for uninvolved lower extremity, trunk, and upper extremities. MMT of amputated limb should be done once healing has occurred. Good strength in the hip extensors and abductors as well as the knee extensors and flexors is required for satisfactory prosthetic ambulation of transtibial amputee. For the transfemoral amputee, good strength of the hip extensors and abductors is mandatory.

UE strength is also important, especially if the patient will use mobility aids for ambulation, and should be included in assessment.

Skin condition, presence of pulses, temperature, edema, pain at rest or at exercise, presence of wounds, ulceration, or any other abnormal status are noted in the uninvolved lower extremity. ADL and mobility skills are also documented. Sitting and standing balance on the remaining extremity is important. Candidates for better prosthetic fitting include those with active lifestyle as compared to individuals with sedentary lifestyle who may face more difficulties.

Change in vital signs during transfers or early mobility training and the time to return to resting baseline values provide information about responsiveness to exercise. Ratings of perceived exertion and dyspnea are useful assessment strategies in the postoperative/preprosthetic period, both to assess how the person with new amputation is tolerating increasing activity and to help the individual target an appropriate level of activity. Treadmill training is inappropriate; hence, arm ergometry, cycling tests, can be used for lower limb amputees. Endurance and physical conditioning are predictors of prosthetic use: The ability to exercise at or above 50% of age-predicted VO_{2max} differentiates between persons with amputation able to walk functional distances (100 m) with a prosthesis and those who were unable to do so. The energy cost of walking increases as the RL length decreases; hence, endurance training is important particularly in transfemoral amputation.

Most of the patients will encounter **phantom limb sensations** (PLS) following amputation which is a sensation of the limb that is no longer there. It may occur initially immediately after surgery or as long as a year after amputation and is often characterized as a tingling, burning, itching, or pressure sensation, or sometimes a numbness. Commonly felt in the distal part of the limb, a patient with phantom limb sensation will feel the presence of whole extremity. It usually does not interfere with prosthetic rehabilitation and it is important for the patient to understand that the sensations are quite normal. **Phantom limb pain** (PLP) is a generalized noxious sensation in the absent limb that is so strong as to interfere with prosthetic fitting. It may be localized or diffuse, continuous or intermittent, and may be triggered by some external stimuli. It may diminish over time or become a permanent and disabling condition. It is necessary to differentiate phantom pain from the more common phantom sensations, RL pain, or neuroma pain. As per a study, PLP was found in 41% and PLS in 14.4% amputated cancer patients in India, following 3 months of amputation.

Sensory reeducation, cognitive behavioral therapy and therapeutic modalities, such as TENS can be useful means of management. A novel serotonin (5-HT) and noradrenaline reuptake inhibitor drug (SNRI), milnacipran is also effective in treating PLP and PLS. PLP

Table 25.4: Landmarks for measurements of transtibial and transfemoral residual limbs.		
Characteristics of residual limb	Transtibial	Transfemoral
Length	From the medial tibial plateau to the end of the bone, then to the end of the skin	From the ischial tuberosity or the greater trochanter to the end of the bone, then to the end of the skin
Measurements	Starting at the medial tibial plateau, taken every 5–8 cm depending on the length of the limb	Starting at the ischial tuberosity or the greater trochanter, whichever is most palpable, taken every 8–10 cm

can be reduced temporarily with injection of steroids or local anesthetic as well. Noninvasive treatments, such as ultrasound, icing, TENS, and massage have been used with varying success. Other techniques that have been used but with inconsistent results include biofeedback, guided imagery, psychotherapy, nerve blocks, and dorsal rhizotomies. Mirror box therapy is a cortical restructuring attempt recreating a body image by performing therapeutic exercise, using a mirror to view the reflection of an anatomical limb in the space occupied by the phantom limb. Acupuncture can also be tried in treating PLS and PLP, wherein a normal afferent input is given to the nervous system through stimulation and an analgesic effect may be elicited. Virtual reality is a latest adjunct therapy in the treatment of PLP, which is particularly effective in chronic PLP. The treatment of phantom pain needs much perseverance as it can be very frustrating for the clinical team as well as the patient.

Psychological distress responses differ in the case of traumatic loss of limb and in amputation resulting from vascular disease. Individual may feel depressed immediately following traumatic loss of the limb. They might experience difficulty in concentration along with insomnia and restlessness. In the early stages, the person's grief may alternate with feelings of hopelessness, despondency, bitterness, and anger. Socially the patient may feel lonely, isolated, and the object of pity. Concerns about the future, body image and sexual function, the responses of family and friends, and employment all affect the individual's reactions. While the amputation may bring relief to the patient against the long painful fight to save the limb in the case of amputation following a vascular disease, the responses may vary among individuals depending on the type of personality traits. The individual goes through several adjustments to the loss and is then reintegrated into a full and active life. Final acceptance stage is achieved after the individual experiences a number of stages including denial, anger, euphoria, and social withdrawal. It is utmost necessary to not give false hopes to the patient while educating them on the rehabilitation process and the steps toward independence.

Psychological distress following any disability increases with age, all other factors being equal. However, the elderly do not show any greater difficulty in psychological adjustment than the adult population as a whole. Assessing psychological component is equally important across all age-groups, and various scales, such as mini-mental state examination, depression scales, such as geriatric depression scale, and beck depression inventory, can be used.

Gait training is an important component of pre-prosthetic phase. All new prosthetic wearers are anxious to get started on walking; hence, basic pregait activities are important components for setting in place good technique, strength, and discipline **(Fig. 25.6)**. Pregait activities focus on weight shifting onto the prosthesis, balance, and breaking down the gait cycle to ensure that the individual does not create bad habits when learning to ambulate.

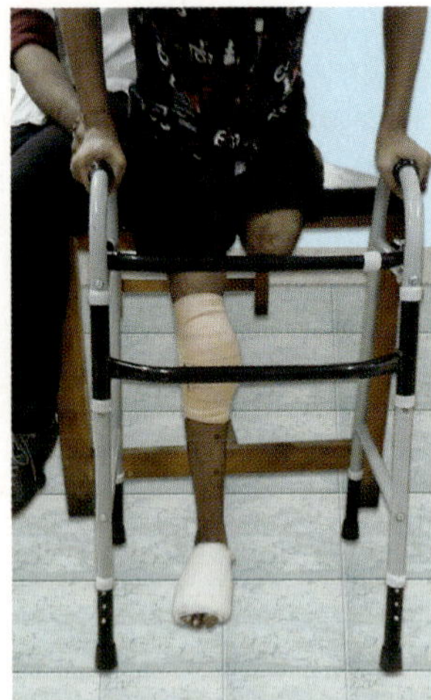

Fig. 25.6: Gait training with walker for a unilateral transfemoral amputee.

Training the patient in **donning** and **doffing** of the prosthesis is equally important. Donning should be taught with the help of socks, liner, lubricant, along with prepositioning the prosthesis in sitting followed by standing and bearing weight through the prosthesis and adjusting the suspension system. Initially the temporary prosthesis is prescribed, and once the leg volume stabilizes, incision is healed which approximately lasts till 6–12 weeks, definitive prosthesis can be prescribed. Prevention of skin breakdown, safe use with the help of prosthesis, positioning with prosthesis, and care of equipment are certain major components that should be addressed adequately.

The patient needs to receive reassurance and understanding from the entire rehabilitation team. An open and receptive environment should be created by the team members. The steps and expectations of rehabilitation should be carefully explained by the surgeon and therapists. Audiovisual media, such as films or photographs may be helpful. Attitudes toward the prosthesis selection also vary among the patients as most of them prefer function and are concerned about regaining the greatest level of function possible, whereas others choose cosmetic appearance of the prosthesis, hoping that it will conceal their disability and give the illusion of an intact body. Active involvement in the entire rehabilitation program and consistent attempts to return to an active lifestyle is considered as a good prognostic factor for recovery. Vocational counseling and training should also be incorporated in order to increase the functional status, improve independence and reduce the impact of participation restriction.

UPPER EXTREMITY PROSTHESES

Prostheses are mechanical devices used to replace an absent limb, in order to restore, and maximize function. Since numerous activities can be accomplished with one hand, most of the individuals with unilateral upper limb

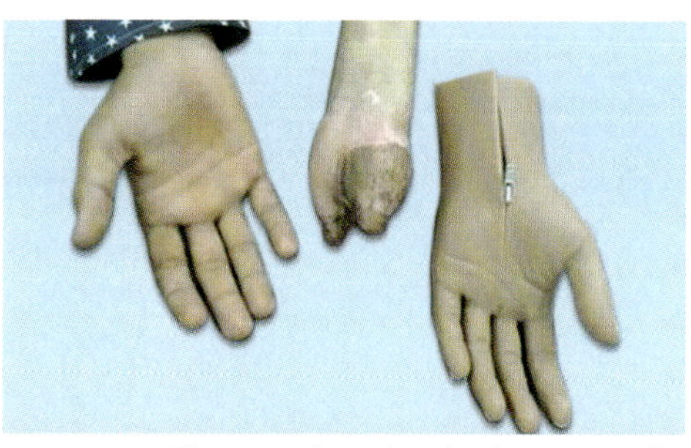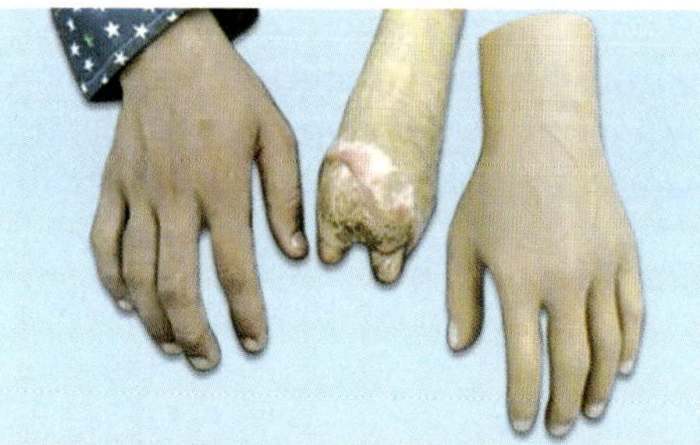

Fig. 25.7: Dorsal and volar aspect of a passive hand resembling normal hand.
Courtesy: Bionis Prosthetics and Orthotics.

amputation prefer not to wear a prosthesis. However, few individuals find that a prosthesis is functionally worthwhile or helps to disguise the amputation. Cosmetic covers made up of PVC, vinyl, or silicone provide a base to an extremely life-like coating that can match the skin tone and characteristics of the intact limb **(Fig. 25.7)**. The covers can also be textured to increase grip and to decrease friction against clothing and material. These covers, however, are not as durable as exposed metal or thermoplastic terminal devices and are not designed for heavy use. Often a more durable cover can be fabricated for use during more demanding tasks and the patient can change the covers as the situation dictates.

Prosthetic replacement for the hand is called a **terminal device** that contributes to patient's self-esteem and functions. Two types of terminal devices are available, namely—the hand and the hook **(Fig. 25.8)**. The hands are further classified as passive and active hands. Both the hands are commercially available in variable sizes and both are covered in flexible plastic glove that resembles the skin tone.

The parts of passive hands cannot be moved. They are lighter in weight, less expensive, more durable, and fingers are made of a flexible wire covered in resilient plastic. They have mainly stabilizing function, such as holding the vegetables, while the other hand does the chopping. Grasp function is unavailable. However, mechanisms in the proximal part of the amputated limb permit the finger control in active hands. Three-jaw chuck is permitted in active hands to hold the objects securely and such hands enable grasping of objects <10 cm (4 inches) in size.

Terminal Devices for Upper Limb Prosthesis

Myoelectrically operated active hands have a socket that has one or more skin electrodes that are in contact with appropriate muscle groups. When the patient contracts the muscle, the microvoltage generated by the muscle is transmitted by the electrode as the electrical signal to a small motor which in turn, enables the hand mechanism to open or close the fingers. A battery worn inside the prosthetic socket powers the motor. Excellent grasp force is provided by the myoelectric hand **(Fig. 25.9)**.

Lighter and less expensive cable operated active hand is attached to a trunk harness. By flexing the shoulder, tension is generated on the cable that, in turn, pulls on the hand mechanism causing the fingers either to open (voluntary opening) or to close (voluntary closing). Releasing the tension on the cable allows the fingers to revert in opposite direction. Therefore in voluntary-opening device, relaxation causes the fingers to close. Grasp force is weak in voluntary-opening device as compared to voluntary-closing device where the force is determined by the force that patient applies to the cable. Some of the patients find difficulty in not only wearing the harness, but also their working space is restricted.

Hooks, either produced from aluminum or steel, have two fingers that the patient can open and close. Most of the patients wear cable-operated hooks that are either voluntary-opening or voluntary-closing devices. Cable-operated hooks carry advantage of more durability, lighter weight and relatively cheaper cost as compared to any other type of hand. The patient can visualize the object to be grasped more easily as the tips of the hook fingers are relatively small. Myoelectrically controlled

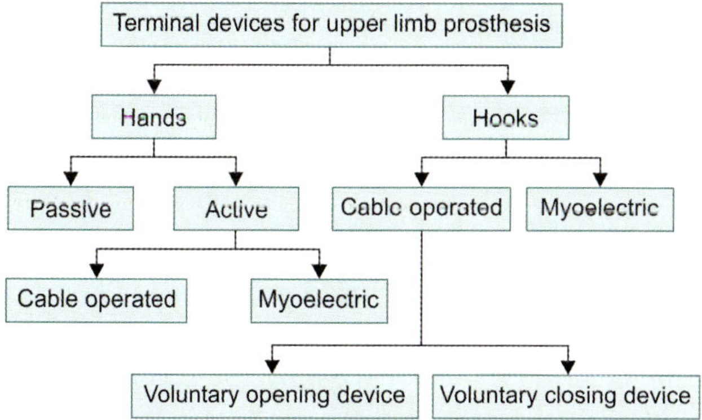

Fig. 25.8: Classification of terminal devices of upper limb.

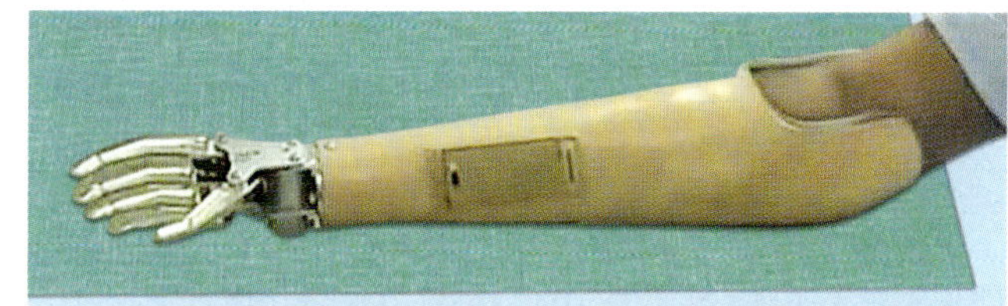

Fig. 25.9: Myoelectric transradial prosthesis.

hooks are manufactured but are less preferred. Although they allow easy grasp of larger, cylindrical, and more irregularly shaped objects, they pose a cosmetic issue. Terminal devices are also designed owing the specific demands of particular occupation or work required, such as construction work which involves specific handling or cooking which requires fine precision.

Terminal Device Selection

The rehabilitation team and patient must consider the relative importance of appearance, weight of the prosthesis, cost, durability, and amount of grasp power needed to arrive at a rational prescription. Vocational and social pursuits play crucial roles in determining the choice of terminal device. For instance, the patient who has a desk job probably will notice that a hand is preferable, whereas individual with very short transradial amputation may become fatigued after repeatedly lifting the relatively heavy myoelectric hand.

Prosthetic Replacements for the Wrist and Forearm

Irrespective of the design, the terminal device is fitted to a wrist unit. The wrist unit replaces forearm motion, allowing the pronation or supination of the terminal device rather than anatomic motions of dorsiflexion, palmar flexion, and radial and ulnar deviation. Flexion unit is a wrist unit, commonly used for patients with bilateral amputations, that allows palmar flexion as well as pronation and supination and enables the wearer to reach the midline of the body, important for eating, buttoning, and toilet activities. Combined myoelectric hand and wrist units are also available nowadays for improved ADL.

Transradial Prosthesis

The wrist unit is attached to the distal end of the socket. The proximal portion of the plastic made, self-suspending transradial socket terminates just near to the humeral epicondyles. The weight of the terminal device and wrist unit is securely held at the epicondyles by the socket, thereby the need for harness suspension is eliminated. Self-suspending sockets **(Fig. 25.10)** are usually applied with myoelectric hands. The silicone and gel suspension, shuttle lock suspension mechanism that is used to suspend the transtibial prosthesis, can also be used to suspend the

Table 25.5: Commonly used wrist and elbow units in upper extremity prostheses.	
Wrist units	*Elbow units*
Friction wrist	Flexible hinge
Constant friction wrist	Rigid hinge
Quick-disconnect unit	Outside locking hinge
Wrist flexion unit	Inside locking elbow unit
Rotational wrists	Flail arm hinge
Ball and socket wrist	Friction unit
	Spring lift assist

transradial prosthesis. The socket is fabricated using carbon graphite that keeps the weight minimal. Suspension is achieved through the support of the humeral condyles and the intimate fit of the sleeve, locking into the forearm socket.

A Dacron web made harness is essential to suspend the socket that is unsupported by the epicondyles or a shuttle lock system, or to transmit shoulder motions to a cable, or for both functions. The conventional design, a figure-of-eight, has a loop around each shoulder that connect in back.

- One strap from the loop on the amputated side is buckled to the cable that controls the terminal device.
- The other strap from the loop on the amputated side is buckled to an inverted "Y" strap that lies on the anterior surface of the upper arm and suspends the prosthesis. The loop on the sound side is known as the axillary loop.

Transhumeral Prosthesis

This prosthesis is indicated for individuals with the elbow disarticulation or higher level amputation. A terminal device, a wrist unit, a forearm shell (to replace the length of the absent forearm), an elbow unit, a socket, and a suspension mechanism are included in this prosthesis. Quick-disconnect wrists used commonly, allow for various options in place of the existing terminal device. A hinge for elbow flexion in all elbow units and a locking mechanism that enables the wearer to retain the desired flexion angle is provided. The elbow unit also includes a turntable that allows the individual to rotate the forearm shell medially and laterally and is commonly applied in transhumeral amputees or amputees with a higher level. Elbow unit is the connecting link between socket and forearm shell. Commonly used wrist and elbow units are mentioned in **Table 25.5**. A figure-of-eight transhumeral harness suspends the prosthesis and transmits shoulder and shoulder girdle motions to the cable system where the terminal device and the elbow hinge are operated by one cable and elbow lock by the second.

Donning and Doffing of Prosthesis

It is very necessary that the patient is capable enough to wear the prosthesis independently. Otherwise, it is quite certain that he might abandon wearing the prosthesis after discharge from the rehabilitation setup.

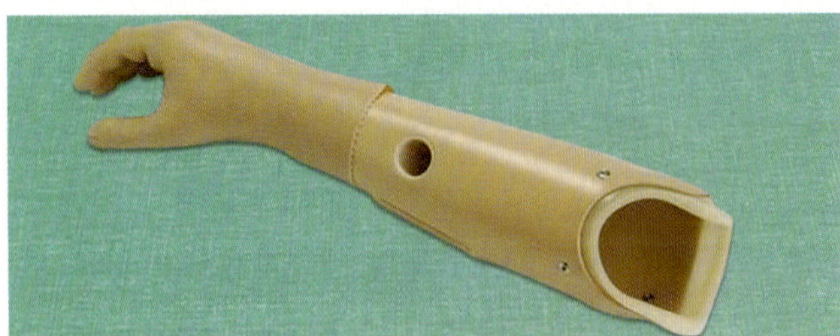

Fig. 25.10: Self-suspending transradial socket (Muenster socket). *Courtesy:* Bionis Prosthetics and Orthotics.

Donning and Doffing of Prosthesis with Figure-of-Eight Harness

Steps involved for donning include:
1. Applying a sock or liner
2. Inserting the amputation limb in the socket
3. Inserting the sound limb through the axillary loop.

Doffing the prosthesis requires the reversed steps.

Donning and Doffing of a Myoelectric-controlled Transradial Prosthesis

Steps involved for donning include:
1. Wearing a cotton stockinette knit tube, taking care that the proximal margin of the stockinette is above the antecubital fossa
2. Applying the socket
3. Pulling the distal end of the stockinette through a hole in the socket, thereby drawing the superficial tissue of the forearm snugly into the socket.

For doffing, the distal part of the prosthesis is gently tugged until it is off the forearm.

Controls Training

Teaching the patient to operate every element of the prosthesis correctly is very essential. A key determinant for long-term prosthetic acceptance is structured training. The two components in the transradial prosthesis that the patient must control include: the terminal device and the wrist unit. The basic principles of controls training for a transhumeral prosthesis shall remain similar to that of transradial prosthesis.

Wrist Unit Training

The patient can change the position of the wrist unit by turning the terminal device with the sound hand or can nudge the terminal device against the edge of a table, the chest, thigh, or contralateral forearm as most of the wrist units are passive. The therapist teaches the patient how to lock and unlock it by means of a lever or rotating rings on the unit if the wrist unit has a locking mechanism. In the case of myoelectric or cable prosthesis, the therapist teaches the correct sequence of motions in the terminal device. The form board consisting of objects of various sizes, shapes, textures, and weights is used to increase skillful use of the prosthesis. The purpose of the prosthesis is to assist the sound hand in complex activities. Grasping of a hard rubber cube is easier as the patient can easily pronate the terminal device and open up the fingers. To grasp the thin metal disk, the patient has to place the terminal device midway between supination and pronation.

The patient has to maintain tension on the control cable with a voluntary-opening terminal device, minimal tension on the control cable with a voluntary-closing device and contract the forearm flexors gently with a myoelectrically controlled device to deform the objects, such as a paper cup or a foam rubber ball.

Terminal Device Training: Myoelectric

To determine the best site for electrode placement, the patient undergoes preliminary training before a prosthesis is made. A surface electrode and a voltmeter are used by the physical therapist to explore the forearm for sites where the patient can produce the greatest electrical response. Most myoelectric prostheses have an electrode on the flexors and another on the extensors. The patient is guided to contract one muscle group isometrically while maintaining relaxation of the antagonists. The patient practices with a test socket that has electrodes, once the sites have been identified. The test socket facilitates alteration in electrode positioning. The permanent socket incorporating electrodes is fabricated once the final electrode positions are determined. The patient then practices contraction of the flexors and extensors to close and open the hand respectively. The person develops proprioceptive inputs of the amount of muscular activity required to achieve the desired amount of finger motion, as they concentrate on the movement of the hand by watching the way the fingers move.

Terminal Device Training: Cable-operated Mechanisms

The patient is instructed to flex the shoulder to operate the terminal device whether voluntary-opening or voluntary-closing. Elbow should be flexed at 90° so that the patient can see the terminal device easily and also note that the cable alignment is optimal. Resistance is often added to shoulder flexion in order to gain enough tension on the cable, to affect the terminal device. Training will make the patient recognize that the same body motion is effective irrespective of the position of the shoulder and elbow. The terminal device is then placed close to the patient's chest by the therapist and the patient is asked to operate the device. Emphasis should be on the scapular abduction as shoulder flexion would cause the terminal device to move away from the chest.

The patient should practice maintaining minimal tension on the control cable to prevent the hand or hook fingers from closing completely while using a voluntary-opening terminal device, as learning this skill shall be helpful when handling fragile objects, whereas the patient should practice to apply a light tension on the control cable while using a voluntary-closing terminal device, which will be effective when dealing with objects that might crush.

Functional Use and Vocational Training

The patient is taught to use the prosthesis to assist the normal hand in the performance of bimanual activities. The therapist must think innovatively in selecting the tasks that are easier to execute bimanually since most of the tasks can be done with single hand. The rule of thumb is that the prosthesis performs the more static part of the task. For instance, when hammering a nail, the prosthetic hand holds the nail while the sound hand strikes the nail with hammer. Other bimanual activities include pulling on socks, folding clothes, and packing up the luggage bag.

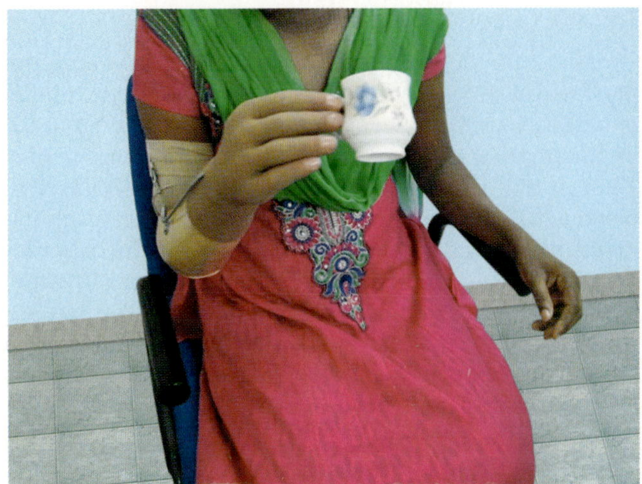

Fig. 25.11: Functional training.

Prerequisites to discharge include a thorough assessment of the patient regarding the practicality and ease of use of the prosthesis, ability to don and doff the prosthesis, and care of the skin. The crucial indicators to the success of rehabilitation include the patient's acceptance, appearance, and effectiveness of the prosthesis.

Apart from functional usage, it is important to look for the vocations that can be pursued with or without a prosthesis as most of the people sustaining upper limb amputation are men of working age. Preparing the patient for return to work is highly motivating for them. Once prevocational evaluation is done, the rehabilitation team should refer the patient to a job training center. Vocational counseling and training can be incorporated to maximize functional abilities. Patients usually tend to change their hand dominance if the amputation involves dominant side. Drawing, craft activities, and computer games can all contribute to developing hand coordination and change of hand dominance **(Fig. 25.11)**.

LOWER LIMB PROSTHESES

Lower Limb Prostheses: Prescription and Factors Affecting Prescription

Lower limb amputations are most common in civilian as well as military populations. Prosthetic devices in the lower limb are commonly resorted to in both of these populations, hugely for functional independence and locomotion. During a prosthetic prescription, prosthetist takes the center stage, whereas the whole rehabilitation team works in unison and complements their role.

Lower limb prosthetic prescription should fit each individual's need for stability, mobility, durability, cosmesis, resources, and cost. Mobility may be of prime importance for the younger individual with an amputation as well as for other patients across a wider age range when the amputation is at the transtibial and more distal levels. On the other hand, for elder population, and for those with more proximal level of amputation, such as transfemoral or hip disarticulation, the goals may often be restricted to

transfers, indoor activities, or short community distances. Hence, prosthetic prescription and fitting should always be matched according to factors, such as comfort, individual needs, acceptable cosmesis, mobility requirements, and, to some extent, personal and psychological concerns. For example, an individual may sometimes find prosthetic foam covers impeding with prosthetic function, whereas some may prefer its cosmetic appearance over function. Another important consideration in prescription is timing of prosthetic device fitting. Immediate postoperative prostheses allow earlier ambulation, but only limited weight-bearing. Customized prostheses can be given 3–6 weeks after amputation, until surgical swelling has resolved and wound healing has been achieved. It allows for full weight-bearing but may predispose to complications, such as pressure ulcers. Later after 6–9 months, when RL volume has been stabilized, a permanent prosthesis can be fit.

In earlier times, digit amputations were fitted by a wood or cork sandal with a leather ankle lacer. Partial foot amputations were sometimes fitted with a socket and keel fashioned from one piece of carefully chosen root wood, the grain of which followed the curve of the ankle. This was referred to as the *natural crook technique*. Another commonly used technique was steel-reinforced leather socket. Recent advances have enabled variety of prosthetic options, such as toe fillers, arch supports, prosthetic boots, and fillers with ankle–foot orthosis (AFO). Cosmetic restoration of silicone and several variations of AFOs are also in common use. Physician, therapist, prosthetist, and everyone involved in the rehabilitation of the amputee must be well versed with wide array of options to best accommodate the individual patient needs.

At present, partial forefoot amputations consist of ray dissections, digits amputation, and metatarsal transections. Midfoot amputations such as Chopart and Lisfranc and hindfoot amputations, such as Pirogoff, Boyd, and Symes are also often included in partial foot amputation. Patients with partial foot amputations are able to ambulate without a prosthesis, if necessary. However, a prosthesis provides protection of distal RL, especially for patients with vascular compromise or neuropathy, as commonly encountered in diabetic foot. Shoes worn without prosthetic replacement of the missing forefoot quickly become disfigured, collapsing at a displaced toe break, further endangering the vulnerable areas of the RL. Most vulnerable areas to tissue damage during walking include the distal end, first and fifth metatarsal heads, navicular, malleoli, and tibial crest. The longitudinal and transverse arches, the heel pad, and the area along the pretibial muscle belly are pressure-tolerant areas for loading in a custom shoe or prosthesis.

As the amputation level becomes more proximal and the length of the residual foot decreases, prostheses are more likely to incorporate supramalleolar containment or more superior support. This is especially important as a patient's activity level increases. At the more distal foot amputation levels and for the less active individual with a transmetatarsal amputation, accommodative shoes with custom insoles, arch supports, and toe fillers are usually adequate. More active individuals with a transmetatarsal amputation may benefit from orthotic modifications that better substitute for the lost anterior foot lever arm. The length and degree of flexibility of the prosthetic forefoot affect the anterior lever arm and consequently foot and ankle motion. The biomechanical goal is to allow anterior support in the area of the lost metatarsals as well as a controlled fulcrum of forward motion as the foot–ankle complex pivots over the area of the lost metatarsal heads in the third rocker of late stance. Other goals include: simulation of missing foot segment; and restoration of functions mainly standing and walking. An additional goal is to minimize pressure at the amputated distal end within the socket or shoe.

Prosthetic/orthotic devices for the individual with a proximal partial foot amputation need to supply medial–lateral stabilization of the hindfoot and substitute for the lost forefoot lever. Options include (1) an extra-depth shoe with toe filler, steel shank, and rocker bottom modifications; (2) custom posterior leaf-spring AFO with toe filler; or (3) a custom prosthetic foot with a self-suspending rear-opening split socket. A major advantage of all partial foot amputations is the ability to be fully end-bearing, allowing ambulation without any devices. Standing will not be affected provided that the metatarsal heads retain.

Prosthetic Types and Parts

The prosthesis may be endoskeletal or exoskeletal in structure. *Endoskeletal prostheses* have a lightweight metal pylon/shank to connect the foot to the socket (transtibial) or knee unit (transfemoral). This shank may be covered by a foam cover that matches the color and configuration of the other leg, giving a more natural appearance. Although the flexible foam cover provides an improved appearance and can be removed for adjustments when necessary, it may not be as durable as the exoskeletal devices. *Exoskeletal prostheses* are constructed of wood or rigid polyurethane covered with a rigid plastic lamination. The rigidity of the shank makes them more durable and more resistant to external wear than the endoskeletal prostheses. Exoskeletal prostheses may be less expensive than endoskeletal devices **(Figs. 25.12A and B)**.

Parts of the lower limb prostheses include:

- Socket
- Body
- Harness/suspension
- Control
- Terminal device

Prostheses for Partial Foot Amputation: Toe Fillers, Spring Shanks, Shoe Inserts

Toe fillers consist of soft foam material, such as room-temperature vulcanized elastomer, which fills the voids in

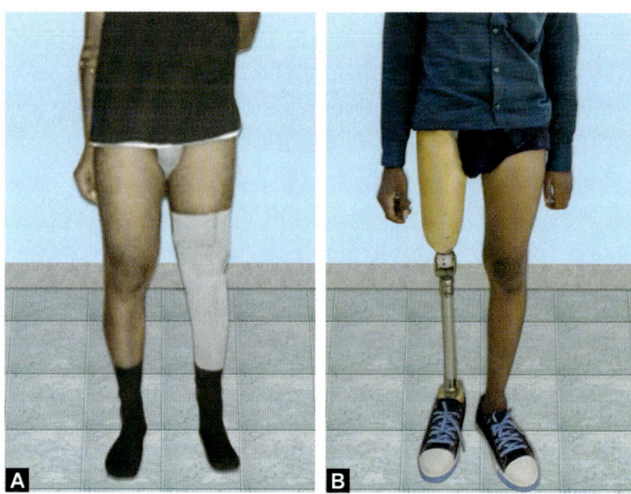

Figs. 25.12A and B: (A) Exoskeletal design; (B) Endoskeletal design.

the toe box of the shoe. They provide limited extension of the shoe life and a moderate degree of cosmesis. They also act as spacers, keeping adjoining toes properly positioned and reducing abnormal motion that can otherwise lead to ulceration. The toe filler alone provides limited mechanical advantage. *Custom insoles* made from sawdust and epoxy resin can also be used instead of foams and thermoplastics.

The patient who has lost one or more toes may simply pad the toe section of the shoe to improve the appearance of the upper portion of the shoe. For a patient with a more complex partial foot amputation, a *rocker bottom shoe modification* distributes force over a greater area and advances stance more quickly and efficiently. A *curved roll* or buildup on the plantar surface of the shoe encourages tibial advancement while minimizing weight-bearing pressures on the distal amputated end. *Spring steel shanks* are another option within the sole to compensate for partial foot loss. It extends from midcalcaneus to metatarsal heads. Another alternative is a *longitudinal support* built into flexible custom insole. Either device must end at metatarsal head, to allow hyperextension of the metatarsophalangeal joints. *University of California Biomechanics Laboratory (UCBL) insert* which is a foot orthosis can also be used, customized into a filler for partial foot amputation.

A prosthesis prevents the shoe from developing an unnatural crease in the forefoot area. The patient bears most weight on the heel and reduces the amount of time spent on the affected foot during walking. A particularly useful prosthesis consists of a plastic socket for the remainder of the foot. The socket is affixed to a *rigid plate* that extends the full length of the inner sole of the shoe. The plate has a cosmetic toe filler. The socket protects the amputated ends of the metatarsals, and the rigid plate restores foot length so that the person can spend more time during the stance phase of gait on the affected side than would otherwise be the case.

Lisfranc-type amputation requires *high-top shoes or boot-type* prosthesis to provide suspension, and it

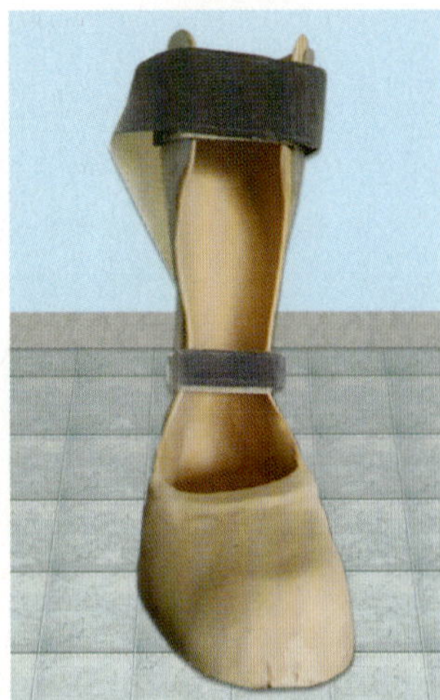

Fig. 25.13: AFO style prosthesis for Chopart amputation.
(AFO: ankle–foot orthosis)

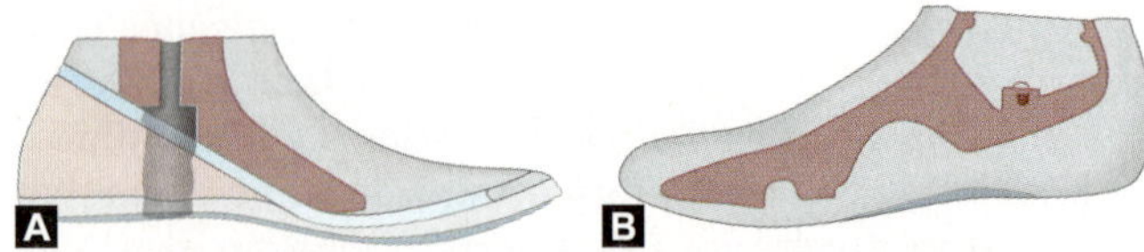

Figs. 25.14A and B: (A) SACH foot and (B) SAFE foot
(SACH: solid ankle cushion heel; SAFE: stationary attachment flexible endoskeleton)

can require an AFO with a filler to provide stability and functional length. In Chopart level of amputation, an *AFO-style prosthesis* is usually required which extends up to the patellar tendon level to distribute the high forces that result from the torques in late stance **(Fig. 25.13)**. With the Chopart amputation, a boot-type device can occasionally be used if the ankle ROM and anterior tissues are good. Prosthetic fittings at both the Lisfranc and the Chopart levels can result in the need for an elevation on the contralateral side to accommodate the height of the prosthesis.

Terminal Devices

Terminal devices in the lower extremity prostheses are prosthetic feet. The prosthetic foot is the interface between the patient and the ground and ideally would emulate the anatomical foot perfectly. Achieving this, however, is difficult. Prosthetic feet range from simple to complex as they attempt to mimic anatomical function. Anatomical articulation at the ankle and midfoot greatly affects gait efficiency and smoothness. It can increase knee stability, and a multiaxial foot can increase the base of support by accommodating uneven terrain. Prosthetic feet comprise the foundation of all lower extremity prostheses, except partial foot amputations. Prosthetic feet should simulate all lower limb activities that a normal foot does. The following functions should be performed by the prosthetic feet:

- Joint motion and activity simulation
- Muscle activity simulation
- Shock absorption
- Stable base of support

Prosthetic feet can be divided into two major categories: dynamic/energy conserving and nondynamic response feet. Nondynamic response feet, such as solid ankle cushion heel (SACH,) stationary attachment flexible endoskeleton (SAFE), Jaipur foot, and single-axis foot, do not store energy, whereas dynamic or energy conserving

feet dynamic response foot incorporate elastic (spring-like) elements that store energy in the foot during limb loading and midstance as the elastic material compresses or flexes. Energy is returned at the time of push-off as the spring component of the foot returns to its normal shape or configuration. This type of design is also referred to as an *energy storage and return design*. Examples include the Flex-foot, the Springlite feet, Seattle foot, and the impulse feet. This type of device can further be classified as articulated or nonarticulated. The dynamic energy characteristics of these prosthetic feet make them particularly suitable for individuals involved in activities requiring running and jumping. This also makes an individual more functional with a dynamic response foot.

SACH foot is a nonarticulated device with solid wood or aluminum keel, sponge rubber heel wedge, and molded cosmetic forefoot with or without individual toes. Plantar flexion is simulated by compression of the heel wedge that is adjusted to the client's weight and activity level. There is no dorsiflexion, eversion, or inversion. Anteriorly, the junction of the keel and the rubber toe sections allows the foot to hyperextend in late stance **(Fig. 25.14A)**.

SAFE foot is a newer version of SACH foot that is heavier and more expensive than SACH foot. It has a rigid ankle block joined to the posterior portion of the keel at a 45° angle, which is comparable to that of the anatomical subtalar joint. The junction permits the wearer to maintain contact with moderately uneven terrain, because of the relatively greater range of medial–lateral motion permitted in the rear foot **(Fig. 25.14B)**.

Jaipur foot is an Indian alternative of SACH foot, which overcomes the limitations of SACH foot. It allows barefoot walking and is water proof and since it is made of uncured rubber, raw material is easily available, making it cost-effective. The elasticity of the rubber provides enough dorsiflexion to permit an amputee to squat, transverse rotation of the foot on the leg to facilitate walking and cross-legged sitting, and sufficient range of inversion–eversion to allow the foot to adapt itself while walking on uneven surfaces. Prof PK Sethi, at SMS medical college, Jaipur, developed this variant along with his team and made it particularly suitable for usage in Indian population where barefoot walking is prevalent in villages, and a practice at places, such as temples. It is also cosmetically acceptable **(Fig. 25.15)**. **Table 25.6** shows the comparison between SACH, SAFE and Jaipur foot.

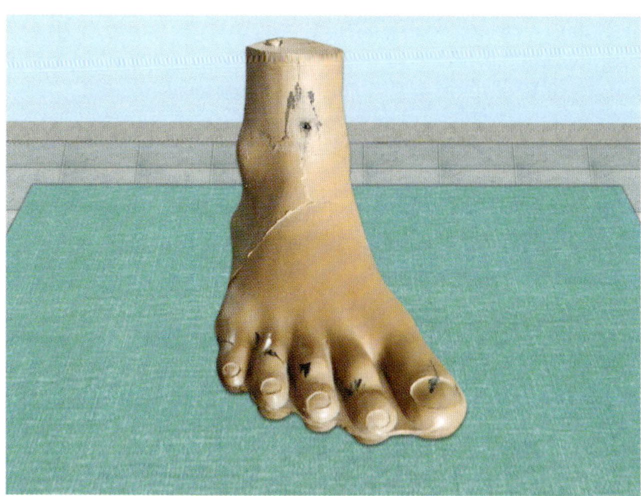

Fig. 25.15: Jaipur foot.

Table 25.6: Comparison between solid ankle cushion heel (SACH), stationary attachment flexible endoskeleton (SAFE), and Jaipur foot.

SACH foot	SAFE foot	Jaipur foot
Requires a closed footwear for protection and hiding	Requires a closed footwear for protection and hiding	Does not require a closed footwear, unless preferred by patient
Squatting and cross-legged sitting not possible	Squatting and cross-legged sitting not possible	Squatting and cross-legged sitting easily possible
No movement at subtalar joint, so inversion and eversion not possible	No movement at subtalar joint, so inversion and eversion not possible	Permits movement at subtalar joint, so inversion and eversion is possible, facilitates uneven ground walking
Barefoot walking is not permissible, hence unacceptable in some cultures	Barefoot walking is not permissible, hence unacceptable in some cultures	Barefoot walking is possible, hence acceptable in India

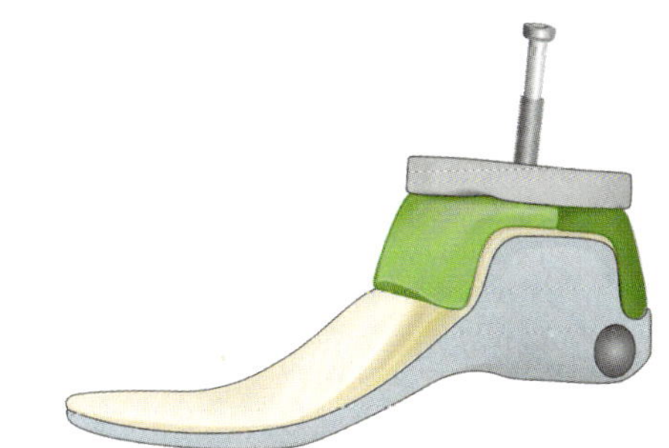

Fig. 25.16: Single-axis foot.

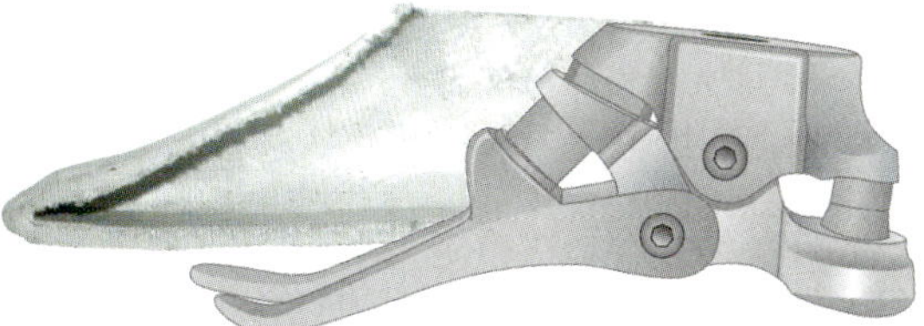

Fig. 25.17: Multiaxis foot.

Articulating prosthetic feet include both single-axis and multiaxis designs. The *single-axis foot* allows controlled movement in the sagittal plane (plantar flexion and dorsiflexion), adjusted by using different durometer bumpers. At heel contact, the plantar flexion bumper compresses, offering a true plantar flexion motion. The rapid foot flat increases knee extension moment and therefore prosthetic stability on stance. The dorsiflexion bumper that is a little firmer than the plantar flexion bumper limits dorsiflexion at midstance and terminal stance. The firmness of bumpers is determined by the client's weight and activity level. The primary advantage of the single-axis foot is its ability to reduce knee bending movements during limb loading, thus improving knee stability. Disadvantages include a greater weight than many other feet and more maintenance to ensure correct function. This foot is primarily used in the individual with a proximal amputation that requires better knee stabilization, such as a short RL **(Fig. 25.16)**.

Multiaxis foot is a type of dynamic response foot, allowing greater mediolateral movement and stability. It is heavier than any other foot, increasing the amount of energy required for ambulation. *Soft keels* have a soft foam shell with an elastic keel that compresses on heel contact, controlling the rate of plantar flexion and the speed of movement to midstance. Inversion and eversion are minimally simulated by cushioning the rubberized heel. These feet provide some adaptation for uneven ground. Seattle foot is an example of soft keel **(Fig. 25.17)**.

Syme's Prosthesis

Ankle disarticulation prosthesis is composed of a socket and a foot; suspension is inherent within the socket because of the configurations of the RL. The Syme's level prosthesis trim lines should extend to the patellar tendon to increase the loading surface. If the trim lines do not extend proximally enough, they can dig into the crest of the tibia. *Conventional Syme's prosthesis* has a medial opening design with a medial window cutout to allow the malleoli to pass. *Modified Syme's prosthesis* has a posterior opening socket, the posterior opening is cut down to the level of the malleoli and is constructed as a removable section that is held with Velcro. This is used for the more bulbous RLs. This is the weakest of the three designs because of the limited material in the sagittal plane. The newer and third design is a *stovepipe construction*, which has no flaps or windows cut in the socket. Instead, a soft insert is built up into a tapered cylinder to slide into a cylindrical socket, or an expandable wall is built into a cylindrical socket to allow passage of the malleoli. If the malleoli are not prominent, suspension is similar to transtibial prostheses.

Socket

In *conventional Syme's prosthesis*, a window is cut along the medial wall of the socket to allow the bulbous end, created by the tibial condyles, to slide down to the end-bearing part of the prosthetic foot. The window is covered by a panel that fits snugly into the opening and is secured by two straps itself. The standard Syme's prosthesis is functional but not very cosmetic with a thick distal end and a strap. *Modified Syme's prosthesis* has a posterior opening socket, and the *stovepipe Syme's* has a closed expandable socket, which is fabricated with a liner attached to the inner wall of the socket. The liner is made of flexible plastic and extends from the distal end of the socket to a point where the diameter of the proximal leg equals the bulbous end distally. A space is created between the inner socket and the outer laminate, and the liner stretches as the end of the RL is inserted into the socket. The liner closes around the length of the residuum to maintain total contact and aid in suspension.

Terminal Device

Ankle disarticulations result in the loss of all ankle–foot motions. Because of the limited space available beneath the socket, foot selection is limited for Syme's level amputations. The two most common designs are—specially designed, low-profile dynamic response feet and specially designed SACH feet. Both of these are made to bolt or bond directly to the bottom of the socket. Also the length of RL precludes the choice of prosthetic feet.

Transtibial Prostheses

Socket

The standard transtibial socket is patellar tendon bearing (PTB) socket **(Fig. 25.18)**. It is a laminated plastic socket fitted with or without a liner. Pressure-tolerant and pressure-sensitive areas of PTB socket are described in **Table 25.7**. Standard PTB design may have several variations. The PTB-supracondylar (PTB-SC) socket has high medial and lateral sidewalls that extend above and over the femoral condyles, providing enhanced mediolateral stability and self-suspension of the prosthesis. The PTB-supracondylar/suprapatellar (PTB-SCSP) socket further extends the PTB-SC socket concept by also extending the anterior aspect of the socket so that the patellar is encompassed within the socket. The PTB-SCSP gives additional stiffness to the mediolateral walls and applies force proximal to the patella during stance to provide sensory feedback to limit genu recurvatum. Both the PTB-SC and PTB-SCSP are primarily used in individuals with transtibial amputation and with short RLs to improve varus/valgus control and to provide greater surface area for weight distribution.

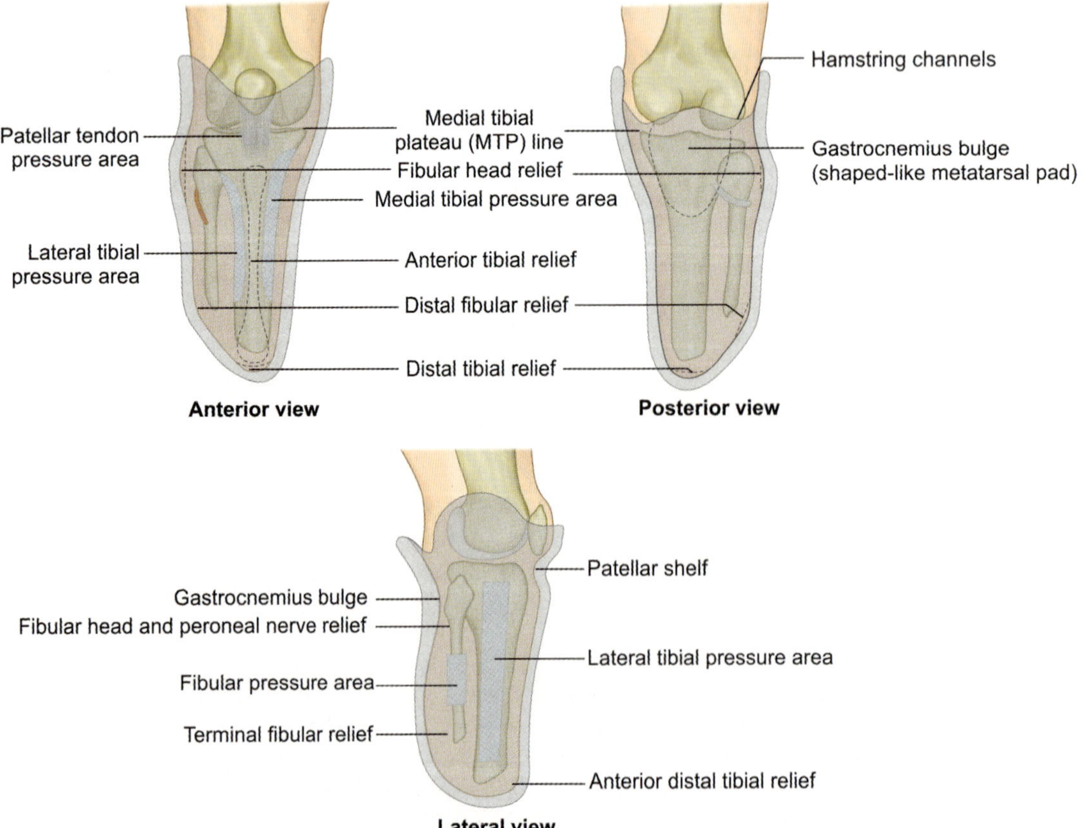

Fig. 25.18: Pressure-tolerant and pressure-sensitive areas of patellar tendon bearing socket.

Table 25.7: Pressure-tolerant and pressure-sensitive areas of patellar tendon bearing socket.

Pressure-tolerant areas	Pressure-sensitive areas
Patellar tendon	Head of fibula with peroneal nerve
Flares of tibial condyles	Distal end tibia–fibula
Areas above femoral condyles	Sharp crest of tibia
Shaft of tibia	
Popliteal fossa	
Distal end of residual limb	

Liners

An alternative socket design for individuals with a transtibial amputation is the total surface bearing (TSB) socket made practical by the development of gel and elastomeric liner systems. The TSB socket is made from a cast of the RL with minimal modifications. When used with gel liners, the TSB socket distributes pressure more evenly within the socket. Other than this type of socket, almost all socket designs require a liner, which is similar to socks, available in various sizes, shapes, and fabric. The liner functions as the primary interface between the RL and the prosthesis. In this role, it must complement socket fit to ensure optimal pressure distribution while also eliminating harmful shear forces and providing a favorable moisture, heat, and chemical environment that prevents skin breakdown.

Fabric liners, pelite liners, silicone liners, nylon liners, and elastomeric gel liners are generally used variety of liners. Each has its own advantage and disadvantage, and the final decision of selecting these should be purely based upon the comfort, fit, cost, and presence of any contraindications, such as open wounds, poor hygiene, and skin conditions like dermatitis. For example, gel liners are thought to enhance comfort and reduce shear, making them the initial choice for RL s with scarring or skin grafts that compromise skin integrity. However, they result in more sweating and are generally less tolerated in warm climates than other liners. Also, gel liners are expensive and require careful maintenance.

Unlined hard sockets that do not use a liner or use a liner made from closed cell foam (more commonly), such as Pe-Lite for improved comfort are often an advantage in the preparatory prosthesis because of the relative ease with which the liner can be modified to accommodate changes in RL volume. A newer advance in such unlined sockets is that they made of thin thermoplastic in a rigid frame. Plastic can be spot heated to facilitate alteration of socket fit. It adheres to the skin better than rigid plastic, thereby providing better suspension, and is relatively comfortable as it dissipates body heat more effectively and responds to changes in amputation limb shape as the patient contracts and relaxes the muscles.

Suspension

Suspension system for the transtibial prosthesis must securely attach the limb during activities, minimize pistoning, and be comfortable when sitting. When working with individuals with an amputation who run, play sports, or are involved in climbing activities, ensuring effective suspension is especially important. Suspension systems can be grouped into categories that include straps, sleeves, gel liners with locking mechanisms, and suction.

Supracondylar cuff is the most commonly used system and is inexpensive, easily applicable and is also comfortable in sitting. It supplies adequate suspension for the low-to-moderate activity-level individual with an amputation and is often the best option when impaired hand function limits grip strength and coordination. It is made of Dacron webbing or leather and attaches via studs to the proximal parts of the socket. It encircles the thigh just above the femoral condyles and patella. The cuff suspends the prosthesis during swing phase. It is designed to hold the prosthesis over the patella, and not circumferentially around the supracondylar aspect of the thigh but accurate suspension is difficult to obtain. It is not frequently used nowadays. *Supracondylar suprapatellar* suspension has its proximal brim extending over the patella and femoral condyles with suspension pressure exerted over the patella and the medial femoral condyle. Suprapatellar suspension is created by an indentation of the socket brim over the soft tissue of the patellar. A cup is created for the patella ensuring that there is no pressure on the patella itself. Pressure over the medial femoral condyle is created by inserting a wedge in the medial portion of the proximal socket. Prostheses with suprapatellar–supracondylar suspension are themselves referred to as patellar-tendon supracondylar (PTS) as described earlier in the transtibial socket.

Sleeve suspension systems consist of rubber, neoprene, or elastic sleeves that are pulled up onto the distal thigh after donning the prosthesis. Sleeves are a general-purpose suspension system that is inexpensive and effective for individuals with an amputation across a wide spectrum of activity levels. Primary disadvantages of sleeves are excessive heat or sweating, the need for good grip strength to pull the sleeve up, and occasional occurrence of contact dermatitis, especially with the use of neoprene-based sleeves, similar to the liner systems. Silicone and elastomeric gel liners are prosthetic sock-shaped sleeves made from a variety of silicone and urethane elastomeric compounds that are rolled onto the RL. They function as both an interface and suspension method.

Shuttle lock suspension requires either a metal pin attached to the distal end of the liner which inserts into a locking mechanism in the bottom of the socket or by a Velcro lanyard strap that passes through a slot in the socket and connects with its counterpart attached to the outside of the socket. The pin locks into a receptacle built into the bottom of the socket as the patient places weight into the prosthesis. It is released by pushing on a button placed on the medial part of the shank of the prosthesis. During swing phase, the pin mechanism prevents the prosthesis from slipping. A lanyard system is available when pin engagement is difficult because of mobile distal tissue or when a low-profile lock is required to avoid making the prosthesis too long and creating a length discrepancy. Lock mechanisms can be very secure and include less cumbersome forms of suspension, avoiding straps, belts, etc. To remove the prosthesis, a release pin is depressed that disengages the lock. A recent advance in this is *osseointegration*, a surgical approach wherein the surgeon implants a metal pin in the distal bone. This pin protrudes through the skin and locks into a mechanism in the prosthesis. It eliminates the need for other suspension apparatus; however, fluid drainage and infection at the skin/pin interface can be sometimes troublesome.

Suction suspension, also known as *vacuum-assisted suspension*, is another option and consists of a one-way air valve ported to the bottom of the socket with an airtight sleeve a partial vacuum is created within the socket effectively suspending the prosthesis during the swing phase. The vacuum needed to hold the RL can be generated through a pistoning action of the RL within the socket or by a vacuum pump built into the prosthetic shank that is activated at heel strike or by an electric-operated vacuum pump attached to the socket. This is not very durable and requires careful maintenance.

Thigh corset or *waist belts* are rarely used nowadays. The leather thigh lacer may be necessary when complete mediolateral stability is required or if a very short or painful RL cannot be suspended any other way. The leather corset attaches by metal side bars and hinged knee joints to the socket. It fits around the distal half of the thigh or may extend to the proximal thigh. It reduces weight-bearing in the socket, limits knee motion, and increases the weight of the appliance. It is also not cosmetic whether worn under or over clothing and is difficult to don. Waist belts with an anterior fork strap that attaches to the socket are a rarely used suspension option. This type of suspension is most commonly used in conjunction with a PTB total contact socket with side joint and a high corset. The weight and bulk of the resulting limb makes it a poor initial choice for a contemporary prosthetic limb, but it does remain a useful option for long-term users of this design of prosthesis.

Shank

Most contemporary transtibial prostheses are endoskeletal in design, which consists of a metal pipe connecting the terminal device to the socket. Shank is a substitute for the human leg and hence should help restore leg length and transmit the body forces from socket to terminal device. Using an *endoskeletal pylon* allows alignment

changes after prosthetic fabrication and enables the use of additional components that can absorb forces or allow motion between the socket and the remainder of RL. Commonly used materials for pylon are carbon graphite, and others include *transverse rotators* that reduce axial torques and *vertical shock absorbers* that cushion impact loading and may reduce oxygen consumption. *Exoskeletal pylon* is made of rigid outer shell, often referred to as *crustacean*, similar in contour to human leg, is durable but does not allow changes in prosthetic alignment. Due to cosmetic deviation from anatomical leg, it is used lesser as compared to endoskeletal design.

Terminal Device

The choice of terminal device in transtibial prosthesis is usually from the types of prosthetic feet described in the previous section the chapter and should rely on factors, such as age, physical activity level, level of ambulation required, and cosmesis. Selecting a prosthetic foot completes the transtibial prosthesis prescription. Nonarticulated type terminal device, i.e. SACH foot is often chosen when prescribing transtibial prosthesis **(Fig. 25.19)**.

Transfemoral Prosthesis

Prescription of a transfemoral prosthesis comprises selection of the socket style initially. Next the RL interface/liner and suspension system are determined. Because liner and suspension options are closely linked at the transfemoral level, they are decided together. Following selection of socket and suspension, the knee unit is selected and finally pylon and foot/ankle components are chosen. Four socket designs are in general use: quadrilateral, ischial containment, contoured ischial containment, and flexible. Transfemoral sockets are designed to emphasize loading on pressure-tolerant structures, such as the gluteal musculature, sides of the thigh, and to a lesser extent, distal end of the amputated limb. Excessive pressure on the pubic symphysis and perineum should be avoided.

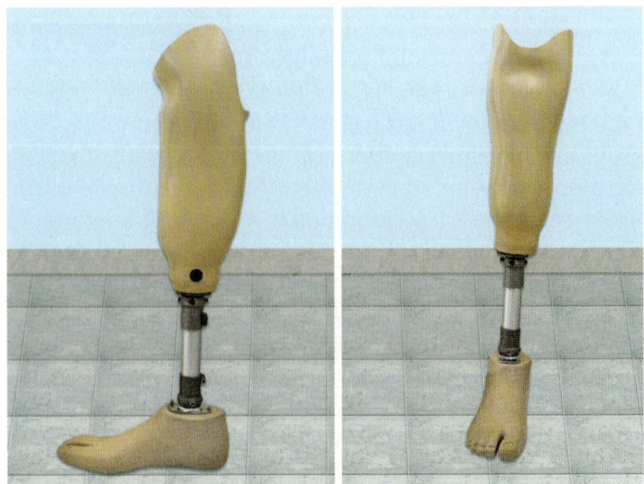

Fig. 25.19: Transtibial prosthesis with supracondylar brim.

Socket

Quadrilateral Socket

More historically, quadrilateral socket refers to the four-sided shape of the socket when viewed transversely. The four walls of the socket are designed to apply pressures and counter pressures to facilitate comfortable load-bearing through soft tissue and underlying structures. The ischial tuberosity and gluteal musculature are used as primary weight-bearing structures and are supported by a posterior shelf. Internally, the wall is contoured for the hamstring muscles, whereas externally, it is flat to prevent rolling in sitting. If the socket is made of rigid plastic, the exterior is padded to absorb sounds and protect clothing. The height of the posterior wall is determined by the position of the ischial tuberosity. Anterior wall is higher than posterior, by about 5 cm, and medially it provides stabilizing pressure to help keep the ischial tuberosity securely on the scat by molding over the femoral triangle. The anterior wall is convex laterally to allow space for the bulk of the rectus femoris muscle. The lateral wall is as high as the anterior wall and inclines medially to set the RL in about 10° of adduction, thereby aiding pelvic control in stance. A relief channel is built into the corner of the medial and anterior walls for the adductor longus tendon. The quadrilateral socket provides minimal mediolateral and little rotational stability. It was considered to be the standard socket of choice, until the emergence of ischial containment socket (ICS). However, quadrilateral sockets are still used for long-term wearers who have not only become accustomed to its weight-bearing and control characteristics but also remain an option for the individual with a transfemoral amputation with a long RL and for individuals who require UE aids for trunk stability **(Fig. 25.20A)**.

Ischial Containment Socket

For the majority of individuals with new transfemoral amputations, the ICS provides a more normal anatomic alignment of the femur inside the prosthesis. This is accomplished by extending the socket trim lines proximally and contouring the medial aspect of the socket to capture the ischial tuberosity inside the socket rather than allowing the tuberosity to sit on the posterior shelf, as in quadrilateral socket **(Fig. 25.20B)**. Weight-bearing forces are distributed through the medial aspect of the ischium and the ramus as well as surrounding soft tissue. This also facilitates rotational stability. Compared to the quadrilateral socket, more of the RL is contained within the ICS, allowing greater force distribution as well as weight-bearing. Lateral wall is extended well over the greater trochanter to add to stance-phase stability of the pelvis, whereas anterior wall is lower than in the quadrilateral socket.

Contoured Ischial Containment

ICS that is contoured around muscle compartments to increase the mediolateral stability of the transfemoral RL in the socket is referred to as contoured ICS. The socket is contoured to lock the pubic ramus and ischium within the socket and provide channels for functioning muscle groups, such as the hip adductors and extensors. The socket itself is made of soft plastic that is meant to fit directly over the RL. However, a gel liner or stump sock interface may be used, although such an interface lessens

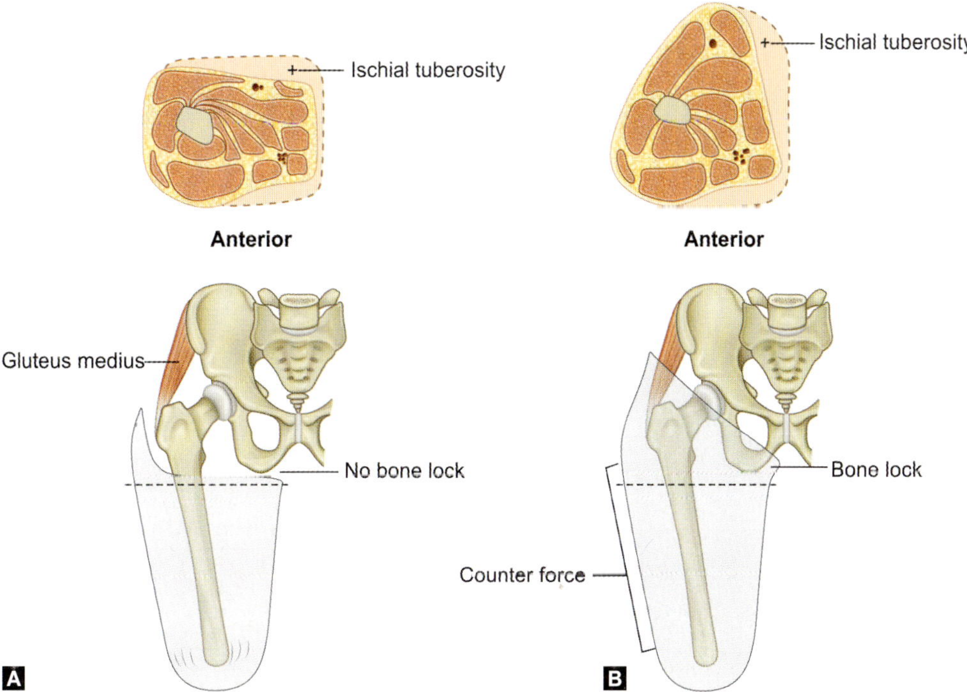

Figs. 25.20A and B: (A) Quadrilateral and (B) ischial containment socket designs.

the degree of proprioceptive feedback. The socket is designed to encourage the individual to use remaining musculature actively within the socket during locomotion. The design is functional for all transfemoral prostheses and all activity levels.

Flexible Socket

Flexible sockets incorporate a malleable thermoplastic socket supported in some type of rigid or semirigid frame. The frame can be of quadrilateral or ischial containment design, although the latter is more frequently used. Flexible sockets are reported to provide better proprioception, better suspension and are more comfortable. ComfortFlex is a type of flexible socket, which is soft and placed in a carbon graphic frame. Carbon fiber provides structural support, and flexible fit socket assures adequate muscle contraction.

Suspension

Suction socket suspension is the second major type of suspension for the individual with a transfemoral amputation and whenever feasible, is generally the preferred option. It provides intimate suspension along with good proprioception and full hip motion. If leg volume fluctuates in a client, suction may not be a feasible choice. There are three ways in which this suspension can be donned: (1) putting on a thin sock, standing, and pushing the RL into the socket while pulling the sock out of the valve hole, (2) spreading a thin layer of lotion over the RL, which is absorbed into the skin and suction is maintained, and (3) without a sock, directly pushing the RL into the socket that pushes the air out of the medial distal hole. The possible problems with this type of suspension are mostly related to perspiration, skin shear and abrasions, along with skin irritation.

Silesian bandage is a soft webbing strap that attaches to the anterior and lateral portions of the proximal prosthetic socket and passes over the opposite iliac crest. Silesian bandage aids in suspension and provides some control of rotation. The bandage is indicated as an auxiliary to suction suspension. *Total elastic suspension (TES)* is made of the same neoprene material used for transtibial suspension sleeves. It slips over the outside of the prosthetic socket and surrounds the waist above the iliac crests to provide suspension. It can be used with suction or as a primary suspension mechanism. Both Silesian and TES suspension systems are simple to don, can be adapted for use by individuals with impaired hand function, and usually provide acceptable prosthetic limb suspension for low-activity-level patients. Disadvantages include some inevitable pistoning of the prosthesis, reduced comfort due to bandage pressure, and heat or occasional dermatitis, especially with the TES belt. **Figure 25.21** shows various suspensions that are used in transfemoral prosthesis.

Other suspension belt options include the *pelvic band*, which uses a single-axis hip joint integrated into the lateral socket wall and belt is closely contoured about the iliac crest. It limits rotation of the prosthesis and is useful for the short RL. It may be made up of metal or leather and is particularly useful when client's weight fluctuates or when client has weak hip abductors.

Knee Unit

The prosthetic knee has several functions, such as sitting, kneeling, and similar activities. It allows for a smooth and controlled movement of the shank and foot during swing phase at any gait speed and on any type of surface and provides stability during stance phase. Generally, knee units may be divided into three categories: those that are only mechanical in control, those that have hydraulic or pneumatic controls, and those that are computerized or controlled by a microprocessor. Functionally, they can be further subdivided into those that provide control only over stance phase of gait, those that provide control of swing phase, and those that provide control of both swing and stance phase.

The most basic knee joint is the *constant friction knee joint*. Prosthetic knee joints should provide stability during stance and smooth, controlled knee extension during the swing phase. A constant friction, single-axis knee has a feature that provides continuous pressure/friction around the knee axis to control the velocity at which the shank and foot can swing to prevent excessive heel rise

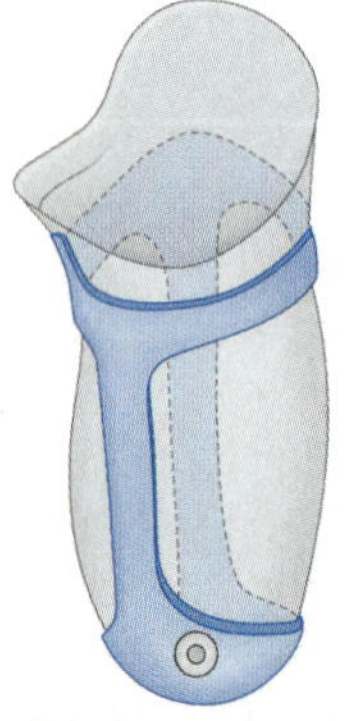
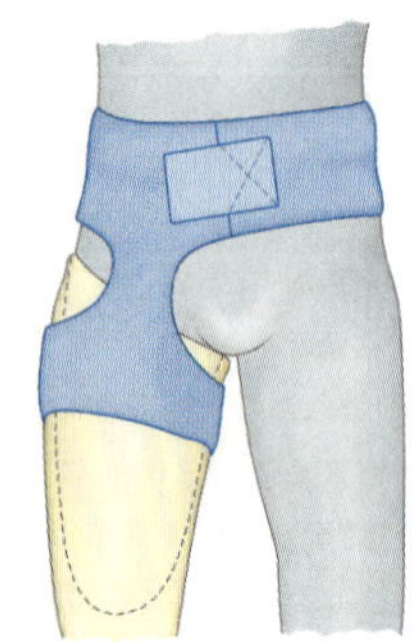
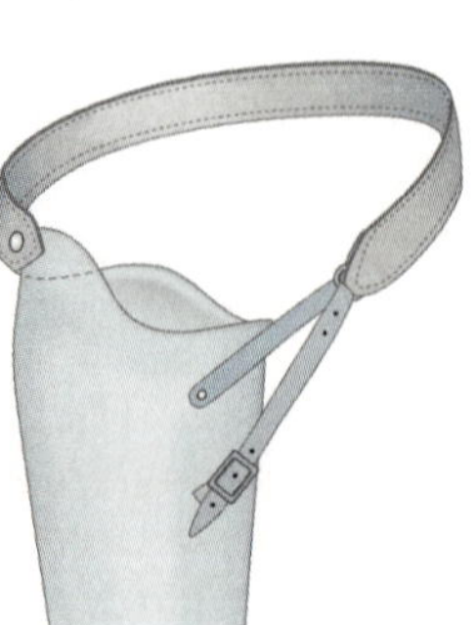
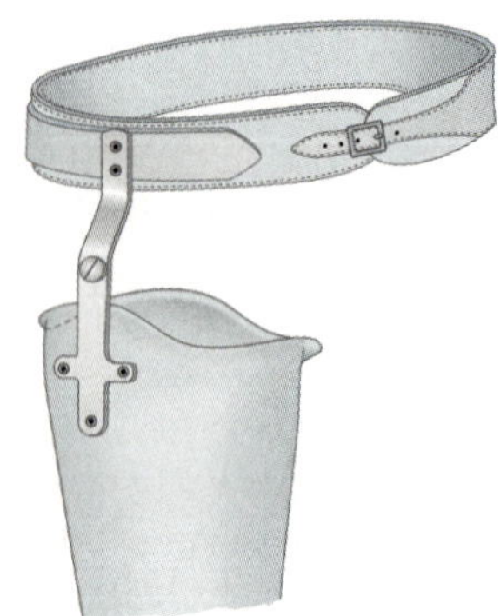

Fig. 25.21: Suspensions used in transfemoral prosthesis.

during flexion and terminal impact at full extension. The resistance to swing is adjustable, but not self-adjusting as velocity changes. For patients who do not alter the speed of their cadence, a constant friction knee is ideal because of its simplicity, durability, and ease of use. However, most individuals walk at varying speeds and will require a more gait-responsive knee.

Polycentric knee joints are usually four bar linkage systems. They have multiple axes of rotation that change during knee motion. These knees provide some response to changing gait speeds and some swing-phase control by shortening the shank during flexion to allow for better toe clearance. They offer some stance-phase control by varying stability through the different axes. In general, the polycentric knee is particularly useful for individuals with long RLs or knee disarticulations (KDs), or for individuals who do not change walking speed a great deal. They are not very effective for usage by active community ambulators or athletes.

There are two basic types of fluid-controlled knees: *pneumatic* and *hydraulic*, both of which provide frictional resistance about the knee axis that will increase proportionally with speed. Fluids include liquids, vapors, and gases. The major difference with fluids in prosthetic knees is that air is more easily compressible, and hydraulic fluids are not. Oil or air is forced through a small orifice or tube. Adjustment screws allow the size of the orifice to be changed to control the rate in which fluid flows through these ports. This permits fine-tuning of swing-phase resistance to individual needs. If air is used, the air under compression within the pneumatic cylinder also acts as an extension assist. The ability of air to compress gives pneumatic knees a springier feel to the patient.

Other types of knee mechanisms comprise microprocessor knee, and motorized knee. *Microprocessor knees* sense the conditions acting on the knee joint and can quickly make internal adjustments to safely meet those conditions. Joint angles and forces on the pylon are measured via sensors and are then sent to the microprocessor for rapid adjustment. Valves open or close electronically to increase or decrease fluid flow through the knee's internal ports, or the viscosity of the fluid changes to vary resistance to knee flexion or extension. Microprocessor knees are better over mechanical knees in that rapid input from the microprocessor makes them significantly more responsive to the patient's activity, whether walking, running, descending stairs, or stumbling. These knees allow for manipulation of the computer program to vary the stability and safety of the knee as the patient progresses through rehabilitation.

Based on microprocessor technology, the *motorized knee* also provides flexion and extension movements, to an externally powered motor-driven knee. The knee replaces lost muscle function, in that it is possible for the user to climb stairs step by step, ascend inclines, and walk longer distances on level ground. Sensors are positioned on the sound side, which accurately measure motion, load, and

position. This information is transmitted to the knee via Bluetooth technology, where the microprocessor analyzes the data and determines the response of the knee to the activity and the amount of power or force needed from the knee to generate the appropriate knee flexion or extension.

A few other advanced knee units are user-activated knee lock, geometric lock, and other knee components, such as positional rotators, combined torsion and vertical shock absorbers, quick release couplings. User-activated lock, also known as manual lock, provides absolute stance-phase control but does not swing because the knee remains locked in extension throughout the gait cycle. *Manual lock knees* have a locking mechanism that is activated by the client, when standing and disengaged when they are about to sit. Occasionally, they are useful in bilateral amputees, or weaker clients, who require complete stance-phase control and are able to walk only a short distance with assistance. Independent torsion and shock-absorbing units are types of advanced knee units, which can be paired with any foot. Interchangeable elastomer rods or adjustable springs provide dampening of vertical and rotational forces, thus reducing the strain on joints and soft tissues. Both torsion absorption and vertical shock dampening are inherent to some prosthetic feet.

Geometric lock, also referred to as a mechanical stance-phase lock, locks the knee on full extension (initial contact) and does not release it until the weight line passes over the forefoot and hyperextension of the knee unit occurs. This clever geometric design is engineered into a polycentric knee and provides excellent stability. The geometric lock can be convenient because it provides reliable stance control. *Positional rotators* permit rotation of the flexed knee and shank of the prosthesis out of the way for ease of movement. It enables cross-legged sitting and also eases tasks, such as changing shoes, or wearing socks with the prosthesis on.

Pylon and Terminal Device

Single-axis foot is commonly used in transfemoral prosthesis, as it achieves the foot-flat position with minimal application of weight-bearing load. However, any foot, including the energy-storing/releasing designs, can be incorporated in a transfemoral prosthesis. As compared with wearers of transtibial prostheses, most wearers of transfemoral prostheses do not load the prosthesis as vigorously. Consequently, less energy would be stored and released in a dynamic response foot (**Fig. 25.22**).

Exoskeletal or endoskeletal design may be used in pylon. The same pylon components (vertical shock pylons and rotators) that are available for the individual with an amputation at the transtibial level are also available at the transfemoral level. In addition, a thigh rotator can be added for the individual with a transfemoral amputation who has a need to cross the prosthetic leg for ADLs. Endoskeleton pylons have better cosmesis and are lighter in weight than exoskeletal shank, and also adjustable in alignment.

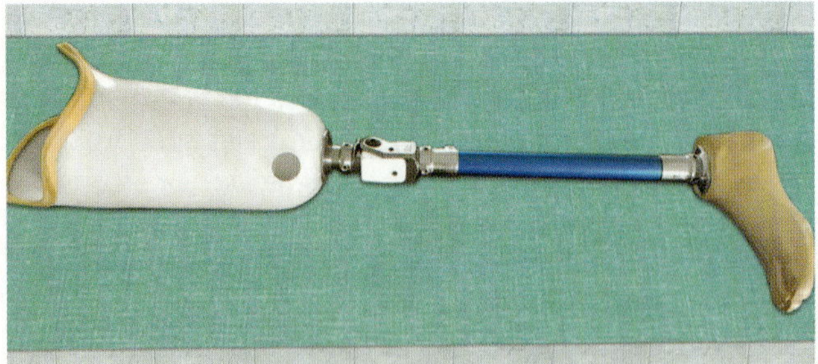

Fig. 25.22: Transfemoral prosthesis with ischial containment socket having suction suspension mechanical knee joint, and solid ankle cushion heel.

Prosthesis for Disarticulation

Prosthesis for Ankle Disarticulation

The ankle disarticulation prosthesis consists of socket and terminal device, suspension being inherent. Syme's prosthesis, used in ankle disarticulation, has been discussed earlier in the chapter.

Prosthesis for Knee Disarticulation

KD also has full weight-bearing on the distal end of the RL, similar to the Syme's amputation. The anatomic flare of the femoral condyles can be used for self-suspension of the prosthesis. Because of the improved distal weight-bearing, the KD amputation does not require an ischial weight-bearing socket leading to enhanced comfort and sitting tolerance as does a transfemoral amputation. The KD has a bulbous distal end, which hampers prosthetic cosmesis. When femoral condyles are not bulbous, roll-on sleeves can be used in combination with air expulsion. Although a pin is not recommended because of space limitations, a lanyard system can be effective. This creates a positive lock that is engaged even if limb volume changes. When the femoral condyles are prominent, a removable door suspension design can be used to suspend the prosthesis. This suspension uses external straps, attached to a door, which can apply variable pressure proximal to the femoral condyles locking them in place. This suspension system is similar to the medial opening door occasionally used for Syme's prosthesis.

The long length of the KD residual improves the prosthetic control and allows a greater degree of dynamic muscular stability. However, the long RL limits the choice of prosthetic knee units that can be used to maintain symmetric knee centers between the amputated and nonamputated side. The knees of choice at this level are those of the polycentric design, and some knees are designed specifically for the KD amputation. They decrease the overall prosthetic length of the thigh section, while decreasing the length of the shin section. In addition, some knees incorporate a linkage that, when flexed to 90°, translates posteriorly under the socket, thereby reducing the thigh section length. As the linkage folds up underneath the prosthetic socket during sitting, the foot will often rise off the floor. The thigh segment will still appear somewhat longer when compared with the sound side. These are common issues, and the patient should be made aware of them during the fitting process. The polycentric design also reduces the length of the shank section during swing, thus facilitating toe clearance.

Prosthesis for Hip Disarticulation/Hemipelvectomy

These levels of amputation are almost always treated with the lighter weight endoskeletal prosthesis, given their lightweight properties, ease of fabrication, and postfabrication adjustability. Knee components, feet, and alignment are selected to enhance stability and ease of use. Energy required to ambulate with these prostheses is 200% times greater than normal.

Canadian hip disarticulation prosthesis is the standard prosthesis of choice for hip disarticulation. The socket of this prosthesis encloses the hemipelvis on the side of the amputation and extends around the hemipelvis of the nonamputated side, leaving an opening for the nonamputated LE. There is a flexible anterior wall with an opening that allows the prosthesis to be donned. Weight is borne on the ischial tuberosity of the amputated side. The medial aspect is cut to provide clearance for the other leg and genitalia. Relief is provided over the anterior and posterior iliac spines. Variations in socket construction include a lateral-opening diagonal socket and a full socket similar to the transpelvic that encloses both iliac crests for stability. Endoskeletal prosthetic components are preferred for this level of amputation to reduce the overall weight. The endoskeletal hip joint has an extension assist, as does the knee unit, which usually is a constant friction knee. Endoskeletal components may be made from aluminum, titanium, or carbon graphite composite materials. Traditionally, a single-axis or SACH foot with a soft heel has been the most common choice for the prosthetic foot. The newer lightweight foot/ankle combination, such as the endolite foot/ankle complex or the endolite ankle with a Seattle lightfoot may be a better option for this level. A cosmetic cover completes the prosthetic prescription. If necessary, locking hip or knee joints can be used.

The *transpelvic socket* is similarly made except that it must include the contralateral iliac crest for proper stabilization and suspension. In the hemipelvectomy, most of the weight is borne by the soft tissues on the amputated side, with some of the weight being borne by the sacrum, the rib cage, and the opposite ischial tuberosity. Care must be taken when constructing both sockets that no excess pressure exists on bony prominences or in the perineum.

Both sockets can be made of rigid or flexible materials and padded for increased comfort on weight-bearing. The socket may also be constructed of flexible silicone rubber in a rigid frame to provide a softer, more intimate fit that increases ROM and comfort. Hip joints are single-axis requiring an extension stop and extension assist. Any knee joint can be used in the hip disarticulation prosthesis. A lightweight polycentric knee or stance-control unit is often utilized to keep the weight of the prosthesis low. Any of the feet discussed at the beginning can be used.

Bilateral Lower Limb Amputation Prosthesis

The loss of both lower limbs complicates the rehabilitation process, especially if the loss occurs simultaneously. The major cause of bilateral lower extremity limb loss is dysvascular disease. Early fitting of prosthesis is strongly recommended. Rehabilitation of persons with bilateral lower limb amputation is similar to that of unilateral amputation, with only major difference being in the advancement which is slower. It should be matched to individual patient's strength, balance, and ability. Breaking down complex skills into small incremental tasks that can be more useful, and wide-based gait pattern should be allowed along with slow and cautious walking.

Patients with bilateral amputation must bear all their body weight on prosthetic devices all the time; hence, components that increase comfort or protect the skin are particularly appropriate. Lessening the weight of the prostheses particularly at the ankle–foot area is also important because lighter weight prostheses are easier to control and increase acceptance of the device. Whenever possible, heavier components should be placed as close to the socket as possible.

Bilateral Transtibial Amputation

An individual with two transtibial amputations uses the same components as an individual with one transtibial amputation. Bilateral transtibial (PTB) prosthesis should be prescribed. The person may require feet with somewhat softer heels for increased stance stability.

Bilateral Transfemoral Amputation

Postural responses are compromised in this population, owing to loss of anatomical ankle and knee on both sides. Hence, stance stability is very important to achieve. Ambulation with bilateral transfemoral prostheses is energy-consuming, slow, and awkward, and most older individuals prefer to use a wheelchair rather than attempt ambulation. It is often unwise to try to fit individuals who do not exhibit considerable strength, endurance, balance, and good ROM of both hips with prostheses. Younger, fit individuals can be prescribed prosthesis, but time to time, even they may require wheelchair. Many patients with bilateral transfemoral amputation use crutches or canes to assist with balance and postural control. However, to be functionally efficient, no more than once cane for external support is recommended. The components of prosthesis are essentially the same, although most are fitted with ICSs for better hip control. The person should be able to don the prosthesis in sitting position. Manual knee locks can be given; however, they make it difficult to come to standing with a locked knee. Hydraulic knee mechanisms with some form of both stance and swing-phase control are more functional.

For many adults with acquired limb losses, an initial fitting with sockets attached to special rocker platforms may facilitate initial gait training. Such "stubby" prosthesis require less energy and provide substantial balance than full-length prosthetic limbs and give the patient new to bilateral prostheses, a best chance for successful ambulation **(Fig. 25.23)**. They can be either be used as temporary prosthesis or permanent prosthesis, for those individuals who are motivated to ambulate but are not candidates for fitting with full-length prostheses. Stubbies may be cosmetically unacceptable, because of the extreme reduction in height. Ambulation in stubbies obligates exaggerated trunk rotation. Short canes or crutches may be needed. Sitting in chair and stair climbing are very difficult because of the shortness of the prostheses. The limbs also protrude in front of the chair when the person is sitting because of the lack of knee joints. However, due considerations to the needs of the patient, their age and physical capacity may necessitate the needed of stubbies, over the highly demand inducing bilateral transfemoral prostheses.

For patients with one transfemoral and one transtibial amputation, the preservation of one biological knee makes prosthetic use much easier and successful ambulation more likely. For most patients, the transtibial side is the propulsive and balances the limb and the transfemoral side supplements these functions. On the basis of these functional differences, the prosthetist may choose to use different prosthetic feet on both sides. When the transfemoral amputation is relatively short, for example, a single-axis foot and stance control knee might be

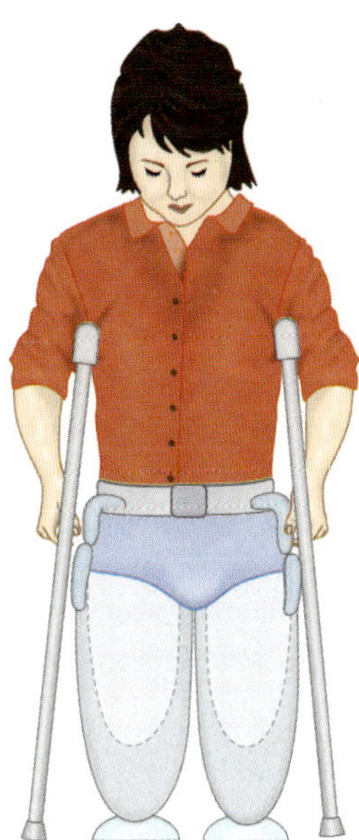

Fig. 25.23: Stubbies.

recommended for the transfemoral prosthesis, whereas a dynamic response foot might be used in the transtibial prosthesis.

PROSTHETIC EXAMINATION

The next step after prosthetic prescription is to assure the fitting of the prosthesis. It is extremely important that the prosthesis is properly aligned and functions well during standing, walking, and while performing other activities, such as sports, if need be. For the same purpose, a static and dynamic prosthetic checkout is required. Energy expenditure is an important consideration, and walking speed affects energy utilization: The faster one walks, the more energy one expends. Hence, most individuals select a walking speed that maintains a comfortable level of oxygen consumption. Individuals with transtibial amputations expend significantly less energy when walking with a prosthesis at a self-selected speed than when walking on crutches without a prosthesis. On the other hand, for individuals using a transfemoral prosthesis, walking with or without a prosthesis does not make much of a difference in their energy expenditure.

Prosthetic Evaluation for Transtibial Prosthesis

Static Analysis for Transtibial Prosthesis

Client is assessed in standing and sitting, and comfort should be asked for. Both heels and feet should be flat on the floor. The points to be checked are highlighted in **Table 25.8**.

Socket Evaluation

PTB socket has 5–8° of socket flexion to allow for better weight-bearing on the patellar tendon and to simulate normal gait. Excessive socket flexion causes knee instability and in order to counteract this instability, anterior distal end of the tibia and the skin come in close approximation with wall of the socket, causing pain and abrasion. Insufficient socket flexion reduces weight-bearing on patellar tendon and medial tibial flares causing RL to press too hard on the bottom of the socket also leading to decreased effectiveness of quadriceps motion.

Dynamic Analysis for Transtibial Prosthesis

Gait analysis is important to identify gait deviations which may in turn cause discomfort in the RL, or may lead to increased energy consumption and can limit functional use of prosthesis. Gait deviations may arise due to an improperly fitting socket, a poorly aligned prosthesis, a painful RL, or poor walking habits. Few terminologies are important in understanding and analyzing these deviations which are as follows:

Toe Lever Arm and Heel Lever Arm

Ideally, center line of the socket falls through the posterior one-third and anterior two-third of the foot. If the foot is set

Table 25.8: Prosthetic checkout for transtibial prosthesis.
Checking of the prosthesis
Is the prosthesis as per prescription?
If fitted with shuttle lock system, does the lock and release pin operate smoothly and easily?
If fitted with suction sleeve, does the mechanism function properly?
Sitting
Is the person comfortable while sitting with sole of the shoe flat on the floor?
Is there adequate flaring of the posterior trim line to accommodate the hamstring tendon?
Are the tissue rolls in the popliteal area excessive?
Is the residual limb forced out of the socket excessively?
Can the patient sit comfortably with knees flexed 10 at least 90° without excessive pressure on knees?
Are the knees level?
Are the color and contour of the prosthesis similar to the sound leg?
Standing
Does the client have any pain or discomfort when bearing weight in the prosthesis?
Is the knee stable? Does the patient have to resist or prevent the knee from being forced into flexion or extension?
Is the pelvis level when weight is borne equally on both feet?
Is the pylon vertical when weight is borne evenly on both feet?
Does the sole of shoe maintain even contact with the floor?
Are tissue rolls around the trim line of the socket excessive?
Is there any gapping at brim of the socket?
Is there evidence of total contact?
If wearing a gel liner, does it fit properly and smoothly?
Is suspension maintained as the foot is lifted off the floor?
If using sleeve suspension, does the sleeve extend over the limb socks?
Walking
Is the gait satisfactory? If the gait is not satisfactory, check the deviations

too far anterior under the socket, the length of the toe lever arm is increased and that of the heel lever arm decreased. This results in posterior displacement of the socket (**Fig. 25.24A**). If the foot is placed too far posteriorly under the socket, the toe lever arm will be shortened resulting in anterior displacement of the socket (**Fig. 25.24B**).

Dynamic Alignment Line

Dynamically, the foot is usually set 1 cm medial to a line from the center of the posterior wall to the floor. This is known as dynamic alignment line. Any deviation in this may result into either an inset or outset foot.

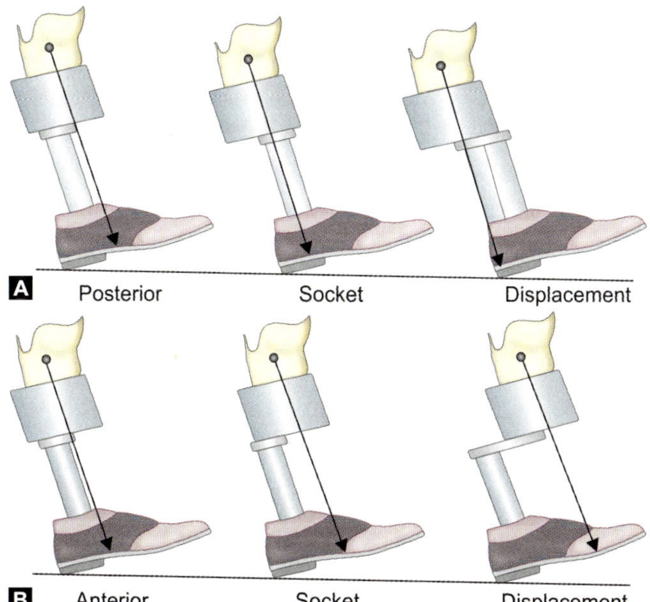

Figs. 25.24A and B: (A) Posterior socket displacement; (B) Anterior socket displacement.

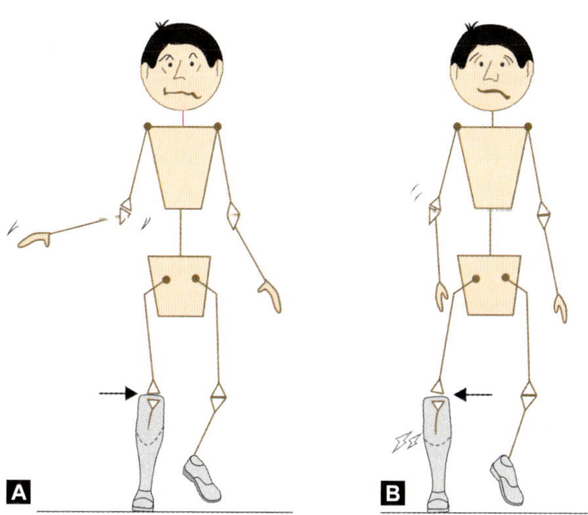

Figs. 25.25A and B: (A) Medial leaning pylon; (B) Lateral leaning pylon.

Proper dynamic alignment places pylon perpendicular to floor, at midstance. Deviations in this may result into medial or lateral leaning pylon. If top of pylon is medial to bottom, it is a medial leaning pylon **(Fig. 25.25A)**, and if top of pylon is lateral to bottom, it is a lateral leaning pylon **(Fig. 25.25B)**. An inset foot results when the prosthetic foot is placed too far medially to the dynamic alignment line, and outset foot results from the foot that is set too far lateral to the line.

Gait Deviations in a Transtibial Prosthesis

For the ease of understanding, the gait deviations are divided as per the gait cycle into the following, as described in **Table 25.9**.

Table 25.9: Gait deviations in a transtibial prosthesis.

Stance phase	
Heel contact to foot flat	Excessive knee extension
	Knee instability
Midstance	Excessive rising and dropping of hip
	Wide-based gait
	Narrow-based gait
	Excessive lateral thrust
Terminal stance	Knee instability
	Knee extension: Vaulting
Swing phase	Pistoning
	Uneven step length
	Circumduction

Stance Phase

- **Heel contact to foot flat:**
  - *Excessive knee extension:* Normally, knee flexes 8–12° during heel strike to midstance. Knee flexion reduces the excursion of the body's center of gravity, allows for absorption of the floor reaction forces generated at heel strike through the joints of the lower limb, and reduces the amount of energy required in gait. If the knee remains extended, the amount of energy expended in walking increases. This deviation can best be seen from the side by observing the prosthetic knee from weight acceptance to midstance. The client reports a sense of walking uphill. Maintaining an extended knee with a socket aligned in flexion may lead to distal anterior pain and skin abrasion. Extension also increases pelvic displacement; it may look as if the prosthesis is too long. Causes of excessive knee extension include:
    - Too soft heel support
    - Too long toe lever arm
    - Shoes with lower heel
    - Plantar-flexed prosthetic foot
    - Weakness of quadriceps
    - Habit
  - *Knee instability:* It refers to buckling of the knee joint while walking and is seen in clients who do not feel stable. The major causes of this include:
    - Too long heel support
    - Too short toe lever arm
    - Dorsiflexed prosthetic foot
    - Shoes with higher heel
- **Midstance:**
  - *Excessive rising and dropping of hip:*
    - Too long prosthesis
    - Too short prosthesis

- *Wide-based gait:* If the base of support is moved laterally, support is lost medially during single foot stance. The client attempts to move the pelvis laterally to reach the support point and exhibits a wide-based gait with the hips and the shoulders dropping laterally during stance phase. Excess pressure will be felt at the proximal lateral brim of the socket and the medial distal end of the RL. Two common causes of this include:
  - Medial leaning pylon
  - Outset foot

  These deviations are best observed from rear and or front view. If the client does not shift the weight properly during stance phase, then also such gait deviation may arise. They can be differentiated from the abovementioned common causes by observing the upper end of the pylon.
- *Narrow-based gait:* The opposite of the above is a narrow-based gait, where support is lost laterally during single foot stance. A narrow-based gait and thrust of the prosthesis laterally away from the knee at midstance often occur together and derive from the tendency of the prosthesis to rotate around the RL. This deviation is best observed from rear and causes include:
  - Lateral leaning pylon
  - Inset foot
- **Terminal stance:**
  - *Knee instability:* The premature loss of support causing the prosthetic knee to flex and the hip to drop sharply just before the end of stance is called "drop-off." Cause include: Short toe lever arm.
  - *Knee extension/vaulting:* When the knee joint remains in extension during the latter part of the stance phase and the client complains of a "walking uphill" sensation, because the center of gravity is carried up and over the extended knee, it is termed "vaulting" and causes include:
    - Long toe lever arm.

Swing Phase

- **Pistoning:** If the suspension mechanism is loose or inadequate, the prosthesis will slip as the foot leaves the ground for swing phase. The toe of the prosthesis can catch on the ground, or the movement of the socket against the skin may cause abrasions.
- **Uneven step length:** Clients may develop the habit of taking a long prosthetic step and a short step with the unamputated leg. This may be the result of a poorly fitting socket causing pain, fear of putting weight on the prosthesis, or a prosthesis that is too long.
- **Circumduction:** If the prosthesis is too long, the suspension is inadequate, or the person has difficulty flexing the hip and knee, then a semicircular swing of the prosthesis may be seen to the side during swing phase.

Prosthetic Evaluation for Transfemoral Prosthesis

Static Analysis for Transfemoral Prosthesis

Client is assessed in standing and sitting, and comfort should be asked for. In addition to the socket fit, suspension, comfort, and leg length, static alignment and knee stability are important to check in the transfemoral limb. The points to be checked are highlighted in **Table 25.10**.

Dynamic Analysis for Transfemoral Prosthesis

A few terminologies are important in understanding and analyzing gait deviations arising in transfemoral prosthesis, which are as follows:

Trochanter-knee-ankle (TKA) line: Knee is placed in a line or slightly posterior to a line drawn from the trochanter to the ankle axis. It allows the body weight line to fall anterior to the knee to create an extension moment on weight-bearing. If the knee axis is on or anterior to the line, the body weight will fall behind the knee, creating a flexion or unstable moment **(Fig. 25.26)**.

Socket flexion: Ideally, the socket is aligned in about 5° of flexion to increase the client's ability to extend the hip without excessively arching the back and to match normal femoral alignment. In clients with a hip flexion contracture, socket must be set in flexion 5° more than the limits of contracture.

Table 25.10: Prosthetic checkout for transfemoral prosthesis.

Checking of the prosthesis
Is the prosthesis as per prescription?
Is the inside of the socket smoothly finished?
Do all joints move freely and smoothly?
Sitting
Is the socket securely on the residual limb?
Do the length of the shin and thigh correspond to the shin and thigh of the unamputated leg?
Can the client sit comfortably without burning or pinching?
Is the client able to lean forward and reach their shoes?
Standing
Does the socket fit properly and comfortably?
Is the knee stable when weight is placed on the prosthesis?
Is the pelvis level when weight is borne evenly on both legs?
Does the socket maintain good contact with the residual limb on all sides as the client shifts his weight?
Is there an adductor roll?
Is there pressure on the pubic ramus?
Walking
Is the gait satisfactory? If the gait is not satisfactory, check the deviations

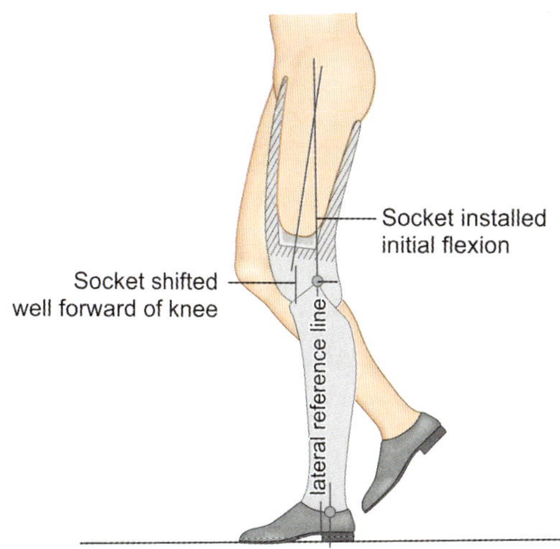

Fig. 25.26: Trochanter-knee-ankle (TKA) line.

Gait Deviations in a Transfemoral Prosthesis

Gait deviations seen in transfemoral prosthesis divided as per the gait cycle are described in **Table 25.11**.

Stance Phase

- **Heel contact to midstance:**
  - *Knee instability:* It is essential for the knee to be extended for the client to feel secure. If it flexes inadvertently, it causes knee instability, causes of which include are as follows:
    - If the knee axis is placed anterior to the TKA line, the line of body weight falls behind the knee, creating a flexion moment. The knee can be poorly aligned if the socket is placed too far anteriorly (long heel lever arm).
    - Knee instability can also be caused by lack of adequate socket flexion, limiting the client's active hip extension.

Table 25.11: Gait deviations in a transfemoral prosthesis.

Stance phase	
Heel contact to midstance	Knee instability
	Terminal impact
	Foot slap
Midstance	Lateral trunk bending
	Abducted gait
	Excessive trunk extension
Terminal stance	Drop-off
	Inadequate heel off
Swing phase	Circumducted gait
	Vaulting
	Medial and lateral whips
	Uneven arm swing and uneven timing

- Heel support that is too hard and does not accept body weight may also create a flexion moment at heel strike.
- A severe hip flexion contracture not accommodated in the socket makes it difficult for the client to control the knee.

- *Terminal impact:* The prosthetic shank comes to a sudden stop with a visible and possibly audible impact as the knee reaches full extension. It occurs most frequently with constant friction knees because the individual uses the sound to indicate that the knee is ready for heel contact. It can also occur due to insufficient friction at the prosthetic knee, too tight an extension aid, absent or worn resilient extension bumper in the knee unit, and fear of buckling causing them to extend the hip abruptly as the knee approaches full extension. This maneuver snaps the shank forward into full extension. It is a difficult habit to change. The impact, if severe, can cause bruising of the distal end of the RL.

- *Foot slap:* The foot plantar flexes too rapidly and strikes the floor with a slap, just after heel strike. It is best observed from side, listening for slap sound. Causes include:
  - Plantar flexion bumper is too soft and does not offer enough resistance to foot motion as weight is transferred to the prosthesis. Client may also be driving the prosthesis into the walking surface too forcibly to ensure extension of the knee. It is not common problem.

- **Midstance:**
  - *Lateral trunk bending:* The amputee leans toward the amputated side when the prosthesis is in stance phase **(Fig. 25.27A)**. It is best observed from posterior view, during midstance, and causes include:
    - Weak hip abductors: By shifting the center of gravity toward the prosthesis, lateral bending counteracts the tendency toward pelvic drop on the sound side.
    - Abducted socket: This alignment fault reduces the effectiveness of the hip abductors in stabilizing the pelvis. The resulting tendency of the pelvis to drop on the sound side is counteracted by lateral trunk bending.
    - Insufficient support by the lateral socket wall: If the lateral wall does not block lateral movement of the femur, the pelvis will tend to drop on the sound side when the prosthesis is in stance phase. To check this tendency, the amputee leans toward the prosthesis.
    - Pain or discomfort particularly on the lateral distal aspect of the femur: By bending to the prosthetic side, the amputee relieves pressure on the lateral aspect.

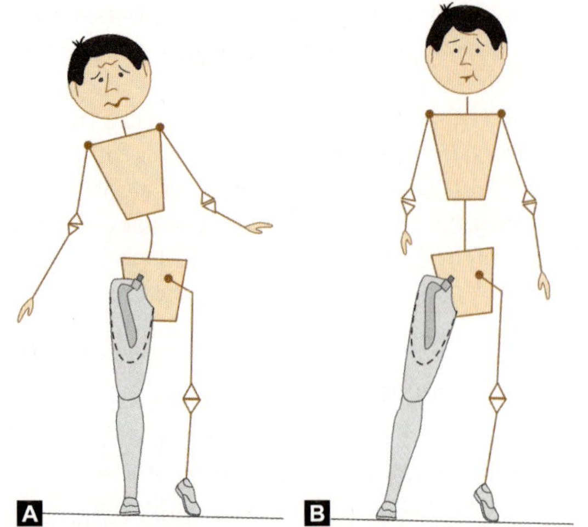

Figs. 25.27A and B: (A) Lateral trunk bending; (B) Abducted gait.

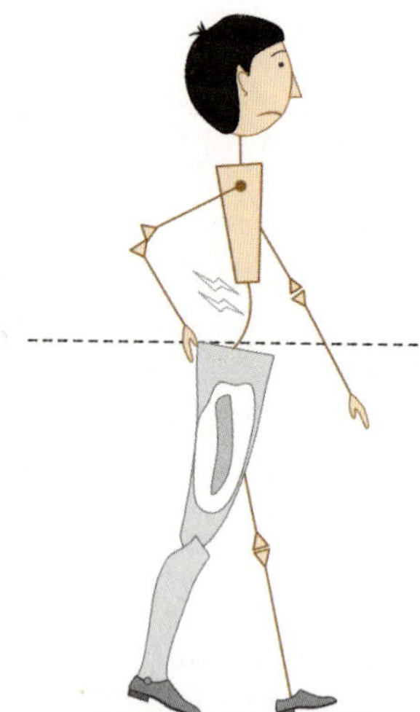

Fig. 25.28: Exaggerated lumbar lordosis.

- ◆ If the medial wall of the socket is too high, the individual may bend laterally to avoid pressure on the pubic ramus.
- ◆ Short prosthesis or inadequate balance to properly shift the weight over the prosthesis.
- *Abducted gait:* It is characterized by a gait with base wider than 5 cm and is best viewed from behind the patient in stance phase **(Fig. 25.27B)**. There is exaggerated displacement of the pelvis and trunk and causes include:
  - ◆ Pain or discomfort in the crotch area: The discomfort may be due to such factors as skin infection, adductor roll, or pressure from the medial socket brim. The amputee tries to gain relief by abducting his prosthesis, thus moving the medial part of the brim away from the painful area.
  - ◆ An improperly shaped lateral wall that fails to provide adequate support for the femur.
  - ◆ A high medial wall that causes the client to hold the prosthesis away to avoid ramus pressure.
  - ◆ Contracted hip abductors.
  - ◆ Prosthesis is too long: Excessive length makes it difficult to place the limb directly under the hip during stance and to clear the floor during swing. Widening the base helps to solve these problems.
  - ◆ Shank aligned in the valgus position with respect to the thigh section.
  - ◆ Mechanical hip joint set so that the socket is abducted.
  - ◆ Feeling of insecurity: The amputee compensates by widening his walking base.
- *Excessive trunk extension:* The lumbar lordosis is exaggerated when the prosthesis is in stance phase, and the trunk may lean posteriorly **(Fig. 25.28)**. This deviation is best viewed from laterally, and causes include:

- ◆ Hip flexion contracture: The pelvis tends to tilt downward and forward because the center of gravity is anterior to the support point (a theoretical point around which the supporting forces are balanced). A flexion contracture aggravates the tendency of the pelvis to tilt anteriorly because the shortened hip flexor muscles exert a downward and forward pull on the pelvis when the femur is at the limit of its extension range.
- ◆ Insufficient socket flexion or insufficient support from the anterior socket brim.
- ◆ Weak hip extensors: The extensors help to restrain the tendency of the pelvis to tilt forward. When this restraining force is lost, the resulting forward pelvic tilt and compensatory backward trunk bending cause increased lordosis. In addition, the amputee may roll his pelvis forward to assist the weak extensors to control knee stability.
- ◆ Weak abdominal muscles: The abdominal muscles restrain the tendency of the pelvis to tilt forward. If the abdominal muscles are weak, some of this restraint is lost, and the amputee will show increased lordosis.

- ■ **Terminal stance:**
  - *Drop-off:* There is a sudden downward movement of the trunk as anterior support is lost prematurely. The main reason is usually a short toe lever arm. It is an unstable deviation because it may cause the knee to buckle prematurely.
  - *Inadequate heel off:* If the client does not feel secure allowing the body weight to shift forward over the toe of the prosthesis, the heel may not come off the floor until the whole foot is brought forward. This deviation is associated with uneven steps that are seen during swing phase.

Swing Phase

- **Circumducted gait:** The prosthesis swings laterally in an arc-like manner during swing phase, and causes include:
  - A prosthesis that is too long.
  - A mechanical knee with too much alignment stability or friction in the knee making it difficult to bend the knee in swing through.
  - The client may lack confidence for flexing the prosthetic knee because of muscle weakness or fear of stubbing the toe.
  - The stance-phase control knee may not be functioning properly.
- **Vaulting:** Client rises on the toe of the sound foot to swing the prosthesis through with little knee flexion. Some individuals use this maneuver temporarily to walk rapidly. Unwanted or continuous vaulting may be caused by:
  - A prosthesis that is too long.
  - Inadequate socket suspension.
  - Excessive stability in the alignment or some limitation of knee flexion.
  - Fear of stubbing the toe or flexing the knee.
  - Manual knee lock, excessive friction, or too tight an extension aid.
  - Inadequate suspension allowing the prosthesis to slip off the stump (piston action).
  - Too small a socket. The ischial tuberosity is above its proper location.
  - Foot set in excessive plantar flexion.
  - Discomfort
- **Medial and lateral whips:** Whips are best assessed when the client walks away from the observer. In medial whip, at toe-off, the heel moves medially on initial flexion at the beginning of swing phase. In lateral whip, at toe-off, the heel moves laterally. Prosthetically, whips are always related to the knee joint as follows:
  - Medial whips result from excessive external rotation of the prosthetic knee.
  - Lateral whips result from excessive internal rotation of the prosthetic knee.
  - Other causes may include a socket that is too tight, thus reflecting RL rotation, or the client may have donned the prosthesis in internal or external rotation.
- **Uneven arm swing and uneven timing:** These two deviations go together. The arm on the prosthetic side is held close to the body, and the individual takes steps of unequal duration and length with a short stance phase on the prosthesis. Poor training and fear of putting weight on the prosthesis are the two major causes of this.

DETERMINING PROSTHETIC POTENTIAL

Medicare, a major funding source for prosthetic limbs in the United States, requires that the functional level of the individual with an amputation be taken into account when prescribing a prosthesis. The functional index is referred to as the Medicare "K" code and limits the components that can be used when fabricating the prosthesis. Although only required for Medicare, the "K" code classification is a simple but useful hierarchical framework for classifying the mobility potential of all individuals with a LE amputation.

K0: Not a potential user for ambulation or transfer

K1: A potential household ambulator including transfers

K2: A potential limited community ambulator

K3: Community ambulator using variable cadence including therapeutic exercise or vocation

K4: High-activity user that exceeds normal ambulation skills.

Apart from this, amputee mobility predictor (AMPPRO/AMPnoPRO) is an important tool of predicting the prosthetic potential. It is a 20-item measure to assess the ability of an amputee to perform functional tasks required for successful ambulation. It is valid, reliable and takes 15–20 minutes to administer. The complexities of potential use of prosthesis for patient with multiple amputations can be reduced with appropriate plan of care and effective implementation of the same **(Fig. 25.29)**.

Functional Outcome Measures

Outcome measures are useful in evaluating the patient progression, effectiveness of treatment interventions and also enhance the quality of care provided. They can be grouped into two: self-report measures and performance-based measures, on the basis of the psychometric properties, such as validity and reliability of the instrument as well as the minimal clinically important difference. One important consideration is whether the instrument allows the use of prosthesis along with ease, time required, and equipment required to administer the outcome measure. **Table 25.12** shows outcome measures that are valid, reliable, responsive to change, and easy to administer in

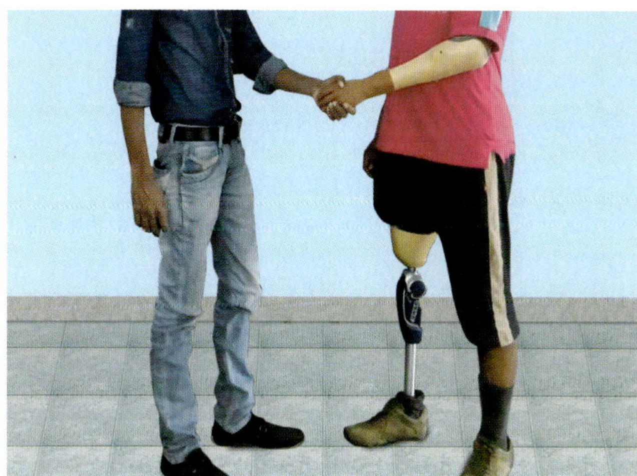

Fig. 25.29: Patient with left transradial and right transtibial prosthesis.

Table 25.12: Outcome measures for persons with amputation.

Self-report measures	Performance-based measures
Prosthetic evaluation questionnaire	Timed Up and Go (TUG)
Locomotor capabilities index	L test
Prosthetic limb users survey of mobility	Six-minute walk test (6-MWT)
Activities-specific balance confidence scale (ABC)	Two-minute walk test (2-MWT)
PROMIS-29	Amputee mobility predictor (AMPPRO/AMPnoPRO)
	Comprehensive high-level activity mobility predictor (CHAMP)

person with amputation. These outcomes are useful in determining the efficacy of treatment and also justify the reimbursement matters.

SUMMARY

Recent advancements in the surgical procedures and prosthetics have generated newer options for those with an unusual but catastrophic UE amputation. Use of prosthesis has alleviated the impact of upper limb amputation on impairments in body functions and the psychological anguish that amputation brings to an individual. The physical therapists concerned with the rehabilitation of such individuals need to take into consideration the surgical approach used, type of dressings done postsurgically, management of the stump and RL, and last but not the least, the knowledge of various prosthesis used in UE amputation while focusing the functional use and vocational training of the patient in mind. Coordination of all team members with prosthetist and physiotherapist as key contributors, is necessary. Lower extremity prosthesis and rehabilitation can be very challenging, especially since the major functional goal of independent ambulation safely under variable environmental settings is the prime concern. However, effective treatment strategies can be incorporated to achieve maximum desired outcome with wide array and advances in prosthetic options available.

Case Scenario

CASE STUDY

History: A 25-year-old male athlete sustained a left transtibial lower extremity amputation, following a road traffic accident. There is no other significant medical or surgical history. Social history suggests that the patient is single, living in a nuclear family.

Examination

- Patient has stable vitals.
- Incision is well healed and mobile.
- Range of motion assessment revealed tightness in left iliopsoas and hamstrings muscle, along with weakness of bilateral lower extremity hip muscles with grade 3 on MMT.

- Sensations are within normal limits; however, there is residual limb pain along with phantom limb pain.

Functionally, the patient is completely independent in bed mobility, transfers, but requires moderate assistance in locomotion. Dressing, and self-care hygiene, also requires moderate assistance.

Guiding Questions:
1. What are the impairments in the patient?
2. Enlist the problems and short- and long-term goals.
3. Describe the postsurgical and preprosthetic management for the patient.
4. Plan a follow-up evaluation and management for long-term.
5. Discuss the role of rehabilitation team for the patient.

Review Questions

1. What are the causes of amputation?
2. Describe the options available for dressings following surgical process after amputation.
3. Discuss the components of physical therapy examination following amputation.
4. What are the goals of management in the preprosthetic phase?
5. Classify terminal devices in upper and lower extremity prostheses.
6. What are the factors affecting lower extremity prosthetic prescription?
7. Discuss the parts of transtibial prosthesis in detail.
8. Describe the gait deviations associated with transfemoral prosthesis
9. What is the functional code classification for classifying the mobility potential of all individuals with a LE amputation?
10. Brief out: (a) Jaipur foot; (b) Stubby prostheses.

BIBLIOGRAPHY

1. Ahmed A, Bhatnagar S, Mishra S, et al. Prevalence of phantom limb pain, stump pain, and phantom limb sensation among the amputated cancer patients in India: a prospective, observational study. Indian J Palliat Care. 2017;23(1):24-35.
2. American Academy of Orthopaedic Surgeons. Orthopedic appliance atlas, vol 2: Artificial limbs. Ann Arbor, MI: J W Edwards; 1960.
3. Atherton R, Robertson N. Psychological adjustment to lower limb amputation amongst prosthetic users. Disabil Rehabil. 2006;28(19):1201-9.
4. Baumgartner RF. Upper extremity amputation and prosthetics. J Rehabil Res Dev. 2001;38(4):vii-x.
5. Beil T, Street G. Comparison of interface pressures with pin and suction suspension systems. J Rehabil Res Dev. 2004;41(6A):821-8.
6. Billock JN. Upper limb terminal devices: hand versus hooks. Clin Prosthet Orthot. 1989;19(2):57-65.
7. Board WJ, Street GM, Caspers C. A comparison of transtibial amputee suction and vacuum socket conditions. Prosthet Orthot Int. 2001;25(3):202-9.
8. Bradbrook D. Acupuncture treatment of phantom limb pain and phantom limb sensation in amputees. Acupunct Med. 2004;22(2):93-7.

9. Brenner CD. Prosthetic principles: wrist disarticulation and transradial amputation. In: Bowker JH, Michael JW (Eds). Atlas of limb prosthetics: surgical, prosthetic, and rehabilitation principles, 2nd edition. St. Louis, MO: Mosby-Year Book: 1992. pp. 241-51.

10. Brånemark R1, Brånemark PI, Rydevik B, et al. Osseointegration in skeletal reconstruction and rehabilitation. J Rehabil Res Dev. 2001;38(2):175-81.

11. Carlson LB, Veatch BD, Frey DD. Technical forum: efficiency of prosthetic cable and housing. J Prosthet Orthot. 1995;7(3):96-9.

12. Cestaro JM. Comments on partial foot amputations. Newsl Prosthet Orthot Clin. 1977;1(3):7.

13. Chin T, Sawamura S, Fujita H, et al. Physical fitness of lower limb amputees. Am J Phys Med Rehabil. 2002;81(5):321-5.

14. Czerniecki JM, Munro CF, Gitter A, et al. A comparison of the power generation/absorption characteristics of prosthetic feet during running (Asttract). Arch Phys Med Rehabil. 1987;68:636.

15. Davidson JH, Jones LE, Cornet J, et al. Management of the multiple limb amputee. Disabil Rehabil. 2002;24(13):688-99.

16. de Boer-Wilzing VG, Bolt A, Geertzen JH, et al. Variation in results of volume measurements of stumps of lower limb amputees: a comparison of 4 methods. Arch Phys Med Rehabil. 2011;92(6):941-6.

17. Dietzen CJ, Harshburger J, Pidikiti RD. Suction sock suspension for above-knee prostheses. J Prosthet Orthot. 1991;3(2):90-3.

18. Dougherty PJ. Long term follow-up study of bilateral above knee amputees from the Vietnam War. J Bone Joint Surg Am.1999; 81A:1384-90.

19. Fillauer C, Pritham C, Fillauer K. Evolution and development of the silicone suction socket (3S) for below-knee prostheses. J Prosthet Orthot. 1989;1:92-103.

20. Foort J. The Canadian type Syme prosthesis. UCBL Tech Rep. 1956;30:75-6.

21. Fortington LV, Rommers GM, Geertzen JH, et al. Mobility in elderly people with a lower limb amputation: a systematic review. J Am Med Dir Assoc. 2011;13(4):319-25.

22. Fraser CM. An evaluation of the use made of cosmetic and functional prostheses by unilateral upper limb amputees. Prosthet Orthot Int. 1998;22:216-23.

23. Gailey R. Functional value of prosthetic foot/ankle systems to the amputee. J Prosthet Orthot. 2005;17(4S):39-41.

24. Gailey RS, Gailey AM. Prosthetic gait training program for lower extremity amputees. Miami, FL: Advanced Rehabilitation Therapy Incorporated; 1989.

25. Gailey RS1, Roach KE, Applegate EB, et al. The amputee mobility predictor: an instrument to assess determinants of the lower-limb amputee's ability to ambulate. Arch Phys Med Rehabil. 2002;83(5):613-27.

26. Gard S, Konz R. The effect of a shock-absorbing pylon on the gait of persons with unilateral transtibial amputation. J Rehabil Res Dev. 2003;40(2):109-24.

27. Goldberg T, Goldberg S, Pollak J. Postoperative management of lower extremity amputation. Phys Med Rehabil Clin N Am. 2000;11(3):559-68.

28. Gottschalk F, Kourosh S, Stills M, et al. Does socket configuration influence the position of the femur in above-knee amputation? J Prosthet Orthot. 1990;2:94-1020.

29. Gutfleisch O. Peg legs and bionic limbs: the development of lower extremity prosthetics. Interdiscip Sci Rev. 2003;28(2):139-49.

30. Hafner BJ, Sanders JE, Czerniecki J, et al. Energy storage and return prostheses: does patient perception correlate with biomechanical analysis? Clin Biomech. 2002;17:325-44.

31. Hafner BJ, Smith DG. Differences in function and safety between Medicare functional classification level-2 and -3 transfemoral amputees and influence of prosthetic knee joint control. J Rehabil Res Dev. 2009;46(3):417-33.

32. Hafner BJ, Willingham LL, Buell NC, et al. Evaluation of function, performance, and preference as transfemoral amputees transition from mechanical to microprocessor control of the prosthetic knee. Arch Phys Med Rehabil. 2007;88(3):207-17.

33. Hakimi KN. Pre-operative rehabilitation evaluation of the dysvascular patient prior to amputation. Phys Med Rehabil Clin N Am. 2009;20(4):677-88.

34. Hamamura S, Chin T, Kuroda R, et al. Factors affecting prosthetic rehabilitation outcomes in amputees of age 60 years and over. J Int Med Res. 2009;37(6):1921-27.

35. Hampton F. A hemipelvectomy prosthesis. Artif Limbs. 1964;8(1):3-27

36. Harrington IJ1, Lexier R, Woods JM, et al. A plaster-pylon technique for below-knee amputation. J Bone Joint Surg Br. 1991;73(1):76-8.

37. Heger H, Millstein S, Hunter GA. Electrically powered prostheses for the adult with an acquired upper limb amputation. J Bone Joint Surg. 1985;67-B:278-81.

38. Hiatt MD, Farmer JM, Teasdall RD. The decision to salvage or amputate a severely injured limb. J South Orthop Assoc. 2000;9(1):72-7.

39. Hoyt C, Littig D, Lundt J, et al. The ischial containment above-knee prosthesis: course manual, 3rd edition, version 1.3. Los Angeles, CA: UCLA Prosthetics Education and Research Program; 1987.

40. Huang CT. Energy cost of ambulation with Canadian hip disarticulation prosthesis. J Med Assoc State Ala. 1983;52(1):47-8.

41. Jelic M, Eldar R. Rehabilitation following major traumatic amputation of lower limbs—a review. Crit Rev Phys Med Rehabil Med. 2003;15(3/4):235-52.

42. Jendrezejczk DJ. Flexible socket systems. Clin Prosthet Orthot. 1985;9:27-30.

43. Kahle J. Conventional and hydrostatic transfemoral interface comparison. J Prosthet Orthot. 1999;11:85-91.

44. Kapp S. Suspension systems for prostheses. Clin Orthop. 1999;361:55-62.

45. Kemp BJ. Motivation, rehabilitation, and aging: a conceptual model. Top Geriatr Rehabil. 1988;3(3):41-51.

46. Klute GK, Glaister BC, Berge JS. Prosthetic liners for lower limb amputees: a review of the literature. Prosthet Orthot Int. 2010;34(2):146-53.

47. Kruger LM. Stubby prostheses in the rehabilitation of infants and children with bilateral lower limb deficiencies. Rehabilitation (Stuttg). 1990;29(1):12-5.

48. Leimkuehler J. Syme's prosthesis—a brief review and a new fabrication technique. Orthot Prosthet. 1980;34(4):3-12.

49. Lim TS, Finlayson A, Thorpe JM, et al. Outcomes of a contemporary amputation series. ANZ J Surg. 2006;76(5):300-5.

50. Lind J1, Kramhoft M, Bodtker S, et al. The influence of smoking on complications after primary amputations of lower limb. Clin Orthop. Relat Res. 1991;267:211-7.

51. Littig DH, Lundt JE. The UCLA anatomical hip disarticulation prosthesis. Clin Prosthet Orthot. 1988;12(3):114-18.

52. Little JM. The use of air splint as immediate prosthesis after below-knee amputation for vascular insufficiency. Med J Aust. 1970;2(19):870-2.

53. Lunsford T. Partial foot amputations: prosthetic and orthotic management. In: American Academy of Orthopaedic Surgeons (Eds). Atlas of limb prosthetics. St. Louis, MO: Mosby; 1981. pp. 320-5.

54. Lusardi MM, Neilson CC. Orthotics and Prosthetics in Rehabilitation, 2nd edition. Saunders Elsevier; 2007.

55. MacLean N, Fick GH. The effect of semirigid dressings on below knee amputations. Phys Ther. 1994;7:668-73.

56. Marx HW. An innovation in Syme's prosthetics. Orthot Prosthet. 1969;23(3):131-8.

57. May B. Amputations and prosthetics. Philadelphia, PA. F. A. Davis. 2002. pp: 169-71.

58. May BJ. Postsurgical management for lower extremity amputation. In: O'Sullivan SB, Schmitz TJ (Eds). Physical rehabilitation: assessment and treatment, 3rd edition. Philadelphia, PA. F A Davis; 1991.

59. Mayfield JA, Reiber GE, Maynard C, et al. Trends in lower limb amputation in the Veterans Health Administration, 1989–1998. J Rehabil Res Dev. 2000;37(1):23-30.

60. McFarlen JM. The Syme prosthesis. Orthot Prosthet. 1966;20(3):23-7.

61. Michael J. Energy storing feet: a clinical comparison. Clin Prosthet Orthot. 1987;11:154-68.

62. Michael JW. Modern prosthetic knee mechanisms. Clin Orthop Relat Res. 1999;361:39-47.

63. Moore TJ. Planning for optimal function in amputation surgery. In: Bowker JH, Michael JW (Ed). Atlas of limb prosthetic surgical, prosthetic and rehabilitation principles, 2nd edition. St. Louis, MO: Mosby Year Book; 1992; p. 59.

64. Ortiz-Catalan M, Sander N, Kristoffersen MB. Treatment of phantom limb pain (PLP) based on augmented reality and gaming controlled by myoelectric pattern recognition: a case study of a chronic PLP patient. Front Neurosci. 2014;8:24.

65. Pinzur MS, Bowker JH, Smith DG, et al. Amputation surgery in peripheral vascular disease. Instr Course Lect. 1999;48:687-91.

66. Pinzur MS, Bowker JH. Knee disarticulation. Clin Orthop. 1999;361:23-8.

67. Pohjolainen T, Alaranta H, Wikstrom J. Primary survival and prosthetic fitting of lower limb amputees. Prosthet Orthot Int. 1989;13(2):63-9.

68. Radcliffe C, Foort J. The patellar-tendon-bearing below-knee prosthesis. Berkeley, CA: Biomechanics Laboratory, Department of Engineering, University of California; 1961.

69. Radcliffe CW. Functional considerations in the fitting of above-knee prostheses. Artif Limbs. 1955;2(1);35-60.

70. Radocy B. Voluntary closing control: a successful new design approach to an old concept. Clin Prosthet Orthot. 1986;10(2):82-6.

71. Rothgangel AS, Braun SM, Beurskens AJ, et al. The clinical aspects of mirror therapy in rehabilitation: a systematic review of the literature. Int J Rehabil Res. 2011;34(1):1-13.

72. Sanders GT. Lower limb amputations: a guide to rehabilitation. FA Davis Company; 1986.

73. Sato K, Higuchi H, Hishikawa Y. Management of phantom limb pain and sensation with milnacipran. J Neuropsychiatry Clin Neurosci. 2008;20(3):368.

74. Schmalz T, Blumentritt S, Jarasch R. Energy expenditure and biomechanical characteristics of lower limb amputee gait: the influence of prosthetic alignment and different prosthetic components. Gait Posture. 2002;16(3):255-63.

75. Schuch CM, Pritham CH. Current transfemoral sockets. Clin Orthop. 1999;361:48-54.

76. Scott M. Jaipur foot: a cost effective prosthetic leg. (Online) We Capable; 2019. Available from https://wecapable.com/jaipur-foot-cost-effective-prosthetic-leg/. (Accessed October 14, 2019).

77. Sears HH, Andrews JT, Jacobsen SC. Experience with the Utah arm, hand and terminal device. In: Atkins DK (Ed). Comprehensive management of the upper limb amputee. New York, NY: Springer Verlag; 1989. pp. 194-210.

78. Sears HH. Approaches to prescription of body powered and myoelectric prostheses. Phys Med Rehabil Clin N Am. 1991;2(2):1047-51.

79. Standard of Care: LE Amputation. Brigham and Women's Hospital; 2001. The Brigham and Women's Hospital, Inc., Department of Rehabilitation Services.

80. Stark G. Overview of knee disarticulation. J Prosthet Orthot. 2004;16(4):130-7.

81. Tang SFT, Chen CPC, Chen MJL, et al. Transmetatarsal amputation prosthesis with carbon-fiber plate enhanced gait function. Am J Phys Med Rehabil. 2004;83(2):124-30.

82. Torres MM, Esquanazi A. Bilateral lower limb rehabilitation: a retrospective review. West J Med. 1991;154(4):583-6.

83. Van der Linde H, Hofstad CJ, Guerts AC, et al. A systematic literature review of the effect of different prosthetic components on human functioning with a lower-limb prosthesis. J Rehabil Res Dev. 2004;41(4):555-70.

84. van de Veen PG. Above Knee Prosthetic Technology. The Netherlands: P.G. van de Veen Consultancy; 2001.

85. Vigier S1, Casillas JM, Dulieu V, et al. Healing of open stump wounds after vascular below-knee amputation: plaster cast socket with silicone sleeve versus elastic compression. Arch Phys Med Rehabil. 1999;80(10):1327-30.

86. Weeks SR, Anderson-Barnes VC, Tsao JW. Phantom limb pain theories and therapies. Neurologist. 2010;16(5):277-86.

87. Williams TW. Use of Boston elbow for high level amputees. In: Atkins DK (Ed). Comprehensive management of the upper limb amputee. New York, NY: Springer Verlag; 1989. pp. 211-26.

88. Working Group of the International Society for Prosthetics and Orthotics. A proposed international terminology for the classification of congenital limb deficiencies (prepared by Kay HW). Orthot Prosthet. 1974;28(2):33-48.

89. Younger AS, Awwad MA, Kalla TP, et al. Risk factors for failure of transmetatarsal amputation in diabetic patients: a cohort study. Foot Ankle Int. 2009;30(12):1177-82.

Stroke

Prakash V

LEARNING OBJECTIVES

After reading this chapter, the readers should be able to:
- Define the stroke and describe the risk factors of stroke
- Understand the types of stroke and pathophysiology of stroke and stroke syndromes
- Gain knowledge on how one can prevent stroke and diagnose stroke
- Understand the medical management of stroke
- Understand the mechanisms of recovery, including neuroplasticity, that drive stroke recovery, as well as the impact of physiotherapy interventions on these underlying mechanisms
- Identify key principles of treatment in stroke rehabilitation
- Design and deliver effective physiotherapy treatment strategies for improving patient-preferred outcomes following stroke

CHAPTER OUTLINE

- Burden of illness
- Risk factors for stroke
- Types of stroke
  - Stroke subtypes
- Pathophysiology
- Stroke syndromes
  - Anterior circulation diseases
  - Posterior circulation diseases
- Sequelae of stroke
- Stroke prevention
- Diagnosis of stroke and investigations
- Management of stroke
  - Medical management of stroke
  - Surgical management of stroke
  - Assessment and examination
- Rehabilitation
  - Recovery of functions following stroke
  - Task-oriented exercises
  - Rehabilitation of sit-to-stand
  - Rehabilitation of walking
  - Rehabilitation of upper limb functions
  - Prevention and management of poststroke shoulder pain and subluxation
- Instructions for patient/caregiver
- Recovery and outcomes

INTRODUCTION

Definition

The World Health Organization defined stroke as: "rapidly developing clinical signs of focal (or global) disturbance of cerebral function, with symptoms lasting 24 hours or longer or leading to death, with no apparent cause other than of vascular origin." This definition excludes transient ischemic attack (TIA), which is defined to last less than 24 hours, and patients with stroke symptoms caused by subdural hemorrhage, tumors, poisoning, or trauma. However, the classic definition has been under criticism due to its primary focus on clinical symptom and its duration.

Recently, the Stroke Council of the American Heart Association (AHA)/American Stroke Association published an updated definition of stroke for the 21st century and recommended that term "stroke" should be broadly used to include all of the following:
- Central nervous system (CNS) infarction
- Ischemic stroke
- Silent CNS infarction
- Stroke caused by intracerebral hemorrhage
- Stroke caused by subarachnoid hemorrhage
- Stroke caused by cerebral venous thrombosis
- Stroke, not otherwise specified.

The updated definition of stroke incorporates clinical and tissue criteria. Definition of each type of stroke is illustrated in **Table 26.1**.

Table 26.1: Definition of stroke.

Definition of CNS infarction: CNS infarction in brain, spinal cord, or retinal cell death attributable to ischemia, based on:
- Pathological, imaging, or other objective evidence of cerebral, spinal cord, or retinal focal ischemic injury in a defined vascular distribution
- Clinical evidence of cerebral, spinal cord, or retinal focal ischemic injury based on symptoms persisting ≥24 h or until death, and other etiologies excluded (*Note:* CNS infarction includes hemorrhagic infarctions, types I and II; *see* "Hemorrhagic Infarction")

Definition of ischemic stroke: An episode of neurological dysfunction caused by focal cerebral, spinal, or retinal infarction (*Note:* Evidence of CNS infarction is defined above)

Definition of silent CNS infarction: Imaging or neuropathological evidence of CNS infarction, without a history of acute neurological dysfunction attributable to the lesion

Definition of intracerebral hemorrhage: A focal collection of blood within the brain parenchyma or ventricular system that is not caused by trauma (*Note:* Intracerebral hemorrhage includes parenchymal hemorrhages after CNS infarction)

Definition of stroke caused by intracerebral hemorrhage: Rapidly developing clinical signs of neurological dysfunction attributable to a focal collection of blood within the brain parenchyma or ventricular system that is not caused by trauma

Definition of silent cerebral hemorrhage: A focal collection of chronic blood products within the brain parenchyma, subarachnoid space, or ventricular system on neuroimaging or neuropathological examination that is not caused by trauma and without a history of acute neurological dysfunction attributable to the lesion

Definition of subarachnoid hemorrhage: Bleeding into the subarachnoid space (the space between the arachnoid membrane and the pia mater of the brain or spinal cord)

Definition of stroke caused by subarachnoid hemorrhage: Rapidly developing signs of neurological dysfunction and/or headache because of bleeding into the subarachnoid space (the space between the arachnoid membrane and the pia mater of the brain or spinal cord), which is not caused by trauma

Definition of stroke caused by cerebral venous thrombosis: Infarction or hemorrhage in the brain, spinal cord, or retina because of thrombosis of a cerebral venous structure. Symptoms or signs caused by reversible edema without infarction or hemorrhage do not qualify as stroke

Definition of stroke, not otherwise specified: An episode of acute neurological dysfunction presumed to be caused by ischemia or hemorrhage, persisting ≥24 h or until death, but without sufficient evidence to be classified as one of the above

(CNS: central nervous system)
Source: Reproduced from Sacco Ralph et al. (2013).

BURDEN OF ILLNESS

Globally, stroke is a leading cause of mortality and disability and there are substantial economic costs for poststroke care. In 2016, there were 5.5 million deaths and 116.4 million disability-adjusted life years (DALYs) due to stroke. There were 80.1 million prevalent cases of stroke globally in 2016; 41.1 million in women and 39.0 million in men. Although the death rates and prevalence of stroke have decreased over time, the overall burden of stroke has remained high.

More than 85% of stroke DALYs can be attributed to known risk factors of stroke. Metabolic risks, such as high systolic blood pressure (BP), high body mass index, high fasting plasma glucose, high total cholesterol, and low glomerular filtration rate, accounted for 72% of stroke DALYs. Behavioral factors (smoking, poor diet, and low physical activity) accounted for 66.3% of attributable DALYs, and environmental risks, such as air pollution and lead exposure contributed to 28% of DALYs.

RISK FACTORS FOR STROKE

Major risk factors for stroke include:
- Hypertension (HTN)
- Heart diseases (HDs), such as ischemic HD, cardiomyopathy, heart failure, and atrial fibrillation, can cause blood clots that can lead to a stroke
- Disorders of heart rhythm
- Diabetes mellitus

Other risk factors include:
- Age: commoner in females with early menopause
- Gender
- Race and ethnicity. Strokes occur more often in African-American, Alaska-Native, and American-Indian adults than in White, Hispanic, or Asian-American adult
- Personal or family history of stroke or TIA
- Cigarette smoking
- Physical inactivity
- Obesity
- Diet

TYPES OF STROKE

Stroke is classified into two main categories based on the pathological mechanism underlying the tissue damage:
1. Ischemic stroke
2. Hemorrhagic stroke

Ischemic stroke is caused by a thrombus or embolism formed in the blood vessels supplying the brain. Hemorrhagic stroke is caused by leakage of blood inside the brain due to rupture of a blood vessel. **Figures 26.1 and 26.2** show how ischemic and hemorrhagic stroke can occur in the brain, respectively. A more extensive subclassification is given below:

Stroke Subtypes

Listed below are stroke subtypes:
1. **Ischemic**
   1.1. Atherothrombotic
      1.1.1. Extracranial
      1.1.2. Intracranial

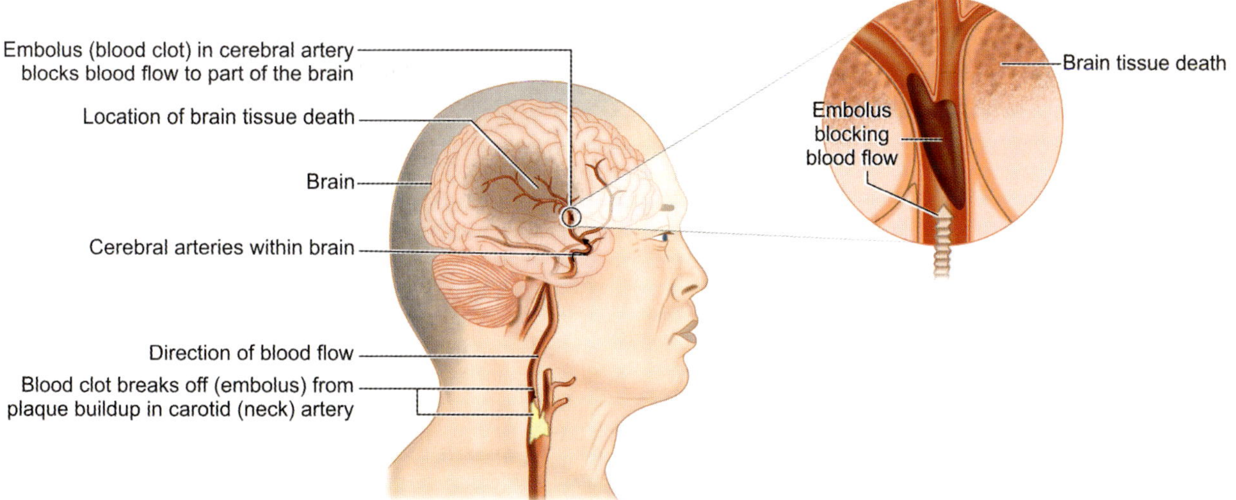

Fig. 26.1: How ischemic stroke can occur in the brain.

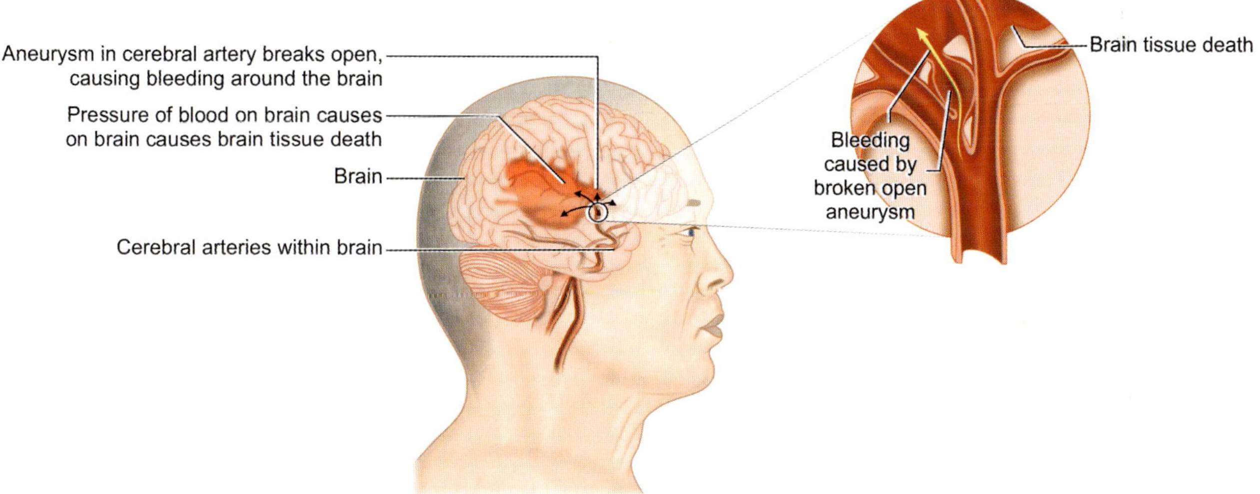

Fig. 26.2: How a hemorrhagic stroke can occur in the brain.

1.2. Small vessel disease (sporadic)

1.3. Cardiac emboli

1.4. Other causes

    1.4.1. Dissection

    1.4.2. Rare or hereditary large- or medium-sized artery disease (e.g., moyamoya disease and fibromuscular dysplasia)

    1.4.3. Rare or hereditary small vessel disease

    1.4.4. Coagulopathy

    1.4.5. Metabolic disease with arteriopathy

    1.4.6. Vasculitis

    1.4.7. Other rare entities

1.5. Coexisting causes

1.6. Unknown

1.7. Unclassifiable

2. **Hemorrhagic**

2.1. HTN-related small vessel disease (hemorrhagic type)

2.2. Cerebral amyloid angiopathy

    2.2.1. Sporadic

    2.2.2. Hereditary

2.3. Bleeding diathesis

    2.3.1. Drugs that decrease clotting

    2.3.2. Other hemostatic or hematologic disorders

2.4. Vascular malformation

    2.4.1. Arteriovenous malformation

    2.4.2. Dural fistula

    2.4.3. Ruptured aneurysm

    2.4.4. Cavernoma

        2.4.4.1. Sporadic

        2.4.4.2. Familial

2.5. Other causes

    2.5.1. Tumor related

    2.5.2. Toxic (e.g., sympathomimetic drugs, cocaine)

2.5.3. Trauma

2.5.4. Arteritis, angiitis, endocarditis (ruptured mycotic aneurysm), and infections

2.5.5. Rare entities (e.g., dissection of intracranial arteries)

2.6. Coexisting cause

2.7. Unknown

2.8. Unclassifiable

3. **Subarachnoid hemorrhage**

3.1. With aneurysm

3.2. With dissection

3.3. Traumatic

3.4. Neoplastic (melanoma)

3.5. Unknown

4. **Cerebral venous thrombosis.**

5. **Spinal cord stroke**

5.1. Ischemic

5.2. Hemorrhagic

5.2.1. Associated with arteriovenous malformation

5.2.2. Associated with coagulopathy

PATHOPHYSIOLOGY

A series of pathophysiological events arises following sudden cessation of blood flow to the major vessels of the brain. The chain of events resulting after ischemia is often referred to as *ischemic cascade* (**Fig. 26.3**).

Ischemic strokes result into cerebral edema, which is an accumulation of fluids within the brain that begins within minutes of the insult and peaks at 3–4 days. It gradually starts subsiding and disappears by almost 2–3 weeks. Significant edema can lead to brainstem herniation, which elevates intracranial pressures, leading to intracranial HTN and neurological deterioration associated with contralateral symptoms and causes caudal shifts of brain structures.

STROKE SYNDROMES

A stroke syndrome is a set of symptoms that helps to identify which part of the brain has been injured in stroke. The earliest classical syndromes were described in the 19th century and since then many new stroke syndromes have been discovered. Recent advances in neuroimaging have allowed many of the classical stroke syndromes previously described on the basis of clinical pathology or during autopsy to be confirmed.

Stroke syndromes are of clinical importance as they could represent the clinical manifestation and consequences of stroke. It is imperative that clinicians are aware of the various stroke syndromes, particularly those with potential devastating effect, which could lead to significant disability and even death. Even if they are not life-threatening, they could pose a great challenge for poststroke treatment and recovery and may delay or prevent aggressive rehabilitation.

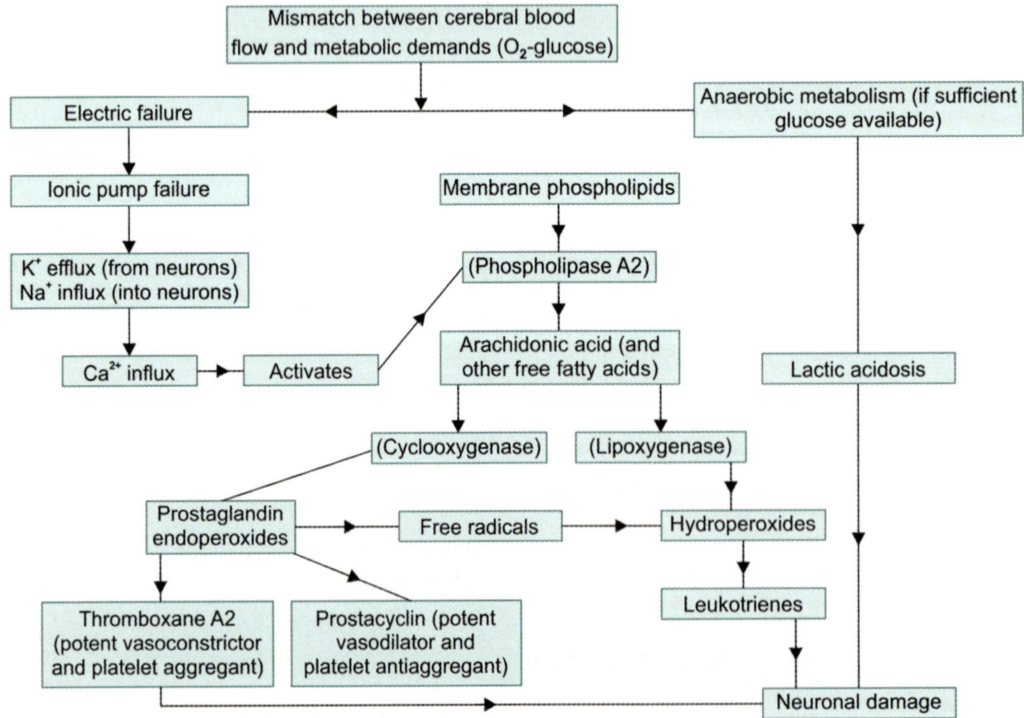

Fig. 26.3: Ischemic cascade.

Anterior Circulation Diseases

Middle Cerebral Artery Diseases

The middle cerebral artery (MCA) is the largest cerebral artery and supplies most of the outer surface of the cerebral cortex, basal ganglia, internal capsule, and corona radiata **(Fig. 26.4)**. Occlusion of the main MCA trunk produces:

- Contralateral hemiparesis
- Hemisensory deficit
- Deviation of eyes toward the side of the infarct
- Hemianopia
- Global aphasia occurs when the dominant hemisphere is severely damaged
- Hemineglect occurs when the infarct develops in the right hemisphere
- Divisional or branch occlusion results in partial or minor neurological deficits
- Occlusion of perforating arteries produces subcortical infarction sparing the cortex and typically yields **lacunar syndrome,** such as pure motor, sensorimotor, ataxic-hemiparesis, or dysarthria clumsy syndromes.

  Patients with MCA atherosclerosis rarely present with a total MCA syndrome; they tend to have lacunar syndromes associated with deep infarcts, whereas cortical symptoms are less common and less severe than in patients with embolism to the MCA from proximal sources.

Anterior Cerebral Artery Disease

Anterior cerebral artery (ACA) territory infarction accounts for less than 3% of ischemic stroke. Clinically, ACA infarction is characterized by the following:

- Limb weakness, worse in the leg than in the arm. A small lesion may produce isolated lower limb weakness. Decreased shoulder shrug and proximal arm weakness often accompany leg weakness in the early stage.
- Sensory dysfunction is usually less severe and occurs almost always in the paretic limbs.

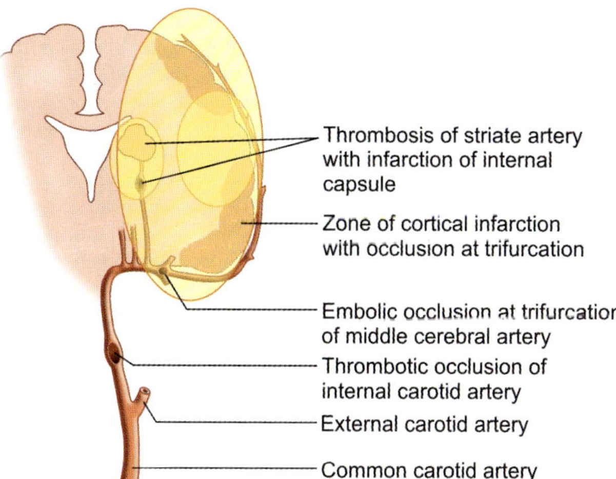

Fig. 26.4: Middle cerebral artery (MCA) infarct.

- Hypobulia/apathy characteristically occurs and has been shown to be related to callosal or anteromedial frontal lobe damage. This finding is more severe and persistent in patients with bilateral than in those with unilateral lesions.
- Other symptoms include urinary incontinence, alien hand sign, and limb apraxia.
- When the infarct involves the left brain, aphasia may develop, transcortical motor aphasia being the most common.
- Other miscellaneous symptoms include emotional lability/incontinence, drowsiness/somnolence, acute confusion/agitation, motor perseveration, amnesia, and Parkinsonian symptoms.

Posterior Circulation Diseases

Lateral Medullary Infarction Syndrome

Lateral medullary infarction (LMI) syndrome is also referred to as **Wallenberg syndrome.**

- Dizziness and gait instability, attributed either to vestibular or cerebellar system dysfunction, occur in more than 90% of the patients. Whirling vertigo occurs in approximately 60%, usually accompanied by nystagmus and nausea/vomiting.
- Gait ataxia is usually more severe than limb incoordination.
- The nystagmus is mostly horizontal rotational to the side opposite to the lesions. Skew deviation, with the ipsilateral eye going down, is also frequent. Ptosis and meiosis (components of a Horner's syndrome) are caused by the involvement of the descending sympathetic fibers in the lateral reticular substance, which occur in about 90% of patients.
- Involvement of the nucleus ambiguous results in dysphagia, dysarthria, and hoarseness. Dysphagia is present in approximately two-thirds of LMI patients, among whom about 60% require nasogastric tube feeding. Dysphagia is distinctly more severe in patients with rostral than in caudal lesions.
- Approximately one-fourth of patients develop hiccup, often days after the stroke onset.
- Headache, most often occurring in the ipsilateral occipital or upper nuchal area, occurs in approximately a half of the patients.

Medial Medullary Infarction Syndrome

Dejerine proposed a triad of medial medullary infarction (MMI) syndrome:

- Contralateral hemiplegia sparing the face
- Contralateral loss of deep sensation
- Ipsilateral hypoglossal paralysis
  - Contralateral hemiparesis sparing the face is the most characteristic sign of MMI.
  - Sensory dysfunction is the second most important symptom/sign of MMI. Unlike LMI patients, MMI patients typically complain of tingling sensation from the onset and show decreased perception of

position and vibration due to selective involvement of the lemniscal sensory fibers. The involved area is usually hemibody/limbs below the ear or neck sparing the face.

Basilar Artery Occlusion Syndrome

The basilar artery occlusion syndrome presents as a subset of the larger category of posterior circulation strokes.

- Although limb weakness is the most common symptom/sign, the clinical features depend upon the degree of involvement of each fiber tract and may manifest as:
  - Pure motor stroke
  - Ataxic-hemiparesis
  - Dysarthria clumsy hand syndromes.
- Ataxia or incoordination is another common finding, observed in the limbs that are not severely paretic
- Dysarthria and dysphagia due to bilateral bulbar muscles paresis are also common and severe. Some patients become totally unable to speak, open their mouth, or protrude their tongue.
- Somatosensory abnormalities should also be common, but they are usually overshadowed by motor dysfunction
- Ocular bobbing, ptosis, and pinpoint pupils may be observed
- Symptoms, such as tinnitus, hearing loss, and auditory hallucination are related to involvement of the central auditory tracts/nuclei or to ischemia of the eighth nerves/fascicles.
- Altered consciousness is an important sign in patients with sudden BA occlusion and is related to bilateral medial tegmental pontine ischemia. Consciousness usually improves overtime.
- Patients may show pathological crying and laughing spells that are triggered by minimal social–emotional stimuli.
- When all voluntary movements are lost, the deficit is referred to as the "locked-in" syndrome.
- Intact vertical eye movements may be used in simple communications.

Box 26.1 summarizes the presentation of different stroke syndromes.

SEQUELAE OF STROKE

Most important areas affected by stroke are motor skills, followed by functional and sensory impairments, immobility, chronic pain, deficits in cognition and perception, coordination or balance deficits, speech, language or communication impairments, and emotional or behavioral issues **(Box 26.2)**.

STROKE PREVENTION

Early warning signs of stroke can help in stroke prevention to a large extent. As identified by the AHA, and National Stroke Association, acronym FAST, can be an important and useful means of identifying these early signs **(Fig. 26.5)**. The significance of recognizing early warning signs rests with prompt initiation of emergency care under the rule that "time is brain." Patients and families are encouraged

---

BOX 26.1: Presentations of stroke syndromes.

- MCA stroke can cause contralateral hemiparesis, sensory loss, hemianopia, and either aphasia or neglect
- ACA stroke can cause contralateral leg weakness and executive dysfunction
- PCA stroke can cause hemianopia, pure sensory infarct (thalamus), memory impairment, and decreased level of consciousness
- Brainstem strokes can cause crossed sensory or motor findings, nystagmus, diplopia, vertigo, and Horner's syndrome
- Cerebellar strokes can cause ataxia, nystagmus, vertigo, nausea, headache, and rapid deterioration in consciousness
- Lacunar strokes often have a characteristic pattern: pure motor, pure sensory, sensorimotor, ataxic-hemiparesis, and clumsy hand–dysarthria

---

BOX 26.2: Impairments associated with stroke.

Altered consciousness: Normal, lethargy, obtundation, stupor, and coma

Disorders of speech and language: aphasia (fluent or nonfluent or global) and dysarthria

Swallowing difficulties: dysphagia and aspiration

Cognitive disorders: higher order functions, executive functions, dementia, and delirium

Perceptual disorders: body image deficits such as unilateral neglect, anosognosia, somatoagnosia, right–left discrimination, finger agnosia, and anosognosia; and spatial disorders, such as figure–ground discrimination, form discrimination, spatial relations, position in space, and topographical disorientation

Emotional issues: emotional lability, emotional dysregulation syndrome, apathy, euphoria, depression; right hemisphere lesions usually lead to difficulty with ability to perceive emotions and difficulty with expression of negative emotions, whereas left hemisphere lesions result in difficulty with expression of positive emotions

Behavioral difficulties: left hemisphere lesions (right hemiplegia) demonstrate difficulties in communication and in processing information in a sequential, linear manner, frequently described as cautious, anxious, and disorganized, whereas individuals with right lesions are described as quick and impulsive, they exhibit poor judgment, unrealistic inability to self-correct, poor insight, awareness of impairments, denial of disability, and increased safety risk

Bowel bladder status: urinary incontinence, urinary tract infections, diarrhea, constipation, and impaction
Cardiovascular and pulmonary dysfunction: coronary artery disease, decreased lung volume, decreased pulmonary perfusion and vital capacity, and altered chest wall excursion

Complications: Deep vein thrombosis (DVT), embolism, seizures, osteoporosis, and fracture risk

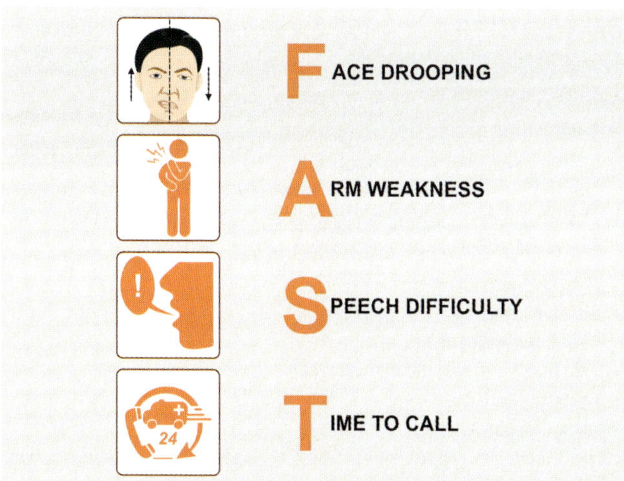

Fig. 26.5: Stroke warning signs and symptoms.

to call "108" immediately, even if these symptoms go away quickly or are not painful.

Early computed tomography (CT) is used to differentiate between atherothrombotic stroke and hemorrhagic stroke. If the stroke is atherothrombotic, clot-dissolving enzymes [e.g., tissue plasminogen activator (tPA)] can be used for thrombolysis. Other thrombolytic therapy, such as tPA must be given within 3 hours of the onset of symptoms and cannot be given with hemorrhagic stroke because the drug may worsen bleeding. Within this duration, the patient must recognize the gravity of situation as a medical emergency, be transported to an appropriate hospital, be evaluated by emergency department (ED) staff (including a CT scan of the brain), and be treated. This is a safe and traditional approach, known to dramatically reduce death and disability; however, fewer than half of individuals experiencing stroke arrive at the ED within 2 hours of symptoms. Women are less likely to arrive in time as compared to men. Major heart and stroke organizations currently promote the use of the term *brain attack*, to help individuals recognize the importance of seeking immediate emergency care **(Box 26.3)**.

DIAGNOSIS OF STROKE AND INVESTIGATIONS

Information regarding the following are obtained from family members of patients:
- Exact time and pattern of symptom onset
- Patient's history, including episodes of TIAs or head trauma

---

BOX 26.3: Significant predictors for stroke prevention and treatment.

- Patients who do receive tPA within 3 hours are at least 33% more likely to recover from their stroke with little or no disability after 3 months as compared to those who do not receive the treatment
- Patients are also less likely to suffer when the spouse or significant other is able to make the decision to seek treatment immediately

---

- The presence of major or minor risk factors, and medications, pertinent family history, and any recent alterations in patient function.

Stroke can mimic various other conditions, which should be ruled out, including seizures, space-occupying lesions (e.g., subdural hematoma, cerebral abscess/infection, and tumor), syncope, somatization, and delirium secondary to sepsis. Vital signs should be checked, and signs of cardiac decompensation, and function of the cerebral hemispheres, cerebellum, cranial nerves, eyes, and sensorimotor system should be noted. Bilateral signs are suggestive of brainstem lesions or massive cerebral involvement; hence, presenting symptoms should be noted, and comparison on both sides should be made. Cerebrovascular imaging techniques are used chiefly to establish the diagnosis of suspected ischemic stroke and to rule out hemorrhagic stroke and other types of CNS lesions (e.g., tumor or abscess) **(Table 26.2)**.

MANAGEMENT OF STROKE

Medical Management of Stroke

Strategies to achieve the following are routinely employed for the medical management of stroke:
- Oxygen therapy via mask or nasal cannula to restore oxygenation and re-establish circulation
- Normalizing elevated BP
- Maintaining cardiac output
- Restoring fluid and electrolyte imbalance
- Maintaining normal blood glucose levels
- Minimizing chances of infections and seizures
- Maintaining bowel bladder function
- Maintaining skin integrity and adequate joint positioning
- Minimizing risk of infections and secondary complications.

Commonly used drugs in the management of stroke and comorbidities associated with stroke are shown in **Table 26.3**.

Surgical Management of Stroke

The surgical management of stroke is as follows:
- In the case of arteriovenous malformation (AVM) resulting in hemorrhagic stroke, repair may be needed to prevent rebleeding and evacuate a clot.
- Mechanical thrombectomy is the removal of large blood clot by sending a stent retriever to the site of blocked blood vessel in the brain.
- Carotid endarterectomy is a surgical procedure used to remove fatty deposits from the carotid artery.

Assessment and Examination

Principles of assessment will be similar to those discussed in chapter on neurological assessment, specific points of assessment are mentioned in **Box 26.4**. Uses of

Table 26.2: Cerebrovascular imaging techniques used in the diagnosis of stroke.

Techniques	Features
CT	• Allows identification of large arteries and veins and venous sinuses • Poor sensitivity for detecting small infarcts and infarction in the posterior fossa • Allows visualization of acute bleeding and hemorrhagic transformation and cerebral edema • Addition of contrast dye allows visualizing areas of decreased density • Allows visualization of long-term parenchymal changes such as scar formation
MRI	• More sensitive in the diagnosis of acute strokes, allowing detection of cerebral ischemia as early as 30 minutes after vascular occlusion and infarction within 2–6 hours • Detects smaller lesions than a CT scan • Allows determination of extent of infarction or hemorrhage • Allows documentation of changes in an infarct over the first 2–3 weeks • Can be used with claustrophobic patients and those with implants
MRA	• Allows identification of vascular abnormalities such as stenosis • Allows identification of alterations in blood flow as a result of embolus or thrombosis
Doppler ultrasound	• Transcranial Doppler is used to examine the posterior circulation of the brain • Carotid Doppler is used to examine the carotid arteries and typically precedes carotid endarterectomy • Also used to examine the peripheral arteries in the diagnosis of PAD
Arteriography	• Invasive and carries a small risk of causing a stroke • Involves X-ray of the carotid artery with a special dye injected into an artery in the leg or arm
DSA	• Invasive and carries a small risk of causing a stroke • Involves X-ray of the carotid artery with less dye used

(CT: computed tomography; DSA: digital subtraction angiography; MRA: magnetic resonance angiography; MRI: magnetic resonance imaging; PAD: peripheral artery disease)

Table 26.3: Commonly used medications in the treatment of stroke.

• Thrombolytics	Angiotensin-II receptor antagonists
• Anticoagulants	Anticholesterol agents/statins
• Antiplatelet therapy	Antispasmodics/spasmolytics
• Antihypertensive agents	Antispastics
• Anticonvulsants	Antidepressants
• GABA receptor antagonists	Neurotoxins

(GABA: gamma amino-butyric acid)

BOX 26.4: Assessment and examination for a patient with stroke.

Patient history
• Goals (emphasis on participation and activity)
• Quick communication and cognition screen (discussed below)
• Demographics, family history, and socioeconomic status
• Preamputation status, work, and leisure activities

Systems review
• Neuromuscular
• Musculoskeletal
• Cardiovascular/pulmonary
• Integumentary

Tests and measures
Participation
• Work, community, and leisure activities: ability to assume/resume activities, safety

Activities
• Postural control and balance
• Gait and locomotion
• Functional status and activity level
• Upper limb use

Body structure and function
• Level of consciousness, arousal, attention, and cognition: mental status, insight, motivation
• Emotional status
• Behavioral style
• Communication and language
• Circulation
• Ventilation and respiration/gas exchange
• Anthropometric characteristics
• Integumentary integrity
• Pain
• Cranial and peripheral nerve integrity
• Sensory integrity and integration
• Perceptual function
• Joint integrity, alignment, and mobility
• Posture
• Motor function
• Muscle performance
• Aerobic capacity and endurance
• Wheelchair management and mobility
• Orthotic, protective and supportive devices

self-reported and performance based outcome measure are shown in **Box 26.5**.

Rehabilitation following stroke considers the patient's history, course, and symptoms, together with impairments, activity limitations, and participation restrictions. Patient's abilities, priorities, and resources, including family, home, and community resources are also important. Interventions can be:

- *Restorative* (aimed at improving impairments, activity limitations, and participation restrictions)
- *Preventive* (aimed at minimizing potential complications and indirect impairments)
- *Compensatory* (aimed at modifying the task, activity, or environment to improve function).

BOX 26.5: Outcome measures commonly used for a patient with stroke.

Self-report measures
- Stroke impact scale
- Goal attainment scale
- Functional independence measure

Performance-based measures
- Functional reach test
- Berg balance scale
- Timed up and go
- 6-Minute walk distance
- Dynamic gait index
- Action research arm test
- Fugl–Meyer motor performance
- Stroke rehabilitation assessment of movement
- Clinical test for sensory interaction in balance
- Performance-oriented mobility assessment (tinetti)
- Trunk impairment scale
- Function in sitting test
- Functional ambulation profile
- Gait abnormality rating scale (GARS) and the modified GARS

REHABILITATION

Traditionally, disability following stroke is viewed as an abnormality or deviation from the "normal" body functioning. Impairments, such as spasticity, abnormal movement coordination have been identified as independent causes of the disability experienced by patients with stroke. Such views are predominant in the doctrines of traditional neurorehabilitation approaches:

- Bobath
- Brunnstrom
- Proprioceptive neuromuscular facilitation

Traditional physiotherapy approaches to stroke rehabilitation assumed normal tone essential for producing normal movement patterns in order to perform functional tasks and equated disappearance of spasticity as a sign of functional recovery. For example, Bobath approach, also known as neurodevelopmental treatment (NDT), emphasized tone as an essential component of functional activity. Similarly, the predominant basis of the Brunnstrom approach is the use of reflexes to develop movement behavior through sensory stimulation to inhibit spasticity.

In summary, the primary goal of traditional stroke rehabilitation approaches is to alleviate impairments, especially spasticity, which is viewed as critical for regaining ability to carry out functional activities, thereby reducing poststroke disability. Patients were discouraged to perform functional tasks especially, during early stage of recovery, based on the belief that abnormal tone and abnormal movement patterns would be reinforced by practicing functional tasks. However, traditional approaches are criticized for placing too much emphasis on normalizing tone and not enough emphasis on the practice of functional activities.

Since the 1950s, the decade in which several traditional neurophysiotherapy approaches were developed, our understanding of how nervous system (NS) produce functional movements and how patients recover following stroke has changed radically. Currently, there is an improved understanding of the mechanisms of functional recovery after stroke. Spasticity is now viewed as an adaptive response of the CNS, and not as a primary impairment. Although spasticity contributes to activity limitations and may be a significant contributor to disability for some patients after stroke, a significant proportion of patients are nonspastic and continue to experience limitations in daily activities. In the past four decades, mounting evidence on the role of spasticity in contributing to disability in patients with stroke strongly supports the view that spasticity management in stroke rehabilitation is less relevant. Therefore, it is inappropriate to routinely focus on reducing or inhibiting spasticity to improve participation in functional activities in stroke rehabilitation. There is a growing body of evidence that problems after stroke may be caused by complex interaction between various biological, personal, and environmental factors other than spasticity.

Recovery of Functions Following Stroke

Modern neurorehabilitation is viewed as a process of facilitating patients in relearning to perform previously learned tasks in a different way by either using compensatory movement strategies or by adaptively recruiting alternative pathways. Recovery is no longer viewed as a linear process of progressing through predetermined and sequential stages of regaining normal tone and normal movement patterns but rather as nonlinear process of skills acquisition. Understanding the recovery after stroke requires knowledge about the time-dependent nature of the mechanisms that reflect neural reorganization, recovery of body functions, and use of behavioral compensation strategies.

Mechanisms of Recovery

Immediately following stroke, a dynamic process of repair and remodeling of remaining neural circuits is initiated. Further, the recovery process is shaped by behavioral experiences that are gained through patients' attempt to reengage in their daily activities. The mechanisms underlying neurological recovery are not fully understood. A number of mechanisms are hypothesized to be involved in recovery:

- Salvation of the penumbra
- Alleviation of diaschisis
- Unmasking of previously present, but functionally inactive connections
- Axonal and dendritic regeneration (i.e., collateral sprouting)
- Synaptogenesis and denervation hypersensitivity.

The mechanisms underlying recovery of function following stroke have been distinguished as involving either restitution or substitution of function. **Restitution** refers to the restoration of a function using prestroke movement patterns through reductions in motor impairments, whereas **substitution** refers to the compensation, or circumvention of, impaired functions, i.e., using new movement patterns to accomplish the desired task or goal.

From the clinical perspective, however, a distinction attributed to these two mechanisms of recovery appears irrelevant. The reasons are:

1. These two mechanisms often overlap in their contributions to performance improvements in such tasks. Thus, it is challenging to distinguish extent of functional gains achieved through the recovery mechanism of restitution (motor recovery of normal patterns) from substitution (compensatory movements of new patterns).
2. Currently, it is not clear whether rehabilitation interventions can specifically promote neural mechanisms of restitution and those of substitution.

Should compensation be encouraged or discouraged during stroke rehabilitation?

Answer to this question is not straightforward. A pragmatic answer would be "it depends." It depends on how and in which context "compensation" is defined and understood.

Compensation

- At the **level of neural connections,** compensation is described in terms of reorganization of synaptic connectivity patterns of surviving neurons in the brain, such as collateral sprouting from neighboring tissue and contralesional hemisphere to compensate for the function of tissues lost due to stroke.
- At the **kinematic level**, compensation is defined as the use of additional or alternate kinematic patterns during task performance, e.g., use of excessive trunk flexion as a compensation to elbow extension deficit while reaching forward, coupling of elbow flexion while lifting the arm as a compensation for a deficit in isolated shoulder flexion.
- At the **level of participation in daily activities**, compensation may involve modifying the task, e.g., using a western toilet, reducing the frequency of engagement or time spent in an activity, and complete abandonment of the participation in previously valued activity.

Traditionally, in stroke rehabilitation compensation is identified at the kinematic level through observation of patients' movement patterns (quality of movements) compared to that of "normal" movement patterns. Compensatory movement patterns are often termed "abnormal synergy." In traditional neurophysiotherapy approaches, interventional strategies were designed and used with the aim of "breaking" or "normalizing" the abnormal synergistic movement patterns. Patients were discouraged to attempt or practice functional activities during the early stages of recovery based on the assumption that such practice may reinforce use of compensatory and, thus, potentially inhibit a return to normal neurological functioning. However, evidence for this assumption is lacking. Current evidence supports the use of function-oriented approaches to achieve their functional goals sooner than traditional approaches, such as NDT or the Bobath approach, which do not allow for behavioral compensation.

- Compensation need not always be viewed as undesirable aspect of recovery. Compensatory strategies can contribute to improvements in patients' functional capacity and their participation in daily activities.
- The use and extent of compensatory movement patterns are related to the degree of severity and the duration of motor impairments. While increased trunk flexion during forward reaching can have negative impact of upper limb recovery in patients with mild impairments, such compensation may be the best available option for using upper limb in patients with severe impairments having limited potential for recovery.
- Compensatory movement strategies can have mixed effects on functional outcome. Thus compensation following stroke should be considered an integral part of recovery; clinicians are encouraged to distinguish more optimal from less optimal ways of compensating.
- Compensatory strategies that counter the remaining capacity for better overall functionality can be considered to be maladaptive and, thus, may be discouraged during rehabilitation. However, the "cutoff point" between adaptive and maladaptive compensatory strategies is unclear at present. In this context, it is worth exploring the views expressed by motor control scientist Mark Latash: "Clinicians are encouraged to view patient-preferred motor patterns that emerge after stroke, as the optimal adaptive behavior for a given state of the system of movement production, rather than as a 'pathologic' behavior to be corrected." The optimal intervention may be the intervention strategy that aims to change the conditions of the state of systems (environmental, perceptual, or behavioral) involved in movement production as favorable for producing functional motor behavior.

Natural Course of Recovery of Motor Functions Following Stroke

Natural course of recovery following stroke has been extensively studied. The following is a summary of what is known about the natural course of recovery following stroke.

- Although individual recovery patterns and outcome differ between patients, several prognostic studies have shown that outcome at 3 or 6 months is highly predictable for upper and lower limb as well as basic activities of daily living (ADLs) in general.

- Though various prognostic indicators have been identified, initial severity of stroke is the strongest predictor of recovery. This means that if recovery takes place early after stroke onset, better outcomes may be expected at 6 months poststroke.
- The recovery rate is highest in the first 3 months after stroke, after which recovery levels off and reaches a plateau.
- After the first 3 months, positive (and at times negative) functional compensation may significantly impact the degree of disability experienced by the patients in the chronic stage.
- At 6 months,
    - 83% of patients recovered independent sitting
    - 60–65% achieved independent walking
    - 33% of the patients were classified as independent in ADL defined as achieving Barthel Index Score of 19 or 20 points.
    - 38% showed some recovery in dexterity of the hemiplegic arm [action research arm test (ARAT) ≥10 points] out of which, 11.6% reached a complete functional recovery in dexterity of the paretic arm (i.e., 57 points on ARAT) at 6 months.

What Makes Therapy Effective?

The following factors are responsible to make therapy effective:

- In the last three decades, several studies have clearly demonstrated that active practice of task-oriented exercises makes physiotherapy effective in improving patient outcomes following stroke.
- Intensive task-oriented rehabilitation programs applied at an early stage influence the natural course of functional recovery better than conventional neurophysiotherapy approaches that discourage early practice of functional activities.
- Task-oriented training involves direct practice of a functional task (e.g., walking, sit to stand, reaching for a cup, and drinking water) with a clear functional goal and may enhance the processes of functional recovery, including spontaneous neurological recovery after stroke.
- Several mechanisms, including the practice-dependent neuronal reorganization (i.e., neuroplasticity) in the affected and nonaffected hemispheres and behavioral compensation strategies, contribute to functional recovery seen as a result of task-oriented training.
- Further, studies have also demonstrated that traditional neurological treatment approaches, including NDT or Bobath Approach and impairment-oriented interventions, such as neuromuscular electrical stimulation, isolated muscle strength training, are less effective when compared to task-specific training.

- There is strong evidence for physiotherapy interventions favoring intensive high repetitive task-oriented training in all phases poststroke and the effects are mostly restricted to the actually trained functions and activities. Thus, across the globe, physiotherapists are encouraged to adopt task-oriented exercise to improve functional recovery of patients following stroke.

The following section outlines the fundamental principles underlying task-oriented interventions and provides general guidelines for designing a task-oriented intervention for addressing patients' limitations in participating in daily activities.

Task-oriented Exercises

There are various descriptions and definitions of task-oriented training exist in the literature. To avoid confusion, the following definition of task-oriented training given by Winstein was adopted for this chapter: "task-oriented training involves practicing real-life tasks (such as walking or pouring water into a cup), with the intention of acquiring or reacquiring a skill (defined by consistency, flexibility and efficiency)." Task-oriented training is also sometimes called **task-specific training, goal-directed training, and functional task practice**.

Task-oriented training is based on the theoretical foundations of dynamic systems theory of motor control, experience-dependent neural plasticity, and principles of motor skill acquisition, i.e., motor learning.

- Dynamic systems theory views functional movements as goal-oriented tasks, such as walking, eating, and dressing. This view posits that functional movements emerge from an interaction between the individual, the task, and the environment in which the task is being carried out **(Fig. 26.6)**. The coordination of multiple joints in producing a goal-oriented movement is not predetermined by the nervous system rather it emerges through the interaction of the person with the environment for a given functional goals. Thus, functional goal and a relevant environment is a precondition for producing functional movement.
- NS cares about functioning, not the movement patterns nor its parameters, i.e., functions and the context in which functions are to be carried out, guiding the characteristics of movement pattern. The movement pattern and its parameters, such as interjoint and interlimb coordination and force

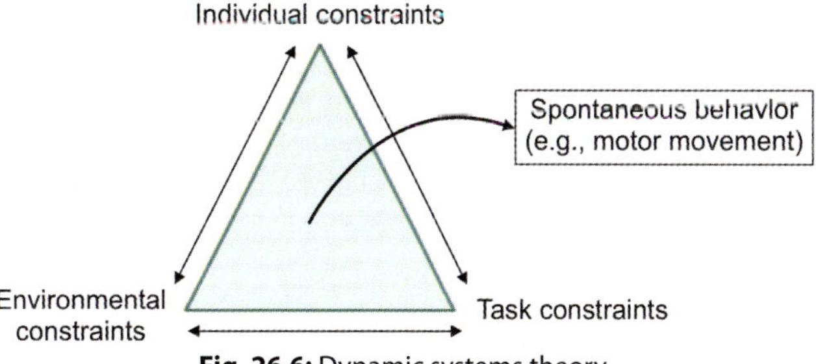

Fig. 26.6: Dynamic systems theory.

production are organized according to the intended goal of the functional movement, the task used, and the environment in which it is done. Movement patterns produced by the NS vary based on the changes in the goal of the task and environmental characteristics. Thus the target of interventions in stroke rehabilitation should be functional activity through practicing relevant tasks within appropriate context not the movement patterns. From this viewpoint, task-oriented exercises were proposed as the most suitable method for promoting functional movements. There is high-quality evidence supporting the benefits of task-oriented exercises in patients with stroke compared to impairment-based or approach-based treatment methods.

Principles of Designing Task-oriented Exercises

Several key principles of designing task-oriented exercises and its components have been identified. There is now sufficient evidence that the acquisition of a new motor skill requires the following especially in the early stages of learning:

- Progressive challenge
- Intensity
- Problem solving
- Sufficient motivation
- Focused attention

Benefits of task-oriented exercises can be maximized when these principles and components of task-oriented training are integrated into the exercises for improving patients' participation in daily activities. These principles are listed below:

1. **Tasks selected for practice should be perceived as meaningful by the patient.**
   - Selection of meaningful task aids functional recovery through promotion of experience-dependent plasticity and coordination of context-specific functional movements.
   - Meaningful tasks are tasks that are relevant and important for participating in daily life activities. For example, within Indian context, sitting on the floor and squatting are important tasks for many daily activities, such as toileting, bathing, and conversing with friends and relatives.
   - Clearly, there will be individual differences in the type of tasks perceived as meaningful. Few tasks that have significant meaning to some patients, e.g., cooking may be perceived as irrelevant by others.
   - Further, tasks such as peg board exercise or sitting on Swiss ball may not be perceived as having any relevance to their daily functions.
   - Thus to design appropriate task-oriented exercise, therapists should discuss with patients to identify tasks that provide opportunities for engagement in the roles and activities considered meaningful and refrain from using tasks that carry little meaning to the patients' daily activities.

2. **Tasks should be challenging and progressively adapted.**
   - The tasks selected for practice during rehabilitation should be perceived by patients as challenging, i.e., not too easy, but also not too difficult enough to facilitate relearning of the functional task.
   - Challenging tasks also aid in engaging the patients' attention and sustain motivation during practice.
   - The level of task difficulty can be adjusted through:
     - Manipulating practice schedules
     - Contextual factors
     - Dual tasking
     - The actual task requirements (e.g., precision, magnitude, and degrees of freedom).

For example, practice of sit-to-stand task can be made more challenging by:

- Reducing chair height
- Placing unaffected foot in front of the affected foot
- Holding a tray with cups filled with water while getting up
- Random practice of multiple sit-to-stand-related tasks as circuit training.

However, therapists should be mindful that the challenge provided should adequately represent challenges of real-life context and perceived as meaningful to the individual patient.

A common practice of sit to stand and reaching while sitting on a Swiss ball is a clear example of challenge that does not represent real-life context, i.e., patients often encounter challenges while getting up from a sofa with deep cushion or a chair without armrest or backrest; obviously, getting up from Swiss ball often not perceived as meaningful by patients. In addition to task and context-related factors, task challenge can also be manipulated by influencing patient perception of the task difficulty through simple statements before practice that have been shown to increase confidence and motivation **(Fig. 26.7)**.

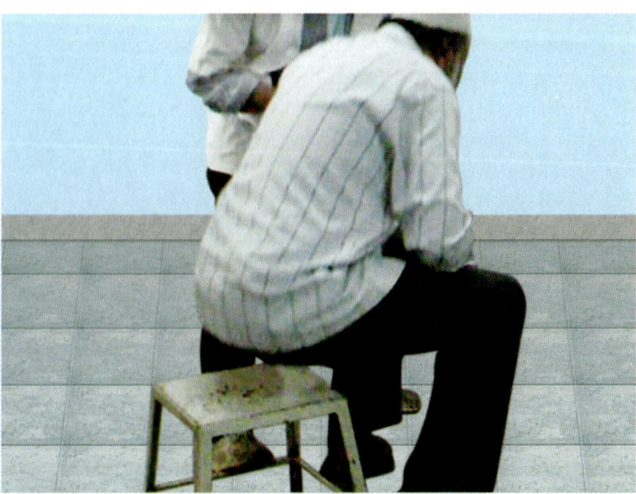

Fig. 26.7: Sit-to-stand task progression by practicing on a chair with low height.

The walking task designed by Lamontagne, et al., for their study, which investigated adaptation to overground walking speed in patients with stroke, is a good example of progressing the challenge of task within functionally relevant context and through influencing patients' perception of difficulty of task. In their study, to encourage to walk faster patients were told to "hurry as much as possible, as if they were trying to catch a bus (a meaningful task within a real-life and relevant context), and reinforced with verbal encouragement and cheering (a useful strategy to positively influence patient perception of difficulty and motivation) throughout the walking trial."

3. **Tasks should be practiced in context-specific environment.**

The practice environment of the task, which includes the following, should be arranged in a way that it equals or mimics the natural environment in which the tasks are routinely performed.
- Supporting surface
- Objects used during practice
- Accompanying people and
- Room

For example, task-oriented exercises for improving upper limb functions shall make use of objects that are handled in normal everyday-life activities **(Fig. 26.8)** such as:
- A cup
- Containers
- Cutlery
- Hairbrush
- Towel
- Practicing over a supporting surface, such as tabletop.

Similarly, exercises targeting walking–related functions shall be carried out on:
- Both even and uneven environment
- With obstacles placed on the ground
- People moving around

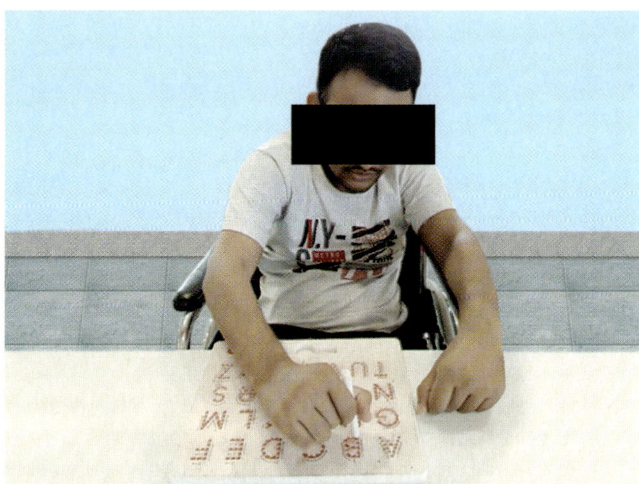

Fig. 26.8: Patient performing task simulating writing function.

4. **Task practice should be done with sufficient intensity.**

To acquire a higher level of skill in task performance, deliberate practice of the task with sufficient intensity is required.
- Intensity is defined as "the amount of physical or mental work put forth by the patient during a particular movement or series of movements, exercise, or activity during a defined period of time."
- Intensity of task practice, which includes a number of repetition, frequency, and duration of task practice, are integral to the design of any effective task-oriented exercise program.

There is considerable evidence supporting the dose–response relationship between extent of practice and levels of task performance. However, what constitutes a "sufficient" level of intensity for a given task is lacking.
- Conceptually, intensity of exercise refers to the amount of effort an individual puts forth during a task practice within a treatment session.
- The effort exerted by the patients during a particular task constitutes both physical and psychological effort.
- Depending on the type of task, the extent or proportion of physical and psychological efforts required to complete a task may vary.

For example, tasks requiring minimal physical effort, such as pouring water into a bottle, threading a needle, and reaching for a container stacked on a kitchen shelf, can involve higher psychological effort and, thus, be considered as high-intensity exercise. Thus, clinically the intensity of task practice can be determined by the extent of work that a patient puts forth in a particular session or exercise.
- Further, therapy time spent on practice of tasks (both supervised and unsupervised practice) is also a significant factor that contributes to recovery of functions. Specifically, more time spent on task practice is more likely to speed up functional recovery after stroke.

5. **Start early, but not very early.**
- Starting active rehabilitation early is a widely accepted principle of care for people affected by stroke.
- Early onset of active task-oriented exercise administered within 3–30 days poststroke is associated with improved functional outcome.
- However, treatment began very early, i.e., within 24–48 hours did not produce favorable outcomes.
- Further, the benefits of early care may not generalize to patients with severe stroke.

Rehabilitation of Sit-to-Stand

Task Characteristics and Requirements

The transition from sitting to standing requires horizontal and vertical momentum generated by movements of the head, arms, trunk, and body segments around the hip, knee, and ankle joints during performance of flexion and extension movements. The sit-to-stand movements have been described in terms of distinct kinematic events that occur during its execution. These events are described as phases. A definition of these phases that is used frequently is the one provided by Schenkman et al. and is marked by four events **(Fig. 26.9)**.

1. Phase I (flexion-momentum phase) starts with initiation of the movement and ends just before the buttocks are lifted from the seat of the chair.
2. Phase II (momentum-transfer phase) begins as the buttocks are lifted and ends when maximal ankle dorsiflexion is achieved.
3. Phase III (extension phase) is initiated just after maximum ankle dorsiflexion and ends when the hips first cease to extend, including leg and trunk extension.
4. Phase IV (stabilization phase) begins after hip extension is reached and ends when all motion associated with stabilization is completed.

The Problem

Following stroke, especially during acute stage, it is common for people to experience limitations in getting up from sitting position. Though majority of the patients (i.e., about 80%) recover independent sit to stand in about 3–6 months, patients may still experience considerable limitations in adapting to various environmental demands, such as getting up from a low chair, a sofa with deep cushion depth, and from transportation vehicle seats, such as bus, car, or auto rickshaw. Additionally, in many nonwestern countries such as India, patients also commonly report problems related to sitting on the floor and squatting.

Problem Analysis

The following steps are taken to analyze the problem:

- During the acute stage, several patients often report poor ability to stand or loss of balance while attempting to get up.

- As a result, patients often prefer to take support by holding the arm of the chair or a person while getting up, which leads to weight-bearing asymmetry.
- Though this strategy helps patient to safely transfer to standing position, it often promotes asymmetry of weight distribution as patients rely on their unaffected side while getting up. Patients commonly adopt weight-bearing asymmetry movement strategy as an adaptation to reduced level of muscle effort while ensuring safety and being independent in sit to stand. However, asymmetric weight distribution is identified as a fall mediator and an indicator of poor mobility.

Common Adaptations Seen During Sit-to-stand (STS) After Stroke

Common adaptations observed during STS after stroke are as follows:

- Increased trunk side flexion toward the unaffected side during flexion and momentum-transfer phase.
- A lack of coordination between the movements of hip, knee, and trunk. For example, knee extension is completed at the end of sit to stand, while their hip joints were still extending.
- Greater body sway in mediolateral direction.
- Use of affected hand to propel the body during extension phase.
- Reduced extension at hip, knee, and ankle at stabilization phase.
- Use of stabilization strategy, i.e., doing increased trunk flexion to bring "nose over toes" then knee extension, and then trunk/hip extension. This strategy often adopted by patients with significant balance deficits and fear of falling.
- Increased movement time

Sit-to-Stand Determinants

Research investigating sit-to-stand performance has identified several key factors as determinants of the limitations experienced by patients with stroke. The literature indicates that chair seat height, use of armrests, and foot position have a major influence on the ability to do an STS movement.

- Lower height of the seat makes the STS movement more demanding or even unsuccessful. Further, chair seat with posterior slant found to have a negative influence because of tilting the body's center of mass farther backward making it difficult to raise the body from sitting position.
- Using the armrests reduced the muscle force needed at the hip by 50%, thus commonly preferred as an adaptive strategy to compensate for deficits in muscular activation especially during the early stages of stroke.
- Positioning of feet prior to the start of the STS movement influences the strategy of the STS movement. A shorter movement time with feet placed posterior was observed as it enables lower muscle force requirements at the hip.

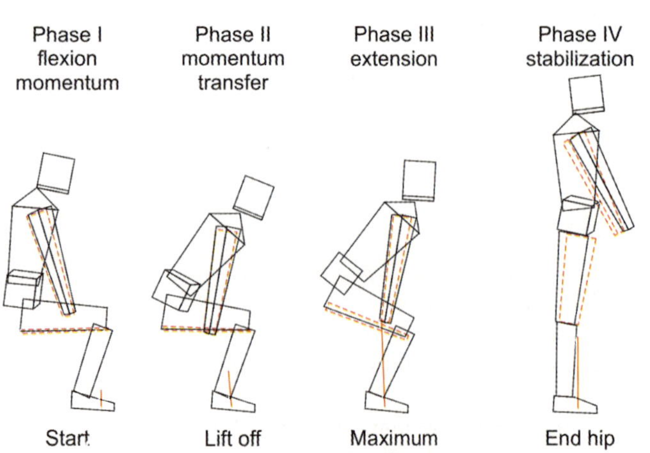

Fig. 26.9: Phases of sit-to-stand movement.

Recommended Treatment Strategies for Improving Sit-to-Stand Performance

To improve sit-to-stand performance, the following treatment strategies are recommended:

- **STS task practice with increased chair height:** Using a higher chair seat, i.e., 100–120% of leg length results in lower muscle force requirement at knee level (up to 60%) and hip level (up to 50%), thus making STS performance less demanding.
- **STS task practice with the paretic foot placed posterior:** Weight-bearing asymmetry during STS can be modified by placing the affected foot placed backward. Liu et al, reported that with the posterior foot position, the asymmetry can be significantly reduced, reaching the levels similar to those reported in healthy subjects.
- **STS task practice with variability:** As a progression in task practice, patients who can independently perform STS task requires practice of STS under varying contextual constraints, which might be more demanding than performing STS in a chair with increased height. In real-life contexts, patients often require to perform STS from chairs with varying seat height and cushion depth, such as low couch, bed, or a stool. Occasionally, patients need to stand from sitting position while balancing an object held in hand, e.g., getting up while holding a hot coffee cup or a food plate in their hand. Thus variability practice is essential for successful performance of STS in real-life contexts. The following tasks can be practiced to improve patients' performance in STS ability in varying contexts:
  - STS task practice with progressively lowered seat height.
  - STS task practice with varying seat cushion depth.
  - STS task practice with varied type of chair such as getting up from a car or auto rickshaw seat and chair with a table placed in front.
  - STS task practice with while holding a glass of water or a plate in their hand.
  - Sit-to-walk practice: Patient can be asked to get up from a chair and walk up to another chair placed at a distance (about 3–5 m).

The variability practice can be delivered in the form of circuit training by having an individual or a group of patients by performing random practice of the tasks listed above.

Avoid

The following are commonly adopted conventional treatment strategies in the management of sit to stand; however, these should be avoided as these strategies do not adhere to contemporary stroke rehabilitation principles outlined in this chapter:

- Overemphasizing the quality of movement
- Part practice or selective movement practice
- Interventions targeting specific impairments, such as spasticity and weakness
- Using meaningless tasks, e.g., getting up from Swiss ball as a chair for progression
- Holding hands while getting up, e.g., clasping hand in front or holding or taking support from arm rest.

Rehabilitation of Walking

Task Characteristics and Requirements

Walking is a primary means of mobility method adopted for moving within indoor environment and for traveling short distances within outdoor environment. Walking in everyday life requires the ability to move from point A to point B safely and also adapting to varying demands of context and task. To carry out mobility-related daily functions, an individual needs ability to adapt walking behavior to meet changing behavioral task goals and demands of the environment. Few daily life examples of changing walking task goals and environmental demands are given below:

- Walking on slippery or uneven surfaces
- Crossing road
- Talking and walk
- Carrying a load and walk
- Walking in a crowded area
- Walking in a cluttered environment with obstacles
- Walking continuously for a long distance or duration

Walking at home and in the community involves interaction of the person with the given environment with the goal of transferring the body in space from one point to another. There are three primary requirements for successful achievement of task goal of walking:

1. **Swing phase:** Forward progression of the swing limb achieved by a forward propulsive force applied at the end of the stance phase, i.e., terminal stance and clearance of the foot off the ground.
2. **Stance phase:** Single limb balance that includes the subtasks transfer of weight to the forward foot and stabilizing the limb through generation of sufficient force to carry the body forward.
3. **Adaptability:** Ability to adapt according to changes in environment and behavioral goals.

The Problem

The following problems are observed:

- During the acute stage, one of the important concerns for patients is independence in walking.
- Although a significant proportion of patients with stroke regain independence in walking within 6 months, many patients report limited ability to adapt to changes in the task and environment, such as walking uneven surface or negotiating an obstacle.

- Patients experience an increased fear of falling when required to walk under these challenging contexts.
- As a result, patients often adopt a "damage control" mode by choosing to avoid walking in these contexts as a safety strategy. Thus, two important goals of poststroke rehabilitation of walking are:
  1. Independent walking inside the home
  2. Independent walking in the community

Problem Analysis

The following steps are taken to analyze the problem:

- Following stroke, patients exhibit several limitations in achieving above-mentioned task goals that lead to poorly coordinated movements often referred to as kinematic deviations.
- Within the perspective of dynamic systems theory of motor control, poorly coordinated movements produced following stroke are viewed as adaptations to system failure not as system (movement) errors that always require correction.
- Stance phase deviations are characterized by poor control of stance limb while transfer of weight from one limb to another and supporting and transferring the stance limb in forward direction.
- Typical kinematic deviations include:
  - Limited ankle dorsiflexion and knee flexion (knee hyperextension) during weight acceptance and initial contact, which often leads to foot contacting the ground with toes or lateral border of foot causing instability in weight transfer.
  - Excessive knee flexion or knee hyperextension during midstance, which leads to inefficient transfer of stance limb and poor balance.
  - Limited hip extension during terminal stance, which results in weak push off. A weak push off during late stance limits the forward displacement of swing limb leading to reduced step length.
- The swing phase of deviations was characterized by poor foot clearance off the ground and poor transfer of swing limb in forward direction.
  - The limited hip and knee flexion and reduced ankle dorsiflexion lead to reduced foot clearance, which often leads to dragging of foot during the swing phase.
  - Stiff knee defined as reduced peak knee flexion angle during the swing phase of the paretic side.
  - Low knee flexion velocity at toe-off is a potential contributor to stiff-knee gait, which is characterized by limited swing-phase knee flexion.
  - Study results indicate that during normal gait, iliopsoas, and gastrocnemius are the largest contributors to peak knee flexion velocity during double support, while vasti, soleus, and rectus femoris are the muscles that act to decrease this velocity. Abnormal force production, i.e., reduced force production in iliopsoas and gastrocnemius

or increased activation of vasti, soleus, and rectus femoris would reduce the knee flexion velocity at the end of stance (terminal stance) thereby contributing to the stiff knee seen during swing phase.

Common Adaptations Seen during Walking

Common adaptations seen during walking are as follows:

- Limited ankle dorsiflexion and knee flexion during swing on the paretic side often result in the use of compensatory strategies (i.e., pelvic hiking and circumduction) to achieve foot clearance.
- Adaptation strategies commonly observed during paretic swing phase include:
  - Pelvic hiking, defined as a frontal plane elevation of the ipsilateral side of the pelvis (i.e., pelvic tilt).
  - Circumduction is defined as excessive hip abduction of the ipsilateral limb. Patients often adopt strategies, such as circumduction of the hip during swing phase.
- Additionally, upward tilt of the affected side pelvis and trunk side flexion toward the unaffected side is also used as an adaptation to ensure foot clearance while transferring the limb forward during the swing phase.
- Patients with stroke also exhibit spatiotemporal adaptations, such as reduced stride/step lengths, increased swing time on the affected side, reduced walking velocity, and reduced cadence.

Environmental Determinants of Walking

As discussed earlier, the primary requirements of walking include ability to adapt walking to environmental circumstances, such as obstacles and targets. Within the perspective of dynamic systems, theory of motor control task functions is achieved via its interaction with the environmental context and behavioral goal. Thus environmental factors are key determinants of task functions. A conceptual framework of environmental nine determinants of walking was proposed by Patla. The nine domains of walking defining dimensions of mobility are described below:

1. **Obstacle negotiation:** Negotiating obstacles in the environment to prevent a collision between the lower limb and the obstacle, such as stepping over an obstacle.
2. **Temporal:** Time constraints imposed on walking, such as needing to walk fast to cross a street or slow in a crowded mall.
3. **Cognitive dual tasking:** Walking while attending to cognitive tasks, such as engaging in conversation while walking.
4. **Terrain demands:** Walking on compliant or uneven surfaces that are not flat and firm, such as stairs, ramps, and grass.
5. **Physical load:** Carrying or interacting with a weighted object while walking, such as carrying a grocery bag and walking to open a heavy door.

6. **Ambient demands:** Factors such as level of lighting, temperature, weather conditions, noise levels, and familiarity with surroundings
7. **Postural transitions**: Varying posture during walking, such as turning and bending down to pick an object while walking
8. **Motor dual-tasking:** Walking while attending to additional motor tasks, such as holding a glass of water while walking and picking up an object from the floor.
9. **Maneuvering in traffic:** Avoiding collision with static and dynamic objects by maneuvering the entire body, such as walking around other people, pets, and vehicles.

Recommended Treatment Strategies for Improving Walking Performance

To improve walking performance, the following treatment strategies are recommended:

- To improve patient's independence in walking, it is critical that patients practice walking and walking-related tasks that represent real-life walking context and demands. Readers are recommended to refer to previous section on recovery of functions and principle of task-oriented exercises.
- Further, physiotherapists are encouraged to not overemphasize the quality of movement or movement errors and refrain from using part practice or selective movement practice, e.g., mat activities or preambulatory training and targeting specific impairments, such as spasticity and weakness.
- Use of non–task-specific exercises, also referred to as preambulatory exercises, for nonambulant patients is commonly recommended practice; however, it should be strongly discouraged as it would adversely affect recovery.

Problem 1: Patient needs one- or two-person support while walking.

The following strategies makes walking more achievable for patients who needs external support for walking:

- Providing manual assistance for supporting the trunk, e.g., by using gait belt or a towel wrapped around their waist and placing the swing limb in front during walking practice.
- Walking within parallel bars during acute stage.
- Frequent encouragement from physiotherapists (PTs) and family.
- Walking close to the wall and having a grab bar fixed on the wall would give patients a sense of safety.

Problem 2: Limitations or inability to adapt to environmental demands associated with "out of home" walking.

Patients report loss of balance, fear of falling, lack of confidence, and fatigue during walking in the community.

The following strategies are recommended to improve ability of patients to adapt to various environment demands of walking outdoors:

- Obstacle avoidance: Stepping over and stepping onto obstacles
- Walking on a narrow path
- Walking in dark environment—dark goggles can be used **(Fig. 26.10)**
- Walking on uneven surface **(Fig. 26.11)**
- Walking on soft/flexible surface
- Walking with frequent change in speed, i.e. fast and slow
- Walking while carrying a load, e.g., grocery bag and bucket filled with water **(Fig. 26.12)**
- Walking while talking
- Walking with frequent turns
- Walk on crowded pathway
- Walking outdoors **(Fig. 26.13)**
- Walking on a slope **(Fig. 26.14)**

Rehabilitation of Upper Limb Functions

Upper Limb Functions

Functions of upper limb are critical for almost all ADLs, such as eating, grooming, toileting, and dressing. Upper limb functions are carried out by the combination of three discrete upper limb tasks:

1. Reaching
2. Grasping
3. Manipulation of objects

The following section provides a brief description and requirements of each task.

Tusk Description

Reaching

The method of reaching can be executed as follows:

- Reaching has been defined as the voluntary positioning of the hand at or near a desired location so that it may interact with the environment.
- Reaching involves continuous movement of the arm, i.e., coordinated movements of shoulder and elbow joints toward the target and contains acceleration and deceleration phase **(Fig. 26.15A)**.
- Reaching to a target within arm's length involves the shoulder, elbow, and wrist.
- Reaching to targets beyond arm's length involves movements at all these joints, as well as trunk and hip motion **(Fig. 26.15B)**.
- The acceleration at each joint is determined by the net torque and the inertia of the object in motion. The net joint torque is produced by the muscle activity and also the effects of gravity, viscoelasticity of the joint and connective tissues, and the externally applied connective forces, e.g., the reaction force of the cup when it is being lifted while drinking water.
- Hand paths during reaching movements are straight or slightly curved.

Grasping

The purpose of reaching is usually grasping. Therefore, two functional requirements are needed:

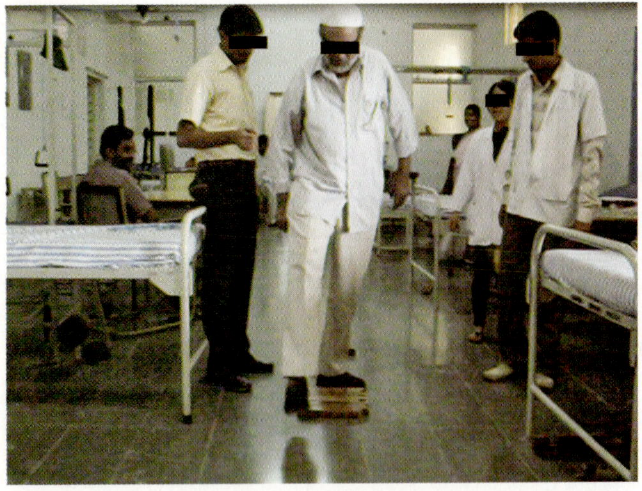

Fig. 26.10: Obstacle avoidance training while wearing a dark glass.

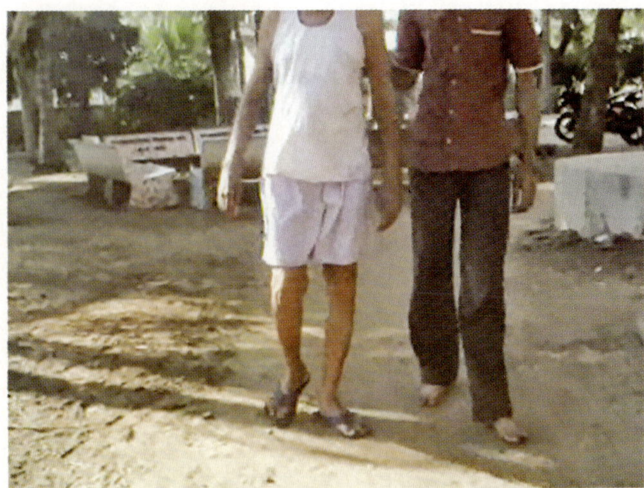

Fig. 26.11: Practice of walking adaptability: walking on uneven surface.

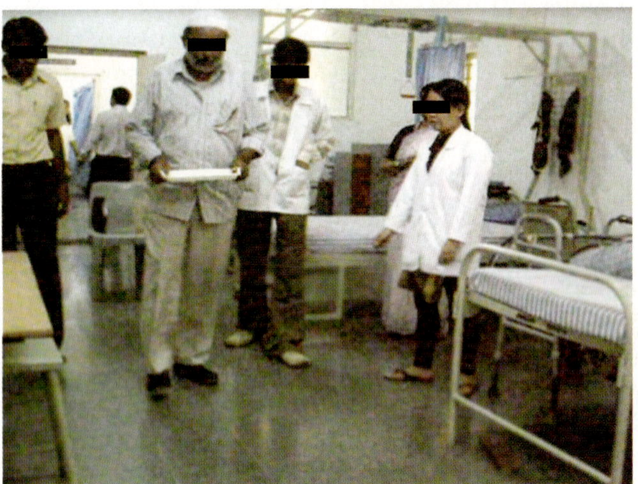

Fig. 26.12: Practice of walking adaptability: walking and carrying a tray.

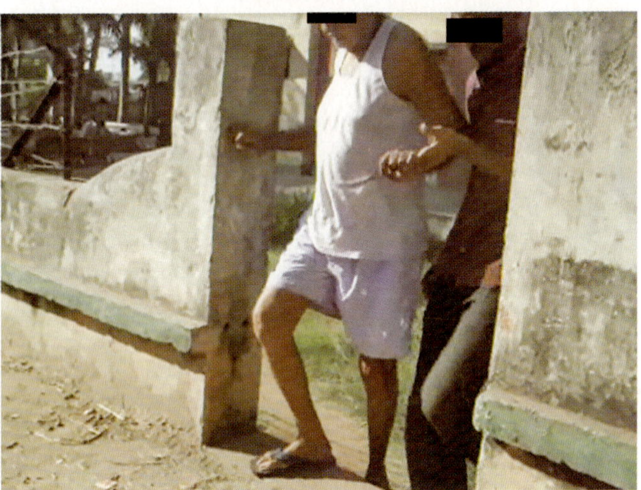

Fig. 26.13: Practice of walking adaptability: walking and negotiating door steps.

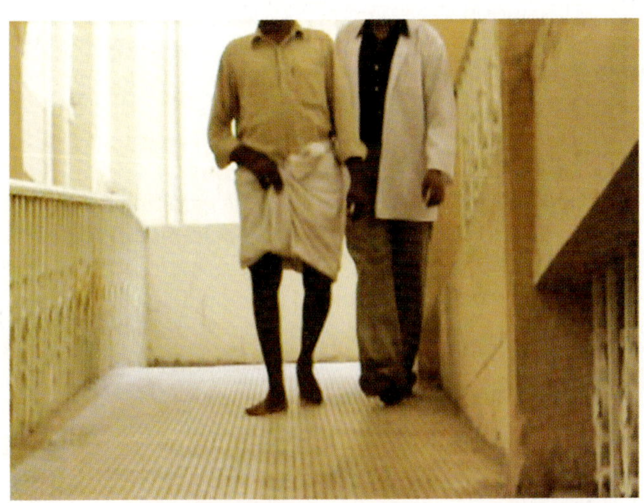

Fig. 26.14: Practice of walking adaptability: walking on inclined surface.

1. Grip must be adapted to size, shape, and use of target object.
2. Timing of finger movements must be coordinated with hand position approaching object, i.e., finger closure that is early or late is ineffective.

- Achievement of first requirement is facilitated by preshaping the grasp according to the orientation, location, whether it has functional asymmetries, e.g., pen and glass; pick up a glass that is upside down on table versus glass that is right side up.
- Preshaping involves anticipating and making the shape and size of the object. Preshaping of the hand, fingers, and thumb begins almost simultaneously with transport of the arm **(Fig. 26.16)**.
- Hand preshaping consists of both an early phase and late phase.

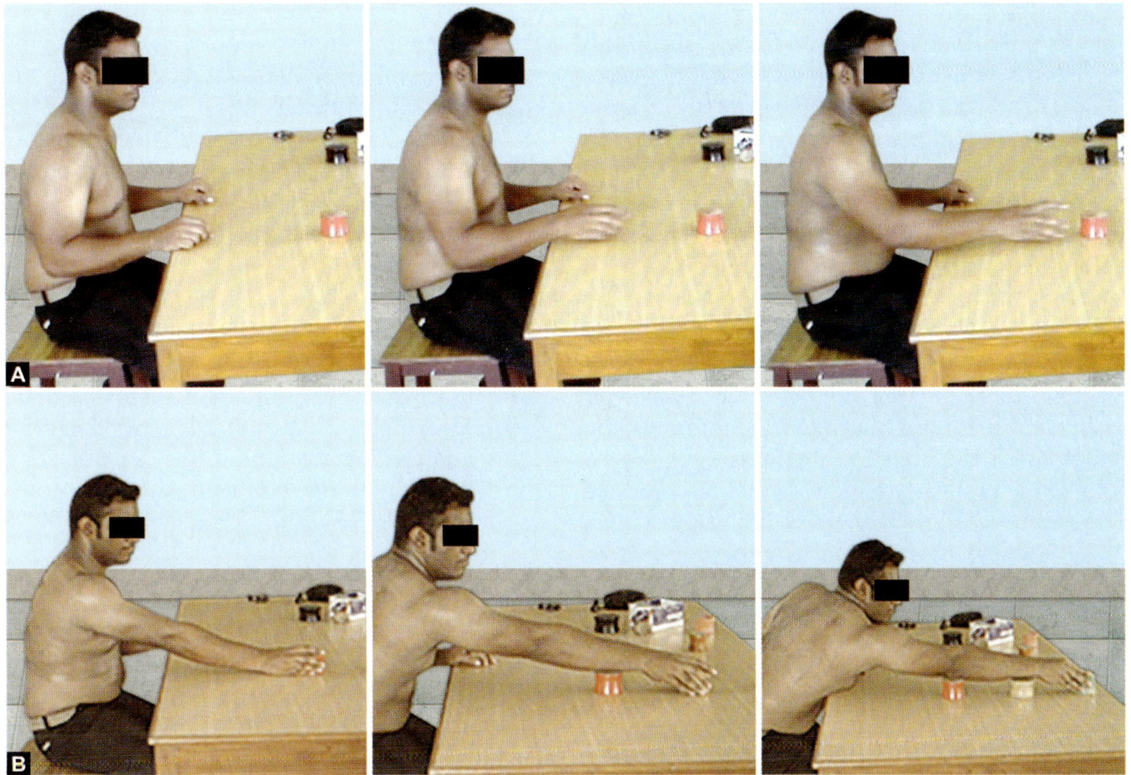

Figs. 26.15A and B: (A) The transport phase of reaching to grasp in a normal individual; (B) Reaching for a target. Target object placed beyond arm's length leads to recruitment of trunk and hip movement in a normal individual.

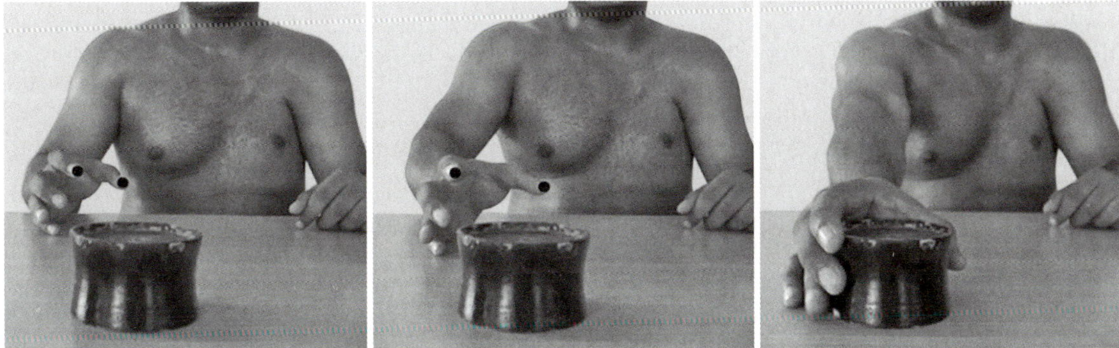

Fig. 26.16: Preshaping, reaching, and grasping involved in grasping task. [Normal subject reaching to grasp an object. Note the opening of the hand in the transportation phase. The distance between the thumb and index (marked with dark dots) is referred to as aperture.

- The early phase is a predictive phase where hand formation is selected, while during the late phase, grasp on the object is optimized.
- During a reaching and grasping task, the fingers initially straighten and the grip aperture increases, and as the hand approaches the object, grip closes in order to match the size of the object.
- During the transport phase, the posture of hand can be discriminated among various shaped objects and gradually evolve.
- The internal forces are mainly involved in maintaining grasp stability: slip prevention, tilt prevention, and resistance to perturbations.

Manipulation

The method of manipulation can be applied as follows:
- When manipulating a hand-held object, for instance, when drinking from a glass, one needs to apply sufficient grip force to prevent the glass from slipping out of the hand. In addition, one needs to control the total torque exerted by all fingers such that the glass remains either vertical (in this case the torque magnitude about the point of thumb contact should equal zero) or at a controlled angle that is suitable for drinking and preventing the liquid from being spilled.
- Usually, the requirements for grip force stabilization allow for some laxity, while the requirements for total torque production are highly specified.

- As in the example of drinking from a glass, the grip force needs only to be larger than the slip threshold and smaller than the force that would break the glass. In contrast, the torque applied to the glass needs to be precisely controlled since any error will lead to rotation of the glass and spilling of the liquid.
- During manipulation of the glass, the fingers may act as force agonists and torque antagonists. To prevent the glass from slipping, the fingers act as agonists; each of them contributes to the total grip force. In contrast, the index and middle fingers and the ring and little fingers exert moments of force in opposite directions about a pivot point created by the thumb. These two pairs of fingers are torque antagonists. To minimize the total finger force, the fingers that generate a moment opposite to the intended moment should not produce any force. At the same time, to prevent the object from slipping they may be required to generate a force that contributes to the total grip force. The CNS must somehow find a balance between these conflicting requirements.

The Problem

The following are the common abnormalities seen upper reaching, grasping, and manipulation following stroke:

- Disruptions in interjoint coordination between shoulder and elbow joint.
- **Use of a compensatory trunk strategy:** Excessive use of the trunk for reaching a target placed well within the range of the arm's reach. Use of excessive trunk movement had prolonged deceleration time.
- Poor ability to open the fingers during a reach-to-grasp movement due to impaired the ability to activate finger muscles and/or selectively activate them in the appropriate temporal patterns.
- Winding fingers around the object, sliding the hand along a surface, and downward grasping are some examples of different compensatory grasping strategies.
- **Altered grip force regulation (grip force overshoots):** Once the fingers are in contact with the object, people with hemiparesis poststroke have difficulty producing appropriate finger forces for object manipulation. Increased grip force for holding, transportation, and cyclical vertical movements has been reported for hemiparetic arm of stroke patients. Excessive grip force has been interpreted as an increase in the safety margin between the applied force and the minimum force necessary to prevent the object from slipping. Increased grip force magnitude may reflect compensatory mechanisms in order to compensate for deficits with sensory feedback mechanisms or motor deficits involving poor rate of force development.
- In people with hemiparesis, hand shaping occurs gradually as the hand is decelerated during the later part of the reach, and not from the initiation of the reach, as happens in healthy individuals.

- Digito-palmar, ulnar and raking grasps could be considered as compensatory alternative strategies for grasping relatively large objects, and the interdigital grasp as a compensatory alternative strategy for lateral pinch or precision grasp for a small object. The common characteristic of these alternative strategies is that they do not involve the thumb.
  - **Digito-palmar:** involves the palm in opposition to one or several fingers.
  - **Raking:** involves the palm and last four fingers. The thumb is not involved.
  - **Ulnar:** involves the ulnar side of the palm and the fourth and fifth finger, which are flexed.
  - **Interdigital:** involves the lateral sides of two fingers, adjacent or not. Often the thumb is not involved, but sometimes, it envelops the object to stabilize the grasp. The palm is not involved.

Exercise Plan for Improving Reaching: Putting the Principles into Practice

In a physiotherapy session with all the above-mentioned principles, how to formulate an exercise program in practice to reduce upper limb dysfunction is the next important question. We know the task should be functional, goal oriented, and preferred by the patient as these types of tasks are easy and patients are willing to execute rather than a nonfunctional task. Exercise can also be selected, which can hold the attention and interest of the patient to encourage novelty and practice. In this section, some practical guidelines are given in implementing this exercise to people with stroke. All these exercises even though are listed for specific dysfunction, they improve not only the stated objective but also the overall competence of upper limb functioning.

Start from an easier task and gradually move toward difficult functional task should be the general theme in developing an exercise regime.

In the acute phase, most persons with stroke cannot move the upper limb or they can move them in a limited way and most of the time, the therapist waits for some activity to return in the affected limb. Rather than waiting the therapist should be proactive and find ways of encouraging either an active movement or active assisted movement. To encourage active functional activity in the earlier stages of stroke is understanding the movement dysfunction in persons with stroke. In person with stroke, the movements against gravity are difficult to perform as well as in the outer range. However, they may be able to perform an activity in the middle range and in a horizontal plane.

- One way to start with an active or active assisted exercise is to keep a board in horizontally in front of the patient and to perform pointing task by sliding the hand on the board as moving against gravity is difficult.
- Rather than having complex activity such as reaching for an objects and holding them, which needs complex coordination, choose semifunctional activity such as pointing toward objects kept on the board in front of them.

- Persons with stroke can be made to touch or point to articles kept on the board on command (semipurposeful movement).
- Keeping the target in the middle range rather than the end range can make the task doable as muscles work better in the middle range.
- Activities that need eccentric muscle action are easy to perform rather than concentric activity. This idea can be used in planning activity in the acute phase by keeping the board slightly lifted downward and instructing the person with stroke to move slowly toward the target.
- All these can make the person with stroke start to move actively rather than doing passive movements. It should also be kept in mind that some parts of the task may need assistance in some patient; hence, active assisted exercise is needed.
- As a progression, moving the target just beyond the ability of the patient to increase joint excursions and working on the outer range can be included.
- Person with stroke can be asked to move against gravity as the ability increases. Pointing toward different objects in the room is a good way to start upper limb movements against gravity.

Choose real-world-like and patient-preferred tasks.
- Reaching for objects such as a glass of water rather than cylindrical blocks or pegs.
- Functional task with grasping should be added along with reaching. Rather than having in-hand manipulation activity such as squeezing a rubber ball, reaching to grasp and then manipulation of hand reflecting a real-life functional activity increases the chances of recovery.
- For patient-preferred activity, if he/she is wearing glasses, reaching for the reading glasses, wearing them, and putting it back in the pouch can be a functional and a patient-preferred activity in many persons with stroke.
- Some exercises chosen by researchers for persons with stroke are washing worktops, opening drawers, putting away dishes, folding towels, closing blinds, counting change, and writing.

Variability in practice to improve movement dysfunction.
- Exercises should not only be on performing functional tasks that are only important to the patient, the practice regiment should be varied.
- Variability can be through modification in different parameters such as changing the properties of the object including position, size, texture, weight, orientation, and goal of the task.
- As explained earlier, functional movements are varied in nature and mastering one task cannot lead to generalization. To have a functional upper limb, the person with stroke should have flexible movement pattern and a good coordination between the joints of the upper limb, both of which are lost in persons with stroke. These can be improved by a variable practice. The task can be arranged in such a way that different combination of movements, which are required to produce flexible movement patterns to do real-life tasks with the hand, is done. Variability in practice can help in reducing movement dysfunction and compensatory movements in poststroke patients.

- Arranging tasks that include different objects the patient and the therapist have selected can be placed in different position in three-dimensional (3D) spaces and ask to randomly pick them or touch those depending on their ability. Having the target objects in different positions in the 3D space puts the upper limb joints in different sets of coordination requirement and they can help in improving joint excursion and movement accuracy and other kinetic and kinematic dysfunctions. In the earlier phase of the disease, the objects can be kept more in a horizontal plane as moving against gravity is difficult and the person with stroke can drag his hand toward the object countering the weight of the arm.
- Increasing the active joint excursion and workspace can also be improved by changing the environment. Objects can be kept just beyond the active functional ROM of the upper limb. For example, making the patient reach to grasp in the ipsilateral side, wherein they have to produce coordinated shoulder abduction and elbow extension.
- When grasping an object, the appropriate grip force should be produced and when picking the article and moving them, the load force has to be appropriately developed. This coordination is also lost in persons with stroke and to improve grasp stability task which consists of lifting and placing objects in different places helps. The properties of the object, such as texture, weight, and goal should again be varied to force the system to produce different behavior for the diverse tasks. Changing the weight and the height of the object to be lifted can help in improving the coordination between the grip force and load force. Gradually increasing the weight of the object can help in improving the force production capacity of the limbs as well as coordination. As we know this coordination happens only when the object is grasped and moved, the exercise should also reflect it. Changing the posture and position of the object during reaching and gasping will also improve the anticipatory postural control too.

  Some practical examples can be:
  - Having half-filled cups, cell phones, remote, etc., and in different places and ask the patient to reach and transport to another place.

- To control tilt force pouring water from a bottle into a cup can be used and lifting different sized books. For varying the task and increasing the difficulty, the water in the bottle can be increased, as it will need more force production and control, decreasing the circumference of the bottle (smaller objects are difficult to hold) and the size of the cup into which the water has to be poured (as it needs more accurately).
- Drinking from the cup in the last phase also needs controlling of the tilt force when emptying water from the cup. The task can be made simpler by having less water, when the weakness is more pronounced to produce sufficient load force. Assistance may be needed for many patients when starting, but as emphasized earlier it should be in the form of active assistance.
- Opening and closing drawers and shelve and doors of houses and cars can all help in pulling and pushing force production while maintaining a standing posture.
- Different texture induces a different friction force between the hand and the object. Grip force and load force are also dependent on friction force; hence, varying it is also important to learn real-life upper limb activities. Having objects made up of different textures such as glass, stainless steel, and paper cups for reaching to transport activities can be used.
- Increasing the weight of the object can be progressively increased by using different cups and bottles with different levels of water in it. This can along with others can be used to improve force production capacity of the muscles.

- Reaching for different objects in different orientation can help in controlling reaching with different orientation of the upper limb. Having the objects in different orientation can induce different joint orientation and coordination. We are all aware of the fact that orienting the hand in a mid-prone position is difficult while reaching in persons with stroke so; to improve activities like that the objects used can be kept in different orientation so as to bring about rotation in the shoulder and forearm. This way the focus of attention can be external and the goal of the task induces rotations and different orientation of the upper limb.
  - Reaching and grasping cups, pens, and bottles can be used for vertical orientation and picking up books from the table can be used to bring about horizontal orientation. This can be a better way to improve activities that need mid-prone orientation rather than reducing supinator spasticity or stretching the muscles.
  - Placing books, small pouches, and boxes and picking them can bring about more horizontal orientation of the forearm.

- Placing books on the table retrieved from the shelf and back on the table. The books can be of different weight, different orientation; hence, this can be a good functional exercise to improve coordination and force production capacity of the muscles and joint excursion. The exercise can be started from keeping the books from a higher point (like the shelf) to a lower point (the table) as it is easier to start with toward gravity movement (which needs more of eccentric muscle contraction) and later moving from the table to shelf as against gravity movement. Keeping the book farther can also bring about shoulder flexion and elbow extension, which is difficult to produce in persons with stroke.

- The goal of the movement can also be changed to increase variability in practice to improve coordination, grasp stability, and generalization of learning upper limb activities.
  - Reaching for the phone, picking it to keep to the ears, and speaking or dialing the numbers
  - Picking the book and keeping in a different place or opening it to read
  - Wearing clothes after picking them, picking a pen, and writing
  - Pouring water and drinking, pouring water into a cup kept near the next person while practicing with the group.
  - Playing games using the computer, etc. can also increase the variability and accuracy of movement and at the same time increase the compliance and attention.

- Picking an object from a group can also induce variability in planning and execution by the patient. This can be done by either having large objects such as cups, kitchen utensils, and bottles and ask them to pick one or it can be a smaller object such as one pen from a collection of it in a stand. This exercise can be akin to obstacle training in gait and it can be helpful in increasing the accuracy of the movement as the other objects should not be disturbed while picking the target object.

- Fine movements should be added as the patient progresses.

As the kinetics and kinematics improve the accuracy and movement optimization occurs more and more, fine movements can be added. Some of the tasks that can be incorporated include:

  - Placing objects in their designated place or holder, such as keeping pens and pencils in the pen holder.
  - Dialing numbers on the phone
  - Placing a lid on the container and screwing them.

Practicing fine movements that are important for specific patient should be added along to improve accuracy of movement, e.g., writing, buttoning the shirt, and wearing a watch. Exercise plan should be made for each patient in a customized fashion depending on his/her ability, goals, and preferences. Rather than teaching them to control or reduce spasticity and synergy, which has been proved to be futile, doing these kinds of goal-oriented exercise can help persons with stroke improve their activities as well as their quality of movements. The exercises and tasks, which have been listed, are just a few of them. The therapist in consultation with the patient should formulate and choose tasks according to the need and ability of the patient.

Feedback

- The first principle to be kept in mind while formulating a treatment plan is feedback. Out-of-phase activities, such as increased shoulder elevation and abduction while reaching forward, excessive trunk movement while reaching forward, as discussed earlier in the chapter are compensatory mechanisms, which also decrease with good shoulder elbow coordination.
- Compensation is a complicated theme in regard to recovery and exercise in the case of persons with stroke. When a person with stroke is starting with his rehabilitation, the therapist concentrates more on reducing the compensation. Persistence of compensatory movements may lead to maladaptive strategies becoming part of the daily movement repertoire.
- Compensatory movement strategies are also very difficult to unlearn. Hence, while practicing the role of therapist is reduced compensatory strategy in the early stages so as to develop an optimal movement strategy while carrying out functional activities.
- In later stages of stroke recovery, if the patient has a good prognosis, compensation is kept to the minimum and motor recovery is emphasized On the other hand, when people with stroke have severe impairments and poor prognosis, compensatory movements should be encouraged to maximize the functional ability of arm and hand. Hence, one should be judicial when the compensation in movement dysfunctions should be given importance or when to be discouraged and when to encourage it.
- When the patients are doing these activities, to improve the accuracy of the movement, and when an error arises, feedback is needed for them. Achieving a goal is important for the patient and it can be achieved through true motor recovery or compensation. For true motor recovery along with practice, the other important factor is to have less compensatory movement, for which feedback is of primary importance. Prescriptive feedback, i.e. information about the error and how to solve them can be used to correct compensatory strategies.

For example, to decrease excessive trunk flexion while reaching forward:

- For excessive compensatory movements such as trunk flexion, feedback should not only be about pointing about the compensatory movement but also how to solve them.
- When trying to correct compensatory movements such as excessive trunk movement, the feedback commonly given is to move the trunk less and concentrate on shoulder flexion and elbow extension. This type of focusing on attention on the body parts' instruction to patients considered as a deterrent to learning. Hence, an optimal way to do it will be to make the patient understand trunk movement is a compensation for the reduced excursion of elbow extension while reaching (information about the error) and to solve it, he has to extend the elbow by having an external focus such as moving the arm fast and thinking as though he is punching (to create sufficient torque in the elbows and shoulder flexors).

To reduce the compensatory elevation of the shoulder, which is brought about by the lack of shoulder flexion and elbow extension and also the height on which the object has to be picked up or placed on. The greater the height, the greater the need for shoulder flexion to raise the arm, which as we know is difficult to produce in many persons with stroke; hence, they compensate with shoulder elevation to achieve it. So to correct it, the therapist can reduce the height on which the object is placed and slowly increase it as the coordination between shoulder flexion and elbow extension is increased.

- To reduce end point inaccuracy, the attention of the patient should be on the external target rather than producing a movement such as shoulder flexion or elbow extension.
- As these tasks inherently have a feedback wherein the person with stroke will know whether he is successful in completion of the task and also errors in the movement; hence, a minimal feedback may suffice and also can act as a positive reinforcement.

Specific exercises can also be designed specifically for some important movement dysfunction. Keep in mind as it has been emphasized elsewhere in the chapter that even though separate exercises are given for each problem, the exercises will have a global effect on all the problems as they are all interconnected.

For opening for the grasp:

- For improving opening of the hand while reaching, the task can be practiced at different speeds and with different-sized objects. These variations can be helpful in producing a larger aperture, which is difficult to achieve in persons with stroke.
- Performing the task faster leads to large aperture formation as a compensation for error during grasping; hence, movement must be done faster by persons with stroke.
- Larger objects also act a feedback to increase the aperture and also help in the person with stroke focus

the attention on the external target rather than on the finger extension.

- As aperture formation happens during the reaching phase itself, while practicing the person with stroke can effectively learn them if they are done in unison rather than separately.

  For improving precise movement when gross movements are possible—decrease the anticipatory grip force:

- Having an increased grip force can lead to early fatigue, handling delicate objects and difficulty doing fine movements.
- To reduce the grip force developing in excess during activity, the person with stroke must be made aware of the increased force developed via feedback.
- As in feedback the focus of attention should be not internally while practicing these activities. Pliable objects can be used, and the deformity of the object can act as the feedback for the patient.
- Commonly used in many rehabilitation centers is the use of disposable paper or Styrofoam cup in practicing. Having water in it and learning to drink from it or transporting it without deforming it and spilling the water can be an effective way to learn to control grip forces. The spilling of the water or deforming of the cup acts as the feedback to control the force. The same idea can be used for smaller objects that were in a roll of paper in the diameter of pens (which collapses when the force is high); flattening methods of shoelaces are some ways the task can inherently have feedback to denote higher grip force.
- It has been suggested that practicing, reaching, and grasping of the object with the unaffected arm before using the affected arm can help the brain in planning the proper grip force required while doing it with the affected hand.
- Asking the patient to image the article to be manipulated as a fragile object can help in reducing the grip force and help in manipulation.

For release of the grasped object:
- Having mildly warm or cold objects, such as warm water– or ice-filled cup of different size and asking the patient to hold and release. Even though it does not mimic real-world activity, the sensory stimulus (warmth) can help in releasing of the grasped object.
- Picking up and placing objects in different position can also be helpful in releasing the grasp. Transporting and releasing is a natural form of activity, which can induce release rather than just closing and releasing of the hand without transport phase.

Bimanual Task Training

Bimanual tasks are also part of the functioning in normal person; hence, they should be also part of the treatment protocol we develop for our patients. When choosing a task either for bimanual or unilateral activities, ask for patents' preference rather than choosing unilaterally. Hence, activities such as playing cards, stacking of cups, and others can be substituted for functional real-world activities given below.

- Folding hand towels (bilateral task), wiping the table, rolling out dough (bilateral task), opening and closing various types of locks, and spooning out dry ingredients are some of the tasks researchers have used on their patients with success.
- Carrying plates and trays, holding large objects and newspaper, and pouring water from a jug are some of the activities we have tried on our patients.

Incorporating gesture while talking

Activities of the arm through the day can also be incorporated by encouraging the patients to use gesture while talking. The therapist should encourage the person with stroke to be more animated while talking, which can bring about upper limb movement.

Prevention and Management of Poststroke Shoulder Pain and Subluxation

For prevention of shoulder pain, emphasis should be on protecting the joint from trauma, especially in the acute stage when the arm is without voluntary control. Trauma here refers to injuries due to moving the flaccid upper limb in an improper manner.

- The upper limb should be carefully handled while moving the patient and other functional activities. Pulling of the affected hand, or letting the hand hang on the side of the bed while lying or sitting should be avoided.
- Vigorous passive movements should be avoided. The shoulder should not be passively moved beyond 90° of flexion and abduction unless the scapula is upwardly rotated and the humerus is externally rotated. As we know, just moving the glenohumeral joint into elevation without consideration for the humeral rotation leads to impingement of the soft tissue and injuries. Thus avoiding the overhead pulley exercise is recommended as it might cause shoulder pain. A gentler and active form of treatment may be helpful in preventing shoulder pain.
- Shoulder pain and subluxation prevention needs mechanical support for the limb especially when muscle activity is lost around the shoulder. This can be done via positioning of the limb while sitting with a lapboard or other supporting devices, such as sling and strapping while sitting and standing **(Fig. 26.17)**. Even though most of these supporting systems have poor evidence in terms of prevention of shoulder pathology, the therapist has to choose a method to support the arm.
- No single intervention has been identified as the gold standard to treat hemiplegic shoulder pain. The therapist needs to manage pain according to each

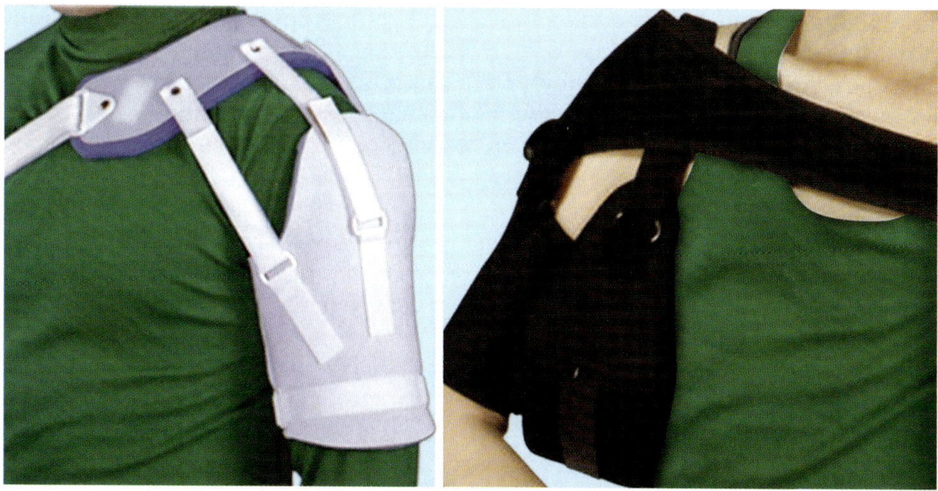

Fig. 26.17: Sling or strapping for shoulder.

patient's needs. Central pain is more stubborn and is difficult to treat with physical modalities and may need stronger drugs, such as intravenous morphine, lamotrigine, and levorphanol.

INSTRUCTIONS FOR PATIENT/CAREGIVER

All those involved in the care of stroke patients are likely to go through a lot of emotional trauma; due to the disability, it tends to leave on the patient. Patients feel depressed, frustrated, isolated, and their caregivers may at times expect, react unwisely, and also exhibit emotional changes. Due to the amount and frequency of contact with the patients and their caregivers, therapist may be in a best position to follow few guidelines while delivering some useful interventions, to ease the influence of such dramatic and emotional events on the patients and caregivers **(Box 26.6)**.

RECOVERY AND OUTCOMES

Patients with stroke, their families, and healthcare team all together can make better decisions for treatment, provided they are aware of the prognosis and outcomes of stroke. Survival, amount of recovery, and extent of residual

---

BOX 26.6: Therapist instructions for intervening patients and caregivers.

- Providing factual and accurate information
- Providing only as much information as needed, in a timely manner
- Considering the educational, cultural, and financial situation of the family and intervening accordingly
- Providing educational resources such as books, pamphlets, brochures, videos, audios, and support group information
- Being supportive, motivating, and maintaining a positive attitude strengthens their outlook
- Providing referrals and alternative therapeutic options when needed

---

disability are the prime concerns of all those involved in the care of person having stroke. Early death following a stroke is usually related to the underlying pathology, the patient's age, and to the severity of the lesion.

Stroke recovery is variable and depends on factors such as physical factors, including severity, emotional factors, such as motivation, mood, and personality; social factors, such as family or peer support; and therapeutic factors, such as how early was the rehabilitation started and the quality and skills of rehabilitation team. Much of the recovery after a stroke occurs early, usually within the first 6 months. The brain can continue to heal for up to 2 years afterward also (i.e., late recovery of function). Even after 2 years, people can continue to slowly improve due to many of the gains after the first year or two that do not depend so much on the healing of the brain, but on the learning of new skills. Patients with chronic stroke (defined as greater than 1-year poststroke) can undergo late recovery of function with the help of extensive task-specific functional training that emphasizes use of the more involved extremities.

Recovery from lacunar strokes is excellent, whereas if the lesion is strategically located, significant deficits are likely to persist. Initial assessment of ADL, age, sitting balance, and pre-existing comorbidities are some of the important predictors of recovery. Independent walking ability is usually achieved within first 3 months in most patients, and also improvement in ADL is seen.

SUMMARY

Stroke occurs when blood flow to the brain is disrupted. Disruption in blood flow is caused when either a blood clot or piece of plaque blocks one of the vital blood vessels in the brain (ischemic stroke), or when a blood vessel in the brain bursts, spilling blood into surrounding tissues (hemorrhagic stroke). Various factors, responsible for the occurrence of stroke, have been discussed in the chapter. Involvement of different cerebral artery can give rise to different syndromes, which result into varied clinical presentation. Stroke persists to be a major cause for neurological disability, and the management involves medical as well as physiotherapy interventions and rarely surgical intervention may be required. Assessment and examination involve the use of various valid and reliable outcome measures, which are also emphasized in the chapter. Management of stroke can employ various approaches, of which task-oriented approach has been elaborated with focus on major primary and secondary impairments.

Case Scenario

CASE STUDY

A 65-year-old man had sudden onset of paralysis on one side of the body since 1 week. Based on the CT scan findings, the patient was diagnosed as having acute ischemic stroke with left MCA artery involvement. Patient has a past history of HTN and diabetes for which he is taking medications since 5 years. Presently, he is admitted to a ward and referred for physiotherapy. During the initial interview, the patient reported that he is unable to lift or move his arm; not able to grasp any objects with his hands; loses balance while getting up from chair; need two-person assistance to walk; dependent on his wife for carrying out all self-care activities, including eating, toileting, dressing, and bathing. He also added that he experiences pain in shoulder when he attempts to move his affected arm.

Steps

1. Rule out any contraindications (red flags) for active rehabilitation, e.g., unstable vital signs and severe cognitive impairments.
2. Determine the baseline status of task performance and function.
3. Perform task analysis through observation and identify the type of task adaptation the patient is currently using to perform the task.
4. Select a task-oriented treatment strategy matching patient current level of performance.
5. Progress treatment program by introducing practice of task adaptation under varying environmental context.

Adhere to principles of designing task-oriented exercises: (a) select a meaningful task, (b) practice in a relevant environment, (c) practice task variability, (d) practice at appropriate intensity: task loading, number of repetitions, and frequency of practice.

Management of Sit-to-Stand

Recommended outcome measures/examination tools:

- Sit-to-stand component of motor assessment scale
- Timed up and go test
- One-minute sit-to-stand repetition test or 30-second sit-to-stand test.

Recommended interventions

- Start practice of sit-to-stand on a chair with higher height
- Provide manual assistance during task practice, if necessary. Caution: avoid holding hands while providing assistance
- Repeat task with sufficient assistance, e.g., during acute stage 5–6 rep/set, 2–3 sets/session can be given. The intensity can be progressed by increasing number of repetitions or number of sets or both.
- Practice task variability: sit to stand with low chair, sit to walk, sit-to-stand while holding a plate and wearing a dark glass.

Management of Walking

Recommended outcome measures/examination tools:

- Functional ambulation categories
- Dynamic gait index
- Rivermead visual gait assessment

Recommended interventions:

- Start early (after 48 hours) practice of walking with manual assistance or within parallel bar or with any form of support.
- Gradually reduce assistance and provide encouragement to walk independently.
- Progress to practicing task variability, such as walking on varied terrain, obstacle avoidance, and carrying a grocery bag while walking.
- Avoid practicing mat activities or preambulatory training as it could delay recovery of walking.

Management of Upper Limb Reaching, Grasping, and Manipulation

Recommended outcome measures/examination tools:
Goal attainment scale.

Recommended interventions

- During initial stage, practice task in which effect of gravity is minimized, i.e., task that involves movements produced in horizontal plane, e.g., wiping a table and folding towel.
- Adapt environment to match patients' ability to facilitate task performance. For example, if patient can only lift their arm up to the hip level, objects used in daily activities, which are usually placed above head, can be rearranged by placing at hip level.
- Devise interventions to keep the arm engaged during nontherapy time, i.e., while at home.
- Practice task variability by using objects with varying size, shape, which are used in daily activities.
- Avoid using squeeze ball or peg board as its use is not relevant to daily activities.

Guiding Questions:

1. Identify common reasons for development of shoulder pain.
2. Identify appropriate measurement tool to determine patients' baseline functional status.
3. State rationale for starting exercise early, i.e., after 48 hours.
4. Describe any three methods of adding task variability for practicing sit to stand.

Review Questions

1. Describe the updated definition of stroke.
2. What are various physiological mechanisms involved in recovery following stroke?
3. Discuss the natural course of recovery for mobility functions after stroke.
4. Enumerate the principles of stroke rehabilitation.
5. List the components of sit-to-stand task.
6. Identify common poststroke adaptations of sit-to-stand task.
7. List the components of walking task.
8. Enumerate various domains of walking.
9. Identify common poststroke adaptations of walking.
10. List the components of reaching, grasping, and manipulation task.
11. Identify common poststroke adaptations of reaching, grasping, and manipulation.

BIBLIOGRAPHY

1. Álvarez AG, Roby-Brami A, Robertson J, et al. Functional classification of grasp strategies used by hemiplegic patients. PLoS One. 2017;12:e0187608. https://doi.org/10.1371/journal.pone.0187608.

2. Cirstea MC, Levin MF. Compensatory strategies for reaching in stroke. Brain. 2000;123:940-53. https://doi.org/10.1093/brain/123.5.940.

3. GBD 2016 Stroke Collaborators. Global, regional, and national burden of stroke, 1990–2016: a systematic analysis for the Global Burden of Disease Study 2016. Lancet Neurol. 2019;18:439. https://doi.org/10.1016/S1474-4422(19)30034-1.

4. Goldberg SR, Anderson FC, Pandy MG, et al. Muscles that influence knee flexion velocity in double support: implications for stiff-knee gait. J Biomech. 2004;37:1189-96. https://doi.org/10.1016/j.jbiomech.2003.12.005.

5. Hawkins KA, Clark DJ, Balasubramanian CK, et al. Walking on uneven terrain in healthy adults and the implications for people after stroke. NeuroRehabilitation. 2017;41:765-74. https://doi.org/10.3233/NRE-172154.

6. Janssen WGM, Bussmann HBJ, Stam HJ. Determinants of the sit-to-stand movement: a review. Phys Ther. 2002;82:866-79.

7. Kang SY, Kim JS. Anterior cerebral artery infarction: stroke mechanism and clinical-imaging study in 100 patients. Neurology. 2008;70(24 Pt. 2):2386-93.

8. Lamontagne A, Fung J. Faster is better: implications for speed-intensive gait training after stroke. Stroke. 2004;35:2543-8. https://doi.org/10.1161/01.STR.0000144685.88760.d7.

9. Lang CE, Wagner JM, Edwards DF, et al. Recovery of grasp versus reach in people with hemiparesis poststroke. Neurorehabil Neural Repair. 2006;20:444-54. https://doi.org/10.1177/1545968306289299.

10. Langhorne P, Wu O, Rodgers H, et al. A Very Early Rehabilitation Trial after stroke (AVERT): a Phase III, multicentre, randomised controlled trial. Health Technol Assess. 2017;21:1-120. https://doi.org/10.3310/hta21540.

11. Latash ML, Anson JG, What are "normal movements" in atypical populations?. Behav Brain Sci. 1996;19:55-68. https://doi.org/10.1017/S0140525X00041467.

12. Levin MF, Liebermann DG, Parmet Y, et al. Compensatory versus noncompensatory shoulder movements used for reaching in stroke. Neurorehabil Neural Repair. 2016;30:635-46. https://doi.org/10.1177/1545968315613863.

13. Liu M, Chen J, Fan W, et al. Effects of modified sit-to-stand training on balance control in hemiplegic stroke patients: a randomized controlled trial. Clin Rehabil. 2016;30:627-36. https://doi.org/10.1177/0269215515600505.

14. Li Z, Zhang X, Wang K, et al. Effects of early mobilization after acute stroke: a meta-analysis of randomized control trials. J Stroke Cerebrovasc Dis. 2018;27:1326-37. https://doi.org/10.1016/j.jstrokecerebrovasdis.2017.12.021.

15. Page SJ, Schmid A, Harris JE. Optimizing terminology for stroke motor rehabilitation: recommendations from the American Congress of Rehabilitation Medicine Stroke Movement Interventions Subcommittee. Arch Phys Med Rehabil. 2012;93:1395-9. https://doi.org/10.1016/j.apmr.2012.03.005.

16. Parry R, Macias SS, Pradat-Diehl P, et al. Effects of hand configuration on the grasping, holding, and placement of an instrumented object in patients with hemiparesis. Front Neurol. 2019;10. https://doi.org/10.3389/fneur.2019.00240.

17. Patla AE, Shumway-Cook A. Dimensions of mobility: defining the complexity and difficulty associated with community mobility. J Aging Phys Act. 1999;7:7-19. https://doi.org/10.1123/japa.7.1.7.

18. Sacco RL, Kasner SE, Broderick JP, et al. An updated definition of stroke for the 21st century. Stroke. 2013;44:2064-89. https://doi.org/10.1161/STR.0b013e318296aeca.

19. Schenkman M, Berger RA, Riley PO, et al. Whole-body movements during rising to standing from sitting. Phys Ther. 1990;70:638-48; discussion 648-651. https://doi.org/10.1093/ptj/70.10.638.

20. Takeuchi N, Izumi SI. Maladaptive plasticity for motor recovery after stroke: mechanisms and approaches. Neural Plasticity 2012;2012. https://doi.org/10.1155/2012/359728.

21. The World Health Organization MONICA Project (monitoring trends and determinants in cardiovascular disease): a major international collaboration. WHO MONICA Project Principal Investigators, 1988. J Clin Epidemiol. 41:105–114.

Vestibular Rehabilitation

Palak Mulji

LEARNING OBJECTIVES

After reading this chapter, the readers should be able to:
- Get an overview of vestibular system, anatomy and physiology
- Understand vestibular disorders
- Describe and perform assessment methods in vestibular disorders
- Decide on treatment options for vestibular disorders.

CHAPTER OUTLINE

- Anatomy and physiology of the vestibular system
  - Peripheral vestibular system
  - Vestibular nerve
  - Central processing of vestibular input
  - Vestibular nucleus complex
  - Vestibulo-ocular reflex gain and phase
  - Cerebellum
  - Motor output of the vestibular system neurons
  - Vestibular reflexes
  - Cervical reflexes
  - Vascular supply
  - Role of the vestibular system in postural control
- Vestibular system disorders
  - Benign paroxysmal positional vertigo
  - Vestibular neuritis
  - Ménière's disease and endolymphatic hydrops
  - Vestibular migraine
  - Vestibular schwannoma
- Vestibular hypofunction assessment
  - Physical therapy evaluation
  - Oculomotor and vestibulo-ocular testing
  - Balance assessment
  - Coordination
  - Range of motion and strength
  - Positional testing assessment
  - Gait assessment
- Treatment for vestibular hypofunction
  - Gaze stabilization exercises
  - Habituation exercises
  - Postural stabilization

INTRODUCTION

The human body's balance is dependent on three key systems:
1. Vision
2. Vestibular system
3. Somatosensory system.

Vestibular system senses body's position and motion. Motion inputs to vestibular system come from the following, which get integrated by vestibular nucleus complex and cerebellum:
- Inner ear
- Visual signals
- Sensory inputs from joints and muscles (proprioception)
- Motor commands.

This eventually creates motor command to eyes and body to create balance and focus.

ANATOMY AND PHYSIOLOGY OF THE VESTIBULAR SYSTEM

Peripheral Vestibular System

The internal ear consists of two parts—the bony labyrinth, a series of cavities within the petrous part of the temporal bone, and the membranous sacs and ducts, contained within the bony cavity (**Fig. 27.1**).

Peripheral vestibular apparatus consists of: Bony labyrinth, and Membranous labyrinth.

Bony labyrinths consist of:
- Three semicircular canals (SCCs)
- Cochlea.

Membranous labyrinth has five sensory organs suspended in the bony labyrinth by perilymphatic fluid and connective tissue. This includes:

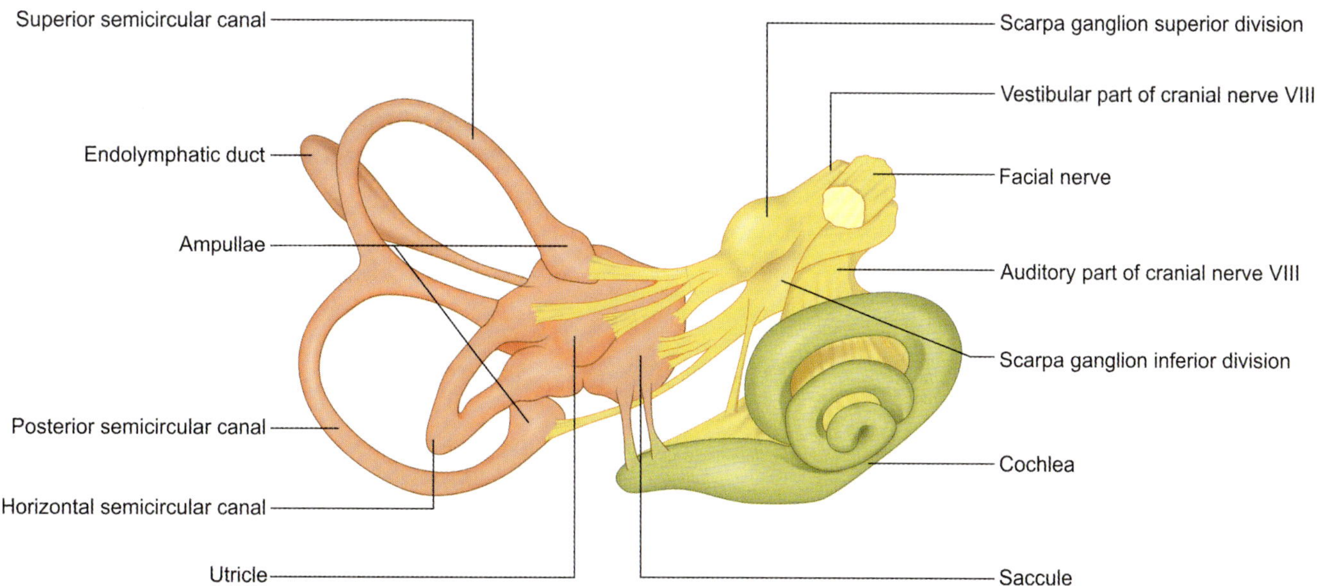

Fig. 27.1: Anatomy of vestibular labyrinth.

- Membranous portion of three SCCs
- Two otolith organs—utricle and saccule.

Note that one end of each SCC is widened in diameter to form an ampulla.

Hair cells are located in otoliths ampullae. The position of SCC and otolith allows hair cells to respond to specific movement of the head. SCCs detect angular motion of the head.

- Horizontal canal detects same side rotation.
- Posterior canal detects posterior rotation of the head.
- Anterior canal detects anterior rotation of the head.

Three important spatial arrangements characterize the alignment of the SCC's loops.

1. First, each canal plane within each labyrinth is perpendicular to the other canal planes.
2. Second, paired planes of the SCCs between the labyrinths conform very closely to each other. The six individual SCCs become three coplanar pairs:
   a. Right and left lateral
   b. Left anterior and right posterior
   c. Left posterior and right anterior.
3. Third, the planes of the canals are close to the planes of the extraocular muscles, thus allowing relatively simple connections between sensory neurons (related to individual canals) and motor output neurons (related to individual ocular muscles).

Coplanar pairing of the canal causes push and pull change in the quantity of SCC output. When angular motion occurs in shared plane, endolymph moves away from ampullae, which causes an increase in neural firing of vestibular nerve of that particular canal and decreases in opposite canal.

There are three main advantages of push and pull arrangements:

1. Sensory redundancy due to information provided from both canals. For example, if one canal of shared pair is unable to send head velocity information to the central nervous system (CNS) due to disease process, it still can receive information from contralateral pair.
2. Brain can ignore changes in neural firing occurring simultaneously on both sides.
3. It allows compensation of sensory overload.

The otolithic membranes are structures similar to the cupulae but are weighted. They contain calcium carbonate (limestone) crystals called otoconia and have substantially more mass than the cupulae. The mass of the otolithic membrane causes the maculae to be sensitive to gravity and linear acceleration. In contrast, the cupulae normally have the same density as the surrounding endolymphatic fluid and are insensitive to gravity.

Otolith organs are utricle and saccule, which respond to linear head motion and static tilt. These two organs can respond to all three dimensions and three linear motions. In an upright individual, the saccule is vertical (parasagittal), whereas the utricle is horizontally oriented (near the plane of the lateral SCC). The saccule senses linear acceleration in the sagittal plane, such as it might be associated with a forward pitch of the head. The utricle senses acceleration in its predominantly horizontal plane, such as it might be provoked by a roll (lateral tilt) of the head. The two organs together can encode all possible vectors of linear acceleration. The labyrinthine artery supplies the peripheral vestibular system. The labyrinthine artery has a variable origin. Most often it is a branch of the anterior inferior cerebellar artery, but occasionally it is a direct branch of the basilar artery.

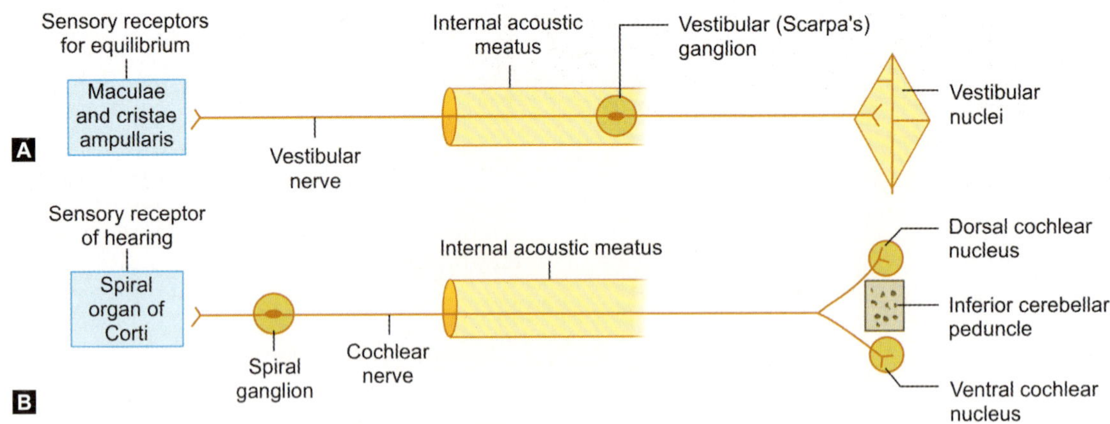

Figs. 27.2A and B: Anatomy of vestibular nerve.

Vestibular Nerve

Vestibular nerve fibers are afferent projection from Scarpa's (vestibular) ganglion **(Figs. 27.2A and B)**. Vestibular nerve transmits afferent signals from labyrinths along the course of internal auditory canal (IAC). It is also joined by the facial nerve, the cochlear nerve (hearing), the facial nerve, the nervus intermedius (a branch of the facial nerve, which carries facial sensation) and the labyrinthine artery.

Central Processing of Vestibular Input

There are two main targets for the vestibular input:
1. Vestibular nucleus complex
2. Cerebellum.

The vestibular nucleus is the main input processor and creates fast connection between efferent input and output motor neuron.

The cerebellum is the main adaptive processor—it monitors vestibular performance and readjusts central vestibular processing if necessary.

At both locations, vestibular sensory input is processed in association with somatosensory and visual sensory input.

Vestibular Nucleus Complex

Vestibular nucleus complex consists of four major nuclei and at least seven minor nuclei. Four major nuclei are superior, medial, lateral, and descending. Vestibular nucleus complex is located in the pons and extends into medulla. Superior and medial vestibular nucleus are main relay for **vestibulo-ocular reflex** (VOR). The medial vestibular nucleus is also involved in vestibulospinal reflexes (VSRs) and coordinates head and eye movements that occur together. The lateral vestibular nucleus is the principal nucleus for the VSR. The descending nucleus is connected to all the other nuclei and the cerebellum but has no primary outflow of its own. The vestibular nuclei between the two sides of the brainstem are laced together via a system of commissures, which are mutually inhibitory.

The commissures allow information to be shared between the two sides of the brainstem and implement the push–pull pairing of canals discussed earlier.

Vestibulo-ocular Reflex Gain and Phase

Normally, as the head moves in one direction, the eyes move in the opposite direction with equal velocity. This relationship of eye velocity to head velocity is expressed as the gain (VOR gain) of the vestibular system. Normal VOR gain is -1. Another useful measurement of vestibular system is VOR phase, which represents amplitude relationship between eye and head. It should represent an equal but opposite head and eye position relationship. When the head and eyes are equally positioned but oppositely directed, this is described as a zero phase shift.

Cerebellum

As discussed earlier, cerebellum is main adaptive processor for vestibular function **(Fig. 27.3)**. It is not required for vestibular reflexes; however, when removed, vestibular reflexes become ineffective and uncalibrated. The cerebellar flocculus is required to adapt the gain of the VOR.

Motor Output of the Vestibular System Neurons

Motor output of the vestibular system neurons includes the following:

- **Output for the vestibulo-ocular reflex:** There are two white matter tracts that carry output from the vestibular nuclear complex to the ocular motor nuclei. The ascending tract of Deiters carries output from the vestibular nucleus to the ipsilateral abducens nucleus (lateral rectus) during the horizontal VOR. All other VOR-related outputs to the ocular motor nuclei are transmitted by the medial longitudinal fasciculus (MLF). Because the MLF is often injured in multiple sclerosis, this connection may account for central vestibular symptoms in these patients.

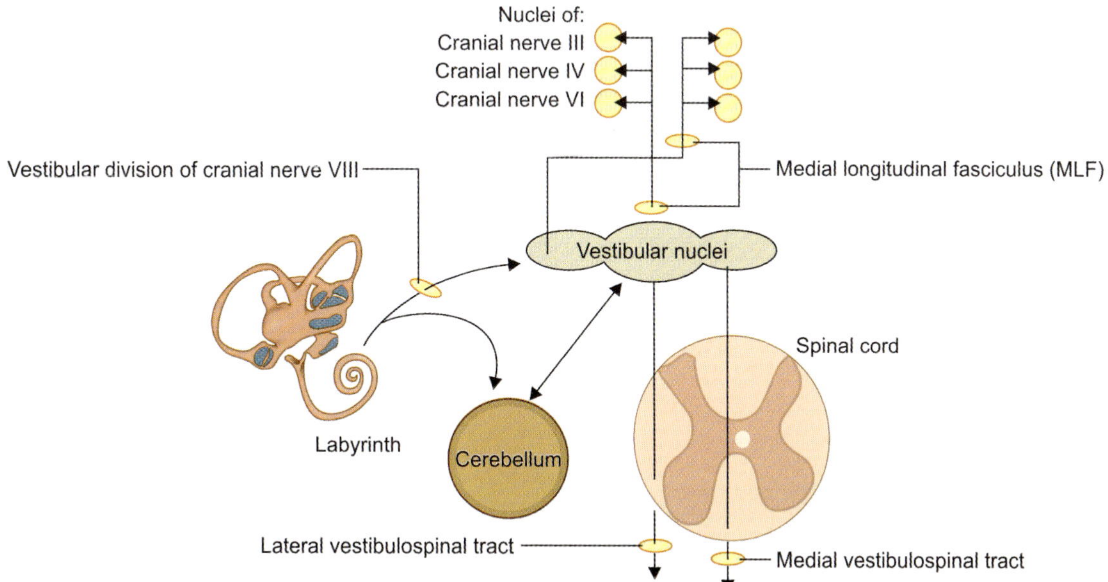

Fig. 27.3: Cerebellum and tracts involved in vestibular system.

- **Output for the vestibulospinal reflex (VSR):** There are three major pathways that connect anterior horn of the spinal cord to vestibular nuclei.
  1. Lateral vestibulospinal tract
  2. Medial vestibulospinal tract
  3. Reticulospinal tract.

Lateral vestibulospinal tract originates from ipsilateral vestibular nucleus and receives most input from cerebellum and otolith. Lateral vestibulospinal tract is responsible for maintaining antigravity postural motor activity or protective extension, primarily in the lower extremities, in response to the head position changes, which occur with respect to gravity.

Medial vestibulospinal tract originates from medial, superior, and descending nuclei and mediates ongoing postural changes or head righting in response to SCC sensory input (angular head motion).

The reticulospinal tract receives sensory input from all vestibular nuclei as well as all the other sensory and motor systems. It is involved in most balance reflex and motor action.

Vestibular Reflexes

Vestibular reflexes can be classified as follows:
- Vestibulo-ocular reflex (VOR) is one of the major reflexes responsible for maintaining gaze stability. Input for this reflex comes from SCC and otoliths. Normal VOR gain is 1 for horizontal head movement.
- VSR stabilizes body with head movement. Input comes from SCC and otolith as well as different sensory and dynamic inputs. Output is generated through vestibulospinal tract.
- Vestibulo-cervical reflex stabilizes head in space.

Cervical Reflexes

Cervical reflexes can be explained as follows:
- Cervico-ocular reflex (COR) causes eye movements driven by neck proprioceptors. COR can supplement the VOR when peripheral vestibular organ is damaged.
- Cervico-spinal reflex stabilizes head and can supplement VSR by altering the tone of the body.
- Cervico-colic reflex (CCR) also stabilizes head over body. CCR with VSR protects head from over rotations.

Vascular Supply

The vertebral–basilar arterial system supplies blood to the peripheral and central vestibular system **(Fig. 27.4)**. The labyrinthine artery supplies the peripheral vestibular system. The labyrinthine artery has a variable origin. Most often it is a branch of the anterior inferior cerebellar artery (AICA), but occasionally it is a direct branch of the basilar artery. The posterior inferior cerebellar arteries (PICA), branch of vertebral arteries are the most important arteries of central vestibular system. They supply the surface of the inferior portions of the cerebellar hemispheres as well as the dorsolateral medulla, which includes the inferior aspects of the vestibular nuclear complex.

Occlusions of the basilar artery, labyrinthine artery, AICA or PICA territory strokes can cause "lateral medullary syndrome," which causes purely central balance symptoms due to damage of vestibular nucleus and inferior cerebellum. AICA territory strokes cause a mixed peripheral/cerebellar pattern because AICA supplies both the labyrinth and part of the cerebellum.

Role of the Vestibular System in Postural Control

Vestibular system is both a sensory and a motor system.
- Sensory system provides CNS with head position and gravity.

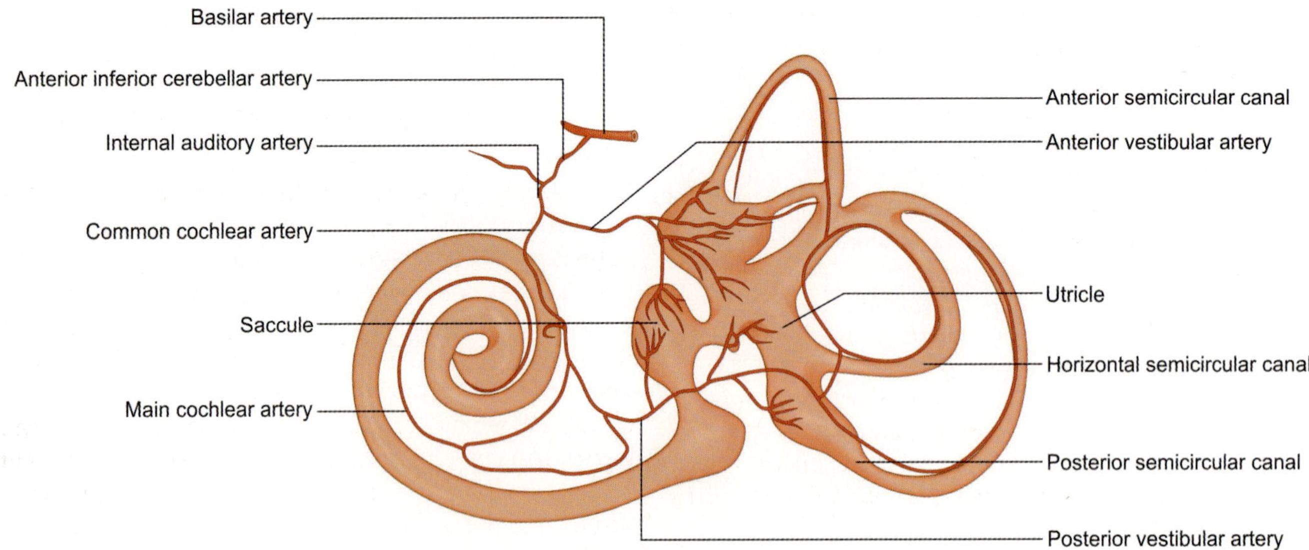

Fig. 27.4: Vascular supply in vestibular system.

- Motor system provides descending motor pathways that control static head and body positions and coordinate postural movements.

Vestibular system has four major roles:
1. Senses body's position and motion
2. Orients the trunk to vertical using sensory orientation and weighting appropriate sensory cues under different sensory environment
3. Controls position of body's center of mass for static and dynamic movements
4. Stabilizes the head during postural movements.

VESTIBULAR SYSTEM DISORDERS

Dysfunction of peripheral vestibular system can create a variety of symptoms. As discussed earlier, peripheral system involves vestibular end organs and vestibular nerve. Detailed evaluation of this system is required to determine specific pathology behind patients complain of dizziness/vertigo or disequilibrium by physician.

Benign Paroxysmal Positional Vertigo

Benign paroxysmal positional vertigo (BPPV) is the most common form of vertigo. It is a mechanical problem of peripheral vestibular system resulting from otoconia being displaced into SCC. Patient complains of true rotational vertigo with change in head positions. In the general population, 64 new cases per 10,000 people are recorded every year.

BPPV is characterized by perception of environment spinning or one's self spinning with change in head position. BPPV can occur spontaneously but it is known to follow head trauma, labyrinthitis or ischemia in the distribution of anterior cerebellar artery. Spontaneous remission is common.

Patients with BPPV commonly report symptoms of spinning vertigo:
- While lying in bed, turning in bed, coming out of bed
- Bending over to pick up things from the floor and looking up.

Patient's activity of daily living is affected, which includes:
- Sleeping and turning in bed
- Waking up in the morning with severe dizziness
- Experience of vertigo while washing hair in the salon
- Gardening and having dental exam.

Other symptoms of BPPV include being off balance while walking.

Two mechanisms have been proposed for occurrence of BPPV.
1. First theory is **canalithiasis,** which was proposed in 1979 by Hall et al. The canalithiasis theory suggests that degenerative debris from the utricle (possibly fragments of otoconia) is free-floating in the long arm of the SCC. Otoconia are more than twice the density of the endolymph in the SCCs. Therefore a positional change of the canals with respect to gravity would result in movement of the otoconia, which in turn would overcome the inertia of the endolymph.

   The movement of the endolymph would deflect the cupula, causing nystagmus and complaints of vertigo. A latency of the response is related to the time needed for the cupula to be deflected by the pull of the endolymph. The intensity of vertigo and nystagmus are related to the degree of deflection of the cupula. Vertigo and nystagmus stop as the position is maintained as a result of cessation of endolymph movement as the otoconia settle in the most dependent portion of the canal.

2. In 1962, Schuknecht attributed the disorder to otoconia crystals adhered to the cupula, which he termed

"**cupulolithiasis**" after noting basophilic staining masses of granular material attached to the cupula of the posterior canal in two patients with a history of BPPV. Presumably, the presence of debris adhering to the cupula significantly increases the density of the cupula and, therefore, produces an inappropriate deflection of the cupula of the posterior canal when the head is positioned with the affected ear below the horizon. The result is vertigo, nystagmus, and nausea. Thus cupulolithiasis is characterized by:

- Immediate onset of vertigo when the patient is moved into the provoking position
- The presence of nystagmus, which appears with the same latency as the complaints of vertigo
- Persistence of the vertigo and nystagmus as long as the person's head is maintained in the provoking position.

Because the cupula remains deflected as long as the patient is in the provoking position, nystagmus and vertigo will persist, although the intensity may decrease slightly because of central adaptation or because the patient may also have canalithiasis. It has been since learned that cupulolithiasis as a cause of BPPV is relatively uncommon.

Cause of Benign Paroxysmal Positional Vertigo

The causes of BPPV are as follows:

- Exact cause of BPPV is unknown.
- More than 50% BPPV are considered to have unknown etiology.
- Head trauma is considered to be the second most cause of BPPV.
- BPPV also occurs in combination with vestibular neuritis.

Assessment of Benign Paroxysmal Positional Vertigo

BPPV assessment is performed by putting patient in different head positions to provoke dizziness and nystagmus. Patient is explained prior to testing about vertigo may occur and they may feel nauseous, as well as to keep eyes open the whole time during testing. If patient has symptoms of severe nausea and vomiting during the testing, antiemetic medications would help. Patient with cervical movement limitation would benefit from using tilt table.

Tests that Identify Benign Paroxysmal Positional Vertigo

Dix–Hallpike testing (Fig. 27.5) is a gold standard for the diagnosis of BPPV. This maneuver is performed by placing patient having head turn to 45° and having head below the table, positioning posterior canal in gravity dependent position. This position would provoke nystagmus and dizziness within a few seconds, this happens because of debris of otoconia moves away from cupula due to pull of gravity. If the patient has BPPV, vertigo and nystagmus will be provoked when the affected ear is inferior. The patient may also experience vertigo upon returning to the sitting position. The test can then be repeated with the patient's head turned to the other side. If the debris is within the posterior SCC, the resultant nystagmus during testing will be upbeating and torsional toward the side being tested. Side lying test can be performed by having the patient go on their side from sitting position with head turn to 45°.

Roll test (Fig. 27.6) is performed to test horizontal canals. Patient is placed in supine position and turns head sideways. The elicited nystagmus is horizontal and may have a torsional component.

- In the canalithiasis form of horizontal SCC BPPV, the nystagmus is geotropic; i.e. the fast phase beats toward the earth and is brief in duration.
- In the cupulolithiasis form of horizontal SCC BPPV, the nystagmus is apogeotropic (the fast phase beats away from the earth) and is prolonged in duration.

The affected side is considered to be the more symptomatic side in canalithiasis and the less symptomatic side in cupulolithiasis. The roll test for horizontal SCC BPPV has only face validity, and its sensitivity and specificity have not been reported.

Treatment for Benign Paroxysmal Positional Vertigo

There are three basic maneuvers used depending on the indication:

1. Canalith repositioning maneuver

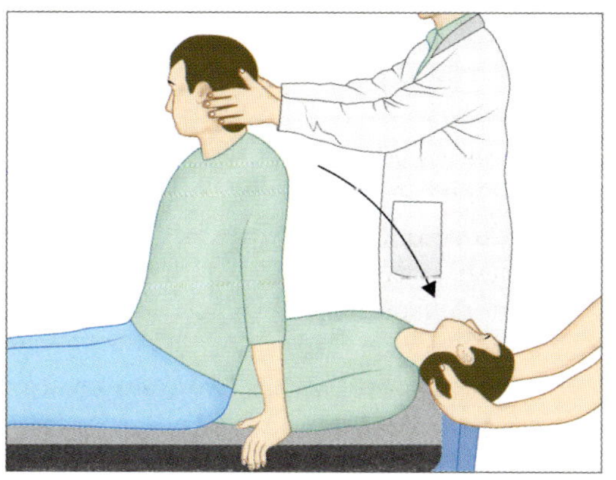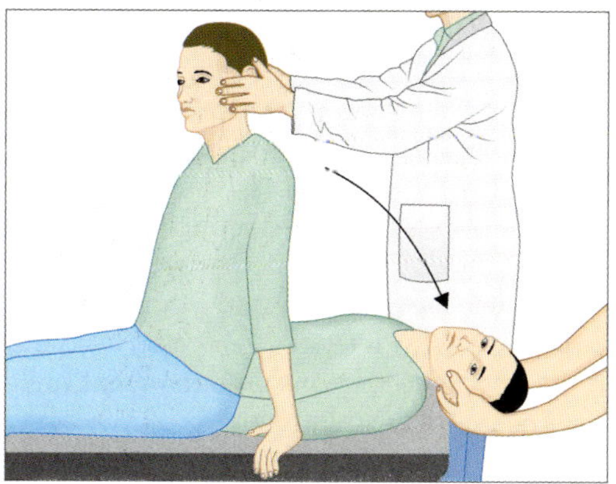

Fig. 27.5: Dix–Hallpike testing.

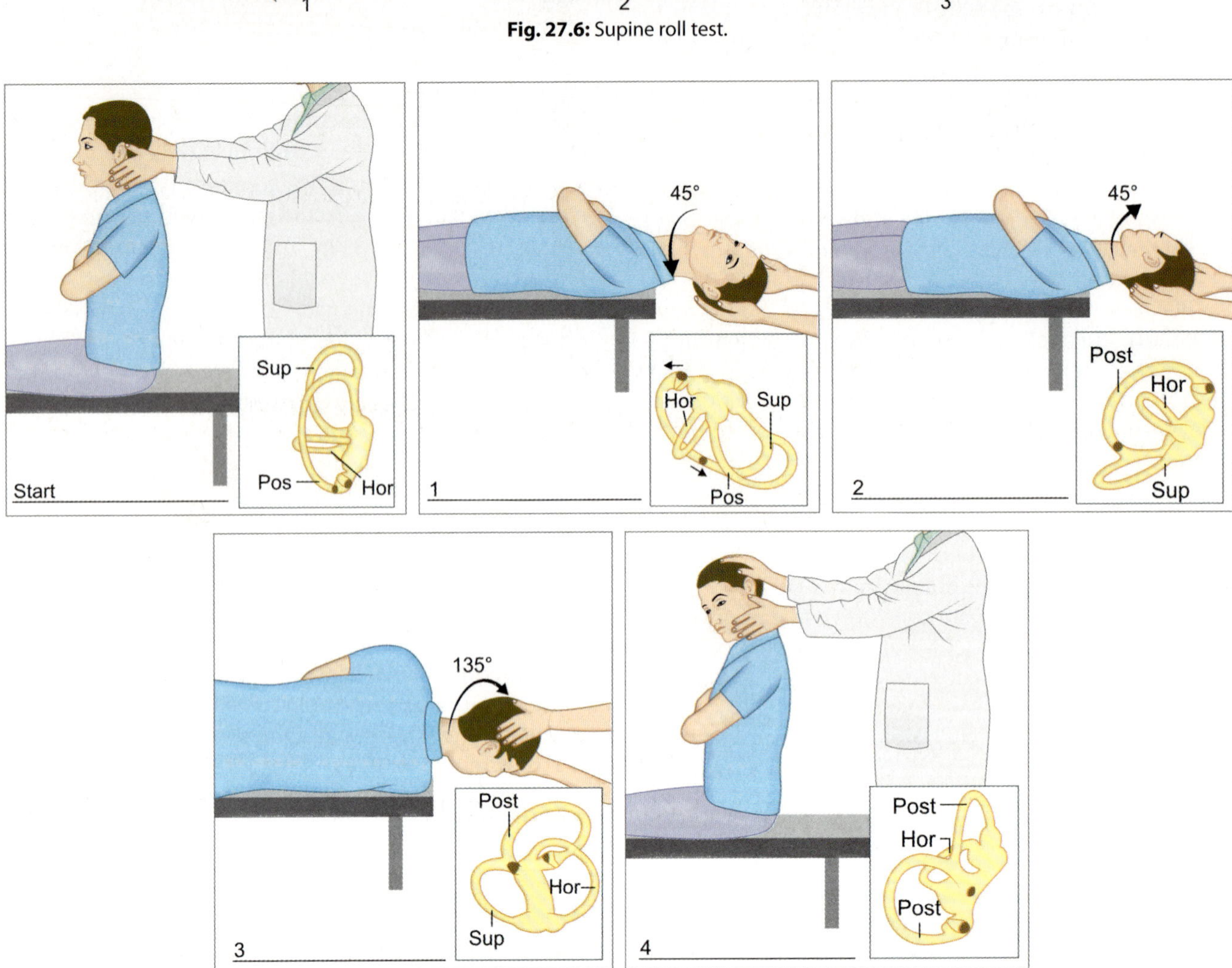

Fig. 27.6: Supine roll test.

Fig. 27.7: Canalith repositioning maneuver.
(Sup: superior; Pos: posterior; Hor: horizontal)

2. Liberatory maneuver
3. Brandt–Daroff habituation exercises.

1. Canalith repositioning maneuver (CRM) (Fig. 27.7): Originally known as Epley maneuver, canalith repositioning treatment (CRT) is performed with positional changes. Clinician helps patient to go in supine with head 45° to the affected side, below the horizontal plane in order to have extension of the neck. After nystagmus and dizziness subsides, the patient's head is turned to 90° increments to the opposite side. Patient is seated from this position. Post-treatment instructions do not appear to be necessary to the success of the treatment.

2. Liberatory maneuver (Figs. 27.8A to D): Liberatory maneuver is mainly used for posterior canal cupulolithiasis;

however, high success rate has been found with posterior canalithiasis.

Bar-B-Que roll treatment for horizontal canalithiasis (Fig. 27.9): The CRM as proposed by Epley for the treatment of posterior SCC canalithiasis has been modified for horizontal SCC BPPV into a treatment referred to as the Bar-B-Que or roll treatment. This treatment is performed as a full 360° roll or as a 270° roll. In both treatments, the patient should be asymptomatic by the time they are in the prone position.

The Casani (or Gufoni) maneuver for horizontal cupulolithiasis: Evidence suggests that horizontal cupulolithiasis is only effectively treated with the Casani maneuver also known as the modified Semont maneuver

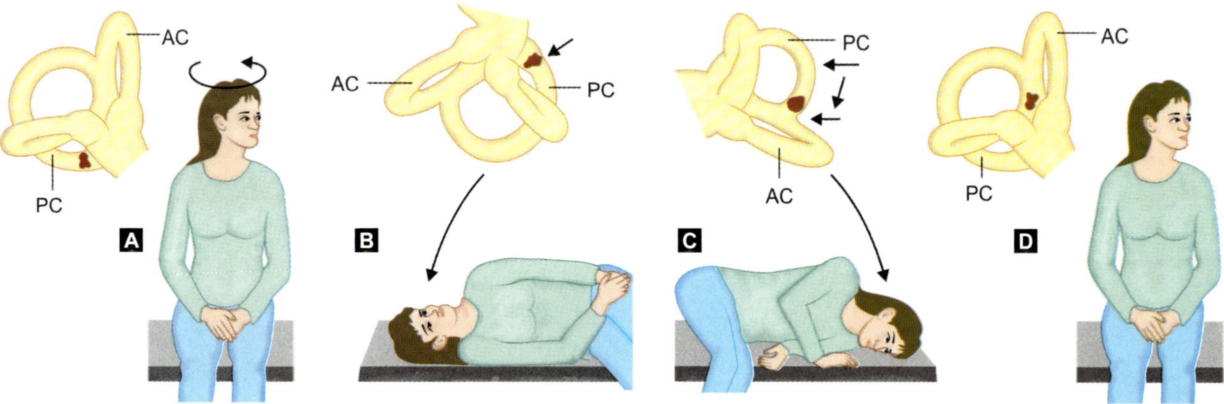

Figs. 27.8A to D: Liberatory maneuver.
(AC: anterior canal; PC: posterior canal)

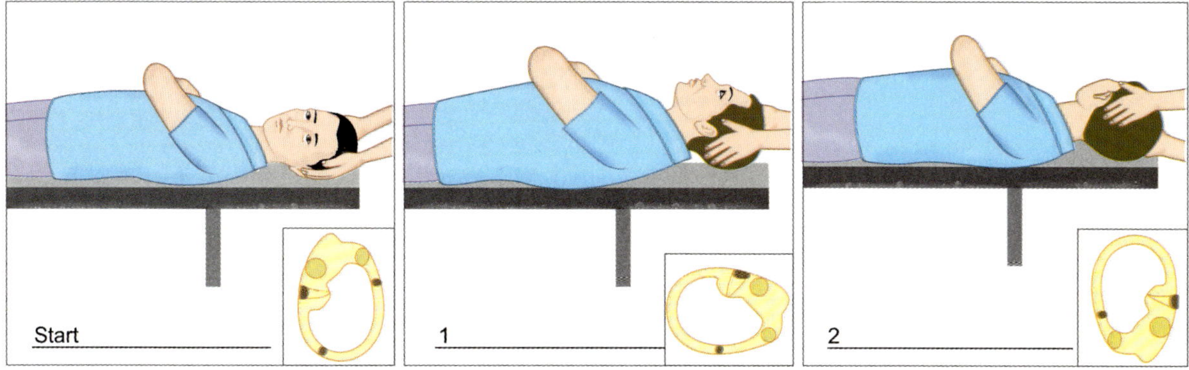

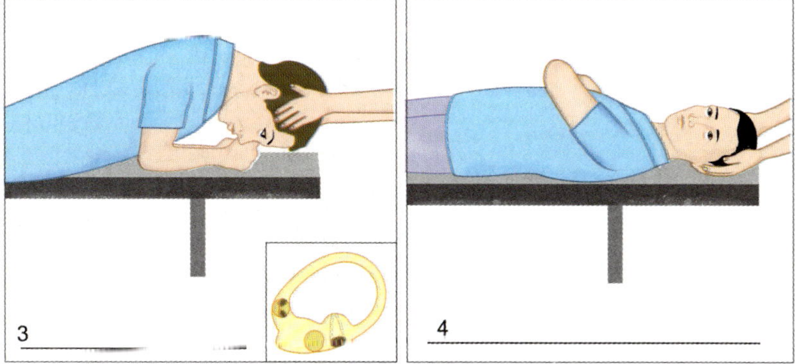

Fig. 27.9: Bar-B-Que roll treatment for horizontal canalithiasis.

for horizontal canal cupulolithiasis. To perform the maneuver, start with sitting position, patient moves quickly to side lying position on affected side. Patient then quickly turns head so that nose is down to 45° and stays in the position for 2–3 minutes before sitting up.

3. Brandt–Daroff exercises (Figs. 27.10A and B): These are habituation exercises performed to habituate the symptoms of dizziness, which are occurring with bed mobility by lying down on one side with head up to 45° angle, then get into sitting position and lie down on the other side with 45° angle so the head is up to the ceiling. This treatment is mostly used when unable to clear the BPPV symptoms with CRMs.

There are multiple treatment options available besides the ones explained above. To discuss all of them here is outside of the scope of this chapter.

Vestibular Neuritis

Vestibular neuritis is the second most common cause of vertigo. Etiology of vestibular neuritis is never proved; evidence supports a viral etiology (similar to Bell's palsy or sudden hearing loss), which comes from histopathological changes of branches of the vestibular nerve in patients who have suffered such an illness and sometimes epidemic occurrence of the condition. It presents with symptoms of acute onset of prolonged severe rotational vertigo that is exacerbated by movement of the head, associated with spontaneous horizontal nystagmus beating toward the good ear, postural imbalance with a tendency to fall toward the affected side, and nausea. Severe symptoms last for 48–72 hours and recovery happens around 6 weeks or more.

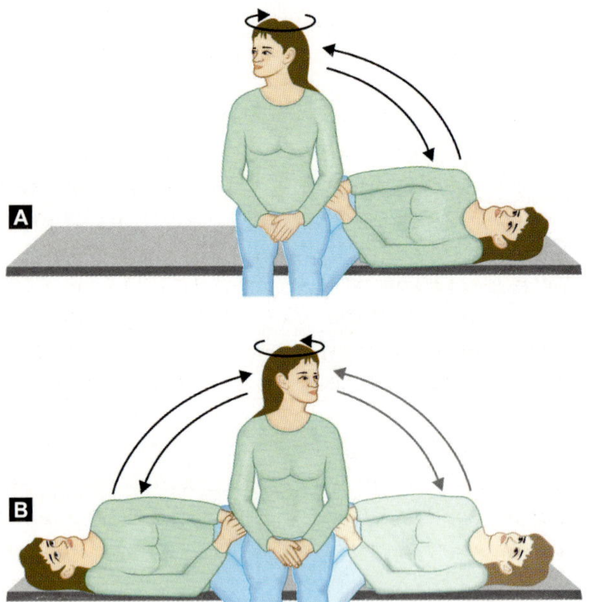

Figs. 27.10A and B: Brandt–Daroff exercises.

Initial treatment of vestibular neuritis includes vestibular suppressants such as the antihistamine. Patient would benefit from bed rest in the beginning for 24–72 hours after that patient can ambulate with assistance and be able to ambulate independently. To further speed up the process of recuperation, vestibular exercises challenge the compensatory mechanisms of the CNS, stimulating adaptation. These exercises are designed to improve both gaze stability and postural stability.

Ménière's Disease and Endolymphatic Hydrops

Ménière's disease is a disorder that affects inner ear function. A phenomenon fundamental to the development of Ménière's disease is endolymphatic hydrops. Whether endolymphatic hydrops itself is the cause of the symptoms characteristic of Ménière's disease or whether it is a pathological change seen in the disease is still unclear. The development of hydrops is generally a function of malabsorption of endolymph in the endolymphatic duct and sac. Malabsorption may itself be a result of disturbed function of components comprising the endolymphatic duct and sac, mechanical obstruction of these structures, or altered anatomy of the temporal bone.

It starts with aural fullness, hearing loss, true rotational vertigo, tinnitus, and postural imbalance. Severe symptoms last anywhere from 30 minutes to 24 hours. Patient slowly gets better and patient generally becomes ambulatory within 72 hours. Patient may experience unsteadiness for days to weeks. Ménière's disease is mostly pharmacologically managed to reduce symptoms of acute vertigo. Decreased balance after Ménière's attack can be treated with vestibular rehabilitation.

Vestibular Migraine

Among migraine headaches, 40% of people suffer from vestibular dysfunction with dizziness. This is also known as migraine-associated vertigo (MAV). Hormonal fluctuations, foods, and weather changes (barometric pressure variations) seem to often exacerbate headaches and dizziness. The clinical presentation of vestibular symptoms that often along with migraine includes—but is not limited to—dizziness; motion intolerance with respect to head, eyes, and/or body; spontaneous vertigo attacks (often accompanied by nausea and vomiting); diminished eye focus with photosensitivity; sound sensitivity and tinnitus; balance loss and ataxia; cervicalgia (neck pain) with associated muscle spasms in the upper cervical spine musculature; confusion with altered cognition; spatial disorientation; and anxiety/panic.

Most effective migraine management is a combination of medications, vestibular rehabilitation, and lifestyle modifications that include limitation of the risk factors associated with migraine (those related to diet, sleep, stress, exercise, and environmental factors). To evaluate patient for the trigger for MAV is the most important aspect of the management. Vestibular deficits are recognized by oculomotor and balance assessment. Vestibular rehabilitation helps with reversing symptoms related to dizziness and balance.

Vestibular Schwannoma

Vestibular schwannoma is also known as acoustic neuroma. Acoustic neuromas are nerve sheath tumors occurring in the IAC or cerebellopontine angle. Most patients with acoustic neuroma starts with loss of sensorineural hearing loss, while some first complain of vestibular symptoms, sudden hearing loss, or occasionally trigeminal symptoms. After diagnosis is made once the diagnosis is established, there are three therapeutic options: watchful waiting, microsurgical removal, and stereotactic radiosurgery. There is moderate evidence which suggests that vestibular rehabilitation is an effective treatment of patients during the acute period onset of vestibular neuritis or after resection of vestibular schwannoma. Patient with vestibular schwannoma is treated as vestibular hypofunction assessment and treatment.

There are other vestibular disorders that are outside of the scope of this chapter, including:

- Bilateral vestibular disorders
- Central disorders
- Chronic subjective dizziness
- Vestibular disorders of central origin.

VESTIBULAR HYPOFUNCTION ASSESSMENT

Peripheral vestibular disorders can cause vestibular hypofunction. Depending on the extent of the vestibular deficit, it can have different clinical course and final level of recovery or deficit. Despite these differences, such patients have many of the same symptoms:

- Dizziness
- Lightheadedness
- Vertigo
- Nystagmus
- Blurred vision
- Postural instability
- Fear of movement
- Gait disturbances
- Occasional falling.

The symptoms of vestibular hypofunction emerge from functional deficits in vestibulo-ocular and vestibulospinal systems and from the results of sensory mismatch and physical deconditioning.

Vestibular ocular reflex (VOR) is a reflex that is responsible for gaze stability with head movement. Peripheral vestibular lesion affects VOR function. During movements of the head, the VOR stabilizes gaze (eye position in space) by producing an eye movement of equal velocity and opposite direction to the head movement. Other eye movements include saccadic eye movements and smooth pursuit.

- Saccadic eye movement is when eye moves back and forth between two targets.
- Pursuit eye movement allows eyes to follow moving objects across the visual field (smooth pursuit). If impaired smooth pursuit or hypermetric saccades are identified during the examination, the clinician should strongly consider that the person has central dysfunction.

Other symptoms of vestibular hypofunction can cause:

- Vertigo due to sensory conflict due to abnormal sensory input by otolith organ
- Postural instability

- Decreased cervical range of motion (ROM)
- Limited activity level causing deconditioning.

Physical Therapy Evaluation

Detailed physical therapy evaluation is required for any dizzy patient since the symptoms can be central, peripheral or both. Central symptoms can be due to acute stroke, tumor, or head injury.

- **Medical history:** Patient's past and current medical history is an important piece of information in determining diagnosis and prognosis. Patients with head and neck injuries, migraines, visual dysfunctions, and peripheral neuropathies are important comorbidities, which can prolong the rehabilitation process. It is important to know about patient's cardiovascular health since orthostatic hypotension can give symptoms of dizziness with change of positions **(Table 27.1)**. Patient's medications need to be reviewed. Some of the medications have their side effects as dizziness as well as some of them are vestibular suppressants.
- **Subjective history:** This should include onset, duration of the symptoms, how long they last and what helps to recover, circumstances in which they occur—positional, spontaneous vs constant. It is important to find out about a patient's prior and current level of function. **The Vestibular Activities of Daily Living Scale** is an excellent example of a tool that will assist the therapist in identifying limitations. Symptoms that trigger dizziness and help to decrease dizziness should be found. Any fall history and use of assistive devices help to determine how patient's balance and gait have been. **Dizziness Handicap Inventory (DHI) questionnaire and activity-specific balance**

Table 27.1: Key items in the history of the dizzy patient.			
Disorder	*Tempo*	*Symptoms*	*Circumstances*
Vestibular neuritis	Acute dizziness	Vertigo, dysequilibrium, nausea and vomiting, oscillopsia	Spontaneous, exacerbated by head movements
Labyrinthitis	Acute dizziness	Vertigo, dysequilibrium, nausea and vomiting, oscillopsia, hearing loss and tinnitus	Spontaneous, exacerbated by head movements
BPPV	Spells: seconds	Vertigo, lightheadedness, nausea	Positional: lying down, sitting up or turning over in bed, bending forward
TIA	Spells: minutes	Vertigo, lightheadedness, disequilibrium	Spontaneous
Migraine	Spells: minutes	Vertigo, dizziness, motion sickness	Usually movement-induced
Panic attack	Spells: minutes	Dizziness, nausea, diaphoresis, fear, palpitations, paresthesias	Spontaneous or situation
Anxiety	Chronic dizziness	Lightheadedness, floating or rocking	Induced by eye movements with head still
Motion sickness	Spells: hours	Nausea, diaphoresis, dizziness	Movement induced, usually visuovestibular mismatch
Ménière's disease	Spells: hours	Vertigo, disequilibrium, ear fullness from hearing loss and tinnitus	Spontaneous, exacerbated by head movements

(BPPV: benign paroxysmal positional vertigo; TIA: transient ischemic attack)

confidence scale can be used prior to evaluating patient, which helps manage times.

- **Clinical examination:** Clinical examination includes oculomotor and vestibulo-ocular testing, balance exam, coordination, ROM and strength assessment, gait assessment, and positional testing.

Oculomotor and Vestibulo-ocular Testing

Patient is assessed for this exam in room light and/or with Frenzel lenses.

- Patient is first observed for spontaneous nystagmus with room light, and for skew deviation. Patient with acute unilateral vestibular loss will have spontaneous nystagmus beating away from the side of the lesion. Patient learns to fixate at room light so spontaneous nystagmus cannot be visible at room light if seen later. Skew deviation is a sign for stroke. Patient's eyeball drops on the side of the lesion and will present with vertical diplopia.
- Infrared goggles or Frenzel lenses are utilized to remove fixation. Patient is assessed with R and L gaze to see nystagmus; patient with unilateral loss presents with nystagmus beating away from the side of the lesion.
- Direction changing gaze-holding nystagmus is consistent with a central lesion, usually in the posterior fossa.
- Patient assessed for smooth pursuit by asking to track the target with eyes and keeping head stationary.
- Abnormal pursuit is never a sign for peripheral disorder.
- Saccadic eye movements are tested by simply asking the patient to look back and forth between two horizontal or two vertical targets.
- VOR cancelation is tested with keeping eye focused on target and moving the head and eye together with the target, hence canceling VOR. VOR cancelation is a sign for CNS involvement.

Patient is then tested for VOR function with visual acuity testing and head thrust tests.

- Patient is asked to read the eye chart and then keep reading while moving the head with speed of 2 Hz. Metronome can be utilized to standardize this. In normal individuals, visual acuity changes by one line in younger individuals or by two lines in older individuals. In patients with uncompensated, unilateral vestibular loss, visual acuity degrades by three or four lines.

Balance Assessment

Static and dynamic balance is assessed by utilizing:

- Modified clinical test of sensory integration and balance (mCTSIB)
- Romberg test with eyes open and closed
- Tandem stance
- Tandem walk testing.

Functional gait assessment (FGA) and Dynamic Gait Index (DGI) testing are utilized to assess balance and have been related to assess fall risk.

Coordination

Finger-to-nose and heel-to-shin movements and the ability to perform rapid alternating movements of fingers or feet are gross tests that may be used to subjectively assess the patient's coordination. Vestibular dysfunctions do not affect coordination.

Range of Motion and Strength

Neck ROM is required to be assessed before testing patient for positional assessment. In older individuals, assessing the range of motion and strength helps determining need of strengthening to prevent risk of falls.

Positional Testing Assessment

Patient with complains of positional vertigo needs to be assessed with Dix-Hallpike testing and roll test to rule out any BPPV-related vertigo. These tests are discussed earlier in this chapter. Patient with motion sensitivity–related positional dizziness can be assessed with motion sensitivity quotient (MSQ) and be able to set a baseline before treating patients with habituation exercises.

Gait Assessment

Patients with possible vestibular dysfunctions:

- Walk with a wider base of support.
- With unilateral vestibular loss they may veer to R or L.
- Difficulty moving head while walking.
- The patient may walk with excessive visual fixation to be able to walk in a straight line.

Dynamic Gait Index is a great tool to screen patients with vestibular dysfunction.

It is possible to have patients referred to physical therapy for vestibular evaluation with undiagnosed central pathology. Patient needs to be screened for the signs and symptoms of CNS and reported to the referring physician. Multiple sclerosis, brainstem transient ischemic attacks, Parkinson's disease, cerebellar disorders, and migraines are but a few of the disorders that have been diagnosed in patients with vestibular dysfunction–like symptoms.

TREATMENT FOR VESTIBULAR HYPOFUNCTION

Patient with vestibular hypofunction can be treated with many different approaches. There are three approaches that are frequently utilized are:

1. Gaze stabilization exercises
2. Habituation exercises to reduce the symptoms
3. Postural stabilization exercises to improve gait and balance.

Gaze Stabilization Exercises

- **VORx1 and VORx2 exercises (Figs. 27.11A to F):** While keeping eyes on target, move the head sideways keeping target in the focus. This slowly improves visual acuity and gaze stability. This exercise can be progressed from sitting to standing to walking.

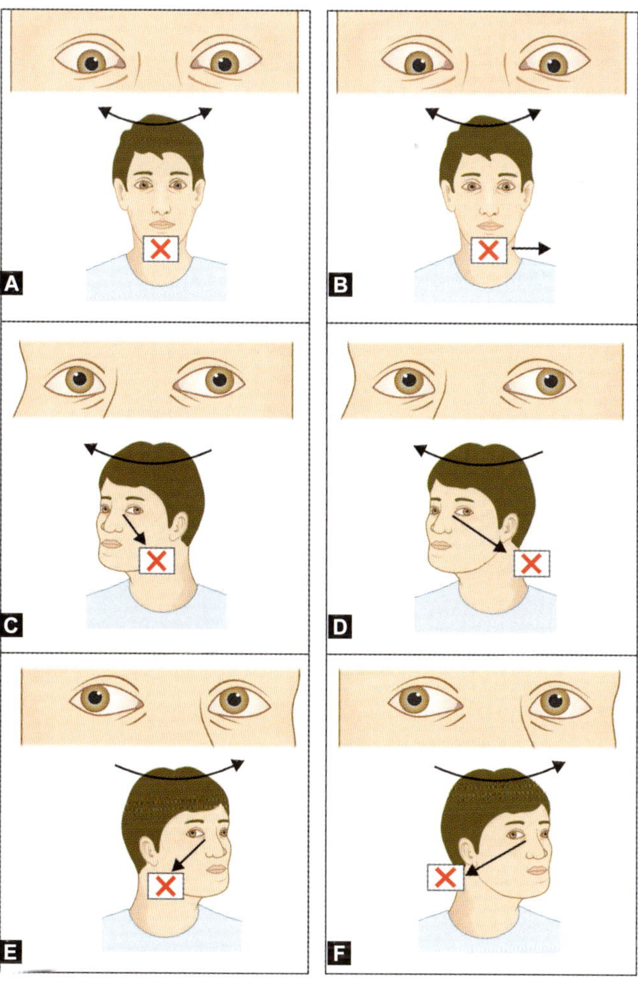

Figs. 27.11A to F: Gaze stabilization exercises.

- **Targets:** This exercise involves repeated eye and then head movement between two targets. Patient is asked to stand against two targets 2 ft apart. When patient is looking at one target, they should be able to see another one from the corner of their eye. When patient looks at the target directly with eye and head in the same line, then the patient is asked to look at the other target with their eyes only and followed by their head.
- **Remembered targets:** In this exercise, patient is asked to look at the target placed right in front of them. Patient is then asked to close their eyes and move their head while imagining to keep eyes on the target. After moving head open eyes to see if the eyes are on the target or moved.

Habituation Exercises

These exercises are based on the concept that repeated exposure to a provocative stimulus will result in a reduction in the pathological response to that treatment. MSQ assessment, along with subjective history, can determine which positions are more symptom-provoking. Patient can be tested for:

- Bed mobility
- Transfers
- Walking without head movement
- Walking with head movements
- Bending over in lying down
- Bending over in sitting
- Bending over in standing.

Patient is started in sitting with repeated movement of provoking position while increasing symptoms minimally to habituate to that particular position. Patient can be progressed from slow to fast movements until asymptomatic. In conjunction with Cooksey, Cawthorne developed a series of exercises that addressed their patients' complaints of vertigo and impaired balance. **The Cawthorne-Cooksey exercises** include pursuit and saccadic eye movements, movements of the head, tasks requiring coordination of eyes with the head, total body movements, and balance tasks.

Postural Stabilization

Postural stabilization exercises are performed while utilizing visual, vestibular and somatosensory cues. Patient having vestibular hypofunction, altering visual and somatosensory cues, would stimulate the system. Examples of these exercises include:

- Standing on foam
- Standing on foam with eyes closed
- Walking on foam
- Walking with eyes closed
- Walking with head turns.

Alternate tapping on the cone progress to single-leg stance improves patient's ability to function with steps and going on and off the curb. Exercises must be updated and progressed to incorporate more challenges **(Fig. 27.12)**.

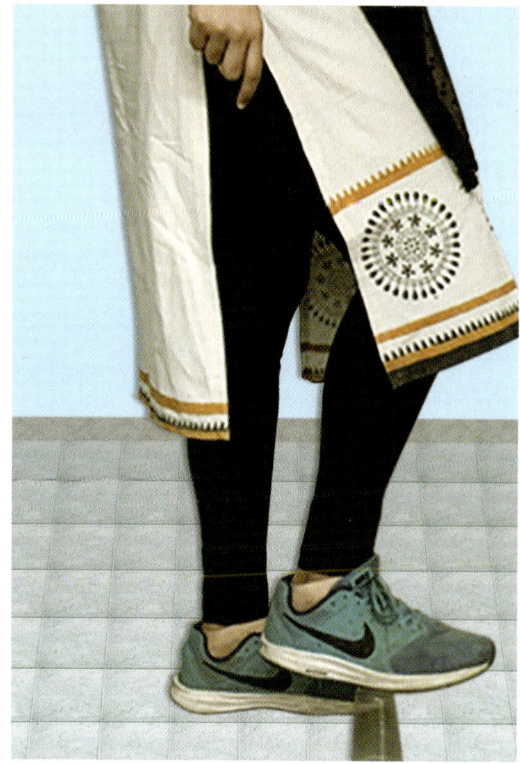

Fig. 27.12: Example of a challenging balance exercise.

The patient is instructed to gently place his or her foot on a plastic cup and maintain his or her balance without crushing the cup. Initially, the patient should be advised to use a handhold that can be progressed to eyes closed, no handhold, or stepping while alternating foot placement on the cup.

Clinical Pearl

The primary concerns when developing an exercise program to improve postural stability is how to challenge the patient's balance without causing the patient to fall. Fall risk should be determined before choosing the most appropriate exercises for a person with postural control deficits.

SUMMARY

While treating patients with vestibular hypofunction, goal should be to have return to prior level of function. Patient with benign paroxysmal vertigo and unilateral vestibular loss recovers from the initial symptoms they experience. Patient with other CNS disorders can delay the recovery. This chapter provides an overview of vestibular system, disorders and treatment strategies. Further reading and specific vestibular rehabilitation training are recommended in order to improve skills to be able to treat patients efficiently.

ACKNOWLEDGMENTS

Some of the information in this chapter is derived from "Herdman S, Clandeil R. Vestibular Rehabilitation. Philadelphia, FA Davis; 2014" More information on vestibular rehabilitation can be found here.

Case Scenario

CASE STUDY 1

A 50-year-old woman developed vertigo a week ago. While coming out of bed she experienced room spinning around her followed by vomiting. The patient went to the emergency room (ER) where she had head CT and MRI done. Due to her history of high blood pressure, she had cardiac workup done in ER. The patient was found negative for all assessment. She was sent home with antivert to manage her vertigo and was referred to a physical therapist. She continued to stay dizzy when she came home and thought she had her Ménière's attack.

Past Medical and Social History

The patient had a history of high blood pressure and hypercholesterolemia, which was controlled with medication. She was diagnosed with Ménière's disease when she was in her 30s and has been on diuretics. The patient denies any head trauma. The patient reports that she ate two or three hot dogs night before which she normally avoids due to high salt content. She lives with her husband and family and works as a program manager in an IT company. She also reported that she has always been sensitive to car rides and boat rides. She never was able to tolerate roller coasters.

Subjective Complaints

Patient's DHI score is 26, her symptoms are with bed mobility, looking up, and bending over. The patient had complained of spinning dizziness, which lasts for less than a minute. Her activity-specific balance confidence scale scores (ABC) is 96%.

Oculomotor and Positional Testing

- The patient had normal visual acuity 20/20 and continued to be normal with horizontal head rotations with 2 HZ.
- Gaze stabilization was normal with slow head turns and had mild complain of dizziness with fast head turns.
- Head thrust was found negative.
- Spontaneous or gaze holding was found negative at room light.
- Gaze holding and head shaking test with infrared goggles was found negative.
- Positional testing—Dix-Hallpike was positive for L side with upbeat torsional nystagmus lasting for 35 seconds. Roll test was found negative.

Balance and Gait Assessment

The patient was able to perform Romberg eyes open and eyes closed on firm surface for a minute. The patient was able to perform Romberg eyes open on foam but had difficulty performing with eyes closed. Patient's FGA was 26/30, had difficulty with walking eyes closed, looking up and down and walking with horizontal head turns.

Comments

The patient's oculomotor exam was negative, which reveals her symptoms were not due to Meniere's or due to vestibular neuritis. Patient was only positive for left Dix-Hallpike lasting less than 60 seconds suggesting left posterior canalithiasis-BPPV. Patient's difficulty with eyes closed activity and low FGA scores could possibly due to her long standing history of Ménière's causing vestibular hypofunction. She also reported about motion sensitivity, which reveals hypersensitive vestibular system. Patient reported that she ate three hot dogs a night before which she could have triggered her Meniere's symptoms causing her to have BPPV.

Problems

The following problems are observed:
- Dizziness/vertigo with bed mobility
- Fear of movement due to vertigo
- Decreased balance.

Guiding Questions:

1. What treatment protocol will be useful to the patient?
2. What plan and reassessment goals should the patient expect?

CASE STUDY 2

A 22-year-old male referred for physical therapy with diagnosis of right peripheral vestibulopathy. Patient started 2 weeks ago with cold, congestion, and sinus infection. Patient started having vertigo symptoms a week ago, which had subsided at the time of evaluation. His complaints included imbalance, especially with head movement, and a sense that his eyes "don't catch up with my head" during head movements. He complained of occasional staggers, stumbles, and side steps when walking. PMH is noncontributory. His medications included prednisone and acyclovir. He has been independent in all activities of daily living. He has not been able to drive and unable to perform his work-related duties as a construction worker.

Diagnostic Assessment

Patient's MRI and audiogram were found negative. Vestibular laboratory testing included an oculomotor screening battery, static positional testing, caloric testing, rotational testing, and posturography. Test results showed a left gaze-evoked nystagmus, a left-beating nystagmus in positional testing, a right vestibular paresis on caloric testing, a left directional preponderance on rotational testing, and abnormal posturography (abnormal response for all six sensory organization conditions and abnormal adaptation to toes-up rotation on movement coordination).

Comments

Patient's diagnostic tests revealed left-beating gaze-evoked nystagmus with left-beating nystagmus in positional testing and directional preponderance reflects right vestibular lesion.

Physical Therapy Assessment

Subjective: He rated his dizziness with head movement as a 3/10, his oscillopsia while walking as a 3/10 and his disequilibrium while walking as a 4/10 (all scores represent decrement associated with movement; score of 10 is worse). His DHI score is 42/100.

Oculomotor Examination

Oculomotor exam shows the following outcomes:

- Patient's oculomotor exam shows negative for spontaneous nystagmus. Infrared goggles assessment was positive for left-beating gaze-evoked nystagmus, and left beating on head shake test. Patient was negative for Dix-Hallpike testing.
- Patient had normal visual acuity and had three line differences with head turns at 2 HZ, suggesting abnormal dynamic visual acuity.
  - Patient had difficulty keeping target in focus with head turns with gaze stability. Positive head thrust on R side.

Balance Examination

Balance exam shows the following results:

- Patient had normal Romberg but had difficulty performing EC on firm. He was able to perform EO on foam but unable to perform with EC on foam.
- Dynamic gait index (DGI) scores were 23/24.

Guiding Questions:

1. What should be the goals for managing this patient?
2. What follow-up assessment should be done?

Review Questions

1. Explain benign paroxysmal positional vertigo (BPPV) in detail.
2. What are the tests used to Identify BPPV?
3. What are Brandt-Daroff habituation exercises?
4. Explain Ménière's disease.
5. What is vestibular ocular reflex (VOR)? How does a physio-therapist conduct vestibulo-ocular examination?
6. Describe gaze stabilization and postural stabilization exercises.

BIBLIOGRAPHY

1. Baloh R, Honrubia V. Clinical neurophysiology of the vestibular system. Philadelphia, PA: FA Davis; 1990.
2. Baloh RW, Honrubia V, Jacobson K. Benign positional vertigo. Clinical and oculographic features in 240 cases. Neurology. 1987;37:371.
3. Baloh RW. Neurotology of migraine. Headache. 1997;37(10):615-21.
4. Barany R. Diagnose von Krankheitserscheinungen im Bereiche des Otolithenapparaten. Acta Otolaryngol Stockholm. 1921;2:434-37. In: Lanska DJ, Remler B. Benign paroxysmal positioning vertigo: classic descriptions, origins of the provocative positioning technique, and conceptual developments. Neurology. 1997;48:1167.
5. Barber H, Stockwell C. Manual of electronystagmography. St Louis, MO: CV Mosby; 1976.
6. Brodal A. Neurological anatomy in relation to clinical medicine. New York, NY: Oxford Press; 1981.
7. Brodal A. Neurological anatomy in relation to clinical medicine. New York, NY: Oxford Press; 1988.
8. Casani AP, Vannucci G, Fattori B, et al. The treatment of horizontal canal positional vertigo: our experience in 66 cases. Laryngoscope. 2002;112:172.
9. Cawthorne T. The physiological basis for head exercises. J Chart Soc Physiother. 1944;30:106.
10. Cooksey FS. Rehabilitation in vestibular injuries. Proc Royal Soc Med. 1946;39:273.
11. Herdman S, Clandeil R. Vestibular rehabilitation. Philadelphia, PA: FA Davis; 2014.
12. Herdman SJ, Blatt P, Schubert MC, et al. Falls in patients with vestibular deficits. Am J Otol. 2000;21:847.
13. Herdman SJ, Tusa RJ, Zee DS, et al. Single treatment approaches to benign paroxysmal positional vertigo. Arch Otolaryngol. 1993;119:450.
14. Highstein SM. Role of the flocculus of the cerebellum in motor learning of the vestibulo-ocular reflex. Otolaryngol Head Neck Surg. 1998;119(3):212-20.
15. Hunt WT, Zimmermann EF, Hilton MP. Modifications of the Epley (canalith repositioning) manoeuvre for posterior canal benign paroxysmal positional vertigo (BPPV). Cochrane Database Syst Rev. 2012;4:CD008675. doi:10.1002/14651858. CD008675.pub2.
16. Massoud EAS, Ireland DJ. Post-treatment instructions in the nonsurgical management of benign paroxysmal positional vertigo. J Otolaryngol. 1996;25:121.
17. Nager GT. Acoustic neurinomas. Acta Otolaryngol (Stockh). 1985;99:245.
18. Nuti D, Nati C, Passali D. Treatment of benign paroxysmal positional vertigo: no need for postmaneuver restrictions. Otol Head Neck Surg. 2000;122:440.
19. Ramadan NM. Epidemiology and impact of migraine. Continuum. 2003;9:9-24.
20. Schuknecht HF, Kitamura K. Vestibular neuritis. Ann Otol Rhinol Laryngol. 1981;90(Suppl 79):1.

21. Schuknecht HF. Positional vertigo: clinical and experimental observations. Trans Am Acad Ophthalmol Otolaryngol. 1962;66:319.
22. Shumway-Cook A, Horak FB. Rehabilitation strategies for patients with vestibular deficits. Neurol Clin. 1990;8:441.
23. Standring S. Gray's anatomy, 40th edition. Elsevier; 2008. p. 1146.
24. Strupp M, Arbusow V, Maag KP, et al. Vestibular exercises improve central vestibulo-spinal compensation after vestibular neuritis. Neurology. 1998;51:838.
25. Thomsen J, Tos M, et al. Acoustic neuromas: progression of hearing impairment and function of the eighth cranial nerve. Am J Otol. 1983;5:20.

Spinal Cord Injuries

Yagna Unmesh Shukla

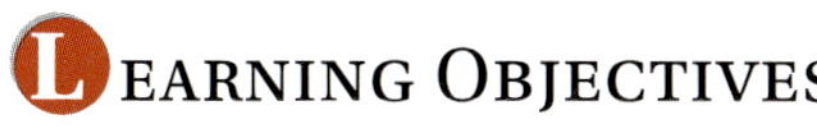 EARNING OBJECTIVES

After reading this chapter, the readers should be able to:
- Describe the etiology and clinical features of spinal cord injury
- Describe the classification of spinal cord injury as per various levels of lesions
- Identify the impairments and complications associated with spinal cord injury
- Describe assessment and test measures in patients with spinal cord injury
- Describe management and different treatment interventions associated with spinal cord injury
- Emphasize the role of rehabilitation in spinal cord injury
- Describe the assessment and management from a physiotherapy perspective along with home care and vocational options, as a rehabilitation team approach

CHAPTER OUTLINE

- Basic anatomy of spinal cord
- Causes of spinal cord injury
- Mechanism of injury
- Classification of spinal cord injury
  - Cauda equina lesions
- Clinical features of spinal cord injury
- Impairments in spinal cord injury
- Assessment and outcome measures
- Prognosis
- Rehabilitation of spinal cord injury
- Medical management of spinal cord injury
- Physiotherapy management
  - Bedside physiotherapy
  - Recovering phase
  - Role of physiotherapy in nonrecovering
  - Home modifications and advices
  - Vocational rehabilitation
- Complications of spinal cord injury
  - Bedsores
  - Deep vein thrombosis
  - Myositis ossificans
  - Renal/bladder calculi and urinary tract infection
  - Osteoporosis
  - Depression and psychosocial issues

Spinal cord injury (SCI) is a devastating event and life-threatening condition, impacting not only the life of the involved individual, but also hugely influencing the family, caregivers, and the society. It poses a serious health burden, as recognized by WHO. Its abrupt onset is tragic, and knowing the epidemiology of the problem helps in planning of resources, adequate treatment, and rehabilitation. The incidence of SCI varies from 9.2 to 56.1 per million. In India, approximately 1.5 million people live with SCI. Approximately 20,000 new cases of SCI are added each year and 60–70% of them comprise illiterate, poor villagers. Majority of them are males in the age-group of 16–30 years, signifying higher incidence in young, active, and productive population of the society.

BASIC ANATOMY OF SPINAL CORD

The spinal cord is made of soft tissues and is surrounded by bones called vertebra. SCI is damage to any part of spinal cord or nerves, which are present at the end of spinal cord. This damage may lead to permanent loss of muscle power, sensations, and bladder—bowel control below the level of lesion. Spinal cord is a long thin tubular structure, which is made up of nervous tissues. It extends from medulla oblongata in brainstem to the lumbar region of vertebral column. There is cerebrospinal fluid in the central canal of spinal cord. The brain and spinal cord comprehend to form central nervous system. The spinal cord ends between first and second lumbar vertebrae. There is protection by vertebral body surrounding the spinal cord. The length of

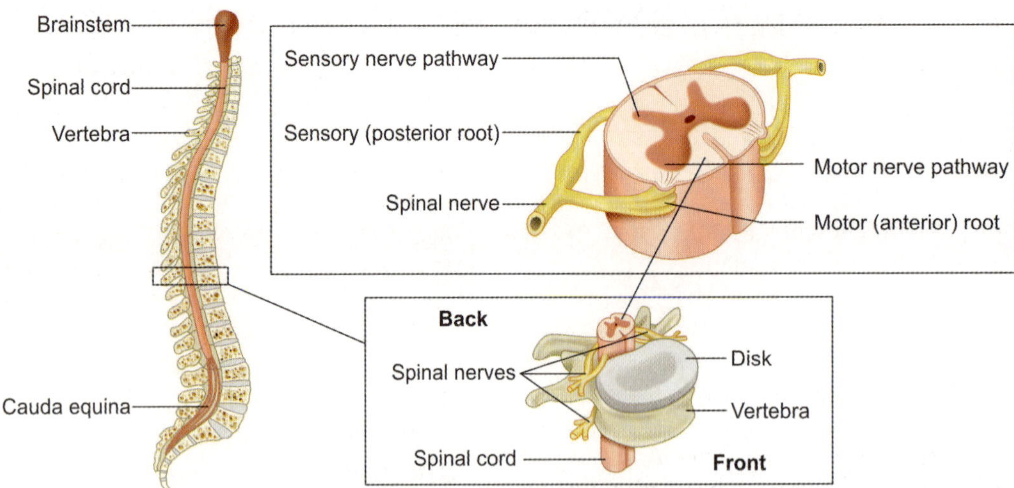

Fig. 28.1: Anatomical structure of spinal cord.

spinal cord is approximately 45 cm (18 inch) in men and 43 cm (17 inch) in women.

The diameter of spinal cord is around 13 mm (1/2 inch) in cervical and lumbar region and around 6.4 mm (1/4 inch) in thoracic region.

The spinal cord transmits nerve signals from motor cortex to different parts of the body and also sensory signals from body to sensory cortex. It also controls reflexes, thus spinal cord is a main pathway for connecting information from brain to peripheral nervous system.

Basically, spinal cord is continuation of caudal portion of medulla. It passes from the base of the skull till the body of first lumbar vertebra. There are 31 vertebral body segments from which one pair of sensory and one pair of motor nerve come out **(Fig. 28.1)**. The spinal cord is covered and protected by three layers of meninges.

1. The dura mater is outermost layer. It is a tough protective layer. The space between dura mater and vertebral bone is called epidural space. It is filled with adipose tissue and there is a network of blood vessels.
2. There is middle protective layer, which has a spider web appearance called arachnoid mater. The space between arachnoid and underlying pia mater is called subarachnoid space, which contains cerebrospinal fluid, which can be taken for examination via spinal tap procedure.
3. The inner most protective layer is pia mater, which is very delicate. In a cross section of spinal cord, the peripheral region has white matter tracts, which contain sensory and motor axons. Inner side of peripheral region is gray matter, which contains nerve cell bodies in a butterfly shape. The central region that contains cerebrospinal fluid is an extension of fourth ventricle. There are 31 pairs of spinal cord nerves in human spinal cord **(Box 28.1)**. Calculation to obtain the relation between vertebral and segmental level can be done as shown in **Table 28.1**.

Spinal cord injury causes paralysis, i.e., inability to move, whereas spinal column injury may or may not be associated with SCI. Functional abilities associated with level of lesion are illustrated in **Table 28.2**.

BOX 28.1: Spinal nerves in human body.

- Eight pairs of cervical nerves
- Twelve pairs of thoracic nerves
- Five pairs of lumbar nerves
- Five pairs of sacral nerves
- One coccygeal segment

Table 28.1: Relation between vertebral and segmental level.

Vertebral level	Segmental level
C2–C7	Add 1 for spinal segmental level
T1–T6	Add 2 for spinal segmental level
T7–T9	Add 3 for spinal segmental level
T10–T12	Add 4 for spinal segmental level
L1	This level has sacral and coccygeal segments
L2	Below this level lies cauda equina

Please note whenever lesion in spine is examined, it is always good to mention level of injury vertebra and spinal segmental level separately

---

Table 28.2: Functional abilities and level of lesion.

Level	Motor functions
C1/C2	Neck flexion/extension
C3	Neck lateral flexion
C4	Shoulder elevation
C5	Shoulder abduction
C6	Elbow flexion/wrist extension
C7	Elbow extension/wrist flexion/finger extension
C8	Finger flexion
T1	Finger abduction
L2	Hip flexion
L3	Knee extension
L4	Ankle dorsiflexion
L5	Great toe extension
S1	Ankle plantar flexion/ankle eversion/hip extension
S2	Knee flexion
S3–S4	Anal wink

CAUSES OF SPINAL CORD INJURY

Spinal cord injury can result from either traumatic or nontraumatic insults.

- **Traumatic injuries:** Direct injury results in dislocation, fracture, and fracture with dislocation of the vertebra.
    - *Accident:* Any road traffic, auto and motorcycle accidents, and earthquake are leading causes of SCI.
    - *Falls:* Fall from height such as trees, fall in well, and fall from terrace or house may cause SCI.
    - *Sports injury:* Athletic activities such as water or sky diving and horse riding may cause SCI.
    - *Stab or gunshot injury:* Around 12% of SCI are a result of stab or gunshot violent encounters.
    - *Whiplash injury:* Any trauma to cervical spine may cause hyperflexion followed by hyperextension, e.g., carrying heavy load on the head or sudden brake of vehicle causes jerk to the neck, which leads to neurological damage to spinal cord without damage to the bone.
- **Nontraumatic injuries:**
    - Tumor
    - Developmental disorders, e.g., spina bifida
    - Ischemia due to blood occlusion, e.g., emboli aneurysm, atherosclerosis
    - Demyelinating diseases, e.g., multiple sclerosis
    - Inflammatory cause
    - Fluorosis, i.e., deposition of flurosis in the spine
    - Vascular malfunctions (arteriorvenous malformations)
    - Infections, e.g., tuberculosis and transverse myelitis
    - Hysterical paralysis

MECHANISM OF INJURY

Spinal cord injury can be classified based on the mechanism of injury **(Figs. 28.2A to E)**.

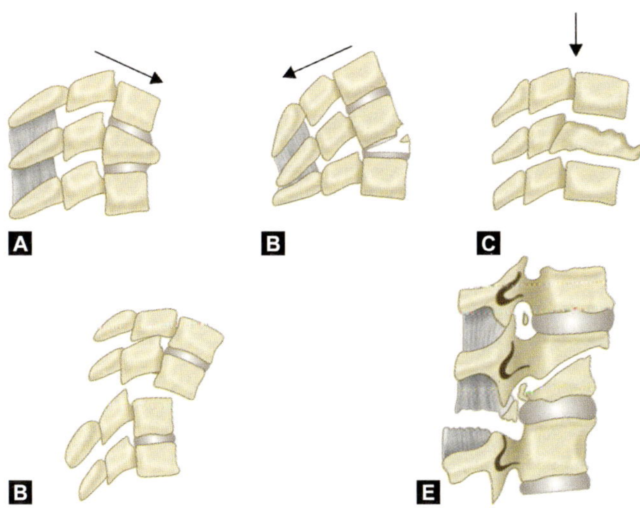

Figs. 28.2A to E: Mechanism of injury: (A) Flexion injury; (B) Extension injury; (C) Compression injury; (D) Flexion-rotation injury; (E) Flexion-distraction injury.

CLASSIFICATION OF SPINAL CORD INJURY

The classification of SCI is as follows:

- The higher the level of injury, the greater is the paralysis and loss of body functions. SCI at the level of the neck results in **tetraplegia (quadriplegia),** i.e., paralysis of all four limbs. The chest and abdomen are also affected with difficulty in breathing and coughing. Injury below the neck usually results in **paraplegia** (paralysis of the lower half of the body).
- However, the extent of injury is also defined by the completeness of injury. Total loss of function below the level of injury is **complete SCI**. No functional recovery is expected. If the spinal cord is partially damaged, signals from the brain can still cross the injured area to reach muscles and skin. This is an **incomplete injury,** and further recovery may be expected with time.
- Incomplete SCI consists of various syndromes, which are classified as per the spared function, which in an important prognostic factor and helps setting realistic rehabilitation goals **(Figs. 28.3A to D)**.

Cauda Equina Lesions

The terminal segment of the spinal cord, conus medullaris, lies at the inferior aspect of the L1 vertebrae. Complete transactions at this level are rare and incomplete lesions typically exhibit areflexia and saddle anesthesia. Cauda equina lesions are nothing but peripheral nerve injuries and hence possess the ability to regenerate just as other peripheral nerves in the body.

CLINICAL FEATURES OF SPINAL CORD INJURY

Spinal shock: It is an immediate symptom that occurs as a result of abrupt cessation of connection between brain centers and spinal cord. It is a short-term temporary physiologic disorganization of spinal cord injury function. It can start between 30 and 60 minutes following and lasts up to 3–6 weeks post-injury or sometimes extend even more. **Box 28.2** describes the stages of spinal shock. Features of spinal shock include:

- Areflexia
- Hypotonia
- Loss of sensations

The trauma causes a sudden loss of background sympathetic stimulation to blood vessels. Loss of neurogenic activities includes loss of:

- Motor
- Sensory
- Reflex
- Autonomic functions

Clinical Pearl

The first reflex to reappear is *bulbocavernosus reflex*

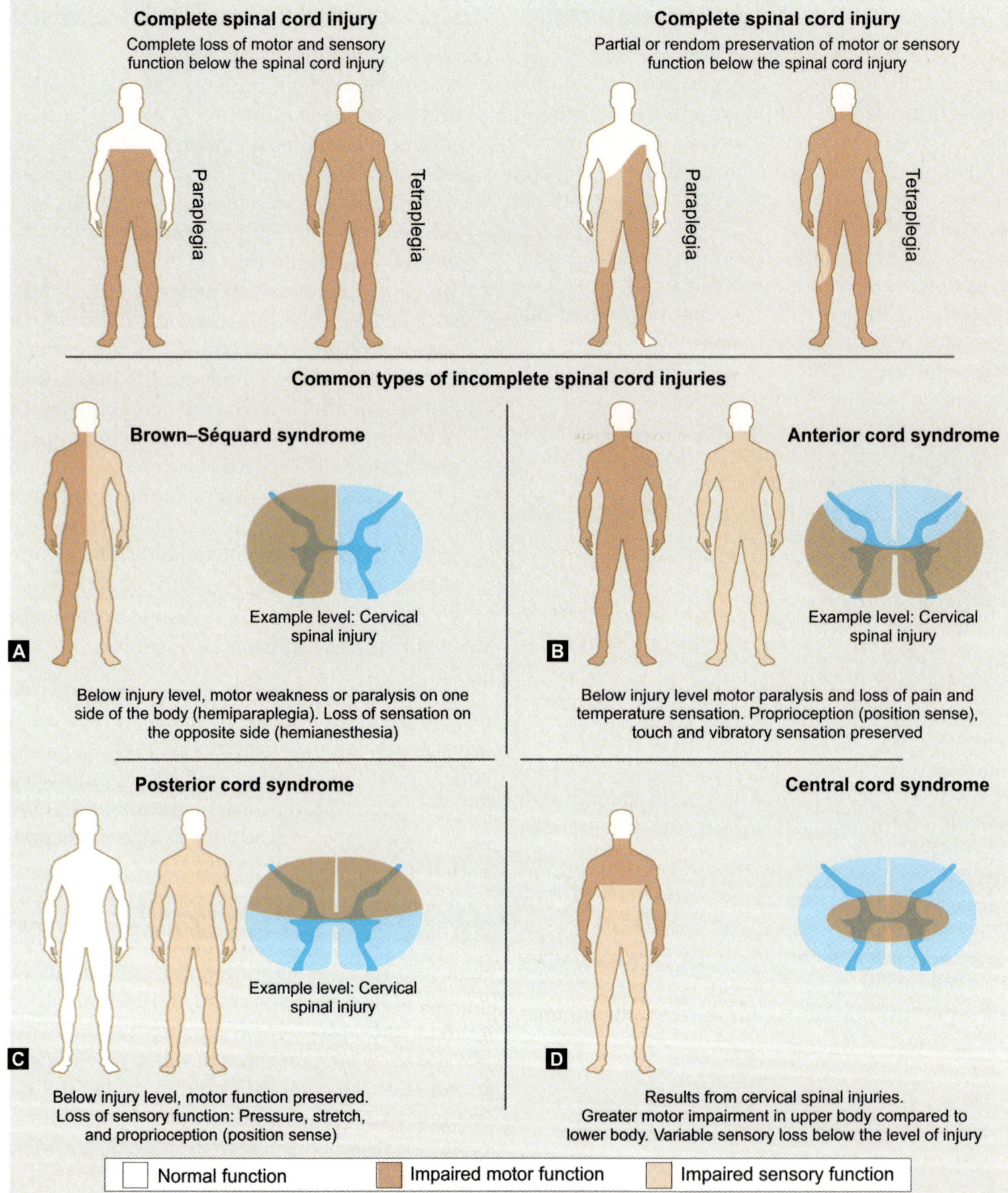

Figs. 28.3A to D: Types of spinal cord syndromes: (A) **Brown–Séquard syndrome:** Ipsilateral paralysis and contralateral loss of pain sensation; (B) **Anterior cord syndrome:** Complete paralysis and anesthesia are seen, but deep pressure and position sense are retained in the lower limbs (dorsal column sparing); (C) **Posterior cord syndrome:** Rarely occurs, only deep pressure and proprioception are lost; (D) **Central cord syndrome:** Commonest, initial flaccid weakness followed by a lower motor neuron (LMN) type of paralysis of the upper limbs and upper motor neuron (spastic) paralysis of the lower limbs, with preservation of bladder control and perianal sensations (sacral sparing).

<table>
<tr><td>

BOX 28.2: Stages of spinal shock include.

- Stage I: Weak or complete loss of all reflexes below the level of lesion. It lasts for a day
- Stage II: There is gradual return of reflex. It may occur over next 2 days
- Stage III: Patient may develop hyperreflexia with minimal stimulation

</td></tr>
</table>

IMPAIRMENTS IN SPINAL CORD INJURY

Table 28.3 shows the list of impairments and complications, which commonly present following an SCI.

Primary impairments

Following are the primary impairments:

- Bradycardia may occur due to unopposed vagal activity following SCI.

Table 28.3: Impairments in spinal cord injury.

Primary impairments	Secondary complications
Bradycardia	Autonomic dysreflexia
Loss of consciousness	Postural hypotension
Extreme backache	Pressure sores
Feeling of pressure in head, back, or neck	Contractures
Deformed or twisted neck or back	Heterotrophic ossification
Weakness or paralysis of any part of the body	Urinary tract infection/renal calculi
Numbness, tingling or loss of sensations	Osteoporosis
Loss of bladder–bowel control	Pain
Impaired breathing	Pneumonia
Difficulty in walking	Deep vein thrombosis

- The patient may or may not be conscious depending on severity and involvement of vital body parts.
- Feeling of extreme pressure in head, neck, or back is often reported.
- Deformed or twisted neck or back may be observed.
- Weakness or paralysis of any part of the body following SCI is common presentation.
- Following SCI there will be either complete (paralysis) or partial (paresis) loss of muscle function below the level of the lesion.
- Disruption of the ascending sensory fibers following SCI results in impaired or absent sensation below the level of the lesion.
- Respiratory function varies considerably, depending on the level of lesion. Paradoxical breathing pattern may be seen in those with muscle imbalance. Those with high level of lesion may have phrenic nerve involvement and loss of spontaneous respiration.
- Similarly, cardiovascular function is affected and may result in secondary complications such as autonomic dysreflexia or postural hypotension, which have been discussed in detail, later in the chapter.
- Gait and balance impairments occur as a result of abnormal tone and muscle weakness.

Bladder dysfunction: Bladder dysfunction following SCI poses a serious medical complication and requires consistent and long-term management. Urinary tract infections (UTIs) are a major cause of mortality and morbidity in people with SCI. SCI alters the complex reflexive and voluntary control of micturition. As a result, people with SCI often require a catheter to drain the bladder.

Type of bladder dysfunction depends on the level of lesion and may result in either:
- Spastic or hyperreflexic bladder or
- Flaccid or areflexic bladder **(Fig. 28.4)**.

Hyperreflexic bladder presents in upper motor neuron (UMN) lesions and areflexic is seen with lower motor neuron (LMN) lesions. The former has intact reflex arc, and detrusor muscle is generally hyperreflexive, whereas the latter has no reflex action of the detrusor muscle.

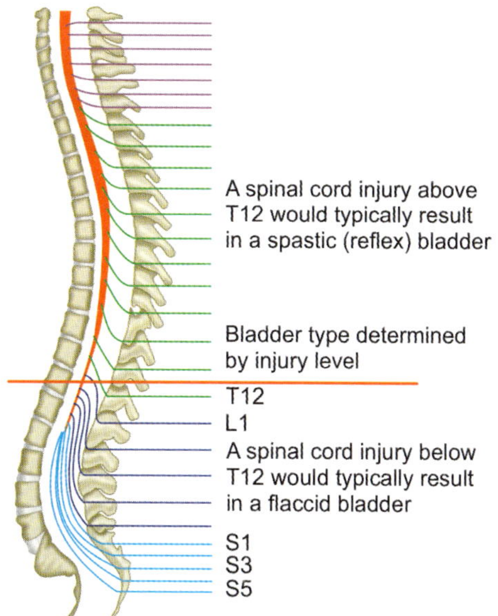

Fig. 28.4: Bladder dysfunction in spinal cord injury.

Bowel dysfunction: Bowel dysfunction in SCI is a major concern and impacts an individuals' quality of life hugely. Two main types of bowel dysfunction are:
1. Spastic or hyperreflexic bowel (UMN lesion)
2. Flaccid or areflexic bowel (LMN lesion).

Evacuation may be difficult and external pressure may be used for voiding. Valsalva maneuver or abdominal massage, manual evacuation programs, suppositories, laxatives, digital stimulation, and devices such as orthotic digital stimulator are generally used for management.

Sexual dysfunction: SCI affects the physical ability of an individual in sexuality, as well as the psychosocial aspect. Sexual response depends on the level and completeness of lesion. Males with LMN lesions have more ability to ejaculate as compared with those with UMN lesions. Erectile capacity is greater in UMN lesions than in LMN lesions and greater in incomplete lesions than in complete lesions. Female sexual responses also follow a pattern related to location of lesion. Fertility may not be affected, and menstrual cycle is interrupted for up to 4–5 months after SCI and may revert thereafter. Childbearing is possible; however, due care must be taken regarding UTIs, anemia, and venous thrombosis. Labor may be affected depending upon neurological level of lesion and hence should be closely monitored.

Secondary complications

Autonomous dysreflexia: It is a dangerous clinical symptom resulting in acute, uncontrolled hypertension. If the neurological level of SCI is at or above sixth thoracic vertebra, there is imbalance in sympathetic discharge that leads to controlled hypertension.

Clinical Pearl

Any painful irritating or even strong stimulus below the level of injury can cause an episode of autonomic dysreflexia. In 75–85% cases, bladder distension or irritation is responsible for this reflex.

If dysreflexia is not treated immediately, then it can cause:

- Seizers
- Retinal hemorrhage
- Pulmonary edema
- Renal insufficiency
- Myocardial infection
- Cerebral hemorrhage
- Death

Clinical Pearl

The role of physiotherapy in autonomous dysreflexia is to first identify the source of painful stimuli, e.g., catheter, restrictive clothing, leg straps, abdominal support, orthosis, and passive stretch. It can be prevented by proper bladder and bowel care.

Postural hypotension: Decreased blood pressure that occurs while assuming upright position is called postural or orthostatic hypotension. It results from a loss of sympathetic vasoconstriction control. Associated with this, is the edema in the lower extremity (LE). These problems can be managed with the help of:

- Compressive stockings
- Abdominal binder
- Pharmacological interventions using diuretics
- Gradual and slow progression from recumbent to vertical or erect position can minimize it.

Pressure sores: Due to constant friction, unrelieved pressure, and shearing forces, some areas of skin undergo breakdown, gradually resulting in pressure sores. They pose serious medical issue, may delay rehabilitation, and occasionally may even result in death. Bony prominences are more prone to undergo this risk, since they are subjected to excessive pressure. Prevention is the most important intervention in their management and involves a coordinated approach by all team members involved in the care of SCI patient.

Contractures: Contractures occur secondary to prolonged shortening of structures across and around a joint, resulting in limited range of motion (ROM). Some of the risk factors associated with occurrence of contractures are:

- Loss of active muscle control
- Spasticity
- Prolonged bed rest
- Improper positioning

All joints are at an equal risk, and occasionally contractures may be painful, resulting in other complications such as skin breakdown. To aid in maintaining ROM and preventing contractures, the following can be done:

- ROM exercises
- Positioning
- Splinting

Heterotrophic ossification (HO): Osteogenesis in soft tissues, usually near joints, below the level of the lesion is known as HO. There is no known cause; however, factors associated with HO include:

- Complete injury
- Trauma
- Severe spasticity
- Urinary tract infection (UTI)
- Pressure sores.

  It most commonly occurs in the hip and knee joints.

Early symptoms of HO are:

- Swelling
- Joint and muscle pain
- Decreased ROM
- Erythema
- Local warmth near a joint

It can result in contractures, pressure sores, and impaired mobility and ability to perform activities of daily living (ADLs). Management involves pharmacological options, surgery, and physiotherapy.

Clinical Pearl

Care should be taken while performing passive range of motion. If it is too vigorous, it may cause trauma, which may be a causative factor for heterotrophic ossification.

Osteoporosis, UTI, and renal calculi: Significant loss of bone mineral density (BMD) may occur, resulting in osteoporosis. Although the exact etiology is not clear, the reduction in BMD is thought to be mainly due to the combination of no (or limited) muscle action and limited (or no) weight bearing.

Due to imbalance in the bone formation and resorption, renal calculi may occur. UTIs are also common in individuals with SCI, due to catheterization, risk of renal calculi, and lack of adequate hygiene.

Pain: Chronic pain is a common finding in individuals with SCI. It may be of neuropathic or nociceptive origin. Causative factors may be:

- Poor posture
- Muscle overuse
- Decreased flexibility
- Incorrect positioning in bed
- Overuse stress injuries due to wheelchair propulsion are also common.

  Neuropathic pain may be of central or peripheral origin and is particularly challenging to treat. It may be treated with approaches similar to those used in the treatment of chronic pain.

Respiratory complications: Pneumonia and atelectasis can occur as a result of inability to clear secretions from the chest. Paralysis or weakness of muscles may result in impaired ventilation and inability to cough will cause accumulation of secretions. Respiratory complications may sometimes result in death of an individual.

Deep vein thrombosis (DVT): Due to lack of mobility and active muscle contraction of the LEs, stasis and hypercoagulability may occur, resulting in DVT. DVT is most likely to occur during the acute stage of recovery, has the potential to convert into emboli, and may pose a life-threatening risk. Thrombus results in inflammation (thrombophlebitis) with characteristic clinical features of local swelling, erythema, and heat. Management chiefly consists of prevention, and nonpharmacological interventions include early mobilization, compression stockings and boots, and pneumatic compression sleeves.

ASSESSMENT AND OUTCOME MEASURES

Assessment of a patient with SCI of is usually done as clinical examination. Few outcome measures can also be used for making the outcomes more objective and can also be useful in documentation, research, and follow-up.

American Spinal Cord Injury Association (ASIA) scale is commonly used to decide the level of injury. The level of injury, severity of affection, and classification of SCI is always confusing, which is why ASIA tried to standardize the language to describe SCI **(Fig. 28.5)**. According to ASIA, SCI can be categorized into five different types of injuries as shown in **Box 28.3**.

It is extremely important to determine the neurological level, which is the most caudal level of the spinal cord, with normal motor and sensory function on both sides of the body. Motor and sensory levels are determined to decide the neurological level. Motor level is the most caudal segment of spinal cord with normal motor function bilaterally and is determined by testing the key muscles, at myotomes adjacent to the suspected level of impairment **(Box 28.4)**. They are rated on a 6-point ordinal scale, ranging from 0 to 5. Sensory level is the most caudal segment of spinal cord, with normal sensory function bilaterally, and is determined by testing the patient's sensitivity to light touch and pinprick on both sides. It is rated on an ordinal scale ranging from 0 to 2, where 0 is absent, 1 is impaired, and 2 is normal **(Fig. 28.6)**.

Sometimes, it is seen that the motor and sensory levels on each of the body may differ significantly in terms of function. In such cases, assigning a single neurological level would seem inappropriate and sensory and motor level may need to be documented separately **(Table 28.4)**.

Nurick scale (Table 28.5): It is based on difficulty in walking scale and most widely used disease-specific severity scale for grading the degree of functional impairment in cervical spondylotic myelopathy.

Various standardized outcome measures can be documented in individuals with SCI. Commonly used tests and measures are mentioned in **Table 28.6**.

PROGNOSIS

Recovering from SCI is a challenging journey and most patients and their families are primarily concerned with this aspect. Predicting the potential for recovery is related to extent of lesion, neurological level of lesion, and completeness of lesion. Following spinal shock, if the sensory and motor components are absent, the lesion is usually considered complete and is a poor

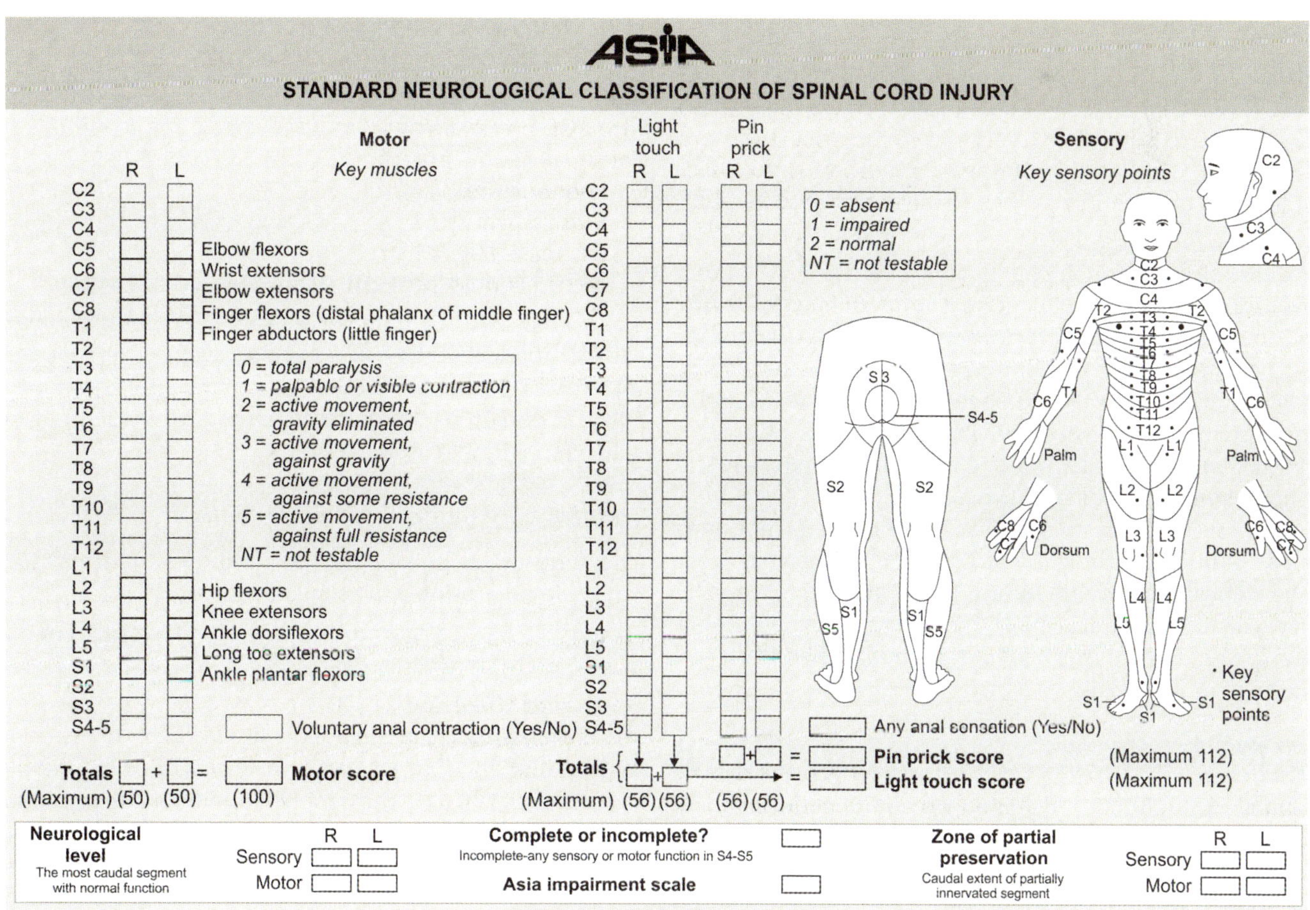

Fig. 28.5: ASIA Impairment Scale.

<table>
<tr><td>

BOX 28.3: ASIA Impairment Scale grades.

A. **Complete:** No sensory or motor function is preserved in the sacral segments S4–S5.
B. **Incomplete:** Sensory but not motor function is preserved below the neurological level and includes the sacral segments S4–S5.
C. **Incomplete:** Motor function is preserved below the neurological level, and more than half of key muscles below the neurological level have a muscle grade less than 3.
D. **Incomplete:** Motor function is preserved below the neurological level, and at least half of key muscles below the neurological level have a muscle grade greater than or equal to 3.
E. **Normal:** Sensory and motor function is normal.

</td><td>

BOX 28.4: Key muscle to be tested to determine motor level.

1. C5: Elbow flexors (biceps, brachialis)
2. C6: Wrist extensors (extensor carpi radialis and brevis)
3. C7: Elbow extensors (triceps)
4. C8: Finger flexors (flexor digitorum profundus) to the middle finger
5. T1: Small finger abductors (abductor digiti minimi)
6. L2: Hip flexors (iliopsoas)
7. L3: Knee extensors (quadriceps)
8. L4: Ankle dorsiflexors (tibialis anterior)
9. L5: Long toe extensors (extensor hallucis longus)
10. S1: Ankle plantar flexors (gastrocnemius, soleus)

</td></tr>
</table>

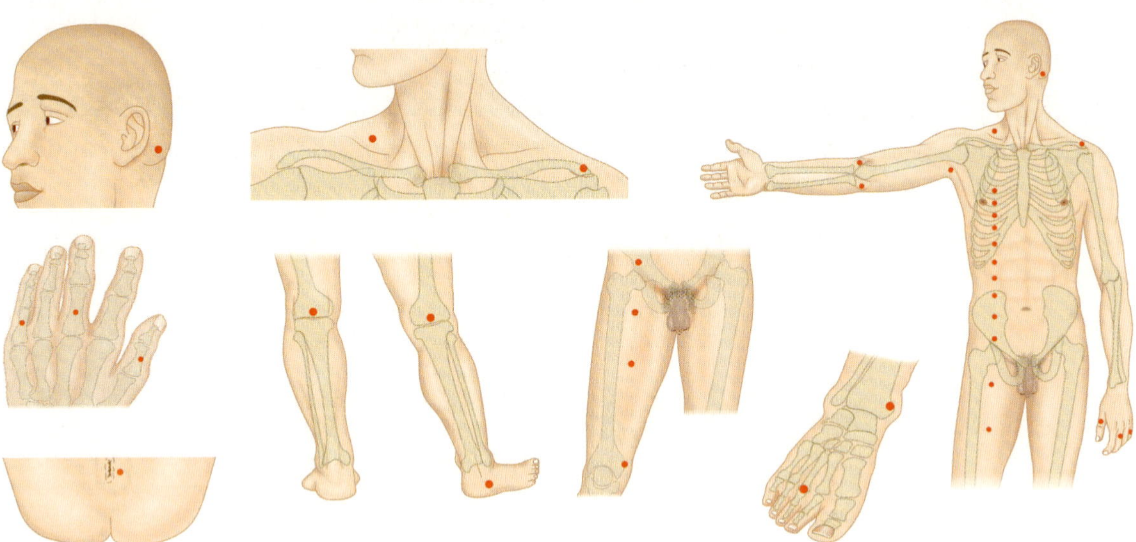

Fig. 28.6: Sensory key points to determine sensory level.

prognostic indicator. Incomplete lesions are good, in that the improvement begins almost immediately following the period of spinal shock. Motor recovery is good in incomplete lesions and ambulation is also better. Eighty percent of individuals with incomplete paraplegia regain antigravity hip flexors and knee extensors at 1 year. Individuals with no LE motor control at 1 month may still show significant return by 1 year.

Apart from this, radiological and diagnostic measures play an important role in confirming the prognosis, after the clinical assessment. Injuries, such as bilateral cervical facet dislocation, transcanal bullet injuries, thoracolumbar flexion rotation injuries, and intramedullary hemorrhages, carry poor prognosis.

REHABILITATION OF SPINAL CORD INJURY

Spinal cord injury is a debilitating condition and requires a meticulous effort from various medical health professionals. A multidisciplinary approach by a rehabilitation team is recommended. **Table 28.7** shows members of the rehabilitation team and their roles in rehabilitation.

Medical Management of Spinal Cord Injury

The spinal cord segment serves very specific motor and sensory regions of the body. Each segment of spinal cord innervates particular area of skin. After any trauma to spine, a person needs immediate medical evaluation to rule out possibility of spinal injury.

Treatment of Spinal Cord Injury Patient

The time taken between injury and treatment can be critical in determining the expected recovery.

Once injury occurs, the following protocol is necessary:
- Not to move the injured person
- Call for "108" (India)
- Ask the person not to move at all
- Stabilize the injured part with the help of any thick, firm material until the patient is shifted to the hospital.
- Basic first aid treatment of bleeding, pain, and distress needs to be taken care of.
- Shifting has to be done like log of wood (i.e., without twisting or bending of spine).

Table 28.4: Sensory key points for examination.

Spinal segments	Corresponding body areas
C2	Occipital protuberance
C3	Supraclavicular fossa
C4	Top of the acromioclavicular joint
C5	Lateral side of the antecubital fossa
C6	Thumb
C7	Middle finger
C8	Little finger
T1	Medial side of antecubital fossa
T2	Apex of axilla
T3	Third IC spine
T4	Fourth IC space (nipple line)
T5	Fifth IC space (midway between T4 and T6)
T6	Sixth IC space (xiphisternum)
T7	Seventh IC space (midway between T6 and T8)
T8	Eighth IC space (midway between T6 and T10)
T9	Ninth IC space (midway between T8 and T 10)
T10	Tenth IC space (umbilicus)
T11	Eleventh IC space (midway between T10 and T12)
T12	Inguinal ligament at midpoint
L1	Half the distance between T12 and L2
L2	Midanterior thigh
L3	Medial femoral condyle
L4	Medial malleolus
L5	Dorsum of the foot at third metatarsophalangeal joint
S1	Lateral heel
S2	Popliteal fossa in the midline
S3	Ischial tuberosity
S4 and S5	Perianal area (taken as one level)

(IC: intercostal)

Table 28.5: Nurick scale.

Grading	Nurick clinical scale
Grade 0	Signs and symptoms of root involvement but without evidence of spinal cord disease
Grade 1	Sign of spinal cord disease but no difficulty walking
Grade 2	Slight difficulty in walking which does not prevent full-time employment
Grade 3	Extreme difficulty in walking that requires assistance and prevents full time employment and occupation
Grade 4	Able to walk only with someone else's help or with the aid of a walker
Grade 5	Chair bound or bedridden

Table 28.6: Outcome measures and tests commonly used in spinal cord injury (SCI).

Variable	Tests and measures
Arousal, attention, and cognition	MMSE
Motor function	MAS
Muscle performance	ASIA, handheld dynamometer, and MMT
Pain	VAS, NPRS, ISCI basic pain data set, Multi-dimensional Pain Inventory, and SCI version
Function	FIM, SCIM III, and QIF
Balance	BBS and TUG
Gait, locomotion	SCI-FAI, Wheelchair Skills Test, WISCI
Aerobic capacity	VC and 6-MAT
Skin	Braden scale
Quality of life	SF-36, SF-12, SIP68, WHOQOL-BREF scale, PQOL, SWLS, QLI, and Global QOL
Community and leisure	CHART and CIQ

(6-MAT: 6-minute arm test; ASIA: American Spinal Cord Injury Association; BBS: Berg Balance Scale; CHART: Craig Handicap Assessment and Reporting Technique; CIQ: Community Integration Questionnaire; FIM: Functional Independence Measure; ISCI: International Spinal Cord Injury; MAS: Modified Ashworth Scale; MMSE: Mini Mental State Examination; MMT: manual muscle test; NPRS: Numeric Pain Rating Scale, PQOL: Perceived Quality of Life; QIF: Quadriplegia Index of Function; QLI: Quality of Life Index; SCI: spinal cord injury; SCI-FAI: Spinal Cord Injury Functional Ambulation Inventory; SCIM III: Spinal Cord Independence Measure III; SF-12: Short-Form 12; SF-36: Short-Form 36; SIP68: Sickness Impact Profile; SWLS: Satisfaction with Life Scale; TUG: Timed Up and Go; VAS: visual analog scale; VC: vital capacity; WHOQOL-BREF: World Health Organization Quality of Life-BREF; WISCI: Walking Index for SCI)

Surgical Management

Surgical management includes the following:

- Reduction and immobilization can be achieved through conservative as well as surgical methods.
- Closed reduction is done with use of traction devices, whereas open reduction is done and stabilized using plate or rod fixation.
- Unstable fractures of spine do require surgical management in order to minimize the risk of further neurological damage.
- Bone grafting, decompression surgeries, and fusion procedures are done in situations where there is a risk of neural element being involved.
- Stable fractures may be treated conservatively and then prescribed an appropriate spinal orthosis.
- Surgeries are also done in the presence of secondary complications such as pressure sores of severe grade.

Table 28.7: Rehabilitation team for management of spinal cord injury.

Team member	Role
Orthopedic surgeon	Performs the surgical process of stabilization of spinal fractures
Neurological surgeon	Decompression of neural elements
Physiotherapist	Evaluation and treatment through postsurgical and conservative management phase, wheelchair and assistive device training, and long-term rehabilitation
Occupational therapist	Evaluation and treatment through postsurgical and conservative management phase and training in activities of daily living
Rehabilitation nurse	In-patient care of the patient, nursing, dressing, and hygiene needs of the patient
Orthotist	Prescription, measurement, and fabrication and fitting of spinal and lower limb orthosis
Psychologist	Counseling of the patient, motivating, and coping through impact of SCI
Nephrologist	In managing patients for prevention and management of secondary complications such as renal calculi
Urologist	Preventing and managing urinary tract infections and catheterizing patients with bladder dysfunction
Plastic surgeon	Grafting of skin, especially in the case of pressure sores; and also in bone graft procedures in patients with unstable spinal fractures
Social worker	Counseling and coordinating with NGOs, GOs, agencies, and community for welfare of patients with SCI
Vocational counselor	Identifying the capacity, educating and training with vocational skills, placement in the appropriate vocation
Nutritionist	Providing advices on maintenance of healthy weight and dietary choices

(SCI: spinal cord injury; NGOs: non-governmental organization)

PHYSIOTHERAPY MANAGEMENT

Physiotherapy protocol is mainly divided into three phases:
1. Bedside physiotherapy
2. Recovering phase physiotherapy
3. Chronic phase/nonrecovering phase physiotherapy

Bedside Physiotherapy

Bedside physiotherapy involves preserving function, airway clearance, and prevention of complications such as pressure sores, contractures, and improving the psychological status of the patient.

In the acute stage, patient is usually managed with:
- Steroids
- Bed rest
- Analgesics
- Traction

The goals of rehabilitation during this acute stage include:
- Prevention of joint contractures and deformities
- Improvement of muscle and respiratory functions
- Prevention of secondary complications

Psychological Support

Rehabilitation in SCI is long and challenging. It is important to explain the course of recovery along with possible outcomes. Patients, their family, and caregivers should be explained about the expectations and psychological support should be adequately provided whenever needed. Understanding all the consequences and aspects associated with SCI is essential. They can also be referred to a clinical psychologist if need be.

Chest Physiotherapy

This involves:
- Maintenance of lung hygiene
- Maximizing ventilation
- Preventing tightness of thoracic cage
- Utilizing effective breathing strategies

Mechanical ventilator support is given to patients with higher level lesion, involving diaphragm. Invasive mechanical ventilation is done through a tracheostomy, whereas noninvasive positive pressure ventilation provides an alternative to invasive mechanical ventilation.

To aid in the preservation of respiratory status, the following techniques can be used **(Figs. 28.7A and B)**:
- Diaphragmatic breathing techniques
- Glossopharyngeal breathing
- Coughing
- Respiratory muscle training
- Chest proprioceptive neuromuscular fascilitation (PNF)
- Assistive devices such as abdominal binder

Passive Movements

Maintaining adequate ROM is one key responsibility of a physiotherapist. Unless contraindicated, they should be carried out several times during the day **(Figs. 28.8A to D)**. Adequate care should be taken to avoid undue movements that may impede the healing process or disrupt the integrity of bony or neural elements.

Clinical Pearl

Full range of motion in all joints may not be required, and allowing tightness in some muscle is rather beneficial to the patient. Hence, selective stretching should be done, and alignment should be maintained across some joints to keep them in a functionally useful state.

Strengthening of Unaffected Muscles

All innervated muscles need to be strengthened maximally. SCI patients will have to rely on assistive devices and

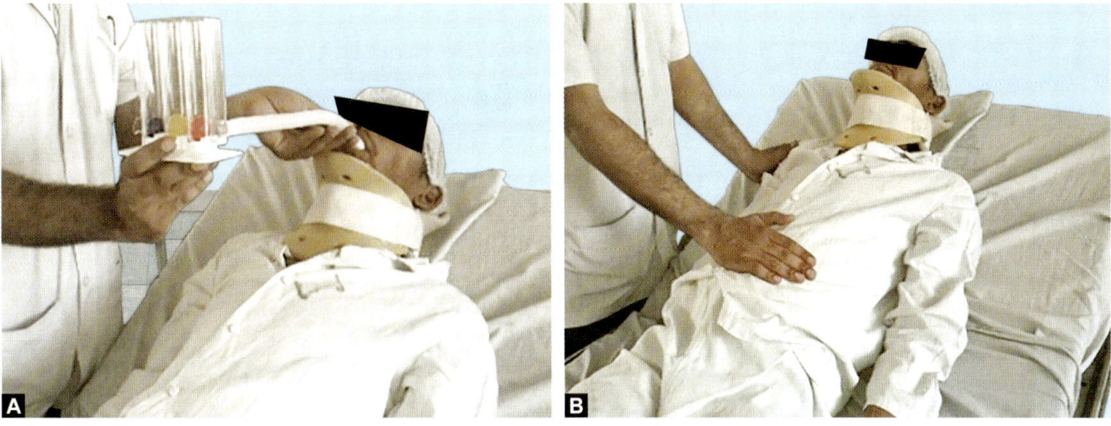

Figs. 28.7A and B: In-patient chest physiotherapy.

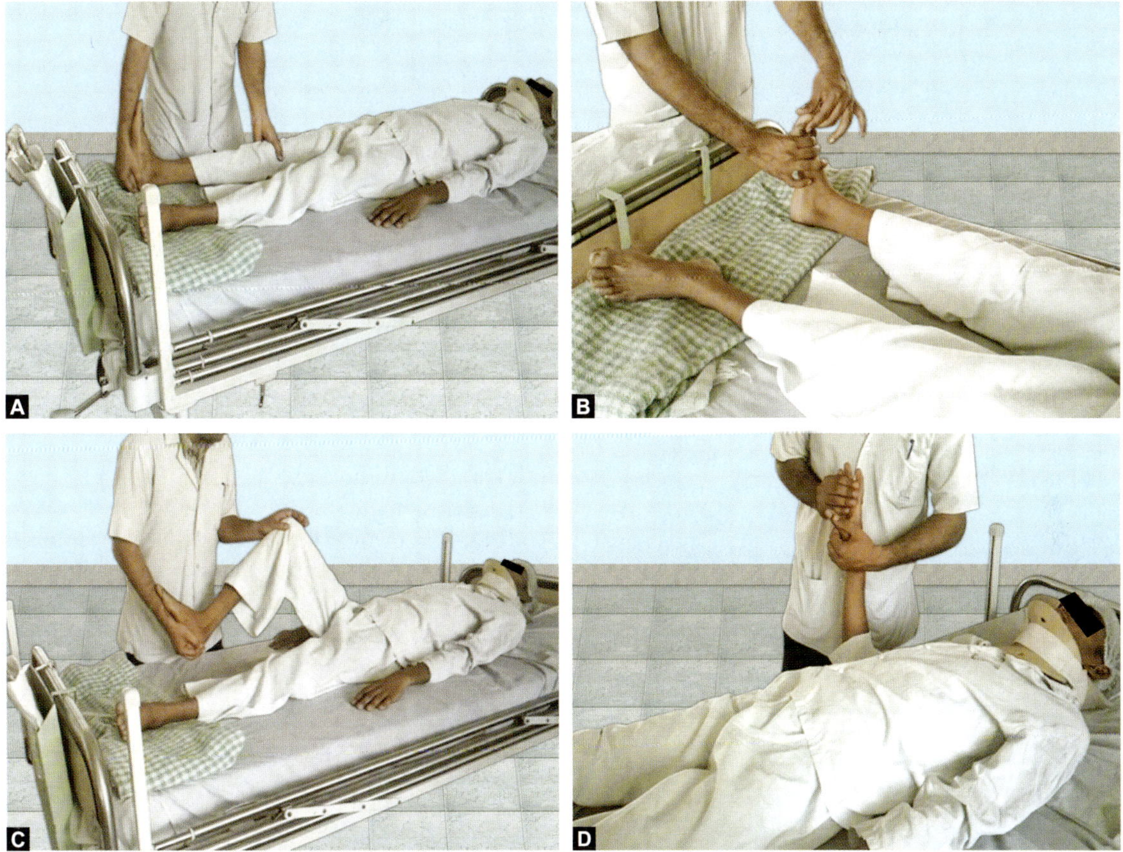

Figs. 28.8A to D: Passive range of motion exercises.

orthoses, during their course of rehabilitation; hence, strengthening should be targeted to such needs **(Figs. 28.9A to D)**. Upper extremity (UE) muscles, as well as, scapular and trunk muscles need to be strengthened. UE muscles that need to be strengthened include:

- Serratus anterior
- Latissimus dorsi
- Pectoralis major
- Rotator cuff muscles
- Triceps brachii

These are important for independent transfer. Due care should be taken to avoid undue stress of fracture sites while resisting any muscle.

Prevention of Bedside Complications

This is an important aspect, and a key role for a physiotherapist to take care of. Most bedside complications such as pressure sores and contractures can be prevented. Positioning prevents development of joint contractures, and also pulmonary complications. Pillows, foams, and positioning devices can be used. Specialized beds such as air beds or water beds can be used. Gloves filled with water or gel can be used if resources are unavailable **(Fig. 28.10)**.

Recovering Phase

After bedside treatment, rehabilitation starts with **tilt table mobilization** (TTM), which prevents orthostatic

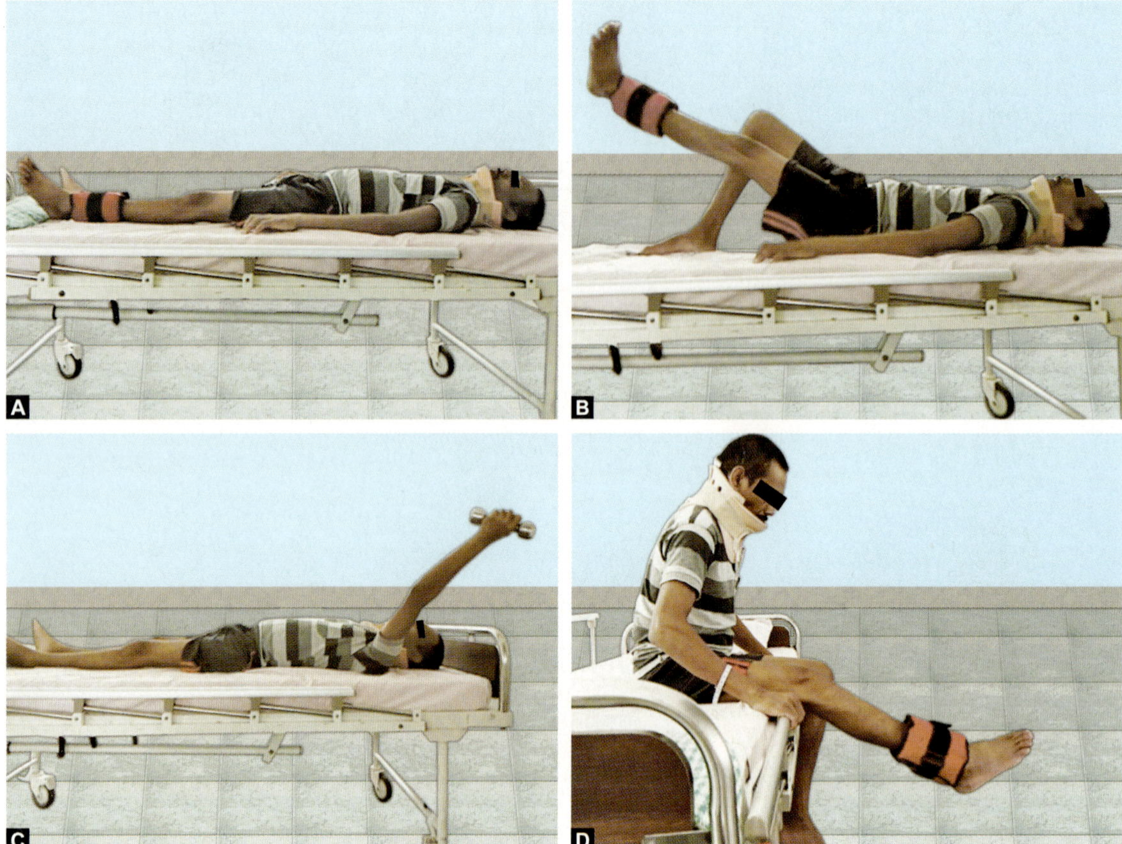

Figs. 28.9A to D: Strengthening exercises.

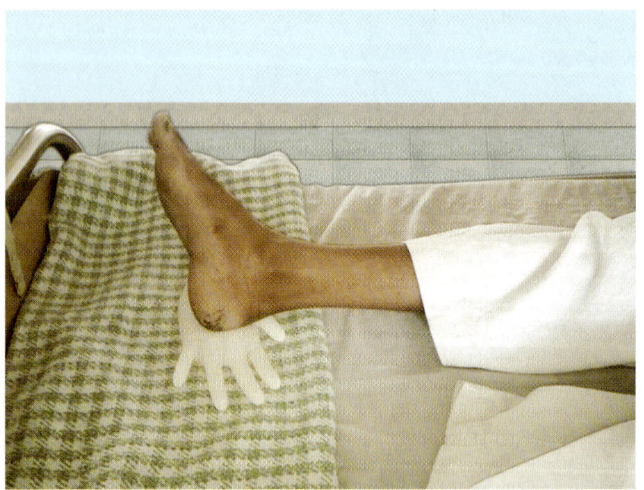

Fig. 28.10: Use of surgical glove filled with water for pressure sore relief.

Mat Exercises

Preparing the patient for independent mobility requires a great deal of motor training. Mat programs should be initiated progressing the patient from rolling to various higher tasks such as sitting **(Figs. 28.12A to C)**. PNF techniques can also be added to exercises, splitting the whole task into subcomponents is the other approach that can facilitate the mobility skills.

Transfer Activities

Transfer from bed to/from wheelchair in a seated position is known as sit-pivot transfer and is divided into three phases: preparatory, lift, and descent. Hand position is very important in transfers and head–hip relationship should be secured correctly. Use of push-up blocks and wrist cuffs can be made to facilitate transfer training. Transfers to/from toilet seat also need to be included in training. Floor to wheelchair transfers, although rare, should be considered and taught accordingly **(Figs. 28.13A to E)**.

Strengthening Exercises

Similar to previous phase, strengthening needs to be incorporated in this phase also. It is important for independent transfers.

- Strengthening exercises should be performed two to four times a week, performing 2–3 sets of 8–12 repetitions at 60–80% of 1 RM.

hypertension **(Figs. 28.11A to C)**. There is gradual weight on spine and limbs. Patients develop confidence. The progress on tilt table is usually 10–15° per day. Sometimes fast TTM is advised so daily patient is kept on progress of 30°, depending on the protocol advised by an orthopedic surgeon. Once patient is allowed sitting, rehabilitation is started with mat exercises, transfer activities, and strengthening with various techniques such as arm ergometer, standing, and balance and gait training.

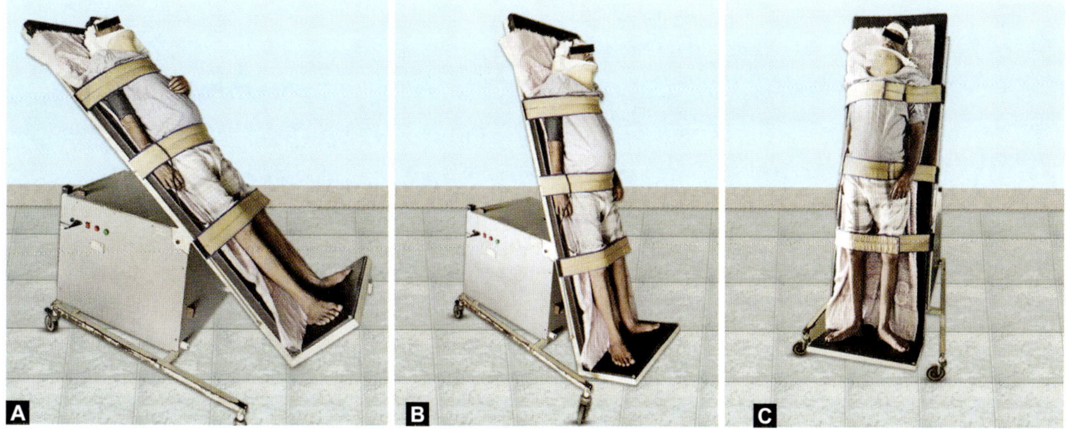

Figs. 28.11A to C: Tilt table mobilization.

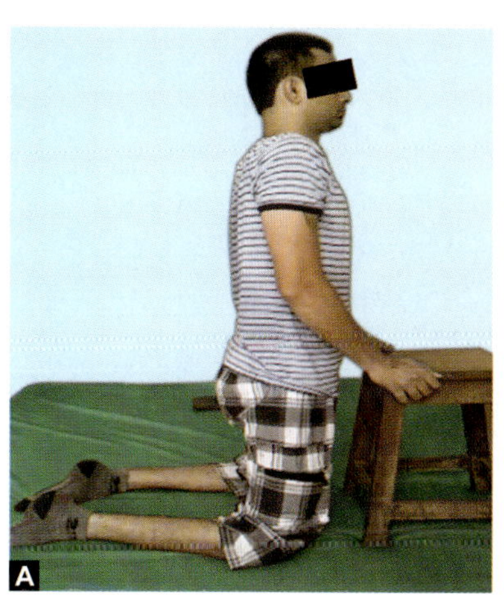 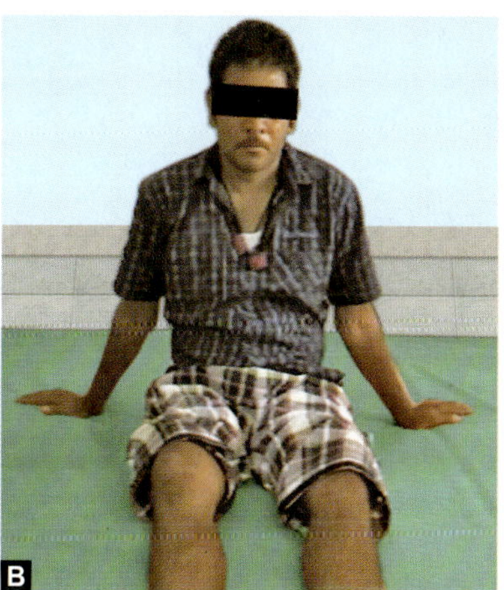 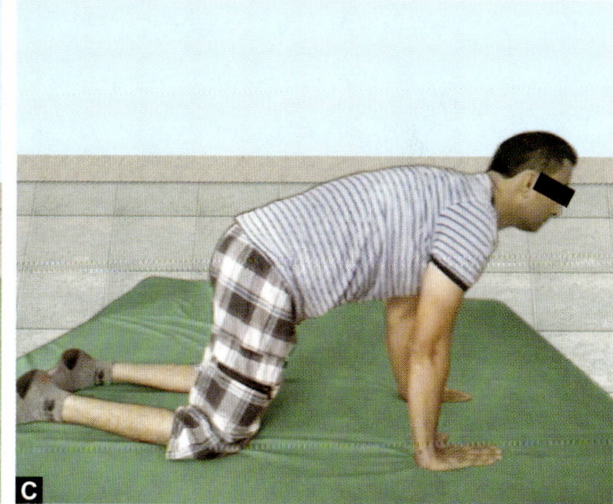

Figs. 28.12A to C: Mat exercises.

- Initially, strengthening exercises may be done daily during early rehabilitation.
- A variety of methods can be used to implement strengthening exercises: pulley systems, free weights, elastic bands, and weight cuffs.
- With very weak muscles (grade ≤2) strengthening can be performed in gravity-reduced positions on a powder board or with active assistive ROM.
- Strengthening can be done in functional postures as well.
- Use of arm ergometer is a means of strengthening as well as developing aerobic endurance in patients with SCI **(Fig. 28.14)**. Speed and resistance can be controlled and heart rate is monitored simultaneously. It also provides a feedback to the patient, which may encourage them to perform better.

Aerobic Training

American College of Sports Medicine recommends endurance training

- 3–5 days a week
- With a total duration per day of 20–60 minutes
- At 50–80% of peak heart rate

- Swimming, arm cycling, and wheelchair propulsion are some ways of challenging the cardiovascular system and developing endurance.

Locomotor training with or without body weight support also helps in endurance training. Since the patient is mostly bedridden during acute rehabilitation phase, their deconditioning effect is large and slightest effort in the form of gait training will also train the aerobic capacity.

Balance Exercises

Sitting balance will largely depend on the level of lesion. Independent sitting balance in short and long sitting is trained first, following which progression is made on various surfaces such as firm mat, bed, and soft foam. Balance on wheelchair should also be trained, since later in community reentry, they will have to face uneven terrains, surfaces, slopes, and even public places that may be crowded. Medicine balls, dumbbells can be added to further challenge the balance.

Standing

Tilt table or standing frames can be used in patients with SCI. Orthosis, such as posterior knee guards, toe-rising

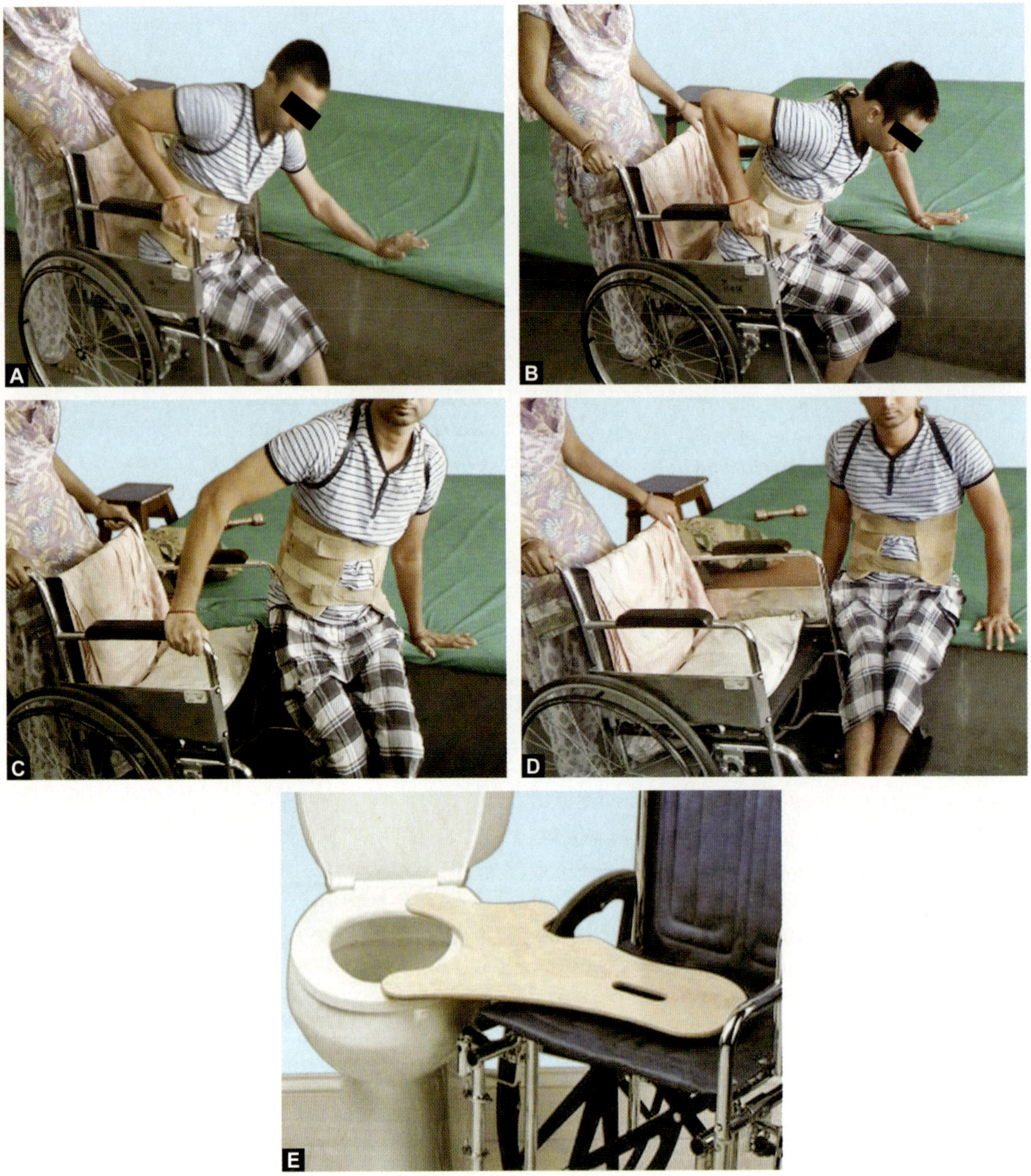

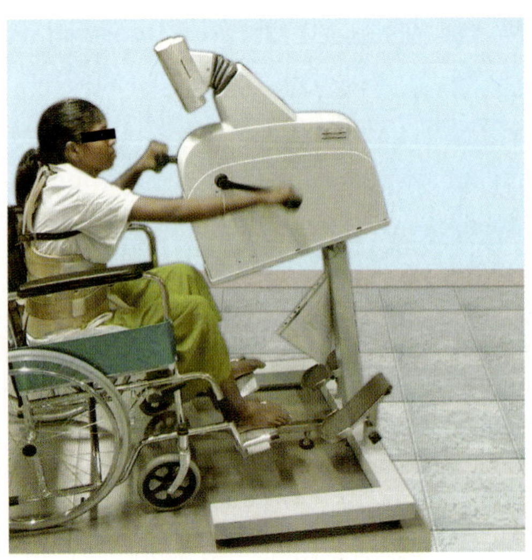

Figs. 28.13A to E: Transfer activities.

Fig. 28.14: Arm ergometer.

splints, stabilizing boots, and Craig–Scott orthoses, can be used, to aid in standing **(Figs. 28.15A and B)**. Standing lessens the risk of hypercalciuria, bone loss and also aids pressure relief while providing weight bearing on joints of spine and LE. However, it should be proceeded with cautions, especially in patients with postural hypotension and autonomic dysreflexia.

Gait Training

Locomotor training is essential for independence of the patient as well as, for preventing complications such as osteoporosis, reducing spasticity, aiding in bowel–bladder function, and it also aids in gaining the psychological benefits such as confidence, and building self-image. Various techniques work in gait training are:

- Body weight supported treadmill training
- Gait trainer with harness **(Fig. 28.16A)**

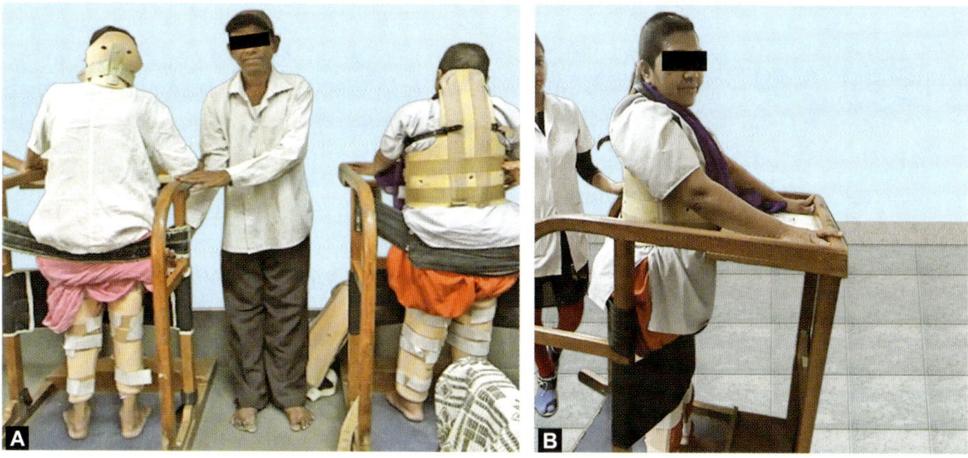

Figs. 28.15A and B: Standing frames used in patients with spinal cord injury.

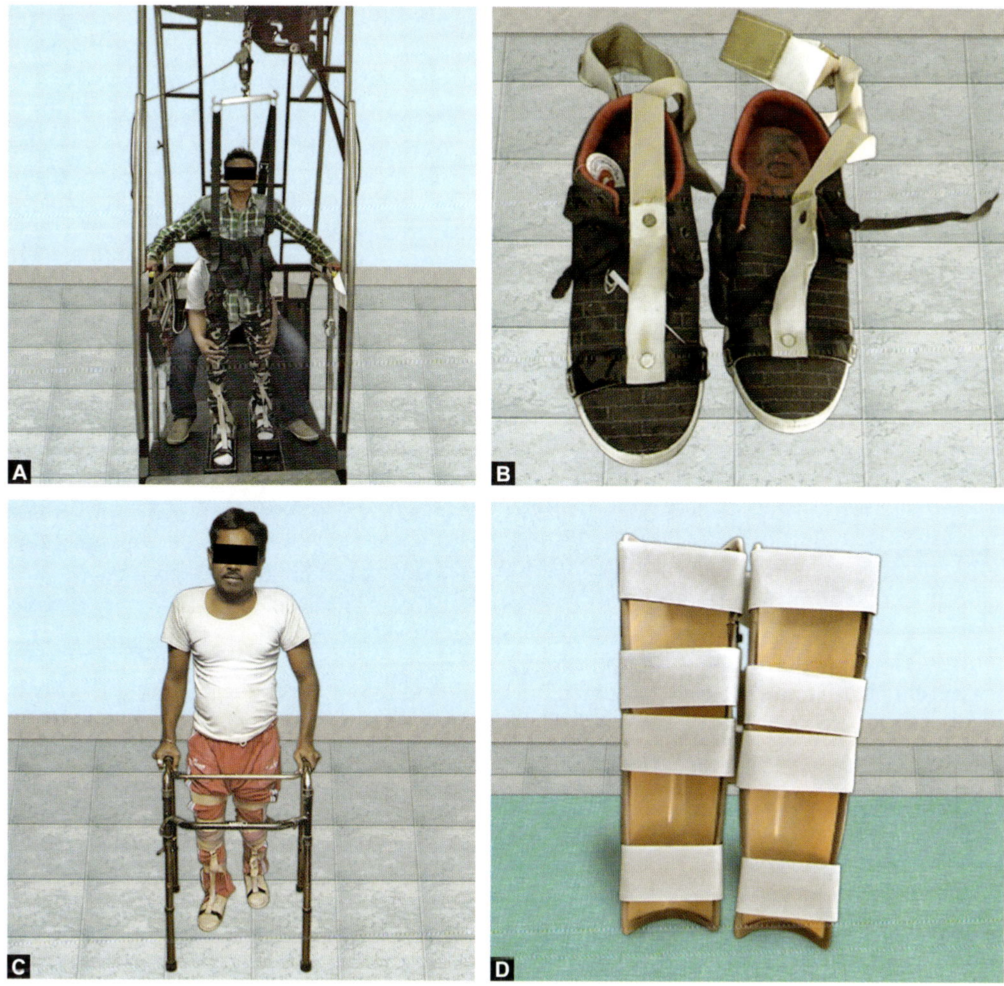

Figs. 28.16A to D: Assistive devices and orthoses commonly used in spinal cord injury patients: (A) Gait trainer with harness; (B) Toe-rising splint; (C) Walker; (D) Posterior knee guard.

- Robotics (Lokomat, Hocoma AG)
- Functional electrical stimulation
- Orthosis can also be provided to assist in ambulation. Knee-ankle-foot orthoses (KAFOs), hip-knee-ankle-foot orthoses (HKAFOs), reciprocating gait orthoses (RGOs), and para-walkers are some widely used options **(Figs. 28.16B to D)**.
- Walking in parallel bars followed by walking with assistive devices such as walkers or crutches should be incorporated in rehabilitation of SCI patients.

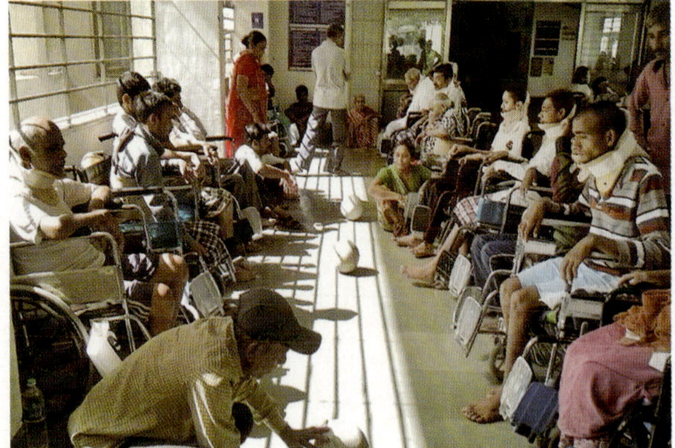

Fig. 28.17: Group therapy enhances confidence and reduces psychological impact of trauma.

Apart from this, patients who have a potential to recover can also be taught the use of ramps, public transportation, and community ambulation. Those who are having poor prognosis should be taught compensatory management strategies, which can preserve the available functions. Group therapy, bowel–bladder management, and wheelchair training are particularly more useful for this set of population **(Fig. 28.17)**. Hydrotherapy has also been shown to have benefits, but due care should be taken in patients at risk/having osteoporosis **(Figs. 28.18A and B)**.

Bladder Management

In early stages of recovery, bladder is flaccid and an **indwelling catheter** is inserted **(Fig. 28.19A)**. Later when the patient is stable during rehabilitation, **intermittent catheterization** is used. Intermittent catheterization is the most common method of bladder management after discharge from the rehabilitation hospital, many males switch to the use of an external, condom catheter. **Self-catheterization** can also be used in some individuals **(Figs. 28.19B and C)**.

- **Flaccid** bladder can be managed by *timed voiding* programs and can be done after establishing a pattern of incontinence in the patient.
- **Spastic** bladder can be managed by the *suprapubic tapping*, in which tapping is done over the bladder with the finger tips. This stimulates the detrusor muscles.
- **Areflexic** bladder can be managed with *Crede's method,* which is done by gently pressing down on the bladder, or *Valsalva maneuver*, which involves leaning forward to increase pressure in the abdomen, thus triggering the detrusor muscles. Other techniques of bladder stimulation include lower abdominal stroking, pinching or hair pulling, clamping of catheter or use of suprapubic catheter.

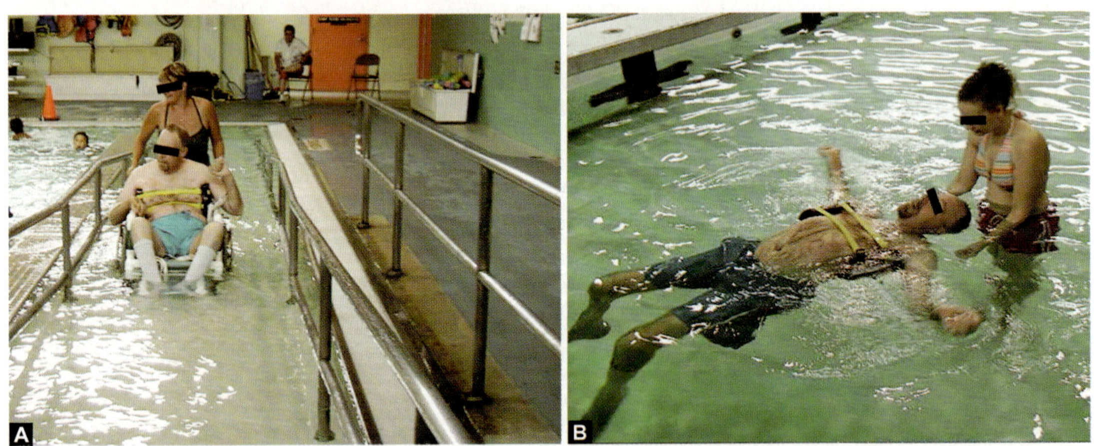

Figs. 28.18A and B: Hydrotherapy.

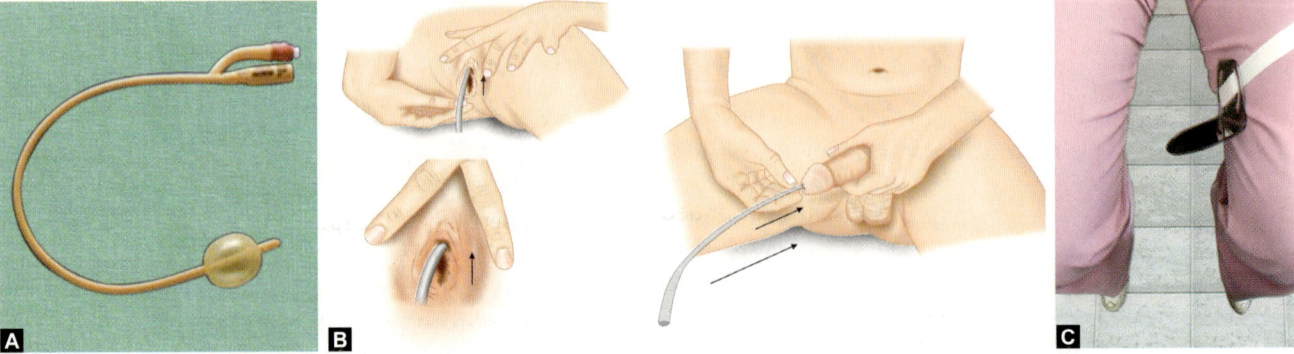

Figs. 28.19A to C: (A) Indwelling catheter; (B) Self-catheterization techniques; (C) position of mirror for visual feedback during self-catheterization.

Role of Physiotherapy in Nonrecovering (Chronic Conditions) of Spinal Cord Injury

Depending upon the neurological status of patient, the physiotherapy treatment protocol is planned.

The basic aims of physiotherapy treatment are as follows:
- Counseling about acceptance of condition
- Chest physiotherapy
- Maintaining joint mobility and prevent contractures
- Maintaining strength of muscles
- Endurance training
- Independence in activities of daily living
- Preventions of complications

Counseling about Acceptance of Condition

Once the fact is established that there will not be further recovery, then it is better to do counseling of patient for gradually accepting the condition in positive way. Routinely 20–30% patients recover fully. Majority of them are living wheelchair or bed ridden life. Vocational training as per the ability of patient plays major role in motivation and self-confidence.

Chest Physiotherapy

It is extremely important to give/do chest physiotherapy daily. Teach the patient to perform deep breathing exercises, segmental and diaphragmatic breathing exercises by themselves; spirometry, pranayam, to maintain/increase vital capacity should also be taught. Due to decrease in mobility, there are chances of getting chest problems, which can be avoided by regular chest physiotherapy.

Maintaining Joint Mobility and Prevent Contractures

Passive movement in full range twice a day prevents joint contracture and thereby prevents deformity. Orthosis like splints well-padded (to prevent soreness in sensory loss cases) helps in maintaining joint position.

Maintaining Strength of Muscles

Residual muscle strength should be preserved through strengthening, repeated resisted exercises, which may play substitute role of paralytic muscles. For example, quadratus lumborum strength helps in hip hiking, which again helps in clearing the ground while walking. Strengthening exercises of latissimus dorsi muscle and all shoulder girdle muscles helps in transfer activities as well as shifting of whole body.

Endurance Training

The expenditure of energy is more in patients with SCI. Endurance training everyday helps in overcoming the energy loss during activities of daily living. Regular, repeated movements and gradual resisted exercises improve endurance of patient.

Independence in Activities of Daily Living

For the benefit and self-respect of patient, it is necessary to teach and encourage independent activities of daily living. As per patients' routine activities of daily living should be taught and if needed modifications can be added. For example, from lying to sitting a rope can be tie on the roof of the room and patient is asked to get up by pulling the rope hence, he may not need any assistance for getting up from bed; teaching of self-catheterization is another example of making patient independent in ADL.

Preventions of Complications

The untimely death occurs in patients with SCI due to complications. Once we know the complications, then it should be prevented from occurring for which patient and his close relatives must be guided. Complications such as bedsores, UTI, and DVT are life-threatening complications that should be prevented.

Home Modifications and Advices

The main areas of home to be evaluated include the entrances, bedroom, bathroom, and kitchen. General safety issues ensuring that there is safe wheelchair access and space to maneuver a wheelchair in the home. The home should be free from fire, health and safety hazards, and an adequate heating, cooling, and electrical supply to meet the needs of additional medical equipment that must be present. Once the patient is discharged, the following advices should be given as found appropriate **(Box 28.5)**.

Vocational Rehabilitation

Vocational rehabilitation helps the person to become financially independent. It improves morale and self-esteem of the person. It helps to maintain the level of physical rehabilitation he/she has achieved. It also improves acceptance of person in the society and by relatives. Help from vocational counselor, evaluator,

---

BOX 28.5: Home advices for individuals with spinal cord injury.

- Take healthy food, leafy vegetables, and fruits so that constipation does not occur
- Take at least 10 glasses of water per day so that urinary infection does not occur
- Maintain healthy body weight
- Protect the skin from extreme cold and hot temperature
- Observe the skin and place where chances of getting bedsore are high
- Turn the body every two hours to prevent bedsores
- Try to be in standing position for as long time as possible
- Cut nails carefully
- Bedsheets should be clean and without wrinkles
- Wear loose, cotton clothes, and wear shoes of your own size

placement officer, and social worker can be sought for fitting the patient into the appropriate vocation as per their functional ability and strengths.

COMPLICATIONS OF SPINAL CORD INJURY

Bedsores

They can be prevented by:

- Frequent change of posture
- Water bed
- Air bed
- Soft water-filled rubber pouch can be kept at suspected pressure areas.

If bedsore has occurred, physiotherapy modalities such as the following can be used:

- LASER
- Ultraviolet radiation (UVR)

Skin grafting is preferred when sores have extended up to deeper tissues or bones. Treatment using maggots can be an option as well. Inspection done at regular intervals, frequent positioning and techniques and equipment relieving pressure are some useful strategies **(Figs. 28.20A to C)**.

Deep Vein Thrombosis

It can be a life-threatening complication. Early identification is extremely necessary. It can be treated by **(Fig. 28.21A)**:

- Rest
- Bandage
- Anticoagulant drugs

Myositis Ossificans

Formation of bone cells in the muscle is commonly seen in quadriceps **(Fig. 28. 21B)**. It can be identified using X-rays and clinical examination. Hard feeling in the muscle, and decreased ROM are some classic features. It can be treated by:

- Rest
- Removal of bony structure

Renal/Bladder Calculi and Urinary Tract Infection

It is better to prevent this complication. Identifying the symptoms clinically is important and diagnosis is usually confirmed by investigations. It is treated and prevented by:

- Asking the patient to drink lots of fluids
- Taking aseptic care of catheter
- Immediately consulting a doctor and starting antibiotics if it occurs

Osteoporosis

Due to nonweight-bearing position, the bone becomes weak **(Fig. 28.21C)**. This complication can be prevented and corrected by:

- Calcium-rich food, e.g., milk and its products, leafy vegetables, and citrous fruits.
- Weight-bearing postures such as standing in frames can help.

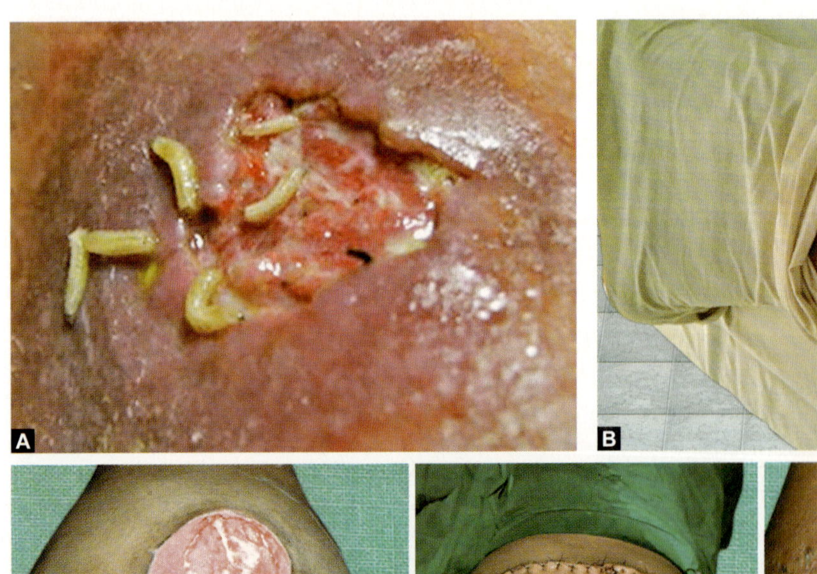
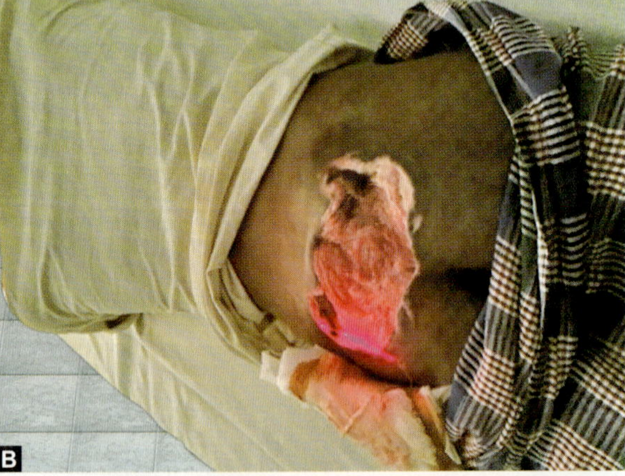
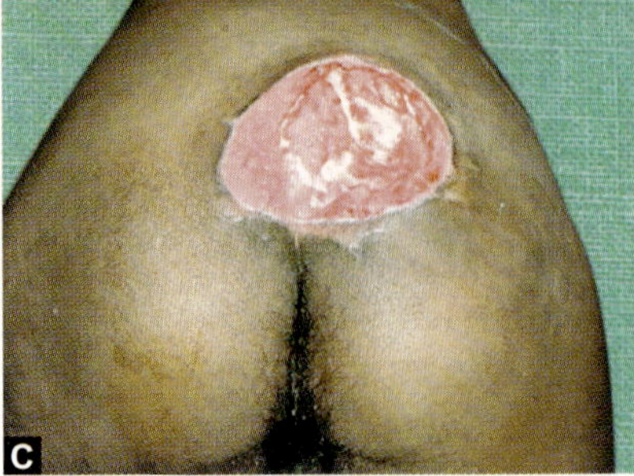
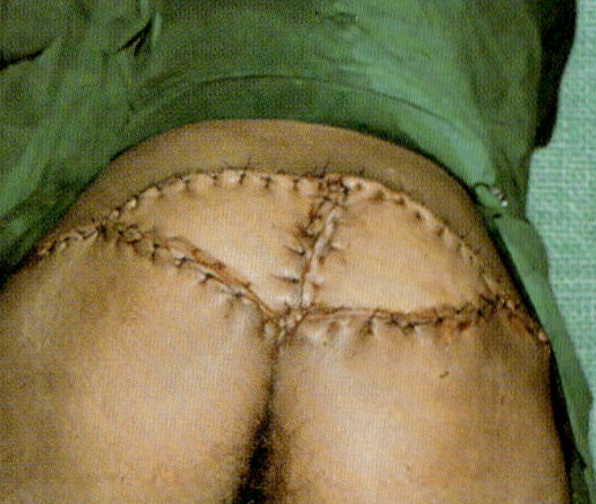
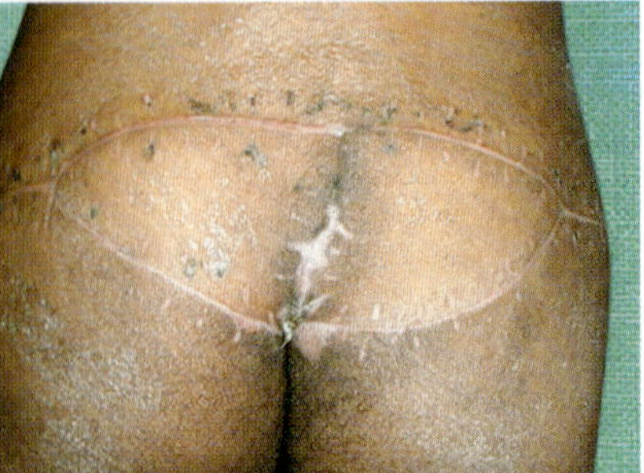

Figs. 28.20A to C: Management of bedsores: (A) Pressure sore treatment using maggots; (B) Physiotherapy management of pressure sore, using LASER; (C) Pressure sore managed surgically, using grafting.

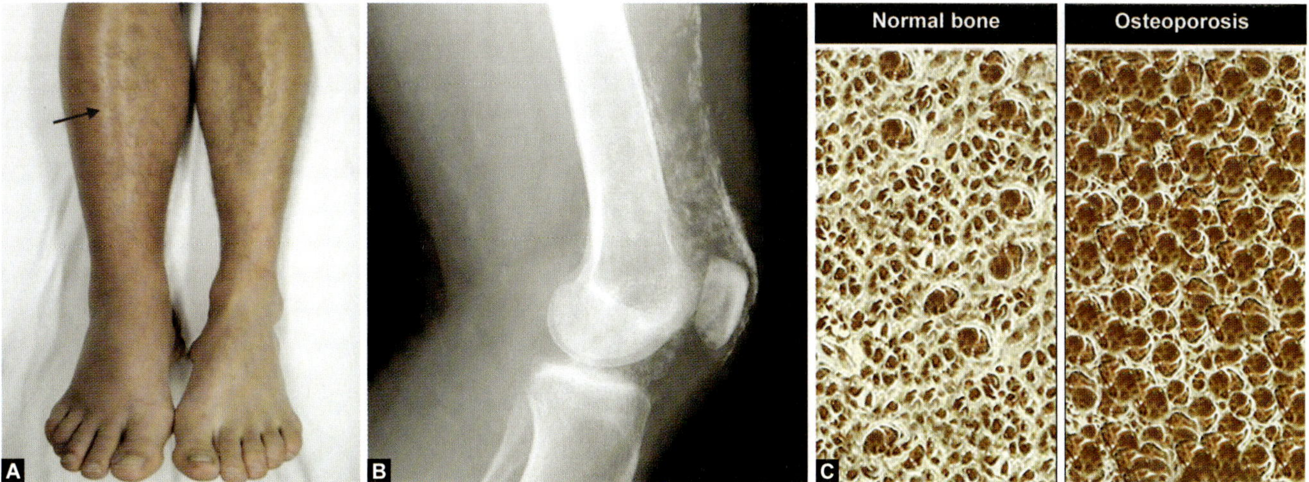

Figs. 28.21A to C: (A) Deep vein thrombosis; (B) Myositis ossificans; (C) Osteoporosis.

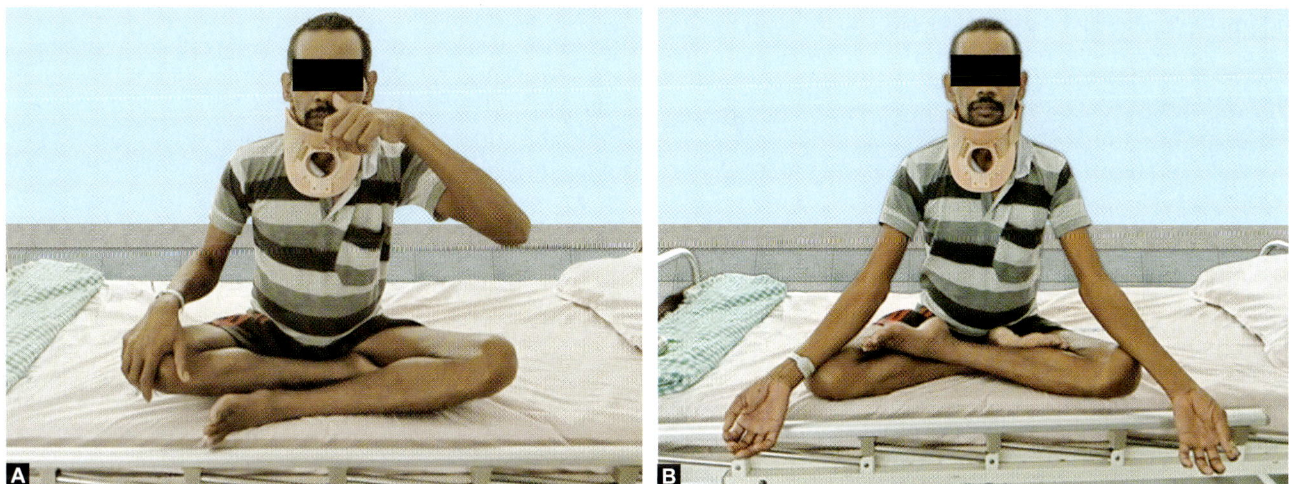

Figs. 28.22A and B: Yoga can help in psychosocial issues.

Depression and Psychosocial Issues

Young patients tend to suffer from depression more often, since they are bread earning members, and some of them are not even married or employed. Depression can be treated by:

- Counseling
- Alternative techniques such as pranayama and yoga have also proven to be beneficial **(Figs. 28.22A and B).**
- Support groups or self-help groups are also some options, which are known to keep the psychological burden of the condition under control.
- Participation in any sports (based on functional ability) or leisure activity can also help combat this aspect.

SUMMARY

Each SCI patient differs, and thorough assessment and appropriate clinical decision-making help in planning a tailor-made physiotherapy protocol. This chapter reviews the clinical features, classification, mechanism as well as impairments in SCI. Physiotherapy across acute as well as chronic phases of recovery have been explained to enable the readers to develop goals and an effective plan of care. Exercises on mat, transfer training, balance as well as gait training, which play a critical component in rehabilitation, are discussed with clinical images for demonstration. Along with physiotherapy, home-based care as well as vocational-based rehabilitation has also been emphasized.

Case Scenario

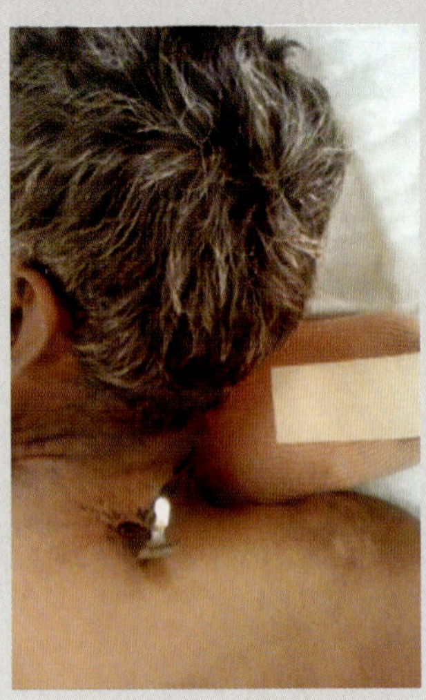

Fig. 28.23: Scar over neck due to sharp instrument assault.

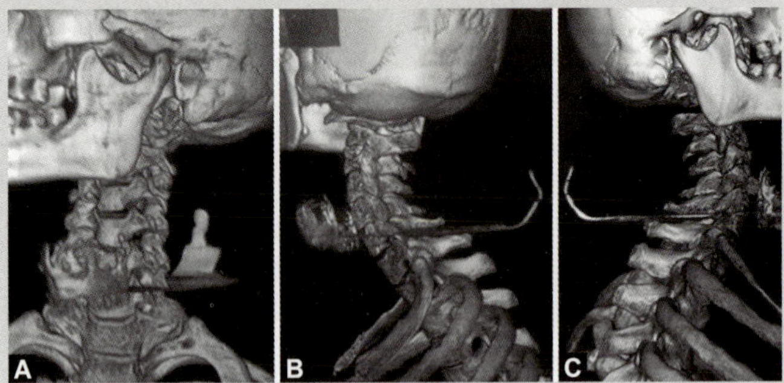

Figs. 28.24A to C: Sharp instrument due to assault as seen during investigations.

History: A 45-year-old male presented with history of assault in the form of sharp instrument inserted in the nape of the neck **(Fig. 28.23)** by someone, while he was working. He was immediately taken to the hospital and was conscious at the time of admission.

Assessment

Neurological status: At the time of admission, he had weakness of all four limbs. The muscle power was around 2/3 except both hands, with left side being more affected than right. He was operated immediately and rehabilitation was initiated. He was dependent in his ADLs, and at the time of discharge he was walking with sticks and orthoses and had functional difficulties in left upper limb.

Patients' vital signs are within normal limit when visiting the outpatient rehabilitation department. No skin breakdown or pressure sores found on observation. Other findings are as follows:

- **MMSE score:** 30/30
- **Sensory examination:** All sensations lost below level of lesion
- **Motor examination:** Hypotonicity in all LE muscles, ROM is within normal limits
- **Bowel:** Incontinence; bladder: indwelling catheter present
- **Balance:** Poor-to-fair sitting balance

Few investigatory and clinical findings are shown in **Figures 28.24A to C**.

Guiding Questions:

1. Make a list of impairments for this patient along with short- and long-term goals.
2. Establish a gait training program for the patient.
3. What preventive measures can be taken to avoid secondary complications?
4. Discuss the role of rehabilitation using specific interventions and strategies for making the patient functionally and vocationally independent.

Review Questions

1. What are the causes of spinal cord injury?
2. Classify spinal cord injuries and discuss various mechanisms associated with spinal cord injury.
3. What is cauda equina lesion?
4. Explain spinal shock in detail.
5. List the primary impairments associated with spinal cord injury.
6. Discuss types of bladder associated with spinal cord injury, and various management techniques for the same.
7. Describe the ASIA scale of classifying SCI.
8. What tests and measures are useful in the assessment of patient with SCI?
9. Discuss the role of rehabilitation in the recovery phase in a patient with SCI.
10. What secondary complications occur following SCI? Discuss the role of physiotherapy in its management.

BIBLIOGRAPHY

1. Birua G, Munda VS, Murmu NN. Epidemiology of spinal injury in North East India: a retrospective study. Asian J Neurosurg. 2018;13(4):1084-6.
2. Chacko V, Joseph B, Mohanty S, et al. Management of spinal cord injury in a general hospital in rural India. Spinal Cord. 1986;24:330-5.
3. Ida B. Tetraplegia and paraplegia. A guide for physiotherapists, 6th edition. Elsevier.
4. Maynard FM, Bracken MB, Creasy G, et al. International standards for neurological and functional classification of spinal cord injury. Spinal Cord. 1997;35(5):266-74.
5. O'Sullivan SB, Schmitz TJ. Physical rehabilitation, 6th edition. Jaypee Publishers.
6. Patel DA, Bhise AR, Shukla YU. Management of spinal cord injury by physiotherapist (site to settlement). Jaypee Brothers Medical Publishers; 2017. ISBN-10: 9789352702695.
7. Singh R, Sharma SC, Mittal R, et al. Traumatic spinal cord injuries in Haryana: an epidemiological study. Indian J Community Med. 2003;XXVIII:4.
8. Waters RL, Adkins RH, Yakura JS, et al. Motor and sensory recovery following incomplete paraplegia. Arch Phys Med Rehabil. 1994;75:67-72.

Parkinson's Disease

Sucheeta Golhar, Chetali Paliwal

LEARNING OBJECTIVES

After reading this chapter, the readers should be able to:

♦ Understand the etiology, pathophysiology, clinical features, and progression of Parkinson's disease
♦ Classify the types of Parkinson's disease and understand the examination procedures used to evaluate patients with Parkinson's disease
♦ Understand the role of a physiotherapist in terms of treating a patient with Parkinson's disease and guidance of family/caregiver for maximum improvement
♦ Gain knowledge regarding the components of the exercise protocol for patients with Parkinson's disease
♦ Identify the neuropsychological effects and social impact of Parkinson's disease
♦ Gain knowledge regarding maintenance of a record of patient details, interpret it, and use it to form practical and achievable goals for patients and formulating a plan of care accordingly.

CHAPTER OUTLINE

- Epidemiology
- Etiology and pathophysiology
- Clinical presentation
  - Motor symptoms
  - Nonmotor symptoms
- Medical diagnosis
- Clinical course
- Management
  - Medical management
  - Physiotherapy assessment
  - Physiotherapy management
- Treatment strategies
  - Exercise
  - Practice
    - Compensatory movement strategy training
- Treatment considerations
  - Patient, family, and caregiver education
- Psycholosocial issues in Parkinson's disease

INTRODUCTION

Parkinson's disease (PD) is a chronic, progressive neurodegenerative disorder, which is characterized by:

- Bradykinesia
- Rigidity
- Tremor
- Postural instability, as its cardinal features along with gradual symptom progression and a sustained response to levodopa therapy.

This condition might also include other:

- Visual features such as decreased eye blinking, ocular surface irritation, altered tear film, visual hallucinations, blepharospasm (involuntary spasms of eyelid muscles), decreased convergence, apraxia of eyelid opening, limitation of upward gaze, and oculogyric crisis (prolonged involuntary upward deviation of eyes)

- Respiratory features such as restrictive or obstructive respiratory disturbances.
- Other features such as dysarthria, hypophonia (soft speech), dysphagia, sialorrhea (excessive salivation).

It also includes nonmotor features such as:

- Autonomic dysfunction
- Cognitive or neurobehavioral disorders
- Sensory abnormalities
- Sleep disturbances.

Pathologically, it is defined as a progressive neurodegenerative disorder characterized by degeneration of the dopaminergic neurons in the substantia nigra and development of Lewy bodies in the residual dopaminergic neurons.

It was first described by Dr James Parkinson, a London-based surgeon, in his *an Essay on the Shaking Palsy* in 1817. He described the term "shaking palsy" (paralysis agitans) as "Involuntary tremulous motion, with lessened muscle power, in parts not in action and even when supported; with a propensity to bend the trunk forward and to pass from a walking to running pace: the senses and intellects being uninjured."

Sixty years after this, Jean-Martin Charcot (1872), a French neurologist, introduced the term "*Maladie de Parkinson*," a name for the disorder characterized by tremor at rest, rigidity, facial immobility, and specific disturbances of gait and posture. He distinguished PD from multiple sclerosis and other disorders characterized by tremor and also classified many cases under Parkinson plus syndromes category. He gave two prototypes: the tremorous and the rigid/akinetic form. He also mentioned about the arthritic changes, dysautonomia (disorder of autonomic nervous system), and pain that might occur along with PD.

In 1888, William Gowers (from London) correctly identified male predominance in this condition and described many joint deformities specific to this condition, in his "Manual of Disease of the Nervous System." Brissaud in 1925 first proposed damage to the substantia nigra as the anatomical center for PD. The most reformed pathological analysis of the condition was performed by Greenfield and Bosanquet in 1953. The morbidity and clinical progression of PD were first studied by Hoehn and Yahr in 1967. He classified key turning points in the disease into unilateral (stage I) disease and bilateral disease (stages II–V) and development of postural reflex impairment (stage III).

EPIDEMIOLOGY

PD is the second most common neurodegenerative disorder with a lifetime risk of developing it, at 2.0% for men and 1.3% for women. There is a rising prevalence with age in this condition—41/100,000 in 40–49 years to 1,087/100,000 in 70–79 years and 1,903/100,000 in >80 years. Lower prevalence rate was found in Asian population (646/100,000) as compared to the Western countries (1,601/100,000) for 70–79 years old individuals. Male-to-female ratio for incidence ranges from 1.3 to 2.0 in maximum studies. A meta-analysis (for individuals older than 40 years) revealed an incidence rate of 61.21/100,000 in males and 37.55/100,000 in females.

ETIOLOGY AND PATHOPHYSIOLOGY

Etiological and pathophysiological factors include:
- PD is caused by deterioration of dopaminergic neurons in the midbrain (mainly extrapyramidal tract).
- It is also accompanied by accumulation of α-synuclein proteins (known as Lewy bodies) in central, peripheral, and autonomic nervous system.
- Thus degeneration of neurons that releases dopamine results in imbalance between acetylcholine (excitatory neurotransmitter) and dopamine (inhibitory neurotransmitter) in the region.
- This imbalance sometimes leads to uncontrolled movements (dyskinesia) and sometimes lack of movements (freezing of gait).

Multiple factors are responsible for precipitation of this condition. These can be a combination of genetic and environmental factors. According to a study by Jon Stoessl, PD was found to be associated with generation of more free radicals and impaired functioning of mitochondrial complex I. According to another study by Karin Wirdefeldt, exposure to pesticides (such as 1-methyl-4-phenyl-1,2,3,6-tetrahydropyridine) may be the reason for precipitation of the disease. It also stated that exposure to metals such as manganese, iron, copper, zinc, and mercury increases the risk of this disease. This study also revealed an association of olfactory dysfunction with increased risk of PD (preceding 2–7 years from PD symptoms). **Table 29.1** reveals various genetic and environmental factors responsible for causing PD. Other than genetic and environmental factors, dietary factors as enlisted in **Table 29.2** also play some role in etiology of PD.

Table 29.1: Factors responsible for Parkinson's disease (PD).

Genetic factors	Environmental factors
Point mutation, duplication, and triplication of SNCA, LRRK2, Parkin, PINK1, DJ-1 gene	Industrial toxins
Mitochondrial dysfunctions	Plant-derived toxins
Alterations in vesicular transport proteins	Well water
Impaired bioenergetics, lipid peroxidation, nuclear RNA deficits, protein–iron and neuromelanin–iron interactions, and transcriptional aSyn dysregulation	Bacterial and viral infections
Disorders of calcium homeostasis, excitotoxicity from increased glutamatergic input and neuroinflammation	Exposure to organic solvents, carbon monoxide, cyanide, carbon disulfide, neurotoxic metal, pollutants, and pesticides
	MPTP

Table 29.2: Dietary factors associated with Parkinson's disease (PD).

Factors	Effects
Vitamin A and carotenoid	Deficiency may lead to PD
Vitamin B_6, B_9, and B_{12}	Deficiency leads to high homocysteine level, which damages DNA and depletes energy reserves, leading to neuron apoptosis
Vitamin D	Deficiency is found in patients with PD
Vitamin E	Deficiency leads to increased sensitivity to MPTP
Flavonoids	Deficiency leads to increased rate of mitochondrial dysfunction
Calorie intake	Reduced calorie intake is associated with increased sensitivity of dopaminergic neurons to MPTP
Unsaturated fatty acid intake	Deficiency may lead to alteration of dopamine mesocorticolimbic pathway (anatomically relevant to PD)
Alcohol intake	Moderate amount of intake reduces PD risk (when not associated with smoking)

(MPTP: 1-methyl-4-phenyl-1,2,3,6-tetrahydropyridine)

To understand the pathophysiology of PD, it is necessary to look into the basal ganglia circuitry, which is the main center of pathology. To explain this, a classical model of basal ganglia function in PD was proposed **(Fig. 29.1A)**. This model was able to explain the reason behind motor features such as bradykinesia, and difficulty in initiation of movements. But it could not explain the presence of tremors and rigidity.

- According to this model, the striatum communicates with output neurons in GPi (globus pallidus pars interna) and SNr (substantia nigra pars reticularis) through a direct pathway and with synaptic connections in the GPe (globus pallidus pars externa) and the STN (subthalamic nucleus) through an indirect pathway. Dopamine is suppose to inhibit neuronal activity in the indirect pathway and to excite neurons in direct pathway.

- In the Parkinsonian state **(Fig. 29.1B)**, dopamine depletion leads to disinhibition of dopamine D2-receptor-bearing striatal neurons in the indirect pathway leading to increased inhibition of the GPe and disinhibition of STN. This resulting increased activity of STN neurons leads to increased excitation of neurons in the GPi/SNr and overinhibition of thalamocortical and brainstem motor centers resulting in Parkinsonism.

- Dyskinesia induced by L-dopa is characterized by reduced activity in the STN **(Fig. 29.1C)**. This model suggests that this is due to dopamine-induced overinhibition of striato-GPe neurons, resulting in excess inhibition of STN and reduced activation of GPi/SNr. So at the end, it reduces inhibition of

thalamocortical neurons with increased drive of cortical motor areas resulting in dyskinesia.

- Thus PD disrupts the normal functioning of dopaminergic nigrostriatal system in basal ganglia. But various other disorders of central nervous system (CNS) may also involve this striatonigral system and so these should be distinguished from PD.

Parkinsonism is a term used to describe disorders related to primary disturbances in dopamine system of basal ganglia. **Table 29.3** shows the classification of Parkinsonism.

- The term "Parkinson's disease" is equated to and has been reserved for what, at present, is considered the *primary or "idiopathic"* form of the disease.

- *Secondary Parkinsonism* is when Parkinsonism is associated with a presumptive etiologic agent and/or signs, which suggest that their Parkinsonism is a fragment of a more diffuse disease of systems not ordinarily involved in the classical syndrome, such as post-encephalitis.

- *Parkinsonism or toxin-induced Parkinsonism:* In a certain number of patients, it is impossible to determine whether the Parkinsonism is primary or secondary. It is associated with other neurologic disease, either by history or by present signs, and there is no indication whether this association is causatively and pathologically determined or whether it is merely coincidental. This is referred to as *indeterminate Parkinsonism.*

- A large number of patients with primary or idiopathic Parkinsonism are present with atypical or additional clinical features. This is referred to as *Parkinsonism*

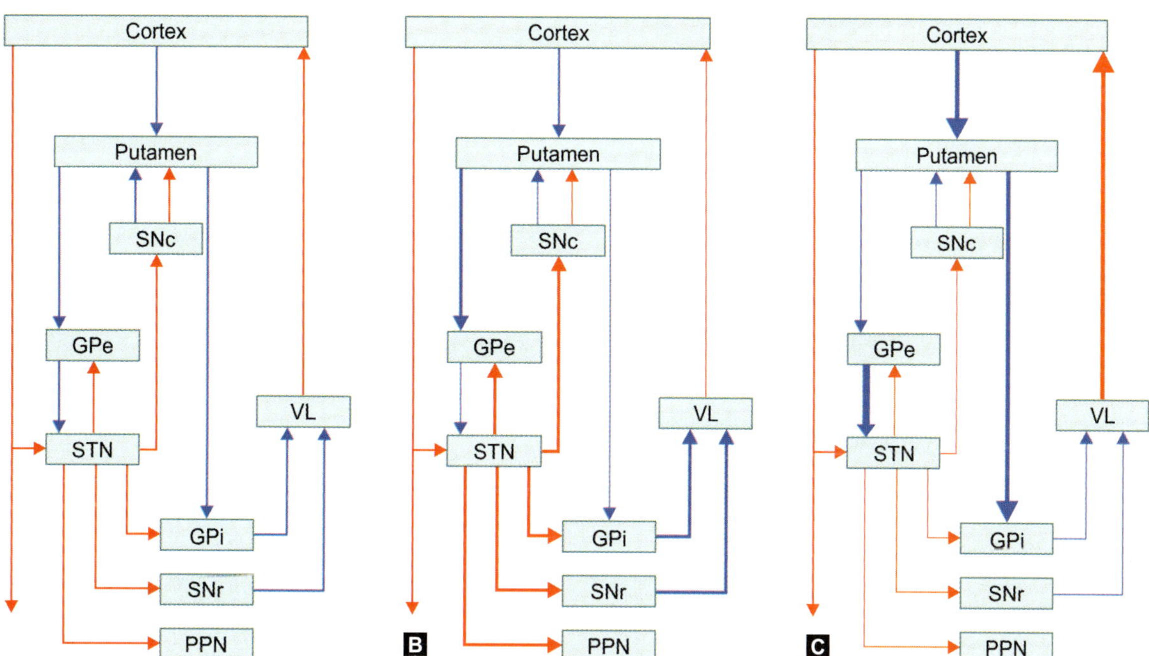

Figs. 29.1A to C: Classical model of basal ganglia circuit: (A) Normal; (B) Parkinsonian; (C) Dyskinetic state. Blue arrows indicate inhibitory projections and red arrows depict excitatory projections. Thickness signifies the degree of activation of each projection. (PPN: pedunculopontine nuclei; SNc: substantia nigra pars compacta; VL: ventralis lateralis; GPi: globus pallidus pars interna; GPe: globus pallidus pars externa; STN: sub-thalamic nucleus; SNr: substantia intra pars reticularis)

Table 29.3: Classification of Parkinsonism.

Primary/idiopathic Parkinsonism
Early onset (<21 years: juvenile; <21 years: young onset)
Late onset (>40 years)
Secondary Parkinsonism
Viral (postencephalitic)
Toxin induced (MPTP, carbon monoxide, manganese)
Drug induced (phenothiazines, reserpine, butyrophenones, metoclopramide)
Space occupying lesions of basal ganglia
Vascular disease (arteriosclerosis)
Metabolic defect
Post-traumatic
Normal pressure hydrocephalus

(MPTP: 1-methyl-4-phenyl-1,2,3,6-tetrahydropyridine)

Table 29.4: Classification of Parkinson's plus syndrome.

Sporadic	*Familial*
• PSP • MSA • CBGD • Olivopontocerebellar atrophy • Shy-Drager syndrome • DLB • Sporadic pallidal degeneration • Bilateral striatopallidodentate calcinosis • Parkinsonism with neuroacanthocytosis	• Associated with dementia, such as familial dementia with corticobasal inclusion bodies or familial DLB • Associated with psychiatric and respiratory disturbances • Associated with other types of movement disorders such as dystonia, myoclonus, seizures • Associated with eye movement abnormalities such as familial PSP • Others

(CBGD: corticobasal ganglionic degeneration; DLB: diffuse Lewy body disease; MSA: multiple system atrophy; PSP: progressive supranuclear palsy)

plus syndrome, which is a group of heterogeneous-degenerative neurological disorders, with certain associated clinical features, poor response to levodopa, distinctive pathological characteristics, and poor prognosis. Associated clinical features include symmetrical onset, infrequent or atypical tremor, prominent rigidity in axial musculature, bradykinesia, early postural instability, supranuclear gaze palsy, early autonomic failure, pyramidal affection, cerebellar involvement, alien limb phenomenon, apraxia, and significant early cognitive dysfunction in some cases.

Table 29.4 shows the various types of Parkinson's plus syndrome, of which progressive supranuclear palsy, multiple system atrophy, and diffuse Lewy body disease are more commonly seen.

According to Braak et al., PD has progressed in six stages **(Table 29.5)**. In stages 1–2 (presymptomatic stage), inclusion bodies are accumulated in medulla oblongata/pontine tegmentum and olfactory bulb/anterior olfactory nucleus. In stages 3–4, substantia nigra and other midbrain and forebrain nuclei become affected. Thus the patient starts developing clinical symptoms now. In the end stage of 5–6, the damage is progressed to neocortex, producing a varying degree of clinical manifestations. **Table 29.5** shows the various stages of PD.

Table 29.5: Stages of Parkinson's disease.

Stage 1	Pathology in dorsal motor nucleus and olfactory bulb causing loss of olfactory function
Stage 2	Lewy body formation in pons and medulla causing symptoms of stage 1 plus lesions in caudal raphe nucleus, gigantocellular reticular nucleus, and coeruleus–subcoeruleus complex
Stage 3	Pathology in midbrain, causing symptoms of stage 2 plus pathology in particular in pars compacta of substantia nigra
Stage 4	Pathology in prosencephalon and mesocortex, causing symptoms of stage 3 plus prosencephalic lesions (clinical motor symptoms) except for neocortex
Stage 5	Pathology in neocortex causing symptoms of stage 4 plus high order sensory association areas of neocortex and prefrontal neocortex
Stage 6	Pathology of stage 5 plus lesions in first-order sensory association areas of neocortex and premotor areas, with occasional mild changes in primary sensory and primary motor field

CLINICAL PRESENTATION

PD is clinically defined by motor and nonmotor symptoms. The disease is usually diagnosed by the first motor symptoms.

Motor Symptoms

Motor symptoms in PD can be divided into:

A. Cardinal motor symptoms—TRAP where:
- T—Tremor (resting tremors of hands, pill-rolling type, generally with occasional involvement of legs is also seen)
- R—Rigidity (axial and limb rigidity with/without cogwheel phenomenon)
- A—Akinesia (bradykinesia)
- P—Postural instability.

B. Other motor symptoms include:
- Hypomimia—Masked-like face **(Fig. 29.2A)**
- Dysarthria—Quiet and hurried speech
- Dysphagia—Swallowing difficulties
- Sialorrhea—Dribbling of saliva (sometimes present)
- Decreased arm swing
- Gait festination—Shuffling of gait along with freezing episodes leading to difficulty in initiating gait and sometimes leading to falls

- Difficulty in rising from chair and turning in bed
- Micrographia **(Fig. 29.3)**—Abnormally small handwriting or handwriting, which becomes progressively smaller
- Difficulty in cutting food
- Feeding difficulty
- Difficulty in maintaining hygiene
- Slowness in activities of daily living
- Presence of glabellar reflex—Blink response is generated on repeatedly tapping the patient between the eyebrows (the glabella area). Normal for infants but abnormally present in adults with frontal lobe pathologies
- Blepharospasm—Involuntary spasms of eyelid muscles
- Dystonia—Dystonia of foot (resulting in equinovarus foot position), upper arm–forearm or forearm–hand flexion, writer's cramp, oromandibular dystonia, torticollis, etc.
- Striatal deformity—Abnormal postures of hand (metacarpophalangeal flexion, interphalangeal extension, ulnar deviation) and foot (extension of metatarsophalangeal joint and flexion of interphalangeal joints)
- Scoliosis
- Camptocormia—Stoop body posture **(Fig. 29.2B)**
- Forward flexion of head and neck (antecollis).

Non-motor Symptoms

These are categorized into:
A. Disturbances in autonomic function
B. Sleep disturbances
C. Cognitive and psychiatric disturbances
D. Sensory symptoms.

Disturbances in Autonomic Function

Disturbances in autonomic function include:
- Orthostatic hypotension

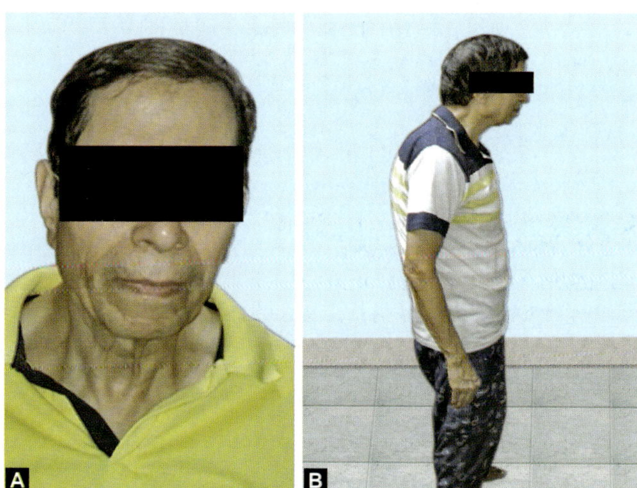

Figs. 29.2A and B: (A) Masked face with reduced facial features; (B) Flexed posture of spine.

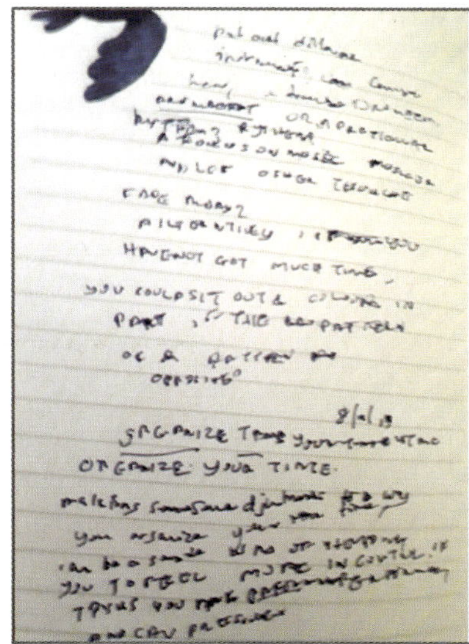

Fig. 29.3: Micrographia (small size of letters).

- Gastrointestinal symptoms such as slowing of gastrointestinal tract motility with postprandial fullness, gastric retention, constipation, and rectal sphincter dysfunction
- Urinary control disturbances including urinary frequency, urgency and incontinence, frequent nocturia, erectile dysfunction in males
- Autonomic dermatological symptoms such as hyperhidrosis
- Dribbling of saliva (sialorrhea)
- Seborrheic keratosis (facial and scalp dermatological disorder)
- Increased fat deposition in central face along with scaling of skin of forehead.

Sleep Disturbances

Sleep disturbances include:
- Most common is fractionated sleep
- Shallow sleep and increased tendency to frequent awakenings in night
- Difficulty in turning around in bed
- Frequent nocturia
- Nocturnal tremor
- Depression
- Excessive daytime sleepiness
- Rapid eye movement behavior sleep disorder
- Restless leg syndrome with or without periodic leg movements in sleep
- Sudden sleep attacks without normal drowsiness as induction to sleep.

Cognitive and Psychiatric Disturbances

The following are cognitive and psychiatric disturbances:
- Visual hallucinations and illusions. These may last from seconds to minutes and may recur over the day.
- Less commonly occurring are olfactory hallucinations, auditory hallucinations and tactile hallucinations.

Table 29.6: Common signs and symptoms of Parkinson's disease.	
Motor signs/symptoms	*Nonmotor signs/symptoms*
Tremor	Staring appearance
Bradykinesia	Flat affect
Falls	Excessive salivation
Shuffling gait	Anosmia
Stooped posture	Depression/anxiety
Dyskinesia	Psychotic symptoms
Muscle rigidity	Sleep disruption
Freezing episodes	Fatigue
Micrographia	Autonomic dysfunction
	Cognitive impairment
	Constipation
	Dysphagia
	Urinary incontinence
	Dysarthria
	Diminished speech volume
	Unexplained pain

Note: Flat affect refers to a lack of response to emotional stimuli, including a neutral facial expression, monotone voice, lack of eye contact

- Psychosis might occur with old age, cognitive impairment, and history of depression.
- Euphoria/hypomania, poor organizational skills, hypersexuality, abnormal hoarding, and risk-taking behavior might occur after dopaminergic treatment.
- Cognitive deterioration and dementia are common, with early symptoms of problems with executive functioning, along with visuospatial dysfunction, impaired speech fluency, and memory impairment.
- Depression and anxiety are also common for PD.

Sensory Symptoms

Sensory symptoms are as follows:
- Reduced or lost sense of smell
- Vague abnormal sensations in body parts may be perceived
- Limb pain is common, but oral, thoracic abdominal, and genital pain may also occur.
  Table 29.6 enlists the common signs and symptoms of PD.

MEDICAL DIAGNOSIS

The diagnosis of PD is based on defined criteria from UK PD Brain Bank **(Table 29.7)**. Slow initiation of voluntary movements with progressive reduction of speed and amplitude of repetitive action, with any one of these (muscular rigidity, resting tremor, or postural instability), are pre-requisite for probable diagnosis of PD.

Differential diagnosis: To diagnose PD correctly, it should be differentiated from its other similar forms, as discussed in **Table 29.8**.

Table 29.7: UK Parkinson's Disease Society Brain Bank clinical diagnostic criteria.
Step 1: Diagnosis of Parkinsonian syndrome

• Bradykinesia (slowness of initiation of voluntary movement with progressive reduction in speed and amplitude of repetitive action)
 • And at least one of the following:
    – Muscular rigidity
    – 4–6 Hz rest tremor
    – Postural instability not caused by primary visual, vestibular, cerebellar or proprioceptive dysfunction

Step 2: Exclusion criteria for Parkinson's disease
• History of repeated strokes with stepwise progression of Parkinsonian features   • History of repeated head injury   • History of definite encephalitis   • Oculogyric crisis (prolonged involuntary upward deviation of eyes)   • Neuroleptic treatment at onset of symptoms   • More than one affected relative   • Sustained remission   • Strictly unilateral features after 3 years   • Supranuclear gaze palsy   • Cerebellar signs   • Early severe autonomic involvement   • Early severe dementia with disturbances of memory, language, and praxis   • Babinski sign   • Presence of cerebral tumor or communicating hydrocephalus on CT scan   • Negative response to large doses of levodopa (if malabsorption excluded)   • 1-methyl-4-phenyl-1,2,3,6-tetrahydropyridine (MPTP) exposure
Step 3: Supportive prospective positive criteria for Parkinson's disease (three or more required for diagnosis of definite Parkinson's disease)
• Unilateral onset   • Rest tremor present   • Progressive disorder   • Persistent asymmetry affecting side of onset more   • Excellent response (70–100%) to levodopa   • Severe levodopa-induced chorea   • Levodopa response for 5 years or more   • Clinical course of 10 years or more

CLINICAL COURSE

PD progresses with great variability among patients. During the early phase of the disease, symptoms are mild in severity and unilateral. These show a good response to the treatment without any variability in motor symptoms during the day. But the symptoms keep on progressing and spread to contralateral side also. The patients still show a good response to drugs and are functioning well. This duration is sometimes called *Honeymoon Period*. With further progression of disease, increased dose of drugs is given, which induces potentially disabling dyskinesias.

Table 29.8: Differential diagnoses of Parkinson's disease.

Diagnosis	Differentiating clinical features
Progressive supranuclear palsy	Oculomotor dysfunctions with vertical gaze abnormalities, axial rigidity, falls during early stages of disease, pseudobulbar palsy, swallowing dysfunction, cognitive impairment, apraxia of eyelid opening, Parkinsonism with lack of or transient response to L-dopa, rapid progression, dysarthria
Multiple system atrophy	Postural hypotension and autonomic dysfunction (Shy-Drager variant), cerebellar dysfunction (olivopontocerebellar atrophy variant), Parkinsonism with lack of or transient response to L-dopa (striatonigral degeneration variant), falls during the early stage of disease, swallowing dysfunction, rapid progression, neck flexion, myoclonus, dysarthria
Vascular Parkinsonism	Lower body presentation with freezing gait during the early stages of disease, pyramidal tract signs, cognitive dysfunction, relative lack of response to L-dopa
Diffuse Lewy body disease	Early dementia, hallucinations with L-dopa therapy, fluctuating level of alertness, sensitivity to extrapyramidal side effects of neuroleptics
Corticobasal degeneration	Apraxia, cortical sensory signs, myoclonus, unilateral presentation, dystonia, cognitive impairment, lack of response to L-dopa

Table 29.9: Comparison between original Hoehn and Yahr and modified Hoehn and Yahr.

Hoehn and Yahr scale	Modified Hoehn and Yahr scale
1. Unilateral involvement only, usually with minimal or no functional disability	0.0: No signs of disease
	1.0: Unilateral involvement only
2. Bilateral or midline involvement without impairment of balance	1.5: Unilateral and axial involvement
3. Bilateral disease; mild-to-moderate disability with impaired postural reflexes; physically independent	2.0: Bilateral involvement without impairment of balance
4. Severely disabling disease; still able to walk or stand unassisted	2.5: Mild bilateral disease with recovery on pull test
5. Confinement to bed or wheelchair unless aided	3.0: Mild-to-moderate bilateral disease; some postural instability; physically independent
	4.0: Severe disability; still able to walk or stand unassisted
	5.0: Wheelchair bound or bedridden unless aided

Gait and balance disturbances, speech, and swallowing difficulties may start appearing and poorly responds to treatment. After a prolonged duration of 10 or more years, many patients start developing some nonmotor symptoms, for which there are limited available treatments. Thus it starts affecting the quality of life and leads to dependent lifestyle in terms of activities of daily living. These patients require earlier and greater need for admission to a nursing home. This causes higher rates of emergency hospital admissions and in-hospital mortality. Mean duration until death ranges from 6.9 to 14.3 years.

Hoehn and Yahr scale or modified Hoehn and Yahr scale are used to categorize stages of PD. **Table 29.9** shows the comparison between the two.

Unified Parkinson's Disease Rating Scale (UPDRS) is another means of measuring progression of PD. It is considered as a gold standard tool and the original version consists of four parts:

Part 1: Mentation, behavior, and mood
Part 2: Activities of daily living
Part 3: Motor examination
Part 4: Complications of therapy.

A modification of this scale, renamed the Movement Disorder Society-UPDRS (MDS-UPDRS), reported by Goetz and colleagues, was developed to improve ability to detect slower and smaller changes in mildly disabled patients and increase focus on non-motor symptoms (**Box 29.1**). It includes a motor evaluation and characterizes the extent and burden of disease across various populations. The scale can be used in a clinical setting as well as in research. The four parts are similar to the original version, in addition to a six item, summing the total items to 65, as compared to 55 in the original version.

Part I concerns *nonmotor experiences of daily living.*
Part II concerns *motor experiences of daily living.*
Part III is retained as the *motor examination.*
Part IV concerns *motor complications.*

BOX 29.1: MDS-UPDRS.

MDS-UPDRS items (each question is anchored with five responses that are linked to commonly accepted clinical terms: 0—normal, 1—slight, 2—mild, 3—moderate, and 4—severe). "Slight" refers to symptoms/signs with sufficiently low frequency or intensity to cause no impact on function; "mild" refers to symptoms/signs of frequency or intensity sufficient to cause a modest impact on function; "moderate" refers to symptoms/signs sufficiently frequent or intense to impact considerably, but not prevent, function; "severe" refers to symptoms/signs that prevent function.

Part I: Non-motor experiences of daily living
• Cognitive impairment
• Hallucinations and psychosis
• Depressed mood
• Anxious mood, apathy
• Features of dopamine dysregulation syndrome
• Nighttime sleep problems

Contd...

Contd...

- Daytime sleepiness
- Pain and other sensations
- Urinary problems
- Constipation problems
- Lightheadedness on standing
- Fatigue

Part II: Motor experiences of daily living
- Speech
- Salivation and drooling
- Chewing and swallowing
- Eating tasks
- Dressing
- Hygiene
- Handwriting
- Doing hobbies and other activities
- Turning in bed
- Tremor
- Getting out of bed, car, or deep chair
- Walking and balance
- Freezing

Part III: Motor examination
- Speech
- Facial expression
- Rigidity of neck and four extremities
- Finger taps
- Hand movements
- Pronation/supination
- Toe tapping
- Leg agility
- Arising from chair
- Gait
- Freezing of gait
- Postural stability
- Posture
- Global spontaneity of movement
- Postural tremor of hands
- Kinetic tremor of hands
- Rest tremor amplitude
- Constancy of rest tremor

Part IV: Motor complications
- Time spent with dyskinesia
- Functional impact of dyskinesias
- Time spent in the OFF state
- Functional impact of fluctuations
- Complexity of motor fluctuations
- Painful OFF state dystonia

MANAGEMENT

Medical Management

There is no definite cure for PD; but treatment is directed toward symptomatic relief and to reduce the dyskinesias appearing. Various drugs are given to control these symptoms, and the effective duration of medicine is called "ON state." While when these symptoms reappear the patient is said to be in "OFF" state. These patients fluctuate between these "ON" and "OFF" periods. Medicines are given to the patients when they start developing disability. This medical treatment depends on age and the symptoms which need to be controlled.

During the early stage, patients are troubled from their tremor, which is controlled by beta-blockers such as propranolol. Anticholinergics, such as benztropine or trihexyphenidyl, and antipsychotics, such as clozapine, have also shown good results in reducing tremor. Motor symptoms usually occur due to lack of dopamine, so dopamine replacements or stimulating the brain through an agonist to release dopamine is the treatment of choice. Levodopa is the most effective form given. However, its prescription is delayed for as long as possible because its effectiveness decreases with time.

Other dopamine agonists that act directly on the dopamine receptors can be prescribed which include ergot derivative (e.g. bromocriptine, pergolide, cabergoline) and nonergot derivative (e.g. pramipexole, ropinirole, rotigotine) dopamine agonists. Inhibitors of monoamine oxidase type B (MAO-B) block central dopamine metabolism and increase synaptic concentrations of the neurotransmitter. They consist of selegiline and rasagiline. Other drugs of choice in PD are catechol O-methyltransferase (COMT) inhibitors, such as tolcapone and entacapone.

Surgical treatment options such as pallidotomy are important but cannot be performed on patients with bilateral involvement. Deep brain stimulation (DBS) is another most commonly utilized surgical procedure, which simulates the effects of a lesion without necessitating a brain lesion. DBS overcomes the limitation of pallidotomy; in that, it does not require making a lesion in the brain and is thus suitable for performing bilateral procedures with relative safety.

Physiotherapy Assessment

An extensive examination of patient is required before planning the management. A thorough assessment needs to be administered, which includes the following points:

1. **Patient history:**
   - Age, gender, ethnicity, primary language, education, address, hand dominance
   - Chief complaint
   - History of present illness: onset, progression
   - Medical/surgical history
   - Personal history
   - Family history
   - Environmental history: home and workplace barriers
   - Social history
   - Medications
   - Medical/laboratory test results
   - Functional status and activity level: earlier to disease onset and current

- General health status: physical, psychological, social, and health habits.
2. **System reviews:**
   - Neuromuscular
   - Musculoskeletal
   - Cardiovascular/pulmonary
   - Integumentary.
3. **Tests and measures:**
   - Cognition: Mental status, memory, hesitation, slowness of thought processes
   - Oromotor function: Communication (fluctuations, reduced volume), swallowing
   - Psychosocial function: Motivation, anxiety, depression
   - Anthropometric characteristics: Body mass index, girth, length, edema
   - Circulation: Orthostatic hypotension
   - Aerobic capacity and endurance: During functional activities and standardized exercise protocols including cardiovascular and pulmonary signs and symptoms
   - Ventilation and gas exchange
   - Integumentary integrity: Skin condition, pressure-sensitive areas; activities, positioning, and posture to relieve pressure
   - Autonomic nervous system integrity: Thermal responses and sweating
   - Sensory integrity and integration
   - Pain: Intensity and location
   - Perceptual function: Visuospatial skills
   - Joint integrity, alignment, and mobility, range of motion (active and passive), muscle length, and soft tissue extensibility
   - Posture: Alignment, position, symmetry (static and dynamic), ergonomics and body mechanics
   - Muscle performance: Strength, power, and endurance
   - Motor function: Motor control and motor learning; tone; voluntary movement patterns; involuntary movements; hesitation, slowness, arrest of movements; poverty of movements
   - Procedural learning for complex and sequential tasks
   - Postural control and balance: Degree of postural instability, balance strategies; safety
   - Gait and locomotion: Gait pattern and speed, safety, and risk of fall
   - Functional status and activity level: Performance-based examination of functional skills, basic and instrumental activities of daily living (ADL); functional mobility skills; home management skills
   - Assistive or adaptive devices: Fit, alignment, function, use, safety
   - Environment, home, and work barriers
   - Work, community, and leisure activities: Ability to participate in activities, safety
   - Disability assessment by using MDS-UPDRS.

Physiotherapy Management

Physical therapy is a vital component of the management of PD. **Table 29.10** presents the aims, working areas, and treatment techniques used for the management of PD.

Table 29.10: Aims, working areas, and treatment of Parkinson's disease (PD).

Aims	Maximizing quality of movement, functional independence, and general fitness
	Minimizing secondary complications
	Optimizing safety
	Supporting self-management and participation
Working areas	Gait (focusing on freezing and correct posture)
	Balance (focusing on prevention of falls, fear of falls, and posture)
	Transfers (inclusive of posture)
	Manual activities
	Physical capacity (in terms of posture and inactivity)
Treatment strategies	Exercise
	Practice
	Movement strategy training
Treatment considerations	Considering fluctuations in daily functioning
	Treatment site (home)
	Multidisciplinary collaboration (with other medical and paramedical staff)
	PD expertise

TREATMENT STRATEGIES

Treatment strategies include:
- Exercise
- Practice
- Compensatory movement strategy training (such as cueing and strategies for complex motor sequences).

Exercise

- Comprises planned, structured, and repetitive physical activity.
- Focuses on physical capacity, functional mobility, balance, transfers, and gait.
- Acts as a symptomatic treatment and helps in motor symptoms particularly.
- It also influences nonmotor symptoms such as depression, apathy, and fatigue.
- When combined with cognitive training, it enhances both motor and cognitive status of patients.
- Cognitive elements can be added to exercise by activities such as gaming.

- Aerobic exercise and strength training exercise improve physical functioning and help in reducing symptoms.
- Technology-assisted training such as robot-assisted treadmills or machines that provide preparatory cues and augmented feedback is the latest method to treat such patients.
- Intensive rehabilitation program (4 weeks, 5 times a week, combined types of exercise) and high amplitude movements, sensory recalibration, and self-cueing are found effective.
- Exercises such as Tai-Chi, hydrotherapy, boxing, and dancing are becoming popular in the present times with increasing evidences.
- Hand functions are found to be improved with the exercises using a therapeutic putty.
- Relaxation techniques: Gentle rocking provides general relaxation and helps in reducing rigidity. Use of a rocking chair can be made to relax the patient as well as for enhancing sit to stand transfers. Jacobson progressive relaxation techniques and meditation along with cognitive-imagining techniques also helps.
- Proprioceptive neuromuscular facilitation (PNF) techniques: PNF techniques can also be useful means of combating the rigidity. Rhythmic initiation, with movements progressing from passive to active assisted to active, can be used. Hold relax and contract relax can also be incorporated for reducing tightness or contractures that develop later in the disease progression.
- Balance training: Weight shifts in both sitting and standing. This can be progressed later by adding upper extremity tasks (e.g., reaching, picking objects off the floor, and tying shoes). Movement transitions such as sit to stand; half kneeling to standing; and stepping can be used to challenge postural control system. Sitting activities on gymnastic ball. Externally induced perturbation for promoting automatic balance reactions. "Kitchen Sink exercise" standing heel raises and toes off, partial wall squats, single limb stance with sidekicks or back kicks can also be useful.

Practice

- It refers to learning a task (old or new) as per the personal goals of the patient.
- Doing a movement repeatedly with increasing complexity and positive feedback can improve the fluency of motor task.
- It might include cognitive role (such as visual or auditory cueing and dual task performance), along with the use of observation of task and mental imagery, related to the context of the task.

Compensatory Movement Strategy Training

- **Cueing and attentional strategies:**
  - External cueing helps in initiating as well as maintaining a movement (such as gait) by activation of external brain networks involving cerebello-parieto-premotor loops, which makes up for the hypoactive basal ganglia.
  - Thus external cues reduce the internal planning and preparation of movements, thereby decreasing cognitive role.
  - Cueing strategy works best on gait (specially initiation and turning), even in patient's home environment, with lower risk of falls.
  - Rhythmic auditory cues can reduce the interference effect of dual task on gait.
  - Visual cues can improve handwriting and self-vocalization.
  - Auditory cues can improve kinematics of reaching.
  - Attentional strategies, such as taking big steps for walking, along with cueing can improve walking speed and stride length in single and dual tasks.
  - Optimal cueing modality and parameter is patient specific and depends on person's abilities, preferences, activity, environment, and problem being faced (initiation or continuation of movement, speed, amplitude of movement, etc.).
  - New devices such as "smart glasses" and "laser walkers" are few user-friendly and personalized devices that should be tried for their effectiveness.
- **Strategies for complex motor sequences:**
  - These are used to improve performances of complex tasks such as transfers and manual activities
  - Complex task is divided into multiple small tasks, which are to be performed in a specific sequence and with conscious control.
  - Approaches such as motor imagery can also be integrated into these strategies for complex tasks.
  - Training should be task specific and should be customized for every individual.
  - In later stages, due to decreased cognitive function, a caregiver can be asked to help in recalling the steps or guiding the movement.
  - **Steps to select a strategy are as follows:**
    1. Therapist observes the patient while performing the activity to find out the limiting component.
    2. Therapist helps the patient in recognizing the activity and selecting the most optimal movement components (4–6 components).
    3. Therapist summarizes the sequence of components in key phrases (may be supported by visuals).
    4. Therapist physically guides the patient while performing.
    5. Patient rehearses the steps aloud.
    6. Patient uses the motor imagery of the consecutive movement components.
    7. Patient carries out the components consecutively, consciously controlled, along with external cues, only if required **(Box 29.2)**.

BOX 29.2: Important points for exercise prescription.
- Treatment approach and exercise protocols should be according to the abilities, needs, motivation, and social context of the patient as well as caregiver.
- Treatment goals and interventions should be discussed with the patient and family before making a final decision to enhance a patient-centered approach.
- Guidance should be given to motivate patients, to be an active participant in adapting to the impact of disease and to apply self-management.
- Patients should be attentive toward preventing, recognizing, and acting adequately toward (new) problems.
- Patients should be motivated to engage in a physically active lifestyle.

TREATMENT CONSIDERATIONS

- **Optimizing day structure and routine:**
  - A daily/weekly schedule can prompt memory and beginning of activities.
  - Prior planning of activities helps in avoiding pressure situations and multitasking.
  - It can help in managing the fluctuations of effects of medicine, bradykinesia, and fatigue.
  - In milder forms of PD, planning might help in getting things done, but in moderate and severe forms, caregiver may have to assist in getting the work done.
  - Planning also helps in energy conservation programs, thereby helping in managing fatigue.
- **Adaptations of physical environment:**
  - Use of assistive devices and environment modification can help in freezing episodes and falls, by increasing independence, safety, and by reducing the effort for activity performance.
  - Devices such as a cane are helpful in mild PD, walkers and walking stabilizers are helpful in moderate disability, and motorized devices can be used for severe forms of PD.
  - But these devices should be used after proper training given by a physical therapist, or else they might worsen the situation.
  - Commonly advised modifications and devices are:
    - Removal of obstacles
    - Rearranging furniture and workspace
    - Improving lighting conditions
    - Optimizing height and support of furniture such as grab rails
    - Nonslippery flooring.
- **Treatment site:**
  - Learning of new task and its practice should be done in patient's home environment.
  - At home, treatment helps in direct evaluation of effect of new strategies and involvement of family and caregiver.
  - Telerehabilitation is a new way of treating patients at home (placed remotely).

- New technologies such as exergaming can be practiced into daily life, when given at home.
- Remote monitoring in patients' own environment through wearable sensors and smartphones is another new approach, for monitoring symptoms such as gait, falls, and voice.
- Technologies such as using virtual coach to promote daily walking in such patients have shown improvement in their mobility performances.

Patient, Family, and Caregiver Education

As a healthcare provider, a physical therapist must provide information regarding various fields related to PD. These can be taken as one-on-one sessions, group interactions, printed formats, and through videos or PowerPoint presentations. Following elements should be included when discussing PD with patient, family, and caregivers:

- PD—clinical presentation, strategies to manage symptoms
- Medications: Purpose, dosage, possible adverse side effects, signs of either over- or undermedication
- Preventive measures to minimize secondary complications and impairments
- Impact of PD on movement and effective strategies to manage movement problems
- Barriers to exercise and effective solutions to regular exercise participation
- Impact of PD on function and techniques to maintain independent function in home, community, or work environments
- Strategies for energy conservation and activity pacing
- Strategies for ensuring activity participation in leisure and family activities
- Community resources for patients such as support groups, in-home interventions, community training programs, and day programs
- Community resources for caregivers such as counseling support groups and exercise programs.

Few activities that can be used to decrease trunk rigidity and to improve strength, coordination, balance, and gait in people with PD are:

- Turning in bed: Turning knees to one side and then to another in a crook lying position (without lifting shoulder blades) as shown in **Figures 29.4 and 29.5**.
- Scooting: Lifting one pelvis at a time to shift it anteriorly or posteriorly in a high sitting position, to move the body anteriorly toward the edge of bed or inside the bed.
- Overhead clapping, catching a light ball with both hands, in a high sitting position with/without back support.
- Sit to stand and back to sitting again, initially with support and later without support, as in **Figures 29.6 and 29.7**.
- Positions to maintain balance in standing—Mini squats with/without support of wall **(Fig. 29.8)**, closed feet standing (with/without support) **(Fig. 29.9)**, tandem

standing (with/without support), one leg standing (with/without support) **(Fig. 29.10)**, on spot marching (with/without support), heel raise, and toe raise (with/without support). Difficulty level can be increased by replacing the firm surface of ground with unstable surfaces like foam mattress.

- Dynamic activities in standing like reach outs in diagonal positions to arms **(Figs. 29.11 and 29.12),** ball catching with both hands, overhead clapping, picking objects from a lower surface/ground, toe touch at different points marked on the floor, stepping one step forward, backward and sideward.

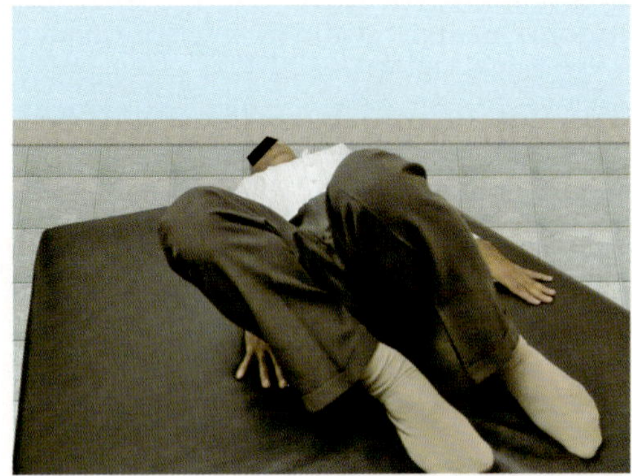

Fig. 29.4: Turning of knees to one side without lifting shoulder blades.

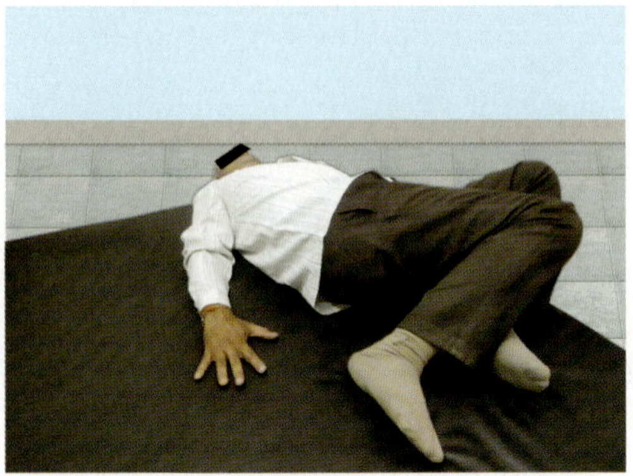

Fig. 29.5: Turning of knees to other side.

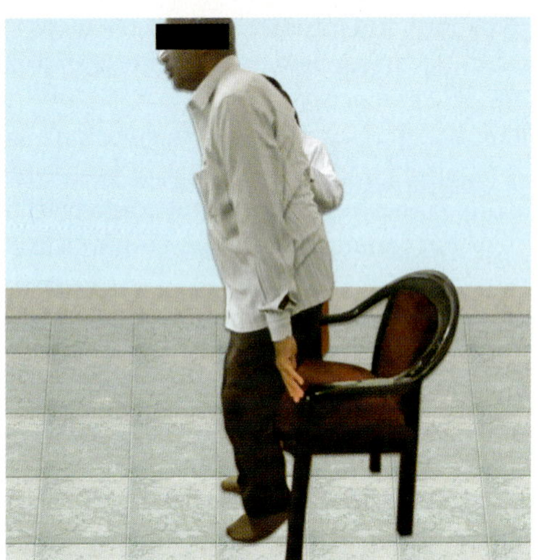

Fig. 29.6: Sit to stand.

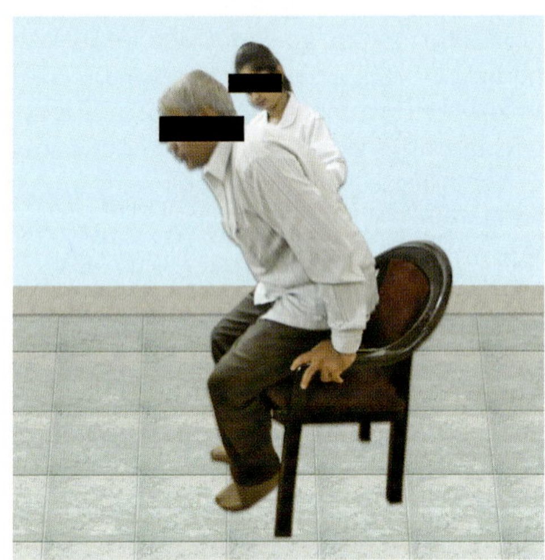

Fig. 29.7: Stand to sit.

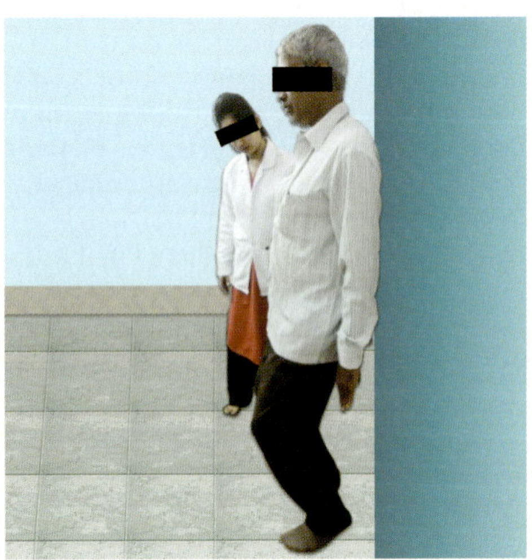

Fig. 29.8: Mini squats.

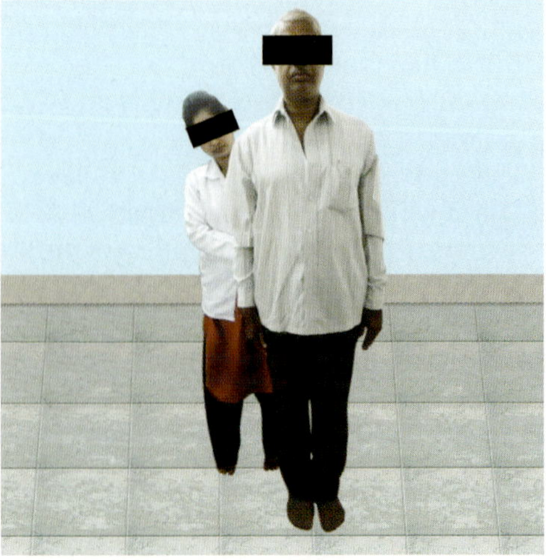

Fig. 29.9: Closed feet standing.

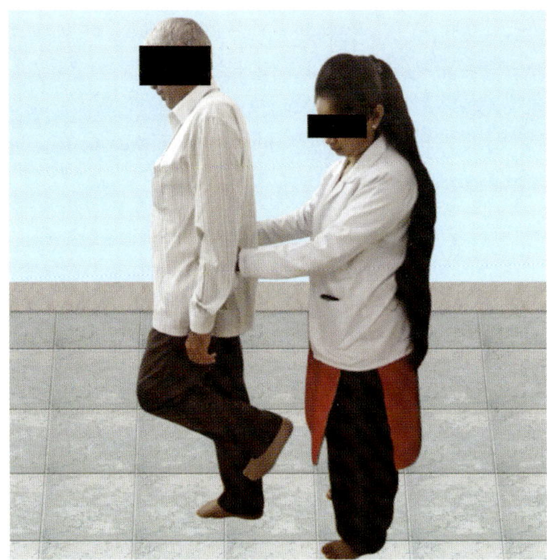

Fig. 29.10: One leg standing.

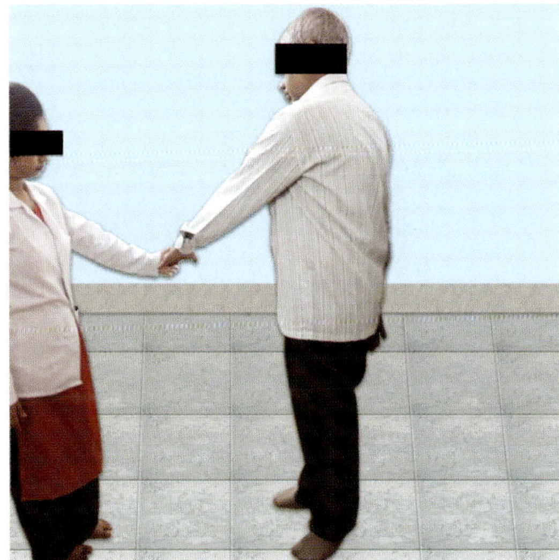

Fig. 29.11: Diagonal reach outs to the right.

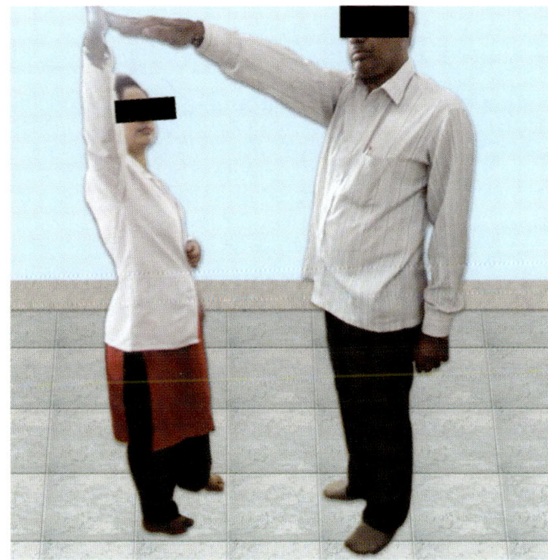

Fig. 29.12: Diagonal reach outs to the left.

■ Walking on a stable surface, later on unstable surface like foam mattress (with/without support), walking on a straight line, tandem walking **(Fig. 29.13)**, walking over obstacles **(Figs. 29.14A and B)**, walking with secondary motor and cognitive task (like head turns, object transfers from one hand to another, digit subtraction task, and walking while talking).

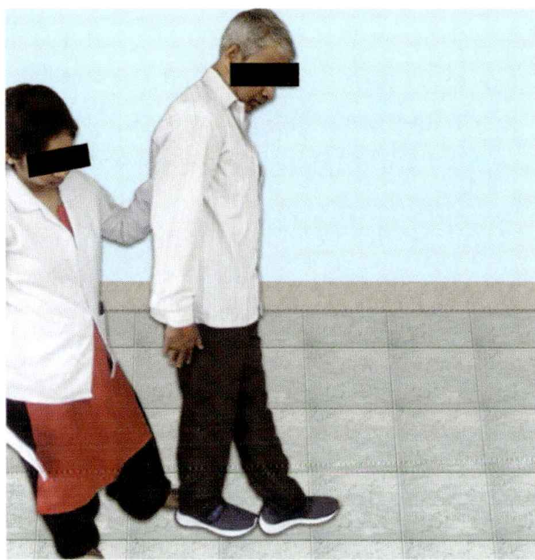

Fig. 29.13: Tandem walking.

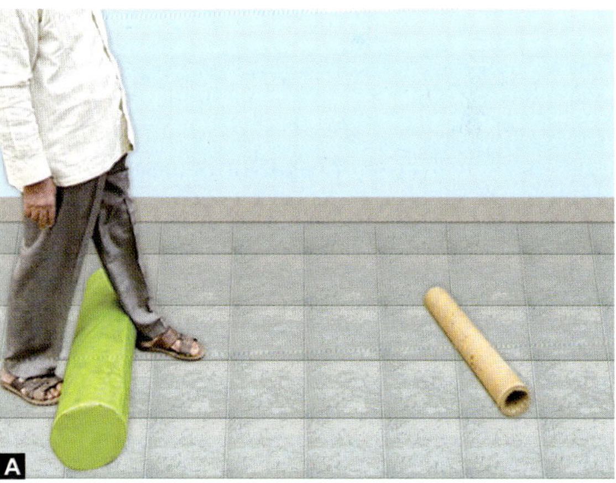

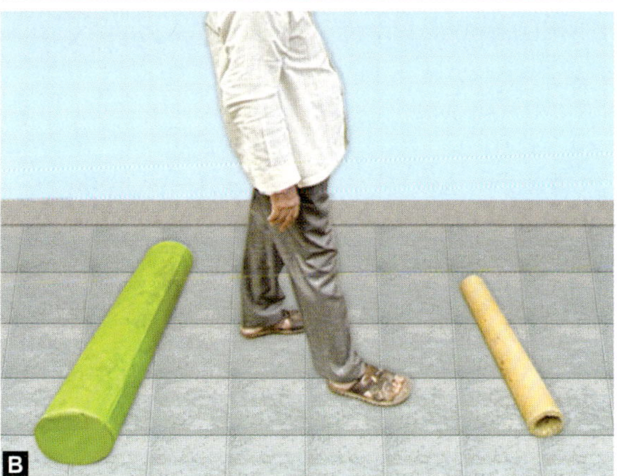

Figs. 29.14A and B: Obstacle walking.

- Activities such as stair climbing and descent, practicing dance forms such as tango and Zumba can be used in milder forms of PD.
- Breathing exercises such as blowing a candle or a paper strip, and deep breathing exercises with chest expansion can be used.

PSYCHOSOCIAL ISSUES IN PARKINSON'S DISEASE

Patients with young-onset PD face more psychosocial problems as compared to their older counterparts. These include anxiety, depression, cognitive disturbances, breakdown of relationships, and unemployment. These problems cause emotional instability in patients as well as in their family members. These issues arise due to lack of understanding of the disease and misinterpretation of character or negative interactions such as staring, avoidance or questioning of people with PD. This causes feeling of shame and fear in such people and creates low self-esteem and leads to reduced social contacts and isolation. These psychosocial problems should be considered important while framing an individual treatment program. Also, changes are required to be done at societal level, by raising public awareness of both visible and invisible symptoms, which can alter the stigma associated with PD.

SUMMARY

PD is a chronic, progressive disorder of the basal ganglia characterized by the cardinal features of rigidity, bradykinesia, tremor, and postural instability. Other than these additional features such as abnormal flexed posture, fatigue, masked face, contractures, festinating gait pattern, swallowing and communication difficulties, visual and sensorimotor disturbances, cognitive and behavioral dysfunctions, autonomic dysfunctions, and cardiopulmonary changes are also seen. Pharmacological treatment provides symptomatic relief but has long-term side effects. Effective rehabilitation depends on patient's stage of disease and symptoms, functional limitations and residual functional abilities. Physical therapy treatment focuses on improvement of strength, range of motion (ROM), functional skills, endurance, etc. Rehabilitation program is designed to prevent or reduce indirect impairments and promote regular exercise, good health, and self-management skills. A comprehensive team approach involving doctor, therapist, patient, family, and caregiver is required during all stages of the disease.

Case Scenario

CASE STUDY

A 67-year-old male presented with tremors in the upper extremities and difficulty in walking since the past 8 months, gradually increasing in intensity. History revealed progression of the abnormal movements from distal to proximal segments of the extremities with aggravation during voluntary movements. The patient had diabetes mellitus type-II since 6 years, but the glucose levels were under control with Metformin 1500 mg/day. The patient had an endomorphic body build, was fully conscious, and had normal higher mental functions. He presented with a stooped posture, a mask-like face, cogwheel rigidity in both the upper and lower extremities with normal muscle strength and bradykinesia, pill-rolling tremors in the upper extremities, normal sensations, dysphagia, drooling of saliva while eating and short, shuffling gait.

Guiding Questions:

1. What is the possible diagnosis?
2. What are the features that point toward the diagnosis?
3. List out the goals of management and formulate a treatment plan.

Review Questions

1. What are the pathophysiological changes associated with Parkinson's disease?
2. What are the factors responsible for Parkinson's disease? Classify Parkinson's disease.
3. Discuss the clinical features involved in Parkinson's disease.
4. Classify the Hoehn and Yahr disability scale.
5. Discuss the medical and surgical options in the treatment of Parkinson's disease.
6. What are the physiotherapy goals in the management of Parkinson's disease?
7. Discuss the physiotherapeutic management in a patient with Parkinson's disease.
8. Enlist the various exercises to treat gait impairments in a patient with Parkinson's disease.

BIBLIOGRAPHY

1. Almeida QJ, Bhatt H. A manipulation of visual feedback during gait training in Parkinson's disease. Park Dis. 2012;2012:508720.
2. Braak H, Tredici K, Riib U, et al. Staging of brain pathology related to sporadic Parkinson's disease. Neurobiol Aging. 2003;24(2):197-211.
3. Caroline H, Gray W, Foltynie, et al. Cognitive deficits and psychosis in Parkinson's disease. CNS Drugs. 2006; 20(6):477-505.
4. Combs SA, Diehl MD, Staples WH, et al. Boxing training for patients with Parkinson disease: a case series. Phys Ther. 2011;91(1):132-42.
5. Connolly BS, Lang AE. Pharmacological treatment of Parkinson disease: a review. JAMA. 2014;311(16):1670-83.

6. Corco DM, Robichaud JA, David FJ, et al. A two-year randomized controlled trial of progressive resistance exercise for Parkinson's disease. Mov Disord. 2013;28(9):1230-40.

7. Cusso ME, Donald KJ, Khoo TK. The impact of physical activity on non-motor symptoms in Parkinson's disease: a systematic review. Front Med. 2016;3:35.

8. Dashtipour K, Johnson E, Kani C, et al. Effect of exercise on motor and non-motor symptoms of Parkinson's disease. Park Dis. 2015;2015:586378. 5 pages.

9. De Bruin N, Doan JB, Turnbull G, et al. Walking with music is a safe and viable tool for gait training in Parkinson's disease: the effect of a 13-week feasibility study on single and dual task walking. Park Dis. 2010;2010:483530.

10. Debaere F, Wenderoth N, Sunaert S, et al. Internal vs external generation of movements: differential neural pathways involved in bimanual coordination performed in the presence or absence of augmented visual feedback. NeuroImage. 2003;19(3):764-76.

11. Ebersbach G, Grust U, Ebersbach A, et al. Amplitude-oriented exercise in Parkinson's disease: a randomized study comparing LSVT-BIG and a short training protocol. J Neural Transm. 2014;122(2):253-6.

12. Fenelon G, Thobois S, Bonnet AM, et al. Tactile hallucinations in Parkinson's disease. J Neurol. 2002;249(12):1699-703.

13. Fischer M, Gemende I, Marsch WC. Skin function and skin disorders in Parkinson's disease. J Neural Transm. 2001;108(2):205-13

14. Foster ER, Golden L, Duncan RP, et al. Community-based argentine tango dance program is associated with increased activity participation among individuals with Parkinson's disease. Arch Phys Med Rehabil. 2013;94(2):240-9.

15. Frazzitta G, Maestri R, Bertotti G. Intensive rehabilitation treatment in early Parkinson's disease: a randomized pilot study with a 2-year follow-up. Neurorehabil Neural Repair. 2014;29(2):123-31.

16. Frazzitta G, Maestri R, Ghilardi MF. Intensive rehabilitation increases BDNF serum levels in Parkinsonian patients: a randomized study. Neurorehabil Neural Repair. 2013;28(2):163-8.

17. Gazewood JD, Richards DR, Clebak K. Parkinson disease: an update. Am Acad Fam Physicians. 2013;87(4):267-73.

18. Goetz C. The history of Parkinson's disease: early clinical descriptions and neurological therapies. Cold Spring Harb Perspect Med. 2011;1(1):a008862.

19. Goetz CG, Tilley BC, Shaftman SR. Movement Disorder Society-sponsored revision of the Unified Parkinson's Disease Rating Scale(MDS-UPDRS): scale presentation and clinimetric testing results. Mov Disord. 2008;23(15):2129-70.

20. Goodwin VA, Richards SH, Taylor RS. The effectiveness of exercise interventions for people with Parkinson's disease: a systematic review and meta-analysis. Mov Disord. 2008;23(5):631-40.

21. Gowers WR. A manual of diseases of the nervous system. London: J and A Churchill; 1888.

22. Hackney ME, Mckee K. Community-based adapted tango dancing for individuals with Parkinson's disease and older adults. J Vis Exp. 2014;(94): e52066.

23. Holroyd S, Currie L, Wooten GF. Prospective study of hallucinations and delusions in Parkinson's disease. J Neurol Neurosurg Psychiatry. 2001;70(6):734-8.

24. Hughes AJ, Daniel SE, Kilford L. Accuracy of clinical diagnosis of idiopathic Parkinson's disease: a clinico-pathological study of 100 cases. J Neurol Neurosurg Psychiatry. 1992;55:181-4.

25. Hui-Ing M, Trombly CA, Tickle-Dengen L. Effect of one single auditory cue on movement kinematics in patients with Parkinson's disease. Am J Phys Med Rehabil. 2004;83(7):530-6.

26. Inzelberg R, Kipervasser S, Korczyn AD. Auditory hallucinations in Parkinson's disease. J Neurol Neurosurg Psychiatry. 1998;64(4):533-5.

27. Jon Stoessl A. Etiology of Parkinson's Disease. Can J Neurol Sci. 1999;30(S1):S10-8.

28. Jost WH. Autonomic dysfunction in idiopathic Parkinson's disease. J Neurol. 2003;250(Suppl 1):i28-30.

29. Kadivar Z, Corcos DM, Foto J. Effect of step training and rhythmic auditory stimulation on functional performance in Parkinson patients. Neurorehabil Neural Repair. 2011;25(7):626-35.

30. Kalia LV, Lang AE. Parkinson disease in 2015: evolving basic, pathological and clinical concepts in PD. Nat Rev Neurol. 2016;12:65-6.

31. Kaur J, Sharma S, Sachdev M, et al. Rehabilitation of patients with Parkinsonism. Delhi Psychiatry J. 2012;15(2):398-401.

32. Keus SHJ, Bloem BR, Hendriks EJM. Evidence-based analysis of physical therapy in Parkinson's disease with recommendations for practice and research. Mov Disord. 2007;22(4):451-60.

33. Koike Y, Takahashi A. Autonomic dysfunction in Parkinson's disease. Eur Neurol. 1997;38(Suppl. 2):8-12.

34. Lahrmann H, Cortelli P, Hilz M. EFNS guidelines on the diagnosis and management of orthostatic hypotension. Eur J Neurol. 2006;13(9):930-6.

35. Larsen JP, Tandberg E. Sleep disorders in patients with Parkinson's disease. Epidemiol Manage. 2001;15(4):267-75.

36. Lee MS, Ernst E. Systematic reviews of Tai Chi: an overview. J Sports Med. 2012;46:713-8.

37. Lotzke D, Ostermann T, Bussing A. Argentine tango in Parkinson disease—a systematic review and meta-analysis. BMC Neurol. 2015;15:226.

38. Macleod AD, Taylor KSM, Counsell CE. Mortality in Parkinson's disease: a systemic review and meta-analysis. Mov Disord. 2014;29(13):1615-22.

39. Maitra KK. Enhancement of reaching performance via self-speech in people with Parkinson's disease. Clin Rehabil. 2007;21(5):418-24.

40. Mak MK, Hui-Chan CW. Cued task-specific training is better than exercise in improving sit-to-stand in patients with Parkinson's disease: a randomized controlled trial. Mov Disord. 2008;23(4):501-9.

41. Mateos-Toset S, Cabrera-Martos I, Torres-Sanchez I, et al. Effects of a single hand–exercise session on manual dexterity and strength in persons with Parkinson disease: a randomized controlled trial. PM&R. 2016;8(2):115-22.

42. Mathers SE, Kempster PA, Law PJ, et al. Anal sphincter dysfunction in Parkinson's disease. Arch Neurol. 1989;46(10):1061-4.

43. McAuley JH, Gregory S. Prevalence and clinical course of olfactory hallucination in idiopathic Parkinson's disease. J Park Dis. 2012;2(3):199-205.

44. Mirelman A, Rochester L, Maidan I, et al. Addition of a nonimmersive virtual reality component to treadmill training to reduce fall risk in older adults (V-TIME): a randomized controlled trial. Lancet. 2016;388(10050):1170-82.

45. Nackaerts E, Nieuwboer A, Broeder S, et al. Opposite effects of visual cueing during writing-like movements of different amplitudes in Parkinson's disease. Neurorehabil Neural Repair. 2016;30(5):431-9.

46. Ni X, Liu S, Shi X, et al. Efficacy and safety of Tai Chi for Parkinson's disease: a systematic review and meta-analysis of randomized controlled trials. PLoS One. 2014;9(6):e99377.

47. Olanow CW, Stern MB, Sethi K. The scientific and clinical basis for the treatment of Parkinson disease. Neurol J. 2009;72(21 Suppl. 4):S1-136.

48. Parashos SA, Maraganore DM, O'Brien PC, et al. Medical services utilization and prognosis in Parkinson disease: a population based study. Mayo Clinic Proc. 2002;77(9):918-25.

49. Petzinger GM, Fisher BE, McEwen S, et al. Exercise-enhanced neuroplasticity targeting motor and cognitive circuitry in Parkinson's disease. Neurology. 2013;12(7):716-26.

50. Picelli A, Melotti C, Origano F, et al. Robot-assisted gait training versus equal intensity treadmill training in patients with mild to moderate Parkinson's disease: a randomized controlled trial. Parkinsonism Relat Disord. 2013;19(6):605-10.

51. Poewe W. The natural history of Parkinson's disease. J Neurol. 2006;253(Suppl 7), vii2-6.

52. Porter B, Macfarlane R, Walker R. The frequency and nature of sleep disorders in a community-based population of patients with Parkinson's disease. Eur J Neurol. 2008;15(1):50-4.

53. Radder DLM, Sturkenboom IH, NImwegen MV, et al. Physical therapy and occupational therapy in Parkinson's disease. Int J Neurosci. 2017;127(10):930-43.

54. Ringenbach SDR, Van Gemmert AWA, Shill HA, et al. Auditory instructional cues benefit unimanual and bimanual drawing in Parkinson's disease patients. Hum Mov Sci. 2011;30(4):770-82.

55. Rochester L, Baker K, Hetherington V, et al. Evidence for motor learning in Parkinson's disease: acquisition, automaticity and retention of cued gait performance after training with external rhythmical cues. Brain Res. 2010;1319:103-11.

56. Rochester L, Hetherington V, Jones D, et al. The effect of external rhythmic cues (auditory and visual) on walking during a functional task in homes of people with Parkinson's disease. Arch Phys Med Rehabil. 2005;86(5):999-1006.

57. Roeder L, Costello JT, Smith SS, et al. Effects of resistance training on measures of muscular strength in people with Parkinson's disease: a systematic review and meta-analysis. PLoS One. 2015;10(7):e0132135.

58. Sakakibara R, Kishi M, Ogawa E, et al. Bladder, bowel and sexual dysfunction in Parkinson's disease. Park Dis. 2011;2011:924605, 21 pages.

59. Shen Xia, Mak MKY. Technology-assisted balance and gait training reduces falls in patients with Parkinson's disease: a randomized controlled trial with 12-month follow-up. Neurorehabil Neural Repair. 2014;29(2):103-11.

60. Shu HF, Yang T, Yu SX, et al. Aerobic exercise for Parkinson's disease: a systematic review and meta-analysis of randomized controlled trials. PLoS One. 2014. https://doi.org/10.1371/journal.pone.0100503.

61. Shulman LM, Katzel LI, Ivey FM, et al. Randomized clinical trial of 3 types of physical exercise for patients with Parkinson disease. JAMA Neurol. 2013;70(2):183-90.

62. Thanvi BR, Lo TCN, Harsh DP. Psychosis in Parkinson's disease. Postgrad Med J. 2005;81:644-6.

63. Van der Kolk NM, Overeem S, De Vries NM, et al. Design of the Park-in-Shape study: a phase II double blind randomized controlled trial evaluating the effects of exercise on motor and non-motor symptoms in Parkinson's disease. BMC Neurol. 2015;15:56.

64. Volpe D, Giantin MG, Maestri R, et al. Comparing the effects of hydrotherapy and land-based therapy on balance in patients with Parkinson's disease: a randomized controlled pilot study. Clin Rehabil. 2014;28(12):1210-17.

65. Waseem S, Gwinn-Hardy K. Pain in Parkinson's disease: common yet seldom recognized symptom is treatable. Postgrad Med. 2001;110(6):33-46.

66. Williams-Gray CH, Foltynie T, Brayne CEG, et al. Evolution of cognitive dysfunction in an incident Parkinson's disease cohort. Brain. 2007;130(7):1787-98.

67. Wirdefeldt K, Adami HO, Cole P, et al. Epidemiology and etiology of Parkinson's disease: a review of the evidence. Eur J Epidemiol. 2011;26(Suppl 1):9581-6.

68. Yang Y, Li XY, Gong L, et al. Tai Chi for improvement of motor function, balance and gait in Parkinson's disease: a systematic review and meta-analysis. PLoS One. 2014;9(7):e102942.

69. Yeo L, Singh R, Gundeti M, et al. Urinary tract dysfunction in Parkinson's disease: a review. Int Urol Nephrol. 2012;44(2):415-24.

70. Yong MH, Fook-Chong S, Pavanni R, et al. Case control of polysomnographic studies of sleep disorders in Parkinson's disease. PLoS One. 2011;6(7):e22511.

71. Zimmermann R, Gschwandtner U, Benz N, et al. Cognitive training in Parkinson disease: cognition-specific vs nonspecific computer training. Neurology. 2014;82(14):1219-26.

Cerebellar Ataxia

Asmita Karajgi

Ⓛ EARNING OBJECTIVES

After reading this chapter, the readers should be able to:

♦ Understand functional anatomy of cerebellum and its role in movement control
♦ Understand the etiology, classification, and differential diagnosis of ataxia
♦ Understand clinical presentation of cerebellar lesion
♦ Gain knowledge regarding the physiotherapy assessment techniques to evaluate the patient with cerebellar ataxia to diagnose impairments and plan the management
♦ Formulate a physiotherapy management in terms of the principles of training and specific exercise prescription
♦ Understand the case study and develop a plan of care.

CHAPTER OUTLINE

- Anatomy of cerebellum
- Functional role of cerebellum
- Etiology
  - Hereditary ataxia
  - Acquired ataxia
- Differential diagnosis
- Clinical presentation
  - Classic signs of cerebellar ataxia
- Physiotherapy assessment
  - Technique
- Assessment of motor skills
  - Coordination
  - Postural control
- Physiotherapy management
  - Goals
  - Stability
- Guidelines for balance training program
  - Training program
  - Precision
  - Mobility
- Psychosocial burden

INTRODUCTION

The researchers have always been fascinated by the little brain, cerebellum as it plays a distinct role in equilibrium, motor planning, movement control, cognition, and motor learning due to its profound connections.

Although the cerebellum constitutes about 10% of the brain's total volume, it contains more than half the total number of neurons in the brain. It functions closely in association with cerebral cortex, brainstem, spinal cord, and vestibular system for movement control.

Ataxia is the umbrella term used to describe clinical features of incoordination of limb movements along with impairment in speech, balance, and eye movements due to cerebellar dysfunction. The word "ataxia," comes from the Greek word, "a taxis" meaning "without order or incoordination."

Clinical Pearl

"Ataxia" is not a disease but a clinical sign.

Cerebellar ataxia can be inherited or acquired. Friedreich's ataxia, spinocerebellar ataxia (SCA) are common examples of hereditary ataxia. Some ataxias are sporadic. Vascular insults, tumors, trauma, and multiple sclerosis are common causes of acquired ataxia. Few ataxias are medically treatable and most are progressive that require symptomatic treatment.

In depth study of ataxia with its diverse nature of etiology and clinical manifestation is important to physical therapists as physical therapy intervention is required in almost all the patients.

ANATOMY OF CEREBELLUM

The cerebellum is located in the posterior cranial fossa behind the pons and the medulla from which it is separated by the fourth ventricle **(Fig. 30.1)**. It consists of the convoluted outer layer of gray matter, **cerebellar cortex** with dense structure of three layers of neurons:

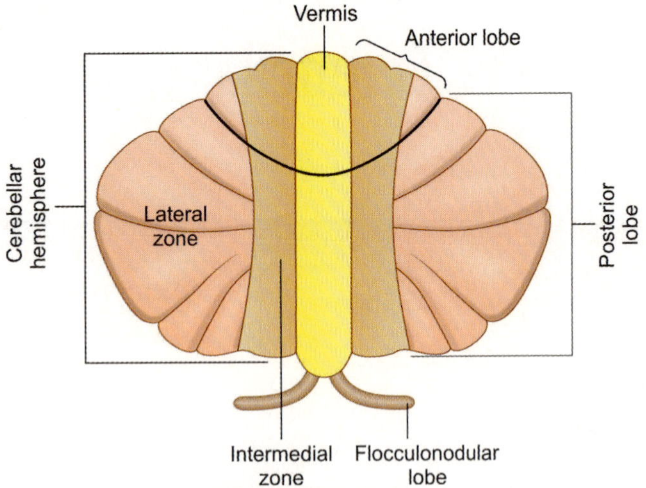

Fig. 30.1: Cerebellum.

1. Molecular layer on the top
2. Purkinje layer in the middle
3. Granular layer at the bottom

The underlying **cerebellar white matter** has three paired **deep cerebellar nuclei:**

1. Dentate
2. Interposed (globus and emboliform)
3. Fastigial

These nuclei send efferent fibers to different parts of the brain.

The **functional unit** of cerebellum essentially consists of a single large Purkinje cell and the corresponding deep cerebellar nuclear cell; both responsible for output signals of the cerebellum.

The superior cerebellar peduncle carries primarily efferent fibers from deep cerebellar nuclei. The middle cerebellar peduncle contains afferent fibers from pons and the inferior cerebellar peduncle contains afferent fibers from medulla.

The afferent information to the cerebellum is passed through mossy and climbing fibers. Mossy fibers carry afferent information from multiple sources, such as cerebral cortex, brainstem, and spinal cord. They stimulate Purkinje cells constantly (simple spikes—weaker short duration action potential) to convey ongoing information. Climbing fibers carry afferent information from the inferior olive and stimulate Purkinje cell with a lesser frequency (complex spikes—prolonged complex action potential). They may be more important for error correction and hence motor learning.

FUNCTIONAL ROLE OF CEREBELLUM

The functional role of cerebellum can be described as follows:

- Morphologically, the cerebellum is classified into lobes and zones.
- Anatomically, the cerebellum has three distinct lobes:
  1. Anterior
  2. Posterior
  3. Flocculonodular lobes separated by two fissures.

Primary fissure separates anterior and posterior lobes. Posterolateral fissure separates posterior and flocculonodular lobes. However, it should be noted that the cerebellum does not function as per the lobes except flocculonodular lobe.

- The cerebellum is identified with the zones divided along the longitudinal axis. Three zones are identified, namely:
  1. Vermis (vermal zone)
  2. Intermediate (paravermal) zone
  3. Lateral zone **(Fig. 30.2)**

The cerebellum has a midline narrow portion, the vermis separated from two large cerebellar hemispheres. Either side of vermis is the intermediate zone and lateral to intermediate zone is the lateral zone. There is a topographical representation of body parts within the cerebellar cortex. Axial body is represented in the vermis, whereas limbs along with face lie in intermediate zone. Lateral zone does not have topographical representation of body. Vermis is responsible for the movement control of neck, trunk, and proximal structures such as shoulders and hips. Intermediate zone is concerned with movement control of distal parts of the extremities such as hands and feet. Lateral zone takes part in motor planning along with cerebral cortex.

- Phylogenetically, the cerebellum is classified into:
  - Archicerebellum (vestibulocerebellum)
  - Paleocerebellum (spinocerebellum)
  - Neocerebellum (cerebrocerebellum)
  - Phylogenetic classification describes the connections and function of various areas of cerebellum.
  - Vestibulocerebellum is the oldest part in evolutionary terms that consists of the flocculonodular lobe and adjacent part of the vermis. Since vestibulocerebellum has primary connections with the vestibular nuclei, it participates in the maintenance of balance mainly during rapid movements and movements of eyes. The flocculonodular lobe is the only part of the cerebellar cortex that does not project to the deep nuclei but has direct connection with the vestibular nuclei.
  - Spinocerebellum is the later part in phylogeny. It consists of intermediate zone of the anterior and posterior lobes. It receives feed forward information of the motor plan from cerebral cortex and proprioceptive feedback from periphery through the spinocerebellar tracts. Thus the spinocerebellum can compare the plan of intended movement with the actual executed movement for error detection. The fastigial and interposed nuclei belong to the spinocerebellum. The interposed nuclei comprise globus nucleus and emboliform nucleus. The efferent fibers from deep cerebellar nuclei project to both the cerebral cortex and the

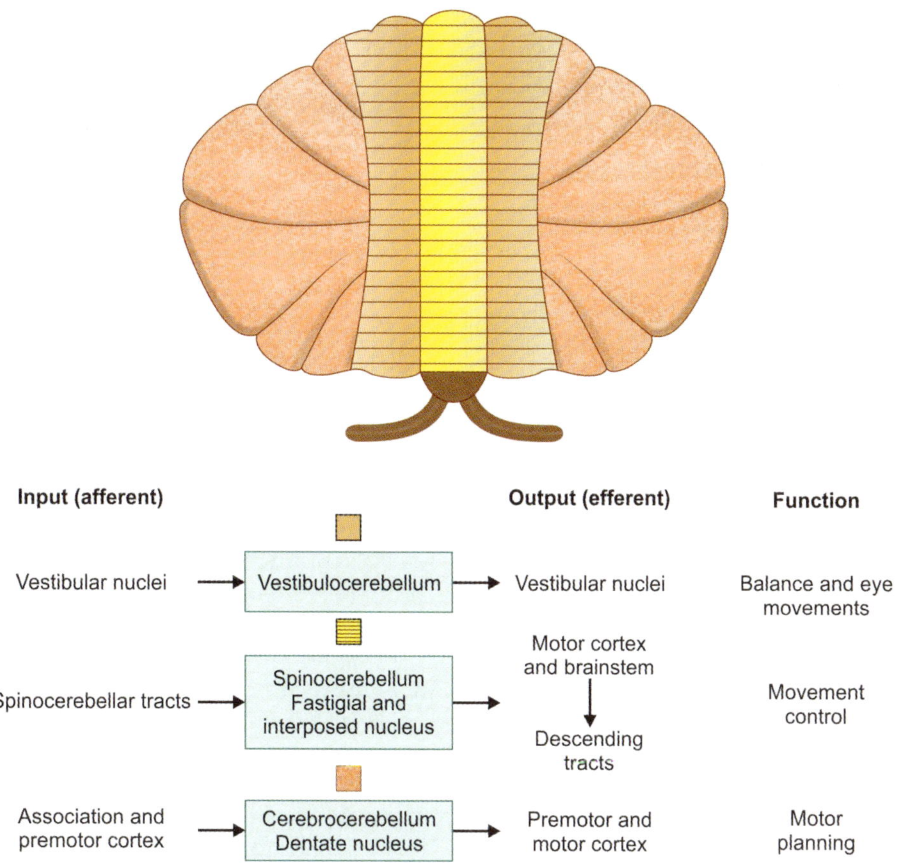

Fig. 30.2: Connections and functions of the cerebellum.

brainstem, thus providing signal modulation of descending motor pathways, such as corticospinal, rubrospinal, and reticulospinal tracts. It modulates muscle tone. It helps to fine-tune muscle activity for performing smooth purposeful movements without overshooting. The cerebellum also plays a role in control of ballistic movements. If there is any difference found between the motor plan and actual movement, cerebellum corrects the error.

- Cerebrocerebellum, also known as neocerebellum, is the phylogenetically the newest part of the cerebellum. It consists of the lateral zone and dentate nucleus. Lateral zone has been found to be large and well developed in humans. It receives input from premotor area and primary and association somatosensory areas of the cerebral cortex via pontine nuclei forming corticopontocerebellar pathways. It sends output mainly to the ventrolateral thalamus, which in turn is connected to the prefrontal cortex, premotor cortex, and primary motor area of the cerebral cortex. The efferent information also goes to the red nucleus. It is thought to be involved in planning and timing of the movement that is about to occur. This planning is especially important for complex, sequential movements. Recent studies have explored its role in motor learning and a number of purely cognitive functions using functional MRI.

ETIOLOGY

The ataxia results due to varied causes.

Some causes are common in children than adults as shown in **Table 30.1**.

The onset could be acute, subacute/chronic as shown in **Table 30.2**.

Ataxia can be categorized into hereditary or acquired.

Hereditary Ataxia

The types of hereditary ataxia are as follows:

- **Autosomal recessive:** Parents are carriers as defective gene comes from both the parents. Mostly they are present in early childhood. Friedreich's ataxia is a common example of early onset ataxia with spinocerebellar degeneration. The structures affected are dorsal root ganglia cells, dorsal column, spinocerebellar tract, dentate nucleus along with systemic manifestations.

Ataxia telangiectasia, SCA with oculomotor apraxia, and infantile SCA are other examples.

Table 30.1: Ataxia seen in children and adults.

Children	Adults
• Ataxic cerebral palsy • Arnold–Chiari malformation • Posterior fossa tumor, such as ependymoma and gliomas • Antiepileptic drug-induced ataxia	• Alcoholism • Stroke • Multiple sclerosis • Vitamin B_1, B_{12}, and E_1 deficiency

Table 30.2: Ataxia according to onset.

Acute onset	Chronic onset
• Stroke • Head injury • Infective (hepatitis A, malaria, etc.)	• Posterior fossa tumors • Vitamins B_1, B_{12}, and E_1 deficiency • Alcoholism • Demyelinating • Degenerative

- **Autosomal dominant**: There are various types of spinocerebellar ataxia (SCA) identified. SCA1, SCA2, SCA6 are common types. Another type is episodic ataxia, which is characterized by transient reversible ataxia.

Acquired Ataxia

There are many causes of acquired ataxia:
- **Congenital anomalies:** Platybasia, Arnold-Chiari malformation, and cerebellar hypoplasia.
- **Developmental disabilities:** Cerebral palsy
- **Vascular:** Stroke involving vertebrobasilar insufficiency.
- **Infection:** Postviral cerebellitis, Lyme disease, malaria, hepatitis A, and enterovirus.
- **Intracranial tumors:** Posterior fossa tumors (glioma, hemangioblastoma, and medulloblastoma).
- **Traumatic:** Head injury
- **Vitamin deficiency:** Vitamin B_1 (Wernicke encephalopathy), vitamin B_{12}, vitamin E deficiency.
- **Demyelinating:** Multiple sclerosis
- **Degenerative:** Paraneoplastic cerebellar degeneration, multisystem atrophy.
- **Toxic reactions:** Alcohol intoxication, heavy metal (lead, mercury) poisoning, and drug (barbiturates, benzodiazepines) toxicity.
- **Metabolic disease:** Myxedema and Wilson disease

DIFFERENTIAL DIAGNOSIS

Ataxia can be caused by pathology of cerebellum (cerebellar ataxia) or lesion of dorsal column (sensory ataxia) or by a combination of both.

Cerebellar ataxia and sensory ataxia can be differentiated as shown in **Table 30.3**.

Table 30.3: Difference between cerebellar and sensory ataxia.

	Cerebellar ataxia	Sensory ataxia
Lesion site	Cerebellum	Dorsal column
Clinical features	• Gait ataxia • Dysmetria • Dysarthria • Dyssynergia • Tremors • Nystagmus	• Ataxia evident in poor visual condition • No associated eye or speech problems
Romberg's test	Sway present with eyes open and closed both	Positive (sway present with eyes closed only)

CLINICAL PRESENTATION

Depending on site, size, and extent of lesion, an individual may have various symptoms of movement dysfunction. Symptoms from unilateral cerebellar damage appear on the ipsilateral side to the injury. Since the cerebellum is not responsible for carrying out movements, damage to it does not lead to paralysis. But cerebellar lesion affects the quality of movement in terms of precision and coordination resulting in "ataxia." There are errors in timing and direction as well as delayed initiation and termination of a movement. There is slowness in agonist activity along with delayed onset latency in antagonist muscle on electromyography (EMG) activity. Ataxia may cause uncoordinated or clumsy balance, speech, or limb movements, mostly resulting in wide-based, unsteady gait. There are some "classic signs" described in cerebellar ataxia.
- Dysmetria
- Dyssynergia (asynergia, decomposition of movement)
- Dysdiadochokinesia
- Hypotonia
- Intention and postural tremors

Rapid ballistic movements are also affected in cerebellar lesion.

Classic Signs of Cerebellar Ataxia

Classic signs of cerebellar ataxia include the following:
- **Dysmetria:** Limb dysmetria can be defined as an error in trajectory due to abnormal range, rate, and/or force of motion. There could be undershooting (hypometria) or overshooting (hypermetria). In hypermetria, a movement does not stop at the required point due to inability to predict distance or loss of movement feedback. Then the cortex tries to correct overshooting by movement in opposite direction to reach the target. Hypometria is seen in slow, small amplitude movements.
- **Tremors:** Intention tremors or kinetic tremors are observed during a voluntary activity. These are rhythmic, alternating, and oscillatory movements of the

limb as it approaches target. First the limb overshoots the target and then oscillates back and forth till reaches the target. It results due to loss of damping effect of cerebellum. Postural or static tremors are observed while maintaining a posture. Titubation of head can also be observed.

- **Hypotonia:** It refers to reduced muscle tone of the muscles. This hypotonia could be due to reduced proprioceptive information from muscle spindles or loss of cerebellar facilitation of motor nuclei in the cerebral cortex, brainstem, and spinal centers. It usually accompanies acute hemispheric lesions due to sudden withdrawal of cerebellar input. It is more noticeable in upper limbs and proximal muscles.
- **Asthenia:** It refers to generalized weakness experienced by the patients. Holmes (1917) suggested that the abnormal fatigability of the affected limbs is associated with and may be regarded as a result of asthenia.
- **Dysdiadochokinesia:** It is inability to perform rapid alternating movements, such as pronation-supination of forearm. There is error in timing and intensity of the antagonist muscle activity to break the movement.
- **Dysarthria:** It refers to the failure in progression in talking due to incoordination of muscles required for articulation. The characteristic speech is "scanning," i.e., one word at a time. The speech is slurred and slow.
- **Dyssynergia:** It is also termed "movement decomposition." Normal flow of movement with smooth, sequential completion of the components is interrupted instead the patient may complete its components or some parts separately. There is defect in timing of the movement at different joints. The lack of synergy of movement is seen especially in complex movements.
- **Cerebellar nystagmus:** It is the tremor of the eyeballs that results as one tries to fix the vision in the peripheral field. The oscillatory movement of the eye back to the midline is observed.
- **Rebound phenomenon:** This is due to loss of check reflex. Normally when resistance to an isometric contraction is suddenly removed, limb remains in the same position due to contraction of the antagonist muscle. Since this check is lost in cerebellar lesion, the patient is unable to stop the movement.
- **Postural instability:** This can be seen in patients whose sitting and standing balance may get affected. The patient feels shaky and uncertain while maintaining a posture. Postural sway is increased. Postural adjustments are affected. It is difficult to maintain equilibrium when center of gravity is shifted outside base of support in many functional activities.
- **Ataxic gait:** It is abnormally wide-based and unsteady ambulation. Typical features of patients with ataxic gait described by Palliyath et al. (1998) are widened base, unsteadiness, irregularity of stepping both in direction and distance, and reduced stride length with a trend to reduced cadence.
- **Vertigo** can be present if vestibulocerebellar system is affected.
- **Cognition** gets affected as the lateral aspect of the neocerebellum and ventral lateral aspect of the dentate nuclei is responsible for cognitive functions.
- **Motor learning** can get hampered in cerebellar lesion as climbing fiber input to Purkinje cell required for error detection is affected. As per Ito M. (2000) the different regions of the lateral hemisphere appear to be particularly important for both motor and cognitive learning that depend on repeated practice.

PHYSIOTHERAPY ASSESSMENT

Preliminary screening in terms of cognition, sensation, range of motion, muscle tone, and strength for impairments should be completed. Pendular knee jerk is another feature where the leg keeps swinging after the initial reflex due to loss of damping.

Environmental assessment in the form of entrance, door, railing, floor, lighting, storage, and furniture should be done to understand participation restriction.

Assessment of ataxia includes evaluation of posture, equilibrium, and movement control. Traditionally, coordination has been assessed with:

- Equilibrium
- Non-equilibrium tests

It is evident that nonequilibrium tests also have the basic requirement of maintenance of equilibrium. Hence, they are not purely nonequilibrium, e.g. in "finger to nose test," the patient needs to maintain sitting balance while touching his finger to nose. Nonequilibrium tests assess upper and lower extremities for dysmetria, intention tremors, dysdiadochokinesia (**Table 30.4**). Nonequilibrium tests assess static postural control (holding a position) or maintain dynamic postural control (during movement) (**Table 30.5**).

Technique

- Environment-coordination examination should be administered in quiet and well-lit environment.
- Patient preparation: The patient is given a comfortable and well-supported position.
- Explanation: The patient is explained the purpose of the examination. The procedure of the coordination tests is also described in brief.
- Demonstration: Each test is demonstrated to the patient before administering it.

Table 30.4: Non-equilibrium tests **(Figs. 30.3A to F).**

Sl. No.	Test	Test position	Instruction/technique	Response
1.	Finger to nose	• Patient in sitting position • Shoulder in 90° flexion or abduction with extended elbow	Touch the tip of the index finger of the hand to the tip of nose	• Difficult/unable to perform • Shows intention tremors • Dysmetria
2.	Finger to finger	• Patient in sitting position • Both shoulders in 90° abduction with extended elbow	Touch the tip of the index finger to the tip of the finger	
3.	Finger to therapist's finger	• Patient in sitting position • Therapist sits in front of the patient	Touch the tip of the index finger to the tip of the therapist's finger	
4.	Alternate nose to finger	• Patient in sitting position	Touch alternately his/her nose and therapist's finger	
5.	Alternate pronation–supination of forearm	• Patient in sitting position • Elbow flexed to 90°, forearm resting on the lap	Turn palm up and down	Difficulty to perform alternate movements
6.	Rebound	• Patient in sitting position	Therapist resists elbow flexion by giving resistance to forearm and suddenly releases	Sudden release of the forearm results in an overshooting of flexion movement
7.	Tapping hand	• Patient in sitting position • Forearm resting on the lap	Tap hand on the knee	Unable to tap rapidly
8.	Heel on shin	Patient in supine position	Run the heel down the contralateral shin	Cannot keep contact of the heel to shin
9.	Heel to knee and toe	Patient in supine or sitting position	Touch opposite knee and toe alternately with heel	Difficult/unable to perform
10.	Tapping foot	Patient in sitting position	Tap forefoot on ground with heel in contact with floor	Unable to tap rapidly
11.	Toe to examiner's finger	Patient in supine position	Touch the toe to the examiner's finger held at different points in space	Difficult/unable to perform
12.	Drawing figures	Patient in sitting position	Draw circle, alphabet, or figure of eight	Unable to draw
13.	Fixation or holding a position of limb	Patient in sitting position	Hold the arm in 90° flexed position/hold the leg straight	Difficult/unable to hold

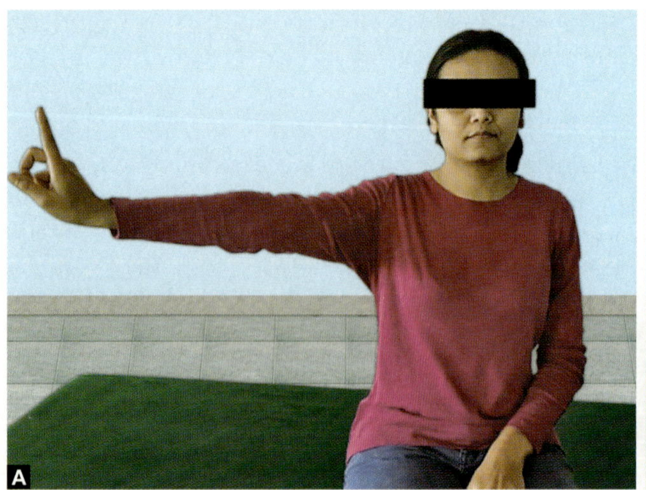
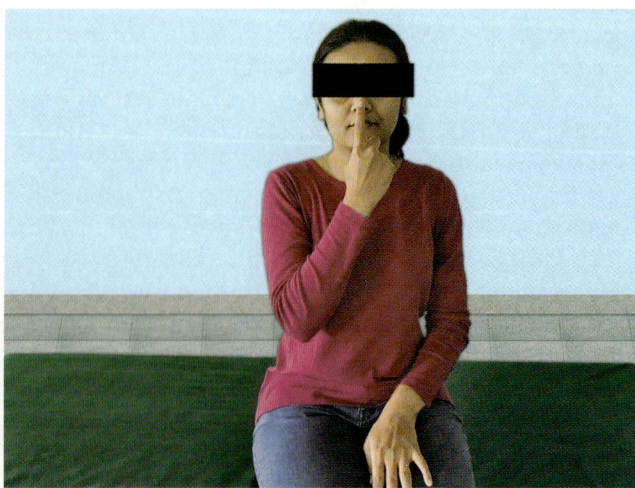

Fig. 30.3A

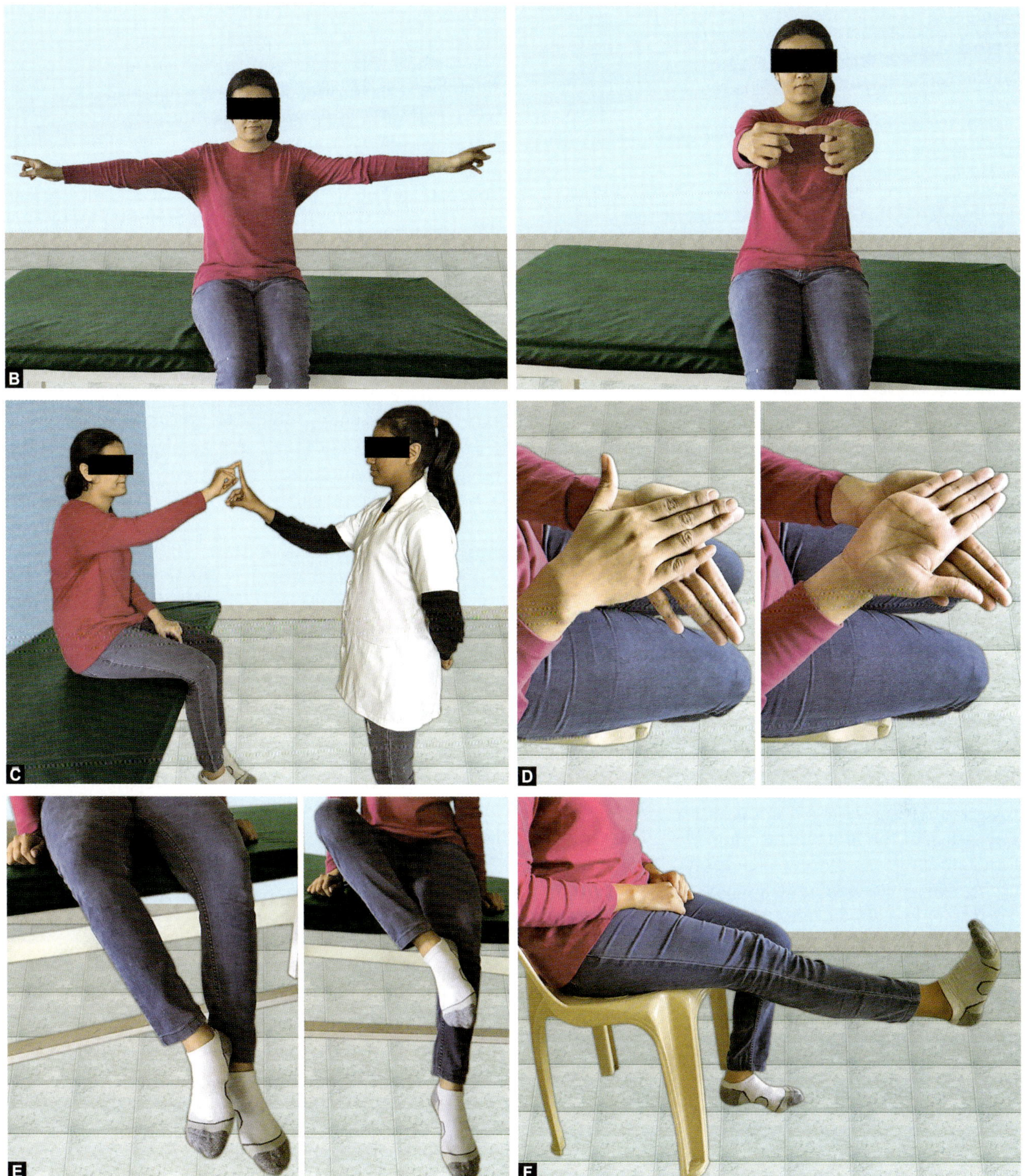

Figs. 30.3B to F

Figs. 30.3A to F: Non-equilibrium tests: (A) Finger to nose; (B) Finger to finger; (C) Finger to therapist's finger; (D) Alternate pronation and supination; (E) Heel on shin; (F) Trying to hold a position.
(*Note:* The pictures show the tests being performed by a normal subject)

ASSESSMENT OF MOTOR SKILLS

Coordination

Coordinated movement is smooth, precise, and purposeful. The muscles need to get activated at appropriate time with optimum force of contraction in a particular sequence for a coordinated movement involving multiple joints. Incoordination of movement leads to participation restriction and affects day-to-day functioning of the patient. Therefore, assessment of functional task is important. Gross motor and fine motor skills are examined for the ability of the patient to initiate, control, and terminate the

Table 30.5: Equilibrium tests **(Figs. 30.4A and B).**

Standing with normal base of support
Standing with feet together (narrow base of support)
Tandem standing
One-leg standing
Standing-forward bending with flexed upper limb, lateral bending
Spot marching
Tandem walking, walking sideways, and backward
Walk on heels/toes
Obstacle walking

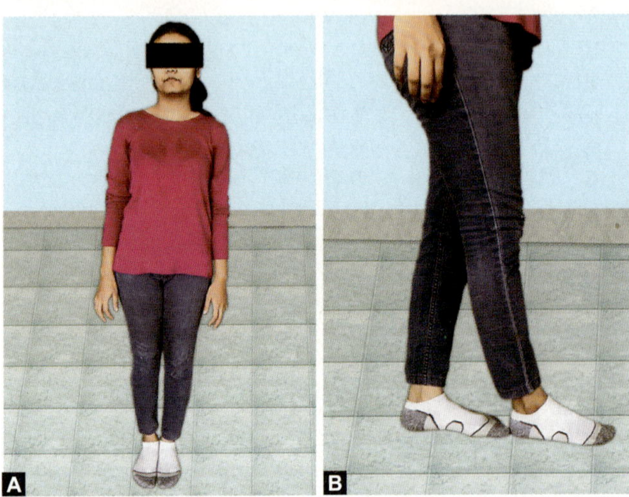

Figs. 30.4A and B: Equilibrium tests: (A) Standing with feet together; (B) Tandem standing.
(*Note:* The pictures show the tests being performed by a normal subject)

movement. Time required to complete the task as well as accuracy of the movement is analyzed. The sequence of movement for a complex task should be observed for dyssynergia or movement decomposition, e.g., getting up from a chair to open the door on the right side. In this task, a smooth flow of movement is expected, but the patient completes it in parts. The patient may take long time to get up from chair, use hands for support, appear stiff to brace him, and stand with wide base of support. Then he/she may prefer to turn to right by taking short steps instead of pivot turn. The patient reaches the door with ataxic gait and shows dysmetria when approaching the door knob.

Dexterity can be assessed by standardized tools, such as Jebsen-Taylor Hand Function Test, Minnesota Manual Dexterity Test, The Purdue Pegboard, and Hand Tool Dexterity Test.

Postural Control

Self-report measures, such as "**Fall Efficacy Scale**" rates confidence in performing activities of daily living and "**Activities-specific Balance Confidence Scale**" quantifies fear of falling. **Single item tools** are useful for quick screening but test only one aspect of balance, e.g., functional reach test, multidirectional reach test, single limb stance, and Get Up and Go test/Timed up and go test.

Sensory test, such as Romberg test helps in differentiating between sensory and cerebellar ataxia. A patient with cerebellar ataxia sways both with eyes open and closed. A patient with sensory ataxia sways only with eyes closed as visual input compensates for loss of proprioceptive sensations. Sensory organization test and clinical test for sensory interaction in balance are also useful to analyze sensory component of ataxia. Multidimensional tools such as Berg Balance Scale, Tinetti's performance oriented mobility assessment (POMA) scale, and Dynamic Gait Index assess balance during functional tasks. It is also important to assess the patient's ability to ambulate with distractions and increased cognitive demands with dual task.

Advanced sophisticated technique with posturography utilizes force platform data of center of pressure to assess postural sway, stability limits, etc. Excessive postural sway may be found in ataxic patients. Dynamic posturography differentiates from static posturography generally by using a special apparatus with a movable horizontal platform.

Clinically ataxia specific scales are also available. International Cooperative Ataxia Rating Scale (ICARS) assesses ataxia in detail but it is time-consuming. Another tool "Scale for the Assessment and Rating of Ataxia (SARA)" **(Appendix)** was developed as an alternative to ICARS developed by Schmitz-Hübsch T et al. (2006) as it is easy to administer and has shown high inter/intrarater reliability. It has eight categories related to gait, stance, sitting, speech, finger-chase test, nose–finger test, fast alternating movements, and heel shin test.

Berg Balance Scale, Timed Up and Go test, stance, and sit subcomponents of the SARA, the posture and gait subcomponent of the ICARS have been recommended for balance assessment in clinical practice for people with cerebellar ataxia.

PHYSIOTHERAPY MANAGEMENT

Physical therapy started early in the disease helps to formulate optimum strategies for the patient. A customized program that includes training of stability and coordination gives beneficial effect. Both remedial and compensatory approach should to be used as per need of the patient. Supportive aids and equipment should be employed when necessary. Treatment should be supported by an appropriate home exercise program and recreational activities.

Goals

The goals of physiotherapy management are as follows:
- Educate the patient and caregivers regarding both motor and non-motor symptoms.
- Improve postural stability, proactive and reactive balance.
- Train control of functional activities such as supine to sit and sit to stand.
- Develop upper extremity coordination for reaching and fine motor skills.

- Develop independent functional gait
- Improve the quality of life of the patient by increasing the patient's independence in performing daily activities of life.

Stability

Hypotonia is a prominent feature leading to lack of axial and proximal joint stability in ataxic patients. Balance abnormalities are characterized by increased postural sway, either excessive or diminished responses to perturbations, poor control of equilibrium during motions of other body parts, and abnormal oscillations of the trunk (titubation). It is important to find the factors responsible for poor balance in the patient. Poor postural control increases risk of falls. It is important to train both postural orientation and equilibrium in order to gain functional independence. **Postural orientation** refers to active alignment of the trunk and head with respect to gravity, support surfaces, the visual surround and internal references. **Postural equilibrium** involves the coordination of movement strategies to stabilize the center of body mass during both self-initiated and externally triggered disturbances of stability. (Shumway-Cook A and Woollacott, MH, 2007)

- Static control (holding) in a number of different weight bearing, antigravity postures improves proximal stability by promoting cocontraction of muscles around the joints. Another way is to increase the number of body segments (degree of freedom) that must be controlled.
- Progression through a series of postures is used to gradually increase postural demand by narrowing the base of support, raising the center of mass and number of body segments to be controlled. Postures such as prone on elbow, sitting, quadruped, kneeling, plantigrade, and standing can be used for this purpose. Postural control requirement of standing position is much more than sitting position.
- Additional proprioceptive input through joint approximation applied through proximal joints (through shoulders or hips) or head or spine is used especially when balance is challenged.
- Special proprioceptive neuromuscular facilitation such as rhythmic stabilization and alternating isometrics is useful in gaining stability. Both the techniques promote an isometric contraction of the agonist followed by an isometric contraction of the antagonist.
- Patient with significant ataxia may not be able to hold steady and may benefit from the technique of slow reversal-hold proprioceptive neuromuscular facilitation (PNF). It involves an isotonic contraction of the agonist followed immediately by an isometric contraction. It can be progressed through decrements of range till midrange holding is achieved.
- Controlled mobility can be trained with weight shifting or rocking from the static postures (quadruped, sitting).
- Movement transitions are trained by moving in and out of postures. Functional movement transitions such as supine to sit and sit to stand are practiced.

- Reactive and proactive balance should be given importance while training balance. Reactive balance is in response to external forces acting on body (feedback). There is either change in center of gravity (COG) or base of support (BOS). Proactive is in anticipation of internally generated, destabilizing forces imposed on body's own movements (feed-forward). Adaptive balance is appropriate modification in response to changing task.
- Somatosensory, visual, and vestibular inputs can be varied, as appropriate.
- Normally central nervous system (CNS) receives sensory information provided by visual, vestibular and somatosensory system. Then processes it in context of previously learned responses and executes a corrective automatic postural response. Anticipatory and ongoing postural adjustments need to be trained.
- Use of force platforms: The patient with ataxia learns to reduce the postural sway (frequency and amplitude) and control center of alignment position. The added biofeedback in form of visual and or auditory feedback display can improve control in some patients.

Guidelines for Balance Training Program

The guidelines for balance training program are as follows:
1. Give supervised, safe, yet challenging exercises
2. Plan exercises sequentially (stable surface-to-dynamic, wide-to-narrow base of support)
3. Stress multiple planes of motion
4. Give emphasis on task specific functional training
5. Train both reactive and proactive balance strategies
6. Incorporate multisensory approach
7. Introduce dual task training
8. Create novel, innovative balance exercises
9. Include home program
10. Progress toward recreational activity

Training Program

There are various activities included in a training program:
- Sitting balance can be trained from supported sitting to unsupported sitting by removing upper extremity support gradually.
- Stability in sitting is achieved by using techniques such as joint compression, rhythmic stabilization, slow reversal-hold in small range, push–pull activities with hands or using a cane, and external perturbation to trunk.
- Anteroposterior and lateral weight shifts in sitting first with hand support and then unsupported is practiced.
- Anticipatory postural adjustments can be trained by adding upper extremity activities one by one, e.g., reaching within arm's length, raising both upper extremities, throwing a ball. This can be followed by reach beyond arm's length to increase limits of stability.
- Change in the supporting surface can be introduced by asking the patient to sit on the vestibular ball. Standing balance can be improved by weight shifts in standing.

- Activities, such as spot marching, stepping, side stepping, and cross-stepping can be practiced first with therapist's assistance or parallel bar support and then independently. Reaching forward or sideways can be practiced.
- Functional activities, such as bending down to pick up a bottle or opening a drawer are trained **(Figs. 30.5A and B)**.
- Ankle, hip, and stepping strategy can be trained.
- The physical therapist supervises and provides support throughout the Balance program. Balance training programs and fall-prevention interventions **(Figs. 30.6A and B)** must include a focus on balance-recovery reactions such as reaching to grab a bar or taking a step.

Precision

Precision is assessed as listed below:
- Emphasis is given on smoothness and accuracy of movements. Frenkel's exercise for upper and lower extremities can be given in supine, sitting, and standing position.
- Progression of exercises is done with range, speed, and complexity. Movements of various amplitudes and speed, stopping and starting at different points in the range (to control agonist–antagonist movements), are practiced.
- Resistance is applied to limbs through PNF diagonal pattern in stabilizing reversals. Elastic resistance bands can be used to provide resistance and reduce ataxic movements **(Figs. 30.7A and B)**.
- Application of light weights provides additional proprioceptive loading.
- Feedback and feed forward tasks, novel movements, and complex task are practiced repeatedly to reduce attention demands of the action.
- Patients with ataxia do better in low-stimulus environment that allows them to concentrate more fully on their movements.

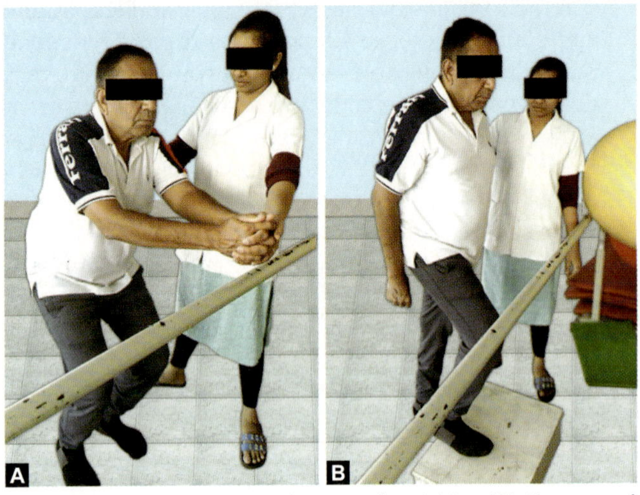

Figs. 30.5A and B: Training functional activities: (A) Sit to stand; (B) Stepping.
Courtesy: Mr Viral Shah (PT), Lakshya Neuro Rehab, Ahmedabad, India.

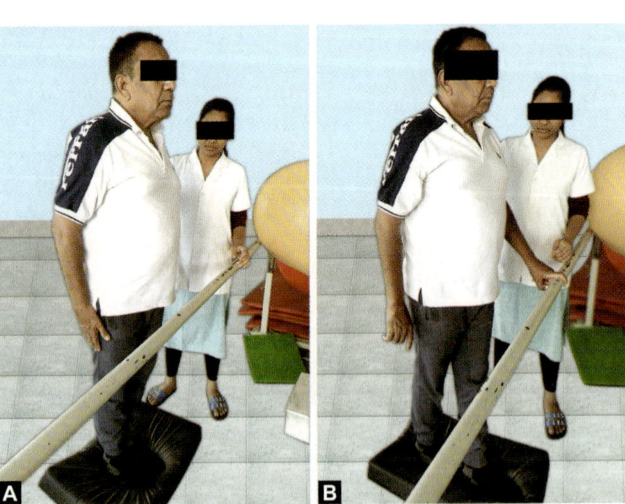

Figs. 30.6A and B: Balance training: (A) Standing with narrow BOS on a soft surface; (B) Tandem standing on a soft surface.
Courtesy: Mr Viral Shah (PT), Lakshya Neuro Rehab, Ahmedabad, India.

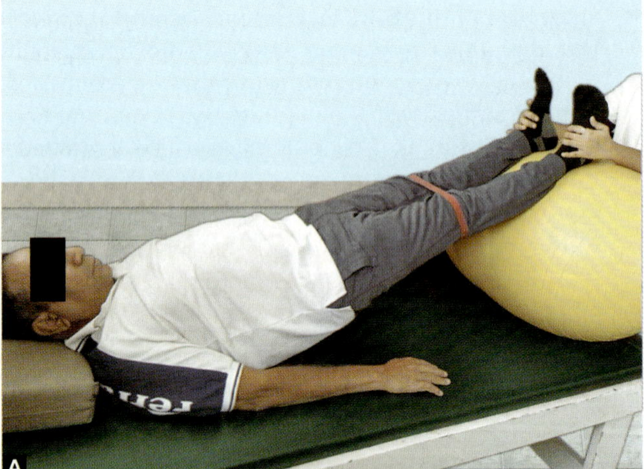

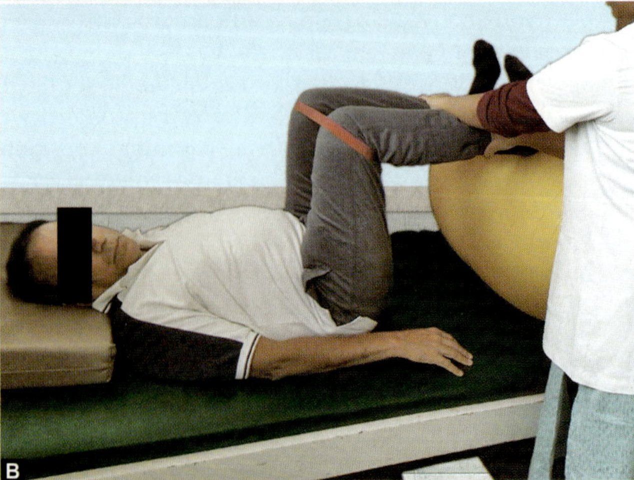

Figs. 30.7A and B: Use of elastic bands to apply resistance in various positions and during various activities.
Courtesy: Mr Viral Shah (PT), Lakshya Neuro Rehab, Ahmedabad, India.

Mobility

Physiotherapy helps in mobility in the following ways:

- If the cerebellar input to the cortex is reduced, problem in automatic movements become apparent. The patient may take a long time to complete the task as cerebral cortex needs to take over. Movement initiation is delayed and timing of muscle activation in synergy is affected.
- Complex motor skills can be broken down into component parts for practice. The component parts are practiced before the whole task is attempted. Control of functional activities, such as supine to sit or sit to stand is trained using tactile/verbal cues, feedback, and practice.
- A practice sequence organized around one task performed repeatedly in blocked, while a variety of tasks are ordered randomly across trials in random practice. Constant practice is useful to repeat the same task till it is learned. A variable practice allows a person to perform significantly better on novel variation of the task as it is performed in variable conditions.
- Gait ataxia is often described as a "drunken gait," with distinctive features including variable foot placement, irregular foot trajectories, a wide base of support, a veering path of movement, and abnormal interjoint coordination patterns. The cerebellum uses both feed forward and feedback mechanisms to maintain balance during locomotion, and when those mechanisms fail, gait ataxia results.
- External support for steadiness during ambulation is provided using a cane or manual support. Walking sideways, obstacle walking, and walking on different surfaces (hard, soft, and inclined surfaces) can be practiced.
- Weighted canes or walkers can be used to reduce ataxic upper limb movements during ambulation. The extra weights will also increase the energy expenditure and must, therefore, be used cautiously in order not to bring about increased fatigue.
- Hydrotherapy can be used where buoyancy of water provides stability and water exerts pressure on the limbs.
- **Advances in treatment:** Virtual reality, biofeedback, treadmill exercises with supported body weight, and torso weighting have shown positive effects in patients with ataxia. Video game–based coordinative exercises are found to be useful. Noninvasive brain stimulation in the form of repetitive transcranial magnetic stimulation and transcranial direct current stimulation over the cerebellum for neuromodulation to facilitate motor learning, and motor function has potential to improve the effect of physical therapy for cerebellar ataxia. Robotic training has also shown promising results.
- Fatigue is a significant problem in ataxic patients. The basic principles of fatigue management are taking regular rest breaks, prioritizing and pacing activities, and maintaining exercise tolerance. In the early stage of disease, distributed practice should be given. In distributed practice, amount of rest time in between a trial is greater than or equal to the amount of practice in the trial. Mental practice is a strategy in which the performance of the motor task is imagined or visualized without physical practice. It should be considered for patients who fatigue easily and are unable to sustain physical practice. When combined with physical practice it showed an increase in the accuracy and efficiency of movement at significantly faster rates than physical practice alone.
- **Evidence:** Physiotherapy can improve gait, balance, and trunk control for people with ataxia and can reduce activity limitations and support increased participation. The prevention of falls is important to consider in patients with progressive ataxia. For people with cerebellar dysfunction, dynamic task practice that challenges stability, explores stability limits, and aims to reduce upper limb weight bearing seems an important intervention to improve gait and balance. Higher training intensities are associated with greater improvements in clinical outcome. Improvement is greater in people with less severe ataxia and it is also related to the ability to learn the task.

PSYCHOSOCIAL BURDEN

Chronic condition such as cerebellar ataxia with functional dependency and psychosocial issues creates additional burden on the patient, family, and the society. There is considerable supporting evidence for cognitive and psychiatric illnesses associated with cerebellar pathology. Schmahmann described the concept of "dysmetria of thought" responsible for cerebellar cognitive affective syndrome (CCAS). Normal function of lateral part of the cerebellar hemisphere (cognitive) and posterior vermis (emotional) is required for behavioral control. The CCAS has been referred to as impairments in executive, visual–spatial, and linguistic abilities, with affective disturbance ranging from emotional blunting and depression, to disinhibition and psychotic features. There is difficulty in managing day-to-day task due to difficulty in multitasking, expressing thoughts along with mood changes such as depression, irritability, and frustration. It is imperative to include management of nonmotor symptoms with medications, cognitive rehabilitation, and counseling to optimize the quality of life in patients.

SUMMARY

Cerebellum makes a very unique and substantial contribution in the movement control by influencing commands of the descending pathways. It has three distinct areas as per the connections: vestibulocerebellum, spinocerebellum, and cerebrocerebellum. Cerebellar damage leads to impairments not only in posture, balance, and movement but also in cognition and motor learning.

Dysmetria, dyssynergia, dysdiadochokinesia, hypotonia, rebound phenomena, and intention and postural tremors are classic signs of cerebellar ataxia. Depending upon etiology, few ataxias are treatable and progressive ataxias require symptomatic medical treatment. Physical therapy intervention aims to maximize function and optimize the quality of life in patients with ataxia. Detail history and clinical examination of coordination and postural control is crucial to understand impairments and formulate treatment goals as per the patient's need. A customized treatment plan includes specific interventions to improve balance during functional tasks, fine motor activities, and gait along with home program and recreational activities. Both restorative and compensatory strategies are utilized to optimize the outcome for benefit of the patient.

Case Scenario

CASE STUDY

A 52-year-old male patient complains of imbalance during standing and walking since last 2 months. He finds difficulty in using right upper limb for personal care and eating. He has stopped going for work due to worsening of the symptoms. There was no family history of ataxia. Personal history reveals chronic alcohol abuse. MRI shows mild cerebellar atrophy. The most probable diagnosis was adult onset, nongenetic, and progressive ataxia due to alcoholic cerebellar degeneration. Treatment in the form of alcohol abstinence and vitamin B_1 supplement is suggested.

Examination

Higher functions: Alert and oriented, mini-mental state score—24 indicating intact cognition, looks depressed

Speech: Slightly slurred and slow

Sensations: Normal

Range of motion: Normal at all the joints except restriction in ankle dorsiflexion

Tone: Hypotonia in the muscles of right arm and bilateral lower limb muscles; muscles look soft and flabby

Balance: Independent sitting is possible. But limits of stability is reduced. Raising both upper limbs in front shows postural tremors. Both reactive and proactive standing balance is affected. Postural sway increases in tandem standing. Considerable gait ataxia is present with a wide base of support and inconsistency in steps

Coordination: Signs of incoordination in finger nose test on right side is present but more marked in heel to shin bilaterally. Berg Balance Score is 45 and SARA score is 26.

Guiding Questions:

1. What is the common clinical presentation of alcoholic cerebellar degeneration? What are the impairments seen in the patient?
2. How do you rule out involvement of any other part of the nervous system that commonly gets affected due to alcoholism?
3. What is multidisciplinary approach for treating ataxia?
4. How do you assess balance and gait with SARA?
5. What are the principles of physical therapy treatment planned for the patient?
6. What strategies can be utilized for improving standing balance?

Review Questions

1. Define "ataxia."
2. What are deep nuclei? What is the role of mossy and climbing fibers?
3. How are the zones of the cerebellum differentiated?
4. Explain the functional anatomy of the cerebellum along with its connections.
5. What are the etiological factors of ataxia?
6. Differentiate between sensory and cerebellar ataxia.
7. What are the clinical features of cerebellar dysfunction?
8. Discuss physiotherapy assessment of coordination. Describe technique of nonequilibrium tests.
9. Discuss various methods of balance assessment and intervention to improve sitting balance.
10. Discuss physiotherapy treatment for ataxic gait.

BIBLIOGRAPHY

1. Adler S, Becker D, Buck M. PNF in practice, 3rd edition. New York, NY: Springer; 2008.
2. Akbar U, Ashizawa T. Ataxia. Neurologic Clin. 2015; 33(1):225-48.
3. Armutlu K, Karabudak R, Nurlu G. Physiotherapy approaches in the treatment of ataxic multiple sclerosis: a pilot study. Int Rehabil Med. 2001;15(3):203-11.
4. Arthur C, Guyton MD and Hall JE. Textbook of medical physiology. Mississippi: Guyton & Hall;2006.
5. Balliet R, Harbst KB, Kim D, et al. Retraining of functional gait through the reduction of upper extremity weight-bearing in chronic cerebellar ataxia. Int Rehabil Med. 1986;8(4):148-53.
6. Carpinella I, Cattaneo D, Abuarqub S, et al. Robot-based rehabilitation of the upper limbs in multiple sclerosis: feasibility and preliminary results. J Rehabil Med. 2009;41(12):966-70.
7. Diener, HC, Dichgans J. Pathophysiology of cerebellar ataxia. Mov Disord. 1992;7(2):95-109.
8. Dow RS. The evolution and anatomy of the cerebellum. Biol Rev. 1942;17(3):179-220.
9. Earhart GM, Bastian AJ. Cerebellar gait ataxia: selection and coordination of human locomotor forms. J Neurophysiol. 2001;85:759-69.
10. Fonteyn EM, Schmitz-Hübsch T, Verstappen CCP, et al. Prospective analysis of falls in dominant ataxias. Eur Neurol. 2013;69(1):53-7.
11. Freund HJ, Barnikol UB, Nolte D, et al. Subthalamic-thalamic DBS in a case with spinocerebellar ataxia type 2 and severe tremor—a unusual clinical benefit. Mov Disord. 2007;22:732-5.
12. Freund JE, Stetts DM. Use of trunk stabilization and locomotor training in an adult with cerebellar ataxia: a single system design. Physiother Theory Pract. 2010;26:447-58.
13. Ghez C. The cerebellum. In: Kandel ER, Schwartz JH, Jessell TM (Eds). Principles of neural science. Norwalk, CT: Appleton and Lange; 1991. pp. 626-46.
14. Gilbert PFC, Thach WT. Purkinje cell activity during motor learning. Brain Res. 1977;128(2):309-28.
15. Grimaldi G, Argyropoulos GP, Boehringer A, et al. Non-invasive cerebellar stimulation—a consensus paper. Cerebellum. 2014;13(1):121-38.
16. Holmes G. The cerebellum of man. Brain. 1939;62(1):1-30.
17. Holmes G. The symptoms of acute cerebellar injuries due to gunshot injuries. Brain. 1917;40:461-535.

18. Ilg W, Schatton C, Schicks J, et al. Video game-based coordinative training improves ataxia in children with degenerative ataxia. Neurology. 2012;79(20):2056-60.

19. Ito M. Mechanisms of motor learning in the cerebellum. Brain Res. 2000;886(1-2):237-45.

20. Jimsheleishvili S, Dididze M. Neuroanatomy, cerebellum. In: StatPearls [Internet]. StatPearls Publishing; 2019.

21. Klein AP, Ulmer JL, Quinet SA, et al. Nonmotor functions of the cerebellum: an introduction. Am J Neuroradiol. 2016;37(6):1005-9.

22. Leiner HC, Leiner AL, Dow RS. Cognitive and language functions of the human cerebellum. Trends Neurosci. 1993;16:444-7.

23. Leiner HC, Leiner AL, Dow RS. The human cerebro-cerebellar system: its computing, cognitive and language skills. Behav Brain Res. 1991;44:113-28.

24. Manto M, Bower JM, Conforto AB, et al. Consensus paper: roles of the cerebellum in motor control—the diversity of ideas on cerebellar involvement in movement. Cerebellum. 2012;11(2):457-87.

25. Marquer A, Barbieri G, Pérennou D. The assessment and treatment of postural disorders in cerebellar ataxia: a systematic review. Ann Phys Rehabil Med. 2014;57(2):67-78.

26. Milne SC, Murphy A, Georgiou-Karistianis N, et al. Psychometric properties of outcome measures evaluating decline in gait in cerebellar ataxia: a systematic review. Gait Posture. 2018;61:149-62.

27. Morton SM, Bastian AJ. Cerebellar control of balance and locomotion. Neuroscientist. 2004;10(3):247-59.

28. Morton SM, Bastian AJ. Mechanisms of cerebellar gait ataxia. Cerebellum. 2007;6(1):79.

29. Oldrati V, Schutter DJ. Targeting the human cerebellum with transcranial direct current stimulation to modulate behavior: a meta-analysis. Cerebellum. 2018;17(2):228-36.

30. O'Sullivan SB, Schmitz TJ, Fulk G. Physical rehabilitation, 6th edition. FA Davis; 2014.

31. Palliyath S, Hallett M, Thomas SL, et al. Gait in patients with cerebellar ataxia. Mov Disord.1998;13(6):958-64.

32. Purves D. Neuroscience. Scholarpedia. 2009;4(8):7204.

33. Roostaei T, Nazeri A, Sahraian MA, et al. The human cerebellum: a review of physiologic neuroanatomy. Neurologic Clinics. 2014;32(4):859-69.

34. Schmahmann JD. Disorders of the cerebellum: ataxia, dysmetria of thought, and the cerebellar cognitive affective syndrome. J Neuropsychiatry Clin Neurosci. 2004;16(3):367-78.

35. Schmitz-Hübsch T, Du Montcel ST, Baliko L, et al. Scale for the assessment and rating of ataxia: development of a new clinical scale. Neurology. 2006;66(11):1717-20.

36. Shumway-Cook A, Woollacott MH. Motor control: translating research into clinical practice. Lippincott Williams & Wilkins; 2007

37. Stoodley CJ. The cerebellum and cognition: evidence from functional imaging studies. Cerebellum. 2012;11(2):352-65.

38. Trobe JD. The human brain. An introduction to its functional anatomy. J Neuroophthalmol. 2010;30(1):107.

39. Trouillas P, Takayanagi T, Hallett M, et al. The ataxia neuropharmacology committee of the world federation of neurology. international cooperative ataxia rating scale for pharmacological assessment of the cerebellar syndrome. J Neurol Sci. 1997;145:205-11.

40. Van Essen DC, Donahue CJ, Glasser MF. Development and evolution of cerebral and cerebellar cortex. Brain Behav Evol. 2018;91:158-69.

41. Winser SJ, Smith CM, Hale LA, et al. Systematic review of the psychometric properties of balance measures for cerebellar ataxia. Clin Rehabil. 2015;29(1):69-79.

42. Witter L, De Zeeuw CI. Regional functionality of the cerebellum. Curr Opin Neurobiol. 2015;33:150-5.

Rater: ________________________________Date: ___________________Patient:________________________________

APPENDIX: SCALE FOR THE ASSESSMENT AND RATING OF ATAXIA

1. **Gait:** Proband is asked (1) to walk at a safe distance parallel to a wall including a half-turn (turn around to face the opposite direction of gait) and (2) to walk in tandem (heels to toes) without support.
   0   Normal, no difficulties in walking, turning and walking tandem (up to one misstep allowed)
   1   Slight difficulties, only visible when walking 10 consecutive steps in tandem
   2   Clearly abnormal, tandem walking >10 steps not possible
   3   Considerable staggering, difficulties in half-turn, but without support
   4   Marked staggering, intermittent support of the wall required
   5   Severe staggering, permanent support of one stick or light support by one arm required
   6   Walking >10 m only with strong support (two special sticks or stroller or accompanying person)
   7   Walking <10 m only with strong support (two special sticks or stroller or accompanying person)
   8   Unable to walk, even supported

   Score ____

2. **Stance:** Proband is asked to stand (1) in natural position, (2) with feet together in parallel (big toes touching each other) and (3) in tandem (both feet on one line, no space between heel and toe). Proband does not wear shoes, eyes are open. For each condition, three trials are allowed. Best trial is rated.
   0   Normal, able to stand in tandem for >10 s
   1   Able to stand with feet together without sway, but not in tandem for >10s
   2   Able to stand with feet together for >10 s, but only with sway
   3   Able to stand for >10 s without support in natural position, but not with feet together
   4   Able to stand for >10 s in natural position only with intermittent support
   5   Able to stand >10 s in natural position only with constant support of one arm
   6   Unable to stand for >10 s even with constant support of one arm

   Score ____

3. **Sitting:** Proband is asked to sit on an examination bed without support of feet, eyes open and arms outstretched to the front.
   0   Normal, no difficulties sitting >10 sec
   1   Slight difficulties, intermittent sway
   2   Constant sway, but able to sit >10 s without support
   3   Able to sit for >10 s only with intermittent support
   4   Unable to sit for >10 s without continuous support

   Score ____

4. **Speech disturbance:** Speech is assessed during normal conversation.
   0   Normal
   1   Suggestion of speech disturbance
   2   Impaired speech, but easy to understand
   3   Occasional words difficult to understand
   4   Many words difficult to understand
   5   Only single words understandable
   6   Speech unintelligible/anarthria

   Score ____

5. **Finger chase (Rated separately for each side):** Proband sits comfortably. If necessary, support of feet and trunk is allowed. Examiner sits in front of proband and performs 5 consecutive sudden and fast pointing movements in unpredictable directions in a frontal plane, at about 50% of proband's reach. Movements have an amplitude of 30 cm and a frequency of 1 movement every 2 s. Proband is asked to follow the movements with his index finger, as fast and precisely as possible. Average performance of last 3 movements is rated.
   0   No dysmetria
   1   Dysmetria, under/overshooting target <5 cm
   2   Dysmetria, under/overshooting target <15 cm
   3   Dysmetria, under/overshooting target >15 cm
   4   Unable to perform 5 pointing movements

   *Score*____________*Right*__________*Left*___________
   Mean of both sides (R+L)/2

6. **Nose-finger test (Rated separately for each side):** Proband sits comfortably. If necessary, support of feet and trunk is allowed. Proband is asked to point repeatedly with his index finger from his nose to examiner's finger which is in front of the proband at about 90% of proband's reach. Movements are performed at moderate speed. Average performance of movements is rated according to the amplitude of the kinetic tremor.
   0   No tremor
   1   Tremor with an amplitude <2 cm
   2   Tremor with an amplitude <5 cm
   3   Tremor with an amplitude >5 cm
   4   Unable to perform 5 pointing movements

   *Score*__________*Right*__________*Left*___________
   Mean of both sides (R+L)/2

7. **Fast alternating hand movements (Rated separately for each side):** Proband sits comfortably. If necessary, support of feet and trunk is allowed. Proband is asked to perform 10 cycles of repetitive alternation of pronations and supinations of the hand on his/her

thigh as fast and as precise as possible. Movement is demonstrated by examiner at a speed of approximately 10 cycles within 7 s. Exact times for movement execution have to be taken.

0   Normal, no irregularities (performs <10 s)
1   Slightly irregular (performs <10 s)
2   Clearly irregular, single movements difficult to distinguish or relevant interruptions, but performs <10 s
3   Very irregular, single movements difficult to distinguish or relevant interruptions, performs >10 s
4   Unable to complete 10 cycles

Score____________Right____________Left______________
Mean of both sides (R+L)/2

8. **Heel-shin slide:** Rated separately for each side Proband lies on examination bed, without sight of his legs. Proband is asked to lift one leg, point with the heel to the opposite knee, slide down along the shin to the ankle, and lay the leg back on the examination bed. The task is performed 3 times. Slide-down movements should be performed within 1 s. If proband slides down without contact to shin in all three trials, rate 4.

0   Normal
1   Slightly abnormal, contact to shin maintained
2   Clearly abnormal, goes off shin up to 3 times during 3 cycles
3   Severely abnormal, goes off shin 4 or more times during 3 cycles
4   Unable to perform the task

Score____________Right____________Left__________
Mean of both sides (R+L)/2

Note: The total score is calculated to determine the severity of ataxia.
For motor activities of the four extremities (items 5–8), assessments are performed bilaterally, and the mean values are used to obtain the total score.
Source: Schmitz-Hübsch T with permission

Motor Neuron Disease

Shivani Verma, Megha S Sheth

LEARNING OBJECTIVES
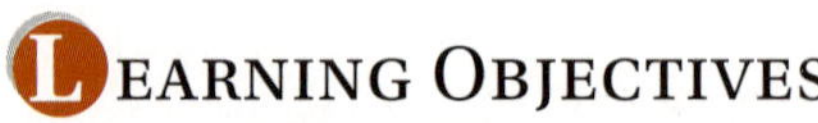

After reading this chapter, the readers should be able to:
- Understand motor neuron diseases (MNDs) and their various types
- Describe the epidemiology and clinical manifestations, and diagnosis of amyotrophic lateral sclerosis
- Differentiate among impairments related to upper motor neuron dysfunction and lower motor neuron dysfunction
- Describe spinal muscular atrophy and its various types
- Describe primary lateral sclerosis and its clinical manifestations
- Describe spastic hereditary paraplegia and its diagnosis along with clinical manifestations
- Differentiate between pseudobulbar palsy and progressive bulbar palsy
- Describe progressive muscular atrophy and its clinical features
- Determine the medical and alternative management of MND
- Understand the role of physiotherapy in MND

CHAPTER OUTLINE

- Amyotrophic lateral sclerosis
  - Epidemiology
  - Etiology
  - Pathophysiology
  - Clinical features
  - Diagnosis
  - Types of amyotrophic lateral sclerosis based on clinical manifestations
  - Disease-specific quality of life measures
- Spinal muscular atrophy
- Primary lateral sclerosis
  - Clinical features
- Hereditary spastic paraplegia
  - Symptom onset
  - Neurologic examination
- Pseudobulbar palsy
- Progressive muscular atrophy
  - Clinical manifestations
- Management
  - Assessment
  - Medical management
  - Alternative management
  - Physiotherapy management
  - Dysarthria, dysphagia, and nutrition management
  - Activity of daily living management
  - Psychological issues

INTRODUCTION

Neurologists in the 19th century recognized that muscle weakness could be due to primary disorders of muscle or secondary to loss of neuromuscular function, for instance when peripheral nerves are cut or when motor neurons degenerate. Furthermore, it was observed that there are forms of motor neuron degeneration that selectively affect upper motor neurons (UMNs) or lower motor neurons (LMNs). A combination of UMN and LMN dysfunction was named amyotrophic lateral sclerosis (ALS) by Charcot and Joffroy.

In the United States, ALS or Lou Gehrig's disease are terms used to describe all forms of the disease, which have the combination of UMN and LMN involvement. In the United Kingdom, the umbrella term "motor neuron disease" (MND) is more common.

Motor neuron disease can be defined as a group of neurodegenerative disorders related to UMN and LMN degeneration which include ALS, spinal muscular atrophy (SMA), hereditary spastic paraplegia (HSP), primary lateral sclerosis (PLS), progressive muscular atrophy (PMA), and pseudobulbar palsy.

AMYOTROPHIC LATERAL SCLEROSIS

Amyotrophic lateral sclerosis was first described in 1869 by a French neurologist, Jean-Martin Charcot. In 1939, Lou

Gehrig, a famous American baseball player, died due to ALS, which had brought international attention to this condition. Since then, ALS is also known as Lou Gehrig's disease.

The disease consists of two parts, namely "amyotrophy" meaning atrophy of the muscles and "lateral sclerosis" meaning hardening of lateral column of spinal cord. ALS is a chronic neurodegenerative disorder of unknown etiology seen in all the ethnic and socioeconomic groups of people in the world.

Epidemiology

Amyotrophic lateral sclerosis has an incidence of 1.5 to 2.7/100,000/year and a prevalence of 3 to 5/100,000 in India. The average age of onset is between 55 and 65 years according to the Western literature; however, the same has been found to be a decade earlier in the Indian population.

There are two different types of ALS, sporadic and familial. Sporadic, which refers to those occurring occasionally (without a significant cause), is the most common form of the disease and accounts for 90–95% of all cases. It may affect anyone, anywhere. Familial ALS (FALS) accounts for 5–10% of all cases. FALS means the disease is inherited.

Mean age at onset is 58–63 years for sporadic ALS and 40–60 years for FALS, with a peak incidence in those aged 70–79 years. The incidence of ALS is higher in men than in women prior to the age of 65–70, but thereafter, the gender incidence is equal. During recent decades, an increasing incidence of or mortality from ALS has been reported in Sweden, Finland, Norway, France, the United States, and other countries.

Etiology

Several studies have shown genetic associations and environmental exposures associated with ALS **(Box 31.1 and Fig. 31.1)**.

Studies show that in 10% of people with ALS, there is a family history of ALS in a first-degree relative and recent detailed genealogical studies extending to more distant relatives and including related diagnoses suggest that more than 20% have a relevant family history.

Gender

Male gender is a factor that is found to be consistently associated with a 1.5 times increased risk of developing ALS compared with female gender. One suggested reason for this association of gender with ALS is that fetal testosterone has been suggested as a risk factor for ALS. Earlier research also suggested that men are more likely to be exposed to many environmental risk factors, including physical activity, head trauma, military service, heavy

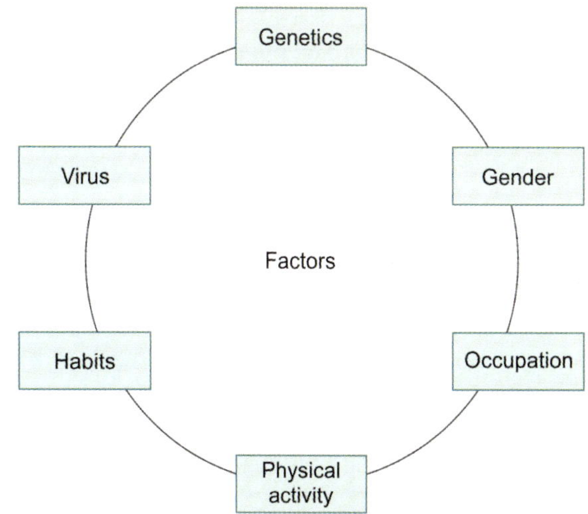

Fig. 31.1: Factors affecting amyotrophic lateral sclerosis.

metal exposure, high field electromagnetic exposure, and other professions that have been the cause of gender being associated with ALS.

Occupation

Recent research has concluded that occupation particularly military service with deployment has been associated with risk of ALS, but the evidence mainly comes from the United States, where there are large military datasets. Sutedja et al. had shown that crafts and related trades work (predominantly in the textile and garment industry) might be a risk factor for developing ALS in women.

Physical Activity

Physical activity is a widely recognized risk factor, because of a number of high-profile sports players who have had ALS (Lou Gehrig). A number of people with ALS are found to have a low BMI on presentation and higher levels of leisure sports participation. It is not clear whether having higher levels of physical activity raises the risk of ALS and, if it does, whether it is the activity itself or being genetically predisposed.

Habits

Various studies have reported smoking to be a causative and risk factor for ALS. A population-based case–control study in Washington state had reported an odds ratio of 2 (95% confidence interval: 1.3–3.2) for the broad smoking category of ever-smokers compared to never smokers who developed ALS. They also found a significant increase in risk of ALS among those with more pack-years of smoking and longer duration of smoking. In a case–control study in New England, cigarette smoking was associated with a significant 70% increase in ALS risk.

Virus

Viral infections have long been suspected as an environmental risk factor and/or a causative pathogen for ALS. Studies of serum and cerebrospinal fluid from ALS

BOX 31.1: Factor affecting amyotrophic lateral sclerosis

- Genetics
- Environmental risk factors.

patients suggested that an activated endogenous retrovirus was associated with ALS. The potential role of enterovirus in ALS has been proposed for decades due to their ability to target motor neurons.

Pathophysiology

Amyotrophic lateral sclerosis is characterized by UMN (corticospinal motor neurons) and LMN (bulbospinal motor neurons) degeneration and death. Along with this, there tends to occur reactive gliosis replacing death neurons. As the corticospinal motor neurons degenerate, the cells suffer from a retrograde axonal loss with secondary myelin pallor and gliosis. These changes are most severe in the brainstem and upper spinal cord. ALS affects spinal motor neurons of the ventral horn and brainstem motor neurons. The ventral roots become thin with loss of large myelinated fibers in motor nerves leading to denervation and atrophy in affected muscles.

Clinical Features

Amyotrophic lateral sclerosis leads to UMN and LMN impairments. It affects LMNs in the medulla and anterior horn of the spinal cord and UMNs in the cerebral cortex. So, the clinical manifestations vary depending on the extent and affection of UMNs and LMNs.

Impairments

Impairments due to lower motor neuron pathology
Degeneration of LMNs causes:
- Fasciculation
- Cramps
- Muscle atrophy
- Marked weakness, which is often more problematic for patients.

The first symptoms are usually unilateral and focal. Early findings include foot drop, difficulty in walking, and loss of hand dexterity or difficulty lifting the arms over the head. ALS begins in the limbs in about two-thirds of patients, most often in the arms. For example at onset difficulty in fine motor movements such as buttoning and writing may be noticed. Eventually, limb function can be lost, leading to dependence on caregivers. Patients may fall or lose the ability to walk all together. Falls are common in patients with ALS (46%).

Recent studies also show that 40% of the patients with ALS had bulbar or generalized symptoms at onset, which is higher than some previously reported. This is further supported by Bryan et al. who reported cases with bulbar onset. In such people with bulbar onset ALS, dysarthria was eight times more common than dysphagia as an initial symptom. Difficulty in moving the tongue, reduced ability to move the lips or open, and close the mouth are some of the features noticed in such individuals with bulbar affection.

An atrophied tongue with fasciculations is so characteristic of bulbar ALS that it is virtually diagnostic of the condition. Axial weakness can cause dropped head

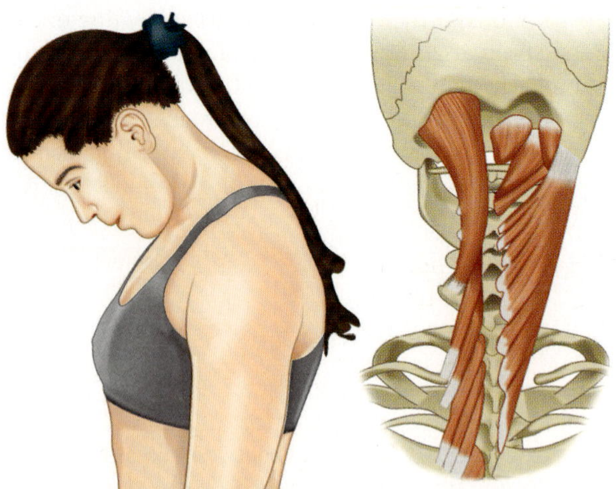

Fig. 31.2: Head drop in amyotrophic lateral sclerosis.

(Fig. 31.2) and kyphosis, features associated with pain and poor balance.

Impairments due to Upper Motor Neuron Pathology
In the early stages of ALS, clinical features of UMN dysfunction may not be easily appreciated in a limb that is concurrently affected by LMN degeneration. The features of UMN involvement include:
- Weakness with slowness
- Spasticity, hyperreflexia
- Pathological reflexes such as Babinski or Hoffman signs

These occur due to degeneration of frontal motor neurons located in the motor strip (*Brodmann area 4*) and their axons traversing the corona radiata, internal capsule, cerebral peduncles, medulla, and the lateral corticospinal tracts of the spinal cord. Studies have confirmed this by the fact that on autopsy the dorsolateral area of the spinal cord, the region containing the lateral corticospinal tract is gliotic and hardened or sclerotic to palpation.

Spasticity over a period of time, if not managed well, causes contractures, deformities as well as dyssynergic movement patterns and loss of dexterity. Due to UMN involvement, loss of motor control and function occurs.

Impairments Related to Bulbar Pathology
Due to brainstem involvement, bulbar symptoms of UMN or LMN type may develop.
- Weakness of the tongue and muscles of the lip, jaw, larynx, and pharynx may result in dysarthria.
- Disease progression may impair speech to an extent where anarthria develops and speech becomes more difficult and unintelligible.
- Impaired swallowing and chewing can lead to dysphagia.
- Due to swallowing, choking issues, and slow eating pattern, the nutrition intake maybe compromised and weight loss or cachexia can also occur.
- Excessive drooling of saliva, referred as sialorrhea, may also be one of the impairments arising due to

absence of automatic spontaneous swallowing to clear excessive saliva or lower facial muscle weakness.

Cognitive Impairments

In the 19th century, Pierre Marie was the first to describe cognitive impairment in ALS. Overt frontotemporal dementia is reported to happen in approximately 15% of patients. This tends to cause:

- Changes in language, judgement, personality, affect, and executive function.
- Patients with ALS and dementia have shorter survival, possibly as a result of poor decision-making ability.
- Depression and anxiety can occur during any stage, from diagnosis to the time of respiratory failure, though patients suffering from ALS often approach the disease philosophically and rates of depression may be lower than expected.
- When present, emotional symptoms impair quality of life (QoL) through poor appetite and sleep, and feelings of hopelessness.

Respiratory Impairments

Respiratory involvement in ALS leads to the following impairments:

- ALS often affects the inspiratory muscles including the diaphragm and external intercostal muscles.
- This leads to a reduction in respiratory muscle strength, restrictive lung disease, and, ultimately, carbon dioxide retention and frank respiratory failure.
- Nocturnal hyperventilation, nocturnal hypoventilation, and sleep apnea are the common problems in MND.
- Vital capacity may decline, and 50% decline is often associated with respiratory symptoms, whereas less than 25–30% of predicted decline shows a significant risk of respiratory failure or death.
- With ventilator support, significant CO_2 retention may occur, resulting in acidosis or coma.

Rare Impairments

Patients with ALS often complain of:

- Sensory symptoms, and a case series has identified objective sensory signs in 2–10% of patients. However, peripheral sensory neuropathy has not been widely recognized as part of the ALS syndrome.
- Various studies have confirmed the presence of bladder and bowel dysfunctions. A study has confirmed that urinary incontinence and especially urge urinary incontinence are common in elderly patients with ALS. Stool incontinence is rarely reported in patients with ALS.
- Eye movements are traditionally regarded as spared from involvement in most cases of ALS, despite progressive weakness of limb, respiratory, and bulbar musculature. A range of oculomotor disorders has been reported in ALS, including ophthalmoplegia, defective pursuit, saccadic impairments, nystagmus, and abnormal Bell phenomenon.

Diagnosis

The diagnosis of ALS and other MND is an exclusion diagnosis, whereby if the history, clinical features, and physical examination are consistent with MND or ALS, a differential diagnosis is prepared and the other possible diagnoses are sequentially ruled out. For the process of exclusion, electrodiagnostic testing, neuroimaging, laboratory test, and muscle biopsies may be used. For some pathologies such as SMA, specific diagnostic tests are available.

El Escorial World Federation of Neurology criteria for the Diagnosis of ALS is the most commonly used criteria for the diagnosis of ALS **(Box 31.2)**.

Electrodiagnosis (EDX) plays an important role in diagnosing MND; however, various forms of MND share several electrodiagnostic features. General EDX characteristics of MND include normal sensory nerve conduction velocity (SNCV), normal or low motor amplitudes depending on disease stage, and normal distal motor latencies and conduction velocities. However, with profound loss of motor amplitude, conduction velocities may drop as low as 25% below the lower limit of normal because of loss of the fastest conducting fibers. The needle electrode examination reveals a decreased recruitment pattern, either normal size or large motor unit action potentials (MUAPs) with or without evidence of remodeling depending on the specific disease process, and abnormal spontaneous activity including positive sharp waves (PSWs), fibrillation potentials, fasciculations, and complex repetitive discharges (CRDs). The prominence of the various forms of spontaneous activity varies with the different forms of MND.

Neuroimaging studies are used to exclude MND from other differential diagnoses. MRI is primarily used; MRI of cervical spine is usually done to rule out presence of syrinx or other spinal cord pathology. The location of symptoms will dictate whether or not other regions of the spinal cord should be screened. Those presenting with bulbar symptoms should also undergo brain MRI to exclude the possibility of stroke, tumor, syringobulbia, etc.

BOX 31.2: El Escorial World Federation of Neurology criteria for the diagnosis of amyotrophic lateral sclerosis (ALS).

The diagnosis of ALS requires the presence of:

- Signs of lower motor neuron (LMN) degeneration by clinical, electrophysiological, or neuropathologic examination
- Signs of upper motor neuron (UMN) degeneration by clinical examination
- Progressive spread of signs within a region or to other regions, together with the absence of:
  - Electrophysiological evidence of other disease processes that might explain the signs of LMN and/or UMN degeneration
  - Neuroimaging evidence of other disease processes that might explain the observed clinical and electrophysiological signs.

Table 31.1: Revised El Escorial research diagnostic criteria for amyotrophic lateral sclerosis (ALS) with the Awaji electrodiagnostic algorithm.

Clinically definite ALS	UMN and LMN clinical signs or electrophysiological evidence in three regions
Clinically definite ALS—laboratory supported	UMN and LMN clinical signs or electrophysiological evidence in one region and the patient is a carrier of a pathogenic SOD1—gene mutation
Clinically probable ALS	UMN and LMN clinical signs or electrophysiological evidence by LMN and UMN signs in two regions with some UMN signs rostral to the LMN signs
Clinically possible ALS	UMN and LMN clinical signs or electrophysiological evidence in one region only, or UMN and LMN clinical signs in two regions with no UMN signs rostral to LMN signs. Neuroimaging and laboratory studies have excluded other diagnoses

(LMN: lower motor neuron; UMN: upper motor neuron; SOD1: superoxide dismutase gene-1)

Types of Amyotrophic Lateral Sclerosis Based on Clinical Manifestations

The revised El Escorial research diagnostic criteria for ALS with the Awaji electrodiagnostic algorithm are shown in **Table 31.1**.

Disease-Specific Quality of Life Measures

The Amyotrophic Lateral Sclerosis Functional Rating Scale (ALSFRS) is an instrument for evaluating the functional status of patients with amyotrophic lateral sclerosis. It can be used to monitor functional change in a patient over time **(Appendix)**. Scores range from 0 to 40, and the higher the score, the more function is retained. It shows close agreement with objective measures of muscle strength and pulmonary function. It shows good construct validity and is sensitive to change in the patient's condition. It shows good test–retest reliability and is consistent.

SPINAL MUSCULAR ATROPHY

Spinal muscular atrophy (SMA) is an autosomal recessive neuromuscular disorder that is characterized by progressive muscle atrophy and weakness. It has an estimated incidence of 1 in 11,000 live births. The main pathological feature of SMA, present in all human patients, is a specific loss of LMNs. Motor neurons are unlikely to be the only neuronal component of the nervous system that is affected in SMA. Disrupted sensory pathways have been described in severe SMA patients. Recent work has identified a range of cells and tissues that are pathological targets out with the traditionally studied neuromuscular system, suggesting that SMA is a multisystem disorder.

- *SMA type I*, also known as *Werdnig-Hoffmann disease.* It is evident when a child is 6 months old. Symptoms tend to be hypotonia, diminished limb movements, lack of tendon reflexes, fasciculations, tremors, swallowing and feeding difficulties, and impaired breathing. Some children also develop scoliosis (curvature of the spine) or other skeletal abnormalities.
- *Symptoms of SMA type II,* the intermediate form, usually begin between 6 and 18 months of age. Children may be able to sit but are unable to stand or walk unaided and may have respiratory difficulties. The progression of disease is variable. Life expectancy is reduced, but some individuals live into adolescence or young adulthood.
- *Symptoms of SMA type III (Kugelberg—Welander disease)* appear between 2 and 17 years of age and include abnormal gait; difficulty running, climbing steps, or rising from a chair; and a fine tremor of the fingers. The lower extremities are most often affected.

PRIMARY LATERAL SCLEROSIS

The term PLS has long been used for the syndrome of progressive UMN dysfunction when no other cause can be identified. PLS is an uncommon diagnosis among patients with MND. Recent series estimate that 2–5% of patients seen in adult neuromuscular clinics will be diagnosed with PLS. The reported mean age of onset ranges from 45 to 53 years, whereas a study has also described a juvenile-onset form of PLS.

Clinical Features

The most common manifestations of PLS are leg weakness and spasticity, and spastic bulbar weakness. **Erb's triad** of spasticity, hyperreflexia, and mild weakness are the most prominent manifestations of PLS. Recent literature shows that several other features also seem to be consistently present in PLS patients. These features include eye movement abnormalities, urinary dysfunction, and cognitive impairment. Unlike ALS in which weakness usually predominates, in PLS spasticity occurs in early stages, which produces most of the limb dysfunction.

HEREDITARY SPASTIC PARAPLEGIA

Hereditary spastic paraplegia (HSP) is a group of hereditary, degenerative, neurological disorders that primarily affect the UMNs. The hallmark feature of HSP is progressive weakness and spasticity (stiffness) of the legs.

Symptom Onset

The onset of symptoms can be classified as follows:
1. *Early onset*: When symptoms begin in very early childhood, they may be nonprogressive and resemble spastic diplegic cerebral palsy.
2. *Later onset*: When symptoms begin in later childhood or after they usually progress slowly and steadily. After a number of years, it is not usual for individuals with progressively worsening gait to experience a "functional plateau" (i.e. the rate of further worsening of gait impairment is similar to that attributable to age).

Neurological Examination

Individuals with HSP demonstrate the following:

- Bilateral lower extremity spasticity (maximal in hamstrings, quadriceps, adductors, and gastrocnemius–soleus muscles) and weakness (maximal in the iliopsoas, hamstring, and tibialis anterior muscles). Spasticity and weakness are variable. Some individuals have spasticity and no demonstrable weakness, whereas others have spasticity and weakness in approximately the same proportions.
- Lower extremity hyperreflexia and extensor plantar responses are common.
- Often, mildly impaired vibration sensation in the distal lower extremities may be seen.

PSEUDOBULBAR PALSY

Psedobulbar palsy is a syndrome characterized by:

- Dysarthria
- Dysphagia
- Dysphonia
- Impairment of voluntary movements of tongue and facial muscles, and emotional lability.

This condition is caused by diseases that affect the motor fibers that travel from the cerebral cortex to the lower brainstem (i.e., corticobulbar tracts).

- Levy noticed that there is frequently intellectual enfeeblement in patients with pseudobulbar palsy.
- Loss of emotional control, manifested as forced laughing or crying, appears in typical cases, but the face in repose shows poverty of expression, sadness being the predominating note.
- A common clinical feature is drooping of saliva from the mouth.
- The jaw jerk is hyperactive.
- The patients eat slowly, owing to difficulties in mastication.

The symptoms may come on suddenly or gradually, the rate of onset influences the clinical picture.

- The coordination between breathing and swallowing is poor, so that food may enter the bronchi and cause bronchopneumonia.
- Since the patients do not swallow readily, saliva accumulates and drips from the mouth.
- Patients with pseudobulbar palsy sometimes show a loss of tone in the palate and absence of the palatal reflexes.
- Studies also show that there is abnormality both in the rhythm and in the timbre of speech. Dissociation between voluntary and automatic speech is manifested as a type of repetition termed palilalia.

Progressive bulbar palsy, also called progressive bulbar atrophy, involves the dysfunction of brainstem that contains LMNs needed for swallowing, speaking, chewing, and other functions. Symptoms include pharyngeal muscle weakness (involved with swallowing), weak jaw and facial muscles, progressive loss of speech, and tongue muscle atrophy. Individuals are at increased risk of choking and aspiration. Affected persons have outbursts of laughing or crying (called emotional lability).

PROGRESSIVE MUSCULAR ATROPHY

In 1850, Aran first reported progressive muscular atrophy (PMA). In 1952, Muller introduced the term progressive SMA. Progressive SMA is an adult-onset, nonhereditary progressive disease of the LMNs. It is clinically characterized by signs of LMN dysfunction. PMA is a rare condition and has been identified in only 2.5% of all patients with adult-onset MND. There are many differences between PMA and ALS. In PMA, the proportion of men was greater than in ALS as per a study (73.6% vs 54.9%).

Clinical Manifestations

Clinical manifestations include:

- Weakness is typically seen first in the hands and then spreads into the lower body, where it can be severe.
- Other symptoms may include:
  - Muscle wasting
  - Clumsy hand movements
  - Fasciculations
  - Muscle cramps
- The trunk muscles and respiration may become affected.
- Exposure to cold can worsen symptoms.

The disease develops into ALS in many instances. More than 20% of patients with PMA develop UMN signs at some time, and among those who do, 50% develop UMN signs within 1 year after LMN symptom onset.

MANAGEMENT

Centralized multidisciplinary care confers a survival advantage for patients with ALS and is superior to devolved community-based care. Palliative care in ALS involves not only physicians but also a large number of different professionals—counselors, dieticians, occupational therapists, physical therapists, speech therapists, nurse practitioners, social workers, hospice personnel, and so forth, not to mention the family members, for whom caring for the patient often becomes a full-time job.

Assessment

Assessment shows:

- Age—40–65 years.
- Gender—males > females.
- History—onset is usually slow and the pattern of motor symptoms is inconsistent, frequently a positive history of smoking and positive family history.
- Nutritional status—reduced appetite.
- Cognition and perception—normal mental status; appearance, emotional affect, language, memory, executive functions are usually impaired; sleep

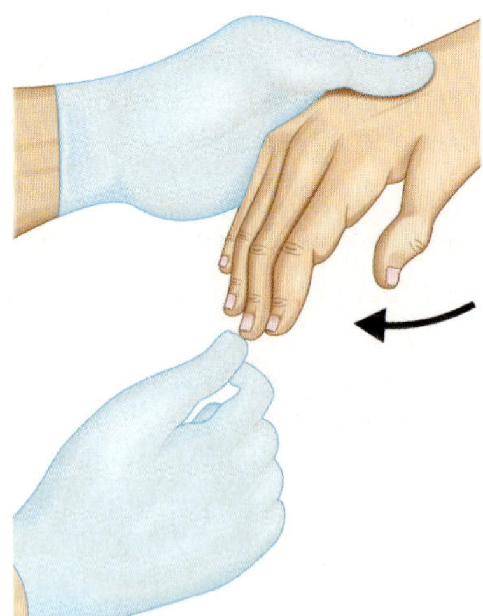

Fig. 31.3: Hoffman sign.

disturbances may be present; patient may have inappropriate laughing or crying occasionally.

- Speech—dysarthria may be seen.
- Swallowing—dysphagia and sialorrhea are seen in most cases.
- Cranial nerve examination—sensory cranial nerves are normal; motor cranial nerves may be affected.
- Sensory examination—normal; very rarely sensory symptoms may be seen.
- Motor examination—in cases of UMN dysfunction, spasticity, hyperreflexia or brisk reflexes, clonus, Babinski's sign, Hoffman sign **(Fig. 31.3)**, and abnormal jaw jerk response are seen; in cases of LMN dysfunction, hyporeflexia, hypotonia, muscle atrophy, fasciculations, and cramps may be present; weakness and reduced dexterity are seen in both UMN and LMN dysfunction; voluntary control may be impaired in UMN dysfunction; cramps in abdominal and trunk muscles prompt a diagnosis of ALS.
- Respiratory assessment—a restrictive lung pathology pattern is usually seen with reduced respiratory muscle strength and vital capacity; nocturnal respiratory failure may be evaluated by the presence of poor sleep pattern accompanied by frequent awakenings at night, morning headaches along with fatigue during the day; adventitious sounds may be heard on auscultation of breath sounds in case of retained secretions; dyspnea on exertion and an obvious use of accessory muscles during respiration may be present.
- Bowel and bladder examination—may be affected in a few cases.
- Posture assessment—head drop and increased kyphosis are found.
- Gait and balance assessment—reduced cadence; gait and balance are both affected.
- Cerebellar examination—normal.
- Psychological assessment—anxiety and depression are very commonly seen; sleep disorders are also common.

- Electrodiagnostic testing—nerve conduction velocity findings: Sensory NCV is normal, motor NCV shows normal or low amplitude with normal distal motor nerve latency and nerve conduction velocity [in case of severe reduction in amplitude, motor conduction velocity (MCV) may be affected]. Electromyography (EMG) findings: Spontaneous activity shows PSWs, fibrillation potentials, fasciculations and CRDs, recruitment pattern is reduced with normal or large MUAP.
- Functional assessment—function is impaired with the patient having difficulty performing fine motor tasks such as writing, buttoning, and eating, inability to walk longer distances or retrieve objects from above the head.

Medical Management

There are limited pharmacological treatment options in MND. Riluzole is the only treatment shown to slow the course of MND and is thought to prolong survival by 2–3 months. The drug should be initiated on diagnosis as it may have little effect in the late stages. Fatigue is reported as a side effect in 26% of patients taking riluzole.

Currently, the main focus in MND is on:
- Symptomatic
- Rehabilitative
- Palliative management
- To maximize lifespan and optimize QoL.

Medications are available which may alleviate symptoms and are shown in **Table 31.2**.

Nocturnal noninvasive positive-pressure ventilation has become the standard treatment for MND patients with respiratory insufficiency. The bilevel intermittent positive-pressure ventilator imitates physiological function; it is triggered by the patient's inspiratory efforts, reduces the work of breathing, and improves gas exchange and sleep quality.

Table 31.2: Medications to alleviate symptoms.	
Symptoms	*Medications*
Muscle spasms and cramps	Quinine sulfate
Spasticity	Baclofen, tizanidine
Sialorrhea	Amitriptyline, atropine, botulinum toxin injection, glycopyrronium, hyoscyamine
Pain	Paracetamol, nonsteroidal anti-inflammatories, anticonvulsant, opiates
Depression	Tricyclic antidepressants or serotonin reuptake inhibitors
Emotional lability	Amitriptyline, fluvoxamine, dextromethorphan-quinidine

Alternative Management

Subjective assessment of the effects of alternative or complementary medicine such as **yoga**, **reflexology**, and **meditation** used in MND populations are positive overall, with **massage** believed to be a useful adjunctive treatment for spasticity and pain in MND.

Energy healing, which also includes spiritual and faith healing, is a branch of alternative medicine where the healer channels healing energy onto a patient in order to cure them from a certain disease. This is usually performed when the healer lays their hands on the patient, although some healers do an "off-hands" method or even do remote healing with the patient being in a different location. There are many different types of energy healing. The most commonly used are spiritual healing and psychic healing, distant healing, intercessory prayer, therapeutic touch, healing touch, esoteric healing, reiki, magnetic healing, qigong healing, pranic healing, and crystal healing. There are no trials on the effect of energy healing in ALS patients. **It needs to be emphasized that there are no scientific evidences proving this.**

Acupuncture is a technique that involves the insertion of thin needles through the skin at specific points with the goal of achieving a therapeutic effect, most often pain reduction. Acupuncture originated in ancient China and is a key component of traditional Chinese medicine. While the underlying mechanisms of acupuncture have not been completely elucidated and may involve a significant placebo component, there is some evidence that it could help relieve two common ALS symptoms: pain and spasticity. More controversial is the possibility that acupuncture could slow, stop or reverse ALS progression. A small, flawed study in a mouse model of ALS showed that acupuncture was associated with improved motor neuron survival and delayed loss of motor performance compared to mice that did not receive any acupuncture.

Patient with ALS often goes for alternative or complementary therapies which they find effective especially diets, nutritional supplements, cannabis, acupuncture, chelation, and energy healing.

Physiotherapy Management

Physical therapy, that is tailored to the individual's needs and goals and is focused on addressing symptoms and maximizing function and participation, enables people with ALS to live their lives to the fullest and with quality. The physical therapist requires a solid understanding of the nature and course of the disease and needs to consider future problems in addition to current status. In order to make appropriate and effective decisions, the nature and significance of the interrelationships among impairments, activity limitations, and participation restrictions need to be determined.

In addition, decision-making involves determining which impairments, activity limitations, and participation restrictions:

- Can be restored
- Require compensatory strategies or interventions
- Require referral to different health care professional(s)
- Cannot be affected by physical therapy interventions at all.

Clinical Pearl

Due to the progressive nature of the condition, the goal of physiotherapy for therapists often in the care of people with MND is not to improve impairment in strength or mobility.

Instead, therapy is usually aimed at assisting the patient to maximize function through provision of aids and appliances, mobility strategies, and respiratory management.

Maintain Mobility, Strength, and Function

Muscle weakness results in limitations in function and mobility in patients with MND. Disuse atrophy and deconditioning, as well as muscle degeneration resulting from the disease process, contribute to the weakness. A recent study suggests resistance exercises of unaffected muscles (and possibly affected muscles with strength of at least grade 3 or above) using a low-to-moderate load and intensity, and aerobic activities, such as swimming, walking, and stationary cycling (mode dependent on safety), at submaximal levels (e.g. between 50 and 65% of heart rate reserve) may be safe and effective in achieving therapeutic goals. Some guidelines suggested for maintaining mobility and function are:

1. Supported treadmill training may be a useful modality in the early stages of MND.
2. Moderate intensity endurance activity may delay the onset of spasticity.
3. Active/passive trainers or unloaded cycling should be considered, ideally for home use, where spasticity is present.
4. Individualized strengthening exercises during the early stage of MND are probably effective in improving the function of patients.
5. Many patients will require an ankle–foot orthosis (AFO). Off-the-shelf AFOs, e.g. Swedish AFO, dictus splint, foot-up splint, will often be sufficient to support gait.
6. Persons with MND often need a collar as their neck muscles become weaker. Rigid and supportive collars may be recommended as the disease progresses to maintain head and neck alignment.

Fatigue Management

Skeletal muscle weakness in MND poses a serious problem to the patients. It can be managed with certain precautions and lifestyle modifications. While exercising, patients should be instructed not to exercise till he/she is exhausted as it can result in muscle damage and dysfunction. Feeling weaker rather than stronger postexercise and postexercise muscle soreness are some warning signs of fatigue, other than muscle cramping, heaviness in the extremities, and prolonged shortness of breath. Aerobic exercises mainly low-impact such as walking, stationary bicycling, pool therapy increase muscle efficiency and help aid fatigue. Energy conservation techniques and activity pacing can be taught to the patient to manage keeping fatigue under control.

Pain Management

Pain is a common problem in MND, with frequency and intensity correlating with a worse functional score and a longer disease duration. Identification of the precipitants leading to pain is the first priority. Much of this relates to neuromuscular weakness, including the effects of posture and immobility. Emotional distress, muscle spasms, cramps, pressure sores, spasticity, and constipation may all cause pain, while the presence of preexisting conditions such as arthritis may be exacerbated by progressive weakness. Severe pain has been reported in up to 20% of patients with MND.

Early training on correct manual handling, positioning, shoulder care, and range of movement exercises may minimize shoulder pain, a common problem in MND. Electrotherapy modalities (e.g. transcutaneous electrical nerve stimulation), splints, or collars should be considered for use to relieve pain. Corticosteroid injections may be indicated to relieve pain where conventional therapy has been unsuccessful. These injections can be accessed through the general practitioner.

Respiratory Symptom Management

Inspiratory, expiratory, and/or bulbar muscle weakness in MND patients has a major prognostic impact. Diaphragmatic dysfunction is associated with dyspnea, impaired QoL, and a shortened survival. The problems can be further complicated by disuse atrophy, shortening and stiffness of chest wall musculature, and reduced lung compliance.

It is important to teach patients and caregivers about signs and symptoms of aspiration and respiratory infection along with it's first line of treatment. Strategies for management of oral secretions and choking episodes should be taught to the patients and caregivers. Manually assisted coughing should be used, and family/care-givers educated in its technique.

Spasticity and Muscle Cramps Management

Slow static stretching sustained for 30 seconds may help in reducing spasticity, especially of muscle groups that are more prone to spasticity such as gastrocnemius, hamstrings. Positional splinting is also helpful; however due precaution should be given to skin breakdown. Cold, passive movements can reduce spasticity and prevent contractures. There are evidences of moderate-intensity exercises being useful in decreasing spasticity in patients with ALS.

Dysarthria, Dysphagia, and Nutrition Management

Due to involvement of brainstem, bulbar symptoms may develop. Dysphagia, dysfunction of lips, tongue, pharyngeal and laryngeal muscles, sialorrhea, and malnutrition are common in MND. A referral to speech therapist can be made for diagnosis and management of speech and swallowing problems. A speech and swallowing therapist will also provide the necessary instructions to patients and families for reducing the risk of aspiration. Dysarthria does not respond well to conventional articulation training. However, some adaptive strategies such as maintaining a slow speaking rate with an emphasis on increasing the precision of speech production may be helpful and can be taught by a speech–language pathologist. Communicative aids, speech synthesizers or multipurpose, multiaccess, and computer-based augmentative communication systems are some recent advances and can be expensive; however, they provide immense benefit in speaking ability of patients who cannot phonate.

In ALS, factors that restrict adequate nutrition develop insidiously and progressively worsen. They lead to functional consequences such as choking, aspiration, weight loss, and dehydration. Dysphagia is a symptom experienced by the patient and is prima facie evidence of swallowing dysfunction. Strategies to maintain oral nutritional intake consist of altering food consistency and using nutritional supplements. In the later course of disease, a percutaneous endoscopic gastrostomy or equivalent device (e.g. radiologically inserted device) may be needed as an alternative route for delivering nutrition.

> Based on an evidence-based review, drug, nutritional, and respiratory therapies practice parameter, an update was established which explains an algorithm that is useful in nutrition and respiratory management, which can be read for further understanding.

Activity of Daily Living Management

Connors et al., in 2017 had done a study of the commonly used equipment's usage according to equipment category in patients with MND, and the findings of which are discussed in **Table 31.3**.

People with MND have high equipment needs to assist them to optimize their QoL. Assistive devices enhance independence in activity of daily living (ADL) and QoL for people living with MND. Pavey interviewed 42 people living with MND and found that a device such as a wheelchair can give a person "my freedom." Power wheelchairs have also been reported as providing those with MND an increased ability to participate in activities and a greater "sense of competence." Assistive communication devices, such as touchscreen tablets with text to speech software, impact positively on QoL in those with MND, and high satisfaction was reported for utility of bathroom adaptive devices, by 63 people with MND in a study by Gruis et al.

Table 31.3: Equipment used to improve activity of daily living (ADL).

Equipment category	Most commonly used equipment item within the category
Communication devices	Natural speech compensations
Transfer devices	Lifting hoist
Mobility devices	Walking frame, orthoses, pressure cushion
ADL equipment	Seating—electric lift recliner chair
Assistive technology	Computer access/tablet (direct access)
Home modification	Major bathroom/toilet modifications

Psychological Issues

Depression is relatively common (prevalence rates up to 50%), as are other forms of psychological distress in the MND population, and is not associated with illness severity and functional status. Depression strongly correlates with QoL. Social support is often limited for MND patients, and this also influences QoL. Hope and hopelessness are important issues for MND patients with hopelessness contributing significantly to suffering and, for some, a desire for hastened death. Depression is common in individuals with MND and also their spouse or caregivers, due to affection in function and independence. Good family, social, and religious support systems, as well as participation in a support group, are helpful.

Referral to a psychiatrist or clinical psychologist with experience in treating depression associated with terminal disease may be required. Group/family counseling may be helpful for caregivers.

SUMMARY

Motor neuron disease gets worse over time and affects muscles of the limbs, speech, swallowing, and breathing. People with MND experience a wide range of symptoms, including a number of physical ability limitations, pain, spasticity, cramps, swallowing problems, and difficulty breathing. Patients with MND should be considered a priority for assessment and offered regular monitoring and review. While therapy is primarily aimed at assisting the patient to optimize functional mobility and respiratory status, symptoms of pain and fatigue should be addressed with a restorative approach. Physiotherapists therefore require a wide range of neurological, musculoskeletal and respiratory skill, and good communication skills.

Case Scenario

CASE STUDY

A 55-year-old man, farmer by occupation, diagnosed with ALS, experienced cramping in his calf, followed by evident slapping of his left foot while walking which caused him to trip a few times. Followed by that, he experienced gradual difficulty in buttoning his *kurta* and tying his *nara dhoti*. He also reported significant fatigue after working for more than half an hour in the farms which he attributed to aging.

Environmental history: He lives in a two-storeyed house with 16 steps to the first floor. His house has an Indian toilet.

Socioeconomic history: He lives with his wife and three sons. Farming is their family occupation.

Examination: Motor examination showed reduced grip strength and weakness of lower limb muscles along with increased muscle tone in upper limb muscles. Hyperreflexia in both upper limbs and hyporeflexia in lower limbs along with positive bilateral Babinski sign were found. No speech or higher mental abnormalities were noted. Respiratory examinations (forced vital capacity and maximal inspiratory volume) were within normal limits.

Guiding Questions

1. What El Escorial Diagnostic criteria would you anticipate were documented in the patient's medical records?
2. What additional tests and examinations should be conducted on the patient and what are the expected findings?
3. What activity limitations and participation restrictions will the patient complain of?
4. What will be the primary focus of physiotherapy in the patient?

Review Questions

1. Explain the term motor neuron disease and its various types.
2. Describe the clinical manifestations seen in amyotrophic lateral sclerosis.
3. Enumerate the ADL assistive equipment which can be used by people with MND.
4. Describe the management of motor neuron disease and elaborate the role of physiotherapist in it.
5. Which physical therapy tests and measures should be included in comprehensive examination of patient with ALS?

BIBLIOGRAPHY

1. Amyotrophic Lateral Sclerosis online Database Available at: http://alsod.iop.kcl.ac.uk.
2. Ashworth NL, Satkunam LE, Deforge D. Treatment for spasticity in amyotrophic lateral sclerosis/motor neuron disease. Cochrane Library. Cochrane Database Syst Rev. 2012 Feb 15;(2):CD004156. doi: 10.1002/14651858.CD004156. pub4.
3. Barnes S, Gardiner C, Gott M, et al. Enhancing patient-professional communication about end-of-life issues in life-limiting conditions: a critical review of the literature. J Pain Symptom Manage. 2012;44(6):866-79.
4. Beard JD, Kamel F. Military service, deployments, and exposures in relation to amyotrophic lateral sclerosis etiology and survival. Epidemiol Rev. 2015;37(1):55-70.
5. Bohannon RW. Results of resistance exercise on a patient with amyotrophic lateral sclerosis. A case report. Phys Ther. 1983;63(6):965-8.
6. Connors KA, Mahony LM, Morgan P. Adaptive equipment use by people with motor neuron disease in Australia: a prospective, observational consecutive cohort study. Disabil Rehabil Assist Technol. Disabil Rehabil Assist Technol. 2019 Jan;14(1):62-7.
7. Coupé C, Gordon PH. Amyotrophic lateral sclerosis—clinical features, pathophysiology and management. European Neurological Review. 2013;8(1):38–44.
8. Das K, Nag C, Ghosh M. Familial, environmental, and occupational risk factors in development of amyotrophic lateral sclerosis. N Am J Med Sci. 2012;4:350-5.
9. Erb WH. Spastic and syphilitic paralysis. Lancet. 1902;ii:969-74.
10. Gordon PH, Delgadillo D, Piquard A, et al. The range and clinical impact of cognitive impairment in French patients with ALS: a cross-sectional study of neuropsychological test performance. Amyotroph Lateral Scler. 2011;12(5):372-8.
11. Gruis K, Wren P, Higgins J. Amyotrophic lateral sclerosis patients' self-reported satisfaction with assistive technology. Muscle Nerve. 2011;43:643-47.
12. Hamilton G, Gillingwater TH. Spinal muscular atrophy: going beyond the motor neuron. Trends Mol Med. 2013;19(1):40-50.
13. Haverkamp LJ, Appel V, Appel SH. Natural history of amyotrophic lateral sclerosis in a database population: validation of a scoring system and a model for survival prediction. Brain. 1995;118:707-71.
14. Hedera P. Hereditary spastic paraplegia overview. 2000 Aug 15 [Updated 2018 Sep 27]. In: Adam MP, Ardinger HH, Pagon RA, et al. (Eds). GeneReviews® [Internet]. Seattle (WA): University of Washington, Seattle; 1993-2020. Available from: https://www.ncbi.nlm.nih.gov/books/NBK1509/
15. Hedera P. Hereditary spastic paraplegia overview. Synonyms: hereditary spastic paraparesis, Strumpell-Lorrain syndrome. GeneReviews.
16. Horowitz S. Evidence-based indications for massage. Altern Complement Ther. 2007;2:30-5.
17. https://www.mda.org/disease/amyotrophic-lateral-sclerosis/causes-inheritance.
18. Huynh W, Simon NG, Grosskreutz J, et al. Assessment of the upper motor neuron in amyotrophic lateral sclerosis. Clin Neurophysiol. 2016;127:2643-60.
19. Kim WK, Liu X, Sandner J, et al. Study of 962 patients indicates progressive muscular atrophy is a form of ALS. Neurology. 2009;73(20):1686–92.
20. Kojan S, Goodwin WE, Bryan WW, et al. Clinical and laboratory features of primary lateral sclerosis. J Child Neurol. 2000;15:200.
21. Lacorte E, Ferrigno L, Leoncini E, et al. Physical activity, and physical activity related to sports, leisure and occupational activity as risk factors for ALS: a systematic review. Neurosci Biobehav Rev. 2016;66:61-79.
22. Langworthy OR. Syndrome of pseudobulbar palsy. Arch Intern Med. 1940;65(1):106.
23. Leigh PN, Garofolo O. The molecular pathology of motor neuron disease. In: Swash M, Leigh PN (Eds). Motor neuron disease. London: Springer Verlag; 1995. pp. 139-61.
24. Levy S. The disorder is speech in the course of des \l=e'\ tatspseudobulbaires. Rev Neurol. 1930;2:289.
25. Logroscino G, Traynor BJ, Hardiman O, et al. Descriptive epidemiology of amyotrophic lateral sclerosis: new evidence and unsolved issues. J Neurol Neurosurg Psychiatry. 2008;79(1):6-11.
26. Miller RG, Jackson CE, Kasarskis EJ, et al. Practice parameter update: the care of the patient with amyotrophic lateral sclerosis: drug, nutritional, and respiratory therapies (an evidence-based review): report of the Quality Standards Subcommittee of the American Academy of Neurology. Neurology. 2009;73(15):1218-26.
27. Morris ME, Perry A, Bilney B, et al. Outcomes of physical therapy, speech pathology, and occupational therapy for people with motor neuron disease: a systematic review. Neurorehabil Neural Repair. 2006;20(3):424-34.
28. Motor Neuron Diseases Fact Sheet, NINDS, Publication date: August 2019. NIH Publication No. 19-NS-5371. Available at: https://www.ninds.nih.gov/Disorders/Patient-Caregiver-Education/Fact-Sheets/Motor-Neuron-Diseases-Fact-Sheet.
29. Narbukera SK, Romitti PA, Campbell KA, et al. Use of complementary medicine and alternative medicine by males with Duchenne or Becker muscular dystrophy. J Child Neurol. 2012;27(6):734-40.
30. National Institute for Health and Clinical Excellence (NICE). Motor neurone disease. The use of non-invasive ventilation in the management of motor neurone disease. Centre for Clinical Practice at NICE. 2010. Available from http://www.nice.org.uk/nicemedia/live/13057/49885/49885.
31. Nelson LM, McGuire V, Longstreth WT, et al. Population-based case-control of amyotrophic lateral sclerosis in Western Washington State, 1. Cigarette smoking and alcohol consumption. Am J Epidemiol. 2000;151:156–73.
32. Newrick PG, Langton-Hewer R. Pain in motor neuron disease. J Neurol Neurosurg Psychiatry. 1985;48(8):838-40.
33. Ng L, Khan F, Mathers S. Multidisciplinary care for adults with amyotrophic lateral sclerosis or motor neuron disease (review). The Cochrane Collaboration. 2009. Available from http://www.thecochranelibrary.com.
34. Pandey S, Sarma N. Commentary: Amyotrophic lateral sclerosis: Ongoing search for prognostic biomarkers of longevity. Neurol India. 2017;65:1155-6.
35. Panzeri C, De Palma C, Martinuzzi A, et al. The first ALS2 missense mutation associated with JPLS reveals new aspects of alsin biological function. Brain. 2006;129:1710-19.
36. Pavey A, Warren N, Allen-Collinson J. "It gives me my freedom": technology and responding to bodily limitations in motor neuron disease. Med Anthropol. 2015;34:442-55.
37. Pringle CE, Hudson AJ, Munoz DG, et al. Primary lateral sclerosis: clinical features, neuropathology and diagnostic criteria. Brain. 1992;115:495-520.

38. Rowland L. How amyotrophic lateral sclerosis got its name the clinical-pathologic genius of Jean-Martin Charcot. Arch Neurol. 2001;58:512-15.
39. Rowland LP. Primary lateral sclerosis: disease, syndrome, both or neither? J Neurol Sci. 1999;170:1-4.
40. Rudnik-Schoneborn S, Goebel HH, Schlote W, et al. Classical infantile spinal muscular atrophy with SMN deficiency causes sensory neuronopathy. Neurology. 2003;60:983-7.
41. Simic G. Pathogenesis of proximal autosomal recessive spinal muscular atrophy. Acta Neuropathol. 2008;116:223-34.
42. Sutedja NA, Veldink JH, Fischer K, et al. Lifetime occupation, education, smoking, and risk of ALS. Neurology. 2007;69(15):1508-14.
43. Swash M. Why are upper motor neuron signs difficult to elicit in amyotrophic lateral sclerosis. J Neurol Neurosurg Psychiatry. 2012;83:659-62.
44. Talbot K. Familial versus sporadic amyotrophic lateral sclerosis—a false dichotomy? Brain. 2011;134(Pt 12):3429-31.
45. The UK Motor Neurone Disease Networking Group. A pathway for the management of pain in motor neurone disease. 2001. Available from http://www.redpublish.co.uk/wpcontent/uploads/2009/03/MND-Pain-Pathway1.
46. Traynor BJ, Codd MB, Corr B, et al. Clinical features of amyotrophic lateral sclerosis according to the El Escorial and Airlie House diagnostic criteria: a population-based study. Arch Neurol. 2000;57(8):1171-76.
47. Visser J. Disease course and prognostic factors of progressive muscular atrophy. Arch Neurol. 2007;64:522-8.
48. Wang H, O'Reilly ÉJ, Weisskopf MG, et al. Smoking and risk of amyotrophic lateral sclerosis: a pooled analysis of five prospective cohorts. Arch Neurol. 2011;68(2):207–13.
49. Wasner M, Klier H, Borasio GD. The use of alternative medicine by patients with amyotrophic lateral sclerosis. J Neurol Sci. 2001;191:151-4.

APPENDIX: THE AMYOTROPHIC LATERAL SCLEROSIS FUNCTIONAL RATING SCALE (ALSFRS)

Overview: The Amyotrophic Lateral Sclerosis Functional Rating Scale (ALSFRS) is an instrument for evaluating the functional status of patients with Amyotrophic Lateral Sclerosis. It can be used to monitor functional change in a patient over time.

Measures:
 1. Speech
 2. Salivation
 3. Swallowing
 4. Handwriting
 5. Cutting food and handling utensils (with or without gastrostomy)
 6. Dressing and hygiene
 7. Turning in bed and adjusting bed clothes
 8. Walking
 9. Climbing stairs
10. Breathing

Measure	Finding	Points
Speech	Normal	4
	Detectable speech disturbance	3
	Intelligible with repeating	2
	Speech combined with nonvocal communications	1
	Loss of useful speech	0
Salivation	Normal	4
	Slight but definite excess of saliva in mouth; may have nighttime drooling	3
	Moderately excessive saliva; may have minimal drooling	2
	Marked excess of saliva with some drooling	1
	Marked drooling; requires constant tissue or handkerchief	0
Swallowing	Normal	4
	Early eating problems; occasional choking	3
	Dietary consistency changes	2
	Needs supplemental tube feedings	1
	Nothing by mouth (NPO); exclusively parenteral or enteral feeding	0
Handwriting	Normal	4
	Slow or sloppy; all words are legible	3
	Not all words are legible	2
	Able to grasp pen but unable to write	1
	Unable to grip pen	0
Cutting food and handling utensils	No gastrostomy/normal	4
	No gastrostomy; somewhat slow and clumsy but no help required	3
	No gastrostomy; can cut most foods although clumsy and slow; some help needed	2
	No gastrostomy; food must be cut by someone but can still feed slowly	1
	No gastrostomy; needs to be bed	0

Contd...

Contd...

Measure	Finding	Points
	With gastrostomy; normal	4
	With gastrostomy; clumsy but able to perform with manipulations independently	3
	With gastrostomy; some help needed with closures and fasteners	2
	With gastrostomy; provides minimal assistance to caregiver	1
	With gastrostomy; unable to perform any aspect of task	0
Dressing and hygiene	Normal	4
	Independent and complete self-care with effort or decreased efficiency	3
	Intermittent assistance or substitute methods	2
	Needs attendant for self-care	1
	Total dependence	0
Turning in bed and adjusting bed clothes	Normal	4
	Somewhat slow and clumsy but no help needed	3
	Can turn alone or adjust sheets but with great difficulty	2
	Can initiate but not turn or adjust sheets alone	1
	Helpless	0
Walking	Normal	4
	Early ambulation difficulties	3
	Walks with assistance	2
	Nonambulatory functional movement only	1
	No purposeful leg movement	0
Climbing stairs	Normal	4
	Slow	3
	Mild unsteadiness or fatigue	2
	Needs assistance	1
	Cannot do	0
Breathing	Normal	4
	Shortness of breath with minimal exertion (walking, talking, etc.)	3
	Shortness of breath at rest	2
	Intermittent (e.g., nocturnal) ventilatory assistance required	1
	Ventilator dependent	0

ALSERS = SUM (points for all 10 measures)

Interpretation:
- Minimum score: 0
- Maximum score: 40
- The higher the score the more function is retained.

Performance:
- It shows close agreement with objective measures of muscle strength and pulmonary function.
- It shows good construct validity and is sensitive to change in the patient's condition.
- It shows test-retest reliability and is consistent.

Bibliography
1. ALS CNTF Treatment Study (ACTS) Phase I-II Study Group. The Amyotrophic Lateral Sclerosis Functional Rating Scale. Assessment of activities of daily living in patients with amyotrophic lateral sclerosis. Arch Neurol. 1996;53:141-7.
2. Cedarbaum JM Stambler N. Performance of the Amyotrophic Lateral Sclerosis Functional Rating Scale (ALSFRS) in multicenter clinical trials. J Neurol Sci. 1997;152(Suppl 1):S1-S9.

Myopathies

R Harihara Prakash

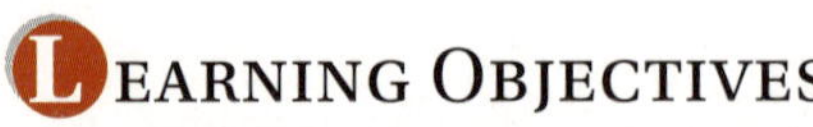 LEARNING OBJECTIVES

After reading this chapter, the readers should be able to:

♦ Define myopathy and classify various types of myopathies
♦ Understand the subtle changes in the clinical manifestation of myopathies
♦ Understand etiopathology and kinesiopathological factors leading to functional disturbance of the patients
♦ Identify the role of various investigative procedures in diagnosing myopathy
♦ Gain knowledge of the available treatment methods, including medical and physiotherapy in treatment of myopathy
♦ Identify the role of physiotherapy rehabilitation in evaluation and intervention of myopathy

CHAPTER OUTLINE

- Classification and types of myopathy
- Common clinical features of myopathies
  - Muscle weakness
  - Muscle atrophy
  - Muscle tone
  - Deep tendon reflexes
  - Pain
  - Myotonic reaction
  - Muscle spasms
  - Contracture
- Muscular dystrophy
  - Types
  - Duchenne's muscular dystrophy
  - Becker's muscular dystrophy
  - Facioscapulohumeral muscular dystrophy (Landouzy-Dejerine disease)
  - Limb-girdle muscular dystrophy
  - Progressive muscular dystrophy of Emery–Dreifuss type
  - Congenital muscular dystrophies
  - Oculopharyngeal muscular dystrophy
- Distal myopathies
- Myotonic muscular dystrophy
- Inflammatory myopathy
  - Polymyositis and dermatomyositis
  - Inclusion body myositis
- Infectious myopathies
- Myopathy in endocrine diseases
- Diagnostic tests
  - Laboratory evaluation
  - Electrodiagnosis
  - Muscle biopsy
  - Genetic studies
- Complications of myopathy
  - Respiratory complications
  - Cardiac complications
  - Obesity
  - Sleep disturbance
  - Osteoporosis
  - Spinal deformity
  - Pressure sores
  - Swallowing difficulty
  - Psychosocial complications
  - Other complications
- Medical management of myopathy
- Physical therapy rehabilitation
  - Physical therapy evaluation
  - Pathomechanics
  - Kinetic analysis
  - Clinical assessment
  - Range of motion assessment
  - Muscle strength assessment
  - Respiratory function tests
- Cardiac assessment
- Functional assessment
- Commonly used outcome measurement scales in myopathic disorders
- Lower limb function tests
- Upper limb function tests
- Functional scales
- Physical therapy management
  - Physiotherapy in early stage
  - Physiotherapy in middle stage
  - Physiotherapy in late stage
  - Role of physical exercises
  - Strengthening exercises
  - Prevent contractures and deformities
  - Promoting ambulation
  - Use of wheelchair
  - Respiratory management
  - Obesity management
  - Managing ADLs
  - Managing sleep
  - Addressing psychosocial issues
  - Facilitating family support
  - Managing pain

INTRODUCTION

Myopathy means muscle disease (Greek: myo—*muscle* + patheia—*pathy*: *suffering*). Myopathies are primarily diseases related to muscles. Children with myopathies are short lived and face a lot of challenges to maintain the function throughout their lifespan. In adults, as seen in certain variants of myopathy, it progresses and hampers most activities of daily living, eventually limiting their longevity. A competent physiotherapist along with other rehab professionals can make their lives productive and less complicated. During the 19th century, a French neurologist, Guillaume Benjamin Amand Duchenne (the disease Duchenne's muscular dystrophy (DMD) is named after him) pioneered on this disease by doing needle biopsy on boys and concluded this disease to be of muscle origin.

Myopathies are a group of disorders that are genetically and clinically heterogeneous in nature affecting the muscles, especially striated muscles throughout the body. This type of muscle disease is caused due to mutations in encoded genes for structural proteins dystrophin linking the cytoskeleton of muscle fibers to the extracellular matrix. These dystrophin encoded genes are required for maintaining muscle integrity. Dystrophin proteins are found in the muscle fiber membrane and function in two ways: Mechanical stabilization and regulated calcium levels. Any alteration or insufficient quantity or absence of these encoded genes will predominantly affect the integrity of the muscles leading to muscle degeneration, progressive weakness, fiber death, and loss of muscle strength. Finally, this results in replacement of muscle by connective tissue and fat and gives a pseudo appearance of muscle hypertrophy called "pseudohypertrophy" **(Figs. 32.1A and B)**.

CLASSIFICATION AND TYPES OF MYOPATHY

There are various forms of myopathies and those that are noticeable at birth are called congenital myopathies which are inherited in nature. Those that develop later in life, such as Becker's muscular dystrophy (BMD) are acquired in nature. Broadly, they can be classified as mentioned in **Figure 32.2**, and in **Table 32.1** which gives its onset.

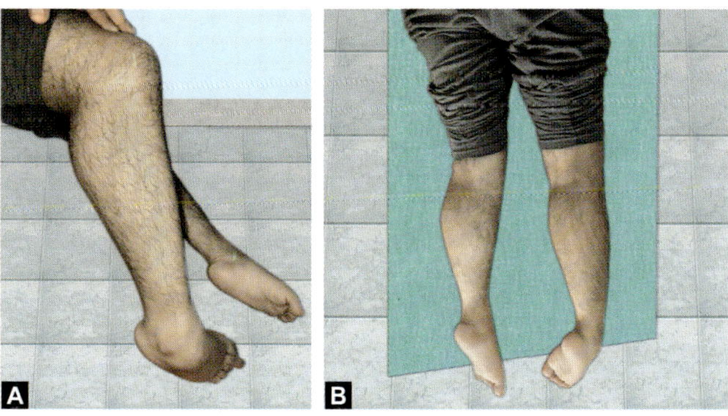

Figs. 32.1A and B: Pseudohypertrophy of bilateral calves.

COMMON CLINICAL FEATURES OF MYOPATHIES

Muscle Weakness

The distribution of muscle weakness is symmetric, affecting proximal more than the distal, also involving the muscles of face, neck, and throat. However, in some cases, distal muscle groups are affected or asymmetric involvement may be noted. This weakness may lead to difficulty in bed mobility; transfer activities such as sit to stand, climbing on to chair, stair climbing, holding an object; grooming such as dressing, undressing, and combing hair; and gait abnormalities. Severe weakness results in patient being dependent on splints, walker or crutches, or manual assistance for daily activities and further leads to either wheelchair dependence or being bed bound in later stages. In most types of myopathy, the muscle weakness is present during all the times; in some however, it is episodic (as in hypo- and hyperkalemic periodic paralyses), exercise induced (as in metabolic myopathies or myasthenia gravis (MG), or progressively severe during course of the day in connection with activity (MG). The age of onset is an important datum for the differential diagnosis in myopathy. The speed of progression is another.

Muscle Atrophy

As the disease progresses, during the later stage, muscle atrophy is seen in a major group of muscles due to weakness and inactivity. Sometimes, muscle atrophy is absent as in MG, or in cases with muscular dystrophy, pseudohypertrophy is noted as the muscle fibers are replaced by connective and fat tissues. In conditions, such as myotonia congenita and other rare forms, due to continuous spontaneous activity of muscle fibers, true hypertrophy can be seen.

Muscle Tone

The tone of the muscle is usually normal or sometimes diminished.

Deep Tendon Reflexes

Except MG, the reflexes are markedly diminished or absent, in direct proportion to the extent of muscle weakness present.

Pain

Though pain is an uncommon feature in myopathy, most infectious myopathies (myositides) and inflammatory myopathies produce continuous pain. Exercise-induced myalgia is a common feature in metabolic myopathy.

Myotonic Reaction

This means inability of the skeletal muscle to relax immediately after a contraction. This can be clinically observed in most forms of myotonia.

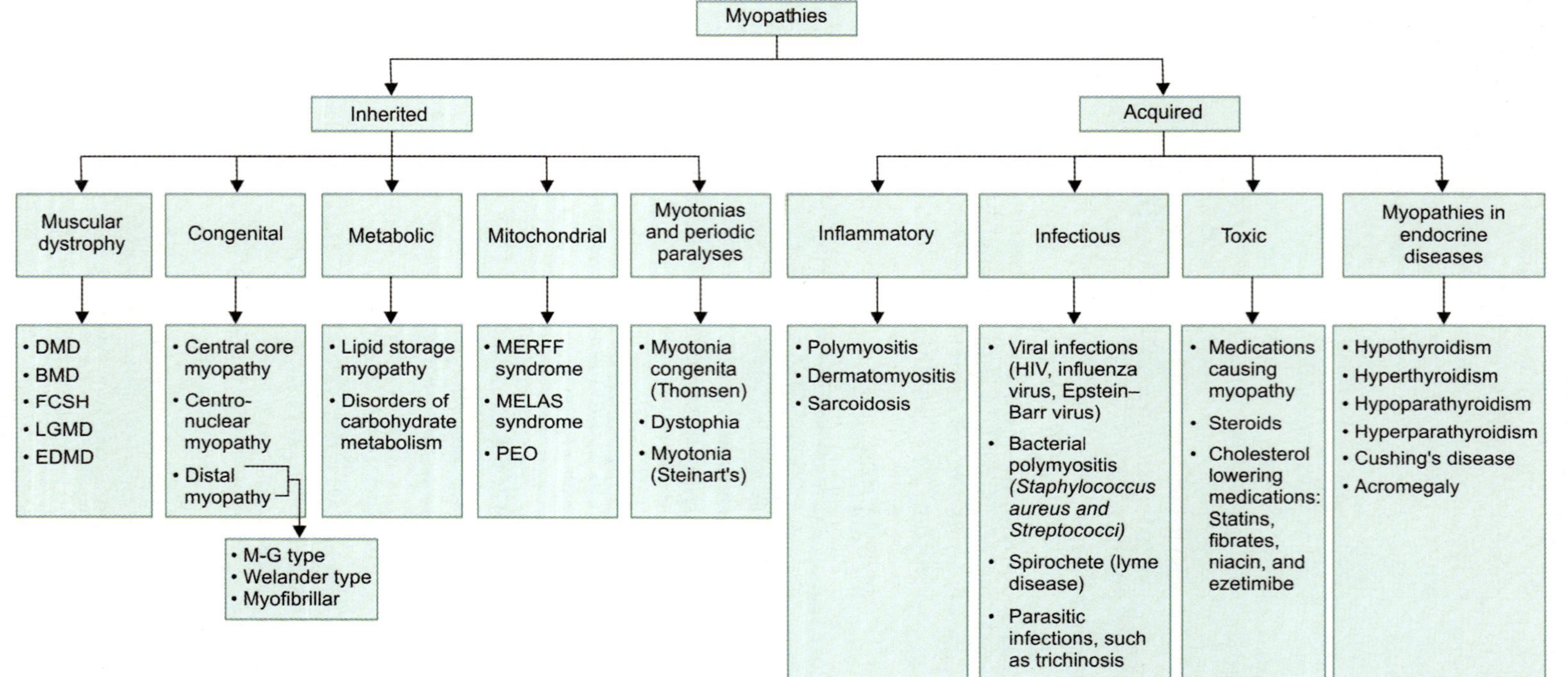

Fig. 32.2: Classification of myopathies.

(DMD: Duchenne muscular dystrophy; BMD: Beckers muscular dystrophy; FCSH: facioscapulohumeral: LGMD: Limb-girdle muscular dystrophy; EDMD: Emery–Dreifuss muscular dystrophy; MERFF: myoclonic epilepsy and ragged–red fibers; MELAS: mitochondrial encephlopathy lactic acidosis and stroke-like episodes; PEO: progressive external ophthalmoplegia; M-G Type: Markesbery–Griggs type)

Table 32.1: Type of myopathy and its onset.	
Type of myopathy	*Onset*
Muscular dystrophies	Early onset, chronic, and progressive
Metabolic myopathies	Occasionally precipitated acutely, may be progressive, fixed or recurrent
Congenital myopathies	Chronic, slowly progressive
Systemic myopathy	Late onset, acute, or subacute
Endocrine myopathies	Adult onset, acute, or subacute
Inflammatory and toxic	Onset in any age, acute, or subacute

Muscle Spasms

The patients with myopathy often complain of constant painful contractions which may be spontaneous or, in some instances, voluntary like those induced by activities. These intermittent states of contractions are termed as muscle spasms. Sometimes, the muscle spasms remain for a longer time leading to a muscle cramp, which can be occasionally seen in this condition.

Contracture

In chronic myopathic disorders, contractures are noted around joints limiting passive movements.

MUSCULAR DYSTROPHY

Types

Muscular dystrophies are classified into nine major types based on the age of onset:
1. Early childhood onset:
   - DMD
   - BMD
   - Congenital muscular dystrophy
   - Emery–Dreifuss muscular dystrophy
2. Youth/adolescent onset:
   - Facioscapulohumeral muscular dystrophy
   - Limb-girdle muscular dystrophy (LGMD)
3. Adult onset:
   - Distal muscular dystrophy
   - Myotonic muscular dystrophy
   - Oculopharyngeal muscular dystrophy

Duchenne's Muscular Dystrophy

Epidemiology and Pathogenesis

It is one of the most common and a rapidly worsening form of muscular dystrophies, affecting 1 in 3,600 male births. Also known as pseudohypertrophic muscular dystrophy or progressive muscular dystrophy, DMD is typically progressive, because the muscles' ability to regenerate is eventually lost, leading to progressive weakness, often leading to use of a wheelchair, and eventually death, usually related to respiratory weakness. DMD results from an abnormal gene on X chromosome (Xp21) that encodes dystrophin where it gets either mutated or deleted leading to no dystrophin protein production. Since DMD has X-linked recessive inheritance, boys are affected whereas girls and women are the carriers of the defective gene. About two-third of the reported cases have a family history where the sisters of the boys suffering from DMD have almost 50% chances of carrying the defective gene. Remaining one-third of the cases are sporadic which is as a result of new mutation.

Clinical Presentation

DMD is the most common and a serious form of muscle disease. Though it is an inherited disease, there will be no noticeable physical presentation until the child learns to stand and walk. Pregnancy and birth are usually normal, except that some mothers report diminished movements during pregnancy. Usually, it is diagnosed between the ages of 3 and 5 when the physical development gradually slows down. In some children with DMD, timing of motor milestones is often delayed (50% of babies with DMD fail to walk until 18 months). Although all skeletal muscles are involved, the para-axial and appendicular postural muscles first formed in the embryo are involved earliest and affected most severely. Facial and extraocular muscles remain clinically intact, although macroglossia and hypertrophy of masseter muscles can be seen.

While reporting, the mother of the child with DMD gives history that the child's movements are clumsy, uncoordinated, and coarse particularly seen while walking, jumping, and climbing stairs. At the onset of the disease, primarily the proximal muscles of the pelvic girdle are prominently and symmetrically involved as compared to shoulder girdle and neck muscles. Due to loss of skeletal muscle fibers, the atrophy will be clinically evident. However, in some muscle groups particularly the calves, buttocks, deltoids, muscles of mastication, and tongue, pseudohypertrophy will be seen as the muscles are gradually replaced by fat and connective tissues. As the disease progresses, the weakness of hip muscle will lead to bilateral Trendelenburg gait, i.e., waddling appearance. Tiptoe walking is commonly noted due to contractures **(Figs. 32.3A and B)**.

Gower's Sign

This is visibly noted when the child tries to stand up from lying position. The children first turn prone then spread the legs or pull them together, raise buttocks, and then climb on their own knees and thighs with their arms and hands up to reach the upright position. This phenomenon is termed as Gower's sign **(Fig. 32.4)**.

Weaknesses in abdominal musculature, paraspinals, and glutei combined with tight hip flexors cause severe lordotic posture. As the child stands, it gives the typical

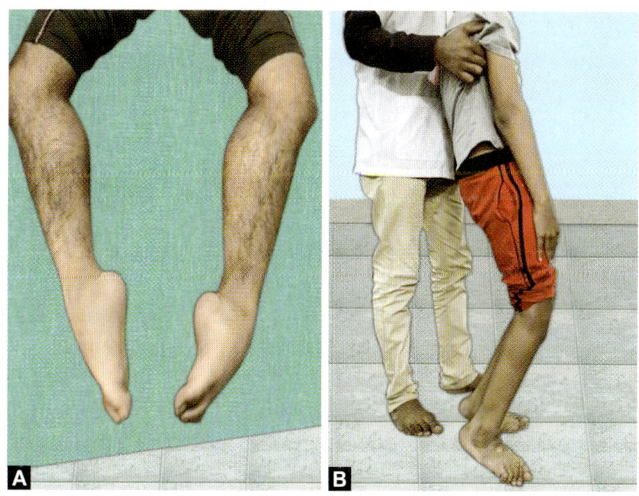

Figs. 32.3A and B: Equinus position of feet resulting in tiptoe walking.

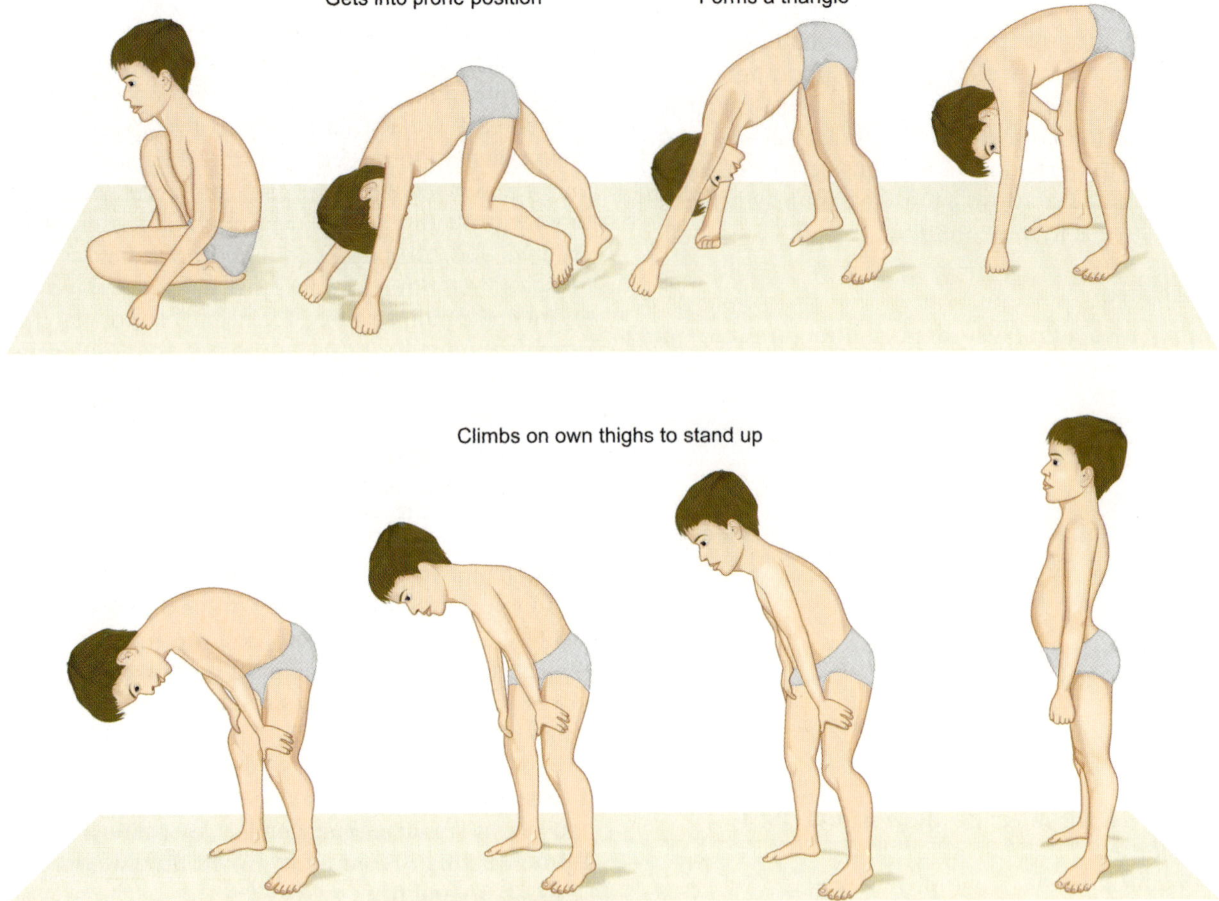

Fig. 32.4: Gower's sign.
Source: Image taken from https://epomedicine.com/clinical-medicine/gowers-sign/)

posture with backward thrust of the shoulders and winging of scapulae. When the clinician tries to lift the child by holding him under the axillae, he slips off his hand, which is termed "Meryon's sign" or "loose shoulder sign." Positional scoliosis develops as the child spends more time sitting, which over the time becomes fixed.

The weakness is steadily progressive with the boys losing strength at 0.322 units per year (SD = 0.318) on a 10-point scale. This average muscle score represents the sum of 34 muscles graded using the Medical Research Council for manual muscle testing (MMT), converted to a 10-point scale.

The range of motion (ROM) of the joints gets limited and patient finds it very difficult to maintain the mechanical alignment necessary for upright posture. The functional activity also gradually declines. These functional activities are considered to be "milestones" and represent significant points in disease progression. The arm grades awarded were developed by Brooke and Associates **(Table 32.2)**, whereas the leg grades are based on a scale developed by Vignos **(Table 32.3)**.

The course of the disease is such that contractures arise at hips, knees, and elbows, and the mobility of the child gets limited. Most of the patients become non-ambulant between the age of 8 and 15 and die between the ages of 18 and 25. The cause of death is usually related to respiratory failure.

Few other organs in the body also get involved. As dystrophin is present in smooth muscles and in brain, patients with advanced DMD will have dystrophic an cardiomyopathy and suffer heart failure, and there can be

Table 32.2: Functional grades—arms and shoulders.	
Grade	**Functional ability**
1	Standing with arms at the sides, the patient can abduct the arms in a full circle until they touch above the head
2	The patient can raise the arms above the head only by flexing the elbow (i.e., by shortening the circumference of the movement) or by using accessory muscles
3	The patient cannot raise hands above the head but can raise an 8-oz glass of water to the mouth (using both hands if necessary)
4	The patient can raise hands to the mouth but cannot raise an 8-oz glass of water to the mouth
5	The patient cannot raise hands to the mouth but can use the hands to hold a pen or to pick up pennies from a table
6	The patient cannot raise hands to the mouth and has no useful function of the hands

Grade	Functional ability
1	Walks and climbs stairs without assistance
2	Walks and climbs stairs with the aid of a railing
3	Walks and climbs stairs slowly (elapsed time of >12 seconds for four standard stairs) with the aid of a railing
4	Walks unassisted and rises from a chair but cannot climb stairs
5	Walks unassisted but cannot rise from a chair or climb stairs
6	Walks only with assistance or walks independently with long-leg braces
7	Walks in long-leg braces but requires assistance for balance
8	Stands in long-leg braces but is unable to walk even with assistance
9	Is in wheelchair
10	Is confined to bed

Table 32.3: Functional grades—hips and legs.

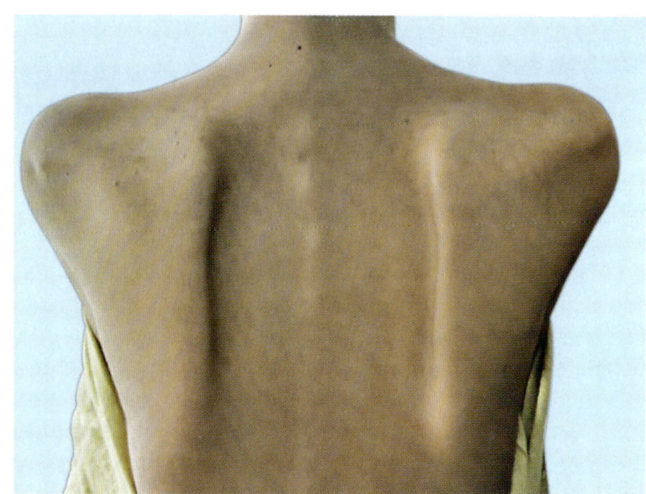

Fig. 32.5: Weakness of serratus anterior.

an occasional finding of intellectual disability. Fortunately, these kids will have intact bladder and bowel; seldom other neurologic signs appear.

Becker's Muscular Dystrophy

This is the milder form and constitutes 10% of DMD and is X linked. BMD has a later onset and the clinical manifestations are visible between ages 10 and 15. The patients are ambulatory in the third decade with longer life expectancy than DMD. The proximal muscle weakness is more prominent, but unlike DMD, the distribution of weakness is asymmetrical. The neck muscle strength is preserved in most of the cases, but patients may develop ambulatory scoliosis because of asymmetrical paraspinal muscle weakness. Approximately 70% of the patients develop cardiac abnormalities by the age of 20. ECG demonstrates left ventricular dilation in 37% of BMD patients, and 63% have subnormal systolic function which is due to cardiac hypokinesia. Mental retardation is uncommon in BMD.

Early symptoms of BMD include tiptoe walking, frequent falls and difficulty rising from chair and other functional movements, such as transfers and self-grooming. Contractures are not a significant early functional problem in BMD becoming problematic only after wheelchair dependence.

Facioscapulohumeral Muscular Dystrophy (Landouzy–Dejerine Disease)

This is identified as a distinctive muscular dystrophy, because of the slow progressive muscular weakness, clinically noted in the facial and shoulder musculature. Prevalence is estimated at 10–20 per million. The chromosomal aberration is identified at *4q35* gene locus and is always inherited as an autosomal-dominant disorder.

The distinctive clinical manifestation is seen in the facial muscles primarily involving orbicularis oris, zygomaticus major, and orbicularis oculi leaving an expressionless face in the patient. The onset of the disease is around adolescence or early adulthood. The patient usually complains of not being able to close the eyes properly, sucking through straw, etc.

Marked weakness will be found in the shoulder girdle musculature especially serratus anterior **(Fig. 32.5)**, latissimus dorsi, rhomboids, and the lower trapezius. This displaces the scapula laterally and superiorly, resulting in winging. Unlike other muscular dystrophies, the weakness is asymmetric and in some cases, the pelvic girdle involvement can be seen. The patients suffering from this muscle disorder usually become wheelchair dependent by late second or third decade.

Cardiac complications are rare, although some studies report cardiac abnormalities including cardiac fibrosis. More than half of the patients suffer from mild restrictive lung disease; however, lifespan does not appear to be affected.

Limb-Girdle Muscular Dystrophy

The mode of inheritance of limb-girdle muscular dystrophy (LGMD) is both autosomal dominant (LGMD type 1) and autosomal recessive (LGMD type 2, more severe). Onset is usually in the second or third decade, and both genders are equally affected. Life expectancy is reduced but variable. Usually, pelvic girdle weakness is more than shoulder girdle with variable progression. Prognosis is better in patients who manifest shoulder weakness first. Sometimes, marked weakness of biceps is seen, but compensatory brachioradialis bulk is seen which gives the appearance of "Popeye arms." These patients may have enlarged and hypertrophied calves. Diaphragm gets involved early which leads to alveolar hypoventilation. No signs of cardiomyopathy are seen, and they may have normal intelligence.

Progressive Muscular Dystrophy of Emery–Dreifuss Type

This muscle disorder is X-linked and rarely autosomal dominant. The chromosomal aberration is at the long arm in the *Xq28* gene. In this condition, *emerin* which is a protein product of the nuclear membrane is absent. This is not alone in the muscle but also in blood and skin.

The onset of this muscular dystrophy is in childhood or during adolescence. In the acute phase, the muscle atrophy is evident in muscle groups, such as triceps, biceps, tibialis anterior, and peroneus. In the later stages, the upper and lower limb-girdle muscles get involved. Contractures appear at prominent muscles particularly in biceps and calves. Most of the patients are ambulant predominantly with equinus gait into the third decade and some throughout their life **(Figs. 32.6A and B)**.

Congenital Muscular Dystrophies

These are muscular dystrophies that affect the child from birth and can lead to various clinical syndromes. Currently, five kinds of congenital muscular dystrophies are commonly found.

1. A relatively congenital nonprogressive muscular dystrophy with or without arthrogryposis multiplex. The latter term refers to congenital joint contractures leading to deformed postures and severely impaired mobility of affected joints.
2. Congenital muscular dystrophy of Fukuyama type. This disorder is usually combined with developmental disorders of brain.
3. Congenital muscular dystrophy of Walker-Warburg type involving muscles, eyes, and brain (MEB disease).
4. Congenital muscular dystrophy of Santavuori type also involving the muscles, eyes, and brain.
5. Rigid spine syndrome which mimics the BMD in the later stage. Here, the contractures of the paraspinal muscles, reduced mobility of the spine, and mainly the pectoral girdle weakness will be present.

Oculopharyngeal Muscular Dystrophy

This type of muscle disease is autosomal dominant inheritance, and the defect is on chromosome 14q11.2-q13.

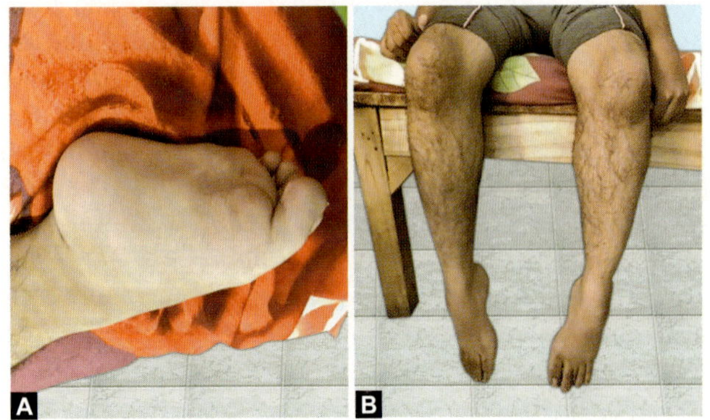

Figs. 32.6A and B: Severe contracture of the bilateral calves including Achilles tendon.

The protein which is defective is poly(A-). Autosomal recessive inheritance of this disease is very rarely reported.

The onset of the disease is somewhere in the middle age and the initial complaint of the patient would be weakness of the extraocular muscle and ptosis. This will be progressive in nature until it leads to ophthalmoplegia. The weakness and atrophy involve facial and bulbar musculature. In many cases, shoulder and hip-muscle involvement are also visible. Patients suffer from severe dysphagia, which leads to cachexia and aspiration pneumonia.

DISTAL MYOPATHIES

There are a number of manifestations of distal myopathies, and few mentioned below can be classified on clinical grounds:

Hereditary tardive distal myopathy of Welander type: This disease is common among Scandinavian people and is first to be described. The genetic defect is located at chromosome 2p13 band. The onset is during middle age and initially affects the hand muscles and gradually the distal muscles of the lower limb. The progression of the disease is slow.

Distal myopathy of Markesbery–Griggs type: This is an autosomal dominant inherent disorder of late onset. In the beginning, the weakness and atrophy are observed in feet and later involve the hands and arms. The genetic defect is on chromosome 2q31 which is the same as in the Finnish variant of this disease. Those with early onset, i.e., adolescence or young adulthood will have autosomal recessive pattern. One variant of this disease, Nonaka type involves the anterior compartment of leg, whereas the Miyoshi type involves the calf muscles first. The genetic defect is located on chromosomes 9p1-q1 and 2p13, respectively. The patients suffering from this disorder usually have difficulty in walking.

Myofibrillar myopathies: This group of disorders is also mainly present with distal muscle involvement. This disorder is clinically diagnosed in young adulthood and can be accompanied by a cardiomyopathy which further leads to heart failure.

MYOTONIC MUSCULAR DYSTROPHY

Myotonic muscular dystrophy is the most common slowly progressive dystrophy due to autosomal dominant inheritance with an incidence of 1 per 8,000. The aberrant chromosome is 19q13.3 coded for the protein kinase, is responsible for this disorder. This disease targets multiple systems in the body affecting smooth muscle, skeletal muscle, myocardium, brain, and ocular structures. The clinical manifestation includes muscle weakness, cardiac conduction defects, swallowing difficulty, and cataract. Patients with this dystrophy often have a typical face. They have long and thin faces with wasting of masseter and temporal muscles. Frontal balding at a young age is indicative of myotonic muscular dystrophy. In contrary to other muscle diseases, the distal muscles including the ankle dorsiflexors, invertors, and evertors, intrinsic muscles of hand are more affected as compared to proximal muscles. This leaves the patient to have foot drop and difficulty in performing fine motor skills. As the disease progresses, the shoulder and pelvic girdle muscles get involved as well. Spinal deformity, especially scoliosis, will be present.

Another distinctive feature of this disease is the presence of myotonia, a state of delayed relaxation or prolonged contraction of muscle. This may be demonstrated by percussion of the thenar eminence with a reflex hammer, causing sustained flexion and adduction of thumb. Grip myotonia is provoked by having the patient sustain a tight grip, then suddenly attempting to relax. Delayed opening of the fingers will occur. Myotonia in all myotonic diseases is often aggravated by cold.

EMG is characterized by high-frequency repetitive discharges that initially increase in frequency and amplitude, then rapidly diminish (dive-bomber effect).

The major forms of myotonic disease are:

- **Myotonia congenita (Thomsen's disease):** In this form, generalized non-progressive muscular hypertrophy with muscle stiffness and weakness, relieved by exercise is classically noted. They occur in two forms:
    1. Autosomal dominant—mild non-progressive myotonia diagnosed in infancy
    2. Autosomal recessive—later onset with subsequent distal atrophy and weakness.

    The patient may present with complaints of garbled speech after eating chilled foods (associated with tongue myotonia induced by cold).

- **Dystrophia myotonica (Steinert's disease):** It is an autosomal dominant multisystem disorder (linked with the *secretor gene*) with poor congruence in affected family members, the most common form of which usually becomes apparent in early adulthood. Expression is variable, and the disease is characterized by:
    a. Stellate cataracts and retinal alterations
    b. Gonadal atrophy

Impotence in males, chronic abortion in females is highly prevalent. Fault tolerance to carbohydrates (diabetic glucose tolerance curve), defective insulin metabolism leads to diabetes. Frontal and/or parietal alopecia in young males is common. Thyroid dysfunction is also one of the features of this muscle disease. Patients with this disease suffer from cardiac dysfunction which may require pacemakers. Many patients suffer pulmonary complications, such as alveolar hypoventilation causing symptoms like night sweats. Progressive psychosocial deterioration along with decrease in higher intellectual functions are seen.

Distal muscle weakness, especially in the forearms and tibialis anterior muscles will be clinically evident. Patient may trip because of weakness, and in attempting to regain balance, provoke a myotonic response that causes a fall. It is the weakness (dystrophy), not the myotonia that troubles these patients the most.

INFLAMMATORY MYOPATHY

These disorders are thought to be due to a viral or autoimmune mechanism:

- Characterized by symmetrical proximal muscle weakness often accompanied by muscular pain and tenderness.
- They occur more frequently in people of African origin.
- Dysphagia is sometimes present.
- Involvement of facial or extraocular muscles is rare.
- Pseudohypertrophy occasionally occurs.
- The deep tendon reflexes may be absent, normal, or hyperactive.
- The heart may be involved.
- Muscle atrophy with contracture and calcinosis is seen late in the course of the disease.

Polymyositis and Dermatomyositis

These are usually generalized, symmetric rapidly progressive inflammatory disease of the muscles. When the inflammation of the skin is noted, it is termed "dermatomyositis." These are rare diseases with an incidence of 5–10 per million per year. The age-specific incidence of dermatomyositis has two peaks, one before puberty and another around the age of 40. Polymyositis occurs after the age of 35 and affects women more than men. It is a non-inherent disorder usually and presumed to be an auto-immune disease.

These patients feel generalized illness, malaise, myalgia, and arthralgia. The affected muscles feel tender and patients do not allow to touch them during clinical examination. The patients face a lot of functional disturbance; even undertaking day-to-day activities, such as lifting objects, getting up from floor, walking and climbing stairs due to progressive muscle weakness. About 20–30% patients suffer dysphagia due to pharyngeal involvement, and this may cause aspiration pneumonia. Patients with dermatomyositis develop patches over the skin. Both these diseases involve the heart and lungs leading to heart failure, arrhythmias, or pulmonary fibrosis. In chronic patient with myositis, Raynaud's phenomenon is not uncommon. Joint involvement ends up in contractures and effusions.

About 10% of the cases of these disorders are associated with carcinoma of lungs, breast, ovary, or stomach and affecting multiple organs in the body. Majority of the patients with dermatomyositis present with scleroderma, which is termed "sclerodermatomyositis."

Inclusion Body Myositis

This disorder which affects commonly men appears after the fifth decade with unknown etiology. It clinically resembles polymyositis but affects both proximal and distal muscles including legs, arms, fingers, and wrists and, sometimes facial muscles. Swallowing difficulty is present. This type of myositis usually progresses unstoppably.

INFECTIOUS MYOPATHIES

These forms of acquired myopathies are uncommon but have a good prognosis. It can be viral, bacterial, and also due to HIV infection. Myalgia like pain in the limbs is a characteristic feature and can be diagnosed by serology and muscle biopsy.

MYOPATHY IN ENDOCRINE DISEASES

This occurs in conditions, such as hypothyroidism, hyperthyroidism, hypoparathyroidism, hyperparathyroidism, acromegaly, Addison's disease, Cushing's disease, and diabetes mellitus. It usually affects the proximal muscles, with preserved deep tendon reflexes. Muscle atrophy will be present in severe cases.

DIAGNOSTIC TESTS

Laboratory Evaluation

The most common and an important blood investigation done for a suspected case of myopathy is serum creatine phosphokinase (CPK) levels. Patients suffering from this disease will have 50–100 times raised CPK levels. This is found mostly in acute inflammatory myopathies and early stages of DMD and BMD. However, CPK is not an ideal screening test for diagnosing a muscle disease because chronic inflammatory muscle disease, slow progressive dystrophies, congenital myopathies, and myopathies arising due to systemic disorders will have CPK within normal limits. So the clinician should be cautious not to overinterpret mildly elevated CPK levels, because it may be elevated in healthy individuals too for several days after vigorous exercise. Conversely, once there is significant muscular atrophy, CPK value may be low or normal based on the paucity of the muscle tissue to release the enzyme.

Electrodiagnosis

The nerve conduction velocity studies of motor and sensory nerves will have normal latencies and conduction velocities. But amplitude of compound muscle action potential (CMAP) decreases as the disease progresses.

EMG studies throw some light in disclosing special findings such as myotonic potentials. Increase in insertional activity can be noted in the early stage of the disease which can decrease in the later stage as fibrotic tissue replaces the muscle. This is characteristic of muscular dystrophy. Patterns of low amplitude, short duration, and polyphasic motor unit action potential will be seen in the EMG. This is the electrical equivalent of clinical myotonia which is manifested as impaired relaxation of muscles after forceful contraction; for example, patients cannot release objects from their grip. Myotonic potentials have the characteristic sound of a dive bomb on EMG and can help point toward the diagnosis of myotonic dystrophy when found in the appropriate muscles. Although integral in the evaluation of a myopathy, the EMG can be normal in mild myopathies, steroid myopathies, and a number of metabolic myopathies. Therefore it is important to remember that a normal EMG does not exclude the presence of a myopathy.

Muscle Biopsy

Under anesthesia, a small tissue is taken from the bulkiest muscle and examined under a microscope. Histopathologic examination of muscle may be helpful in determining the specific type of muscle disease, especially in patients with a suspected inflammatory or infectious myopathy. Selecting the optimal muscle to biopsy is very important because factors, such as severe weakness and technical artifacts can hamper an accurate histologic diagnosis. The ideal muscle that should be sampled is one that is clinically involved but still antigravity in strength, because more severe weakness can lead to unhelpful, nonspecific findings of fibrosis. Avoid muscles that have been examined by an EMG as the needle portion of the electrical study might have caused local damage which can result in spurious findings. Common biopsy sites include the *biceps* and *deltoid* muscles in the upper extremity and the *quadriceps* and *gastrocnemius* muscles in the lower extremity.

Genetic Studies

Genetic testing is another form of investigation for some inherited myopathies. It is important to have genetic confirmation as it will help the family to take decision regarding prenatal diagnosis and future planning of pregnancies. If mother is found to be the carrier, genetic counseling should be advised for other female relatives of the child.

Tables 32.4 and 32.5 give a quick review on most common and less common forms of myopathy, respectively.

COMPLICATIONS OF MYOPATHY

Respiratory Complications

Breathing complications mostly occur only after the patient stops walking. But in the case of *congenital muscular dystrophy*, breathlessness is noticed even when the patient is still walking. This is due to the indirect involvement of the respiratory muscles due to the spinal musculature weakness and restricted thoracic mobility due to spinal deformity.

Table 32.4: The most common forms of myopathy (muscular dystrophy).

Type	Onset	Clinical manifestations	Involvement of other body part
Duchenne's muscular dystrophy	Before 4–5 years of age	1. Weak hip and shoulder muscles 2. Stops walking around the age of 10–12 years 3. Kyphosis and scoliosis of spine 4. Weak respiratory muscles	Cardiomyopathy (heart becomes large in size and weak in pumping action)
Becker's muscular dystrophy	Early childhood to adult	1. Weak hip and shoulder muscles 2. Can walk even beyond the age of 15 years 3. Muscles of respiration also become weak but at a very later stage	Same as above
Limb-girdle muscular dystrophy	Early childhood to adult	Muscles of hip and shoulder become weak	Same as above

Table 32.5: Less common forms of myopathy (muscular dystrophy).

Type	Onset	Clinical manifestations	Involvement of other body part
Facioscapulohumeral muscular dystrophy	Before the age of 19–20	Weakness of shoulder, face, and upper arm muscles, but slowly	None
Congenital muscular dystrophy	At birth or within the first few months	1. Low tone or floppy 2. Muscle contractures 3. Delayed milestones 4. Weak respiratory muscles	Mentally retarded and problems with the eyes
Myotonic muscular dystrophy	Starts between 11 and 20 years of age	Weakness of shoulder, face, and upper arm muscles but slowly	Mental retardation, cataract. Gonadal atrophy, heart problems
Oculopharyngeal dystrophy	Between 40 and 60 years	Slow weakness of the extraocular and throat muscles	None
Emery–Dreifuss muscular dystrophy	Childhood to adult	1. Weakness of shoulder and upper arm 2. Contractures	Cardiomyopathy
Distal myopathy	40–50 years	Weakness of hand, arm, and foot muscles	None

Breathing complications in muscular dystrophy majorly include reduced lung expansion leading to collapse of lung tissue, which in turn causes chest infections. It also causes difficulty in coughing which increases the accumulation of mucus in the lungs. In *myotonic dystrophy*, due to dysphagia, aspiration pneumonia is very common. In about 90% of persons with DMD, death results due to respiratory complications.

Cardiac Complications

In myopathy, the skeletal muscle weakness is not alone evident; the disease involves cardiac muscle also, resulting in cardiac complications, such as cardiomyopathy and heart failure. Heart problems in BMD are worse than in DMD patients. Myotonic muscular dystrophy type 1 has more than one system affected with prominent heart problems leading to an increased incidence of sudden death. Approximately 70% of boys with BMD have cardiac involvement by age 20.

Obesity

People with muscular dystrophy often are overweight due to lack of physical activity. It adds strain to weak muscles due to which the person can approach non-walking stage faster.

Sleep Disturbance

Due to muscle weakness, the patient's bed mobility gets lost which results in inability to take turns while in the bed. This disturbs patients as well as the caretaker's sleep. Moreover, due to breathing issues, the patients suffer sleepless nights.

Osteoporosis

The risk of osteoporosis in children with myopathy increases with age and disease progression. As they become non-ambulant, the bones become brittle and osteoporotic as the bones are not subjected to normal weight bearing. Fractures of the long bones in the lower limbs occur frequently which also results in immobility.

Spinal Deformity

Scoliosis (S-shaped curvature) in the spine is commonly seen due to poor sitting tolerance. The trunk musculature weakness, as it prolongs, results in contracture leading to this deformity (**Figs. 32.7A and B**). Because of the hip and the pelvic girdle muscle weakness, excessive lordosis is prominent as the patient stands.

Pressure Sores

Staying for prolonged periods in any particular position in muscular dystrophy could result in pressure or bedsore.

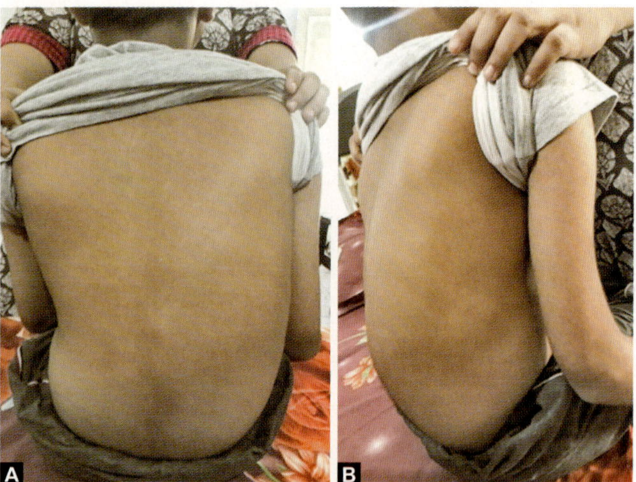

Figs. 32.7A and B: Noticeable spinal deformity in an 11-year-old boy, suffering from Duchenne's muscular dystrophy.

Although sensation is generally not affected, individuals with muscular dystrophy (MD) are at risk of developing pressure sores as they are unable to reposition themselves on their own. Also, being overweight can increase the risk considerably. Pressure sores develop mainly on bony prominences, such as occiput, interscapular area, sacrum, ischium, greater trochanter, and lateral malleolus depending upon the position of the patient.

Swallowing Difficulty

In some variants of myopathic disorders, swallowing difficulty is seen. Due to the pseudohypertrophy of the tongue, there will be poor sucking phenomenon, difficulty in making bolus and swallowing. Dysphagia leads to complication of aspiration pneumonia.

Psychosocial Complications

These individuals, due to lack of mobility, will not be able to move out or participate in social gatherings, and in children it may even result in stopping their school. This has a huge impact on the psychosocial aspects of a kid. This leads to various psychological and social abnormalities, such as aloofness, anxiety, depression, reduced self-esteem, and many times they are seen irritated, non-cooperative, and throw tantrums. They feel helpless as they are dependent on others. Associated conditions, such as Attention Deficit Hyperactivity Disorder (ADHD), learning difficulties, or autism spectrum disorders should be identified early to reduce psychological issues.

Other Complications

As the kids with muscle disease are mostly on long-term steroid intake, complications, such as cataracts, retarded bone growth, constipation, and even hypertension may be seen. Conditions, such as ADHD, intellectual disability are seen in some children. Prevalence of early diabetes is not uncommon among children with endocrine myopathy.

MEDICAL MANAGEMENT OF MYOPATHY

The treatment of myopathy needs a multidisciplinary approach, and it depends on the type of myopathy. Immunosuppressant agents (e.g., prednisone) and intravenous immunoglobulin (IVIg) are the choice of drug for treating certain types of myopathy, such as dermatomyositis and polymyositis. Enzyme replacement therapy is life-saving in infantile-onset Pompe disease and improves pulmonary function. A Cochrane review concluded that creatine monohydrate (3–20 g/day) slightly increased strength and function in dystrophinopathies. However, the side effects caused by pharmacologic management should be aggressively managed.

Effective management of myopathy requires a multimodal approach with the use of supportive services, such as physical and occupational therapy, pulmonary medicine, cardiology, dietary management, and speech/swallowing therapists. Surgical treatment of spine and limb deformities is used in long-standing cases.

PHYSICAL THERAPY REHABILITATION

Physical Therapy Evaluation

Each patient suffering from any variant of myopathic disorder needs to undergo a detailed physiotherapy assessment. As there is no cure to the disease, rehabilitation, especially physiotherapy helps the patients undertake functional tasks and thereby they can lead a fairly independent life till they are alive. Such an evaluation involves the gathering of information that can directly attribute to the plan of care. Most of the findings should have functional significance and the plan of treatment will be based on it.

Pathomechanics

As the muscles are involved in this disorder, understanding the pathomechanics of the disease will help the physiotherapist to assess the patient in detail. Here, DMD being a rapidly progressive disorder with its severe disability is taken as a model for discussion and analysis of those forces that create an imbalance of the body are discussed. The pathomechanics and the findings of postural dynamics can, by and large, be applied to any other muscle disease.

Most major axial or appendicular musculature loses at least 30–40% of their original strength before clinical weakness manifests. Spurt muscles, such as the biceps brachii, tend to atrophy earlier in myopathy than shunt muscles, such as the brachioradialis. Muscles that get shortened due to contracture fatigue easily and frequently. The antigravity muscles are first targeted, e.g. psoas is more affected than the iliacus. As the weakness progresses, it leads to alteration in the maintenance of posture. As gravity is constantly acting upon the body, it inhibits the upright posture of the patient, due to contracture and fatigue of muscles. Muscles become vulnerable to deforming forces caused by postural or supportive stress due to loss of elasticity and contractibility. Trunk has 70% of the body weight. Due to girdle muscle weakness, the hips and the legs may not be able to bear the torso upon themselves, which leads to imbalance and instability.

Kinetic Analysis

This is very important for better clinical understanding. Assessment of biokinetics helps to deal with the patients in a better way. Though the weakness is symmetrical, the contractures are noticed more on the dominant side. Especially, tensor fasciae latae (TFL), hip flexors, triceps surae are more affected.

Some changes in joint lever systems occur. For instance, the hip is a first-class lever with force exerted by the abductors over the fulcrum of the articulated femoral head to balance body weight. As hip abductors weaken, hip hikers (quadratus lumborum) are called upon to elevate the hip during swing, thus creating a third-class lever, where power is sacrificed for a wider arc of movement. Hip adductors perform the knee extension as the quadriceps muscle goes for insufficiency.

Lumbar lordosis exaggerates secondary to weakness of hip extensors and this is accompanied by hip flexor contracture. Abdominal muscle weakness allows the pelvis to drop anteriorly, augmenting this deformity. The loss of power in the scapular stabilizers causes the shoulder to position forward thus contributing the lordotic posture. Due to this posture, the center of gravity (COG) is shifted posteriorly. They keep the hips abducted so as to widen the base of support and thereby line of gravity within it.

Clinical Assessment

Assessment starts with history taking. History taking is an art. During the early stage of disease evaluation, the parent or the caretaker may be the informant, and during later stages, the patient themselves can share the history of the onset of the disease. Careful history taking which includes the age of onset of the disease; progression of the symptoms; developmental age-appropriate milestones, such as head, neck, and trunk control; sitting; crawling; standing; and walking will help in diagnosing the myopathic disorder. Genetic history should be part of the assessment as it gives the clinician, information about the inheritance pattern of the disease.

Assessing a child suffering from any myopathic disorder on regular interval is essential in order to check the degree of severity. It should not be conducted in such a way that it upsets the child or the family members. The examination and the findings should not appear as if to confirm the increase in the disability level.

Range of Motion Assessment

Joint ROM, especially the lower limbs joints, should be tested periodically with the use of goniometer. Goniometer has shown to have high intratester reliability but variable intertester values. Due to contractures around the joint, the children with DMD and other muscle disorders develop joint range restriction. This may lead to restricted functional movements and the child gradually becomes wheelchair bound. Periodic joint range analysis helps in taking decision of whether to choose conservative management, such as stretching, augmented stretching, or to opt for surgical corrections, such as tenotomy. Achilles tenotomy is usually performed for keeping the joint stable or to prescribe shoes to maximize the mobility.

Muscle Strength Assessment

Though the Medical Research Council (MRC) Manual Muscle Testing (MMT) is the commonly used tool in the clinical setting, it is controversial, having poor inter, tester reliability, as it is purely a subjective examination. Considering the quickness in the method of assessment, MMT is still a clinical tool used by physiotherapists globally. A myometer in the form of hand-held dynamometer has been suggested as means of obtaining quantitative data on muscle force production, although there are some disadvantages such as lack of sensitivity to disease progression at some stages in the course of DMD, ALS, and Spinal Muscular Atrophy (SMA). An electronic strain gauge is reported as a measure of isometric force.

Group muscle testing in the form of break test is also considered to be helpful in assessing the progressive muscle weakness. Regular muscle charting helps to track the progress in muscle weakness and the degree of disability so that an adequate plan of care can be delivered to the patients to maintain the functional status.

Respiratory Function Tests

Respiratory complications that arise in these individuals are life threatening. Hence, it is very important to assess the respiratory functions, effectiveness of cough, and frequent auscultation.

Cardiac Assessment

As cardiac involvement is a frequent finding in various kinds of myopathies, risk assessment for the cardiac involvement is essential right from the early stage so that appropriate cardiac therapy can be given since management of these patients is influenced by the degree of cardiac involvement.

Functional Assessment

As the aim of the treatment protocol is always focused on improving the functional abilities of a child, viz. dressing and undressing, self-care activities, grooming, walking short distances, and climbing stairs up and down, functional assessment forms an integral and important area to be assessed in order to quantify the quality of life of individuals suffering from myopathic disorders.

Commonly Used Outcome Measurement Scales in Myopathic Disorders

Apart from the Brooke and Vignos scales mentioned in **Tables 32.1 and 32.2**, there are many simple, reproducible functional scales that can be used by the physiotherapists for measuring the prognosis and functional status of the patients. Few commonly used upper and lower limb scales are mentioned here for quick reference.

Lower Limb Function Tests

The below-mentioned tests are limited to ambulatory patients.

Timed Function Tests

Walk/run 10 m, to get up from the floor (supine-to-stand test), and to climb four stairs.

In the 10-m walk/run test, the patient is asked to either walk or run for 10 m, whichever they think is faster, while the time is recorded. In the climbing four stairs test, the patient is asked to climb four stairs either with/without the use of railings, while the time is recorded. In the supine-to-stand test, the patient is asked to get up from a lying down position on the floor and the time is recorded until he/she is standing upright with their hands at their sides. Qualitative grades ranging from 1 to 6 are used to assess each timed function test (TFT), with grade 1 being an inability to perform the test and grade 6 indicating an ability to perform the test without any compensatory movement. If the time taken to walk/run 10 m is >12 seconds or the time taken to climb four stairs is greater than 8 seconds, then the patient has a higher chance of losing ambulation within 12 months.

Upper Limb Function Tests

Upper limb functions are essential to carry out daily routine activities, such as brushing, dressing/undressing, bathing, and eating. In the disease course, it is noted that upper limb muscle functions are maintained for a period of time after a patient with myopathy loses his ambulation. The following scales will be of great help for the physiotherapists in their clinical practice.

Performance of Upper Limb

The performance of upper limb test is used to evaluate the function of upper limbs in the patients suffering from myopathy. This is a reliable and valid scale that can be used for both ambulatory and nonambulatory patients from the age of 5 and above. It has the ability to assess the extent and the severity of the disease. It consists of 22 items, divided into three level dimensions—shoulder, elbow, and wrist, which can help in tracking impairments in upper limb function. The scores can vary from 0 to 1 or from 0 to 6, depending upon the item being evaluated.

Jebsen Hand Function Test

Jebsen hand function test is a timed test, which can be used in evaluating hand function in patients with myopathy. In this test, the individual will be asked to perform seven tasks that include activities that are commonly used in daily living. The tasks include "writing a sentence, turning over cards, picking up small common objects, simulating eating, stacking checkers, moving large light objects, and moving large heavy objects," which are commonly used in the activities of daily living. However, it does not include tasks that measure the function of proximal muscles of the upper limb which are important for activities, such as bathing and grooming.

Microsoft Kinect Gaming

Microsoft Kinect gaming is a newly developed outcome measure for assessing upper limbs in DMD. It is a reliable and valid test that has the ability to evaluate upper limb impairment in both ambulatory and nonambulatory patients with DMD or BMD. Kinect gaming can be used to determine the reachable workspace or the functional reaching volume, the velocity of movement, and the fatigue rate while playing video games. However, the major disadvantages of this outcome measure are the cost and the complexity of the setup. The complexity of the setup makes it harder for physiotherapists and clinicians to easily use this tool in clinics for assessing upper limb function in the DMD population.

Functional Scales

The functional scales are used to determine the quality of movements. They are very easy to use in clinics by physiotherapists and give a quick assessment of the quality of movements of both upper and lower limbs. Below are some of the functional scales used in DMD.

North Star Ambulatory Assessment

The North Star Ambulatory Assessment (NSAA) is a relatively new scale, developed in Europe over the last decade to assess activity of daily livings (ADLs) in patients with myopathy. This clinical outcome measure contains 17 activities involving lower limbs, varying from easy tasks such as standing; to difficult tasks such as running a distance of 10 m. Each activity is scored from 0 to 2, with a score of 0 indicating an inability to perform the activity and a score of 2 indicating that the activity is performed normally, without any compensatory movement which sums up to the maximum score of 34. This scale has the disadvantage of being age dependent. It has been shown that NSAA scores tend to increase for DMD patients who are <7 years old and decrease for those who are of 7 years of age or will become older than that age within 1 year. Therefore this scale might not be useful for younger DMD patients.

Egen–Klassifikation Scale

The Egen-Klassifikation (EK) scale can be used for nonambulatory patients. This scale comprises 10 categories ranging from the use of a wheelchair to overall physical well-being. Each category is scored from 0 to 3 and the total score ranges from 0 to 30. A higher score indicates a lower functional level in a patient.

Muscular Dystrophy Functional Rating Scale

The muscular dystrophy functional rating scale (MDFRS) was developed to evaluate function in muscular dystrophy patients of age 6 years and above. This scale comprises 33 items which are further subdivided into the 4 domains of mobility, basic daily living activities, arm function, and impairment.

Barthel Index

The Barthel index (BI) is a reliable and valid scale that is used for determining function in personal care and mobility domains in muscular dystrophy patients. This scale consists of 10 items with the total score varying from 0 (inability to perform any activity) to 100 (ability to perform all activities without any assistance).

Bayley-III Scale of Infant and Toddler Development

Since there are delayed developmental milestones in DMD, neither 6 MWT nor NSAA is suitable for DMD patients under the age of four. Therefore the Bayley-III scale of infant and toddler development could be an appropriate alternative in very young patients with DMD. This scale evaluates cognitive function, language, and motor function skills. It is a reliable measure to evaluate development in infants and very young patients with DMD over a period of time.

PHYSICAL THERAPY MANAGEMENT

It is fairly understood that physiotherapy deals with treating the symptoms and associated problems and not the disease. The primary problems encountered by the patients with myopathy include the following:

- Weakness
- Decreased active and passive ROM
- Loss of ambulation
- Decreased functional ability
- Decreased cardiopulmonary function
- Emotional trauma—individual and family
- Progressive spinal deformity

The above are the gross findings, and the problems vary from child to child based on the severity. The sequence of managing the problems also differs as per the detailed assessment the physiotherapist does. Again here, for the sake of convenience, DMD is taken into consideration for discussion as the problems encountered by them, by and large, represent the myopathic diseases. The areas of concern while goal setting by a physiotherapist for the management are:

- Improve the muscle power, thereby compensating the progressive reduction of muscle mass.
- Prevent and manage cardiopulmonary complications time to time.
- Maintain the joint ROM.
- Prevent and manage contractures and deformity and correct postural alignment. Prolong the functional capacity and help to perform activities of daily living.
- Create barrier free, accessible physical environment to promote mobility.
- Counsel the individual and family members and strengthen the support system.

Physiotherapy in Early Stage

The primary goal of the physiotherapist is to educate the family members and in some cases, the patient themselves and teach them coping strategies. Further goals include:

- Prevention of contractures and deformity
- Maintain or improve muscle strength
- Maintenance of maximal functional capabilities
- Use of any adaptive devices
- Teach home management strategies
- Promote mobility
- Prevent increase in weight

Physiotherapy in Middle Stage

This stage is classified when the patient becomes nonambulant. The primary goals include the following:

- Continue the early stage PT program as and where applicable
- Care of spine to manage and/or to prevent further deformity
- Respiratory care to avoid pulmonary complications
- Teach transfers to patients and family members
- Teach proper positioning on bed/chair to prevent further contractures/deformity
- Adaptive devices to modify self-care activities.

Physiotherapy in Late Stage

Physiotherapy in the late stage is as follows:

- Continue all the above program wherever possible.
- Evaluate the fatigue level of the patient.
- Teach less energy consuming endurance exercises to promote activities.
- Maximize upper limb function.

Role of Physical Exercises

Exercises are the mainstay in keeping the patients fit in this condition. They help in multiple ways, viz. maintaining the muscle mass, strengthening the muscle groups, maintaining the length and tension, flexibility and further prevention of contractures, deformity, and increase in weight and promoting mobility and functional capability.

Strengthening Exercises

This can be achieved by performing the exercise in an optimal position, thereby gaining the mechanical advantage of the particular muscle that is being worked out. By using proper alignment, the muscle work can be maximized.

In the early stage, the patient remains functional and so the power of the muscles would be grade 3 and above. The patient might find difficulty in climbing stairs, getting up from the floor, and in maintaining upright posture. The following exercises would benefit the patient: bed mobility/mat exercises, such as rolling, bridging **(Fig. 32.8)**, quadruped **(Fig. 32.9)**, kneeling, kneel walking, spinal extension exercises **(Fig. 32.10)** and abdominal strengthening exercises **(Fig. 32.11)**. Exercises on the Swiss ball **(Fig. 32.12)** particularly for the strengthening of trunk muscles and abdominal muscles can/may be of great use.

Mat exercises such as side sitting facilitation **(Fig. 32.13)**, from either side lying or prone-kneeling can also be used. Kneeling position can also be trained intermediately on mat **(Fig. 32.14)**.

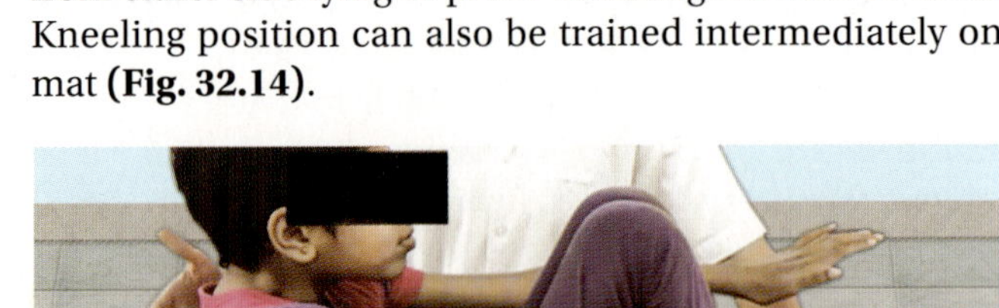

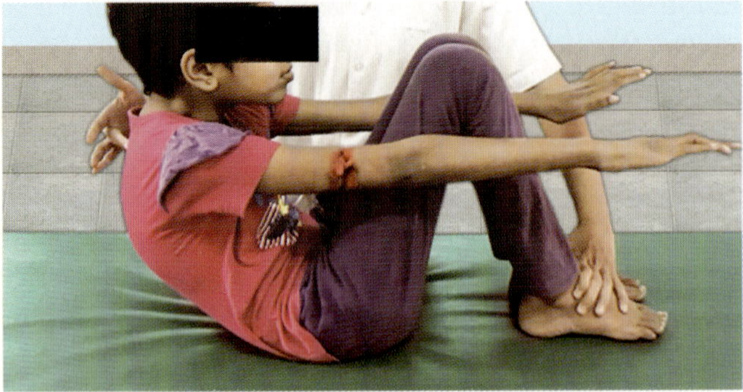

Fig. 32.11: Strengthening of abdominal muscle.

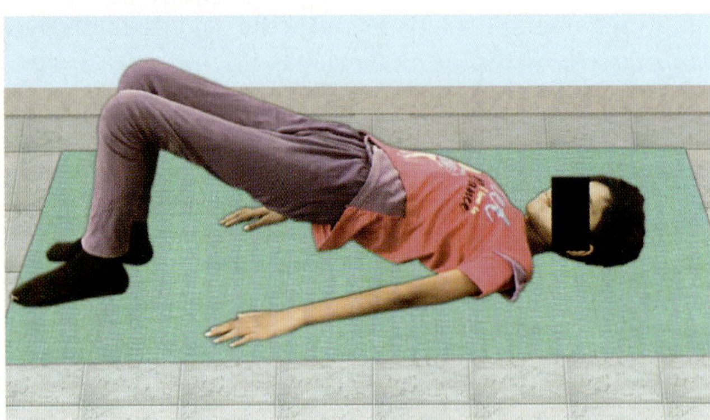

Fig. 32.8: Bridging exercise.

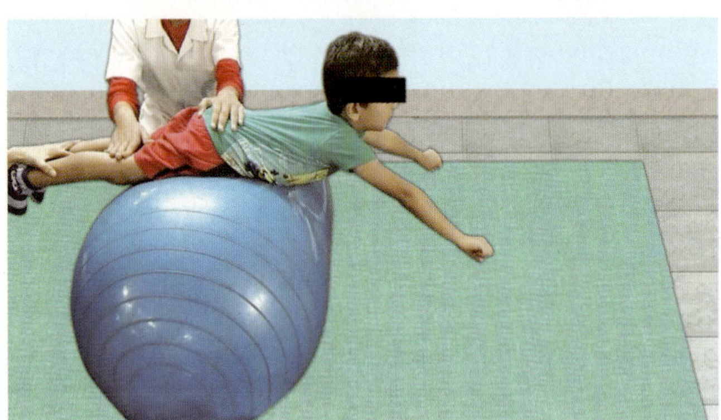

Fig. 32.12: Spinal extension on swiss ball.

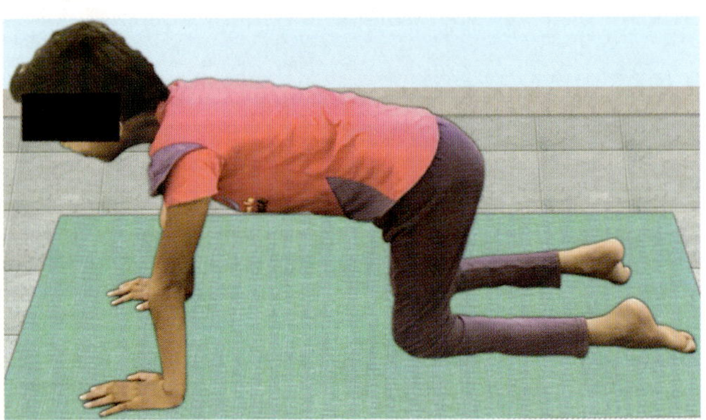

Fig. 32.9: Quadruped position.

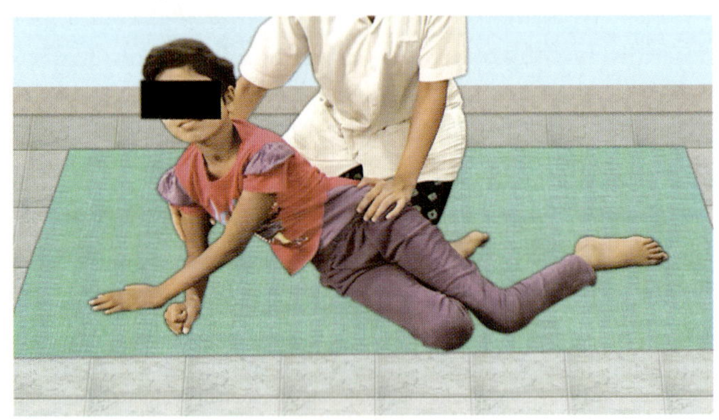

Fig. 32.13: Transitional sitting.

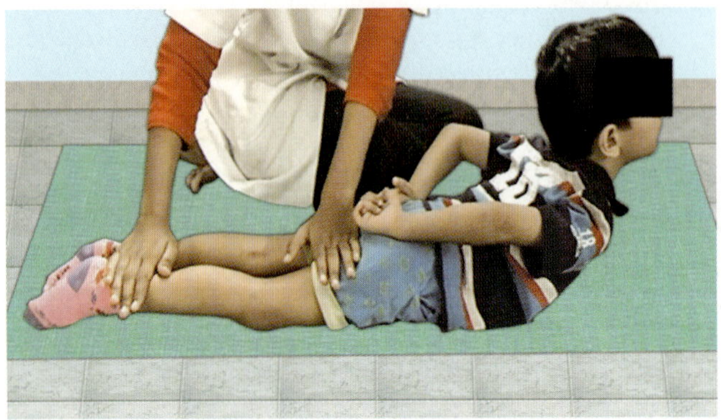

Fig. 32.10: Strengthening of back extensors.

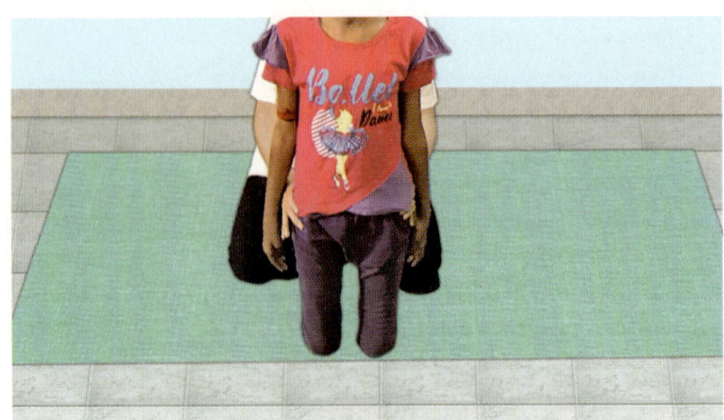

Fig. 32.14: Kneeling position.

Strength training can also be done with the use of weights, sandbags, and resistive springs. Care should be taken that the exercises should be in the graded form. In the later stage, endurance exercises should be carried out wherein patient will be made to do more repetitions of movement with less weight. Crutch muscle strengthening should be incorporated right from the beginning, anticipating the progressiveness in the muscle weakness leading to immobility.

If the muscle power drops down to < 3 or 2, suspension therapy can be initiated for strengthening the hip, knee, and trunk muscles. If the muscle grading progresses to 2 or 1, electrical stimulation can be an option to re-educate the muscle as well as to maintain the muscle properties. Passive movements should also be incorporated on a regular basis, and the caretaker should be instructed to perform passive movements of all the joints with adequate repetition at least twice a day. Cryotherapy in the form of excitatory cold on the affected muscles, proprioceptive neuromuscular facilitation (PNF), quick stretch, and muscle tapping also serves the purpose during the acute or the middle stage.

Prevent Contractures and Deformities

Traditional method of stretching still holds good to maintain the length and flexibility of the muscle **(Figs. 32.14 to 32.18)**. No studies are available upon which to base a passive stretching prescription, but the regimen often prescribed is between 10 and 30 repetitions, held

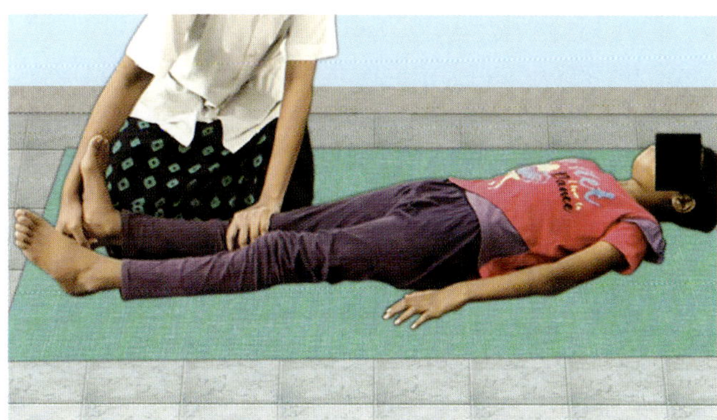

Fig. 32.17: Stretching of calf muscle.

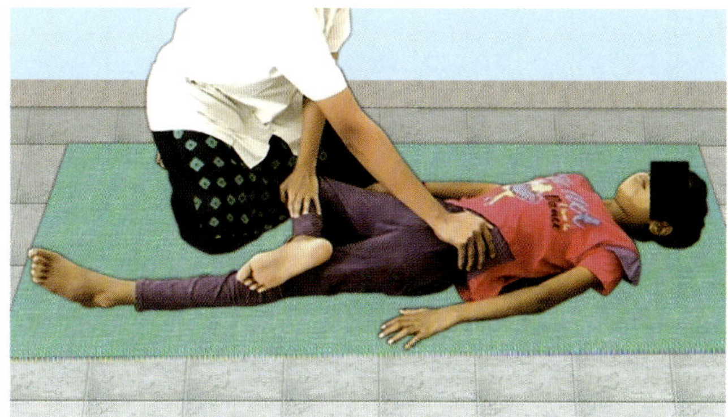

Fig. 32.18: Stretching of hip adductor muscle.

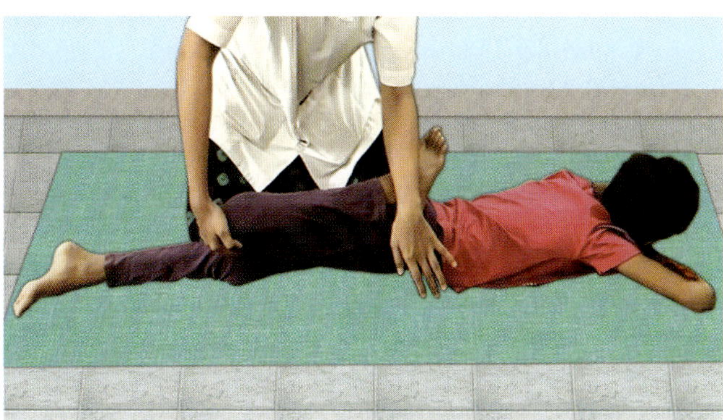

Fig. 32.15: Stretching of rectus femoris muscle.

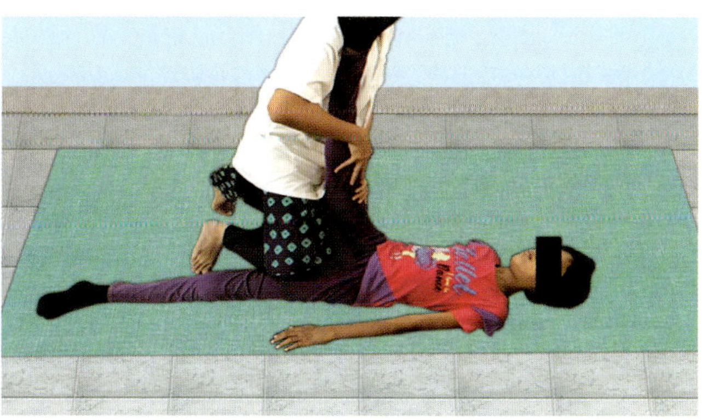

Fig. 32.16: Stretching of hamstring muscle.

for 5–10 seconds each, at least once a day or twice. The commonly affected muscles either due to weakness or static position are:

- Rectus femoris muscle
- Hip adductors
- Hamstrings
- Calves
- Achilles tendon
- Hip flexors
- The iliotibial band
- Foot evertors
- Paraspinal musculature

Since the lower limb muscles are more involved, missing the periodical check-up for ROM assessment will lead to early stage of nonambulation. Other techniques that can be included are:

- PNF contract relax
- Joint mobilization in the form of traction to all the joints
- Myofascial release technique

Moist heat can be given prior to these exercises in order to avoid pain during stretching.

Splinting the affected joints especially night splints in the stretched position maybe of great help. Serial casting is also one form of management for keeping the muscle in lengthened position. In some non-yielding cases to the conservative management, subcutaneous release of Achilles tendon and hamstring muscles and fasciotomy of iliotibial band are performed.

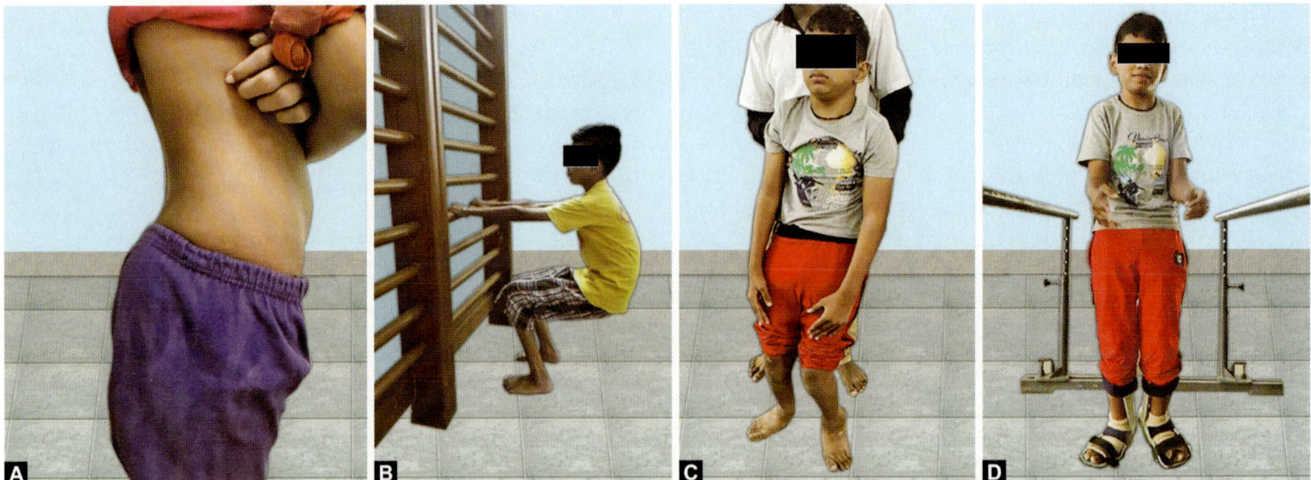

Figs. 32.19A to D: (A) In standing hyper-lordosis; (B) Squatting; (C) Standing; (D) Standing with AFO.

Promoting Ambulation

A patient with DMD alters his/her gait pattern to maintain the stability as the muscles progressively weaken. Decrease in stride length, speed, and cadence will be noticed. Due to gluteal muscle weakness, the child typically adopts waddling gait. Pronounced lordotic curvature leads to an abnormal posture while standing by shifting the center of gravity (COG) posterior to hip joint, and in order to maintain the stability, the child retracts the arm backward and further increases the lordosis **(Fig. 32.19A)**. Primarily, the iliofemoral ligament provides the stability passively. Mobility becomes impossible for the child even with mild knee flexion contracture at this stage. Exercises such as squatting **(Fig. 32.19B)** can be used to aid in functional transfers. Independent standing facilitation can also be incorporated before working on ambulation **(Fig. 32.19C)**.

Treatment protocol includes stretching of the tightened structures, lower extremity braces **(Fig. 32.19D)**, such as ankle–foot orthoses (AFO) and knee–ankle foot orthoses (KAFO). Push knee splint will help the child to stand and can reduce the rate of progression of contracture and can prolong the ambulation. Night splints to some extent also prevent the muscles getting tightened. Training on balance board improves proprioception **(Fig. 32.20A)**, helps in aligning the COG, and thereby promotes balance. Once when the child starts balancing, obstacle walking can be started which will improve the dynamic balance and as well help to meet the challenges while walking in real-life situations **(Fig. 32.20B)**.

Various surgical interventions including lengthening of Achilles tendon and Ober-Yount fasciotomies, tibialis posterior transpositions, and percutaneous tenotomies in combination with vigorous physiotherapy and orthotic intervention can have a lasting effect and is reported to improve and prolong ambulation. However, it is mandatory that postoperative physiotherapy aimed at making the patient stand up and ambulate is highly recommended, whatever the surgical procedures the patient undergoes. There should be a minimum of 3–5

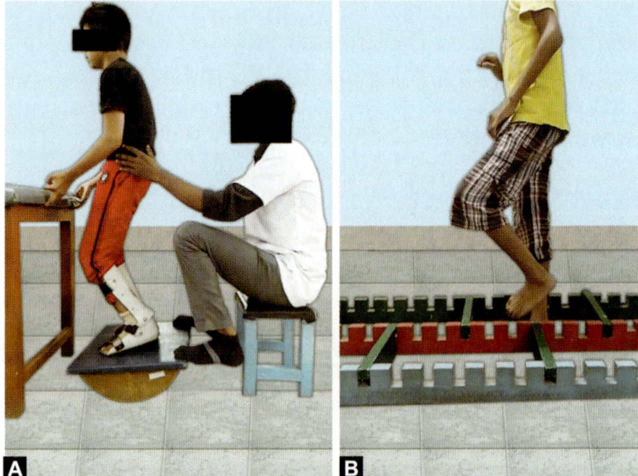

Figs. 32.20A and B: (A) Balance training on balance board; (B) Obstacle walking.

hours of standing, and ambulatory training is essential for the program to be successful. The ROM exercises along with active stretching should be incorporated after the surgical release techniques.

Use of Wheelchair

Wheelchairs are essential forms of transport for persons with muscular dystrophy when they reach the nonambulatory stage. This will help them to participate in routine day-to-day life when they have ambulatory issues. Various kinds of wheelchairs are available for mobility purpose at different stages of disease. Appropriate assessment and identifying the need of the patient are the key to prescribe the right model for the patient. The therapist should recommend adequate postural support and other pressure relieving accessories while making the patient use the wheelchair.

The therapists will have to train the patient and the caretaker as well, about the use of wheelchair in their routine life. They should also teach them the transfer techniques with the use of transfer boards, hoists and slings, sliding sheets, and handling belts. This will help the patient, therapist, and the caretaker to avoid unnecessary strain and injuries while handling.

Respiratory Management

Due to the involvement of respiratory muscles, the respiratory functions are highly compromised. Further due to the spinal deformities that the child suffers, function gets deteriorated still further and many a times becomes the cause for death. Hence, respiratory management has to be incorporated right from the early stage of muscle disease. The main focus will be to:

- Improve and maintain the thoracic wall mobility
- Improve and maintain the strength and the endurance of respiratory muscles
- Maintain or establish proper breathing pattern.

The interventions can be in the form of breathing exercises, viz. diaphragmatic and segmental exercises. The same can be done with minimal to maximal resistance in order to improve the respiratory muscle power. Inspiratory muscle training will help the patient to maintain the respiratory capacity. Devices, such as incentive spirometer can be regularly used by the patient. Proprioceptive neuromuscular facilitation can be incorporated along with breathing that helps in thoracic wall mobility and as well to ventilate the lungs adequately. During the early stage of the disease, swimming should be advised as it will help in improving the endurance and breathing patterns.

The child should be taught to cough and huff effectively that will maintain the bronchial hygiene in the long run. Postural drainage should be done and can be taught to the patients/caretaker lobe-wise which will help in removing the lung secretions. In addition to this, chest manipulative techniques, such as percussion, shaking, and vibration can be performed at regular intervals, if secretions are present in the lobes of the lung. Therapeutic vibrator will be of great help to mobilize thick sputum.

During the later stage of the disease, nocturnal or daytime intermittent positive pressure ventilator (IPPV) can be used as and when required. Oxygen support can be provided when indicated. Suctioning should be done when patients lose the muscle endurance to cough effectively.

Aerobic exercise combined with a supervised submaximal strength training program is considered safe. Low-impact aerobic exercise (swimming, stationary bicycling) improves cardiovascular performance, increases muscle efficiency, and lessens fatigue in certain types of dystrophies. However, it is important to counsel patients with muscular dystrophy to hydrate adequately, not to exercise to exhaustion, and to avoid supramaximal, high-intensity exercise. Educating patients with muscular dystrophy who are participating in an exercise program about the warning signs of overwork weakness and myoglobinuria is critical. It includes feeling weaker rather than stronger within 30 minutes after exercise, excessive muscle soreness 24–48 hours following exercise, severe muscle cramping, heaviness in the extremities, and prolonged shortness of breath.

Obesity Management

The children with muscular dystrophy are prone to put on weight due to lack of mobility. Hence weight management also forms an important aspect while treating these children. Regular exercise and physical activity, such as self-care tasks, involving them in some sort of sports in the beginning stage of the disease, would help the child to check putting on more weight. The steroids intake as part of the treatment protocol can also produce weight gain by means of fluid retention, increasing appetite, and body fat redistribution. Hence, introducing a strict diet regimen and restriction on binge/snack eating would help in controlling the weight gain.

Edwards and associates have demonstrated that controlled weight reduction in obese children with DMD is a safe and practical way to improve mobility and self-esteem. However, as the saying goes "Prevention is better than cure," preventing excessive weight gain in a child who is ambulatory is easier as compared to reducing the excessive weight in an obese child who is nonambulatory. For unsuccessful cases, use of hydraulic lift becomes important. Family members should be trained in using this device to handle the patient safe.

Managing ADLs

The child's ability to perform the daily routine activities, such as feeding self, bathing, personal hygiene, and turning the pages of the book should be assessed periodically. If deterioration is noticed, it should be addressed adequately so as to avoid dependency. Occupational therapy will also be helpful to address such issues. If needed, home visits may be arranged in identifying any architectural barriers and need for any adaptive equipment.

Managing Sleep

Due to deterioration of disease, patient in the chronic stage becomes confined to bed. The child will find difficulty in positioning in the bed as well as taking turns. This will lead to pressure ulcers at the vulnerable points. Provision of air or water beds will provide relief from this issue and also to family members who otherwise have to be up every 2–3 hours in the night to change the position of the child. Provision of hospital beds in the later stage will help in adjusting the heights while transfers. These beds will also help in keeping the head end elevated during the time the child suffers respiratory distress that can occur during sleep.

Addressing Psychosocial Issues

The mental and social stress faced by families and caregivers of children suffering from myopathy are tremendous. The difficulties that are faced by the caregivers are commonly referred to as "family burden" and are classified as psychological and social burdens. The psychological burdens are the ones that describe the reactions that family members experience, e.g., feeling of loss, sadness, tension, and feeling unable to cope with the situation. Whereas the social burdens describe the issues related to isolation, problems performing leisure and work activities strain in the family relationships and financial difficulties.

To address this need, coordinators form the bridge between the family and the medical consultants who deal with the child. Routine mental health screening is to be done at frequent intervals. This can be done by using standardized questionnaires. An appropriate tool for pediatric patients is the Strengths and Difficulties Questionnaire. This questionnaire is available in multiple languages. For adult patients, the Patient Health Questionnaire is recommended (Patient Health Questionnaire-9 for depression and Generalized Anxiety Disorder-7 for anxiety). For parents of patients aged 5–17 years, the Personal Adjustment and Role Skills Scale is recommended. The screening can be done by any health-care provider including the care coordinator. If screening is positive, a referral should be made to a psychologist and psychiatrist for further assessment or treatment. The emotional adjustment of the family members should be carefully monitored and intervention should be provided at appropriate times. Siblings of the child with myopathy should be provided with opportunities to establish connection with siblings of other children with myopathy which can be of great help in providing mental support. Informal counseling is of great help in enriching the life of the children with myopathy and their families to live rich, fulfilling lives. Standard, evidence-based practices should be used for those who need more formal mental health treatment.

Facilitating Family Support

Diseases, such as myopathy affect not only the child but also all members of the family. The quality of life of the child directly depends on the family support system. Hence, it is very important to address this need. As the disease is progressive in nature, the physiotherapists are of great help in treating, motivating, and counseling the patient and their family members. The parents/caretakers should be involved from the early stage.

Though not psychotherapists, as physiotherapy is the mainstay in the treatment, the physiotherapists share a strong bondage with the patients and their relatives. They can educate them and can be a pillar of support in keeping up the spirit and resilience to fight against the disease during the course of time. Home program can be taught to the family members and can be executed at frequent intervals during the day.

The physiotherapist should assess the social situation of the family during the visits. Apart from the therapy, a simple gesture of talking to the child and the parents for a few minutes showing positivity is as important as preventing any secondary complications of the disease.

Managing Pain

The child will experience pain around the joints where the ROM is restricted due to contractures. This can overall be prevented if the aforementioned goals are achieved. However, if pain is a chief complaint, hot/cold compress, sometimes electromodalities, such as infrared (IR), TENS, or interferential currents help in alleviating the pain. Proper positioning and by keeping the muscle in adequate length many times do the magic.

SUMMARY

As there are no standalone medicines for curing the disease, physiotherapy is the mainstay in preventing and managing the symptoms and complications. The quality of life of the patient can be very well achieved by physiotherapy. Proper timely assessment, appropriate goal setting at different stages of the disease, and adequate treatment program that aims at maintaining the functional capacity of the individual and prevents secondary complications are very essential. The treatment program is deemed successful when it promotes additional years of independent ambulation, improved resilience, capacity to undertake ADLs, self-sufficiency, and community participation. Physiotherapists, apart from providing the routine physical care, should play an important role as an educator, counselor, motivator, facilitator, and pillar of moral support to the patient and the family members in achieving the desired results.

Case Scenario

CASE STUDY

A 9-year-old boy presented to the department with difficulty in walking. His parents gave a medical history of repeated falls, fatigue, and muscle weakness with difficulty in climbing stairs. He also had decreased strength and endurance. His parents did not have a consanguineous marriage and have one daughter who is healthy. No other members of the family were similarly affected. His intelligence quotient was claimed to be in the normal range.

On examination: He had difficulty getting onto the examination table. The boy had an obese appearance, proximal weakness of pectoral and pelvic girdle muscles, calf hypertrophy, hamstring muscle contracture, and positive Gower's sign (a sequence of maneuvers for rising from the floor). He had hyperlordotic spine at the lumbar level. He walked with waddling gait and had tight heel cords. There was no thinning and twitching of muscles. Muscle tone and cranial nerve examination were also found to be normal.

Investigations: The patient was asked for serological, electromyogram (EMG), and nerve conduction study (NCS) investigations. His serum creatine kinase and aldolase levels were 50-fold higher than normal. Motor nerve conduction studies revealed low amplitude CMAPs throughout, with normal conduction velocities. EMG showed myopathic pattern in the right vastus lateralis suggestive of primary muscle disease. The boy was advised to consult a pediatrician regarding his general and physical health status. He was counseled to undergo daily physiotherapy, steroid therapy, and regular assessment for progressive muscle and cardiac/respiratory damage.

Guiding Questions:

1. What are the classical features of DMD?
2. What is the normal range for serum CPK?
3. How is the EMG and NCS pattern seen in myopathy?
4. What is the role of splinting?
5. What is the role of physiotherapy in acute stage and in chronic stage?

Review Questions

1. Classify myopathic disorders.
2. Discuss the etiopathological model of myopathy.
3. Compare and contrast DMD with BMD.
4. Enumerate the clinical features of congenital myopathies.
5. List down the investigatory procedures commonly used to diagnose muscle disease.
6. What are the EMG findings in myotonic dystrophy?
7. Explain the physiotherapy assessment for a case of DMD.
8. List down the short- and long-term goals in the management of DMD.
9. Mention the various scales used to measure the outcomes in case of myopathic disorders.
10. Describe the role of physiotherapy in rehabilitating a 9-year-old wheelchair-bound child suffering from DMD.

BIBLIOGRAPHY

1. Archibald DC, Vignos PJ Jr. A study of contractures in muscular dystrophy. Arch Phys Med Rehabil. 1959;40:150-7.
2. Brooke MH, Fenichel G, Griggs R, et al. Clinical investigations in Duchenne dystrophy. Part 2. Determination of the 'power' of therapeutic trials based on the natural history. Muscle Nerve. 1983;6:91-103.
3. Brussock CM, Haley SM, Musat TL, et al. Measurement of isometric force in children with and without Duchenne muscular dystrophy. Phys Ther. 1992;72:105-14.
4. Bushby K, Connor E. Clinical outcome measures for trials in Duchenne muscular dystrophy: report from International Working Group meetings. Clin Investig (Lond). 2011;1:1217-35.
5. Bushby K, Muntoni F, Urtizberea A, et al. Report on the 124th ENMC International Workshop. Treatment of Duchenne muscular dystrophy; defining the gold standards of management in the use of corticosteroids, The Netherlands. Neuromuscul Disord. 2004;14:526-34.
6. Connolly AM, Florence JM, Cradock MM, et al. One year outcome of boys with Duchenne muscular dystrophy using the Bayley-III scales of infant and toddler development. Pediatr Neurol. 2014;50:557-63.
7. Connolly AM, Malkus EC, Mendell JR, et al. Outcome reliability in non-ambulatory boys/men with Duchenne muscular dystrophy. Muscle Nerve. 2015;51:522-32.
8. Delisa JA, Gans BM, Walsh NE, et al. Physical medicine and rehabilitation principles and practice, vol. q, 4th edition. Philadelphia, PA: Lippincott Williams & Wilkins; 2005. pp. 915-21.
9. Edwards RHT, Hyde S. Methods of measuring muscle strength and fatigue. Physiotherapy. 1977;63(2):52-5.
10. Edwards RHT. Weight reduction in boys with muscular dystrophy. Dev Med Child Neurol. 1984;26:384-90.
11. Emery AE. Population frequencies of inherited neuromuscular diseases: a world survey. Neuromuscul Disord. 1991;1:19-29.
12. Florence JM, Pandya S, King W, et al. Clinical trial in muscular dystrophy. Standardization and reliability of evaluation procedures. Phys Ther. 1984;64:41-5.
13. Han JJ, de Bie E, Nicorici A, et al. Reachable workspace and performance of upper limb (PUL) in Duchenne muscular dystrophy. Muscle Nerve. 2016;53:545-54.
14. Han JJ, Kurillo G, Abresch RT, et al. Upper extremity 3-dimensional reachable workspace analysis in dystrophinopathy using Kinect. Muscle Nerve. 2015;52:344-55.
15. Heckmatt JZ, Dubowitz V, Hyde SA, et al. Prolongation of walking in Duchenne muscular dystrophy with lightweight orthoses. Review of 57 cases. Dev Med Child Neurol. 2015;27:149-54.
16. Jacob VC, Biju H, Sharma A. Neuro-rehabilitation: a multidisciplinary approach. Mumbai: NeuroGen, Brain and Spine Institute; 2012.
17. Jebsen RH, Taylor N, Trieschmann RB, et al. An objective and standardized test of hand function. Arch Phys Med Rehabil. 1969;50:311-9.
18. Kley R, Tarnopolsky M, Vorgerd M. Creatine for treating muscle disorders. Cochrane Database Syst Rev. 2013;(6).
19. Kliegman RM, Behrman R, Jenson H, et al. Nelson textbook of paediatrics. Philadelphia, PA: Saunders Elsevier; 2007. Chap 608.

20. Lowes LP, Alfano LN, Yetter BA, et al. Proof of concept of the ability of the Kinect to quantify upper extremity function in dystrophinopathy. PLoS Curr. 2013, Available from doi: 10.1371/currents.md. 9ab5d872bbb944c6035c9f9bfd314ee2.

21. Lue YJ, Lin RF, Chen SS, et al. Measurement of the functional status of patients with different types of muscular dystrophy. Kaohsiung J Med Sci. 2009;25:325-33.

22. Mayhew A, Mazzone ES, Eagle M, et al. Development of the performance of the upper limb module for Duchenne muscular dystrophy. Dev Med Child Neurol. 2013;55:1038-45.

23. Mazzone ES, Messina S, Vasco G, et al. Reliability of the North Star Ambulatory Assessment in a multicentric setting. Neuromuscul Disord. 2009;19:458-61.

24. McDonald CM, Abresch RT, Carter GT, et al. Profiles of neuromuscular diseases: Becker's muscular dystrophy. Am J Phys Med Rehabil. 1995;74:S93-103.

25. Medical Research Council of the United Kingdom. Aids to examination of the peripheral nervous system. In: Memorandum no. 45. Palo Alto, CA: Pendragon House; 1978.

26. Mumenthaler M, Mattle H, Taub E. Neurology. Georg Thieme Verlag, Stuttgart, Germany; 2004, 873, 902.

27. Olsen D, Orngreen M, Vissing J. Aerobic training improves exercise performance in facioscapulohumeral muscular dystrophy. Neurology. 2005;64(6): 1064-66.

28. Pandya S, Florence JM, King W, et al. Reliability of goniometric measurements in patients with Duchenne muscular dystrophy. Phys Ther. 1985;65:1339-42.

29. Pane M, Mazzone ES, Fanelli L, et al. Reliability of the performance of upper limb assessment in Duchenne muscular dystrophy. Neuromuscul Disord. 2014;24:201-6.

30. Roy L, Gibson DA. Pseudohypertrophic muscular dystrophy and its surgical management: review of 30 patients. Can J Surg. 1970;13:13-20.

31. Sharma A, Badhe P, Chandran NG, et al. Stem cell therapy and other recent advances in muscular dystrophy. Mumbai: NeuroGen Brain and Spine Institute; 2011.

32. Siegel IM. Management of musculoskeletal complications in neuromuscular disease. Enhancing mobility and the role of bracing and surgery. In: Fowler WM Jr (Ed). Advances in the rehabilitation of neuromuscular diseases: state of the art reviews, vol. 4. Philadelphia, PA: Hanley & Belfus; 1988. pp. 553-75.

33. Spencer GE. Orthopaedic care of progressive muscular dystrophy. J Bone Joint Surg (Am). 1967;49:1201-04.

34. Steare SE, Benatar A, Dubowitz V. Subclinical cardiomyopathy in Becker muscular dystrophy. Br Heart J. 1992;68:304-8.

35. Steffensen B, Hyde S, Lyager S, et al. Validity of the EK scale: a functional assessment of non-ambulatory individuals with Duchenne muscular dystrophy or spinal muscular atrophy. Physiother Res Int. 2001;6(3):119-34.

36. Stuberg WA, Metcalf WK. Reliability of quantitative muscle testing in healthy children with DMD using Hand Held Dynamometer. Phys. Ther. 1988;68:977-82.

37. Tecklin JS. Paediatric physical therapy. Philadelphia, PA: JB Lippincott Company; 1994.

38. Vignos PJ, Spencer GE, Archibald KC. Management of progressive muscular dystrophy of childhood. JAMA. 1963;184;89-96.

39. Vignos PJ. Management of musculoskeletal complications in neuromuscular disease: Limb contractures and the role of stretching, braces and surgery. In: Fowler WM Jr (Ed). Advances in the rehabilitation of neuromuscular diseases: state of the art reviews, vol. 4. Philadelphia, PA: Hanley & Belfus; 1988. pp. 509-36.

40. Yamamoto S, Matsushima H, Suzuki A, et al. A comparative study of thallium—201 single photon emission computed tomography and electrocardiography in Duchenne and other types of muscular dystrophy. Am J Cardiol. 1988;61:836-43.

41. Ziter FA, Allsop KG. The value of orthoses for patients with Duchenne muscular dystrophy. Phys Ther. 1979;59:1361-5.

Peripheral Neuropathies

Shivani Verma, Megha S Sheth, Srishti S Sharma

Ⓛ EARNING OBJECTIVES

After reading this chapter, the readers should be able to:
- Understand polyneuropathy and its various types
- Describe the epidemiology and clinical manifestations, and diagnosis of Guillain-Barré syndrome along with its clinical variants
- Describe diabetic peripheral neuropathy and it's classification along with clinical manifestations and medical management
- Describe chemotherapy-induced polyneuropathy, it's clinical manifestations, diagnosis, and medical management
- Describe alcohol-induced polyneuropathy and it's diagnosis along with clinical manifestations
- Describe HIV-associated polyneuropathy and it's clinical features
- Determine the psychosocial aspects of polyneuropathy
- Describe the assessment of polyneuropathy
- Describe the medical, physiotherapy, and alternative management in the course of polyneuropathy.
- Discuss the role of physiotherapy in management of polyneuropathy.

CHAPTER OUTLINE

- Epidemiology
- Classification of polyneuropathy
  - Based on etiology
  - Based on clinical pattern of presentation and duration of presentation
  - Based on pathology
- Immune-mediated neuropathies
  - Guillain–Barre syndrome
- Chronic inflammatory polyradiculoneuropathy
  - Charcot–Marie–Tooth
  - Paranodopathies

- Diabetic neuropathy
- Autonomic impairments
- Chemotherapy-induced neuropathy
  - Clinical features
  - Diagnosis
  - Medical management
- Other toxic neuropathies
  - Alcohol-induced polyneuropathy
  - Nutritional neuropathy
  - Overdose neuropathy
- Human immunodeficiency virus-related neuropathy
  - Clinical features

- Psychosocial aspects of polyneuropathy
- Assessment
- Examination
- Investigations
  - Electrodiagnostic testing
- Management
  - General medical management
  - Physiotherapy management
  - Alternative management

INTRODUCTION

Peripheral nerves are made up of motor, sensory, and autonomic elements. Peripheral neuropathies can impair sensory, motor or autonomic function, either alone or in combination. Polyneuropathy (PN) occurs when several nerves in different parts of the body are affected at the same time, whereas in mononeuropathy, only one nerve is affected. In simple terms, PN is said to be damage of multiple peripheral nerves, it is also commonly called peripheral neuropathy. PN is defined as a generalized pathological process involving primary degeneration of parenchyma of multiple peripheral nerves. PNs are a major cause of neurological disabilities, and as per National Institute of Neurological Disorders and Stroke, approximately 20 million people in the United States have some form of peripheral neuropathy, and most of them have PN.

EPIDEMIOLOGY

Epidemiological studies from India from various regions show the overall prevalence of PN varied from 5 to 2,400 per 10,000 population in various community studies. The prevalence of Guillain-Barré syndrome (GBS) increases linearly with age, and men are about 1.5 times more affected than women. Diabetes mellitus (DM) is a common cause of neuropathy worldwide. Prevalence of PN in diabetic patients ranges from around 10.5 to 32.2% in various studies across India. Most PNs are chronic and usually develop over several months.

CLASSIFICATION OF POLYNEUROPATHY

PNs may be classified in different ways, based on etiology, pathology, clinical presentation, location of lesion, and time since injury. **Table 33.1** summarizes the types of PN briefly.

Based on Etiology

The causes of PN can be divided into hereditary and acquired and comprise the following:

- **Hereditary** causes are inherited in nature and consist of hereditary peripheral neuropathies, including hereditary motor and sensory neuropathies, Charcot-Marie-Tooth (CMT) disease, Dejerine-Sottas disease, Refsum's disease, and pressure-sensitive hereditary neuropathy (i.e. with liability to pressure palsy).
- **Acquired** causes are usually secondary to a primary medical condition and contracted during course of adult life. They may consist of those due to endocrine pathologies such as DM, thyroid; metabolic disease, collagen-vascular neuropathy; due to alcohol abuse; nutritional deficiency such as vitamin B_{12} deficiency and those due to variety of toxins.

The other classification is based on primary condition, which leads to PN as a complication, which are:

1. **Endocrine-related neuropathy:** Diabetic neuropathy (DN) is the most commonly seen PN. It is estimated that 60–70% of diabetics have diabetic PN (DPN). Hypothyroidism commonly predisposes patients to entrapment neuropathies, such as carpal tunnel syndrome, but rarely it can cause generalized sensory neuropathy, characterized by painful paresthesia and numbness in distal limbs. Parathyroid disorders can also induce pathologies of peripheral nerve axon.

2. **Infection-associated neuropathies:** Human immunodeficiency virus (HIV) or AIDS are often accompanied by the development of peripheral neuropathic conditions. Of all HIV/AIDS patients, 33% have PN. Diphteritic neuropathy is also an infection-associated neuropathy.

3. **Chemotherapy-induced peripheral neuropathy (CIPN):** Around 30–40% of all cancer patients have CIPN. CIPN is caused by chemotherapy drugs used in cancer treatments. Chemotherapy is hardest on the nervous system due to the fact the nerve cells are more sensitive than other cells. Sensory nerves are at an increased risk to chemotherapy-associated damage compared to motor nerves.

4. **Toxic neuropathy:** Numerous drugs and environmental toxins are capable of causing PN.

5. **Immune-mediated neuropathy:** GBS is the most common example of this type.

6. **Uremic neuropathy** refers to neuropathy that is associated with renal failure. Approximately 60% of patients with chronic renal failure develop distal symmetrical sensory-motor neuropathy (DSPN).

7. **Chronic liver disease** is another cause of neuropathy. DSPN and autonomic neuropathy are both common in patients with liver disease.

8. **Nutritional neuropathies:** Due to B_1, thiamine (beriberi or pellagra), riboflavin (B_2), pyridoxine (B_6), B_{12} (pernicious anemia), and protein or calorie deficiency. They are commonly seen in patients with inflammatory bowel disease, fat malabsorption, chronic liver disease, pancreatic disease, gastritis, and small bowel resections. Neuropathies associated with gastric surgeries are also often included in this. Alcoholic neuropathy is also considered in nutritional or beriberi or vitamin B-deficiency neuropathy.

Based on Clinical Pattern of Presentation and Duration of Presentation

On the basis of clinical pattern and duration of presentation, three main patterns of PN can be distinguished:

1. **Chronic symmetrical peripheral neuropathy:** The largest group of PNs, they develop gradually over time and affect nerves throughout the body.

2. **Acute symmetrical peripheral neuropathy:** Rare but severe, rapidly developing form of PN affects nerves throughout the body and is most often seen in GBS, an autoimmune disorder that attacks the peripheral nervous system and can be fatal.

3. **Multiple mononeuropathy:** Involving damage to at least two distinct nerve areas, this form of PN can result from vasculitis (inflammation of the blood vessels), sarcoidosis, and some forms of cancer. In this both peripheral and cranial nerves are affected.

Table 33.1: Classification of polyneuropathy.

Based on etiology	Hereditary Acquired Endocrine related Infection associated Chemotherapy induced Toxic neuropathy Immune mediated Uremic neuropathy Chronic liver disease Nutritional neuropathies
Based on clinical presentation and duration of symptoms	Chronic symmetrical peripheral neuropathy Acute symmetrical peripheral neuropathy Multiple mononeuropathy
Based on pathology	Axonal Demyelinating

Based on Pathology

This classification is based on which part of the nerve cell is affected mainly: the axon, the myelin sheath or the cell body **(Fig. 33.1)**. **Figure 33.2** shows the broad approach to diagnosis of type of polyneuropathy.

1. **Axonal neuropathy**: Axonal neuropathy is a neurological disorder that involves degeneration. The axonal type of neuropathy can be further classified as acute motor axonal neuropathy (AMAN) and acute motor and sensory axonal neuropathy (AMSAN).
2. **Demyelinating neuropathy**: In this type of PN degeneration of myelin (fatty layer of insulating substance), surrounding axons of neurons occurs. It is believed that if demyelinating diseases are not treated in time, then they will eventually damage the axons too.

IMMUNE-MEDIATED NEUROPATHIES

Guillain-Barré Syndrome

It can be defined as an acute inflammatory demyelinating disease of the peripheral nerves. It is a generalized, usually symmetrical disorder, which tends to affect motor nerves predominantly; sensory system and autonomic manifestations are rarely seen. It may involve facial and other cranial nerves. In China and Japan, axonal variants, either AMAN or AMSAN, are commonly seen.

Etiology

According to the Centers for Disease Control and Prevention (CDC), about two-thirds of people with Guillain-Barré develop it soon after they have been sick with respiratory infection or diarrhea (particularly *Campylobacter jejuni*). Campylobacter is often found in undercooked food, especially poultry. Recent reports have shown that some other infections have also been found to be associated with Guillain-Barré. These are:

- Influenza
- Cytomegalovirus (CMV), which is a strain of the herpes virus

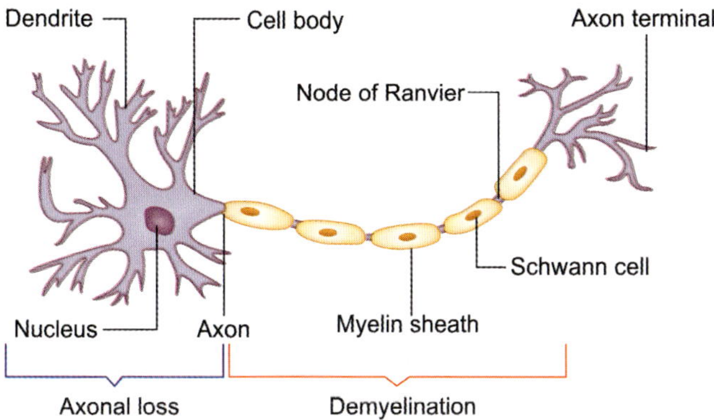

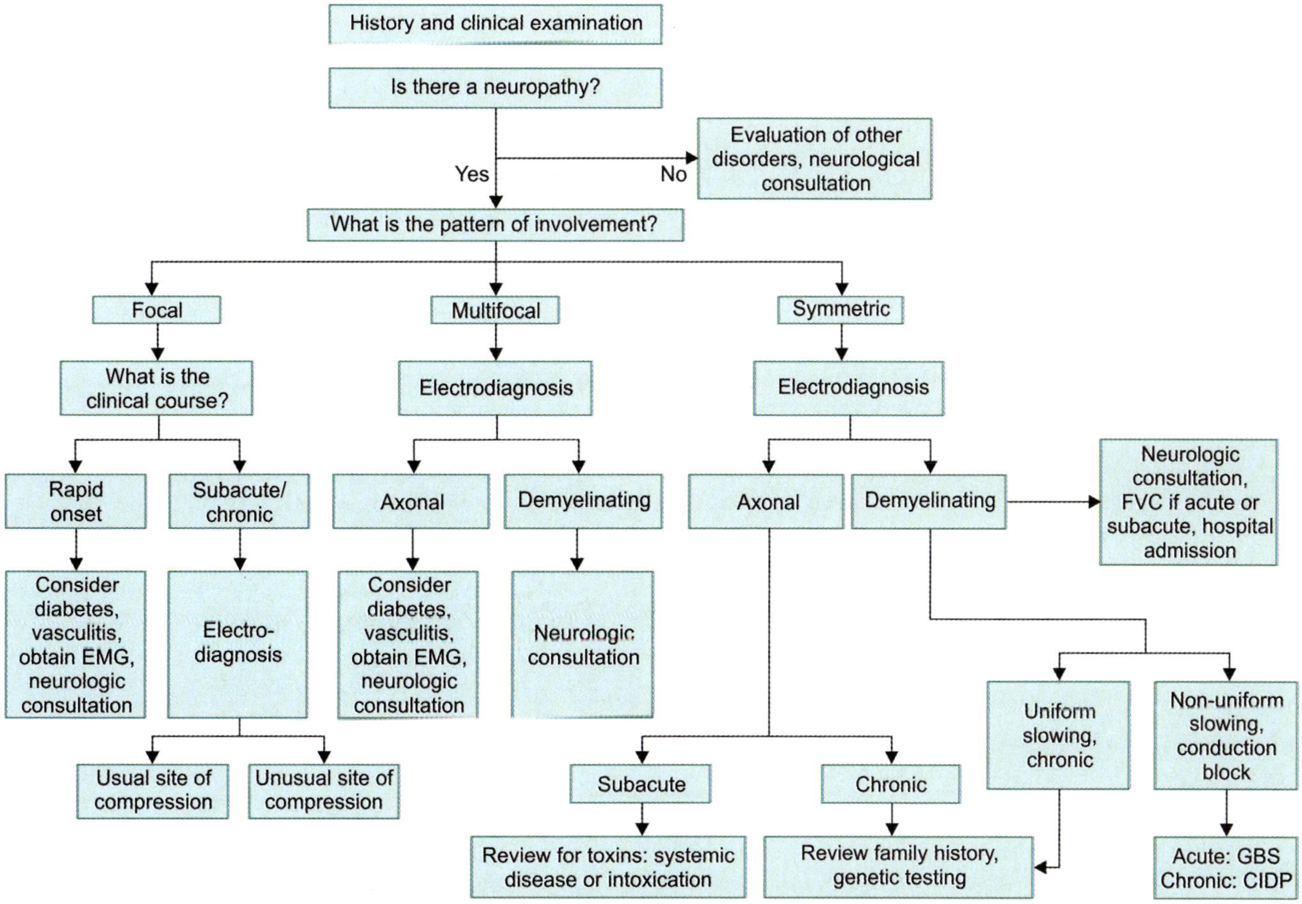

Fig. 33.1: Affection of the part of neuron in axonal and demyelinating neuropathy.

Fig. 33.2: Approach to evaluation of polyneuropathy.
(GBS: Gullain-Barré syndrome; CIDP: chronic inflammatory demyelinating polyneuropathy; FVC: forced vital capacity; EMG: Electromyography)

- Epstein-Barr virus infection or mononucleosis
- Mycoplasma pneumonia, which is an atypical pneumonia caused by bacteria-like organisms.
- HIV or AIDS

Pathophysiology

The pathophysiology of GBS is complex. GBS is considered to be an autoimmune disease triggered by a preceding bacterial or viral infection.

- In the AMAN form of GBS, the infecting organisms probably share homologous epitopes to a component of the peripheral nerves (molecular mimicry) and, therefore, the immune responses cross-react with the nerves causing axonal degeneration.
- In the AMSAN form, pathology is similar to AMAN, but it also affects sensory nerves and roots; axonal damage is usually severe.
- In the acute inflammatory demyelinating PN form, immune system reactions against target epitopes in Schwann cells or myelin result in demyelination.

Clinical Features

The most common symptoms reported before onset of GBS are fever, cough, sore throat, and other upper respiratory symptoms. Gastrointestinal symptoms may be more likely to precede the acute motor or motor–sensory axonal neuropathy subtypes that are related to slower recovery and higher risk of residual disability **(Box 33.1)**.

Impairments

Motor Impairments

Motor impairments can be described as follows:

- Muscle weakness is the most common motor impairment, which is seen in all patients of GBS. This muscle weakness is characteristically symmetrical and usually involves the lower limbs first.
- The most common motor manifestation of GBS is proximal limb muscle weakness, which usually rapidly ascends from lower limb to upper limb muscles and gradually affects the distal muscle groups. Weakness is always bilateral, although some asymmetry in onset and severity is common.
- Slowly and gradually weakness of facial, ocular, and oropharyngeal muscles also tends to develop.
- Once respiratory muscle weakness becomes established, the person requires ventilatory support, which occurs in 20% of cases. Recent studies suggest that in most people with GBS weakness progresses for 1–3 weeks but rapid deterioration to respiratory failure can develop within hours.

Sensory Impairments

Sensory impairments seen in GBS are:

- Sensory symptoms frequently appear before or at the onset of weakness. Patients complain of a tingling or pricking sensation (paresthesia) in their hands and feet. Characteristically this is very symmetrical and generally progressive.
- Distal numbness and limb or back pains are also common.
- About 50% will present with symmetric distal limb paresthesia, before clinically evident limb weakness. Early finger paresthesia suggests a patchy process, unlike the pattern seen with distal axonopathies.
- Paresthesia of trunk or face unusual, but sensory loss over the trunk is frequent.

Autonomic Impairments

The common autonomic impairments seen in GBS are as follows:

- Dysautonomia is seen in 65% of people with GBS. Dysautonomia refers to autonomic dysfunction, which is basically a condition in which the autonomic nervous system does not work properly. This may affect the functioning of the heart, bladder, intestines, sweat glands, pupils, and blood vessels.
- Most common manifestations include cardiac dysfunction such as sinus tachycardia, sinus bradycardia, sinus arrest and other supraventricular arrhythmias, paroxysmal hypertension, and hypotension (especially postural).
- Some other rarely occurring autonomic impairments are ileus, urinary retention (one-fourth cases), altered sweating, and mild orthostatic hypotension.

Impairments Related to Cranial Nerve Involvement

- GBS is associated in 45–75% of cases with cranial nerve involvement. Facial nerve is the most common to be involved followed by extraocular muscles and lower cranial nerve involvement. Twelfth cranial nerve involvement is extremely rare in GBS. Only two cases have been reported till date with GBS with total paresis of motor cranial nerves.
- The common clinical manifestations due to cranial nerve involvement are:
  - Diplopia
  - Dysarthria
  - Dysphagia
  - Ophthalmoplegia
  - Pupillary disturbances
  - Facial palsy.

Diagnosis

Diagnostic criteria for GBS include:

- The presence of progressive weakness and areflexia
- Relative symmetry
- Mild sensory involvement

BOX 33.1: GBS presentation.

Guillain-Barré syndrome is an acute, predominantly motor neuropathy presenting with distal limb paresthesia, relatively symmetric leg weakness, and frequent gait ataxia.

- Cranial nerve involvement
- At least partial recovery
- Autonomic dysfunction, and absence of fever:
  - Cerebrospinal fluid features that strongly support the diagnosis are an increase in protein beyond the first week, cell count <10 (albuminocytological dissociation).
  - Electrophysiologic evidence of conduction slowing, block, prolonged distal latency or F-wave latencies are also strongly supportive (80% of the case), though these abnormalities may be delayed for several weeks.
  - Marked persistent asymmetry of weakness, the presence of a sensory level, bowel/bladder involvement at onset, and a prominent pleocytosis often cast doubt on the diagnosis.
  - Imaging studies, such as magnetic resonance imaging (MRI) and computed tomography (CT) scanning of the spine, may be helpful in excluding mechanical causes of myelopathy.

WHO has recommended using Brighton criteria (**Table 33.2**) as the case definition of GBS, so that standardized information may be available for epidemiologic purposes (not as a criterion for treatment). This criterion is based on presenting clinical findings and ancillary testing, including neurophysiology and lumbar puncture findings (www. brightoncollaboration.org). Brighton criteria also account for the level of diagnostic certainty based on the presenting findings at clinical and additional examinations, ranging from level 1 (highest level of diagnostic certainty) to level 4 (reported as GBS, possibly due to insufficient data for further classification).

Disease-Specific Quality of Life Measure

The GBS disability score is a widely accepted scoring system to assess the functional status of patients with GBS. It was originally described in Hughes et al. (1978) and since then, various iterations have appeared in the literature. The criteria require that the patient's level of disability be documented using the scale from 0 to 6 as given in **Table 33.3**.

Miller Fisher Syndrome

Miller Fisher syndrome (MFS) is named after Dr C Miller Fisher who described it in 1956 as a limited variant of ascending paralysis, GBS. It is a rare, acquired nerve disease that is considered to be a variant of GBS. MFS variant represents a tiny subset of the cases (1 to 2 in 1,000,000). It affects more men than women with an approximate gender ratio of 2:1 and a mean age of 43.6 years at the onset of disease.

Clinical Features

Listed below are the clinical features of MFS:

- The clinical hallmark of MFS is a triad presentation of acute ophthalmoplegia, areflexia, and ataxia in the setting of a preceding bacterial or viral illness.
- People with this condition have a rapid decrease in vision over days and/or difficulty in walking. These changes are frequently preceded by a viral or diarrheal illness 1–4 weeks earlier.
- Slurred speech, difficulty swallowing, and abnormal facial expression with inability to smile or whistle may also occur.
- Examination shows poor balance and coordination of the hands as well as loss of deep tendon reflexes and eye muscle weakness.
- Facial weakness, enlarged or dilated pupils, and a decreased gag reflex on stimulation of the throat can be present in some patients.
- Distal paresthesia with or without weakness is also present.

Table 33.2: Key diagnostic criteria and Brighton case definitions for Guillain-Barré syndrome (GBS).

Diagnostic criteria	Level of diagnostic certainty			
	1	2	3	4
Bilateral and flaccid weakness of limbs	+	+	+	+/−
Decreased or absent deep tendon reflexes in weak limbs	+	+	+	+/−
Monophasic course and time between onset and nadir 12 h to 28 days	+	+	+	+/−
CSF cell count <50/µL	+	+[a]	−	+/−
CSF protein concentration>normal value	+	+/−[a]	−	+/−
NCS findings consistent with one of the subtypes of GBS	+	+/−	−	+/−
Absence of alternative diagnosis for weakness	+	+	+	+

Keynote: + present; − absent; +/− present or absent.
(CSF: cerebrospinal fluid; NCS: nerve conduction studies)
[a]If CSF is not collected or results not available, nerve electrophysiology results must be consistent with the diagnosis GBS.

Table 33.3: Guillain-Barré Syndrome disability scale.

Score	Description
1	A healthy state
2	Minor symptoms and capable of running
3	Able to walk 10 m or more without assistance but unable to run
4	Able to walk 10 m across an open space with help
5	Bedridden or chair bound
6	Requiring assisted ventilation for at least part of the day
7	Dead

Diagnosis

Diagnosis should be made as follows:

- Tests of nerve conduction may show diminished activity of nerves that carry sensory information to the spinal cord and brain.
- MRI or other imaging studies of the brain and/or spinal cord are usually normal in Miller Fisher Syndrome (MFS).
- Lumbar puncture may reveal that spinal fluid protein is elevated.
- Pure Fisher syndrome is uncommon, with many patients going on to develop the prominent widespread weakness of GBS.

Management of Guillain-Barré Syndrome

Clinical Pearl

The treatment of Guillain-Barré syndrome aims to accelerate recovery as well as reduce complications in acute phase of illness and occurrence of long-term neurological residual disability.

Medical Management

Medical management is classified as follows:

- **Respiratory management:** Respiratory status should be monitored in all patients. Up to 30% of patients need ventilatory support or airway protection **(Fig. 33.3)**.
- **Cardiovascular management:** Hemodynamic monitoring of pulse and blood pressure should be started early. Hypotensive/hypertensive episodes may be managed accordingly.
- **Prophylaxis for prevention of deep vein thrombosis (DVT):** There is increased risk of DVT (formation of blood clots) in deep brain stimulation (DBS) patients due to immobility and hypercoagulability [(increased tendency toward blood clotting from treatments such as intravenous immunoglobulin (IVIg)]. Medication and support stockings may be used in nonambulatory patients until they are able to walk independently.

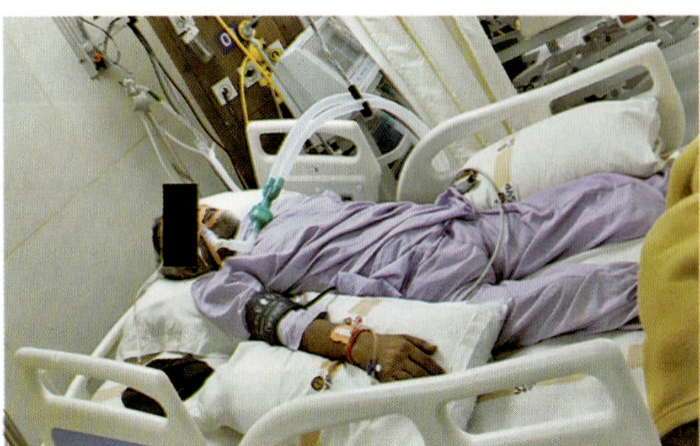

Fig. 33.3: A patient with GBS on ventilator support in ICU.
(GBS: Guillain-Barré syndrome)

- **Pain management:** Safe and effective drugs are required for pain management in acute phase.

Immunotherapy: Immunotherapy comprises IVIg or plasma exchange.

- **IVIgs:** High doses of immunoglobulin can help to block the antibodies causing GBS. Immunoglobulin contains normal, healthy antibodies from donors. It should begin within 2 weeks from the onset of symptoms.
- **Plasmapheresis (plasma exchange):** Plasmapheresis is a process that filters the blood and removes harmful antibodies. Plasma exchange is most beneficial when initiated within 7–14 days from the onset of the disease.

Physiotherapy Goals

Physiotherapy management goals should be as follows:

- Maintain clear airways to prevent respiratory complications
- Prevent lung infections
- Regain the patient's independence with everyday tasks
- Improve the balance and coordination
- Maintain joint range of motion (ROM)
- Support joint in functional position to minimize damage or deformity
- Prevention of pressure sores
- Maintain peripheral circulation
- Provide psychological support for the patient and relatives.

CHRONIC INFLAMMATORY POLYRADICULONEUROPATHY

In contrast to GBS, which, by definition, reaches its peak by 4 weeks, chronic inflammatory demyelinating polyneuropathy (CIDP) is a chronic autoimmune disease that develops within 8 weeks. Its prevalence is reported at 2–3/100,000. It generally follows a chronic progressive course and only rarely a relapsing–remitting course. It has symmetric and at times asymmetric distribution. Sensory, motor, or autonomic nerves can be involved. Individual presence of sensory and motor impairments is often reported in this.

Many inherited chronic demyelinating neuropathies are also known. CMT disease is one of them. Motor involvement causing distal weakness ("stork legs") is common.

Charcot–Marie–Tooth

Charcot–Marie–Tooth (CMT) disease is named after the three doctors who first identified it. It is one of the most common inherited chronic PN, which affects motor and sensory nerves.

Clinical Features

Typically, the earliest symptoms of CMT disease result from motor nerve involvement, which causes weakness and gradual muscle atrophy in the feet. Affected individuals may have foot abnormalities, such as high arches (pes cavus), flat feet (pes planus) or curled toes (hammer toes).

They often have difficulty flexing the foot or walking on the heel of the foot. These difficulties may cause a higher than normal step (high steppage gait).

Affected individuals may gradually also develop weakness in the hands, causing difficulty with daily activities, such as writing, fastening buttons, and turning doorknobs.

Sensory impairments are also very common in this condition. People with CMT disease typically experience a decreased sensitivity to touch, heat, and cold in the feet and lower legs.

In rare cases, affected individuals have loss of vision or gradual hearing loss that sometimes leads to deafness.

Medical Management

Research suggests that 60–80% of patients that are treated with IVIg, corticosteroids, or plasma exchange have improvements in their condition, but the long-term prognosis varies according to when the therapy is initiated and the degree of associated axonal loss.

Paranodopathies

Paranodium is the portion of the nerve fiber directly adjoining the sides of the node of Ranvier. It demarcates the node, on which the odium channels important for the saltatorial excitation are localized, from the juxtaparanode, where potassium channels are located. The term "paranodopathies" was coined after autoantibodies against paranodal proteins on the nodes of Ranvier were discovered in patients exhibiting the clinical picture of CIDP. Hence, this condition can be defined as neuropathies with autoantibodies to paranodal proteins. They usually have an acute onset, as in GBS.

Clinical Features

Clinically, one sees acute, severe, and predominantly motor neuropathy that is usually axonal on electrophysiology and often accompanied by action tremor and ataxia.

Medical Management

Rituximab is considered the treatment of first choice in this generally.

Diabetic Neuropathy

Diabetic neuropathy (DN) is a common disorder and is defined as signs and symptoms of peripheral nerve dysfunction in a patient with DM in whom other causes of peripheral nerve dysfunction have been excluded. According to an estimate, two thirds of diabetic patients have clinical or subclinical neuropathy. All types of diabetic patients—insulin-dependent DM (IDDM), non-IDDM, and secondary diabetic patients—can develop neuropathy. The presence of DN is directly associated with the duration of diabetes and the amount of metabolic control. The cause of DN though remains unknown but ischemic and metabolic components are implicated.

Hyperglycemia induces rheological changes, which increase endothelial vascular resistance and reduce nerve blood flow. In majority of patients, this condition is symptomless. Motor, sensory, and autonomic nerves maybe involved in varying combinations so usually a clinically mixed picture is seen.

Clinical classifications of DNs include the following:

- *Symmetric:*
  - DPN
  - Painful autonomic neuropathy
  - Painful distal neuropathy with weight loss "diabetic cachexia"
  - Insulin neuritis
  - PN after ketoacidosis
  - PN with glucose impairment
  - Chronic inflammatory demyelinating PN with DM.
- *Asymmetric:*
  - Radiculoplexoneuropathies—lumbosacral, thoracic, and cervical
  - Mononeuropathies
  - Median neuropathy at wrist
  - Ulnar neuropathy at the elbow
  - Peroneal neuropathy at the fibular head
  - Cranial neuropathy

Clinical Features

DN usually affects the nerves of lower limbs. In rare cases, affection of the nerves in the arms, abdomen, and back occur. Commonly seen symptoms include:

- Tingling
- Numbness (which may become permanent)
- Burning (especially in the evening)
- Pain

Autonomic Impairments

This type usually affects the digestive system, especially the stomach. It can also affect the blood vessels, urinary system, and sex organs. The system-wise manifestation is as discussed in the following section:

Digestive System

Symptoms include:

- Bloating
- Diarrhea
- Constipation
- Heartburn
- Nausea
- Vomiting
- Feeling full after small meals.

Genitourinary System

Symptoms include:

- Bloating
- Incontinence
- Vaginal dryness
- Erectile dysfunction.

Diagnosis

The American Academy of Neurology (AAN) recommends that DN is diagnosed in the presence of somatic or autonomic neuropathy when other causes of neuropathy have been excluded. At least one of each of the five criteria is needed:

1. Symptoms
2. Signs
3. Electrodiagnostic tests
4. Quantitative sensory
5. Autonomic testing.

This may be necessary in research protocols. However, in clinical practice two of five criteria have been recommended.

Medical Management

The following medical management is to be done:

- *N*-acetylcysteine, an amino acid, is a potent antioxidant. *N*-acetylcysteine application is found helpful in the prevention or treatment of neuropathy. Rats with experimentally induced diabetes for 2 months had a 20% reduction in nerve conduction velocity and 48% reduction in endoneurial blood flow. Both were largely corrected by *N*-acetylcysteine supplementation.
- Lacosamide, a new anticonvulsant drug, had a small but significant pain relieving effect on painful DN.
- Vitamin E is used to refer to a group of fat-soluble compounds that include both tocopherols and tocotrienols.
- Myo-inositol is an important constituent of the phospholipids that make up nerve cell membranes. Because low nerve myo-inositol concentrations have been observed in the pathogenesis of DN, which suggests the effectiveness of it management of DN.

Physiotherapy Management Goals

Unlike GBS, in DN sensory symptoms are more established; hence, the approach varies. The main goals are:

- Care of anesthetic part
- Relief of pain and paresthesia
- Prevention of postural hypotension
- Physical therapists can also recommend braces and/or splints to enhance balance and posture
- Splinting is often used in the treatment of compression mononeuropathies.

American Diabetes Association (ADA) recommends moderate-to-vigorous exercise for patients with diabetes to help manage the disease.

Clinical Pearl

Diabetic clients must tightly monitor their blood sugar levels during exercise to prevent major fluctuations. This may involve educating clients and monitoring blood sugars, ideally through a multidisciplined approach in rehabilitation.

CHEMOTHERAPY-INDUCED NEUROPATHY

Chemotherapy-induced neuropathy (CIN) is the most frequent neurological side effect of tumor therapy with cytostatic drugs, such as platinum derivatives, vinca alkaloids, taxanes, proteasome inhibitors, as well as modern antibody-based therapies. Due to the rise in cancer and higher long-term survival rates, the incidence of CIN is increasing. Due to its high prevalence among cancer patients, CIN constitutes a major problem for both cancer patients and survivors as well as for their health-care providers, especially because, at the moment, there is no single effective method of preventing CIN.

Clinical Features

In comparison to other peripheral neuropathies patients with CIPN may present more fulminant symptoms, affecting at the same time the feet and hands, with predominant pain, and symptoms have a faster progression as well. CIN is a predominantly sensory neuropathy that may be accompanied by motor and autonomic changes. It typically starts with sensory deficit symptoms and pain within the first 2 months of therapy and can stabilize or resolve once treatment has been discontinued. Sensory symptoms usually develop first, involve the feet and hands, and commonly present as a typical "glove and stocking" neuropathy **(Fig. 33.4)**. The most distal parts of the limbs exhibit the greatest deficits. The symptoms comprise:

- Numbness
- Tingling
- Altered touch sensation
- Impaired vibration
- Paresthesia
- Dysesthesia induced by touch and warm or cool temperatures.

Moreover, painful sensations, including spontaneous burning, shooting or electric shock-like pain as well as mechanical or thermal allodynia or hyperalgesia is

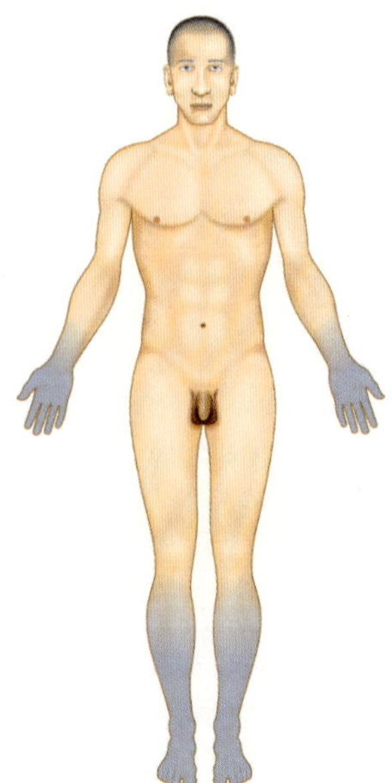

Fig. 33.4: Glove and stocking type of sensory symptoms.

frequently seen. In severe cases, these symptoms can progress to a loss of sensory perception.

Motor symptoms occur less frequently than sensory symptoms and, as a rule, they assume the form of distal weakness, gait and balance disturbances, and impaired movements. In severe cases, CIPN can lead to paresis, complete patient immobilization, and severe disability. Very rarely autonomic symptoms, which usually involve orthostatic hypotension, constipation, and altered sexual or urinary function, can occur.

Diagnosis

Research suggests that CIN is characterized as an axonal sensorimotor neuropathy by electrodiagnostic studies. Other causes of neuropathy (i.e. DN) should also be excluded in a patient with symptoms. Subjective assessments of CIN can be done by The National Cancer Institute-Common Terminology Criteria for Adverse Events (NCI-CTCAE) grading scale and patient-reported outcome measures. NCI-CTCAE version 4.03 is a subjective method to evaluate CIPN, which is performed by a healthcare professional, who grades adverse events that include:

- Peripheral sensory or motor neuropathy
- Dysesthesia
- Paresthesia
- Neuralgia

All of these are graded on a scale of 1–5, depending on the severity. The advantage of the NCI-CTCAE is that the assessment is quick and easy for providers to perform **(Table 33.4)**. However, it is limited by the subjectivity of interpretation; lack of detail about location, type, and severity of impairment; and a narrow scoring range.

Medical Management

American Society of Clinical Oncology (ASCO) recommends the use of duloxetine for painful CIN.

Acetyl-L-carnitine—It has been tested in clinical and animal studies for the treatment of CIPN. The decreases in nerve conduction velocity were significantly less in groups supplemented with acetyl-L-carnitine. In addition, acetyl-L-carnitine is found to not interfere with the antitumor effects of the drugs.

Table 33.4: Grades of assessment of chemotherapy-induced neuropathy using NCI-CTCAE.

Grade	NCI-CTCAE
1	Asymptomatic; loss of deep tendon reflexes or paresthesia (including tingling), but not interfering with function
2	Sensory alteration or paresthesia (including tingling) interfering with function, but not interfering with activities of daily living (ADL)
3	Sensory alteration or paresthesia interfering with ADL
4	Disability
5	Death

The use of topical menthol for CIPN is also found to show improvement in CIPN pain and function with a 6-week course of twice-daily application of 1% topical menthol to affected areas.

OTHER TOXIC NEUROPATHIES

Other than toxic neuropathies secondary to chemotherapy, various other toxic neuropathies can develop as a result of drug or environmental exposure. Chloroquine and hydroxychloroquine can cause a toxic myopathy characterized by slowly progressive, painless, and proximal weakness and atrophy, which is worse in the legs than the arms. Amiodarone can cause a neuromyopathy similar to chloroquine and hydroxychloroquine. Colchicine can also cause a neuromyopathy, which usually presents as proximal weakness and numbness and tingling in the distal extremities. Thalidomide is associated with severe teratogenic effects as well as peripheral neuropathy that can be dose-limiting.

Exposure to heavy metals can also induce peripheral neuropathy. Lead neurotoxicity may present as a combination of motor-predominant peripheral neuropathy (classically described as wrist drop) and encephalopathy. Chelation therapy is used in the treatment of lead toxicity. Inorganic arsenic neurotoxicity may occur from well water contamination, accidental exposure to industrial or agricultural agents, or in the setting of homicidal/suicidal intent. Organic arsenic neurotoxicity from acute poisoning often occurs 1 to 2 weeks after a severe acute systemic syndrome characterized by nausea, vomiting, and diarrhea. Thallium or mercury poisoning can also result in peripheral neuropathic presentation.

Alcohol-Induced Polyneuropathy

The prevalence of alcohol-induced PNP among chronic alcoholics is 22–66%. The duration of alcohol abuse and the lifetime quantity of alcohol consumed are the factors associated with the presence of the condition. In Victor's (1984) study of hundreds of cases of neuropathy associated with alcoholism, dietary deficiency was always found to be present. Alcohol-induced neuropathy is found to be associated with several risk factors, such as malnutrition, thiamine deficiency, direct toxicity of alcohol and a family history of alcoholism.

Pathophysiology

The pathogenesis of alcoholic neuropathy is still under debate. Current literature does show a strong association of nutritional, especially thiamine, deficiencies seen in alcoholics with alcohol neuropathy. Thiamine deficiency is closely related to chronic alcoholism and can induce neuropathy in alcoholic patients. It has been found that ethanol diminishes thiamine absorption in the intestine, reduces hepatic stores of thiamine, and affects the phosphorylation of thiamine, which converts it to its active form. Deficiency of vitamins other than thiamine may also contribute to clinical features of alcoholic neuropathy. Chronic alcoholism can alter the intake, absorption, and utilization of various nutrients (nicotinic acid, vitamin B_2, vitamin B_6, vitamin B_{12}, folate, or vitamin E). In addition, patients with chronic alcoholism tend to consume smaller amounts of essential nutrients and vitamins and/or exhibit impaired gastrointestinal absorption of these nutrients secondary to the direct effects of alcohol. These relationships make chronic alcoholism a risk factor for thiamine deficiency. In addition to thiamine deficiency, recent studies indicate a direct neurotoxic effect of ethanol or its metabolites.

Clinical Features

In most cases of alcoholic neuropathy, the onset of the PN is insidious and prolonged, but some cases have been associated with acute, rapidly progressive onset. Symptoms of alcoholic neuropathy, like those of many of the other axonal mixed PNs, manifest initially in the distal lower extremities.

Sensory Symptoms

Sensory symptoms include:

- Numbness
- Paresthesia
- Dysesthesias
- Allodynia
- Loss of vibration and position sense.

All these symptoms generally manifest prior to motor symptoms (e.g., weakness). However, patients may present with both motor and sensory symptoms at initial presentation. If abstinence is maintained, neuropathy can resolve within months to years.

Medical Management

Treatment is directed toward halting further damage to the peripheral nerves and returning to normal functioning.

Clinical Pearl

Further damage can be prevented by alcohol abstinence, a nutritionally balanced diet supplemented by all B vitamins, and rehabilitation.

Painful dysesthesias associated with alcoholic neuropathy can be treated using gabapentin or amitriptyline with other over-the-counter pain medications, such as aspirin or acetaminophen.

Alpha-lipoic acid, the most researched nutrient for peripheral neuropathy, has been used as a treatment for peripheral neuropathy. It is found to have a potential benefit in the treatment of patients with alcoholic neuropathy.

Topical application with capsaicin is also found to provide symptomatic relief from neuropathic pain in patients suffering from alcoholic neuropathy.

Nutritional Neuropathy

Deficiencies of various vitamins can result into peripheral neuropathy. Pernicious anemia is the most common cause of cobalamin (vitamin B_{12}) deficiency. Occasionally, it may be associated with cognitive dysfunction. On electrodiagnosis, it will reveal axonal sensorimotor neuropathy. Central nervous system (CNS) involvement produces abnormal somatosensory and visual evoked potential latencies.

Thiamine (vitamin B_1) deficiency is uncommon, but in the case of chronic alcohol abuse, recurrent vomiting, total parenteral nutrition, and bariatric surgery, it can arise as a secondary condition. Vitamin B_6 or pyridoxine deficiency can also result into peripheral neuropathic manifestations. The PN of vitamin B_6 is non-specific, manifesting as a generalized axonal sensorimotor PN. Vitamin B_6 deficiency can be detected by direct assay.

Another deficiency is that of niacin, which results in pellagra. It is a common problem in the developed areas also, such as Asia or Africa where corn is the main source of carbohydrate. Neurologic manifestations are variable; abnormalities can develop in the brain and spinal cord as well as peripheral nerves. When peripheral nerves are involved, the neuropathy is usually mild and resembles beriberi.

Vitamin E deficiency usually occurs secondary to lipid malabsorption or in uncommon disorders of vitamin E transport. Clinical features may not appear until many years after the onset of deficiency. The onset of symptoms tends to be insidious, and progression is slow. The main clinical features are spinocerebellar ataxia and PN, thus resembling Friedreich ataxia or other spinocerebellar ataxias. Patients manifest progressive ataxia and signs of posterior column dysfunction, such as impaired joint position and vibratory sensation. Because of the PN, there is hyporeflexia, other neurologic manifestations may include ophthalmoplegia, pigmented retinopathy, night blindness, dysarthria, pseudoathetosis, dystonia, and tremor.

Overdose Neuropathy

Pyridoxine is an essential vitamin that serves as a co-enzyme for transamination and decarboxylation. However, at high doses (116 mg/dL), a severe sensory neuropathy with dysesthesias and sensory ataxia can develop. NCV reveals absent or markedly reduced SNAP amplitudes with relatively preserved CMAPs. Nerve biopsy reveals axonal loss of fiber at all diameters. Medical management will consist of reverting the effects of toxicity due to vitamin overdose.

HUMAN IMMUNODEFICIENCY VIRUS-RELATED NEUROPATHY

HIV-related peripheral neuropathies are among the most prevalent chronic neurological disorders affecting persons living with HIV and AIDS. HIV-related peripheral neuropathies are classified into six different types, depending on the symptoms and the time of onset:

1. Distal symmetric polyneuropathy (DSPN)

2. Inflammatory demyelinating PN (including both GBS and CIDP)
3. Multiple mononeuropathies (e.g., vasculitis, CMV-related)
4. Polyradiculopathy (usually CMV-related)
5. Autonomic neuropathy
6. Sensory ganglionitis.

Of these, distal sensory PN (HIV-DSPN) is the most common type, affecting more than one-third of the people living with HIV and AIDS.

Clinical Features

The clinical manifestation of HIV-SN presents as symmetrical symptoms of:
- Pain (burning or shooting)
- Numbness
- Paresthesia (pins and needles)
- Hyperesthesia (increased contact sensitivity)
- Weakness of the muscles in the feet and legs and sometimes in the hands and arms, leading to functional limitation and disturbance of sleep.

PSYCHOSOCIAL ASPECTS OF POLYNEUROPATHY

Growing body of evidence indicates that DPN is a risk factor for depression predicting both the severity and increments in depression over time. Various studies have provided evidence that indicates that depression, anxiety, low quality of life (QoL), and poor sleep are associated with pain in painful DPN.

Numerous studies have evaluated the effect of pain on QoL and consistently found that those with painful DPN have an impaired QoL, particularly in relation to their reduced physical activity. It has been established that patients with higher pain intensity experienced the worse QoL. Sleeping disorders are common in painful DPN. A vicious cycle is established, as a lack of sleep can worsen the perception of pain, which as a result leads to an increased burden of disease.

Fatigue, pain, and anxiety/depression are increasingly being recognized in patients with GBS and CIDP, although their pathophysiological provenance remains unknown. A study also showed that GBS had a clear impact on psychological distress, particularly in the first month. Three months after the onset of GBS, psychological distress was higher than normal, but it improved significantly at 6 months.

Both physical recovery and the perceived physical condition are important with respect to the level of psychological distress, health status, and psychosocial health status. The perceived disruption of the physical residual at 12 months is found to be related not only to a decrement in health status and psychosocial health status and increased psychological distress but also to depressive symptoms. These findings confirm that the patient's perspective is of central importance. With respect to psychological distress, social function is most consistently disturbed at 12 months. More physical residual and perceived disruption can be the cause of more limitations in being able to go to social events or to work, or enjoying leisure activities.

ASSESSMENT

Following factors are assessed:
- Age—15–25 years (common for GBS).
- Sex—females (though alcohol-induced PN is more commonly seen in males as compared to females, whereas for all other kinds, data shows females are more predisposed than males).
- History—history of viral or bacterial infection is common in patients with GBS or MFS.
- Medical history—(usually uncontrolled) diabetes in DPN.
- Vaccination of rabies, tetanus, or influenzas may precipitate GBS.
- History of chemotherapy or anti-cancer drugs.
- Prolonged use of antidepressants, such as zimelidine or other neurotoxins are found to cause GBS.
- Family history is generally positive.
- Personal history—alcohol addiction.
- Nutritional status—reduced appetite.

Observation: Atrophy of muscles may be seen **(Fig. 33.5)**.

EXAMINATION

The following are to be examined:
- Vitals: blood pressure—hypo/hypertension is common in the case of autonomic neuropathy. Postural hypotension could also be present.
- Sensory examination—reduced or absent sensations. The pattern of sensory involvement reflects peripheral nerve distributions.

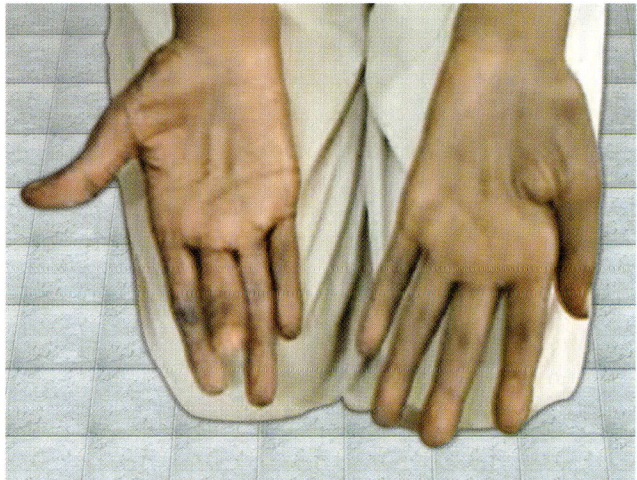

Fig. 33.5: Atrophy of hands.

- Motor examination—reduced muscle strength.
- Postural examination—abnormal posture due to muscle weakness is common.
- Gait examination—gait disturbances in the form of high steppage gait or waddling gait.
- Reflex examination—diminished or absent.
- Bladder/bowel affection—in autonomic affection, urinary incontinence or retention is often present

INVESTIGATIONS

Blood tests should be done for:
- Vitamin B_{12} and folate levels
- Thyroid, liver, and kidney functions
- Vasculitis evaluation
- Oral glucose tolerance test
- Antibodies to nerve components [e.g., anti-myelin-associated glycoprotein (MAG) antibody]
- Antibodies related to celiac disease
- Lyme disease
- HIV/AIDS
- Hepatitis C and B

Electrodiagnostic Testing

Nerve conduction velocity studies usually show slowing of conduction velocity (slower than 75% of the lower limit of normal), marked prolongation of distal latency (longer than 130% of the upper limit of normal) or both. Amplitude changes can also occur with demyelination due to secondary axonal loss.

Demyelinating neuropathy characteristically shows a reduction in conduction velocity and prolongation of distal and F-wave latencies, whereas axonal neuropathy shows a reduction in amplitude.

Electromyography studies show long duration and large amplitude and polyphasic motor unit potentials are seen in chronic axonal neuropathies, due to uninjured motor axons innervating denervated muscle fibers.

MANAGEMENT

General Medical Management

- Tricyclic antidepressants (TCAs) are often the first-line drugs to alleviate neuropathic pain symptoms. They have central effects on pain transmission and block the active reuptake of norepinephrine and serotonin.
- Antiepileptic drugs, such as the gamma aminobutyric acid analog (gabapentin) have proven helpful in some cases of neuropathic pain. These drugs have central and peripheral anticholinergic effects, as well as sedative effects, and they block the active reuptake of norepinephrine and serotonin. Recently, extended release gabapentin relieved symptoms of painful PN.
- Benfotiamine, alpha-lipoic acid, acetyl-L-carnitine, and methylcobalamin are among the well-researched

alternative options for the treatment of peripheral neuropathy. Other potential nutrient or botanical therapies include vitamin E, myo-inositol, *N*-acetyl-cysteine, and topical capsaicin.

Physiotherapy Management

Clinical Pearl

The main role of physiotherapy is to restore, or maintain muscle strength, and prevent muscle shortening and deformity.

Rehabilitation in PN utilizes an interdisciplinary team approach (e.g., physiotherapist, occupational therapist, nurse, and social worker) encouraging active patient and family education and participation using a time-based, goal-focused, functional approach to minimize disability and maximize function and community participation.

In Acute Stage

During the acute stage, when the weakness is more significant, attention is directed towards preventing complications as well as ensuring the symptomatic relief. Body positioning, bracing, pressure relief, frequent position changes, maintaining chest hygiene, and preventing muscle contractures should be ascertained.

- Participation in active movements may not be possible during this stage; hence, passive ROM exercises should be emphasized.
- Breathing exercises and cough clearance techniques should be incorporated.
- A tilt table for immobilized patients can be effectively used in rehabilitation units.
- Patients may be wheelchair dependent initially; hence, wheelchair transfers and locomotion in wheelchair should be taught for functional independence. Safety should be ensured during each step, since the patient may be having significant weakness during this stage.

Respiratory Symptom Management

Most of the patients are very disabled and usually require ventilator support during the acute stage. Initially, the patients are closely monitored for the signs of respiratory distress in the rehabilitation setting. Intubation becomes necessary when the vital capacity decreases to <18 mL/kg.

Respiratory complications commonly encountered in patients with GBS include chronic obstructive pulmonary disease, restrictive respiratory disease resulting from pulmonary scarring and pneumonia, and tracheitis due to chronic intubation and respiratory muscle insufficiency.

Physical therapy measures (chest percussion, breathing exercises, inspiratory muscle training exercises, and body positioning) are used to facilitate airway clearance; optimize the mechanical position of diaphragm, ventilation and perfusion matching, optimizing pH, peripheral circulation, and tissue perfusion; eliminate carbon-dioxide; and thereby reduce the work of breathing and of the heart.

Patients who have cranial nerve involvement are more susceptible to aspiration and pulmonary complications. Therefore they require frequent suctioning from artificial airway; however, it should be done only when indicated as this procedure can cause significant desaturation (up to 60%) particularly in the ventilated patient. Mobilization and ambulation of the ventilated patient should be the priority whenever possible.

In Recovery Stage

As the patient regains some muscle control, efforts should be directed toward active movements, gradually progressing to strengthening.

Studies have shown that the exercise interventions are associated with significant improvements in muscle strength, functional ability, and fatigue. For patients with peripheral neuropathy the recent recommendation of exercises includes a combination of aerobic and functional exercises as well as therapeutic exercises, including progressive resisted exercises utilizing repetitions of specific muscle contraction and strengthening exercises to target specific weak muscle groups with care to avoid overexertion.

- **Strengthening exercise:** Strengthening exercises for peripheral neuropathy are shown to moderately improve muscle strength **(Figs. 33.6 and 33.7)**.
  - Exercising can help when done regularly. Research shows that strengthening exercises can also reduce the neuropathic pain and also help in controlling the blood sugar levels.
  - Peripheral neuropathies often create muscle atrophy particularly distally in the feet and legs, which ultimately leads to limited ankle ROM. While it is doubtful whether major increases in strength can occur in muscle fibers affected by axonal degeneration, muscle fibers that have not yet been affected by neuropathy should respond to strength training.
  - Chetlin et al. administered a strengthening exercise program to a cohort of 20 individuals with a diagnosis of chemotherapy-induced PN. They observed improvements in strength in both men and women, but the final measures of strength after the 24-week program remained less than the standards established for healthy, age-matched individuals. Nevertheless, these strength changes had a positive effect on activities of daily

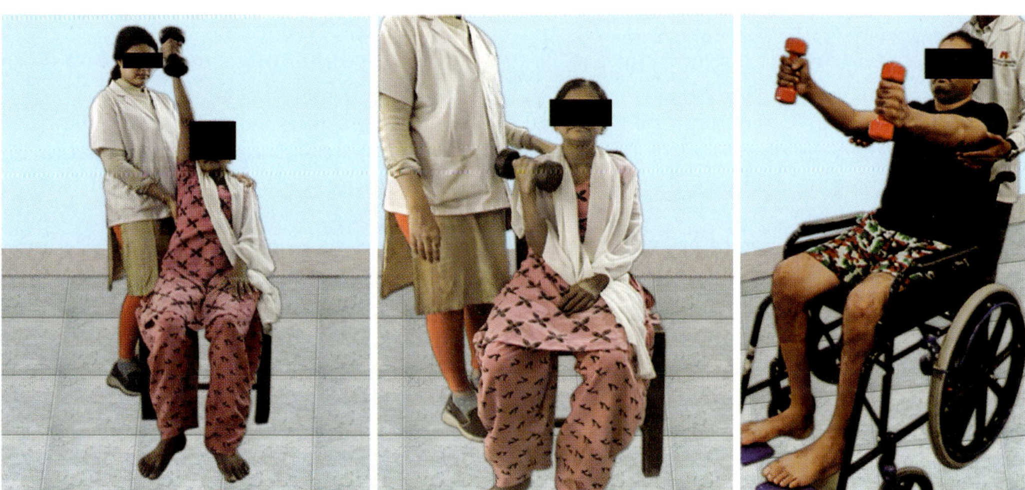

Fig. 33.6: Strengthening exercises of upper extremity in recovery stage.

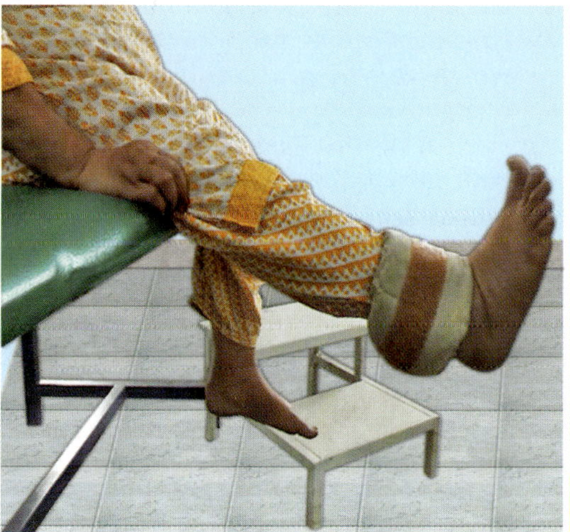
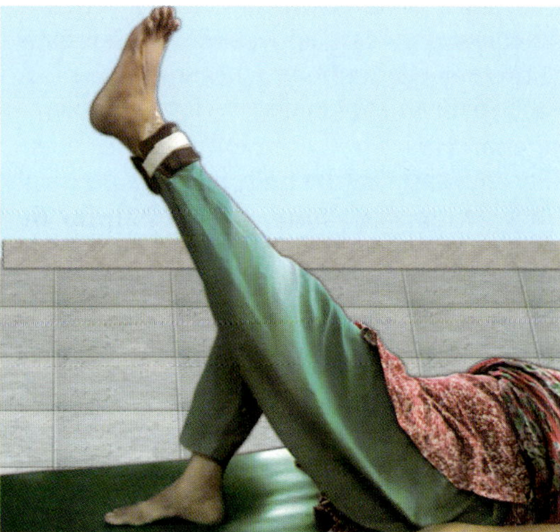

Fig. 33.7: Strengthening of lower extremity muscles in diabetic neuropathy.

living (ADL), sit to stand, rising from the supine position, and climbing stairs, with performance improvements.

- Steady gait requires strength and coordination of the larger muscles of the lower extremities, which are diminished in patients with neuropathy. Progressive resistance training is considered to be the most effective intervention for building muscle strength in older adults.

■ **Aerobic exercise:**

- A recent randomized controlled trail conducted by Dixit et al. showed that moderate-intensity aerobic exercises can play a valuable role to disrupt the normal progression of DPN in type 2 diabetes. Various other studies show that improvements in neuropathic and cutaneous nerve fiber branching following supervised exercise in people with DPN is seen. It is recommended that for any type of neuropathy best practices for aerobic exercising include routine activity for about 30 minutes a day, at least 3 days a week.

  Some examples of aerobic exercises are:
  - Brisk walking
  - Swimming
  - Bicycling

- Aerobic exercise delays the onset of DPN. In patients with diabetes who had not developed DPN, Balducci et al. reported that a supervised 4-hour per week brisk walk at 50–85% of heart rate reserve significantly impacted development of DPN in a 4-year study when compared with controls who did not exercise aerobically.

- Individuals with GBS who have recovered normal strength on clinical testing continue to report fatigue as a major residual symptom. Sixteen subjects with relatively good recovery from GBS, but with continued fatigue issues, were compared with 10 healthy, age- and sex-matched adults in a 12-week cycling program to assess its effect on fatigue, muscle strength, ADL, and QoL. Researchers reported significant improvement in fatigue.

- A literature review by Johnson and Takemoto indicated that in patients who have been inactive or cannot achieve such intensity levels, low-intensity aerobic therapy can improve sensation in the feet and reduce pain and tingling in the lower limbs.

■ **Stretching exercises:** Stretching exercises increase the flexibility and warm up the body for other physical activity. They are especially important after the acute stage, to prevent contractures and to combat the effects of immobilization period. Hip and knee muscles may be more prone to tightness; hence, stretching of these muscles should be ensured. Ankle plantarflexors may also be likely to tightness; hence, attention should be given to minimize the tightness of this muscle group. Heterotopic ossification (periarticular bone formation in the muscle planes) is a known complication of conditions, which require prolonged immobilization.

This can be prevented by early aggressive joint ROM exercise, stretching, and mobilization exercises. Self-stretching can be advised for home exercise, especially in those with DN **(Fig. 33.8)**.

■ **Balance training:**

- Several studies have described risk for postural instability, falls, and fall-related injury in patients with PN. This suggests the inclusion of balance training in patients with PN **(Fig. 33.9A)**.

- Numerous studies, primarily in the physical therapy and geriatric literature, support the use of balance training exercises among community-dwelling adults with postural instability or at high risk for falls due to peripheral neuropathy.

- Research has been done to check effects of weight-bearing exercise on lower extremity strength, balance, and falls. Although few differences in balance, muscle strength, fall or fear of falling were identified, the intervention was determined to be safe and well tolerated in patients with diabetes with peripheral neuropathy.

- Recent research now supports the incorporation of balance training programs, which includes double-limb standing activities and single-limb balance activities.

- The effect of vision on balance can be addressed by incorporating components of reduced-vision or eyes-closed to exercise.

- Progressions can be made in walking maneuvers, by making them more complex by adding surface variation and dual- or multitasking activities. Walking on different texture land surfaces is also found to improve balance and provide sensory re-education. **(Fig. 33.9B and C)**.

■ **For pain relief:** Evidence has been provided for relief of pain:
  - Transcutaneous electrical nerve stimulation (TENS)
  - Static magnetic field therapy
  - Low-intensity LASER therapy
  - Monochromatic infrared light

■ **Prevention of postural hypotension:** If the person is found to be developing signs and symptoms of autonomic affection, abdominal binders, and elastic stockings can be given to prevent pooling of blood, which will help prevent development of postural hypotension.

■ **Care of anesthetic part:** Once the person is diagnosed with sensory neuropathy, self-care regarding regular inspection of part of the limb is to be taught. Minor cuts could lead to ulcerations in parts with anesthesia; hence, regular inspection and avoiding use of sharp equipment is recommended. Sensory desensitization techniques should be inculcated into exercise protocols.

■ **Functional independence:** To make the patient functionally independent, functional training and use of adaptive equipment can be given. Equipment such as grabbers, sock donners, and plate guards can be advised for the patient to facilitate personal care. Home

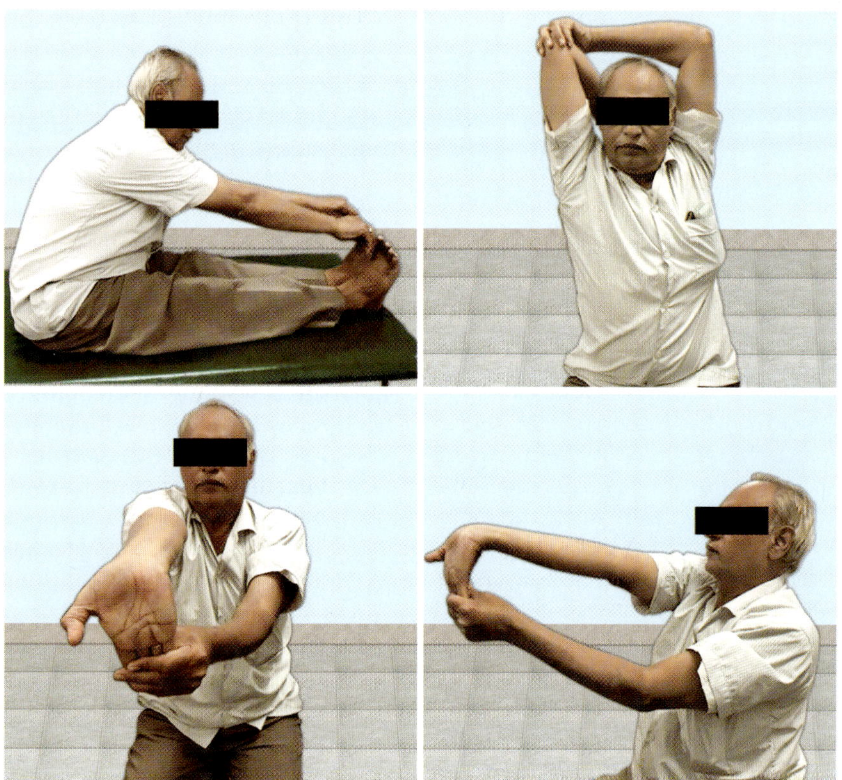

Fig. 33.8: Self-stretching exercises for home exercise programs.

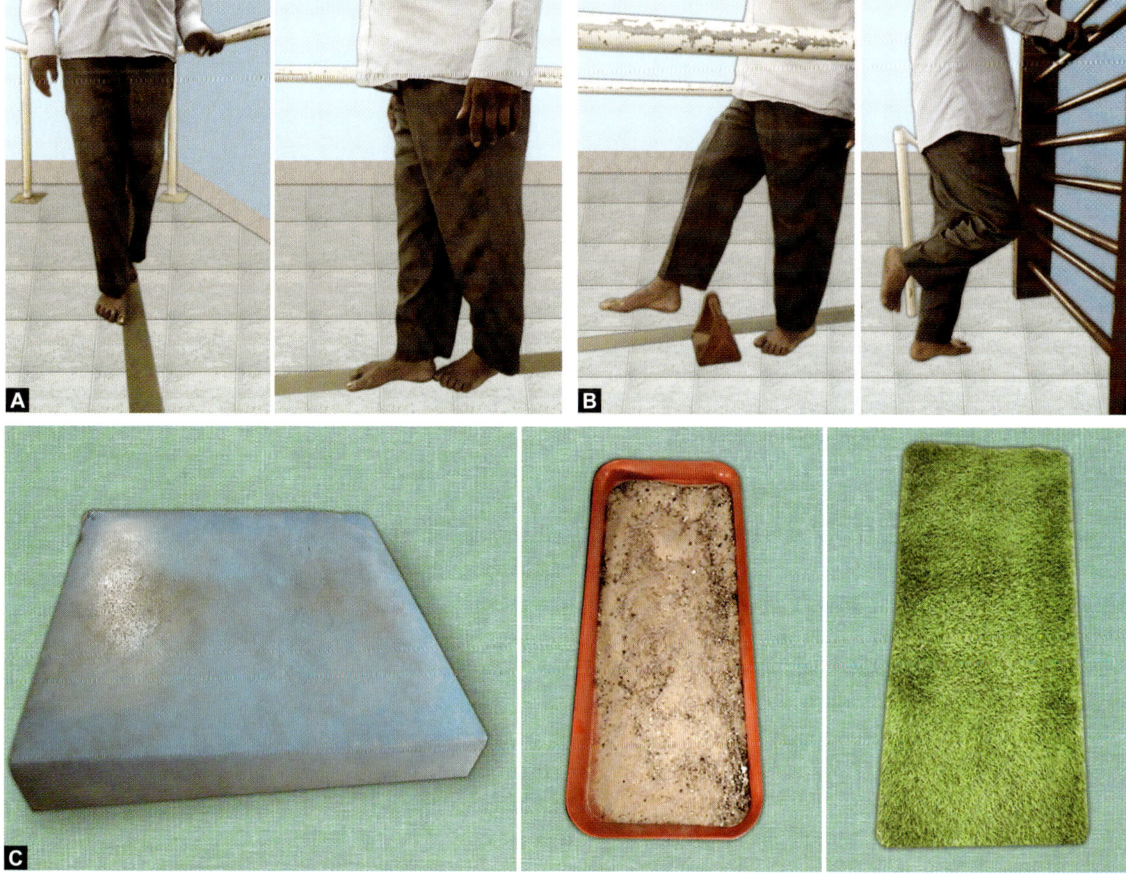

Figs. 33.9A to C: (A) Tandem walking as a part of balance training in parallel bar; (B) Obstacle walking and one-leg standing in diabetic neuropathy; (C) Different textures used for balance training in diabetic neuropathy.

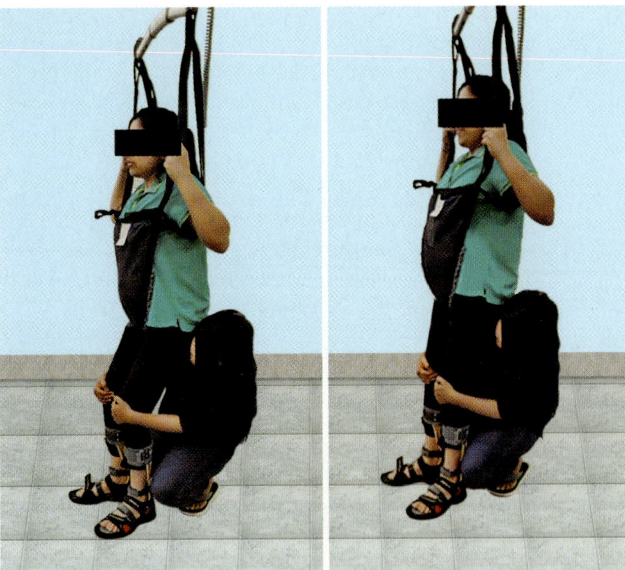

Fig. 33.10: Training for functional independence (using orthoses and harness).
Courtsey: Mission Health, Ahmedabad, India.

modifications are also undertaken to make the environment safer and accessible (e.g. non-skid mats, proper lighting, and grab rails). Use of assistive devices for ambulation should be made, as per the status of the individual patient. Orthoses and resting splints like ankle foot orthoses when needed should be prescribed to prevent contractures and restore muscle length **(Fig. 33.10)**.

Alternative Management

Alternative management includes the following:

- **Acupuncture,** one of the oldest and most commonly used forms of alternative medicine, has existed for more than 2,500 years. Acupuncture is a meridian-based therapy. In traditional acupuncture, needles are inserted into precisely defined, specific points on the body, each of which has distinct therapeutic actions. Various studies have supported the claim that acupuncture treatment improved not only nerve conduction velocity decreased by DPN improved a variety of subjective symptoms associated with this progressive disabling disorder.
- **Yoga** can help in the prevention of peripheral neuropathy by lowering inflammation, oxidative stress and mitigating the causes of neuropathy. Yogic practice can improve the mental health of neuropathy patients. It has been reported that yoga offers several benefits with regards to DPN. Its regular practice can control oxidative stress and improve balance and muscular movement in affected patients. Yoga is shown to provide a constructive rehabilitation activity for patients suffering from neuropathy especially in chemotherapy or HIV infection–induced peripheral neuropathy. Their QoL, stress levels, and pain sensitivity have shown favorable change post regular yoga practice.
- **Lifestyle modifications**—regular exercise, proper balanced diet with all nutrients especially vitamin B_{12} supplements, and abstinence from alcohol help in prevention of PN. Teaching energy conservation techniques (e.g., pacing and breaking tasks into steps) are essential in patients with fatigue and endurance problems.

SUMMARY

There are numerous PNs that are now identified and classified in various ways. Proper assessment and timely diagnosis helps in preventing complications such as diabetic foot or total dependency. Physiotherapy management along with lifestyle modifications is essential in management of PNs. As functional improvement is a goal of rehabilitation combining strength and functional training, focused on the needs and demands of each individual is important.

Case Scenario

CASE STUDY

A 60-year-old male with a previous history of type 2 DM for more than 20 years, treated with antidiabetic agents initially and insulin for the last 5 years and with poor metabolic control visited the physiotherapy department with complaints of tingling and numbness in bilateral sole of feet. He is also a known alcoholic.

On physical examination: The patient was in good general condition and was conscious and oriented in time, place, and person. Blood pressure was 160/110 mm Hg; heart rate was 90 beats/min.

His sensory examination revealed hyperesthesia of both feet as well as decreased vibratory sensation. His reflexes were normal. Motor examination was normal.

Special tests for radiculopathy were negative.

Laboratory studies revealed normal chemistries.

A review of his blood glucose log revealed fasting blood glucose levels—130 mg/dL. Postprandial glucose levels—150 mg/dL. His HbA1c was 7.2% (normal 4.0–6.0%), up from 6.1%, 6 months earlier.

Electrophysiological testing revealed decrease in amplitudes of compound sensory action potential of bilateral median and sural nerves with other motor nerve conduction velocities, latencies, and amplitude within normal limits.

Guiding Questions:

1. What are the possible causes for his complaints?
2. List out the impairments for physiotherapy management in the patient.
3. Describe an exercise program to manage the symptoms of neuropathy.
4. How can his sensory symptoms be managed?
5. Discuss the role of rehabilitation in the overall recovery of the patient.

Review Questions

1. What do you understand by the term "polyneuropathy"? Enumerate the various types of polyneuropathies
2. Discuss Guillain-Barré syndrome in detail along with its clinical variants.
3. Explain in detail management of diabetic neuropathy.
4. What does the term "paranodopathies" stand for?
5. Write a case assessment of polyneuropathy along with physiotherapy goals.
6. Describe in detail physiotherapy management of polyneuropathy.

BIBLIOGRAPHY

1. Balducci S, Iacobellis G, Parisi L, et al. Exercise training can modify the natural history of diabetic peripheral neuropathy. J Diabetes Complications. 2006;20(4):216-23.
2. Bansal V, Kalita J, Misra UK. Diabetic neuropathy. Postgrad Med J. 2006;82(964):95-100.
3. Chopra K, Tiwari V. Alcoholic neuropathy: possible mechanisms and future treatment possibilities. Br J Clin Pharmacol. 2012;73(3):348-62.
4. Dixit S, Maiya AG, Shastry BA. Effect of aerobic exercise on peripheral nerve functions of population with diabetic peripheral neuropathy in type 2 diabetes: a single blind, parallel group randomized controlled trial. J Diabetes Complications. 2014;28(3):332-9.
5. Doppler K, Appeltshauser L, Wilhelmi K, et al. Destruction of paranodal architecture in inflammatory neuropathy with anticontactin-1 autoantibodies. J Neurol Neurosurg Psychiatry. 2015;86:720-8.
6. Dubinsky RM, Miyasaki J. Assessment: efficacy of transcutaneous electric nerve stimulation in the treatment of pain in neurologic disorders (an evidence-based review): Report of the Therapeutics and Technology Assessment Subcommittee of the American Academy of Neurology. Neurology. 2010;74(2):173-6.
7. Ferri A, Scaglioni G, Pousson M, et al. Strength and power changes of the human plantar flexors and knee extensors in response to resistance training in old age. Acta Physiol Scand. 2003;177:69-78.
8. http://www.differencebetween.net/science/health/disease-health/difference-between-axonal-neuropathy-and-demyelinating-neuropathy/
9. https://patient.info/doctor/Polyneuropathies
10. https://www.healthline.com/health/guillain-barre-syndrome#treatmen
11. Hughes RA, Newsom-Davis JM, Perkin GD, et al. Controlled trial of prednisolone in acute polyneuropathy. Lancet. 1978;2(8093):750-3.
12. Joint Task Force of the European Federation of Neurological Societies (EFNS) and the Peripheral Nerve Society (PNS). European Federation of Neurological Societies/Peripheral Nerve Society guideline on management of multifocal motor neuropathy. Report of a joint task force of the European Federation of Neurological Societies and the Peripheral Nerve Society—first revision. J Peripher Nerv Syst. 2010;15:295-301.
13. Kautio AL, Haanpaa M, Kautiainen H, et al. Burden of chemotherapy-induced neuropathy—a cross-sectional study. Support Care Cancer. 2011;19:1991-6.
14. Koike H, Iijima M, Sugiura M, et al. Alcoholic neuropathy is clinicopathologically distinct from thiamine-deficiency neuropathy. Ann Neurol. 2003;54:19-29.
15. Krajewski KM. Neurological dysfunction and axonal degeneration in Charcot–Marie–Tooth disease type 1A. Brain. 2000;123(7):1516-27.
16. Kruse RL, Lemaster JW, Madsen RW. Fall and balance outcomes after an intervention to promote leg strength, balance, and walking in people with diabetic peripheral neuropathy: "Feet First" randomized controlled trial. Phys Ther. 2010;90:1568-79.
17. Mori M, Kuwabara S, Fukutake T, et al. Clinical features and prognosis of Miller Fisher syndrome. Neurology. 2001;56(8):1104-6.
18. Morrison S, Colberg SR, Mariano M, et al. Balance training reduces falls risk in older individuals with type 2 diabetes. Diabetes Care. 2010;33:748-50.
19. Nanda SK, Jayalakshmi S, Ruikar D, et al. Twelfth cranial nerve involvement in Guillain Barré syndrome. J Neurosci Rural Pract. 2013;4(3):338-40.
20. National Institute of Neurological Disorders and Stroke. Charcot-Marie-Tooth disease fact sheet. Available from www.ninds.nih.gov. [Retrieved July 24, 2017].
21. Paterson DH, Jones GR, Rice CL. Ageing and physical activity: evidence to develop exercise recommendations for older adults. Can J Public Health. 2007;98(Suppl 2):S69-108.
22. Quan D, Lin HC. Diabetic neuropathy clinical presentation. Available from http://emedicine.medscape.com/article/1170337-clinical#a0256. Updated: Jan 17, 2020.
23. Querol L, Illa I. Paranodal and other autoantibodies in chronic inflammatory neuropathies. Curr Opin Neurol. 2015;28:474-479
24. Shaw JE, Zimmet PZ. The epidemiology of diabetic neuropathy. Diab Rev. 1999;7:245-52.
25. Sommer C, Geber C, Young P, et al. Polyneuropathies—etiology, diagnosis, and treatment options. Dtsch Arztebl Int. 2018;115:83-90.
26. Soykan I, McCallum RW. Gastrointestinal involvement in neurologic disorders: Stiff-man and Charcot–Marie–Tooth syndromes. Am J Med Sci. 1997;313(1):70-3.
27. Thomas PK. Classification, differential diagnosis, and staging of diabetic peripheral neuropathy. Diabetes. 1997;46(Suppl 2):S54-7.
28. Tofthagen C, Visovsky C, Berry DL. Strength and balance training for adults with peripheral neuropathy and high risk of fall: current evidence and implications for future research. Oncol Nurs Forum. 2012;39(5):E416-24.
29. Tong Y, Guo H, Han B. Fifteen-day acupuncture treatment relieves diabetic peripheral neuropathy. J Acupunct Meridian Stud. 2010;3(2):95-103.
30. Trivedi S, Pandit A, Ganguly G, et al. Epidemiology of peripheral neuropathy: an Indian perspective. Ann Indian Acad Neurol. 2017;20(3):173-84.
31. Van der Meché FG, Van Doorn PA, Meulstee J, et al.; GBS-Consensus Group of the Dutch Neuromuscular Research Support Centre. Diagnostic and classification criteria for the Guillain-Barré syndrome. Eur Neurol. 2001;45(3):133-9.
32. Vittadini G, Buonocore M, Colli G, et al. Alcoholic polyneuropathy: a clinical and epidemiological study. Alcohol Alcohol. 2001;36(5):393-400.

Multiple Sclerosis

Zarna Ronak Shah

LEARNING OBJECTIVES

After reading this chapter, the readers should be able to:
- Describe the epidemiology, etiology, and pathogenesis of multiple sclerosis (MS)
- Describe the clinical presentation of a patient with multiple sclerosis
- Evaluate, conclude the diagnosis, and discuss the prognosis of the patient with multiple sclerosis
- Understand the literature regarding multiple sclerosis and formulate a plan of care to manage the patient
- Describe the role of physical therapist in the management of multiple sclerosis
- Understand the elements of exercise prescription for patient with MS
- Identify the psychosocial impact of MS

CHAPTER OUTLINE

- Epidemlology
- Pathophysiology
  - Pathological hallmarks of multiple sclerosis
  - Pathophysiology of multiple sclerosis
- Clinical features
  - Onset
  - Common symptoms
  - Paroxysmal symptoms
  - Physical signs
- Classification
- Investigations
- Differential diagnosis
- Medical management
- Physiotherapy assessment
- Fatigue assessment
- Disease-specific measures
- Physiotherapy management
  - Aims of physiotherapy treatment
  - General preventive measures
  - Physiotherapy treatment
- Psychosocial issues

INTRODUCTION

Multiple sclerosis (MS), also known as *disseminated sclerosis,* is an autoimmune central nervous system (CNS) disorder affecting the brain, spinal cord, and optic nerves. It is a disorder of myelin sheaths where nerve axons are affected in a secondary manner. Myelin is derived from oligodendroglia. It allows passage of ions and functions as an insulation of the nerve. Passage of ions is needed for transmission of impulses. Thus myelin sheath helps in normal propagation and conduction of impulse. Affection of the myelin sheath leads to abnormalities in the conduction of impulses.

Jean–Martin Charcot first described MS as a clinical pathology in 1868. He found hardened, patchy areas disseminated in the CNS during autopsy. MS was characterized by the pathological findings of paralysis and Charcot's triad (intention tremor, nystagmus, and scanning speech). He termed the disease *"sclerose en plaques"* due to the presence of these plaques. These plaques are patchy areas of demyelination found in a widespread manner in the CNS and form the characteristic feature of MS. Later on, gliosis can follow this demyelination. It was due to the widespread nature of the plaques that the pathology was named "multiple sclerosis."

Bharucha, Ramamurthy and Singh were the ones who first described the disease in India in the 1950s and early 1960s.

EPIDEMIOLOGY

Epidemiology is as follows:
- Gender incidence: Female>male
- Prevalence: 7–10/100,000
- Hereditary: There is around 20 times higher risk of occurrence in siblings than in the general population.

- Age onset: MS affects people between the ages of 20 and 50 years. The average age of onset is approximately 34 years.

PATHOPHYSIOLOGY

Pathological Hallmarks of Multiple Sclerosis

Pathological hallmarks of MS are as follows:
- Multiple plaques within the CNS gray and white matter
- Relative preservation of axons
- Inflammation
- Variable amount of gliosis

Pathophysiology of Multiple Sclerosis

The immunodysregulation in MS is an amalgamated activity of the innate and adaptive immune responses **(Box 34.1)**. Activation of dendritic cells (innate immune cells) by the binding of antigen to their cell surface in turn activates the adaptive immune response by means of CD8+ T cells, CD4+ T cells, B cells, etc. These adaptive immune cells cross the blood–brain barrier, enter the CNS, and activate autoantigens that produce autoimmune cytotoxic effects causing demyelination of the axonal tissue. As discussed previously, myelin sheath acts as an insulation of the nerve, hence conserving energy, and also increases the speed of conduction. Due to demyelination, the conduction slows down and a lot of energy is lost in the process, leading to fatigue of the nerves and subsequent loss of function.

This local pathology causes an acute inflammatory reaction, which heightens up to a mass effect, thus reducing the conduction even further. Gradually, the inflammation subsides as the antiinflammatory response catches up. The oligodendrocytes remyelinate the demyelinated tissue. With progressing pathology, anti-inflammatory reactions fail to repair the damage done by the inflammatory cells as the oligodendrocytes are also affected and the symptoms worsen. These demyelinated areas are filled, with time, with fibrous astrocytes and other neuroglial tissue. This process is called *gliosis* and consequently forms the plaques. After gliosis, the axon undergoes degeneration and causes permanent neurological deficit **(Fig. 34.1)**.

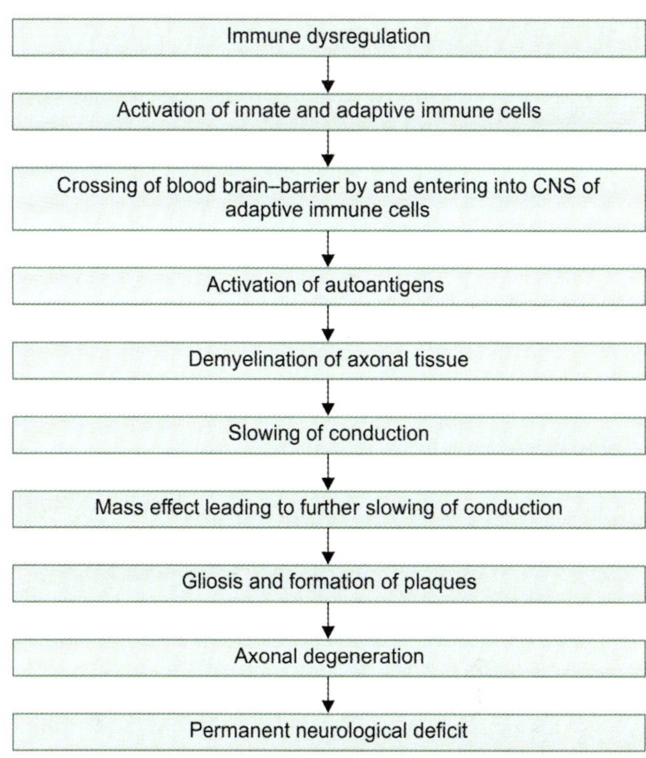

Fig. 34.1: Pathophysiology of multiple sclerosis.

CLINICAL FEATURES

Onset

It can be sudden or insidious. Initially, it starts with a single lesion in the white matter giving symptoms of disability of one or more limbs. This can be accompanied by visual symptoms such as impaired vision in one eye or diplopia. Paresthesia may or may not accompany.

Common Symptoms

The common symptoms of MS can be as follows:
1. **Spasticity:** It indicates sign of upper motor neuron (UMN) involvement. It can be present in upper limb and lower limb and also in trunk muscles. Spasticity can result in impaired voluntary control and thus can affect muscle work.
2. **Blurred vision:** Involvement of optic nerve results in impaired visual acuity. Blindness can be seen in rare cases. The light reflex can also be affected on examination.
3. **Diplopia:** This can be due to impaired gaze. Third and fourth cranial nerve palsy can give rise to double vision known as diplopia. The main reason behind this is the affected motor coordination of muscles of both eyes.
4. **Limb weakness:** Patients with UMN syndrome will show altered muscle performance, which can lead to secondary muscle weakness. Spastic muscles consume more energy to perform any action. Lack of energy will make the patient feel weak, which ultimately leads to loss of muscle performance, weakness due to disuse. The patients with cerebellar involvement will show generalized weakness known as asthenia.

BOX 34.1: Pathophysiology of multiple sclerosis.

Multiple sclerosis is believed to be autoimmune in nature. The autoimmune reaction is mediated by autoreactive lymphocytes. These lymphocytes cross the blood–brain barrier to enter the central nervous system and cause local inflammation, leading ultimately to the characteristic demyelination, gliotic scarring, axonal damage, and eventual axonal loss. What causes the initial inflammatory response is still unclear. The immune dysregulation is believed to be multifactorial—a combination of genetic susceptibility, epigenetic, and postgenomic events and environmental factors such as Epstein-Barr virus and other similar viral pathogens, sun exposure (vitamin D levels), smoking, diet, and chemicals.

5. **Pain:** Patient can show acute and chronic pain. Trigeminal neuralgia, headache, and limb pains are some of the common pains. Altered muscle coordination and control can lead to unnecessary stress on few muscles, which can give spasm and pain. Chronic neuropathic pain can be due to demyelination in the sensory tracts.

6. **Sensory impairments:** Complete loss of any sensation known as anesthesia is very rare, whereas patients with MS show paresthesia (burning or tingling numbness), hyperesthesia or hypoesthesia.

7. **Ataxia:** It is a cerebellar sign, which is present with dysmetria, dysdiadochokinesia, and tremors. Patients with ataxia show incoordination and impaired balance. Incoordination is a sign of cerebellar disorder. Equilibrium and nonequilibrium tests will show the exact problem. Loss of proprioceptors or altered inputs from the proprioceptors can lead to incoordination.

8. **Intentional tremors:** While attempting to reach a particular object, patient shows tremors at hand known as intentional tremors. It again indicates positive cerebellar signs. Tremors are absent at rest.

9. **Dysarthria and dysphagia:** Incoordination of bulbar muscles either due to cerebellar involvement or due to the cranial nerve palsy can lead to difficulty in speech known as dysarthria and difficulty in swallowing known as dysphagia. The cranial nerves, which can be considered responsible, are ninth and tenth.

10. **Urinary incontinence:** Urinary bladder dysfunction occurs due to demyclinating lesions affecting lateral and posterior spinal tracts. Spastic bladder is very commonly seen, which causes dribbling incontinence. Apart from this, dyssynergic and flaccid bladders are also seen. Dyssynergia is seen due to loss of coordination between bladder and sphincter.

11. **Fatigue:** It is a lack of mental or physical energy, which affects patient's day-to-day performance. Altered muscle tone, weakness, and incoordination can all result in unnecessary energy consumption, leading to decrease in the overall capacity to work. Emotional disturbances can aggravate the symptoms.

12. **Emotional and psychological changes:** A lot of emotional changes can happen in patient with MS. Pseudobulbar palsy can lead to uncontrolled crying or laughing and emotional lability. Fatigue, urinary incontinence, and generalized disability can all make the patient depressed and psychologically unstable.

Paroxysmal Symptoms

These symptoms may last for seconds to minutes. They can be trigeminal neuralgia, seizures, ataxia, and dysarthria. Presence of Lhermitte's sign which is an electric shock-like feeling that goes down to the back is seen while flexion of the neck is performed. Few patients also experience tingling and vibration in limbs with neck flexion. Several patients may exhibit Uhthoff's syndrome. It is worsening of neurologic symptoms in MS when the body gets overheated from hot weather, exercise, fever or sauna and hot tubs.

Physical Signs

The signs of MS are very vague and varied due to its scattered lesions in the CNS white matter. The symptoms are generally unilateral and asymmetrical if present bilaterally.

CLASSIFICATION

Multiple sclerosis can be phenotypically classified as benign or malignant. This classification only takes into account the disease's severity and overlooks other factors such as recovery from relapses and drug responsiveness.

- Benign MS is the mildest form of MS. There is a wide variation in the reported incidence of benign form of MS (5–40%). A patient with benign MS usually has very few symptoms and mild disability, even with >10 years of affection. The Expanded Disability Status Scale (EDSS) score **(Appendix A)** is usually low (≤3, which indicates that the patient has mild disability but can walk). The patient, very often, is without significant disability even after 15 years of affection and there are no relapses.

- Malignant MS is a rare occurrence and highly aggressive in nature. There is rapid symptom onset and progression. The patient may become so disabled that they may require assistance for locomotion within 5 years of onset.

There are four clinical variants of MS based on the disease course **(Figs. 34.2A to D)**:

1. Relapsing–remitting MS (RRMS):
   - Episodic attacks of neurological deficits (relapse) where symptoms develop over a few days and remain for several weeks with either complete or partial recovery.
   - No progression of disease between two relapses.
   - Stable patient shows local inflammatory activity, which is symptom-free.
   - About 85% of people have such type of MS.

2. Secondary progressive MS (SPMS):
   - Gradual worsening of signs or symptoms between relapses with or without acute attack.
   - There is a progressive axonal loss, which shows an increase in neurological disability.
   - Different pathophysiologies are responsible for SPMS than RRMS.

3. Primary progressive MS (PPMS):
   - There are disease progression and continuous decline in functions from onset without any relapse or remission.
   - It occurs at a late age (mean age 40 years) and there is equal gender distribution.
   - Affects 10% of cases.

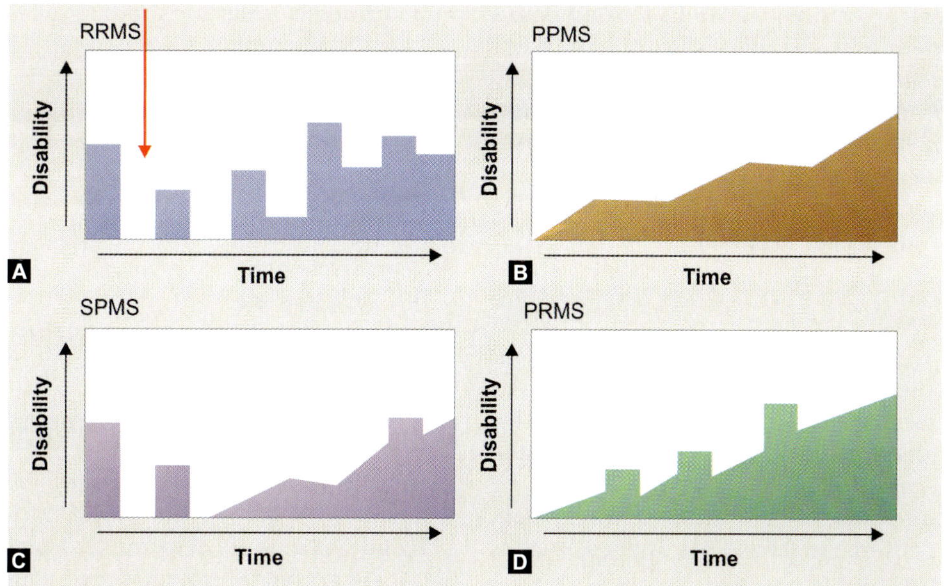

Figs. 34.2A to D: Clinical variants of multiple sclerosis (MS): (A) Relapsing–remitting MS; (B) Primary progressive MS; (C) Secondary progressive MS; (D) Progressive relapsing MS.

(RRMS: Relapsing–remitting MS; PPMS: Primary progressive MS; SPMS: Secondary progressive MS; PRMS: Progressive relapsing MS)

4. Progressive relapsing MS (PRMS):
   - Continuous deterioration in disease from onset with occasional relapse.
   - Intervals between relapses are characterized by continuing disease progression.
   - Affects 5% of cases.

INVESTIGATIONS

Investigations are as follows:
- **Laboratory:** Lumbar puncture and CSF examination will show increased gamma globulins. The IgG/albumin ratio may be altered. Oligoclonal bands are present in electrophoresis.
- **Electrodiagnoses:** Abnormal visual evoked potentials are seen in majority of cases (70–80%). Somatosensory and auditory evoked potentials are also seen as abnormal in many cases. Electromyography and nerve conduction studies are usually not affected as MS does not affect the peripheral nervous system.
- **CT brain scan:** Old plaques will show low density, whereas recent demyelination will show high density.
- **Nuclear magnetic resonance:** It seems effective in showing subcortical lesion in CNS.

The revised 2017 McDonald Criteria for the Diagnosis of MS can be used to make an early diagnosis of MS. The inclusion of oligoclonal bands in the diagnostic criteria helps in a rapid diagnosis as opposed to the previous inclusion of dissemination in time.

DIFFERENTIAL DIAGNOSIS

Multiple sclerosis can be misinterpreted with many diseases, depending on the level of the nervous system involved.

- **Spinal cord site lesion:** Can be misdiagnosed with spinal tumor, spondylosis, Friedreich's ataxia, motor neuron disease, vitamin B_{12} neuropathy, and syringomyelia.
- **Optic nerve lesion:** Can be misdiagnosed with optic neuritis or optic nerve glioma.
- **Third and fourth cranial nerve lesion:** Can be misdiagnosed with aneurysm of circle of Willis, myasthenia gravis, and intracranial tumor.
- **Cerebellum lesion:** Can be misdiagnosed with tumor, abscess of cerebellum, alcohol-induced ataxia or Friedreich's ataxia.

MEDICAL MANAGEMENT

Medical management of MS is three-fold focusing on prevention of relapses, symptomatic relief, and slowing the progression of the disease. Management of acute relapses is done by the use of corticosteroids. In patients who do not respond to corticosteroids, plasmapheresis may be used. Disease-modifying agents help in reducing the progression of the disease **(Table 34.1)**.

Table 34.1: Medical management of multiple sclerosis.

Drug group	Name of the drug
Antiviral agents	Amantadine, acyclovir, interferon
Immunosuppressive therapy	Corticotrophin (ACTH), corticosteroids, cyclophosphamide, antilymphocyte serum, plasmapheresis
Immunopotentiating therapy	Interferon
Others	Low-fat diet Vitamin B_{12} Hyperbaric oxygen

The symptomatic treatment of MS is decided based on the variety, extent, and severity of the symptoms. For spasticity, antispastic drugs such as baclofen, dantrolene, diazepam, and phenol can be given. Urinary catheterization and subtrigonal phenol injections can be given for urinary incontinence. Paroxysmal symptoms can be well managed with carbamazepine and clonazepam. Depression can be treated with amitriptyline and imipramine.

PHYSIOTHERAPY ASSESSMENT

The physiotherapy management starts with proper and detailed assessment as described in the previous chapter of neurological assessment. As the disease is progressive and the signs and symptoms may vary throughout the course of the disease, follow-up assessments must be taken at regular intervals so that effective management strategies can be delivered to the patient. The major areas of assessment are as follows:

- Higher functions examination:
  - Cognition
  - Perception
  - Speech
  - Memory
  - Behavior and intellectual functions
- Cranial nerve examination (all cranial nerves should be examined in detail):
  - Visual examination:
  - Impaired vision
  - Nystagmus
  - Diplopia
- Musculoskeletal examination:
  - Joint ranges: Active and passive
  - Muscle power
  - Contracture, deformity and tightness assessment
- Sensory examination
  - Check superficial, deep, and cortical sensations
  - Check for paresthesia, its severity, and distribution
- Tone examination:
  - Hypertonia: Spasticity or rigidity
  - Hypotonia
- Involuntary movement:
  - Generalized or isolated to one joint or limb
  - Ataxia
  - Tremors
  - Chorea
  - Athetosis
- Posture examination:
  - Attitude of the body
  - Alignment of the joints
- Balance examination:
  - Static and dynamic balance
  - Anticipatory and reactive balance
- Coordination examination: Equilibrium and non-equilibrium tests
- Gait examination—type of gait: Spastic, ataxic, or mixed gait can be found out.

- Cardiovascular and pulmonary examination: Endurance evaluation.
- Functional examination:
  - Activities of daily living (ADL)
  - Instrumental ADL
- Environment examination:
  - Work-place evaluation
  - Home environment
- Pain assessment:
  - Type and site
  - Aggravating and relieving factors
  - Severity and frequency

FATIGUE ASSESSMENT

Fatigue assessment plays a major part in the overall assessment of MS. Frequency, duration, and severity of fatigue have to be documented properly so that the physiotherapist (PT) can plan the treatment accordingly. The aggravating and relieving factors should be asked in detail to avoid unnecessary episodes of fatigue during the course of the disease. The Modified Fatigue Impact Scale (MFIS) **(Appendix B)** and the Fatigue Scale for Motor and Cognitive (FSMC) Functions are developed to objectify fatigue during examination. Apart from this, Visual Analogue Scale (VAS) can also be taken.

DISEASE-SPECIFIC MEASURES

Disease-specific measures include:
- MFIS
- EDSS for MS
- The Minimum Record of Disability
- Multiple Sclerosis Functional Composite
- Multiple Sclerosis Quality of Life-54
- MS Quality of Life Inventory
- Functional Assessment of MS
- Multiple Sclerosis Impact Scale-29
- Numeric Pain Rating Scale or VAS for pain

PHYSIOTHERAPY MANAGEMENT

Aims of Physiotherapy Treatment

A detailed assessment of the patient will help in planning the treatment protocol for physiotherapy. The major goal is to make the patient functionally active and to prevent secondary disability. The aims of rehabilitation are to:
- Gain the confidence of the patient and to give psychological support
- Reduce the pain
- Manage any abnormal tone
- Improve and maintain voluntary control
- Improve and maintain all sensory inputs
- Improve and maintain a full range of motion (ROM) of all joints
- Improve and maintain full length of muscles and soft tissues

- Improve and maintain normal posture and movement
- Improve and maintain the strength of weak muscles
- Improve and maintain coordination and balance
- Improve the gait and locomotor ability
- Teach energy-saving techniques and fatigue management
- Improve aerobic capacity
- Manage the speech and swallowing difficulties
- Improve cognitive function
- Improve psychological well-being and functional ability

General Preventive Measures

The treatment of MS can never be generalized but must be tailor made. There are certain issues of patients which can be prevented:

- Prevention of tightness of tendo Achilles can be done by proper positioning and exercises. All measures have to be taken to maintain the length of the muscle by giving slow stretching.
- A predominant pattern of extension and adduction in the lower extremity can be prevented by training the patient for correct weight bearing through a mobile knee. Proper positions and postural correction have to be taught. Biofeedback can be of use.
- Knee flexion contracture can be prevented by self-stretching techniques of hamstrings muscle group. Patient is made to touch the toes in long sitting.
- Hip flexor contractures can be prevented by ensuring good hip extension while walking and standing. Daily prone lying should be encouraged.
- Flexed thoracic spine can be avoided by active thoracic extension in sitting and prone position.
- Shoulder flexors and internal rotators can be lengthened by self-assisted full ROM exercises.
- Neck flexors can be stretched actively and passively by extending neck in sitting or prone.

Physiotherapy Treatment

Strengthening of Muscles

Apart from stretching of spastic and tight muscles, it is essential to strengthen the weak muscles with progressive resisted exercise training. Initially, manual resistance can be used for weak muscles. Later therabands, sandbags, weight cuffs, dumbbells, and other mechanical resistance can be used under observation of a physical therapist. Strengthening exercises will help in maintaining and increasing the power of the muscles and thus will help in functional independency **(Fig. 34.3)**.

Pain Management

This needs proper assessment and finding the exact etiology behind the presence of pain. Removal of cause may reduce pain, e.g., patients with altered posture may land up into musculoskeletal pain. In such cases, postural

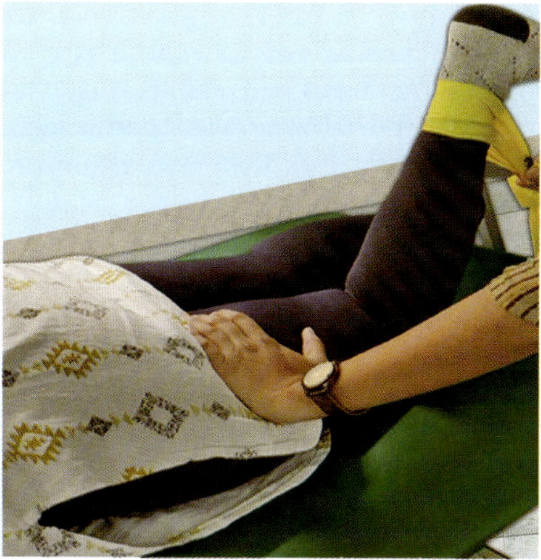

Fig. 34.3: Strengthening of hamstring muscles with therabands.

correction will relieve pain. Regular stretching of tight structures, strengthening of weak muscles, and postural retraining will indirectly relieve pain.

Resting pain can be relieved by physical modalities such as:

- Ice pack or hot pack
- Ultrasound therapy
- Interferential therapy (IFT) or transcutaneous electrical nerve stimulation (TENS) (after proper examination)

Following can help in reducing anxiety and pain.

- Relaxation
- Meditation
- Biofeedback

Spasticity Management

Proper positioning and stretching during the preventive phase can delay or prevent the secondary issues such as tightness and contractures. Spasticity can never be treated completely but should be managed properly so that the functions of the patient are not affected.

Severe spasticity can be managed by Rood's approach such as slow icing and scrubbing. Slow relaxed passive stretching and Myofascial release techniques can help in maintaining the length of the muscle. The muscle must be stretched in a functional position.

Sensory Deficit and Skin-care Management

The physiotherapist should plan strategies to increase awareness of sensory deficits and to compensate for sensory loss. Compensatory strategies can be used when one system is working better and has negligible impairments, e.g., the patient can be asked to use visual stimuli when proprioceptors are not working and there is imbalance due to that.

Tapping, verbal cueing, and biofeedback can also help. Risk of fall due to visual loss can be decreased by:

- Adequate lights at home
- Use of bright light at night
- Color contrast at stairs
  Double vision can be managed by patching one eye.

Somatosensory loss can lead to hypoaesthesia. There is an increased risk of pressure ulcers in such cases. The skin at the bony prominences will lead to skin break down. Following measures should be taken to reduce it:

- Regular inspection of skin
- Maintaining moisture level
- Prevention of secondary skin infection
- Comfortable and breathable cotton clothings
- Regular pressure relieving techniques

Fatigue Management

Proper assessment of fatigue will help in managing the symptoms. The PT should teach energy saving techniques or energy effectiveness strategies (EES). Expected exercise-related fatigue and the MS fatigue must be well differentiated. MS-related fatigue during exercise is often associated with thermal stress, which can be managed with adequate rest and the use of cooling and precooling treatments during exercise.

Well-planned aerobic conditioning program will help in building endurance and reduce the fatigue level. The patient must also be taught to use work and environment ergonomics in their day-to-day life. Patients should be advised to keep a record of their day-to-day schedule in a diary that can provide the insight to the therapist about energy costing of each activity which patient does. For each activity, they can be advised to record the importance, fatigue level, and perception of satisfaction after performing it. According to this, the PT can modify or can change the activity and plan the routine of patient.

Based on the information from the diary, the PT can start training sessions of EES. This includes modification of either the task or the environment. Activities that are difficult or have high energy consumption can be broken down into components. Activity pacing that involves planning proper rest intervals in between two activities may be tried. Rest–activity ratio should be developed for patients with chronic fatigue.

Exercise Training

MS patients usually exhibit loss of muscle power and endurance. In addition to this, they tend to have a sedentary lifestyle, and so, it becomes essential to introduce a well-planned strength and endurance training to them. Physiotherapy should focus on the following aspects of training:

- Strength and conditioning
- Aerobic conditioning
- Flexibility exercises

Management of Coordination and Balance

Cerebellar ataxia and postural instability are very common symptoms of MS. Following intervention and strategies may help in improving the balance and coordination:

- Postural control **(Fig. 34.4)**
- Rhythmic stabilization at shoulder and pelvic girdle

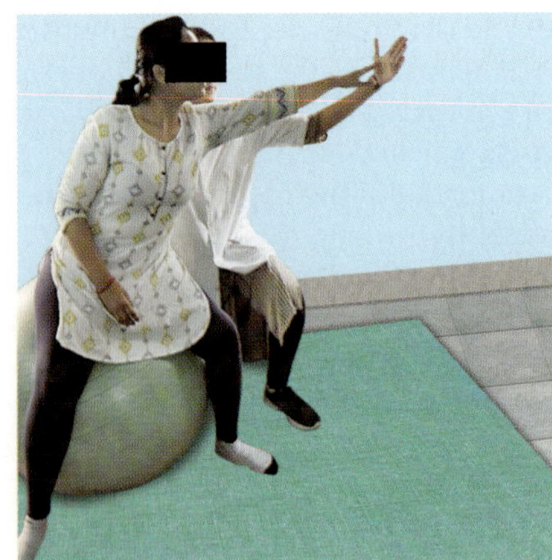

Fig. 34.4: Dynamic postural control in sitting on vestibular ball.

- Weight shifting in the static posture
- Dynamic balance exercises on physioball or balance board
- Change of the surface such as foam and hard
- Proprioceptive neuromuscular facilitation (PNF) chop and lift pattern
- Movable platform

Patients with central vestibular dysfunction may benefit from vestibular rehabilitation (Described in Chapter 27: Vestibular Rehabilitation).

Hydrotherapy can also be used effectively to improve balance. Resistance by water slows down the ataxic movement. Buoyancy will be added in upright position and will improve the balance of the patient. Hydrotherapy will also help in building the endurance.

Biofeedback aids in improving balance and posture in a variety of ways.

Control of ataxic movement can be done with the following strategies:

- Increasing proprioceptive loading
- PNF techniques such as rhythmic stabilization
- Light weights (weight cuffs) added to the distal parts of extremities
- Latex resistance bands
- Weighted boots, jackets, and belts
- Weighted canes and walkers
- Weighted spoons and forks while eating
- External devices such as splints
- Air splints and soft cervical collars

It is to be kept in mind that the added weight may increase the energy expenditure and so must be used with precautions. These strategies can make patient independent in their day-to-day life but they are compensatory and temporary. As unwanted and uncontrolled movements such as ataxia are worst when stress and anxiety are present, one must learn relaxation and stress management techniques.

Locomotor Training

Poor balance and coordination will lead to impaired locomotion. Many of the patients report heaviness in limb and foot drop. Apart from this, Trendelenburg gait is also commonly seen.

Following techniques can be used to improve the locomotor ability:
- Tone management
- Stretching of tight and spastic muscles
- Strengthening of weak muscles
- Practice and feedback while gait training
- Verbal and manual cues
- Functional training
- Body weight supported treadmill training
- Robot-assisted treadmill training

Orthotics and Assistive Devices

Following orthoses can be used as per the requirement of an individual:
- **Ankle–foot orthosis:** For foot drop, poor knee control, minimal-to-moderate spasticity, and poor somatosensation.
- **Functional electrical stimulation:** For treatment and compensation of foot drop. This will improve locomotor ability.
- **Knee–ankle–foot orthosis:** Rarely used for poor knee control. Increased energy expenditure presents as a disadvantage.

    Proper wearing on (donning) and off (doffing) methods must be taught.

Following assistive devices can be used:
- Canes
- Crutches
- Walkers

    These devices will help in improving balance and locomotion, but patient usually tends to become overdependent on them so their use should be done strictly as indicated. Care must be taken so that the patient does not get fatigue as these devices will increase the energy expenditure. In later stages of the disease wheelchair can be prescribed. The choice of assistive device and wheelchair depends on patient's physical status, will power, and cultural scenario.

Functional Training

Patient must be assessed for their functional independence using different clinical tools. Proper assessment will help in proper decision making of which ADL must be practiced. Instrumental ADL should also be practiced as well. Training in the use of the adaptive devices should be given. The goal is to make the patient functionally independent.

Management of Speech and Swallowing

MS patients show dysphagia and dysarthria as a symptom due to respiratory issues, incoordination, and weakness of muscles. The role of a therapist is as under:
- To improve posture and provide proper sitting control
- To improve head control

- To use neuromuscular electrical stimulation (NMES) to affected muscles
- Facilitation of swallowing manually or by electrical stimulation
- Further referral to speech and language pathologist

    Often, to solve feeding issues, nasogastric tube is given to patient. If the problem of dysphagia continues, percutaneous endoscopic gastrostomy can be done.

Cognitive Training

Cognitive training includes:
- Referral to neuropsychologist
- Compensatory strategies for memory deficits such as keeping a diary and noting down important things in it
- Personal digital assistance device to improve functional task
- Pill dispenser to help patient take medicine at a scheduled time
- Cueing device such as alarm clock
- Direction for functional task should be written in the environment
- Additional cognitive strategies:
  - Mental rehearsal
  - Requesting assistance
  - Maximizing alertness
  - Avoidance of difficult situation
  - Mental exercises
- Cognitive–behavioral therapy (CBT) can give excellent results.

PSYCHOSOCIAL ISSUES

Disability in MS progresses with the disease, so the psychological issues too will increase. Anger, denial, and depression can be considered a few amongst them. Because of the relapsing and remitting nature of the disease, the patient has to adjust every time with the new environment and circumstances, and so many times it is seen that a patient well set in one stage behaves differently in another. This gives significantly emotional and psychological disturbances. Fluctuation in the symptoms, physical dependency, architectural, and environmental barriers add to this. Fatigue also plays a major role in overall low psychological status.

Such psychological disturbances cannot be correlated to the severity of disease as it is a totally subjective feeling of an individual. Yoga, meditation, and counseling play a major role in dealing with such situations. In addition to this, positive feedback on signs of recovery or independency in ADL has to be highlighted to the patient. The therapist must be hopeful and realistic. False hope may aggravate psychological issues if the goals are not achieved. Making the patient aware about the prognosis and teaching positive dealing with MS seeks skill of a therapist. CBT can also help in such cases.

Patient and caregiver's education also play a major role. The caregivers must be educated about the psychological disturbances going on with the patient and also how to deal with them patiently as they are the ones going to stay with the patient the whole day. Positive reinforcement and support from the family members and caregivers can help in resolving such issues easily.

SUMMARY

Multiple sclerosis is a disorder of myelin sheath and a pathology that affects CNS in a wide spread manner. The main clinical features include spasticity, diplopia, ataxia, dysarthria, and dysphagia. These symptoms end up making the patient functionally dependent. Physiotherapy rehabilitation can work on the impairments and activity limitations and can make the patient as much functionally independent as possible so that they can participate in the society as earlier.

Case Scenario

CASE STUDY

A 37-year-old woman, housewife having complaint of imbalance while walking, difficulty in manipulating objects with hands, weakness in all four limbs, and occasional blurring of vision reported to the neurologist 6 months back. She had gradual worsening of the symptoms since last 6 months which started with the inability to lift heavy objects but later on progressed to difficulty in manipulating objects in the hand, tingling and numbness in the hands and legs. Later, she developed a loss of balance that caused difficulty in walking. While asking in detail, she revealed of a loss of control on urination and extreme tiredness. Doctor has done several lab tests and prescribed medicines. She was then referred to the PT for further management.

Observation: She is an overweight female with near-normal posture in supine and sitting except excessive plantar flexion at both ankles. She seems to be very low emotionally and cries while giving history. Standing balance seems to be affected with increased sways mainly anterior and posterior indicating loss of ankle strategies. Ataxia was observed while walking when she walks with broad base of support and imbalance. She further has to look down on the surface while walking and dual task seems quite impossible for her.

Objective Examination: While testing the cranial nerves, the second nerve showed some delayed response on light reflex. Rest cranial nerves seemed normal. Other higher functions were also found within normal limits. The speech was dysarthric and swallowing difficulties were also present.

The tonal examination revealed spasticity in the following group of muscle with given grades on Modified Ashworth Scale (MAS).

Group of muscles	MAS grade
B/L shoulder flexors	1
B/L elbow flexors	1+
Right pronators	2
Left pronators	1+
B/L long finger flexors	1
B/L hams	1
B/L calves	2

The manual muscle testing (MMT) of all four limbs showed around four grade.

Coordination examination showed dysmetria and dysdiadochokinesia of both upper limbs. The equilibrium tests were positive showing imbalance while standing.

The Berg balance score was found to be 36/56 showing a moderate risk of fall.

Specific scales: The Modified Fatigue Impact Scale scores are as follows:

Subset	Scores
Physical	20/36
Cognitive	12/40
Psychosocial	6/8
Total	38/84

The interpretation shows that fatigue is moderately affecting the patient as a whole but the psychosocial subset is more severely affected.

The EDSS score shows 6.0, which means intermittent or unilateral constant assistance is required to walk about 100 m with or without resting.

Guiding Questions:
1. What can be the possible diagnosis of the patient? Justify the answer with appropriate positive signs and symptoms.
2. List the primary and secondary impairments of the patient.
3. Formulate a plan of care for the patient.
4. Based on the occupation of the patient, what can be the possible modifications that may be required?

Review Questions

1. What is the pathophysiology responsible for multiple sclerosis?
2. What are the clinical subtypes of MS?
3. Enumerate the clinical signs and symptoms of MS.
4. Discuss the plan of care for rehabilitation of MS patient.
5. Discuss the assessment and management of fatigue in MS patient.
6. Discuss the strategies to improve postural control and balance in MS patient.
7. Enumerate the functional goals and its management strategies of MS patients.

BIBLIOGRAPHY

1. Bharucha EP, Umarji RM. Disseminated sclerosis in India. Int J Neurol. 1961:2:182-8.
2. Charcot J. Histologie de la sclerose en plaques. Gaz Hop, Paris. 1868;41:554-5.
3. Didonna A, Oksenberg JR. The genetics of multiple sclerosis. In: Zagon IS, McLaughlin PJ (Eds). Multiple sclerosis: perspectives in treatment and pathogenesis. Brisbane, AU: Codon Publications; 2017. Chapter 1. [Internet] Available from https://www.ncbi.nlm.nih.gov/books/NBK470155/.
4. Downie PA. Cash's textbook of neurology for physiotherapists, 1st Indian edition. Philadelphia, PA: JB Lippincott Company; 1992. pp. 383-417.

5. Grigoriadisa N, van Pesch V. A basic overview of multiple sclerosis immunopathology. Eur J Neurol. 2015;22(Suppl. 2):3-13.

6. Hawkins SA, McDonnell GV. Benign multiple sclerosis? Clinical course, long term follow up, and assessment of prognostic factors. J Neurol Neurosurg Psychiatry. 1999;67:148-52.

7. Huang WJ, Chen WW, Zhang X. Multiple sclerosis: pathology, diagnosis and treatments. Exp Ther Med. 2017;13(6):3163-6.

8. Popescu BF, Pirko I, Lucchinetti CF. Pathology of multiple sclerosis: where do we stand?. Continuum (Minneapolis, MN). 2013;19(4 Multiple Sclerosis):901-21.

9. Ramamurthy B. Disseminated sclerosis. In: Paper presented at International Congress of Neurological Sciences. Brussels; 1957.

10. Singhal BS, Advani H. Multiple sclerosis in India: an overview. Ann Indian Acad Neurol. 2015;18(Suppl 1):S2-5.

11. Singh B, Isaiah P, Chandy J. Multiple sclerosis (studies on sixteen cases). Neurology. 1954;1:49-59.

12. Susan B, O'Sullivan, Thomas J, et al. Physical rehabilitation, 6th edition. FA Davis Company; 2014. pp. 721-69.

13. Thompson AJ, Banwell BL, Barkhof F, et al. Diagnosis of multiple sclerosis: 2017 revisions of the McDonald criteria. Lancet Neurol. 2018;17(2):162-73.

APPENDIX A: KURTZKE EXPANDED DISABILITY STATUS SCALE (EDSS)

0.0 – Normal neurological examination (all grade 0 in all Functional System (FS) scores*).

1.0 – No disability, minimal signs in one FS* (i.e., grade 1).

1.5 – No disability, minimal signs in more than one FS* (more than 1 FS grade 1).

2.0 – Minimal disability in one FS (one FS grade 2, others 0 or 1).

2.5 – Minimal disability in two FS (two FS grade 2, others 0 or 1).

3.0 – Moderate disability in one FS (one FS grade 3, others 0 or 1) or mild disability in three or four FS (three or four FS grade 2, others 0 or 1) though fully ambulatory.

3.5 – Fully ambulatory but with moderate disability in one FS (one grade 3) and one or two FS grade 2; or two FS grade 3 (others 0 or 1) or five grade 2 (others 0 or 1).

4.0 – Fully ambulatory without aid, self-sufficient, up and about some 12 hours a day despite relatively severe disability consisting of one FS grade 4 (others 0 or 1), or combination of lesser grades exceeding limits of previous steps; able to walk without aid or rest some 500 meters.

4.5 – Fully ambulatory without aid, up and about much of the day, able to work a full day, may otherwise have some limitation of full activity or require minimal assistance; characterized by relatively severe disability usually consisting of one FS grade 4 (others or 1) or combinations of lesser grades exceeding limits of previous steps; able to walk without aid or rest some 300 meters.

5.0 – Ambulatory without aid or rest for about 200 meters; disability severe enough to impair full daily activities (e.g., to work a full day without special provisions); (usual FS equivalents are one grade 5 alone, others 0 or 1; or combinations of lesser grades usually exceeding specifications for step 4.0).

5.5 – Ambulatory without aid for about 100 meters; disability severe enough to preclude full daily activities; (usual FS equivalents are one grade 5 alone, others 0 or 1; or combination of lesser grades usually exceeding those for step 4.0).

6.0 – Intermittent or unilateral constant assistance (cane, crutch, brace) required to walk about 100 meters with or without resting; (usual FS equivalents are combinations with more than two FS grade 3+).

6.5 – Constant bilateral assistance (canes, crutches, braces) required to walk about 20 meters without resting; (Usual FS equivalents are combinations with more than two FS grade 3+).

7.0 – Unable to walk beyond approximately 5 meters even with aid, essentially restricted to wheelchair; wheels self in standard wheelchair and transfers alone; up and about in wheelchair some 12 hours a day; (usual FS equivalents are combinations with more than one FS grade 4+; very rarely pyramidal grade 5 alone).

7.5 – Unable to take more than a few steps; restricted to wheelchair; may need aid in transfer; wheels self but cannot carry on in standard wheelchair a full day; May require motorized wheelchair; (usual FS equivalents are combinations with more than one FS grade 4+).

8.0 – Essentially restricted to bed or chair or perambulated in wheelchair, but may be out of bed itself much of the day; retains many self-care functions; generally has effective use of arms; (usual FS equivalents are combinations, generally grade 4+ in several systems).

8.5 – Essentially restricted to bed much of day; has some effective use of arm(s); retains some self-care functions; (usual FS equivalents are combinations, generally 4+ in several systems).

9.0 – Helpless bed patient; can communicate and eat; (usual FS equivalents are combinations, mostly grade 4+).

9.5 – Totally helpless bed patient; unable to communicate effectively or eat/swallow; (usual FS equivalents are combinations, almost all grade 4+).

10.0 – Death due to MS.

***Excludes cerebral function grade 1.**

Note 1: EDSS steps 1.0 to 4.5 refer to patients who are fully ambulatory and the precise step number is defined by the Functional System score(s). EDSS steps 5.0 to 9.5 are defined by the impairment to ambulation and usual equivalents in Functional Systems scores are provided.

Note 2: EDSS should not change by 1.0 step unless there is a change in the same direction of at least one step in at least one FS.

Bibliography

1. Haber A, LaRocca NG (Eds). Minimal record of disability for multiple sclerosis. New York: National Multiple Sclerosis Society; 1985.

2. Kurtzke JF. Rating neurologic impairment in multiple sclerosis: An expanded disability status scale (EDSS). Neurology. 1983;33(11):1444-52.

APPENDIX B: MODIFIED FATIGUE IMPACT SCALE (MFIS)

Fatigue is a feeling of physical tiredness and lack of energy that many people experience from time to time. But people who have medical conditions like MS experience stronger feelings of fatigue more often and with greater impact than others.

Following is a list of statements that describe the effects of fatigue. Please read each statement carefully, circle the one number that best indicates how often fatigue has affected you in this way during the past 4 weeks. (If you need help in marking your responses, tell the interviewer the number of the best response.) Please answer every question. If you are not sure which answer to select choose the one answer that comes closest to describing you. Ask the interviewer to explain any words or phrases that you do not understand.

Because of my fatigue during the past 4 weeks

		Never	Rarely	Sometimes	Often	Almost always
1.	I have been less alert	0	1	2	3	4
2.	I have had difficulty paying attention for long periods of time	0	1	2	3	4
3.	I have been unable to think clearly	0	1	2	3	4
4.	I have been clumsy and uncoordinated	0	1	2	3	4
5.	I have been forgetful	0	1	2	3	4
6.	I have had to pace myself in my physical activities	0	1	2	3	4
7.	I have been less motivated to do anything that requires physical effort	0	1	2	3	4
8.	I have been less motivated to participate in social activities	0	1	2	3	4
9.	I have been limited in my ability to do things away from home	0	1	2	3	4
10.	I have trouble maintaining physical effort for long periods	0	1	2	3	4
11.	I have had difficulty making decisions	0	1	2	3	4
12.	I have been less motivated to do anything that requires thinking	0	1	2	3	4
13.	My muscles have felt weak	0	1	2	3	4
14.	I have been physically uncomfortable	0	1	2	3	4
15.	I have had trouble finishing tasks that require thinking	0	1	2	3	4
16.	I have had difficulty organizing my thoughts when doing things at home or at work	0	1	2	3	4
17.	I have been less able to complete tasks that require physical effort	0	1	2	3	4
18.	My thinking has been slowed down	0	1	2	3	4
19.	I have had trouble concentrating	0	1	2	3	4
20.	I have limited my physical activities	0	1	2	3	4
21.	I have needed to rest more often or for longer periods	0	1	2	3	4

Instructions for scoring the MFIS

Items on the MFIS can be aggregated into three subscales (physical, cognitive, and psychosocial), as well as into a total MFIS score. All items are scaled so that higher scores indicate a greater impact of fatigue on a person's activities.   0

Physical subscale: This scale can range from 0 to 36. It is computed by adding raw scores on the following items: 4+6+7+10+13+14+17+20+21.   0

Cognitive subscale: This scale can range from 0 to 40. It is computed by adding raw scores on the following items: 1+2+3+5+11+12+15+16+18+19.   0

Psychosocial subscale: This scale can range from 0 to 8. It is computed by adding raw scores on the following items: 8+9.   0

Total MFIS score: The total MFIS score can range from 0 to 84. It is computed by adding scores on the physical, cognitive, and psychosocial subscales.   0

Head Injury

Dhara Sharma

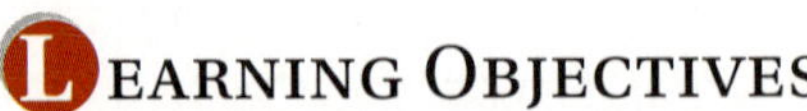 LEARNING OBJECTIVES

At the end of this chapter, the readers will be able to:

♦ Describe the types and mechanism of head injury
♦ Analyze the impact of cognitive, behavioral, motor, and sensory impairments on a patient with head injury
♦ Assess an individual with head injury by identifying the key components and choosing the right outcome measure
♦ Plan a management for individual with severe, moderate, or mild head injury
♦ Gain knowledge of medical and surgical interventions used commonly
♦ Discuss the role of physiotherapist in the rehabilitation of an individual with head injury.

CHAPTER OUTLINE

- Prevalence and impact
- Classification and mechanism of injury
  - Classification based on type of trauma
  - Classification based on severity of trauma
  - Classification based on mechanism of injury
- Clinical presentation
  - Primary impairments
  - Secondary complications
  - Activity limitations and participation restrictions
- Diagnostic procedures
- Prognosis
- Interventions
  - Medical intervention
  - Surgical intervention
- Rehabilitation
  - Physiotherapy evaluation
  - Physiotherapy interventions
  - Active rehabilitation

PREVALENCE AND IMPACT

Head injury or traumatic brain injury (TBI) is defined as an acquired injury to the brain causing nonprogressive impairments of brain functions. It is always caused by an external force. The external force can be in the form of a blow, jolt or penetrating wound. If the force is mild enough, it may not cause damage to the brain but only to the skull bones. This milder form of brain injury is called **concussion**. Head injury causes death or hospitalization of over 10 million people every year across the globe. In India, this number is over 1 million per year.

The individuals with head injury experience a wide variety of symptoms, and their rehabilitation start usually in intensive care unit and continue to progress gradually at an in-patient department; out-patient department; out-patient rehabilitation unit; and then at school, community or vocational rehabilitation center. Therapists having versatile skills are preferred for individuals with brain injury as they show multiple system involvement. Expert communication skills are required to encounter the difficulties faced during the rehabilitation because of cognitive and communication impairments.

CLASSIFICATION AND MECHANISM OF INJURY

Head injury can be classified into various types. Based on the type of trauma, the injury can be classified as primary injury and secondary injury. Based on the severity of the trauma, the injury can be classified as severe, moderate, and mild injury. According to the mechanism of injury, it can also be classified as closed head injury, open head injury, contrecoup injury, and blast injury. It is important to understand that these varieties of injuries do not occur in isolation and may overlap each other. Due to this, the individual affected with head injury may have a wide spectrum of impairments.

Classification Based on Type of Trauma

Primary Injury

The primary injury results from direct trauma to the parenchyma. The trauma can be penetrating injuries causing laceration or contusion. This type of injury causes more focal damage. It involves areas such as anterior temporal poles, frontal poles, lateral and inferior temporal cortices, and orbital frontal cortices. Acceleration deceleration injury causes concussion or diffuse axonal injury (DAI). Due to shear, tensile, and compressive forces, widespread axons are damaged in the brain, causing DAI which in turn causes Wallerian degeneration of the damaged axons. The most affected regions in DAI are parasagittal white matter of the cerebral cortex, corpus callosum, and pontine mesencephalic junction adjacent to superior cerebellar peduncles. Sometimes, direct injuries can also cause hematomas.

Secondary Injury

It results due to surge of events occurring at cellular level following the injury. Hypotension, increased intracranial pressure (ICP), hypoxemia, ischemia, and edema cause secondary damage to the tissues that may occur hours or days after injury. There is a release of excitatory neurotransmitters such as glutamate which causes neurotoxicity. Increased influx of calcium ions and cytokines causes increased inflammatory response and swelling and ultimately causes cell death. Increased swelling causes increased ICP. Normal ICP is 5–20 cm H_2O. Abnormally high ICP leads to herniation of the brain. Uncal, central or tonsillar herniation may commonly occur due to increased ICP.

Sometimes, following injury, there might be intracranial hemorrhage or rupture of meningeal vessels. It will lead to either extra- or intracranial hematoma. Hematoma can further compress the vessels and structures of the brain, causing vasospasm and cerebral ischemia. Seizures also can occur as a consequence of hematoma and, if not controlled, can cause cerebral hypoxia causing further damage. Other common causes of secondary injury can be acid–base imbalance and infections.

Classification Based on Severity of Trauma

Head injuries can also be classified based on the severity of symptoms.

Severe Head Injury

Following head injury, if the period of loss of consciousness (LOC) or alteration of consciousness (AOC) lasts for more than 24 hours, post-traumatic amnesia (PTA) is for more than 7 days, Glasgow Coma Scale (GCS) shows score of less than 9, with abnormal neuroimaging findings; it is classified as severe head injury. The GCS, developed by Teasdale and Jennet, has three components: eye opening, motor response, and verbal response. It has a maximum score of 15 and a minimum score of 3.

Moderate Head Injury

Moderate head injury is when period of LOC or AOC is between 30 minutes and 24 hours, PTA is between 1 and 7 days, GCS is between 9 and 12 with abnormal or normal neuroimaging findings.

The person who suffers from moderate-to-severe brain injury faces life-long disabilities and widespread cognitive and psychological problems. The physical disabilities are challenging but psychobehavioral issues following head injury affect the quality of life (QoL) more than the physical disabilities.

Mild Head Injury

Mild head injury or concussion has less-severe symptoms, with either no LOC and AOC or less than 30 minutes of LOC or AOC. There may be no PTA or it may last for less than a day. GCS is between 13 and 15 with normal neuroimaging findings. Individual, who suffers mild head injury, often recovers fully. About 10–15% of the cases suffer from post-traumatic psychological or cognitive dysfunctions. Some may also suffer from symptoms such as headache, vestibular problems, fatigue, or sleep disturbances. Collectively, these symptoms are called postconcussion syndrome.

Classification Based on Mechanism of Injury

Closed Head Injury

When the head gets injured but the skull is not penetrated, it is termed as closed head injury. Though the skull is not penetrated, it might be fractured often. It most frequently occurs due to road-traffic accidents (RTAs) or a blow to the head or fall. It may lead to both focal as well as diffuse head injury.

Open Head Injury

In contrast to closed head injury, open head injury is where the skull is penetrated. It often leads to focal brain damage. Usually, stab injury or bullet injury causes open head injury.

Coup–Contrecoup Injury

Coup injury occurs beneath the contact point of the force and may be associated with the fracture of the skull. Contrecoup injury occurs when the force is sufficient enough to cause the movement of the brain within the skull, causing injury to the opposite end of the brain to the point of impact. Coup–contrecoup injury occurs where both the ends of the brain get injured.

Blast Injury

Head injuries that are sustained due to detonation of an explosive device, e.g., missile are coined as blast injuries. There are three consequences of blast injury. **Primary blast injury** occurs due to direct effect of the blast causing transient shock and overpressure of the brain. **Secondary injury** occurs when the sharp objects are hurdled toward the brain and cause penetrating injuries. **Tertiary injury** is where the individual is tossed due to the blast hitting his head with an object.

CLINICAL PRESENTATION

Injury to the brain causes a broad range of impairments, including neuromuscular, cognitive, neurobehavioral, sensory, communication and swallowing. Though physiotherapy addresses mainly physical impairments, the associated impairments may bring challenges in the process of rehabilitation.

Primary Impairments

Neuromuscular Impairments

Due to devastating nature of head injury, the impairments are seen on both sides of the body. It impairs motor functions per se muscle tone, strength, endurance, and length of muscles of the trunk, upper and lower extremities. Approximately 12% of individuals with craniocerebral trauma will develop decorticate rigidity. It is an abnormal fixed flexion posture of upper limb. Those individuals, who develop decerebrate rigidity, abnormal extension of upper limb as well lower limb, are considered more severe than decorticate rigidity; have reduced chances of survival from 79 to 28%. These symptoms might be present unilaterally or bilaterally. Individuals might as well have hyporeflexia initially in the state of shock, followed by hyperreflexia. As a consequence of these, motor control is impaired which will also cause impaired postural control. Coordination impairment and ataxia are seen quite often too. As a result of these primary impairments, balance and gait get persistently affected. Individuals with head injury may also show sensory impairments depending on the lesion

site. Involuntary movements such as tremors or chorea are seen in about 20% of individuals with head injury. These dyskinesias are often transient and drug-induced, but in some cases, they persist for a longer period of time. The dyskinesia might also occur in the case of deep brain injury involving basal nuclei. Intentional tremors may be transient and are more obvious when an individual is more active.

Cognitive Impairments

Cognition is a method used by brain to process information. It includes, but is not limited to, memory, attention, vocabulary and language, information retention, recalling and manipulation, executive functions, planning, problem solving, and calculations. The wide variety of cognitive functions is controlled by various parts of the brain, but many of the functions are controlled by the frontal lobe. Situated anteriorly in the brain, the frontal lobe is the most susceptible area during head injury. Hence, individuals with head injury show a wide spectrum of cognitive dysfunctions.

Alteration in Level of Consciousness

The consciousness is altered in most of the cases of head injury. It can be classified as coma, vegetative state, and minimally conscious state **(Table 35.1)**.

Coma is a state of unarousable unresponsiveness. Other altered levels of consciousness are stupor, obtundation, and lethargy. **Stupor** can be defined as a state where only vigorous and repetitive stimuli will arouse the individual, when left undisturbed the individual will fall back to unresponsive state. **Obtundation** is where an individual is less interested in environment, slowed response to stimulation, and tends to sleep more than normal with drowsiness in between sleep states. **Lethargy** is a state of severe drowsiness where the individual will be aroused only by moderate stimuli and then drift back to sleep. **State of confusion** is where the individual is disoriented, bewilderment, and has difficulty in following commands. **Locked-in syndrome** is also described as pseudocoma state; it is often seen due to damage to the

Table 35.1: Characteristics of different altered levels of consciousness seen in head injury subjects.

Condition	Coma	Vegetative state	Minimally conscious state
Symptoms			
Sleep/wake cycle	No sleep/wake cycle (eyes are closed)	Sleep/wake cycle is present	Sleep/wake cycle is present
Breathing	Ventilator dependent	Can be weaned from ventilator	Spontaneous breathing
Sensory and communicative functions	No auditory, visual, cognitive, or communicative functions	May startle to or is briefly oriented to auditory or visual stimuli, no cognitive or communicative functions	May localize sound location or sustained visual fixation and visual pursuit are present
Motor responses	Abnormal motor and postural reflexes	Movements are nonpurposeful, reflexive and not reproducible	Localizes noxious stimuli and produces inconsistent movements
Prognosis	May become brain dead, enter vegetative or minimally conscious state	Complete absence of awareness after a period of greater than 1 year in the absence of stimulating environment	May show inconsistent motor recovery with minimal impairments

ventral portion of the pons below the level of third nuclei. The individual will be able to open, elevate, and depress their eyes but cannot move them horizontally. The individual lacks other voluntary movements or speech. Here, consciousness of an individual is not affected.

Neurobehavioral Impairments

Head injury can cause debilitating behavioral problems in the victim. Frontal lobe of the brain is largely responsible for the behavior of an individual. Damage to frontal lobe can result in behavioral problems, and it is closely linked to cognitive dysfunction. The common behavioral impairments seen in individuals with head injury are lower tolerance to frustration, anxiety, depression, emotional lability, aggression, self-centered behavior, agitation, disinhibition, etc.

Communication Impairments

Communication deficit commonly occurs in individuals with brain injury. Often, individuals suffer from expressive aphasia, receptive aphasia or dysarthria. Most of the deficits occur because of the cognitive involvement. Sometimes, the language is imprecise and socially unacceptable. These communication impairments may persist after 3 years of injury or longer. Difficulty heightens in open environments. Individuals fail to show adjustments in language according to the situations. These deficits affect their relationships, employability, as well as QoL. Over 75% individuals with head injury reported that they are understood with difficulty by the people outside their family.

Vision, Hearing, Smell and Taste

Head injury may lead to blindness, partial blindness, blurred vision, double vision, photophobia or light sensitivity. Individual may suffer from deafness or tinnitus; sometimes, they may develop hypersensitivity to sounds. There are chances of developing hyposensitivity toward sense of taste and smell, which might lead to reduction in appetite. This may be a result of cranial nerve damage, especially olfactory, optic, oculomotor, and trochlear which are commonly injured with head trauma.

Dysautonomia

Increased sympathetic activity following an injury is termed "dysautonomia." Individual presents with symptoms such as increased heart rate, respiratory rate, blood pressure, sweating, and hypertonia. Approximately 10–33% individuals with head injury suffer from dysautonomia. It is most frequently experienced in individuals with DAI.

Post-traumatic Seizures

Individuals with penetrating head injuries or depressed skull fractures are most likely to have post-traumatic seizures. Children less than 7 years of age are more likely to

suffer from post-traumatic epilepsy than the adults. Older adults are less likely to experience posttraumatic seizures. Phenytoin is the drug of choice for the prevention of early post-traumatic seizures.

Secondary Complications

Prolonged immobility following injury causes increased risk for secondary complications in individuals with head injury. Some of the most common complications following head injury are as follows:

- Deep vein thrombosis (DVT)
- Heterotrophic ossification
- Pressure ulcer
- Pneumonia
- Contractures
- Decreased endurance
- Muscle atrophy
- Fracture
- Peripheral nerve damage
- Urinary incontinence
- Bowel incontinence
- Chronic pain
- Hydrocephalus
- Elevated ICP
- Uncal herniation
- Hypertension
- Cranial neuropathies
- Endocrine complications such as syndrome of inappropriate antidiuretic hormone secretion, diabetes insipidus, and cerebral salt wasting syndrome.

In the longer run, the individuals with TBI may have feeding difficulties due to either impairment of chewing or swallowing, inappropriate head and trunk control. These impairments may lead to feeding difficulties which may further lead to nutritional deficiency and further complications such as decreased immunity.

Impaired motor learning is one of the most challenging complications followed by head injury. It hinders the process of rehabilitation and causes difficulty in coping up with activities of daily living (ADL).

Activity Limitations and Participation Restrictions

Devastating and broad-spectrum effects of head injury cause wide varieties of activity limitations such as feeding, bathing, toileting, grooming, and other ADL and instrumental ADL. Participation restrictions may include employment, homemaking, attending school or college, participating in social events, etc.

DIAGNOSTIC PROCEDURES

Almost all cases of head injury are referred for computerized tomography (CT) scan and/or magnetic resonance imaging (MRI). CT scan can be useful in the early stages of postinjury. It reveals fractures, hemorrhages, hematomas, contusions, or swelling in the brain. MRI is often suggested in the later stages once an individual is medically stable. MRI helps to understand the damage to the brain tissues. Other diagnostic procedures that may be used are monitoring of ICP, X-rays of the skull as well as extremities to rule out fractures, positron emission tomography (PET) scans, and electroencephalography. Routine MRI scans sometimes may not rule out the mild TBI. Diffuse tensor imaging helps scanning the white matter of the brain and tracts that may detect the mild brain injury.

PROGNOSIS

Table 35.2 describes Glasgow Outcome Scale (GOS) and GOS Extended (GOSE). The prognosis depends on several factors such as demographic factors (age), severity and type of the injury, premorbid status of an individual, duration of coma, time elapsed since injury, dose and use of phenytoin, and secondary impairments or complications. The severity of the injury is decided by GCS and GOS and GOSE. For GCS score of 13–15 indicates mild injury, 9–12 defines moderate and 3–8 defines severe brain injury **(Table 35.3)**.

Other than GCS, Corticosteroid Randomization After Significant Head Injury (CRASH) and International Mission for Prognosis and Analysis of Clinical Trials in TBI (IMPACT) models give an accurate prognosis and also predict functional ability. Dead, vegetative state or severe disabilities are considered to be unfavorable outcomes. Another predictor of the prognosis can be PTA. The duration between the injury and time when the patient is able to remember current events consistently helps predict

Table 35.3: Glasgow Coma Scale.

Activity	Score
Eye opening	
Spontaneous	4
To speech	3
To pain	2
No response	1
Best motor response	
Follows motor commands	6
Localizes	5
Withdraws	4
Abnormal flexion	3
Extensor response	2
No response	1
Verbal response	
Oriented	5
Confused conversation	4
Inappropriate words	3
Incomprehensible sounds	2
No response	1

the recovery of an individual. PTA can predict functional status, employment, over all recovery after 1 year of injury. Individual with PTA of 48.5 days or lesser is going to have higher functional independence at the time of discharge, PTA less than 34 days will have an overall good recovery, PTA less than 53 days will not require any assistance.

Ranchos Los Amigos Scale (RLAS) for cognition and behavior for individuals with head injury is often used with GCS to monitor the recovery from head injury. But, unlike GCS, the RLAS can be used even in the later stages to determine the cognition and behavioral recovery of an individual to know how efficiently he will be able to carry out the cognitive and physical tasks. The original RLAS had 8 levels; the revised scale, RLAS-R has 10 levels that give more comprehensive information especially with the higher levels of recovery **(Table 35.4)**.

INTERVENTIONS

Medical Intervention

The early care starts at the site of the accident by the mean of resuscitation. The purpose of giving this maneuver is to maintain the oxygen supply and blood flow to the brain. It will also help prevent secondary trauma to the brain. Once the individual arrives at the trauma center or medical emergency department, the vitals are stabilized first. The saturation of oxygen is kept above 90% and systolic blood pressure is maintained above 90 mm Hg. The cervical spine should be stabilized with the collar and the head is positioned at 30° elevation to prevent the rise in the ICP. Mannitol may be given as a drug of choice for raised ICP. The GCS is monitored regularly.

ICP monitoring not only helps to monitor ICP but also quantifies the cerebral perfusion pressure (CPP). ICP monitoring is indicated when the CT scan shows evidence

Table 35.2: Glasgow Outcome Scale and Glasgow Outcome Scale Extended.

GOS	GOSE	Interpretation
1 = Dead	1 = Dead	Dead
2 = Vegetative state	2 = Vegetative state	Absence of awareness of self and environment
3 = Severe disability	3 = Lower severe disability	Needs full assistance in ADL
	4 = Upper severe disability	Needs partial assistance in ADL
4 = Moderate disability	5 = Lower moderate disability	Independent, but cannot resume work/school or all previous social activities
	6 = Upper moderate disability	Some disability exists, but can partly resume work or previous activities
5 = Good recovery	7 = Lower good recovery	Minor physical or mental deficits that affects daily life
	8 = Upper good recovery	Full recovery or minor symptoms that do not affect daily life

(ADL: activities of daily living; GOS: Glasgow Outcome Scale, GOSE: Glasgow Outcome Scale Extended)

Table 35.4: Ranchos Los Amigos Scale—Revised.

Level	Response
Level I: No response: Total assistance	No response to external stimuli
Level II: Generalized response: Total assistance	• Responds inconsistently and nonpurposefully to external stimuli • Responses are often the same regardless of the stimulus
Level III: Localized response: Total assistance	• Responds inconsistently and specifically to external stimuli • Responses are directly related to the stimulus, e.g. patient withdraws or vocalizes to painful stimuli • Responds more to familiar people (friends and family) versus strangers
Level IV: Confused/agitated: Maximal assistance	• The individual is in a hyperactive state with bizarre and nonpurposeful behavior • Demonstrates agitated behavior that originates more from internal confusion than the external environment • Absent short-term memory
Level V: Confused, inappropriate nonagitated: Maximal assistance	• Shows increase in consistency with following and responding to simple commands • Responses are nonpurposeful and random to more complex commands • Behavior and verbalization are often inappropriate, and individual appears confused and often confabulates • If action or tasks is demonstrated, individual can perform but does not initiate tasks on own • Memory is severely impaired and learning new information is difficult • Different from level IV in that individual does not demonstrate agitation to internal stimuli. However, they can show agitation to unpleasant external stimuli
Level VI: Confused, appropriate: Moderate assistance	• Able to follow simple commands consistently • Able to retain learning for familiar tasks they performed preinjury (brushing teeth, washing face), however unable to retain learning for new tasks • Demonstrates increased awareness of self, situation, and environment but unaware of specific impairments and safety concerns • Responses may be incorrect secondary to memory impairments but appropriate to the situation
Level VII: Automatic, appropriate: Minimal assistance for daily living skills	• Oriented in familiar settings • Able to perform daily routine automatically with minimal to absent confusion • Demonstrates carry over for new tasks and learning in addition to familiar tasks • Superficially aware of one's diagnosis but unaware of specific impairments • Continues to demonstrate lack of insight, decreased judgment, and safety awareness • Beginning to show interest in social and recreational activities in structured settings • Requires at least minimal supervision for learning and safety purposes
Level VIII: Purposeful, appropriate: Standby assistance	• Consistently oriented to person, place, and time • Independently carries out familiar tasks in a nondistracting environment • Beginning to show awareness of specific impairments and how they interfere with tasks, however requires standing by assistance to compensate • Able to use assistive memory devices to recall daily schedule • Acknowledges other's emotional states and requires only minimal assistance to respond appropriately • Demonstrates improvement of memory and ability to consolidate the past and future events • Often depressed, irritable, and with low frustration threshold
Level IX: Purposeful, appropriate: Standby assistance on request	• Able to shift between different tasks and complete them independently • Aware of and acknowledges impairments when they interfere with tasks and able to use compensatory strategies to cope • Unable to independently anticipate obstacles that may arise secondary to impairment • With assistance able to think about consequences of actions and decisions • Acknowledges the emotional needs of others with standby assistance • Continues to demonstrate depression and low frustration threshold
Level X: Purposeful, appropriate: Modified independent	• Able to multitask in many different environments with extra time or devices to assist • Able to create own methods and tools for memory retention • Independently anticipates obstacles that may occur as a result of impairments and take corrective actions • Able to independently make decisions and act appropriately but may require more time or compensatory strategies • Demonstrate intermittent periods of depression and low frustration threshold when under stress • Able to appropriately interact with others in social situations

of brain swelling and large bifrontal contusion. It is also recommended when sedation is interrupted in order to examine the neurological functioning. It is recommended in individuals where neurological examinations are not as much reliable, e.g., maxillofacial trauma or spinal cord injury. It is also recommended in individuals who are already hypertensive and are to undergo craniotomy.

Any medical maneuver will not be able to reverse the changes caused by intracranial injury, but it can limit to a certain extent the secondary trauma resulting in inflammatory changes, expanding hematomas, cellular swelling, seizures, and systemic complications (i.e., hemodynamic or pulmonary changes, fever, pain). These issues can be addressed by analgesics, sedatives, anticonvulsants, hyperosmotic agents, etc. Tranexamic acid has been proven to be most effective in limiting the growth of hematomas following intracranial hemorrhage. Coagulopathy is one of the most common complications that may arise following traumatic head injury. Fresh frozen plasma, platelets, tranexamic acid, hypertonic saline (osmotic therapy) dextran, recombinant factor VIIa, etc., can be probable treatment options. Usage of corticosteroids is not recommended anymore for individuals with TBI. Hypothermia can be one of the complications following head injury, which can be effectively treated with diuretics and barbiturates.

If ICP is not controlled, coma-inducing drugs are given as brain in the state of coma requires less oxygen. Often following brain injury, the increased ICP compresses the blood vessels, hampering the blood supply to the brain. If the brain is put to the state of coma, it will be beneficial. Diuretics are another choice of drugs. They help reduce the swelling, which, in turn, reduces ICP by draining the fluid from the soft tissues. To prevent post-traumatic seizures, antiepileptic medicines are prescribed to individuals following head injury. Appropriate medicines for spasticity management and improvement of cognition can be added.

Surgical Intervention

Emergency surgery is often executed for head injury in order to prevent concomitant damage. The surgery is indicated in the presence of:

- Hematoma—removal of hematoma reduces pressure on the brain tissues
- Increased ICP—removal of part of skull to relieve pressure
- Skull fractures—removal of remains of fractured skull from brain tissues.

The surgical intervention in the form of craniotomy, craniectomy, burr hole surgery, or shunting is chosen depending on the ICP and CPP. Generally, ICP should be maintained <20 mm Hg and CPP should be maintained at ≥60 mm Hg. Ventriculostomy allows drainage of CSF and reduces ICP **(Box 35.1)**.

<table>
<tr><td>BOX 35.1: Cerebral perfusion pressure (CPP).</td></tr>
<tr><td>CPP is usually defined as the difference between mean arterial pressure and increased intracranial pressure (ICP) or central venous pressure, whichever is higher. CPP is easily monitored, and maintaining CPP to sustain adequate cerebral blood flow is crucial in traumatic brain injury management. Its level is up to 11 mm Hg in 30° head elevation, and increases with head elevation at higher angles. Reduced CPP leads to increased ischemia, vasodilation, ICP, and further reductions in CPP, a cycle leading to further neurologic injury.</td></tr>
</table>

REHABILITATION

The rehabilitation of head injury begins in the hospital, continues at an out-patient department (OPD) and in the community. Those with severe injuries and persistent vegetative state receive medical care and rehabilitation for longer period of time in hospital. Those who recover or who have less severe injuries continue their rehabilitation in different community settings.

The key is to have a holistic approach for the rehabilitation to attain maximum functional recovery. Since the condition includes spectrum of symptoms, the rehabilitation must include interdisciplinary team approach. The rehabilitation team should include the individual and the family, physician, speech and language pathologist, nurse, neuropsychologist, physiotherapist, occupational therapist, recreational therapist, and social worker. The role of physiotherapist in the initial stages of rehabilitation is to prevent secondary complications which can occur following prolonged immobilization. In the later stages, the therapist will focus on improving the level of arousal followed by functional recovery.

Physiotherapy Evaluation

The physiotherapy evaluation plays a vital role in deciding the management of an individual; hence, it is very important to first evaluate an individual thoroughly **(Table 35.2)**. It is of utmost importance to go through an individual's medical records. The individual may not be fully conscious or medically stable. Reviewing the medical records may give the therapist an idea about any nonneurological injuries such as musculoskeletal injuries or open wounds. Considering the complexity of the ailment, it may not be possible to assess entirely in a single session and consecutive therapy sessions as well might include continuum of the assessment.

The physiotherapy examination must include:

- Assessment of level of consciousness
- Vital signs
- Cognitive examination
- Communication
- Speech and language
- Integumentary integrity

Clinical Pearl

It is in the best interest of the individual with head injury that a therapist consults the team before beginning the assessment and change in the position of the individual, especially unconscious individuals. Slight change in the position also can lead to major variations in blood pressure.

- Sensory and motor functions
- Ventilation and respiratory status
- Status of bowel and bladder
- Functional status
- Changes in the functions of autonomic nervous system have to be taken into consideration such as hypotension/hypertension, excessive sweating, and dry scaly skin.
- Motor functions such as tone and strength get affected the most.
- Other movement disorders such as ataxia, apraxia, and dyskinesia also may be seen.
- Balance and vestibular functions will be affected.
- Almost 50% of individuals with brain injury experience pain and the most common site of pain is the head.

Physiotherapy Interventions

In the initial stage of injury, the goal of physiotherapy intervention is to improve the level of consciousness and improve the functional autonomy of the individual. As the rehabilitation progresses to the later stages, the goals become more precise based on individual's premorbid condition, vocation, environmental constraints, their family members' expectations, and wishes **(Box 35.2)**.

The outcome of the rehabilitation depends on age, intensity, duration, specificity and transfer of training, etc.

The interventions can be categorized mainly into three sets:

1. Restorative
2. Compensatory
3. Preventive.

In the initial stage of injury, where the individual may not be able move, the interventions are largely preventive.

Prevention of Secondary Complications

Contractures, pressure sores, deep vein thrombosis (DVT), pneumonia, etc., can hinder progress in the rehabilitation and so it is important to prevent them. Proper positioning can prevent the skin breakdown, contractures, respiratory complications and help improve the muscle tone. The head should be kept in neutral position, and hips and knees should be kept in slightly flexed position. The range of motion (ROM) of all the joints should be monitored regularly in order to prevent contractures. Regular relaxed

passive movements can help in maintaining the properties of the muscles. If required, splinting can be used for positioning. The signs of DVT should be monitored. If there are signs of inflammation such as swelling, redness, pain appearing only on one leg, the individual can be suspected for DVT. The part should be immobilized and the anticoagulation therapy can be started. To prevent respiratory complications, regular chest physiotherapy and bronchial hygiene can be given. Modifying postural drainage positioning for head injury should be given as in most of the cases, the head-down position is contraindicated till an individual is medical stable and has regularized ICP.

Skin breakdown can be prevented by frequent turning in the bed. It is recommended that the individual should be repositioned every 2 hours in order to prevent pressure sores. Additionally, air bed or water bed can also be used. The skin should be kept clean and dry. And if there is bowel or bladder incontinence, the individual should be catheterized. Soiling leads to maceration of the skin which can lead to pressure ulcer.

If the individual has to be positioned in the wheelchair, the position of the head and neck has to be maintained in neutral position. A cushion can be used in the wheelchair to prevent the pressure in the pelvic region. Mobilizing of the individual as early as possible should be aimed at, considering the benefits of early mobilization of improved alertness, circulation, and ROM. Tilt table can be used to prevent orthostatic hypotension. The measures taken for the prevention of secondary complications are continued in the active rehabilitation phase.

Sensory Stimulation

Individuals with coma or decreased arousal are provided with multisensory stimulation in order to activate the reticular formation and in turn improve their level of consciousness. Various sensory stimuli to stimulate olfactory, gustatory, auditory, visual, kinesthetic, tactile, and vestibular senses are used in disciplined manner to arouse an individual. There is a lack of concrete evidence to provide a protocol to be used for sensory stimulation for individuals with head injury. If the individual remains to be in low level of arousal even at the time of discharge, the sensory stimulation has to be continued by the caregivers.

Active Rehabilitation

The examination of an individual continues as the individual enters the active rehabilitation stage. At this stage, there are chances of individuals having disorientation, confusion, memory deficits, aggression, lack of attention, etc. The examination and intervention have to be carried out considering the above deficits. The tests and measures used for individuals with head injury are listed in **Table 35.5**.

BOX 35.2: Goals of management.

While setting the goal, the therapist should keep the goals: **S**pecific, **M**easurable, **A**chievable, **R**elevant and **T**imed (SMART)

Table 35.5: Outcome measures and tests used for individuals with head injury.

Area of assessment	Outcome measure/test
Balance and mobility	Berg Balance Scale Community Balance and Mobility Scale Functional Independence Measure
Cognition	Moss Attention Rating Scale Trail Making test—B
Orientation and memory	Galveston Orientation and Amnesia Test
Safety	Supervision Rating Scale
Behavior	Neurobehavioral Rating Scale
Gait	Observational Gait Analysis Rancho Los Amigos Observational gait Analysis
Endurance	6-Minute Walk Test
Dual-task performance	Modified Walking and Remembering Test

The goals of active rehabilitation phase will depend on:

- If the individual is able to follow one step, two steps or multistep commands?
- Is he oriented to time, place, person, and circumstances?

The rehabilitation will start by educating the individual and the family about the current condition and the prognosis.

Education of the Individual with Head Injury, Caregivers and Family

The nature of ailment and its complexity has to be explained to the individual, caregivers, and family. If an individual has a cognitive deficit, he may not understand or learn the new information conveyed to them. In such scenarios, it becomes important to educate family members and caregivers. It is sometimes difficult for the family members to understand why the individual is behaving in a certain way. He may show aggression or lack of interest or attention. They may not be able to carry over the information which is conveyed to them. One must also make them understand to take care of the individual's safety. Lack of neuromotor control and sufficient insight from individual may put him at additional risk of injury.

Joint Integrity and Mobility

It is maintained by different mobilization, manipulation, and other musculoskeletal techniques. The joints that are prone to contractures are stretched regularly such as hip, knee, and ankle. Ankles are stretched to the maximum available ROM in order to prevent contracture. Serial casting can be used as an effective treatment for maintaining ROM of the joint **(Fig. 35.1)**. The resting splints can be used for maintenance for joint ROM and prevention of contractures for individuals with head injury.

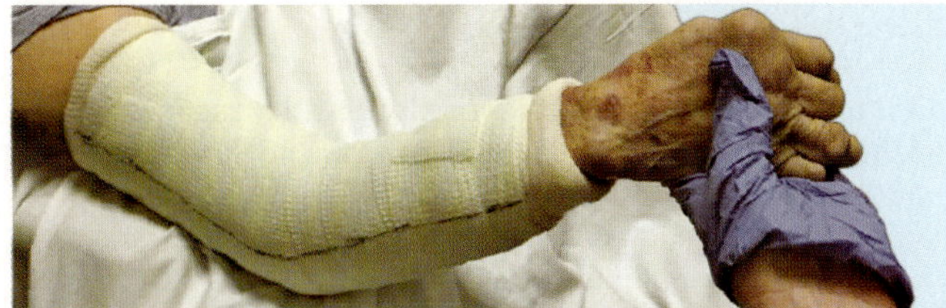

Fig. 35.1: Serial casting to maintain joint ROM and prevent contractures.

Muscle Tone

Spasticity is a common occurrence following head injury. It can be managed with the combination of pharmacological and nonpharmacological interventions. Pharmacological interventions include baclofen, botulinum toxin A, clonidine, dantrolene sodium, tizanidine, and phenol injection, whereas nonpharmacological interventions include casting, splinting, stretching, strengthening, transcutaneous electric nerve stimulation (TENS), Bobath technique, weight bearing, gait training, and seating. These interventions aim to relax the muscle by reducing overactivity of the muscle and lengthen them.

Motor Function (Motor Control and Motor Learning)

To reestablish the motor learning, initially a distributed model of learning is implemented. The sessions are well planned with several practice sets distributed across the session. In the initial stages, mental as well as physical fatigue hinders the performance of an individual, and hence, the signs of fatigue have to be identified and enough rest periods should be given. Signs of physical fatigue can be deteriorated performance, whereas signs of mental fatigue can be irritability, aggression, lack of attention, and delay in initiation.

The feedback should be given at regular intervals. Knowledge of performance is more effective in the initial stages of learning compared to knowledge of result. Visual feedback in the form of video performance of an individual performing activity can provide an insight into an individual on how he is currently performing an activity. These self-generated insights help in better learning. If the individual has cognitive deficits, augmented feedback should be provided to an individual. As the learning improves, the frequency of feedback should be reduced to make sure the individual does not develop feedback dependency.

In the initial stages, the restorative approach can be focused upon but if the injury is severe, and there are less chances of an individual becoming functionally independent, the compensatory approach is adapted. Most of the cases will require balanced approach between compensatory and restorative strategies, as most recent evidences suggest that opting for compensatory approach may cause "nonuse" of affected arm, which may lessen the potential of recovery in an individual. Choosing an approach will also depend on individual's physical capabilities, and environment barriers and facilitators.

In restorative approaches, the task-oriented approach has proven to be beneficial in individuals with brain injury. It is in line with current motor control and learning theories. The task that is important and meaningful for an individual serves to be more beneficial in inducing neuroplastic changes. Locomotor training using body-weight support **(Fig. 35.2)** has proven to be effective in individuals with stroke, and it does have very sound theatrical base, but the discrete strictures are not available for the individuals with head injury. The locomotor training using body-weight support system did not prove to be more beneficial than conventional gait training. The locomotor training using body-weight support can also be used for cardiovascular endurance training. It can be done using a treadmill as well **(Fig. 35.3)**. Functional electrical stimulation (FES) can be given with locomotor training using body-weight

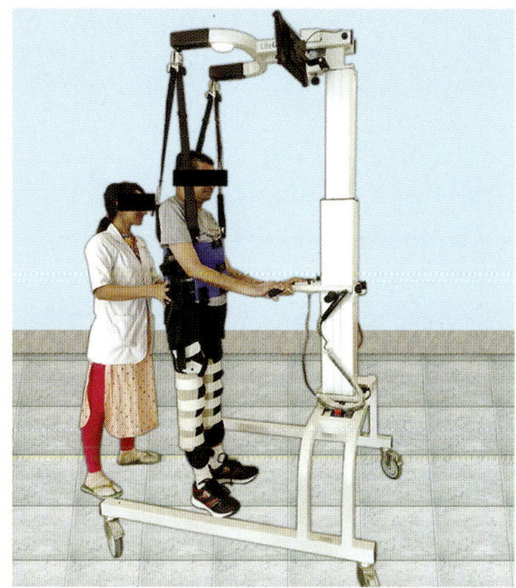

Fig. 35.2: Locomotor training using body-weight support.
Courtesy: Mission Health, Ahmedabad

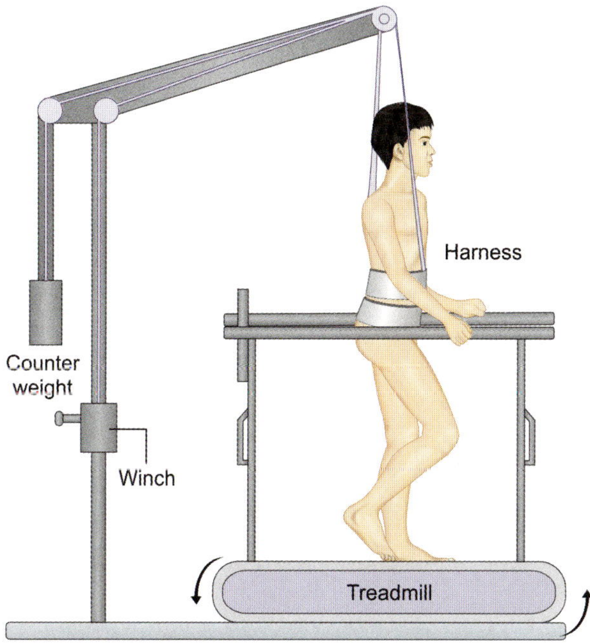

Fig. 35.3: Body-weight support treadmill training.

support as an adjunct to task-oriented approach. FES can be used for grasping, locomotor training, sit to stand training, bladder voiding, etc.

Constraint-induced movement therapy is an approach used most frequently for individuals with stroke. Following its theoretical principles, the same can be used for individuals with head injury. It requires constraining the unaffected upper extremity for almost 90% of the awake time for a period of 2–3 weeks. When using this approach for an individual with brain injury, cognitive impairment has to be considered by the caregivers.

Aerobic Capacity and General Fitness

The protocol should be designed after considering the individual's physical and cognitive capabilities. Traditional ways of endurance training such as jogging, cycling, running, swimming, and elliptical training can be used. Circuit training can also be beneficial. The intensity can be kept between 60 and 90% according to the age-predicted maximum heart rate; duration can vary from 20 to 40 minutes per session for three to four times a week. or it can be modified as per the rate of perceived exertion, maintaining it at mild to moderate.

Muscle Performance (Strength, Power, Endurance)

There are not enough evidences providing effects of strength and power training for individuals with head injury. Strength training improves force production capacity of the muscle in individuals with stroke and Parkinson's disease. It is also useful for postural correction and balance. With the same line of thought, it is implemented in individuals with head injury also. Strength training should be given as three sets of 8–12 repetitions with 10 repetitions maximum, two to three times a week.

Postural Control and Balance

The aim of postural control and balance training is to achieve symmetrical balanced weight bearing for a longer duration. Due to head injury, the individuals might show more weight bearing toward one side compared to the other which also makes them prone for falls. The weight bearing can be corrected by making them focus in the center and shifting their weight to the affected side. Stability can be induced by rhythmic stabilization of proprioceptive neuromuscular facilitation (PNF) technique.

The weak muscles can be strengthened to promote the postural control. Elastic resistance bands can be used to enhance proprioceptive loading. For modified plantigrade position **(Fig. 35.4)**, the bands can be used around forearm, which promotes contraction of shoulder stabilizers. While standing, the bands can be tied around ankle to promote greater contractions of proximal muscles.

For dynamic control, weight shifting and perturbations can be practiced. Challenging the limits of stability in all directions, while shifting the weight **(Figs. 35.5A and B)** enhances the dynamic postural control. Progression can be made by reach outs **(Fig. 35.6)** and stepping activities.

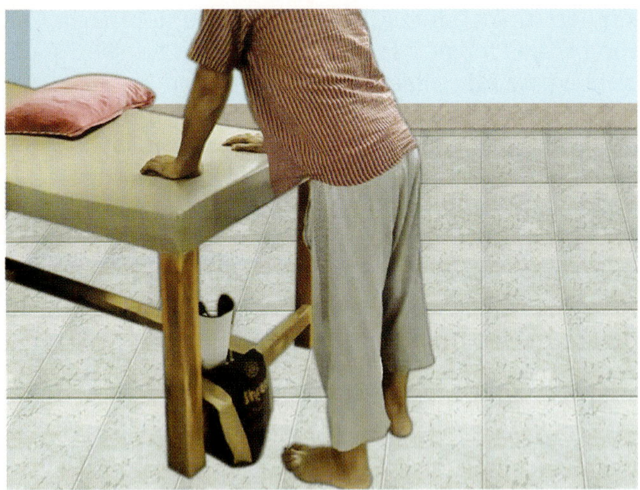

Fig. 35.4: Modified plantigrade position.

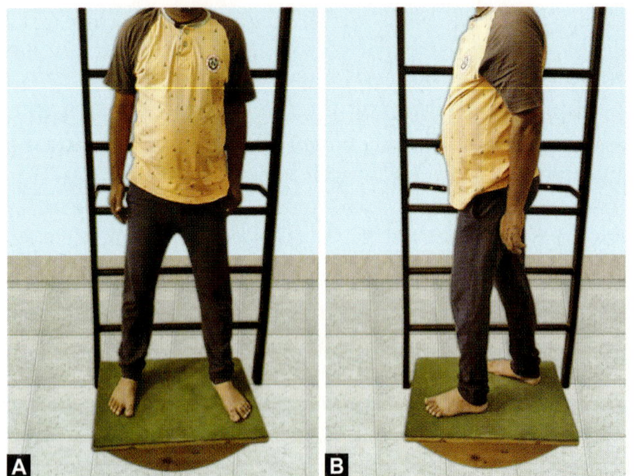

Figs. 35.5A and B: Dynamic balance training on balance board:
(A) Lateral weight shifts; (B) Anteroposterior weight shifts.

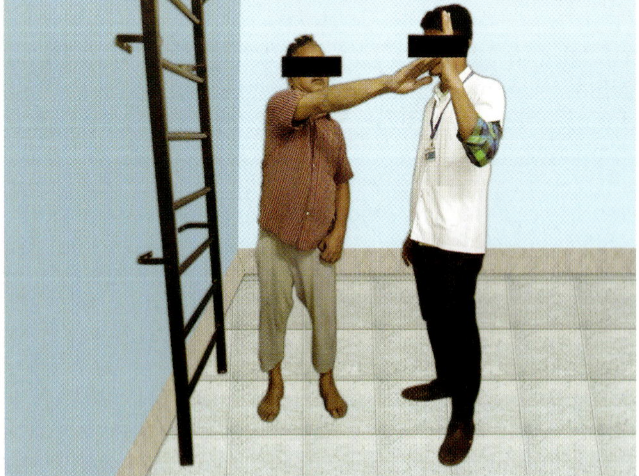

Fig. 35.6: Reach outs in standing for balance training.

In sitting, an individual can be made to practice chopping and reverse chopping pattern of PNF to promote upper limb motor control as well as dynamic postural control. Sitting on therapy ball and gently moving in front-back

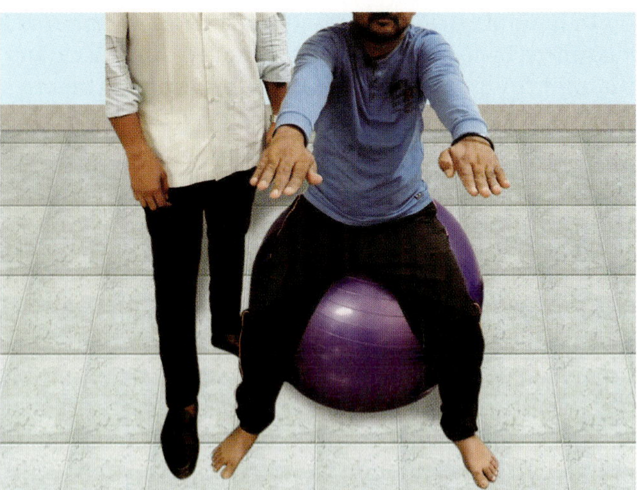

Fig. 35.7: Balance training on vestibular ball.

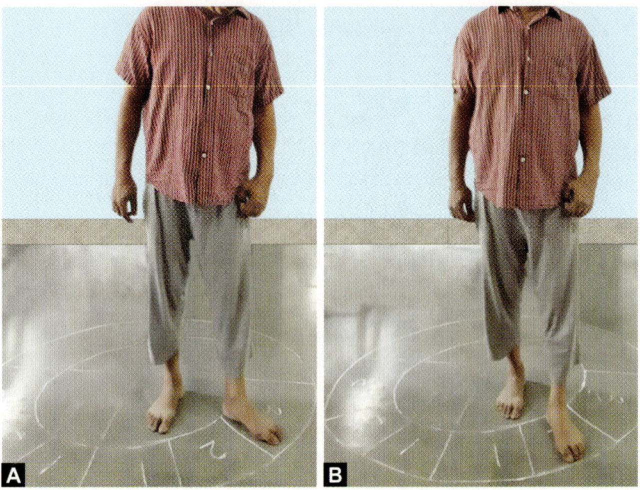

Figs. 35.8A and B: Frenkel exercises.

and side-to-side directions promotes recruitment of trunk muscles **(Fig. 35.7)**. Other activities such as catching and throwing the ball, kicking a ball can be practiced as a progression. While performing the activities, making the patient learn the number forward or backward, or counting backward can be practiced to promote dual-task training, or training for cognitive functions. Other techniques such as Frenkel exercises, obstacle training, and one-leg standing can also be used **(Figs. 35.8 to 35.10)**.

The equilibrium tests for coordination can be used to assess the equilibrium in an individual, such as standing with narrow base of support with eyes open and then close, tandem standing, tandem walking, walking sideways, and braiding. These same tests can be used as repetitive exercises for enhancing equilibrium.

Sensory Awareness and Skin Integrity

The sensory deficits are drawn attention to and individuals are asked to compensate it by vision. Patients with proprioceptive losses tend to develop impairments in balance, movement control, and motor learning. Tapping, verbal cueing, or biofeedback can be given as an adjunct.

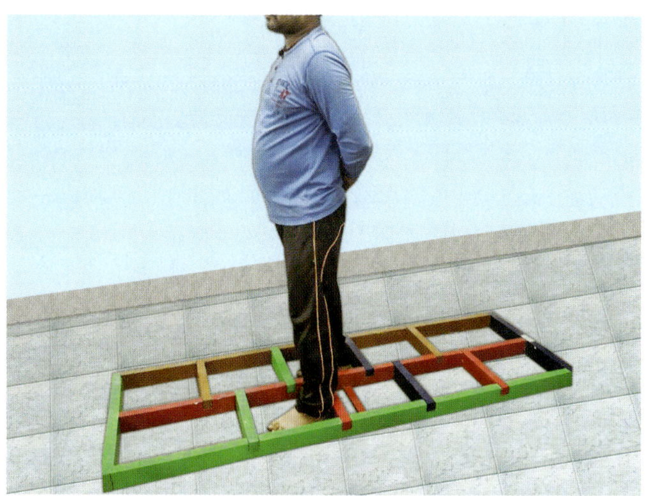

Fig. 35.9: Obstacle walking.

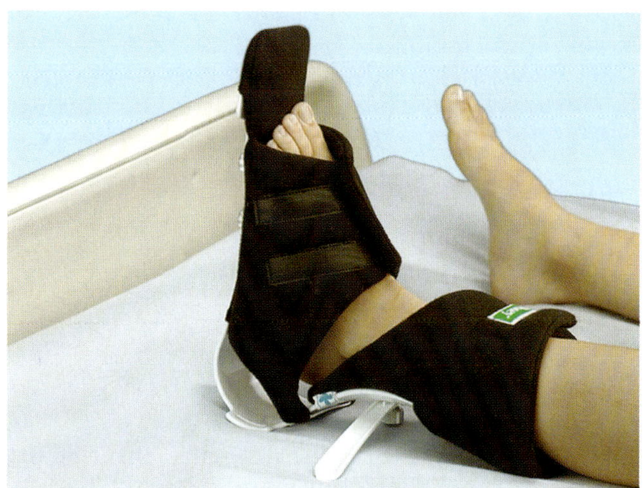

Fig. 35.11: Multipodus boot.

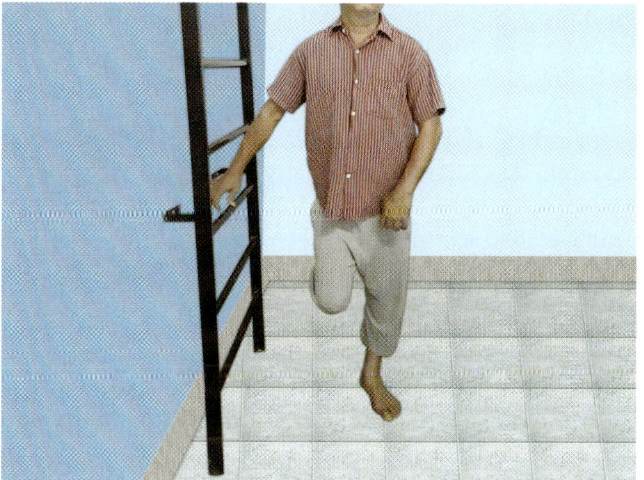

Fig. 35.10: One-leg standing.

Individuals with visual impairment may experience exacerbation of symptoms in low light. They are instructed to maintain sufficient light at all times. Double vision can be managed by providing an eye patch to the individual, but it may prevent the adaptation by the nervous system and disturb the depth perception, so it should not be used for prolonged time. Usage of strong contrast colors can be utilized for stairs.

For tactile deficits, the skin should be kept clean and dry. Soiling should be prevented and, if occurs, should be cleaned immediately. Regular inspection of the skin should be carried out. Multipodus boots are often used to prevent skin breakdown at heel (**Fig. 35.11**). Clothing should be loose and comfortable, and the seams, buttons, or pockets should not compress the pressure prone areas. The individual should be made aware about the tactile deficit and asked to be cautious about touching sharp and hot objects.

Cognitive and Behavioral Training

The purpose of cognitive therapy following head injury is to enhance the cognitive abilities of an individual for him to process the information and carry out mental tasks with ease. The cognitive therapy has two types of approach—the remedial (restorative) and compensatory. Remedial approach includes practicing the task repetitively with gradually increasing difficulty until it is mastered. Compensatory approach includes by-passing the lost function. The functions that are lost are specifically trained with task-specific approach. For attention, attention-training programs are given which include all types of attention such as focused, sustained, divided, and alternating. The training consists of visual and auditory inputs with varying degrees of attention requirements. For memory, mnemonics, memory drills, computer-assisted memory programs, mobile applications–assisted programs can be given. For language, constraint-induced aphasia therapy, computer-assisted therapy, melodic intonation therapy, and neurostimulation techniques, such as transcranial direct current stimulation, have proven to be effective for dysarthria and aphasia following head injury. Certain dopaminergic agents such as bromocriptine and amantadine have proven benefits for cognitive functions. Cognitive–behavioral therapy, dialectical behavior, mind-fulness, and acceptance and commitment therapies can be used for the behavioral issues of individuals with head injury.

Bladder and Bowel Training

When in active phase, intermittent catheterization is considered to be a gold standard treatment for bladder incontinence as compared to the other methods of catheterization, as it has less chances of infection. Fluid management, micturition schedule, and positive reinforcement establish better bladder management program. During 24 hours approximately 2,500 cm^3 of fluid is required, unless otherwise indicated. During morning and early afternoon, from 7 AM to 3 PM, overhydration by the fluid intake of 1,300 cm^3 allows the feeling of fullness of bladder to an individual. This helps in establishing frequency and satisfaction. From late afternoon to early evening, 3 PM to 7 PM, 1,000 cm^3 fluid is given. About 200 cm^3 is given between 7 PM and 7 AM ensuring undisturbed

Date	Void	7A	9A	11A	1P	3P	5P	7P	9P	11P	3A	Comments
	Incontinent											
	Positive reinforcement											
	Void											
	Incontinent											
	Positive reinforcement											
	Void											
	Incontinent											
	Positive reinforcement											

Table 35.6: Micturition schedule.

rest. Voiding is scheduled every 2 hours, ensuring the documentation of the voiding in the chart **(Table 35.6)**, also documenting any episode of incontinence in between the voiding schedule. **Table 35.6** can be used for this. With every successful effort of voiding on schedule, a positive reinforcement can be given in verbal or nonverbal form. Verbal reinforcements can be "good job," "nice," etc. Nonverbal forms can be gentle smile, or a nod, sticker on the schedule chart, favorite dish or candy. Though these reinforcements feel little for the caregivers, it may mean more to an individual with head injury.

At the time of admission approximately, 82% of individuals face bowel incontinence, and at the time of discharge, 36% still have some bowel impairment. Like bladder program, an effective bowel program can be made to establish a routine. Documentation of bowel evacuation should be done. Few of the steps an individual can follow for effective bowel management are:

1. Setting a routine for bowel evacuation, using toilet at the same time everyday, like after a shower or after a meal.
2. Using toilet for 15–45 minutes, and gently rubbing the lower abdominal area which can help in movement of the stool in colon.
3. Using suppositories in beginning help in establishing bowel movement.
4. Taking fiber-rich food and staying active as much as possible also helps prevent constipation.

Return to Play/Activity

Cognitive rest is required till the time an individual recovers from the symptoms. Like physical activities, cognitive activities can aggravate the symptoms. The activities should be gradually progressed as one step at a time and 24 hours should be given to recover from the activity; in the meantime, if an individual experiences worsening of the symptoms, the activity is stopped and the individual is allowed to recover further.

Community Reentry

Individuals with good motor and cognitive recovery are progressed to community reentry programs. The individuals are made to stay in the community environment such as school or workplace for 4–5 days in a week and return home in the afternoon. Providing cognitive, social, and physical training to the individual in the same environment where they are expected to be can bring better recovery and build self-responsibility in an individual that improves his decision-making capabilities.

If the modifications at home are required, then it can be done with the instructions of the therapists such as installing elevators or lifts, enlarging doorways to allow wheelchair passage, modifying kitchens for easier meal preparation, and installing emergency communication systems. Assistive devices such as canes, crutches, walker, or wheelchair can be prescribed to an individual as per their requirements to aid mobility **(Fig. 35.12)**. A magnifying glass to assist with reading; a touch-fastener grip attached to a pen or fork for eating or writing; a special telephone to help with speech and hearing problems; braces or splints to support weak joints or to limit joint contractures; calendar, memory notebook, or other memory aid for tracking appointments, planning, and organizing; eye patches or prism glasses to help with vision problems; and special beds to help limit skin breakdown and pressure sores, or to help with improving circulation, etc. can be prescribed to make an individual functionally independent.

The smartphones can be used as an aid for individuals with head injury. The memory apps/organizational apps and higher communication apps can be used for the better functional outcomes. The smartphone apps can also help

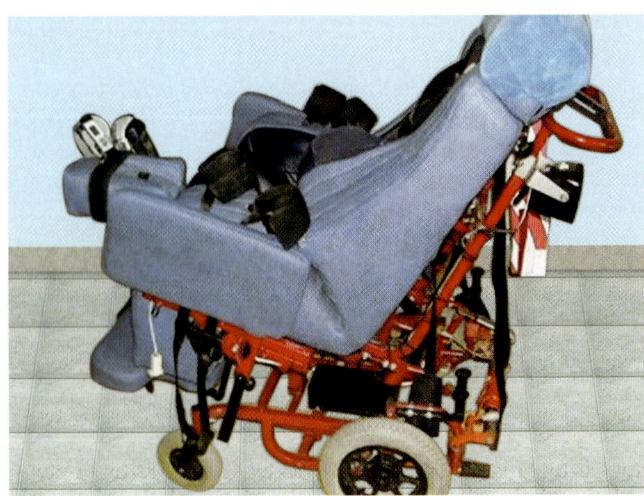

Fig. 35.12: Power-control wheelchair for an individual with head injury.

an individual in setting up a reminder for taking medicines, managing appointments, etc. The therapists can instruct the individual on using smartphone and can as well help the user to learn to use certain applications if the user interface is difficult. The therapists can as well instruct individuals on using apps that can help in improving their functions. The social media apps can provide a better opportunity for social interaction.

SUMMARY

Head injury is a devastating condition affecting physical, cognitive, social, and psychological aspects of an individual's life to a great extent. The role of a physiotherapist is to maximize the potential of an individual in collaboration with his family, caregivers, and other team members to improve the QoL of an individual and that of the caregivers and family members. Maximizing the physical activities and social participation can be rewarding to an individual with head injury and will encourage him further for community participation.

Case Scenario

CASE STUDY

Aditya, a 35-year-old software engineer, met with a RTA. His motorbike was hit by a car that propelled Aditya off the bike. He was thrown to the road divider and his helmet broke due to the impact. At accident site, GCS is 6 (E1 V2 M3). He lives with his wife and son (age 4 years), in a two storied house. He is a sports enthusiast, plays cricket with his friends weekly, and in his spare time enjoys biking. No significant past medical history. Investigation showed mild subdural hematoma, moderate right intracranial bleed, large depressed right skull fracture, right clavicle fracture, and fourth rib fracture. Diffuse brain swelling. He was operated with right hemicraniectomy for removal of hematoma. Tracheostomy tube placed 4 days following injury.

Two months post injury, tracheostomy tube was removed, GCS is 10 (E4 V2 M4). The tone was decreased on the left side; he was unable to participate in manual muscle testing, coordination, range of motion (ROM), and sensory examination. Reflexes were diminished, and plantar response was upgoing on the left side. Six months post injury, on the left side, the tone has increased, muscle power is 2/5, coordination is impaired, restricted shoulder ROM flexion 110, abduction 90, and both external and internal rotations 40. Elbow and wrist have full ROM. Reacts to tactile stimulation but does not participate in formal sensory examination. Reflexes are increased. The blood pressure stays within normal limits, needs supervision with bed mobility, contact guard with transfers and gait.

Guiding Questions:

1. Considering the information you have, list out the impairments, activity limitation, and participation restrictions.
2. What outcome measures will you use for Aditya? Why?
3. Considering family support, environment, equipment, and further rehabilitation needs, plan a discharge for Aditya.
4. Plan out management for Aditya during his active rehabilitation phase.
5. What home-care plan would you give to Aditya?

Review Questions

1. List out the various classifications of head injury.
2. List out primary and secondary impairments of head injury.
3. How will you assess the level of consciousness in individuals in head injury?
4. How will you monitor the recovery in individuals' head injury?
5. Discuss the importance of interdisciplinary management for individual with head injury.
6. What measures will you take to prevent secondary complications in individuals with head injury?
7. How will you draw a plan of care for individuals with head injury?

BIBLIOGRAPHY

1. Al-Hassani A, Strandvik GF, El-Menyar A, et al. Functional outcomes in moderate-to-severe traumatic brain injury survivors. J Emerg Trauma Shock. 2018;11(3):197-204.
2. Alderson P, Roberts I. Corticosteroids for acute traumatic brain injury. Cochrane Database Syst Rev. 2005;(1):CD000196.
3. Arumugam A, A Rahman NA, Theophilus SC, et al. Tranexamic acid as antifibrinolytic agent in non traumatic intracerebral hemorrhages. Malays J Med Sci. 2015;22(Spec Issue):62-71.
4. Asikainen I, Kaste M, Sarna S. Early and late posttraumatic seizures in traumatic brain injury rehabilitation patients: brain injury factors causing late seizures and influence of seizures on long-term outcome. Epilepsia. 1999;40(5):504-9.
5. Barman A, Chatterjee A, Bhide R. Cognitive impairment and rehabilitation strategies after traumatic brain injury. Indian J Psychol Med. 2016;38(3):172-81.
6. Bricolo A, Turazzi S, Alexandre A, et al. Decerebrate rigidity in acute head injury. J Neurosurg. 1977;47(5):680-9.
7. Brwon TH, Mount J, Rouland BL, et al. Body weight-supported treadmill training versus conventional gait training for people with chronic traumatic brain injury. J Head Trauma Rehabil. 2005;20(5):402-15.
8. Budashevski BG, Balashov AN. Decerebrate rigidity in craniocerebral injuries (clinico-statistical analysis), Zh Vopr Neirokhir Im N N Burdenko. 1986;(4):14-19.
9. Chang B, Lowenstein D. Practice parameter: antiepileptic drug prophylaxis in severe traumatic brain injury: report of the quality standards subcommittee of the American Academy of Neurology. Neurology. 2003;60(1):10-6.
10. Clement M. Imaging of brain trauma. Radiol Clin North Am. 2019;57(4):733-44.
11. Copley J, Kuipers K, Fleming J, et al. Individualised resting hand splints for adults with acquired brain injury: a randomized, single blinded, single case design. NeuroRehabilitation. 2013;32(4):885-98.
12. Dhandapani S, Manju D, Sharma B, et al. Prognostic significance of age in traumatic brain injury. J Neurosci Rural Pract. 2012;3(2):131.
13. Doolin Carver M. Adaptive equipment to assist with one-handed intermittent self-catheterization: a case study of a patient with multiple brain injuries. Am J Occup Ther. 2009;63(3):333-6.

14. Grinspun D. Bladder management for adults following head injury. Rehabil Nurs. 1993;18:300-5.

15. Gururaj G. Epidemiology of traumatic brain injuries: Indian scenario. Neurol Res. 2002;24(1):24-8.

16. Gómez-de-Regil L, Estrella-Castillo DF, Vega-Cauich J. Psychological intervention in traumatic brain injury patients. Behav Neurol. 2019;2019:6937832.

17. Hammond FM, Meghen MJ. Venous thromboembolism in the patient with acute traumatic brain injury: screening, diagnosis, prophylaxis and treatment issues. J Head Trauma Rehabil. 1998;13(1):36.

18. Han J, King N, Neilson S, et al. External validation of the CRASH and IMPACT prognostic models in severe traumatic brain injury. J Neurotrauma. 2014;31(13):1146-52.

19. Head injuries: mechanisms, diagnosis and management. Ann Intern Med. 1959;50(1):241.

20. Hellweg S, Johannes S. Physiotherapy after traumatic brain injury: a systematic review of the literature. Brain Inj. 2008;22(5):365-73.

21. Hendricks H, Heeren A, Vos P. Dysautonomia after severe traumatic brain injury. Eur J Neurol. 2010;17(9):1172-7.

22. Jaffrey R. Management of head and neck injury, 1st edition, Churchill Livingstone, Australia: Elsevier; 2012. pp. 150-76.

23. Kalisky Z, Morrison DP, Meyers CA, et al. Medical problems encountered during rehabilitation of patients with head injury. Arch Phys Med Rehabil. 1985;66(1):25-9.

24. Leary SM, Liu C, Cheesman AL, et al. Incontinence after brain injury: prevalence, outcome and multidisciplinary management on a neurological rehabilitation unit. Clin Rehabil. 2006;20(12):1094-9. https://doi.org/10.1177/0269215506071258.

25. Le Roux P. Chapter 15: Intracranial pressure monitoring and management. In: Laskowitz D, Grant G (Eds). Translational research in traumatic brain injury. Boca Raton, FL: CRC Press/Taylor and Francis Group; 2016. Available from https://www.ncbi.nlm.nih.gov/books/NBK326713/.

26. Lin K, Wroten M. Ranchos Los Amigos. [Updated 2019 May 29]. In: StatPearls [Internet]. Treasure Island, FL: StatPearls Publishing; 2019. Available from https://www.ncbi.nlm.nih.gov/books/NBK448151/.

27. Lombardi F, Taricco M, De Tabti A, et al. Sensory stimulation for brain injured individuals in coma and vegetative state. Cochrane Database Syst Rev. 2002;(2):CD001427.

28. Losiniecki A, Shutter L. Curr Treat Options Neurol. 2010;12:142. https://doi.org/10.1007/s11940-010-0063-z.

29. Maegele M. Coagulopathy after traumatic brain injury: incidence, pathogenesis, and treatment options. Transfusion. 2013;53:28S-37S.

30. Main KL, Soman S, Pestilli F, et al. DTI measures identify mild and moderate TBI cases among patients with complex health problems: a receiver operating characteristic analysis of US veterans. NeuroImage: Clinical. 2017;16:1-16.

31. McCrory P, Meeuwisse W, Johnston K, et al. Consensus statement on concussion in sports. The 3rd international conference on concussion in sports held in Zurich, November 2008. Br J Sports Med. 2009;43 (Suppl. 1):76.

32. Morris DM, Taub E, Mark VW. Contraint induced movement therapy: characterizing the intervention protocol. Eura Medicophys. 2006;42(3):257.

33. Mossberg KA, Amonette WE, Masel BE. Endurance training and cardiorespiratory conditioning after traumatic brain injury. J Head Trauma Rehabil. 2010;25(3):173.

34. Murthy TVSP, Bhatia P, Sandhu K, et al. Secondary brain injury: prevention and intensive care management. Indian J Neurotrauma (IJNT). 2005;2(1):7-12.

35. Nampiaparampil DE. Prevalence of chronic pain after traumatic brain injury: a systematic review. JAMA. 2008;300(6):711.

36. Ozer AB, Demirel I, Bayar MK, et al. Locked-in syndrome caused by the pressure exerted by the sound gun. Saudi J Anaesth. 2014;8(Suppl 1):S109-12.

37. O'Suilleabhain P, Dewey RB Jr. Movement disorders after head injury: diagnosis and management. J Head Trauma Rehabil. 2004;19(4):305-13.

38. O'Sullivan S, Schmitz T, Fulk G. Physical rehabilitation, 6th edition. Philadelphia, PA: FA Davis; 2014. pp. 859-88.

39. Palmer-McLean K, Harbst KB. Stroke and brain injury. In: Durstine JL, Moore GE (Eds). ACSM's exercise management for persons with chronic diseases and disabilities. Champaign, IL: American College of Sports Medicine; 2003.

40. Safaz I, Alaca R, Yasar E, et al. Medical complications, physical function and communication skills in patients with traumatic brain injury: a single centre 5-year experience. Brain Inj. 2008;22(10):733-9.

41. Satyajit Toshniwal S, Amey Joshi N. Residual speech impairment in patients with traumatic brain injury. Indian J Neurotrauma. 2010;7(1):61-6.

42. Shaefi S, Mittel AM, Hyam JA, et al. Hypothermia for severe traumatic brain injury in adults: recent lessons from randomized controlled trials. Surg Neurol Int. 2016;7:103.

43. Sharma DA, Chevidikunnan MF, Khan FR, et al. Effectiveness of knowledge of result and knowledge of performance in the learning of a skilled motor activity by healthy young adults. Phys Ther Sci. 2016;28(5):1482-6.

44. Shumway-Cook A, Woolacott MH. Motor control: translating research into practice, 4th edition. Philadelphia, PA: Lippincott Williams & Wilkins; 2012.

45. Stein R, Everaert D, Thompson A, et al. Long-term therapeutic and orthotic effects of a foot drop stimulator on walking performance in progressive and nonprogressive neurological disorders. Neurorehabil Neural Repair. 2009;24(2):152-67.

46. Synnot A, Chau M, Pitt V, et al. Interventions for managing skeletal muscle spasticity following traumatic brain injury. Cochrane Database Syst Rev. 2017;11(11):CD008929.

47. Tindall SC. Chapter 57: Level of consciousness. In: Walker HK, Hall WD, Hurst JW (Eds). Clinical methods: the history, physical, and laboratory examinations, 3rd edition. Boston, MA: Butterworths; 1990. Available from https://www.ncbi.nlm.nih.gov/books/NBK380/.

48. Wakai A, McCabe A, Roberts I, et al. Mannitol for acute traumatic brain injury. Cochrane Database Syst Rev. 2013;(8):CD001049.

49. Wong D, Sinclair K, Seabrook E, et al. Smartphones as assistive technology following traumatic brain injury: a preliminary study of what helps and what hinders. Disabil Rehabil. 2016;39(23):2387-94.

Post-polio Syndrome

Megha S Sheth, Srishti S Sharma

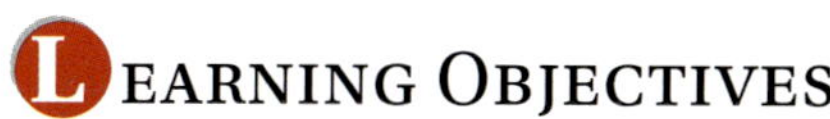 LEARNING OBJECTIVES

After reading this chapter, the readers should be able to:
- Gain knowledge about poliomyelitis
- Learn the definition of post-polio syndrome (PPS) and various theories associated with its etiology
- Understand the clinical features associated with PPS
- Develop clinical reasoning to confirm its diagnosis
- Learn the medical management options in PPS
- Understand the role of physiotherapy in PPS and to enable the formulation of an effective plan of care for a subject with PPS.

CHAPTER OUTLINE

- Acute poliomyelitis
- History of post-polio syndrome
- Pathophysiology of post-polio syndrome
- Diagnosing post-polio syndrome
  - Step 1: evaluating the symptoms
- Step 2: elimination of other possible diseases
- Step 3: fulfilling the diagnostic criteria
- Assessment of post-polio syndrome
- Management of post-polio syndrome
- Medical management
- Rehabilitative management
- Aerobic training
- Hydrotherapy
- Chest physiotherapy
- Orthoses/assistive devices

ACUTE POLIOMYELITIS

Polio, or poliomyelitis, is an infectious viral disease caused by an enterovirus of the picornavirus family—poliovirus that can strike at any age and affect a person's nervous system. Between the late 1940s and early 1950s, polio crippled around 35,000 people each year in the United States alone, making it one of the most feared diseases of the twentieth century. The polio vaccine was first introduced in 1955; its use since then has eradicated polio from the United States. As a result of the global effort to eradicate the disease, only three countries (Afghanistan, Nigeria, and Pakistan) remain polio-endemic as of February 2012, down from more than 125 in 1988. Nigeria was also declared polio-free in 2015.

The three strains (serotypes of wild poliovirus—types 1, 2, and 3—each with a slightly different capsid protein) of paralytic poliomyelitis spread primarily through feco–oral route, entering through mouth, and replicates in pharynx and gastrointestinal tract, invading local lymphatic tissue. **Table 36.1** shows the phases of polio. It generally presents as fever, sore throat, diarrhea, and vomiting caused by the virus's invasion of the gastrointestinal tract. In few cases, the virus attacks the anterior horn cells and invades the spinal cord, causing inflammation in the spinal cord and sometimes also in the motor neurons of the brainstem, asymmetric flaccid paresis or paralysis with varying degrees of severity, reaching its peak in 48 hours, and sometimes associated to a respiratory and bulbar affection causing breathing and swallowing disorders.

Following this acute infection, there is a slow and progressive "recovery" phase. The recovery phase, optimized by physical rehabilitation, leads to a "sequel-related impairment" with residual muscular atrophy that can vary according to the individual subject and topography. These impairments are considered stable. This is the stage of residual poliomyelitis **(Table 36.1)**.

Clinically, polio is divided into four types—*paralytic, non-paralytic, subclinical, and abortive.*
- The most severely affected individuals usually die because of the bulbar affection.

Table 36.1: Phases of acute poliomyelitis.

Phases of acute poliomyelitis	Presentation
Acute phase	Sudden, requires bed rest, asymmetric muscle paralysis
Recovery phase	Reinnervation of orphaned muscles
Stable disability	Chronic period of stable disability, variable in severity

- This is followed by people with *paralytic polio* who survive and recover. However, they are inflicted with the most severe damage to the ventral horn of the lower motor neurons of the spinal cord, which results in muscle tremors, flaccid paresis, paralysis, weakness, subsequent atrophy, fatigue, and pain.
- A second clinical presentation is *non-paralytic polio*. Despite the name, muscle paralysis and weakness do occur, both early in the course of the disease and later again after many years of acute infection.
- Two other less severe forms of polio are the *subclinical* and *abortive* types. A person with subclinical polio is unaware of the infection, this form occurs in very young children and there are no physical signs or symptoms of the disease.
- *Abortive* polio primarily affects the respiratory and gastrointestinal systems. However, no physical or skeletal muscle problems other than short-lived symptoms are reported.

HISTORY OF POST-POLIO SYNDROME

History of post-polio syndrome (PPS) is as follows:
- Starting around 1970, reports began to appear in medical literature that persons who had paralytic poliomyelitis were experiencing new health problems similar to the symptoms of an individual who has lived with chronic neuromuscular conditions.
- By the mid-1980s, clinicians began to realize that there was a fourth stage characterized by the onset of new symptoms related to original polio attack.
- The existence was first suggested by Charcot and Raymond (1875).
- The word "PPS" was first coined by Wiecher and Hubbell (1980).

Post-polio syndrome (PPS) is a condition that affects polio survivor's years after recovery from an initial acute attack of the poliomyelitis virus. Most often, polio survivors start to experience gradual new weakening in muscles that were previously affected by the polio infection. Some individuals experience only minor symptoms, while others develop visible muscle weakness and atrophy. More worrying is the fact that PPS may also affect the non-paralytic polio victims who may be misdiagnosed and mistreated as chronic fatigue syndrome (Epidemiological data suggest that for each paralytic polio case, there may have been 100 persons infected with poliovirus). This may further add to the real number of PPS victims.

For most polio survivors, the approximate 15-year recovery period is uneventful, and they perform their activities of daily livings (ADLs) without undue strain or fatigue. However, at some point, the remaining motor neurons fail to generate new sprouts and denervation exceeds reinnervation. This stage, considered as stage four, following the recovery phase is known as PPS, which is experienced by not all, but a large number of polio survivors.

Post-polio syndrome is a clinical entity affecting polio survivors with the onset of new neuromuscular symptoms several years after the initial polio attack, which was followed by a period of stability. Common symptoms are:
- Fatigue
- Pain
- New and unusual muscular deficits, on healthy muscles as well as deficient muscles initially affected by the poliovirus
- Muscle atrophy
- Cold intolerance
- Sleep disorders
- Dysphonia
- Dysphagia
- Respiratory insufficiency

All these symptoms are not necessarily present in all the cases.

Two subtypes of PPS are also known. Post-polio myelitis progressive muscle atrophy usually is regarded as encompassing neurologic symptoms. Post-polio myelitis muscle dysfunction or musculoskeletal post-poliomyelitis syndrome refers to local signs of new or increased muscle weakness and/or muscle atrophy and does not include weakness and atrophy from neurologic decline. The prevalence of PPS has been reported to be between 20% and 85% of people who have had poliomyelitis. One of the few Indian studies showed that the prevalence of PPS in Gujarat can be estimated to be 86.53%.

PATHOPHYSIOLOGY OF POST-POLIO SYNDROME

Pathophysiology of PPS is obscure, and while many theories have been proposed pertaining to it, it is better considered multifactorial since many factors at a time influence the disease process.

The most commonly accepted hypothesis is that of an ongoing denervation–reinnervation process, called by the term **neuron fatigue theory**. This theory assumes that many motor neurons that were destroyed by the original infection leave small numbers of overworked neurons behind to innervate many (orphaned) muscle fibers. With time and overuse, these few working neurons simply wear out leaving muscles denervated.

This is probably initiated after acute poliomyelitis, and over time it leads to increased motor unit areas caused by collateral sprouting of adjacent motor neurons in the spinal cord in patients with PPS; a process also evident

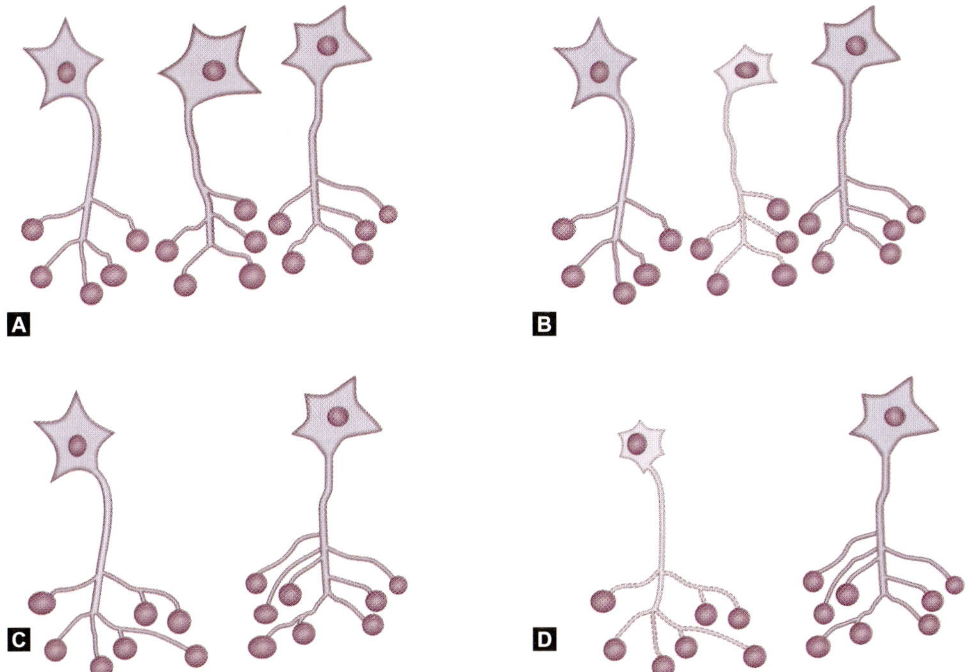

Figs. 36.1A to D: Pathogenesis of PPS: (A) Normal motor units; (B) Acute polio; (C) Reinnervation and recovery; (D) Post-polio syndrome.

during normal aging, although not until the seventh decade of life. The motor unit area might increase by up to 20 times, reaching a level at which further reinnervation is no longer possible. Uncompensated denervation causes atrophy of muscle fibers and subsequently loss of muscle strength. The underlying cause of the ongoing denervation resulting in the motor symptoms of PPS is unclear.

Figures 36.1A to D depict the pictorial representation of the pathogenesis of PPS. Other proposed etiologies include premature degeneration of surviving motor neurons, stress-induced degeneration of surviving neurons, persistent poliovirus replication or reactivation and immune-mediated damage, active cellular inflammation, genetical alterations, such as mutation of poliovirus sequences in cerebrospinal fluid, autoimmunity, and normal aging.

DIAGNOSING POST-POLIO SYNDROME

Goals of evaluating PPS can vary and usually consist of:

- Problem-oriented evaluation is common and typically used in clinical setup where it is important to provide urgent attention and care to the presenting problem.
- Prevention-oriented evaluation may be less common as it involves getting one self-evaluated to know if anything can be done to maintain current health status and avoid experiencing problems related to PPS.
- Diagnosis-oriented evaluation is also rare and involves one who wants to come to a specific diagnosis, irrespective of not experiencing any problems, but rather based on the findings of other polio survivors.
- Lastly, comprehensive evaluation, which is the most important of all, comprises a detailed assessment

based on a number of problems being experienced all at once.

A syndrome is a collection of symptoms, which occur together; hence, by definition, it has no single test to identify it. Most commonly, a threefold procedure is employed for coming to a definite diagnosis **(Table 36.2)**.

Table 36.2: Steps to diagnose post-polio syndrome.
Step 1: Evaluating the symptoms
Fatigue, new muscle weakness, muscle/joint pain, cold intolerance, swallowing problems, breathing difficulties, and sleep disorders
Step 2: Elimination of all other possible diseases
Fibromyalgia, radiculopathy, amyotrophic lateral sclerosis, multifocal motor neuropathy, cramp fasciculation syndrome, and chronic fatigue syndrome
Step 3: Fulfilling the diagnostic criteria
Halstead criteria (1985), revised Halstead criteria (1991), Dalakas criteria (1995), and March of Dimes (2001)

Step 1: Evaluating the Symptoms

Post-polio syndrome (PPS) is a neurological disease, and the presenting symptoms in an individual must be consistent with those of the syndrome. New muscle weakness is a cardinal symptom. Following symptoms are enlisted, and not all of these need to be manifested to come to a diagnosis. However, if a polio survivor complains of symptoms not listed below, other diagnoses should be considered.

- New muscle weakness
- Fatigue
- Muscle/joint pain

- Muscle atrophy
- Cold intolerance
- New swallowing difficulties
- New breathing difficulties
- New difficulties in activities of daily living, particularly mobility-related activities.
- Sleep impairment

A few associated or secondary symptoms, such as weight gain, osteoporosis, psychological problems, such as depression may also be seen. It is also important to remember that many individuals may also have comorbid conditions, such as hypothyroidism, diabetes, and hypertension along with PPS. And it becomes even more critical to rule out the secondary health aspects associated with comorbidities such as diabetic neuropathy, metabolic syndrome due to hypothyroidism.

Step 2: Elimination of Other Possible Diseases

Steps for elimination are as follows:
- There is no laboratory test for PPS and in making a diagnosis all other causes of these symptoms must be excluded.
- Therefore, careful clinical evaluation using history, observation, and examination are the diagnostic tools required to eliminate other disease entities.
- Since this is a diagnosis of exclusion, laboratory tests, such as complete blood counts among others will be important.
- Diagnostic imaging, such as joint X-rays or MRI scans of spinal cord may be useful in ruling out other causes.
- Referral to a consultant neurologist is usually essential for electromyography (EMG) (single-fiber EMG), confirmation of the diagnosis and exclusion of other neurological and muscle disorders. It may be impractical to rule out all diseases that may be causing the symptoms, and considering alternative diagnoses that manifest the same clinical presentation may help to delineate a few specific possibilities.

Step 3: Fulfilling the Diagnostic Criteria

Post-polio syndrome was initially defined as the clinical syndrome of new weakness, pain, and fatigue in patients who have recovered from acute polio.
- New criteria for PPS have been developed, but fatigue and new weakness are essential elements.
- The term "PPS" was introduced by Halstead in 1985 to cover medical, orthopedic, and psychological problems possibly or indirectly related to the long-term disability occurring many years after the acute episode. This is the most widely accepted criteria **(Table 36.3)**.
- However, Halstead revised his own criteria in 1991 and added gradual or abrupt onset of new neurogenic weakness as a necessary criterion for PPS, with or without other coexisting symptoms.
- Dalakas redefined and narrowed the use of PPS in 1995 with an additional criterion of neurological examination on EMG and/or MRI. According to

Table 36.3: Diagnostic criteria of post-polio syndrome.

Halstead criteria, 1985
- Confirmed medical history of poliomyelitis
- Partial or almost complete neurological recovery after the acute period
- A period of neurological stability that lasted for at least 15 years
- A recent muscular weakness with a sudden onset and quick progressive deterioration
- At least two new symptoms among the following ones: excessive fatigue, muscle or joint pain, muscle atrophy, cold intolerance, no other medical explanation

Dalakas criteria, 1996
- History of paralytic polio: Confirmed or not confirmed, partially or fairly complete functional recovery
- After a period of functional stability of at least 15 years' development of new muscle dysfunction: Muscle weakness, muscle atrophy, and muscle pain and fatigue
- Neurological examination compatible with prior polio: Lower motor neuron lesion, decreased or absent tendon reflexes, no sensory loss, and compatible findings on EMG and/or magnetic resonance imaging

March of Dimes, 2001
- Confirmed medical history of poliomyelitis
- A period of partially to fairly complete recovery after acute polio, followed by neurological and functional stability for at least 15 years
- New or increased muscle weakness or abnormal muscle fatigue, with or without generalized fatigue, muscle atrophy, and muscle/joint pain
- Symptoms usually have a gradual but sometimes sudden onset and should persist for at least 1 year
- No other medical diagnosis to explain the symptoms

(EMG: electromyography)

Kimura, on EMG, fibrillation potentials develop as the motor axons degenerate. Reinnervation will result in diminution of spontaneous discharges and the appearance of motor unit potentials of large amplitude and long duration. Weak muscles may only have few extremely large motor unit potentials.
- A newly proposed addition to the current criteria consists of a gradual or abrupt onset of progressive new weakness with a duration of at least 12 months. Since 2017, PPS is also included in the ICD-10 diagnostic criteria under the code G-14.

ASSESSMENT OF POST-POLIO SYNDROME

Physiotherapy is a cornerstone of management of prior polio and PPS. There is increasing evidence for the effectiveness of physiotherapy in alleviating PPS-associated physical problems. Patients with prior polio or PPS should have access to regular physiotherapy assessment, and treatment should be made available when needs are identified. These needs are likely to change with time, thus patient-centered, lifelong physiotherapy is recommended. A comprehensive and detailed assessment by the physiotherapist is necessary at the first consultation to establish a baseline from which future changes can be evaluated and a treatment plan developed.

An assessment will usually have three components:

1. Neurological
2. Musculoskeletal
3. Cardiorespiratory

A detailed subjective history should be taken first and important aspects of the physical examination are shown in **Table 36.4.** Subjective and objective findings by the therapist, along with clinical reasoning, guide the therapist in clinical decision-making of diagnosis and management. Along with this, few valid and reliable tools for measuring the problems seen in PPS are mentioned in **Table 36.5.**

History of surgeries may include:

- Osteotomy
- Arthrodesis
- Epiphyseodesis
- Tendon transfers
- Myofascial releases

Common postural deviations seen are:

- Scoliosis
- Kyphosis
- Limb length discrepancy
- Genu recurvatum
- Flail knee
- Knee flexion contracture

Foot deformities are common and include:

- Equinus
- Equinovarus
- Equinovalgus
- Cavovarus
- Claw toes
- Bunions

Gait deviations following poliomyelitis include:

- Hand to knee gait (due to quadriceps paralysis)

Table 36.4: Essential components of assessment.

History	Chief complaint, polio history, past general medical and surgical history, current health, family and social history
Examination	• Observation: Posture, gait • Motor examination: ROM, MMT, and LLD • Neurological examination: Tone, DTR, and sensation (which are normal in polio, and their affection may guide in other possible disease) • Pain examination: Type, intensity, and diurnal variation • Functional examination: Gait and transfers
Diagnosis and goal planning	Need for any other investigations, such as laboratory studies, imaging, electrodiagnostic tests, and sleep studies

(ROM: range of motion; MMT: manual muscle testing; LLD: limb length discrepancy; DTR: deep tendon reflexes)

Table 36.5: Outcome measures/assessment tools commonly used in post-polio syndrome (PPS).

Pain	• Numerical pain rating scale (NPRS) • Visual analogue scale (VAS) • Brief pain inventory (BPI)
Fatigue	• Fatigue impact scale (FIS) • Fatigue severity scale (FSS) • Multidimensional fatigue inventory (MFI) • Piper Fatigue Scale
Impairments	• Self-reported impairments in person with post-polio syndrome (SIPP) • Index of post-polio sequelae (IPPS)
Cardiorespiratory function	• Physiologic cost index (PCI), • 6-minute walk distance (6-MWD), • 2-minute walk distance (2-MWD), • VO_2 max
Physical activity	Physical activity and disability survey (PADS), pedometers, accelerometers
Mobility	• Walking speed • Walk-12
Falls	Fall efficacy scale (FES)
Function and quality of life	• Patient reported outcome measurement information system-physical function (PROMIS-PF), • SF-12/36, • Nottingham health profile

- High steppage gait (due to tibialis anterior paralysis)
- Trendelenburg gait (due to gluteus medius paralysis)
- Posterior lurching gait (due to gluteus maximus paralysis).

MANAGEMENT OF POST-POLIO SYNDROME

Best practices in the care of PPS are still evolving. However, the goals should be directed at:

- Treatment of primary symptoms
- Optimizing health and function
- Promoting wellness

All individuals presenting with PPS are unique and do not follow a fixed pattern of problems. Hence, the management of these problems cannot be the same. Individualized plan of care, tailor-made as per the needs of each person, should be used.

Medical Management

Several different types of medications can be prescribed, most of which are aimed at symptom reduction. These range from:

- Nonsteroidal anti-inflammatory drugs
- Muscle relaxants
- Steroids
- Immunoglobulins
- Coenzymes

Detailed description of medications along with their mechanism of action is shown in **Table 36.6**. There are a few drugs that may aggravate the symptoms of PPS; hence, necessary precautions should be taken in prescribing them.

Table 36.6: Pharmacological approach commonly prescribed for persons with post-polio syndrome.

Drug	Action	Indication	Side effects
NSAIDs	Inhibit prostaglandin synthesis	Muscle or joint pain	Muscle cramps, weakness, and fluid retention
Muscle relaxants	Suppress nociceptive nerve impulses	Muscle stiffness/pain	GI distress, headache, and dizziness
Prednisone	Inhibits inflammatory and immunologic responses	Reduces inflammation or block immunologic actions	Osteoporosis, edema, weight gain, decalcification of bone, loss of strength, and increased blood pressure
Pyridostigmine	Stimulates nicotinic receptors at neuromuscular junction and inactivates cholinesterase	Weakness of skeletal muscles	GI distress, cramps, salivation, and sweating
Immunoglobulin	Inhibits inflammatory and immunologic responses	Fatigue and pain	Muscle cramps and weakness
Co-enzyme Q10	Inhibit inflammatory and immunologic responses	Fatigue and pain	Muscle cramps and weakness

(NSAIDs: nonsteroidal anti-inflammatory drugs; GI: gastrointestinal)

Benzodiazepines and beta-blockers are contra-indicated; certain antiepileptic drugs, such as phenytoin are also to be avoided.

Due care should also be given when prescribing opiates which may precipitate respiratory depression.

Anesthetists should use smaller doses of anesthetic agents during surgeries, and also in use of muscle relaxants, as compared to general population.

- No specific curative treatment is available for PPS. Rehabilitation is considered the mainstay of management in PPS, with an emphasis on physical therapy. This rehabilitation differs largely from the approach employed to provide relief in the recovery phase of poliomyelitis.
- The aim is to reach a functional balance by increasing capacities and reducing demands. Several different approaches can be applied.

Rehabilitative Management

Figure 36.2 shows the core components of physiotherapy management.

1. Energy conservation:
Muscular aching and cramping are thought to be as a result of muscle overuse and should be avoided. Reduction in activity levels, regular rest periods (pacing), weight reduction, and use of assistive devices can help.

- It is recommended to intersperse activity with short intervals of rest to avoid overworking a muscle.
- Activity levels have been shown to correlate highly with pain and therefore a reduction may be of benefit.
- Maintaining a healthy weight is advisable as one study demonstrated that a higher body mass index (BMI) was associated with a higher risk of joint pain.
- Activity pacing is nothing but balancing of daily activities with rest periods incorporated and breakdown of larger activities into smaller frequent bouts. Energy conservation is the adoption of energy-efficient

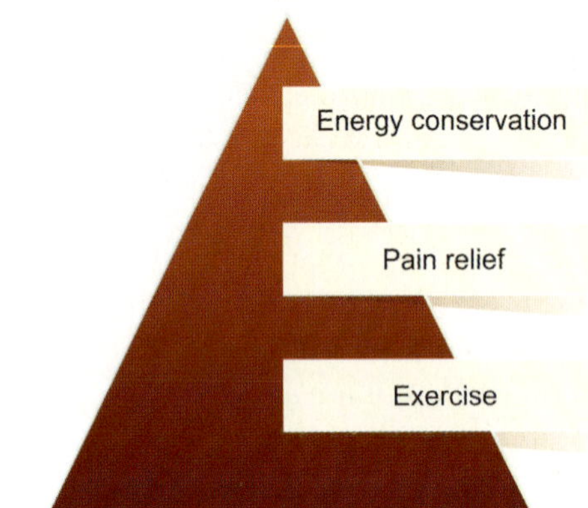

Fig. 36.2: Core components of physiotherapy management.

strategies that reduce the overall requirement of task and consequently fatigue.

- Simple advises, such as maintaining a healthy body weight and sleep hours can also be beneficial.

All these health benefits are also supported by research-based evidences, and no matter how massive the health risk may be, trivial and consistent efforts toward the same, along with the appropriate guidance of the physiotherapist can turn out to be favorable.

- Education about posture and back care may help to minimize aggravating factors.

2. Pain relief:
Pain-relieving measures may be necessary in the form of analgesic preparations combined with the following:

- Heat treatment—heat has been shown to help to relieve pain.
- Transcutaneous stimulation of the nerves—transcutaneous electrical nerve stimulation (TENS) is also recommended.
- Acupuncture
- Stretching can be helpful but should be used carefully as particular patients may have better function because

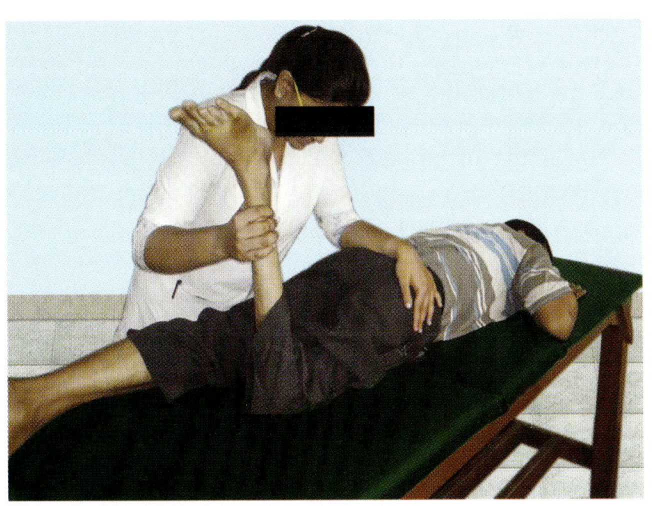

Fig. 36.3: Passive stretching of tight muscle being performed by the therapist.

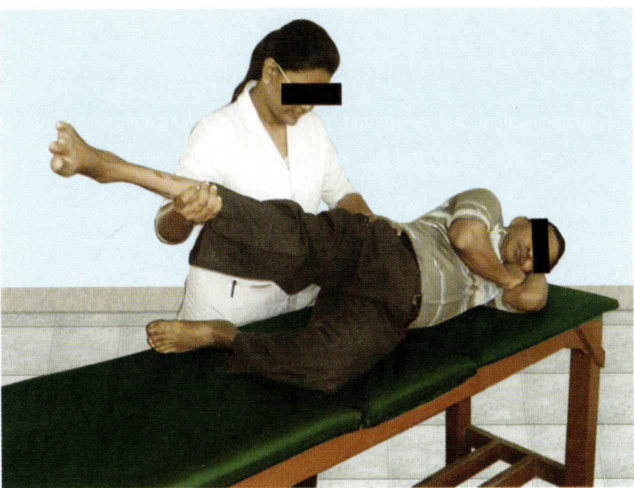

Fig. 36.4: Active-assisted range of motion exercises as a means of warm-up phase.

of shorter muscle length and associated reduced range of movement that improves stability **(Fig. 36.3)**.

3. Exercise:

Once energy management techniques have been effectively learned, and pain is controlled as far as possible, exercise programs can be considered. Exercises may be useful in PPS in serving two purposes: one is for strengthening and the other is for secondary prevention. Exercises may also help in improving overall cardiovascular health and promoting relaxation and sleep quality.

Residual effects in PPS may vary; hence, physical exercise programs should be adapted based on the needs of each individual **(Fig. 36.4)**.

- Aerobic exercises improve cardiovascular health, and resistance training improves muscle strength.
- Hence, strengthening regimes for weakest muscles or muscle groups, along with aerobic and anaerobic training of the body as a whole should be incorporated.

Functional training may also be useful to improve the efficiency of ambulation.

European guidelines are available and updated routinely for exercise recommendations in post-polio syndrome. They suggest that exercise is a safe and effective mean to prevent further decline in muscle activity, and additionally it helps in reducing symptoms of muscle weakness, pain, and fatigue. Precautions to avoid muscular overuse should be taken with intermittent breaks, periods of rest between series of exercises; and submaximal workload should always be taken.

Resistance training using load of the body itself, together with low-intensity training is known to increase the strength of individual muscles or muscle groups **(Figs. 36.5A and B)**. However, careful supervision is recommended, especially when it involves elderly population.

- Resistance training is inadvisable for people with very weak or fatigued muscles who are already using all their strength for activities of daily life.
- Endurance training can also be incorporated as spontaneous adaptations appear to prioritize strength before endurance.

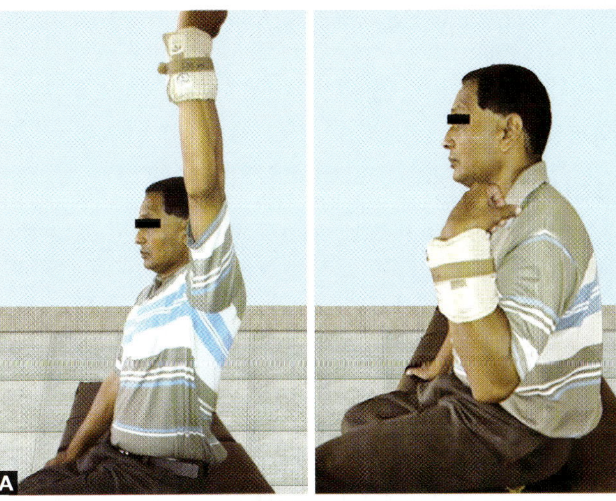

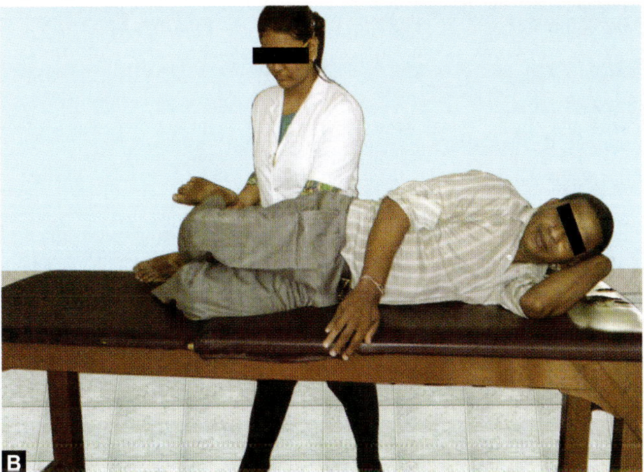

Figs. 36.5A and B: (A) Strengthening exercises of upper extremity using weight cuffs; (B) Strengthening of weaker muscle groups in gravity-eliminated plane.

As a basic guide, if the patient struggles to move their limb against gravity (and this is not due to a period of disuse), or has chronic injuries in the limb, then they will already be using the available muscle maximally during daily living **(Figs. 36.6A and B)**.

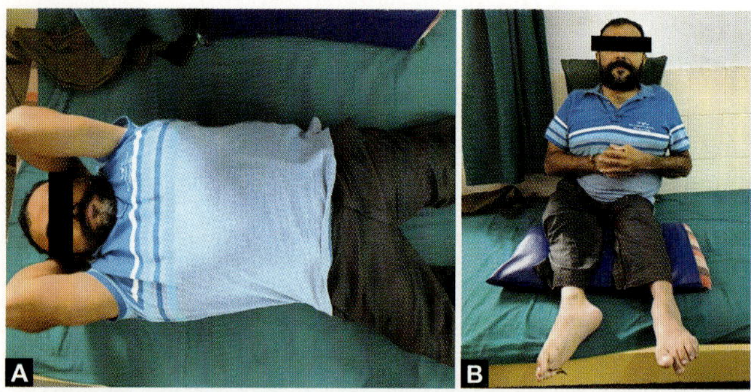

Figs. 36.6A and B: A patient with post-polio syndrome performing breathing exercises in supine and sitting.

Exercises should be nonfatiguing and performed at submaximal levels to avoid overloading the limited muscle capacity.

Initial aerobic intensity levels at a rate of perceived exertion of 11 on the Borg scale or 50–75% of three repetitions maximum are advised. All strengthening programs should be implemented in the context of an individual's ventilatory, circulatory, and respiratory function **(Table 36.7)**.

General Rules

Clinical Pearl

The patient's response acts as the most important training guideline.

Initially, the training should be carefully monitored with shorter than normal training sessions. Several short sessions of training are better than one session of a long duration. A long duration of pain or tiredness (24 hours or more) after training is an indication that the muscle load needs to be reduced. A perceived exertion scale can be used to stop the patient from exceeding a certain level during training. People affected by polio have a longer post-exercise muscle recovery period than people with a normal muscular system. Consequently, a training frequency of more than twice a week is not recommended.

Precautions

Following are the precautions to be taken:

Overuse: The cause of the ongoing denervation leading to PPS has not been proven, but the stress or overuse of the neuromuscular system has been proposed as a possible factor. Hence, it is important that any exercise program is nonfatiguing and does not cause pain or increased weakness. For people with severe weakness and/or neuromuscular fatigue, exercise may not be appropriate as they may be using their muscles maximally in everyday life.

Symptom aggravation: Instruction in self-monitoring should be given by the therapist. Therapists should teach their patients how to recognize and attend to excessive fatigue and pain during exercise. Patients should also be taught to identify and attend to those activities that cause

Table 36.7: Studies on rehabilitation for persons with post-polio syndrome with evidences.

Author	Mode of training	Activity	Intensity	Conclusions
Dean (1988)	Submaximal aerobic training	Treadmill walking	• 0–40 minutes • 3 times/week • 8 weeks	Decrease of HR_{max}, endurance improvement (+28%)
Jones (1989)	Submaximal aerobic training	Bicycle ergometer	• 13–30 minutes • 3 times/week • 16 weeks	Improvement of capacity (+20 W), endurance (+50%), $VO2_{max}$ (+15%), and $Ve2_{max}$
Kritz (1992)	Submaximal aerobic training	Bicycle ergometer and arms	• 20 minutes • 3 days/week • 16 weeks	Improvement of the cardiovascular parameters during effort without loss of muscular strength
Agre (1997)	Low-intensity isotonic strengthening	Quads strengthening	• 4 times/week • 12 weeks	No dynamometric strength increase, improvement of the amount of weight lifted, and no harmful side effects
Willen (2001)	Aquatic exercises	Knee flexion and extension in a pool heated at 33°	• 40 minutes • 2 days/week • 5 months	Improvement of HR_{max} during effort and pain and no improvement for strength or gait parameters
Strumse (2003)	Aquatic exercises	–	–	Improvement for pain and gait parameters in the aquatic therapy group
Chan (2003)	Muscular strengthening (submaximal resistance)	Thenar muscles	• 3 days/week • 12 weeks	Improvement of the motor command in the trained group
Oncu (2009)	Aerobic training	–	• 8 weeks, 3/week 90 minutes	Improvement in fatigue, functional capacity, and health profile scores
Sharma (2015)	Exercises and lifestyle modification	–	• 40 minutes • 4 days/week • 4 weeks	Improvement in fatigue and functional capacity

BOX 36.1: Recommendations for safe, effective exercise protocol.

- Assessing the capacity of an individual carefully
- Exercise program should be individually tailored, started gradually, with periods of rest, and taken into account the longer recovery times required
- It should be pain-free and nonfatiguing
- Close monitoring to identify aggravation of symptoms
- Slower progression to high intensity

an increase in the level of pain and fatigue and modify their activities accordingly **(Box 36.1)**.

Isometric exercises may be useful for muscles grading 2/5 to promote circulation in that part. It may also help retain some stability of joints in body parts with this degree of weakness.

Aerobic Training

Aerobic training includes the following:

- Low-level cycle ergometer for upper limb/lower limb seems to be best tolerated.
- In general, 15–20 minutes of total aerobics (including warm-up, cool-down) three times a week is maximum recommended **(Fig. 36.7)**.
- Interspersing 2–5 bouts of exercise intervals assists to avoid muscle fatigue, pain, and quivering.
- A good balance is vital and there is an increased risk of falling when mounting and dismounting the bicycle due to a reduced muscle function. Outdoor cycling should be restricted to those with very good muscle function. Cycling uphill is not recommended.
- Walking is less recommended due to the trauma produced by gait abnormalities. Nordic pole walking is a safer way of walking, but it requires good function of the upper extremities to avoid injuries due to overloading. Walking with poles unloads the lower extremities, which is advantageous; however, evidence on this is limited.

Hydrotherapy

Swimming and exercise in warm water has proved both enjoyable and beneficial for many polio survivors. With new problems from PPS, a course of hydrotherapy may help relieve symptoms and also be useful in discovering how to safely exercise in water. Water provides resistance but minimizes stress on muscles and joints. The properties of water allow assisted, resisted, or supported exercise, often enabling those limited by weakness on land to exercise with minimal assistance. The heat in hydrotherapy pool may also be beneficial. It results in a positive functional impact, less pain, and a lower heart rate at a submaximal work level as per a controlled trial, lending evidence to this form of treatment (CSP Hydrotherapy Standards). Warm water can also provide an environment that reduces concerns, such as falling, and the buoyancy can offer more movements to limbs, which are constrained by the load of gravity and mechanisms of the limb on land. Anecdotally, the main barrier to exercising in water is difficulty in accessing a pool. If this can be overcome, most patients find this an enjoyable and feasible way to exercise. Hydrotherapy may also result in increased strength without exacerbating fatigue or pain. It is essential that the individual's overall physical condition is assessed prior to commencing a hydrotherapy program.

Chest Physiotherapy

The aims of respiratory care are to avoid hospitalization, tracheal intubation, and respiratory infections although it should be emphasized that these are rare occurrences. Chest physiotherapy can be provided to assist with the removal of secretions, and teach manual and assisted cough techniques.

Orthoses/Assistive Devices

It is imperative that pain caused by a relatively high level of activity, specific loading on unstable joints or biomechanical conditions are alleviated **(Figs. 36.8A and B)**. The patient should be given guidance on the

Fig. 36.7: A post-polio syndrome patient performing static cycling as a form of aerobic training.

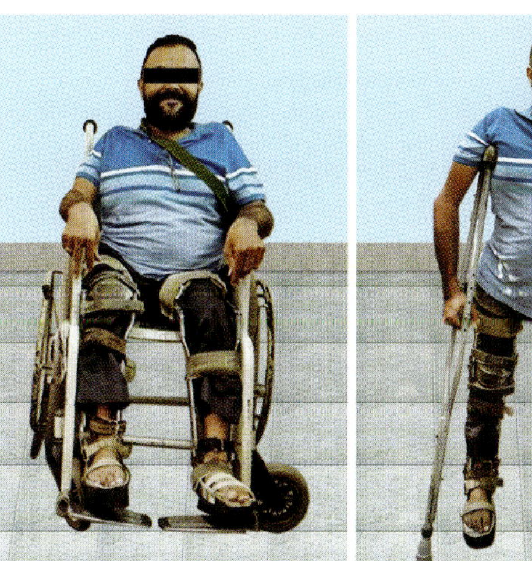

Figs. 36.8A and B: Use of wheelchair, assistive aids, and orthoses in post-polio syndrome.

appropriate level of activity and the use of mobility aids, and orthotic devices should be prescribed and adjusted. Aids and appliances should be provided with the aim of improving abnormal body mechanics, and correcting and minimizing postural and gait deviations mechanically. An appropriate orthosis has been shown to significantly reduce overall pain levels. A "comfy" grip crutch may improve the wrist and hand position. Wheelchairs when found suitable should be advised to improve the mobility and quality of life of the polio survivor.

SUMMARY

Polio comes in three phases, namely acute viral infection phase, recovery phase, and a lifelong stable phase. However, recently over the past few decades many polio survivors have reported new symptoms, such as muscle/joint pain, weakness, muscular or generalized fatigue, decline in physical function of healthy muscles or deficient muscles previously affected by polio, and this has been termed a fourth phase known as PPS. Diagnosing PPS can be difficult since it heavily relies on the exclusion of other conditions. Previous history of polio, long recovery following, and gradual onset of new physical problems guide its confirmation. Various pharmacological interventions can be helpful in alleviating the symptoms. Physiotherapy is known to provide a substantial relief in this condition, with the main emphasis on simple exercises and lifestyle modifications. Exercises in the form of active exercises, passive gentle stretches, arm or leg cycling (depending on the involvement), all in sets of few repetitions interspersed with rest breaks to avoid undue fatigue over already weak muscles. Overall aim is to use the muscles, but judiciously. For those who cannot follow exercises, can be advised lifestyle modifications, which consist of energy conservation techniques and activity pacing, both causing decreased physical demands and building adequate energy reserves to prevent problems of muscle as well as generalized fatigue.

Case Scenario

CASE STUDY

A 63-year-old male patient (retired bank officer) presents with pain in the left shoulder following trauma, right upper extremity weakness, and difficulties in accomplishing activities of daily living. He has a history of bilateral lower extremity poliomyelitis with a stabilization period of more than 60 years but manages his ambulation without the need of assistive devices. Gradually, he noted weakness of right upper extremity, and day by day, managing ADLs was getting difficult, with complaints of fatigue after even a few bouts of movement.

Contd...

Contd...

Clinical assessment: It was suggestive of right upper extremity muscle weakness, pain, and limited ROM of left shoulder, with no sensory involvement, and provocative tests for neck and cervical radiculopathy were negative. No involuntary movements were noted, and balance and coordination was found to be within normal limits.

Investigations: Before 8 months, he sustained trauma of the left shoulder, which was later diagnosed as subscapularis tear on MRI.

Electrodiagnostic findings revealed ongoing axonal degeneration in right deltoid, biceps brachii, and bilateral soleus muscles with regeneration.

Guiding Questions:
1. What is the probable diagnosis of the patient?
2. Enlist the impairments present.
3. Develop an appropriate plan of care with short-term and long-term goals.
4. Explain the role of physiotherapy in the rehabilitation of this patient.

Review Questions

1. Define post-polio syndrome.
2. Describe the clinical features of post-polio syndrome.
3. Discuss the steps involved in the diagnosis of post-polio syndrome.
4. Enlist the diagnostic criteria of March of Dimes, 2001.
5. What are the core components in the management of post-polio syndrome?
6. Identify the tests and measures used in the rehabilitation of post-polio syndrome.
7. Describe the goals and interventions for the management of fatigue in post-polio syndrome.
8. Discuss the role of exercises in the management of problems in post-polio syndrome.

BIBLIOGRAPHY

1. Agre JC, Rodriquez AA. Muscular function in late polio and the role of exercise in post-polio patients. Neurorehabilitation. 1997;8:107-18.
2. Agre J, Sliva J. Neuromuscular rehabilitation and electro-diagnosis 4. Specialized neuropathy. Arch Phys Med Rehabil. 2000;81(3):S27-31.
3. Bach JR. Management of post-polio respiratory sequelae. Ann NY Acad Sci. 1995;753:96-102.
4. Bartels M, Omura A. Aging in polio. Phys Med Rehabil Clin N Am. 2005;16(1):197-218.
5. Chan KM, Amirjani N, Sumrain M, et al. Randomized controlled trial of strength training in post-polio patients. Muscle Nerve. 2003;27(3):332-8.
6. CSP Hydrotherapy Standards. Available from http://www.csp.org.uk/director/groupandnetworks/ciogs/skillsgroups/hydrotherapy.cfm.
7. Dean E, Ross J. Effect of modified aerobic training on movement energetic in polio survivors. Orthopaedics. 1991;14(11):1243-6.

8. Falconer M, Bollenbach E. Late functional loss in nonparalytic polio. Am J Phys Med Rehabil. 2000;79(1):19-23.

9. Farbu E, Gilhus N, Barnes M, et al. EFNS guideline on diagnosis and management of post-polio syndrome. Report of an EFNS task force. Eur J Neurol. 2006;13(8):795-801.

10. Halstead L. Post-polio syndrome. Sci Am. 1998;278(4):42-7.

11. Jones DR, Speier J, Canine K. Cardiorespiratory responses to aerobic training by patients with postpoliomyelitis sequelae. JAMA. 1989;261:3255-8.

12. Kimura J. Electrodiagnosis in disease of nerve and muscle, principles and practice, 2nd edition. Philadelphia, PA: FA Davis Company; 1989. pp. 440-1.

13. Koopman FS, Beelen A, Gilhus NE, et al. Treatment for postpolio syndrome. Cochrane Database of Systematic Reviews 2015, Issue 5. Art. No.: CD007818. DOI: 10.1002/14651858.CD007818.pub3.

14. Kritz JL, Jones DR, Speier JL. Cardiorespiratory responses to upper extremity aerobic training by post-polio subjects. Arch Phys Med Rehabil. 1992;5:29-39.

15. March of Dimes Steering Committee on Post-Polio Syndrome. March of dimes international conference on post-polio syndrome: identifying best practices in diagnosis and care. White Plains, NY; 2002.

16. Nollet F, Beelen A, Prins M, et al. Disability and functional assessment in former polio patients with and without postpolio syndrome. Arch Phys Med Rehabil. 1999;80(2):136-43.

17. Oncu J, Durmaz B, Karapolat H. Short-term effects of aerobic exercise on functional capacity, fatigue, and quality of life in patients with post-polio syndrome. Clin Rehabil. 2009;23:155-63.

18. Post-Polio Task Force: Post-polio Syndrome Update. (1997) Bioscience Rep 5.

19. Sheth M, Sharma S, Jadav R, et al. Prevalence of post polio syndrome in Gujarat and the correlation of pain and fatigue with functioning in subjects with post polio syndrome. Indian J Physiother Occup Ther. 2014;8(4):230.

20. Sharma S, Sheth M, Vyas N. Fatigue and functional capacity in persons with post-polio syndrome: short-term effects of exercise and lifestyle modification compared to lifestyle modification alone. Disabil CBR Inclusive Dev. 2014;25(3):78.

21. Spector S, Gordon P, Feuerstein I, et al. Strength gains without muscle injury after strength training in patients with postpolio muscular atrophy. Muscle Nerve. 1996;19(10):1282-90.

22. Strumse Y, Stanghelle J, Utne L, et al. Treatment of patients with postpolio syndrome in a warm climate. Disabil Rehabil. 2003;25(2):77-84.

23. Tiffreau V, Rapin A, Serafi R, et al. Post-polio syndrome and rehabilitation. Ann Phys Rehabil Med. 2010;53(1):42-50.

24. Trojan D. Pathophysiology and diagnosis of post-polio syndrome. Neurorehabilitation. 1997;8(2):83-92.

25. Vasiliadis H, Collet J, Shapiro S, et al. Predictive factors and correlates for pain in postpoliomyelitis syndrome patients. Arch Phys Med Rehabil. 2002;83(8):1109-15.

26. Webster J, Miknevich M, Stevens P et al., Lower extremity orthotic management in neurologic rehabilitation. Crit Rev Phys Rehabil Med. 2009;21(1):1-23.

27. Wiechers D, Hubbell S. Late changes in the motor unit after acute poliomyelitis. Muscle Nerve. 1981;4(6):524-8.

28. Wills AK, Black S, Cooper R, et al. Life course body mass index and risk of knee osteoarthritis at the age of 53 years: evidence from the 1946 British birth cohort study. Ann Rheum Dis. 2012;71(5):655 60.

29. Willén C, Grimby G. Pain, physical activity, and disability in individuals with late effects of polio. Arch Phys Med Rehabil. 1998;79(8):915-19.

30. Willen C, Sunnerhagen KS, Grimby G. Dynamic water exercise in individuals with late poliomyelitis. Arch Phys Med Rehabil. 2001;82:66-72.

37
CHAPTER

Cancer

Jaini Patel, Aashish Contractor

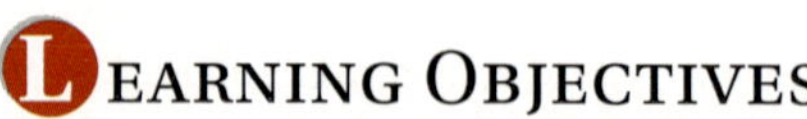 LEARNING OBJECTIVES

After reading this chapter, the readers should be able to:

- Know about various types of cancers occurring in India and their usual therapies
- Understand the immediate, late, and delayed side effects associated with cancer and cancer therapy
- Understand the role of each team member involved in the comprehensive cancer care
- Understand important aspects of assessing patient and designing a plan of care using different physical rehabilitation therapies and modifying the care in relation to ongoing, planned or completed cancer treatment
- Improvise knowledge on use of different outcome tools for cancer patients
- Understand how health-related quality of life is impacted by cancer and cancer therapy and the role of rehabilitation in lowering the impact
- Explore certain international guidelines currently available on cancer care and their implications

CHAPTER OUTLINE

- Epidemiology (cancer incidence and survival)
- Risk factors for cancer in India
  - Dietary habits
  - Tobacco use
  - Alcohol
  - Radiation
  - Carcinogenic viruses
  - Pollutants
  - Obesity
- Exercise/physical activity and primary cancer prevention
- Medical and clinical considerations
  - Cancer screening
  - Signs and symptoms
  - Diagnostic testing
  - Cancer staging
- Common cancers and their treatment
  - Local therapy
  - Systemic therapy
  - Breast cancer
  - Head and neck cancer
  - Lung cancer
  - Cervix cancer
  - Colorectal cancer
  - Prostate cancer
- Cancer recurrence warning signs
- Side effects of cancer or cancer therapy
  - Fatigue
  - Cardiovascular changes
  - Pulmonary changes
  - Neurological changes
  - Musculoskeletal changes
  - Lymphedema
  - Pain
  - Oral complications
  - Sleep disturbance
  - Issues with body image and confidence
  - Nausea and vomiting
  - Increased risk of infections
  - Chemotherapy-induced neutropenia and thrombocytopenia
  - Gastrointestinal changes
  - Endocrine changes
  - Sexual dysfunction
  - Psychological issues
  - Health-related quality of life
- Cancer rehabilitation
  - Assessment
  - Goals of rehabilitation program
- Precautions or contraindications to exercise for patients with cancer
  - Contraindication for exercise testing
  - Precautions to exercise in patients with cancer
- Program implementation
  - Management of fatigue
  - Management of pain
  - Cardiorespiratory fitness/exercise and physical activity prescription
  - Muscle strength and endurance
  - Resistance training
  - Addressing musculoskeletal impairments
  - Addressing neurological impairments
  - Lymphedema management
  - Management of incontinence
  - Speech and swallowing rehabilitation
  - Nutrition education and planning
  - Psychological counseling
  - Mindfulness-based exercise

INTRODUCTION

"Cancer" is a term for diseases in which abnormal cells divide without control and can invade nearby tissues. Cancer cells can also spread to other parts of the body through the blood and lymph systems.

Cancer is broadly categorized into the following types:

- *Carcinoma* is a type of cancer that begins in the skin or in tissues that line or cover internal organs.
- *Sarcoma* is a type of cancer that begins in bone, cartilage, fat, muscle, blood vessels or other connective, or supportive tissue.
- *Leukemia* is a type of cancer that starts in blood-forming tissue, such as the bone marrow, and causes large numbers of abnormal blood cells to be produced and enter the blood.
- *Lymphoma* and multiple myeloma are types of cancers that begin in the cells of the immune system.
- *Central nervous system cancers* are types of cancers that begin in the tissues of the brain and spinal cord. Also called malignancy.

EPIDEMIOLOGY (CANCER INCIDENCE AND SURVIVAL)

Cancer is one of the leading causes of death amongst adults in the world and in India **(Fig. 37.1)**. In 2012, the International Agency for Research on Cancer (IARC) GLOBOCAN-project estimated 14 million new cases of cancer worldwide and more than 8 million deaths due to cancer. Out of which about 1,157,294 new cases and 634,000 deaths occurred in India, which is 17% of the global population. The GLOBOCAN has predicted that India's cancer burden will reach approximately 1,700,000 new cases and 1,200,000 deaths by 2035.

RISK FACTORS FOR CANCER IN INDIA

The causes of cancer in India are almost the same as in other parts of the world. The causes for cancers can be either internal factors such as inherited mutations, hormones, and immune conditions or external factors such as tobacco, diet, radiation, and other infectious agents.

Dietary Habits

Improper diet is one of the main causes of cancer prevalence in India. About 70% of colorectal cancer cases are believed to be due to imbalanced diet.

- The heavy consumption of red meat is the main cause of several cancers, including gastrointestinal tract (GIT) and colorectal, prostate, bladder, breast, gastric, and oral cancers.
- A low intake of fresh fruits and high cooking temperatures may cause low levels of vitamin C, resulting in higher risks of stomach, mouth, pharyngeal, esophageal cancer.
- Beans, chickpeas and lentils, and pulses have been significantly associated with a lower risk of cancer.
- The Indian diet containing adequate quantities of vegetables, fruits, and fiber-rich grains provides protection against the increased risk of colon and breast cancers.

Tobacco Use

Tobacco use is a leading cause of cancer because of the addictive nature of nicotine.

- Data from the Global Adult Tobacco Survey, which conducted surveys in 14 low- and middle-income

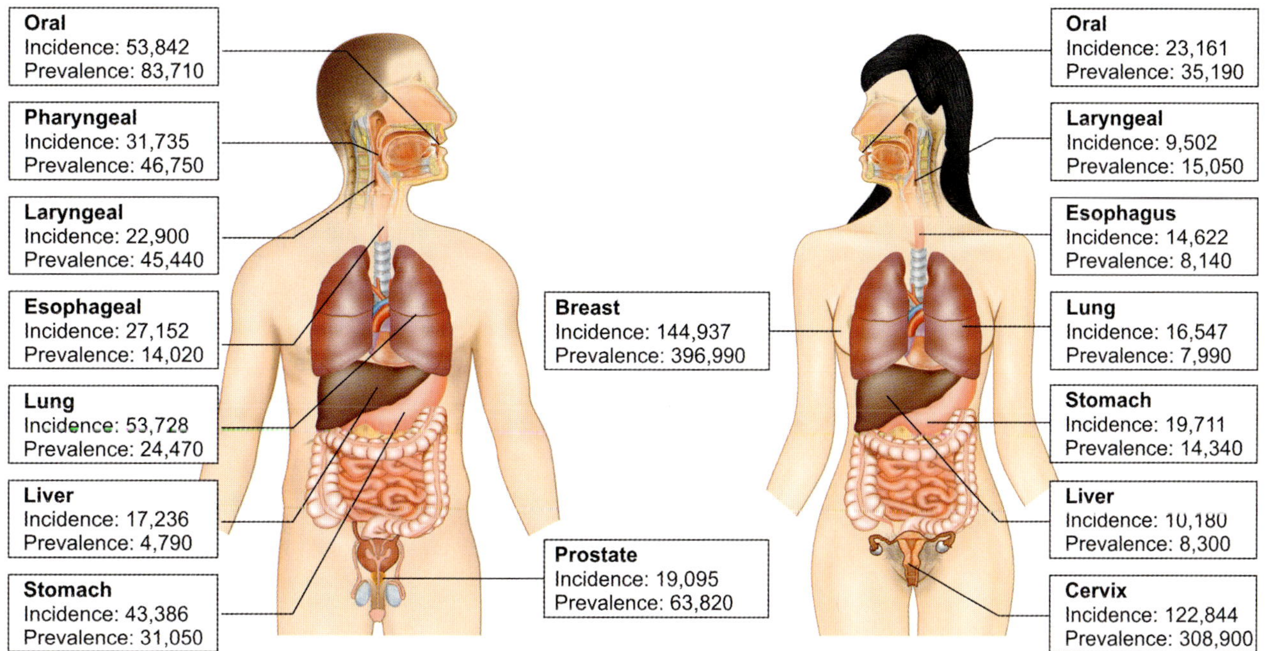

Fig. 37.1: Schematic diagram of most common sites for cancer along with annual incidence and deaths in India.

countries, including India, suggest 41% of men and 5% of women across these countries currently smoke compared to approximately 16% of men and 13% of women in the United States in 2015.

- India has regular use of tobacco via smoking, chewing, snuffing, etc. The various cancers produced by the use of tobacco are of oral cavity, pharynx, esophagus, larynx, lungs, and urinary bladder.
- The IARC has classified both cigarette smoke and smokeless tobacco as Group 1 carcinogens. Smokeless tobacco products, although they are not burned, nonetheless contain substantial levels of carcinogens.
- Although each cigarette or tobacco product may contain seemingly low levels of a given carcinogen, via repeated exposure per day over decades, a mixture of numerous carcinogens is administered. It leads to the formation of carcinogen–DNA adducts, which then cause mutations that, if not repaired or removed, will give rise to cell-transformation processes that can lead to cancer.
- Approximately 90% of all lung cancers are related to smoking, with a strong dose–response relationship. Risk decreases with smoking cessation, but former smokers are still at higher risk of lung cancer than nonsmokers.

Alcohol

Alcohol is classified as a carcinogen by the IARC, attributing to 600,000 cancer deaths per year globally.

- Consumption of alcohol increases the risk of the liver, esophagus, pharynx, oral cavity, larynx, breast, and colorectum in a dose-dependent fashion.
- At least in the developed world, about 75% of cancers of the esophagus, pharynx, oral cavity, and larynx are attributable to alcohol and tobacco, with a marked increase in risk among drinkers who also smoke, suggesting a multiplicative effect.

Radiation

Ionizing radiation is defined as radiation that has sufficient energy to ionize molecules by displacing electrons from atoms.

- Ionizing radiation can be electromagnetic, such as X-rays and gamma rays, or consist of particles, such as electrons, protons, neutrons, alpha particles, or carbon ions. The increased medical use of diagnostic X-rays and computed tomography (CT) scanning procedures as well as airport screenings translates into higher incidences of cancer.
- The main series of cancers induced by exposure to the adequate doses of the carcinogenic radiations include thyroid, skin, leukemia, lymphoma, lung, and breast carcinomas.

Carcinogenic Viruses

Viral infections play a causal role in at least 10% of all new cancer diagnoses worldwide. A vast majority of cases (>85%) occur in developing countries, where poor sanitation, high rates of cocarcinogenic factors such as HIV/AIDS, and lack of access to vaccines and cancer screening all contribute to increased rates of virally induced cancers.

- Even in developed countries, where effective counter-measures are widely available, cancers attributable to viral infection account for at least 4% of new cases.
- Following are the most common viruses associated with direct (hit and run) or indirect carcinogenic properties:
  - High-risk human papillomavirus (HPV) types
  - Hepatitis B and C virus
  - Epstein–Barr virus (HHV–4)
  - Kaposi sarcoma herpesvirus (HHV–8)
  - Merkel cell polyomavirus
  - Human T-cell leukemia virus
  - BK polyomavirus

Pollutants

It is estimated that about 90% of cancer is owing to the environmental contaminants. Various types of cancers are believed to be due to ill effects of the polluted environment. Outdoor pollutants such as polyaromatic hydrocarbons increase risk of lung cancer while indoor environmental pollutants such as volatile organic compounds and pesticides increase the risk of leukemia and lymphoma, brain tumors, Wilms tumors, Ewing's sarcoma, and germ-cell tumors.

Obesity

Overweight, obesity, and inactivity are the major contributors to cancer risk.

- In 2016, the IARC reviewed more than 1,000 studies and determined that obesity is associated with an increased risk of developing 13 different types of cancers.
- In 2003, a landmark study of 900,000 US adults demonstrated that obese men and women were up to 52 and 62% more likely to develop and die from cancer, as compared to their normal-weight counterparts, respectively.
- Weight gain of 10 kg or more is associated with a significant increase in postmenopausal breast cancer incidence among women who never used hormone replacement therapy, whereas weight loss of comparable magnitude after menopause is associated with a substantially lower risk of breast cancer.
- Apart from that, individuals who are obese at the time of cancer diagnosis are at increased risk of cancer recurrence, complications from cancer-directed therapy and mortality, compared to individuals of normal body weight. It is estimated that 20% of new cancer cases and 17% of cancer-related deaths are attributable to obesity.

EXERCISE/PHYSICAL ACTIVITY AND PRIMARY CANCER PREVENTION

It is estimated that 10% of all new cancer cases and 9% of cancer-related deaths are attributable to physical inactivity.

- In 2011, the American Cancer Society (ACS) published a report stating that physical activity and dietary interventions are strategies to successfully help reduce the overall incidence, morbidity, and mortality from certain kinds of cancer.
- World Cancer Research Fund International panel determined that physical activity is associated with a decreased risk of developing colon cancer; breast and endometrial cancer in postmenopausal women.
- About 48 studies on 40,000 patients showed a reduced risk of colon cancer, while 41 studies on 108,321 women suggested a reduced risk of breast cancer in physically active individuals.
- A research published in JAMA analyzed the association of leisure-time physical activity with 23 types of cancers from data of 12 prospective cohorts on 1.44 million participants. Results suggested statistically significant association of leisure-time physical activity with lower risk of 13 types of cancer. It is to be noted that most of these associations were evident regardless of body size or smoking history.
- In breast, colorectal, and prostate cancer, participation in physical activity is associated with a lower risk of cancer-specific mortality.
- Promotion of physical activity is important for population-wide cancer prevention; however, the amount of physical activity required to reduce the risk of cancer is yet to be determined.

MEDICAL AND CLINICAL CONSIDERATIONS

Cancer Screening

Cancer screening is done to detect a cancer at an asymptomatic stage in average risk, asymptomatic people (primary) or to detect a reoccurrence or new cancer in a survivor (secondary). Detection of cancer at an early stage can lead to reduction in mortality. Currently, ACS has recommended primary screening for breast and cervical cancer in women, prostate cancer in men, and colorectal cancer in men and women.

Signs and Symptoms

At an early stage, patient may experience nonspecific symptoms such as fatigue, weight loss, nausea, and malaise. Later, patient may develop symptoms specific to the involved organ.

Diagnostic Testing

An accurate diagnosis is key to decide appropriate care for cancer. Diagnostic tests include imaging, laboratory, and pathology techniques, in addition to physical examination.

Imaging tests: X-rays, ultrasonography, magnetic resonance imaging (MRI) scan, CT scan, PET scan, or SPECT scans.

Laboratory tests: Tests on blood, urine, other fluids, and tissues. Specimens are collected by phlebotomy (blood drawing), fine-needle aspiration cytology or fine-needle-biopsy, and surgical procedures.

Pathology tests: Pathologic examination for most solid tumors requires surgically excising a sample of the tumor, a biopsy.

Cancer Staging

A staging system is a standardized way to describe the extent to which a cancer has spread. It is done with the help of clinical or pathological information and helps to determine the expected morbidity and mortality and treatment regimen most suited for that patient. Each cancer has a unique staging system, but the principles are common to all cancers. The common elements of staging are:

- Location of primary tumor
- Tumor size and number
- Spread to lymph nodes (LNs)
- Cell type and grade of tumor
- Spread to distant sites

For solid tumors, AJCC (American Joint Committee on Cancer) TNM (Tumor, Node, metastasis) classification system (0–IV stages) is being widely used, where T denotes size of the tumor, N denotes degree of LN involvement, and M describes extent of metastasis. Stage 0 refers to noninvasive or in situ cancer. Early stage (I and II) generally represents disease that is confined to the site of origin or locoregional area. Advanced stage (III and IV) suggests spread of disease to distant sites and is more likely to result in mortality than early stage.

Similarly, there are REAL (Revised European-American Classification of Lymphoid Neoplasms) and WHO (World Health Organization) classification systems. The staging system varies for various types of cancers.

COMMON CANCERS AND THEIR TREATMENT

Cancer treatment is vast and includes different regimens, therapies depending on the type, stage, and clinical state of the patient. The top five commonly occurring cancers in India are breast cancer, oral cavity, gastric, cervix, and lung cancer. However, this chapter describes more about breast, head and neck (which includes oral cavity, larynx, and pharynx), lung, cervix, colorectal, and prostate cancer where rehabilitation plays a major role in all stages of cancer care. To cover other types of cancer is beyond the scope of this chapter.

The term "*adjuvant therapy*" refers to treatment that occurs after the main treatment of cancer; it is aimed at preventing recurrence of disease. The term "*neoadjuvant therapy*" is used for a therapy given as a first step to shrink a tumor before the main treatment.

Cancer treatment has advanced a lot in the past few years and includes a variety of regimen. Patient may be given one or a combination of therapies as mentioned below, in various sequences depending on the stage and clinical status **(Table 37.1)**.

Table 37.1: Common cancer therapy regimen (may include one or combination of therapies).

	Surgery	Evaluation/dissection of lymph nodes	Radiation therapy	Chemotherapy	Hormone therapy	Targeted therapy
Breast	• Lumpectomy • Breast conservation surgery • Mastectomy—modified or radical with/without breast reconstruction and implant	• Sentinel lymph node dissection (SLND) • Axillary lymph node dissection (ALND)	• For patients with breast conservative surgery and some patients with mastectomy • Dosage: 52.5–65 Gy • Frequency: 5 days a week for 4–6 weeks	• Neoadjuvant or adjuvant • Commonly used drugs: Adriamycin, cyclophosphamide, paclitaxel, docetaxel, methotrexate, 5-fluorouracil • Given at an interval of 2–4 weeks 4–6 cycles for 12–24 weeks	• For tumors expressing estrogen or progesterone receptors (ER or PR positive) • Reduce risk of recurrence by 40% • Drugs: Tamoxifen or aromatase inhibitors	• For tumors expressing HER2 protein (HER2 positive), e.g., Trastuzumab (Herceptin)

Head and neck	• Simple or complex e.g., simple removal of tumor
	• Commando surgery (removal of major part of face including mandible, muscle, tongue, and reconstruction with bone graft, myocutaneous graft, etc.)
	• Laryngectomy or pharyngectomy (may lead to loss of speech)
		• Selective neck lymph node dissection (SNLND)
		• Radical neck dissection (RND): removal of all the ipsilateral cervical lymph node groups, spinal accessory nerve, internal jugular vein, and sternocleidomastoid muscle
		• Modified radical neck dissection (MRND): preservation of at least one of the nonlymphatic structures
			• Irradiation of involved area
			• Dosage: 60–70 Gy
			• Frequency: 5 days a week for 5–6 weeks
				• Usually given with radiotherapy
				• Common drugs:
				  – Methotrexate, cisplatin, carboplatin, 5-fluorouracil, paclitaxel, and docetaxel
				  – Usually given at intervals of 1–4 weeks
						• Occasionally combined with chemotherapy
						• Common drugs: Cetuximab, panitumumab, etc.

Lung cancer	Surgical removal of tumor may include segmentectomy, lobectomy, bilobectomy, or pneumonectomy		• Adjuvant radiation therapy to thorax • In SCLC, due to higher chances of brain metastasis, frequently prophylactic cranial irradiation • Every 3–4 week cycle, 4–6 such cycles	• Adjuvant or neoadjuvant • Common drugs: Cisplatin, carboplatin, paclitaxel, docetaxel, gemcitabine, and etoposide		Common drugs: Gefitinib, crizotinib, or erlotinib
Cervix cancer	• For smaller lesions: Cryosurgery, LEEP (loop electrosurgical excision procedure), hysterectomy with bilateral salpingo-oophorectomy • For larger lesions: Trachelectomy, radical hysterectomy, occasionally pelvic exenteration	Laparoscopic evaluation/dissection of pelvic and retroperitoneal lymph nodes	• Reserved for cancers that have spread beyond the cervix or very large lesions • Dosage: 46–50 Gy 23–25 fractions with external radiotherapy • Followed by 3–4 sessions of internal brachytherapy	Common drug: Cisplatin—given every week along with the course of radiation therapy		

Contd...

Contd...

	Surgery	Evaluation/dissection of lymph nodes	Radiation therapy	Chemotherapy	Hormone therapy	Targeted therapy
Colorectal	• Open or laparoscopic polypectomy, local excision, colectomy (hemi, partial, segmental or total colectomy) • Local transanal resection • Transanal endoscopic microsurgery (TEM) • Low anterior resection (LAR) • Proctectomy with coloanal anastomosis • Abdominoperineal resection (APR) • Pelvic exenteration • Resection of rectal tumors (sphincter sparing approach if possible) • Colostomy or ileostomy may be required in few cases	Evaluation/dissection of retroperitoneal lymph nodes	• For colon tumors invading or perforating muscles of the bowel wall or those with positive surgical resection margins: Postoperative radiotherapy Dosage: 59–63 Gy for 30–35 fractions • For rectal cancers, it can be concurrently, before or after surgery Dose is 50 Gy in 25 fractions	• For colon cancer, usually offered when tumor has involved lymph nodes or adjacent muscles • For rectal cancers, it is concurrent, before or after surgery • Common drugs: 5-Fluorouracil, capecitabine, oxaliplatin, irinotecan		Common drugs: Cetuximab or bevacizumab
Prostate cancer	• Open radical prostatectomy or minimally invasive laparoscopic robotic surgery • Surgery may include removal of prostate, both seminal vesicles, short segment of urethra passing through prostate, neurovascular bundle	Evaluation/dissection of pelvic or retroperitoneal lymph nodes	• External beam radiation therapy or brachytherapy or combination • Dosage: 65–78 Gy for 25–39 fractions	• Reserved for patient with metastasis or not responding to hormone therapy • Commonly used drugs: Docetaxel and cisplatin	• Androgen deprivation therapy: reduces testosterone levels, commonly used in locally advanced and metastatic prostate cancer • It may include orchiectomy (surgical removal of testes) • LHRH (luteinizing hormone-releasing hormone) agonists (via subcutaneous injections at certain intervals) or antiandrogen oral medications (flutamide or bicalutamide)	

Local Therapy

Local therapy includes:

1. **Surgical removal of tumor:** Surgery is the oldest and most definitive treatment of cancer. It can be curative or palliative. Surgery may include removal of tumor along with adjacent tissues depending on the margin and extent of involvement. Major surgical procedures may include removal of involved muscle, fascia, bone, nerve, vessels, etc., and may also involve grafting of tissues (bone, myocutaneous, skin graft) to restore or cover the deficit. This may lead to mild-to-severe musculoskeletal dysfunction at the local as well as at donor region.

2. **Evaluation/dissection of LNs:** It is done to see the presence of metastasis.
   Sentinel LNs are the nodes that directly drain in the area of tumor or axillary or submandibular or supraclavicular etc.

3. **Radiation therapy (RT):** About half the patients undergo ionizing radiation treatments pre- or postoperatively. It is thought to damage DNA within the cell and thus to stop growth of malignant cells. It can be given from external machines or from implanted internal source (brachytherapy). Common schedule involves frequent appointments (5 days a week) over a defined time period (4–6 weeks).
   Modern techniques such as IMRT (intensity modulated RT), RapidArc RT, SRS (stereotactic radiosurgery), and SBRT (stereotactic body RT) have reduced the acute and late toxicities to significant extent, which has in turn improved the quality of life of the patients.

Systemic Therapy

The necessity of and options for systematic treatment are based on a number of characteristics of tumor, including size, grade, the presence or absence of LN involvement, and the expression of certain receptors that can guide the use of specific therapies.

1. **Chemotherapy:** Majority of cancer patients also receive chemotherapy. It is effective on cells that grow faster, and it interferes with the cell-replication process. It can be given orally or delivered intravenously on cyclical schedules (e.g., 1 day or cycle, followed by recovery of 2–3 weeks, such 6–8 cycles). It may last for duration of few months or even longer. There are numerous chemotherapy regimens where drugs are given concurrently or in sequence.

2. **Biotherapy:** Biotherapy stimulates immune response of the body to distinct protein antigens that are present in cancer cells.
   - *Hormonal therapy:* Mostly used to treat certain types of breast or prostate cancer, in the form of drugs to be taken every day for few years or it is done in form of surgery (oophorectomy or orchiectomy).
   - *Targeted therapy:* Targeted therapies are developed for specific tumors that have expression of certain receptors in the cancer cells.

Breast Cancer

Most of the breast cancers are detected by abnormal screening mammogram or a lump palpated by the patient or physician. Few of the patients present with local symptoms, e.g., breast pain, breast enlargement, nipple retraction or nipple discharge, or thickening of the skin, resulting in an orange-peel texture.

- Most breast cancers have been classified as either ductal or lobular depending on where they originate from, i.e., milk-producing lobules or milk ducts.
- There are three major receptors identified on cancer cell surface that play important roles in the patient's prognosis and treatment: human epidermal growth factor receptor-2 (HER2)-positive breast cancer, progesterone receptor (PR)-positive/estrogen receptor (ER)-positive breast cancer, or triple-negative breast cancer.
- Usual investigations involved are mammography, biopsy, MRI, and LN examination.

Head and Neck Cancer

The term "head and neck cancer" (HNC) refers to cancers of the upper aerodigestive tract, which includes oral cavity (lips, tongue, the gums, the lining inside the cheeks and lips, the floor of the mouth, the hard palate), pharynx, larynx, sinonasal cavities, and salivary glands.

- Squamous cell carcinoma is the most common type and usually affects males with heavy tobacco use, alcohol abuse, poor diet, and bad dentition.
- Depending on the site of lesion, the symptoms may include a nonhealing lump, white or red patch in the mouth, long-term sore throat, difficult swallowing or hoarseness of voice. In very few patients, oral submucosal fibrosis can be the first presenting subclinical symptom in a tobacco chewer.
- HNCs are known to have very high mortality rates as the disease progresses to advanced stage by the time the patient reaches the doctor.

Clinical Pearl

Patients who are in poor nutritional condition may require a nasogastric tube or a percutaneous gastrostomy (PEG) before, during, or after the completion of cancer therapy.

Patients operated for larynx or pharyngeal tumor may undergo surgeries which require laryngectomy or pharyngectomy, may have temporary or permanent tracheostomy tube or laryngeal valve tube, and may be candidates for artificial larynx or other modified speech devices and may need extensive speech and swallowing therapy.

Lung Cancer

Symptoms may vary depending on the location and extent of tumor.

- Patient may experience cough, shortness of breath, or hemoptysis if the tumor is in major airways, lung tissue, or surrounding blood vessels.

- Patient may present with chest pain, pleural effusion, or shoulder and arm pain if the tumor is invading surrounding structures of lungs.
- Some patients may present with symptoms of bone pain, neurological symptoms, or others if the tumor has metastasized in distant organs.

Lung cancer is divided into two types depending on the histopathological findings:

1. SCLC: Small cell lung cancer—20% (usually advanced disease)
2. NSCLC: Non-SCLC—80% (squamous cell, large cell, or adenocarcinoma).

Cervix Cancer

It usually affects women between age of 20 and 50 years. Most cases of cervical cancer are caused by infection with HPV, which usually is passed from person to person by sexual contact. Introduction of PAP smear test for screening and HPV vaccination has reduced the mortality rates.

- Cervical cell carcinoma can be mostly of following types—squamous cell cancer, adenocarcinoma or mixed carcinoma.
- Common presenting symptoms are abnormal vaginal discharge or bleeding after sexual intercourse, after menopause or between menstrual periods; or excessively heavy periods, urinary frequency, or dyspareunia.
- Additional specific diagnostic tests may include colposcopy, cystoscopy, proctoscopy or endocervical curettage.

Colorectal Cancer

Colon cancers can be asymptomatic or may have vague abdominal complaints such as pain, bloating, blood in stool, nausea, or vomiting. Lesions in rectal regions may cause feelings of urgency to pass stool or rectal fullness.

- Apart from usual biopsy, tissue examination and CT scan, digital rectal examination (DRE), colonoscopy, and carcinoembryonic antigen marker are useful investigations for colorectal cancers.
- Adenocarcinoma is the most common type of colorectal cancer while carcinoid tumors, gastrointestinal stromal tumors, lymphoma, and sarcoma are less common.

Prostate Cancer

Prostate cancer affects older men and many times are detected incidentally or during routine screening, and in early stages, it can be asymptomatic.

- Few common symptoms may include painful or burning urination, inability or difficulty in urination, blood in the urine or semen, continual pain in the lower back, pelvis, hips or thighs or difficulty having an erection.
- Many men with prostate cancer die of other illnesses before the cancer can cause any disability.

- Almost all prostate cancers begin in the glandular cells of the prostate and are known as adenocarcinomas.
- To determine the prognosis of the tumor and make therapeutic decisions, in addition to routine cancer investigations, DRE, prostate-specific antigen test, Gleason score (classification scoring system used to determine aggressiveness of prostate cancer), patient age, and comorbid conditions are considered.

CANCER RECURRENCE WARNING SIGNS

Signs are generally related to the site and extent of the disease. For example, metastatic disease in lung may present with breathlessness or hemoptysis, while bony metastasis generally presents with pain. Therefore any new or progressive symptoms in cancer survivors should be addressed aggressively and should be evaluated by patient's primary doctor.

SIDE EFFECTS OF CANCER OR CANCER THERAPY

Despite advances in cancer therapy and efforts directed toward optimizing efficacy and minimizing toxicity, therapies may result in significant side effects that can result in long-term morbidity and even mortality. Side effects can be acute, short-term (lasting for days or weeks), long-term or persistent (lasting for years after treatment), and late (appearing months or years after treatment completion). Apart from the type of surgery and treatment received, side effects may vary in individual patients depending on their age, gender, comorbidities, and fitness levels prior to cancer diagnosis.

Fatigue

Cancer-related fatigue is defined as distressing, persistent sense of tiredness, or exhaustion that is related to cancer or its treatment and is one of the most common symptoms experienced by cancer patients.

It is a multifaceted condition characterized by:

- Diminished energy.
- An increased need to rest, disproportionate to any recent change in activity level.
- Accompanied by a range of other characteristics, including generalized weakness, diminished mental concentration, insomnia or hypersomnia, and emotional reactivity.
- It is usually out of proportion to the level of recent activity and interferes with functioning, affects 70–100% of patients undergoing treatment and may last for months to years after finishing therapy.

There may be factors contributing to fatigue. The reversible factors (e.g., anemia, insomnia) are managed with medicines.

In the absence of these factors, nonpharmacological interventions such as exercise, psychological counseling to reduce stress and anxiety, nutrition counseling, and sleep therapy are helpful.

Cardiovascular Changes

There are multiple reasons for a cancer patient to have higher chances of developing cardiovascular disease. Primarily, predisposing factors for cancer also promote cardiovascular problems. Furthermore, cancer causes immune-suppression; prolonged and extensive surgical trauma has additional effects.

Cancer therapy may cause direct as well as indirect damage to the cardiovascular system. For example RT to the chest wall (radiation-induced heart damage) in patients with breast, Hodgkin's or non-Hodgkin's lymphoma or drugs such as anthracyclines and taxanes can damage the muscle, electric systems or valves of heart; or may cause pericarditis, pericardial effusion, and this is usually called cardiotoxicity. This can occur as acute or late side effect of the cancer therapy. Indirect effects may result due to decreased physical activity levels, stress, sleep disturbances, fatigue, etc. Patients at risk are scheduled for routine 2D ECHO by their doctor.

Pulmonary Changes

They are commonly seen in patients with lung cancer, breast cancer, Hodgkin's lymphoma, etc.

- Most common changes are pneumonitis or pulmonary fibrosis and are related to RT or chemotherapy.
- Patients with HNC are at risk of developing aspiration pneumonia when swallowing is compromised.

Symptoms of acute radiation pneumonitis usually become evident 2–3 months after the completion of therapy; rarely, they occur within the first month and occasionally as late as 6 months after irradiation. Patient may experience dyspnea and nonproductive cough; it may be self-limiting or may progress to severe respiratory distress. They are usually detected by chest X-ray or high-resolution computed tomography (HRCT).

Neurological Changes

Neurological impairments may occur due to cancer itself or as a result of cancer therapy (e.g., surgery, radiation or chemotherapy). Patient may experience symptoms such as:

- Tingling
- Numbness
- Weakness
- Burning
- Radiating pain that may increase with dose and duration of therapy
- Chemotherapy may lead to problems with fine movements and balance.

These symptoms may or may not resolve after completion of therapy.

Peripheral neuropathy is one of the most common chronic complications of cancer and its treatment, especially due to certain chemotherapeutic drugs (e.g., taxanes) or postsurgery. The clinical manifestations of neuropathy may include any combination of weakness, sensory deficits, pain, and autonomic dysfunction with resultant gait and other functional deficits.

- Injuries to lateral thoracic nerve to serratus anterior or transection of medial or lateral pectoral nerve are the complications associated with breast cancer surgery.
- Injury to or dissection of recurrent laryngeal nerve or superior laryngeal nerve in HNC patients may result in vocal cord palsy or may require tracheostomy.
- Involvement of facial nerve due to direct tumor invasion or surgical insult is less common, but not rare.

Spinal cord injury (SCI): At times, symptoms are due to SCI as a result of metastasis (5% of all cancers). Cancer-related SCI most often occurs as a late complication and has poor prognosis.

Compressive radiculopathy/plexopathy resulting directly from cancer most commonly results from tumors arising from spinal cord, epidural space, vertebral body or paravertebral structures while noncompressive radiculopathy/ plexopathy results from radiation, chemotherapy, and paraneoplastic syndromes, e.g., brachial plexopathy after breast irradiation, lumbosacral plexopathy after pelvic irradiation.

Radiation myelopathy may manifest as an early and essentially reversible "transient radiation myelopathy" (after 1–6 months) or late and irreversible "delayed radiation myelopathy" (6–10 years after radiation). It is associated with RT to head and neck, lung, mediastinum, Hodgkin's disease, and metastatic tumors of spinal cord.

Musculoskeletal Changes

They can appear as a result of surgical damage, RT, or chemotherapy. Direct surgical insult results in impairment of local function due to resection, removal or relocation of muscle, nerve or connecting tissue. RT may lead to muscle fibrosis or neuralgia as late or persistent side effects. Certain chemotherapy drugs lead to arthralgia of small joints along with joint stiffness which may last even after completion of therapy. Cancer and also its therapy result in a decrease in lean muscle mass.

- *Bony metastasis* is a common complication of cancer (e.g., 69% of patients with advanced breast cancer) and has a risk of fracture resulting in pain and disability.
- *Radiation fibrosis* can damage any tissue type including skin, muscle, ligament, tendon, nerve, viscera, and bone. The effects of radiation can be acutely experienced during or immediately after treatment (up to 3 months), delayed (after 3 months), or late (years after completion of radiation). It can be localized or extensive, depending on the extent of radiation field. Common examples of localized fibrosis are shoulder

dysfunction, pain, axillary web syndrome, muscular tightness or fibrosis, neuropathy or lymphedema. Radiation fibrosis leading to brachial or lumbosacral plexopathy is most commonly seen in Hodgkin's lymphoma.

- *Shoulder pain and dysfunction* is one of the commonly seen complications in head and neck carcinoma patients, more associated with radical LN dissection. It usually results due to injury to spinal accessory nerve, cervical plexus or nerve supplying to rhomboids, levator scapulae, and scalenes. It is associated with pain, drooping of shoulder, decreased range of motion (ROM) (abduction affected the most), tipping of scapula, at times sternoclavicular subluxation, and adhesive capsulitis.
- *Axillary web syndrome* is characterized by palpable cords in the breast, underarm, medial arm, antecubital fossa, and/or forearm that develop after axillary LN dissection (38 to 72%) or sentinel LN biopsy (20%). It is associated with pain and shoulder ROM limitations (especially abduction) is often self-limited.
- The prevalence of *trismus* in HNC patients ranges from 5 to 38% and is a result of tumor invasion into critical structures of mastication. It is a common side effect of surgery or RT (worsens with increasing dosage of RT). Impairment in mouth opening may have an adverse effect on quality of life by compromising functions such as chewing, swallowing, respiratory function, oral hygiene and health, intimacy with partner and ability to self-examine for recurrence.

Lymphedema

Lymphedema is the abnormal accumulation of protein-rich lymphatic fluid in extremity, face, neck, trunk, or genitalia. It is usually diagnosed clinically with patient's history of cancer, surgery, LN dissection, or RT along with clinical signs and symptoms of edema, not reducing with elevation and positive Stemmer's sign. A positive Stemmer's sign is inability to pinch and lift a skinfold at the base of the second toe or middle finger. Common investigative tools, though rarely required, are lymphography, lymphoscintigraphy, and near-infrared fluorescence imaging.

Risk factors for lymphedema include:

- The extent of surgery and LN dissection (e.g., 3–5% incidence with Sentinel vs. 16–19% with axillary LN dissection)
- Radiation therapy
- Certain chemotherapy drugs (e.g., taxanes)
- Being overweight or obese

It is most commonly seen in patients with breast cancer and sometimes in patients with head and neck, cervix, prostate, and colorectal cancer. In patients with HNC, it can also affect the area of face and neck and at times can affect internally, which can be dangerous as it may compress on to trachea or esophagus.

If untreated, the accumulation of protein rich fluid can lead to fibrosis and worsening of lymphedema and may result in elephantiasis or lymphangiosarcoma. It is associated with limb heaviness, decreased sensation or numbness, aching, chronic pain, and increased chances of infection. Lymphedema can occur as acute, long-term, or late (at times after years) side effect of the treatment. At times, patient may also develop seroma, a fluid-filled pocket, after mastectomy and axillary surgery which may require aspiration or drain.

Pain

There are varieties of factors leading to pain such as:

- Tissue or nerve damage from original tumor
- Treatment-related injury from surgery
- Postural changes
- Radiation or chemotherapy

At times, pain may be caused due to noncancer conditions resulting from cancer treatment. Irradiation of pelvis in cervix or colorectal cancer patients may result in pelvic inflammatory disease which may lead to chronic pelvic pain syndrome.

Oral Complications

Chemotherapy or radiation-induced oral *mucositis* is an inflammation of the mucous membranes of the oral cavity and oropharynx characterized by tissue erythema, edema, and atrophy, often progressing to ulceration. Approximately 40% of patients receiving chemotherapy and almost all patients undergoing radiation to oropharyngeal area develop oral mucositis. It leads to oropharyngeal pain which in turn interferes with patient's mouth opening, speech, swallowing, and food intake.

Xerostomia is a major clinical problem experienced by patients who receive head and neck RT, with severity dependent on RT dosage and volume of exposed salivary glands and occasionally increased by chemotherapy. It is defined as dry mouth resulting from reduced or absent saliva flow, can be transient or permanent. It causes pain, discomfort, minimal and thickened saliva, difficulty in speaking and swallowing, oral infection or dental caries, decreased nutrition intake, and, therefore, reduced body weight.

Sleep Disturbance

Patients may complain of difficulty falling asleep, difficulty staying asleep, or early morning awakening. Apart from pharmacological therapy, exercise and yoga may improve sleep quality.

Issues with Body Image and Confidence

Surgical procedures in breast and HNC patients lead to issues with body image and identity of patients as their body or face does not preserve their previous own identity. RT may lead to skin erythema, dry desquamation, moist desquamation, darkening, and ulceration which may last for a few weeks, but usually is reversible. Chemotherapy on the other hand leads to darkening of toenails and hair loss which may take a long time to recover. Hair loss or alopecia can be an immense burden, serving as a stressful visible reminder of the patient's disease and negatively impacting social function; it also results in a loss of privacy because it reveals the patient's medical condition.

Nausea and Vomiting

Nausea and vomiting are the most common side effects resulting due to complications directly or indirectly related to cancer itself or its therapy, especially related to chemotherapy (70–80% patients undergoing chemotherapy). If treated inadequately, they impair functional activity, increase the use of other health resources, and at times reduce adherence to cancer treatment (~20% patients).

Increased Risk of Infections

Cancer patients are at increased risk for infection because of their disease and its treatment. It can be due to intrinsic host factors (e.g., tumor itself or hematological malignancies), treatment-related factors (e.g., mucositis, chemotherapy-induced neutropenia) or immunomodulatory agents (e.g., corticosteroids).

Chemotherapy-induced Neutropenia and Thrombocytopenia

They are the most frequent manifestations of cytotoxic chemotherapy-induced myelosuppression and may last several weeks. There is an increased risk of mortality from infection and bleeding, more frequent hospitalizations, increased treatment cost, reduction in dose intensity of chemotherapy, and treatment discontinuation.

Gastrointestinal Changes

Radiation to head and neck can cause esophageal stricture and to abdomen or pelvis may cause malabsorption, adhesions, and diarrhea. Surgical resection in colorectal cancer patient may lead to diarrhea, fecal incontinence, urgency, etc. These effects may last for years. Chemotherapy, RT, and certain targeted therapy may also lead to diarrhea or constipation.

Endocrine Changes

In pediatric population, effect to endocrine system results in growth and developmental abnormalities. In adult population, changes are specific to location of tumor and treatment involved. For example HNC radiation may result in hypothyroidism. Patient may experience fatigue, weight gain, weakness, depression, etc. Chemotherapy drug cyclophosphamide may result in infertility in both genders.

Sexual Dysfunction

Despite widespread acknowledgment that sexual function is often profoundly disrupted by cancer treatment, it is still a least acknowledged and addressed problem, especially in India. It is commonly affecting patients with prostate, testicles, bladder, head and neck, bone, bone marrow, lymphatic system, colorectal, breast, and gynecological cancers. Apart from direct sexual dysfunction, there are factors affecting intimacy between the partners due to fear of transmission of disease, problems with self-body image and acceptance (e.g., disfigurement of face in HNC, mastectomy or lymphedema in breast cancer patients).

Psychological Issues

The diagnosis of cancer is a life-altering experience for patients and their families. A wide range of psychiatric and psychological problems affect patients and families before, during, and after cancer care and treatment due to anxiety about survival, relapse and treatment effects, medical isolation, helplessness, disruption of social roles, truncated future, and loss of social contacts. The problems may clinically vary from depression, anxiety, stress-related disorders (e.g., panic, phobias, post-traumatic stress disorder), adjustment disorders, delirium to other neurocognitive disorders.

Health-related Quality of Life

Health-related quality of life (HRQoL) is a multidimensional concept that includes domains related to physical, mental, emotional, and social functioning and focuses on the impact health status has on these domains. It is important to assess how a patient feels rather than just addressing clinical findings. Cancer and its treatment cause a significant decline in HRQoL during and may affect for months to years after completion of therapy. Most of the research on HRQoL in cancer patients have concluded that the physical well-being is the most commonly and intensively negatively affected aspect followed by emotional well-being.

CANCER REHABILITATION

Cancer rehabilitation is a process that helps cancer survivors obtain and maintain the maximal possible physical, social, psychological, and vocational functioning within the limits created by cancer and its treatments. Comprehensive cancer rehabilitation team includes medical oncologist, radiation oncologist, oncosurgeon, rehabilitation physician (physiatrist), physical therapist, occupational therapist, speech–language pathologist, nutritionist, psychologist, yoga therapist, and others. The major part of rehabilitation is aimed at addressing side effects of cancer and cancer therapy in addition to treating cancer impairments.

Cancer-related symptoms and side effects have a negative impact on patient's physical, emotional, functional, and social well-being and thus decline in HRQoL. The effects may be short-term or may last for months to years. Certain delayed side effects may arise after years of completing cancer treatment.

A detailed mindful assessment is of key role/importance to make appropriate rehabilitation program for patients.

Assessment

History and Diagnosis

- Type of cancer e.g., sarcoma, carcinoma
- Area affected (Location/body part) e.g., breast/head and neck
- Side (left or right) if applicable

Stage of Cancer

Treatment—completed, current, or planned

Treatment for cancer includes:

- **Surgery:** Date of surgery, details of surgical notes, tissues removed/dissected, LNs dissected, grafts taken
- **RT:** Targeted area, number of sessions and dosage, start date
- **Chemo/hormonal/targeted therapy:** Drug name, frequency, intervals, number of cycles, and total duration.

Medication Review

Patient's current medication list needs to be reviewed as there may be few medicines which may require more attention or may need modification or caution while prescribing exercises. For example, beta-blockers, hormonal therapy drugs, steroids, chemotherapy medicines, etc.

Medical History or Comorbidities

It is important to know if patient has any preexisting medical problems such as hypertension, diabetes, known cardiovascular disease, cholesterol, osteoarthritis, and joint pain which will require modification in the rehabilitation program.

Family History of Cancer

Personal history

Tobacco chewing or smoking: Current or ex consumer, duration, pack years

Alcohol: Current or ex consumer, amount.

Review of reports

Following reports are analyzed:

- Routine blood investigations—hemoglobin, neutrophil, thrombocyte counts, lipid and sugar profile
- Biopsy report
- USG
- CT/MRI/PET/SPECT scan
- Other relevant reports, e.g., 2D ECHO, PFT, etc.

Symptoms

The past as well as current symptoms include—Onset, intensity, aggravating and relieving factors, relation of symptom to certain therapy if cyclic, and duration for which they last.

Physical Assessment

- Height, weight, BMI
- Fat and muscle mass: Bioimpedance
- Vitals: Heart rate, blood pressure, etc.
- Blood sugar, if diabetic.

Fatigue Assessment

It should be assessed in detail at the beginning, during, and post rehabilitation.

- Onset of fatigue
- Aggravating and relieving factors
- Diurnal variations
- Variation in relation to certain cancer therapy
- Based on National Comprehensive Cancer Network (NCCN) guidelines, fatigue should be assessed quantitatively on a 0–10 scale (0 = no fatigue and 10 = worst fatigue imaginable); patients with a severity of >4 should be further evaluated by history and physical examination.
- Brief measures do not fully capture the following various dimensions of fatigue:
  - Sensory dimension (fatigue severity, persistence).
  - Physiologic dimension (e.g., leg weakness, diminished mental concentration), performance dimension (reduction in performance of needed or valued activities).
  - There are various tools available to measure fatigue for cancer patients.
  - For example, FACT—Fatigue questionnaire, Fatigue inventory, Fatigue assessment scale.

Cardiovascular System Assessment

A close monitoring of vitals (heart rate and blood pressure) and patient symptoms is important for those at higher risk of developing cardiotoxicity.

- Regular vital assessment at rest and during exercise sessions
- Reviewing ECG or 2D echo reports
- Submaximal or symptom-limited tests, e.g., 6-minute walk test (6MWT).

Neurological Assessment

Neurological assessment includes:

- Examination of sensation
- Tone assessment
- Manual muscle testing
- Balance assessment
- Peripheral or central nervous system assessment
- There are few tools that can be used to evaluate the impact of neurotoxicity on patient, e.g., FACT_NTx13.

Musculoskeletal System Assessment

The accurate assessment of musculoskeletal disorders, including the differentiation of benign from malignant etiologies of pain, is an important component of the cancer rehabilitation assessment.

- Postural changes
- Range of motion and tissue tightness
- Manual muscle testing
- Pain assessment—a detailed pain assessment including intensity, location, aggravating and relieving factors, variation in relation to certain drugs/therapy:
  - **Type:** It can be somatic, visceral, or neuropathic
  - **Temporal aspect:** Acute, subacute, episodic, or chronic
  - **Intensity of pain:** Numeric rating scale or visual analog scale

  Measurement schema: Brief pain inventory, McGill pain questionnaire.
- Mouth opening for HNC patients
- Temporomandibular joint assessment, evaluation for trismus
- Shoulder, spine, or other assessment

Lymphedema Assessment

- Regular screening (if absent at the time of assessment)
- Associated symptom assessment: Skin condition, pain, vascular system, range of motion, tissue tightness, and manual muscle testing
- Objective assessment: A relative change of 10% in circumference or volume compared to the initial (preoperative) or unaffected side is defined as lymphedema.
- Volumetric assessment **(Figs. 37.2A and B):** Water displacement method relies on measuring the amount of water that is displaced from a container when the limb or part of the limb is submerged. This provides information on the volume of the whole limb, including the hand or foot, and can be used to accurately measure the hand or foot alone. The total volume of each limb can be used to calculate the excess and percentage excess volume of the whole limb, hand, or foot. It is most reliable and recommended, but time consuming and is generally not practical for clinical use.
  - Absolute circumference measurements: Most commonly, the limb is marked and measured at 4-cm intervals. There are formulas available based on which limb volume from the measurement values can be calculated, though less reliable.
    a. Herpertz method
    b. Kuhnke method
  - Bioimpedance spectroscopy (BIS): It measures extracellular fluid by resistance to a small electrical current. BIS appears to be more sensitive than traditional diagnostic methods in potentially detecting early changes before physically measurable changes in limb volume are observed.
  - Infrared perometry: It uses infrared light and optoelectronic sensors to calculate limb volume from the three-dimensional silhouette of the limb.
  - Moisture meter
- Severity: Difference between volume of affected and unaffected extremity
  - Subclinical or no lymphedema (less than 10% difference)
  - Minimal (less than 20% difference)
  - Moderate (20–40% difference)
  - Severe (more than 40% difference)
- Staging (International Guidelines on Lymphedema and Lymphatic Disorders by European Society of Lymphology) **(Figs. 37.3A to D)**
  - 0: Subclinical or latent
  - I: Swelling reduces with limb elevation, pitting edema
  - II: Early stage—Limb elevation rarely reduces swelling, edema is still pitting
  - II: Late stage—Nonpitting edema due to tissue fibrosis
  - III: Lymphostatic elephantiasis.

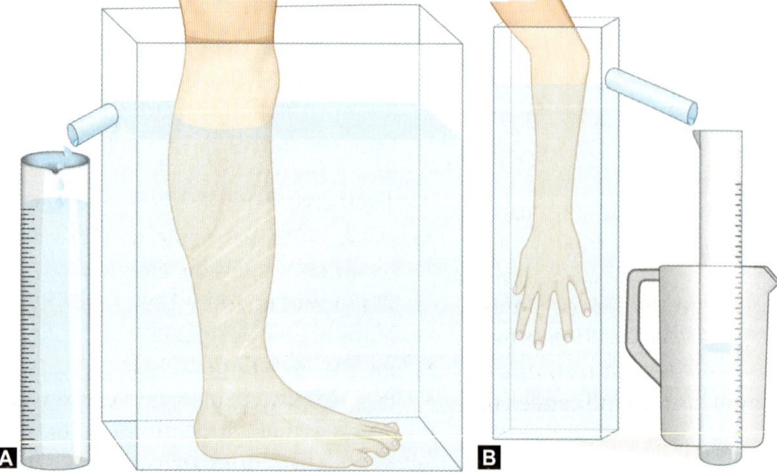

Figs. 37.2A and B: Volumetric assessment of lymphedema.

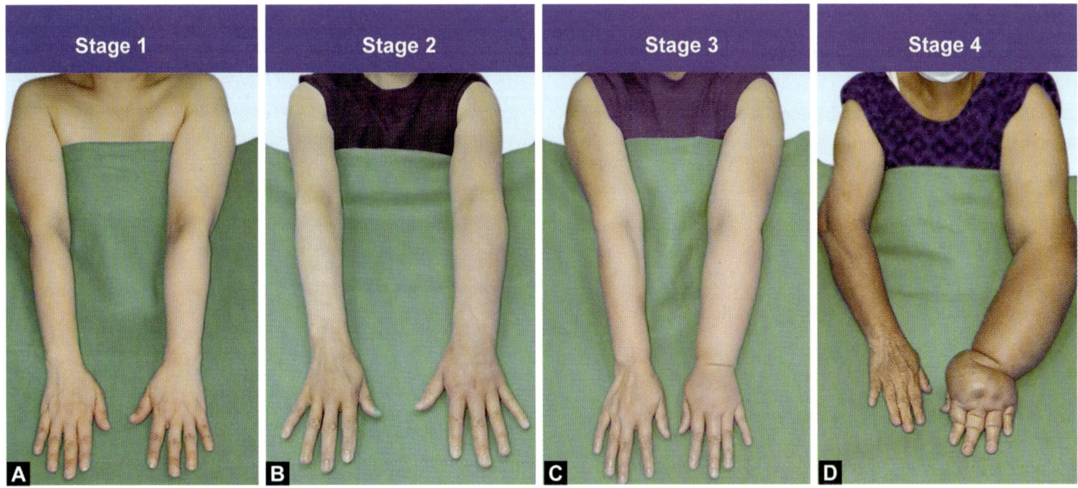

Figs. 37.3A to D: Stages of lymphedema by the European Society of Lymphology.

Health-Related Quality of Life Assessment

There are numerous patient-reported questionnaires which are developed to assess different aspects of quality of life of cancer patients such as physical, emotional, social, and functional.

- Functional Assessment of Cancer Therapy (FACT), now called Functional Assessment of Chronic Illness Therapy (FACIT)
- European Organization for the Research and Treatment of Cancer Quality of Life Questionnaire (EORTC QLQ-C30)
- SF-36 (short form-36) Health Survey
- The Memorial Symptom Assessment Scale (MSAS)
- Edmonton Symptom Assessment Scale
- Performance Status Scale (PSS) for head and neck patients
- There are many other questionnaires that can be used to assess impairment specific problems.
  For example Disabilities of the Arm, Shoulder, and Hand (DASH) questionnaire or The Shoulder Pain and Disability Index (SPADI)—to assess pain and disability in breast/head/neck cancer patients.

Nutritional Assessment

- All of the major modalities of cancer treatment, including surgery, radiation, and chemotherapy, can significantly impact nutritional needs, alter regular eating habits, and adversely affect how the body digests, absorbs, and uses food.
- Symptoms such as anorexia, early satiety, changes in taste and smell, and disturbances of the gastrointestinal tract are common side effects of cancer treatment and can lead to inadequate nutrient intake and subsequent malnutrition, reported in more than 50% of patients. However, overnutrition also affects cancer pathogenesis and prognosis and influences the effectiveness of cancer therapy.
- Detailed nutrition assessment by a dietitian since the time of diagnosis and during and after cancer treatment is crucial to maintain adequate weight and protein intake of patients.
- Physical therapists should pay attention to patient's complaints of reduced food intake, nausea, vomiting, diarrhea and seek dietitian's help immediately. If left un-addressed, they can lead to a drastic reduction in weight and may impact the treatment plan.

Assessment of Speech and Swallowing

It is usually done by speech and swallowing pathologist for HNC patients.

- Speech assessment includes the assessment of respiration, phonation, resonance, and articulation which decides understandability of speech and requirement of assistive devices (e.g., trial of a trache-esophageal voice prosthesis: TEP).
- Swallowing assessment includes an evaluation of oral sphincter competence, the patient's ability to handle secretions, tongue to premaxillary/palatal contact, anterior–posterior movement of the tongue, location of sensate tissue, and identification of areas where food will collect (i.e., dead space) which is done by assessing patient's ability to remove the bolus from an eating utensil (e.g., a spoon), create a labial seal, manipulate the bolus, control the bolus, and clear the bolus is assessed.
- Fiberoptic endoscopic evaluation of swallowing (FEES) or videofluoroscopic swallow study (VFSS) can be used to objectively assess swallowing.
- Their assessment also includes normalcy of diet, i.e., solid, semisolid, liquid, and requirement to have food orally or need for feeding tube insertion [nasogastric or percutaneous endoscopic gastrostomy (PEG) tube].

Cognitive and Psychological Assessment

- It is usually done by a psychologist on various issues such as fear of death, acceptance of disease, depression screening, stress and anxiety evaluation, sleep disturbance, and family support and expectations.

- It also involves assessing the nature of the patient's response to diagnosis and effects of cancer and its therapy as it will affect patient's mood, adherence to treatment, and the quality of his or her social support.

Goals of Rehabilitation Program

Goals of rehabilitation may vary if patient is currently undergoing cancer treatment or has completed or is going to undergo in future. Setting goals for cancer rehabilitation is a critical task as it involves clinical knowledge about current patient problems, variation in problems in relation to cancer treatment, and managing patient expectations. It needs regular reassessments and revision, especially if the patient is on active cancer therapy.

Goals should be SMART (specific, measurable, achievable, realistic, and timely). They can be short-term and long-term. Goals should be framed keeping in mind the patient's goals and not only therapy directed, e.g., improve physical fitness, weight loss, lymphedema management and starting new activity.

Developing Plan of Care

Plan of care focuses on two aspects: cancer specific and general. It is more appropriate to use words as "symptom specific" rather than "cancer specific," where the plan is made to address current symptoms of patients, e.g., pain, restricted range of motion, muscle weakness, restricted mouth opening, and lymphedema. It is more focused on to cancer-affected area. General plan of care involves overall fitness levels of patient, fatigue, nutrition, emotional well-being, etc.

Plans have to be made keeping in mind that cancer patients have relatively lower levels of energy due to fatiguability, muscle wasting, cardiovascular side effects, depression, fear, or anxiety. Therefore planning an exercise program is to be done with high caution and at relatively lower intensity levels as compared to other patients. Exercise progression should be slow too and should be modified with repeated reassessments.

It is important to discuss with patients if their expected goal is achievable or not and to draw attention to other therapy goals which are important for their health but not present on their list. For example an obese patient having stage III lymphedema may have a goal of reducing swelling through manual lymphatic drainage (MLD) alone. Though actual goal needs additional weight loss to optimize benefits and the plan of care needs complete or complex decongestive therapy (CDT) to achieve reduction in swelling. It is important to discuss therapy goal with reasons (e.g., not explaining patients about effects of weight loss on lymphedema, may have low compliance related to weight management therapy), explaining plan of care [e.g., doing MLD alone is not going to achieve benefit for stage III lymphedema, patient may need CDT, i.e., intermittent pneumatic compression (IPC), exercise and multilayer lymphedema bandaging (MLLB) in addition to MLD] and being realistic (e.g., doing CDT is time-consuming,

difficult to manage, expensive, will reduce lymphedema to great extent but will not cure completely).

This will help therapist to build a comprehensive program to achieve multiple goals, keeping in mind what patient wants to achieve the most and thus having higher patient satisfaction and better compliance.

PRECAUTIONS OR CONTRAINDICATIONS TO EXERCISE FOR PATIENTS WITH CANCER

Contraindication for Exercise Testing

The absolute and relative contraindication for exercise testing for cancer patients remain the same as for other patients as recommended by exercise testing and prescription guidelines by different bodies, e.g., American Cancer Society (ACS), American College of Sports Medicine (ACSM), American Thoracic Society (ATS), American College of Chest Physicians (ACCP), and American Association of Cardiovascular and Pulmonary Rehabilitation (AACVPR).

Some of the absolute contraindications to exercise testing suggested by the ACS are as follows:
- Acute myocardial infarction (3–5 days)
- Unstable angina
- Uncontrolled cardiac dysrhythmias causing symptoms or hemodynamic compromise
- Symptomatic severe aortic stenosis
- Uncontrolled symptomatic heart failure
- Acute pulmonary embolus or pulmonary infarction
- Acute myocarditis or pericarditis
- Acute systemic infection, accompanied by fever, body aches, or swollen lymph glands
- Uncontrolled asthma
- Pulmonary edema
- Resting SpO_2 levels below 85%
- Respiratory failure
- Evidence of extensive visceral or skeletal metastasis or both

Precautions to Exercise in Patients with Cancer

The following precautions need to be taken by patients with cancer while exercising:
- Thrombocytopenia: Less than $20,000/\mu L \rightarrow$ no aerobic exercise
- Anemia: Hematocrit <25%, hemoglobin <8 mg/dL $\rightarrow$ avoid aerobics
- Neutropenia: Absolute neutrophil count <500/μL $\rightarrow$ high risk of infection to patient; strict hygiene should be followed
- Pulmonary dysfunction: FEV_1 or diffusion capacity between 50 and 75% of predicted $\rightarrow$ light aerobics, consider supplemental oxygen if needed
- Large pleural effusion or pericardial effusions $\rightarrow$ No aerobics without consulting cardiologist/oncologist
- Cardiac dysfunction: Recent premature ventricular contractions, fast atrial arrhythmias, ventricular arrhythmia, ischemic pattern $\rightarrow$ no aerobics without consulting cardiologist/oncologist

- Electrolyte abnormalities: Sodium <130 mEq/L → no exercise
- Electrolyte abnormalities: Potassium <3.0 mEq/L or >6.0 mEq/L → no exercise
- Extensive skeletal metastasis
- Severe nausea.

PROGRAM IMPLEMENTATION

Multiple reviews published till now have found evidence supportive of role of exercise in attenuating cancer-related symptoms and side effects. Studies also suggest that exercise in cancer patients receiving radiation or chemotherapy helps to improve physical fitness, fatigue, health-related quality of life, depression, lymphedema, muscle atrophy, bone loss, cardiopulmonary toxicity, neurotoxicity, balance issues, and nausea.

Cancer rehabilitation can be helpful during as well as after completion of cancer treatment. In certain patients, rehabilitation is recommended before starting the cancer therapy to have a better outcome. When exercise is undertaken after completion of cancer treatment, there are chances of achieving greater benefits. However, it does not mean delivering rehabilitation care during cancer treatment is not advisable. There are various studies that suggest that providing rehabilitation during cancer treatment reduces decline in the physical health and reduces the side effects associated with cancer treatment. Exercise during cancer treatment helps to prevent the decline in cardiorespiratory fitness, muscle strength and endurance and thus health-related quality of life. So, it is important to remember the fact that during active cancer therapy, rehabilitation may not show positive impact on patient but it may lessen the negative effects.

The major areas where rehabilitation can help are fatigue, pain, cardiovascular and pulmonary toxicity, neurological impairments, musculoskeletal problems, lymphedema, incontinence, speech and swallowing difficulties, maintaining nutrition, and maintaining emotional well-being.

Management of Fatigue

A structured rehabilitation program that includes physical activity interventions, yoga, energy conservation and activity management, management of concurrent symptoms, nutrition education, supportive counseling, and measures to optimize sleep quality has shown supportive evidence for reducing fatigue levels.

The goal of physical activity interventions is to maintain or improve physical function by means of aerobic exercises. Regular exercises focusing on improving cardiorespiratory fitness have the maximum positive effects on fatigue levels both during and following treatment (*see* the "Cardiorespiratory Fitness/Exercise and Physical Activity Prescription" section for details of aerobic exercise prescription).

Other complimentary therapies such as acupuncture, massage, corticosteroids, ginseng, bright light therapy, and mindfulness-based stress reduction have shown some supporting evidence in fatigue management.

Clinical Pearl

In patients with significant fatigue levels, exercise needs multiple breaks and slower progression with a close check on fatigue levels by use of patient-reported outcome measures. Activities or session needs to be planned at the time of day when patient feels more energetic.

Management of Pain

Pain arising from musculoskeletal impairments, e.g., surgical insult and postural changes, is easier to manage. Usual treatment includes therapeutic massage, therapeutic heat, therapeutic cold, patient education (advice on activity modification), transcutaneous electrical nerve stimulation (TENS), range of motion and strengthening exercise, training ambulation using assistive devices, environmental modification, energy conservation, and work-simplification techniques.

Hypersensitive skin can be treated with desensitization measures with other alternative sensory stimuli that are tolerated fairly by the patient. A hyposensitive skin can be treated with sensory re-education methods using various forms and textures of materials.

A variety of physiotherapy treatment methods such as electrical simulation, magnetic therapy, pulsed electromagnetic energy, photon stimulation, and monochromatic near-infrared therapy for peripheral neuropathic pain are used. Cognitive behavioral therapy (CBT) intervention comprising education, distraction, relaxation, positive mood development, and self-coping strategies for pain helps the patient develop acceptance toward symptom persistence and enables them to lead a functionally active life.

Note: While active RT, application of any physical agents or touching or stroking of skin of the area being exposed to radiation, is contraindicated.

Dry needling can be done on the site that is not affected by cancer and there is evidence of no possible metastasis.

Cardiorespiratory Fitness/Exercise and Physical Activity Prescription

Currently, there is no evidence supporting a different response to exercise in patients with cancer from that in other population. Exercise prescription guidelines are followed as recommended by the ACSM and ACS.

It has been proven that aerobic exercise improves cardiorespiratory fitness in breast, prostate, hematologic cancers, while in other cancers, it has shown to have possible benefits and require more extensive research. Aerobic and resistance training exercise interventions can be given during active cancer treatment as well as after completion of cancer therapy.

Aerobic Exercise (Figs. 37.4A to C)

- Frequency—2–5 days a week
- Intensity—50–75% of maximum heart rate
- Type—walking, cycling, swimming, cross-trainer, etc.
- Time—10–60 minutes (continuous or multiple interrupted bouts of exercise throughout the day)
- Duration—6–26 weeks.

Clinical Pearl

Pool activities are not advised for patients with intravenous catheter or those who are receiving radiation therapy or chemotherapy (within 48 hours of drug administration).

Clinical Pearl

For some patients who are under active cancer treatment, exercise progression needs to be slow. At times, despite regular rehabilitation, there may be a need to reduce the intensity and duration of exercise, instead of gradual increase. It should not be disappointing to the therapist or patient. Sometimes not getting decline in patient's health or getting lesser decline is also an achievement.

The exercise program for cancer patients does not typically require electrocardiographic monitoring, although regular monitoring of heart rate and blood pressure is useful. Recent statement from the American Heart Association recommends the use of cardiac rehabilitation to provide structured exercise and ancillary services to cancer patients and survivors which is termed as **cardio-oncology rehabilitation**. It is proposed to identify patients at high risk of cardiovascular disease (CVD) including cardiotoxicity related to cancer therapies and use the multimodal approach of cardiac rehabilitation (e.g., exercise plus nutritional counseling and cardiovascular risk factor assessment) to prevent or mitigate cardiovascular events.

6MWT gives a lot of insight in deciding the intensity of exercise. For example a patient could walk 120 m on 6MWT, and it was somewhat hard on Borg scale 6–20 [rate of perceived exertion (RPE) 13], can do 60–70-m walking (with breaks if needed) as aerobic exercise to begin with (keeping RPE levels between 9 and 11).

Physical activity suggestions for cancer survivors by US Department of Health and Human Services and ACSM round table guidelines are as follows:

- 150 minutes per week for moderate intensity
- 75 minutes per week of vigorous intensity
- If cancer survivors are unable to meet these recommendations, they should be as active as their abilities and conditions allow and avoid inactivity.

Clinical Pearl

It is important to understand that prescribing exercise in the expected intensity or duration may not be possible in all the patients. For some patients, doing simple mobility exercise may also be tiring, and for some doing 45 minutes, aerobic exercise may be light-intensity exercise. While we aim to prescribe exercise in the recommended framework, it is extremely important to give priority to patient symptoms and to keep a check on their fatigue levels and rate of perceived exertion (RPE) every single time. Remember "DO NO HARM".

Muscle Strength and Endurance

Resistance training is effective in improving muscle strength and endurance, especially in breast, head and neck, and prostate cancer patients. ACSM and ACS guidelines also recommend strength training for all cancer patients (caution for metastatic bone cancer patients and patients with severe osteoporosis). Strength training of large muscle groups of the body (not specific to cancer affected area) adds to the benefits achieved by aerobic exercise.

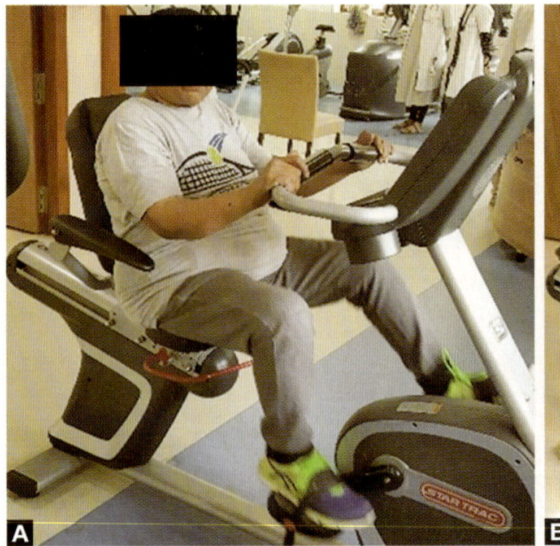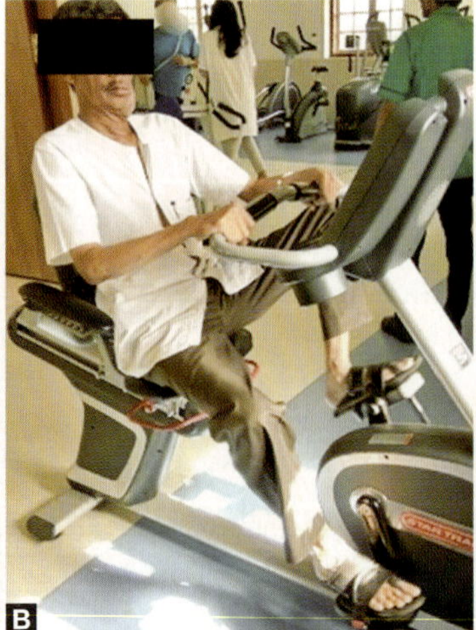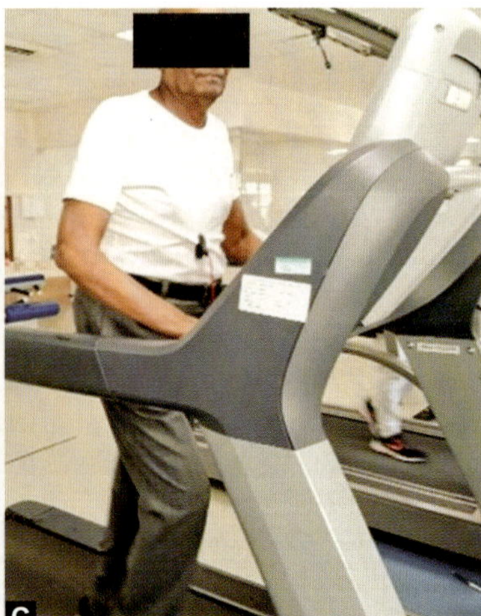

Figs. 37.4A to C: Aerobic exercise on (A and B) Stationary bicycle; (C) Treadmill.
Courtesy: Sir HN Reliance Foundation Hospital, Mumbai.

Resistance Training

- Frequency—1–5 days a week (at least 48 hours break for the same muscle group) **(Figs. 37.5A to C)**
- Intensity—25–85% of 1RM
- Type—large muscle groups (five to nine different muscle groups)
- Sets—1–3
- Repetitions—8–10
- Duration of program—3–52 weeks

For postoperative patients, resistance training of the muscles involved in the surgery should be started after 4–6 weeks.

Clinical Pearl

In case the patient is too fragile to do 1RM testing in view of possible chances of injury, it is easier to start with gentle Theraband exercises for large muscle groups and use free weights as light as half kilogram and progress them slowly in consecutive sessions as per their tolerance. Current recommendations suggest to begin with very light resistance and progress resistance gradually after two consecutive "pain-free" sessions.

Addressing Musculoskeletal Impairments

Specific rehabilitation interventions depend on the combination of deficits and are generally similar to those used in patients with other etiologies of musculoskeletal disorders or impairments. Restricted range of movements and tightness of tissues are common result of surgery as well as RT. Flexibility exercise should be used in routine as per clinical allowable time frames for postsurgical patients.

In postsurgical patients, if the drains are in situ, range of motion exercise of the immediate joint, proximal and distal, should be done as permitted by the surgeon. After removal of drains, gentle active, active-assisted ROM exercises should begin. Slow sustained passive stretching should be commenced after removal of sutures, but the time frame should be adjusted depending on the type of surgery, structures involved, graft taken, and surgeon's preference.

Clinical Pearl

To begin exercises of affected or surrounding areas (around recipient site) in patients with graft surgeries, it is necessary to wait till the graft is "accepted" which can be only confirmed by the surgeon and a therapist will need to wait for a green signal from the surgeon.

In subacute or chronic phase postsurgery or postradiation therapy, various physical therapy techniques can be used, e.g., passive stretching, mobilization, tissue release techniques, dry needling, and heat or ice modalities unless contraindicated.

Clinical Pearl

During active radiation therapy, due to side effects on the skin over irradiated area, any kind of stroking or touching of skin and application of heat or ice therapies directly to the irradiated area is contraindicated as it can lead to inflammation, ulceration, infection or bleeding.

Postradiation muscle fibrosis is not very common but possible, at times irreversible, complication of RT. Therapist needs to have realistic goals and can work on maintaining the remaining range by preventing further tightening and improving flexibility of surrounding muscles. Major role of rehabilitation lies in preventing it by starting early rehabilitation.

According to Cochrane database review, shoulder pain and dysfunction in head and neck carcinoma respond better with progressive resistance exercises in addition to other treatment modalities in comparison to traditional physiotherapy regimen.

Combination of physical therapy and speech-swallowing therapy is the mainstay of trismus treatment

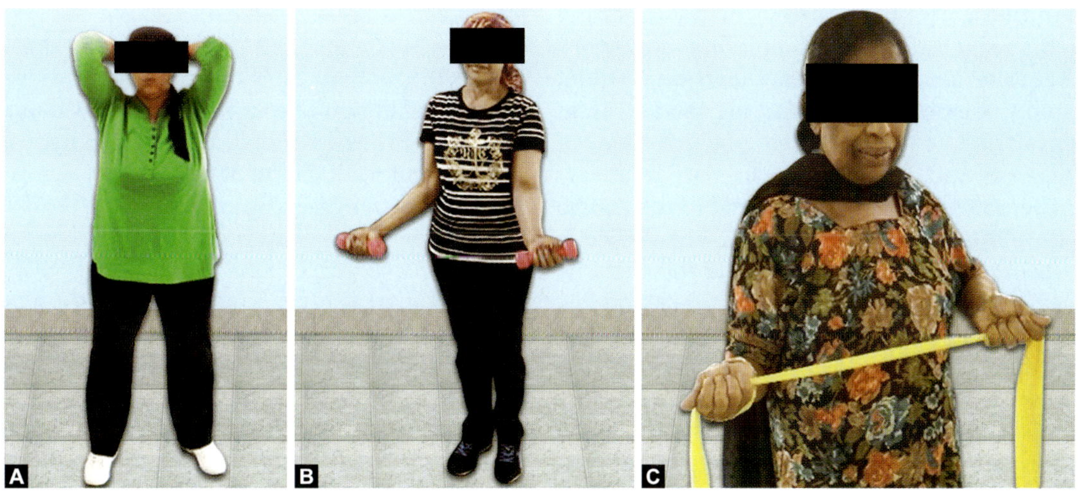

Figs. 37.5A to C: (A) Breathing exercise; (B and C) Strength training.
Courtesy: Sir HN Reliance Foundation Hospital, Mumbai.

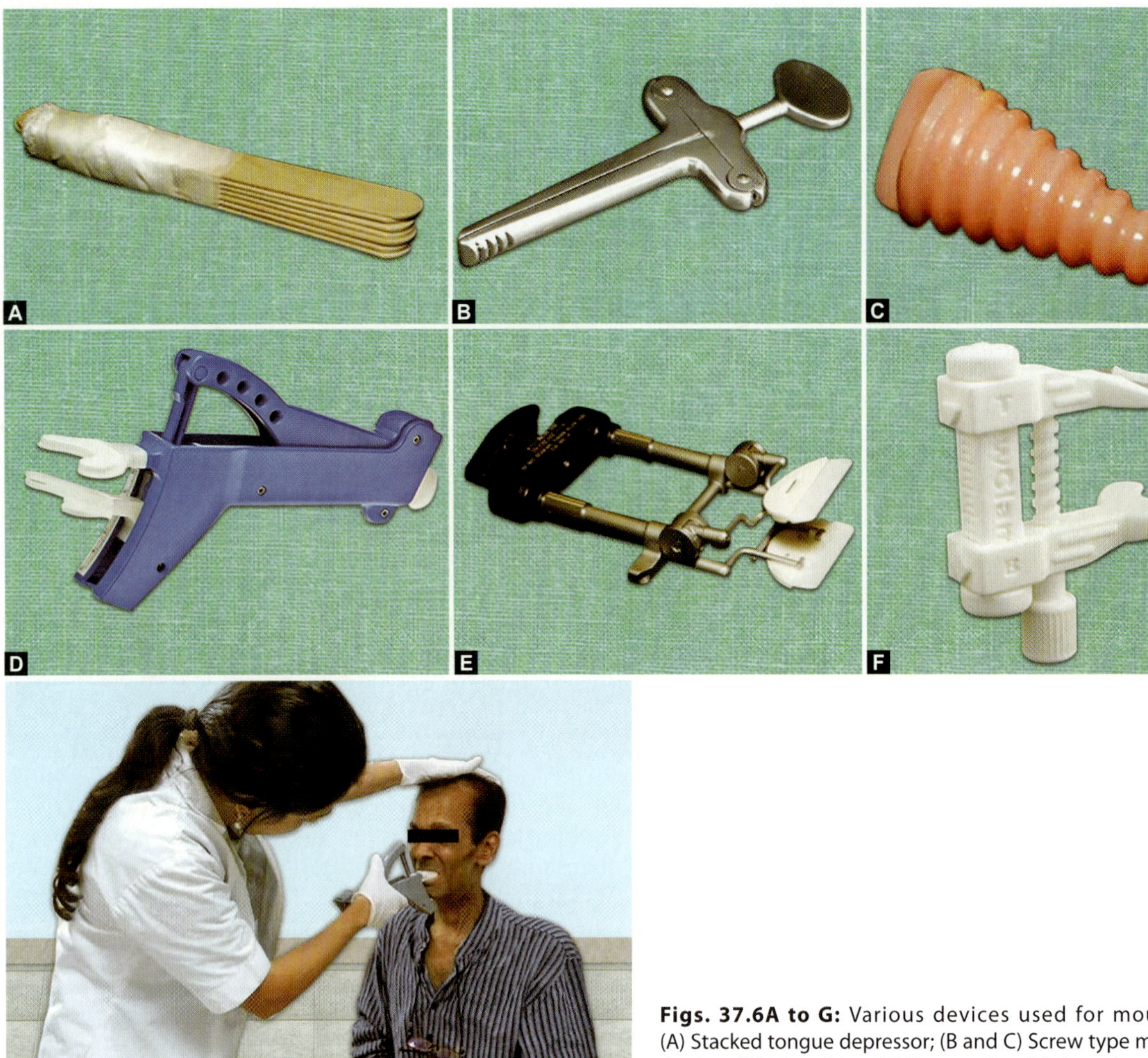

Figs. 37.6A to G: Various devices used for mouth opening: (A) Stacked tongue depressor; (B and C) Screw type mouth opening device; (D) Therabite; (E) Dynasplint; (F) Jaw clamp; (G) Patient practicing mouth opening with Therabite with speech therapist. *Courtesy:* Sir HN Reliance Foundation Hospital, Mumbai.

for patients with HNC. Apart from mouth opening and stretching exercises, passive mobilization of temporomandibular joint, a variety of jaw-opening devices such as stacked tongue depressors, corkscrew devices, TheraBite Jaw Motion Rehabilitation System, and Dynasplint Trismus System can be used to treat trismus **(Figs. 37.6A to G)**. In clinical practice, stacked tongue depressors and corkscrew devices are relatively ineffective. TheraBite may be effective early in the course of trismus development and easy to use. The device is inserted in the mouth and activated to near tolerance by squeezing leveraged handles for few repetitions and few seconds hold. This is usually repeated several times per day. It may cause rebound spasm of the masseter and pterygoid muscles. If the patient has had trismus for more than 3 months, the Dynasplint Trismus System may be a better option because it works on the principle of low-torque, prolonged stretch. It is kept in an open position in the mouth for several minutes and is repeated 2–3 times

a day. At times, therapy may only be able to reduce the progression of trismus and possibly may not be able to stop progression or reverse it.

Muscle strength can also be affected due to surgical insults (retraction, excision, grafting, or nerve damage), and rehabilitation of it may involve activation, isometric, isotonic, concentric or eccentric strength training of muscle, and reeducation of new muscle action apart from the regular strengthening guidelines.

Addressing Neurological Impairments

Rehabilitation interventions depend on the types of deficit and are generally similar to those used in patients with other etiologies of neurological disorders. For example, rehabilitation of brain tumors is having the same principles and practices as rehabilitation for traumatic brain injury or stroke.

Rehabilitation efforts are directed toward goals such as improving bed mobility, transfers, self-care, and ambulation (may vary from patient to patient, e.g., wheelchair training or gait training), prescription and use of assistive devices and/or orthosis (e.g., ankle–foot orthosis), achieving bowel and bladder continence, safe swallowing, adequate nutritional intake, optimal sensory input (including vision and hearing), and restorative sleep. Pharmacologic and nonpharmacologic therapies to address pain, spasticity, mood, bowel and bladder, and sleep and wake issues are often indicated.

Treatment of peripheral neuropathy may include desensitization techniques to deal with pain, maintaining range of motion and flexibility, improving strength of weak muscles, and prescription and use of splints and braces.

Rehabilitation of cancer survivors with spinal-cord dysfunction is a challenging endeavor and is similar to other etiologies of SCI (e.g., trauma from a motor vehicle accident). But, the degree of functional recovery anticipated in a patient with a malignant cause of SCI is generally lower as compared to nonmalignant SCI. This is because patients with cancer tend to develop SCI later in their disease and usually progress in their cancer and other medical comorbidities.

Lymphedema Management

Lymphedema is not curable and must be managed as a chronic condition. At-risk patients should be educated about lymphedema and its complications, especially cellulitis. Risk reduction strategies include skin care and protection, avoiding venipuncture, blood pressure measurements, and constricting clothing or dependent positioning of the affected region.

Current standard therapeutic modalities are designed to serve as an external transport assist mechanism to help move fluid from affected areas to unaffected areas of lymphatic system. There are various therapies that can be tried for the management of lymphedema including complete decongestive therapy, exercise, low-level laser therapy (650–1,000 nm wavelength is believed to stimulate lymphatic motricity, lymphangiogenesis, and macrophage activity), weight reduction if overweight or obese, pharmacotherapy, LN transplant, and microscopic surgeries.

Complex Decongestive Therapy

Complex decongestive therapy (CDT) or combined physical therapy is by far the most commonly used and most effective modality. It comprises of multiple therapies: MLLB, MLD, IPC and exercise. It is divided in two phases: initial tntensive therapy phase and maintenance phase. It should be administered by a specialty trained therapist with the goal of reducing swelling and fibrosis in the affected area.

- The first phase (initial intensive therapy) consists of skin care, manual lymph drainage, ROM exercise, and compression typically applied with multilayered bandage-wrapping. It lasts 2–12 weeks depending on the amount of swelling and tissue firmness, and compression is maintained for 21–23 hours per day. Phase 2 (maintenance phase), initiated promptly after Phase 1, aims to conserve and optimize the results obtained in Phase 1. It consists of compression by a low-stretch elastic stocking or sleeve, skin care, continued "remedial" exercise, and repeated light massage as needed.

- *MLD* is a specific light manual scientific massage which activates the lymphatic channels and thus stimulates absorption and movement of lymph fluid from affected to unaffected area. There are various school of techniques available across the world: Vodder, Leduc, Foldi, Casley-Smith, LDI–Alan Hudson, and Asdonk are the known ones.

- *MLLB* **(Figs. 37.7A and B)** is the integral and most important part of lymphedema management, especially in stages II and III. It consists of finger or toe bandaging, foam roll to give conical shape to the extremity and nonelastic/short-stretch bandages. The aim is to create pressure gradient to facilitate movement of lymph fluid from distal to proximal area.

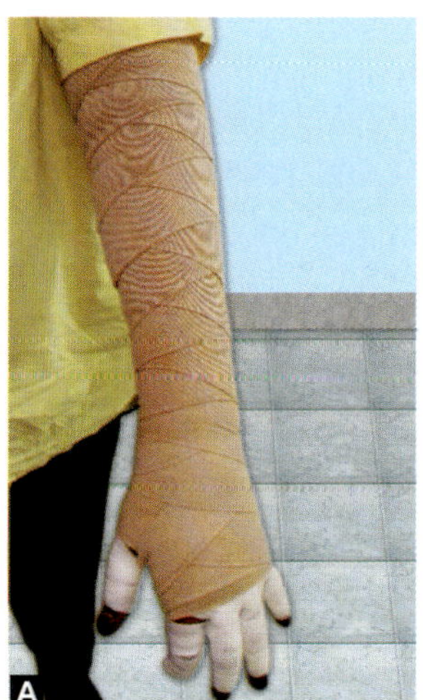
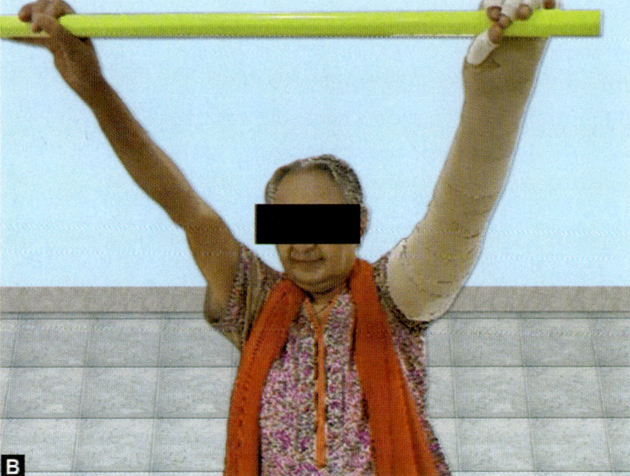

Figs. 37.7A and B: (A) Multilayer lymphedema bandaging (MLLB); (B) Patient exercising with MLLB.
Courtesy: Sir HN Reliance Foundation Hospital, Mumbai.

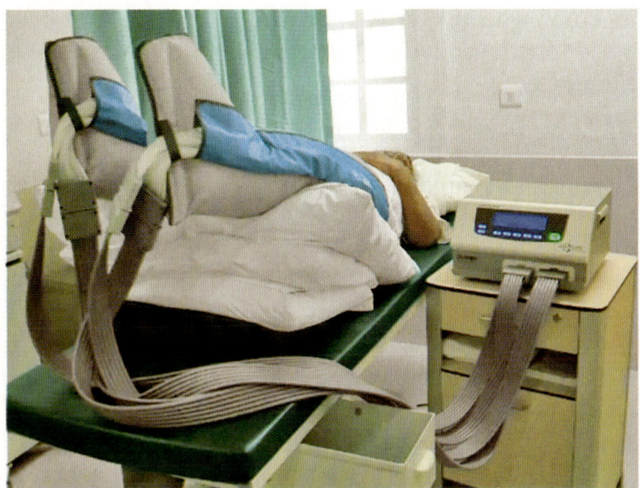

Fig. 37.8: Intermittent pneumatic compression device.
Source: Sir HN Reliance Foundation Hospital, Mumbai.

- *IPC devices* **(Fig. 37.8)** are assumed to reduce capillary filtration. The recommended range of pressure is 30–60 mm Hg for 30–120 minutes duration. Due to the lack of consensus regarding the recommended IPC treatment parameters or frequency, a systematic review finding indicates that IPC may be appropriate as a part of a supervised multimodality approach for home-based management in select patients.

Skin care consists of using pH neutral soap and skin-care products, regular inspection, avoiding injury (e.g., cuts, mosquito bites, burns, and scratches), avoiding potential allergic products such as scents, avoiding punctures or blood pressure measurements on the affected side, and reporting immediately to the treating doctor in case of signs of infection.

Clinical Pearl

> Therapists should keep in mind that applying pressures higher than 60 mm Hg is not recommended as it may cause underlying lymphatic vessel to collapse and may achieve no benefit.

Compression garments **(Table 37.2 and Figs. 37.9A to D)** are elastic garments used in the maintenance phase of lymphedema management or in patients where there is minimal to no distortion in the shape of the extremity and edema is pitting. It is not useful in patients with nonpitting

Table 37.2: Different class of compression garments and their pressure ranges.

Class	British standard (mm Hg)	French standard (mm Hg)	German (RAL) standard (mm Hg)
I	14–17	10–15	18–21
II	18–24	15–20	23–32
III	25–35	20–36	34–46
IV	NA	>36	>49

edema or distorted shape of extremity. Depending on the pressure support they provide, they can be classified into class I (15–21 mm Hg), class II (23–32 mm Hg), or class III (34–46 mm Hg). Flat-knit stockings provide a high degree of stiffness, while circular knit provides low degree of stiffness. Upper limb lymphedema is usually dealt with class I and II garments, while for lymphedema of the legs, usually class II or III garments are required. The decision is made based on clinical judgment, staging, and severity of lymphedema.

Role of Resistance Exercise in Lymphedema

Considerable high-quality data are now available to affirm that resistance exercise including weight lifting does not increase the risk of or exacerbate symptoms of lymphedema. In contradiction to the long-held belief, patients doing resistance training demonstrated a decreased incidence of exacerbation of lymphedema as well as reduced symptoms and increased strength. Another randomized prospective trial demonstrated that with resistance training program, women in the highest risk group actually saw a decreased risk of lymphedema compared with the control group. Comprehensive treatment of lymphedema should address weight control because of the association between increased body mass and lymphedema.

Management of Incontinence

Management of pelvic floor dysfunction (mainly bladder/bowel incontinence) includes pelvic floor protocols, functional retraining, voiding dynamics, defecation dynamics, biofeedback, bladder retraining, management of fluids and fiber, electrical stimulation (ES), and general advice. Physical therapy interventions for urinary incontinence after prostatectomy are the first choice of treatment and may include pelvic floor exercises (PFE), ES, biofeedback (BFB) training, and also behavioral therapy (BT). PFE or pelvic floor muscle training (PFMT) are the main physical therapy interventions with grade A recommendation in several countries with good results for the treatment of urinary incontinence. Better improvements are expected in patients who were enrolled earlier in rehab and attended supervised sessions for longer duration of time. The chances for complete recovery of continence decreased considerably with increasing interval between surgery and beginning of rehabilitation.

Speech and Swallowing Rehabilitation

The objective of swallowing rehabilitation is to maximize and maintain mobility of the tongue, mouth opening and focusing on the use of the remaining native tissue. The patient is trained on swallowing strategies to improve laryngeal closure in an attempt to prevent aspiration. Implementation of swallowing maneuvers, such as the supra- and super-supraglottic swallow maneuvers, is helpful in facilitating airway protection **(Figs. 37.10A and B)**.

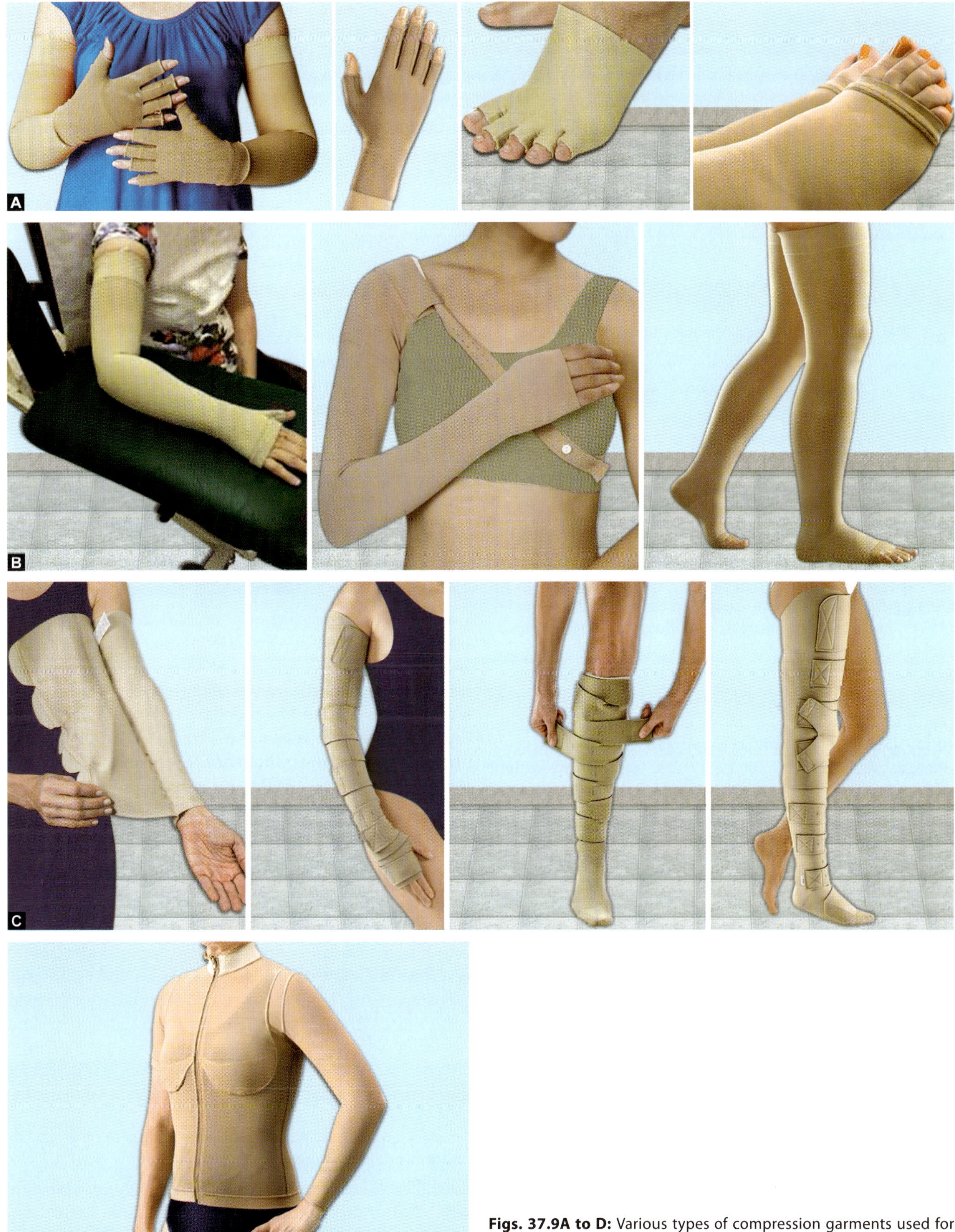

Figs. 37.9A to D: Various types of compression garments used for lymphedema management: (A) Hand glove and foot sleeves; (B) Simple compression garment sleeves; (C) Circaid wrap or farrow wraps; (D) Vest for truncal edema.

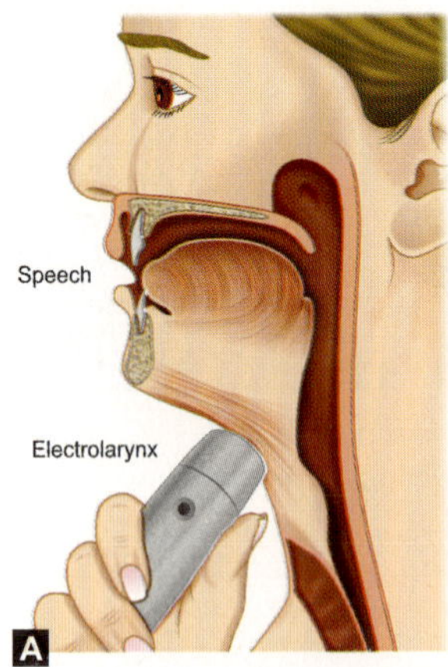

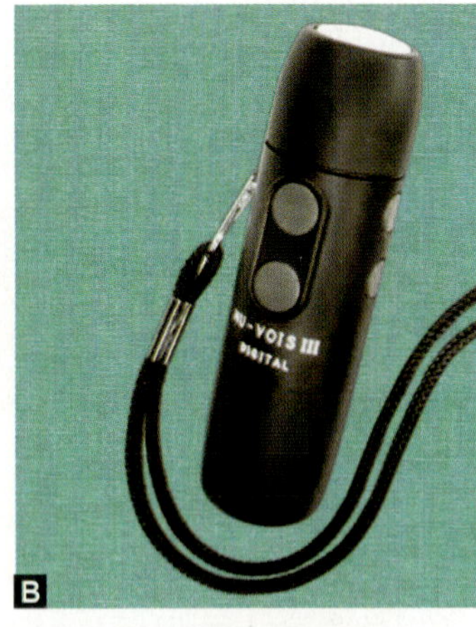

Figs. 37.10A and B: Alaryngeal communication devices: (A) Artificial larynx; (B) Artificial larynx stimulator.

In patients with total laryngectomy, therapist decides and trains the patient for alaryngeal communication via tracheoesophageal voice, voice generated by artificial larynx, and esophageal voice. Speech and swallowing rehabilitation is extensive, comprehensive, and individual patient-based care that plays a very important part of rehabilitation of HNC patients.

Nutrition Education and Planning

During the active cancer therapy, nutritionist screens the patient for signs of malnutrition, evaluates the daily calorie requirement for individual patient, and designs a diet plan in order to balance calorie needs and preserve lean body mass to counteract protein break down. The plan is also made in reference to patient's ability to swallow solid, semisolid, or liquid and the route of food intake, i.e., oral, nasogastric (NG) tube, or PEG tube. It is also modified with reference to side effects such as inability to tolerate certain food smells/taste, nausea, vomiting, and diarrhea. Regular appointments with the nutritionist are important during the active cancer therapy as the patient's calorie demand may vary a lot depending on the symptoms and progression of treatment. As with exercise prescription, diet prescription varies a lot after completion of cancer treatment and needs fresh setting of goals and plans for the patient.

The ACS and NCCN have published recommendations on nutrition for cancer survivors. These guidelines recommend that individuals eat a healthy diet with an emphasis on plant foods (e.g., limiting how much processed meat and red meat consumed, consuming ≥2.5 cups of fruits and vegetables each day, choosing whole grains instead of refined-grain products) and limit alcohol intake (e.g., no more than one drink per day for women and no more than two per day for men).

Psychological Counseling

Effective coping with the diagnosis of cancer involves dealing with its direct and indirect effects, ranging from managing the details of medical appointments to handling existential dread. Facing the illness and its consequences requires acknowledging and managing strong but inevitable emotions that can interfere with medical care, vocational engagement, sleep, diet, sexual intimacy, and exercise.

Therapy includes psychoeducational interventions such as coping skills training, mindfulness training, CBT, and group psychotherapy. A psychologist uses adaptive-coping techniques that help to handle stressors by following principles: facing rather than fleeing, altering perception, coping actively, expressing emotion, and social support. Some patients may require pharmacological interventions.

Mindfulness-based Exercise

Mindfulness-based modes of exercise such as yoga and tai chi can provide substantial benefits for cancer survivors by decreasing side effects and improving function and QoL. Yoga intervention consists of simple yoga—relaxation exercises, postures, breathing, and visualization. Multiple studies have suggested that yoga and tai chi performed 1–3 times a week for 60–90 minutes, at a moderate intensity level, can reduce side effects and improve QoL.

SUMMARY

Evidence suggests physical activity or exercise may play a pivotal role at all points of cancer survivorship. Participation in physical activity is associated with a reduced likelihood of developing cancer. Despite the success of a variety of cancer treatments, many result in deleterious symptoms and side effects which can be attenuated by physical activity. Exercise prescriptions for cancer survivors need to be individualized and to be tailored considering the disease site and stage, planned treatments, individual's current fitness level along with past and present exercise participation and preferences. After the discharge from rehabilitation, a detailed home-care program should be given and explained to patients with a list of warning signs, indicating an early visit to oncology health-care provider. All cancer survivors should be educated about risk factors and signs and symptoms recurrence and benefits of engaging in healthy lifestyle habits such as weight management, physical activity, and nutrition with a goal to achieve and maintain a healthy weight throughout life, be physically active, eat a healthy diet with an emphasis on plant foods, limit alcohol intake, and restrain from smoking.

To conclude, comprehensive rehabilitation program consists of physical-therapy interventions such as cancer-specific exercises, aerobic exercise, strength training, addressal of physical symptoms, nutritional education, psychological intervention, speech and swallowing therapy, and mindfulness-based exercise aimed at improving physical, functional, and psychological outcomes in patients with cancer.

Case Scenario

CASE STUDY 1
Head and Neck Cancer

Patient seen on July 1, 2019. Mr ABC is a 46-year-old overweight (BMI—27.52) gentleman, had complaints of nonhealing ulcer over tongue for 3 months. No neck swelling, dysphagia. He consulted Dr XYZ, who after examination suggested a biopsy that showed positive results. He was diagnosed with carcinoma base of tongue and underwent surgery (total glossectomy with bilateral modified neck dissection) on July 31, 2019. Graft was taken from left thigh.

TNM scoring: pT4N3bM0

Type: Biopsy suggested moderately differentiated squamous cell carcinoma (MDSCC)

Radiation therapy: 30 sessions planned (started on August 31, 2019; 5 days/week)

Chemotherapy: 5 cycles (once in two weeks, started on September 7, 2019)

Comorbidities: Known case of DM since 4 years and on medication for the same. No H/O CVD or HTN.

He has started with RT on August 31, 2019, and is referred for comprehensive oncology rehabilitation today. Currently, he has complaint of pain over the suture sight and mild level of fatigue. He has a PEG tube in situ.

Investigations: PET CT and MRI head and neck reports are reviewed and noted down.

Social history: Ex–tobacco chewer, quit before 3 months after the diagnosis. He was having oral tobacco for 30 years, 2 sachets a day. No use of alcohol or recreational drugs.

Medications: Galvus MET 50/1,000 OD, glynase OD.

Assessment

Local examination: C-shaped scar present on to the right side of face, extending from below mandible to chin up to center of the lip. Healed, slightly adherent over chin area, nontender. Skin over left thigh region, healed, nontender.

6MWT distance: 416 m

ROM: Neck range of motion moderately restricted due to tightness of sternocleidomastoid, scaleni, trapezius, pectorals. Bilaterally shoulder end-range restricted due to tissue tightness. Tightness of quadriceps and rectus femoris of left thigh (graft donor area) present.
Muscle strength full.

Functional Assessment of Cancer therapy (FACT) for Head and Neck (H&N): Quality of Life scale
- FACT_Physical: 14
- FACT_Social: 23
- FACT_Emotional: 12
- FACT_Functional: 8
- FACT_Additional: 24
- FACT_Total: 81
- FACT_Fatigue: 25
- FACT_NTx13: 39

Guiding Questions:
1. What are the goals of rehabilitation for this patient?
2. What can be the plan of care now and after completion of radiation therapy?
3. How frequently would you like to see the patient and till what time period would you like them to follow-up?

CASE STUDY 2:
Breast Cancer

Patient seen on May 28, 2019. She has complaint of right breast pain and swelling with blood discharge from nipple in the past 15 days. She underwent mammography, PET CT, and biopsy after which she was diagnosed to have right breast carcinoma. She underwent surgery—right modified radical mastectomy with axillary clearance on May 29, 2019.

TNM scoring: pT4N2M0

Type: Invasive ductal carcinoma Grade III, ER/PR negative, Her2 positive

Radiation therapy: 15 sessions (started on June 25, 2019, for 5 days/week)

Chemotherapy: Adjuvant chemotherapy 12 weekly cycles of paclitaxel and trastuzumab last dose on September 6, 2019.

Comorbidities: Postmenopausal, HTN since 2013, hypothyroidism 2013, IHD (angioplasty done twice) 2013 and 2017, bilateral knee osteoarthritis.

She has started with RT on September 25, 2019, and is referred for comprehensive oncology rehabilitation. She has complaint of right shoulder pain and edema since 1 month.

Investigations: Mammography, PET CT, and biopsy reports available.

Social History
Medication List

Tablet Clopitab	75	1-0-0
Tablet Atorva	10	0-0-1
Tablet Covance	25	1-0-0
Tablet Angispan TR	2.5	1-0-0
Tablet Thyronorm	50	1-0-0
Tablet Polybion C	25	1-0-0
Tablet Gemcal	1-0-0	
Tablet Esoz D		

Assessment

Local examination: Healed, nonadherent, nontender scar.

6MWT distance: 160 m (patient walked with walker support, uses walker since 2 years due to knee pain).

ROM: Neck range of full. Right shoulder flexion and abduction restricted (muscle tightness), no joint pain, end feel—tissue stretch with tightness of pectorals.
Muscle strength full.

Lymphedema Assessment

Stage 2, pitting edema of a moderate severity. Limb girth measurement shows 3–4 cm difference between right and left upper limb circumference measurements.
- *FACT Breast + Lymphedema: Quality of Life Scores*
- FACT_Physical: 16
- FACT_Social: 28
- FACT_Emotional: 20
- FACT_Functional: 28
- FACT_Additional: 25
- FACT_Total: 117
- FACT_Fatigue: 37
- FACT_NTx13: 36

Guiding Questions:
1. What are the goals of rehabilitation for this patient?
2. What can be the plan of care now and after completion of radiation therapy?
3. How frequently would you like to see the patient and till what time period would you like them to follow-up?

BIBLIOGRAPHY

1. Abrams P, et al. Fourth international consultation on incontinence recommendations of the international scientific committee: evaluation and treatment of urinary incontinence, pelvic organ prolapse, and fecal incontinence. Neurourol Urodyn. 2010;29:213.

2. Ahmed RL, et al. Randomized controlled trial of weight training and lymphedema in breast cancer survivors. J Clin Oncol. 2006;24(18):2765-72.

3. Alzabaidey F. Quality of life assessment for patients with breast cancer receiving adjuvant therapy. J Cancer Sci Ther. 2012.

4. American Cancer Society. Cancer facts and figures. Atlanta, GA: American Cancer Society; 2011.

5. American Institute for Cancer Research. Tobacco smoke and involuntary smoking, vol 83. Lyon, France: World Health Organization; 2004.

6. Anand P. Cancer is a preventable disease that requires major lifestyle changes. Pharm Res. 2008;25:2097-116.

7. Arathuzik D. Effects of cognitive-behavioral strategies on pain in cancer patients. Cancer Nurs. 1994;17:207-14.

8. Backer D. Resistance training in cancer survivors: a systematic review. Int J Sports Med. 2009;30(10):703-12.

9. Bao T, et al. Long-term chemotherapy-induced peripheral neuropathy among breast cancer survivors: prevalence, risk factors, and fall risk. Breast Cancer Res Treat. 2016;159(2):327-33.

10. Belpomme D, et al. The multitude and diversity of environmental carcinogens. Environ Res. 2007;105:414-29.

11. Bingham SA, et al. Effect of white versus red meat on endogenous N-nitrosation in the human colon and further evidence of a dose response. J Nutr. 2002;132:3522S–5S.

12. Blot WJ, et al. Smoking and drinking in relation to oral and pharyngeal cancer. Cancer Res. 1988;48(11):3282-87.

13. Bodensteiner, et al. Adverse hematologic complications of anticancer drugs. Clinical presentation, management, and avoidance. Drug Saf. 1993;8(3):213-24.

14. Bray F, et al. Global cancer statistics 2018: GLOBOCAN estimates of incidence and mortality worldwide for 36 cancers in 185 countries. CA Cancer J Clin. 2018:1-31.

15. Brown JC, et al. Obesity and energy balance in GI cancer. J Clin Oncol. 2016;34(35):4217-24.

16. Calle EE, et al. Overweight, obesity, and mortality from cancer in a prospectively studied cohort of US adults. N Engl J Med. 2003;348(17):1625-38.

17. Campbell A, et al. A pilot study of supervised group exercise program as a rehabilitation treatment for women with breast cancer receiving adjuvant treatment. Eur J Oncol Nurs. 2005;9(1):56-63.

18. Campbell KL, Winters Stone KM, Wiskemkann J, et al. Exercise guidelines for cancer survivors: consensus statement from International Multidisciplinary Roundtable. Medicine and Science in Sports and Exercise; 2019;51(11):2375-90.

19. Cao Y, et al. Body mass index, prostate cancer-specific mortality, and biochemical recurrence: a systematic review and meta-analysis. Cancer Prev Res (Phila). 2011;4(4):486-501.

20. Carvalho A, et al. Exercise interventions for shoulder dysfunction in patients treated for head and neck cancer. Cochrane Database Syst Rev. 2012;(4):CD008693.

21. Carver JR, et al. American Society of Clinical Oncology clinical evidence review on the ongoing care of adult cancer survivors: cardiac & pulmonary late effects. J Clin Oncol. 2007;25(25):3991-4008.

22. Chan DS, et al. Body mass index and survival in women with breast cancer-systematic literature review and meta-analysis of 82 follow-up studies. Ann Oncol. 2014;(10):1901-14.

23. Cohen EE, et al. American Cancer Society head and neck cancer survivorship care guideline. CA Cancer J Clin. 2016;66(3):203-39.

24. Cohen L, et al. Psychological adjustment and sleep quality in randomized trial of the effects of a Tibetan yoga intervention in patients with lymphoma. Cancer. 2004;100(10):2253-60.

25. Coleman RE, et al. The clinical course of bone metastases from breast cancer. Br J Cancer. 1987;55(1):61-6.

26. Courneya KS, et al. Randomised controlled trial of exercise training in postmenopausal breast cancer survivors: cardiopulmonary and quality of life outcomes. J Clin Oncol. 2003;1660-68.

27. Cousins N, et al. A systematic review of interventions for eating and drinking problems following treatment for head and neck cancer suggests a need to look beyond swallowing and trismus. Oral Oncol. 2013;49(5):387-400.

28. Crew KD, et al. Prevalence of joint symptoms in postmenopausal women taking aromatase inhibitors for early stage breast cancer. J Clin Oncol. 2007;25(25):3877-83.

29. Curt G, et al. Impact of cancer related fatigue on the lives of patients: new findings from fatigue coalition. Oncologist. 2000;5(5):353-60.

30. Damstra RK. Multidisciplinary guidelines for early diagnosis and management. J Lymphoedema. 2007;2(1).

31. de Raaf PJ, et al. Elucidating the behavior of physical fatigue and mental fatigue in cancer patients: a review of the literature. Psycho-Oncology. 2013;22(9):1919-29.

32. DeVitta, et al. Cancer principles and practice of oncology. Philadelphia, PA; Baltimore, MD; London; New York; NY: Wolters Kluwer; 2019.

33. Dijkstra PU, et al. Incidence of shoulder pain after neck dissection: a clinical explorative study for risk factors. Head Neck. 2001;23(11):947-53.

34. Dijkstra PU, et al. Trismus in head and neck oncology: a systematic review. Oral Oncol. 2004;40(9):879-89.

35. Dimeo F, et al. Effects of aerobic exercise on the physical performance and incidence of treatment-related complications after high dose chemotherapy. Blood. 1997;3390-4.

36. DiSipio T, et al. Incidence of unilateral arm lymphoedema after breast cancer: a systematic review and meta-analysis. Lancet Oncol. 2013;14(6):500-15.

37. Doyle C, et al. Nutrition and physical activity during and after cancer treatment: an American Cancer Society guide for informed choices. CA Cancer J Clin. 2006;56(6):323-53.

38. D'Cruz AK, et al. Guidelines for complications of cancer treatment, vol VIII, part B. Mumbai, India: Tata Memorial Hospital; 2008.

39. Ehrman JE, et al. Clinical exercise physiology, 3rd edition. USA: Human Kinetics; 2013.

40. Eliassen AH, et al. Adult weight change and risk of postmenopausal breast cancer. JAMA. 2006;296(2):193-201.

41. Ellenhorn JD, et al. Colorectal and anal cancers. In: Cancer management: a multidisciplinary approach. New York, NY: Healthcare Media; 2004. pp. 323-55.

42. Elliott P, et al. Mobile phone base stations and early childhood cancers: case-control study. BMJ. 2010;340:c3077.

43. Feldman JL, et al. Intermittent pneumatic compression therapy: a systematic review. Lymphology. 2012;45(1): 13-25.

44. Ferlay J, et al. GLOBOCAN 2012 v1.0, Cancer incidence and mortality worldwide: IARC CancerBase no.11. Lyon, France: International Agency for Research on Cancer; 2013.

45. Friedenreich CM, et al. Physical activity and cancer outcomes: a precision medicine approach. Clin Cancer Res. 2016;22(19):4766-75.

46. Furmaniak A, et al. Exercise for women receiving adjuvant therapy for breast cancer (review). Cochrane Database Syst Rev. 2016;9:CD005001.

47. Gao C, et al. Mendelian randomization study of adiposity-related traits and risk of breast, ovarian, prostate, lung and colorectal cancer. Int J Epidemiol. 2016;45(3):896-908.

48. Gelband F, et al. Cancer control opportunities in low- and middle-income countries. Washington, DC: The National Academies Press; 2007.

49. Gilchrist, et al. Cardio-oncology rehabilitation to manage cardiovascular outcomes in cancer patients and survivors. a scientific statement from the American Heart Association. Circulation. 2019;139.

50. Giovino GA, et al. Tobacco use in 3 billion individuals from 16 countries: an analysis of nationally representative cross-sectional household surveys. Lancet. 2012;380(9842):668-79.

51. Gittes R. Carcinoma of the prostate. N Engl J Med. 1991;324(4):236-45.

52. Griffin A, et al. On the receiving end. V: Patient perceptions of the side effects of cancer chemotherapy in 1993. Ann Oncol. 1996;7(2):189-95.

53. Guenancia C, et al. Obesity as a risk factor for anthracyclines and trastuzumab cardiotoxicity in breast cancer: a systematic review and meta-analysis. J Clin Oncol. 2016;34(26):3157-65.

54. Hardell L, et al. Biological effects from electromagnetic field exposure and public exposure standards. Biomed Pharmacother. 2008;62(2):104-9.

55. Headley JA, et al. The effects of seated exercise on fatigue and quality of life in women with advanced breast cancer. Oncol Nurs Forum. 2004;31:977-83.

56. Hecht SS, et al. Tobacco smoke biomarkers and cancer risk among male smokers in the Shanghai Cohort Study. Cancer Lett. 2013;334(1):34-8.

57. Hecht SS. Lung carcinogenesis by tobacco smoke. Int J Cancer. 2012;131(12):2724-32.

58. Hewitt ME, et al. From cancer patient to cancer survivor: lost in transition. Washington, DC, National Academies Press; 2006. p. 189.

59. Huo J, et al. Post-mastectomy breast reconstruction and its subsequent complications: a comparison between obese and non-obese women with breast cancer. Breast Cancer Res Treat. 2016;157(2):373-83.

60. IARC (International Agency for Research on Cancer). Smokeless tobacco and tobacco-specific nitrosamines, vol 89, Lyon, France: World Health Organization; 2007.

61. Imran Ali, et al. Cancer scenario in India with future perspectives. Cancer Ther. 2011;8:56-70.

62. Irwin ML. ACSM's guide to exercise and cancer survivorship. USA: Human Kinetics; 2012.

63. Jamal A, et al. Current cigarette smoking among adults—United States, 2005-2015. MMWR Morb Mortal Wkly Rep. 2016;65(44):1205-11.

64. Jane M, et al. Best practice guidelines in assessment, risk reduction, management, and surveillance for post-breast cancer lymphedema. Curr Breast Cancer Rep. 2013;5(2):134-44.

65. Joshu CE, et al. Weight gain is associated with an increased risk of prostate cancer recurrence after prostatectomy in the PSA era. Cancer Prev Res (Phila). 2011;4(4):544-51.

66. Karen Mustian, et al. Exercise for the management of side effects and quality of life among cancer survivors. Curr Sports Med Rep. 2009;8(6):325-30.

67. Kerrigan D, et al. Cancer. In: Clinical exercise physiology. USA: Human Kinetics; 2003. p. 388.

68. Khurana VG, et al. Epidemiological evidence for a health risk from mobile phone base stations. Int J Occup Environ Health. 2010;16(3):263-67.

69. Kumar SP, et al. Physiotherapy management of painful diabetic peripheral neuropathy: a current concepts review of treatment methods for clinical decision-making in practice and research. Int J Curr Res Rev. 2010;2:29-39.

70. Lacy AM, et al. Laparoscopy-assisted colectomy versus open colectomy for treatment of non-metastatic colon cancer: a randomized trial. Lancet. 2002;359(9325):2224-29.

71. Langer I, et al. Morbidity of sentinel lymph node biopsy alone versus SLN and completion axillary lymph node dissection after breast cancer surgery: a prospective Swiss multicenter study on 659 patients. Ann Surg. 2007;245(3):452-61.

72. Langstein HN. Mechanisms of cancer cachexia. Hematol Oncol Clin North Am. 1991;5:103-23.

73. Lauby-Secretan B, et al. Body fatness and cancer—viewpoint of the IARC working group. N Engl J Med. 2016;375(8):794-8.

74. Lee IM, et al. Effect of physical inactivity on major non-communicable diseases worldwide: an analysis of burden of disease and life expectancy. Lancet. 2012;380(9838): 219-29.

75. Ligibel JA, et al. American Society of Clinical Oncology position statement on obesity and cancer. J Clin Oncol. 2014;32(31):3568-74.

76. Lyden D, et al. Rehabilitation after treatment of head and neck cancer, 11th edition. In: Cancer: principles and practice of oncology. Philadelphia, PA; Baltimore, MD; New York, NY; London: Wolters Kluwer; 2019. pp. 1009-24.

77. Mallath M, et al. The growing burden of cancer in India: epidemiology and social context. Lancet Oncol. 2014:S1470-2045.

78. Marchiori D, et al. Pelvic floor rehabilitation for continence recovery after radical prostatectomy: role of a personal training re-educational program. Anticancer Res. 2010;30:553.

79. McMahon K, et al. Integrating proactive nutritional assessment in clinical practices to prevent complications and cost. Semin Oncol. 1998;5(Suppl. 6):20-7.

80. McNeely ML, et al. Effects of exercise on breast cancer patients and survivors: a systematic review and meta-analysis. CMAJ. 2006;175(1):34-41.

81. Mitchell SA, et al. Putting evidence into practice: an update of evidence-based interventions for cancer-related fatigue during and following treatment. Clin J Oncol Nurs. 2014;18(Suppl):38-58.

82. Mock V, et al. Exercise manages fatigue during breast cancer treatment: a randomised controlled trail. Psycho-Oncology. 2005;14(6):464-77.

83. Mock V, et al. NCCN practice guidelines for cancer related fatigue. Oncology. 2000;14(11A):151-61.

84. Moore SC, et al. Association of leisure-time physical activity with risk of 26 types of cancer in 1.44 million adults. JAMA Intern Med. 2016;176(6).

85. Moos RH, et al. The crisis of physical illness: an overview and conceptual approach. In: Coping with physical illness: 2: New perspectives. New York, NY: Plenum Press; 1987. pp. 3-25.

86. Munn LL, et al. Imaging the lymphatic system. Microvasc Res. 2014;96:55-63.

87. Mustian KM, et al. Comparison of pharmaceutical, psychological, and exercise treatments for cancer-related fatigue: a meta-analysis. JAMA Oncol. 2017;3(7):961-68.

88. Mustian KM, et al. Integrative nonpharmacologic behavioural interventions for the management of cancer related fatigue. Oncologist. 2007;(Suppl. 1):52-67.

89. Network N. et al. Cancer-related fatigue (version 2.2018). Jenkintown, PA: National Comprehensive Cancer Network; 2018.

90. Newton D, et al. Review of exercise intervention studies in cancer patients. J Clin Oncol. 2005;23(4).

91. Nicolussi A, et al. Health-related quality of life of cancer patients undergoing chemotherapy. Rev Rene. 2014;15(1):132-40.

92. Nitenberg GR, et al. Nutritional support of the cancer patient: issues and dilemmas. Crit Rev Oncol Hematol. 2000;34:137-68.

93. NMA Committee. Position statement of the National Lymphoedema Network. San Francisco, CA: National Lymphoedema Network; 2012.

94. O'Brien, et al. Impact of chemotherapy-associated nausea and vomiting on patients' functional status and on costs: survey of five Canadian centers. CMAJ. 1993;149(3):296-302.

95. PAGA Committee. Physical activity guidelines advisory committee report. Washington DC: UDHHS; 2008.

96. Paice JA, et al. Clinical challenges: chemotherapy induced peripheral neuropathy. Semin Oncol Nurs. 2009;25(2 Suppl. 1):S8-19.

97. Palmore T, et al. Infections in the cancer patients. In: Principles and practice of oncology, 11th edition. Philadelphia, PA; Baltimore, MD; New York, NY; London: Wolters Kluwer; 2019. pp. 3481-534.

98. Parsch D, et al. Postacute management of patients with spinal cord injury due to metastatic tumour disease: survival and efficacy of rehabilitation. Spinal Cord. 2003;41(4):205-10.

99. Paskett ED, et al. Cancer-related lymphedema risk factors, diagnosis, treatment, and impact: a review. J Clin Oncol. 2012;30(30):3726-33.

100. Paula JM, et al. Health-related quality of life of cancer patients undergoing radiotherapy. Rev Rene. 2015;16(1):106-13.

101. Pearson EJM, et al. Interventions for cancer-related fatigue: a scoping review. Eur J Cancer Care (Engl). 2018;27:1.

102. Pescatello LS. ACSM's guidelines for exercise testing and prescription, 10th edition. Wolters Kluwer; 2018.

103. Peto R, et al. Smoking, smoking cessation, and lung cancer in UK since 1950: combination of national statistics with two case control studies. BMJ. 2000;321(7257):323-9.

104. Petrek J. et al. Lymphoedema in a cohort of breast carcinoma survivors 20 years after diagnosis. Cancer. 2001;92(6):1368-77.

105. Plummer M, et al. Global burden of cancers attributable to infections in 2012: a synthetic analysis. Lancet Glob Health. 2016;4(9):e609-16.

106. Raber-Durlacher, et al. Oral mucositis. Oral Oncol. 2010;46(6):52-456.

107. Ramsey S, et al. Quality of life in long term survivors of colorectal cancer. Am J Gastroenterol. 2002;97(5):1228-34.

108. Riba D. Psychological issues. In: Cancer principles and practice of Oncology. Philadelphia, PA; Baltimore, MD; New York, NY; London: Wolters Kluwer; 2019. pp. 3809-24.

109. Ridner SH, et al. Body mass index and breast cancer treatment-related lymphedema. Support Care Cancer. 2011;19(6):853-7.

110. Sagen A, et al. Physical activity for the affected limb and arm lymphedema after breast cancer surgery. A prospective, randomized controlled trial with two years follow-up. Acta Oncol. 2009;48(8):1102-10.

111. Santiago-Palma J, et al. Palliative care and rehabilitation. Cancer. 2001;92:1049-52.

112. Schiller JT, et al. Virus infection and human cancer: an overview. Recent Results. Cancer Res. 2014;193:1-10.

113. Schmitz KH, et al. American College of Sports Medicine roundtable on exercise guidelines for cancer survivors. Med Sci Sports Exerc. 2010;42:1409-26.

114. Schmitz KH, et al. Weight lifting for women at risk for breast cancer-related lymphedema: a randomized trial. JAMA. 2010;304(24):2699-705.

115. Schmitz KH, et al. Weight lifting in women with breast-cancer-related lymphedema. N Engl J Med. 2009;361(7):664-73.

116. Schmitz KH. American College of Sports Medicine roundtable on exercise guidelines for cancer survivors. Med Sci Sports Exerc. 2010;42(7):1409-26.

117. Secord AA, et al. Body mass index and mortality in endometrial cancer: a systematic review and meta-analysis. Gynecol Oncol. 2016;140(1):184-90.

118. Shah C, et al. Breast-cancer related lymphedema: a review of procedure-specific incidence rates, clinical assessment AIDS, treatment paradigms, and risk reduction. Breast J. 2012;18(4):357-61.

119. Shen D, et al. Sedentary behavior and incident cancer: a meta-analysis of prospective studies. PLoS One. 2014;9(8):e105709.

120. Shi H, et al. Titanium dioxide nanoparticles: a review of current toxicological data. Part Fibre Toxicol. 2013;10:15.

121. Smith G, et al. Hypothyroidism in older patients with head and neck cancer after treatment with radiation: a population based study. Head Neck. 2009;31(8):1031-38.

122. Sobel-Fox RM, et al. Assessment of daily and weekly fatigue among African American cancer survivors. J Psychosoc Oncol. 2013;31(4):413-29.

123. Sonis S. Oral complications of cancer therapy. In: H. S. R. S. e. DeVita VT (Eds). Cancer: principles and practice of oncology, 4th edition. Philadelphia: PA: J.B. Lippincott; 2019. pp. 1993-2385.

124. Steinherz, et al. Cardiac toxicity 4 to 20 years after completing anthracycline therapy. JAMA. 1991;266(12):1672-77.

125. Straif K, et al. Carcinogenicity of polycyclic aromatic hydrocarbons. Lancet Oncol. 2005;6(12):931-2.

126. Stubblefield MD. Cancer rehabilitation: principles and practices. Demos Medical; 1st edition, 2009.

127. Stubblefield MD. Rehabilitation of the cancer patient. In: Cancer principle and practice of oncology. Baltimore, MD; Philadelphia, PA; New York, NY; London: Wolters Kluwer; 2019. pp. 3842-76.

128. Swedborg I. Effects of treatment with an elastic sleeve and intermittent pneumatic compression in post-mastectomy patients with lymphedema of the arm. Scand J Rehab Med. 1984; 16:35-41.

129. Tapple A. Heme of consumed red meat can act as a catalyst of oxidative damage and could initiate colon, breast and prostate cancers, heart disease and other diseases. Med Hypotheses. 2007; 68:562-4.

130. Texas T, et al. Cancer algorithms. Texas: MD Anderson Cancer Center; 2015.

131. Thune I, et al. Physical activity and cancer risk: dose response and cancer, all sites and site specific. Med Sci Sports Exerc. 2001;33:S530-50.

132. Todd M. Selecting compression hosiery. Br J Nurs. 2015;24(4):210-12.

133. Toporcov TN, et al. Fat food habitual intake and risk of oral cancer. Oral Oncol. 2004;40:925-31.

134. Twycross R. Factors associated with difficult-to-manage pain. Indian J Palliat Care. 2004;10:67-78.

135. Usuba M, et al. Experimental joint contracture correction with low torque: long duration repeated stretching. Clin Orthop Relat Res. 2007;456:70-8.

136. Van Cutsem, et al. Cetuximab and chemotherapy as initial treatment for metastatic colorectal cancer. N Engl J Med. 2009;360(14):1408-17.

137. van Dam RM, et al. Combined impact of lifestyle factors on mortality: prospective cohort study in US women. BMJ. 2008;337:a1440.

138. Wagner, et al. Psychosocial issues in oncology: clinical management of psychosocial distress, health-related quality of life, and special considerations in dermatologic oncology. In: Dermatologic principles and practice in oncology: conditions of the skin, hair, and nails in cancer patients. New York, NY: John Wiley & Sons; 2013. pp. 60-8.

139. WCRF/AICR (World Cancer Research Fund/ American Institute for Cancer Research): Food, nutrition, physical activity, and the prevention of cancer: a global perspective. Washington, DC: American Institute for Cancer Research; 2007.

140. Williams AF. Measuring change in limb volume to evaluate lymphoedema treatment outcome. EWMA J. 2015;15(1).

141. Wolin KY, et al. Obesity and cancer. Oncologist. 2010;15(6):556-65.

142. World Cancer Research Fund. Food, nutrition, physical activity, and the prevention of cancer: a global perspective. Washington, DC: American Institute for Cancer Research; 2007.

143. World Cancer Research Fund: Food, nutrition and the prevention of cancer: a global perspective/world cancer research fund, in association with American Institute for Cancer Research. Washington, DC: American Institute for Cancer Research; 1997.

38
CHAPTER

Burns

Harita Pultsya Vyas

ⓛEARNING OBJECTIVES

After reading this chapter, the readers should be able to:
- Describe in detail about anatomy and physiology of the skin in healthy state as well as in the damaged condition that occurs with a burn injury
- Discuss pathology, etiology, signs and symptoms of burn injuries
- Discuss the sequelae of the burn injuries
- Describe the treatment according to depth and extent of burn injury in form of medical, surgical, and physiotherapy management
- Identify consequences of contracture formation after burn injury and treatment of the condition
- Discuss the management of hypertrophic scar
- Develop a physical therapy plan of care that appropriately incorporates positioning, splinting, and exercise
- Analyze and interpret patient data, formulate goals and outcomes, and make plan of care in the case of burns
- Understand different types of skin grafting and management for the same

CHAPTER OUTLINE

- Epidemiology
- Risk factors
- Skin anatomy
  - Epidermis
  - Dermal–epidermal junction
  - Dermis
- Etiology
- Classification
  - Classification according to depth of burns
  - Classification according to the size of burns
  - Electrical burn

- Pathological changes
- Clinical features
  - Inhalation injury
  - Features at the site
  - During shock: up to 3 days postburn
  - About 4 weeks later
  - Long-term (depends on site and extent of burn)
- Complications
- Burn wound healing
  - Epidermal healing
  - Dermal healing

- Management of burns
  - First aid
  - Medical management for burns
  - Wound care
  - Physiotherapy assessment
  - Physiotherapy management
  - Surgical management
- Follow-up care

INTRODUCTION

Burn is a wound following coagulative necrosis of the tissue, resulting in loss of skin with impairment of skin functions. Effect of the burn depends on the extent and site of damage. The World Health Organization (WHO) defines burns as damage caused due to heat (in the form of flames, hot objects, or gases), chemicals, electricity or lightning, friction, or radiation. Burn injuries form one of the largest health burdens of the modern world. Annually, burns cause 7.1 million injuries and around 250,000 deaths throughout the world. Of these, 90% burns occur in low- and middle-income countries with Eastern Mediterranean Region, the South East Asian Region, and the African Region having the maximum burden. About 50% burns occur in South East Asian region.

There has been a significant decline in the number of burn cases reported each year within the past decade. The survival rate has improved annually owing to improved resuscitation techniques; the acute medical and surgical care now practiced and continued research into the management and care of the patient with the burns.

The American Burn Association (ABA) reported an overall survival rate of 94.8% from 2000 to 2009. As a result of an improvement in care, treatment and survival of patient with burns, more physical therapists will become responsible for treating these patients for a significant portion of their rehabilitation in settings other than a hospital burn center.

EPIDEMIOLOGY

Around 96% of the death-causing fire-related burns occur in low- and middle-income countries. India not only has a very high incidence of burns but also exceeds other countries in the mean body surface area (BSA) of burns. Around 1,000,000 people suffer moderate-to-severe burns each year in India (https://www.who.int/news-room/fact-sheets/detail/burns). Studies have reported a decline in the number of burns cases and the female-to-male ratio, but the mortality rate (40.20%) as well as the total burn surface area (44.39%) still remains high. Around 48.8% of the burn victims fall in the 20–40 years age-group category. Flame burns (65.16%) are the most common types of burns seen.

WHO reported that fire-related burns are among the leading causes of death in children, with the highest incidence in 15–19 years age group (seventh leading cause). Fire-related burns form the 11th leading cause of death in children within 1–9 years of age. Fire burns account for 3.9 deaths per 100,000 children globally and 4.3 deaths per 100,000 children in low- and middle-income countries. The most common cause of burn injury in children 1–5 years of age is from scalds from hot liquids. The primary cause of burn injury in adolescents and adults is accidents with hot liquids. Men, especially those between ages 16 and 40, have the highest incidence of injury. Most of the deaths associated with home or structure fires are due to inhalation injury.

A major reason for the improved prognosis and survival of patients with severe burn injury is the availability of specialized burn centers. The advent of the burn center and the concentrated team care and focused research that has been generated by these facilities has improved the outcome of the most severely burned patient as well as reduced the average hospital stay in most of the cases.

The ABA has established criteria for admission to a designated burn center as follows:
- Partial-thickness burns greater than 10% of total BSA (TBSA)
- Full-thickness burns in any age group
- Burns that involve the hands, feet, face, perineum, genitalia, or skin overlying major joints
- Electrical burns including lightning injury
- Chemical burns
- Inhalation injury
- Burn injury in patients with pre-existing illness that could complicate management
- Patients with a burn and coexistent trauma (e.g., fractures)
- Patients who require special social, emotional, or long-term rehabilitation including cases involving suspected child abuse
- Children with burns in hospital settings without qualified burn management personnel or equipment.

A burn center is staffed by specialists from multiple disciplines—physicians, nurses, physical therapists, occupational therapists, dieticians, psychiatrists, psychologists, social workers, child life therapists, chaplains, pharmacists, vocational rehabilitation specialists, and other support personnel—who direct their professional expertise toward the care, treatment, and rehabilitation of the patient with a burn injury.

Each member is an integral part of the team, and the most effective burn centers are successful because of their team approach to the care of each patient.

RISK FACTORS

There are several factors that may lead to an increased incidence of burns:
- **Gender:** Females are at a greater risk of burns than males due to working in the kitchen that forms one of the most common places where burns occur. Self-directed or interpersonal violence directed toward female also contributes to an increased risk.
- **Age:** Children are specifically at higher risk of burns due to inappropriate adult supervision.
- **Regional factors:** Individuals living in low- and middle-income countries, such as Africa are at higher risk than children living in high-income countries that are poor, overcrowded and lack the basic fire safety measures.
- **Socioeconomic factors:** People belonging to the lower strata of the economic chain are at higher risk due to lack of awareness and improper living situations.
- **Occupation:** Several occupations are at higher risk of exposure to burns, e.g., working in a mine and fire safety department.
- **Comorbidities:** Medical conditions, such as epilepsy and physical and mental disabilities increase the risk of sustaining burns.
- **Personal factors:** Alcohol abuse and smoking

SKIN ANATOMY

The skin is the largest organ of the body comprising approximately 15% of total body weight. It covers the entire BSA. It is responsible for several functions of the body including protection of the underlying tissues from external physical, biological, and chemical injuries, prevention of excessive dehydration and homeostasis. Anatomically, the skin consists of two distinct layers of tissue:
1. Epidermis which is the outermost layer of the skin and made of specialized cells called keratinocytes

2. Deeper layer termed the dermis is made up of collagen (subdivided into the papillary and reticular dermis)
3. A third layer involved in the anatomical consideration of the skin is the subcutaneous fat cell layer directly under the dermis and above muscle fascial layers. This layer is also called the panniculus or the hypodermis and is composed of lipocytes **(Fig. 38.1)**.

The thickness of the skin and individual layers of the skin varies depending on the geographic location on the body, e.g., epidermis is thinnest on the eyelids, around 0.1 mm, and thickest at the soles and palms around 1.5 mm (the epidermis at the soles and palms consists of an extra layer called the stratum lucidum); the upper back has the thickest skin due to thickest dermal layer but very thin epidermal layer due to an absent stratum lucidum (30–40:1 dermal:epidermal thickness ratio).

Epidermis

The epidermis composed of multiple layers is avascular and performs several vital functions. The layers of the epidermis include:

- Stratum corneum—uppermost 20–30 cell layer, consisting of keratin and scales made of dead keratin cells, which secrete defensin (part of the first immune defense); gives the skin its waterproof characteristic and serves the role of protection from infection.
- Stratum granulosum—a three to five cell layer containing diamond shaped cells with keratohyalin granules (keratin precursors); responsible for water retention.
- Stratum spinosum—an 8–10 cell layer; also called prickle cell layer due to the presence of cells having spine-like processes used for contact with neighboring cells; adds a layer of protection and also contains dendritic cells.
- Stratum basale layer—the deepest layer; also called stratum germinativum; separated from the dermis by the basal lamina; contains mitotically active cells that enable the epidermis to regenerate through production of keratinocytes, as well as melanocytes, the cells responsible for skin pigmentation **(Box 38.1)**.

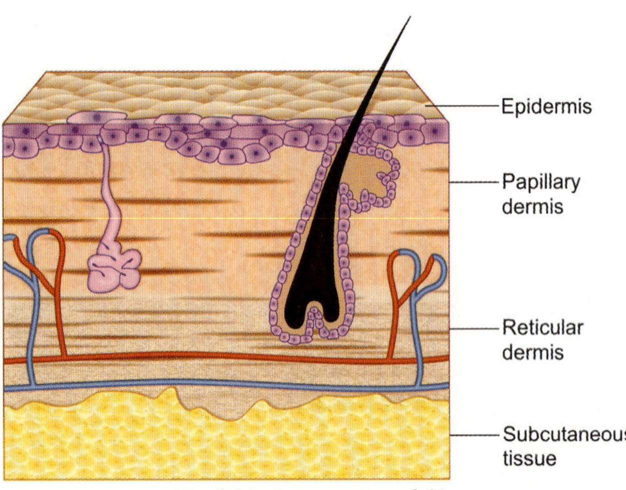

Fig. 38.1: Cross-section of skin.

> **BOX 38.1:** Stratum lucidum.
>
> A fifth layer called stratum lucidum may exist in thicker skin (at the palms and soles) between the stratum granulosum and stratum corneum. It is a clear thin two to three cell layers made up of eleidin, which is a product of keratohyalin.

Dermal–Epidermal Junction

The interface between the epidermis and the dermis is termed the rete peg region. This area consists of an extensive series of epidermal–dermal ridges and valleys that serve to increase the surface area between the epidermis and the dermis. The dermal-epidermal junction plays a role in the exchange of cells and fluids between the two layers along with holding them together.

Dermis

The dermis is subdivided into two layers:
1. Superficial papillary layer
2. Deep reticular layer

The papillae of the papillary layer project upward and interlock with the epidermis. The papillae are vascular plexuses that serve, in part, to nourish the epidermis through osmosis. Morphologically, this layer is composed of a loose basket-weave network of collagen fibers.

The reticular dermis lies below the papillary dermis and is composed of densely interwoven collagen fibers. The reticular dermis attaches to the subcutaneous tissue by an irregular interlacing network of fibrous connective tissue. It contains sweat glands, hairs, hair follicles, muscles, blood vessels, and sensory neurons.

Skin is important in **temperature regulation** through the emission of sweat and electrolytes, secretion of oils from the sebaceous glands to lubricate the skin, vitamin D synthesis, contributes to cosmetic appearance and identity.

The amount of skin destruction due to burns is based on temperature and length of time the tissue is exposed to heat. The type of insult (i.e., flame, liquid, chemical, or electrical) will also affect the amount of tissue destruction. While evaluating the depth of the burn, the sensory receptors might prove to be an important factor to be considered **(Table 38.1)**. Depending on the findings of sensory assessment, the depth of the burn can be estimated.

Table 38.1: Sensory receptors found in different layers of skin.

Sensory receptor	Location	Sensation mediated
Bare nerve ending	Epidermis	Nociception, thermal sensation
Bare nerve ending	Dermis	Nociception
Merkel's discs (slowly adapting mechanoreceptors)	Stratum spinosum	Maintained deformation or sustained touch
Meissner's corpuscle (rapidly adapting mechanoreceptors)	Papillary dermis	Moving touch
Ruffini's corpuscle	Papillary dermis	Warmth, continuous pressure or stretch
Krause's end bulb	Papillary dermis	Cold, touch
Pacinian corpuscle	Reticular dermis	Pressure, vibration

ETIOLOGY

Following are the types of etiology for burns:
1. **Flame:** It occurs when patient gets caught by fire in a house or car; partial- or full-thickness burn can occur
2. **Chemicals:** Strong acid or base, or caustic substances, such as strong acids and alkali can cause deep burns
3. **Scalds:** By moist heat—hot drinks and boiling fluid from a pan or kettle commonly seen in elder people
4. **Radiation:** X-rays or radium
5. **Cold burns:** Exposure to cold—frostbite seen
6. **Inhalation:** By flames, hot gases, or steam
7. **Electrical:** High-voltage electric current, contact with live wire.

CLASSIFICATION

Classification According to Depth of Burns

Burns can be classified according to depth as follows:
1. Superficial burn
2. Superficial partial thickness
3. Deep partial thickness
4. Full thickness
5. Subdermal burn

Table 38.2 shows the burn wound classification for differential diagnosis.

Superficial Burn

The features of superficial burn are as follows:
- An epidermal burn **(Fig. 38.2)**, cell damage only to the epidermis, irritated dermis, and intact skin
- Clinically skin appears red or erythematous
- Surface of burn is dry, slight edema may be seen, delayed pain, tender to touch, and no blister formation
- Healing is spontaneous, skin will heal on its own with no scarring, for example, sunburn.

Superficial Partial-thickness Burn

The features, consequence, effects of superficial partial-thickness burns are as follows:

- Damage through epidermis and into papillary layer of dermis **(Fig. 38.3)**
- Blister formation seen, moist surface, and inflamed dermis
- Wound will be bright red, moderate edema can be seen
- Extremely painful due to irritation of nerve endings contained in the dermis
- Discoloration of the skin can be seen
- Spontaneous healing, minimal scarring. When the wound is open it is sensitive to change in temperature, light touch, and air
- Superficial partial-thickness burns heal without surgical intervention by means of epithelial cell production and migration from the wound's periphery and surviving skin appendages. Coverage by new epithelium resumes the barrier function of the skin, and complete healing should occur in 7–10 days.

Deep Partial-thickness Burn

The features of deep partial-thickness burn are as follows:
- Destruction of epidermis with damage to dermis down into reticular layer **(Fig. 38.4)**.
- Appear as a mixed red or waxy white color, broken blisters, and wet surface.
- Sensitive to deep pressure, but insensitive to light touch, or soft pinprick. Marked edema can be seen.
- Slow healing, excessive scarring; Heals in 3–5 weeks, if it does not become infected. It is critical to keep the wound free of infection because infection can convert a deep partial-thickness burn into a deeper injury.
- Hypertrophic and keloid scars are seen.

Full-thickness Burn

The characteristics of full-thickness burn are as follows:
- Epidermal and dermal layers are destroyed completely, with subcutaneous fat layer, all the nerves ending in the dermal tissue are destroyed, so wound will be insensate **(Fig. 38.5)**.
- Poor distal circulation.
- Hard, parchment-like eschar covering area is seen **(Box 38.2)**.

Table 38.2: Burn wound classification: Differential diagnosis.

	Appearance	Capillary refill	Sensations	Swelling	Healing duration	Scarring
Epidermal	Dry and pink or red skin, no blister formation	Blanches	Present	Minimal	Within 7–10 days	Absent
Superficial partial thickness	Bright pink or red, intact blisters present	Blanches with brisk capillary refill	Very painful	Moderate	Within 14 days	Minimal scarring; pigmentation change
Deep partial thickness	Red and fixed stained, waxy white; broken blisters	Blanches with slow refill	Reduced	Marked	>21 days	Excessive scarring; increased chances of hypertrophic scarring
Full thickness	White charred/black	Absent	Absent	Area depressed	Requires skin grafting	Excessive scarring
Subdermal	Charred	Absent	Absent	Tissue defects	Requires skin grafting or flap	Excessive scarring

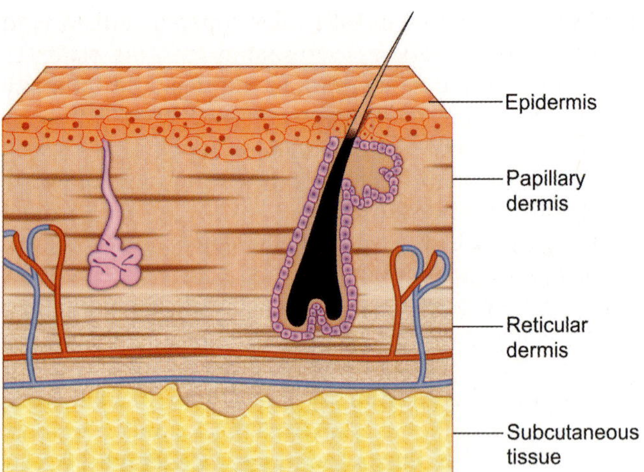

Fig. 38.2: Damage in an epidermal burn (red shaded layers show the damage).

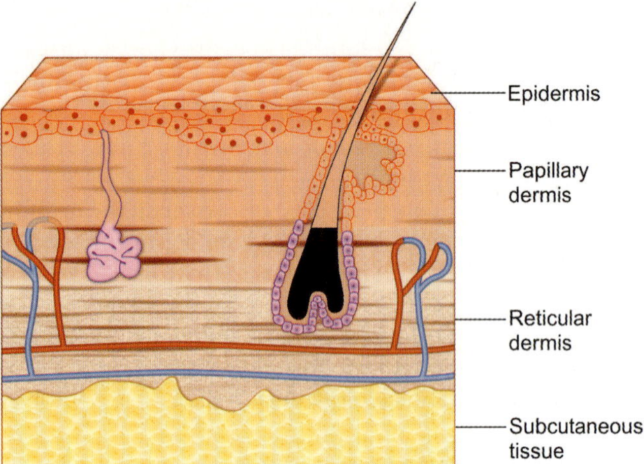

Fig. 38.3: Damage in a superficial partial-thickness burn.

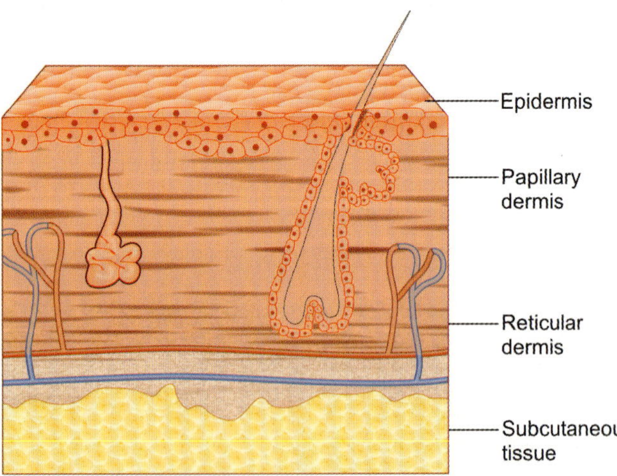

Fig. 38.4: Deep partial-thickness burn.

A major problem that arises from deep burns is the damage to the peripheral vascular system. Because large amounts of fluid leak into the interstitial space beneath unyielding eschar, the pressure in the extravascular space increases, potentially constricting the deep circulation to the point of occlusion, so poor distal circulation is seen.

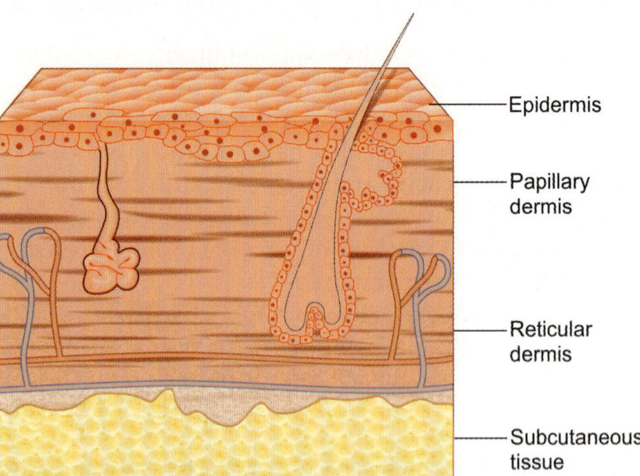

Fig. 38.5: Full-thickness burns.

> **BOX 38.2:** Eschar.
>
> Eschar is devitalized tissue with necrotic cells, which feels dry, leathery, and rigid (latter indicates ischemia of the area).

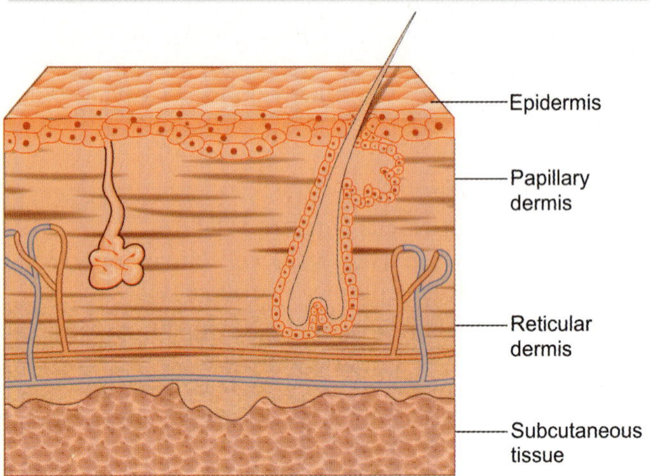

Fig. 38.6: Subdermal burns.

No sites are available for re-epithelialization of the wound, all epithelial cells have been destroyed, and skin grafting is necessary. Scarring can be seen.

Subdermal Burn

Listed below are the features of subdermal burn:
- Destruction of all tissue from the epidermis down to and through the subcutaneous tissue **(Fig. 38.6)**.
- It occurs with prolonged contact with flame or hot liquid, and contact with electricity.
- Muscle damage and neurological involvement is present.
- Heals with skin grafting. Scarring can be seen.

Methods to determine depth of burn are given in **Box 38.3**.

Classification According to the Size of Burns

It was established in the late 19th century that a relationship exists between the size of the burn and mortality. Berkow

BOX 38.3: Determination of the depth of burns.

> **BOX 38.3:** Determination of the depth of burns.
>
> Accurate determination of the depth of burns is essential for determining the optimal line of treatment and also to predict the rate and extent of healing. The most commonly used method is the clinical assessment method, but it has been found to be less accurate (<75% accuracy). A range of other methods exist, e.g., thermography, vital dyes, radioactive isotopes, ultrasound, magnetic resonance imaging, and photometry. Scanning LASER Doppler imaging (LDI) is the most commonly used investigative method for the determination of burn depth. It is much more accurate (96–10%) and feasible. However, it is expensive, large in size and takes long time for image acquisition. Duration for image acquisition can be reduced by using fast LDI or the LASER Doppler line scanner (LDLS), which is 300 cm^2 in 4 seconds and has a higher use in the pediatric population. Infrared thermography—both static and active—dynamic is been used now to assess the burn depth. Dermoscopy is a method whereby microanatomy skin vasculature is visualized and burn depth is estimated. Spectrophotometry is another inexpensive method that may be used.

used the calculation of the BSA as a function of height and weight and calculated the surface area of various body parts in relation to the TBSA. However, his calculations could not be used for a pediatric population. Later on, in 1944, Lund and Browder modified Berkow's calculations by adding an age correction factor to them and divided the BSA into 12 different regions, so that it could be used for both pediatric and adult populations **(Fig. 38.7)**. This method provides a more accurate estimate of the size of the burns; however, another method called the Rule of Nines (also called Wallace Rule of Nines, since it was first published by Wallace in 1951), developed by Pulaski and Tennison in 1947 (and first presented at a symposium in 1950) carries more importance in situations of emergency triage as it is more practical **(Fig. 38.8)**. The rule of nines estimates the surface area of the patient's hand as 1% and divides the rest of the body areas into areas of either 9% or multiples of 9%. Assessment of the size of burns is crucial to the diagnostic, prognostic, and treatment (for fluid replacement therapy) processes.

Calculation of extent of burns by the rule of nines:

- Divides body surface in 11 areas, each constituting 9% and perineum—1%.
  - Adult above 10 years
    Chance of survival = 100 – (age + % of body area involved), e.g., if an adult aged 60 years, has 30% burns, his chance of survival can be calculated as:
    100 – (60 years + 30%) = 10%.
- Greater extent—poorer prognosis: age >70, <10 years—has poor prognosis.
- TBSA cannot be considered alone—site and depth of injury affect the prognosis:
  - 4% of superficial burn on back
  - 4% of burn on face with an inhalation injury.

So, if the affection is on the face by inhalation injury, then prognosis is poor than on the back, though the percentage of the burns are same.

Electrical Burn

Electrical burn can be described as follows:

- Signs and symptoms vary according to the type of current, intensity of current, area of the body the electric current passes through.

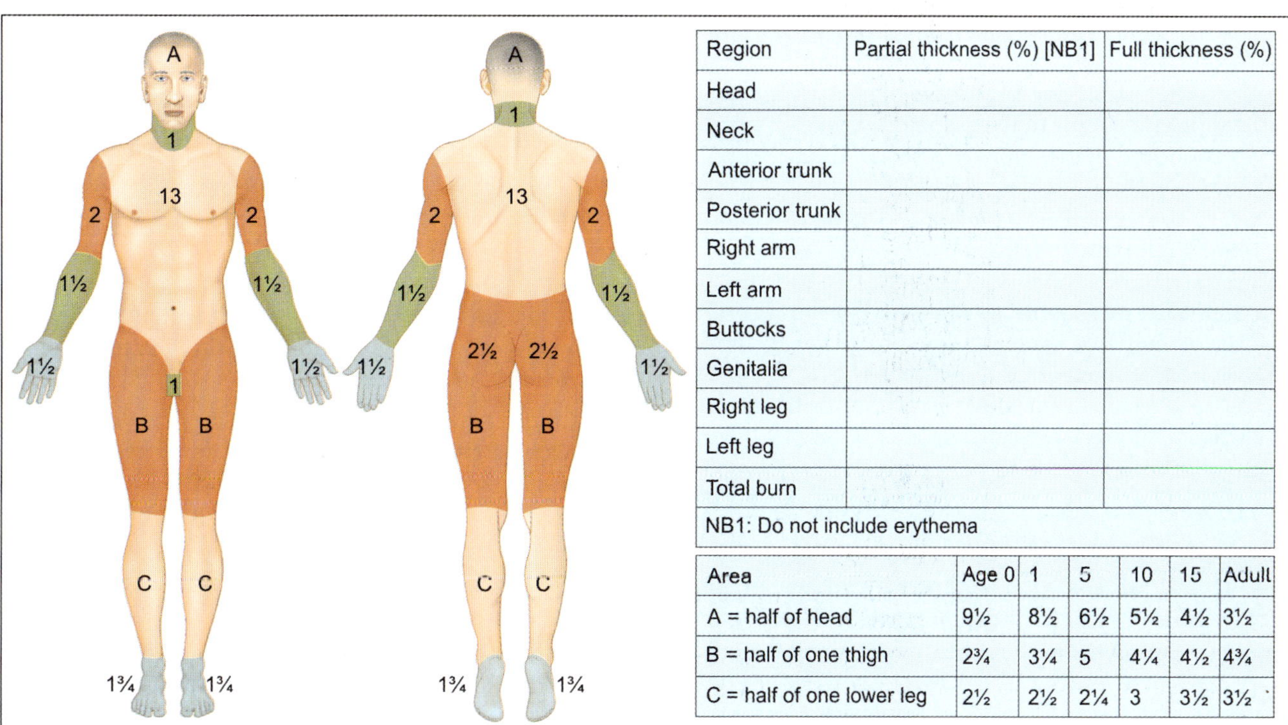

Region	Partial thickness (%) [NB1]	Full thickness (%)
Head		
Neck		
Anterior trunk		
Posterior trunk		
Right arm		
Left arm		
Buttocks		
Genitalia		
Right leg		
Left leg		
Total burn		
NB1: Do not include erythema		

Area	Age 0	1	5	10	15	Adult
A = half of head	9½	8½	6½	5½	4½	3½
B = half of one thigh	2¾	3¼	5	4¼	4½	4¾
C = half of one lower leg	2½	2½	2¼	3	3½	3½

Fig. 38.7: Lund–Browder chart for estimation of size of burns.

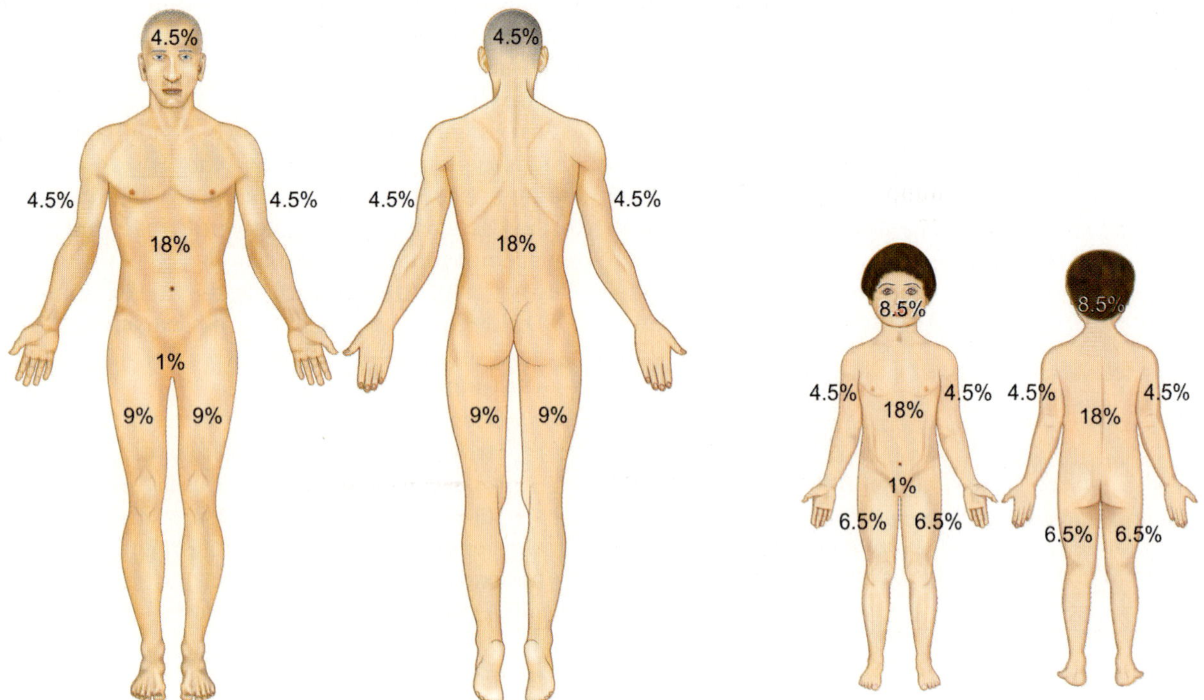

Fig. 38.8: Rule of nines (adult and child).

- Electric current follows the course of least resistance offered by tissues. (Nerves offer the least resistance, muscles are more resistant than nerves but less than bone, bone offers the highest resistance.)
- Contact site—at the site of contact with the electricity [at site where first contact was made (entrance wound) and the site where the current exited the body (exit wound)]; skin at entrance wound appears charred, whereas at the exit wound, it appears dry.
- Tissues lying between the entrance and exit wound also suffer burns due to passage of the current and the heat produced due to the tissue resistance.
- Surrounding tissues may be affected due to impaired blood supply.
- Other consequences—cardiac arrhythmias and acute renal failure can be seen.
- Complication—spinal cord damage, vertebral fracture. (Clinically, these patients will have spastic paresis but may or may not have any sensory pathway changes over concomitant areas of spasticity.)
- Cause of death—ventricular fibrillation and respiratory arrest.

PATHOLOGICAL CHANGES

The events that ensure any burn injury depend on the age and the location, duration and intensity of heat exposure in the case of thermal injuries. **Figure 38.9** explains the cascade of physiologic events that occurs postburn injury.

In cases of severe burns, due to release of inflammatory mediators, there is compromised cardiovascular function, and burn shock ensues, causing intravascular hypovolemia

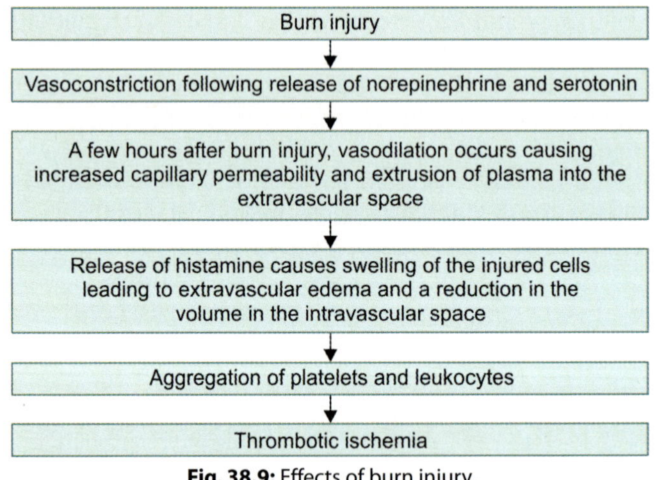

Fig. 38.9: Effects of burn injury.

and an increase in the systemic vascular resistance. This results in a decreased cardiac output which causes end-organ ischemia and metabolic acidosis. Resuscitation can help reverse these effects.

Local changes that can be seen at the site of the damage part:

- **Vascular changes**—dilatation of small vessels due to direct injury causes increased blood flow to the injured part, in turn, causing increased inflammation and capillary permeability.
- **Infection**—at the site of the damage.

Systemic changes:

- **Shock**—it is defined as inability of the circulatory system to meet the needs of tissues for oxygen and nutrients and the removal of their metabolites. It can last for 2–3 days.

- Neurogenic shock—due to pain and apprehension
- Cardiogenic shock—fall in cardiac output and increase heart rate
- Bacteremic shock—due to infection and release of toxins.
- **Biochemical changes:**
  - Electrolyte imbalance due to low sodium, chloride
  - Hypoproteinemia, hyperglycemia, and hypovolemia.
- **Changes in blood**—anemia can be seen.
- **Systemic lesions**—liver failure, renal failure, alteration in the pulmonary function, neurogenic changes, and immunologic impairment.

CLINICAL FEATURES

Inhalation Injury

The causes and symptoms of inhalation injury are as follows:

- It can be due to smoke, steam, or fire.
- Burned lips and nose, sore throat, cough, hoarseness of voice, injury to alveoli, abnormal breath sound, respiratory distress, and hypoxemia could be present. Hypoxia can result from alveolar damage, causing ventricular insufficiency, impairment of the circulation, and reduced oxygen transport.
- It affects mainly upper airway causing edema of larynx, pharynx, and trachea.

Features at the Site

The signs include:

- Redness
- Blisters
- White/yellow skin
- Weeping of plasma
- Limb edema
- Blackened tissue

During Shock: Up to 3 Days Postburn

The symptoms during shock (up to 3 days postburn):

- Restlessness and disorientation
- Coldness, paleness of the skin
- Sweating
- Reduced blood pressure
- Tachycardia
- Cyanosis
- Hypotension
- Rapid breathing
- Thirst and dehydration
- Gastric dilation, gastrointestinal ileus
- Immune function impaired (making the burn victim susceptible to infection).

About 4 Weeks Later

The symptoms about 4 weeks later are:

- Scar
- Pain

- Limitation of joint range of movement
- Joint deformities
- Loss of function.

Long-term (Depends on Site and Extent of Burn)

Long-term effects include:

- Amputation of limb
- Emotional trauma for both patient and relatives
- Social rejection
- Loss of independence and loss of employment.

COMPLICATIONS

Depending on the extent, the depth, and the type of burn injury, there may be secondary systemic complications.

- Pulmonary complications:
  - Pneumonia
  - Carbon monoxide poisoning
  - Tracheal damage
  - Upper airway obstruction
  - Pulmonary edema
  - Acute respiratory distress syndrome
  - Inhalation—facial burn, patient who has burned in closed space should be suspected of having an inhalation injury causing carbon monoxide inhalation, tracheal damage, pulmonary edema, and upper airway obstruction.
- Cardiac complications:
  - Congestive cardiac failure
  - Cardiac arrhythmias
  - Ventricular failure
  - Decrease cardiac output
- Infections—it is a leading cause of mortality of burn at wound site and other infections seen are:
  - Urinary tract infection
  - Respiratory tract infection
- Metabolic complications:
  - Increase in core temperature
  - Decrease body weight
  - Decrease in energy stores
    (It is recommended that room temperature be kept at 86°F (30°C), which will significantly reduce the metabolic rate).
- Peripheral neuropathy: **Two forms**—polyneuropathy and local neuropathy.
  1. Polyneuropathy following burns is rare
  2. Local neuropathy—it can be due to prolonged position, tightly or poorly fitted splint, or compression bandage.
  Common sites of involvement are brachial plexus, ulnar nerve, and common peroneal nerve
- Scar: Hypertrophic scar formation is seen, contraction of scar tissue causing joint deformity.
- Heterotopic ossification: Commonly seen in full-thickness burn; common areas—elbow, hip, and shoulder; symptoms are decreased range of motion and pain
- Septicemia, gastric dilatation, renal and liver failure

- Joint effusion, periarticular swelling
- Calcification of periarticular tissue
- Atrophy of the involved muscle
- Psychological trauma to the patient

BURN WOUND HEALING

Wound healing starts just after the injury and continues for several months continuing with the scar remodeling, depending on the extent and depth of the burns. The two layers of the skin—the epidermis and dermis—differ morphologically, and they heal by separate mechanisms **(Box 38.4)**.

Epidermal Healing

When a burn injures just the epidermis, or if there are viable cells lining the skin appendages, epithelial healing can occur on the surface of a wound. The process of epithelialization is most evident clinically in the partial-thickness wound that has intact hair follicles and glands.

The stimulus for epithelial growth is the presence of an open wound exposing subepithelial tissue to the environment. The intact epithelium attempts to cover an exposed wound through mitosis and the ameboid movement of cells from the basal layer of the surrounding epidermis into the wound.

Damage to sebaceous glands may cause dryness and itching of a healing wound. Lubrication can be a problem, and newly healed skin is characteristically dry and may split.

Dermal Healing

When an injury involves tissue deeper than the epidermis, dermal healing, or scar formation occurs. Scar formation can be divided into three phases: inflammatory, proliferative, and maturation phase.

Inflammatory Phase

The primary reaction of viable tissue to a burn wound is inflammation, which prepares the wound for healing through hemostatic, vascular, and cellular events. Inflammation begins at the time of injury, ends in about 3–5 days, and is characterized by redness, edema, warmth, pain, and decreased range of motion. Initially, when a blood vessel is ruptured, the wall of the vessel contracts to decrease blood flow. Platelets aggregate, and fibrin is deposited to form a clot over the area.

Proliferative Phase

During this phase, re-epithelialization is occurring at the surface of the wound, while deep within the wound, fibroblasts are migrating and proliferating. Fibroblasts are the cells that synthesize scar tissue which is composed of collagen and protein polysaccharides in the form of a viscous ground substance that surrounds the collagen strands.

During this period of fibroplasia, the tensile strength of the wound increases at a rate proportional to the rate of collagen synthesis. In conjunction with collagen deposition, granulation tissue is formed during this phase. Granulation tissue consists of macrophages, fibroblasts, collagen, and blood vessels. Newly formed blood vessels bring a rich blood supply to the area and encourage further wound healing.

During the proliferative phase, wound contraction occurs. Wound contraction is an active process in which the body attempts to close a wound where a loss of tissue has occurred.

Maturation Phase

During the maturation phase, there is a reduction in the number of fibroblasts, a decrease in vascularity due to a lesser metabolic demand, and remodeling of collagen, which becomes more parallel in arrangement and forms stronger bonds.

The ratio of collagen breakdown to production determines the type of scar that forms. If the rate of breakdown equals or slightly exceeds the rate of production, maturation results in a pale, flat, and pliable scar. If the rate of collagen production exceeds breakdown, then a hypertrophic scar may result.

The active process of scar contraction during both this maturation phase and the proliferative phase creates a risk of contracture formation.

MANAGEMENT OF BURNS

First Aid

The first aid management for different burns includes the following:

> **BOX 38.4:** Zones of burn wound.
>
> The burn wound can be divided into three different zones based on the severity of the tissue damage and the changes in the blood supply—zone of coagulation, zone of stasis, and zone of hyperemia. **Zone of the coagulation** is the most central zone, which has suffered the maximum amount of heat and is the most damaged. Excessive heat leads to denaturation, degradation, and coagulation of proteins causing tissue necrosis. It can be considered equivalent to a full-thickness burn and, hence, may require skin grafting. There is increased risk of infection and so, the patient needs to be carefully monitored in a specialized burn unit and antibiotics need to be administered. The **zone of stasis or the zone of ischemia** surrounds the zone of coagulation and contains damaged cells, which can be salvaged through appropriate treatment within 24–48 hours of injury. Any infection or inadequate perfusion (e.g., tight compression bandages or splints) can result in the death of these salvageable cells and broaden the zone of coagulation. The **zone of hyperemia** is the outermost zone and has an increased blood supply by virtue of inflammatory vasodilation. This zone recovers completely in a few days in the absence of any infection or another injury.

- Flame burn—cold water should be poured because it relieves pain and limits the depth of burn.
- Chemical burn—clothing must be removed and running water should be applied to the affected area.
- Scald—running cold water should be applied.
- Electrical—cardiopulmonary resuscitation can be needed.

Remove contaminated clothing and cover the part with a towel or sheet.

Minor burn: <10% TBSA, hands and feet in child, and 15% in adult, patient can stay at home and cover the part with bactericidal nonstick dressing regularly.

Major burn: >10% TBSA in child and >15% TBSA in adult, patient should be admitted to burns unit or intensive care unit.

Medical Management for Burns

Initial Management of Burns

Transportation is directly to a burn center, rather than to a hospital emergency room. The goals of treatment in transit are to stabilize the patient and maintain an airway. During the initial transportation phase, patient history and personal data are gathered when possible. The type of agent causing the burn is noted, and initial examination of the burn injury takes place.

Emergency medical personnel may use the rule of nines to estimate the percent of burn injury. In addition, they will prepare the individual for triage at the burn center by removing all burned clothing and jewelry and initiating the administration of fluid through an intravenous line.

Goals of initial management:

- Transfer the patient to burns ward
- Maintain airway and breathing by O_2, suction, and ventilator
- Maintain fluid balance
- Removal of clothing and cover with sterile cotton
- Prevention of cyanosis, shock, and hemorrhage
- Documentation of baseline data—extent and depth of the burn should be noted
- Cleaning of wounds (debridement)
- Prevention of pulmonary and cardiac complications
- Admission to a warm room—to reduce metabolic demand
- Proper position **(Fig. 38.10)**
- Pain relief and control edema
- High-protein diet
- Prevent infection by isolation and sterilization
- Examine other injuries near the burn area
- Prevention of contractures and scarring
- Maintaining strength and function.

Deep skin burns are rather inelastic in nature and they fail to accommodate the rising fluid buildup due to edema postinjury. This causes the so-called **tourniquet effect** where the inelastic accumulated fluid starts compressing the surrounding tissues, blocking their blood supply, eventually

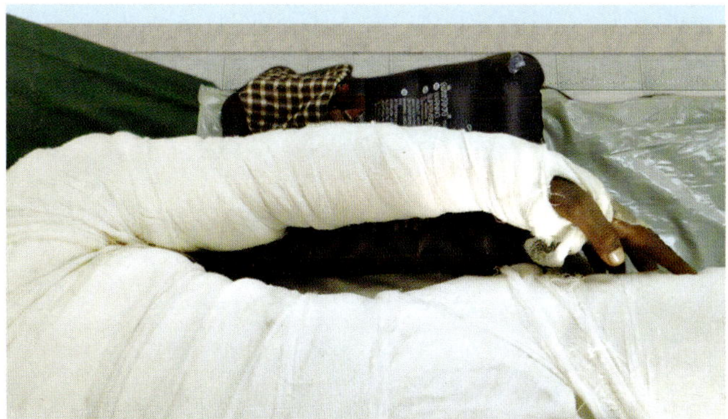

Fig. 38.10: Placing a water bag under the bony prominences to reduce risk of pressure sores.

leading to their necrosis. This phenomenon is called **compartment syndrome**. Escharotomy or fasciotomy may be required to relieve the pressure developed on the tissues and avoid necrosis of the underlying tissues.

Wound Care

Examination of the wound is crucial since it is susceptible to infection. The wound should be assessed for location, size, depth, odor, and exudate. The wound should be cleaned (debridement) to prevent infection and enhance healing.

Open Method

The technique of applying a topical cream or ointment without dressings is called the open technique and allows for ongoing inspection of the wound and examination of the healing process. Silver sulfadiazine, mafenide acetate, silver nitrate, and collagenase are some of the medications used topically for the treatment of burn wounds.

Closed Method

The closed technique consists of applying dressings over a topical agent **(Figs. 38.11A and B)**. Dressings serve several purposes:

- They hold topical antimicrobial agents on the wound.
- They reduce fluid loss from the wound.
- They protect the wound.

Physiotherapy Assessment

Physiotherapy assessment includes:

- Personal data
- History—type of agent causing burn
- Past history regarding previous injuries and functional limitations.
- First aid management at site of burns
- Check extent of burns by rule of nines
- Presence of other injury like fracture, contusion
- Examination of the burn wound, pain, and edema
- Motor assessment
- Sensory assessment
- Respiratory and cardiovascular assessment

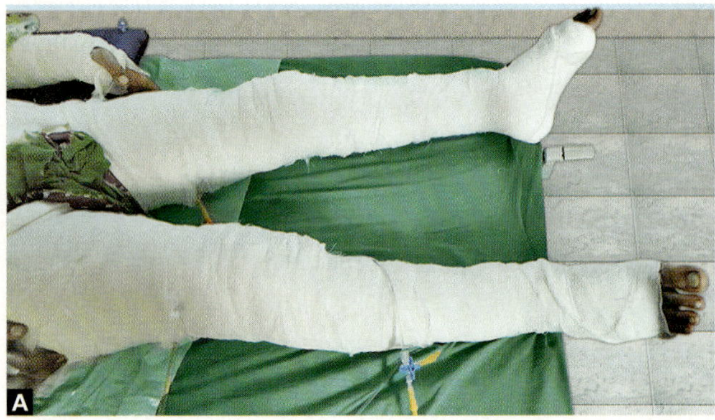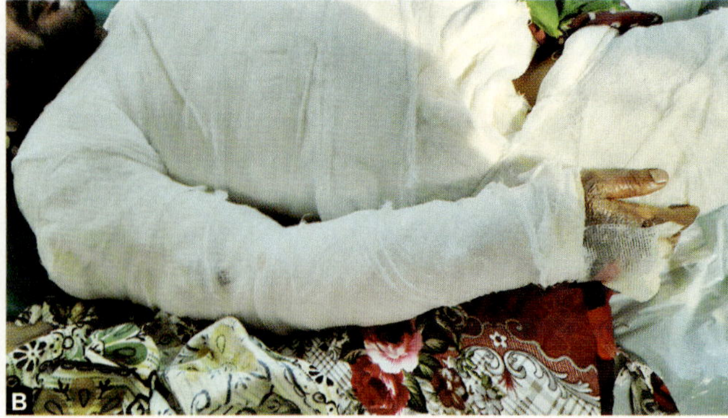

Figs. 38.11A and B: Closed method of wound care.

- Speech and swallowing assessment (in the case of large injuries, inhalation injuries, or injuries to the upper part of the body).
- Depth of the burn
- Functional assessment

Physiotherapy Management

Aims

Aims of physiotherapy management are to:
- Provide psychological support
- Achieve a clear airway and so prevent respiratory complications
- Minimize scarring
- Maintain soft tissue length
- Maintain joint range of movement, and prevent contracture and deformities
- Maintain muscle strength
- Regain maximum function and cardiopulmonary endurance
- Help the patient to gain independence and return to an active lifestyle.

Techniques

Prevent Respiratory Complications

Prevention is required for following cases:
- In the case of elderly patient, if they have any associated medical history
- Inhalation or facial burn—in the case of facial edema, patient may lie supine or on either side, tipping is contraindicated
- For an immobile patient
- Pre- and postoperatively to maintain the clear airway.

Interventions that may be used:
- Chest expansion exercises for ventilation of all lung areas
- In the case of full-thickness burns to chest—breathing exercises should be given
- Chest physiotherapy in the form of clapping, vibration, suctioning, huffing, and coughing to clear secretions depending on status of the patient. If the patient has chest burns then a piece of foam may be used under the hands.

Maintain Full Range of Motion

Active and passive exercises can be used to maintain full range of motion (ROM).
- Active exercise begins on the day of admission.
- Patient should perform active exercises of all extremities and trunk including unburnt areas.
- Slow sustained stretch to the affected area.
- Active-assisted or passive movement to affected part
- Free active exercises to the adjacent joints.
- Trunk movement, such as flexion, extension, and rotation to prevent robot-type posture.
- Paraffin wax bath and ultrasound—to increase pliability of tissue before the exercise.
- Hold-relax exercises, if possible in later stages.

Resistive and Conditioning Exercises

Resistive and conditioning exercises can also be performed.
- According to patient's condition and stage of wound healing.
- Isotonic, isokinetic, or with free weights, rubber exercise bands, springs and pulley can be done for the parts which do not have burns.
- Patients should be encouraged to participate in exercises that will stress the cardiovascular system, e.g., walking, cycling, treadmill walking, and stair climbing—to increase cardiovascular endurance and also strengthen and maintain the range of motion of the extremities.
- Monitoring of vitals before, during, and after exercise should be done.

Prevent Deformity/Contracture

Positioning—it should start from the day of admission **(Table 38.3)**.
- Head and neck—small roll behind the neck or pillow under the shoulder for extension of cervical spine
- Facial burn—half lying
- Upper limb—elevation, 90° shoulder abduction, slight flexion, external rotation; elbow, wrist—extension; metacarpophalangeal joint—flexion; interphalangeal joint—extension, thumb abduction. Lower limb—elevation, raise the end of bed; hip—extension, abduction, knee extension, ankle-90° dorsiflexion.

Table 38.3: Positioning required for burn victims.

Joint	Common deformity	Difficulty experienced	Movements to be stressed	Anti-contracture approaches
Anterior aspect of neck	Flexion	Neck contours are lost, chin is pulled towards the chest region making neck movements difficult	Hyperextension	Use of double mattress; positioning neck in extension; in cases of healing burns—use rigid cervical orthosis; avoid using pillow below neck, use of roll below neck is preferred
Posterior aspect of neck	Extension	Difficult neck flexion	Flexion	Position the patient in sitting with neck in flexion or in lying with pillow below the head
Shoulder-axilla (anterior and posterior folds)	Adduction and internal rotation	Abduction and protraction (in cases of burns also over anterior region of chest)	Abduction, flexion, and external rotation	Position in lying or sitting with shoulder flexed and abducted to 90 degrees with support using pillows or foam blocks between the chest and the arms; use of figure of eight bandaging or airplane splint
Anterior aspect of elbows	Flexion and pronation	Stretch on the anterior aspect of elbows, restricted movement leading to difficulty in ADL	Extension and supination	Splint in extension
Hand	Claw hand (also known as intrinsic minus position)	Difficulty in ADL like eating, grooming, toileting, etc.	Wrist extension; metacarpophalangeal flexion, both interphalangeal joints extension; thumb abduction	Wrapping of individual fingers separately; elevation for relieving edema; positioning in intrinsic plus position—wrist extension, metacarpophalangeal flexion, proximal interphalangeal and distal interphalangeal extension, thumb abduction
Hip (groin)	Hip flexion and adduction	Hip stretched towards abdomen restricting hip movements and impairing gait	All movements emphasizing hip extension and abduction	Positioning in prone lying—hip neutral (zero degrees of flexion/extension), with slight abduction; avoid side lying and sitting; supine lying with hips extended—no pillow beneath knees
Knee	Flexion	Restricted knee extension—impairing gait	Extension	Posterior knee splint; position with knees extended in lying and sitting
Ankle	Plantar flexion	Limit standing and walking	All motions (especially dorsiflexion)	Maintain ankles at 90 degrees using pillows; encourage standing with feet flat on the ground if edema is absent; plastic ankle-foot orthosis with cutout at Achilles tendon and ankle positioned in neutral

Positioning is important to minimize edema, prevent tissue destruction, and maintain soft tissue in elongated state and preserve function.

Splinting—maintain anatomical position of the joints.

Splints are usually worn at night, when a patient is resting, or continuously to maintain the same positioning for several days following skin grafting. Splints should conform to the body part, and care must be taken to ensure that there are no pressure points that may cause a breakdown in healing or normal skin. Splints should be checked routinely for proper fit and revised if necessary.

Active motion is important, splints and positioning are intended to serve as adjuncts to the therapy program until full active motion can be achieved.

Static splint: Mainly used to hold the position. Use in night → to prevent soft tissue tightening—hand resting splint, foot drop splint. These type of splints have no moveable parts and maintains a position or immobilizes an area following skin grafting.

Dynamic splint: For controlled movement of joint—intermittent use.

These splints have moveable parts that allow joint movement. At the same time, dynamic splints apply a low-load, prolonged stress that can be adjusted to a patient's tolerance, they offer great potential for correcting a developing contracture and the early return of active function in areas of extensive burn and grafting.

Following are a few commonly used splints:

- Neck—collar
- Shoulder—abduction–external rotation brace
- Axilla—figure-of-eight clavicle brace
- Elbow, knees—gutter splint
- Ankle foot—foot drop stop, shoes with soft inserts.

Splinting is used to prevent contracture, maintain ROM, correction of contracture, protection of joint or tendon, and reduce overall pain experience.

Stretching Exercises

Stretching exercises should be prescribed in cases of abnormal ROM. Skin and muscle, being two biomechanically different structures, should be stretched in different manners. Muscle stretching should be performed in the conventional manner. However, skin stretching should be performed with a slow, sustained stretch till the point of tissue blanching. However, care should be taken that the tissue does not blanch beyond a point, since it may be at risk of tearing.

Prevent Edema

Elevation, active exercises, bandaging, and massage help in relieving edema. Elevation helps in draining the excess fluid by means of gravity. Active exercises and massage mobilize the fluid. Bandaging uses compression to increase the extravascular pressure and push the fluid back into the intravascular space.

Maintain Muscle Strength, Endurance

Resisted exercises using manual resistance, free weights, and springs help in maintaining and improving muscle strength and endurance.

Scar Management

Hypertrophic scar formation needs to be minimized to regain function as much as possible. Pressure helps in enhancing scar maturation and minimizing hypertrophic scar formation. Pressure alters the biochemical structure of the scar tissue and helps in reorganizing the collagen structures. Pressure is usually indicated for deep partial-thickness burns.

Silicone gel sheets may be used, but the patient should first be examined for allergic reactions as it tends to form rashes. Deep friction massage is thought to loosen scar tissue by mobilizing cutaneous tissue from underlying tissue and acting to break up adhesions. Ultrasound therapy can be used to mobilize the scar.

Pressure Dressings

Compression therapy or pressure therapy forms an important component of the burn rehabilitation program. Pressure can be applied through elastic bandages or compression garments. The pressure generated interferes with the production of collagen and realigns the few collagen fibers that are produced, hence, effectively minimizing scar formation. Along with reducing scar formation, the pressure dressings:

- Protect the fragile skin
- Improve the circulation of damaged tissues
- Reduce pain
- Reduce the dryness of skin, making the skin less itchy and irritated
- Improve the extensibility of skin.

Types of pressure garments:

- Elastic wrap bandages: Used in the initial phase of management to provide pressure on the extremities till the burn area can tolerate the shearing force of a pressure garment. It is applied in a figure-of-eight pattern in the lower extremities, a spiral pattern in the upper extremities and a circular pattern on the trunk. Self-adherent elastic bandage for hands and toes are available.
- Tubular pressure bandages (tubigrip): Used in the initial phase of management to provide gentle pressure. They are more useful for growing children as they need frequent garment alterations.
- Interim care garments: Available off the shelf and used in the interim phase until custom-made garments are made available.
- Custom-made garments: Manufactured according to the patient's measurements using nylon and spandex.

Pressure garments should be worn 23 hours a day, 7 days a week. They can be removed for bathing and applying lotion or any other moisturizer. The use of pressure garments needs to be continued till the scars mature (become soft, pliable and the color seems similar to the color of the surrounding normal skin). It may take around 8 months to a year depending on the depth of the burns and genetic factors.

Camouflage Makeup

Burns often lead to hypo- or hyperpigmentation of skin, which may be cosmetically disapproving to the patient. The patients usually feel psychologically depressed due to this and may be advised to use camouflage makeup. Skin camouflage or camouflage makeup is the application of highly pigmented creams and lotions to mask the skin pigmentation and scarring. These cosmetics are usually water resistant and hence allow use throughout the day without the fear of removal by sweat or water. It can be used before the maturation of scar to allow the patient to visit outdoors without having to don the pressure garments.

Ambulation

It should be started as early as possible. After skin grafting, the lower limb should be wrapped in elastic bandage in figure-of-eight pattern to support the new graft and promote venous return.

- If patient cannot tolerate upright position, then tilt table can be used for standing.
- Initially assistive device can be used.
- Encourage walking, cycling, treadmill, and stair climbing to improve aerobic capacity.
- Regain maximum function, prepare for activity of daily living (ADL)—skipping, jumping a height, and achieving grip strength by a given time.

Surgical Management

Primary Excision

Primary excision is the removal of eschar to increase the survival rate. Excision generally includes removal of peripheral layers of eschar until vascular, viable tissue is exposed as the site for skin graft placement. Early excision reduces infection, scarring and promotes rapid healing, than repeated debridement.

Skin Grafting

- **Autograft:**
  - Patient's own skin from unburnt part
  - Provides permanent coverage of wound
  - No rejection by patient's skin.
- **Allograft (homograft):**
  - Same species are used for allograft
  - Usually cadaver skin
  - It provides temporary coverage of wound. It is used until there is sufficient normal skin available for an autograph
  - Rejection—3–4 weeks
  - Provides protection to the area.
- **Xenograft (heterograft):**
  - Another species, usually a pig is used
  - Rejection in 3–4 weeks
  - Provides protection and is used until there is sufficient normal skin available for an autograft.
- **Advancement—"skin substitutes" for coverage of wound:**
  - Biopsy of patient's own skin or cadaver skin grown in lab
  - Use large area of burn, coverage is necessary for patient's survival
  - Range of motion exercise should delay and shearing forces must be avoided
  - Expensive intervention for wound coverage.

Types of Grafts:
Free grafts
- Partial thickness/split thickness skin graft
- Whole thickness

Flaps:
- Fasciocutaneous—skin and fascia
- Myocutaneous—muscle and skin (latissimus dorsi muscle used in reconstruction of breast)
- Cutaneous—full-thickness skin
- Osteomyocutaneous—bone, muscle, and skin (taken from forearm and used for maxillofacial reconstruction)
- Random pattern—for local repair of adjacent defect, usually face.

Pedicle grafts:
- Direct pedicle
- Bridge pedicle
- Tube pedicle

Free grafts: Skin is removed from one part of the body and applied to another part.

According to the thickness:
- *Split skin graft*—the epidermis and part of is present dermis, transferred without blood supply. It is used in the case of traumatic injury when large area of skin loss is present

- Usually performed from volar aspect of thigh and medial aspect of upper arm
- *Whole thickness*—full dermis excludes superficial fascia, requires better blood supply for survival → face, hand, supraclavicular area and eyelids
- Donor sites heal in 12–14 days depending on thickness
- Common donor sites—thigh, buttocks, back, and medial aspect of upper arm
- For first 48 hours, nutrition is obtained from recipient site
- Thicker graft—better cosmetic results
- Thinner graft—better adherence, a thin graft will contract more than a thick skin graft once it has adhered to the wound bed.

"Dermatome" is an instrument which allows large amount of skin to be taken of consistent thickness. The dermatome is adjusted to remove a predetermined thickness of skin for a split-thickness skin graft. For graft to adhere, vascularity is important; it cannot adhere to poorly vascularized area, such as tendon.

Survival of graft depends on various factors:
- Circulation—which provides a nutritive supply to the graft
- Nutrition
- Penetration of host vessels into the graft site.

Mesh graft— the meshing of a graft consists of processing the sheet graft through a device that makes tiny parallel incisions in a linear manner, to cover large area when limited donor skin is available and once the graft adheres, the interstices heal through re-epithelialization. Autograft is used.

Sheet graft—a sheet graft is a skin graft applied to a recipient bed without alteration following harvesting from a donor site.

Face, neck, and hands are covered with this type of graft for cosmesis, preservation, and function.

Flaps and Pedicles

Flap: Flap includes the following:
- Skin to be transferred remains attached by one end to the donor area and other to recipient site.
- Blood supply of flap remains as it is.
- Skin of trunk is used to cover wound of upper limb, and skin of lower limb is used to cover wound of other lower limb.
- As flaps have their own blood supply, they can be used to cover avascular defects, e.g., open joints, exposed bone, cartilage, or tendon.
- For example, abdominal forearm skin flap.

Pedicle: Pedicle includes the following:
- Intermediate as well as final recipient site
- It connects the recipient area to donor area
- It is used to cover bare tendons, bone, and cartilage
- Blood supply is preserved throughout the procedure
- Free flaps are used; skin is taken with its blood vessels and then anastomosed with vessels of recipient site.

Direct pedicle: Donor area can brought near the recipient wound, i.e., skin of the trunk can be used to cover the skin of the upper limb **(Fig. 38.12)**

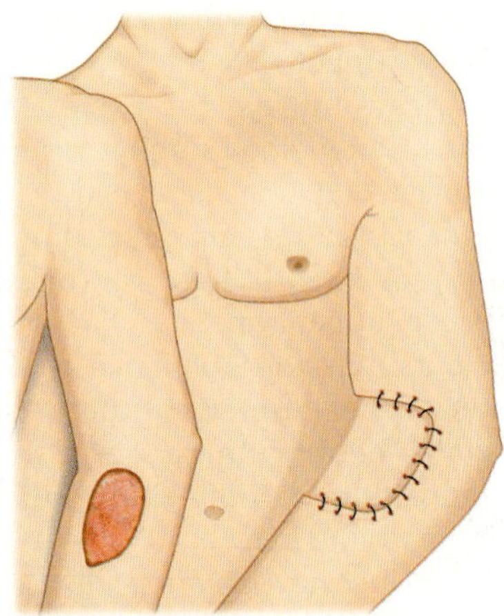

Fig. 38.12: Direct pedicle graft.
Courtesy: S Das, Textbook of Surgery, 6th edition

Bridge pedicle (**Fig. 38.13**)
- Used for wound of palm
- Flap raised from donor area with its both the ends attached to area and recipient wound pushed beneath the flap and attached to it, i.e., skin from thigh to cover the wound of palm.

Tube pedicle (**Fig. 38.14***)*
- Used for face
- Flap is taken from abdomen-forearm-neck-forearm. It is then free and can be attached to the final recipient site like the neck (tube pedicle).

Pressure garments: Lycra should be worn nearly 24 hours a day.
- It helps to reduce hypertrophic scarring.
- Used for 2 years, to reduce hypertrophic scarring.
- Gloves, sleeves, tights, vest, and high-waist pants are available.

Escharotomy
- Removal of dead, burnt skin

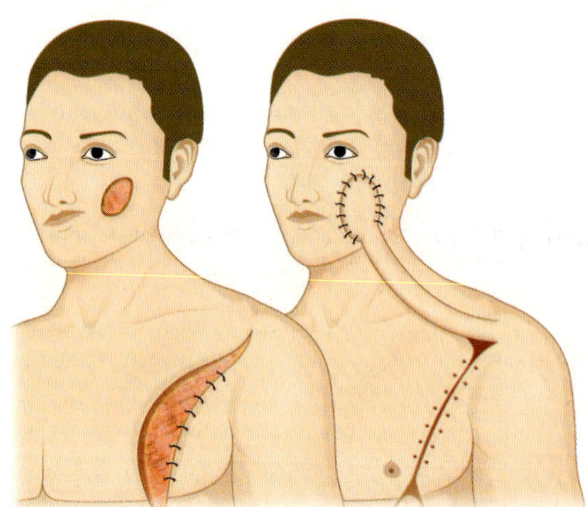

Fig. 38.14: Tube pedicle graft.
Courtesy: S Das, Textbook of Surgery, 6th edition

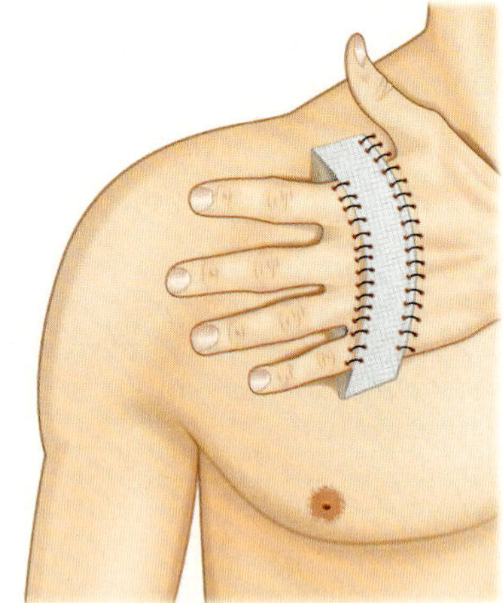

Fig. 38.13: Bridge pedicle graft.
Courtesy: S Das, Textbook of Surgery, 6th edition

- Midlateral incision of eschar
- Slit made in the skin which restricts the movement
- Around chest where respiration can be impaired.

Tissue Expansion
- Gradual stretching of marginal skin by implanting expander balloons under adjacent normal skin, then enlarging the expander and stretching overlying skin.
- Expander is removed and excess skin stretched to grafted area for reconstruction.
- Useful in burn alopecia, missing eyebrows, eyelids, lips, and nose.
- Z-plasty (**Fig. 38.15**) and V-Y plasty (**Fig. 38.16**) are used to lengthen the scar, whereas Y-V plasty (**Fig. 38.17**) is used to broaden the scar.

Physiotherapy Management for Skin Grafting, Flaps, and Pedicles

Physiotherapy management for skin grafting, flaps, and pedicles are as follows:
- For donor area—ultraviolet radiation → E1 dose for healing
- For scar—kneading, passive stretches, passive and active movement
- Splinting to prevent contracture of graft and prevent joint deformities
- After 7 days—exercise adjacent joints
- After 14 days—kneading over scar/around wound
- LASER—for wound healing and to reduce pain
- High-protein and high-calorie diet to improve nutritional status
- Chest—chest physiotherapy in form of breathing exercises, huffing, and coughing—especially after administration of anesthesia when surgery is performed.

Rest of the management remains similar to nonoperative management.

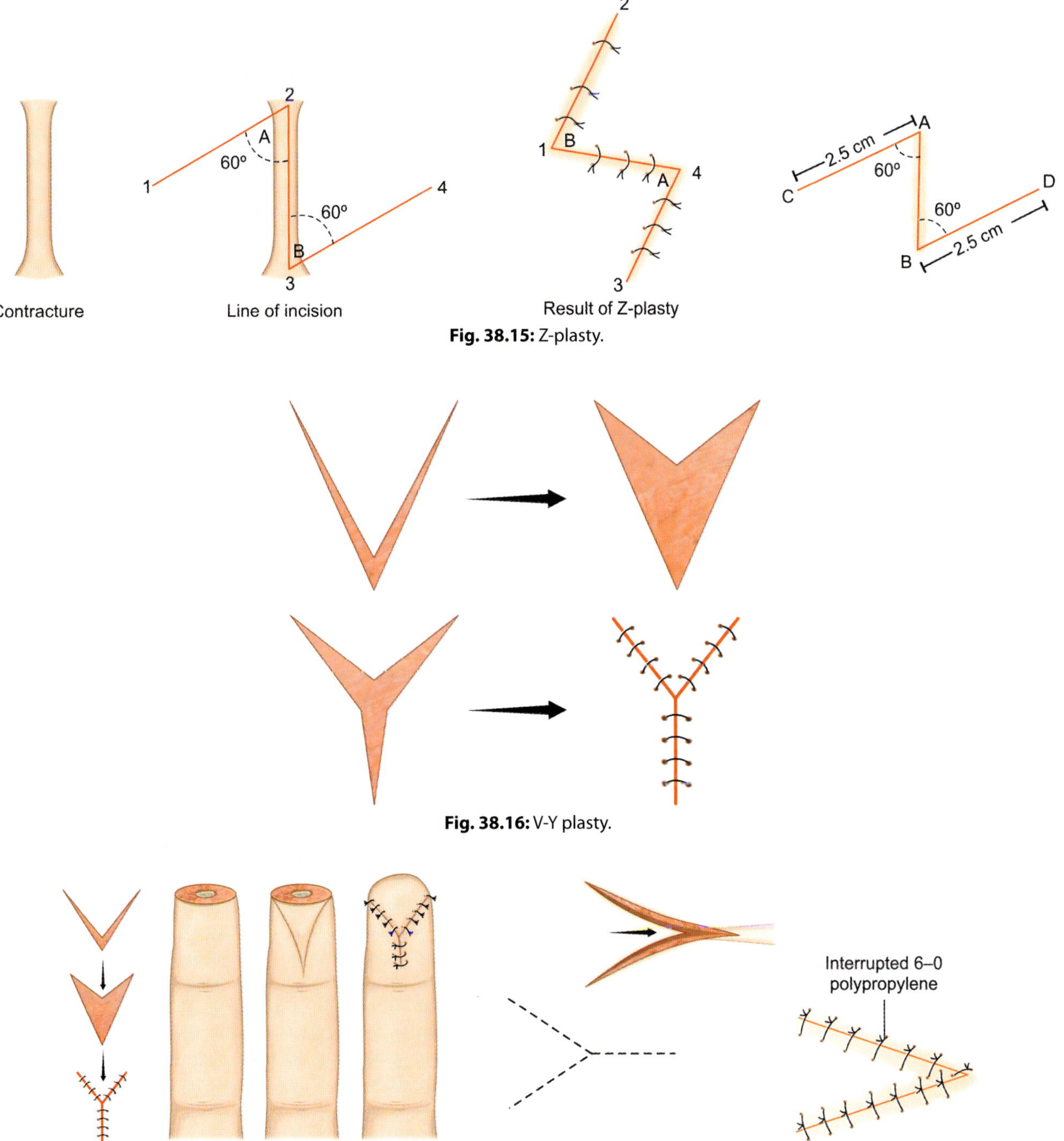

Fig. 38.15: Z-plasty.

Fig. 38.16: V-Y plasty.

Fig. 38.17: Y-V plasty.

FOLLOW-UP CARE

Discharge from the rehabilitation center does not mean that life goes back to normal for a burns patient. The rehabilitation professional should provide the patient with a detailed and individualized home care regime. The patient should be taught exercises that are to be performed at home. They should be educated about appropriate splinting procedures and positioning to prevent contractures and scars. They should be given proper skin care advices to prevent skin damage. The therapist should guide the patient about going back to routine activities and gradually moving towards independence. It may not be possible for all patients to be completely functional and that should not demotivate the patient. The patient should try to gain as much functional independence as possible.

Patient compliance post-discharge remains a huge setback in the rehabilitation of burn patients. Regular follow-up sessions should be scheduled to maintain compliance and the patient can be requested to maintain a log diary of the exercise sessions at home. Several patients may report forgetfulness and inability to correctly perform the exercises without the therapeutic equipment. Video recording of the exercise session is a good method to allow the patient to remember the correct technique and sequence of movements and exercises. The patient and the family members should be taught techniques using minimal equipment so that they can be reproduced at home.

Before discharge, the patient and the family members should be able to apply and remove splints and pressure dressings independently. The patient should be educated about the importance of compliance to the home care program and should be given written information in the form of pamphlets, information booklet, etc. Advices regarding when to consult a medical professional should also be given.

SUMMARY

Burn injury represents a major health problem in terms of management and care of surviving patients. Impairments and complications vary according to extent and depth of burns. Classification of burn injuries is based on the depth of the tissue destroyed. Rule of nines formula was developed for initial determination of extent of injury. Clinical signs and symptoms and pathological changes vary according to the depth of the injury. Complication is also seen according to the site of the burn injury. Initial management at the site of the burn and medical management in the early period are important. Physiotherapy examination and management and surgical management including skin grafting, flaps, and pedicles help in rehabilitation of the patient. Although burn trauma and subsequent recovery can be a devastating life occurrence, there are treatment facilities and medical professionals to assist patient with burn injuries and their families return to as normal a lifestyle as possible.

Case Scenario

CASE STUDY

A 26-year-old male, autorickshaw driver by occupation, was caught in a house fire and got burns over his face, arms, legs, and upper chest. After first aid management with running cold water, he was admitted to the regional burns unit. The face and leg burns were superficial partial-thickness and upper chest and arms were deep partial-thickness burns. The patient was initially treated in the regional burn unit and is now referred to the local hospital at the follow-up outpatient physical therapy. Ten days after his discharge from hospital, he presented with the pressure garments as he was instructed.

Examination

Pain: Patient complains of pain over the burnt area and has a feeling of stretching pain over the upper chest region.

ROM: He has a decreased range of motion of right upper extremity in form of flexion of shoulder limited to 0–140° of flexion and abduction and a lack of 20° of elbow flexion. Range of motion was affected for the legs as well.

Strength of the patient is within the functional limit in available range for the affected part

ADL: Patient states that he has difficulties in eating, combing, and wearing clothes. All the facial muscles are working properly and he is able to chew the food. His wounds have healed properly and he is discharged from the hospital.

Guiding Questions:
1. How will you assess the percentage of burns?
2. Write down the late complications according to the involvement of the body parts.
3. What are the pathological changes around the burnt area?
4. Establish the plan of care in the form of short-term and long-term goals.
5. How will you manage the hypertrophic scar due to burn over the upper limb?
6. Describe physical rehabilitation emphasizing the occupation of the patient.

Review Questions

1. Enumerate the layers of the skin with its functions.
2. Discuss the first aid management of a patient having flame burn over the right upper limb.
3. Describe the clinical features and management of inhalation burns in detail.
4. Write in detail about etiology, clinical features, and complications of burns.
5. Write in detail about burn wound healing.
6. Write down the management of a person having electrical burns affecting right upper and lower limb.
7. Write down the clinical features and management of a 65-year-old male having burns at the anterior chest region and face.
8. Write a short note on skin grafting and other reconstructive surgeries.
9. Write a short note on scar management.
10. What are the pathological changes in the skin due to burn?
11. What are the complications of the burns?

BIBLIOGRAPHY

1. Ahuja RB, Bhattacharya S, Rai A. Changing trends of an endemic trauma. Burns. 2009;35(5):650-6.
2. Apfel L. Approaches to positioning the burn patient. In: Richard RL, Staley MJ (Eds.). Burn care and rehabilitation: principles and practice. Philadelphia, PA: FA Davis; 1994. p. 221.
3. Boyea BL,Hubert temmen,David J Bariillo. Use of the tilt table for postural reconditioning of burn patients prior to ambulation. Presented at 30th annual meeting. American Born Asoociation, Chicago:1998.
4. Chern PL, Baum CL, Arpey, CJ. Biologic dressings: current applications and limitations in dermatologic surgery. Dermatol Surg. 2009;35(6):891-906.
5. Covey MH, Dutcher K,Marvin JA. Efficacy of continuous passive motion (CPM) devices with hand burns. J Burn Care Rehabil. 1988;(4):397-400.
6. Cuono C,Langdon R,McGuire J. Use of cultured epidermal autografts and dermal allografts as skin replacement after burn injury. Lancet. 1986;1(8490):1123-4.
7. Das S. Textbook of surgery, 6th edition. 2010.

8. Daugherty M, Carr-Collins J. Splinting techniques for the burn patient. In: Richard RL, Staley MJ (Eds.). Burn care and rehabilitation: principles and practice. Philadelphia, PA: FA Davis; 1994. p. 242.

9. Dersh J, Polatin PB, Gatchel RJ. Chronic pain and psychopathology: research findings and theoretical considerations. Psychosom Med. 2002; 64(5):773-86.

10. Dutcher K, Johnson C. Neuromuscular and musculoskeletal complications. In: Richard RL, Staley MJ (Eds.). Burn care and rehabilitation: principles and practice. Philadelphia, PA: FA Davis; 1994. p. 576.

11. Fohn M, Bannasch H. Artificial skin. Methods Mol Med. 2007;140:167-82.

12. Goswami P, Singodia P, Sinha AK, et al. Five-year epidemiological study of burn patients admitted in burns care unit, Tata Main Hospital, Jamshedpur, Jharkhand, India. Indian J Burns. 2016;24(1):41-6.

13. Greenhalgh DG, Staley MJ. Burn wound healing. In: Richard RL, Staley MJ (Eds.). Burn care and rehabilitation: principles and practice. Philadelphia, PA: FA Davis; 1994. p. 70.

14. Grigsby de Linde L. Rehabilitation of the child with burns. In: Tecklin JS (Ed.). Pediatric physical therapy, 3rd edition. Philadelphia, PA: Lippincott; 1999. p. 468.

15. Hansbrough JF, mozingo DW, Kealey GP, Davis M. Clinical trials of a biosynthetic temporary skin replacement, dermagraft-transitional covering, compared with cryopreserved human cadaver skin for temporary coverage of excised burn wounds. J Burn Care Rehabil. 1997;18(1 pt 1):43-51.

16. Heimbach D, Luterman A, Burke J. Artificial dermis for major burns: a multicenter, randomized clinical trial. Ann Surg. 1988;208(3):313-20.

17. Institute of Medicine Committee on Advancing Pain Research, Care, and Education. Relieving pain in America: a blueprint for transforming prevention, care, education, and research. Washington, DC: National Academy of Sciences; 2011.

18. International Association for the Study of Pain (IASP). Neuropathic pain. In: Charlton JE (Ed). Core curriculum for professional education in pain, 3rd edition. Seattle, WA: IASP Press; 2005.

19. Kolarsick PA, Kolarsick MA, Goodwin C. Anatomy and physiology of the skin. J Dermatol Nurs Assoc. 2011;3(4):203-13.

20. Lee KC, Joory K, Moiemen NS. History of burns: the past, present and the future. Burns Trauma. 2014;2(4):169-80.

21. Mayday Fund Special Committee on Pain and the Practice of Medicine. A call to revolutionize chronic pain care in America: an opportunity in health care reform. New York, NY: Mayday Fund; 2009.

22. Miller SF, et al. Triage and resuscitation of the burn patient. In: Richard RL, Staley MJ (Eds.). Burn care and rehabilitation: principles and practice. Philadelphia, PA: FA Davis; 1994. p. 107.

23. Miller SF. Surgical management of the burn patient. In: Richard RL, Staley, MJ (Eds.). Burn care and rehabilitation: principles and practice. Philadelphia, PA: FA Davis; 1994. p. 180.

24. Moore ML, Palmgren LA, Yenne-Laker CJ. The burn unit. In: Campbell SK, Palisano RJ, Orlin MN (Eds.). Physical therapy for children, 4th edition. St. Louis, MO: Elsevier/Saunders; 2012. p. 1008.

25. Mozingo DW. Surgical management. In: Carrougher GJ (Ed.). Burn care and therapy, St. Louis, MO: Mosby; 1998. p. 233.

26. Munster AM. Cultured epidermal autographs in the management of burn patients. J Burn Care Rehabil. 1992;13:121.

27. O'Sullivan SB, Schmitz TJ, Fulk GD. Physical rehabilitation, 6th edition. 2014. pp. 1090-117.

28. O'Sullivan SB, Schmitz TJ, Fulk GD. Physical rehabilitation, 6th edition. Philadelphia, PA: FA Davis Company; 2014.

29. Peden M, Oyegbite K, Ozanne-Smith. World report on child injury and prevention. Geneva: World Health Organization; 2008. pp. 79-98. Chapter 1.

30. Porter S. Tidy's physiotherapy, 13th edition. 2003. pp. 96-104.

31. Purdue Gf, Hunt JL, Still JM Jr. A multicenter clinical trial of a biosynthetic skin replacement, Dermagraft-TC, compared with cryopreserved human cadaver skin for temporary coverage of excised burn wounds. J Burn Care Rehabil. 1997;18 (1 pt 1):52-7.

32. Reid KJ, Harker J Bala MM, Truyers C, Kellen E, Bekkering GE, Kleijnen J. Epidemiology of chronic non-cancer pain in Europe: narrative review of prevalence, pain treatments and pain impact. Curr Med Res Opin. 2011;27(2):449-62.

33. Richard R, Miller S, Staley M, Johnson RM. Multimodal versus progressive treatment techniques to correct burn scar contractures. J Burn Care Rehabil. 2000;21(6):506-12.

34. Richard R, Miller SF, Steinlage R Finley RK Jr. A comparison of the tanner and bioplasty skin mesher systems for maximal skin graft expansion. J Burn Care Rehabil. 1993;14(6):690-5.

35. Richard R, Ward RS. Splinting strategies and controversies. J Burn Care Rehabil. 2005;26(5):392-6.

36. Richard RL, Miller SF, staley MJ. The physiologic response of a patient with critical burns to continuous passive motion. J Burn Care Rehabil. 1990;11(6):554-6.

37. Rybarczyk MM, Schafer JM, Elm CM, et al. A systematic review of burn injuries in low- and middle-income countries: epidemiology in the WHO-defined African Region. Afr J Emerg Med. 2017;7(1):30-7.

38. Sauer SE, Burris JL, Carlson CR. New directions in the management of chronic pain: self-regulation theory as a model for integrative clinical psychology practice. Clin Psychol Rev. 2010;30(6):805-14.

39. Schneider JC. Contractures in burn injury: defining the problem. J Burn Care Res. 2006;27(4):508.

40. Serghiou M, Cowan A, Whitehead C. Rehabilitation after a burn injury. Clin Plast Surg. 2009;36(4):675-86.

41. Sheridan R. Closure of the excised burn wound: autografts, semipermanent skin substitutes, and permanent skin substitutes. Clin Plast Surg. 2009;36(4):643-51.

42. Singer AJ, Boyce ST. Burn wound healing and tissue engineering. J Burn Care Res. 2017;38(3):e605-13.

43. Sluka KA. Definitions, concepts, and models of pain. In: Sluka KA (Ed.). Mechanisms and management of pain for the physical therapist. Seattle, WA: IASP Press; 2009. pp. 3-18.

44. Temmen HJ, BL Boyea, DJ Barillo DT harrington. Tilt table exercise guidelines for burn patients: are cardiac exercise parameters appropriate?. Proc Am Burn Assoc. 1998;30:221.

45. Trees DW, Ketelsen CA, Hobbs JA. Use of a modified tilt table for preambulation strength training as an adjunct to burn rehabilitation: a case series. J Burn Care Rehabil. 2003;24(2):97-103.

46. Ward RS. the rehabilitation of burn patients. Crit Rev Phys Rehabil Med. 1991;2:121.

47. Yousef H, Alhajj M, Sharma S. Anatomy, skin (integument), epidermis. In: StatPearls. Treasure Island, FL: StatPearls Publishing; 2019. [Internet] Available from https://www.ncbi.nlm.nih.gov/books/NBK470464/. [Updated Jun 12, 2019].

Organ Transplant

Jaini Patel, Bijal Dodia, Aashish Contractor

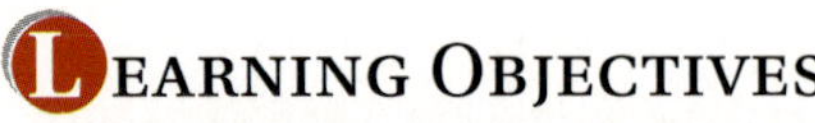

LEARNING OBJECTIVES

After reading this chapter, the readers should be able to:
- Understand the brief historical review of heart, lung, liver, and kidney transplantation
- Understand an overview of the recipient evaluation process, surgical procedures, frequently used medications, and general complications that affect the management of transplant recipients
- Understand the physical therapy evaluation and management of organ transplant recipients, ranging from prehab to in-patient rehabilitation and outpatient rehabilitation.
- Discuss the similarities and differences in the treatment of various organ transplantation recipients.

CHAPTER OUTLINE

- Indications
- Contraindications
- Eligibility and candidacy
  - Heart transplant
  - Lung transplant
  - Liver transplant
  - Kidney transplant
- Pretransplant period
- Transplant surgery types
- Transplant surgery
  - Heart transplant
  - Lung transplant
  - Liver transplant
  - Kidney transplant
- Transplant surgery outcomes
- Immunosuppressive agents
  - Side effects of immunosuppressant drugs
- Rehabilitation
  - Patient limitations
  - Effects of exercise
  - Barriers to enrolment for rehabilitation
  - Transplant and rehabilitation team
  - Rehabilitation program
  - Inpatient rehabilitation
  - Outpatient rehabilitation

INTRODUCTION

Organ transplantation is the treatment of choice for many patients with end-stage organ failure if optimal therapy as recommended by guidelines has failed to improve symptoms or halt progression of the underlying pathology. For carefully selected patients, organ transplantation offers markedly improved survival and quality of life.

There are various kinds of transplant of vital organs of the body, single organ as well as multiple organ transplant is possible. A few examples of single and multiple organ transplantation procedures are shown in **Table 39.1**.

According to the data published by WHO from records in 2008 for 104 countries, representing nearly 90% of the worldwide population, it is shown that around 100,800 solid organ transplants are performed every year worldwide: 69,400 are kidney transplants (46% from living donors), 20,200 liver transplants (14.6% from living donors), 5,400 heart transplants, 3,400 lung transplants, and 2,400 pancreas transplants.

This chapter will describe the single organ transplantation for heart, lung, liver, and kidney. Covering other types of transplantation and rehabilitation is beyond the scope of this chapter.

Table 39.1: Single- and multiple-organ transplantation procedures.

Single-organ transplant	Multiple-organ transplant
• Heart transplant	• Heart–lung transplant
• Lung transplant	• Heart–kidney–pancreas transplant
• Liver transplant	• Heart–liver transplant
• Kidney transplant	• Heart–liver–kidney transplant
• Pancreas transplant	• Heart–lung–liver transplant
• Intestine transplant	• Lung–kidney transplant
	• Lung–liver transplant

INDICATIONS

The primary indication for organ transplantation is a progressive terminal disease, which causes irreversible loss of organ function, leading to limited life expectancy. The majority of patients with end-stage organ disease present with numerous cardiopulmonary, metabolic, musculoskeletal, and/or neurological abnormalities, resulting in difficulty in carrying out activities of daily living **(Table 39.2)**.

Table 39.2: Indications for organ transplant.

Heart transplant	Refractory cardiogenic shock requiring intra-aortic balloon pump counter pulsation or left ventricular assist device (LVAD)
	Cardiogenic shock requiring continuous intravenous inotropic therapy
	Peak VO_2 (VO_{2max}) less than 10 mL/kg/min in cardiomyopathy or heart failure patient
	NYHA class of III or IV despite maximized medical and resynchronization therapy
	Recurrent life-threatening left ventricular arrhythmias despite an implantable cardiac defibrillator, antiarrhythmic therapy, or catheter-based ablation
	End-stage congenital HF with no evidence of pulmonary hypertension
	Refractory angina without potential medical or surgical therapeutic options
Lung transplant	Severe chronic obstructive pulmonary disease BODE index of 7–10 and any of the following: • FEV1<20% and DLCO of <20% or homogeneous distribution of emphysema • Pulmonary hypertension or cor pulmonale
	Idiopathic pulmonary fibrosis Evidence of usual interstitial pneumonitis and any of the following: • DLCO <39% predicted • 10% or greater decrease in FVC during 6 months of follow-up • <88% oxygen saturation during 6-MWT • Honeycombing on HRCT
	Cystic fibrosis FEV1<30% and any of the following: • Increasing oxygen requirements or hypercapnia or pulmonary hypertension
	Pulmonary hypertension • Persistent NYHA class III or IV • 350 m (low) or declining 6-MWT • Failing therapy with epoprostenol • Cardiac index of 0.2 L/min/m^2 • Right atrial pressure >15 mm Hg
	Sarcoidosis NYHA class III or IV and any of the following: • Hypoxemia at rest • Pulmonary hypertension • Right atrial pressure >15 mm Hg

Contd...

Contd...

Liver transplantation	Acute liver failure • Hepatitis A and autoimmune hepatitis • Hepatitis B, hepatitis C, hepatitis D, and nonalcoholic liver disease • Wilson's disease • Budd–Chiari syndrome
	Cirrhosis from chronic liver disease • Chronic hepatitis B or C virus infection • Alcoholic liver disease • Cryptogenic liver disease
	Malignant diseases of the liver • Hepatocellular carcinoma or carcinoid tumor or islet cell tumor
	Metabolic liver diseases • Alpha 1 antitrypsin deficiency • Glycogen storage disease 1 and 4 • Hemophilia A and B • Veno-occlusive diseases
	Cholestatic liver disease • Primary biliary cirrhosis • Biliary atresia • Primary sclerosing cholangitis
	Miscellaneous • Adult polycystic liver disease • Amyloidosis • Sarcoidosis • Hepatic trauma • Chronic hepatic encephalopathy
Kidney transplant	Patients with end-stage kidney disease on dialysis
	Patients with advanced chronic kidney disease (stage IV or V with calculated or estimated GFR <20 mL/min
	Patients with chronic kidney disease (stage IV with GFR <30 mL/min) who also need another organ transplant
	Patients with chronic kidney disease who have type 1 diabetes that has not responded to medical treatment may also be considered for a combined kidney–pancreas transplant

(HF: heart failure; BODE: Body-mass index, airflow Obstruction, Dyspnea, and Exercise; DLCO: diffusing capacity of the lung for carbon monoxide; FEV1: forced expiratory volume in 1 second; HRCT: high resolution computed tomography; NYHA: New York Heart Association; 6-MWT: 6-minute walk test; GFR: glomerular filtration rate)

CONTRAINDICATIONS

The absolute contraindications remain the same for all type of transplants. Any disease condition that may aggravate due to transplant surgery or its therapy, jeopardizing the patient's life and long-term success of the transplant, is considered as contraindication. **Table 39.3** gives the list of absolute contraindications for all types of organ transplant.

The relative contraindications for each organ and can be referred in detail for heart, lung, liver, and kidney from bibliography section.

Table 39.3: Absolute contraindications for organ transplant.
• Advanced irreversible failure of more than one organ, without plans for concurrent transplant • History of solid organ or hematologic malignancy within the last 5 years (due to probability of recurrence) • Active infection • Severe comorbidity

ELIGIBILITY AND CANDIDACY

The transplant team determines a patient's eligibility for transplantation after weighing all the facts from:
- Medical history
- Physical examination
- Tests

Evaluation consists of:
- Mental health evaluation (to assess recipient's ability to comply with post-transplant care).
- Detailed blood investigations (for blood typing, tissue typing, crossmatching, serology, etc.).
- Multiple diagnostic tests for multiple systems (include X-rays, ultrasound, and biopsy).

At a given point of time, there are far more eligible candidates than suitable donor organs across the world. Therefore, detailed risk stratification and eligibility criteria are designed for each organ transplant for the donor as well as recipient. A formal procedure is managed by Scientific Registry in each country who maintains the record and listing of patients waiting for transplant.

Clinical Pearl

The organ donation process in India is administered by the National Organ and Tissue Transplant Organization (NOTTO) in addition to state and district level bodies.

The tools to improve risk stratification of patients for transplant are critical to ensure that only patients with a high probability of benefit are subjected to the risks of organ transplant. Few risk scores have been developed to help clinicians identify patients whose severity of illness is sufficient to merit consideration for transplant. The best known and most widely used scores are listed below:

Heart Transplant

The widely used scores for heart transplant are:
- Heart Failure Survival Score
- Seattle Heart Failure Model
- Index for Mortality Prediction after Cardiac Transplantation Score

Lung Transplant

The widely used score for lung transplant is:
Lung allocation score.

Liver Transplant

The widely used score for liver transplant is:
Model for end-stage liver disease Score

Kidney Transplant

The widely used scores for kidney transplant are:
- Kidney allocation system
- Estimated post-transplant survival score
- Calculated panel reactive antibodies score

PRETRANSPLANT PERIOD

For a deceased organ donor, patients have to wait for invariable period of time till the organ is available for transplant. Depending on the patient's clinical state, they are managed with frequent outpatient department (OPD) consultations medically or are admitted in hospital if critically ill. Some patients may undergo regular frequent hospital procedures (e.g., dialysis), while some may undergo pretransplant surgery (e.g., lung volume reduction surgery or nephrectomy).

For a critically ill heart or lung-failure patient, mechanical circulatory support such as left ventricular assist device or extracorporeal membrane oxygenator is used while waiting for transplant to keep them alive and functioning.

Dialysis is a process by which wastes and excess water from the body are removed using an external filter called a dialyzer, which contains a semipermeable membrane. Hemodialysis is the most common type of dialysis practiced across the globe. It requires a patient to have frequent visits to the hospital (2–3 days/week) for a period of 4–8 hours depending on the need.

TRANSPLANT SURGERY TYPES

The types of organ transplant surgeries are shown in **Table 39.4**.

Table 39.4: Types of organ transplant surgeries.	
Organ	*Types of organ transplant*
Heart	Orthotopic heart transplant
Lung	• SLTx • Bilateral or DLTx: both lungs are sequentially transplanted
Liver	• OLT • LDLT • SLT • Auxiliary liver transplantation
Kidney	• Deceased donor kidney transplant • Double kidney transplants (duals) • Living donor kidney transplant • Preemptive kidney transplant • Crossover renal transplantation or a paired kidney-exchange transplant

(DLTx: double lung transplantation; LDLT: living donor liver transplantation; OLT: orthotopic liver transplantation; SLT: split type of liver transplantation; SLTx: single lung transplantation)

TRANSPLANT SURGERY

All transplant surgeries are done under general anesthesia. The patient is kept on heart-lung machine and/or mechanical ventilator as required.

Heart Transplant

The following discusses the relevant points for heart transplantation:

- Open-heart procedure, median sternotomy incision.
- The orthotopic transplantation involves removing the native heart at the level of atrioventricular junction, leaving an atrial cuff, and transecting the aorta and pulmonary artery just above the semilunar valves. Therefore, it is important to note that the native atria remain innervated, but across the suture line, there is no conduction and the donor heart is denervated **(Fig. 39.1)**.

Lung Transplant

The following discusses the relevant points for lung transplantation:

- Bilateral anterior thoracotomies or a trans-sternal bilateral thoracotomy or clamshell incision, which provides better exposure than the previously preferred median sternotomy. For single lung transplantation posterolateral thoracotomy incision or axillary thoracotomy is preferred. **(Fig. 39.2)**.
- The lungs are harvested while pulmonary veins are detached from the heart along with a cuff from the left atrium; the pulmonary arteries are transected; and the lungs removed en bloc, divided into separate right and left lungs for implantation. For a single lung transplantation, the side chosen is related to prior surgery, the desire to replace the worst recipient lung, and the best donor side.

Liver Transplant

The following discusses the relevant points for liver transplantation:

- Mercedes incision
- Depending on the type of liver transplant, a part or entire liver is transplanted in the recipient **(Fig. 39.3)**.

Kidney Transplant

The following discusses the relevant points for kidney transplantation:

- Paramedian, hockey stick incision

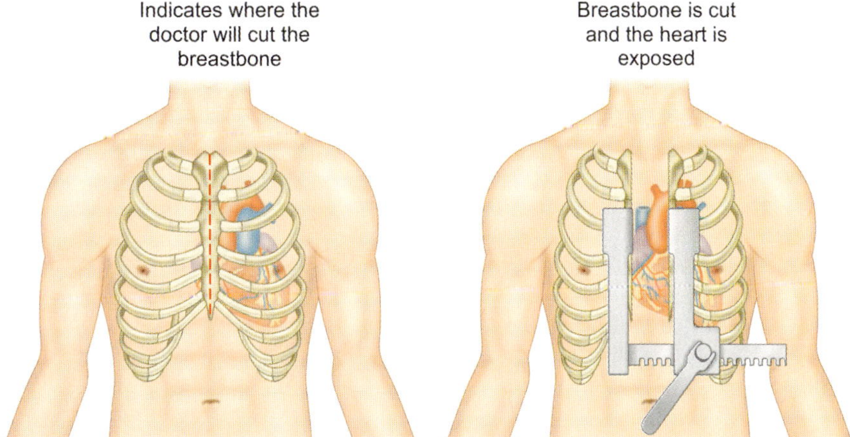

Fig. 39.1: Median sternotomy.

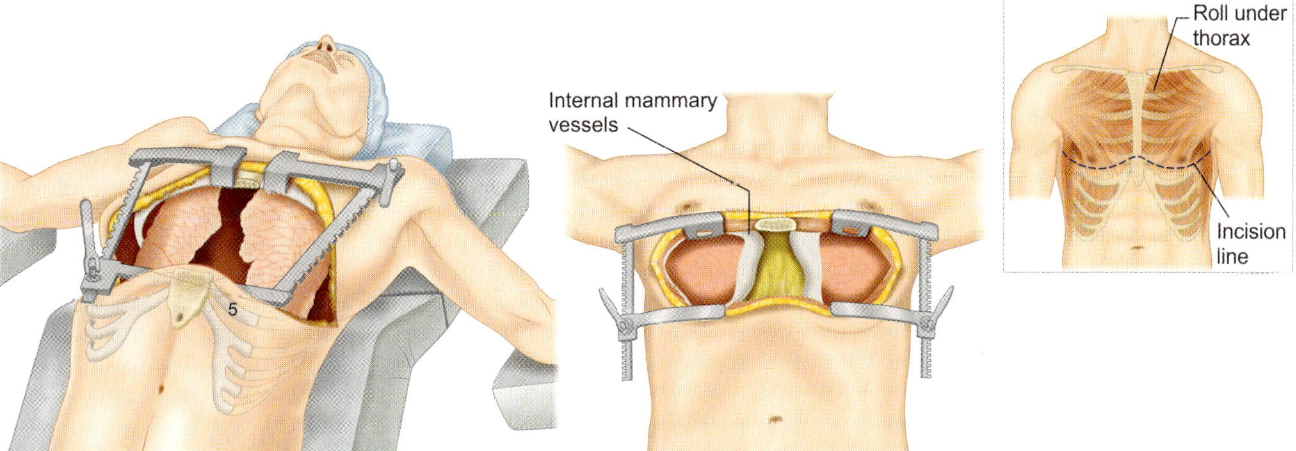

Fig. 39.2: Clamshell incision.

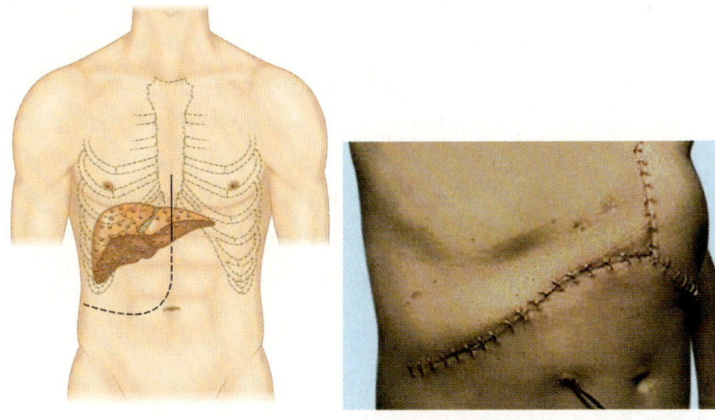

Fig. 39.3: Mercedes incision.

- If there are no complications, recipient kidneys are not removed. A left donor kidney is implanted on right side and a right donor kidney is implanted on left side to allow the ureter to be accessed easily for connection to the bladder. As the kidney is placed in a different location than the existing kidneys, it is called heterotopic transplant **(Fig. 39.4)**.

TRANSPLANT SURGERY OUTCOMES

Table 39.5 shows average survival rates for people who have had organ transplantation across the globe.

IMMUNOSUPPRESSIVE AGENTS

The organ transplant recipients are put on multiple medications for life after the surgery to achieve optimal level of immunosuppression. **Table 39.6** shows the most commonly prescribed drugs.

Side Effects of Immunosuppressant Drugs

Most common side effects of immunosuppressant drugs:
- Weight gain
- Osteoporosis or osteonecrosis
- Hypertension
- Hypercholesterolemia
- Increased risk of infection
- A higher risk of developing certain skin cancers and non-Hodgkin's lymphoma.

REHABILITATION

Patients with end-stage organ failure suffer from a number of comorbidities, including malnutrition, loss of muscle mass, decreased exercise capacity, and decreased muscle strength. Because of the sequelae of the transplantation procedure and alteration in patients' physical performance, physical therapists have become key members of

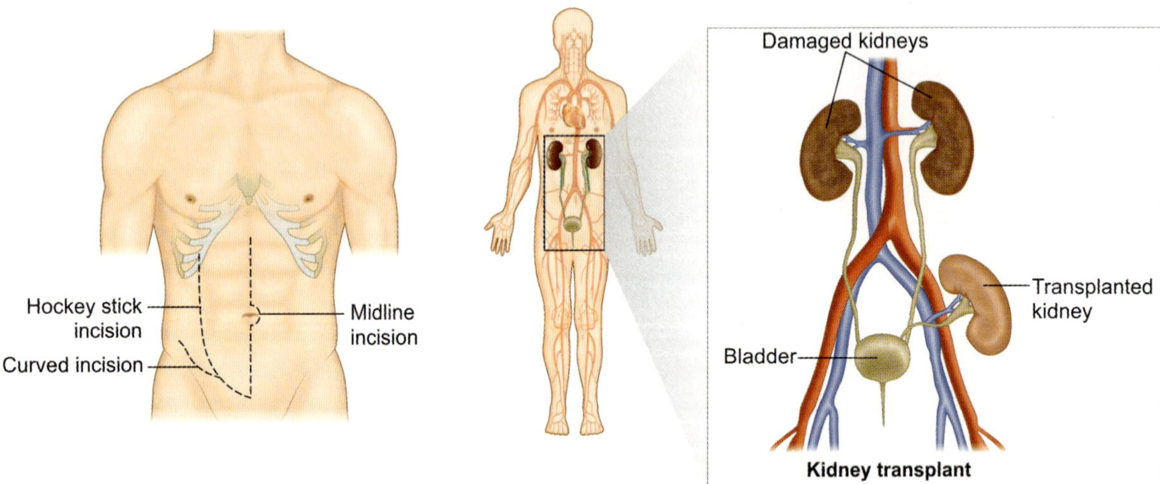

Fig. 39.4: Incision for kidney transplant.

Table 39.5: Average Survival Rates for Organ Transplant Recipients.

	1-year survival (%)	3-year survival (%)	5-year survival (%)	10-year survival (%)	20-year survival (%)
Heart[*]	90	–	70	–	20
Lung[†]	80	65	54	32	–
Liver[‡]	86	78	72	–	53
Kidney[§]	97	90	84	48	–

[*]Russo MJ, Rana A, Chen JM, et al. Pretransplantation patient characteristics and survival following combined heart and kidney transplantation: an analysis of the united network for organ sharing database. Arch Surg. 2009;144(3):241-6.
[†]Thabut G, Mal H. Outcomes after lung transplantation. J Thorac Dis. 2017;9(8):2684-91.
[‡]The National Institute of Diabetes and Digestive and Kidney Diseases (NIDDK); 2018.
[§]The Global Role of Kidney Transplantation: Kidney Transplantation. 2012;81:425-7. Adv Chronic Kidney Dis. 2016;23(5):281-6 (numbers are averages out between living donor and diseased donor values).

Table 39.6: Commonly prescribed drugs and their adverse effects following transplant surgery.

Drug	Drug class	Significant adverse effects
Corticosteroids	• Prednisone • Prednisolone • Methylprednisolone	Hypertension, glaucoma, adrenal suppression, cataracts, thinning skin, hyperglycemia, osteopenia, myopathy, dyslipidemia
Calcineurin inhibitors	Cyclosporine	Nephrotoxicity, hypertension, neurotoxicity, increased infections, gingival hyperplasia
	Tacrolimus (TAC or FK506)	Inhibits interleukin-2 and T lymphocytes
Antiproliferative agents	Azathioprine	Nephrotoxicity, hyperglycemia, neurotoxicity, gastrointestinal disturbances
	MMF	Bone disorders, gastrointestinal problems, hypertension, dysrhythmias
M-TOR inhibitors	Sirolimus and everolimus	Blood disorders, dyslipidemia, delayed postsurgical healing

(MMF: mycophenolate mofetil; M-TOR: mammalian-target of rapamycin)

transplantation teams, providing expertise in examination and rehabilitation of transplant recipients and donors both before and after surgery.

Physical and Functional Limitations

Patients may have following physical or functional limitation after transplant:
- Decreased exercise capacity
- Increased risk of mortality due to cardiovascular disease.
- Decreased muscle mass due to protein energy wasting (has combination of malnutrition and wasting).
- Fatigue and weakness
- Muscle cramps
- Reduced immunity, increased risk of infections/rejection/graft failure.
- Osteoporosis
- Steroid-induced myopathy or neuropathy.
- Depression, anxiety, and social withdrawal.

Effects of Exercise

- Improves cardiorespiratory fitness
- Improves graft function:
  - Greater physical activity leads to improved cardiovascular function which may improve perfusion and oxygen delivery to the graft.
  - Increased physical activity is a statistically significant predictor of improved graft function over a 1-year period.
- Reduces the need for pharmacological therapy of hypertension in transplant patients.
- **Decrease the levels of homocysteine:** Homocysteine level is relatively high in transplant patients as compared to age matched normal and is associated with higher prevalence of cardiovascular disease and poorer outcomes.
- **Improves immunity:** An 8-week aerobic exercise program enhances T-helper cell count, CD4+ to CD8+ ratio, natural killer cells activity and IgG and IgM levels without causing graft dysfunction in the short-term.

- **Reduces levels of interleukin-6 (IL-6):** IL-6 is responsible for trigger of inflammatory reactions, which may lead to increased chances of glomerulonephritis or cardiovascular disease.
- Decreases anxiety and depression

Clinical Pearl

There is a difference in the interleukin-6 (IL-6) production depending on the dose of physical training. This can lead to the conclusion that if strenuous exercise increases IL-6 production as seen in "overtraining syndrome," it results in "under performance." Therefore, it is very important to prescribe appropriate and well-regulated amount of exercise, which will produce the positive result (i.e., a reduction of IL-6 levels).

Barriers to Enrollment for Rehabilitation

Despite these many proven benefits of exercise, there are very few patients who enroll for the rehabilitation program. Following are the barriers to enrollment:
- Lower awareness and confidence about rehabilitation in transplant professionals and patients.
- Low referral by the transplant surgeons due to fear of injuring the transplanted graft.
- Inadequate emphasis and education by transplant professional on benefits of exercise.
- Protective attitude of the family members and friends.
- Diverse ethnic and cultural backgrounds may place differential values on exercise and self-care.
- Absence of structural support: No availability of rehabilitation center or trained staff.

Transplant and Rehabilitation Team

The transplant team includes a transplant surgeon, a transplant physician, one or more transplant nurses, a social worker, a psychiatrist, or psychologist. The rehabilitation team comprises of physical therapist, exercise physiologist, nutritionist, and psychologist (**Figs. 39.5 and 39.6**).

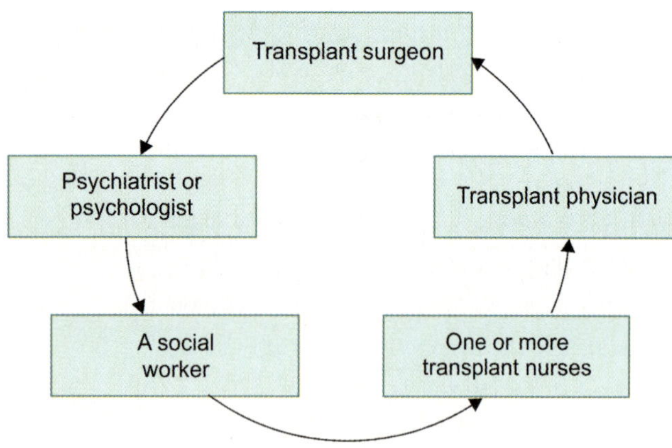

Fig. 39.5: Transplant team.

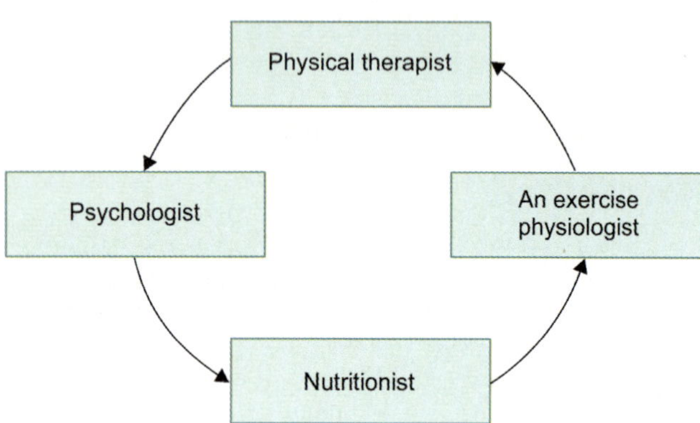

Fig. 39.6: Rehabilitation team.

Rehabilitation Program

It can be divided broadly into two categories:

1. **Pretransplant rehabilitation:** Most of the patients with end-stage organ failure who are awaiting organ transplant should be subjected to prehabilitation (unless contraindicated).

   Goals of prehabilitation:
   - Effective chest clearance and lung-expansion techniques
   - Maintaining or improving physical activity levels
   - Maintaining or improving cardiorespiratory fitness
   - Preparing patient for transplant.

   These potential benefits of pretransplant rehabilitation are also acknowledged in the latest joint American Thoracic Society/European Respiratory Society official statement on pulmonary rehabilitation. In spite of the high disease severity in candidates for organ transplantation, pretransplant rehabilitation has consistently been shown to be feasible and capable of improving functional exercise capacity and quality of life (QOL) if offered appropriately.

   If the patient is admitted to the hospital before transplant due to his critical health, the rehabilitation plan mentioned under "inpatient rehabilitation" should be followed. For relatively stable patient who does not require hospital admission till they are

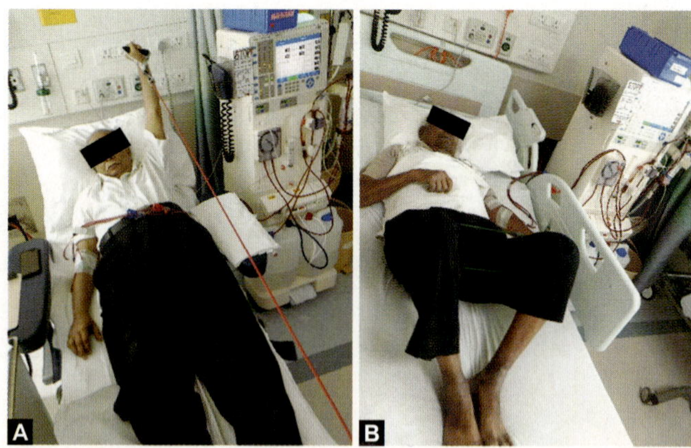

Figs. 39.7A and B: Patients doing upper and lower limb strength exercise (intradialysis rehabilitation).
Courtesy: Sir HN Reliance Foundation Hospital, Mumbai

awaiting transplantation, "outpatient rehabilitation" program should be prescribed.

Patients awaiting renal transplant may require to undergo regular hemodialysis (2–3 days/week). Rehabilitation during this period is divided into two parts: intradialysis rehabilitation and inter- or extradialysis rehabilitation. Extradialysis rehabilitation is carried out on the outpatient basis and is done on non-dialysis days. Intradialysis rehabilitation is done preferably during the first hour of dialysis which includes symptom management, aerobic exercise and strength training **(Figs. 39.7A and B)**.

2. **Rehabilitation after transplant**

Inpatient Rehabilitation

Early Postoperative Physical Therapy

Rehabilitation after solid organ transplant starts immediately after surgery, where the initial focus is on maintenance of bodily systems, as well as pulmonary hygiene and chest wall mobility in order to assist with the ventilator/supplemental oxygen weaning process. This phase is divided into two stages:

1. Physical therapy in the intensive care unit (ICU)
2. Physical therapy in wards

Assessment

Table 39.7 gives some components in the assessment of early post-transplant patient.

Physical Therapy in the Intensive Care Unit

Typically, intensive care physical therapy should begin as early as possible and/or at least 24 hours later postsurgery and after extubation. It should first start with respiratory physiotherapy and should prioritize upright positioning (e.g., sitting) and mobilization (e.g., out of the bed).

Table 39.7: Components of physical therapy examination in early phase of post-transplant rehabilitation.

Components	Physical therapy examination item	Special considerations
Chart review	• Mental health and current history • Laboratory results • Medical test results • Organ biopsy • Echocardiogram • Ejection fraction • PFTs • ABGs • Medication list • Baseline vital signs	• Typical for the patient to have demonstrated a decline in function over the previous 6–12 months • Provide an overview of the patient's status. If the status is critical, before proceeding with the examination, it will be important to discuss the acceptable limits of activity with physician
Appearance	Skin • Color • Presence of edema Posture: Breathing pattern (at rest and with activity) • Use of accessory muscles • Depth of breathing • Areas of decreased chest expansion • Work of breathing Sputum • Color, consistency, quantity, odor	
Vital signs	• At rest and with exercise/activity testing • Auscultation of lung and heart sounds	Monitor vital signs and oxygen saturation levels; important to correlate oxygen saturation levels with hematocrit and hemoglobin levels to ensure patient safety
Musculoskeletal	• Pain • Joint integrity and mobility • Muscle strength, 1RM, respiratory muscles: MIP/MEP • Bed mobility, transfers, and gait • Balance	The musculoskeletal examination is typical of that for any other patients but should emphasize the thoracic area. This part of the examination will be useful to create an individualized strengthening and flexibility program for the patient
Physical performance and mobility	• Sit–stand tests (e.g., 30 s sit to stand; five times sit to stand), short physical performance battery, timed-up and go, balance tests (e.g., Berg's balance scale, BESTest), functional independence measure • Tests specifically for ICU: Egress test, various ICU physical function tests	
Exercise capacity	Laboratory-based test: Cardiopulmonary exercise test on cycle or treadmill Field based walk tests: 6MWT, 2MWT Upper extremity endurance testing	

(1RM: 1-repetition maximum; 2MWT: 2-minute walk test; 6MWT: 6-minute walk test; ABGs: arterial blood gases; ICU: intensive care unit; MEP: maximal expiratory pressure; MIP: maximal inspiratory pressure; PFTs: pulmonary function tests; BESTest: balance evaluation systems Test)

The rehabilitation **goals** in the early phase post-transplantation are to improve:

■ Pulmonary hygiene and lung capacity
■ General mobility
■ Functional capacity
■ Muscle strength and endurance
■ Facilitate discharge from the ICU

Clinical Pearl

Intensive care unit acquired weakness (ICUAW) can occur after organ transplantation. ICUAW can be caused by the following three entities:

1. Critical illness polyneuropathy
2. Critical illness myopathy
3. Critical illness polyneuromyopathy

If there is no other cause of muscle weakness, early diagnosis and suspicion of ICUAW is necessary and essential in establishing a rehabilitation plan.

Table 39.8: Overview of intensive care physical therapy.

Patient's clinical condition	Goals and treatment	Special considerations
Intubated and ventilated	• **V/Q optimization** by secretion clearance techniques (chest wall percussions and vibrations), lung recruitment and positioning, reassessing supplemental oxygen requirements • Frequent change of position • **Maintenance of muscle strength and joint mobility:** Positioning and passive limb mobility exercises • **Upright positioning**	• Avoid Trendelenburg position in heart and lung transplant patients • Neuromuscular electrical stimulation may be a safe, low cost treatment for early intervention in critically ill patients
Extubated (close coordination with medical team/pain management team to optimize pain relief)	• Active limb mobility exercises • Deep breathing and thoracic expansion exercises, incentive spirometry • Supported cough/forced expiratory techniques • Early mobilization	• Because of incisional pain and the denervated cough reflex of the donor lung, patients require direction and encouragement to cough In lung transplant patients
Prolonged weaning	• Lung recruitment and secretion management • Inspiratory muscle training • Encourage gradual progressive mobilization	

Intensive care unit (ICU) acquired weakness is a highly prevalent problem that is related to the duration of mechanical ventilation, use of sedative agents, neuromuscular blockers, corticosteroid, and reduced physical activity resulting from immobilization in patients admitted to the ICU.

Table 39.8 gives an overview of physiotherapy required in intensive care.

Common Complications and Barriers

Common complications and barriers to rehabilitation in ICU are shown in **Box 39.1**.

Graded Functional Retraining in Intensive Care Unit

Following are the steps to promote gradual progressive mobilization in ICU **(Figs. 39.8 and 39.9)**.

BOX 39.1: Common complications and barriers to rehabilitation in intensive care unit (ICU).

• Encephalopathy
• Acute respiratory distress syndrome
• ICU acquired weakness
• Delirium
• Hemodynamic instability
• Bleeding and coagulopathy

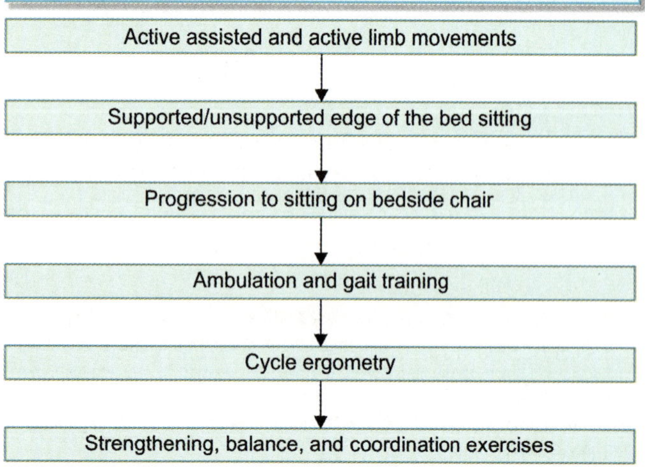

Fig. 39.8: Flowchart for gradual progressive mobilization in ICU.

There should be constant monitoring and recording of vital signs such as:

■ Blood pressure
■ Pulse rate
■ Respiratory rate
■ SpO_2
■ Pattern of breathing
■ Dizziness
■ Fatigue
■ Perspiration
■ Fainting, if any

Although the heart rate provides an accurate measure of exercise intensity (except for heart transplant patients), it is helpful to use the ventilatory index, rating of perceived exertion (RPE) scale, and respiratory rate for additional information to guide activities of daily living and activity progression from bed mobility, to sitting up in a chair and finally to ambulation.

Supplemental oxygen should be titrated as needed to keep oxygen saturation levels above 90%.

In critically ill patients, even passive or active exercise training sessions for 20 min/day (continuously or with breaks) using bedside ergometer is able to increase short-term functional recovery.

Rehabilitation in Wards

Majority of the patients when extubated and mobilized early, transfer to the wards after 48–72 hours postoperatively.

After the patient is moved out of the intensive care setting, rehabilitation continues to focus on ventilation and airway clearance for optimal oxygen transport and gradual progressive mobilization.

By the time patients are shifted to ward, they are already walking for few minutes; they can begin with a cycle ergometer.

The exercise program is designed based on FITT (frequency, intensity, time, and type) principle as shown in **Table 39.9**.

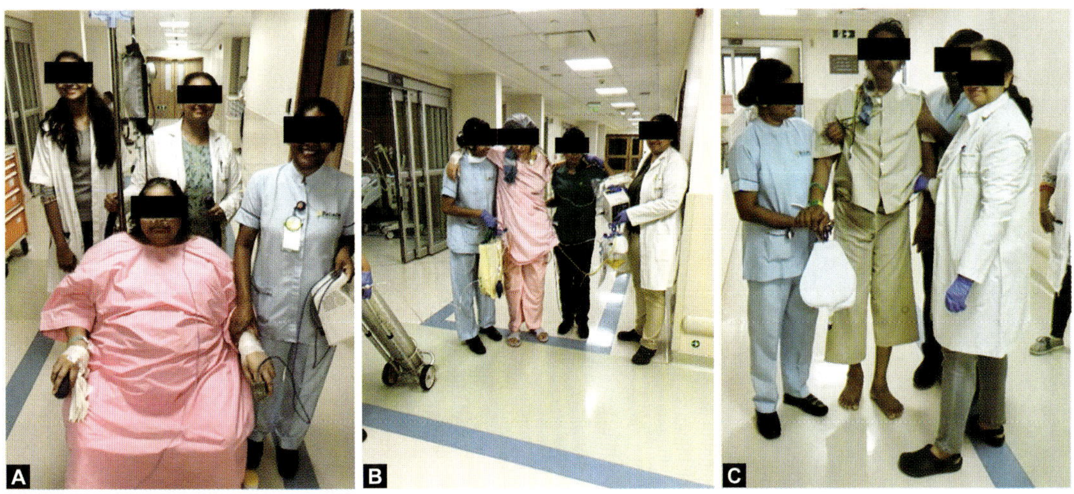

Figs. 39.9A to C: Patient mobilization in Intensive care unit.
Courtesy: Sir HN Reliance Foundation Hospital, Mumbai.

Table 39.9: FITT principles for exercise.

Frequency	Mobilization: 2–4 times per day for the first 3 days of the hospital stay
Intensity	Resting heart rate (HRrest) + 20 beats/min Upper limit of 120 beats/min that corresponds to an rating of perceived exertion (RPE) = 13 on a Borg scale of 6–20
Time	Begin with intermittent walking bouts lasting 3–5 min as tolerated with exercise bouts of progressively increasing duration The rest period may be a slower walk (or complete rest at the patient's discretion)
Type	Walking or cycle ergometer Stair climbing
Progression	When continuous exercise duration reaches 10–15 min, increase intensity as tolerated within the recommended rating of perceived exertion (RPE) and HR limits as applicable
Resistance training (except for heart transplant patients)	• Up to 2–2.5 kg (1 set × 10 reps) • Education regarding: Lifting restrictions • Postural correction/reeducation • Oxygen titration: Maintain SpO_2 >90% on exertion

Medical issues that may be encountered in this early post-transplant phase that can impact exercise include:

- Infection
- Acute rejection
- Anxiety
- Depression
- Postsurgical pain at the incision or drain insertion site
- Arrhythmias
- Venothrombotic events
- Infections requiring isolation
- Postural hypotension
- Skin ulcers
- Poor wound healing

Clinical Pearl

It is important to keep in mind that therapist should follow all sterile precautions while seeing the patient as patient would be on immunosuppressive drugs. Extra vigilance is necessary in early postoperative weeks to monitor development of transplant rejection, infection, arrhythmias, neurological deficits, or renal dysfunction.

Activity Pacing and Fatigue Management

- Fatigue is a common sequela of end-stage organ failure, transplant surgery, and post ICU stay. Hence it is very important for a physical therapist to teach patients how to pace and optimize energy consumption.
- Overactivity → Longer periods of rest and inactivity → deconditioning → Fatigue
- Frequent short bouts of activities are recommended.
- Slow, steady increase in activity/exercise is advised for allowing body to adapt to the activity/exercise stress.

Prior to Discharge

By the time of discharge, patient should be prepared and prescribed possible physical activity requirement at home and should be educated on necessary home modifications.

A predischarge low-level submaximal exercise test is useful for exercise prescription and physical activity counseling. If an exercise test is not conducted or patient has not joined a clinically supervised outpatient rehabilitation program, the upper limit of exercise intensity should not exceed those levels observed during the inpatient program.

Patients should be educated about following and should be referred and counseled for outpatient rehabilitation program **(Box 39.2).**

> **BOX 39.2:** Patient education topics.
>
> - Secretion management
> - Controlled coughing techniques and wound splinting techniques
> - Incentive spirometry
> - Chest tubes
> - Wound and pain management
> - Importance of early mobilization
> - Recognizing signs and symptoms of rejection
> - Importance and proper use of supplemental oxygen therapy
> - Importance of physical rehabilitation
> - Management of daily activities: pacing, energy conservation, and when to stop exercise.

Outpatient Rehabilitation

Due to preexisting organ failure, the physical activity levels of patients who undergo transplant are limited resulting in deconditioning. Multiple systematic reviews and randomized controlled trials published till now have found moderate quality evidence suggesting that supervised OPD-based rehabilitation improves exercise capacity and appears to be safe in transplant recipients. It has shown to improve physical fitness levels (as indicated by increased VO_2 peak levels) and health-related quality of life in transplant patients on self-reported questionnaires.

Studies also suggest that inclusion of exercise professionals in the treatment to facilitate a supervised exercise intervention has more benefits as compared to prescription of unsupervised exercise. It also has greater adherence to the prescribed exercise.

Rehabilitation of the patient with transplant is aimed at attenuating the many possible adverse effects of immunosuppressive therapy.

Outpatient rehabilitation programs may begin as soon as possible after hospital discharge. The goal setting has to be done by therapist with patient's goals in mind, and it has to be tailor-made for each patient. A detailed clinical assessment is very crucial to design exercise program for each patient.

Assessment

- **History and diagnosis**
- **Treatment:**
  - Medically managed, awaiting transplant, or post-transplant
  - Immunosuppressant drugs: Type, dosage, etc.
  - Surgery: Date of surgery, details of surgical notes, tissues dissected, complications if any.
- **Medication review**: Patient's current medication list.
- **Medical history or comorbidities:** It is important to know if patient has any preexisting medical problems, such as hypertension, diabetes, known cardiovascular disease, cholesterol, osteoarthritis, and joint pain which will require modification in the rehabilitation program.
- **Personal history:**
  - Tobacco chewing or smoking: Current or ex-consumer, duration, pack years
  - Alcohol: Current or ex-consumer, amount.

- **Review of reports/investigations:**
  - Routine blood Investigations: Hemoglobin, lipid, and sugar profile
  - Two-dimensional echocardiography (2D ECHO), pulmonary function test (PFT), arterial blood gas analysis (ABGA), etc.
  - Special relevant tests
- **Symptoms:** Past as well as current symptoms: Onset, intensity, aggravating and relieving factors, diurnal variations.
- **Physical assessment:**
  - Height, weight, BMI
  - Vitals: Heart rate, blood pressure, etc.
  - Blood sugar if diabetic
  - Auscultation
  - Girth measurement for extremities.
- **Fatigue assessment:**
  - Onset of fatigue, aggravating and relieving factors, diurnal variations
  - Intensity (on a scale of 0–10)
  - Brief measures do not fully capture following various dimensions of fatigue:
    - Sensory dimension (fatigue severity, persistence)
    - Physiologic dimension (e.g., leg weakness and diminished mental concentration)
    - Performance dimension (reduction in performance of needed or valued activities).
  - There are various tools available to measure fatigue, e.g., fatigue symptom inventory, and fatigue assessment scale.
- **Cardiovascular system assessment:**
  - A close monitoring of vitals (heart rate and blood pressure) and patient symptoms is important as these patients are at higher risk of developing cardiovascular disease
  - Regular vital assessment at rest and during exercise sessions
  - Reviewing ECG or 2D ECHO reports
  - Submaximal or symptom limited tests, e.g., 6-minute walk test.
- **Musculoskeletal system assessment:** Most common complaints of patients are pain or stiffness in joints, at times muscle cramps, weakness of leg muscles.
  - Postural changes
  - Range of motion restriction if any and tissue tightness
  - Manual muscle testing
  - Pain assessment: A detailed pain assessment including intensity, location, aggravating and relieving factors, variation in relation to certain drugs/therapy.
  - Intensity of pain: Numeric rating scale or visual analogue scale.

Clinical Pearl

Any new complain of pain in high intensity should be dealt with caution as osteoporosis may lead to stress fractures which at times remain undiagnosed and lead to further problem with time.

- **Health-related quality of life assessment:** There are numerous patient-reported questionnaires that are developed to assess different aspects of quality of life, such as physical, emotional, social, functional, etc.
  - SF-36, psychosocial adjustment to illness scale, EuroQOL, EuroQOL 5-D can be used for all transplant types.
  - Heart specific: Kansas City Cardiomyopathy Questionnaire.
  - Lung specific: Baseline Dyspnea Index, the Medical Research Council Dyspnea Scale, and the UCSD Shortness of Breath Questionnaire, St George Respiratory Questionnaire.
  - Liver specific: National Institute of Diabetes and Digestive and Kidney Diseases (NIDDK) Quality of Life questionnaire, the Liver Disease Quality of Life questionnaire, and the chronic liver disease questionnaire.
  - Kidney specific: Kidney transplant questionnaire, the kidney disease questionnaire (KDQ), the kidney disease-quality of life (KDQOL), chronic KDQ (CKDQ), Dialysis Symptom Index.
- **Assessment of physical activity levels:** Patient's current and past physical activity level evaluation is important to prescribe a program for them. It can be assessed by certain tools, such as:
  - Physical activity readiness questionnaire
  - Physical activity scale for the elderly
  - Duke activity status index
  - International physical activity questionnaire
  - It can also be objectively assessed by monitoring number of steps walked in a day using smart devices (pedometer, app in the mobile phone, smart watch, etc.).
- **Exercise testing:** Discussed in detail later.
- **Assessment of patient's work demands and environment:**
  - Nature of work
  - Muscle groups used at work
  - Work demands that primarily involve muscular strength and endurance.
  - Primary movements performed during work
  - Periods of high metabolic demands versus periods of low metabolic demands.
  - Environmental factors, including temperature, humidity, and altitude.
- **Nutritional assessment:** Detailed nutrition assessment by a dietician since the time of diagnosiss, before transplant and post-transplant is crucial.
- **Psychological assessment:** The emotional reaction to the transplantation process is complex and intense. There are various stressors that the transplant recipient and their caretaker go through even before transplant and continue to have after the transplant is done.
  - Coping with disabling or life-threatening illness.
  - Making financial arrangements required for enrolment.
  - Fear of being unsuitable for transplantation.

- Travel or moving to area of transplantation program.
- Organizing an adequate support system.
- Fear of transplantation rejection.
- Onset of medical complications pre- or post-operatively.

These stressors are assessed by the psychologist to determine the nature of the patient's response to diagnosis and readiness for transplant as well as adherence to post-transplant care.

Goals of Rehabilitation Program

Goals of rehabilitation may be divided in two parts where one part is focused on minimizing patient's symptoms related to disease and its therapy, while other part on general well-being of patient. Therapist should discuss patient goals and modify the therapy goals accordingly to achieve a unique goal set for that particular patient. For some patients, goal may be to return to a level of physical fitness they had prior to the onset of the primary disease in couple of months, while some patients may want to even exceed their previous level of fitness on longer time run. Based on the clinical knowledge and patient's expectations, therapist needs to set goal which is SMART (specific, measurable, achievable, realistic, and timely).

Monitored graded exercise training should be safe and effective for most patients; however, all patients should be stratified based on their risk for occurrence of a cardiac related event during exercise training.

Clinical Pearl

Routine preexercise assessment of risk for exercise should be performed before, during, and after each rehabilitation session, as deemed appropriate by the qualified staff and include the following:
- Heart rate
- Blood pressure (BP)
- Body weight (weekly)
- Symptoms or evidence of change in clinical status
- Symptoms or evidence of exercise intolerance
- Change in medications and adherence to the prescribed medication regimen
- For heart transplant patients, consideration of ECG surveillance that may consist of telemetry or hardwire monitoring, "quick-look" monitoring using defibrillator paddles, or periodic rhythm strips depending on the risk status of the patient and the need for accurate rhythm detection.

Exercise Testing

A low-level incremental maximal exercise test on cycle or treadmill may be helpful for exercise prescription, 4–8 weeks after the transplant. Most commonly used protocols on treadmill are modified Bruce or modified Naughton protocol where there is progressive increment by 1–2 METs (metabolic equivalent) per stage until peak and it lasts between 10 and 14 minutes. A common incremental cycle ergometer protocol for testing involves 16.4 W power output every minute, at times 8.2 W for severely deconditioned individuals **(Figs. 39.10 and 39.11)**.

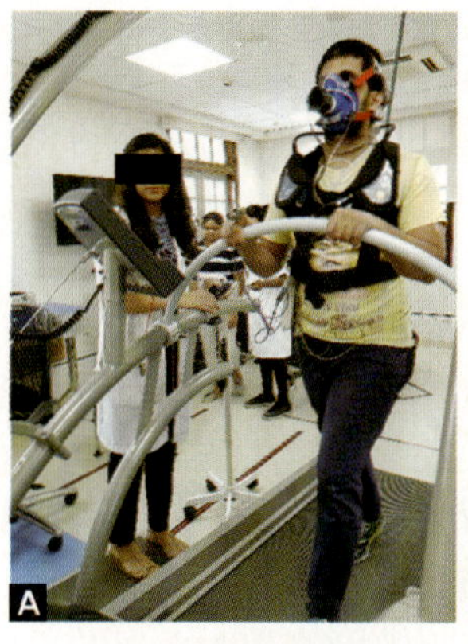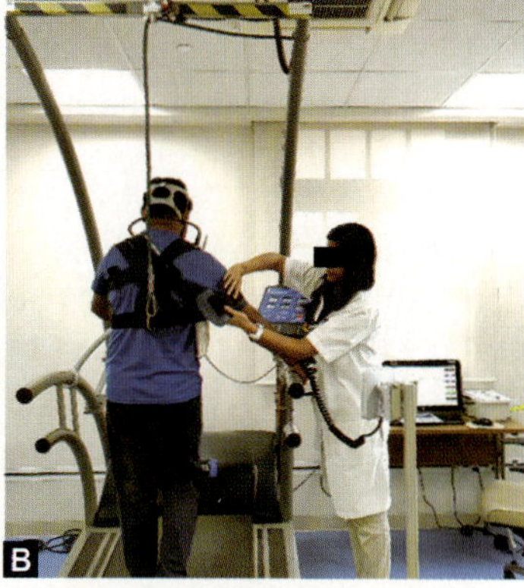

Figs. 39.10A and B: VO$_{2max}$ test on modified Bruce protocol.
Courtesy: Sir HN Reliance Foundation Hospital.

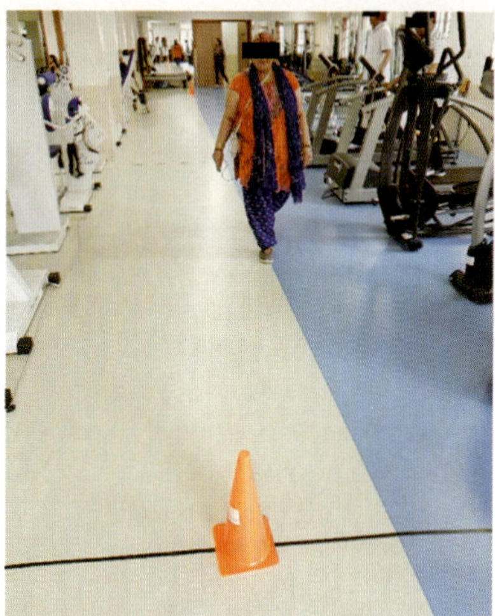

Fig. 39.11: 6-minute walk test on 16 m long walkway.
Courtesy: Sir HN Reliance Foundation Hospital.

However, it is not mandatory to conduct a maximal exercise test to prescribe exercise. A submaximal exercise test like 6-minute walk test should be sufficient to begin with. In very fragile patients, a timed up and go test or a 2-minute walk test or a symptom limited walk test can be conducted. Choice of test depends on patient's estimated fitness levels, risk stratification (based on history and assessment), and therapist's clinical knowledge and skills.

Clinical Pearl

Special consideration
In heart transplant patients, it is important to do direct measurement of VO$_2$ (oxygen consumption) levels at peak exercise because predicting VO$_2$ value from heart rate will be inaccurate due to atypical heart rate response to exercise. Expired air is collected and analyzed to measure oxygen intake, carbon dioxide production, ventilation and ventilatory threshold.
The ventilatory threshold (noninvasive) is a ventilatory determinant of anaerobic threshold (invasive) and occurs at the same level of VO$_2$ even in heart transplant patients. It is attainable even by patients who are unable or unwilling to exert maximal effort and occurs at 50–65% of maximal oxygen intake. It is an important parameter to prescribe exercise in cardiac transplantation patients.

Exercise Prescription and Training

A detailed assessment and testing should follow a discussion with patient about their goals. Patient's earlier and current fitness levels, complexities of the procedure, current cardiac risk stratification level (low, moderate, or high), comorbidities, and their own goals with regards to their fitness levels are analyzed by therapist to formulate short-term and long-term goals with rehabilitation.

For example, a 40-year old physically active male, who used to play lawn tennis every day for years, had a decline in physical activity for 2–3 months because of heart failure. After heart transplant, his goals would be to get back to playing tennis within allowable medical parameters. On the other hand, a 60-year-old male patient who had sedentary lifestyle would have a goal to be able to walk 30 minutes without any breathlessness or just return to desk job work. The therapist would have to design different plans for each of them keeping in mind their goals and progress accordingly.

Clinical Pearl

There are no specific guidelines available for exercise prescription for transplant patients. Clinicians may follow ACSM guidelines for exercise testing and prescription, Systematic reviews on transplant rehabilitation published in World Transplant Journal, ATS guidelines and AACVPR cardiac rehabilitation resource manual. The content below has been taken from these guidelines.
Prescription of exercise for a heart transplant patient requires a detailed knowledge of altered physiology after transplant. It is described in detail at the end of the chapter.

The SMART (specific, measurable, achievable, realistic, and time-bound) plan of care is designed using FITT principle.

Aerobic Exercise
Points to be considered when advocating aerobic exercise.
Frequency: 3–6 days/week.
Intensity:
- At 50–80% HR reserve or <85% age-predicted HR$_{max}$
- At peak power output occurring at 50–75% of peak oxygen intake or equivalent METs (for heart transplant).
- At ventilatory threshold (for heart transplant)
- Upper limit of RPE between 12 and 14 (on Borg scale 6–20) or (3–4 on Borg's scale 0–10).
- 75–100% of 6 MWT speed for walking
- SpO$_2$ > 88% (without supplemental oxygen)
- SpO$_2$ > 90% (with supplemental oxygen)

Type:
- Walking, stationary cycling, rowing machine, and stair stepping.
- Avoid arm ergometry in first 3 months to allow for incision healing.

Time:
- Warm-up and cool-down activities of 5–10 minutes, including static stretching and range of motion exercise, should be a component of each exercise session and precede and follow the conditioning phase.
- The goal for the duration of the aerobic conditioning phase is generally 20–60 min/session. Patients may begin with as little as 5–10 minutes of aerobic

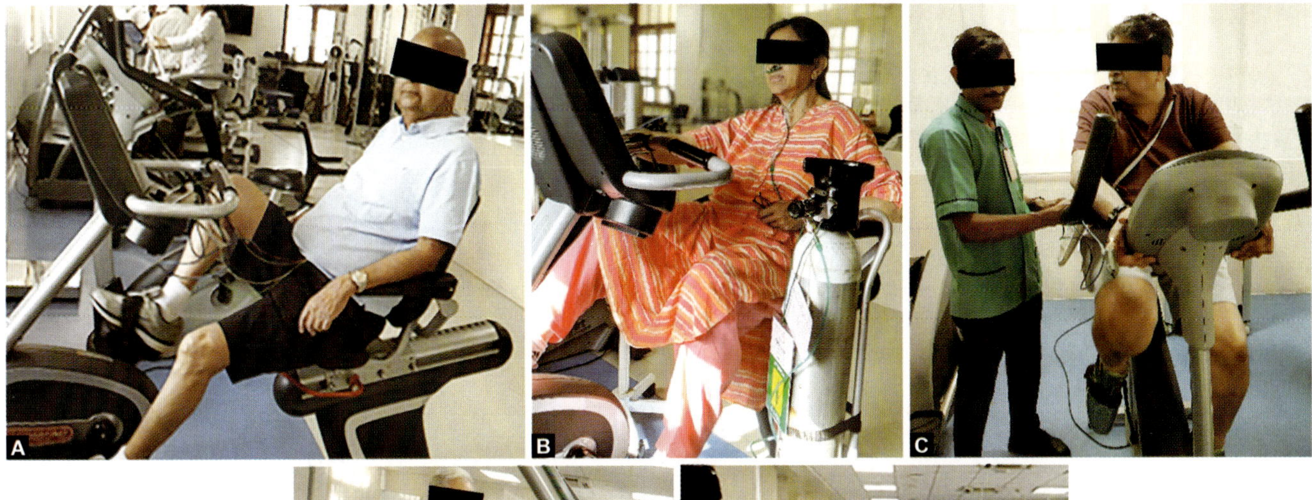

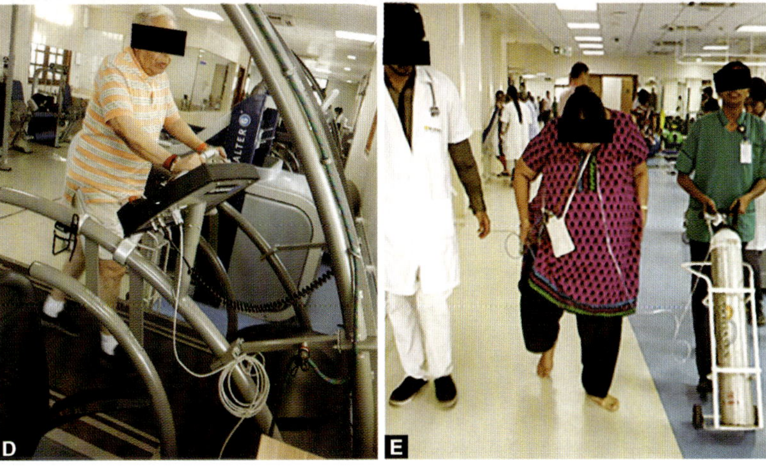

Figs. 39.12A to E: Patients at various level of rehabilitation (pre- or post-transplant) doing aerobic exercise.
Courtesy: Sir HN Reliance Foundation Hospital.

conditioning with a gradual increase in aerobic exercise time of 1–5 min/session or an increase in time per session of 10–20%/week **(Figs. 39.12A to E)**.

Clinical Pearl

- It is customary to monitor the exercise electrocardiogram (for heart transplant), heart rate, blood pressure, and rate of perceived exertion on Borg scale (6–20) regardless of protocol.
- Heart rate cannot be used to prescribe exercise for patients with heart transplantation due to atypical response to effort for initial 6–12 months. At 1 year after surgery, approximately one-third of patients exhibit a partially normalized HR response to exercise and may be given a target heart rate based on results from an exercise test.
- It is also important to remember at all the times that cardiac transplantation patient will need a longer warm-up and cool-down period due to physiologic alterations discussed earlier.
- Allograft coronary artery disease is common complication following organ transplant. Patient should be thoroughly educated for the concept of perceived exertion levels and correct interpretation of symptoms of myocardial ischemia such as excessive dyspnea, lightheadedness, unusual fatigue or development of any kind of arrhythmias. Angina or exercise-induced ST segment changes are not reliable indicators of ischemia in patients with heart transplant.
- Rejection episodes or intercurrent infections may interrupt training.

Resistance Training

Resistance training is an integral part of a rehabilitation program. It helps to improve lean body mass and improved skeletal muscle metabolism.

Frequency: 2–3 days/week with at least 48 hours separating training sessions for the same muscle group.

Intensity:
- ~30–40% one repetition maximum (1-RM) for the upper body
- No upper extremity lifting > 4-5 kg/pulling/pushing for first 3 months (for patients with median sternotomy or clamshell incision).
- Extra restrictions if signs of sternal instability
- ~50–60% 1-RM for the lower body
- A RPE of 11–14 ("light" to "somewhat hard") on a Borg Scale of 6–20 may be used as a subjective guide to effort.

Type:
- Elastic bands, cuff and hand weights, free weights, wall pulleys, body weight exercises, machines (dependent on weight of lever arms and range of motion).
- Each major muscle group (i.e., chest, shoulders, arms, abdomen, back, hips, and legs) should be trained.
- Avoid abdominal muscle strength training for 3 months **(Figs. 39.13A to C)**.

Repetitions: 1–3 sets, 8–15 repetitions.

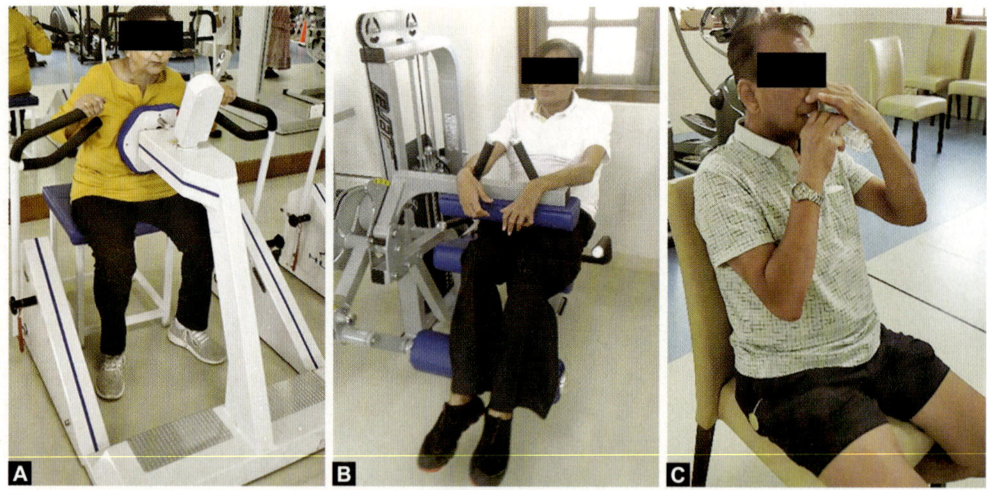

Figs. 39.13A to C: Strength training exercise for latissimus dorsi, hamstrings, and inspiratory muscles.
Courtesy: Sir HN Reliance Foundation Hospital, Mumbai, India.

Progression:
- Exercise dosage can be progressed by increasing the number of repetitions, increasing the resistance, or decreasing the rest period between sets or exercises.
- Increase loads by 5% increments when the patient can comfortably achieve the upper limit of the prescribed repetition range (e.g., 12–15 repetitions).

Cautions:
- Raising and lowering weights should be slow and controlled to full extension.
- Patient should avoid breath holding or straining.
- Patient should avoid sustained tight gripping which may evoke an excessive blood pressure response.
- Exercise should be terminated if warning signs or symptoms occur, including dizziness, arrhythmias, unusual shortness of breath, or anginal discomfort.

Clinical Pearl

In heart-transplant patients, there is a possibility of transient hypotension during resistance training, exaggerated when lifting above heart level. Therefore, it is advisable to conduct resistance training when muscles are warm enough and have a dedicated cool down for 5–10 min post-training.
It is important to include inspiratory muscle strength training for post lung transplant patients.

Flexibility Exercise
Points to be followed in flexibility exercises are:

Frequency: 3–5 days/week concentrating on exercising muscle group and muscle imbalance if any postsurgery. All tight muscles should be stretched unless contraindicated.

Intensity: Hold stretches to point of tightness/slight discomfort for the count of 30–60 seconds.

Type:
- Dynamic stretches are preferred over static before and after exercise
- Major muscle groups of upper and lower body
- Thoracic cage and chest wall mobility
- Postural reeducation.

Repetitions: Hold up to 10–30 seconds each, repeat 2–4 times.

Caution: Extra restrictions if sternal instability (e.g., avoid chest-expansion stretches).

Exercise Prescription for Returning to Work
When prescribing exercises following points should be considered:
- In addition to formal outpatient exercise sessions, patients should be encouraged to gradually return to general activities of daily living, such as household chores, shopping, routine employment job, and hobbies as evaluated and appropriately modified by the rehabilitation staff.
- A therapist should:
  - Emphasize exercise modalities that use muscle groups involved in work tasks.
  - If possible, use exercises that mimic movement patterns used during work tasks.
  - Balance resistance v/s aerobic training relative to work tasks.
- The patient should be educated about appropriate precautions including avoidance if need be while performing activities at work.
- If work includes high stress levels, education on stress management strategies should be done by a psychologist.

The comprehensive rehabilitation program following transplant maximizes the benefits of surgery and can induce a good training effect. It is important that therapist eventually transition patient from a medically supervised OPD program to an independent (i.e., self-monitored and unsupervised) home exercise program.

Long-term adherence to exercise may be greater if individuals participate or resume activities they enjoy. Thinking beyond the traditional gym protocol and exploring individuals' interest, access, and resources can be helpful when counseling individuals about increasing and maintaining physical activity in their home community. Group therapy classes and activities also encourage

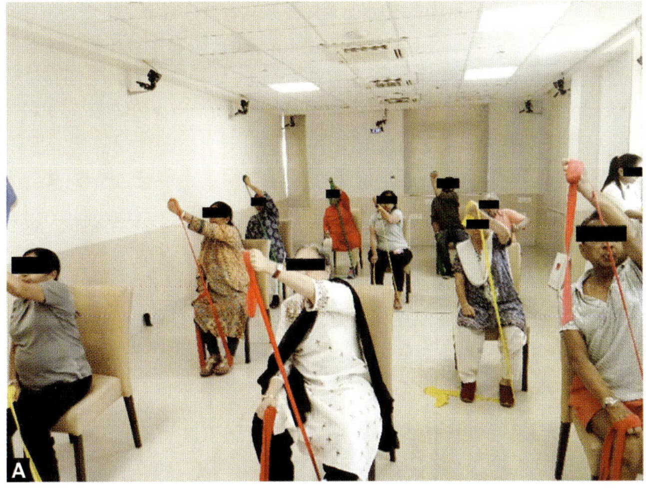
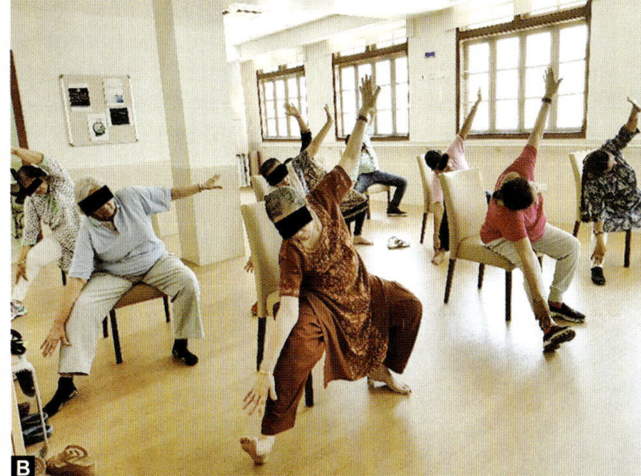
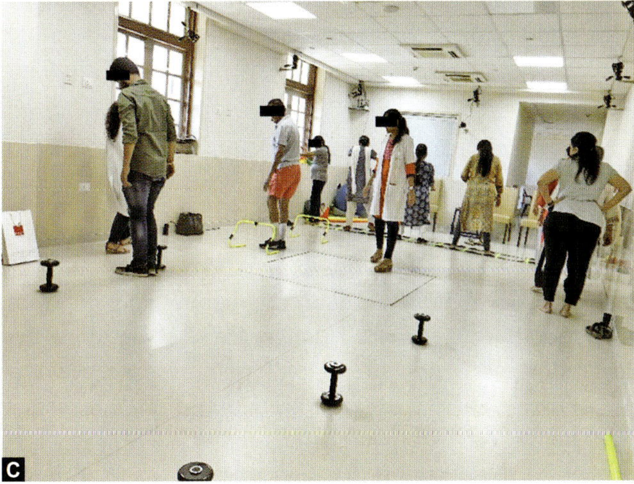
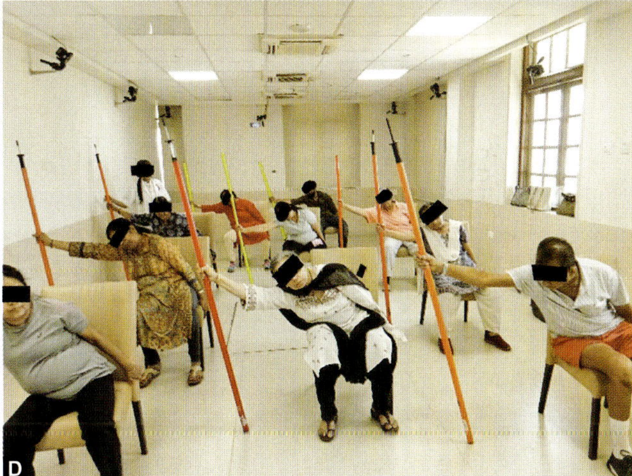

Figs. 39.14A to D: Group therapy class and activity sessions.
Courtesy: Sir HN Reliance Foundation Hospital, Mumbai, India.

patients for long-term adherence to exercise in addition to providing support. Inexpensive speedometers, activity watches, fitness monitors, and smartphone applications can be used to track daily steps and activity levels and set targets to increase physical activity **(Figs. 39.14A to D)**.

Additional activities such as yoga, Tai Chi, dance, and seasonal activities such a swimming, paddling, outdoor cycling, hiking, or skating can be done in a social setting with family and friends after clearance and training by physiotherapist and transplant professional.

It would be interesting and surprising for readers to know that since 1978, the World Transplant Games Federation organizes World Transplant Games event every two years in different countries across the world. The events have been held to promote amateur sports amongst organ-transplant recipients, living donors, and their families and showcase the athletic achievements of patients who have undergone organ transplantation. The games include athletics, swimming, cycling, kayak, badminton, table tennis, paddle tennis, squash, triathlon, bowling, darts, golf, basketball, in-door volleyball, skiing, and snowboarding. Till now many organ transplant patients have participated in long distance running like half and full marathons successfully.

Special Considerations

Physiology of the Denervated Heart

It is very important to have basic knowledge about normal physiology of cardiac circulation and its response to exercise. This physiology gets altered in transplanted heart at rest as well during exercise. Thus there is a strong need for any clinician to understand these changes to incorporate appropriate exercise and physical activity program.

Resting tachycardia: No vagal inhibition on intrinsic rate of sinoatrial node of transplanted heart leads to resting heart rate 15–25 beats/min above age and sex matched controls → resting tachycardia.

Resting hypertension: The resting blood pressure can be on a higher side in a heart transplant patient due to elevated peripheral vascular resistance, cyclosporine therapy, and/or use of steroids.

Response to Exercise

Chronotropic incompetence:

- When physical activity is initiated, the transplanted heart relies entirely on Frank–Starling's mechanism to increase cardiac output in response to physical exertion. Exercise causes skeletal muscle pumping which results in increased venous return, increased left ventricular end-diastolic volume and thus increased contractility of myocardium resulting in increased stroke volume.

- If exercise or physical activity continues beyond few minutes, catecholamines are released which has direct effect on sinoatrial node and myocardium of transplanted heart resulting in increase in heart rate, contractility, and ejection fraction. After cessation of exercise, there is a delay in decline of catecholamine levels and, therefore, the heart rate may continue to increase for a while in the recovery period, followed by late and gradual return to resting levels.
- Thus a heart transplant patient is dependent on preload at the beginning of exercise and on catecholamines when exercise is prolonged. While for normal heart, these two mechanisms operate simultaneously.

Reduced peak heart rate and peak blood pressure:
- As there is no sympathetic control on sinoatrial node of transplanted heart and decreased myocardial contractility, the peak heart rate and blood pressure are reduced to approximately 80% of normal, resulting in reduction in cardiac output by 25%.
- Higher resting heart rate and lower peak heart rate limits in heart rate reserve to 30–50 beats/min, instead of 90–110 beats/min normally.

Reduced peak work rate and oxygen consumption: The physiological limitations, such as chronotropic incompetence, reduced heart rate reserve, decreased cardiac output, in addition to reduced arteriovenous oxygen difference, may result in lower peak work rate and lower peak oxygen uptakes with exercise in heart transplant patients as compared to age matched controls.

Peripheral system abnormalities: Prolonged period of physical inactivity and side effects of immunosuppressant steroids or cyclosporine therapy leads to reduction in skeletal muscle mass by 15–20%. Preexisting heart failure state is also related to skeletal muscle metabolism abnormalities which improves with exercise, but do not match to age matched normal levels even after months of rehabilitation. These abnormalities may include decreased phosphocreatine re-synthesis rate, altered ratio of type I to type II fibers, decreased cross-sectional area of all fiber types, decreased levels of oxidative and glycolytic enzymes.

Early onset of anaerobiosis: Higher or normal lactate levels are achieved during submaximal efforts, with increased breathing frequency. The absolute ventilatory threshold is lower than normal, but because of lower peak oxygen intake, relative ventilatory threshold is similar to age-matched controls.

SUMMARY

Organ transplantation has become a common procedure for managing patients with failing organs. Because of the sequelae of the transplantation procedure and alterations in patients' physical performance, physical therapists have become key members of transplantation team, providing expertise in examination and rehabilitation of transplant recipients both before and after surgery.

Although many similarities exist in the treatment of patients undergoing organ transplantation and other cardiothoracic or abdominal surgeries, certain differences significantly affect physical therapy interventions and progression of activity.

Case Scenario

CASE STUDY 1

Mr ABC, 46-year-old overweight male, was diagnosed with hypertension in 2002, which was uncontrolled even with optimal medications. In 2003, his creatinine level rose from 2.7 to 9 mg/dL; further investigations revealed membranoproliferative glomerular nephritis leading to stage 5 CKD. He was started with hemodialysis through arteriovenous (AV) fistula at wrist level 3 days/week since then. He underwent living donor (mother) kidney transplantation on June 27, 2019.
- Past history of hepatitis C (2005). He underwent antiviral therapy from 2018 to 2019 before transplant. Past history of severe parathyroidism underwent parathyroidectomy in 2018. No history of diabetes mellitus (DM) or cardiac diseases. No history of tobacco/smoking/alcohol.
- No family history of cardiac or renal disease.
- Currently, he presented wearing a mask and had complaints of reduced physical activity levels, weakness of leg and arm muscles, and reduced confidence to perform certain physical activities.

Investigations Available

Following investigations are available:
- Preoperative 2D ECHO (March 8, 2019) revealed no significant abnormalities and LVEF = 60%. Dobutamine stress echocardiography (March 8, 2019) was negative for stress inducible ischemia. ECG showed normal sinus rhythm with T wave inversion in lead I and aVL which did not change with drug infusion.
- Postoperative (October 13, 2019) blood investigations: Hb—12 g/dL, FBS—102 mg/dL, creatinine—1.18 mg/dL, eGFR—74 mL/min/1.73 m^2.

Exercise history: He used to exercise regularly before surgery; 30 minutes walking 4 days/week and strength training on nondialysis days. He used to go for trekking once in every 2 months without any difficulties on nondialysis day.

List of Medications
- Tablet Tacroren 0.5 mg 1.5-0-1.5 (immunosuppressant)
- Tablet Wysolone 10 mg 1-0-0 (corticosteroid—anti-inflammatory)
- Tablet Immuntil S (A/D) 360 1-0-1 (immunosuppressant)
- Capsule Eido 0-0-1 (multivitamin)
- Tablet Bactrim DS (antibiotic).

His upper and lower limb girth measured and noted down along with 10 RM strength.

On **6-minute walk test,** ECG monitor showed similar resting changes at rest as recorded previously, and there were no fresh changes during exercise.

	Pre	Peak	Post
Heart rate (bpm)	109	131	108
Blood pressure (mm Hg)	128/82	162/82	128/82
SpO_2 (%)	99	100	100
Respiratory rate (bpm)	16	32	20
Rating of perceived exertion (Borg scale 6–20)	6	13	9
Distance	352 m		

The **health-related quality of life** was assessed using KDQOL Questionnaire. Scores were as listed below:
- Physical component summary: 36.6; mental component summary: 49.0; burden of kidney disease: 51.3; symptoms and problems of kidney disease: 78.1; effects of kidney disease: 43.0
- Patient goals: Patient wants to get back to trekking.

Guiding Questions:
1. What will be the goals of his rehabilitation program?
2. How will you plan his rehabilitation?
3. What complications can occur in this case?

CASE STUDY 2

Mr XYZ, 52-year-old malnourished male, was diagnosed with liver cirrhosis in 2018. He was a chronic alcoholic and had uncontrolled diabetes as well. He was initially managed conservatively with medications but showed no improvement in liver function and had deteriorated. He underwent living donor liver transplantation after 3 months of initiation of medical therapy. The liver was donated by his son. Post-transplantation, he was on ventilator for 5 days in view of difficult weaning and hemodynamic instability. Post-transplantation, his liver function test and blood investigations improved. He found intensive care rehabilitation fatiguing and required frequent break periods.
- He was shifted to wards on postoperative day 8 with drains. His goal was to get back to his job which included frequent, intermittent walking.
- No family history of cardiac or hepatic disease.
- Currently, his primary complaints are easy fatigability while performing basic personal care and being dependent on care givers for the same, weakness of both upper and lower limb, and lack of self-confidence.

Investigations Available
- Postoperative blood investigations: Hb—10 g/dL, FBS—182 mg/dL, chest X-ray: suggestive of bilateral pleural effusion (right > left).

Exercise history: Not exercising regularly.

List of Medications
- Tablet Prograf (immunosuppressant)
- Tablet Wysolone (corticosteroid—anti-inflammatory)
- Tablet Cyclosporine (immunosuppressant)
- Broad-spectrum antibiotic.

Guiding Questions:
1. What will be the goals of his rehabilitation program?
2. How will you plan his rehabilitation?
3. What are the precautions that he needs to take?

Review Questions

1. What are the indications and contraindications of transplant surgeries?
2. What are the types of transplant surgeries?
3. What medications are advised post-transplant surgeries and what are their complications?
4. What is the role of physiotherapy during the rehabilitation phase post-renal transplant?
5. What is the role of physiotherapy during the rehabilitation phase post-liver transplant?
6. What is the role of physiotherapy during the rehabilitation phase post-heart transplant?
7. Who are the members of the rehabilitation team?
8. What are the complications post-transplant surgeries?
9. What is the role of physiotherapy immediately post-transplant surgeries?

BIBLIOGRAPHY

1. 2017 ACC/AHA/HFSA/ISHLT/ACP advanced training statement on advanced heart failure and transplant cardiology (revision of the ACCF/AHA/ACP/HFSA/ISHLT 2010 clinical competence statement on management of patients with advanced heart failure and cardiac transplant): a report of the ACC Competency Management Committee. J Am Coll Cardiol. 2017;69(24):2977-3001. http://www.onlinejacc.org/content/accj/69/24/2977.full.pdf.

2. Aaronson KD, et al. Development and prospective validation of a clinical index to predict survival in ambulatory patients referred for cardiac transplant evaluation. Circulation. 1997;95:2660-7.

3. ACSM's guidelines for exercise testing and prescription, 9th edition. Baltimore, MD: Wolters Kluwer/Lippincott Williams and Wilkins; 2014.

4. Anderson L, et al. Exercise-based cardiac rehabilitation in heart transplant recipients (review). Cochrane Database Syst Rev. 2017;(4): CD012264.

5. Basha M, Mowafy Z, Morsy E. Sarcopenic obesity and dyslipidemia response to selective exercise program after liver transplantation. Egypt J Med Hum Genet. 2015;16:263-8.

6. Beck W, et al. Heart rate after cardiac transplantation. Am J Physiol. 1969;218:475-84.

7. Borow KM, et al. Left ventricular contractility and contractive reserve in humans after cardiac transplantation. Circulation. 1985;71:866-72.

8. Braith RW, et al. Cardiac output responses during exercise in volume expanded hear transplantation recipients. Am J Cardiol. 1998;81:1-5.

9. Braith RW, et al. Resistance exercise training restores bone mineral density in heart transplant recipients. Am J Coll Cardiol. 1996;28:1471-7.

10. Braith RW, et al. Resistance training prevents glucocorticoid induced myopathy in heart transplant recipients. Med Sci Sports Exerc. 1998;30:483-9.

11. Braith RW, et al. Reta responsive pacing improves exercise tolerance in heart transplant recipients. J Cardiopulm Rehabil. 2000;20:377-82.

12. Braith RW, et al. Role of Cardiac rehabilitation in heart failure and cardiac transplantation. In: Z. R. Weisman EM (Ed). Clinical exercise testing. Basel, Switzerland: Karger; 2002. pp. 120-38. (it is a book reference: Z.R. Weisman is editor's name)

13. Brubaker P, et al. Relationship of lactate and ventilatory thresholds in cardiac transplant patients. Med Sci Sports Exerc. 1993;25:191-6.

14. Burlis TV, e. a. Thoracic organ transplantation: heart, heart-lung and lung. In: Hillegas E (Ed). Essentials of cardiopulmonary physical therapy. Georgia:; 2003. pp. 410-41.

15. Busch M, et al. Potential cardiovascular risk factors in chronic kidney disease: AGEs, total homocysteine and metabolites, and the C-reactive protein. Kidney Int. 2004;66:338-47.

16. Bussieres LM, et al. Changes in skeletal muscle morphology and biochemistry after cardiac transplantation. Am J of Cardiol. 1997;79:630-4.

17. Cardiac transplantation. In: AACVPR cardiac rehabilitation resource manual. Champaign, IL, USA. Human Kinetics; 2006.

18. Carleton RA, et al. Hemodynamic performance of a transplanted human heart. Circulation. 1969;40:447-52.

19. Chadi-Alraies M, et al. Adult heart transplant: indications and outcomes. J Thorac Dis. 2014;6(8):1120-8.

20. Chambers D C, et al. The registry of the International Society for Heart and Lung Transplantation: thirty-fourth adult lung and heart-lung transplantation report-2017; focus theme: allograft ischemic time. J Heart Lung Transplant. 2017;36(10):1047-59.

21. Christopher G, et al. Chronic renal failure: renal replacement therapy. In: Morris PJ (Ed). Kidney transplantation: principles and practices. Philadelphia, PA: WB Saunders Company; 2001. pp. 32-44

22. Craven J, et al. Psychiatric, psychosocial and rehabilitative aspects of lung transplantation. Clin Chest Med. 1990;11(2):247-57.

23. Dempsey PJ, Cooper T: Supersensitivity of the chronically denervated feline heart. Am J Physiol. 1968;215:1245-1249.

24. Dressendorfer R. Lung transplantation and exercise. Clinical Rev. 2015.,www.ebscohost.com

25. Ehrman JK, et al. Exercise stress tests after cardiac transplantations. Am J Cardiol. 1993;71:1372-3.

26. Englesbe M, Patel S, He K. Sarcopenia and mortality after liver transplantation. J Am Coll Surg. Aug 2010, 211 (2), 271-78

27. Fernandes I, Cruz M, Castillo B, et al, Solid organ transplant rehabilitation., PM&R Now, American Academy of Physical Medicine and Rehabilitation. 2016.

28. Gaer J, et al. Physiological consequences of complete cardiac denervation. Br J Hosp Med. 1992;48:220-4.

29. Gibbons RJ, et al. ACC/AHA 2002 guideline update for exercise testing: summary article. A report of the American College of Cardiology/American Heart Association Task Force on Practice Guidelines (Committee to Update the 1997 Exercise Testing Guidelines). J Am Coll Cardiol. 2002;40(8):1531-40.

30. Giulio Romano, et al. Effects of exercise in renal transplant recipients. World J Transplant. 2012 (24):46-50.

31. Giulio Romano, et al. Effects of exercise in renal transplant recipients. World J Transplant. 2012;24:46-50.

32. Gordon EJ, et al. L. Longitudinal analysis of physical activity, fluid intake, and graft function among kidney transplant recipients. Transpl Int. 2009;22:990-8.

33. Gordon EJ, Prahaska T, Siminoff LA.Needed: tailored exercise regimens for kidney transplant recipients. Am J Kidney Disc. 2005;45(4):769-74.

34. Gottlieb J, et al. Update on lung transplantation. Ther Adv Respir Dis. 2008;2(4):237-347.

35. Graziadei I, Zoller H, Fickert P, et al, Indications for liver transplantation in adults. Recommendations of the Austrian Society for Gastroenterology and Hepatology (ÖGGH) in cooperation with the Austrian Society for Transplantation, Transfusion and Genetics (ATX), Wein kiln wochenschr, October 2016;128(19-20):679-90, Epub 2016, Sep 2

36. G Thabut, et al. Outcomes after lung transplantation. J Thorac Dis. 2017;9(8):2684-91.

37. Heiwe S, et al. Exercise training for adults with chronic kidney disease. Cochrane Database Syst Rev. 2011;10:CD003236.

38. Heiwe S, et al. Exercise training in adults with CKD: a systematic review and meta-analysis. Am J Kidney Dis. 2014;64(3):383-93.

39. Horii Y, et al. Role of interleukin-6 in the progression of mesangial proliferative glomerulonephritis. Kidney Int Suppl. 1993;39:S71-5.

40. Jessup M, et al. 2009 focused update: ACCF/AHA guidelines for the diagnosis and management of heart failure in adults: A report of the American College of Cardiology Foundation/ American Heart Association Task Force on practice guidelines. Circulation. 2009;119:1977-2016.

41. Juskowa J, et al. Physical rehabilitation and risk of atherosclerosis after successful kidney transplantation. Transplant Proc. 2006;38:157-60.

42. Kao AC, et al. Central and peripheral limitations to upright exercise in untrained cardiac transplant recipients. Circulation. 1994;89:2605-15.

43. Karam G, et al. Guidelines on renal transplantation. Eur Assoc Urol. 2014:1-88.

44. Kavanagh T, et al. Cardiorespiratory responses to exercise training after orthotopic cardiac transplantation. Circulation. 1988;77:162-71.

45. Kaye DM, et al. Functional and neurochemical evidence for partial cardiac sympathetic reinnervation after orthotopic cardiac transplantation in humans. Circulation. 1993;88:1110-8.

46. Kilic A, et al. Validation of the united states-derived index for mortality prediction after cardiac transplantation (IMPACT) using international registry data. J Heart Lung Transplant. 2013;32:492-8.

47. Kirsten A, et al. A structured exercise programme during haemodialysis for patients with chronic kidney disease: clinical benefit and long-term adherence. BMJ Open. 2015;5:e008709.

48. Kobashingawa JA, et al. A controlled trial of exercise rehabilitation after heart transplantation. N Eng J Med. 1999;75:40-3.

49. Kreider M, et al. Selection of candidates for lung transplantation. Proc Am Thorac Soc. 2009;6:20-7.

50. Kristen P, et al. Intradialytic exercise is medicine for hemodialysis patients. Exerc Med. 2016;15(4).

51. Langer D. Rehabilitation in patients before and after lung transplantation. Respiration. 2015;89:353-62.

52. L Beekman, A Berzigotti, V Banz; Physical Activity in Liver Transplantation: A patient's and physician's Experience, Advances in Therapy, 35 (11), October 2018

53. Lerman J, et al. Low level dynamic exercises for earlier cardiac rehabilitation: aerobic and hemodynamic responses. Arch Phys Med Rehabil. 1976;57:355-60.

54. Levy WC, et al. The Seattle Heart Failure Model: Prediction of survival in heart failure. Circulation. 2006;113:1424-33.

55. Lipkin DP, et al. The role of exercise training in chronic heart failure. Br Heart J. 1987;58:559-66.

56. Locklear C, Golabi P, Gerber L, et al. Exercise as an intervention for patients with end-stage liver disease. Medicine. 2018;97:42.

57. Locklear C ,Golabi P, Younossi ZM, Exercise as an intervention for patients with end-stage liver disease: systematic review. Medicine (Baltimore), 2018;97(42);e12774.

58. Loor G, Simpson L, Parulekar A. Bridging to lung transplantation with extracorporeal circulatory support: when or when not? J Thorac Dis. 2017;9(9):3352-61.

59. Luk WS, et al. The HRQoL of renal transplant patients. J Clin Nurs. 2004;13:201-9.

60. Mancini D, et al. Selection of cardiac transplantation candidates in 2010. Circulation. 2010;173(83):122.

61. Mandal Λ, et al. Types of liver transplantation. Med News Life Sci. 2019.

62. Maury G, Langer D, Verleden G, et al. Skeletal muscle force and functional exercise tolerance before and after lung transplantation: a cohort study. Am J Transplantat. 2008; 8:1275-81.

63. Mehra MR, et al. Listing criteria for heart transplantation: International society for heart and lung transplantation guidelines for the care of cardiac transplant candidates—2006. J Heart Lung Transplant. 2006;25:1024-42.

64. Meric S, at al. Hemodynamic effects of physiotherapy program in intensive care unit after liver transplantation. Disabil Rehabil. 2010;1461-6.

65. Naughton P, et al. Methods of exercise testing. In: H. H. Naughton JP (Eds). Exercise testing and exercise training in coronary heart disease. New York, NY: Academic Press; 1973. pp. 79-91.

66. Needed: tailored exercise regimens for kidney transplant recipients. Am J Kidney Dis. 2005;45(4):769-74.

67. Parker K, et al. An early cardiac access clinic significantly improves cardiac rehabilitation participation and completion rates in low risk STEMI patients. Can J Cardiol. 2011;27(5):619-27.

68. Pieber K, Crevenna R. Nuhr MJ et al, Aerobic capacity, muscle strength and health related quality of life before and after orthotopic liver transplantation: Preliminary data of an Australian transplantation centre. J Rehabil Med. Sept 2006; 38 (5), 322-8.

69. Romano G, et al. Physical training effects in renal transplant recipients. Clin Transplant. 2010;24:510-14.

70. Rongies W, Stepniewska S, Lewandowska M, et al, Physical activity long-term after liver transplantation yields better quality of life. Annals of Transplantation.Jul-Sep 2011, 16 (3),126-31.

71. Russo MJ, et al. Pretransplantation patient characteristics and survival following combined heart and kidney transplantation: an analysis of the united network for organ sharing database. Arch Surg. 2009;144:241-6.

72. Savin WM, et al. Cardiorespiratory responses of cardiac transplant patients to graded, symptom limited exercise. Circulation. 1980;62:55-60.

73. Schuler S, et al. Endocrine responses to exercise in cardiac transplant patients. Transplant Proc. 1987;19:2506-9.

74. Senduran M, Yurdalan SU. Physiotherapy in Liver Transplantation, Inter Open Publishers. London; 2012. pp. 445-55.

75. Services, et al. Clinical practice guideline no: 17: Cardiac rehabilitation, 90-0672 edition. Washington DC: Agency for Health Care Policy & Research; 1995.

76. Squires R, et al. Cardiac rehabilitation issues for heart transplantation patients. J Cardiopulm Rehabil. 1990;10:159-68.

77. Squires RW, et al. Partial normalization of the heart rate response to exercise after cardiac transplantation: frequency and relationship to exercise capacity. Mayo Clin Proc. 2002;77(12):1295-300.

78. Stratton JR, et al. Training partially reverses muscle metabolic abnormalities during exercise in heart failure. J Appl Physiol. 1994;76:1575-82.

79. Surgit O, et al. Effects of exercise training on specific immune parameters in transplant recipients. Transplant Proc. 2001;33:3298.

80. Surgit O, et al. Effects of exercise training on specific immune parameters in transplant recipients. Transplant Proc. 2001;33:3298. (repeated, can be removed)

81. Tudor-Locke C, et al. In their own voices: definitions and interpretations of physical activity. Womens Health Issues. 2003;13:134-99.

82. Vadakedath S, et al. Dialysis: a review of the mechanisms underlying complications in the management of chronic renal failure. Cureus. 2017;9(8):1603.

83. Varma V, Mehta N, Kumaran V, et al, Indications and contraindications for liver transplant. International Journal of Hepatology, vol 2011, Article ID 121862, pg 1-9

84. Veeranna V, et al. Homocysteine and reclassification of cardiovascular disease risk. J Am Coll Cardiol. 2011;58:1025-33.

85. Wharton J, et al. Immunohistochemical demonstration of human cardiac innervation before and after transplantation. Circ Res. 1990;66:900-12.

86. Wickerson L, et al. Physical rehabilitation for lung transplantation candidates and recipients: an evidence-informed clinical approach. World J Transplant. 2016;6(3):517-31.

87. Yamagata K. Clinical practice guideline for renal rehabilitation: systematic reviews and recommendations of exercise therapies in patients with kidney diseases. Ren Replace Ther. 2019;(5)28.

88. Yancy CW, et al. 2013 ACCF/AHA guideline for the management of heart failure: A report of the American College of Cardiology Foundation/American Heart Association Task Force on practice guidelines. J Am Coll Cardiol. 2013;62(e):147-239.

89. Yusuf S, et al. Increased sensitivity of the denervated transplanted human heart to isoprenaline both before and after beta-adrenergic blockade. Circulation. 1987;75:696-704.

90. Yusuf SA, et al. Interrelation between donor and recipient heart rates during exercise after heterotopic cardiac transplantation. Br Heart J. 1985;54:173-8.

91. Zhong R, et al. Mutation of SAC1, an Arabidopsis SAC domain phosphoinositide phosphatase, causes alterations in cell morphogenesis, cell wall synthesis, and actin organization. Plant Cell. 2005;17:1449-66.

Diabetes Mellitus

Dhruv Dave

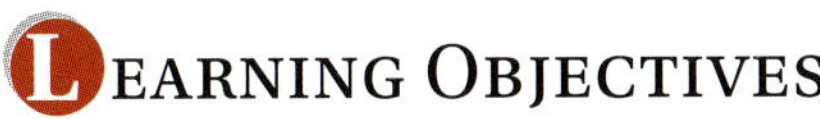

LEARNING OBJECTIVES

After reading this chapter, the readers should be able to:
♦ Explain the pathophysiology, signs, and symptoms of diabetes mellitus
♦ Understand the diagnosis
♦ Learn the treatment and complications of diabetes mellitus
♦ State various guidelines for framing exercise planning and prescription
♦ Plan and execute various forms of therapeutic modalities for diabetes mellitus.

CHAPTER OUTLINE

- Etiology of diabetes mellitus
- Pathophysiology of diabetes mellitus
- Risk factors for development of diabetes mellitus
- Clinical classification of diabetes mellitus
- Signs and symptoms of diabetes mellitus
- Diagnosis of diabetes mellitus
- Treatment modality in type 2 diabetes mellitus
  - Classification of antidiabetic drugs
- Management of type 2 diabetes mellitus
  - First-line therapy
  - Second-line therapy
  - Third-line therapy
  - Fourth-line therapy
- Complications of diabetes mellitus
- Glycemic control in diabetes
  - Targets for glycemic control
  - Factors affecting glycemic control
- Physiotherapy evaluation
  - Measurement of adiposity
- Role of exercises in diabetes mellitus
  - Impact of aerobic exercise on type 2 diabetes mellitus
  - Effect of resistance exercise in type 2 diabetes mellitus
  - Exercise prescription in type 2 diabetes mellitus
  - Other forms of exercises in type 2 diabetes mellitus
  - Impact of physical exercise on blood pressure among diabetic patients
  - Impact of physical exercise on waist circumference and basal metabolic rate among diabetic patients
- Management of diabetic foot
- Management of diabetic neuropathy
- Management of musculoskeletal complications
- Prevention guidelines
- Psychosocial burden of diabetes mellitus

INTRODUCTION

Diabetes mellitus is a group of metabolic diseases in which primarily hyperglycemia occurs due to defects in insulin secretion, insulin action, or both. Chronic hyperglycemia in diabetes is associated with long-term damage, dysfunction, and failure of vital organs, especially eyes, kidneys, nerves, heart, and blood vessels. The global burden of this disease is magnifying day by day, and it is one of the four major types of noncommunicable diseases (cardiovascular disease, diabetes, cancer, and chronic respiratory diseases). If not managed, it can lead to some serious complications by damaging the major organs of the body. Early detection and management along with prevention is the key to reduce its impact.

Box 40.1 shows a brief history of origin of diabetes mellitus.

ETIOLOGY OF DIABETES MELLITUS

Type 1 diabetes is caused by autoimmune destruction of the β cells of the pancreas. This process occurs in genetically susceptible people and is (presumably) triggered by an environmental factor. When the majority (approximately

> **BOX 40.1:** History of diabetes mellitus.
>
> Diabetes mellitus was described some 3000 years ago by the ancient Egyptians. The term "diabetes" was first coined by Araetus of Cappadocia (AD 81–133). Later, the word mellitus (honey sweet) was added by *Thomas Willis* (Britain) in 1675. Sweetness of urine in patients was first noticed by the Indian physicians. Diabetes mellitus was classified as *madhumeha* or *honey urine* noting that the urine would attract ants. Type 1 and 2 diabetes were identified as separate conditions for the first time by the Indian physicians *Sushruta* and *Charaka* in 400–500 CE with type 1 associated with young adults and type 2 with obesity. It was only in 1776 that Dobson (Britain) first confirmed the presence of excessive sugar in urine and blood as a cause of sweetness. In modern times, the history of diabetes coincided with the emergence of experimental medicine.
>
> An important milestone in the history of diabetes is the establishment of the role of the liver in glycogens and the concept that diabetes is caused due to excess glucose production by Claude Bernard (France) in 1857. The role of the pancreas in pathogenesis of diabetes was discovered by Mering and Minkowski (Austria) in 1889. Credit for the discovery of insulin is given to Banting and Best (Canada) who extracted the active principle from pancreas and demonstrated its therapeutic effect in diabetic dogs and human subjects in the years 1921 and 1922. The first patient to receive active extracts was Leonard Thompson, age 14, on January 11, 1922, in Toronto. Abelin (1926) prepared crystalline form and Sangerin (1960) established amino acid sequence of polypeptide hormone.
>
> Another milestone in the history of diabetes mellitus treatment was the introduction of orally effective hypoglycemic agents. Franke and Fuchs demonstrated the usefulness of antibiotic *carbutamide* in lowering the blood sugar in patients treated for infectious disease. Soon thereafter, *tolbutamide* was introduced which was from class sulfonylureas, Ungar in 1957 found *phenformin* as a member of biguanide series. Frederick Sanger established the amino acid sequence of insulin and received the Nobel Prize in 1958. Dorothy Hodgkin et al. (Nobel Prize for chemistry, 1964), elucidated insulin's three-dimensional structure.
>
> **Diabetes mellitus: Indian scenario**
> Diabetes is fast gaining the status of a potential epidemic in India with more than 62 million individuals currently diagnosed with the disease. In 2000, India (31.7 million) topped the world with the highest number of people with diabetes mellitus followed by China (20.8 million) with the United States (17.7 million) in second and third place, respectively. According to Wild et al., the prevalence of diabetes is predicted to double globally from 171 million in 2000 to 366 million in 2030 with a maximum increase in India. It is predicted that by 2030 diabetes mellitus may afflict up to 79.4 million individuals in India.

80–90%) of the β cells have been destroyed, a normal level of serum glucose cannot be maintained and signs and symptoms of type 1 diabetes will become evident.

Type 2 diabetes is characterized by insulin resistance and a progressive decline in pancreatic β cell insulin production. Insulin resistance is a condition in which insulin is produced but is not used properly, given amount of insulin does not produce the expected result.

In people who are obese, it may be that the chronic inflammation associated with obesity affects the function of the insulin receptors on the cells in the liver, muscles, etc., decreases the number of insulin receptors, affects insulin signaling pathways, or inactivates insulin receptors.

- **Genetic factors:** There are susceptibility genes that definitely play a role in the development of type 2 diabetes, but their contribution appears to be small.
- **Lifestyle factors/demographics:** Obesity is definitely a major risk factor for the development of type 2 diabetes and the greater the degree of obesity, the higher the risk. Excess adipose tissue is typically in a state of chronic inflammation, and this inflammation is thought to cause insulin resistance in the adipose tissue and in other organs. Other factors that increase the risk of developing type 2 diabetes are the presence of the metabolic syndrome, age, and sedentary lifestyle. Type 2 diabetes is much more common in African-Americans than other ethnic groups. There may be a genetic explanation for this, but socioeconomic factors are also probably to blame.

PATHOPHYSIOLOGY OF DIABETES MELLITUS

The pathophysiology of diabetes is related to the levels of insulin within the body, and the body's ability to utilize insulin. There is a total lack of insulin in type 1 diabetes, while in type 2 diabetes, the peripheral tissues resist the effects of insulin. Normally, the pancreatic beta cells release insulin due to increased blood glucose concentrations. Glucose is required continuously for normal functioning of the brain. Hypoglycemia, or low plasma glucose (PG) levels, is usually caused by drugs used in the treatment of diabetes, including insulin and oral antihyperglycemics. The pathophysiology of diabetes involves plasma concentrations of glucose signaling the central nervous system to mobilize energy reserves. It is based on cerebral blood flow and tissue integrity, arterial PG, the speed that PG concentrations fall, and other available metabolic fuels. Low PG causes a surge in autonomic activity. Diagnosis of hypoglycemia requires verification of low PG levels. Immediate line of treatment is the intake of glucose.

The responses to hypoglycemia include:
- Decreased insulin secretion
- Increased secretion of glucose counter-regulatory hormones such as glucagon and epinephrine
- An increased sympathoadrenal response, related symptoms, and finally
- Cognitive dysfunction, seizures; or
- Coma.

India is known as the diabetic capital of the world. Indians are more prone to develop the disease because of their "Asian Indian Phenotype." The "Asian Indian Phenotype" refers to certain unique biochemical and clinical abnormalities in Indians. This includes increase in insulin resistance, higher waist circumference (WC) in spite of lower body mass index (BMI) (greater abdominal adiposity), lower adiponectin values, and high levels of highly sensitive C-reactive protein levels.

The primary goal in the management of diabetes mellitus is the attainment of near-normal glycemia. Glycosylated hemoglobin (HbA1c) is the primary target of glycemic control. HbA1c is formed by nonenzymatic covalent addition of glucose moieties to hemoglobin in red cells. Unlike blood glucose levels, HbA1c is the index that indicates the average blood glucose during the past 3 months and hardly varies by the day-to-day variations. Glycemic control remains the major therapeutic objective for prevention of target organ damage and other complications arising from diabetes. Despite the evidence from large randomized controlled trials establishing the benefit of improved glycemic control in reducing microvascular and macrovascular complications, large proportion of diabetic patients remain poorly controlled. Therefore, recognizing the determinants of poor glycemic control will contribute to a clearer understanding of modifiable antecedents of diabetes-related complications and help to achieve improved diabetic control. In clinical practice, optimal glycemic control is difficult to obtain on a long-term basis because the reasons for poor glycemic control in type 2 diabetes are complex.

RISK FACTORS FOR DEVELOPMENT OF DIABETES MELLITUS

A variety of factors **(Fig. 40.1)** are identified in influencing glycemic control which include:

- Age
- Sex
- Education
- Body mass index
- Smoking
- Diabetes duration
- Type of medications.

Factors predominantly associated with poor glycemic control among type 2 diabetics attending any particular hospital setup are warranted so that appropriate interventions can be planned at the level of the patient, healthcare professionals, and medical institute or hospitals.

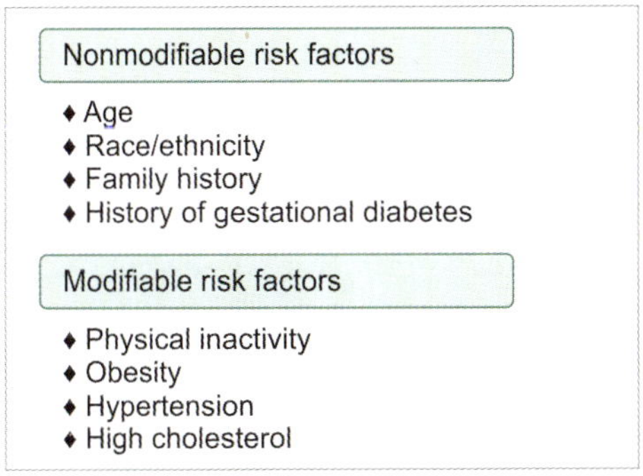

Nonmodifiable risk factors

- ♦ Age
- ♦ Race/ethnicity
- ♦ Family history
- ♦ History of gestational diabetes

Modifiable risk factors

- ♦ Physical inactivity
- ♦ Obesity
- ♦ Hypertension
- ♦ High cholesterol

Fig. 40.1: Risk factors of diabetes mellitus.

CLINICAL CLASSIFICATION OF DIABETES MELLITUS

The four clinical categories of diabetes mellitus are listed in **Table 40.1**.

Table 40.1: Clinical categories of diabetes mellitus.

1. **Type 1 diabetes** (cell destruction, usually leading to absolute insulin deficiency)
   - Immune-mediated
   - Idiopathic

2. **Type 2 diabetes** (may range from predominantly insulin resistance with relative insulin deficiency to a predominantly insulin secretory defect with insulin resistance)

3. **Other specific types of diabetes**
   - Besides type I and II there are other types of diabetes as follows:
     - Hepatocyte nuclear transcription factor (HNF-4) (maturity onset diabetes of the young—MODY 1)
     - Glucokinase (MODY 2)
     - HNF-1 (MODY 3)
     - Insulin promoter factor-1 (IPF-1; MODY 4)
     - HNF-1 (MODY 5)
     - Neuro D1 (MODY 6)
     - Mitochondrial DNA
     - Subunits of ATP-sensitive K^+ channel
     - Proinsulin or insulin sequence conversion
   - Genetic defects in insulin action
     - Type A insulin resistance
     - Leprechaunism
     - Rabson–Mendenhall syndrome
     - Lipodystrophy syndromes
   - Diseases of the exocrine pancreas—pancreatitis, pancreatectomy, neoplasia, cystic fibrosis, hemochromatosis, fibrocalculous pancreatopathy, mutations in carboxyl ester lipase
   - Endocrinopathies—acromegaly, Cushing's syndrome, glucagonoma, pheochromocytoma, hyperthyroidism, somatostatinoma, aldosteronoma
   - Drug or chemical induced—Vacor (rodenticide)
   - Infections—congenital rubella, cytomegalovirus
   - Uncommon forms of immune-mediated diabetes—"stiff-person" syndrome, anti-insulin receptor antibodies
   - Other genetic syndromes sometimes associated with diabetes—Wolfram's syndrome, Down's syndrome, Klinefelter's syndrome, Turner's syndrome, Friedreich's ataxia, Huntington's chorea, Laurence–Moon–Biedl syndrome, myotonic dystrophy, porphyria, Prader–Willi syndrome

4. **Gestational diabetes mellitus (GDM)**

(HNF: hepatocyte nuclear factor; MODY: maturity onset diabetes of the young; DNA: deoxyribonucleic acid; ATP: adenosine triphosphate)

SIGNS AND SYMPTOMS OF DIABETES MELLITUS

The signs and symptoms of diabetes mellitus are as follows:

- Increased thirst
- Frequent urination
- Extreme hunger
- Unexplained weight loss

- Presence of ketones in the urine
- Fatigue
- Irritability
- Blurred vision
- Slow wound healing or slowly healing sores
- Frequent infections, such as gums or skin infections and vaginal infections.

DIAGNOSIS OF DIABETES MELLITUS

Diabetes is usually diagnosed based on PG criteria, either the fasting PG (FPG) or the 2-hour PG (2-hour PG) value after a 75-g oral glucose tolerance test. Recently, an International Expert Committee added the HbA1c (threshold ≥6.5%) as a third option to diagnose diabetes **(Box 40.2)**.

TREATMENT MODALITY IN TYPE 2 DIABETES MELLITUS

Diabetes care is best provided by a multidisciplinary team of health professionals with expertise in diabetes, working in collaboration with the patient and family. Management includes the following **(Fig. 40.2)**:
- Appropriate goal setting
- Dietary and exercise modifications

Classification of Antidiabetic Drugs

Antidiabetic drugs can be classified into the following:
I. **Oral hypoglycemic agents:** The following are the classes of oral hypoglycemic agents used for the management of type 2 diabetes mellitus (T2DM):
  A. **Enhance insulin secretion:**
    1. Sulfonylureas (KATP channel blockers): *First generation*: tolbutamide; *Second generation*: glibenclamide (glyburide), glipizide, gliclazide, and glimepiride

    2. Meglitinide/phenyl alanine analogs: Repaglinide and nateglinide
    3. Glucagon-like peptide-1 (GLP-1) receptor agonists (injectable drugs): Exenatide and liraglutide
    4. Dipeptidyl peptidase-4 (DPP-4) inhibitors: Sitagliptin, vildagliptin, saxagliptin, alogliptin, and linagliptin.
  B. **Overcome insulin resistance:**
    1. Biguanide (AMPK activator): Metformin
    2. Thiazolidinediones (PPARγ activator): Pioglitazone.
  C. **Miscellaneous antidiabetic drugs**
    1. α-Glucosidase inhibitors: Acarbose, miglitol, and voglibose
    2. Amylinanalogue: Pramlintide
    3. Dopamine-D2 receptor agonist: Bromocriptine
    4. Sodium-glucose cotransport-2 (SGLT-2) inhibitor: Dapagliflozin.
II. **Insulin:** The various preparations of insulin used in the management of T2DM are summarized in **Table 40.2.**

MANAGEMENT OF TYPE 2 DIABETES MELLITUS

First-line Therapy

Following discusses the first-line therapy:
- Therapy is usually started with metformin, unless there is evidence of renal impairment or any other contraindication.
- Other options include a sulfonylurea for rapid response where glucose levels are high, oral glucosidase inhibitors in some populations; these agents can also be used initially where metformin cannot be used.
- In some circumstances dual therapy may be indicated initially if it is considered unlikely that single agent therapy will achieve glucose targets.

Second-line Therapy

Following discusses the second-line therapy:
- When glucose control targets are not being achieved by first line treatment drugs, a sulfonylurea needs to be added.
- Other options include adding metformin if not used first line, an α-glucosidase inhibitor, a DPP-4 inhibitor, or a thiazolidinedione.
- A rapid acting insulin secretagogue is an alternative option to sulfonylureas.

BOX 40.2: American Diabetes Association—criteria for the diagnosis of diabetes.

- HbA1c≥6.5% OR
- Fasting plasma glucose (PG) ≥126 mg/dL (7.0 mmol/L). Fasting is defined as no caloric intake for at least 8 hours OR
- 2 hours PG ≥200 mg/dL (11.1 mmol/L) during an oral glucose tolerance test. The test should be performed as described by the WHO, using a glucose load containing the equivalent of 75 g anhydrous glucose dissolved in water OR
- In a patient with classic symptoms of hyperglycemia or hyperglycemic crisis, random PG ≥200 mg/dL (11.1 mmol/L).

Glycemic control	Treatment of underlying conditions	Screening for complications
♦ Diet/lifestyle ♦ Exercise ♦ Medication	♦ Dyslipidemia ♦ Hypertension ♦ Obesity ♦ Coronary heart disease	♦ Retinopathy ♦ Cardiovascular disease ♦ Nephropathy ♦ Neuropathy ♦ Other complications

Fig. 40.2: Management of type 2 diabetes mellitus.

Table 40.2: Properties of insulin preparations.

Preparation		Onset (h)	Peak (h)	Effective duration (h)
			Time of action	
Short-acting	Aspart	<0.25	0.5–1.5	3–4
	Glulisine	<0.25	0.5–1.5	3–4
	Lispro	<0.25	0.5–1.5	3–4
	Regular	0.5–1.0	2–3	4–6
Long-acting	Detemir	1–4	–*	20–24
	Glargine	1–4	–*	20–24
	Neutral protamine Hagedorn (NPH)	1–4	6–10	10–16
Insulin combinations	75/25–75% protamine lispro, 25% lispro	<0.25	1.5	Up to 10–16
	70/30–70% protamine aspart, 30% aspart	<0.25	1.5	Up to 10–16
	50/50–50% protamine lispro, 50% lispro	<0.25	1.5	Up to 10–16
	70/30–70% NPH, 30%	0.5–1	Dual[†]	10–16

*Glargine and detemir have minimal peak activity.
[†]Dual: two peaks—on eat 2–3 hours; the second one several hours later.

Third-line Therapy

Following discusses the third-line therapy:
- When glucose control targets are no longer being achieved, insulin should be started or a third oral agent should be added.
- If insulin is started, adding basal insulin or using premixed insulin is suggested.
- Third oral hypoglycemic agent options include an α-glucosidase inhibitor, a DPP-4 inhibitor or a thiazolidinedione.
- Another option is to add a glucagon-like peptide-1 receptor agonist (GLP-1RA).

Fourth-line Therapy

Following discusses the fourth-line therapy:
Begin insulin therapy when optimized oral blood glucose lowering medications (and/or GLP-1RA) and lifestyle interventions are unable to maintain target glucose control.

COMPLICATIONS OF DIABETES MELLITUS

Long-term complications of diabetes develop gradually. The longer one has diabetes—and the less controlled blood sugar—the higher the risk of complications. Eventually, diabetes complications may be disabling or even life-threatening. Possible complications include:
- **Cardiovascular disease:**
  - Coronary artery disease with chest pain (angina)
  - Heart attack
  - Stroke
  - Narrowing of arteries (atherosclerosis)
- **Nerve damage (neuropathy):** Excess sugar can injure the walls of the tiny blood vessels (capillaries) that nourish nerves, especially in legs. This can cause:
  - Tingling
  - Numbness
  - Burning
  - Pain that usually begins at the tips of the toes or fingers and gradually spreads upward.

  Damage to the nerves related to digestion can cause problems with:
  - Nausea
  - Vomiting
  - Diarrhea
  - Constipation

  For men, it may lead to erectile dysfunction.
- **Kidney damage (nephropathy):** Severe damage can lead to kidney failure or irreversible end-stage kidney disease, which may require dialysis or a kidney transplant.
- **Eye damage (retinopathy)**
  - Diabetes can damage the blood vessels of the retina (diabetic retinopathy), potentially leading to blindness.
  - Diabetes also increases the risk of other serious vision conditions, such as cataracts and glaucoma.
- **Foot damage:** Cuts and blisters healing poorly can lead to serious infections. These infections may ultimately require toe, foot, or leg amputation.
- **Skin conditions:** Diabetes may leave one more susceptible to skin problems, including bacterial and fungal infections.
- **Hearing impairment:** Hearing problems are more common in people with diabetes.
- **Alzheimer's disease:** Type 2 diabetes may increase the risk of dementia, such as Alzheimer's disease.

GLYCEMIC CONTROL IN DIABETES

The following discusses glycemic control in diabetes:

- Glycemic control is a medical term referring to the typical levels of blood sugar (glucose) in a person with diabetes mellitus. Glycemic control is essential in diabetes management. Since lower level of blood glucose leads to decreased rates of morbidity and mortality, maintaining glycemic control is a goal for all patients with diabetes.
- Various studies have shown that glycemic control is related with reduced rates of retinopathy, nephropathy, neuropathy, and cardiovascular diseases. Glycemic control is considered as the main therapeutic goal for prevention of organ damage and other complications of diabetes. In various epidemiological analyses, glycosylated hemoglobin (HbA1c) levels >7.0% was associated with a significantly increased risk of both microvascular and macrovascular complications, regardless of underlying treatment.
- Glycemic targets should be individualized based on the individual's age, duration of diabetes, risk of severe hypoglycemia, presence or absence of cardiovascular disease, and life expectancy.

Glycemic control is central to the management of diabetes mellitus as:

- Even mild sustained elevations in HbA1c, as a reflection of overall blood glucose control, are associated with increased risks of complications and, in particular, the risk of myocardial infarction.
- Every effort should be made to lower HbA1c, because any reduction in HbA1c will translate into a reduction in the risk of complications.
- The individuals who are most likely to benefit from risk reduction are those with the highest initial blood glucose values.

Physicians caring for patients with type 2 diabetes should aim for the best possible glycemic control. Unless contraindications exist, a near-normal or normal level of glycemia, as manifested in a normal HbA1c, should be the goal of diabetic therapy.

Targets for Glycemic Control

According to American Diabetes Association guidelines, the following have been established as targets for glycemic control **(Table 40.3)**.

Targets may be individualized based on:

- Age/life expectancy
- Comorbid conditions
- Diabetes duration
- Hypoglycemia status
- Individual patient considerations.

Lowering HbA1c below or around 7.0% has been shown to reduce:

- Microvascular complications

Table 40.3: Blood glucose targets for nonpregnant adults with diabetes.

HbA1c	<7.0% (53 mmol/L)
Preprandial capillary PG	80–130 mg/dL (4.4–7.2 mmol/L)
Peak postprandial capillary PG	<180 mg/dL (<10.0 mmol/L)

More or less stringent targets may be appropriate for individual patients if achieved without significant hypoglycemia or adverse events

More stringent target (<6.5%)	**Less stringent target (<8.0%)**
• Short diabetes duration • Long-life expectancy • Type 2 diabetes treated with lifestyle or metformin only • No significant CVD/vascular complications	• Severe hypoglycemia history • Limited life expectancy • Advanced microvascular or macrovascular complications • Extensive comorbidities • Long-term diabetes in whom general HbA1c targets are difficult to attain

(PG: plasma glucose; CVD: cardiovascular disease)

- Macrovascular disease (if implemented soon after diagnosis)
- Mortality (individuals with type 1 diabetes only)

According to Canadian Diabetes Association guidelines:

1. Glycemic targets should be individualized based on age, duration of diabetes, risk of severe hypoglycemia, presence or absence of cardiovascular disease, and life expectancy.
2. Therapy in most individuals with type 1 or type 2 diabetes should be targeted to achieve an HbA1c ≤7.0% in order to reduce the risk of micro vascular.
3. HbA1c ≤6.5% may be targeted in some patients with type 2 diabetes to further lower the risk of nephropathy.
4. Less stringent HbA1c targets (7.1–8.5% in most cases) may be appropriate in patients with type 1 or type 2 diabetes with any of the following:
   a. Limited life expectancy
   b. High level of functional dependency
   c. Extensive coronary artery disease at high risk of ischemic events
   d. Multiple comorbidities
   e. History of recurrent severe hypoglycemia
   f. Hypoglycemia unawareness
   g. Long-standing diabetes for which it is difficult to achieve HbA1c ≤7.0% despite effective doses of multiple antihyperglycemic agents, including intensified basal-bolus insulin therapy.

In order to achieve HbA1c ≤7.0%, people with diabetes should aim for: Fasting plasma glucose (FPG) or preprandial plasma glucose (PG) target of 4.0–7.0 mmol/L and a 2-hour postprandial plasma glucose (PPG) target of 5.0–10.0 mmol/L. If HbA1c target ≤7.0% cannot be achieved with a PPG target of 5.0–10.0 mmol/L, further PPG lowering to 5.0–8.0 mmol/L should be achieved.

Table 40.4: Indian Council of Medical Research guidelines for glycemic control.

	Ideal	Satisfactory	Unsatisfactory
FPG	80–110	111–125	>125
2-h PPG	120–140	140–180	>180
BP	<130/80	<140/90	>140/90
BMI	20–23		
WHR	Men <0.90, women <0.85		
HbA1c	<7	7–8	>8

(BMI: body mass index; BP: blood pressure; FPG: fasting plasma glucose; WHR: waist–hip ratio; PPG: post-prandial glucose)

Table 40.5: The IWGDF Risk Classification System 2015 and preventative screening frequency.

Category	Characteristics	Frequency
0	No peripheral neuropathy	Once a year
1	Peripheral neuropathy	Once every 6 months
2	Peripheral neuropathy with peripheral artery disease and/or a foot deformity	Once every 3–6 months
3	Peripheral neuropathy and a history of foot ulcer or lower extremity amputation	Once every 1–3 months

According to Indian Council of Medical Research (ICMR) guidelines: HbA1c value in percent for ideal control should be <7 for satisfactory control 7–8 and >8 would be unsatisfactory control. These are only general guidelines and individualized target are to be established **(Table 40.4)**.

Factors Affecting Glycemic Control

In clinical practice, the recommended glycemic control target is very difficult to achieve. It is important, therefore, to identify factors that influence the outcomes of glycemia in order to improve the quality of diabetic management. Factors which influence glycemic control are as follows:

- Treatment modality
- Adherence to medication
- Presence of complications of diabetes
- Study showed that longer duration of diabetes was associated significantly with poor glycemic control
- Effective educational and therapeutic approaches on management of hyperglycemia.
- Abdominal obesity
- Physical exercise and weight control

PHYSIOTHERAPY EVALUATION

An individual's comprehensive assessment should be done before any treatment protocol is advised or undertaken. History should be taken at depth to identify the modifiable risk factors, along with family history and personal habits which have the potential of influencing the treatment outcome. Systems review should consist of reviewing presence of any other comorbid conditions. This will consist of evaluating the lifestyle, physical activity participation, and determining exercise tolerance with the help of exercise tolerance tests. All medical records should be gathered and investigations undertaken should be thoroughly studied to plan a therapeutic intervention. Assessment should comprise of use of both subjective and objective tools of measurement depending on both availability and resources.

Foot care is an important domain that requires individualized evaluation. Previous ulcer/amputation, end stage renal disease, previous foot education, social isolation, poor access to health care and barefoot walking are asked in history additionally. History of claudication, rest pain and palpation of pedal pulses is done, callus, color, temperature, and edema are checked for. Footwear/socks (those worn when at home and when outside) including assessment of both their inside and outside is done. Following examination of the foot, each patient can be assigned to a risk category that should guide subsequent preventative management. The International Working Group on Diabetic Foot (IWGDF) risk classification categories 2015 can be found in **Table 40.5**.

Measurement of Adiposity

The standard measurements of adiposity include BMI, WC, and skin fold thickness:

- WC is an index of central fatness. WC is known to be a better predictor than total fat of adverse outcomes such as insulin resistance.
- Waist–hip ratio is independently associated with morbidity in adults. However, the association between abdominal fat and waist–hip ratio is inconsistent.
- Skin fold thickness and bioelectric impedance measurements are used by predictive techniques to assess body composition. Skin fold thickness has been traditionally used to assess individual's fatness or size of specific subcutaneous fat depots. Skin fold thickness is also used as an index of regional fatness. Among South Asians, obesity related comorbidities at lower cut off BMI and WC has been used as their body fat is higher compared to white Caucasians.
- For Asian populations, it has been debated whether BMI cutoffs should be lower as compared to the available international guidelines (25.0–29.0 kg/m^2 as overweight, 30–34.9 kg/m^2 as obesity). A WHO expert Consultative Committee in 2004 suggested BMI cutoffs as $\geq$23–24.9 kg/m^2 for overweight and $\geq$25 kg/m^2 for

obesity, respectively. WHO group left the decision for guidelines for BMI to the governments of respective Asian countries. Thereafter, Consensus Group from India formulated revised guidelines for BMI for Asian Indians. Although BMI positively correlates with adiposity it does not discriminate fat from lean mass or distribution of body fat.

- Cutoff points of WC (for men: ≥94 cm and women: ≥80 cm) are based on selection of international obesity data derived from white Caucasians. WHO Expert Committee on Obesity in Asian and Pacific populations suggested revised cutoff points for WC: 90 cm for men and 80 cm for women for Asians. Indian expert group proposed for adult Asian Indians; men ≥78 cm, women ≥72 cm as cutoff points.

ROLE OF EXERCISES IN DIABETES MELLITUS

Macrovascular and microvascular complications of diabetes mellitus are a well-known cause of morbidity and mortality seen among diabetic patients. The healthcare cost burden due to the complications of diabetes mellitus is increasing worldwide. Besides pharmacological therapy, nonpharmacological approach for effective management of diabetes mellitus is the corner stone of treatment.

Nonpharmacological management such as exercise training programs is an alternative therapeutic approach for both type 1 diabetes mellitus and in T2DM. Exercise promotes increased peripheral glucose utilization via glucose transporter 4 (GLUT4) to the skeletal muscle. This brings down glucose levels and is responsible for reducing the elevated blood sugar level in patients of T2DM. Different forms of exercise have been reported to have favorable effects in patients of T2DM:

- Aerobic exercise
- Endurance type exercise
- Passive exercise
- Resistance exercises.

Impact of Aerobic Exercise on Type 2 Diabetes Mellitus

Aerobic exercises comprise of:

- Swimming
- Cycling
- Treadmill
- Walking
- Rowing
- Running
- Jumping rope

Aerobic exercise is known to have beneficial effects in the patients of T2DM by increasing the functioning of the cardiovascular and respiratory systems and increasing oxygen consumption **(Figs. 40.3A to F)**. Aerobic exercise has favorable effects on reducing the metabolic risk factors in insulin resistance among patients of T2DM and also has known beneficial effects on physiological parameters.

Several studies have shown the benefits of aerobic exercise in T2DM. There is accumulating evidence that aerobic exercise improves:

- Insulin sensitivity
- Glycemic control
- Fasting blood-glucose level
- Lipid profile
- Aids in weight loss
- Additionally, the arterial stiffness is reduced.
- Also, endothelial function, a positive denominator for developing cardiovascular complications in diabetes mellitus, is improved.

Increase glucose uptake into skeletal muscle via the glucose transporter (GLUT4) is mediated by aerobic exercise just like the physiological function of insulin. Studies have documented that diabetes mellitus is associated with deficiencies in the insulin receptors which result in impaired glucose uptake and GLUT4 translocation. Exercise therapy promotes GLUT4 translocation and can partly restore the defects of insulin signaling.

Effect of Resistance Exercise in Type 2 Diabetes Mellitus

Resistance exercise leads to the development of proper glucose control and less insulin resistance among T2DM. Exercises that have to be performed against resistance are called resistance exercises. Weight lifting is an example of resistance exercises **(Figs. 40.4A to D)**. Some form of equipment or one's own body weight can be used for performing resistance exercises. High and moderate intensities of resistance exercise range between 50 and 75% of 1-repetition maximum (1-RM). Various studies have documented the potential benefits of resistance exercises in the therapeutic regimen in patients with T2DM. In addition, it is also proven to be safe and effective for the population with insulin resistant diabetes patients. Studies have shown that resistance training improves:

- Insulin sensitivity
- Quality of life
- Daily energy expenditure

Moreover, an increase in muscle strength, lean muscle mass, and bone mineral density is observed with resistance training. Therefore, resistance exercise has the potential to improve glycemic control and assists in the prevention of osteoporosis.

Exercise Prescription in Type 2 Diabetes Mellitus

The American College of Sports Medicine recommends accumulating 150 minutes of moderate intensity or 60 minutes of vigorous intensity aerobic exercise per week. It also recommends performing 2–3 nonconsecutive days of resistance training per week at intensities between 50 and 80% of 1-RM and targeting all major muscle groups using a scheme of 1–4 sets of 8–15 repetitions per exercise. Progression should be gradual and not sudden to avoid injuries and increase patient compliance.

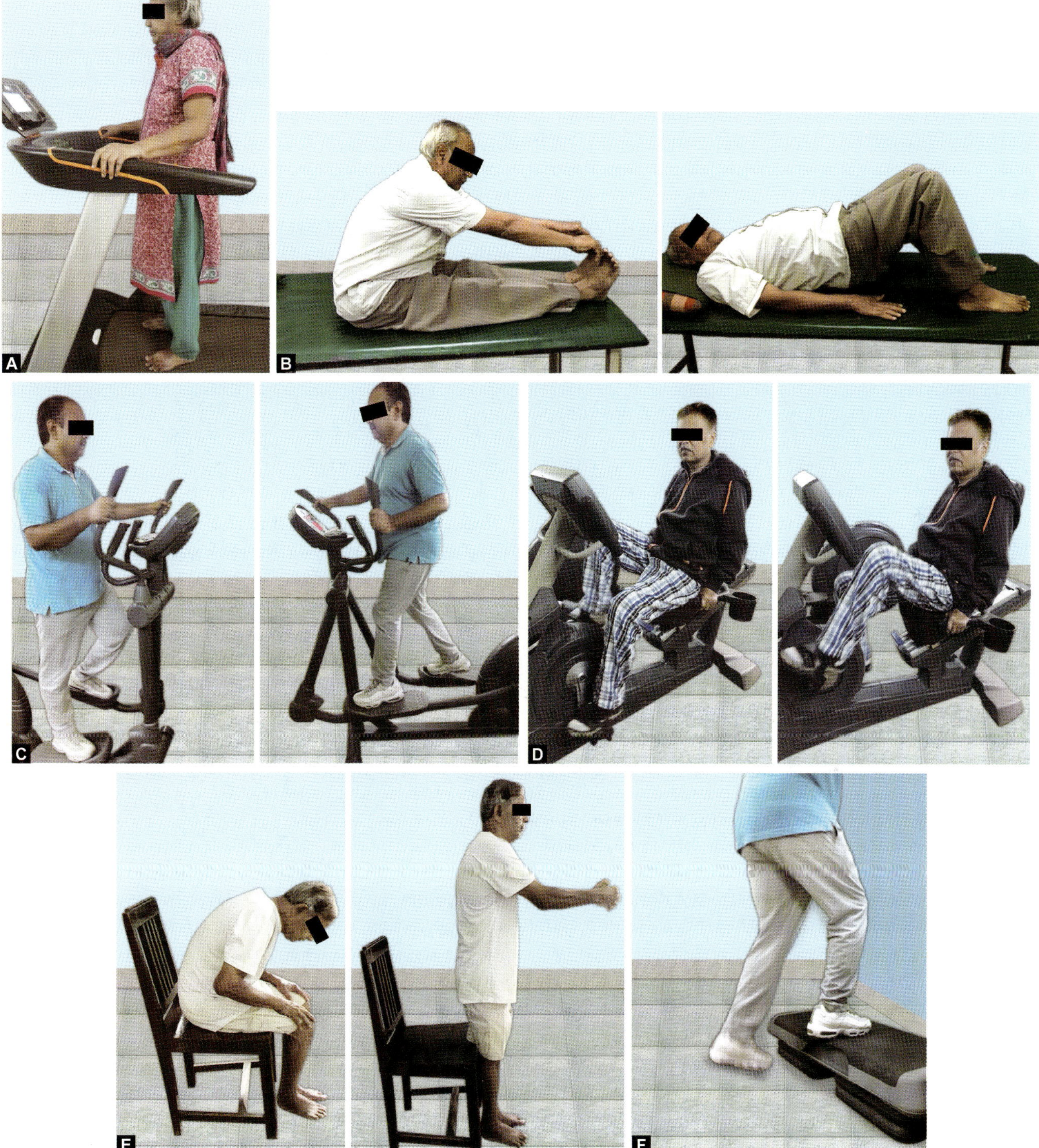

Figs. 40.3A to F: (A) Diabetic patient performing treadmill form of aerobic exercises; (B) Diabetic patient performing warm-up exercises; (C) Diabetic patient performing cross-training form of aerobic exercises; (D) Diabetic patient performing cycling form of aerobic exercises; (E) Diabetic patient performing trunk flexion and sit to stand exercises; (F) Diabetic patient performing exercises on stepper.

Other Forms of Exercises in Type 2 Diabetes Mellitus

Endurance and passive exercise are other types of exercise which are beneficial in chronic diseases like T2DM. Several large groups of muscles are used in endurance exercise. Endurance exercise relies on the delivery of oxygen to the muscles by the cardiovascular system. On the other hand, another person or outside force is used in passive exercise or produced by voluntary effort of another segment of the patient's own body. A large segment of studies support the aerobic and resistance training program because of their beneficial effects. However, there is paucity of studies on endurance and passive exercise training in treating T2DM

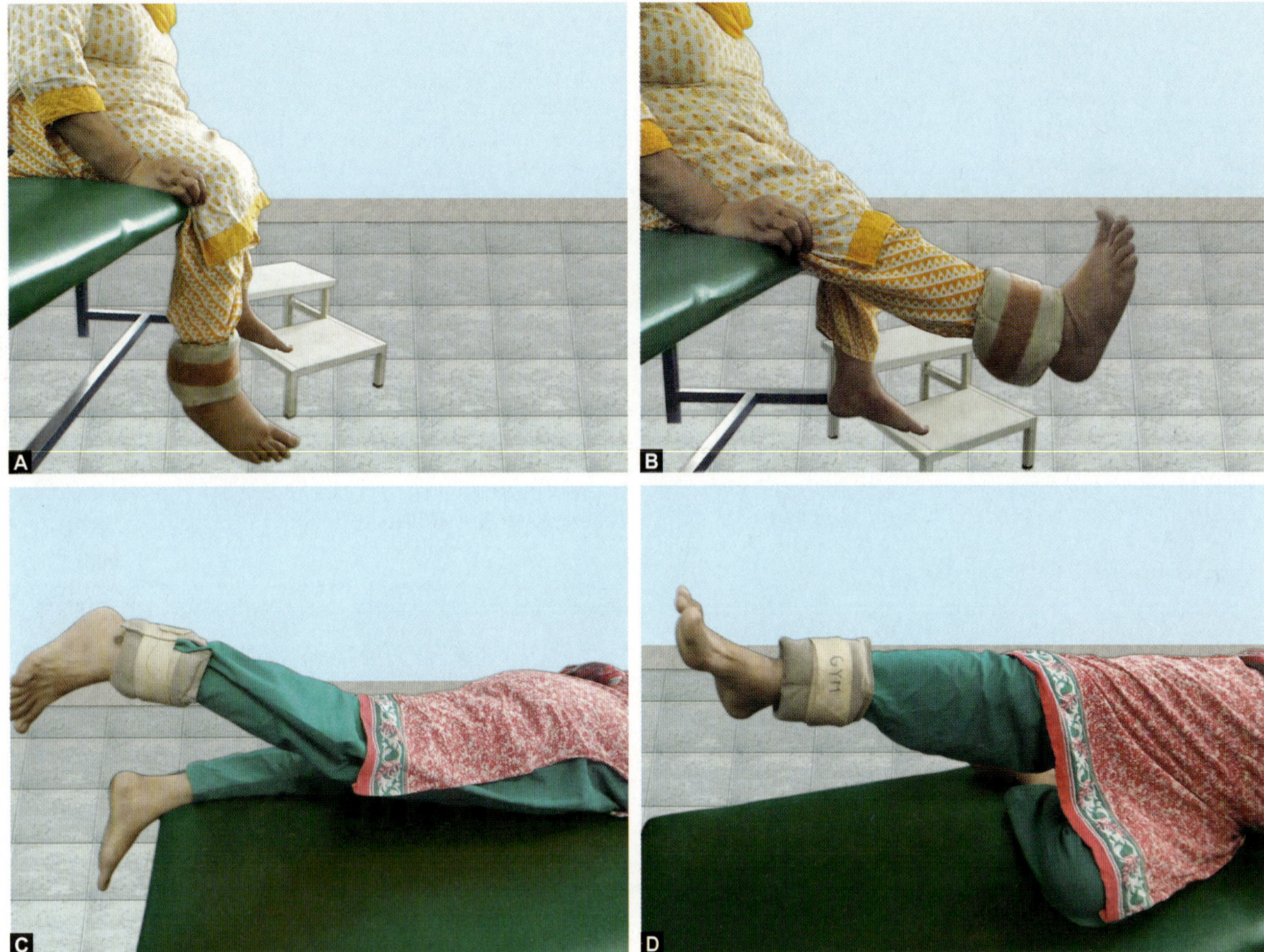

Figs. 40.4A to D: Diabetic patient performing resisted exercise of lower extremity.

patients. Endurance training is also reported to reduce postprandial hyperglycemia in T2DM patients.

Other forms of exercise includes yoga that has shown to have a positive impact in patients of T2DM. Joba horseback riding has shown to improve insulin sensitivity in T2DM patients. Yoga has also been reported to improve the glycemic control in diabetic patients.

Exercise is an important nonpharmacological component in the clinical management of patients with T2DM. There are no clear cut recommendations or guidelines on the various types of exercise as well as its benefits in the effective management of patients with type 2 diabetes. Studies have shown that both endurance and resistance types of exercise have benefits in the effective management and metabolic control of patients with type 2 diabetes. Attention should be paid to the avoidance of cardiovascular and musculoskeletal deconditioning.

Impact of Physical Exercise on Blood Pressure Among Diabetic Patients

Several studies have reported that exercise may slightly reduce systolic blood pressure (SBP) in people with T2DM. Reduction in diastolic BP (DBP) is less common among diabetic patients. Dobrosielski et al., conducted a randomized controlled trial and found no reductions in resting SBP or DBP among exercisers after 6 months of training. The authors, however, found a training effect as an increase in fitness level, glycemic control, and improved body composition was seen. The lack of change in BP was explained based on several factors.

Diabetes mellitus results in metabolic abnormalities that are associated with impaired vascular function, inhibition of vasodilatation, and augmentation of vasoconstriction responses. These reasons predispose to arterial structural remodeling and stiffness, resulting in increase in SBP. Exercise training did not translate in reduction in aortic stiffness perhaps because of limited plasticity in diabetic vasculature. It was also speculated that among diabetics, adverse vascular changes reflect end-organ damage that exercise alone may not be able to reverse. Physicians must consider drug therapy, with exercise as an adjunct treatment for elevated BP in T2DM. The effect of exercise training over and above conventional treatment as practiced in the community was evaluated. A significant reduction in SBP at 6 months, regardless

Current Status of Research

Zaghlol et al.

Studied impact of aerobic and resisted exercise on glycated hemoglobin in 30 subjects with prediabetes and concluded that both aerobic and resisted exercise prevents or delays type 2 diabetes mellitus (T2DM). Resisted exercise was found to be more effective than aerobic exercise in reducing the glycated hemoglobin values

Elsisi et al.

Studied the impact of 12 weeks high-intensity interval training (HIIT) on glycated hemoglobin (HbA1c) in patients of T2DM and concluded that HIIT is an effective training method as compared to only aerobic training in improving HbA1c in T2DM

Bose et al.

Studied the effect of progressive resistance training along with aerobic exercise on glycemic control in type 2 diabetes and concluded that progressive resisted training along with aerobic training is effective method for glycemic control in type 2 diabetes

Najafipour et al.

Studied the long-term effects of regular exercise training on hemoglobin A1c (HbA1c), body mass index (BMI), and VO_{2max} in 65 patients with type 2 diabetes, and concluded that among patients with T2DM, regular physical activity training improved glycemic control, body composition, and cardiovascular fitness. Training program included aerobic exercise three sessions per week, 90 min, 50–80% VO_{2max}

Yang et al.

Studied the effectiveness and safety of aerobic exercise and resistance exercise in people with type 2 diabetes by assessing its impact on glycemic control, blood lipids, anthropometric measures, blood pressure, fitness, health status, and adverse events. They concluded a greater reduction in glycosylated hemoglobin, BMI, peak oxygen consumption, and maximum heart rate

Eskandary et al.

Studied the impact of 8 weeks of aerobic training, resistance training, and concurrent training (combined of aerobic and resistance training) on glycated hemoglobin (HbA1c) and the metabolic syndrome in men diagnosed with type 2 diabetes

Concluded a decrease in blood HbA1c level in the concurrent group and reduced serum LDL levels and increase in the HDL level was observed in the resistance training group

of group assignment or current use of antihypertensive medications was observed.

Jackson et al. investigated if risk of developing hypertension was modified by nonpharmacological intervention of physical activity carried out on a continuous long-term basis. At 3-year interval, BMI, physical activity, and hypertension were measured at base line and after 14 years. Risk of hypertension correlated with an increase in BMI and decrease in physical activity. Physical activity attenuated the positive association between weight and risk of hypertension, especially for obese women. Lower risk of hypertension was associated with an increase in physical activity and maintenance of a healthy body weight. The effect of obesity on hypertension risk was reduced by increase in physical activity.

Impact of Physical Exercise on Waist Circumference and Basal Metabolic Rate Among Diabetic Patients

Maintaining normal adiposity is a concern in the management of T2DM. Asians are more prone to central obesity with high visceral adiposity. Central obesity is known to cause low-grade systemic inflammation by inflammatory mediators such as adipokines, adiponectin, and tumor necrosis factor-α. These inflammatory mediators are known to cause the development of insulin resistance, T2DM and cardiovascular disease.

MANAGEMENT OF DIABETIC FOOT

With respect to prevention, all healthcare professionals have a duty of care to identify the at-risk foot in patients with diabetes by routinely carrying out foot inspection. As a result of damage to the nervous system, foot neuropathy is common in diabetic patients and hence a major role of physiotherapist would also consist of diabetic foot care. Numbness and tingling of the feet can cause foot injury and wounds to go unnoticed, which may lead to breakdown and skin infections or wounds eventually. Damage to the nervous system also impairs sweat secretion and oil production of the foot. If proper lubrication of the foot does not occur, this leads to abnormal pressure on the skin, bones, and joints during walking and will also result in skin breakdown and sores on the foot.

Patients should be educated regarding how to prevent foot problems before they happen. Treatment for diabetic foot problems have recently improved, but prevention remains the best approach to prevent complications. Educating the patients how to properly examine their own feet and be able to recognize early signs and symptoms of diabetic foot problems is crucial. They should be educated on proper footwear. Protective footwear is an important element of prevention of diabetic foot complications. The most important aim is to achieve a substantial reduction of peak pressure over the plantar surface of the feet. This is also known as *offloading*.

The *five key elements* used for prevention of diabetic foot problems are:

1. Identification of the at-risk foot
2. Regular inspection and examination of the at-risk foot
3. Education of patient, family, and healthcare providers
4. Routine wearing of appropriate footwear
5. Treatment of preulcerative signs (abundant callus, cracks and fissures, blisters, ingrown or thickened nails, and fungal infections).

There are *seven key elements* that underlie ulcer treatment:

1. Relief of pressure and protection of the ulcer
2. Restoration of skin perfusion
3. Treatment of infection
4. Metabolic control and treatment of comorbidity
5. Local wound care
6. Education for patient and relatives
7. Prevention of recurrence

All people with diabetes should have their feet examined at least once a year to identify those at risk for foot ulceration. Patients found to have a risk factor should be examined more often as per **Table 40.5.** Those at risk should be educated along with family and healthcare providers involved in the treatment of diabetic individuals.

Items that should be covered when instructing the patient at-risk for foot ulceration:

- Determine if the person with diabetes is able to perform a daily foot inspection. If not, discuss who can assist the person in this task. A substantially visually impaired person cannot adequately do the inspection.
- Perform daily foot inspection, including areas between the toes.
- Notify the appropriate healthcare provider at once if foot temperature is markedly increased, or if a blister, cut, scratch, or ulcer has developed.
- Avoid walking barefoot, in socks without footwear, or in thin-soled standard slippers, whether at home or outside.
- Do not wear shoes that are too tight, have rough edges, or uneven seams.
- Inspect and feel inside all shoes before you put them on.
- Wear socks/stocking without seams (or with the seams inside out), do not wear tight or knee-high socks and change socks daily.
- Wash feet daily (with water temperature always below 37°C) and dry them carefully, especially between the toes.
- Do not use any kind of heater or a hot-water bottle to warm feet.
- Do not use chemical agents or plasters to remove corns and calluses; see the appropriate healthcare provider for these problems.
- Use emollients to lubricate dry skin, but not between the toes.
- Cut toenails straight across
- Have your feet examined regularly by a healthcare provider.

Footwear advices should also be given such as:

- The shoe should neither be too tight nor too loose.
- The inside of the shoe should be 1–2 cm longer than the foot.
- The internal width should equal the width of the foot at the metatarsophalangeal joints (or the widest part of the foot), and the height should allow enough room for all the toes.
- Evaluate the fit with the patient in the standing position, preferably at the end of the day.
- If the fit is poor because of foot deformities, or if there are signs of abnormal loading of the foot (e.g., hyperemia, callus, and ulceration), refer the patient for special footwear (advice and/or construction), including insoles and orthoses.
- If possible, demonstrate that there is reduced plantar pressure of this special footwear to prevent a recurrent plantar foot ulcer.

Those people who develop ulcers may require medical or surgical interventions such as debridement, or in severe cases, amputation may be indicated. However, relief of pressure and protection of the ulcer is a cornerstone in treating an ulcer associated with increased biomechanical stress. This can be achieved with physiotherapy rehabilitation. Hence, a nonremovable knee-high offloading device, either total contact cast (TCC) or removable walker rendered irremovable is useful.

- When a nonremovable TCC or walker is contraindicated, use a removable device.
- When these devices are contraindicated, use footwear that best offloads the ulcer.
- In nonplantar ulcers, consider offloading with shoe modifications, temporary footwear, toe spacers, or orthoses.
- If other forms of biomechanical relief are not available, consider felted foam, in combination with appropriate footwear.
- Instruct the patient to limit standing and walking and to use crutches if necessary.

Negative pressure therapy, systemic hyperbaric oxygen treatments are some options for ulcer treatment. Electrical stimulation, given daily with a short pulsed, asymmetric biphasic waveform, is also effective for enhancement of healing rates for patients with diabetes and open ulcers. Other therapeutic modalities, such as LASER and high-voltage pulsed galvanic stimulation (HVPGS), should be checked for contraindications before applying to a diabetic patient as per the wound status and its healing.

MANAGEMENT OF DIABETIC NEUROPATHY

Details of diabetic neuropaties are described in Chapter 33: Peripheral Neuropathies.

MANAGEMENT OF MUSCULOSKELETAL COMPLICATIONS

Adhesive capsulitis is described in Chapter 19: Shoulder Conditions.

PREVENTION GUIDELINES

Evidence suggests that type 1 diabetes cannot be prevented. However, a number of factors that influence the development of type 2 diabetes are mainly related to lifestyle and can hence be modified.

Current recommendations consist of advices on the following as key components in prevention of T2DM:

- Maintenance of healthy weight
- Proper and healthy nutrition intake
- Participation in aerobic and resistance exercise programs.

Comprehensive management strategies include:

- Addressing behavioral component such as maintaining diaries, or attending diabetes education classes.
- Participation in regular physical activity at least 30 min/day for 5 days in a week is recommended for adults at high risk of diabetes.
- Limiting screen time to less than 60 minutes daily and inclusion of at least 60 min/day of physical activity for adolescents and youth are helpful in preventative role.

PSYCHOSOCIAL BURDEN OF DIABETES MELLITUS

The psychosocial burden of diabetes mellitus can be described as follows:

- Patients with diabetes mellitus need psychological support throughout their life span from the time of diagnosis.
- The psychological makeup of the patients with diabetes mellitus plays a central role in self-management behaviors. Without patient's adherence to the effective therapies, there would be persistent suboptimal control of diseases, increase diabetes-related complications, causing deterioration in quality of life, resulting in increased healthcare utilization and burden on healthcare systems.
- Positive psychological health may sustain long-term coping efforts and protect patients from the negative consequences of prolonged emotional disorders, illness perception and thus facilitating diabetes self-management behaviors, and better physical health.
- Having patients acquire valued personal beliefs and achievable standards of performance could strengthen self-regulation and self-efficacy leading to more positive experience and healthy behaviors. Furthermore, improved personal resources such as resilience would lead to better functioning of cognition and stronger will power, quality of life, and disease control in patients with diabetes mellitus.

SUMMARY

Diabetes mellitus is rising to an alarming epidemic level. Early diagnosis of diabetes and prediabetes is essential using recommended glycated hemoglobin (HbA1c) criteria for different types except for gestational diabetes. Screening for diabetes especially in developing and underdeveloped countries is essential to reduce the complications related to diabetes. Diabetes development

involves the interaction between genetic and nongenetic factors. Biomedical research continues to provide new insights in our understanding of the mechanism of diabetes development that is reviewed here. Recent studies may provide tools for the use of several genes as targets for

Case Scenario

CASE STUDY 1

Miss D was diagnosed with T2DM at the age of 54. At the time of diagnosis, she was obese, preferred high calorie junk food was having a sedentary lifestyle. Her mother and sister also had diabetes in their late 60s. Weight loss, appropriate exercise, and diet with medications were advised to reduce blood glucose levels. At 60, she developed tingling and numbness in right foot and blister on sole of left great toe. Regular foot care was advised to her. She was diagnosed with hypertension at 62 years of age, and BMI was 23.5 kg/m^2. At present her vitals are within normal limits. Sensory examination revealed hypoesthesia on bilateral plantar aspect of feet. Range of motion of all joints was within normal limits.

Guiding Questions:

1. List the factors contributing to diabetes in this case. Classify them as modifiable and non-modifiable factors.
2. What investigative procedures can be done in this case?
3. How will the prescription be revised from age 54 to 62?
4. What are the possible complications that can happen in this case?
5. How will the exercises be beneficial in this case?

CASE STUDY 2

Mr W is a 40-year-old male with HbA1c level has HbA1c reading of 8.2%. He lives in a nuclear family with his wife and two kids. He does not prefer exercise at gymnasium. His hobby is badminton which he plays every weekend for 2 hours. His BP readings were 136/90 mm Hg. Sensory and motor examination did not reveal any significant findings. His BMI was 24.2 kg/m^2 and waist–hip ratio is greater than 1. His dietary habits consist of long meal intervals and occasional nonvegetarian food consumption.

Guiding Questions:

1. Plan the exercise for Mr W with possible complexities which may arise during exercise.
2. Briefly review the effects of various types of exercise in this case.
3. How will you overcome the problems you may face during execution of exercise planning?

Review Questions

1. What are the risk factors in the development of diabetes mellitus?
2. What is glycemic control and what is its importance?
3. What is the medical management of diabetes?
4. What are the prevention guidelines for diabetes?
5. What complications can be seen in diabetes?
6. What is the role of physiotherapy in a patient of diabetes?

risk assessment, therapeutic strategies, and prediction of complications.

BIBLIOGRAPHY

1. Ahmed AM. History of diabetes mellitus. Saudi Med J. 2002;23(4):373-8.
2. Ali Imran S, Rabasa R, Ross S, et al. Canadian Diabetes Association 2013 clinical practice guidelines for the prevention and management of diabetes in Canada: pharmacologic management of type 2 diabetes. Can J Diabetes. 2013;37(Suppl. 1):S61-8.
3. American Diabetes Association. Standards of medical care in diabetes—2016. [serial online]. http://care. diabetes journals. org/content/39/Supplement_1. S13. full. pdf [22 Mar 2016]. 2016.
4. American Diabetes Association Guidelines. Classification and Diagnosis of Diabetes: Standards of Medical Care in Diabetes: 2018. Diabetes Care. 2018;41(Suppl. 1):S13-27
5. Birke JA, Pavich MA, Patout Jr. CA, et al. Comparison of forefoot ulcer healing using alternative offloading methods in patients with diabetes mellitus. Adv Skin Wound Care. 2002;15(5):210-5.
6. Brochu M, Tchernof A, Dionne IJ, et al. What are the physical characteristics associated with a normal metabolic profile despite a high level of obesity in postmenopausal women? J Clin Endocrinol Metab. 2001;86:1020-5.
7. Burt Solorzano CM, McCartney CR. Obesity and the pubertal transition in girls and boys. Reproduction. 2010;140:399-410.
8. Colberg SR, Sigal RJ, Fernhall B, et al.; American Diabetes Association. Exercise and type 2 diabetes: The American College of Sports Medicine and the American Diabetes Association: joint position statement. Diabetes Care. 2010;33(12):e147-67.
9. Coutinho M, Gerstein HC, Wang Y, et al. The relationship between glucose and incident cardiovascular events. A meta regression analysis of published data from 20 studies of 95,783 individuals followed for 12.4 years. Diabetes Care. 1999;22:233-40.
10. Despres JP. Is visceral obesity the cause of the metabolic syndrome? Ann Med. 2006;38:52-63.
11. Doelle GC. The clinical picture of metabolic syndrome. An update on this complex of conditions and risk factors. Postgrad Med. 2004;116:30-2, 35-8.
12. Ebrahim S, Papacosta O, Whincup P, et al. Carotid plaque, intima media thickness, cardiovascular risk factors, and prevalent cardiovascular disease in men and women: the British Regional Heart Study. Stroke. 1999;30:841-50.
13. Executive Summary of The Third Report of The National Cholesterol Education Program (NCEP) Expert Panel on Detection, Evaluation and Treatment of High Blood Cholesterol in Adults (Adult Treatment Panel III). JAMA. 2001;285:2486-97.
14. Ferrannini E. Is insulin resistance the cause of the metabolic syndrome? Ann Med. 2006;38:42-51.
15. Ghazanfari Z, Niknami S, Ghofranipour F, et al. Determinants of glycemic control in female diabetic patients: a study from Iran. Lipids Health Dis. 2010;9(1):1 [Internet]. 2016 [cited 17 November 2016]. Available from: https://www.pharmacists. ca/education-practice-resources/patient-care/diabetes-practice-tools-and-resources/diabetes-practice-guidelines/ cpg-highlights-chapter-8/.
16. Goldbourt U, Yaari S, Medalie JH. Isolated low HDL cholesterol as a risk factor for coronary heart disease mortality. A 21-year follow-up of 8000 men. Arterioscler Thromb Vasc Biol. 1997;17:107-13.
17. Goodman L, Gilman A. Goodman & Gilman's the pharmacological basis of therapeutics, 12th edition. New York, NY: McGraw-Hill; 2012.
18. Goodman L, Gilman A. The pharmacological basis of therapeutics, 5th edition. New York, NY: Macmillan; 1975.
19. Goudswaard AN, Stolk RP, Zuithoff P, et al. Patient characteristics do not predict poor glycaemic control in type 2 diabetes patients treated in primary care. Eur J Epidemiol. 2004;19:541-5.
20. Hassinen M. Predictors and consequences of the metabolic syndrome population-based studies in aging men and women (doctoral thesis). Institute of Clinical Medicine, Unit of Clinical Physiology and Nuclear Medicine, University of Kuopio.
21. Jeppesen J, Hein HO, Suadicani P, et al. Low triglycerides—high high-density lipoprotein cholesterol and risk of ischemic heart disease. Arch Intern Med. 2001;161:361-6.
22. Kannel WB. Elevated systolic blood pressure as a cardiovascular risk factor. Am J Cardiol. 2000;85:251-5.
23. Laakso M. How good a marker is insulin level for insulin resistance? Am J Epidemiol. 1993;137:959-65.
24. Lambert E, Sari CI, Dawood T, et al. Sympathetic nervous system activity is associated with obesity-induced subclinical organ damage in young adults. Hypertension. 2010;56(3):351-8.
25. Lean ME, Han TS, Morrison CE. Waist circumference as a measure for indicating need for weight management. BMJ. 1995;311:158-61.
26. Lean ME, Han TS, Morrison CE. Waist circumference as a measure for indicating need for weight management. BMJ. 1995;311:158-61.
27. Ligtenberg PC, Hoekstra JB, Bol E, et al. Effects of physical training on metabolic control in elderly type 2 diabetes mellitus patients. Clin Sci (Lond). 1997;93:127-35.
28. Lipsky BA, Aragón-Sánchez J, Diggle M, et al. IWGDF guidance on the diagnosis and management of foot infections in persons with diabetes. Diabetes Metab Res Rev. 2016;32(S1):45-74.
29. Longo D, Harrison T. Harrison's principles of internal medicine, 18th edition. New York, NY: McGraw-Hill, Medical; 2012.
30. Magliano DJ, Shaw JE, Zimmet PZ. How to best define the metabolic syndrome. Ann Med. 2006;38:34-41.
31. Masuo K, Lambert GW, Esler MD, et al. The role of sympathetic nervous activity in renal injury and end-stage renal disease. Hypertension Res. 2010;33(6):521-8.
32. Masuo K, Tuck ML, Lambert GW. Hypertension and diabetes in obesity. Int J Hypertens. 2011;2011:695869.
33. McLaughlin T, Abbasi F, Cheal K, et al. Use of metabolic markers to identify overweight individuals who are insulin resistant. Ann Intern Med. 2003;139:802-9.
34. Mikines KJ, Sonne B, Farrell PA, et al. Effect of physical exercise on sensitivity and responsiveness to insulin in humans. Am J Physiol. 1988;254(3 Pt 1):E248-59.
35. Mogensen CE, Ruderman N, Devlin JT, et al. (Eds). Nephropathy: early. In: Handbook of exercise in diabetes, 2nd edition. American Diabetes Association; 2002. pp. 433-49.
36. Mokdad AH, Ford ES, Bowman BA, et al. Prevalence of obesity, diabetes, and obesity-related health risk factors, 2001. J Am Med Assoc. 2003;289(1):76-9.

37. Okosun IS, Tedders SH, Choi S, Dever GE. Abdominal adiposity values associated with established body mass indexes in white, black and Hispanic Americans. A study from the Third National Health and Nutrition Examination Survey. Int J Obes Relat Metab Disord. 2000;24:1279-85.

38. Poretsky L (Ed). Principles of diabetes mellitus. Springer New York; 2010.

39. Pouliot MC, Despres JP, Lemieux S, et al. Waist circumference and abdominal sagittal diameter: best simple anthropometric indexes of abdominal visceral adipose tissue accumulation and related cardiovascular risk in men and women. Am J Cardiol. 1994;73:460-8.

40. Reaven GM, Chen YD, Jeppesen J, et al. Insulin resistance and hyperinsulinemia in individuals with small, dense low density lipoprotein particles. J Clin Invest. 1993;92:141-6.

41. Ross R, Dagnone D, Jones PJ, et al. Reduction in obesity and related comorbid conditions after diet-induced weight loss or exercise-induced weight loss in men: a randomized, controlled trial. Ann Intern Med. 2000;133:92-103.

42. Saad MF, Rewers M, Selby J, et al. Insulin resistance and hypertension: the Insulin Resistance Atherosclerosis study. Hypertension. 2004;43:1324-31.

43. Schaper NC, Van Netten JJ, Apelqvist J, et al. Prevention and management of foot problems in diabetes: a summary guidance for daily practice 2015, based on the IWGDF guidance documents. Diabetes Metab Res. 2016;32(Suppl. 1):7-15.

44. Segal KR, Edano A, Abalos A, et al. Effect of exercise training on insulin sensitivity and glucose metabolism in lean, obese, and diabetic men. J Appl Physiol. 1991;71:2402-11.

45. Seidell JC, Perusse L, Despres JP, et al. Waist and hip circumferences have independent and opposite effects on cardiovascular disease risk factors: the Quebec Family Study. Am J Clin Nutr. 2001;74:315-21.

46. Stevens J, Juhaeri J, Cai J, Evans GW. Impact of body mass index on changes in common carotid artery wall thickness. Obes Res. 2002;10:1000-7.

47. Stewart KJ. Exercise training and the cardiovascular consequences of type 2 diabetes and hypertension: plausible mechanisms for improving cardiovascular health. JAMA. 2002;288:1622-31.

48. Targets of glycemic control [Internet]. ICMR Guidelines for Management of Type 2 Diabetes-2005 [cited 17 November 2016]. Available from: http://icmr.nic.in/guidelines_diabetes/section4.pdf.

49. Thent ZC, Das S, Henry LJ. Role of exercise in the management of diabetes mellitus: the global scenario. PLoS One. 2013;8(11):e80436.

50. Tripathi K. Essentials of medical pharmacology, 7th edition. New Delhi: Jaypee Brothers; 2013. pp. 259-79.

51. Unwin N, Shaw J, Zimmet P, et al. Impaired glucose tolerance and impaired fasting glycaemia: the current status on definition and intervention. Diabet Med. 2002;19:708-23.

52. van Deursen RWM, Bouwman EFH. Diabetic foot care within the context of rehabilitation: keeping people with diabetic neuropathy on their feet. A narrative review. Phys Ther Rev. 2017;22:3-4, 177-85.

53. Wallace TM, Matthews DR. Poor glycemic control in Type 2 diabetes, conspiracy of disease, suboptimal therapy and attitude. Q J Med. 2000;93:369-74.

54. Wild S, Roglic G, Green A, et al. Global prevalence of diabetes: estimates for the year 2000 and projections for 2030. Diabetes Care. 2004;27(5):1047-53.

55. Willerson JT, Ridker PM. Inflammation as a cardiovascular risk factor. Circulation. 2004;109:II2-10.

56. World Health Organization. Definition, diagnosis and classification of diabetes mellitus and its complications: report of a WHO Consultation. Part 1: Diagnosis and classification of diabetes mellitus. Geneva. 1999;WHO/NCD/NCS/99.2.

57. Yamanouchi K, Shinozaki T, Chikada K, et al. Daily walking combined with diet therapy is a useful means for obese NIDDM patients not only to reduce body weight but also to improve insulin sensitivity. Diabetes Care. 1995;18(6):775-8.

58. Yokoyama H, Emoto M, Fujiwara S, et al. Short-term aerobic exercise improves arterial stiffness in type 2 diabetes. Diabetes Res Clin Pract. 2004;65:85-93.

Obesity

Anjali Bhise

LEARNING OBJECTIVES

After reading this chapter, the readers should be able to:
- Describe obesity and metabolic syndrome
- Describe the recent global changes in terms of obesity
- Understand the causes and complications of obesity
- Describe the techniques for diagnosis of obesity
- Describe the management and rehabilitation for patients with obesity
- Prescribe a fitness program for overweight and obese patients

CHAPTER OUTLINE

- Definition
- Classification
- Prevalence
- Causes
- Physiological changes
  - Cardiovascular system
  - Respiratory system
  - Musculoskeletal system
  - Nervous system
  - Endocrine system
  - Gastrointestinal system
  - Malnutrition
  - Psychological changes
- Complications
- Measurement
  - Body weight
  - Anthropometry
  - Field Methods
  - Laboratory Methods
- Management
  - Dietary changes
  - Increased physical activity
  - Behavior modification
  - Pharmacotherapy
  - Bariatric surgery
  - Management of secondary causes

INTRODUCTION

Obesity is currently an important public health problem of epidemic proportions (globesity). Rehabilitation interventions that aim at improving weight loss, reducing obesity-related complications, and changing dysfunctional behavior, should ideally be carried out.

Physical therapists, as exercise experts, join the worldwide concern for the evergrowing epidemic of obesity, which is probably one of the greatest challenges to our health systems around the world in this 21st century.

DEFINITION

Overweight and obesity are defined as abnormal or excessive fat accumulation that poses a risk to health. In medical terms, **overweight** refers to an overfat condition relative to other individuals of the same age or height despite the absence of accompanying body fat measures and **obesity** refers to individuals at the extreme of the overfat continuum that accompanies a constellation of comorbidities that include one or all of the following components of the **metabolic syndrome:**

- Glucose intolerance
- Insulin resistance
- Dyslipidemia
- Type 2 diabetes
- Hypertension
- Elevated plasma leptin concentrations
- Increased visceral adipose tissue
- Increased risk of coronary heart disease (CHD) and some cancers.

Person's fat content can be measured by three appropriate approaches:
1. Percentage of body mass composed of fat
2. Distribution or patterning of fat at different anatomic regions
3. Size and number of individual fat cells.

CLASSIFICATION

Obesity can be classified based on fat cells and fat distribution **(Fig. 41.1)**:

A. Obesity may be exogenous or endogenous. Hyperplastic (exogenous) obesity is an increase in the number of fat cells in the increased adipose tissue mass and hypertrophic (endogenous) obesity is an increase in the size of the fat cells in the increased adipose tissue mass.

B. Central or android-type obesity is fat deposition in the abdominal area whereas peripheral or gynoid-type obesity is fat in the gluteal and femoral regions **(Figs. 41.2A and B)**. Increases in central fat more readily support processes that cause heart disease. Central fat deposition, independent of fat storage in other anatomic areas, reflects an altered metabolic profile that increases any of the following medical conditions:

1. Hyperinsulinemia (insulin resistance)
2. Glucose intolerance
3. Type 2 diabetes mellitus (DM)
4. Endometrial cancer
5. Hypertriglyceridemia
6. Hypercholesterolemia and negatively altered lipoprotein profile
7. Hypertension
8. Atherosclerosis

In obesity, increased weight of adipose tissue over the thoracic cavity leads to alveolar hypoventilation, impaired PaO_2, and gas exchange. Diaphragmatic descent can be restricted due to large abdomen and can cause abdominal content impingement on diaphragmatic motion. Obesity can lead to obstructive sleep apnea (OSA) or **obesity hypoventilation syndrome** (OHS), which can cause restrictive lung pathology.

PREVALENCE

According to recent World Health Organization (WHO) global estimates:

- In 2016, more than 1.9 billion adults aged 18 years and older were overweight. Of these over 650 million adults were obese. In 2016, 39% of adults aged 18 years and over (39% of men and 40% of women) were overweight. Overall, about 13% of the world's adult population (11% of men and 15% of women) was found to be obese in 2016. The worldwide prevalence of obesity nearly tripled between 1975 and 2016.

- In 2016, an estimated 41 million children under the age of 5 years were overweight or obese. Once considered a high-income country problem, overweight and obesity are now on the rise in low- and middle-income countries, particularly in urban settings. In Africa, the number of overweight children under 5 has increased by nearly 50% since 2000. Nearly half of the children under 5 years of age who were overweight or obese in 2016 lived in Asia. Over 340 million children and adolescents aged 5–19 were overweight or obese in 2016.

- The prevalence of overweight and obesity among children and adolescents aged 5–19 has risen dramatically from just 4% in 1975 to just over 18% in 2016. The rise has occurred similarly among both boys and girls: in 2016, 18% of girls and 19% of boys were overweight. While just less than 1% of children and adolescents aged 5–19 were obese in 1975, more 124 million children and adolescents (6% of girls and 8% of boys) were obese in 2016.

- In India, the prevalence of obesity is higher among the urban populations, high socioeconomic states, and also in South India. From 1998 to 2018, the prevalence of obesity is rapidly spurting due to sedentary lifestyle and consumption of high-calorie food.

- The prevalence of obesity in India is varying from rural to urban areas and state wise also, which is due to various factors. The main factors for variation in obesity are geographical conditions, lifestyle, and dietary pattern, e.g., population in high socioeconomic states (such as Chandigarh and Goa) where the sedentary lifestyle and high-calorie food intake are the main reasons for

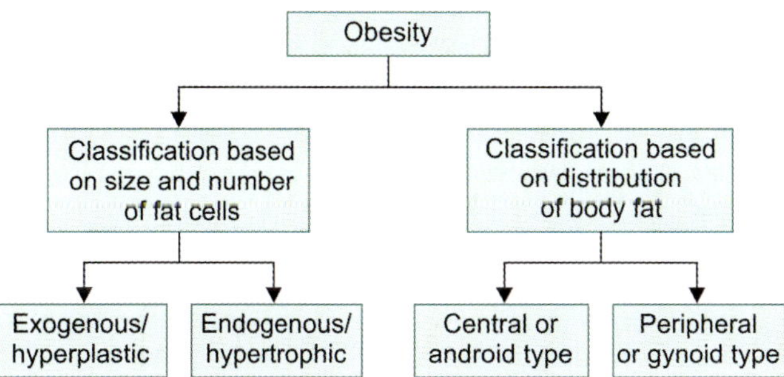

Fig. 41.1: Classification of obesity.

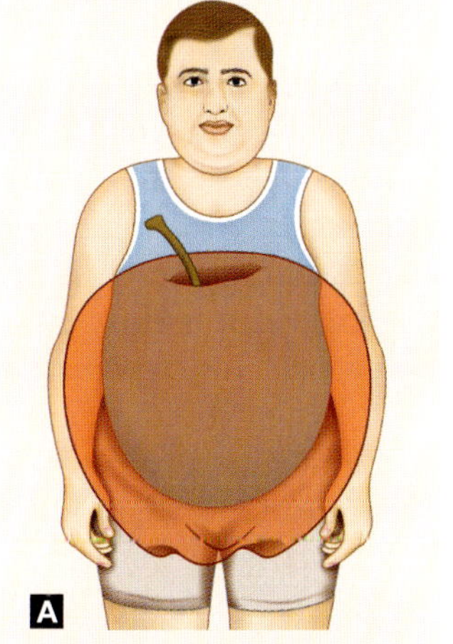
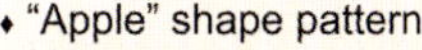
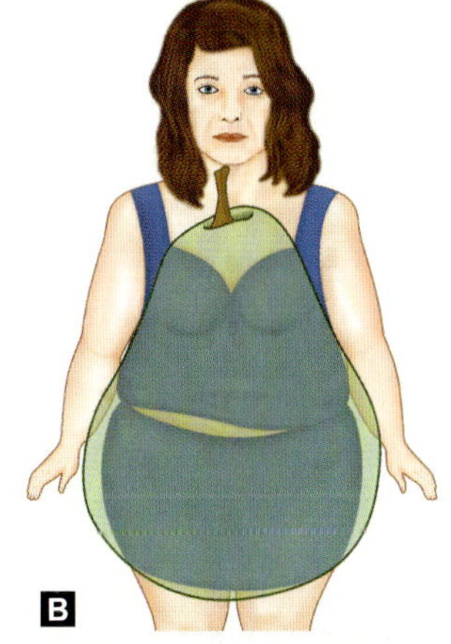

- "Apple" shape pattern
- More common in men
- Fat deposition above the waist
- Greater risk of heart disease, hypertension, diabetes and stroke

- "Pear" shape pattern
- More common in women
- Fat deposition below the waist

Figs. 41.2A and B: Types of obesity. (A) Android; (B) Gynoid.

higher frequency obesity (i.e., >30% in both the sexes) as compared to lower socioeconomic states (such as Jharkhand, Chhattisgarh, Madhya Pradesh, and Bihar). In South India (i.e., Andhra Pradesh, Kerala, and Puducherry), populations have higher prevalence (i.e., > 25%) of obesity compared to other states.

CAUSES

The causes of obesity are multifactorial which include:
- Excessive caloric intake
- Reduced physical activity (PA)
- Genetic/constitutional susceptibility
- Environmental factors

Secondary causes for obesity are:
- Medications that cause weight gain
- Underlying diseases (particularly endocrinopathies, such as Cushing's syndrome, insulinoma, and hypothyroidism)
- Psychological consequence of sexual, physical, and emotional abuse, especially if experienced during childhood or adolescence
- Racial differences that also exist in diet and exercise habits.

When obesity begins in childhood, the chances of becoming obese adults increase threefold compared with normal body weight children. Obese parents likely give birth to children who become overweight and whose offsprings also often become overweight.

PHYSIOLOGICAL CHANGES

Cardiovascular System

Cardiovascular system undergoes changes due to the adaptations required by the body in response to an increased body mass and metabolic demand **(Fig. 41.3)**. Individuals with extreme obesity usually develop *obesity cardiomyopathy* in the later stages.
- *OSA* is very commonly seen in obese subjects. OSA causes intermittent airway obstruction that leads to repeated cyclic nocturnal hypoxia and hypercarbia. This, along with other cardiotoxic factors such as

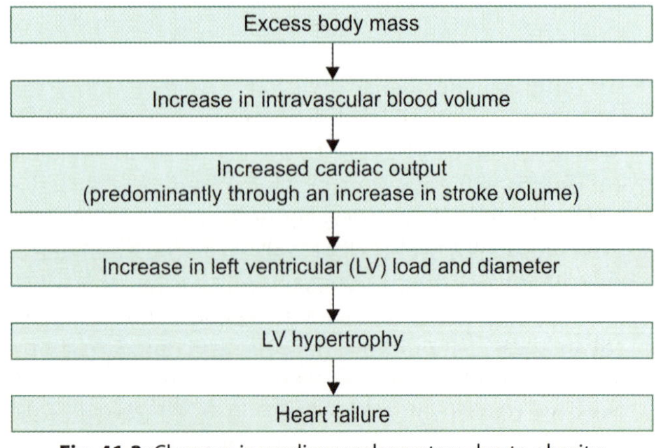

Fig. 41.3: Changes in cardiovascular system due to obesity.

insulin resistance and steatosis, leads to structural remodeling and eventually mechanical impairment in the cardiovascular system.
- Another common feature that is seen in obese subjects is *hypertension*. Excess body weight and elevated blood pressure have a direct relationship. It is impacted by multiple factors such as genetics, insulin resistance, and sodium retention. The activation of sympathetic nervous system and renin–angiotensin–aldosterone axis also plays a crucial role. Angiotensin-converting enzyme inhibitors and angiotensin receptor blockers have been found to be favorable due to their ability to increase insulin sensitivity in the management of obesity-related hypertension along with weight reduction.
- *Arrhythmias* also occur in obese subjects due to precipitating factors such as hypoxemia, hypercarbia, left atrial and left ventricular (LV) hypertrophy, and electrolyte disturbances due to various medications used for weight loss (diuretic therapy).

Respiratory System

The physiological changes in respiratory system are as follows:
- Respiratory function reduces with an increase in the body mass index (BMI) (especially after BMI crosses 45). The impairment in the respiratory function depends more on the pattern of weight distribution rather than the BMI itself.
- The work of breathing is increased.
- Obesity-related changes are seen in the pulmonary function test as well. There is a reduction in the functional residual capacity, expiratory reserve volume, and vital capacity (VC). Severe obesity might lead to reduction in the total lung capacity, forced expiratory volume in 1 second (FEV_1), forced VC (FVC), and FEV_1/FVC ratio. In cases of class I and II obesity, they remain unchanged.

With increased deposition of adipose tissue, the pharyngeal structures increase in size and there is an increase in the airway resistance. These anatomical changes along with an alteration in the control of ventilation lead to OSA. A significant majority of the obese individuals will be able to maintain eucapnia but many would develop *OHS*. The hypoxia and hypercarbia that result from OSA can cause sleep fragmentation and reduced energy levels and motivation to perform any activity. The anatomical changes that occur in the respiratory pathway also increase the risk of developing asthma. The risk of developing *pulmonary hypertension* is also increased due to OSA, OHS, and LV dysfunction.

Musculoskeletal System

The low-grade systemic inflammation, increased loading due to excess body weight and reduced load bearing capacity due to sarcopenia that are seen in

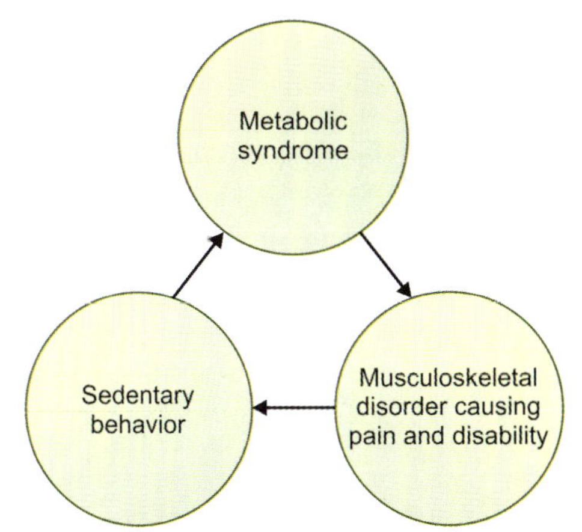

Fig. 41.4: Vicious cycle of metabolic syndrome, musculoskeletal disorder, and sedentary behavior.

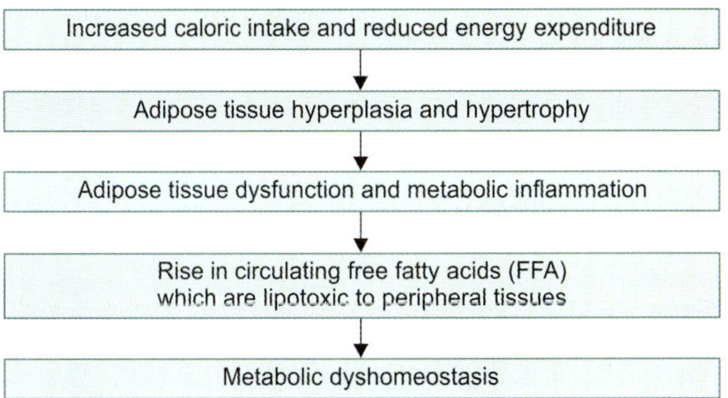

Fig. 41.5: Changes in nervous system due to obesity.

metabolic syndrome, usually increase the risk of certain musculoskeletal disorders (MSDs), such as osteoarthritis, sarcopenic obesity (muscle loss in obesity), tendon pathologies, soft tissue pathologies, and osteoporosis. MSDs carry significant importance since they create a vicious cycle that increases the morbidity **(Fig. 41.4)**.

Nervous System

This metabolic dyshomeostasis **(Fig. 41.5)** leads to Alzheimer's disease and mild cognitive impairment in the central nervous system (CNS) and autonomic and peripheral neuropathy in the autonomic and peripheral nervous system **(Box 41.1)**.

Endocrine System

A BMI of ≥40 increases the risk of developing *DM* seven-fold compared to a normal-weight person.

- Obesity leads to a series of comorbidities such as DM, hypertension, and dyslipidemia.
- A positive association is seen between obesity and alterations in the reproductive system and reproductive hormone levels. It is yet unclear whether this alteration is seen due to changes associated with obesity or as a direct impact of the comorbidities.
- Increased levels of insulin and insulin resistance lead to reduced levels of testosterone among males; increased levels of estradiol and estrone are also

BOX 41.1: Neurological changes seen with obesity.

- **Central nervous system:**
  - Brain atrophy
  - Cerebral ischemia and hypoperfusion
  - Reduced brain metabolism and nerve function.
- **Peripheral nervous system:**
  - Overactivation of the sympathetic nervous system leads to damage to the organ.
  - Reduction in number of peripheral sensory neurons.
  - Sensory polyneuropathy symptoms such as pain, paresthesia, allodynia, and hyperalgesia, which may progress to complete sensory loss (stocking glove distribution).
  - Increased activation of the sympathetic tone may lead to increase in efferent muscle activity, release of adrenaline, cardiac output, liver gluconeogenesis, and reduction in the amount of pancreatic insulin released.
  - Reduced gastric and intestinal motility.
  - Reduced motor and sensory neural function.

found. In females, the increased levels of insulin and insulin resistance lead to increased levels of androgens and leptin.

- Growth hormone (GH) and insulin-like growth factor-binding proteins (IGFBP) are decreased.
- The neural regulation of the hypothalamic pituitary axis is affected, leading to impaired ovulatory function and eventual impairment of the reproductive function. It also causes reduced levels of sex hormone binding globulin (SHBG) in both males and females. Obesity may change the expected time course of puberty. It results in anovulation, menstrual abnormalities, infertility or subfertility, difficulty in assisted reproduction technology (ART), and increased rates of miscarriages and negative pregnancy outcomes due to increased maternal and fetal complications.
- A similar impact is seen among males where reduced reproductive potential results by virtue of increased rates of failure of ART and increased number of nonviable pregnancies. The reason for this reduced fertility among males is unclear since the sperm parameters such as ejaculation volume and concentration and sperm motility are similar to normal-weight males.

Gastrointestinal System

Individuals with metabolic syndrome should be suspected of associated *nonalcoholic fatty liver disease*. Steatosis (fatty infiltration) can progress to nonalcoholic steatohepatitis, which can in turn progress to cirrhosis, increasing the vulnerability to develop liver cancer, portal hypertension, and liver failure.

Mechanical and hormonal changes that occur with obesity make the individual more susceptible to develop *gastroesophageal reflux disorder* (GERD). Frequent GERD episodes can increase the chances of developing esophageal cancer or Barrett's esophagus.

> **BOX 41.2:** Psychological changes with obesity.
> - Anxiety
> - Depression
> - Panic disorders
> - Phobia
> - Mania
> - Personality disorders

Malnutrition

Since most of the obese individuals are stress and unhealthy eaters, the diet they have does not contain adequate nutrients. They lack intake of nutrient-rich food. Also, altered metabolism and other comorbidities, such as secondary hyperparathyroidism contribute to nutritional deficiencies.

Psychological Changes

High BMI is associated with psychological problems as shown in **Box 41.2**.

COMPLICATIONS

Obesity is associated with a number of complications because of abovementioned changes:
- Cardiovascular disease (CVD), e.g., hypertension and coronary artery disease
- Osteoarthritis
- Gastrointestinal disorders
- Cancer, i.e., increased risk of breast and endometrial cancer in women, increased mortality with prostate and colon cancer in men
- Pulmonary disorders
- Insulin resistance and type 2 DM
- Dyslipidemia, i.e., increased triglycerides, low-density lipoprotein (LDL), and very LDL; and decreased high-density lipoprotein (HDL) and cholesterol.

Obesity in older persons can exacerbate the age-related decline in physical function and lead to frailty.

MEASUREMENT

The assessment of obesity can be thought of as being two fold:
1. Measurement of body weight
2. Measurement of body dimensions (anthropometry).

Body Weight

Body weight is the most common method of assessment of obesity. Body weight is measured by various techniques and a variety of scales are available. Body weight depends on the amount of body fat, bone density, muscle mass and other lean tissues, body water, etc. Changes in body weight may correspond to a change in amount of body fat, body water content, or muscle mass. Since it does not very accurately indicate the source of weight change, it is considered to be a very crude method of assessment.

Technique

Body weight is usually measured clinically using a bathroom scale. The subject can keep their clothes on but all other items, such as shoes, wallets, and accessories need to be removed. The subject is asked to stand on the weighing scale with minimal movement and the weight is measured to the most accurate figure.

Anthropometry

Anthropometry is the science of systematically measuring the human body. It is used to measure size, structure, and composition of the human body. Various tools can be used for anthropometric measurements—stadiometers, anthropometers, bicondylar calipers, skinfold calipers, etc.

The following techniques can be used to measure the body composition **(Box 41.3)**:

Field Methods

Body Mass Index

Body mass index (BMI) is a person's weight (in kilograms) divided by the square of their height (in meters). The criteria for classification of overweight and obesity in adults and children according to WHO are given in **Boxes 41.4, 41.5 and Fig. 41.6**.

> **BOX 41.3:** Techniques to measure body composition.
> - Field methods:
>   - Body mass index
>   - Waist-to-hip ratio
>   - Waist circumference
>   - Waist-to-height ratio
>   - Skinfold thickness assessment
>   - Bioimpedance analysis
> - Laboratory methods:
>   - Densitometry
>   - Dual-energy X-ray absorptiometry
>   - Computed tomography scanning
>   - Near-infrared scanning
>   - Isotope dilution method (hydrometry)

> **BOX 41.4:** Classification according to body mass index (BMI) (WHO guidelines).
> - Adults:
>   - Overweight is a BMI $\geq$25.
>   - Obesity is a BMI $\geq$30.
> - Children under 5 years of age:
>   - Overweight is weight for height >2 standard deviations above WHO Child Growth Standards median.
>   - Obesity is weight for height >3 standard deviations above the WHO Child Growth Standards median.
> - Children aged between 5 and 19 years:
>   - Overweight is BMI-for-age >1 standard deviation above the WHO Growth Reference median.
>   - Obesity is >2 standard deviations above the WHO Growth Reference median.

BOX 41.5: Classification according to body mass index (BMI) (Asia-Pacific guidelines).

Adults:
- Overweight is a BMI >23 and <24.9
- Obesity is a BMI ≥25.

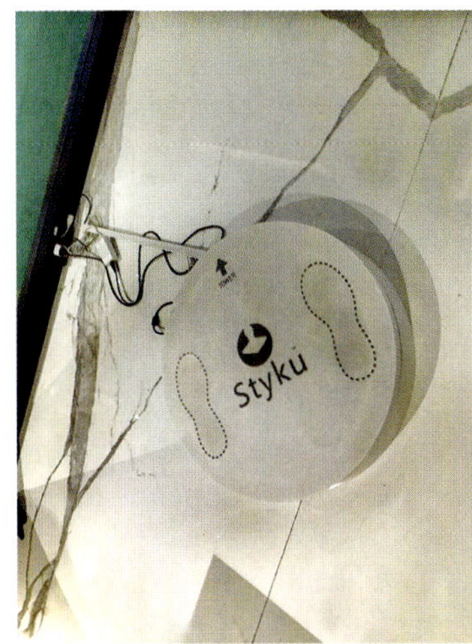

Fig. 41.6: 3D scanner for analysis of BMI and body composition. *Courtesy:* Mission Health, Ahmedabad

Waist Circumference

- Waist circumference (WC) is a measure to assess central obesity. Central obesity is associated with an increased risk of obesity-related complications such as metabolic syndrome, coronary artery disease, hypertension, dyslipidemia, and diabetes.
- WC is a better measure to evaluate central obesity than BMI or waist-to-hip ratio (WHR).
- Two methods exist to measure the WC: WC-mid (mid way between lower ribs and iliac crest) and WC-IC (at superior border of iliac crest). The WHO and International Diabetes Federation (IDF) recommend the WC-mid technique. The recommended cutoff values varies from one ethnic group to another. Asians tend to accumulate more body fat per BMI; hence, they are at higher risk of developing obesity-related complications at lesser BMI values.

- Ethnic differences in the BMI cutoff values were reviewed by the 2002 WHO expert consultation on appropriate BMI for Asian population **(Table 41.1)**. The consultation recommended that in population with a predisposition to central (i.e., abdominal or visceral) obesity, WC should be used.

Technique

WC-mid: Measure the circumference of the waist midway between the lowest margin of the ribs and the superior border of the iliac crest **(Fig. 41.7)**.

WC-IC: Measure the circumference of the waist at the superior border of the iliac crest.

For both the techniques, the measurement needs to be made at the end of normal expiration to the nearest 0.1 cm. The therapist needs to ensure that the tape is snug and no creases or bends are present in the tape. The tape should not pinch the skin. It should be parallel to the floor.

Waist-to-Hip Ratio

- WHR is also a strong predictor of noncommunicable diseases (NCDs) such as CVD or DM.
- WHO recommends WHR, WC, or waist-to-height ratio (WHtR) over BMI for evaluating the risk of obesity-related complications.
- The cutoff values for the Asian population have been suggested as 0.89 for men and 0.82 for women.

Technique

- Measure the WC using the WC-mid technique **(Fig. 41.8A)**.
- Measure the hip circumference at a level parallel to the floor, at the largest circumference of the buttocks **(Fig. 41.8B)**.
- Make both measurements with a stretch-resistant tape that is wrapped snugly around the subject, but not to the point that the tape is constricting. Keep the tape level parallel to the floor at the point of measurement.

Table 41.1: Classification of overweight and obesity by body mass index (BMI), waist circumference, and associated disease risk.

	BMI (kg/m²)	Obesity class	Disease risk* relative to normal weight and waist circumference	
			Men 102 cm (40 inches) Women 88 cm (35 inches)	Men >102 cm (>40 inches) Women >88 cm (>35 inches)
Underweight	<18.5			
Normal†	18.5–24.9			
Overweight	25.0–29.9		Increases	High
Obesity	30.0–34.9	I	High	Very high
	35.0–39.9	II	Very high	Very high
Extreme obesity	40	III	Extremely high	Extremely high

*Disease risk for type 2 diabetes, hypertension and coronary heart disease (CHD).
†Increased waist circumference can also be a marker for increased risk even in persons of normal weight.
Source: Adapted from Preventing and Managing the Global Epidemic of Obesity. Report of the World Health Organization Consultation of Obesity. Geneva: WHO; June 1997.

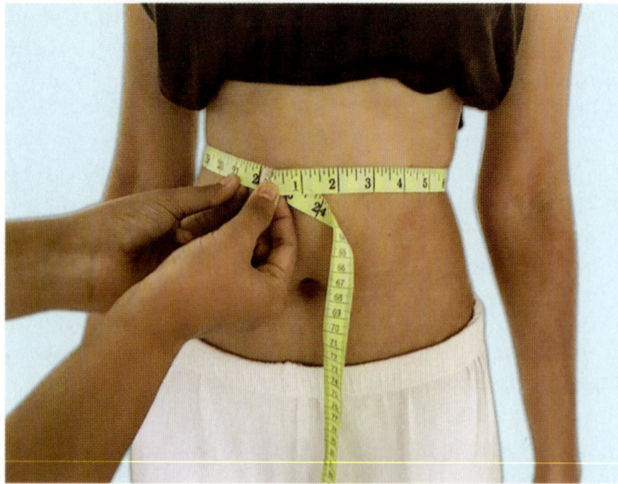

Fig. 41.7: Waist circumference at midway between lower costal margin and iliac crest.

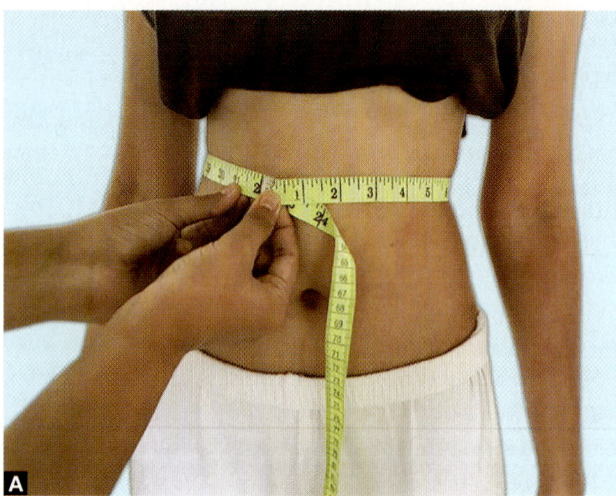

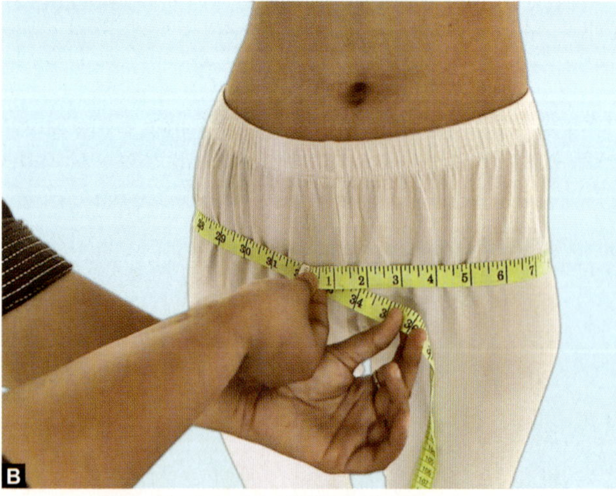

Figs. 41.8A and B: (A) Waist circumference-mid; (B) Hip circumference.

For both measurements, the subject should stand with feet close together, arms at the side and body weight evenly distributed, and should wear little clothing. The subject should be relaxed, and the measurements should be taken at the end of a normal expiration. Each measurement

> **BOX 41.6:** World Health Organization's report on metabolic syndrome.
>
> According to this report, the working definition of **metabolic syndrome** is a condition characterized by "glucose intolerance, IGT (impaired glucose tolerance) or diabetes mellitus, and/or insulin resistance together with two or more components listed below," which includes abdominal obesity in addition to raised arterial pressure, raised plasma triglycerides, and microalbuminuria. Abdominal obesity is further defined as waist–hip ratio above 0.90 for males and above 0.85 for females, or a body mass index above 30.0.

should be repeated twice; if the measurements are within 1 cm of one another, the average should be calculated. If the difference between the two measurements exceeds 1 cm, the two measurements should be repeated.

There is substantial evidence of gender and age variations in WC and WHR, and some evidence for ethnic differences. Compared to Europeans, Asian populations have greater visceral adipose tissue, and African populations and, possibly, Pacific Islanders have less visceral adipose tissue or percentage of body fat at any given WC. It has been suggested that WC, WHR, and WHtR, which reflect abdominal adiposity, are superior to BMI in predicting CVD risk. Both generalized and abdominal obesity are associated with increased risk of morbidity and mortality.

Recommendations about abdominal obesity and WC have been made as one of the components of metabolic syndrome in a report on DM, under the definition of metabolic syndrome **(Box 41.6)**.

The definition for metabolic syndrome has been proposed by the new International Diabetes Federation (IDF). Metabolically healthy or unhealthy obesity (MHO or MUO, respectively) was defined as the absence or the presence of the metabolic syndrome, respectively, as defined below.

According to the new IDF definition, for a person to be defined as having the metabolic syndrome they must have:

- Central obesity (defined as WC* with ethnicity-specific values) plus any two of the following four factors.
- Increased WC (population specific) plus any two of the following factors.

Component criteria	Criteria
Triglycerides	>150 mg/dL Or on triglyceride treatment
HDL cholesterol	Or on HDL-C treatment
Men	<40 mg/dL
Women	<50 mg/dL
Blood pressure	Or on antihypertensive drugs
Systolic BP	>130 mm Hg
Diastolic BP	>85 mm Hg
Fasting glucose	>100 mg/dL (includes diabetes)

*Ethnicity-specific values for WC.

South Asians based on a Chinese, Malay, and Asian-Indian population
- Male ≥90 cm
- Female ≥80 cm

Despite increased adiposity, the so-called MHO subjects are characterized by a favorable metabolic profile (high levels of insulin sensitivity, a low prevalence of hypertension, and favorable lipid and inflammation profiles) and show similar risk of all-cause mortality and mortality for CVDs when compared to metabolically healthy normal-weight individuals. In a large prospective study, the risks of all-cause and CVD mortality were 57 and 76% lower in MHO compared with MUO subjects, respectively. Furthermore, the clinical phenotype of obese subjects is not limited to metabolic and cardiorespiratory aspects.

Waist-to-Height Ratio

Waist-to-height ratio (WHtR) is also a measure of central obesity. WC-mid is used here. Height is measured using a stadiometer. Both measurements are converted to cm and then the ratio is calculated.

Skinfold Thickness Assessment

- Skinfold thickness describes the amount of subcutaneous fat that lies beneath the skin, measured using a specialized caliper **(Fig. 41.9)** by lifting the skinfold.
- The skinfold should comprise a double layer of skin along with underlying adipose tissue.
- The sum of skinfolds obtained from eight standardized sites (given by the International Society for the Advancement of Kinanthropometry) is used to compare with the general population norms or to monitor changes in the same subject with time.
- All measurements need to be recorded to the nearest 0.1 mm and should always be taken on the right side of the body except in the case of loss of body part when they are taken on the left side.

- The most commonly used sites are biceps, triceps, subscapular, and suprailiac. Other sites include supraspinale, abdominal, medial calf, and anterior thigh.

Technique

Before measuring the skinfold, the appropriate point should be marked using a cosmetic pencil. The examiner should next grasp and pull the skinfold between the thumb and index finger approximately 2 cm above the measurement point. The sides of the fold should be parallel. With the other hand, the caliper should be placed perpendicular to the length of the fold. The handle of the caliper should then be released to apply full tension on the fold. This position should be held for approximately 3 seconds to allow the needle on the caliper dial to settle, and then the measurement needs to be recorded. Three measurements should preferably be taken at each site and then averaged to get the final measurement.

- **Triceps:** At the midpoint of the posterior surface of right upper arm
- **Subscapular:** At the inferior angle of the right scapula
- **Biceps:** At the midpoint of anterior surface of right upper arm **(Fig. 41.10)**
- **Suprailiac:** At the iliac crest on the lateral surface
- **Supraspinale:** At the intersection of a line joining front of axilla to spinale (on anterior surface of iliac crest) and another line horizontal to iliac crest
- **Anterior thigh:** At midpoint of anterior thigh
- **Medial calf:** At the largest circumference of the calf, on the medial aspect
- **Abdominal:** At a point 5 cm lateral to the umbilicus.

The triceps measurement is the most reliable one, as it there is usually no edema in that part. Skinfold thickness is dependent on age, gender, race, and the state of hydration of the individual. Older people tend to have less reliable readings since they have less firm soft tissues. Moreover, skinfolds have a constant compressibility; hence, the readings may differ if the technique is not followed accurately by the examiner.

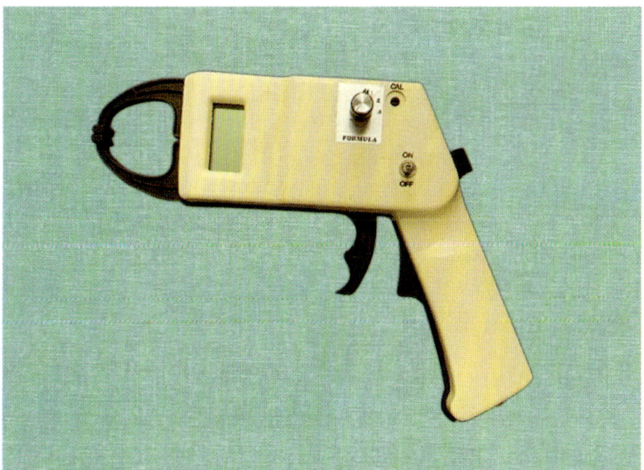

Fig. 41.9: Skinfold caliper.

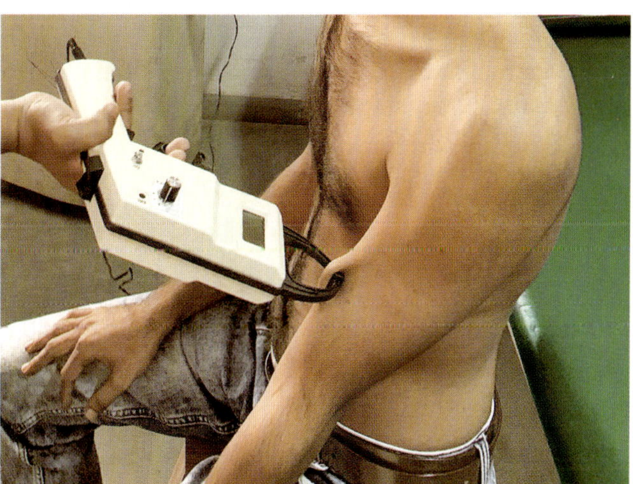

Fig. 41.10: Skinfold thickness measurement at biceps.

Bioimpedance Analysis

- Bioimpedance or bioelectric impedance analysis is based on measurement of the electrical resistance of the body by applying an imperceptible amount of current.
- The electrical resistance depends on the body shape and volume of the tissues from where the current passes.
- Several equations exist that estimate the total body water (TBW) by using the height and the bioelectrical resistance.
- One of the limitations is the rather tedious calculation. First, the electrical resistance needs to be measured. Then putting the values in the equation, the TBW is obtained, the TBW, in turn, gives an estimate of the fat-free mass (FFM).

Laboratory Methods

Densitometry

Densitometry can be described as follows:
- Densitometry is a technique that uses calculation of total body density as a measure for the estimation of the body composition.
- The most commonly used technique is called hydrodensitometry or hydrostatic weighing or underwater weighing. A hydrostatic stainless steel weighing tank is used, with water filled in it. The volume of water in the tank is known. The subject is asked to sit on a chair and their position is secured with weighted belts. The subject needs to exhale all the air out from the lungs and then a nose clip is applied to the nose of the subject. The subject is then slowly lowered in the tank. The amount of water displaced is noted as the body volume. The body density of the subject is calculated by dividing the body mass by the body volume. This method uses the Archimedes' principle to calculate the body fat using an equation containing the total body density and the specific densities of fat (0.9 g/mL) and FFM (1.1 g/mL).
- The technique has several disadvantages. It uses a huge tank that is filled with water, which makes it difficult to maintain and expensive. The subject needs to be lowered inside water, which makes it a difficult technique to administer especially for people having hydrophobia. It is also difficult for the subject to remain immersed inside water, holding breath for several seconds.
- To overcome these disadvantages, the BodPod® has been developed. It is an air displacement plethysmograph, which can be used for body composition analysis. The assessment takes about 3–5 minutes and it is highly accurate. It has the accuracy as hydrostatic weighing but is much easier and quicker.

Dual-energy X-ray Absorptiometry

Dual-energy X-ray absorptiometry can be described as follows:

- Dual-energy X-ray absorptiometry can be used for whole body or regional assessments of bone mass, lean mass, and fat mass. Photons are emitted at two different energy levels over the body. Absorption of these photons takes place in an exponential manner by the body tissues. Based on this exponential attenuation, body weight is resolved in to bone mass, lean mass, and fat mass.
- This technique is rather expensive and, hence, not available at all facilities. It uses low radiation doses and, therefore, is not harmful. It has a relatively quick scan time (≤20 seconds).

Computed Tomography Scanning

Computed tomography scanning can be explained as follows:
- The measurement of body fat distribution is equally important as the measurement of total body fat.
- In vivo imaging techniques, such as computed tomography scanning or magnetic resonance imaging can be used to estimate the distribution of body fat.
- It is more often used to estimate the abdominal fat distribution. Males tend to have more distribution in the abdominal region than females.
- Body fat distribution also depends on the age and ethnicity of the individual.
- The disadvantages include the cost, radiation exposure, and research-based use (it cannot be used commercially).

Near-infrared Scanning

Near-infrared scanning can be explained as follows:
- Near-infrared (IR) scanning or near-IR interactance uses a computerized spectrophotometer containing a single, rapid scanning monochromator and a fiber optic probe.
- It is based on the principles of reflection and absorption of radiations.

Technique

The monochromator emits low-energy near-IR radiations into the appropriate tested site (usually the biceps on the dominant side). The near-IR radiations penetrate into the underlying tissues up to a depth of 1 cm. The other rays are either reflected or refracted. The reflected rays are detected by the fiber optic probe. The probe measures the intensity of the radiations reflected back. The change in the wavelengths of the emitted and reflected rays is used to measure body fat.

The technique requires less expertise and is safe and portable. However, it cannot be used for large areas of the body.

Isotope Dilution Method (Hydrometry)

Isotope dilution method (hydrometry) is detailed as follows:
- Based on the dilution principle, the TBW is calculated if the concentration and amount of the isotope is measured.

- Isotope dilution techniques are the gold standard techniques of measurement of TBW.
- The isotopes or tracers usually used are D_2O (deuterium oxide) or oxygen-18 because they are stable.
- Hydrometry works on the principle that all body tissues contain water except fat.

Technique

Body fluid samples such as saliva, urine, or blood are collected before the test to know the baseline levels. A known dose of the isotope is then administered to the subject. After 3–4 hours, another sample of the same body fluid is taken and the concentration of the tracer is measured. This can be done using either isotope ratio mass spectrometry or infrared spectrophotometry. TBW that is calculated can be used to measure FFM.

This technique though being accurate is very expensive and the technical expertise that is required is quite high. Often, there may be errors in the initial measurement of concentration or there may be contamination or dilution of the isotopes.

MANAGEMENT

Overweight and obesity are largely preventable. Their management requires a multiprong approach. Healthier foods and regular PA, supportive environments and communication are fundamental in preventing overweight and obesity.

The energy balance equation can be unbalanced by:
- Reducing caloric intake below daily energy requirements
- Maintaining caloric intake and increasing energy expenditure through additional PA above daily energy requirements **(Box 41.7)**.

Dietary Changes

The following dietary changes can be made:
- People at individual level can restrict energy consumption from total fats and sugar **(Fig. 41.11)** and increase intake of fruits and vegetables, legumes, whole grains, and nuts.
- Dietary therapy consists, in large part, of instructing patients on how to modify their diets to achieve a decrease in caloric intake. A key element of the current recommendation is the use of a moderate reduction in caloric intake to achieve a slow but progressive weight loss. Ideally, caloric intake should be reduced only to the level required to maintain weight at the desired

level. If this level of caloric intake is achieved, excess weight will gradually disappear. In practice, somewhat greater caloric deficits are used in the period of active weight loss, but diets with very low calories are to be avoided. Alcohol intake should also be reduced. **Table 41.2** gives the average recommended intake of various nutrients.

Increased Physical Activity

Physical activity should be monitored in the following way:
- Regular PA in the form of recreational or occupational activity effectively restricts weight gain and the adverse changes in body composition.
- Individuals who maintain weight loss over longer time period show greater muscle strength and engage in more PA than who regained lost weight.
- The normal pattern of fat gain in adulthood can be reduced by physically active lifestyles. For young and middle-aged men who exercise regularly, PA time inversely relates to body fat level.

The total energy expenditure of infants from age 3 months to 1 year who later become overweight averaged 21% lower than infants with normal weight gain. For 6–9-year-old children, percentage body fat inversely related to PA level in boys but not in girls. Obese preadolescent and adolescent children generally spend less time engaging in PA or engage in lower intensity PA than normal-weight children. Many girls do not engage in PA by the time they attain adolescence.

Physical inactivity has been identified as the fourth leading risk factor for global mortality. The global recommended levels of PA for health for different age-groups are discussed in the following sections.

5–17 Years Old

Play, games, sports, transportation, recreation, physical education or planned exercise, in the context of family, school, and community activities are the PAs of this age-group.

To improve cardiorespiratory and muscular fitness, bone health, cardiovascular and metabolic health biomarkers and reduced symptoms of anxiety and depression, the following are recommended:
- Children and young people aged 5–17 years should accumulate at least 60 minutes of moderate-to-vigorous-intensity PA daily.
- PA of amounts greater than 60 minutes daily will provide additional health benefits.
- Most of daily PA should be aerobic. Vigorous-intensity activities should be incorporated, including those that strengthen muscle and bone, at least three times per week.

18–64 Years Old

Recreational or leisure-time PA, transportation (e.g., walking or cycling), occupational (i.e., work), household

---

BOX 41.7: Management of obesity.

- Dietary changes
- Increased physical activity
- Behavior modification
- Medications
- Bariatric surgery
- Management of secondary causes

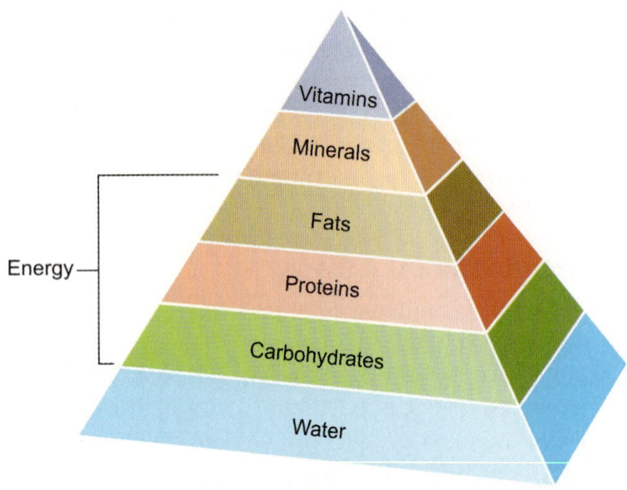

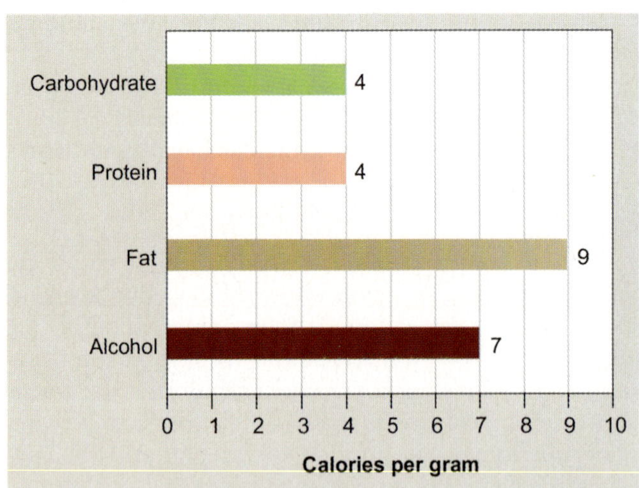

Fig. 41.11: Energy centers and energy values of various macronutrients of food.

Table 41.2: Recommended intake of various nutrients.

Nutrient	Recommended intake
Calories	Approximately 500–1,000 kcal/day reduction from usual intake
Total fat	30% or less of total calories
Saturated fatty acids	8–10% of total calories
Monounsaturated fatty acids	Up to 15% of total calories
Polyunsaturated fatty acids	Up to 10% of total calories
Cholesterol	300 mg/day
Protein	Approximately 15% of total calories
Carbohydrate	55% or more of total calories
Sodium chloride	No more than 100 mmol/day (approximately 2.4 g of sodium or approximately 6 g of sodium chloride)
Calcium	1,000–1,500 mg
Fiber	20–30 g

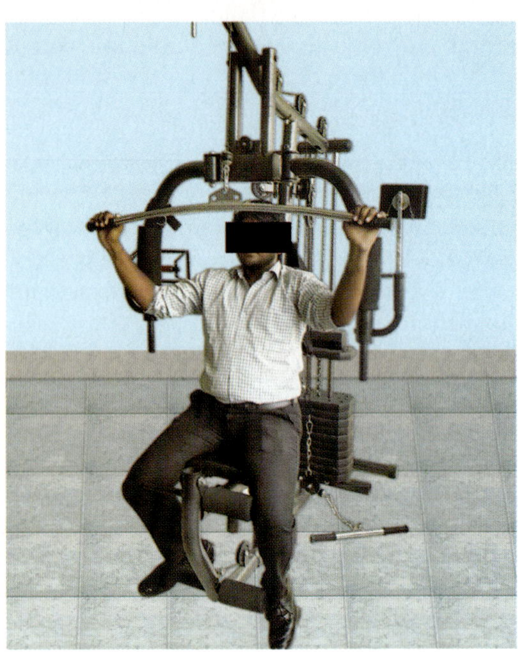

Fig. 41.12: Resisted exercises.

chores, play, games, sports or planned exercise, in the context of daily, family, and community activities, are the PAs of this age-group.

In order to improve cardiorespiratory and muscular fitness, bone health and reduce the risk of NCDs and depression, the following are recommended:

- Adults aged 18–64 years should do at least 150 minutes of moderate-intensity aerobic PA throughout the week or do at least 75 minutes of vigorous-intensity aerobic PA throughout the week, or an equivalent combination of moderate- and vigorous-intensity activity.
- Aerobic activity should be performed in bouts of at least 10-minute duration.
- For additional health benefits, adults should increase their moderate-intensity aerobic PA to 300 min/week or engage in 150 minutes of vigorous-intensity aerobic PA per week, or an equivalent combination of moderate- and vigorous-intensity activity.

- Muscle-strengthening activities should be done involving major muscle groups on 2 or more days a week **(Fig. 41.12)**.

65 Years Old and above

For adults of this age-group, PA includes recreational or leisure-time PA, transportation (e.g., walking or cycling), occupational (if the person is still engaged in work), household chores, play, games, sports or planned exercise, in the context of daily, family, and community activities.

In order to improve cardiorespiratory and muscular fitness, bone, and functional health and reduce the risk of NCDs, depression, and cognitive decline, the following are recommended:

- Adults aged 65 years and above should do at least 150 minutes of moderate-intensity aerobic PA throughout the week or do at least 75 minutes of vigorous-intensity aerobic PA throughout the week, or an equivalent combination of moderate- and vigorous-intensity activity.

- Aerobic activity should be performed in bouts of at least 10-minute duration.
- For additional health benefits, adults aged 65 years and above should increase their moderate-intensity aerobic PA to 300 min/week or engage in 150 minutes of vigorous-intensity aerobic PA per week, or an equivalent combination of moderate-and vigorous-intensity activity.
- Adults of this age group with poor mobility should perform PA to enhance balance and prevent falls on 3 or more days/week.
- Muscle-strengthening activities should be done involving major muscle groups on 2 or more days a week.
- When adults of this age-group cannot do the recommended amounts of PA due to health conditions, they should be as physically active as their abilities and conditions allow.

Frequency, Intensity, Time, and Type Framework

To avoid musculoskeletal injuries, PA should be progressed from moderate to higher level. The following is the recommended minimal frequency, intensity, time, type framework for people who are overweight and obese:

Frequency: 5 days/week to maximize caloric expenditure.

Intensity: Moderate-to-vigorous-intensity PA should be encouraged. Initial exercise training intensity should be moderate [i.e., 40–60% VO_2 reserve (VO_2R) or heart rate reserve (HRR)]. Eventual progression to more vigorous-intensity exercise (i.e., 50–75% VO_2R or HRR) may result in further health/fitness benefits.

Time: 30–60 min/day to total 150 min/week, progressing to 300 min/week, of moderate PA; 150 minutes of vigorous PA; or an equivalent combination of moderate and vigorous PA.

Performance of intermittent exercise of at least 10 minutes in duration; accumulating these duration recommendations is an effective alternative to continuous exercise.

Type: The primary mode should be aerobic PAs that involve the large muscle groups. As part of a balanced exercise program, resistance-training exercise should be incorporated.

- Overweight and obese adults may benefit from progression to approximately 250–300 min/week or 50–60 minutes on 5 days/week as this magnitude of PA appears to enhance long-term weight loss maintenance. For some individuals to promote or maintain weight loss, progression to 60–90 min/day of daily exercise may be necessary.
- Adequate amounts of PA should be performed 5–7 days/week.
- The duration of moderate-to-vigorous intensity PA should initially progress to at least 30 min/day and when appropriate progress to 50–60 min/day or more

to enhance long-term weight control. Adults with overweight and obesity may accumulate this amount of PA in multiple daily bouts of at least 10 minutes in duration or through increases in other forms of moderate-intensity lifestyle activities.

- The addition of resistance exercise to energy restriction does not appear to prevent the loss of FFM or the observed reduction in resting energy expenditure (REE). However, resistance exercise may enhance muscular strength and physical function in people with overweight and obesity. Moreover, there may be additional health benefits of participating in resistance exercise in this population.

Behavior Modification

The management of body weight is dependent on energy balance, which is affected by energy intake and energy expenditure. For a person who is overweight or obese to reduce body weight, energy expenditure must exceed energy intake. A weight loss of 5–10% provides significant health benefits, and these benefits are more likely to be sustained through the maintenance of weight loss and/or participation in habitual PA. Weight loss maintenance is challenging, with weight regain averaging approximately 33–50% of initial weight loss within 1 year of terminating treatment.

Lifestyle interventions for weight loss that combine reductions in energy intake with increases in energy expenditure through exercise and other forms of PA typically result in an initial 9–10% reduction in body weight. However, PA appears to have little impact on the magnitude of weight loss observed across the initial 6-month intervention compared with reductions in energy intake. Thus the combination of modest reductions in energy intake with adequate levels of PA is necessary to maximize weight loss in people with overweight and obesity. Despite the minimal impact of PA for initial weight loss periods of 6 months in duration, PA appears to be important for sustaining significant weight loss and to prevent weight regain.

An effective behavioral weight loss program should include reductions in energy intake and increases in energy expenditure through PA. Thus American College of Sports Medicine makes the following recommendations for weight loss programs.

- Target adults with a BMI 25 kg/m^2 and children exceeding the 95th percentile of BMI based on age and sex.
- Target a minimal reduction in body weight of at least 5–10% of initial body weight over a 3–6-month period.
- Incorporate opportunities to enhance communication between healthcare professionals, dietitians, and exercise professionals and people with overweight and obesity following the initial weight loss period.
- Target changing eating and exercise behaviors, as sustained changes in both behaviors result in significant long-term weight loss.

- Target reducing current energy intake by 500–1,000 kcal/day to achieve weight loss. This reduced energy intake should be combined with a reduction in dietary fat to 30% of total energy intake.
- Target progressively increasing to a minimum of 150 min/week of moderate-intensity PA to optimize health/fitness benefits for overweight and obese adults.
- Progress to higher amounts of exercise (i.e., 200–300 min/week or 2,000 kcal/week) of PA to promote long-term weight control.
- Consider resistance exercise as a supplement to the combination of aerobic exercise and modest reductions in energy intake to lose weight.
- Incorporate behavioral modification strategies to facilitate the adoption and maintenance of the desired changes in behavior

Clinical Pearl

A 100 kcal reduction in daily metabolism translates to nearly 1 pound of body fat gained each month.

An increased level of regular PA combined with dietary restraint maintains weight loss more effectively than long-term caloric restriction alone. A negative energy balance induced by increased caloric expenditure, through either lifestyle activities or formal exercise programs, unbalances the energy balance equation for weight loss, improves physical fitness and the health risk profile, and favorably alters body composition and body fat distribution for children and adults. Regular exercise produces less accumulation of central adipose tissue associated with aging **(Fig. 41.13)**.

The effectiveness of regular PA for weight loss relates closely to the degree of excess body fat. Obese persons generally lose weight and fat more readily with increased PA than normal-weight persons.

Clinical Pearl

In addition, aerobic exercise and resistance training even without dietary restriction provide positive spin-off to the weight loss effort.

Aerobic exercise and resistance training alter body composition favorably (reduced body fat with a small increase in FFM) for otherwise healthy overweight children, adolescents, and adults; postmenopausal women; cardiac patients; and physically challenged individuals.

Clinical Pearl

Scientific evidence suggests that the combination of diet modification and exercise is the most effective behavioral approach for achieving weight loss, and continued exercise participation appears to be one of the best predictors of long-term weight maintenance.

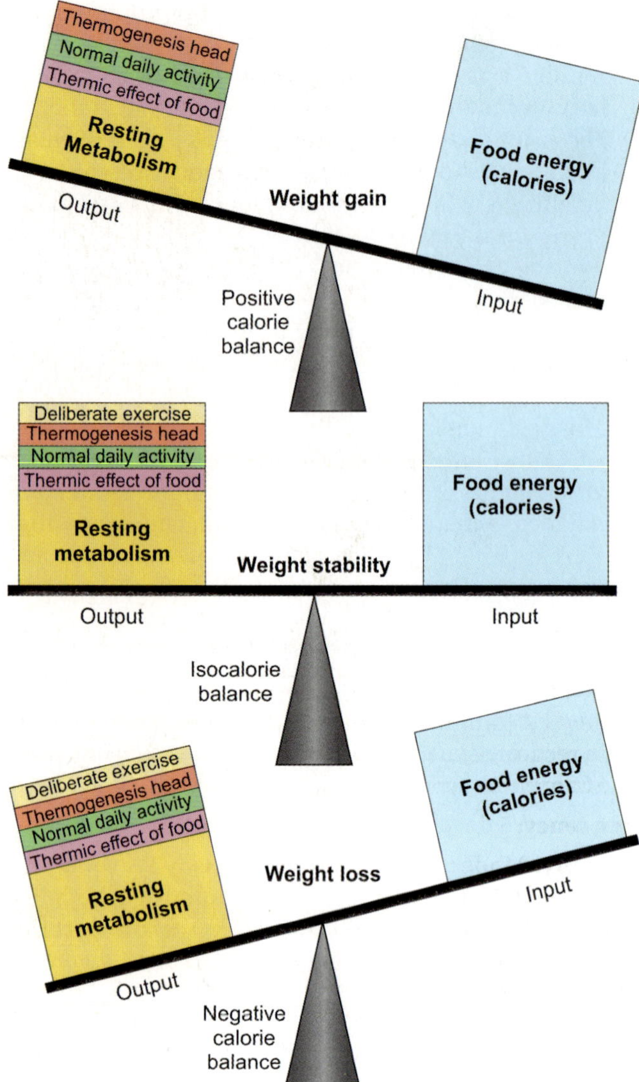

Fig. 41.13: Energy balance.

Clinical Pearl

Importantly, even modest reductions in weight (5–10%) will significantly improve health, while long-term health benefits may be maximized with sustained weight loss of at least 10% of initial body weight.

The goal of behavior therapy is to alter the eating and activity habits of an obese patient. Behavioral strategies to reinforce changes in diet and PA can produce a weight loss in obese adults in the range of 10% of baseline weight over 4 months to 1 year. Unless a patient acquires a new set of eating and PA habits, long-term weight reduction is unlikely to succeed. The acquisition of new habits is particularly important for long-term weight maintenance at a lower weight. Most patients return to baseline weights in the absence of continued intervention.

- **Self-monitoring of both eating habits and PA:** Objectifying one's own behavior through observation and recording is a key step in behavior therapy. Patients should be taught to record the amount and types of food

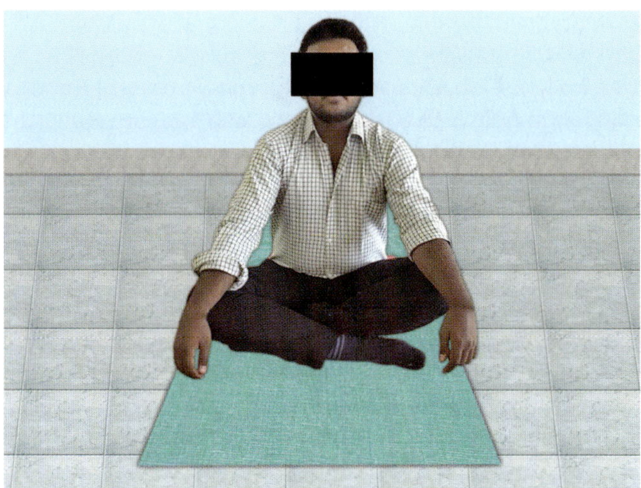

Fig. 41.14: Meditation for stress management.

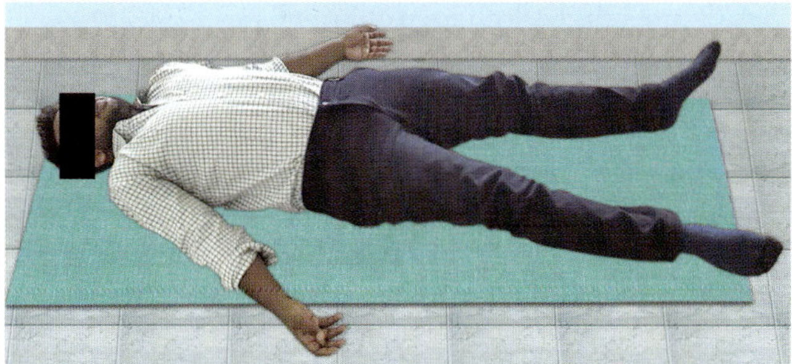

Fig. 41.15: Relaxation (Savasana) for stress management.

they eat, the caloric values, and nutrient composition. Keeping a record of the frequency, intensity, and type of PA likewise will add insight to personal behavior.

- **Stress management:** Stress can trigger dysfunctional eating patterns, and stress management can defuse situations leading to overeating. Coping strategies, meditation **(Fig. 41.14)**, and relaxation techniques **(Fig. 41.15)** all have been successfully employed to reduce stress.
- **Stimulus control:** Identifying stimuli that may encourage incidental eating enables individuals to limit their exposure to high-risk situations. Examples of stimulus control strategies include learning to shop carefully for healthy foods, keeping high-calorie foods out of the house, limiting the times and places of eating, and consciously avoiding situations in which overeating occurs.
- **Problem-solving:** Self-corrections of problem areas related to eating and PA. Approaches to problem-solving include identifying weight-related problems, generating or brainstorming possible solutions and choosing one, planning and implementing the healthier alternative, and evaluating the outcome of possible changes in behavior.
- **Contingency management:** Behavior can be changed by the use of rewards for specific actions, such as increasing time spent walking or reducing consumption of specific foods. Rewards can come from either the professional team or from the patients themselves. For example, self-rewards can be monetary or social and should be encouraged.
- **Cognitive restructuring:** Unrealistic goals and inaccurate beliefs about weight loss and body image need to be modified to help change self-defeating thoughts and feelings that undermine weight loss efforts. Rational responses designed to replace negative thoughts are encouraged.
- **Social support:** A strong system of social support can facilitate weight reduction. Family members, friends, or colleagues can assist an individual in maintaining motivation and providing positive reinforcement.

Pharmacotherapy

The role of pharmacotherapy is as follows:
- Major role of medications is to help patients stay on a diet and PA plan while losing weight.
- Medication cannot be expected to continue to be effective in weight loss or weight maintenance once it has been stopped.
- Therefore an initial trial period of several weeks with a given drug or combination of drugs may help determine their efficacy in a given patient. If a patient does not respond to a drug with reasonable weight loss, the physician should reassess the patient to determine adherence to the medication regimen and adjunctive therapies or consider the need for dosage adjustment. If the patient continues to be unresponsive to the medication, or serious adverse effects occur, the physician should consider its discontinuation.
- Medications are to be used in conjunction with lifestyle modification (i.e., dietary interventions, behavioral therapy, and increased PA).

Clinical Pearl

Pharmacotherapy is recommended for individuals with a body mass index (BMI) >30 kg/m^2 or a waist circumference >35 inches (women) or 40 inches (men) and for patients with a BMI >27 kg/m^2 with the presence of an additional comorbid condition or more than one risk factor for "weight-related" disease, such as hypercholesterolemia, diabetes, and hypertension.

Medications used are mostly appetite suppressants and intestinal lipase inhibitors such as:
- Benzphetamine (Didrex)
- Phendimetrazine (Bontril, Prelu-2, Melfiat-105 Unicelles)
- Phentermine (Adipex-P)
- Phentermine resin (Ionamin)
- Diethylpropion (Tenuate, Tenuate Dospan)

Bariatric Surgery

Bariatric surgery is quickly emerging as a standard treatment for severely obese (BMI ≥40kg/m^2) individuals, because of its significant long-term effects on body weight,

> **BOX 41.8: Bariatric surgeries.**
>
> Bariatric surgeries routinely performed are:
> - Roux-en-Y gastric bypass
> - Gastroplasty
> - Vertical stapling
> - Vertical banded gastroplasty
> - Gastric banding

obesity-related comorbidities, and health-related quality of life (HRQoL). Surgical success, however, is dependent on more than the procedure that is employed and the proficiency with which a particular technique is performed. Several nonsurgical factors, including demographic and weight-related characteristics, eating patterns, and psychosocial factors, may contribute to variability in postoperative weight loss and HRQoL improvement **(Box 41.8)**.

Bariatric surgical procedures **(Figs. 41.16A to E)** generate substantial weight loss primarily by reducing energy availability through decreased intake and/or reduced absorption of macronutrients. Studies of nonsurgical weight loss have confirmed that improved weight loss outcomes can be achieved when an exercise program is combined with reduced energy intake, compared with reduced intake alone.

It seems intuitive that exercise should benefit the postbariatric surgery patient in several ways. Total daily energy expenditure is the sum of resting energy expenditure (REE), the thermic effects of food and the thermic effects of activity. The most obvious primary role of exercise is to increase the thermic effect of activity. A 30-minute period of moderate-intensity exercise, such as brisk walking, is estimated to use 150–300 kcal depending on body weight. This would represent an average of 20% of energy intake in a typical postweight loss surgery patient.

In any weight loss program, it is important to focus on fat loss while maintaining the FFM as the muscle component is responsible for the majority of the REE. The REE accounts for 60–70% of total energy expenditure, so the loss of muscle mass that inevitably accompanies any weight loss has a negative influence on energy balance. A recent systematic review shows that the loss of FFM was a significant component of weight loss for all bariatric procedures and that the extent of loss varies for the different procedures. Biliopancreatic diversion (BPD) was associated with 26%, Roux-en-Y gastric bypass (RYGB) 31% and laparoscopic adjustable gastric banding (LAGB) 18% loss of FFM. Mitigation of this loss of muscle through exercise should lead to a more favorable outcome in terms of body composition.

Cross-sectional studies suggest that postoperative PA is associated with enhanced weight loss and maintenance following bariatric surgery. Two studies comprising samples of >1,000 patients—one conducted in the United States following RYGB and the other in France following LAGB—found that categorical endorsement of participation in regular PA postoperatively was related to better weight loss maintenance at 2 years postoperatively. More recently, postoperative participation in ≥150 minutes of moderate–vigorous-intensity activity, as assessed by the International Physical Activity Questionnaire, was shown to be associated with greater weight loss and BMI change at both 6 months and 1 year following RYGB.

Individuals who progressed from being inactive before bariatric surgery to being highly active at 1 year following their surgery had better weight loss outcomes than those who continued to be inactive after their surgery. Individuals who became or continued to be highly active after surgery had greater improvements in mental HRQoL than those who remained inactive postoperatively.

Improvement in PA has been reported after bariatric surgery for severe obesity, and individuals who are physically active after surgery lose more weight and experience better quality of life compared to those who stay inactive.

Management of Secondary Causes

Obesity can be managed using the abovementioned approaches. However, when the cause of the obesity is some other underlying pathology or physiology, the approach needs to be changed. Several medications such as antidiabetic, antipsychotic, and antidepressant drugs may cause weight gain as a side effect. All underlying pathologies that may be the cause of obesity, e.g., neurological or endocrine diseases should be managed accordingly. The subject should be evaluated for the presence of any psychological disorders and managed with medications, psychological counseling, and exercise.

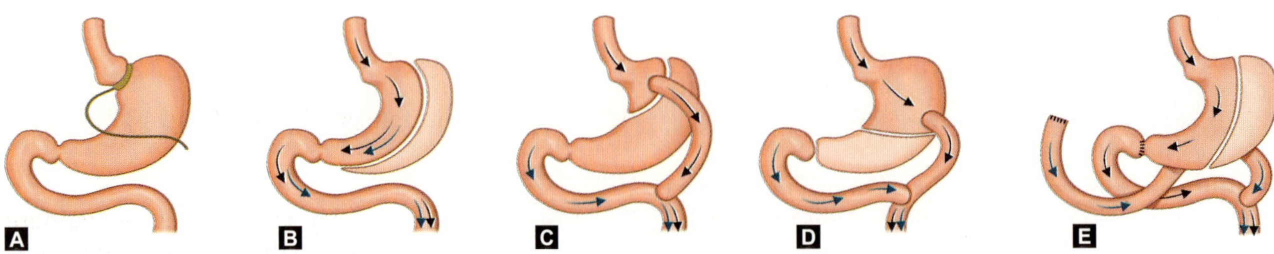

Figs. 41.16A to E: Various types of bariatric surgeries. (A) Adjustable gastric band; (B) Vertical sleeve gastrectomy; (C) Roux-en-Y gastric bypass; (D) Biliopancreatic diversion; (E) Biliopancreatic diversion with a duodenal switch.

SUMMARY

Obesity is currently an important public health problem of epidemic proportions (globesity). In India, the prevalence of obesity is higher among the urban populations, high socioeconomic states, and also in South India. The causes of obesity are multifactorial and include excessive caloric intake, reduced physical, genetic/constitutional susceptibility, and environmental factors. Overweight and obesity are largely preventable. Healthier foods and regular PA, behavior modification, and supportive environments and communication are fundamental in preventing overweight and obesity.

Case Scenario

CASE STUDY

A 45-year-old woman consulted a physician at outdoor clinic for abdominal pain. The physician referred her to a general surgeon for further evaluation where she was diagnosed with abdominal hernia and a BMI of 37.2 kg/m^2. But she could not be referred for surgery since she was extremely obese. The general surgeon referred her to physiotherapy for evaluation and management to attain a BMI of 30 kg/m^2 to get the surgery done.

- Body weight—86 kg
- Body height   1.52 m
- BMI—37.2 kg/m^2

History of present illness—the subject reported onset of weight gain post her pregnancy (she has a 6-year-old son). Her weight was 52 kg before the pregnancy.

Medical history—diabetes (since 3 years; on medication and under control) and hypertension (since 4.5 years; on medication and under control).

Drug history—antihypertensives and antidiabetics.

Personal history—subject is an occasional drinker, does no substantial PA during the day, has a sedentary lifestyle, and stress eater.

Dietary details—daily calorie intake—4,270 kcal; diet high in fat and calories; overeating with multiple bingeing sessions during the day.

Vitals examination—normal.

Bioelectrical impedance analysis revealed 47% fat mass

Investigations:
- Serum cholesterol—243 mg/dL
- Glucose—125 mg/dL

Guiding Questions:
1. Which category of obesity does the subject fall in?
2. What different measurement techniques can be used for this patient?
3. What are the different management options available for this patient?

Review Questions

1. Define obesity and metabolic syndrome.
2. Classify obesity. Mention the causes of obesity and overweight.
3. What are the WHO criteria for obesity and overweight in adults and children?
4. Explain the physiological changes associated with obesity in detail.
5. Explain the different anthropometric techniques used for the measurement of body composition.
6. Write a short note on skinfold thickness assessment.
7. Describe the management of obesity in detail.
8. Write a short note on the dietary changes that can be advised to an obese subject.

BIBLIOGRAPHY

1. Ahmad N, Adam SI, Nawi AM, et al. Abdominal obesity indicators: waist circumference or waist-to-hip ratio in Malaysian adults population. Int J Prev Med. 2016;7:82. doi:10.4103/2008-7802.183654.
2. American College of Sports Medicine. Position stand. Appropriate intervention strategies for weight loss and prevention of weight regain for adults. Med Sci Sports Exerc. 2001;33:2145-56.
3. Bond DS, Phelan S, Wolfe LG, et al. Becoming physically active after bariatric surgery is associated with improved weight loss and health-related quality of life. Obesity. 2009;17(1):78-83.
4. Bray GA. Obesity and reproduction. Eur Soc Hum Reprod Embryol. 1997;12(1):26-32.
5. Campbell JM, Lane M, Owens JA, et al. Paternal obesity negatively affects male fertility and assisted reproduction outcomes: a systematic review and meta-analysis. Reprod Biomed Online. 2015;31(5):593-604.
6. Clinical guidelines on the identification, evaluation, and treatment of overweight and obesity in adults—the evidence report. National Institute of Health ObesRes. 1998;6(Suppl. 2):51S-209S.
7. Collins KH, Herzog W, MacDonald GZ, et al. Obesity, metabolic syndrome, and musculoskeletal disease: common inflammatory pathways suggest a central role for loss of muscle integrity. Front Physiol. 2018;9:112. Available from https://www.frontiersin.org/article/10.3389/fphys.2018.00112. doi:10.3389/fphys.2018.00112.
8. Dağ ZÖ, Dilbaz B. Impact of obesity on infertility in women. J Turk Ger Gynecol Assoc. 2015;16(2):111-7. doi:10.5152/jtgga.2015.15232.
9. Dietz WH. Health consequences of obesity in youth: childhood predictors of adult disease. Pediatrics. 1998;101:518.
10. Dorsey KB, Wells C, Krumbolz HM, et al. Diagnosis, evaluation, and treatment of childhood obesity in pediatric practice. Arch Pediatr Adolesc Med. 2005;159:632-8.

11. Egberts K, Brown WA, Brennan L, et al. Does exercise improve weight loss after bariatric surgery? A systematic review. Obes Surg. 2012;22(2):335-41.

12. Goran MI. Measurement issues related to studies of childhood obesity: assessment of body composition, body fat distribution, physical activity, and food intake. Pediatrics. 1998;101:505-18.

13. Hirsch J, Hudgins LC, Leibel RL, et al. Diet composition and energy balance in humans. Am J Clin Nutr. 1998;67(Suppl. 3):551S-555S.

14. https://www.cdc.gov/obesity/index.html

15. https://www.who.int/topics/obesity/en/

16. Lim JU, Lee JH, Kim JS, et al. Comparison of World Health Organization and Asia-Pacific body mass index classifications in COPD patients. Int J Chron Obstruct Pulm Dis. 2017;12:2465-75. doi:10.2147/COPD.S141295.

17. Maud PJ, Foster C. Physiological assessment of human fitness. Human Kinetics, 2nd edition. Champaign, IL; 2006.

18. Ma WY, Yang CY, Shih SR, et al. Measurement of waist circumference: midabdominal or iliac crest?. Diabetes Care. 2013;36(6):1660-6. doi:10.2337/dc12-1452.

19. National Institutes of Health and National Heart, Lung, and Blood Institute. Clinical guidelines on the identification, evaluation, and treatment of overweight and obesity in adults—the evidence report. Obes Res. 1998;6(Suppl. 2):515-2095.

20. NHLBI Obesity Education Initiative Expert Panel on the Identification, Evaluation, and Treatment of Obesity in Adults (US). Clinical Guidelines on the Identification, Evaluation, and Treatment of Overweight and Obesity in Adults: The Evidence Report. Bethesda (MD): National Heart, Lung, and Blood Institute; 1998 Sep. Available from: https://www.ncbi.nlm.nih.gov/books/NBK2003/.

21. Ortiz VE, Kwo J. Obesity: physiologic changes and implications for preoperative management. BMC Anesthesiol. 2015;15:97. doi:10.1186/s12871-015-0079-8.

22. O'Brien PD, Hinder LM, Callaghan BC, et al. Neurological consequences of obesity. Lancet Neurol. 2017;16(6):465-77. doi:10.1016/S1474-4422(17)30084-4.

23. Report of the World Health Organization Consultation of Obesity. Preventing and managing the global epidemic of obesity. Geneva: WHO; 1997.

24. Wareham NJ, van Sluijs EM, Ekelund U. Physical activity and obesity prevention: a review of the current evidence. Proc Nutr Soc. 2005;64(2):229-47.

25. Wouters EJ, Larsen JK, Zijlstra H, et al. Physical activity after surgery for severe obesity: the role of exercise cognitions. Obes Surg. 2011;21(12):1894-9.

Pregnancy

Payal Gahlot

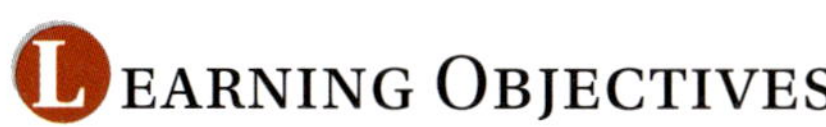 LEARNING OBJECTIVES

After reading this chapter, the readers should be able to:
♦ Understand the physiology and changes that take place during pregnancy
♦ Understand the postural changes that happen during pregnancy
♦ Understand the benefits of exercises during pregnancy
♦ Know the complications of pregnancy and the contraindications of exercises
♦ Assess and formulate an exercise program during pregnancy
♦ Understand the role of physiotherapy during labor
♦ Assess and formulate an exercise program after normal delivery and cesarean section

CHAPTER OUTLINE

- Trimesters
  - First trimester
  - Second trimester
  - Third trimester
- Complications of pregnancy
- Postural changes associated with pregnancy
  - Spinal instability during pregnancy
  - Pelvic pain provocation test
- Benefits of exercising during pregnancy
- Assessment
  - Antenatal assessment
  - Postnatal assessment
- Exercises during pregnancy
  - Antenatal classes/early bird classes
  - General instructions for exercises
  - Contraindications of exercises during pregnancy
  - Diet during pregnancy
- Labor
  - Stages of labor
  - Preparation for labor
  - Physiotherapy during labor
  - Positions in labor
  - Massage during labor
  - Massage during pregnancy
  - Pain-relieving strategies
- Postnatal period
  - Postpartum physical/mental condition
  - Postnatal problems
  - First 6 weeks after the birth
  - Postnatal physiotherapy
  - Diastasis recti
  - Ergonomic principles
- Cesarean section
  - Role of physiotherapy

INTRODUCTION

Pregnancy, also known as gestation, is the time during which one or more offspring develops inside a woman. Conception takes place around the time of ovulation, approximately day 10–16 in the menstrual cycle. Childbirth typically occurs around 40 weeks from the last menstrual period. An embryo then develops as an offspring during the first 8 weeks following fertilization, after which the term fetus is used until birth. Four elements for successful conception are a healthy egg, a healthy sperm, a prepared woman, and timing.

During pregnancy, there are progressive anatomical, physiological, and biochemical changes, not only confined to the genital organs but also to all systems of the body. It is the process of maternal adaptation to the increasing demands of the growing fetus.

The common symptoms of pregnancy are:
- Amenorrhea
- Morning sickness
- Nausea, vomiting, mental irritability, sleeplessness
- Breast tenderness and secretions
- Cutaneous changes such as pigmentation
- Weight gain
- Tiredness/fatigability
- Increased urinary frequency
- Blood volume increases
- Cardiac output increases

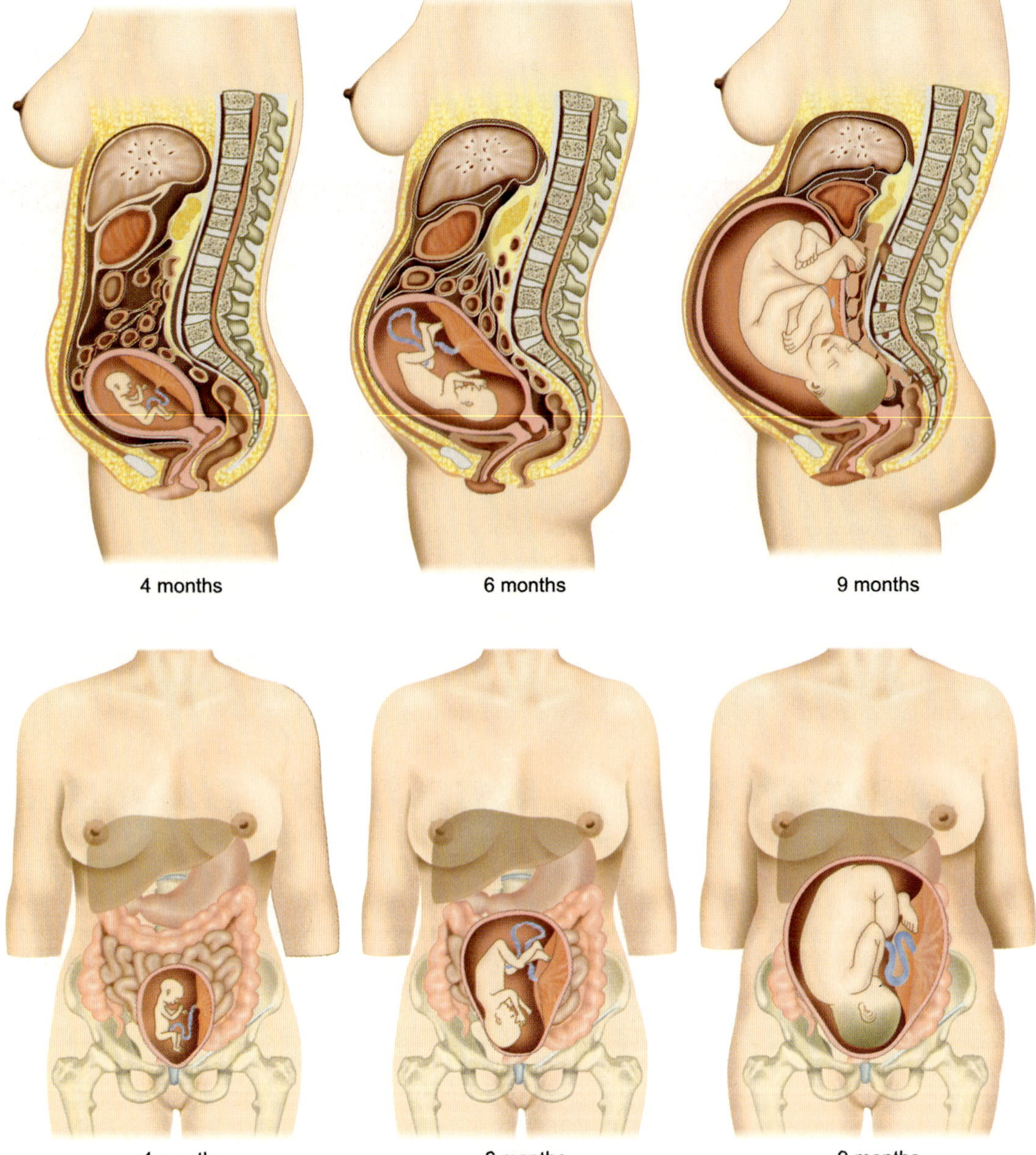

Fig. 42.1: Development of fetus in utero during gestation.

- Metabolic changes such as increase in plasma insulin
- Hyperventilation
- Glomerular filtration rate increases
- Musculoskeletal changes such as carpal tunnel syndrome (CTS) and exaggerated lumbar lordosis.

Development of fetus in utero during gestation is shown in **Figure 42.1**.

TRIMESTERS

Pregnancy itself is often divided into "trimesters," each equating to approximately 3 months. A simplistic view of the child-bearing year can be seen as four trimesters—9 months of pregnancy plus the first 3 months after the birth of the baby. Period between the fertilization to childbirth is called antenatal period.

First Trimester

The first 3 months of pregnancy include a period of adjustment to the fact of having a baby and to the physical changes beginning in the body. Nausea and vomiting are the most frequent and troublesome symptoms. Nausea and vomiting of intense severity is termed "hyperemesis gravidarum." It may result in electrolyte disturbance and weight loss.

Second Trimester

The second 3 months are usually more comfortable, though the changes include development of stretch marks, production of colostrum, heartburn, indigestion and constipation, urinary infections, varicose veins, and backache. Mother may also experience fetal movements.

Third Trimester

This is the time of marked growth for the baby and expansion of abdomen. The changes noted are breathlessness; swelling in legs and feet, cramps, muscle, and nerve twinges; mixed emotions including anticipation and anxiety and "Braxton Hicks contractions." Women may be aware of "lightening" sensation in the last weeks, when baby's head settles into the pelvis and takes pressure away from diaphragm and ribs.

COMPLICATIONS OF PREGNANCY

Following are the complications generally faced during pregnancy:

- Ectopic pregnancy
- Abortion
- Premature rupture of membranes
- Pregnancy-induced hypertension
- Placenta previa
- Polyhydramnios
- Hyperemesis gravidarum
- Pre-eclampsia
- Maternal obesity
- Gestational diabetes mellitus
- Contracted pelvis
- Antepartum hemorrhage
- Multiple pregnancies
- Prolonged pregnancy
- Hepatitis
- Jaundice
- Rupture of uterus
- Stillbirth

POSTURAL CHANGES ASSOCIATED WITH PREGNANCY

Following are the postural changes associated with pregnancy:

- Postural adaptations **(Fig. 42.2)** appear to be a natural consequence of pregnancy. The most obvious physical features in pregnancy influencing the woman's posture are the alterations in body mass and consequent changes in center of gravity.
- Increased anterior displacement of line of gravity occurs. This would result in increased activation of gastrocnemius and soleus muscles, and an active posterior displacement of upper trunk, along with increased extension of hip joint.
- This would increase the lumbosacral angle, an increase of lumbar curvature or a displacement of pelvis anteriorly with simultaneous displacement of shoulders posteriorly.

Marcel Betsch et al., in 2015 found a significant increase in thoracic kyphosis during the course of pregnancy, but no increased lumbar lordosis. The lateral deviation of the spine also decreased significantly. However, they did not

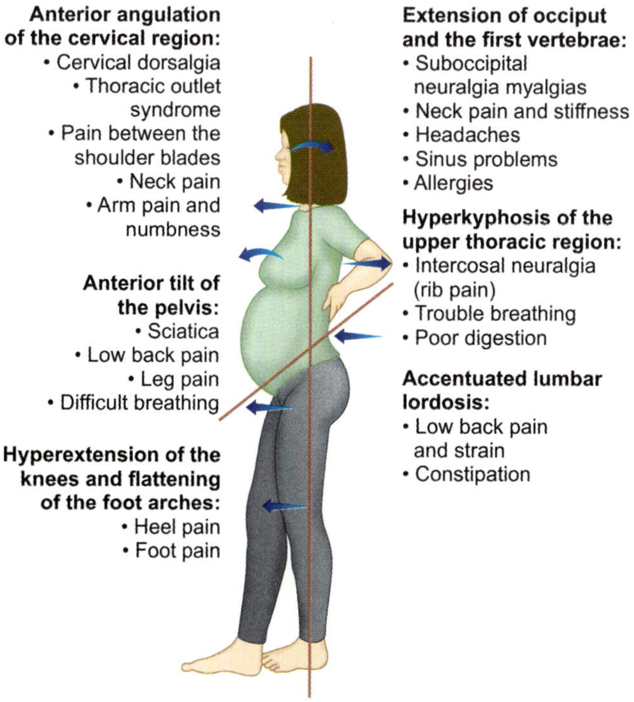

Fig. 42.2: Postural changes during pregnancy leading to different musculoskeletal disorders.

measure significant changes of the pelvic position during or after pregnancy.

Spinal Instability during Pregnancy

The spinal instability is dependent on the coordinated interaction of three subsystems:

1. **Control subsystem:** Neural feedback from various force and motion transducers located in ligaments, tendons and muscles, and the neural control centers.
2. **Passive subsystem:** Vertebrae, facet articulations, intervertebral disks, spinal ligaments, and joint capsules, as well as passive mechanical properties of the muscle.
3. **Active subsystem:** Muscles and tendons surrounding the vertebral column.

In pregnancy, there is a rapid change in passive subsystem due to changes in circulating hormones. Spinal stability is thus affected due to changes in ligament restraints, lengthening of abdominal muscles and consequential change in their ability to generate tension. The spinal stability may be a factor to consider in development of low back pain in pregnant women. In women with chronic low back pain, the activation of transversus abdominis (TAs) is significantly delayed. It no longer acts in anticipation of movement, but rather responds to the movement. Hence, training the subjects to activate TAs leads to decrease in symptoms. A few authors emphasize early rehabilitation of multifidus and TAs so that the establishment of motor plan incorporating their appropriate and early activation may be encouraged. This can be achieved by cocontraction of multifidus, TA, and pelvic floor. The isolated activation of TA is achieved by asking subject to slowly and gently draw in abdominal muscles. Often, there is simultaneous isometric contraction of multifidus posteriorly that helps to maintain neutral spine posture.

There are various causative factors for low back pain (LBP) and sacroiliac pain during pregnancy. Few of them are:

- Weight gain during pregnancy
- Rapid postural changes
- Vascular effects
- Previous back pain during menstruation or previous pregnancies
- Repetitive lifting/bending
- Pelvic insufficiency due to hormonal changes

Relaxin plays a significant role in laxity of symphysis pubis as well as collagenous ligamentous structures of the pelvis. Radicular symptoms are thought to be most probably due to mechanical pressure of ligaments, spinal structures, or nerve roots and also due to effect of "lightening" in the final weeks of pregnancy. Some women may also complain of stabbing pain in buttocks distal and lateral to L5–S1 area, with or without radiation to posterior thigh. This pain is exacerbated by posterior pelvic pain provocation test.

Figure 42.3 shows correct and incorrect posture during pregnancy.

Pelvic Pain Provocation Test

It is carried out with the patient lying supine and tested leg flexed at hip and knee with hip at 90° flexion. Therapist applies light longitudinal compression down the length of femur while stabilizing the other side of pelvis with second hand. The test is positive when patient reports a familiar well-localized pain deep in gluteal area.

The important feature differentiating between LBP and posterior pelvic pain seems to be that posterior pelvic pain often becomes worse during back muscle training, which may be a treatment offered to low back patients.

BENEFITS OF EXERCISING DURING PREGNANCY

Box 42.1 lists some of the benefits of exercises. Detail of benefits is as follows:

1. **Reduce maternal weight gain and fat accumulation:** The US Institute of Medicine has issued guidelines for weight gain during pregnancy based on the body mass index (BMI) of the female preconception. Underweight

---

BOX 42.1: Benefits of exercising during pregnancy.

Benefits of exercising during pregnancy are as follows:
1. Promotes healthy weight gain and reduces fat accumulation
2. Reduces musculoskeletal pains
3. Less maternal discomfort and injury
4. Labor and delivery benefits
5. Effects on potential pregnancy complications
6. Maternal fitness and physical performance
7. Boost up energy
8. Sleep better
9. Prepare for childbirth
10. Reduce stress
11. Improves self-image

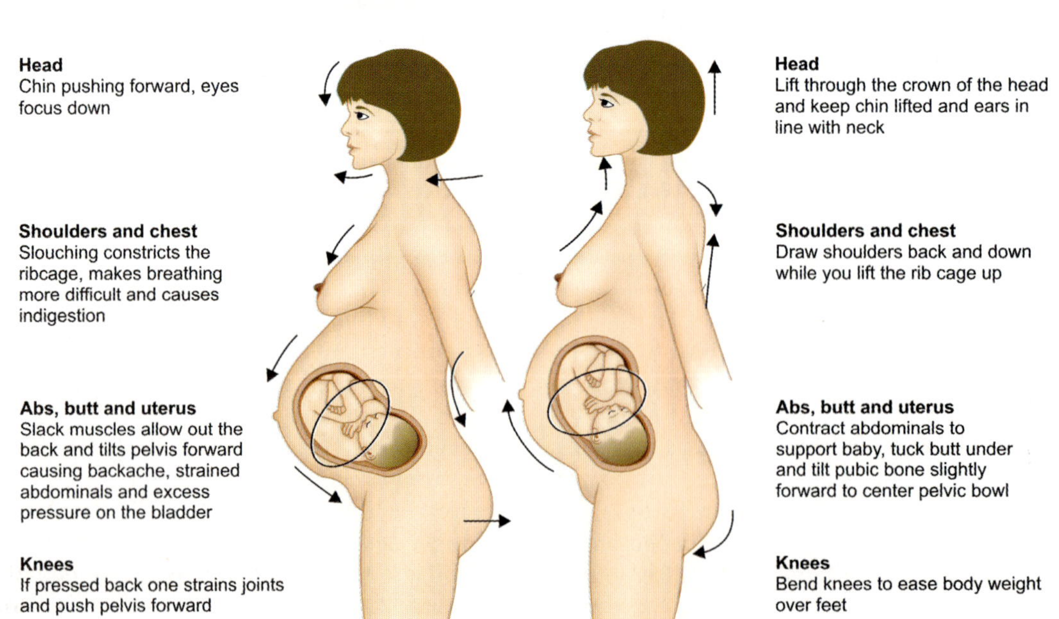

Fig. 42.3: Correct and incorrect posture during pregnancy.

women (BMI<18.5 kg/m^2) need to gain around 12.5–18 kg of weight during pregnancy, normal-weight females (BMI between 18.5 and 24.9 kg/m^2) need to gain 11.5–16 kg, overweight women (BMI between 25 and 29.9 kg/m^2) should gain 7–11.5 kg weight and those who are obese (BMI >30 kg/m^2) should gain 5–9 kg of weight during pregnancy.

Too much weight gain puts the woman at risk of developing certain health problems and complications during delivery and would probably require a cesarean section (CS). Also, weight loss after delivery becomes difficult. Weight of women who exercised averaged about 3.6 kg less than who continued to exercise throughout pregnancy and 15 mm reduced skin-fold thickness than nonexercising mothers. Regular exercises reduced pregnancy weight gain and fat deposition during pregnancy. Women appear leaner than physically active controls. This does not mean that they are malnourished or underfed. Average increase in weight is 13 kg/29 lb and skin-fold thickness of 10 mm during pregnancy **(Figs. 42.4 and 42.5)**.

Does continuing regular exercise after birth have the same effect on postpartum weight and fat?

This depends on caloric intake and caloric expenditure of breastfeeding women. If caloric intake increases to match demand, weight does not change.

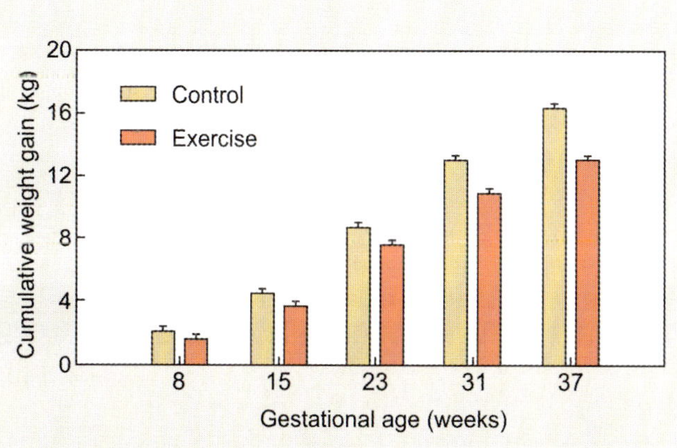

Fig. 42.4: Benefits of maternal exercises week wise.

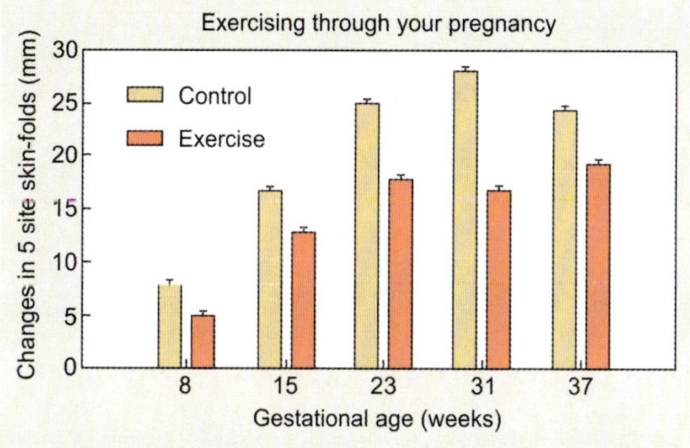

Fig. 42.5: Skin-fold changes during pregnancy.

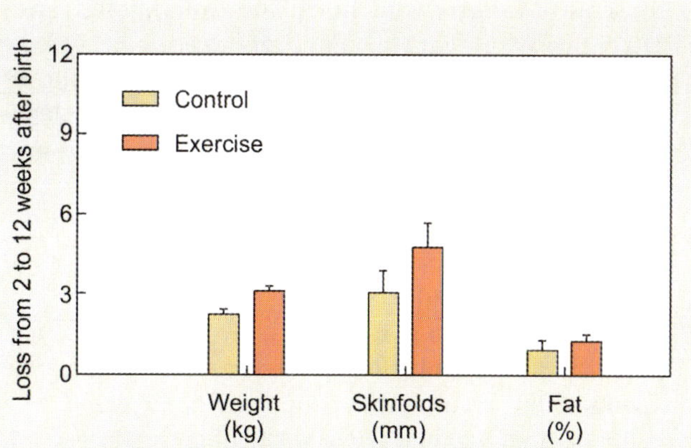

Fig. 42.6: Caloric expenditure with and without exercises.

Amount of exercise required to modify weight gain or fat is greater for women who start exercising in the third month compared to exercise threshold for one who is already fit/exercising before pregnancy. Caloric expenditure of untrained woman exercising at 55% of her maximal capacity is less than that of a fit one exercising at same intensity as shown in **Figure 42.6**.

2. **Less maternal discomforts and injuries:**
   - Regular exercise stretches and strengthens muscles
   - Helps cope up with aches and pains
   - Eases back pain
   - Walking improves overall circulation and fitness
   - Swimming stretches and strengthens back and abdominal muscles

3. **Labor and delivery benefits:** On an average,
   - 35% decrease in need of pain-relieving drugs
   - 75% decrease in maternal exhaustion
   - 50% decrease in need of artificially rupture of membrane
   - 50% decrease in need to intervene due to abnormal fetal heart rate
   - 55% decrease in episiotomy
   - 75% decrease in need of forceps or cesarean section
   - 30% increase in uncomplicated, spontaneous delivery
   - Decrease duration of active labor

4. **Effects on potential pregnancy complications:** With exercises, water bag bursting well before contractions start is lowered. Possible reduction in risk of gestational diabetes and developing pre-eclampsia.

5. **Maternal fitness and physical performance:** There is a 10% increase in maximum aerobic capacity if pregnant women perform low-volume exercise programs for 20 min/day, 3–5 times/week; moderate to hard according to rate of perceived exertion (RPE), hence this will increase the efficiency and decrease time to fatigue. A woman may have a positive attitude to life and the pregnancy, feel proud of her physical abilities, and be fit and ready for challenges of labor, delivery, and lactation.

6. **Reduces fatigue and increase energy efficiency:** Exercises help get through daily tasks, e.g., grocery shopping, coping with demanding schedule, viz. meetings in offices. It strengthens the cardiovascular system, hence women feel less fatigue. Pregnancy gives a mixed feeling of simultaneously being ecstatic, overwhelmed, and anxious. Exercise boosts level of serotonin responsible for mood changes, hence puts women in better spirits.

7. **Regularizes sleep pattern:** Many women experience a disturbance in their sleep pattern as their pregnancies progress. Comfortable sleeping position is very challenging. Exercises help work off any excess energy and tire a woman such that a woman lulls into deeper and more restful sleep.

8. **Improves self-image:** A woman would look leaner and feel fitter and lighter with exercises. It gives her the opportunity for social interaction.

9. **Reduces pain of musculoskeletal origin:** Exercises prevent/reduce low back, pelvic pain/SI joint pain due to exaggerated lumbar lordosis, prevent urinary incontinence and pelvic organ prolapse with Kegel's exercises, abdominal exercises and pelvic floor exercises during pregnancy, improve coordination, balance and rhythm of the body, and also help reduce pedal and hand edema, hence reducing symptoms of CTS.

ASSESSMENT

Antenatal Assessment

The PARmed-X for Pregnancy is a four-page guideline for health screening prior to participation in a prenatal fitness class or other exercise for use by health-care providers and fitness professionals **(Fig. 42.7)**.

Postnatal Assessment

- Obstetric record
  Surname _________
  Name ____________ DOB ________
  Doctor _____________________
- Obstetric history **(Table 42.1)**
- Relevant medical history:
- Antenatal complications this pregnancy:
- Delivery summary: date of delivery
  Stages of labor (time)
- Descriptions of delivery:
  - Labor—spontaneous/induced
  - Type of delivery—
  - Reason—
  - Complications if any—
  - Perineum—episotomy/lacerations
  - Pain relief—
- History—intrapartum history
  - Place of birth
  - Outcome of pregnancy

- Gestational age at confinement
- Mode of delivery
- Appearance, Pulse, Grimace, Activity, Respiration (APGAR) score
- Weight of newborn and sex
- Complications
- Feeding and illness
- Discomfort from sutures
- Breast engorgement and pain
- Nipple soreness
- Emotional state
- Wound infection
- Hemorrhage
- Leg or calf pain
- Problems in defecation and urination
- Fever
- Lochia
- Previous level of activity
- Physical assessment
  - General appearance—pale, sad, fatigued, relaxed, anxious
  - Temperature—
  - Weight
  - Chest and heart
  - Look for signs of thrombosis in lower extremities
  - Abdomen for diastasis recti
  - Pelvic floor
  - Lower back, upper back, neck/shoulders
  - Breasts
  - Neurological examination
  - Inspect pad and perineum
  - Maternal danger signs—heavy bleeding, fever, pain
  - Care of the newborn
  - Sleeping habits, urination, stool, and cord

EXERCISES DURING PREGNANCY

Antenatal Classes/Early Bird Classes

Antenatal preparation for parenthood classes is designed to fulfill the parent expressed needs. The class should not have a didactic lecturer–student image and should be replaced with adult teaching approach. It should be encouraging, self-learning, and problem solving. Antenatal education is successful when it is parent centered, with everyone involved contributing fully.

The classes can offer two or three visits that should be attended by women at around 6–8 weeks pregnancy of early physiotherapy advice and instructions. Then, there is usually a course of six classes of 2 hours each, once per week during the third trimester. The physiotherapist takes 1 hour of each class and the other hour taken by various member of team, e.g., midwives, health visitor, or dental hygienist, etc. These may be held in hospitals, but increasingly are held in the community. Women are encouraged to bring their partners.

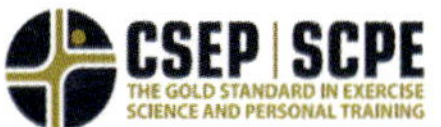

PARmed-X FOR PREGNANCY

Physical Activity Readiness Medical Examination

PARmed-X for PREGNANCY is a guideline for health screening prior to participation in a prenatal fitness class or other exercise.

Healthy women with uncomplicated pregnancies can integrate physical activity into their daily living and can participate without significant risks either to themselves or to their unborn child. Postulated benefits of such programs include improved aerobic and muscular fitness, promotion of appropriate weight gain, and facilitation of labour. Regular exercise may also help to prevent gestational glucose intolerance and pregnancy-induced hypertension.

The safety of prenatal exercise programs depends on an adequate level of maternal-fetal physiological reserve. PARmed-X for PREGNANCY is a convenient checklist and prescription for use by health care providers to evaluate pregnant patients who want to enter a prenatal fitness program and for ongoing medical surveillance of exercising pregnant patients.

Instructions for use of the 4-page PARmed-X for PREGNANCY are the following:

1 The patient should fill out the section on PATIENT INFORMATION and the PRE-EXERCISE HEALTH CHECKLIST (PART 1, 2, 3, and 4 on p. 1) and give the form to the health care provider monitoring her pregnancy.

2 The health care provider should check the information provided by the patient for accuracy and fill out SECTION C on CONTRAINDICATIONS (p. 2) based on current medical information.

3 If no exercise contraindications exist, the HEALTH EVALUATION FORM (p. 3) should be completed, signed by the health care provider, and given by the patient to her prenatal fitness professional.

In addition to prudent medical care, participation in appropriate types, intensities and amounts of exercise is recommended to increase the likelihood of a beneficial pregnancy outcome. PARmed-X for PREGNANCY provides recommendations for individualized exercise prescription (p. 3) and program safety (p. 4).

Note: **Sections A and B** should be completed by the patient before the appointment with the health care provider.

A PATIENT INFORMATION

NAME _______________________   ADDRESS _______________________

PHONE _______________   BIRTHDATE __MM__ / __DD__ / __YEAR__   HEALTH INSURANCE No. _______________

NAME OF PRENATAL FITNESS PROFESSIONAL _______________   PHONE NUMBER OF PRENATAL FITNESS PROFESSIONAL _______________

B PRE-EXERCISE HEALTH CHECKLIST

PART 1: GENERAL HEALTH STATUS

In the past, have you experienced: Y N

1 Miscarriage in an earlier pregnancy?   ☐ ☐
2 Other pregnancy complications?   ☐ ☐
3 I have completed a PAR-Q within the last 30 days.   ☐ ☐

If you answered YES to question 1 or 2, please explain:

____

Number of previous pregnancies: _______________

PART 2: STATUS OF CURRENT PREGNANCY

Due Date: _____ / _____ / _______

During this prenancy, have you experienced: Y N

1 Marked fatigue?   ☐ ☐
2 Bleeding from the vagina ("spotting")?   ☐ ☐
3 Unexplained faintness or dizziness?   ☐ ☐
4 Unexplained abdominal pain?   ☐ ☐
5 Sudden swelling of ankles, hands or face?   ☐ ☐
6 Persistent headaches or problems with headaches?   ☐ ☐
7 Swelling, pain or redness in the calf of one leg?   ☐ ☐
8 Absence of fetal movement after 6th month?   ☐ ☐
9 Failure to gain weight after 5th month?   ☐ ☐

If you answered YES to any of the above questions, please explain:

____

PART 3: ACTIVITY HABITS DURING THE PAST MONTH

1 List only regular fitness/recreational activities:

INTENSITY	FREQUENCY (times/week)			TIME (minutes/day)		
	1-2	2-4	4+	<20	20-40	40+
Heavy						
Medium						
Light						

2 Does your regular occupation (job/home) activity involve: Y N

Heavy lifting?   ☐ ☐
Frequent walking/stair climbing?   ☐ ☐
Occasional walking (> once/hr)?   ☐ ☐
Prolonged standing?   ☐ ☐
Mainly sitting?   ☐ ☐
Normal daily activity?   ☐ ☐

3 Do you currently smoke tobacco?*   ☐ ☐
4 Do you consume alcohol?*   ☐ ☐

PART 4: PHYSICAL ACTIVITY INTENTIONS

What physical activity do you intend to do?

Is this a change from what you currently do?   ☐ YES   ☐ NO

*Note: Pregnant women are strongly advised not to smoke or consume alcohol during pregnancy and during lactation.

Fig. 42.7: PARmed-X.

Table 42.1: Obstetric history.

Obstetric history		Complications	Gravida	Para						
No	Date	Type of delivery	Gestation	Pregnancy	Labor	Puerperium	Sex	Birth weight	Fetal outcome method of feeding
1.									
2.									
3.									

SECTION 3: Management Strategies

The antenatal classes aim to:

- Help couples check and increase knowledge of physiological changes of pregnancy, labor, and puerperium.
- Monitor and promote well-being of a mother and her developing baby.
- Show ways useful for coping with physical changes of pregnancy and their associated discomforts.
- Guide toward realistic understanding of labor.
- Encourage to consider profound change in lifestyle that parenthood brings emotional maturity, etc.
- Encourage to talk and air any fears, ask questions, and help them obtain satisfactory answers.
- Add to their knowledge about physiological changes of pregnancy, labor, and puerperium.
- Encourage to consider profound change in lifestyle that parenthood brings, emotional maturity necessary and additional responsibilities explained.
- Encourage to talk and air any fears, ask questions, and helped with satisfactory answers.
- Incorporate ergonomic principles of back care in moving and changing positions, gentle stretches for muscles, practice of relaxation, and breath awareness.

Class Design

These can be designed as follows:

- A small group up to 10 is ideal.
- Well-ventilated, air-conditioned room.
- Low impact movements.
- Slow music with strong beat.
- Mirror for visual feedback.
- Participant is encouraged to wear loose comfortable clothes, supportive shoes and under clothes.
- Water should be available.
- Emergency services should be available.

Class Structure

In the following way, the class can be structured:

- At the beginning of a class, the physiotherapist introduces herself and gives guidelines for exercises.
- Safety aspects are also explained along with risks and warnings signs for exercise.
- A woman should be encouraged to take lots of fluid while in the session. She is encouraged to drink water to maintain hydration. Liberal consumption of liquids before, during and after exercise helps to prevent hyperthermia and dehydration.
- Basic vitals should be monitored prior to beginning the exercises.
- A detailed assessment related to pregnancy, musculoskeletal conditions, and other medical conditions is required.
- A warm-up, modified cardiovascular section and a cool down is the exercise protocol to be followed.
- The class can also include strengthening, stability and toning exercises, lengthening of tight soft-tissue structures, and relaxation exercises.

- Adequate breaks are allowed in between the session wherein heart rate is monitored.

General Instructions for Exercises

Instructions and Safety

Following are the list of instructions that should be taken care of while exercising:

- Education
- Necessary loose clothing
- Appropriate footwear (sports shoes)
- Safe and cool environment
- Speed of exercise
- Eating pattern (exercise 1–2 hours post meals)
- Rest–activity cycle
- Proper hydration and salt intake
- Avoid excessive fatigue
- Avoid overheating of body
- Consult for medical help immediately

Exercise Guidelines

Following are the guidelines that should be kept in mind while exercising:

- Prenatal exercise prescription is individualized according to health status, interests, and fitness level.
- **Frequency:** Moderate exercise at least 3 times/week.
- **Intensity:** 10–14 RPE on Borg rating scale or heart rate as shown in **Table 42.2**.
- **Time/duration:** 30 minutes or more.
- **Type:** Aerobic exercise, yoga, circuit interval training with warm up and cool down 10–15 minutes.
- Exercise requiring lying on back should be avoided after first trimester.
- Exercise intensity should be light enough to allow conversation and prevent shortness of breath, fatigue, pain, and exhaustion; strength training should be limited to 2–3 times/week with low resistance.

Exercise Program

Exercises are tailor made for each individual. They are individualized or conducted in antenatal class.

Begin with warm-up/stretching exercises (**Figs. 42.8A and B**):

- Neck stretch
- Upper back stretch
- Calf stretch

Table 42.2: Heart rate target zone according to maternal age.

Maternal age	HR target zone (beats/min)
<20	140–155
20–29	135–150
30–39	130–145
40 or more	124–140

Source: American College of Obstetricians and Gynecologists (ACOG), 2015.

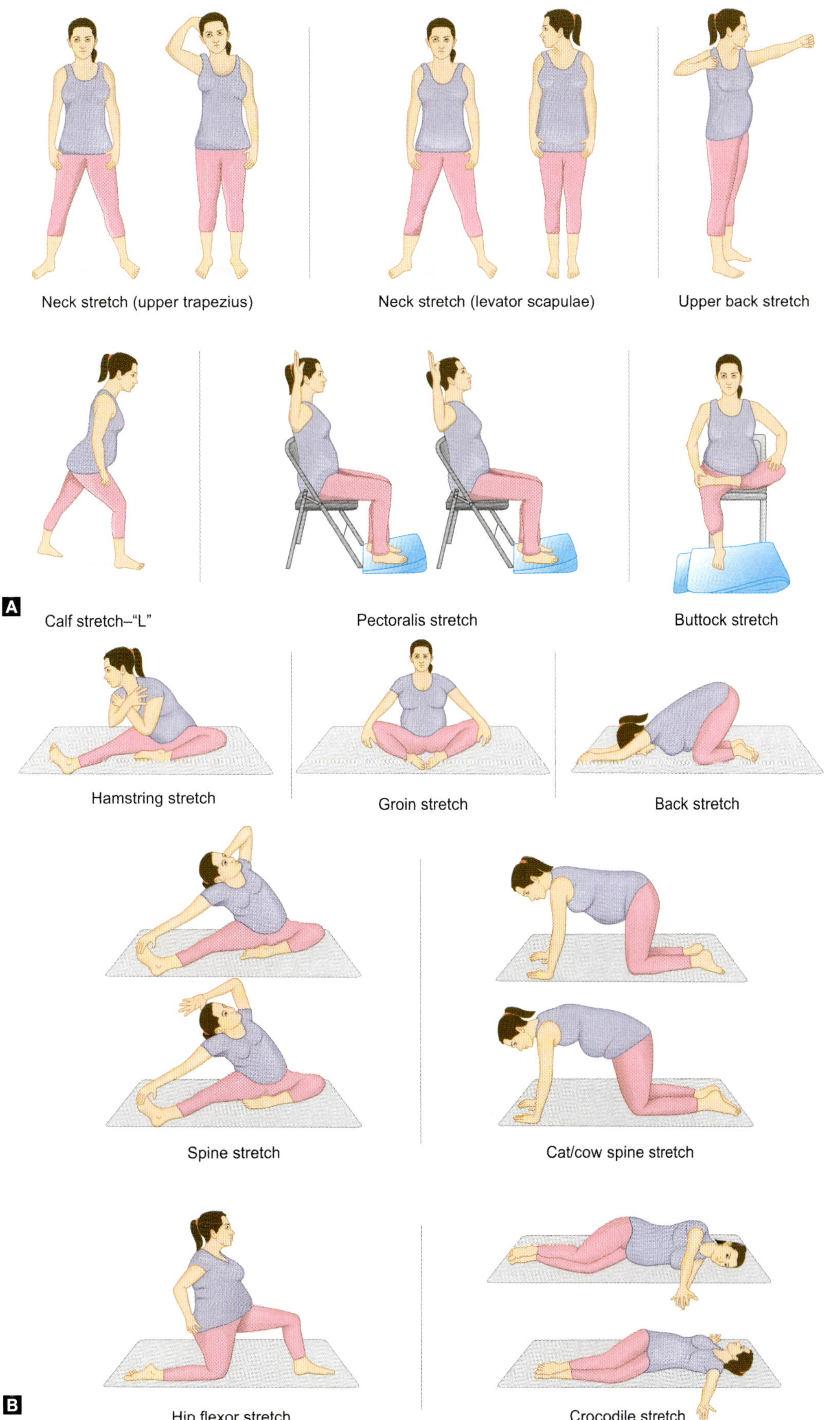

Figs. 42.8A and B: Stretching exercises during pregnancy.
Courtesy: Purvi K Changela, Role of Physiotherapist in Obstetric and Gynecological Conditions, 1st edition, Jaypee Brothers.

- Pectoralis stretch
- Buttock stretch
- Hamstring stretch
- Groin stretch
- Back stretch
- Spine stretch
- Cat/cow/spine stretch
- Hip flexor stretch
- Crocodile stretch
- Upper backstretch

Exercises for First Trimester

Following exercises are recommended for the first trimester:

- Stretching exercises
- Breathing exercises
- Anulom vilom
- Chin tucks
- Simple basic yogasanas—matsyasana, virabhadrasana, tadasana
- Upper chest mobility exercises
- No exercises which increase intra-abdominal pressure
- No breath holding

Exercises for Second and Third Trimester

Following exercises are recommended for the second and third trimester:

- Semirecumbent curls with ball support
- TA on all fours
- Sacroiliac and low back exercises
- Exercises for edema
- Postural correction exercises
- Perineal strengthening
- Pelvic floor exercises (Kegel's exercises)
- Pelvic circles
- Pelvic tilting exercises **(Figs. 42.9 to 42.11)**
- Exercises to support and strengthen back and abdominal muscles
- Quadruped with 2/3 point weight bearing **(Fig. 42.12)**
- Heel slides
- Half squats/full squats/sumo squats **(Figs. 42.13 and 42.14)**
- Lamaze technique
- Massages
- Mother aerobic exercises

Physioball Exercises during Pregnancy

One of the biggest benefits of using a pregnancy ball is that it helps open up your hips to make room for baby to descend into the pelvis. Following exercises can be performed **(Figs. 42.15 and 42.16)**:

- Ball bouncing in sitting
- Pelvic tilting
- Pelvic circles on ball
- Semirecumbent curls

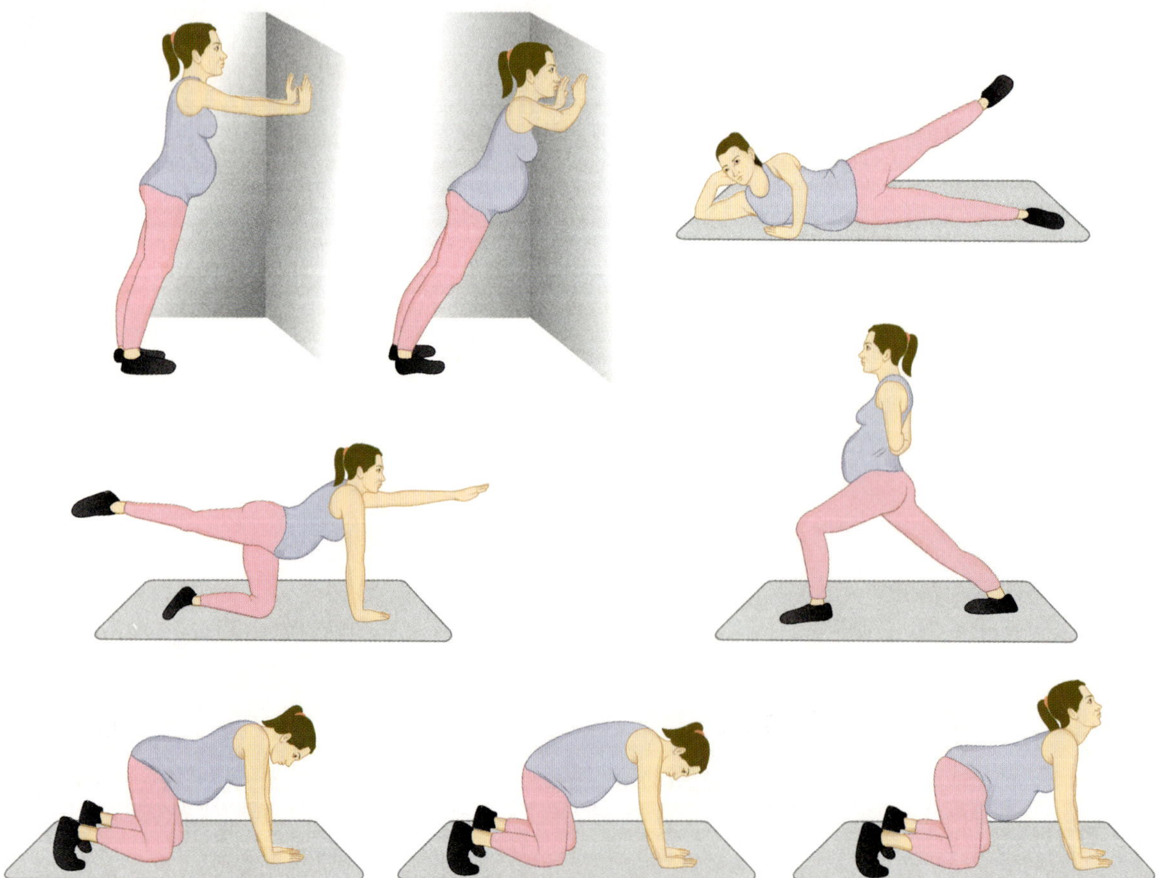

Fig. 42.9: Pelvic tilting exercises.

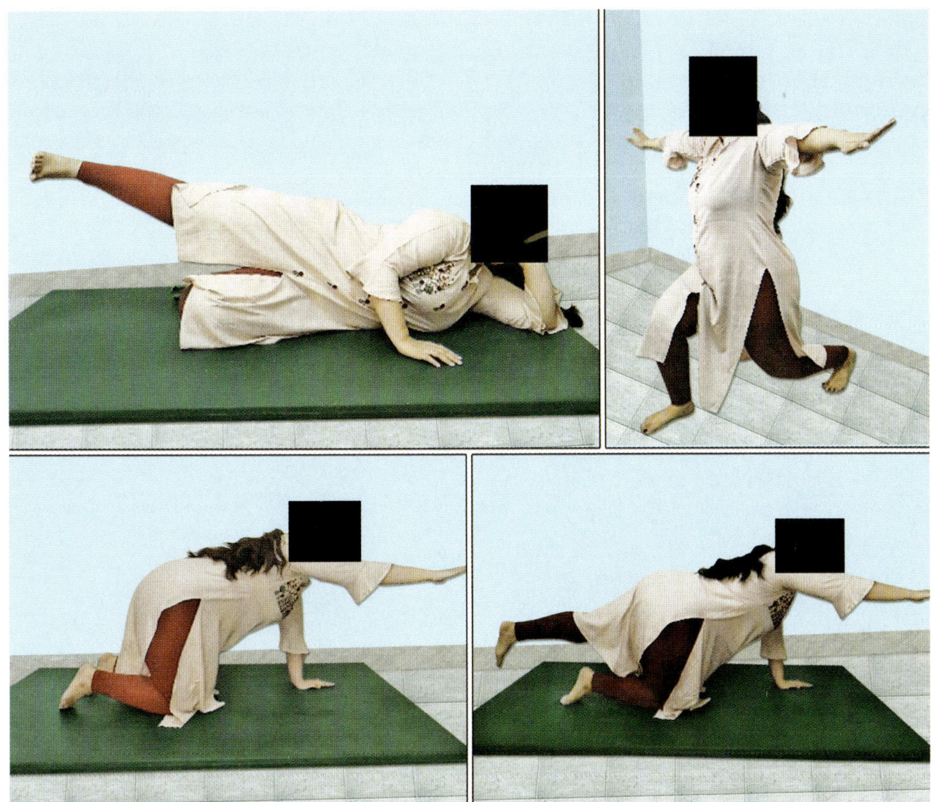

Fig. 42.10: Lower extremity and quadruped exercises (during second and third trimester).

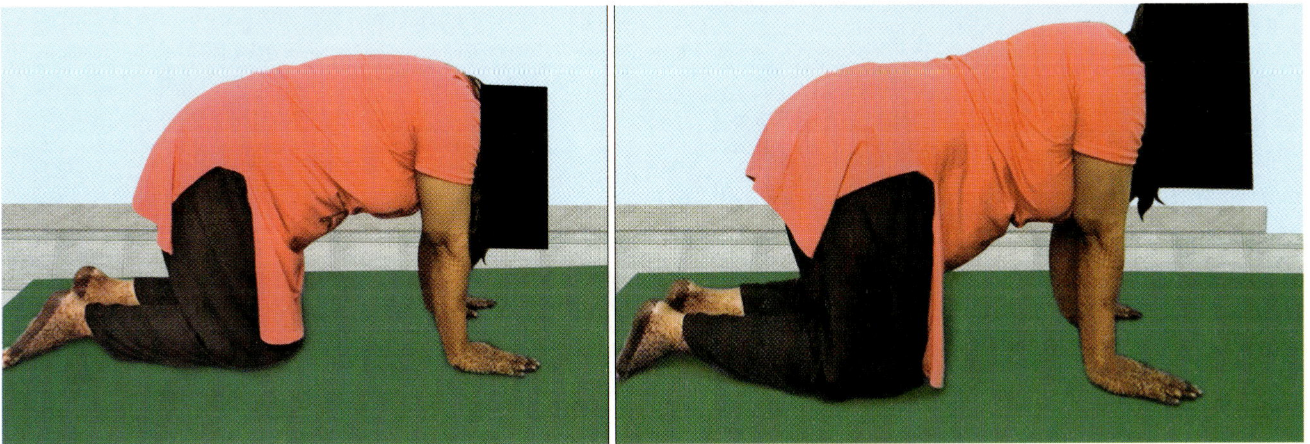

Fig. 42.11: Cat and camel exercises (during second trimester).

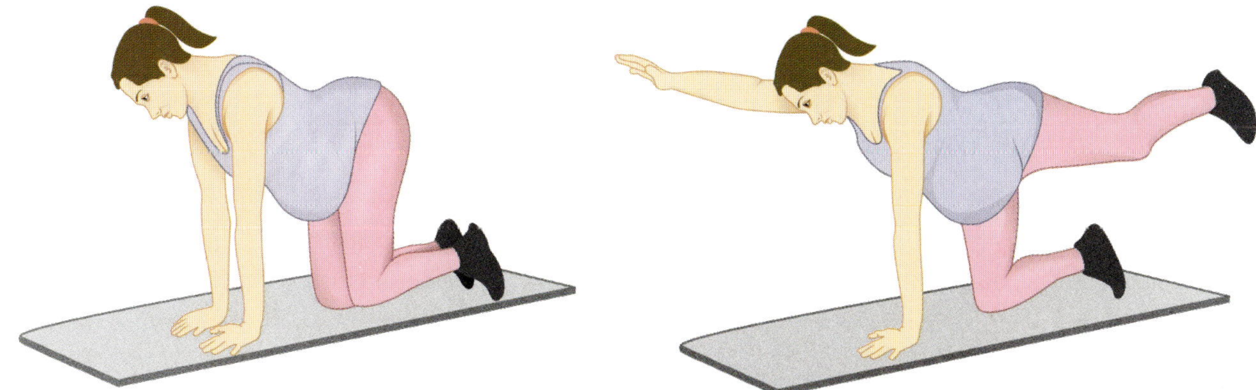

Fig. 42.12: Quadruped with 2 and 3 point weight bearing.

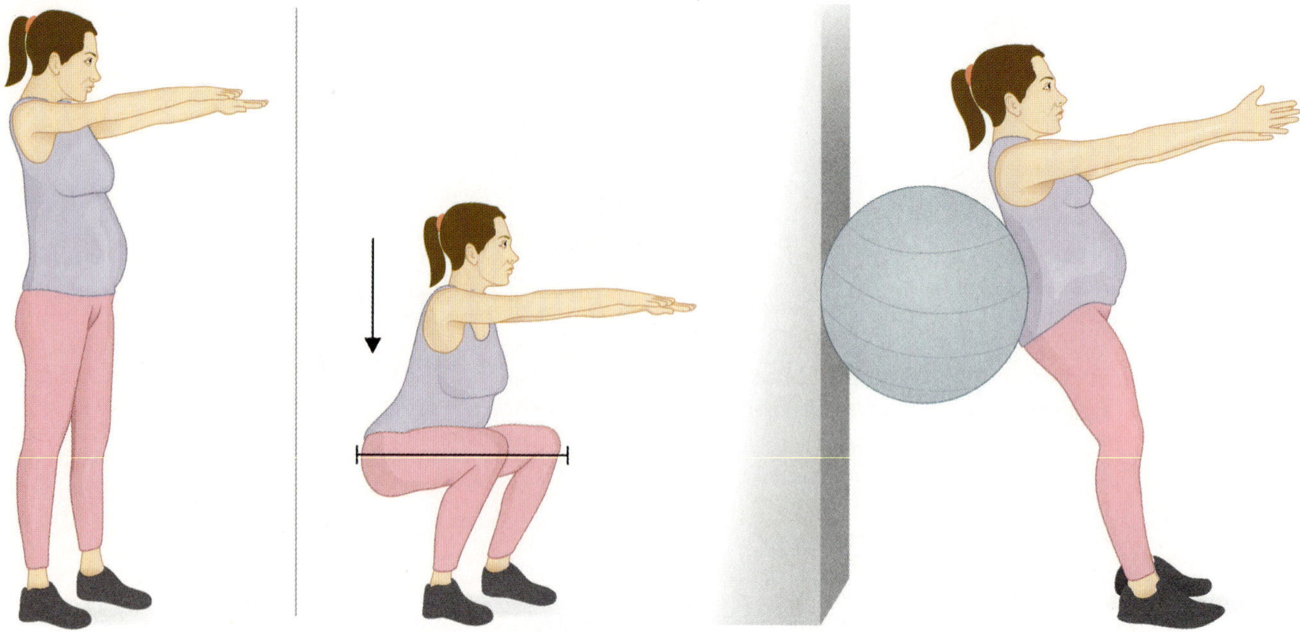

Fig. 42.13: Squatting exercises.

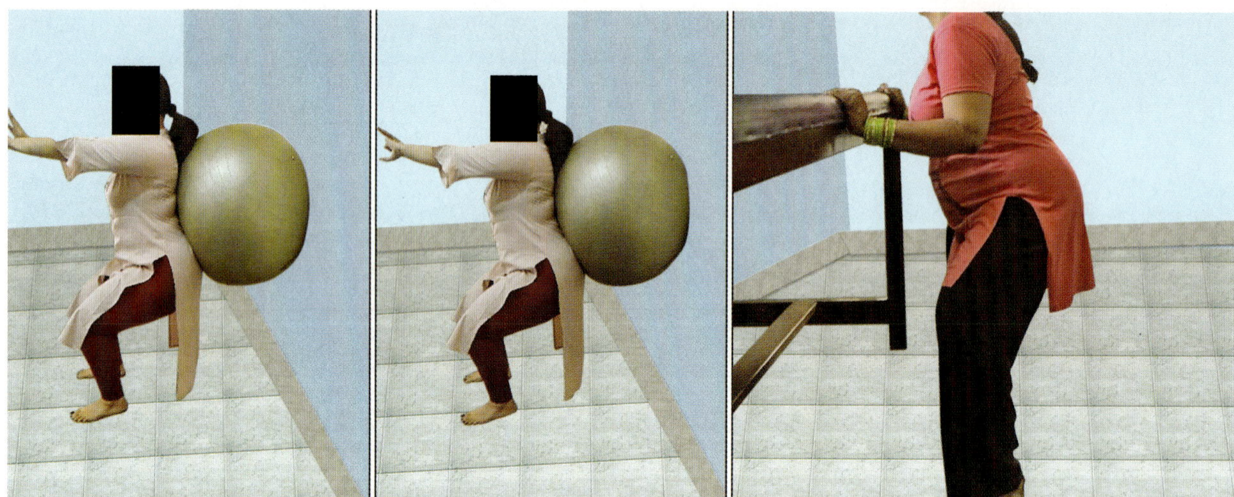

Fig. 42.14: Squatting exercises (during second and third trimester).

- Pelvic bridging
- Trunk stretches
- Knee extension on ball
- Cat and camel
- Wagging tail with ball

Strengthening Exercises during Pregnancy

Following are the strengthening exercises:
- Rowing exercise
- Thoracic traction
- Arm slide on wall
- Shoulder abduction exercise
- Biceps curls
- Lunges
- Modified push-ups
- Wall squats

- Heel raises
- Static abdominals
- Cat and camel
- Side bending
- Abdominal crunch
- Side crunch
- Bridging
- Pelvic clock exercises
- Heel slide

Yoga during Pregnancy

Below is the list of asanas that can be done during pregnancy **(Figs. 42.17 to 42.19)**:
- Matsyasana
- Tadasana
- Virabhadrasana

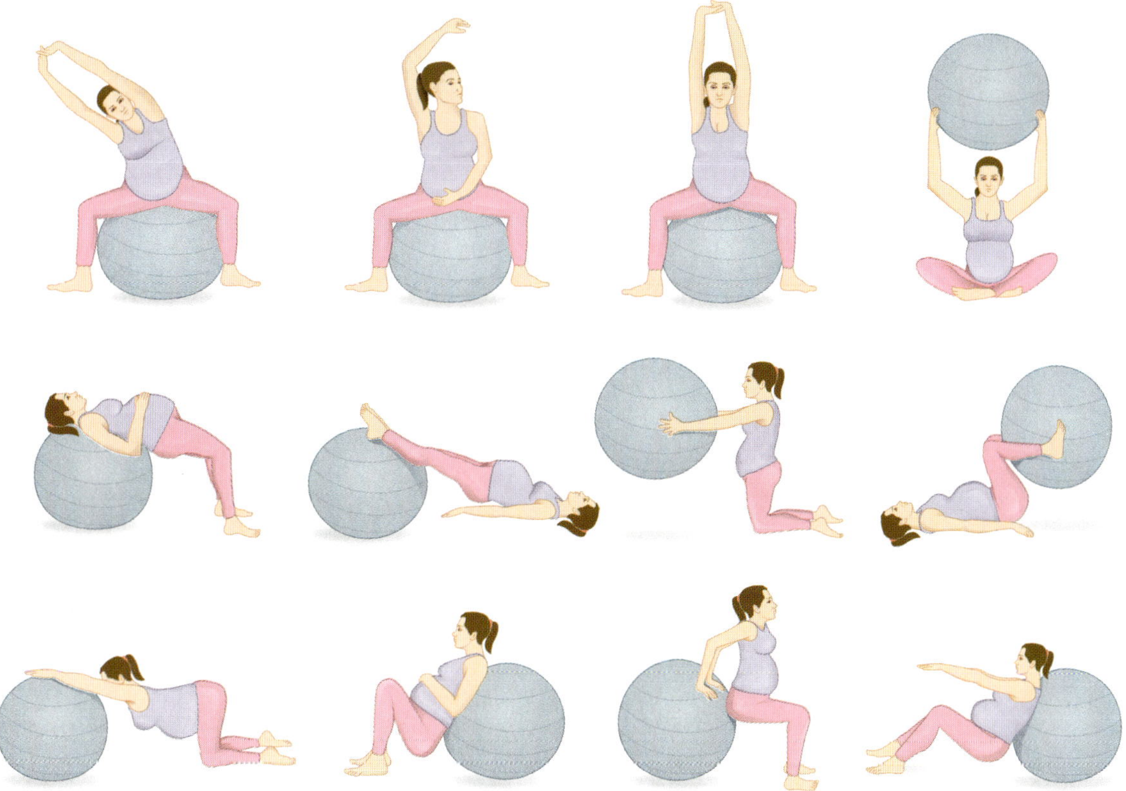

Fig. 42.15: Exercises with swiss ball.

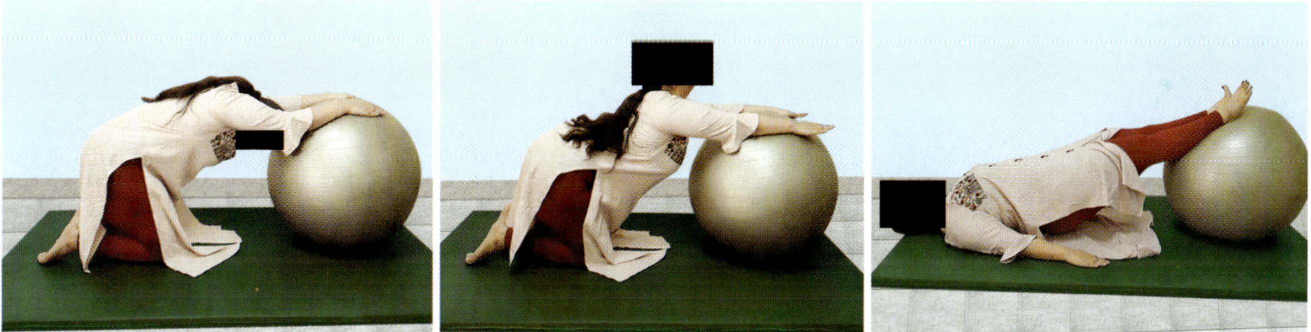

Fig. 42.16: Exercises using swiss ball (during second trimester).

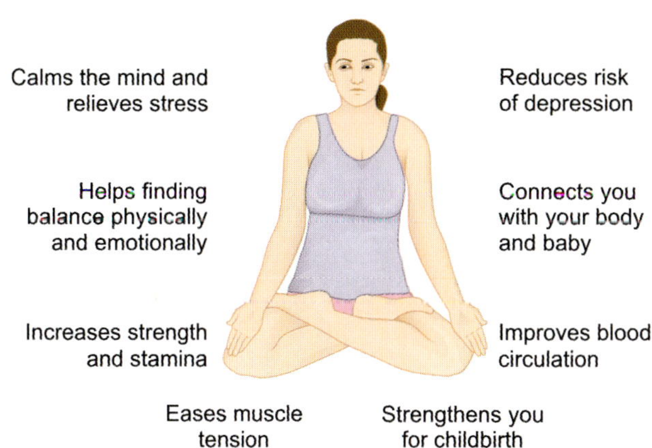

Fig. 42.17: Benefits of yoga during pregnancy.

- Bhadrasana
- Marjariasana
- Konasana 1 and 2
- Trikonasana
- Savasana

Contraindications of Exercises during Pregnancy

The contraindications of exercises given by American College of Obstetricians and Gynecologists during pregnancy are listed as follows:

- Heart disease
- Lung disease

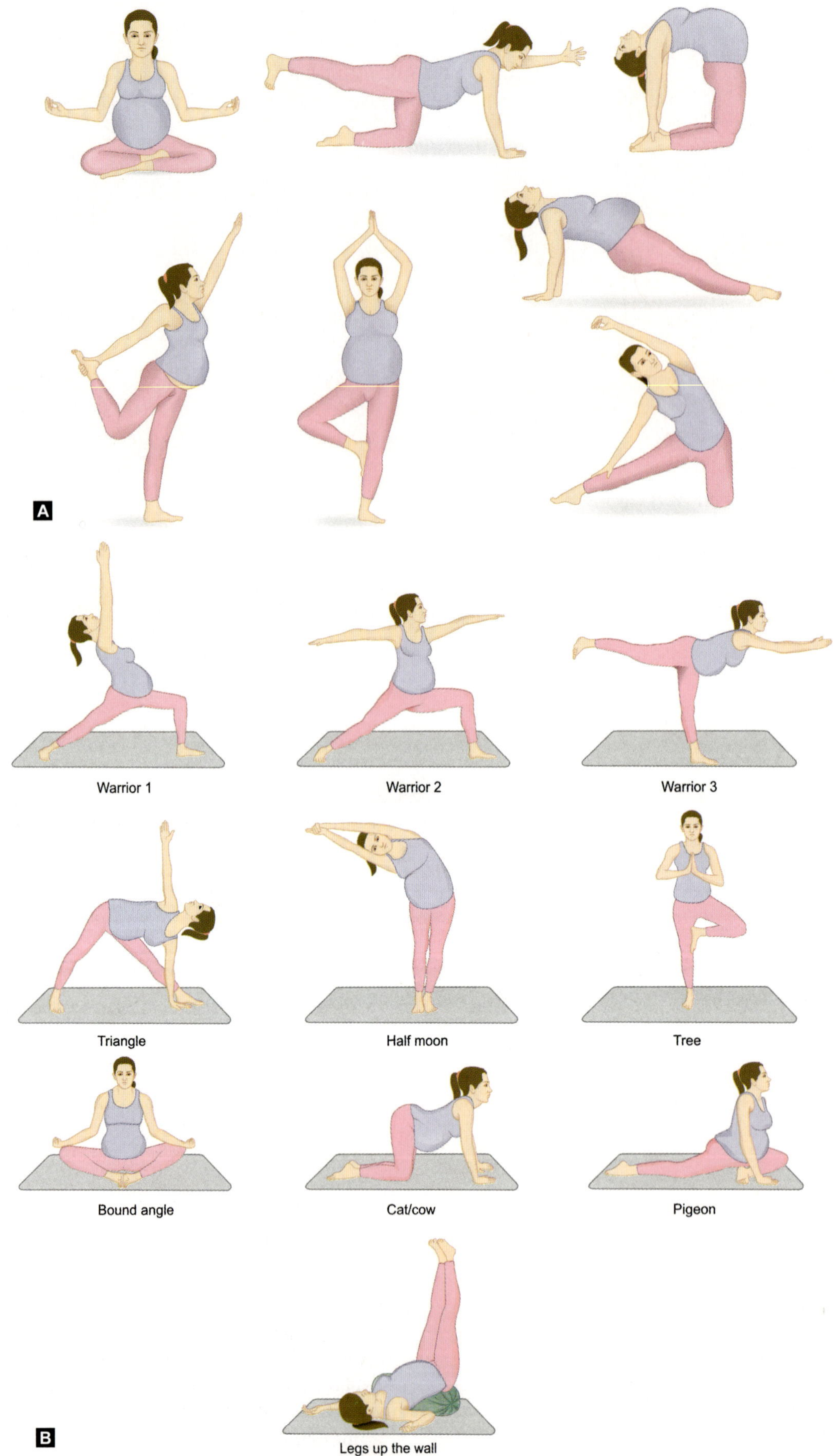

Figs. 42.18A and B: Different yoga poses during pregnancy.

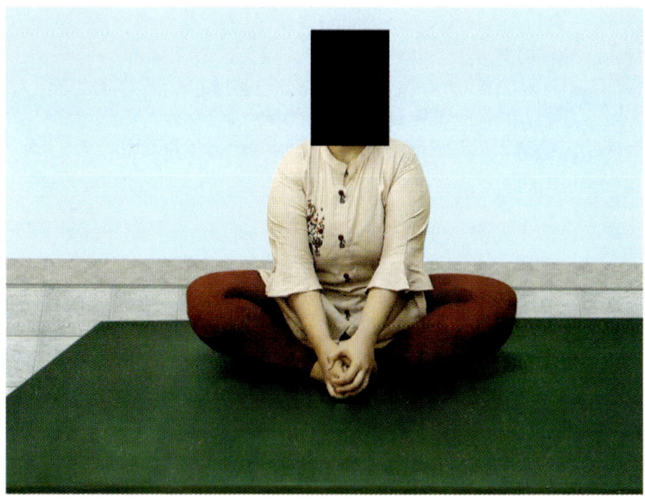

Fig. 42.19: Yoga—bhadrasana (butterfly pose).

- Cervical insufficiency
- Multiple gestations (at risk)
- Persistent second and third trimester bleeding
- Abnormal placental function or position
- Preterm labor
- Ruptured membrane
- Pre-eclampsia
- Chronic hypertension (HTN)
- Severe anemia
- Breech presentation in the third trimester

Warning signs to stop exercising (is given in **Box 42.2**):

Diet during Pregnancy

The First Trimester

During this period of fertilization, there is a formation of individual organs and skeleton. The heart and blood vessels continue to develop. Apart from fetal growth, development of placenta takes place providing nourishment to the growing fetus. Undernourishment of mother during this phase leads to smaller placental size and lack of nutrients and oxygen to fetus leading to lower birth weight **(Tables 42.3 and 42.4)**.

BOX 42.2: The warning signs to discontinue exercises in a class.

- Tachycardia
- Palpitation
- Shortness of breath
- Dizziness
- Faintness
- Headache
- Chest pain
- Muscle weakness
- Calf pain or swelling
- Severe back or pelvic pain
- Contractions preterm labor
- ↓ Fetal movement
- Vaginal fluid loss/bleeding
- Any other pain.

Table 42.3: Macronutrients (normal + addition for pregnancy).	
Energy (kcal/day)	1,875 + 300 (2,175)
Protein (g/day)	50 + 15 (65)
Fat (g/day)	20 + 10 (30)

Table 42.4: Micronutrients (normal + addition for pregnancy).	
Iron (mg/day)	30 + 8 (38)
Folic acid (µg/day)	100 + 300 (400)
Vitamin B_{12} (µg/day)	1 + 0.5 (1.5)
Calcium (mg/day)	400 + 600 (1,000)
Thiamine (mg/day)	0.9 + 0.2 (1.1)
Riboflavin (mg/day)	1.1 + 0.2 (1.3)
Niacin (mg/day)	12 + 2 (14)
Pyridoxine (mg/day)	2 + 0.5 (2.5)
Vitamin A (µg/day)	(600)
Vitamin C (µg/day)	(40)

Nutrients such as folic acid and vitamin B_{12} are very crucial during this phase. Deficiency can lead to neural tube defects such as spina bifida, anencephaly. Rich sources of folic acid and vitamin B_{12} such as dark green leafy vegetables, nuts, whole grains, legumes, and organ meats must be included in diet.

Nutrient Requirements during Second and Third Trimesters

During this period, there is an additional requirement for energy to meet the need for increased BMR. Feeding pattern should be five to six meals per day, which includes some healthy snacks in between the main meals.

These nutrients such as calcium, iron, B group vitamins (thiamine, riboflavin, folic acid, vitamin B_{12}) need to be taken in diet. Additional iron needs can be inclusion of whole grain cereals, whole pulses, leafy vegetables, dried foods, and organ meats. Milk and milk products, dark green leafy vegetables, legumes, ragi, and til (black) seeds are excellent sources of calcium.

LABOR

Labor is defined as the process in which the fetus, placenta, and secundines are expelled from the uterus via the birth canal after a minimum period of 20 weeks.

WHO defines normal birth as "spontaneous in onset, low-risk at the start of labor and remaining so throughout labor and delivery, the infant is born spontaneously in the vertex position between 37 and 42 completed weeks of pregnancy. After birth, mother and infant are in good condition." During labor, the uterus, a hollow structure, has the ability to contract and relax, progressively causing the descent of the fetus, the effacing and dilation of the cervix, and finally the passive movement of the fetus through the birth canal. Cervical dilation and effacement may also be present before labor. Labor starts when the cervical dilation progresses beyond 2 cm; however, some women in labor experience intense painful sensations even through the cervix is not dilated to this level.

Signs that indicate the labor is imminent:
- Mucoid discharge and "show"
- Spontaneous rupture of membranes
- Rhythmic regular contractions

Stages of Labor

Labor can be classified into three stages:
1. Stage 1 is from onset of labor until full dilation of the cervix.
2. Stage 2 is from full cervical dilation to the expulsion of the fetus from the vagina.
3. Stage 3 is the expulsion of the placenta and membranes.

Preparation for Labor

Following is the list by which labor is prepared:
- Prenatal visits to educate and prepare the future parents about normal labor, delivery, pain relief and possible complications, breastfeeding, normal newborn care, and postpartum adjustments.
- Information about physiology of labor and birth process, explanation of medical procedures, advice on relaxation techniques and stress management, guide to relief pain, etc., should be taught.
- Women should be taught massage skills, breathing techniques, breastfeeding techniques, and coping skills for pregnancy-induced discomforts.

Physiotherapy during Labor

Relaxation Techniques

Relaxation helps conserve energy and helps the mother adjust herself to labor with special breathing, positioning, and relaxation techniques. A soft-spoken, positive attitude, affirming, and creating calm atmosphere through lighting, music, comfortable positioning, and being around supportive people helps mother to relax.
- Breathing exercises—deep breathing, diaphragmatic breathing, costal breathing **(Table 42.5)**.
- Relaxation positions—supine, side lying, sitting with head and feet supported on table **(Figs. 42.20A and B)**.
- Jacobson relaxation technique
- Mitchell relaxation technique
- Pelvic rocking exercises
- Cat and camel exercises
- Relaxation massage—light to firm touch stroking in circular motion over some muscles along with use of heat or cold with lotion over back or SI gives relaxation.
- Guided imagery or visualization—technique that depends on imagination, relive the sounds, touch, emotions, and all sensations pertaining to that memory. For example, mother may visualize a scenery beach, mountains, calm ocean, sounds of birds chirping, feeling of the wind on her face, etc. to feel relaxed.

Table 42.5: Breathing exercises.	
Cleaning breath	Relaxed breath in through nose and out mouth. Used at the beginning and end of each contraction
Slow-paced breathing	Approximately 6–8 breaths/min, not less than half normal breathing rate (no. breaths/min divided by 2) in-2-3-4/out-2-3-4/in-2-3-4/out-2-3-4
Modified paced breathing	Approximately 32–40 breaths/min, also can combine slow and modified breathing by using slow breathing for beginnings and ends of contractions and modified breathing for more intense peaks. This conserves energy and reduces the risk for hyperventilation
Patterned paced breathing (same as modified)	To a repeated phrase, or in pyramid pattern such as 1:1, 2:1, 3:1, 4:1, 5:1-5:1, 4:1, 3:1, 2:1, 1:1

Source: Shaprio et al., 1997.

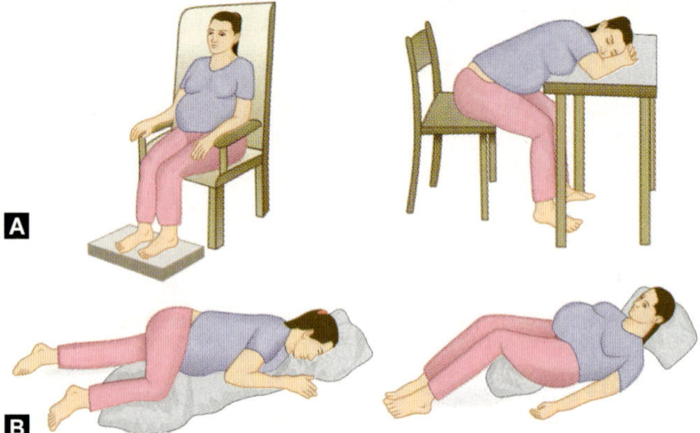

Figs. 42.20A and B: Relaxation positions. (A) Sitting; (B) Lying. *Courtesy*: Purvi K Changela, Role of Physiotherapist in Obstetric and Gynecological Conditions, 1st edition, Jaypee Brothers.

- Music
- Physical exercise—gentle walking or movement is helpful during labor and delivery. Physical activity releases tension and promotes relaxation.

Lamaze Technique

The Lamaze method of childbirth was introduced by a French obstetrician, Dr Fernand Lamaze in the early 1950s. It trains a woman's body to be prepared for natural delivery. It also helps her to cope with pains related to childbirth. Lamaze techniques emphasize on following the right breathing methodology during childbirth. The controlled breathing exercise helps a woman to take her mind off stress and relaxes her mentally and physically.

Positions in Labor

It refers to various physical postures the pregnant mother may assume during the process of childbirth. Commonly used by many obstetricians, positions **(Fig. 42.21)** that are successfully used by midwives and traditional birth-attendants include squatting, standing, kneeling, on all

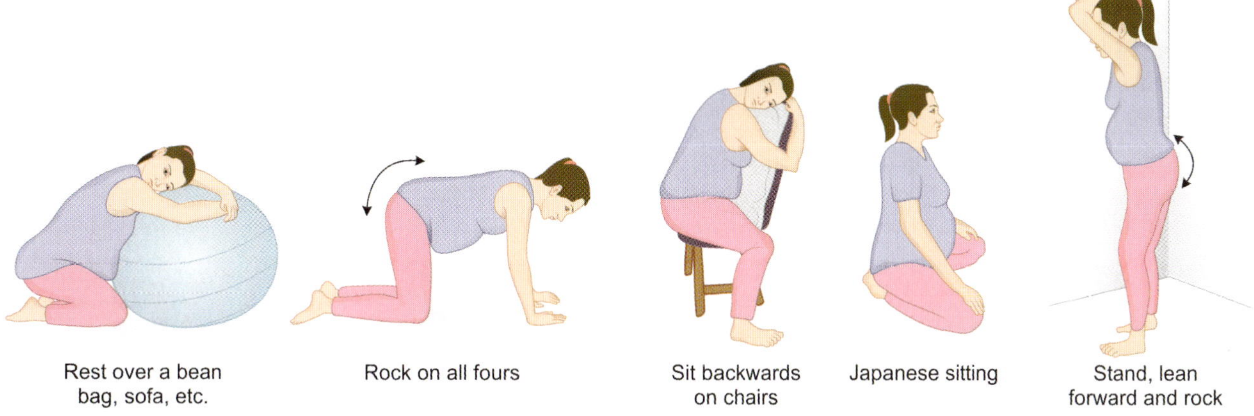

Fig. 42.21: Positions during labor.
Courtesy: Purvi K Changela, Role of Physiotherapist in Obstetric and Gynecological Conditions, 1st edition, Jaypee Brothers.

fours. These positions use gravity, reduce risk of aorto-caval compression, better align the fetus, and increase pelvic outlet.

- **First stage:** Avoid lying flat and assume upright position, can include walking. Forward lean sitting is the best position when uterus is anteverted.

  Patient should not bear down during this stage as it is useless and exhausts the patient and predisposes to genital prolapse.
- **Second stage:** Upright positions include sitting more than 45° from horizontal, squatting, or kneeling and being on hands and knees. Recumbent positions include supine, lateral, lithotomy, and semirecumbent with wedges **(Fig. 42.22)**.

Massage during Labor

Massages can be helpful for relaxation during antenatal class or in labor room. Massages can be applied to various parts such as face, arm, low back, leg, foot, para scapular kneading with heel of hands, and knuckle massage at low back **(Figs. 42.23 and 42.24)**.

Massage during Pregnancy

The erector spinae work hard to maintain a mother's erect posture during pregnancy while a heavy anterior load pulls her forward. Back massage will help to alleviate this general stress. Holding pressure on either side of the spinal vertebrae brings a mother's awareness to her spine, helps the therapist to locate areas of particular tension, and release this tension with the relaxing touch and compression on areas of restriction. These points are also the location of acupressure points on the bladder meridian. Effleurage and Petrissage to the back are the techniques used frequently.

Belly rubs offer time for the client and therapist to connect with the baby. They can be wonderfully relaxing and nurturing and help a mother feel more united in

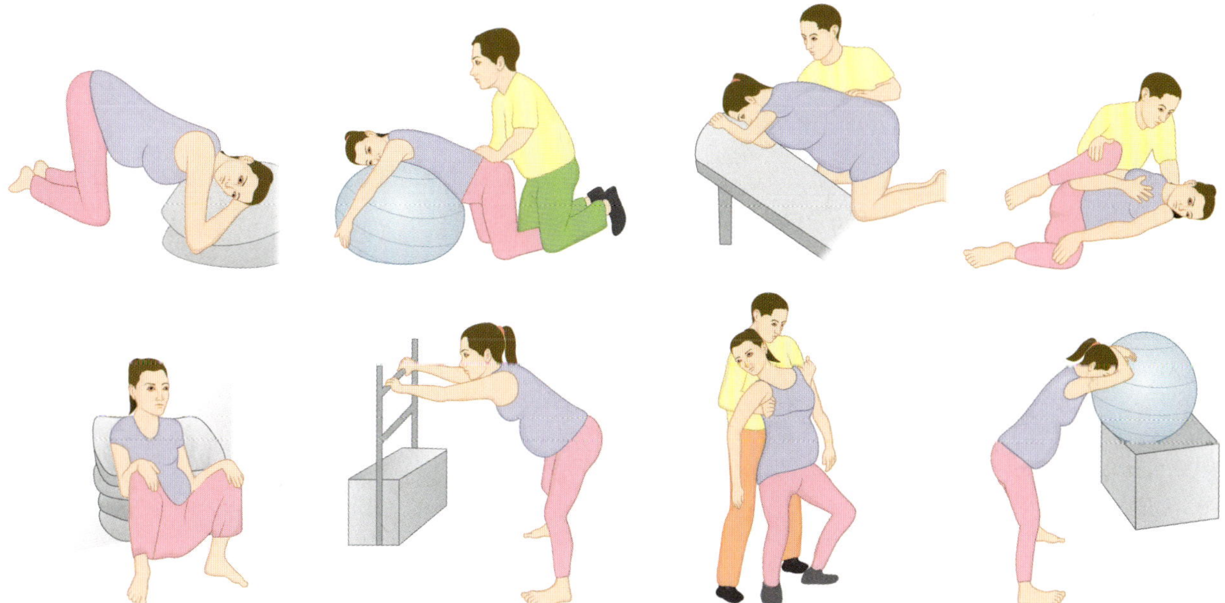

Fig. 42.22: Positions for the second stage of labor.
Courtesy: Purvi K Changela. Role of Physiotherapist in Obstetric and Gynecological Conditions, 1st edition, Jaypee Brothers.

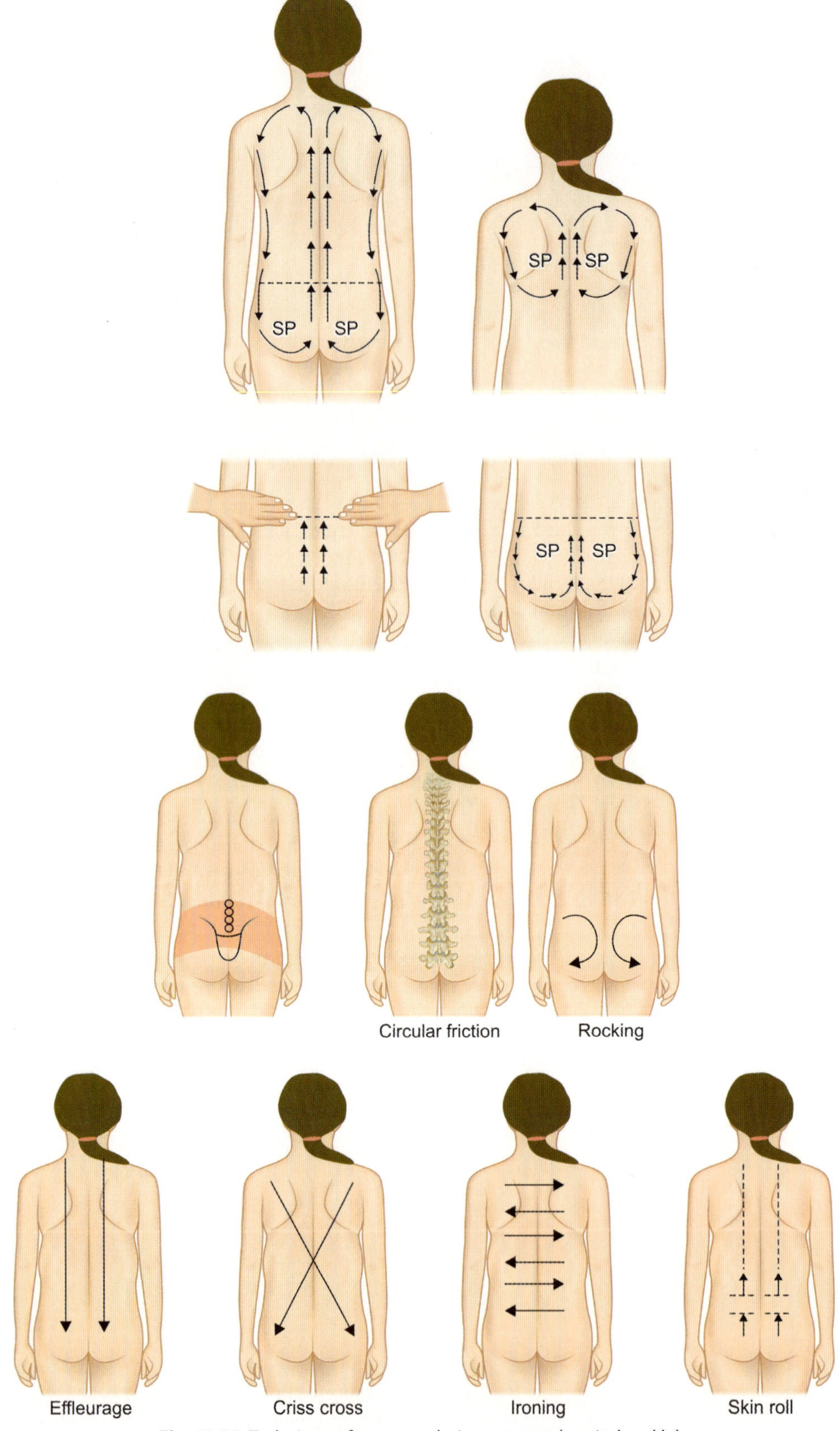

Fig. 42.23: Technique of massage during antenatal period and labor.
Courtesy: Purvi K Changela. Role of Physiotherapist in Obstetric and Gynecological Conditions, 1st edition, Jaypee Brothers.

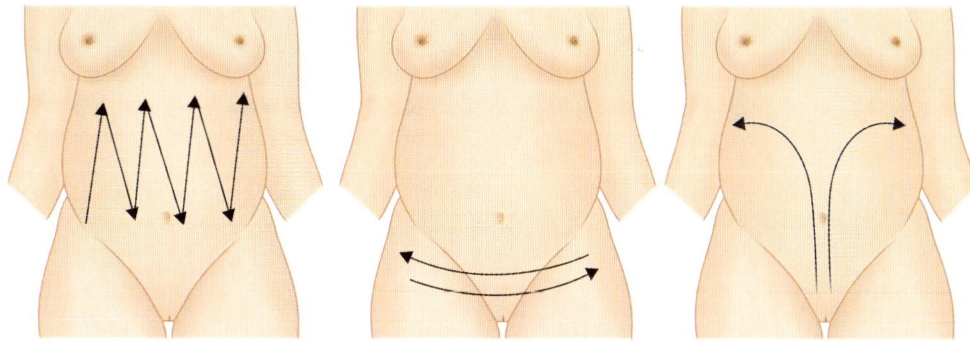

Fig. 42.24: Massage for lower abdomen.
Courtesy: Purvi K Changela, Role of Physiotherapist in Obstetric and Gynecological Conditions, 1st edition, Jaypee Brothers.

her body, as both the belly and back can be massaged simultaneously. Both side-lying and semi-reclining positioning are excellent for giving and receiving belly rubs.

Pain-relieving Strategies

Following are the pain-relieving strategies:
- Immersion in water
- Aromatherapy
- Acupuncture or acupressure
- Application of heat and cold
- Hypnosis
- Intracutaneous or subcutaneous sterile water injection
- Biofeedback
- Transcutaneous electrical nerve stimulation (TENS): Electrodes of TENS are placed on either side of the spinal column, one pair covering either side of spinous processes of T10–L1 and other pair covering either side of the spinous processes of S2–S4.
  - The mode of TENS used is burst TENS which is used all the time during labor and brief TENS when the women experiences the beginnings of a contraction.
  - The ideal time to start use of TENS is in the first stage of labor when contractions begin and start becoming painful. A minimum of 30 minutes throughout birth and up to several hours afterward can be the duration of treatment with labor TENS.
  - **Benefits of labor TENS:**
  - No harm to baby
  - Drug-free pain control
  - Instant long-lasting pain relief
  - No side effects or drowsiness
  - Fully controllable
  - Used at home when contractions start
  - Can be used with other methods/drugs
  - Safe and easy to use at home or in hospital

POSTNATAL PERIOD

It is the period immediately after delivery when a new mother's body begins its period of recovery and its return to "normal." In the first few postpartum hours, she may be thrilled with the softness and relative flatness of her abdomen, but sooner she will be confronted with a different image—empty, sagging, and still enlarged abdomen. She soon realizes complete lack of abdominal muscle control, painful perineum, and difficulty in initiating micturition or may experience retention of urine. She may also experience leakage when intra-abdominal pressure increases on coughing, sneezing, or laughing.

Not only physical but her emotional state may also be "labile," varying from euphoric exhilaration to inability to sleep or disillusioned disappointment accompanied by total exhaustion.

Postpartum Physical/Mental Condition

- The muscle, ligaments, and collagenous connective tissues are soft, more elastic, stretched, and elongated. There may be a separation between the two recti abdominis muscles varying from a small vertical gap of 2–3 cm wide and 12–15 cm long to space measuring 12–20 cm in width and extending nearly the whole length of recti muscles, known as diastasis recti. Hence, the entire abdominal corset weakens with little mechanical control.
- The pelvic floor muscles will certainly be weaker prior to pregnancy and during perineum also it will be considerably stretched.
- A woman may complain of heavy, edematous, aching legs, swollen feet and ankles immediately postpartum, the cause being prolonged pushing during labor, pelvic congestion, dysfunctional urinary tract, or temperature of the postnatal ward.
- The passage of the fetus through pelvis and resultant stretching and movement of the lax joints, epidural anesthesia, lithotomy position, poor feeding or nappy changing postures, tension, and fatigue may cause back pain.
- Breasts become more engorged, hot, full, and painful when lactation begins on the third or fourth postnatal day.
- Psychologically, the mother's attention is fixed on her baby. Her initial elation can change after a few days to a flattening of her mood. She may well be more concerned with her baby than she is for herself.

Postnatal Problems

Following are the postnatal problems:
- Postpartum hemorrhage
- Painful perineum
- Stress incontinence/retention of urine
- Constipation
- Varicose veins/deep vein thrombosis (DVT)
- Edema
- Breast engorgement
- Diastasis recti abdominal muscles
- Spinal pains
- Pubic symphysis pain
- Fatigue
- Concern for the baby
- Carpel tunnel syndrome
- Headaches
- Coccydynia
- De Quervain's tendonitis
- Postpartum depression: Depression can be assessed using the Edinburgh Postnatal Depression Scale.

First 6 Weeks after the Birth

Education

Following are exercise education:
- Exercise education should be quick and to the point. Time away from baby and house can keep women from feeling overwhelmed that can become the first step toward postpartum depression; at the same time, many find the exercise a way to be sure they get that time away.
- Paying attention to the baby and herself during this time is important, as a few ignore this. During this hectic time, exercise provides time to relax and think.
- The easiest way to avoid fatigue is to sleep when the baby sleeps.
- Drinking a lot of fluid and eating at regular intervals as well, both are important. A good rule is 8 oz of fluid and a piece of fruit, salad, or half a sandwich (or small bowl of upma, poha, idli, cereals, oats) for the mother each time she nurses the baby. The same applies to after exercise.
- Nursing women should wear a double bra during exercise sessions to compress and stabilize the breasts on the chest wall. It should be tight enough to support but not enough to create discomfort during workout.

Postnatal Classes

Following are the instructions for postnatal classes:
- It is difficult for women to exercise with new demands of caring for a baby. This is why specialized classes with child-caring facilities facilitate postnatal exercise. This class would be shorter in duration and consists of a warm-up period, simple low-impact movements, gentle stretches, posture correction, specific strengthening exercises, and relaxation.
- The class can be attended on the second day after a normal delivery and fifth day after a CS. Exercises and movement patterns should be modified for women with pain.
- An individualized assessment is needed to tailor postnatal exercises to each woman's presentation and muscle strength, muscle length, pain, and posture.
- It facilitates social interaction for new mothers and gives an opportunity to meet women with a similar situation where they could exchange experiences about the new role of motherhood, its difficulties and uncertainties, and to exercise safely.
- Some classes actively involve the baby in exercises which provide interaction with baby. A therapist can provide education about normal baby development and facilitation of development through everyday handling, play, and touch. It creates bonding between mother and baby and can use baby as a weight to increase resistance.
- Physiotherapist can advise on ergonomic problems that women may be experiencing such as back pain, in activities such as feeding, bathing, and carrying.

Postnatal Physiotherapy

A detailed assessment of the new mother should be conducted postdelivery to determine her priority needs.

Pelvic Floor Dysfunction

The pelvic floor dysfunctions are as follows:
- The new mother is encouraged to perform deep breathing and vigorous circulatory exercises so as to reduce the risk of circulatory and respiratory dysfunction.
- Pelvic floor muscle exercises are valuable for their strengthening and pain-relieving properties. They will speed healing by reducing edema and encourage good circulation. Slow, progressive, controlled contractions along with fast, short, sharp contractions can be practiced little and often. A right starting position for exercise will be the key to effectiveness (e.g., sitting on gymnastic ball, crook lying, standing, prone kneeling). A more efficient contraction may be obtained by contracting the TA before engaging the pelvic floor.
- Kegel's exercises—it entails gaining awareness of muscles of pelvic floor and learning how to consciously contact and release them. Women are taught to stop and start the flow of urine midstream during urination by using the sphincters, gently yet firmly, several times.
- For the first week, at least six repetitions are done slowly, maintaining tension for at least 5 seconds each time followed by release. It should be progressed to 10-second duration with a rest–work ratio of 2:1, graduate to 1:1 as quality and endurance improve. Slow twitch muscle repetitions: individualize dosage, starting with 3s/5–10 repetition. Fast twitch muscle repetitions: contractions are held less than 2 seconds. This is done several times throughout the day, 30–80 contractions per day. Graduate exercises from horizontal to standing and functional activity.

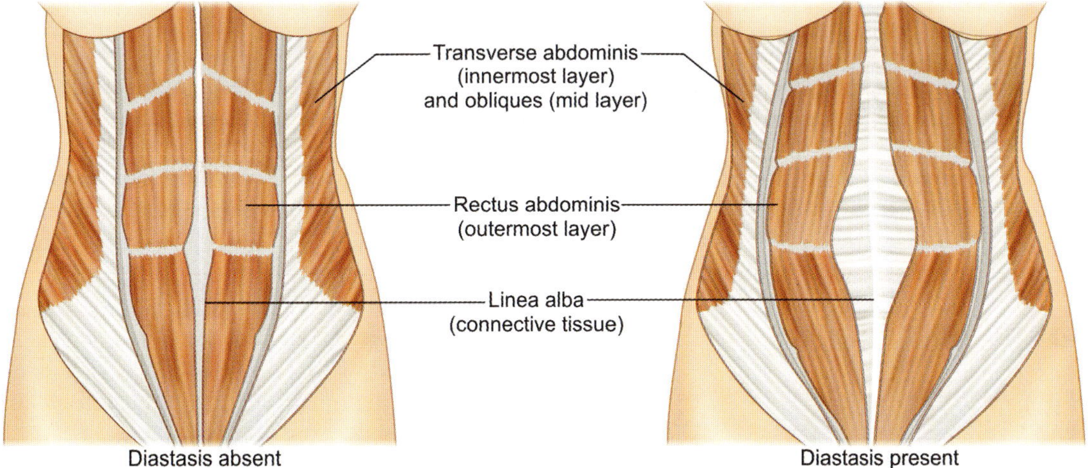

Fig. 42.25: Diastasis recti: Separation of the abdominal muscles at the linea alba.

Diastasis Recti

Diastasis recti **(Fig. 42.25)** is separation of the rectus abdominis muscles in the midline at linea alba. The integrity and continuity of the abdominal musculature are disrupted. Any separation larger than two finger width is considered significant. It may occur in pregnancy as a result of hormonal effects on the connective tissue and the biomechanical changes of pregnancy, it may also develop during labor, especially with excessive breath-holding during the second stage. It appears to be less common in women with good abdominal tone before pregnancy.

Symptoms

Following are the symptoms of diastasis recti:
- It may produce musculoskeletal complaints such as low back pain, as a result of decreased ability of the abdominal musculature and thoracolumbar fascia to stabilize the pelvis and lumbar spine.
- Inability to perform independent supine-to-sitting transitions.
- If it occurs in antenatal period, in case of severe separation, the remaining midline layers of abdominal wall tissue are skin, fascia, subcutaneous fat, and peritoneum, which lead to less protection for the fetus.
- There may be herniation of abdominal viscera through separated linea alba.

Examination of Diastasis Recti

Technique of examination of diastasis recti is as follows:
- The test can be performed during pregnancy and after the third postpartum day for optimal accuracy. The patient is in hook lying position. Ask the patient slowly raise her head and shoulders off the floor, reaching her hands toward the knees, until the spines of scapulae leave the floor.
- Place the fingers of one hand horizontally across the midline of the abdomen at the umbilicus **(Fig. 42.26)**. If a separation exists, the fingers will sink into the gap

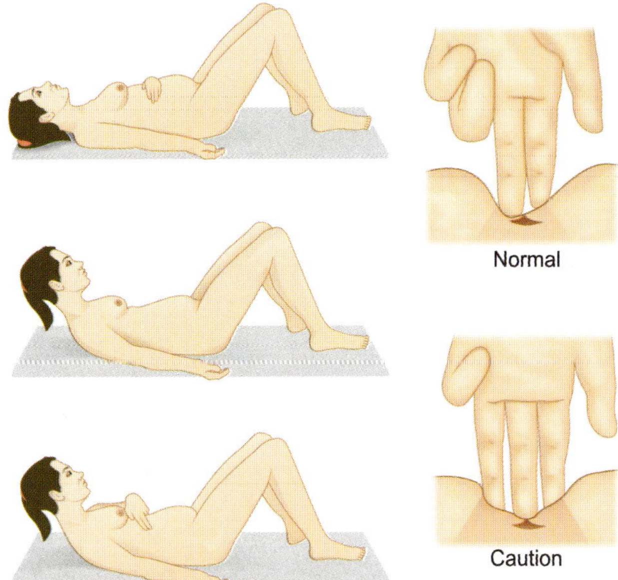

Fig. 42.26: Examination of diastasis recti.

between the rectus muscles, or a visible bulge between the rectus bellies may be appreciated. The number of fingers that can be placed between the muscles bellies is noted.

Intervention

Following interventions need to be made:
- Corrective exercise for diastasis recti until the separation is decreased to 2 cm or less is encouraged.
- Head lifts and head lifts with pelvic tilting are advised.
- TA exercises may be incorporated with a caution against breath-holding.
- Strengthening of obliques and more advanced abdominal work can be resumed.

Postural Awareness and Control

The growing fetus places added stress on postural muscles as center of gravity shifts forward and upward and spine

888

shifts to compensate and maintain stability. Activities involving holding and caring the baby stress postural muscles. Muscles that require emphasis for strengthening (low intensity) are upper neck flexors, lower neck and upper thoracic extensors, scapular retractors and depressors, shoulder external rotators, trunk flexors particularly lower abdominals, hip extensors, knee extensors, and ankle dorsiflexors.

Muscles that require stretching (with caution) and strengthening are (figure as shown in antenatal and **Fig. 42.27**):

- Upper neck extensors
- Scalene
- Scapular protractors
- Shoulder internal rotators
- Levator scapulae
- Low back extensors
- Hip flexors
- Adductors
- Hamstrings
- Ankle plantar flexors

Ergonomic Principles

Feeding

The new mother may be feeding her baby eight or more times each day. Inappropriate positioning may result in musculoskeletal symptoms; hence, a therapist should teach the mother with regard to "good" positioning which best reinforces and benefits the mother.

The therapist should teach a new mother regarding:

- Learning proper posture, lifting and carrying techniques while feeding, napping changing, and baby caring **(Figs. 42.28 and 42.29)**.
- Become aware of body position during all activities.
- Alter habits, positions, or environment to provide a safe and efficient work area.
- Rebuilding or maintaining a healthy back consists of a healthier lifestyle, safe body mechanics, and regular exercise.
- Each position used should have trunk fully supported, maintaining natural spinal curves, supported by pillows—head, knees, low back, legs should not be

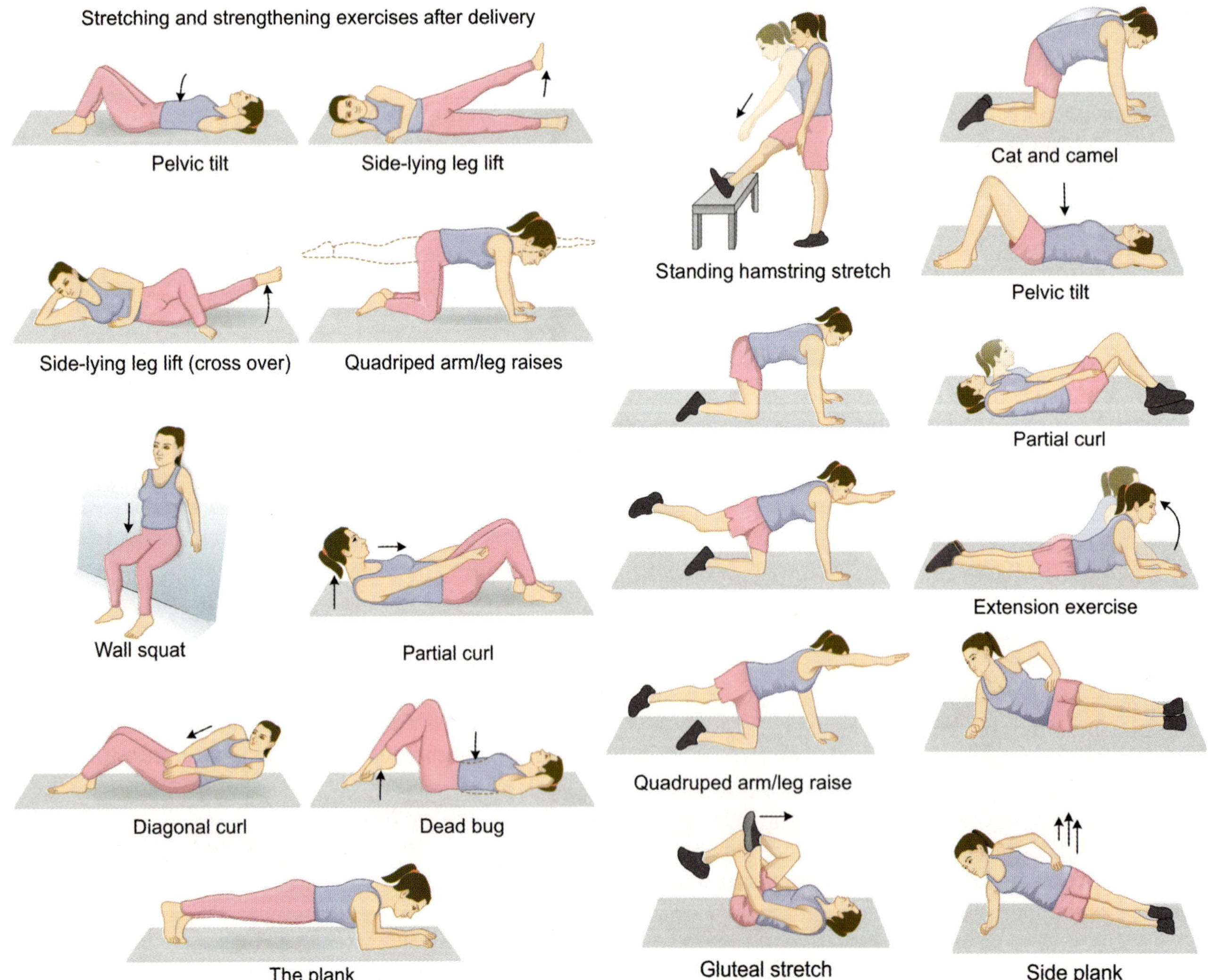

Fig. 42.27: Exercises in postnatal period of pregnancy.

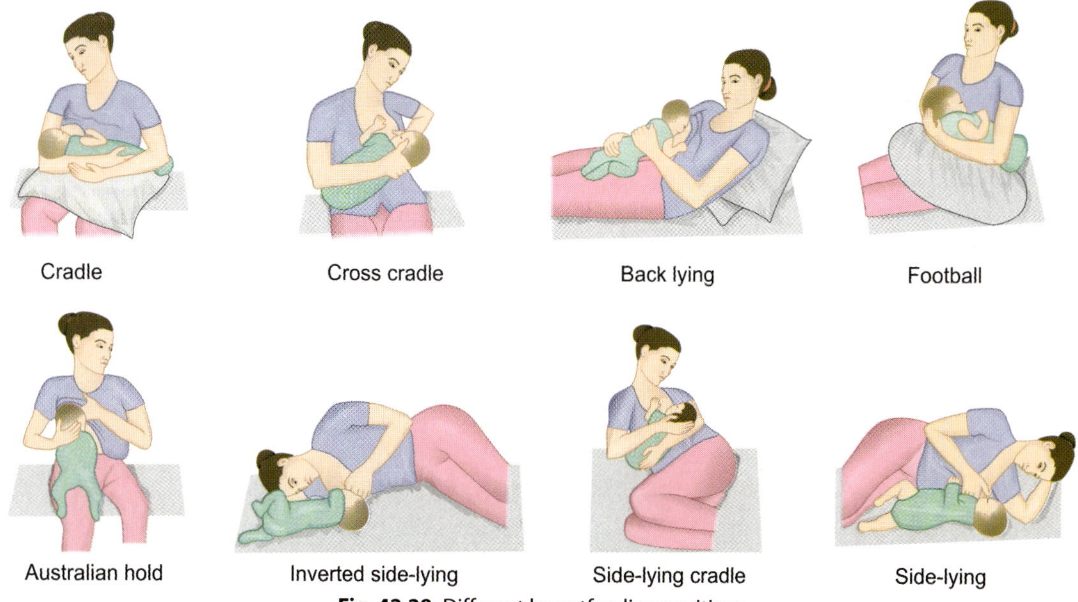

Fig. 42.28: Different breastfeeding positions.

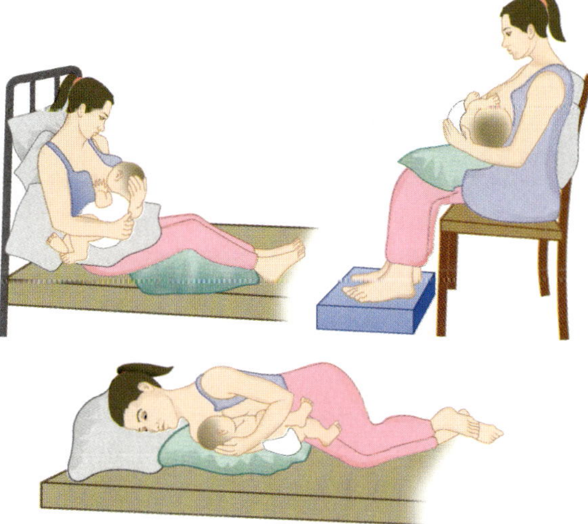

Fig. 42.29: Breastfeeding positions.

crossed, weight evenly distributed over both buttocks, sitting surface should be depressible to allow for pressure distribution.

Nappy Changing

Nappy changing is another activity that can result in incapacitating pain. A mother may change a nappy 10 times a day or more which becomes a frequent activity and at risk to musculoskeletal problems. Positions that increase risk to mother should be avoided (e.g., standing, knees extended, trunk flexed, and twisted). Mothers should be encouraged to follow certain positions such as sitting and changing on the lap, standing and changing on a surface of appropriate height, kneeling and changing on the floor or surface of appropriate height **(Fig. 42.30)**. Bath time should be fun for both. Bathing area should be selected such that it suits most requirements, e.g., bathtubs

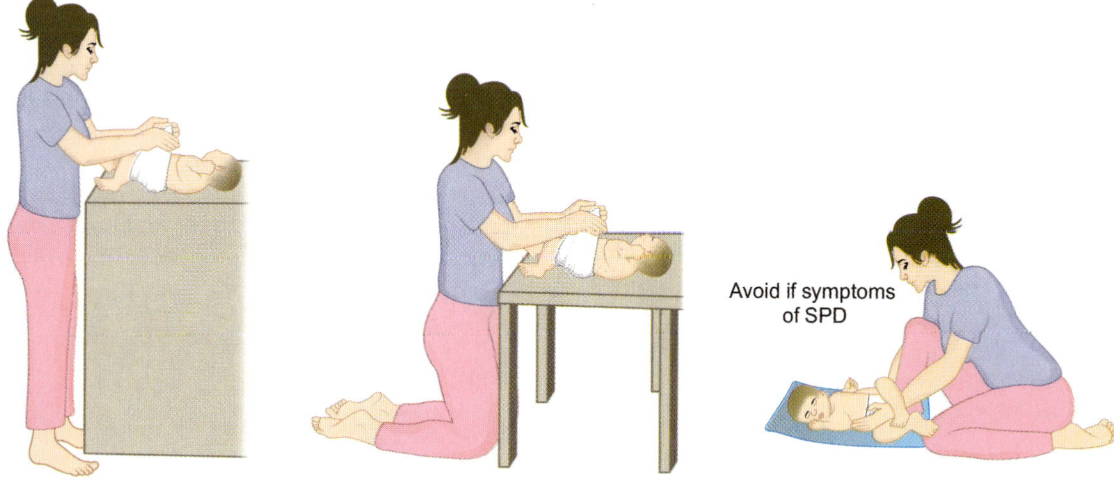

Fig. 42.30: Napping changing positions.
(SPD: symphysis pubis dysfunction)

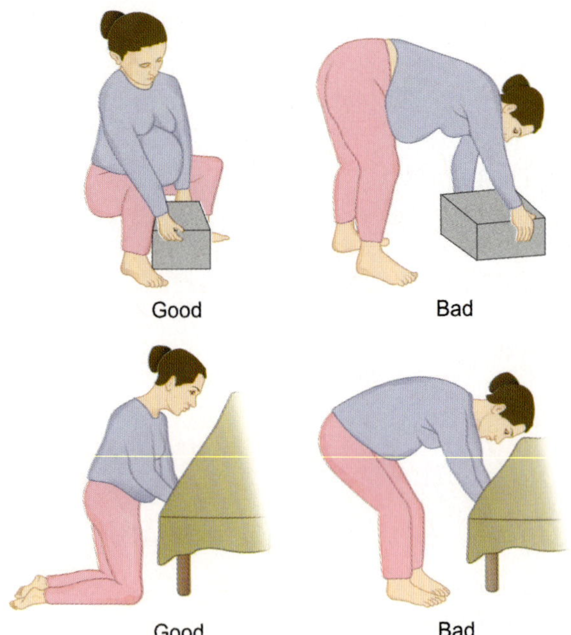

Fig. 42.31: Proper lifting techniques during pregnancy.

of the infant that can rest over an adult-sized bath so that the mother can kneel alongside, or traditionally make the baby lie on mother's legs with head on higher side for bathing. Special washing-up bowl (nonslip) on the kitchen draining board, or well-cleaned bathroom hand basin may be used.

Ergonomics and Proper Lifting Techniques

Following ergonomics and proper lifting techniques should be followed:

Teaching points a therapist should remember (**Figs. 42.30 and 42.31**):

- Well-supported back and comfortable perineum
- Exercises in sitting position for posture, abdominals, pelvic floor muscle (PFM)
- Appropriate footwear
- Stable base of support in standing
- Use of pillows or wedges for support in lying
- Checking of diastasis recti (separation of recti abdominis) muscle
- Posture awareness in mirror

CESAREAN SECTION

Cesarean section is a surgical technique whereby the fetus is delivered through incisions in the uterus and the abdomen. The surgical approach is usually made transversely through the uterine segment [lower segment CS (LSCS)]. Rarely, a vertical incision is made in upper body of uterus (classic cesarean). The procedure can be carried out under general anesthesia, spinal, or epidural analgesia.

Cesarean births are on an increase resulting in increase in maternal mortality rate as a result from surgery-related complications. CS may be performed as a planned procedure (elective) or an emergency procedure prior to

Table 42.6: Main indications of cesarean section (CS).	
Elective	*Emergency*
<ul><li>Cephalic disproportion</li><li>Placenta previa</li><li>Malpresentation, e.g., breech</li><li>Previous CS depending on its indication</li><li>Active genital herpes</li><li>Pre-eclampsia and eclampsia</li><li>Multiple births</li><li>Low birth weight</li></ul>	<ul><li>Obstructed labor</li><li>Fetal and maternal distress</li><li>Antepartum hemorrhage</li><li>Placental abruption</li><li>Prolapsed cord</li><li>Failed trial of forceps</li><li>Failed trial of previous CS scar</li></ul>

or during labor. **Table 42.6** shows the main indications of a CS.

Role of Physiotherapy

Physiotherapy assessment following CS includes mainly degree and site of pain and patient's mobility in the immediate stage. A supervised program within the first 24 hours is advisable and should be reinforced every 2 hours.

- Assisted active and active movements of limbs especially ankle–toe to help prevent venous stasis, joint stiffness, and peripheral edema.
- Encourage movement around bed, using crook lying, feet placement, bottom lift techniques (**Fig. 42.32**).
- Encourage gentle exercises, such as crook lying/pelvic rock, crook lying/knee rolls from side to side, hip hitching, abdominal contraction on expiration, gluteal contractions, and pelvic floor exercises.
- Deep breathing, huffing, and effective coughing are encouraged to prevent respiratory problems.
- Ambulation is encouraged after removal of drains and IV lines.
- Appropriate abdominal support may be given for comfort of patient. Towel "binder" or a pillow may be firmly supported at the lower abdomen during activities involving increasing intra-abdominal pressure such as coughing.
- Active exercise program to strengthen the abdominal muscles is cautiously introduced; its intensity depends on the recovery of the patient.
- Lower limb movement especially dorsi and planter flexion and gluteal contractions, early mobilization, application of compression stocking, and encouragement of deep breathing should be enhanced to prevent risks of deep vein thrombus.
- Correct positioning, general back mobility exercises (rolling in and out of the bed) and application of heat are often efficacious for back pain post C-section (**Figs. 42.33 and 42.34**).

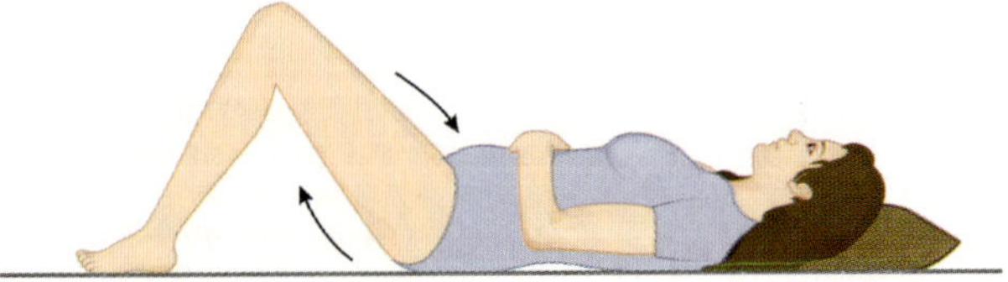

Fig. 42.32: Abdominal drawing in and lift-bottom technique.

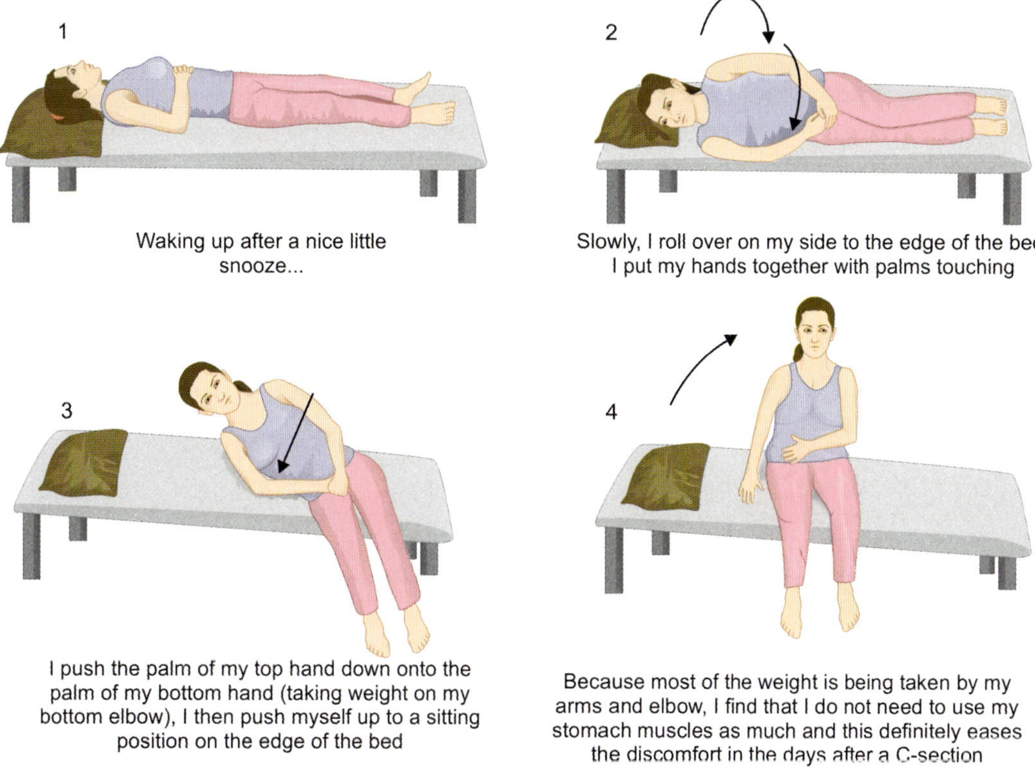

Fig. 42.33: Rolling out of bed after lower segment cesarean section (LSCS).

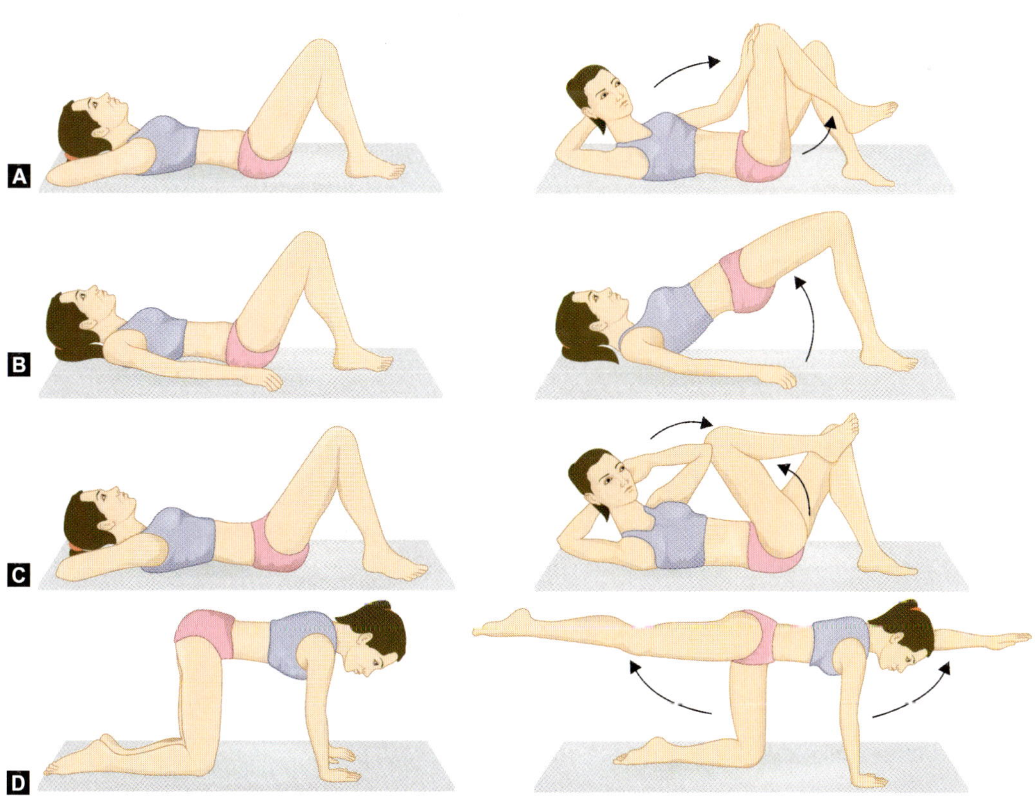

Figs. 42.34A to D: Exercises after lower segment cesarean section (LSCS).

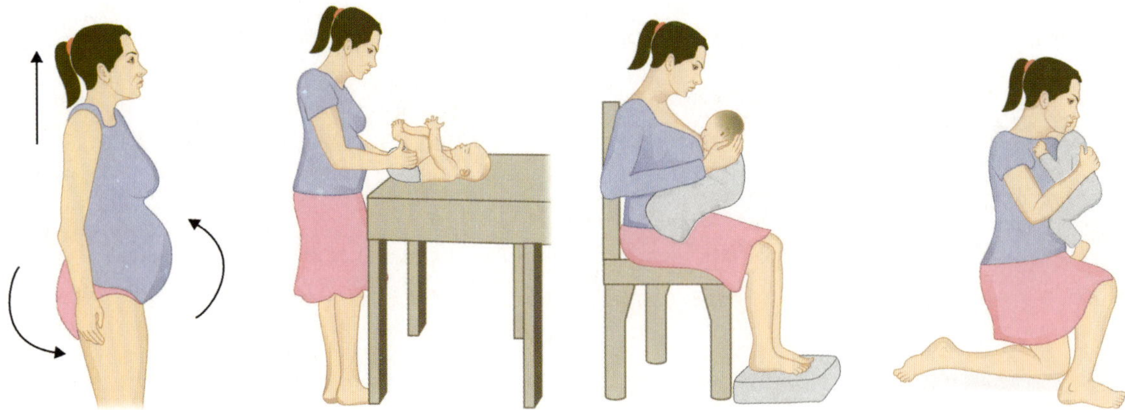

Fig. 42.35: Nappy changing, feeding and carrying after lower segment cesarean section (LSCS).

- Self-administered massage following abdominal exercise—For example vibration/stroking over the wind pain site (a severe intermittent colic type pain, where abdomen is usually very distended and painful to touch) single or two-handed abdominal effleurage following line of colon or double-handed kneading if a woman can withstand have very positive results.
- While feeding, the baby can be positioned in such a way as to allay her fears, such as tucking the baby's feet under her arm to avoid potential kicking or positioning pillows to protect the wound **(Fig. 42.35)**.
- Posture post LSCS can be of protective flexion, complicated by weak abdominal muscles and possible backache; hence, women should be encouraged to rediscover their prepregnancy posture.

SUMMARY

Pregnancy is not a disease but a stage of the women's life during which various physiological, hormonal biomechanical alterations are taking place in the women's body to accommodate the needs of the growing fetus. Physiotherapy during the antenatal period consists of teaching ways to avoid any pregnancy-related problems, correcting postures, avoiding complications, and exercise to wade symptoms of musculoskeletal changes focusing and preparing for labor and childbirth. A thorough assessment of the physiological, physical, and mental condition is carried out; certain specific exercise prescription is prepared catering to the all needs taking precautions of any hazards of exercises that may need restriction to some individuals. The exercises focus on making the mother physically and mentally stress free at the same time active and fit to be prepared for childbirth and nursing. A balanced diet along with physiotherapy in the form of exercises, yoga, aerobics, etc., plays an important role to achieve the prepregnant state of a mother. Customized exercises program helps combat problems during and after pregnancy whether normally delivered or surgically with C-section. A woman's health physiotherapist need to make knowledge and skill to strengthen a role in education, evaluation, prevention, treatment, and wellness to contribute to movement in health care of a woman.

Case Scenario

CASE STUDY 1

A 27-year-old pregnant woman—primigravida has a complaint of low back and SI joint pain at 30 weeks of pregnancy. She is a homemaker and has difficulties in doing all household activities such as sweeping, mopping, and washing. Her weight gain at the eighth month is 11 kg from prepregnancy and has developed an abnormal posture and an altered gait.

Guiding Questions:

1. Assess her for the complaints of low back, SI joint pain and altered musculoskeletal problems.
2. Design a treatment plan to reduce her pain, correct her posture and gait, and make her independent in her activities.
3. Guide her on the required nutrients and weight gain during pregnancy.
4. Educate her regarding the benefits of exercises and ergonomics that she needs to follow while working and lifting.

CASE STUDY 2

Jaya is a multigravida, 37 years old who delivered her third child before 25 days. Her previous delivery histories include one normal delivery and the other LSCS due to complications during the last trimester. The third delivery was a planned LSCS at the end of 37 weeks of pregnancy. Her chief complains include pain at the incision site and in whole back and left shoulder. Mentally also, she seems to be disturbed due to her pain, her newborn, and responsibility of her two earlier children. She has a forward bent posture and a small step gait.

Guiding Questions:

1. Assess Jaya for the incisional scar and advise her proper physiotherapy and wound care for the same.

2. Educate her about the importance of wound care, methods of pain relief, and exercises to follow after LSCS.
3. Guide her about the do's and dont's post–cesarean section and how she can remain stress free and mentally relaxed after the LSCS with already two elder children.

CASE STUDY 3

Mrinal is going to be a first-time mother. She is 26 years old and is physically quite active and works in an MNC. Her job profile includes that of a manager and involves 8 hours of desk work on computer. Occasionally, she has a complaint of low back pain. She is in her third trimester and is aware about the importance of exercises and its benefits during pregnancy. Her only problem is the fear of going through the process of labor and childbirth.

Guiding Questions:

1. Assess Mrinal for her posture and gait, her back, and SI joint complaints, if any.
2. Educate her about antenatal classes and importance of attending it with partner.
3. Educate her about preparing her for labor and childbirth both physically and mentally, various positions to assume during labor, relaxation techniques, and pain-relief strategies.

Review Questions

1. What are the various musculoskeletal problems and complications that a woman comes across during the second and third trimester of pregnancy?
2. How will you explain to a pregnant woman about the benefits of exercises on the women's body and the fetus during pregnancy?
3. How will you in detail assess the women in her antenatal period and on what basis will the exercises be prescribed?
4. What is the role of a physiotherapist during labor and at the time of childbirth?
5. How will you justify the role of physiotherapy after surgical cesarean section?
6. What are the ergonomic advices explained to the mother during pregnancy and after childbirth?

BIBLIOGRAPHY

1. Aua RS, Bullock-Saxton J. Women's health—a textbook for physiotherapist; 1998.
2. Betsch M1, Wehrle R, Dor L, et al. Spinal Posture and Pelvic Position During Pregnancy: A Prospective Rasterstereographic Pilot Study. Eur Spine J. 2014;24(6):1282-8.
3. Bunevicius A, Kusminskas L, Pop VJ, et al. Screening for antenatal depression with the Edinburg Depression scale. Journal of Psychosomatic Obstetric and Gynaecology. 2009;4:238-43.
4. Changela PK. Role of physiotherapist in obstetric and gynecological conditions, 1st edition; 2016.
5. Chauhan R, Sahu B, Singh N ,et al, Enhancing normal labor by adapting antenatal physiotherapy. Int J Reprod Contracept Obstet Gynaecol. 2016;5(8) 2672-6.
6. InformedHealth.org. Pregnancy and birth: Weight gain in pregnancy. Cologne, Germany: Institute for Quality and Efficiency in Health Care (IQWiG); 2006. 2009 Jun 17. [Internet] Available from https://www.ncbi.nlm.nih.gov/books/NBK279575/. [Updated Mar 22; 2018].
7. Jahdi F, Sheikhan F, Haghani H, et al. Yoga during pregnancy: the effects on labor pain and delivery outcomes (a randomized controlled trial). Complement Ther Clin Pract. 2017;27:1-4.
8. James F, Clapp I. A compelling case for exercise before, during and after pregnancy. In: Catherine cram—exercising through your pregnancy, 2nd edition; 2012.
9. Kisner C. Therapeutic exercise—foundations and techniques, 6th edition; 2012.
10. Konar H (Ed.). D.C. Dutta's textbook of obstetrics, 7th edition; 2011.
11. Linda I, Lubis R, Siregar Y, et al. Prenatal yoga are more effective than pregnancy gymnastics in shortening total duration of normal childbirth. Health Nations. 2017;1(2) 113-7.
12. Mantle J, Haslam J. Physiotherapy in obstetrics and gynecology, 2nd edition; 2005.
13. Saxena R. Bedside obstetrics and gynecology, 1st edition; 2010.
14. Shaprio H, et al. 1997.

Psychosocial Issues in Rehabilitation

Srishti S Sharma, Priyasingh Rangey, Neeta J Vyas, Megha S Sheth

LEARNING OBJECTIVES

After reading this chapter, the readers should be able to:

♦ Understand the psychosocial factors that influence rehabilitation
♦ Describe the psychosocial adaptations that people with chronic illness and disability go through
♦ Determine the various types of personality
♦ Develop the understanding of dealing with people having personality disorders
♦ Understand the coping styles
♦ Describe the clinical manifestations and management of patients having depression and anxiety
♦ Understand acute and post-traumatic stress disorders along with their assessment
♦ Determine psychosocial wellness
♦ Apply psychosocial techniques to facilitate patient/client-centered intervention.

CHAPTER OUTLINE

- Epidemiology
- Psychosocial adaptation
  - Phase models of psychosocial adaptation
- Personality and coping styles
  - Personality types
  - Personality disorders
  - Coping styles
- Depression and anxiety
  - Types of depression
    - Assessment of depression
    - Depression and rehabilitation
- Anxiety
  - Anxiety and rehabilitation
- Acute stress disorder and post-traumatic stress disorder
  - Clinical features
  - Assessment of post-traumatic stress disorder and acute stress disorder
- Psychosocial wellness
  - Wellness in rehabilitation
    - Influence of psychosocial factors on rehabilitation
    - Psychosocial techniques and strategies to facilitate rehabilitation
- Substance abuse, agitation and violence, and hypersexuality
  - Substance abuse
  - Agitation and violence
  - Hypersexuality

INTRODUCTION

There is a growing contribution of mental health problems to the global burden of disease. The concept of psychological well-being is related to the positive dimensions of mental health, while the negative dimensions include psychological distress and psychiatric disorders. Adverse psychosocial exposure is associated with physical disease. Adverse psychosocial conditions are found to erode people's quality of life. Current report does suggest that psychosocial interventions are needed to improve population physical health.

Wickramasekera et al., found that >50% of all visits to primary care doctors involved somatic complaints resulting from psychosocial problems. Patients with physical disabilities may fail to respond to treatment if a prominent psychosocial issue is affecting them as well.

EPIDEMIOLOGY

According to a 2017 study, 197 million Indians (14.3% of the total population) were suffering from mental disorders, of whom 46 million had depression and 45 million had anxiety disorders. Depression and anxiety disorders are the most common mental disorders and their prevalence is increasing across India and is relatively higher in the southern states and in women. The prevalence of depression is the highest in older adults, which has significant impact

Table 43.1: Phases of psychosocial adaptation.

Phase	Features
Shock	Initial reaction to a psychological trauma or severe and sudden physical injury, usually short lived
Anxiety	Usually presents once the traumatic event has subsided and is characterized by panic-like feature, accompanied by confused thinking, cognitive flooding, and a multitude of physiological symptoms, including rapid heart rate, hyperventilation, excess perspiration, and irritable stomach
Denial	Regarded as defense mechanism, it involves minimal or sometimes complete negation of the traumatic event
Depression	As denial lessens, depression develops increasing the overall awareness of loss
Internalized anger	Self-directed feelings and behaviors of resentment, bitterness, guilt, and self-blame are common manifestations
Externalized hostility	Other or environment-directed retaliatory feelings and behaviors include passive aggressive behaviors, hypercriticism, antagonistic behaviors, and abusive accusations
Acknowledgment	First indication of acceptance of condition and future implications, including reconciliations, affective acceptance, internalization, sense of self-concept, and a continued search for new meaning
Final adjustment	Final phase of adaptation, consists of restored sense of self-worth, renewed life values along with pursuit of new goals, negotiations, and overcoming obstacles

on the geriatric population of our country. The prevalence of childhood onset mental disorders, such as idiopathic developmental intellectual disability, conduct disorders, and autism, was found to be high. Burden of depression is maximized due to its impact not only on the individual but also on the families and societies.

PSYCHOSOCIAL ADAPTATION

Psychosocial adaptation is defined as the process of putting oneself in harmony with the changing circumstances of life so as to enhance one's sense of well-being and long-term survivorship.

Adaptation is the dynamic process that a person with chronic illness and disability experiences in order to achieve the final state of maximal person–environment congruence known as adjustment. Simply put, adaptation is the path on which one travels in his or her journey to adjustment. In adjustment, the person places value on existing abilities and moves beyond physical losses and experiences an optimal level of congruence between the subjective world and the external environment.

When adjustment is successfully attained, the person demonstrates:
- Psychosocial equilibrium or reintegration
- Awareness of remaining assets and existing functional limitations
- Positive self-esteem, self-concept, and sense of personal mastery
- Successful negotiation of the environment
- Active participation in social, vocational, and recreational activities.

Phase Models of Psychosocial Adaptation

Phase models suggest that a patient's reaction to chronic disability or illness follows a stable sequence of phases, or stages, that are hierarchically and temporally ordered. This progression is gradual, linear, and involves the psychological assimilation of changes to one's body image and self-concept **(Table 43.1)**. In the adaptation to chronic disability and disease, the following phases are most commonly seen:
- Shock
- Anxiety
- Denial
- Depression
- Internalized anger
- Externalized hostility
- Acknowledgment
- Final adjustment.

PERSONALITY AND COPING STYLES

Chronic illnesses and disabling conditions are common occurrences in the lives of many individuals. How one copes and survives through it depends a lot on their innate personality and coping skills. Personality is the dynamic organization within the person of the psychological and physical systems that underlie that person's patterns of actions, thoughts, and feelings. On the other hand, coping skill is a type of psychological strategy that one uses to decrease, modify, or diffuse the impact of stress generating life events.

Personality Types

Although each personality is unique, personalities have been categorized into different types, such as:
- Type A
- Perfectionistic
- Authoritative
- Passive-aggressive.

Type A people are high achievers. They tend to be competitive, ambitious, and very well organized. Physiotherapists can use these qualities in patients with type A personalities to motivate their interest in rehabilitation.

Because they are often self-starters and take initiative for their own learning, they are suitable candidates for practicing home exercise programs.

Individuals with *perfectionistic* personalities uphold high standards in order to maintain self-esteem. They judge themselves by inflexible and possibly unachievable criteria and may not be able to tolerate slow progress during rehabilitation. Such set of individuals can be aided in physiotherapy by helping them derive pleasure from simple things.

Patients with *authoritative* personalities have difficulty adapting to disability, which often requires acceptance and compromise. They may require alternative strategies to solve what may have been perceived as an unsolvable problem. Engaging such patients in problem-solving to generate strategies to meet their goals serves a meaningful role in their rehabilitation.

Those with *passive-aggressive* personalities express hostility by using passive techniques such as procrastination, resistance, stubbornness, and intentional inefficiency. They react to authority negatively and have difficulty working with others. They can be best addressed in physiotherapy by placing the responsibility for progress onto them.

Clinical Pearl

Physical therapists should engage patients in problem-solving to generate strategies to meet their goals. Awareness of their patients' personality styles better enables therapists at strategizing interventions, developing a plan of care, and motivating and guiding patients through rehabilitation.

Personality Disorders

A personality disorder:
- A way of thinking, feeling, and behaving that deviates from the expectations of the culture
- Causes distress or problems functioning
- Lasts over time.

Personality disorders are long-term patterns of behavior and inner experiences that differs significantly from what is expected. The pattern of experience and behavior begins by late adolescence or early adulthood and causes distress or problems in functioning. Without treatment, personality disorders can be long-lasting.

Types of Personality Disorders

Antisocial Personality Disorder

The features of antisocial personality disorders and their treatments are as follows:
- It is a pattern of disregarding or violating the rights of others.
- A person with antisocial personality disorder may not conform to social norms, may repeatedly lie or deceive others, or may act impulsively.
- While dealing with such patients, a physiotherapist has to be aware of their dishonest ways. Therapist should

take care about the fact that such patients frequently cause disruption to others in rehabilitation.
- These patients require a cohesive team approach with immediate and strong intercommunication to minimize disruptive behaviors and refocus on rehabilitation goals.

Borderline Personality Disorder

Listed below are the features of borderline personality disorder and their treatments:
- This is a pattern of instability in personal relationships, intense emotions, poor self-image, and impulsivity.
- A person with borderline personality disorder may go to great lengths to avoid being abandoned, have repeated suicide attempts, display inappropriate intense anger, or have ongoing feelings of emptiness.
- While dealing with such patient's, physiotherapists should respond with understanding and empathy instead of anger and should emphasize strengths and strategies for ongoing work. Self-mutilating behaviors, such as repetitive cutting with razor blades, pinpricking, or cigarette burning, should be immediately reported to a doctor and referral made to psychiatrist.

Paranoid Personality Disorder

The features of paranoid personality disorder and its treatments are as follows:
- It is a pattern of being suspicious of others and seeing them as mean or spiteful. People with paranoid personality disorder often assume that people will harm or deceive them and do not confide in others or become close to them
- Physical therapists should look for behaviors that indicate paranoid thoughts, such as hostile reactions, guardedness, argumentation, and stubbornness, and encourage patients to express their thoughts at that moment. If the patient seems paranoid, the physical therapist should help him or her to better understand the reality of a specific situation.

Obsessive–compulsive Personality Disorder

The features of obsessive–compulsive personality disorder and the remedies are as follows:
- It is a pattern of preoccupation with orderliness, perfection, and control.
- A person with obsessive–compulsive personality disorder may be overly focused on details or schedules, may work excessively not allowing time for leisure or friends, or may be inflexible in their morality and values.
- For such patients, the physiotherapist should provide rehabilitative activities that promote a sense of control and predictability, and consider allowing patients to set treatment goals, and then monitor their daily progress.

Standardized Assessment of Personality Disorders

Many standardized tools are available for assessment of personality disorders.

Minnesota Multiphasic Personality Inventory-2

Minnesota Multiphasic Personality Inventory-2 (MMPI-2) is the most widely used and thoroughly researched objective measure of personality.

The Strong Interest Inventory

The Strong Interest Inventory (SII) is traditionally considered a measure of vocational interests; however, research has supported its use as a valid non-pathology-oriented measure of personality. First published in 1927, the SII is one of the most thoroughly researched, highly respected, and frequently used psychological tests. It was revised in 2004. Improvements include more focus on business and technology occupations, number of items reduced from 317 to 291, representative sampling of ethnic, racial, and demographic workforce diversity, and an expanded number of scales.

Coping Styles

Coping strategies have been found to be of great importance in rehabilitation. Patients with higher level coping skills can more easily:

- Identify and report symptoms
- Make treatment decisions
- Comply with intervention
- Accept support.

Patients with good problem-solving skills and positive attitudes have been found to make more positive adjustments to their disabilities than patients with low self-esteem and poor self-concept. Coping styles often determine whether or not patients seek medical help and follow advice.

Mainly, the coping strategies identified in literature include planning, problem-solving, wishful thinking, avoiding, minimizing, seeking social support, searching for meaning, emoting feelings, blaming, accepting, negotiating, disengaging, and turning to religion. Based on this, they are chiefly categorized into three different types:

1. Seeking versus avoiding control and information
2. Expressing versus repressing emotional reactions
3. Seeking versus withdrawing from social interactions and networks.

Coping styles that result in positive outcomes for people with disabilities utilize positive, direct, and active problem-solving, social support seeking, and information seeking and comprise adaptive or positive styles of coping. The ones that lead to unfavorable adaptation outcomes include self-blame; nondirect, passive, and escape/avoidance modes of coping; and substance abuse that constitutes nonadaptive or negative styles of coping **(Fig. 43.1)**.

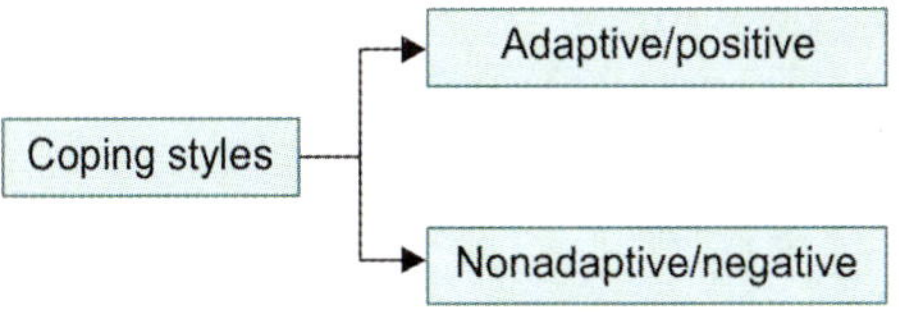

Fig. 43.1: Types of coping styles.

DEPRESSION AND ANXIETY

Response mechanisms used by a person against a major catastrophic event such as death or disability are nothing but defenses against internal and external stressors. They are spontaneous and unconscious in effort, and sometimes a person may use one or more than one techniques to cope. Diagnostic and Statistical Manual of Mental Disorders (DSM-III) identifies a list of various such defense mechanisms **(Box 43.1)**. Anxiety is the apprehensive anticipation of future danger or misfortune accompanied by feelings of tension and agitation. On the other hand, depression refers to feelings of despair and hopelessness, negative shifts in perception, and decreased interest in activities that once provided pleasure. Anxiety and Depression Association of America (ADAA) reports that depression occurs more often in women than men. Some differences in the manner in which the depressed mood manifests has been found based on sex and age.

- In men, it manifests often as tiredness, irritability, and anger. They may show more reckless behavior and abuse drugs and alcohol. They also tend to not recognize that they are depressed and fail to seek help.
- In women, depression tends to manifest as sadness, worthlessness, and guilt.
- In younger children, depression is more likely to manifest as school refusal, anxiety when separated from parents, and worry about parents dying.
- Depressed teenagers tend to be irritable, sulky, and get into trouble in school. They also frequently have comorbid anxiety, eating disorders, or substance abuse.
- In older adults, depression may manifest more subtly as they tend to be less likely to admit to feelings of sadness or grief and medical illnesses, which are more common in this population, also contribute or cause the depression.

Types of Depression

Types of depression are as follows:

- The most commonly diagnosed form of depression is **major depressive disorder**. It is characterized by at least five of the diagnostic symptoms of which at

BOX 43.1: Common defense mechanisms.	
• Acting out	• Intellectualization
• Altruism	• Isolation of affect
• Autistic fantasy	• Omnipotence
• Denial	• Projection
• Devaluation	• Rationalization
• Displacement	• Repression
• Dissociation	• Splitting
• Help-rejecting	• Sublimation
• Humor	• Suppression
• Idealization	• Undoing

least one of the symptoms is either an overwhelming feeling of sadness or a loss of interest and pleasure in most usual activities. The other symptoms that are associated with major depression include:

- Decrease or increase in appetite
- Insomnia or hypersomnia
- Psychomotor agitation or retardation
- Constant fatigue
- Feelings of worthlessness
- Excessive and inappropriate guilt
- Recurrent thoughts of death and suicidal ideation with or without specific plans for committing suicide
- Cognitive difficulties, such as, diminished ability to think, concentrate, and take decisions.

- Another type of depression is called **persistent depressive disorder (dysthymia)**. The essential feature of this mood disorder is a low, dark, or sad mood that is persistently present for most of the day and on most days, for at least 2 years (children and adolescents may experience predominantly irritability and the mood persist for at least 1 year).
- **Premenstrual dysphoric disorder** is another manifestation of depression, which is a severe and sometimes disabling extension of premenstrual syndrome.

Assessment of Depression

The assessment of depression is as follows:

- The Hamilton Depression Rating Scale was designed by psychiatrist Max Hamilton in 1960. It includes 21 questions with between 3 and 5 possible responses, which increase in severity. The clinician must choose the possible responses to each question by interviewing the patient and by observing the patient's symptoms.
- The Beck Depression Inventory was originally designed by psychiatrist Aaron T Beck. It is a 21-question self-report inventory that covers symptoms such as irritability, fatigue, weight loss, lack of interest in sex, and feelings of guilt, hopelessness, or fear of being punished. The scale is completed by patients to identify the presence and severity of symptoms consistent with the DSM-IV diagnostic criteria.
- The Geriatric Depression Scale (GDS) is another self-administered scale, but in this case it is used for older patients, and for patients with mild-to-moderate dementia. Instead of presenting a five-category response set, the GDS questions are answered with a simple "yes" or "no."

Depression and Rehabilitation

Several studies show that patients with higher levels of depressive symptoms used rehabilitation services less efficiently than those with lesser symptoms. Recovery from minor trauma or musculoskeletal disorders is also

impacted by depression. A recent study done on geriatric population showed that depression and cognitive impairment are predictive of negative outcomes in elderly patients' rehabilitation from skeletal fractures. Depression, and its impact on acute rehabilitation, is significantly related to functional recovery but does not differ in its frequency or impact for stroke patients. Because depressive symptoms do not appear to discriminate across diagnostic groups, routine screening for depression is recommended for all rehabilitation inpatients.

Depressed patients require assistance with motivation. Physical therapists can facilitate motivation by:

- Providing encouragement
- Emphasizing strengths
- Offering positive feedback
- Addressing values
- Mobilizing guilt into goal acquisition.

Empowering patients by providing activities that offer opportunities for self-control and success has been shown to decrease depression.

ANXIETY

Anxiety is the apprehensive anticipation of future danger or misfortune accompanied by feelings of tension and agitation. The anticipated danger may be real or imagined but is experienced both psychologically and physiologically. Cultural factors have influenced the presentation, diagnoses, and treatment of anxiety disorders in India for several centuries. The symptoms can include excessive worry, difficulty in concentration, and sleep disturbances. Causes of anxiety include major life events as stressors, life events that refer to major changes in lifestyle, status, role, or situation.

Anxiety and Rehabilitation

An anxious patient's thought and energy are focused on the anxiety instead of physiotherapy; hence, they may concentrate less. Due to this, they will be unable to concentrate on the therapist's instructions resulting in decreased learning. Performing motor tasks that require multiple-step directions thus becomes difficult. This can also lead to safety risks as the patient's attention may be alternating between the anxiety and the demands of rehabilitation.

Anxiety often can cause misperception, which leads to patients perceiving their level of dysfunction and improvement very differently as compared to their therapists. Patients with anxiety often leave therapy sessions with an unrealistic opinion concerning any progress or gains made.

- Physical therapists should make use of a purposeful activity with the patient's anxiety in mind.
- Some anxious patients have been known to respond to activities that consist of one repetitive motor action, as rhythmic motion helps to calm them.

- Gross motor movements help decrease the physical symptoms of anxiety such as muscle aches, agitation, and restlessness.
- Therapists should begin by involving patients in a therapeutic activity that is easily performed and then increase the complexity of the task once the patient has gained confidence.

ACUTE STRESS DISORDER AND POST-TRAUMATIC STRESS DISORDER

Both post-traumatic stress disorder (PTSD) and acute stress disorder (ASD) are specific forms or subsets of anxiety disorders. The term "post-traumatic stress disorder" came into use in the 1970s in large part due to the diagnoses of US military veterans of the Vietnam War. It was officially recognized by the American Psychiatric Association in 1980 in the third edition of the Diagnostic and Statistical Manual of Mental Disorders (DSM-III).

- PTSD is a common and often chronic and disabling anxiety disorder that can develop after exposure to highly stressful events characterized by actual or threatened harm to the self or others.
- ASD involves symptoms that must range in duration between 2 days to a maximum of 4 weeks. If symptoms of ASD persist longer than 4 weeks, the diagnosis of ASD is discontinued and changed to PTSD.
- PTSD is differentiated as acute PTSD if symptoms last >4 weeks but <3 months and as chronic PTSD if symptoms last 3 months or longer.

Clinical Features

Symptoms of ASD and PTSD are similar and generally involve a combination of the following:

Intrusion Symptoms

Intrusion symptoms are described as follows:

- Recurrent, involuntary, and distressing memories or dreams of the traumatic event (in children <6 years, it may not be clear whether their distressing dreams are related to the event)
- Dissociative reactions (typically flashbacks in which patients reexperience the trauma, although young children may frequently reenact the event in play)
- Distress at internal or external cues that resemble some aspect of the trauma (e.g., seeing a dog or someone who resembles a perpetrator).

Avoidance Symptoms

Avoidance symptoms include persistent avoidance of memories, feelings, or external reminders of the trauma.

Negative Effects on Cognition and/or Mood

Following are the negative effects on cognition and/or mood:

- Inability to remember important aspects of the traumatic event
- Distorted thinking about the causes and/or consequences of the trauma (e.g., that they are to blame or could have avoided the event by certain actions)
- A decrease in positive emotions and an increase in negative emotions (fear, guilt, sadness, shame, and confusion)
- General lack of interest
- Social withdrawal
- A subjective sense of feeling numb
- A foreshortened expectation of the future (e.g., thinking "I will not live to see 20").

Altered Arousal and/or Reactivity (e.g., Hyperarousal)

The signs and symptoms of altered arousal and/or reactivity are:

- Jitteriness
- Difficulty relaxing
- Difficulty concentrating
- Disrupted sleep (sometimes with frequent nightmares)
- Aggressive or reckless behavior.

Dissociative Symptoms

Dissociative symptoms include feeling detached from one's body as if in a dream and feeling that the world is unreal.

Several recent investigations have attempted to identify biological markers or risk factors for the development of PTSD, with the two most promising being:

1. Low cortisol levels in the acute aftermath of the trauma
2. Elevated resting heart rate shortly after the trauma.

Assessment of Post-traumatic Stress Disorder and Acute Stress Disorder

The assessment of PTSD and ASD requires, at minimum, of:

- The person's trauma history
- Obtaining information on both the objective features of the trauma(s) (i.e., Was the person exposed to an event involving real or threatened injury or death to self or others?)
- The person's subjective reaction (i.e., Did the person respond to the event with intense fear, terror, horror, or helplessness?)
- The person's current symptoms (i.e., Given a qualifying traumatic event, does the person meet the remaining symptom, duration, and functional impairment criteria for ASD or PTSD?).

  Also, there is the presumed etiological role of trauma in the development of PTSD, the temporal relationship between the traumatic event and the person's symptoms (i.e., Did the trauma precede onset or exacerbation of the patient's symptoms?).
- The Acute Stress Disorder Interview and the Acute Stress Disorder Scale are useful for the assessment of ASD.

- The PTSD Symptom Scale Interview (PSS-I) and PTSD Symptom Scale Self-Report are a pair of measures used for the assessment of PTSD.

PSYCHOSOCIAL WELLNESS

Psychosocial well-being is when individuals, families, or communities have cognitive, emotional, and spiritual strengths combined with positive social relationships. Wellness is defined as a dynamic process in which people attempt to fully develop their emotional, environmental, physical, spiritual, and intellectual health.

Wellness in Rehabilitation

Psychosocial wellness requires that patients experience success in both rehabilitation activities and long-term relationships and roles. Rehabilitation activities focus on improving functional outcomes, involvement in meaningful events that foster socialization (e.g., playing wheelchair basketball with other patients), and community reintegration. Maintaining a daily balance of work, leisure, and social activities is important to sustain psychosocial wellness. Therapists can help patients to engage in leisure activities along with exercises.

A negative outlook inhibits psychosocial wellness. Thus therapists should help patients with negative perspectives to positively alter their expectations through:
- Goal setting
- Identifying optimistic options
- Using cognitive behavioral techniques that challenge the validity of negative perceptions
- Referring the patient to a psychologist for longer term intervention.

Influence of Psychosocial Factors on Rehabilitation

Studies have shown that clinicians need to be more sensitive toward patients' psychological concerns. Psychological assessment and assistance from a mental health professional should be considered during the hospital stay and rehabilitation period. Emotional problems and weak social support systems can diminish the effect of a good treatment session.

Emotional factors can include anxiety, depression, and stress and **social support issues** might be mental or physical, which have direct influence on the outcomes of rehabilitation. Hence as a practicing physiotherapist, one must have some knowledge pertaining to a patient's outlook and "personality type" as it relates to these factors.

Psychosocial Techniques and Strategies to Facilitate Rehabilitation

Global clinical interventions emphasize the need to provide the client and his or her family and significant others with emotional, cognitive, and behavioral support.

These interventions have been successfully adapting to their condition and its impact on their lives. They aim at:
- Assisting clients to explore the personal meaning of the chronic illness and disability (CID)
- Providing clients with relevant medical information
- Providing clients with supportive family and group experiences
- Teaching clients adaptive coping skills for successful community functioning.

Optimizing Patient Involvement

The process of optimizing patient involvement can be performed as follows:
- Allowing patients to maintain a passive role fosters helplessness, encourages dependency, and slows progress in the long-term.
- Hence, patients should be actively involved in their own treatment to the best of their ability.
- This includes involvement in goal setting, treatment planning and in the ongoing evaluation of progress.
- Patient cooperation is also dependent on the therapist's clear explanation of the patient's situation, anticipated goals and expected outcomes, and interventions.

Use of Jargon and Labels

A therapist should keep the following in mind regarding the use of jargon and labels:
- Patient–therapist communication should be simple and easy to match the cognitive level of the patient.
- The use of scientific jargon and labels should be avoided when speaking with patients, because it impedes patient understanding and bridges the patients from therapists emotionally.

Self-awareness

The self-awareness of a therapist plays a role in the following way:
- Therapists need to be aware of their own feelings, motivations, and responses.
- Such self-awareness is critical for therapists to understand their own reactions to patients.

SUBSTANCE ABUSE, AGITATION AND VIOLENCE, AND HYPERSEXUALITY

Substance Abuse

Substance abuse refers to the harmful or hazardous use of psychoactive substances, including alcohol and illicit drugs. The use of psychoactive substances causes significant health and social problems for the people who use them, and also for others in their families and communities. Substances of abuse include alcohol, opiates, cocaine, amphetamines, hallucinogens, prescription, and over-the-counter drug abuse (Psychoactive substances are substances that, when taken in or administered into one's system, affect mental processes).

The commonly abused opioids in India include heroin ("smack"/"brown sugar") as well as pharmaceutical opioids (such as buprenorphine, pentazocine, and dextropropoxyphene). In the north-eastern region, heroin and dextropropoxyphene are the most commonly used opioids; impure heroin (smack) and buprenorphine are the most commonly used opioids in metropolitan cities such as Delhi, Mumbai, Chennai, and Kolkata. Pentazocine is the most commonly injected opioid in Karnataka, Andhra Pradesh, and Chhattisgarh. In the states of Punjab and Haryana, buprenorphine is commonly used by injectors.

Treating Patients Who Abuse Substances

Physiotherapists can help patients in recovery by providing opportunities that allow them to control addiction. Such assistance can be given by providing opportunities to practice setting boundaries, regulating emotions, and tolerating frustration.

Physical therapists can emphasize healthy activities that provide pleasure and decrease cravings. Stress management, time management, activities of daily living (ADL), and social skills are usually necessary skills to promote recovery.

Agitation and Violence

Agitation is defined as increased verbal and/or motor activity as well as restlessness, anxiety, tension, and fear, whereas aggression means self-assertive verbal or physical behavior arising from innate drives and/or a response to frustration that may manifest by cursing/threats and/or destructive and attacking behavior toward objects or people. These symptoms are commonly present in patients with central nervous system disorders.

Epidemiological evidence points to an increased risk for violence among individuals with a mental disorder compared with the general population. Role of physiotherapy is to create a calm environment and remove stressors:

- Avoid environmental triggers. Noise, glare, and background distraction (such as having the television on) can act as triggers
- Monitor personal comfort
- Simplify tasks and routines
- Addressing the underlying circumstance causing the agitation may help to defuse it. If the source of agitation is unknown, the physical therapist should acknowledge to the patient, in a nonaccusatory manner, that he or she seems upset. Many people are unaware of their agitation and calm down once it is brought to their attention.

Hypersexuality

Sexual addiction or hypersexuality is defined as a dysfunctional preoccupation with sexual fantasy, often in combination with the obsessive pursuit of casual or nonintimate sex, pornography, compulsive masturbation, romantic

intensity, and objectified sex partner for a period of at least 6 months.

If a physiotherapist realizes the presence of hypersexuality in patient, he/she is treating and feels threatened by it, he or she should leave the area and obtain assistance. If the patient's hypersexual behavior is a newly observed behavior, the therapist must firmly state that the behavior exhibited is inappropriate and will not be tolerated. Referral to psychiatrist can be made if the behavior doesn't seem to be in control of the patient.

SUMMARY

Successful intervention depends on the following:

- Understanding the psychosocial factors affecting each patient
- Knowing each patient's personality styles and coping skills
- Distinguishing the stages of psychosocial adaptation to disability and helping patients' progress in their own adjustment
- Understanding how to identify anxiety, depression, and other psychological issues
- Knowing when to send such patients for medical assistance
- Integrating a patient/client-centered approach that emphasizes respect, empathy, and compassion
- Empowering patients and families through psychosocial education, and wellness and prevention strategies
- Collaborating with patients and team members to establish and implement appropriate interventions
- Developing a team approach and providing referrals as necessary.

It is important for physical therapists to identify and understand the individual psychosocial factors that enhance or inhibit the rehabilitation of their patients and intervene accordingly.

Review Questions

1. Identify and describe the phases of psychosocial adaptation to disability.
2. What are the signs and symptoms of post-traumatic stress disorder?
3. Describe the general adaptation syndrome.
4. Describe the assessment and management of patients with depression.
5. Explain the term anxiety and its effect on rehabilitation.

BIBLIOGRAPHY

1. American Physical therapy Association. Guide to physical therapist practice, 2 edition. Phys Ther. 2001;81:1.
2. Beck AT. Depression: causes and treatment. Philadelphia, PA: University of Pennsylvania Press; 1972. p. 333. ISBN 978-0-8122-1032-3.

3. Bryant RA, Harvey AG. Avoidant coping style and PTS following motor vehicle accidents. Behav Res Ther. 1995;33:631.

4. Camara WJ, Nathan JS, Puente AE. Psychological test usage: implications in professional psychology. Prof Psychol Res Pract. 2000;31(2):141-54. doi:10.1037/0735-7028.31.2.141.

5. Chan F, Da Silva Cardoso E, Chronister JA (Eds). Understanding Psychosocial Adjustment to Chronic Illness and Disability: A Handbook for Evidence-Based Practitioners in Rehabilitation. Springer, New York; 2019. pp.51-68.

6. Craven J, Rodin G, Littlefield C. The Beck Depression Inventory as a screening device for major depression in renal dialysis patients. Int J Psychiatry Med. 1988;18(4):365-74.

7. economictimes.indiatimes.com/articleshow/72950200.cms?utm_source=contentofinterest&utm_medium=text&utm_campaign=cppst

8. Frank RG, Rosenthal M, Caplan B (Eds). Handbook of rehabilitation psychology, 2nd edition. Washington, DC: American Psychological Association; 2009.

9. Hardy CJ, Richman JM, Rosenfeld LB. The Role of Social Support in the Life Stress/Injury Relationship. The Sport Psychologist. 1991;5:128-39.

10. https://psychcentral.com/lib/hypersexuality-symptoms-of-sexual-addiction/

11. https://www.nhp.gov.in/disease/non-communicable-disease/substance-abuse

12. https://www.psychiatry.org/patients-families/personality-disorders/what-are-personality-disorders

13. Kaplan SP. Psychosocial adjustment three years after traumatic brain injury. Clin Neuropsychol. 1991;5:360.

14. Krause JS, Rohe DE. Personality and life adjustment after spinal cord injury: an exploratory study. Rehabil Psychol. 1998;43:118.

15. Livneh H, Martz E, Bodner T. Psychosocial Adaptation to Chronic Illness and Disability: A Preliminary Study of its Factorial Structure. Journal of Clinical Psychology in Medical Settings. 2006;13:250-60.

16. Loy DP, Dattilo J, Kleiber DA, et al. Dimensions of leisure and depression symptoms after spinal cord injury. Annu Ther Recreat. 2002;11:43.

17. Mayou RA, Smith KA. Post-traumatic symptoms following medical illness and treatment. J Psychosom Res. 1997;43:121.

18. McFarlane J, Hughes R, Nosek MA, et al. Abuse Assessment Screen-Disability (AAS-D): Measuring Frequency, Type, and Perpetrator of Abuse toward Women with Physical Disabilities. Journal of women's health & gender-based medicine. 2001;10:861-6.

19. Merriam New World Dictionary of American English, 2nd edition. Upper Saddle River, NJ: Prentice-Hall; 1988.

20. Nemeroff CB. The molecular neurobiology of depression. Psychiatr Clin North Am. 2007;30(1):1-11.

21. Precin P. Living skills recovery workbook. Woburn, MA: Butterworth-Heinemann; 1999.

22. Reker GT, Woo LC. Personal Meaning Orientations and Psychosocial Adaptation in Older Adults. SAGE Open; 2011.

23. Rintala DH, Young ME, Har KA, et al. Social support and the well-being of persons with spinal cord injury living in the community. Rehabil Psychol. 1992;37:155.

24. Sahler OJZ, Carr JE. Developmental–behavioral pediatrics, 8th edition. Elsevier; 2009.

25. Schiele BC, Baker AB, Hathaway SR. The Minnesota Multiphasic Personality Inventory. J Lancet. 1943;63:292-7. ISSN 0096-0233.

26. Sheth HC, Gandhi Z, Vankar GK. Indian anxiety disorders in ancient Indian literature. J Psychiatry. 2010;52(3):289-91.

27. US Department of Health and Human Services. Healthy people 2020. Understanding and improving health, 3rd edition. Washington, DC: US Government Printing Office; 2010.

28. Vaillant GE. Adaptation to life. Little, Boston: Brown; 1977.

29. Wickramasekera I, et al. Applied psychophysiology: a bridge between the biomedical model and the biopsychosocial model family medicine. Prof Psychol Res Pract. 1996;27:221.

30. World Health Organization (WHO). Towards a Common Language for Functioning, Disability and Health: ICF. Geneva, Switzerland: WHO; 2002. Available from www.who.int/classifications/icf/training/icfbeginnersguide.pdf.

31. Yesavage JA. Geriatric Depression Scale. Psychopharmacol Bull. 1988;24(4):709-11. PMID 3249773.

32. Zagaria MAE. Agitation and aggression in the elderly individualized therapy is key. US Pharm. 2006;11:20-8.

Disorders of Speech

Srishti S Sharma, Neeta J Vyas, Megha S Sheth, Priyasingh Rangey

LEARNING OBJECTIVES

After reading this chapter, the readers should be able to:
- Understand the production of speech
- Classify speech and language disorders
- Discuss and characterize various types of aphasia
- Understand recent development in treatment of aphasia
- Describe the primary types of dysarthria and rationale for dysarthria treatment
- Describe apraxia of speech and its treatment
- Understand basics of swallowing disorders
- Understand the psychosocial factors affecting speech
- Understand implications of speech disorders for physiotherapy.

CHAPTER OUTLINE

- Production of speech
- Epidemiology
- Classification of speech disorders
- Aphasia
  - Classification of aphasia
  - Aphasia assessment
  - Treatment of aphasia
- Dysarthria
  - Types of dysarthria
  - Treatment
- Apraxia of speech
  - Clinical features
- Swallowing impairment
- Cognitive communication disorders
- Treatment of cognitive communication disorders
- Psychosocial aspects of communication disorders
- Implications of speech disorder on physiotherapy

INTRODUCTION

Human communication is often described as a well-coordinated, timed, and multidimensional group of processes used to share thoughts, ideas, and emotions. The processes include speech, language, cognition, and hearing. Speech is the system that produces individual sounds, which, when placed together, develop meaningful messages. It is the verbal means of communication often thought of as the motor vehicle for message delivery. It is thought that the study of speech communication is one of the oldest academic disciplines with roots dating back to the time of Aristotle.

PRODUCTION OF SPEECH

Speech is one of the most *natural* forms of communication for human beings. It is a complex feedback process in which hearing, perception, and information processing in the brain are also involved. The five systems comprising speech production include:
1. Respiration
2. Phonation
3. Resonation
4. Articulation
5. Hearing.

Speaking is in essence the by-product of a necessary bodily process, the expulsion from the lungs of air charged with carbon dioxide after it has fulfilled its function in respiration. Most of the time, one breathes out silently; but it is possible, by contracting and relaxing the vocal tract, to change the characteristics of the air expelled from the lungs.

The phonatory process, or voicing occurs when air is expelled from the lungs through the glottis (space between the vocal folds). A normal voice is best described

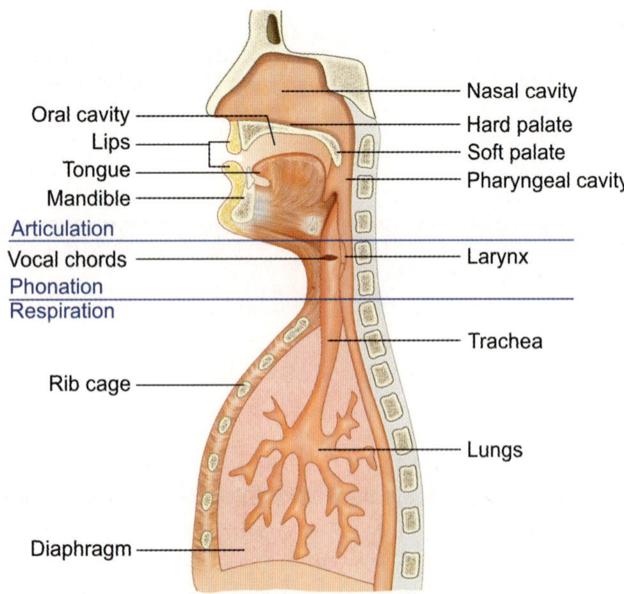

Fig. 44.1: Speech organs.

as the product of a controlled exhalation of air, steady maintenance of subglottic air pressures, and delicately balanced vocal folds movement. The raw vocal tone is modified and amplified by *resonance* within the pharyngeal, oral, and nasal cavities which are referred to collectively as the vocal tract. The final production of sound occurs as air is expelled through and manipulated within the oral cavity by the movements of the lips, teeth, and tongue. Coordinated actions of the tongue, lips, jaw, and soft palate regulate the air stream and produce the meaningful sounds of speech called phonemes. These structures are often referred to as articulators as shown in **Figure 44.1**.

EPIDEMIOLOGY

All India Institute of Speech and Hearing, in a recent report, had stated that 68.24% of the population are found to have communication disorders. The same report also stated that males showed a higher prevalence of communication disorders compared to females. Child language disorders and reading/writing difficulties were the most prevalent problems among speech and language disorders. Prevalence of communication disorders in India is found to be higher in comparison to that of developed countries. In their study, Konadath et al. has revealed prevalence of at-risk population for communication disorders to be 6.07% in the rural part of India in a population size of 15,441.

CLASSIFICATION OF SPEECH DISORDERS

There are three general classes of speech disorders **(Fig. 44.2)**:
1. Disorders of rhythm in verbal expression
2. Disorders of articulation and vocalization
3. Disorders of symbolic formulation and expression.

There are guidelines by the American Speech–Language–Hearing Association (ASHA), which provide guidance on definitions of communication disorders and variations.

Clinical Pearl

A communication disorder is impairment in the ability to receive, send, process, and comprehend concepts or verbal, nonverbal, and graphic symbol systems.

- A communication disorder may be evident in the processes of hearing, language, and/or speech. A communication disorder may range in severity from mild to profound.
- It may be developmental or acquired. Individuals may demonstrate one or any combination of communication disorders.
- A communication disorder may be a primary disability or it may be secondary to other disabilities.

I. A **speech disorder** is an impairment of the articulation of speech sounds, fluency, and/or voice:
   1. An **articulation disorder** is the atypical production of speech sounds characterized by substitutions, omissions, additions, or distortions that may interfere with intelligibility.
   2. A **fluency disorder** is an interruption in the flow of speaking characterized by atypical rate, rhythm, and repetitions in sounds, syllables, words, and phrases. This may be accompanied by excessive tension, struggle behavior, and secondary mannerisms.
   3. A **voice disorder** is characterized by the abnormal production and/or absences of vocal quality, pitch, loudness, resonance, and/or duration, which is inappropriate for an individual's age and/or sex.

II. A **language disorder** is an impaired comprehension and/or use of spoken, written, and/or other symbol systems. The disorder may involve:
   1. The form of language (phonology, morphology, and syntax)
   2. The content of language (semantics)
   3. The function of language in communication (pragmatics) in any combination.

   Form of language:
   - **Phonology** is the sound system of a language and the rules that govern the sound combinations.
   - **Morphology** is the system that governs the structure of words and the construction of word forms.

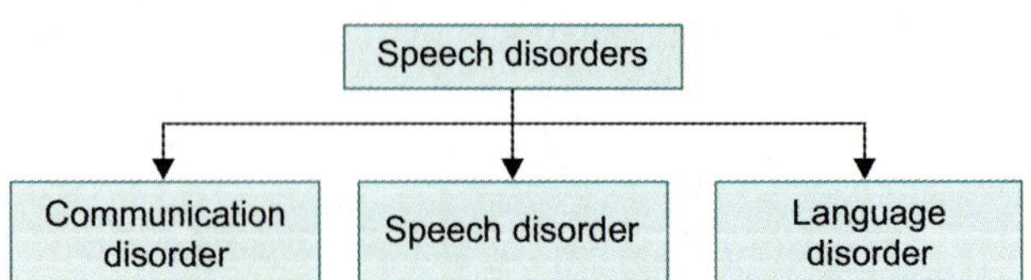

Fig. 44.2: Classification of speech disorders.

- **Syntax** is the system governing the order and combination of words to form sentences, and the relationships among the elements within a sentence.

Content of language: **Semantics** is the system that governs the meanings of words and sentences.

Function of language: **Pragmatics** is the system that combines the above language components in functional and socially appropriate communication.

APHASIA

According to the National Aphasia Association, aphasia is defined as an impairment of language, affecting the production or comprehension of speech and the ability to read or write. Aphasia is often associated with focal disease, usually of the left hemisphere.

Classification of Aphasia

The Boston classification system is easy to understand clinically. It standardizes terminology by classifying disorders into those in which expressive skills are predominantly fluent and those in which they are predominantly nonfluent (**Box 44.1, Figs. 44.3A and B**).

> **BOX 44.1:** Classification of aphasia.
>
> The eight major types of aphasia in the Boston system include the more common forms of Broca's aphasia, Wernicke's aphasia, anomia, conduction aphasia, and global aphasia, as well as the less frequent transcortical types, transcortical motor and transcortical sensory (**Figs. 44.3A and B**).

A. **Nonfluent aphasias:**
1. **Broca's aphasia:** Broca's aphasia is one of the classic aphasias according to the localization theory of aphasias with site of lesion in Broca's area (or area 44). Localization of function (LOF)is the theory that explains that the certain areas of the brain correspond to certain functions and reflects the notion that behavior, emotions, and thoughts originate in the brain in specific locations. In 1861, Paul Broca deduced from localized brain lesions that the speech center of the brain is in the left frontal lobe (see Broca's area). This Broca's area is located in the third frontal convolution anterior to the precentral gyrus.

Another term commonly used for this type of aphasia is "expressive aphasia." In this, expressive skill is more greatly impaired than receptive skills. Agrammatic

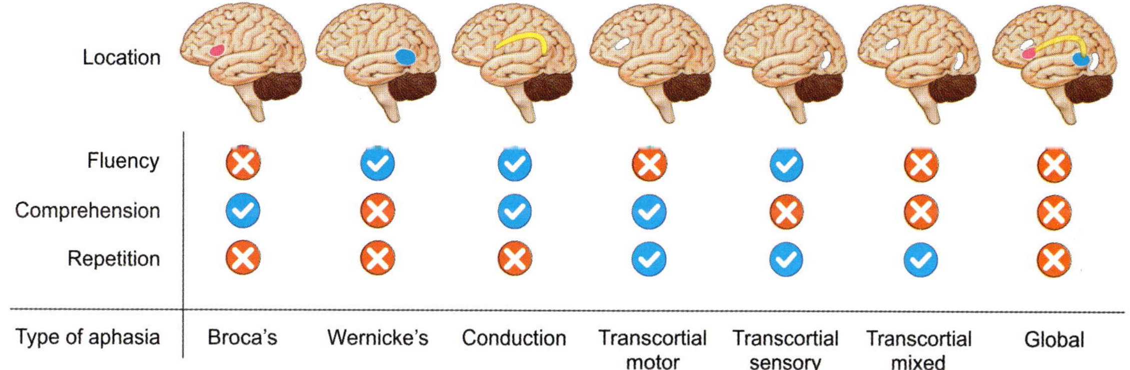

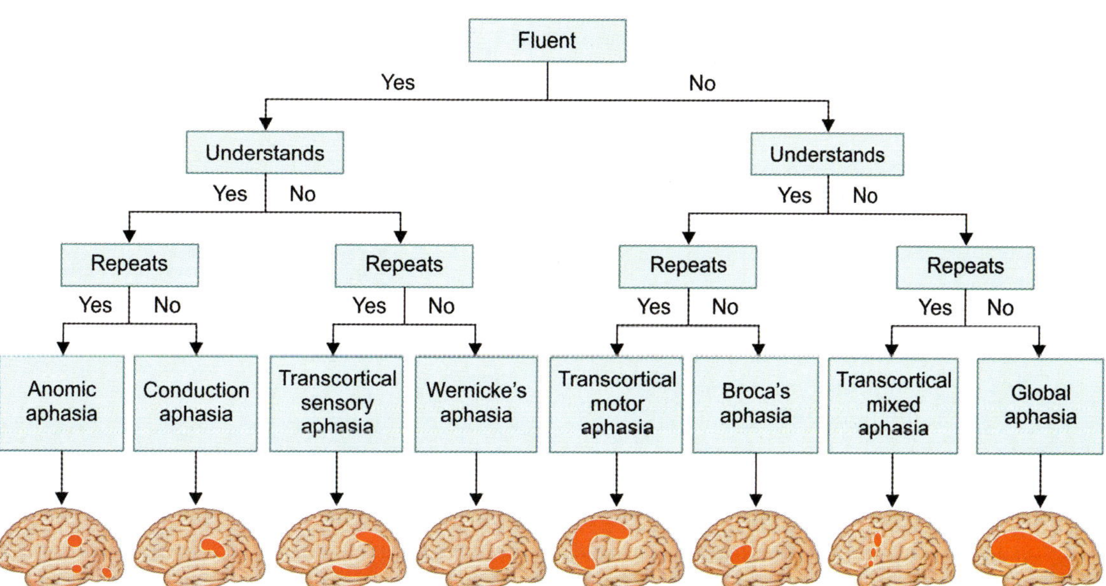

Figs. 44.3A and B: (A) Types of aphasia; (B) Classification of aphasias.

verbal output is a hallmark symptom. In this, the patient is a relatively good communicator, as compared with those with other types of aphasias; however, repetition is typically poor.

2. **Transcortical motor aphasia:** Currently, this type of aphasia is believed to be of a smaller site of lesion, located in the frontal lobe, superior and anterior to Broca's area. Language function is similar to those of Broca's aphasia. The only differentiating feature is that in this repetition is relatively preserved.

3. **Global aphasia:** This is commonly associated with a large left hemisphere lesion, typically, including both Broca's and Wernicke's areas. It is considered the most severe aphasia with significant deficits in all language modalities. In this, automatic expressions, such as counting or profanity are preserved. Patients often tend to use other modalities of communication, such as facial expression and/or gesture to communicate basic wants, needs, or feelings.

B. **Fluent aphasias:**

1. **Wernicke's aphasia:** As the name suggests, this aphasia is associated with lesion in the Wernicke's area (area 22), which is the posterior portion of the superior temporal gyrus. It also known as "receptive aphasia." The hallmark feature of this aphasia is receptive skills are more impaired than expressive skills. Patients with this type of aphasia often produce sentences with intact grammar and rhythm of speech but frequent paraphasias of both types and/or frequent neologisms or jargon. Due to poor auditory comprehension, error awareness is also poor, usually making for a less effective communicator than one with Broca's aphasia. Repetition is also impaired.

2. **Transcortical sensory aphasia:** This aphasia is due to lesion in the inferior temporo-occipital border area of the brain. It is similar to Wernicke's aphasia, but differentiating feature is that repetition is relatively preserved.

3. **Conduction aphasia:** It is found to be associated with subcortical lesions in the arcuate fasciculus, an association tract running beneath the cortex, connecting temporal and parietal lobes and carrying impulses between Wernicke's area and Broca's area. In conduction aphasia, repetition is disproportionately impaired compared to auditory comprehension and verbal expression. Verbal output is generally grammatically correct and fluent but has episodes of halting speech during moments because of difficulty in word retrieval.

4. **Anomic aphasia:** It is associated with lesion of the temporal and parietal lobes. It is typically the mildest form of aphasias. Its clinical features are word retrieval difficulties, with syntax and fluency generally intact. Verbal output is characterized by frequent semantic paraphasias or overgeneralizations for the intended words. Comprehension impairment is mild.

C. **Primary progressive aphasia:** Primary progressive aphasia (PPA) is a neurological syndrome in which language capabilities become slowly and progressively impaired. Unlike other forms of aphasia that result from stroke or brain injury, PPA is caused by neurodegenerative diseases, such as Alzheimer's disease or frontotemporal lobar degeneration. PPA results from deterioration of brain tissue important for speech and language. Although the initial symptoms are difficulties with speech and language, other issues associated with the underlying disease, such as memory loss, often also happen later.

PPA commonly begins as a subtle disorder of language, progressing to a nearly total inability to speak, in its most severe stage. The type or pattern of the language deficit may differ from patient to patient. The initial language disturbance may be fluent aphasia (i.e., the person may have normal or even increased rate of word production) or nonfluent aphasia (speech becomes effortful and the person produces fewer words). A less common variety begins with impaired word finding and progressive deterioration of naming and comprehension, with relatively preserved articulation.

Aphasia Assessment

Tests for aphasia measure the patient's receptive and expressive language capacities by sampling different types of language skills through systematically controlled channels. Some of the more commonly utilized aphasia assessments include:

- Western aphasia battery-revised (WAB-R)
- Boston diagnostic aphasia examination (BDAE)
- Communication activities of daily living-2 (CADL-2)
- Boston naming test (BNT)
- Reading comprehension battery of aphasia-2 (RCBA-2)
- Neurosensory center comprehensive examination for aphasia (NCCEA).

Clinical Pearl

These assessments are rarely given in their entirety. Depending on the degree of the patient's impairment and the area of deficit, the evaluating clinician gathers information regarding patient's function, and specific subtests are then selected and administered.

Treatment of Aphasia

Word retrieval difficulty is a characteristic present in all people with aphasia regardless of the applicable aphasia classification system. Therefore treatment of word retrieval is a common focus of intervention by nearly all clinicians implementing an impairment-based treatment approach.

Constraint-induced language treatment (CILT) is a behavioral treatment approach for aphasia with theoretical underpinnings based on knowledge about the brain mechanism. CILT is modeled after constraint-induced movement treatment (CIMT) which encourages forced use of the hemiparetic hand and arm in order to promote neuroplastic changes in the lesioned hemisphere contralateral to the weak arm/hand, with the ultimate goal of improved movement. CILT is an intervention strategy aimed at improving the quality and quantity of verbal linguistic output of people with aphasia. The treatment focuses on reducing the reliance on compensatory (substitutive) communication strategies, such as writing and gesturing, in order to force the individual to utilize more extensive verbal means to communicate. It is possible that practicing oral language can promote neuroplastic changes in the left hemisphere and support improved language function. Oral verbal expression is required (and actually promoted using constrained techniques) for people with aphasia, who may previously have made extensive use of nonverbal strategies or reading/writing to enhance communication effectiveness.

DYSARTHRIA

The ASHA has defined dysarthria as a group of neurogenic speech disorders characterized by "abnormalities in the strength, speed, range, steadiness, tone, or accuracy of movements required for breathing, phonatory, resonator, articulatory, or prosodic aspects of speech production."

Types of Dysarthria

The various types of dysarthria are:
1. Flaccid
2. Spastic
3. Ataxic
4. Hypokinetic
5. Hyperkinetic
6. Unilateral upper motor neuron
7. Mixed: Various combinations of dysarthria types (e.g., spastic–ataxic and flaccid–spastic)
8. Undetermined

1. **Flaccid dysarthria:** Flaccid dysarthria is due to weakness in cranial or spinal column nerve innervations to the speech systems. Most common characteristics of the speech in this are diplophonia, hypernasality, breathiness, nasal emission, audible inspiration (stridor), short phrases, and rapid deterioration, and recovery with rest. Brainstem stroke or brain injury is a common cause of flaccid dysarthria.
2. **Spastic dysarthria:** Spastic dysarthria is found to be linked with bilateral lesions of upper motor neuron pathways that innervate the relevant cranial nerve and spinal nerve. Its characteristics include a harsh, strained vocal quality, slow speech, pitch breaks, and variable loudness. All speech systems are typically affected in spastic dysarthria.
3. **Ataxic dysarthria:** Ataxic dysarthria is associated with dysfunctions of the cerebellum. This type of dysarthria has also been known as "drunken speech." The common characteristics seen in this type are irregular articulatory breakdowns, distorted vowels, and inappropriate variations in pitch, loudness, and stress. Ataxic dysarthria is often caused by cerebellar stroke or spinocerebellar ataxia.
4. **Hypokinetic dysarthria:** Hypokinetic dysarthria is associated with pathology of basal ganglia. The notable characteristics are reduced loudness, short rushes of speech, breathy–tight dysphonia, and monopitch. Often dysfluency and word repetition are reported. Parkinson's disease and its syndromes are the most common causes of hypokinetic dysarthria.
5. **Hyperkinetic dysarthria:** Hyperkinetic dysarthria is also associated with basal ganglia pathology. Some of the common characteristics are distorted vowels, excess loudness variations, sudden forced inspiration/expiration, voice stoppages/arrests, transient breathiness, intermittent hypernasality, and inappropriate vocal noises. It is commonly associated with Huntington's chorea, Tourette's syndrome, cerebral palsy, and side effects of neuroleptic drugs.
6. **Unilateral upper motor neuron dysarthria:** This dysarthria has an anatomical rather than a patho-physiological label. It typically results from stroke affecting upper neuron pathways. Often its character-istics overlap with flaccid, spastic, or ataxic dysarthria.
7. **Mixed dysarthria:** Mixed dysarthria is a combination of two or more of the single dysarthria. It occurs more frequently than any single dysarthria type. A common diagnosis involving mixed dysarthria is amyotrophic lateral sclerosis which has characteristics of both flaccid and spastic dysarthria.
8. **Undetermined:** Perceptual features are consistent with a dysarthria but do not clearly fit into any of the identified dysarthria types.

Treatment

Recent evidence obtained shows that patients with progressive neurological disease and severe hypokinetic dysarthria aided in improving speech intelligibility through the use of delayed auditory feedback (DAF) produced by a small instrument which they carried in their shirt pockets. Equally important is the finding that the positive effects of DAF were maintained over a period of 3 months, during which the subject continued to wear the instrument daily. The instrument is a miniature, solid-state, battery-powered unit that provides controlled DAF.

Mechanism of Delayed Auditory Feedback

The device receives incoming audio signals from a microphone positioned near the patient's mouth and delays these signals, a user-selected length of time (ranging from a minimum of 20 to a maximum of 200 ms), delivering the delayed speech to earphones located in (or on) the user's ears. The device has a variable gain control, and the body of the instrument fits easily into a shirt pocket.

An EMG biofeedback technique was developed for the treatment of dysarthria. It aims at increasing the quantity of information about the myofascial system, which can be used by the patients to improve the control of their musculature and speech production.

APRAXIA OF SPEECH

National Institute on Deafness and Other Communication Disorders defines apraxia of speech (AOS) as a neurological disorder that affects the brain pathways involved in planning the sequence of movements involved in producing speech. The brain knows what it wants to say but cannot properly plan and sequence the required speech sound movements.

Clinical Features

Clinical features of AOS are as follows:
- **Distorting sounds:** People with AOS may have difficulty in pronouncing words correctly. Sounds, especially vowels are often distorted. Because the speaker may not place the speech structures (e.g., tongue, jaw) quite in the right place, the sound comes out wrong. Longer or more complex words are usually harder to say than shorter or simpler words. Sound substitutions might also occur when AOS is accompanied by aphasia.
- **Making inconsistent errors in speech:** For example, someone with AOS may say a difficult word correctly but then have trouble repeating it or may be able to say a particular sound one day and have trouble with the same sound on the next day.
- **Groping for sounds:** People with AOS often appear to be groping for the right sound or word and may try saying a word several times before they say it correctly.
- **Making errors in tone, stress, or rhythm:** Another common characteristic of AOS is the incorrect use of prosody. Prosody is the rhythm and inflection of speech that one uses to help express meaning. Someone who has trouble with prosody might use equal stress, segment syllables in a word, omit syllables in words and phrases, or pause inappropriately while speaking.

SWALLOWING IMPAIRMENT

Swallowing is an essential life function that begins in utero. It is essential for the survival of both because it is the source of hydration and alimentation and as it has an important role in maintaining airway integrity by clearing residue from the oral cavity and pharyngeal tract. American College of Gastroenterology has defined dysphagia as the medical term, which is used to describe difficulty in swallowing.

Dysphagia includes difficulty starting a swallow (called *oropharyngeal dysphagia)* and the sensation of food being stuck in the neck or chest (called *esophageal dysphagia*). Oropharyngeal dysphagia results from abnormal functioning of the nerves and muscles of the mouth, pharynx, and upper esophageal sphincter. When a patient is being evaluated for dysphagia, it is important for the doctor to determine which type of dysphagia is more likely, oropharyngeal or esophageal, as different tests are ordered for each type.

COGNITIVE COMMUNICATION DISORDERS

The ASHA defines cognitive communication disorders as difficulty with any aspect of communication that is affected by disruption of cognition.

Various commonly observed conditions which often lead to cognitive communication disorders are:
- Traumatic brain injury (TBI)
- Stroke (especially right hemisphere damage)
- Dementia
- Brain tumors
- Aging
- Degenerative neurological diseases
- Alcohol/drug abuse
- Medications

Cognitive dysfunctions, such as impaired memory can also affect word retrieval, topic maintenance, a person's ability to recall and integrate which leads to communication disorder information, and the speed of processing information which leads to communication disorders.

Treatment of Cognitive Communication Disorders

Intervention depends on the type and severity of the cognitive communication disorder and is usually based on a combination of behavioral, metacognitive, and counseling approaches. The management of patients with cognitive communication disorders begins with determining environmental factors, if any, which can be modified to provide the least visual or auditory distraction.

PSYCHOSOCIAL ASPECTS OF COMMUNICATION DISORDERS

Children with speech disorders are found to have:
- Poorer peer relationships
- Increased victimization
- More problems in social competence
- Problems in adaptive functioning
- Emotional problems
- More self-regulatory problems compared to their peers.

Children with language impairments are also at risk for:
- Mental health difficulties (e.g., somatic symptoms or problems with depressed, anxious, or angry mood), which may contribute to:
  - Higher rates of unemployment
  - Lesser educational attainment in adulthood.

A recent research conducted on subjects with aphasia showed that the middle adult group with age range 41–65 years indicated their career was greatly impacted by aphasia resulting in job loss. A recent study suggests good psychosocial outcomes for adolescents and adults with histories of early childhood communication disorders especially if no other comorbid conditions are present.

IMPLICATIONS OF SPEECH DISORDER ON PHYSIOTHERAPY

Implications of speech disorder on physiotherapy are as follows:

- The treatment of voice disorders includes physiotherapy and complementary therapies. However, research to support these treatments is scarce.
- Physiotherapy which consists of a systematic approach of manual therapy, education, and therapeutic exercises is shown to have good results as voice therapy, i.e., improving voice handicap index scores.
- The knowledge of the relationship between body posture, laryngeal muscles, voice production, and dysphonia is of paramount importance because a transdisciplinary action can optimize evaluation and treatment in order to provide clinically significant benefits to patients with speech problems.
- Based on this association of muscle tension and speech, studies have shown that TENS, and acupuncture, may be useful as either a unique therapy or as an adjunct therapy to other established treatments for voice disorders.
- The evidence from the various recent studies suggest that manual therapy through laryngeal massage and massage of the neck or shoulder girdle is an effective treatment to improve vocalization.
- A physiotherapist can encourage patients to produce single word or repetitive speech which coincides with movements, as a means of providing supplemental practice of speaking to patients with neurological speech disorders.
- While dealing with people with any sort of speech disorder, due care should be taken to reduce or eliminate any kind of excessive background noises, competing voices and any other sort of distraction, which could hinder proper communication.
- A physiotherapist should make sure to refer the patient to a proper speech–language pathologist or speech therapist as per the nature and degree of impairment caused by the speech pathology.

SUMMARY

Speech pathology began to get recognition in the 1920s when the American Academy of Speech Correction was formed in 1926. It began to develop over the next 20 years as speech therapy approaches became more widespread. At this time, World war II was going on, and soldiers were returning home with brain injuries. This was becoming a concern, so it was speech pathology researchers who worked with them through therapy. Currently, aphasia and dysarthria are common neurogenic speech

disorders which are seen in the rehabilitation setting. Auditory comprehension is also often compromised in patients with aphasia. There is a huge negative impact of communication disorders on the sociovocational life of a person. As a rehabilitation team member, one must make an effort to provide necessary support and not "talk down" and avoid open-ended questions while dealing with people with speech disorders.

Case Scenario

CASE STUDY

A 68-year-old housewife sustained right hemiplegia and difficulty in communication due to hemorrhagic stroke, 6 months ago. She is able to perform her ADL independently and ambulation is with a cane. She has labored and awkward articulation. Inability to join her *bhajan group* because of inability to speak and sing properly is her chief compliant. Her family believes that she has curtailed her social life due to the communication impairments. Her caregivers and family also report that she tends to become frustrated while expressing herself.

Guiding Questions:

1. What communication strategy can be used in this patient?
2. Which are the diagnostic assessment scales one take in this patient?
3. As a physiotherapist, how can you help the patient manage communication impairment?
4. What are the management strategies her family and caregiver can adapt to reinforce communication?

Review Questions

1. What is aphasia? Explain the various types of aphasia.
2. Describe the negative effects of communication disorders from the psychosocial perspective.
3. Explain clinical manifestations of apraxia of speech.
4. Define dysarthria.
5. How will a physiotherapist manage a patient with aphasia?

BIBLIOGRAPHY

1. Baker L, Cantwell DP. Psychiatric disorder in children with different types of communication disorders. J Commun Disord. 1982;15(2):113-26.
2. Cardoso R, Meneses RF, Lumini-Oliveira J. The effectiveness of physiotherapy and complementary therapies on voice disorders: a systematic review of randomized controlled trials. Front Med (Lausanne) 2017; 4: 45.
3. Docio-Fernandez L, Mateo CG. Speech Production. In: Li SZ, Jain AK. (eds) Encyclopedia of Biometrics. Springer, Boston, MA, 2015.
4. Dronkers NF, Plaisant O, Iba-Zizen MT, et al. Paul Broca's historic cases: high resolution MR imaging of the brains of Leborgne and Lelong. Brain. 2007;130(Pt. 5):1432-41.
5. Duffy JR. Motor speech disorders: substrates, differential diagnosis, and management, 2nd edition. Saint Louis, MO: C.V. Mosby; 2005.
6. Gyawali CP, Washington University School of Medicine, St. Louis, MO – Published November 2010. American College

of Gastroentrology. Available from: https://www.nidcd.nifi. gov/health/aprfaxie-speech//gi.org/topics/d.

7. Hanson WR, Metter EJ. DAF as instrumental treatment for dysarthria in progressive supranuclear palsy: a case report. J Speech Hear Disord. 1980;45(2):268-76.

8. Hustad KC. A closer look at transcription intelligibility for speakers with dysarthria: evaluation of scoring paradigms and linguistic errors made by listeners. Am J Speech Lang Pathol. 2006;15(3):268-77.

9. Konadath S, Chatni S, Jayaram G, et al. Prevalence of communication disorders in rural population of India. J Hearing Sci. 2013;3(2):41-9.

10. Lechtenberg R, Gilman S. Speech disorders in cerebellar disease. Ann Neurol. 1978;3(4):285-90.

11. Lewis BA, Patton E, Freebrim L, et. al. Psychosocial co-morbidities in adolescents and adults with histories of communication disorders. J Commun Disord. 2016;61:60-70.

12. National Institute on Deafness and other communication disorders (NIDCD). Apraxia of speech. Available from: https:// www.nidcd.nih.gov/health/apraxia-speech.

13. Pedersen PM, Jørgensen HS, Nakayama H, et al. Aphasia in acute stroke: incidence, determinants, and recovery. Ann Neurol. 1995;38(4):659-66.

14. Shriberg LD, Tomblin JB, McSweeny JL. Prevalence of speech delay in 6-year-old children and comorbidity with language impairment. J Speech Lang Hearing Res. 1999;42(6):1461-81.

15. Spencer K, Slocomb D. The neural basis of ataxic dysarthria. Cerebellum. 2007;6(1):58-65.

16. Sreeraj Konadath, Suma C, Jayaram G. et al. Prevalence of Communication Disorders in a Rural Population of India. Journal of Hearing Science. 2013;3 pp. 41-50.

Health and Wellness

Neeta J Vyas, Srishti S Sharma

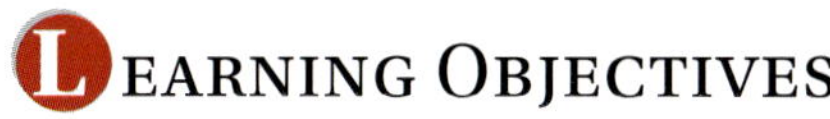 EARNING OBJECTIVES

After reading this chapter, the readers should be able to:
- Explain the importance of health promotion and wellness initiative
- Explain communicable and noncommunicable diseases
- Describe the role of physiotherapist in health promotion
- Discuss the evolution of models of health
- Identify measures of health and wellness, health behaviors, and quality of life
- Explain the role of physical therapists in health promotion and wellness concepts into the plan of care for individuals with impairments and disabilities.

CHAPTER OUTLINE

- Importance of health promotion and wellness
- Communicable and noncommunicable diseases
- Factors affecting health and wellness
- Health promotion and health education
- International classification of functioning, disability and health, health and health promotion
- Role of physiotherapist in health promotion

- Terms used in health promotion
- Theories of behavior change
    - Health belief model
    - Theory of reasoned action and theory of planned behavior
    - Transtheoretical model (stages of change)
    - Social–cognitive theory
- Physical activity model for people with a disability
- Community models

- Health promotion models
- Motivational interviewing
- Measures of health, wellness, quality of life, and health behaviors
- Role of physiotherapist in health and wellness among people with disability and wellness
    - Physiotherapists as advocates

IMPORTANCE OF HEALTH PROMOTION AND WELLNESS

According to the latest World Health Organization (WHO) data published in 2018, life expectancy in India is:
- For males—67.4 years
- For females—70.3 years
- Total life expectancy—68.8 years.

This gives India a World Life Expectancy ranking of 125. According to the World Bank, infant mortality in India fell from 66 to 38 per 1,000 live births from 2000 to 2015, and the maternal mortality ratio has fallen from 374 to 174 per 100,000 live births over the same period. Latest reports show India has improved in terms of life expectancy and health in the last one decade. The life expectancy at birth in 1969 was 47 years, growing to 60 years in 1994 and 69 years in 2019.

COMMUNICABLE AND NONCOMMUNICABLE DISEASES

Global burden of diseases study examines 333 health conditions and 84 risk factors. This, and other similar studies, classifies the burden of diseases in three broad groups: communicable, noncommunicable diseases (NCDs), and injuries.

Within communicable diseases are included the following conditions: diseases of infectious etiology (diarrhea, pneumonia, tuberculosis, HIV being the most common ones), all maternal and neonatal deaths (irrespective of the cause), and all deaths due to nutritional deficiencies (deaths due to undernutrition).

Within the broad group of NCDs are included the following conditions: cardiac conditions, diabetes, cancers, chronic pulmonary diseases, mental health conditions, and many others. The third type of condition is injury, which includes: injuries due to trauma, drowning, poisonings, and bites.

India is a populous country of about 1.3 billion people. NCDs contribute to around 5.87 million (60%) of all deaths in India. Four NCDs which are responsible for the total NCD mortality and morbidity are cardiovascular diseases, chronic respiratory disease, cancers, and diabetes, contributing to about 82% of all NCD deaths. Between 1990 and 2016, India has seen an epidemiological transition in disease burden and deaths, with a steady rise in NCD burden.

The most common NCD seen in India is diabetes. India has the highest number of diabetes cases in the world, with 72 million reported in 2017. Prevalence of the disease is rapidly increasing in India, at a much higher rate than the global average. Between 1990 and 2013, the rate of diabetes increased by 123% in India compared to a global increase of 45%.

Tobacco use is a significant lifestyle factor leading to the development of various NCDs including several forms of cancer, respiratory disease, cardiovascular ailments, and strokes. Though on the bright side, tobacco use in India is on the decline, its prevalence falling by 6% between 2009–2010 and 2016–2017.

Many of the so-called NCD, such as cancer cervix and hepatocellular cancers are caused by infectious agents, which primarily cause communicable diseases. Chronic obstructive pulmonary diseases are also often a result of or are exacerbated by chest infections, such as bacterial pneumonias and past tuberculosis. Similarly, rheumatic heart disease is classified as NCD, but it has its origins in streptococcal throat infection, an infectious disease.

In India, the most commonly encountered communicable diseases are malaria, typhoid, tuberculosis, HIV, hepatitis, influenza, and diarrheal diseases. So, in response to that, the Indian government has established some forums or programs, such as:

- Human immunodeficiency virus infection/acquired immunodeficiency syndrome (HIV/AIDS)—Department of AIDS Control
- Revised National TB Control Programme (RNTCP)
- National Vector Borne Disease Control Programme (NVBDCP)
- Integrated Disease Surveillance Project (IDSP)
- National Leprosy Eradication Programme (NLEP)

FACTORS AFFECTING HEALTH AND WELLNESS

The factors that influence the health of an individual can be classified as external and internal factors.
The *external factors* affecting health are:
- Social and economic environment
- Physical environment
- Availability of proper resources.

Internal factors include:
- Person's own choice of habits
- Lifestyle
- Personality characteristics

There are many commonly accepted determinants of health, but there is no single definite data for India. The Global Burden of Disease Study for 2016, an observational epidemiological study of risk to health and life from diseases, injuries, and risk factors, found common determinants to be bad diets, tobacco use, and high blood pressure. Unhealthy diet alone is a risk factor in one in five global deaths, raising the risk of heart disease, diabetes, obesity, high blood pressure among others.

India accounts for 2.8 million of the 10.4 million new tuberculosis (TB) cases globally, according to the WHO's Global TB Report 2016. India's National Programme provides free medicines and treatment to all, but many patients do not complete the full course of medicine, which must be taken for 6–8 months for uncomplicated disease. This leads to drug-resistant infection which takes longer to treat using more toxic and expensive medicines.

Approximately 2.8 million deaths around the world are reported as a result of being overweight or obese. Overweight and obesity are the major public health issues in developing as well as developed countries. Current report for the prevalence of obesity in the Indian population suggests that from 1998 to 2018, the prevalence of obesity has been rapidly increasing which could be due to sedentary lifestyle and consumption of high calorie food. In India, more than 135 million individuals are obese; this is a result of spurt in urbanization and industrialization. Physical activity (PA) is an important and essential aspect of our life to achieve optimum health and well-being nowadays. PA simply means movement of the body that consumes energy. According to the WHO, PA is defined as "Any movement of the body by skeletal muscles that requires energy expenditure."

A recent study which was conducted on 14,227 individuals showed that 54.4% ($n = 7,737$) were inactive (male: 41.7%). The region-wise prevalence of physical inactivity was as follows: Chandigarh—66.8%, Tamil Nadu—60.0%, Maharashtra—55.2% and Jharkhand—34.9%. When extrapolated to the whole country, the estimated number of inactive individuals in India would be 392 million.

The International Diabetes Federation estimates that more than 382 million people worldwide have diabetes as of 2013, and this number is projected to increase to 592 million by the year 2035. Low- and middle-income countries are expected to contribute to most of this increase with China and India alone contributing to 163.5 million individuals with diabetes globally.

HEALTH PROMOTION AND HEALTH EDUCATION

Health promotion is universally regarded as a significant tool in dealing with lifestyle conditions, in the literature.

It is defined by the WHO as "Process which enables people to increase control over and to improve their health." Green and Kreuter describe health promotion as a planned combined political, regulatory, educational and organizational activity which supports actions and conditions for improvement of health of community.

Health education is one of the many components of health promotion. Green and Kreuter define health education as "any planned combination of learning experiences designed to predispose, enable, and reinforce voluntary behavior conducive to health in individuals, groups, or communities." Health education interventions aim at providing information to individuals and groups about health, actions associated with it and the impact of negative health behaviors. This in turn makes a connection between voluntary behaviors and health. Awareness about the relationship between behavior and disease and injury is the primary step toward positive health behavior change.

INTERNATIONAL CLASSIFICATION OF FUNCTIONING, DISABILITY AND HEALTH, AND HEALTH PROMOTION

The prevailing model of health and wellness in the 20th century medicine was the biomedical model. This was a model that was based on the biological sciences and conceptualized health as the absence of disease. Healthcare providers hold the locus of control in this, and the patient is provided necessary medical care by them. It was an effective model for managing acute and infectious diseases and illnesses but proved less effective for managing chronic disease or in addressing the psychological, social, or behavioral dimensions of illness.

As the limitations of using a purely biomedical framework to understand the concept of health became apparent, the biopsychosocial model evolved. The various biopsychosocial models used today to explain health and illness incorporate those domains missing from the biomedical model namely the psychological and social domains. An example of this is the Nagi disablement model. In 2001, the WHO endorsed the ICF biopsychosocial model. ICF provides a common language to describe health, function, and disability to facilitate scientific communication within and across health professions. In this model, the complex interrelationships of biological, environmental, and personal factors and the impact of these variables on health, activity, and function are recognized. This has been discussed in depth in the Chapter 8: Assessment of Function.

ROLE OF PHYSIOTHERAPIST IN HEALTH PROMOTION

Today, physiotherapists are broadening their clinical role to include health-promotion strategies in their clinical practice. This is because of increased emphasis on reducing the global burden of NCD, health professionals who traditionally focused on the individual are being encouraged to address population-level health problems. There been a recent suggestion that physical therapists should be "birth to death" health practitioners, providing regular consultations on exercise and PA that has to be geared toward prevention and health promotion. Recent reports from the United States do suggest that physical therapists provide prevention services that forestall or prevent functional decline. Physical therapists also are involved in promoting health, wellness, and fitness initiatives including education and service provision that stimulate the public to engage in healthy behaviors.

TERMS USED IN HEALTH PROMOTION

Terms like health, disease, quality of life that are used in health promotion are described in **Table 45.1.**

Term	Definition
Health	"A state of complete physical, mental and social well-being and not merely the absence of disease." Health is a dynamic balance of physical, emotional, social, spiritual, and intellectual health
Disease	Often considered the opposite of health. Defined as a pathological condition affecting the body
Wellness	Individual's sense of growth and balance across the physical, spiritual, emotional, intellectual, social, and psychological domains **(Fig. 45.1)**
Illness	It is the opposite of wellness. It is multidimensional and has been defined as a social construct where individuals are not achieving balance in their lives and are unable to create a higher quality of life
Quality of life	The perception of individuals or groups that their needs are being satisfied and that they are not being denied opportunities to achieve happiness or fulfillment

Table 45.1: Terms used in health promotion.

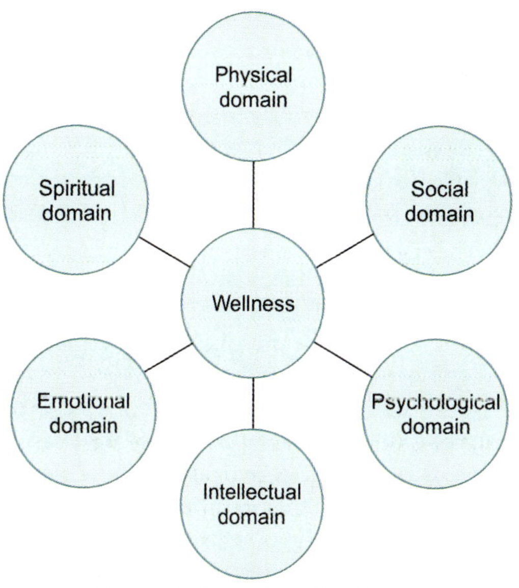

Fig. 45.1: Dimensions of wellness.

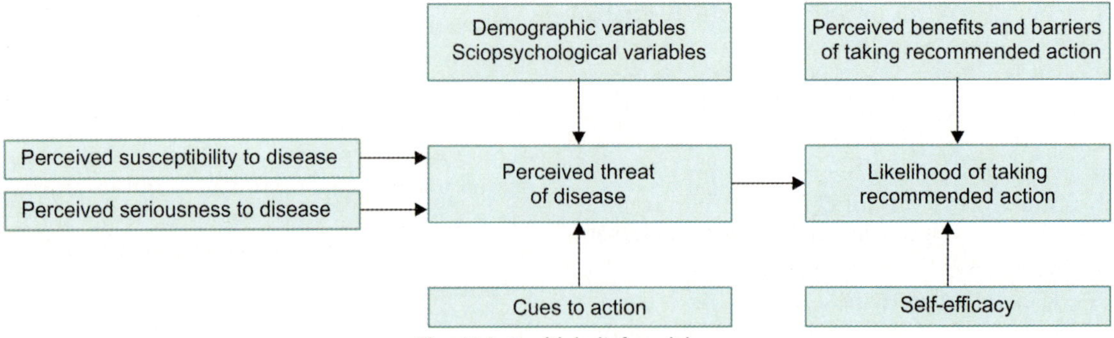

Fig. 45.2: Health belief model.

THEORIES OF BEHAVIOR CHANGE

Health Belief Model

The *Health belief model* (HBM) is one of the earliest theoretical models developed to explain health behaviors. It was developed and articulated in the 1950s. This theory hypothesizes that an individual's perceptions about his or her susceptibility to and the severity of the disease, along with beliefs about the benefits and barriers of taking the recommended action will influence the decision to act **(Fig. 45.2)**.

When using this model in the clinical setting to promote healthy behaviors, the clinician first assesses the individual's beliefs and perceptions relative to his or her health condition and the recommended health actions. Based on this assessment, the clinician would then provide appropriate interventions, e.g., educating the individual about his or her susceptibility to the disease or the effectiveness of recommended health behavior.

Theory of Reasoned Action and Theory of Planned Behavior

In 1967 Fishbein proposed the *Theory of Reasoned Action*, in which he hypothesized that an individual's attitudes and beliefs about a particular behavior directly influence the intention to engage in the behavior which then leads to change in the actual behavior.

The *Theory of Planned Behavior*, along with its predecessor, the theory of reasoned action, is an individual model of health behavior that emphasizes the importance of and relationship between cognitions (thought processes) and behavioral intention **(Fig. 45.3 and Table 45.2)**.

Clinical studies that have examined a variety of health-related behaviors have provided empirical support for the constructs and the relationships articulated in this theory. A clinician using this theoretical model to design a clinical intervention to change a behavior should begin by assessing the individual's attitude toward the behavior and the individual's perceptions regarding how significantly others think about the behavior. The individual's perceived behavioral control can be ascertained by inquiring about any personal, social, or environmental barriers that might limit the ability to successfully engage in the behavior.

Table 45.2: Key constructs in the theory of planned behavior.

Construct	Definition
Attitude toward behavior	Individual's overall attitude toward the behavior
Subjective norm	Individual's beliefs about whether others approve or disapprove of the behavior
Perceived behavioral control	Individual's perception about the level of control he/she has over the behavior
Behavioral intention	Individual's intention to engage in the behavior, the direct precursor to engage in the behavior

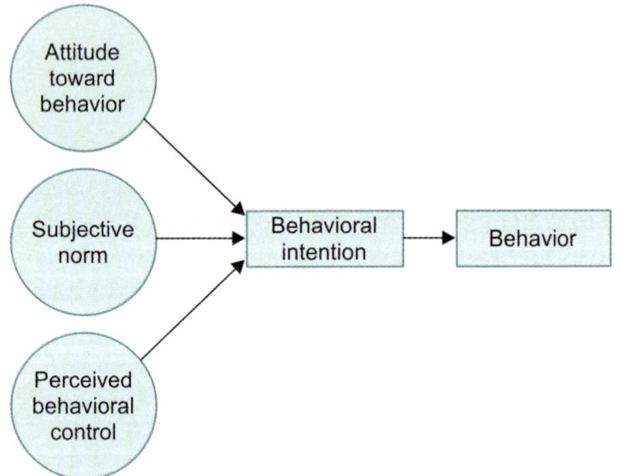

Fig. 45.3: Theory of planned behavior.

Transtheoretical Model (Stages of Change)

The transtheoretical model (TTM) was developed by Prochaska in 1979. Key constructs within the TTM includes stages of change, decisional balance, self-efficacy, and processes of change **(Table 45.3)**.

Prochaska had hypothesized that there are five stages of change **(Box 45.1)**:

1. Precontemplation
2. Contemplation
3. Preparation
4. Action
5. Maintenance.

Table 45.3: Key constructs of transtheoretical model.

Construct	Definition
Stages of change	The stages an individual moves through when changing a behavior
Decisional balance	The process of weighing the pros and cons of changing a behavior
Self-efficacy	The confidence the individual has that he/she can successfully engage in the behavior
Processes of change	Activities used to support progress through stages

BOX 45.1: Stages of change in transtheoretical model.

Precontemplation: Individual does not intend to take action within the next 6 months

Contemplation: Individual intends to take action within the next 6 months

Preparation: Individual intends to take action within the next 30 days and has taken some preliminary steps

Action: Individual has engaged in the behavior for <6 months

Maintenance: Individual has engaged in the behavior for >6 months

Termination: Individual engages in the behavior, has high self-efficacy for the behavior and is no longer tempted to return to the unhealthy behavior

A sixth stage called termination is occasionally included as the final stage of change. It is defined as the stage when an individual has engaged in the behavior for >6 months, is no longer susceptible to temptation, and has high levels of self-efficacy for maintaining the behavior. An individual cycles through the first five stages as he/she makes changes in a particular behavior. Decisional balance and self-efficacy influence an individual's decision to move from one stage to another.

Clinical interventions based on this theoretical model have been successful in changing behaviors, particularly in the areas of smoking, diet, and PA. TTM has also been examined in a study looking specifically at the exercise behaviors of adults with physical disabilities, and the key constructs and relationships hypothesized in this theoretical model of behavior were supported by the researchers' findings.

Social–Cognitive Theory

The previous models with the emphasis on the cognitions and behaviors of the individual can be categorized as individual models of health behavior **(Fig. 45.4)**. *Social-cognitive theory*, with its additional emphasis on the individual's physical and social environment, is an example of a model of interpersonal health behavior.

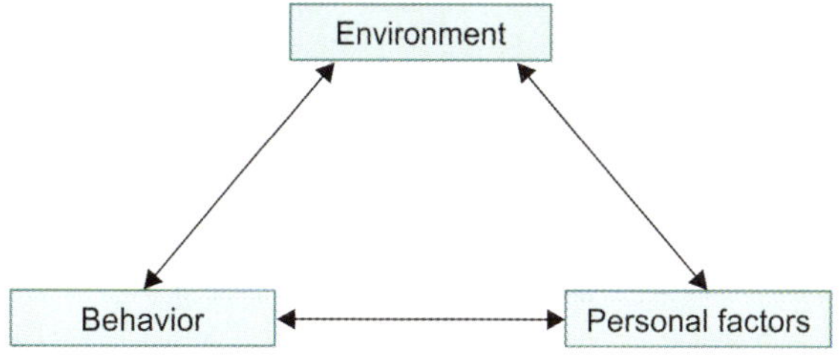

Fig. 45.4: Social–cognitive theory.

PHYSICAL ACTIVITY MODEL FOR PEOPLE WITH A DISABILITY

The recently proposed *physical activity for people with a disability* (PAD) model has been developed to explain the behavior of PA in a population of people with a disability. It integrates behavioral theoretical models with disability models and uses the ICF framework and terminology. In this model, environmental factors and personal factors interact to influence an individual's intention to engage in PA.

Environmental factors include such variables as transportation, availability and accessibility of facilities, and assistance from others. Environmental factors also encompass social influence variables, such as the opinion of family, friends, or health professionals. Personal factors include attitude, self-efficacy, health condition, and facilitators or barriers, such as energy level, time, motivation, and skills.

COMMUNITY MODELS

A number of behavior change theoretical models have been developed to explain behavior change at a community level. Physical therapists interested in changing the health behaviors of a group or community would gain benefit if they familiarize themselves with community and group models of health behavior change, ecological models of health behavior, and intervention planning models, such as the *PRECEDE-PROCEED planning model*.

HEALTH PROMOTION MODELS

The health protection/disease prevention model is one of the most accepted models. Within this model, health is hypothesized as the absence of disease/pathology, and health promotion is therefore aimed at preventing disease. Interventions in this model are categorized as primary, secondary, or tertiary prevention **(Table 45.4)**.

Primary prevention includes activities designed to prevent injury or the onset of illness or disease. The use of bicycle helmets and seat belts, water fluoridation, and immunizations are all examples of primary prevention.

Secondary prevention is where interventions take place following the development of pathology. Physical therapists engage in secondary prevention when they

Table. 45.4: Health promotion models.

Prepathology	Pathology present	
Goals: Protect health Prevent disease Promote health	Goal: Early diagnosis and intervention to limit impairment and disability	Goal: Rehabilitation following significant impairment or disability
Primary prevention	Secondary prevention	Tertiary prevention

treat a patient/client with a recent injury or who has been recently diagnosed in the early stages of a chronic condition or disease, e.g., when giving regular passive movement to prevent contracture in bed-ridden patients.

Tertiary prevention activities are designed to:
- Slow progression of the disease
- Improve quality of life.

Physical therapists engage in tertiary prevention when they work with patients/clients who have chronic disease or have sustained an irreversible injury, e.g., regular exercises prescribed for patient suffering from rheumatoid arthritis.

MOTIVATIONAL INTERVIEWING

Motivational interviewing is a way of being with a client, not just a set of techniques for doing counseling. Motivational interviewing is a client-centered counseling method designed to facilitate a client's internal motivation to change by identifying dissonance between behaviors and values and resolving ambivalence. It is a way to interact with substance-using clients, not merely as an adjunct to other therapeutic approaches, and a style of counseling that can help resolve the ambivalence that prevents clients from realizing personal goals. Motivational interviewing builds on Carl Rogers' optimistic and humanistic theories about people's capabilities for exercising free choice and changing through a process of self-actualization. Motivational interviewing is a counseling style based on the following assumptions:
- Ambivalence about substance use (and change) is normal and constitutes an important motivational obstacle in recovery.
- Ambivalence can be resolved by working with your client's intrinsic motivations and values.
- The alliance between you and your client is a collaborative partnership to which you each bring important expertise.
- An empathic, supportive, yet directive, counseling style provides conditions under which change can occur. (Direct argument and aggressive confrontation may tend to increase client defensiveness and reduce the likelihood of behavioral change.)

BOX 45.2: Key principles of motivational interviewing.
1. Express empathy through reflective listening
2. Develop discrepancy between clients' goals or values and their current behavior
3. Avoid argument and direct confrontation
4. Adjust to client resistance rather than opposing it directly
5. Support self-efficacy and optimism

The clinician practices motivational interviewing keeping five general principles in mind **(Box 45.2)**.

MEASURES OF HEALTH, WELLNESS, QUALITY OF LIFE, AND HEALTH BEHAVIORS

There is no one standard tool for measuring health, wellness, health behaviors, or quality of life. Some tools have been specifically designed to measure the health or health behaviors of a population, whereas other tools are used to measure health and personal health behaviors at the level of the individual patient. Some self-report measures of perceived health, wellness, and quality of life are generic and can be completed by clients with a variety of conditions. Some of the most commonly used measures of self-perceived health are shown in **Box 45.3.**

One of the most commonly used measures of self-perceived health and quality of life is the *Medical Outcomes Study 36-Item Short-Form Health Survey (SF-36)*. The SF-36 measures self-perceived health and function across eight scales that include physical, psychological, social, and emotional domains. It has been used in general populations and in specific populations, and normative scores for various groups and populations have been documented.

The *perceived wellness survey* (PWS) measures self-perceived wellness across psychological, physical, emotional, spiritual, social, and intellectual domains. The survey consists of 36 statements with six items for each of the six domains. This tool has been tested and found to be valid and reliable for use with different populations.

The *arthritis impact measurement scale (AIMS)* and *AIMS2* were developed to measure the physical, mental, and social domains of health in persons with rheumatic diseases.

The *child health questionnaire* measures the physical and psychosocial well-being of children and has been

BOX 45.3: Measures of self-perceived health.
- Medical Outcomes Study 36-Item Short-Form Health Survey (SF-36)
- Nottingham Health Profile
- Sickness Impact Profile (SIP)
- Dartmouth Cooperative
- Functional Assessment Charts (Dartmouth COOP charts)
- Duke Health Profile
- Perceived Wellness Survey (PWS)

found to be a valid and reliable measure of health status across a variety of conditions and disorders.

ROLE OF PHYSIOTHERAPIST IN HEALTH AND WELLNESS AMONG PEOPLE WITH DISABILITY AND WELLNESS

A physically active lifestyle is accompanied by several fitness and health benefits. Individuals with a disability can particularly benefit from an active lifestyle: not only does it reduce the risk for secondary health problems but all levels of functioning can also be influenced positively.

The aims of a health promotion program for people with disabilities are to:

- Reduce secondary conditions (e.g., obesity, hypertension, and pressure sores)
- Maintain functional independence
- Provide an opportunity for leisure and enjoyment
- Enhance the overall quality of life by reducing environmental barriers to good health.

A greater emphasis must be placed on community-based health promotion initiatives for people with disabilities in order to achieve these objectives.

Current reports show lower levels of PA/exercise by the population with disability or impairments that may be due to a host of factors including:

- Limited mobility
- Chronic pain
- Fatigue
- Fear of aggravating their condition or
- Limited access to fitness facilities that have the necessary equipment and personnel to enable safe and effective PA.

Hence, the role of physiotherapist while dealing with health promotion and wellness of such population is to:

- Consider individual's environment, personal skills, and attitudes when developing strategies to incorporate PA in daily life.
- Consider how to incorporate physical support in order to maintain a physically active lifestyle.
- Correct misperceptions about the environment and the behaviors of others.
- Provide education and skills training.
- PA recommendations should be tailored to ensure safety and effectiveness of the patient's unique medical condition.
- Physical therapists must consider not only the patient's conditions but also any comorbidities and potential side effects or limitations associated with medical treatments when prescribing a PA program.

Physiotherapists as Advocates

Healthy People 2020 is a nationwide drive with an agenda to improve health and achieve health equity. One of the goals of it is the need for increased health promotion programs for individuals with disabilities. Physiotherapists can make a meaningful contribution to the health by providing health and wellness to this population within their own practices globally as well as nationally. Physiotherapists are well-versed and most commonly encounter the needs and challenges faced by individuals with chronic disease and disability. With the agenda of Healthy People 2020, they should participate in both the community and national levels to ensure that this population is provided the same access to health promotion and wellness programming.

SUMMARY

With the advancement in science and technology the life expectancy of people in India is increasing. Along with this it is now essential to drive the focus to quality of life as well. For this various health promotion models can be used. Not only for normal people but even people with disability and impairment should be encouraged to take up regular PA. Physical therapists have the knowledge, the skill set, and the opportunity to engage in health promotion practice.

Review Questions

1. What factors contribute to the health of an individual?
2. How does the World Health Organization define *health*?
3. Explain the *primary*, *secondary*, and *tertiary* prevention for health promotion.
4. Describe the health belief model.
5. Explain the role of physiotherapist in health promotion for people with disability and impairments.
6. State the difference between the terms "illness" and "disease."

BIBLIOGRAPHY

1. Ahirwar R, Mondal PR. Prevalence of obesity in India: a systematic review. Diabetes Metab Syndr Clin Res Rev. 2019;13(1):318-21.
2. Ajzen I. The theory of planned behavior. Organ Behav Hum Decis Process. 1991;50(2):179-211.
3. American Physical Therapy Association. Guide to physical therapist practice, 2nd edition. American physical therapy association. Phys Ther.2001;81(1):9-746.
4. Anjana RM, Pradeepa R, Das AK, et al. Physical activity and inactivity patterns in India—results from the ICMR-INDIAB study (Phase-1 [ICMR-INDIAB-5]. Int J Behav Nutr Phys Act. 2014;11(1):26.
5. Bergner M, Bobbitt RA, Kressel S, et al. The sickness impact profile: conceptual formulation and methodology for the development of a health status measure. Int J Health Serv. 1976;6(3):393-415.
6. Campbell HM, Khan N, Cone C, et al. Relationship between diet, exercise habits, and health status among patients with diabetes. Res Social Adm Pharm. 2011;7(2):151-6.
7. De Vries H, Dijkstra M, Kuhlman P. Self-efficacy: the third factor besides attitude and subjective norm as a predictor of behavioral intentions. Health Educ Res. 1988;3(3):273-82.
8. Duke health profile. Durham, NC: Department of Community and Family Medicine, Duke University Medical Center.

Available from http://healthmeasures.mc.duke.edu/images/DukeForm.pdf.

9. Glanz K, Rimer BK, Lewis FM (Eds). Health behavior and health education, 3rd edition. San Francisco, CA: Jossey-Bass; 2002.

10. Global status report on non-communicable diseases 2014. Available from: http://www.who.int/nmh/publications/ncd-status-report-2014/en/. [Accessed February 25, 2018].

11. Godin G, Kik G. The theory of planned behavior: a review of its applications to health-related behaviors. Am J Health Promot. 1996;11(2):87.

12. Higgs J, Refshauge K, Ellis E. Portrait of the physiotherapy profession. J Interprof Care. 2001;15(1):79-89.

13. Hunt SM, McEwen J. The development of a subjective health indicator. Social Health Illn. 1980;2:231-46.

14. International Diabetes Federation. IDF diabetes atlas, 6th edition. Brussels, Belgium: International Diabetes Federation; 2013. Available from http://www.idf.org/diabetesatlas.

15. Junker L, Carlberg EB. Factors that affect exercise participation among people with physical disabilities. Adv Physiother. 2011;13(1):18.

16. Kigin CM, Rodgers MM, Wolf SL. The physical therapy and society summit (PASS) meeting: observations and opportunities. Phys Ther. 2010;90(11):1555-67.

17. McKenzie JF, Neiger BL, Smeltzer JL. Planning, implementing and evaluating health promotion programs: a primer, 4th edition. San Francisco, CA: Benjamin Cummings; 2005.

18. National Family Health Survey, India. Key findings. 2015–16. Available from http://rchiips.org/NFHS/factsheet_NFHS-4.shtml.

19. National Health Commission update about noncommunicable disease. Available from: https://www.healthissuesindia.com/noncommunicable-diseases/.

20. Nethan S, Sinha D, Mehrotra R. Non communicable disease risk factors and their trends in India. Asian Pac J Cancer Prev. 2017;18(7):2005-10.

21. Prochaska JO. Systems of psychotherapy: a transtheoretical analysis. Pacific Grove, CA: Brooks-Cole; 1979.

22. Rimmer JH. Health promotion for people with disabilities: the emerging paradigm shift from disability prevention to prevention of secondary conditions. Phys Ther. 1999;79(5):495-502.

23. Sahrmann S. Ask an expert. Today in PT. 2009;2:20.

24. The common causes of death in India. Available from: https://www.hindustantimes.com/health/the-top-10-causes-of-death-in-india/story-lFLxCFVHmF7svw2RK-Cl70K.html.

25. World Health Organization. Ottawa charter for health promotion. Ottawa: World Health Organization; 1986. Available from http://www.who.int/healthpromotion/conferences/previous/ottawa/en/.

26. World Health Organization: Noncommunicable Diseases (NCD) Country Profiles, 2018. Available from: https://www.who.int/countries/ind/en/.

INDEX

Page numbers followed by *b* refer to box, *f* refer to figure, and *t* refer to table.

A

Abdomen 93, 191
Abdominal bracing 373
Abdominal drawing 890*f*
Abdominal endurance test 370*f*
Abdominal movement 80
Abdominal muscle
    separation of 887*f*
    strengthening of 706*f*
Abdominal obesity 292
Abdominal test, isometric 369
Abduction pillow 536*f*
Abductors strengthening, horizontal 415*f*
Accessory movements 369
Acetaminophen 722
Acetylcholine 115
Achilles heel sleeve 525*f*
Achilles tendinitis 524, 524*f*, 525*f*
Achilles tendon 698*f*, 707
Acrocyanosis 335
Action research arm test 39
Activity of daily living 24, 44, 143, 148, 210, 263, 299,
        300, 322, 643, 686, 687*t*, 704, 746
    basic 158
    instrumental 210
    Katz index of 146
    scale, Lawton instrumental 146
Acupuncture 205, 685
Acute exacerbations
    classification of 314*t*
    episodes of 315
    management of 314
Adams' theory 275
Adaptive behavior skills 211
Addison's disease 700
Adductor contracture 441*f*
Adenosine triphosphate 296, 346, 837
Adho Mukha Virasana 257
Adiposity, measurement of 841
Adjuvant analgesics 201, 201*t*
Adjuvant therapy 771
Advanced balance training 282*f*
Adventitious sounds, continuous 85
Aerobic capacity 751
Aerobic exercise 709, 726, 784, 784*f*, 826, 827*f*, 842,
        843*f*
Aerobic training 298, 299*t*, 317, 318*f*, 639, 765
Afferent pain fibers 182
Agitation 901
Agnosia 47, 49
Ahimsa 245
Air plethysmography 343
Air pollution
    indoor 307
    outdoor 307
Airflow obstruction 308*t*, 322, 815
Airplane splint 228, 228*f*
Airway 78, 78*f*
    hyperreactivity 307
    obstruction 85
        causes of 78*b*
Alabdha bhumikatva 245
Alcohol 770
Alcoholic neuropathy 126, 721
    pathogenesis of 721
Alcoholism, chronic 283
Algometry testing 197
Allodynia 182
Alpha-lipoic acid 722

Alprazolam 201
Alveolar cell carcinoma 74
Alveolar ducts 306
Alveolar sacs 306
Alzheimer's disease 839
Amenorrhea 867
Amitriptyline 201
Amnesia 46
Amplifiers 130, 131*f*, 140
Amputation 212, 551, 582*t*
    level of 552
Amputees, management of 556*b*
Amyotrophic lateral sclerosis 52, 134, 278, 280, 678-
        680, 680*f*
    diagnosis of 681*b*
Amyotrophy 679
Anaerobiosis, early onset of 830
Analgesia 182
Analgesics 201*t*
Analog oscilloscope 131, 131*f*
Anavashthitattva 245
Anemia 89, 775
Aneurysm 335
Angina 191, 292, 294*b*
Anginal symptoms refractory 295
Angiotensin-converting enzyme 75, 294, 345
Angular acceleration 100
Angular velocity sensor 100, 108
Ankle 34
    and foot conditions 509
    brachial index 341, 341*t*, 342
    complex 510*f*
    control 232
    cushion heel
        foot, solid 566*f*, 574*f*
        solid 567*t*
    disarticulation prosthesis 567
    dorsiflexors, manual strengthening of 520*f*
    foot orthosis 229, 232, 232*f*, 233*f*, 566*f*, 708, 737
    instability, chronic 522
    joint 525, 526, 526*f*
    sprain 518
        ice pack for 204*f*
    strategies 64
Ankle to brachial
    index, measurement of 341*f*
    pressure 341
Ankle toe movements 493*f*
Ankle-foot orthosis
    solid 234*f*
    spiral 234*f*
Ankylosing spondylitis 381
Anomic aphasia 906
Anorexia 781
Anosognosia 48
Anoxia 87
Anterior cruciate ligament
    injury 477, 478*f*
        causes of 477*b*
    reconstruction 504*t*
    rehabilitation, phases of 478*t*
Anterograde amnesia 46
Anthropometry 854
Anti-citrullinated protein antibodies 435
Anticonvulsants 201
Antidiabetic drugs
    classification of 838
    miscellaneous 838
Antidromic conduction 124, 124*f*, 127

Antiepileptic drugs 724
Antiplatelet therapy 345
Antiproliferative agents 819
Anxiety 89, 191, 192, 322, 897, 898
Anxiolytics 201
Aortic aneurysm 75
Aortoiliac disease 334
Aparigraha 245
Aphasia 905
    assessment 906
    classification of 905, 905*b*, 905*f*
    global 906
    primary progressive 906
    treatment of 906
    types of 905*f*
Aplasia 338
Apley's scratch test 38
Apoptosis, activation of 334
Appendicitis 191
Apraxia 47, 49
Archicerebellum 664
Ardha paschimottanasana 258
Arm and hand, movement of 67
Arm ergometer 640*f*
Arnold-Chiari malformation 666
Arrhythmias 699, 716, 852
Arterial blood gases 87
    normal 88*t*
Arterial disease 332, 333*f*, 334*f*
Arterial disorders, management of 344
Arterial dysfunction, test for 340
Arterial emboli 333
Arterial insufficiency 332, 334
Arterial occlusion, acute 339
Arterial system 331
    vessel walls of 333
Arteriosclerosis obliterans 333
Artery 332*t*, 333*f*
    palpation of 340, 340*f*
Arthritic hip joint 458*f*
Arthritic knee joint 539*f*
Arthritis 33, 190, 191, 212, 255, 260
Arthrodesis 761
Arthrokinematics 37
Arthroscopic procedures 504
Arthroscopy 483*f*
Articulation disorder 904
Asana 245
Ashtanga namashkara 249, 249*f*
Ashwa sanchalasana 248, 248*f*, 250, 250*f*
Ashworth scale, modified 57*b*, 269
Asia impairment scale 633*f*, 634*b*
Aspiration 74
Aspirin 722
Assistive technology 211, 240, 262-264, 269, 272
    role of 268*t*
    types of 264, 264*t*
Astereognosis 49
Asthenia 283, 307, 667
Asthma
    acute 73
    bronchial 74
Asymmetrical tonic neck reflex 59
Asynergia 666
Ataxia 281, 302, 663, 665, 666, 666*t*, 732, 738
    acquired 666
    assessment of 667, 676
    telangiectasia 665
Ataxic dysarthria 907